MW00989983

Langenscheidt

Merriam-Webster

Medical Dictionary

Merriam-Webster's
Medical
Dictionary

Merriam-Webster, Incorporated
Springfield, Massachusetts, U.S.A.

A GENUINE MERRIAM-WEBSTER

The name *Webster* alone is no guarantee of excellence. It is used by a number of publishers and may serve mainly to mislead an unwary buyer.

Merriam-Webster™ is the name you should look for when you consider the purchase of dictionaries or other fine reference books. It carries the reputation of a company that has been publishing since 1831 and is your assurance of quality and authority.

Copyright © 2006 by Merriam-Webster, Incorporated

ISBN-13: 978-0-87779-853-8
ISBN-10: 0-87779-853-2

MADE IN THE UNITED STATES OF AMERICA

1 2 3 4 5 6 7 8 9 10 NK:QWB 10 09 08 07 06

CONTENTS

PREFACE

This new edition of MERRIAM-WEBSTER'S MEDICAL DICTIONARY follows the tradition established in 1995 by the first edition in providing a concise guide to the essential language of medicine. It is an abridged version of *Merriam-Webster's Medical Desk Dictionary,* and it shares many of the features of its parent volume. These are features that are standard for most desk dictionaries of the English language but are often missing from medical dictionaries. For example, users of this book will find how to pronounce *CABG, NSAID,* and *RU-486;* how to spell and pronounce the plurals of *arthritis, chlamydia,* and *uterus;* where to divide *arteriosclerosis* and *thrombolytic* at the end of a line; and the part-of-speech labels of *spermicide, spermicidal,* and *spermicidally.*

The 37,000 vocabulary entries include the most frequently used words of human and veterinary medicine. The reader will find entries for human diseases such as *AIDS, Lyme disease,* and *chronic fatigue syndrome* and also for those of domestic animals such as *heartworm* of dogs, *panleukopenia* of cats, and *foot-and-mouth disease* of cattle. The new entries for *bird flu, bovine spongiform encephalopathy* (less technically known as *mad cow disease*), and *SARS* define diseases that have become major threats to human and/or animal health since publication of the first edition. Every word used in a definition in this book appears as a boldface vocabulary entry either in this dictionary or in its companion general paperback, *The Merriam-Webster Dictionary.*

New for this edition is an updated treatment of the taxonomic nomenclature of viruses, based on two monumental reports published in 2000 and 2005 by the International Committee on Taxonomy of Viruses (ICTV). These reports, the seventh and eighth in a series, extended the classification of viruses down to the species level. In the eighth report, the entire corpus of viruses is divided into 73 families, 298 genera, and about 1,950 species. (For more information on virus classification, see the section on Virus Taxonomy in the Explanatory Notes of this dictionary.) In this new edition of this dictionary, the previously used phrase "any of a group" has been replaced with a more specific phrase such as "any of a family" or "any of a genus," and when a specific virus is entered and defined (as *Epstein-Barr virus*) or referred to in the context of a definition (as in the entry for *mumps*), the species name is usually given. Typical of the taxonomic findings in the series of reports by the ICTV are the discovery that the arboviruses are not a natural taxon but a collection of various RNA viruses now assigned to several different families; the recognition that the three primary kinds of hepatitis (hepatitis A, hepatitis B, and hepatitis C) are each caused by a different virus species in a different genus and in a different family from the other two; and the determination that the three basic kinds of influenza are caused by three different species of virus in one family (*Orthomyxoviridae*) but in three different genera.

This dictionary is designed to serve as an interface between the language of doctor and the language of patient, between sports medicine and the sports page, between the technical New Latin names of plants and animals and their common names, and between the old and the new in medical terminology. The user of this dictionary will find, for example, that the *abs, delts, glutes, lats,* and *pecs* of the physical fitness enthusiast are the *abdominal muscles, deltoidei, glutei, latissimi dorsi,* and *pectorales* of the anatomist. In more technical anatomical writing, the *eustachian tubes* may be called the *auditory tubes* or *pharyngotympanic tubes* and the *fallopian tubes* may be called the *uterine tubes.* All of these words are entered and defined in this dictionary with mention of synonymous or former terminology when appropriate.

Entries known to be trademarks or service marks are so labeled and are treated in accordance with a formula approved by the United States Trademark Association. No entry in this dictionary, however, should be regarded as affecting the validity of any trademark or service mark.

When a trademark or service mark for a drug is entered in this dictionary, it is also mentioned in a cross-reference following the definition of its generic equivalent, so that, for example, from either of the entries for *atorvastatin* and *Lipitor, fluoxetine* and *Prozac,* or *sildenafil* and *Viagra,* the reader can determine which is a generic name and which is a proprietary name for the same drug.

This dictionary contains material from its parent work supplemented by new material from the research files in the Merriam-Webster editorial offices which now include more than 15,700,000 citations (examples of English words used in context).

Another important feature of this book is that words occurring only as part of compound terms are entered at their own place in alphabetical sequence with a cross-reference to the compound terms themselves. Thus, *herpetiformis* has a cross-reference to *dermatitis herpetiformis,* and *longus* is followed by a list of 11 compound terms of which it is part. These lists may help the reader unfamiliar with medical terminology to find the place of definition of compound terms.

The biographical information following words derived from the names of persons has been limited to the person's name, birth and death dates, nationality, and occupation or status. Such information is entered only for historical figures, not for fictional or mythical characters.

It is the intent of the editors that this dictionary serve the purposes of all those who seek information about medical English as it is currently spoken and written, whether in the context of a clinical setting, in correctly rendering spoken and written text, or from the perspective of lexicography as an art and science.

Merriam-Webster's Medical Dictionary is the result of collective effort by the staff of Merriam-Webster, Incorporated. The editor was assisted by Joan I. Narmontas in preparing definitions for the original 1995 edition and by Joan I. Narmontas and Christopher C. Connor for the 2006 edition. For the 2006 edition, Joshua S. Guenter, Ph.D., was responsible for pronunciations, building on the previous work of Brian M. Sietsema, Ph.D. Biographical information was researched by Michael G. Belanger. Cross-reference work for the 2006 edition was performed by Adrienne M. Scholz, building on the previous work of Maria A. Sansalone and Donna L. Rickerby. The manuscript for the 1995 edition was copyedited by Stephen J. Perrault, and this edition was copyedited by Joan I. Narmontas. For this edition, other specialized editorial assistance was provided by Daniel B. Brandon, Robert D. Copeland, Ilya A. Davidovich, Kathleen M. Doherty, Mary M. Dunn, Carol A. Fugiel, Stacy-Ann S. Lall, E. Louise Langford, Anne P. Miller, Donna L. Rickerby, Maria A. Sansalone, and Paul S. Wood. Thomas F. Pitoniak, Ph.D. managed production, and Madeline L. Novak coordinated all editorial operations.

Roger W. Pease, Jr., Ph.D.
Editor

EXPLANATORY NOTES

This section provides information on the conventions used throughout the dictionary, from the styling of entries and pronunciation to how we present information on usage and meaning. An understanding of the information contained in these notes will make the dictionary both easier and more rewarding to use.

ENTRIES

MAIN ENTRIES

A boldface letter or a combination of such letters, including punctuation marks and diacritics where needed, that is set flush with the left-hand margin of each column of type is a main entry or entry word. The main entry may consist of letters set solid, of letters joined by a hyphen, or of letters separated by one or more spaces:

> al·ler·gy . . . n
> ¹an·ti–in·flam·ma·to·ry . . . adj
> blood vessel n
> non–A, non–B hepatitis . . . n

The material in lightface type that follows each main entry explains and justifies its inclusion in the dictionary.

Variation in the styling of compound words in English is frequent and widespread. It is often completely acceptable to choose freely among open, hyphenated, and closed alternatives. To save space for other information, this dictionary usually limits itself to a single styling for a compound. When a compound is widely used and one styling predominates, that styling is shown. When a compound is uncommon or when the evidence indicates that two or three stylings are approximately equal in frequency, the styling shown is based on the treatment of parallel compounds.

ORDER OF MAIN ENTRIES

The main entries follow one another in alphabetical order letter by letter without regard to intervening spaces or hyphens: *luteinizing hormone* follows *luteinization* and *heart-healthy* follows *heart failure*. Words that often begin with the abbreviation *St.* in common usage have the abbreviation spelled out: *Saint Anthony's fire, Saint Vitus' dance*.

Full words come before parts of words made up of the same letters. Parts of words with no hyphen in front but followed by a hyphen come before parts of words preceded by a hyphen. Solid words come first and are followed by hyphenated compounds and then by open compounds. Lowercase entries come before entries that begin with a capital letter:

> path . . . abbr
> path- . . . comb form

    -path . . . *n comb form*
    work·up . . . *n*
    work up . . . *vb*
    tri·chi·na . . . *n*
    Trichina *n*

Entries containing an Arabic numeral within or at the end of the word are alphabetized as if the number were spelled out: *glucose phosphate* comes after *glucose-1= phosphate* and before *glucose-6= phosphate* while *LD50* is between *LD* and *LDH*. Some chemical terms are preceded by one or more Arabic numerals or by a chemical prefix abbreviated to a Roman or Greek letter or by a combination of the two usually set off by a hyphen. In general, the numerical or abbreviated prefix is ignored in determining the word's alphabetical place: *N-allylnormorphine* is entered in the letter *a*, *5-hydroxytryptamine* in the letter *h*, and

β₂-microglobulin in the letter *m*. However, if the prefix is spelled out, it is used in alphabetizing the word: *beta globulin* is entered in the letter *b*, and *levo-dihydroxyphenylalanine* in the letter *l*. In a few cases, entries have been made at more than one place to assist the reader in finding the place of definition, especially when the prefix has variants: *gamma-aminobutyric acid*, defined in the letter *g*, is often written with a Greek letter as *γ= aminobutyric acid*, and an entry has been made in the letter *a* to direct the reader to the place of definition.

  If the names of two chemical substances differ only in their prefixes, the terms are alphabetized first by the main part of the word and then in relation to each other according to the prefix: *L-PAM* immediately precedes *2-PAM* in the letter *p*.

GUIDE WORDS

A pair of guide words is printed at the top of each page. The entries that fall alphabetically between the guide words are found on that page.

  It is important to remember that alphabetical order rather than position of an entry on the page determines the selection of guide words. The first guide word is the alphabetically first entry on the page. The second guide word is usually the alphabetically last entry on the page:

    artifactual · ascites

The entry need not be a main entry. Another boldface word—a variant, an inflected form, or a defined or undefined run-on—may be selected as a guide word. For this reason the last main entry on a page is not always the last entry alphabetically.

  All guide words must themselves be in alphabetical order from page to page throughout the dictionary; thus, the alphabetically last entry on a page is not used if it follows alphabetically the first guide word on the next page.

HOMOGRAPHS

When main entries are spelled alike, they are distinguished by superscript numerals preceding each word:

    ¹ano·rex·ic . . . *adj*
    ²anorexic *n*

    ¹se·rum . . . *n*
    ²serum *adj*

Although homographs are spelled alike, they may differ in pronunciation, derivation, or functional classification (as part of speech). The order of homographs is historical: the one first used in English is entered first. In this dictionary abbreviations and symbols are listed last in a series of homographs and are not given superscripts. Abbreviations appear before symbols when both are present.

END-OF-LINE DIVISION

The centered dots within entry words indicate division points at which a hyphen may be put at the end of a line of print or writing. Centered dots are not shown after a single initial letter or before a single terminal letter because printers seldom cut off a single letter:

> **abort** . . . *vb*
> **body** . . . *n*

Nor are they shown at second and succeeding homographs unless these differ among themselves in division or pronunciation:

> **¹mu·tant** . . . *adj*
> **²mutant** *n*
> **¹pre·cip·i·tate** \pri-'si-pə-,tāt\ *vb*
> **²pre·cip·i·tate** \pri-'si-pə-tət, -,tāt\ *n*

There are acceptable alternative end-of-line divisions just as there are acceptable variant spellings and pronunciations. No more than one division is, however, shown for an entry in this dictionary.

Many words have two or more common pronunciation variants, and the same end-of-line division is not always appropriate for each of them. The division *ho·me·op·a·thy*, for example, best fits the variant \,hō-mē-'ä-pə-thē\ whereas the division *hom·e·op·a·thy* best fits the variant \,hä-mē-'ä-pə-thē\. In instances like this, the division falling farther to the left is used, regardless of the order of the pronunciations:

> **ho·me·op·a·thy**   \,hō-mē-'ä-pə-thē, ,hä-\

A double hyphen at the end of a line in this dictionary stands for a hyphen that belongs at that point in a hyphenated word and that is retained when the word is written as a unit on one line:

> **DNA polymerase** *n* : any of several polymerases that promote replication . . . of DNA usu. using single-stranded DNA as a template

VARIANTS

When a main entry is followed by the word *or* and another spelling, the two spellings are equal variants:

> **¹neu·tro·phil** . . . *or* **neu·tro·phil·ic**

If two variants joined by *or* are out of alphabetical order, they remain equal variants. The one printed first is, however, slightly more common than the second:

> **phys·i·o·log·i·cal** . . . *or* **phys·i·o·log·ic**

When another spelling is joined to the main entry by the word *also,* the spelling after *also* is a secondary

variant and occurs less frequently than the first:

> **lip·id** . . . *also* **lip·ide**

If there are two secondary variants, the second is joined to the first by *or.* Once the word *also* is used to signal a secondary variant, all following variants are joined by *or:*

> **taen-** *or* **taeni-** *also* **ten-** *or* **teni-**

A variant whose own alphabetical place is at some distance from the main entry is also entered at its own place with a cross-reference to the main entry. Such variants at consecutive or nearly consecutive entries are listed together:

tendonitis *var of* TENDINITIS
anchylose, anchylosis *var of* AN-KYLOSE, ANKYLOSIS

Variants having a usage label (as *Brit* or *chiefly Brit*) appear only at their own alphabetical places:

-aemia *also* **-haemia** *chiefly Brit var of* -EMIA
anae·mia *chiefly Brit var of* ANEMIA
haem- *or* **haemo-** *chiefly Brit var of* HEM-

hae·mo·glo·bin *chiefly Brit var of* HEMOGLOBIN

When long lists of such variants would be generated by entering all those at consecutive entries, only one or a few are given. The rest can be deduced by analogy with those which are entered. For example, the chiefly British variant *haemoglobinaemia* is formed analogously with *haemoglobin* and *anaemia* (it might also be recognized from the combining forms *-aemia* and *haem-* or *haemo-*).

RUN-ON ENTRIES

A main entry may be followed by one or more derivatives or by a homograph with a different functional label. These are run-on entries. Each is introduced by a boldface dash and each has a functional label. They are not defined, however, since their meanings can readily be derived from the meaning of the root word:

healthy . . . *adj* . . . — **health·i·ly** . . . *adv* — **health·i·ness** . . . *n*
drift . . . *n* . . . — **drift** *vb*

A main entry may be followed by one or more phrases containing the entry word. These are also run-on entries. Each is introduced by a boldface dash but there is no functional label. They are, however, defined since their meanings are more than the sum of the meanings of their elements:

²couch *n* . . . — **on the couch** : . . .
risk . . . *n* . . . — **at risk** : . . .

A run-on entry is an independent entry with respect to function and status. Labels at the main entry do not apply unless they are repeated.

PRONUNCIATION

The matter between a pair of reversed virgules \ \ following the entry word indicates the pronunciation. The symbols used are listed in the chart printed on the page facing the first page of the dictionary proper and on the inside of the back cover.

SYLLABLES

A hyphen is used in the pronunciation to show syllabic division. These hyphens sometimes coincide with the centered dots in the entry word that indicate end-of-line division; sometimes they do not:

ab·scess \'ab-₁ses\
met·ric \'me-trik\

STRESS

A high-set mark \\'\\ indicates primary (strongest) stress or accent; a low-set mark \\,\\ indicates secondary (medium) stress or accent:

ear·ache \\'ir-,āk\\
The stress mark stands at the beginning of the syllable that receives the stress.

VARIANT PRONUNCIATIONS

The presence of variant pronunciations indicates that not all educated speakers pronounce words the same way. A second-place variant is not to be regarded as less acceptable than the pronunciation that is given first. It may, in fact, be used by as many educated speakers as the first variant, but the requirements of the printed page are such that one must precede the other:

oral \\'ōr-əl, 'är-\\
um·bi·li·cus \\,əm-bə-'lī-kəs, ,əm-'bi-li-\\

PARENTHESES IN PRONUNCIATIONS

Symbols enclosed by parentheses represent elements that are present in the pronunciation of some speakers but are absent from the pronunciation of other speakers:

de·sen·si·tize \\(,)dē-'sen-sə-tīz\\
RNA \\,är-(,)en-'ā\\

PARTIAL AND ABSENT PRONUNCIATIONS

When a main entry has less than a full pronunciation, the missing part is to be supplied from a pronunciation in a preceding entry or within the same pair of reversed virgules:

psy·chol·o·gy \\-jē\\
vit·i·li·go \\,vi-tə-'lī-,gō, -'lē-\\

The pronunciation of the first two syllables of *psychology* is found at the main entry *psychologist*:

psy·chol·o·gist \\sī-'kä-lə-jist\\

The hyphens before and after \\-'lē-\\ in the pronunciation of *vitiligo* indicate that both the first and the last parts of the pronunciation are to be taken from the immediately preceding pronunciation.

When a variation of stress is involved, a partial pronunciation may be terminated at the stress mark which stands at the beginning of a syllable not shown:

li·gate \\'lī-,gāt, lī-'\\

In general, no pronunciation is indicated for open compounds consisting of two or more English words that have own-place entry:

lateral collateral ligament *n*

A pronunciation is shown, however, for any unentered element of an open compound:

Meiss·ner's corpuscle \\'mīs-nərz-\\

Only the first entry in a sequence of numbered homographs is given a pronunciation if their pronunciations are the same:

¹sig·moid \\'sig-,mȯid\\ *adj*
²sigmoid *n*

The pronunciation of unpronounced derivatives run on at a main entry is a combination of the pronunciation at the main entry and the pronunciation of the suffix or final element.

ABBREVIATIONS, ACRONYMS, AND SYMBOLS

Pronunciations are not usually shown for entries with the functional labels *abbr* or *symbol* since they are usually spoken by saying the individual letters in sequence or by giving the expansion. The pronunciation is given only if there is an unusual and unexpected way of saying the abbreviation or symbol:

ICU *abbr* intensive care unit
Al *symbol* aluminum
CABG \'ka-bij\ *abbr* coronary artery bypass graft

Acronyms (as *DNA* and *HEPA*) and compounds (as *ACE inhibitor*) consisting of an acronym and a word element which have one of the traditional parts of speech labels (usually *n, adj, adv,* or *vb* in this book) are given a pronunciation even when the word is spoken by pronouncing the letters in sequence:

DNA \ˌdē-(ˌ)en-'ā\ *n*
ACE inhibitor \'ās-, ˌā-(ˌ)sē-'ē-\ *n*
HEPA \'hē-pə\ *adj*

FUNCTIONAL LABELS

An italic label indicating a part of speech or some other functional classification follows the pronunciation or, if no pronunciation is given, the main entry. Of the eight traditional parts of speech, five appear in this dictionary as follows:

healthy . . . *adj*
psy·cho·log·i·cal·ly . . . *adv*
hos·pi·tal . . . *n*
per . . . *prep*
pre·scribe . . . *vb*

Other italic labels used to indicate functional classifications that are not traditional parts of speech include:

tid *abbr*
pleur- *or* **pleuro-** *comb form*
-poi·e·sis . . . *n comb form*
-poi·et·ic . . . *adj comb form*
dys- *prefix*
-lyt·ic . . . *adj suffix*
-i·a·sis . . . *n suffix*
Rolf·ing . . . *service mark*
Ca *symbol*
Val·ium . . . *trademark*

Two functional labels are sometimes combined:

calm·ative . . . *n or adj*
cold turkey *n* . . . — **cold turkey** *adv or vb*

INFLECTED FORMS

The inflected forms recorded in this dictionary include the plurals of nouns; the past tense, the past participle when it differs from the past tense, and the present participle of verbs; and the comparative and superlative forms of adjectives and adverbs. When these inflected forms are created in a manner considered regular in English (as by adding -*s* or -*es* to nouns, -*ed* and -*ing* to verbs, and -*er* and -*est* to adjectives and adverbs) and when it seems that there is nothing about the formation to give the dictionary user doubts, the inflected form is not shown in order to save space for information more likely to be sought.

If the inflected form is created in an irregular way or if the dictionary user is likely to have doubts about it (even if it is formed regularly), the inflected form is shown in bold-face either in full or, especially when the word has three or more syllables, cut back to a convenient and easily recognizable point.

The inflected forms of nouns, verbs, adjectives, and adverbs are shown in this dictionary when suffixation brings about a change in final *y* to *i*, when the word ends in *-ey*, when there are variant inflected forms, and when the dictionary user might have doubts about the spelling of the inflected form:

> **scaly** . . . *adj* **scal·i·er; -est**
> ²**atrophy** . . . *vb* **-phied; -phy·ing**
> **kid·ney** . . . *n, pl* **kidneys**
> **sar·co·ma** . . . *n, pl* **-mas** *also* **-ma·ta**
> ¹**burn** . . . *vb* **burned** . . . *or* **burnt** . . . ;
>   **burn·ing**
> **sta·tus** . . . *n, pl* **sta·tus·es**

A plural is also shown for a noun when it ends in a consonant plus *o* or in a double *oo*, and when its plural is identical with the singular. Many nouns in medical English have highly irregular plurals modeled after their language of origin. Sometimes more than one element of a compound term is pluralized:

> **ego** . . . *n, pl* **egos**
> **HMO** . . . *n, pl* **HMOs**
> **tattoo** *n, pl* **tattoos**
> ¹**pu·bes** . . . *n, pl* **pubes**
> **en·ceph·a·li·tis** . . . *n, pl* **-lit·i·des**
> **cor pul·mo·na·le** . . . *n, pl* **cor·dia**
>   **pul·mo·na·lia**

Nouns that are plural in form and that are regularly used with a plural verb are labeled *n pl:*

> **in·nards** . . . *n pl*

If nouns that are plural in form are regularly used with a singular verb, they are labeled *n* or if they are used with either a singular or plural verb, they are labeled *n sing or pl:*

> **rick·ets** . . . *n*
> **blind stag·gers** . . . *n sing or pl*

The inflected forms of verbs, adjectives, and adverbs are also shown whenever suffixation brings about a doubling of a final consonant, elision of a final *e*, or a radical change in the base word itself. The principal parts of a verb are shown when a final *-c* changes to *-ck* in suffixation:

> **re·fer** *vb* **re·ferred; re·fer·ring**
> **hot** . . . *adj* **hot·ter; hot·test**
> **op·er·ate** . . . *vb* **-at·ed; -at·ing**
> **sane** . . . *adj* **san·er; san·est**
> ¹**break** . . . *vb* **broke** . . . ; **bro·ken**
>   . . . ; **break·ing**
> ¹**ill** . . . *adj* **worse** . . . ; **worst**
> **mim·ic** . . . *vb* **mim·icked** . . . ; **mim·**
>   **ick·ing**

Inflected forms are not shown at undefined run-ons.

CAPITALIZATION

Most entries in this dictionary begin with a lowercase letter, indicating that the word is not ordinarily capitalized. A few entries have an italic label *often cap,* indicating that the word is as likely to begin with a capital letter as not and is equally

acceptable either way. Some entries begin with an uppercase letter, which indicates that the word is usually capitalized:

> **pan·cre·as** . . . *n*
> **braille** . . . *n, often cap*
> **Gol·gi** . . . *adj*

The capitalization of entries that are open or hyphenated compounds is similarly indicated by the form of the entry or by an italic label:

> **heart attack** *n*
> ¹**neo–Freud·ian** . . . *adj, often cap N*
> **Agent Orange** . . . *n*

Many acronyms are written entirely or partly in capitals, and this fact is shown by the form of the entry or by an italic label:

> **DNA** . . . *n*
> **cgs** *adj, often cap C&G&S*

A word that is capitalized in some senses and lowercase in others shows variations from the form of the main entry by the use of italic labels at the appropriate senses:

> **strep·to·coc·cus** . . . *n* **1** *cap*
> **pill** . . . *n* . . . **2** *often cap*

ATTRIBUTIVE NOUNS

The italicized label *often attrib* placed after the functional label *n* indicates that the noun is often used as an adjective equivalent in attributive position before another noun:

> **blood** . . . *n, often attrib*
> **hos·pi·tal** . . . *n, often attrib*

Examples of the attributive use of these nouns are *blood clot, blood disorder, hospital patient,* and *hospital ward.*

While any noun may occasionally be used in attribution, the label *often attrib* is limited to those having broad attributive use. This label is not used when an adjective homograph (as *serum*) is entered. And it is not used at open compounds that are used in attribution with an inserted hyphen.

ETYMOLOGY

Etymologies showing the origin of particular words are given in this dictionary only for some abbreviations and acronyms and for all eponyms.

If an entry for an abbreviation is followed by the expansion from which it is derived, no etymology is given. However, if the abbreviation is derived from a phrase in a foreign language or in English that is not mentioned elsewhere in the entry, that phrase and its language of origin (if other than English) are given in square brackets following the functional label:

> **IFN** *abbr* interferon
> **bid** *abbr* [Latin *bis in die*] twice a day

Words derived from the names of persons are called eponyms. Eponymous entries in this dictionary that are derived from the names of one or more real persons are followed by the last name, personal name, birth and death dates where known, nationality, and occupation or status of the person (or persons) from whose name the term is derived:

> **pas·teu·rel·la** . . . *n* . . .
> **Pas·teur** . . . **Louis (1822–1895),** French chemist and bacteriologist.

Doubtful dates are followed by a question mark, and approximate dates are preceded by *ca* (circa). In some instances only the years of principal activity are given, preceded by the abbreviation *fl* (flourished):

> **Gard·ner·el·la** . . . *n* . . .
> **Gard·ner** . . . **Herman L. (*fl* 1955–80),** American physician.

If a series of main entries is derived from the name of one person, the data usually follow the first entry. The dictionary user who turns, for example, to *pasteurellosis, pasteurization,* or *Pasteur treatment* and seeks biographical information is expected to glance back to the first entry in the sequence, *pasteurella.*

If an eponymous entry is defined by a synonymous cross-reference to the entry where the biographical data appear, no other cross-reference is made. However, if the definition of an eponymous entry contains no clue as to the location of the data, the name of the individual is given following the entry and a directional cross-reference is made to the appropriate entry:

> **gland of Bartholin** *n* : BAR-THOLIN'S GLAND
>
> **Rolandic area** . . . *n* : the motor area of the cerebral cortex lying just anterior to the central sulcus . . .
> **L. Rolando** — see FISSURE OF ROLANDO

The data for C. T. Bartholin can be found at *Bartholin's gland* and that for Luigi Rolando at *fissure of Rolando.*

USAGE

USAGE LABELS

Status labels are used in this dictionary to signal that a word or a sense of a word is restricted in usage.

A word or sense limited in use to a specific region of the English-speaking world has an appropriate label. The adverb *chiefly* precedes a label when the word has some currency outside the specified region, and a double label is used to indicate currency in each of two specific regions:

> **red bug** . . . *n, Southern & Midland*
> **ap·pen·di·cec·to·my** . . . *n* . . . *Brit*
> **fru·se·mide** . . . *n, chiefly Brit*

The stylistic label *slang* is used with words or senses that are especially appropriate in contexts of extreme informality, that usually have a currency not limited to a particular region or area of interest, and that are composed typically of shortened forms or

extravagant or facetious figures of speech. Words with the label *slang* are entered if they have been or in the opinion of the editors are likely to be encountered in communicating with patients especially in emergencies. A few words from the huge informal argot of medicine are entered with the label *med slang* because they have appeared in general context or have been the subject of discussion in medical journals:

> **ben·ny** . . . *n* . . . *slang*
> **go·mer** . . . *n, med slang*

Subject orientation is generally given in the definition; however, a guide phrase is sometimes used to indicate a specific application of a word or sense:

> **¹drug** . . . *n* **1** . . . **b** *according to the Food, Drug, and Cosmetic Act*
> **erupt** . . . *vb* **1** *of a tooth*

ILLUSTRATIONS OF USAGE

Definitions are sometimes followed by verbal illustrations that show a typical use of the word in context. These illustrations are enclosed in angle brackets, and the word being illustrated is usually replaced by a lightface swung dash. The swung dash stands for the boldface entry word, and it may be followed by an italicized suffix:

ab·er·rant ... *adj* ... **2** ... ⟨∼ salivary tissue⟩

treat ... *vb* ... ⟨∼*ed* their diseases⟩

The swung dash is not used when the form of the boldface entry word is changed in suffixation, and it is not used for open compounds:

tu·ber·os·i·ty ... *n* ... ⟨ischial *tuberosities*⟩

tie off *vb* ... ⟨*tie off* a bleeding vessel⟩

USAGE NOTES

Definitions are sometimes followed by usage notes that give supplementary information about such matters as idiom, syntax, semantic relationship, and status. For trademarks and service marks, a usage note is used in place of a definition. A usage note is introduced by a lightface dash:

pill ... *n* ... **2** ... : ... — usu. used with *the*

bug ... *n* **1 a** : ... — not used technically

hs *abbr* ... — used esp. in writing prescriptions

pec ... *n* ... — usu. used in pl.

Val·ium ... *trademark* — used for a preparation of diazepam

Sometimes a usage note calls attention to one or more terms that mean the same thing as the main entry:

lep·ro·sy ... *n* ... : a chronic disease caused by infection with an acid-fast bacillus of the genus *Mycobacterium* (*M. leprae*) ... — called also *Hansen's disease, lepra*

The called-also terms are shown in italic type. If the called-also term falls alphabetically at some distance from the principal entry, the called-also term is entered in alphabetical sequence with the sole definition being a synonymous cross-reference to the entry where it appears in the usage note:

Hansen's disease *n* : LEPROSY

lep·ra ... *n* : LEPROSY

Two or more usage notes are separated by a semicolon:

parathyroid hormone *n* : a hormone of the parathyroid gland that ... — abbr. *PTH;* called also *parathormone*

SENSE DIVISION

A boldface colon is used in this dictionary to introduce a definition:

pul·mo·nary ... *adj* : relating to, functioning like, associated with, or carried on by the lungs

It is also used to separate two or more definitions of a single sense:

mal·func·tion ... *vb* : to function imperfectly or badly : fail to operate in the normal or usual manner

Boldface Arabic numerals separate the senses of a word that has more than one sense:

nerve ... *n* **1** : any of the filamentous bands of nervous tissue that connect parts of the nervous system with other organs ... **2 nerves** *pl* : a state or condition of nervous agitation or irritability **3** : the sensitive pulp of a tooth

Boldface lowercase letters separate the subsenses of a word:

¹dose ... *n* **1 a** : the measured quantity of a therapeutic agent to be taken at one time **b** : the quantity of radiation administered or absorbed **2** : a gonorrheal infection

Lightface numerals in parentheses indicate a further division of subsenses:

ra·di·a·tion . . . *n* . . . **2 a :** . . . **b** (1)
: the process of emitting radiant
energy . . . (2) : the combined
processes of emission, transmission, and absorption of radiant energy

A lightface colon following a definition and immediately preceding
two or more subsenses indicates
that the subsenses are subsumed by
the preceding definition:

mac·u·la . . . *n* . . . **2** : an anatomical
structure having the form of a spot
differentiated from surrounding
tissues: as **a :** MACULA ACUSTICA
b : MACULA LUTEA

extensor ret·i·nac·u·lum . . . *n* **1**
: either of two fibrous bands of fascia crossing the front of the ankle:
a : a lower band . . . **b :** an upper
band . . .

The word *as* may or may not follow
the lightface colon. Its presence (as
at *macula*) indicates that the following subsenses are typical or significant examples. Its absence (as at
extensor retinaculum) indicates that
the subsenses which follow are ex-
haustive.

Sometimes a particular semantic
relationship between senses is suggested by the use of one of four
italic sense dividers: *esp, specif,
also,* or *broadly.* The sense divider
esp (for *especially*) is used to introduce the most common meaning
subsumed in the more general preceding definition. The sense divider

specif (for *specifically*) is used to introduce a common but highly restricted meaning subsumed in the
more general preceding definition.
The sense divider *also* is used to introduce a meaning that is closely
related to but may be considered
less important than the preceding
sense. The sense divider *broadly* is
used to introduce an extended or
wider meaning of the preceding
definition.

The order of senses within an entry is historical: the sense known to
have been first used in English is
entered first. This is not to be taken
to mean, however, that each sense
of a multisense word developed
from the immediately preceding
sense. It is altogether possible that
sense 1 of a word has given rise to
sense 2 and sense 2 to sense 3, but
frequently sense 2 and sense 3 may
have arisen independently of one
another from sense 1.

Information coming between the
entry word and the first definition
of a multisense word applies to all
senses and subsenses. Information
applicable only to some senses or
subsenses is given between the appropriate boldface numeral or letter and the symbolic colon.

bur . . . *n* **1** *usu* **burr**
chla·myd·ia . . . *n* **1** *cap* . . . **2** *pl* **-iae**
also **-ias**

NAMES OF PLANTS, ANIMALS, & MICROORGANISMS

The most familiar names of living
and formerly living things are the
common or vernacular names (as
mosquito, poison ivy, and *AIDS
virus*) that are determined by popular usage.

In contrast, the scientific names of
biological classification are gov-
erned by four highly prescriptive,
internationally recognized codes of
nomenclature for zoology, botany,
bacteriology, and virology. These

systems of names classify each kind
of organism into a hierarchy of
groups—taxa—with each kind of
organism having one—and only
one—correct name and belonging
to one—and only one—taxon at
each level of classification in the hierarchy.

The taxonomic names of biological nomenclature are used in this
dictionary in the definitions of the
common names of plants, animals,

and microorganisms and in the definitions of diseases and products relating to specific plants, animals, and microorganisms when those organisms do not have entries of their own. Some genus names appear as dictionary entries in the book but they are the only taxonomic names that have their own entries. Taxonomic names that are not given own-place entry will appear only within parentheses when used in a definition:

> **dust mite** *n* : any of various mites (esp. family Pyroglyphidae) commonly found in dust . . .

If a genus name is used in a definition and is not inside parentheses, there is an entry for it at its own alphabetical place:

> **Rocky Mountain spotted fever** . . . *n* : an acute bacterial disease . . . that is caused by a bacterium of the genus *Rickettsia* (*R. rickettsii*) usu. transmitted by ixodid ticks and esp. by the American dog tick and Rocky Mountain wood tick

The use of the genus name *Rickettsia* outside of parentheses indicates that a definition of this genus is entered its own place. The scientific names of the *American dog tick* and *Rocky Mountain wood tick* will be found at the entries for these organisms. The name of the family (Ixodidae) to which the two ticks belong will be found in parentheses at the entry for *ixodid*.

Many common names are derived directly from the names of taxa, and especially genera, with little or no modification. The genus name (as *Acarus* or *Chlamydia* or *Lentivirus*) is capitalized and italicized but is never pluralized. In contrast, the common or vernacular name (as acarus or chlamydia or lentivirus) is not usually capitalized or italicized but does take a plural (as acari or chlamydiae or lentiviruses). In many cases both the systematic taxonomic name and the common name derived from it are entered in this dictionary:

> **giar·dia** . . . *n* **1** *cap* : a genus of flagellate protozoans inhabiting the intestines of various mammals and including one (*G. lamblia*) that is associated with diarrhea in humans   **2** : any flagellate of the genus *Giardia*

> **strep·to·coc·cus** . . . *n* **1** *cap* : a genus of . . . gram-positive bacteria (family Streptococcaceae) that . . . include important pathogens of humans and domestic animals **2** *pl* **-coc·ci** . . . : any bacterium of the genus *Streptococcus*; *broadly* : a coccus occurring in chains

> **co·ro·na·vi·rus** . . . *n* **1** *cap* : a genus of single-stranded RNA viruses (family *Coronaviridae*) that infect birds and many mammals including humans . . . **2** : any virus of the genus *Coronavirus* or of the family (*Coronaviridae*) to which it belongs

LINNAEAN NOMENCLATURE OF PLANTS, ANIMALS, & BACTERIA

The nomenclatural codes for botany, zoology, and bacteriology follow the binomial nomenclature of Carolus Linnaeus, who employed a New Latin vocabulary for the names of organisms and the ranks in the hierarchy of classification.

The fundamental taxon is the genus. It includes a group of closely related kinds of plants (as the genus *Digitalis,* which contains the foxgloves), a group of closely related kinds of animals (as the genus *Plasmodium,* which includes the protozoans causing malaria in humans), or a group of closely related kinds of bacteria (as the genus *Borrelia,* which includes the causative agents of relapsing fever and Lyme disease). The genus name is an italicized and capitalized singular noun.

The unique name of each kind of organism or species in the Linnaean system is the binomial or species name which consists of two parts: a genus name and an italicized lowercase word—the specific epithet—denoting the species. The name for a variety or subspecies—the trinomial, variety name, or subspecies name—adds a similar varietal or subspecific epithet. For example, the head louse (*Pediculus humanus capitis*) and the body louse (*Pediculus humanus humanus*) are subspecies of a species (*Pediculus humanus*) infesting humans.

The genus name in a binomial may be abbreviated to its initial letter if it has been previously spelled out in full within the same text. In this dictionary, a genus name will be found abbreviated before a specific epithet when the genus is spelled out in full earlier within the same sense or within a group of senses that fall under a single boldface sense number:

> **scar·let fever** . . . *n* : an acute contagious febrile disease caused by Group A bacteria of the genus *Streptococcus* (esp. various strains

of *S. pyogenes*) and characterized
. . .

In Linnaean nomenclature, the names of taxa higher than the genus (as family, order, and class) are capitalized plural nouns that are often used with singular verbs and are not abbreviated in normal use. They are not italicized.

Sometimes two or more different New Latin names can be found used in current literature for the same organism or group. This may happen, for example, when old monographs and field guides are kept in print after name changes occur or when there are legitimate differences of opinion about the validity of the names. To help the reader in recognizing an organism or group in such cases, some alternate names are shown as synonyms in this dictionary:

> **Ro·cha·li·maea** . . . *n, syn of* BAR-TONELLA
>
> **plague** . . . *n* . . . **2** : a virulent contagious febrile disease that is caused by a bacterium of the genus *Yersinia* (*Y. pestis* syn. *Pasteurella pestis*) . . .

VIRUS NOMENCLATURE

The system of naming viruses evolved in a series of reports by a committee of the International Union of Microbiological Societies. The report published in 2005 with the title *Virus Taxonomy: Eighth Report of the International Committee on Taxonomy of Viruses (8th Rept. of the ICTV)* is the one followed in this dictionary. The code of nomenclature developed there is independent of the three Linnaean systems governing the taxonomy of plants, animals, and bacteria and differs in the way names are constructed and written.

The names for species, genera, and families of viruses used in this dictionary are those that are recognized as valid by the *8th Rept. of the ICTV*. Such names appear in italics and are preceded by the name of the taxon ("species," "genus," or "family") in roman before the italicized name. No two valid taxa in virus classification are permitted to have the same name even if they are assigned to different higher taxa. Thus, each valid taxonomic name is unique no matter where it occurs in the taxonomic hierarchy.

In the nomenclature of viruses, the names of all valid taxa at the species or higher level are written in italics. The name of a species consists of an italicized phrase in which the first word is capitalized, other words are lowercase unless derived from a proper name, and the last word is *virus* or ends in

-*virus,* sometimes followed by a number or letter or combination of both (as in species *Human herpesvirus 3,* the causative agent of chicken pox). The name of a genus is a single capitalized word ending in -*virus* sometimes followed by a capital letter (as in genus *Influenzavirus A* which contains species *Influenza A virus*). The name of a family is a single capitalized word ending in -*viridae* (as in family *Herpesviridae* or family *Poxviridae*):

> **small·pox** . . . *n* : an acute contagious febrile disease of humans that is caused by a poxvirus of the genus *Orthopoxvirus* (species *Variola virus*) . . .
>
> **pox·vi·rus** . . . *n* : any of a family (*Poxviridae*) of large brick-shaped

or ovoid double-stranded DNA viruses . . .

Italics are not used for the names of strains or subtypes or for synonyms or former names that are no longer valid:

> **pa·po·va·vi·rus** . . . *n* : any of a former family (Papovaviridae) that included the papillomaviruses and the polyomaviruses

The rejected family name Papovaviridae is written in roman. The names of the two valid families (*Papillomaviridae* and *Polyomaviridae*) into which the family Papovaviridae has been split are mentioned in parentheses at the entries for *papillomavirus* and *polyomavirus.*

CROSS-REFERENCE

Four different kinds of cross-references are used in this dictionary: directional, synonymous, cognate, and inflectional. In each instance the cross-reference is readily recognized by the lightface small capitals in which it is printed.

A cross-reference usually following a lightface dash and beginning with *see* or *compare* is a directional cross-reference. It directs the dictionary user to look elsewhere for further information. A *compare* cross-reference is regularly appended to a definition; a *see* cross-reference may stand alone:

> **heart attack** *n* . . . — compare ANGINA PECTORIS, CORONARY INSUFFICIENCY, HEART FAILURE 1
>
> **iron** . . . *n* **1** . . . — symbol *Fe;* see ELEMENT table
>
> **mammary artery** — see INTERNAL THORACIC ARTERY

A *see* cross-reference may be used to indicate the place of definition of an entry containing one or more Arabic numerals or abbreviated chemical prefixes that might cause doubt. Examples of chemical names are given above at "Order of Main

Entries." The entry below follows the entry for the abbreviation *GP:*

> **G₁ phase, G₂ phase** — see entries alphabetized as G ONE PHASE, G TWO PHASE

A *see* cross-reference may follow a main entry that consists of a single word which does not stand alone but appears only in a compound term or terms; the *see* cross-reference at such entries indicates the compound term or terms in which the single word appears:

> **herpetiformis** — see DERMATITIS HERPETIFORMIS
>
> **dorsi** — see ILIOCOSTALIS DORSI, LATISSIMUS DORSI, LONGISSIMUS DORSI

A *see* cross-reference may appear after the definition of the name of a generic drug to refer the reader to a trademark used for a preparation of the drug:

> **di·az·e·pam** . . . *n* . . . — see VALIUM

A cross-reference immediately following a boldface colon is a synonymous cross-reference. It may stand alone as the only definitional matter, it may follow an analytical definition, or it may be one of two synonymous cross-references separated by a comma:

> **serum hepatitis** *n* : HEPATITIS B
> **liv·id** . . . *adj* : discolored by bruising : BLACK-AND-BLUE
> **af·fec·tion** . . . *n* . . . **2** . . . **b** : DISEASE, MALADY

A synonymous cross-reference indicates that a definition at the entry cross-referred to can be substituted as a definition for the entry or the sense or subsense in which the cross-reference appears.

A cross-reference following an italic *var of* is a cognate cross-reference:

> **procaryote** *var of* PROKARYOTE
> **ma·noeu·vre** *chiefly Brit var of* MANEUVER

A cross-reference following an italic label that identifies an entry as an inflected form is an inflectional cross-reference. Inflectional cross-references appear only when the inflected form falls alphabetically at some distance from the main entry:

> **corpora** *pl of* CORPUS
> **broke** *past of* BREAK

When guidance seems needed as to which one of several homographs or which sense of a multisense word is being referred to, a superscript numeral may precede the cross-reference or a sense number may follow it or both:

> **ossa** *pl of* ¹OS
> **lateral cuneiform bone** *n* : CUNEIFORM BONE 1c

COMBINING FORMS, PREFIXES & SUFFIXES

An entry that begins or ends with a hyphen is a word element that forms part of an English compound:

> **pharmaco-** *comb form* . . . ⟨*pharmaco*logy⟩
> **dys-** *prefix* **1** : . . . ⟨*dys*plasia⟩
> **-i·a·sis** *n suffix, pl* **-i·a·ses** . . . ⟨ame*biasis*⟩

Combining forms, prefixes, and suffixes are entered in this dictionary for two reasons: to make understandable the meaning of many undefined run-ons and to make recognizable the meaningful elements of words that are not entered in the dictionary.

ABBREVIATIONS & SYMBOLS

Abbreviations and symbols for chemical elements are included as main entries in the vocabulary:

> **RQ** *abbr* respiratory quotient
> **Al** *symbol* aluminum

Abbreviations are entered without periods and have been normalized to one form of capitalization. In practice, however, there is considerable variation, and stylings other than those given in this dictionary are often acceptable.

The more common abbreviations and the symbols of chemical elements also appear after the definition at the entries for the terms they represent:

> **respiratory quotient** *n* : . . . — *abbr. RQ*

Symbols that are not capable of being alphabetized are included in a separate section in the back of this book headed "Signs and Symbols."

ABBREVIATIONS USED IN THIS WORK

abbr	abbreviation
AD	anno Domini
adj	adjective
adv	adverb
attrib	attributive
b	born
BC	before Christ
Brit	British
C	Celsius
ca	circa
Canad	Canadian
cap	capitalized
comb	combining
d	died
esp	especially
F	Fahrenheit
fl	flourished
n	noun
No	North
n pl	noun plural
occas	occasionally
orig	originally
part	participle
pl	plural
pres	present
prob	probably
sing	singular
So	South
SoAfr	South African
specif	specifically
spp	species (*pl*)
syn	synonym
U.S.	United States
usu	usually
var	variant
vb	verb

PRONUNCIATION SYMBOLS

ə	abut, collect, suppose	ȯi	toy
ˈə, ˌə	humdrum	p	pepper, lip
ə	(in ᵊl, ᵊn) battle, cotton; (in lᵊ, mᵊ, rᵊ) French table, prisme, titre	r	rarity
		s	source, less
		sh	shy, mission
ər	further	t	tie, attack
a	map, patch	th	thin, ether
ā	day, fate	th	then, either
ä	bother, cot, father	ü	boot, few \ˈfyü\
à	a sound between \a\ and \ä\, as in an Eastern New England pronunciation of aunt, ask	u̇	put, pure \ˈpyu̇r\
		ue	German füllen
		ǖ	French rue, German fühlen
au̇	now, out	v	vivid, give
b	baby, rib	w	we, away
ch	chin, catch	y	yard, cue \ˈkyü\
d	did, adder	ʸ	indicates that a preceding \l\, \n\, or \w\ is modified by having the tongue approximate the position for \y\, as in French digne \dēnʸ\
e	set, red		
ē	beat, easy		
f	fifty, cuff		
g	go, big	z	zone, raise
h	hat, ahead	zh	vision, pleasure
hw	whale	\	slant line used in pairs to mark the beginning and end of a transcription: \ˈpen\
i	tip, banish		
ī	site, buy	ˈ	mark at the beginning of a syllable that has primary (strongest) stress: \ˈshə-fəl-ˌbȯrd\
j	job, edge		
k	kin, cook		
ḵ	German Bach, Scots loch	ˌ	mark at the beginning of a syllable that has secondary (next-strongest) stress: \ˈshə-fəl-ˌbȯrd\
l	lily, cool		
m	murmur, dim		
n	nine, own	-	mark of syllable division in pronunciations (the mark of end-of-line division in boldface entries is a centered dot ·)
ⁿ	indicates that a preceding vowel is pronounced through both nose and mouth, as in French bon \bōⁿ\		
		( )	indicate that what is symbolized between sometimes occurs and sometimes does not occur in the pronunciation of the word: bakery \ˈbā-k(ə-)rē\ = \ˈbā-kə-rē, ˈbā-krē\
ŋ	sing, singer, finger, ink		
ō	bone, hollow		
ȯ	saw		
œ	French bœuf, German Hölle		
œ̄	French feu, German Höhle		

A \'ā\ *n* : one of the four ABO blood groups characterized by the presence of antigens designated by the letter A and by the presence of antibodies against the antigens present in the B blood group

A *abbr* **1** adenine **2** ampere

Å *symbol* angstrom

a- *or* **an-** *prefix* : not : without ⟨*asex*ual⟩ — *a-* before consonants other than *h* and sometimes even before *h*, *an-* before vowels and usu. before *h* ⟨*achromatic*⟩ ⟨*an*hydrous⟩

āā *also* **aa** *abbr* [Latin *ana*] of each — used at the end of a list of two or more substances in a prescription to indicate that equal quantities of each are to be taken

AA *abbr* Alcoholics Anonymous

ab \'ab\ *n* : ABDOMINAL — usu. used in pl. ⟨highly developed ∼*s*⟩

AB \'ā-'bē\ *n* : the one of the four ABO blood groups characterized by the presence of antigens designated by the letters A and B and by the absence of antibodies against these antigens

ab- *prefix* : from : away : off ⟨*ab*oral⟩

abac·te·ri·al \ˌā-(ˌ)bak-'tir-ē-əl\ *adj* : not caused by or characterized by the presence of bacteria ⟨∼ prostatitis⟩

A band *n* : one of the cross striations in striated muscle that contain myosin filaments and appear dark under the light microscope and light in polarized light

aba·sia \ə-'bā-zhə, -zhē-ə\ *n* : inability to walk caused by a defect in muscular coordination — compare ASTASIA

Ab-be–Est·lan·der operation \'a-bē-'äst-ˌlän-dər-, -'est-ˌlan-\ *n* : the grafting of a flap of tissue from one lip of the oral cavity to the other lip to correct a defect using a pedicle with an arterial supply

    Abbe, Robert (1851–1928), American surgeon.

    Estlander, Jakob August (1831–1881), Finnish surgeon.

ab·cix·i·mab \ˌab-'sik-si-mab\ *n* : an anticlotting drug that inhibits platelet aggregation — see REOPRO

abdom *abbr* abdomen; abdominal

ab·do·men \'ab-də-mən, (ˌ)ab-'dō-\ *n* **1 a** : the part of the body between the thorax and the pelvis with the exception of the back — called also *belly* **b** : the cavity of this part of the trunk lined by the peritoneum, enclosed by the body walls, the diaphragm, and the pelvic floor, and containing the visceral organs (as the stomach, intestines, and liver) **c** : the portion of this cavity between the diaphragm and the brim of the pelvis **2** : the posterior often elongated region of the body behind the thorax in arthropods

abdomin- *or* **abdomino-** *comb form* **1** : abdomen ⟨*abdomino*plasty⟩ **2** : abdominal and ⟨*abdomino*perineal⟩

¹ab·dom·i·nal \ab-'dä-mən-əl\ *adj* **1** : of, belonging to, or affecting the abdomen **2** : performed by entry through the abdominal wall — **ab·dom·i·nal·ly** *adv*

²abdominal *n* : an abdominal muscle — usu. used in pl.

abdominal aorta *n* : the portion of the aorta between the diaphragm and the bifurcation into the right and left common iliac arteries

abdominal cavity *n* : ABDOMEN 1b

abdominal hernia *n* : any of various hernias (as an inguinal hernia, umbilical hernia, or spigelian hernia) in which an anatomical part (as a section of the intestine) protrudes through an opening, tear, or weakness in the abdominal wall musculature

abdominal reflex *n* : contraction of the muscles of the abdominal wall in response to stimulation of the overlying skin

abdominal region *n* : any of the nine areas into which the abdomen is divided by four imaginary planes of which two are vertical passing through the middle of the inguinal ligament on each side and two are horizontal passing respectively through the junction of the ninth rib and costal cartilage and through the top of the iliac crest — see EPIGASTRIC 2b, HYPOCHONDRIAC 2b, HYPOGASTRIC 1, ILIAC 2, LUMBAR 2, UMBILICAL 2

abdominis — see OBLIQUUS EXTERNUS ABDOMINIS, OBLIQUUS INTERNUS ABDOMINIS, RECTUS ABDOMINIS, TRANSVERSUS ABDOMINIS

ab·dom·i·no·pel·vic \(ˌ)ab-ˌdä-mə-nō-'pel-vik\ *adj* : relating to or being the abdominal and pelvic cavities of the body

ab·dom·i·no·per·i·ne·al \-ˌper-ə-'nē-əl\ *adj* : relating to the abdominal and perineal regions

abdominoperineal resection *n* : resection of a part of the lower bowel together with adjacent lymph nodes through abdominal and perineal incisions

ab·dom·i·no·plas·ty \ab-'dä-mə-nō-ˌplas-tē\ *n, pl* **-ties** : cosmetic surgery of the abdomen that typically involves the removal of excess skin and fat and tightening of the abdominal muscles — called also *tummy tuck*

ab·du·cens nerve \ab-'dü-ˌsenz-, -'dyü-\ *n* : either of the sixth pair of cranial nerves which are motor nerves, arise beneath the floor of the fourth ventricle, and supply the lateral rectus muscle of each eye —

called also *abducens, sixth cranial nerve*

ab·du·cent nerve \-sənt-\ *n* : ABDUCENS NERVE

ab·duct \ab-'dəkt *also* 'ab-,\ *vb* : to draw or spread away (as a limb or the fingers) from a position near or parallel to the median axis of the body or from the axis of a limb — **ab·duc·tion** \ab-'dək-shən\ *n*

ab·duc·tor \ab-'dək-tər\ *n, pl* **ab·duc·to·res** \,ab-,dək-'tōr-(,)ēz\ *or* **abductors** : a muscle that draws a part away from the median line of the body or from the axis of an extremity

abductor dig·i·ti min·i·mi \-'di-jə-(,)tē-'mi-nə-(,)mē\ *n* **1** : a muscle of the hand that abducts the little finger and flexes the phalanx nearest the hand **2** : a muscle of the foot that abducts the little toe

abductor hal·lu·cis \-'hal-yə-səs; -'ha-lə-səs, -kəs\ *n* : a muscle of the foot that abducts the big toe

abductor pol·li·cis brev·is \-'pä-lə-səs-'bre-vəs, -lə-kəs-\ *n* : a thin flat muscle of the hand that abducts the thumb at right angles to the plane of the palm

abductor pollicis lon·gus \-'lȯŋ-gəs\ *n* : a muscle of the forearm that abducts the thumb and wrist

ab·er·rant \a-'ber-ənt; 'a-bə-rənt, -,ber-ənt\ *adj* **1** : straying from the right or normal way ⟨∼ behavior⟩ **2** : deviating from the usual or natural type : ATYPICAL ⟨∼ salivary tissue⟩

ab·er·ra·tion \,a-bə-'rā-shən\ *n* **1** : failure of a mirror, refracting surface, or lens to produce exact point-to-point correspondence between an object and its image **2** : unsoundness or disorder of the mind **3** : an aberrant organ or individual — **ab·er·ra·tion·al** \-sh(ə)-nəl\ *adj*

abey·ance \ə-'bā-əns\ *n* : temporary inactivity or suspension

ABFP *abbr* American Board of Family Practice

ab·i·ence \'a-bē-əns\ *n* : a tendency to withdraw from a stimulus object or situation — compare ADIENCE — **abi·ent** \-ənt\ *adj*

abi·ot·ro·phy \,ā-(,)bī-'ä-trə-fē\ *n, pl* **-phies** : degeneration or loss of function or vitality in an organism or in cells or tissues not due to any apparent injury

ab·late \a-'blāt\ *vb* **ab·lat·ed; ab·lat·ing** : to remove or destroy esp. by cutting — **ablative** *adj*

ab·la·tion \a-'blā-shən\ *n* : the process of ablating; *esp* : surgical removal

ab·la·tio pla·cen·tae \a-'blä-shē-ō-plə-'sen-(,)tē\ *n* : ABRUPTIO PLACENTAE

abled \'ā-bəld\ *adj* : capable of unimpaired function — compare DIFFERENTLY ABLED

¹ab·nor·mal \(,)ab-'nȯr-məl\ *adj* : deviating from the normal or average ⟨∼ behavior⟩ ⟨∼ development⟩ — **ab·nor·mal·ly** *adv*

²abnormal *n* : an abnormal person

ab·nor·mal·i·ty \,ab-nȯr-'ma-lə-tē\ *n, pl* **-ties** **1** : the quality or state of being abnormal **2** : something abnormal

abnormal psychology *n* : a branch of psychology concerned with mental and emotional disorders (as neuroses and psychoses) and with certain incompletely understood normal phenomena (as dreams)

ABO blood group \,ā-(,)bē-'ō-\ *n* : one of the four blood groups A, B, AB, or O comprising the ABO system

ab·oma·sum \,a-bō-'mā-səm\ *n, pl* **-sa** \-sə\ : the fourth compartment of the ruminant stomach that follows the omasum and has a true digestive function — compare RUMEN, RETICULUM — **ab·oma·sal** \-səl\ *adj*

ab·oral \(,)a-'bȯr-əl, -'bōr-\ *adj* : situated opposite to or away from the mouth — **aborally** *adv*

abort \ə-'bȯrt\ *vb* **1** : to cause or undergo abortion **2** : to stop in the early stages ⟨∼ a disease⟩ — **abort·er** *n*

¹abor·ti·fa·cient \ə-,bȯr-tə-'fā-shənt\ *adj* : inducing abortion

²abortifacient *n* : an agent (as a drug) that induces abortion

abor·tion \ə-'bȯr-shən\ *n* **1** : the termination of a pregnancy after, accompanied by, resulting in, or closely followed by the death of the embryo or fetus: **a** : spontaneous expulsion of a human fetus during the first 12 weeks of gestation — compare MISCARRIAGE **b** : induced expulsion of a human fetus **c** : expulsion of a fetus of a domestic animal often due to infection at any time before completion of pregnancy — see CONTAGIOUS ABORTION **2** : arrest of development of an organ so that it remains imperfect or is absorbed **3** : the arrest of a disease in its earliest stage

abor·tion·ist \-sh(ə)nist\ *n* : one who induces abortion

abortion pill *n* : a drug taken orally to induce abortion esp. early in pregnancy; *esp* : RU-486

abor·tive \ə-'bȯr-tiv\ *adj* **1** : imperfectly formed or developed : RUDIMENTARY **2 a** : ABORTIFACIENT **b** : cutting short ⟨∼ treatment of pneumonia⟩ **c** : failing to develop completely or typically

abor·tus \ə-'bȯr-təs\ *n* : an aborted fetus; *specif* : a human fetus less than 12 weeks old or weighing at birth less than 17 ounces

ABO system \,ā-(,)bē-'ō-\ *n* : the basic system of antigens of human blood behaving in heredity as an allelic unit to produce any of the ABO blood groups

aboulia *var of* ABULIA

abrade \ə-'brād\ *vb* **abrad·ed; abrad·ing** : to irritate or roughen by rubbing : CHAFE

abra·sion \ə-'brā-zhən\ *n* **1** : wearing, grinding, or rubbing away by friction **2 a** : the rubbing or scraping of the surface layer of cells or tissue from an area of the skin or mucous membrane; *also* : a place so abraded   **b** : the mechanical wearing away of the tooth surfaces by chewing

¹abra·sive \ə-'brā-siv, -ziv\ *adj* : tending to abrade ⟨an ∼ substance⟩ — **abra·sive·ness** *n*

²abrasive *n* : a substance used for abrading, smoothing, or polishing

ab·re·ac·tion \ₐa-brē-'ak-shən\ *n* : the expression and emotional discharge of unconscious material (as a repressed idea or emotion) by verbalization esp. in the presence of a therapist — compare CATHARSIS 2 — **ab·re·act** \-'akt\ *vb* — **ab·re·ac·tive** \-'ak-tiv\ *adj*

ab·rup·tion \ə-'brəp-shən\ *n* : a sudden breaking off : detachment of portions from a mass ⟨placental ∼⟩

ab·rup·tio pla·cen·tae \ə-'brəp-shē-ˌō-plə-'sen-(ˌ)tē, -tē-ˌō-\ *n* : premature detachment of the placenta from the wall of the uterus — called also *ablatio placentae*

abs \'abz\ *pl of* AB

ab·scess \'ab-ˌses\ *n, pl* **ab·scess·es** \'ab-sə-ˌsēz, -(ˌ)se-səz\ : a localized collection of pus surrounded by inflamed tissue — **ab·scessed** \-ˌsest\ *adj*

ab·scis·sion \ab-'si-zhən\ *n* : the act or process of cutting off : ABLATION

ab·sco·pal \ab-'skō-pəl\ *adj* : relating to or being an effect on a nonirradiated part of the body that results from irradiation of another part

ab·sence seizure \'ab-sᵊns-\ *n* : a nonconvulsive generalized seizure that is marked by the transient loss or impairment of consciousness usu. with a blank stare, that begins and ends abruptly, and is usu. unremembered afterward, and that is seen chiefly in mild types of epilepsy — called also *petit mal*

ab·so·lute \ˌab-sə-'lüt\ *adj* **1** : pure or relatively free from mixture ⟨∼ alcohol⟩ **2** : relating to, measured on, or being a temperature scale based on absolute zero ⟨∼ temperature⟩

absolute humidity *n* : the amount of water vapor present in a unit volume of air — compare RELATIVE HUMIDITY

absolute refractory period *n* : the period immediately following the firing of a nerve fiber when it cannot be stimulated no matter how great a stimulus is applied — called also *absolute refractory phase;* compare RELATIVE REFRACTORY PERIOD

absolute zero *n* : a theoretical temperature characterized by complete absence of heat and equivalent to exactly −273.15°C or −459.67°F

ab·sorb \ab-'sȯrb, -'zȯrb\ *vb* **1** : to take up esp. by capillary, osmotic, solvent, or chemical action **2** : to transform (radiant energy) into a different form usu. with a resulting rise in temperature — **ab·sorb·able** \ab-'sȯr-bə-bəl, -'zȯr-\ *adj* — **ab·sorb·er** *n*

ab·sor·bent *also* **ab·sor·bant** \-bənt\ *adj* : able to absorb — **ab·sor·ben·cy** \-bən-sē\ *n* — **absorbent** *also* **sorbant** *n*

ab·sorp·ti·om·e·try \əb-ˌsȯrp-shē-'äm-ə-trē\ *n, pl* **-tries** : measurement of the amount of radiation absorbed (as by living tissue) esp. to determine density — see DUAL-ENERGY X-RAY ABSORPTIOMETRY

ab·sorp·tion \əb-'sȯrp-shən, -'zȯrp-\ *n* : the process of absorbing or of being absorbed — compare ADSORPTION — **ab·sorp·tive** \-tiv\ *adj*

ab·stain \ab-'stān\ *vb* : to refrain deliberately and often with an effort of self-denial from an action or practice — **ab·stain·er** *n*

ab·sti·nence \'ab-stə-nəns\ *n* : the act or practice of abstaining esp. from engagement in sexual intercourse or consumption of intoxicating beverages — **ab·sti·nent** \-nənt\ *adj*

ab·stract \'ab-ˌstrakt\ *n* **1** : a written summary of the key points esp. of a scientific paper **2** : a pharmaceutical preparation made by mixing a powdered solid extract of a vegetable substance with lactose in such proportions that one part of the final product represents two parts of the original drug from which the extract was made — **ab·stract** \'ab-ˌstrakt, ab-'\ *vb*

abu·lia *or* **abou·lia** \ā-'bü-lē-ə, ə-, -'byü\ *n* : abnormal lack of ability to act or to make decisions that is characteristic of certain psychotic and neurotic conditions — **abu·lic** *also* **abou·lic** \-lik\ *adj*

¹abuse \ə-'byüs\ *n* **1** : improper or excessive use or treatment ⟨drug ∼⟩ **2** : physical maltreatment: as **a** : the act of violating sexually : RAPE **b** *under some statutes* : rape or indecent assault not amounting to rape

²abuse \ə-'byüz\ *vb* **abused; abus·ing 1** : to put to a wrong or improper use ⟨∼ drugs⟩ **2** : to treat so as to injure or damage ⟨∼ a child⟩ : as **a** : MASTURBATE **b** : to subject to abuse and esp. to rape or indecent assault — **abus·able** \-'byü-zə-bəl\ *adj* — **abus·er** *n*

abut·ment \ə-'bət-mənt\ *n* : a tooth to which a prosthetic appliance (as a denture) is attached for support

ac *abbr* **1** acute **2** [Latin *ante cibum*] before meals — used in writing prescriptions

Ac *symbol* actinium

aca·cia \ə-'kā-shə\ *n* : GUM ARABIC

acal·cu·lia \ˌā-ˌkal-'kyü-lē-ə\ *n* : lack or loss of the ability to perform simple arithmetic tasks

acal·cu·lous \ā-'kal-kyə-ləs\ *adj* : not affected with, caused by, or associated with gallstones ⟨an ∼ gallbladder⟩

acanth- *or* **acantho-** *comb form* **1** : spine : prickle : projection ⟨acanthocyte⟩ **2** : prickle cell layer ⟨*acan-thoma*⟩

acanth·amoe·ba \ə-ˌkanth-əˈmē-bə\ *n* **1** *cap* : a genus of free-living amoebas (family Acanthamoebidae) found esp. in soil and freshwater and including several which are pathogenic in humans causing infections of the skin, respiratory tract, eyes, and brain **2** : any amoeba of the genus *Acanthamoeba*

acan·tho·ceph·a·lan \ə-ˌkan-thəˈse-fə-lən\ *n* : any of a small phylum (Acanthocephala) of unsegmented parasitic worms that have a proboscis bearing hooks by which attachment is made to the intestinal wall of the host — **acanthocephalan** *adj*

acan·tho·cyte \ə-ˈkan-thə-ˌsīt\ *n* : an abnormal red blood cell characterized by variously shaped protoplasmic projections

ac·an·tho·ma \ˌa-(ˌ)kan-ˈthō-mə, ˌā-\ *n, pl* **-mas** \-məz\ *also* **-ma·ta** \-mə-tə\ : a tumor originating in the skin and developing through excessive growth of skin cells esp. of the stratum spinosum

ac·an·tho·sis \-ˈthō-səs\ *n, pl* **-tho·ses** \-ˌsēz\ : a benign overgrowth of the stratum spinosum of the skin — **ac·an·thot·ic** \-ˈthä-tik\ *adj*

acanthosis ni·gri·cans \-ˈni-grə-ˌkanz, -ˈnī-\ *n* : a skin disease characterized by gray-black warty patches usu. situated in the axilla or groin or on elbows or knees and sometimes associated with cancer of abdominal viscera

acap·nia \ə-ˈkap-nē-ə, (ˌ)ā-\ *n* : a condition of carbon dioxide deficiency in blood and tissues

acar- *or* **acari-** *or* **acaro-** *comb form* : mite ⟨*acariasis*⟩ ⟨*acaricide*⟩

ac·a·ri·a·sis \ˌa-kə-ˈrī-ə-səs\ *n, pl* **-a·ses** \-ˌsēz\ : infestation with or disease caused by mites

acar·i·cide \ə-ˈkar-ə-ˌsīd\ *n* : a pesticide that kills mites and ticks — **acar·i·cid·al** \ə-ˌkar-ə-ˈsid-ᵊl\ *adj*

ac·a·rid \ˈa-kə-rəd\ *n* : any of an order (Acari syn. Acarina) of arachnids comprising the mites and ticks; *esp* : any of a family (Acaridae) of mites that feed on organic substances and are sometimes responsible for dermatitis in persons exposed to repeated contacts with infested products — compare GROCER'S ITCH — **acarid** *adj*

ac·a·rine \ˈa-kə-ˌrīn, -ˌrēn, -rən\ *adj* : of, relating to, or caused by mites or ticks ⟨∼ dermatitis⟩ — **acarine** *n*

ac·a·rus \ˈa-kə-rəs\ *n, pl* **-ri** \-ˌrī, -ˌrē\ : MITE; *esp* : one of a formerly extensive genus (*Acarus*)

ac·cel·er·ate \ik-ˈse-lə-ˌrāt, ak-\ *vb* **-at·ed; -at·ing** : to speed up; *also* : to undergo or cause to undergo acceleration

ac·cel·er·a·tion \ik-ˌse-lə-ˈrā-shən, ak-\ *n* **1** : the act or process of accelerat-

ing : the state of being accelerated **2** : change of velocity; *also* : the rate of this change **3** : advancement in mental growth or achievement beyond the average for one's age

ac·cel·er·a·tor \ik-ˈse-lə-ˌrā-tər, ak-\ *n* : a muscle or nerve that speeds the performance of an action

accelerator globulin *n* : FACTOR V

accelerator nerve *n* : a nerve whose impulses increase the rate of the heart

ac·cep·tor \ik-ˈsep-tər, ak-\ *n* : an atom, molecule, or subatomic particle capable of receiving another entity (as an electron) esp. to form a compound — compare DONOR 2

¹ac·ces·so·ry \ik-ˈse-sə-rē, ak-, -ˈses-rē\ *adj* **1** : aiding, contributing, or associated in a secondary way: as **a** : being or functioning as a vitamin **b** : associated in position or function with something (as an organ or lesion) usu. of more importance **2** : SUPERNUMERARY ⟨∼ spleens⟩

²accessory *n, pl* **-ries** : ACCESSORY NERVE

accessory hemiazygos vein *n* : a vein that drains the upper left side of the thoracic wall, descends along the left side of the spinal column, and empties into the azygos or hemiazygos veins near the middle of the thorax

accessory nerve *n* : either of a pair of motor nerves that are the 11th cranial nerves, arise from the medulla and the upper part of the spinal cord, and supply chiefly the pharynx and muscles of the upper chest, back, and shoulders — called also *accessory, spinal accessory nerve*

accessory olivary nucleus *n* : any of several small masses or layers of gray matter that are situated adjacent to the inferior olive and of which there are typically two on each side

accessory pancreatic duct *n* : a duct of the pancreas that branches from the chief pancreatic duct and opens into the duodenum above it — called also *duct of Santorini*

ac·ci·dent \ˈak-sə-dənt, -ˌdent\ *n* **1** : an unfortunate event resulting from carelessness, unawareness, ignorance, or a combination of causes **2** : an unexpected bodily event of medical importance esp. when injurious ⟨a cerebrovascular ∼⟩ **3** : an unexpected happening causing loss or injury which is not due to any fault or misconduct on the part of the person injured but for which legal relief may be sought — **ac·ci·den·tal** \ˌak-sə-ˈdent-ᵊl\ *adj* — **ac·ci·den·tal·ly** \-ˈdent-lē, -ᵊl-ē\ *also* **ac·ci·dent·ly** \-ˈdent-lē\ *adv*

accident–prone *adj* **1** : having a greater than average number of accidents **2** : having personality traits that predispose to accidents

ac·cli·mate \ˈa-klə-ˌmāt; ə-ˈklī-mət, -ˌmāt\ *vb* **-mat·ed; -mat·ing** : ACCLIMATIZE

ac·cli·ma·tion \ˌa-klə-ˈmā-shən, -ˌklī-\ n : acclimatization esp. by physiological adjustment of an organism to environmental change

ac·cli·ma·tize \ə-ˈklī-mə-ˌtīz\ vb **-tized; -tiz·ing** : to adapt to a new temperature, altitude, climate, environment, or situation — **ac·cli·ma·ti·za·tion** \ə-ˌklī-mə-tə-ˈzā-shən\ n

ac·com·mo·date \ə-ˈkä-mə-ˌdāt\ vb **-dat·ed; -dat·ing** : to adapt oneself; also : to undergo visual accommodation — **ac·com·mo·da·tive** \-ˌdā-tiv\ adj

ac·com·mo·da·tion \ə-ˌkä-mə-ˈdā-shən\ n : an adaptation or adjustment esp. of a bodily part (as an organ): as **a** : the automatic adjustment of the eye for seeing at different distances effected chiefly by changes in the convexity of the crystalline lens **b** : the range over which such adjustment is possible

ac·couche·ment \ˌa-ˌküsh-ˈmäⁿ, ə-ˈküsh-ˌ\ n : the time or act of giving birth

ac·cou·cheur \ˌa-ˌkü-ˈshər\ n : one that assists at a birth; esp : OBSTETRICIAN

ac·cou·cheuse \ˌa-ˌkü-ˈshərz, -ˈshüz\ n : MIDWIFE

ac·cre·tio cor·dis \ə-ˈkrē-shē-ō-ˈkȯr-dəs\ n : adhesive pericarditis in which there are adhesions extending from the pericardium to the mediastinum, pleurae, diaphragm, and chest wall

ac·cre·tion \ə-ˈkrē-shən\ n : the process of growth or enlargement; esp : increase by external addition or accumulation — compare APPOSITION 1 — **ac·cre·tion·ary** \-shə-ˌner-ē\ adj

accumbens — see NUCLEUS ACCUMBENS

Ac·cu·pril \ˈa-kyu-ˌpril\ trademark — used for a preparation of the hydrochloride of quinapril

Ac·cu·tane \ˈa-kyu-ˌtān\ trademark — used for a preparation of isotretinoin

Ace \ˈās\ trademark — used for a bandage with elastic properties

ACE inhibitor \ˈās-, ˌā-(ˌ)sē-ˈē-\ n : any of a group of antihypertensive drugs (as captopril) that relax arteries and promote renal excretion of salt and water by inhibiting the activity of angiotensin converting enzyme

acel·lu·lar \(ˌ)ā-ˈsel-yə-lər\ adj **1** : containing no cells (∼ vaccines) **2** : not divided into cells : consisting of a single complex cell — used esp. of protozoa and ciliates

acen·tric \(ˌ)ā-ˈsen-trik\ adj : lacking a centromere (∼ chromosomes)

ace·sul·fame-K \ˈā-sē-ˌsȯl-ˌfäm-ˈkä\ n : a white crystalline powder C₄H₄KNO₄S that is much sweeter than sucrose and is used as a noncaloric sweetener — called also acesulfame potassium

acetabular notch \-ˈnäch\ n : a notch in the rim of the acetabulum through which blood vessels and nerves pass

ac·e·tab·u·lo·plas·ty \ˌa-sə-ˈta-byə-(ˌ)lō-ˌplas-tē\ n, pl **-ties** : plastic surgery on the acetabulum intended to restore its normal state

ac·e·tab·u·lum \-ˈta-byə-ləm\ n, pl **-lums** or **-la** \-lə\ : the cup-shaped socket in the hip bone — **ac·e·tab·u·lar** \-lər\ adj

ac·et·al·de·hyde \ˌa-sə-ˈtal-də-ˌhīd\ n : a colorless volatile water-soluble liquid aldehyde C₂H₄O used chiefly in organic synthesis that can cause irritation to mucous membranes

acet·amin·o·phen \ə-ˌsēt-ə-ˈmi-nə-fən, -ˌset-, -ˈmē-, ˌa-sə-tə-\ n : a crystalline compound C₈H₉NO₂ used in medicine instead of aspirin to relieve pain and fever — called also paracetamol; see LIQUIPRIN, TYLENOL

ac·et·an·i·lide or **ac·et·an·i·lid** \ˌa-sə-ˈtan-ᵊl-ˌīd, -əd\ n : a white crystalline compound C₈H₉NO used esp. to relieve pain or fever

ace·tate \ˈa-sə-ˌtāt\ n : a salt or ester of acetic acid

ac·et·azol·amide \ˌa-sə-tə-ˈzō-lə-ˌmīd, -ˈzä-, -məd\ n : a diuretic drug C₄H₆N₄O₃S₂ used esp. to treat edema associated with congestive heart failure, control epileptic seizures, prevent and treat altitude sickness, and treat glaucoma

ace·tic acid \ə-ˈsē-tik-\ n : a colorless pungent acid C₂H₄O₂ that is the chief acid of vinegar and is used occas. in medicine as an astringent and styptic

ace·to·ace·tic acid \ˌa-sə-ō-(ˌ)tō-ə-ˌsē-tik-, ə-ˌsē-tō-\ n : an unstable acid C₄H₆O₃ that is one of the ketone bodies found in abnormal amounts in the blood and urine in certain conditions of impaired metabolism (as in starvation and diabetes mellitus) — called also diacetic acid

ace·to·hex·amide \ˌa-sə-tō-ˈhek-sə-ˌməd, ə-ˌsē-tō-, -ˌmīd\ n : a sulfonylurea drug C₁₅H₂₀N₂O₄S used in the oral treatment of some of the milder forms of diabetes in adults to lower the level of glucose in the blood

ace·to·me·roc·tol \ˌa-sə-tō-(ˌ)tō-mə-ˈräk-ˌtȯl, ə-ˌsē-tō-, -ˌtȯl\ n : a white crystalline mercury derivative C₁₆H₂₄HgO₃ of phenol used in solution as a topical antiseptic

ac·e·ton·ae·mia chiefly Brit var of ACETONEMIA

ace·tone \ˈa-sə-ˌtōn\ n : a volatile fragrant flammable liquid ketone C₃H₆O found in abnormal quantities in diabetic urine

acetone body n : KETONE BODY

ac·e·to·ne·mia \ˌa-sə-tō-ˈnē-mē-ə\ n : KETOSIS 2; also : KETONEMIA 1

acetonide — see FLUOCINOLONE ACETONIDE

ac·e·to·nu·ria \ˌa-sə-tō-ˈnu̇r-ē-ə, -ˈnyu̇r-\ n : KETONURIA

ace·to·phe·net·i·din \ˌa-sə-tō-(ˌ)tō-fə-ˈne-tə-dən, ə-ˌsē-tō-\ n : PHENACETIN

ace·tyl \ə-ˈsēt-ᵊl, ˈa-sət-; ˈa-sə-ˌtēl\ n : the radical CH₃CO of acetic acid

acet·y·lase \ə-'set-ᵊl-ˌās\ *n* : any of a class of enzymes that accelerate the synthesis of esters of acetic acid

acet·y·late \ə-'set-ᵊl-ˌāt\ *vb* **-lat·ed; -lat·ing** : to introduce the acetyl radical into (a compound) — **acet·y·la·tion** \-ˌset-ᵊl-'ā-shən\ *n*

ace·tyl·cho·line \ə-ˌset-ᵊl-'kō-ˌlēn, -ˌsēt-; ˌa-sə-ˌtēl-\ *n* : a neurotransmitter C₇H₁₇NO₃ released at autonomic synapses and neuromuscular junctions, active in the transmission of nerve impulses, and formed enzymatically in the tissues from choline

ace·tyl·cho·lin·es·ter·ase \-ˌkō-lə-'nes-tə-ˌrās, -ˌrāz\ *n* : an enzyme that occurs esp. in some nerve endings and in the blood and promotes the hydrolysis of acetylcholine

acetyl CoA \-ˌkō-'ā\ *n* : ACETYL COENZYME A

acetyl coenzyme A *n* : a compound C₂₅H₃₈N₇O₁₇P₃S formed as an intermediate in metabolism and active as a coenzyme in biological acetylations

ace·tyl·cys·te·ine \ə-ˌsēt-ᵊl-'sis-tə-ˌēn, -ˌset-; ˌa-sə-ˌtēl-, ˌa-sət-ᵊl-\ *n* : a mucolytic agent C₅H₉NO₃S used esp. to reduce the viscosity of abnormally viscid respiratory tract secretions — see MUCOMYST

ace·tyl·phenyl·hy·dra·zine \-ˌfen-ᵊl-'hī-drə-ˌzēn, -ˌfēn-\ *n* : a white crystalline compound C₈H₁₀ON₂ used in the symptomatic treatment of polycythemia

ace·tyl·sa·lic·y·late \ə-ˌsēt-ᵊl-sə-'li-sə-ˌlāt\ *n* : a salt or ester of acetylsalicylic acid

ace·tyl·sal·i·cyl·ic acid \ə-ˌsēt-ᵊl-ˌsa-lə-ˌsi-lik-\ *n* : ASPIRIN 1

AcG *abbr* [accelerator globulin] factor V

ACh *abbr* acetylcholine

acha·la·sia \ˌā-kə-'lā-zhē-ə, -zhə\ *n* : failure of a ring of muscle (as a sphincter) to relax — compare CARDIOSPASM

¹ache \'āk\ *vb* **ached; ach·ing** : to suffer a usu. dull persistent pain

²ache *n* **1** : a usu. dull persistent pain **2** : a condition marked by aching

achieve·ment age \ə-'chēv-mənt-\ *n* : the level of an individual's educational achievement as measured by a standardized test and expressed as the age for which the test score would be the average score — compare CHRONOLOGICAL AGE

achievement test *n* : a standardized test for measuring the skill or knowledge attained by an individual in one or more fields of work or study

Achil·les reflex \ə-'ki-lēz-\ *n* : ANKLE JERK

Achilles tendon *n* : the strong tendon joining the muscles in the calf of the leg to the bone of the heel — called also *tendon of Achilles*

achlor·hy·dria \ˌā-ˌklōr-'hī-drē-ə\ *n* : absence of hydrochloric acid from the gastric juice — compare HYPER-

CHLORHYDRIA, HYPOCHLORHYDRIA — **achlor·hy·dric** \-'hī-drik\ *adj*

acho·lia \(ˌ)ā-'kō-lē-ə, -'kä-\ *n* : deficiency or absence of bile

achol·ic \(ˌ)ā-'kä-lik\ *or* **acho·lous** \-'kō-ləs\ *adj* : exhibiting deficiency of bile ⟨∼ stools⟩

achol·uria \ˌā-kō-'lür-ē-ə, -kä-, -lyúr-\ *n* : absence of bile pigment from the urine — **achol·uric** \-'lúr-ik, -'lyúr-\ *adj*

achon·dro·pla·sia \ˌā-ˌkän-drə-'plā-zhē-ə, -zhə\ *n* : a genetic disorder disturbing normal growth of cartilage, resulting in a form of dwarfism characterized by a usu. normal torso and shortened limbs, and usu. inherited as an autosomal dominant — compare ATELIOSIS — **achon·dro·plas·tic** \-'plas-tik\ *adj or n*

achromat- *or* **achromato-** *comb form* : uncolored except for shades of black, gray, and white ⟨*achromato*psia⟩

ach·ro·mat·ic \ˌa-krə-'ma-tik\ *adj* **1** : not readily colored by the usual staining agents **2** : possessing or involving no hue : being or involving only black, gray, or white ⟨∼ visual sensations⟩ — **ach·ro·mat·i·cal·ly** \-ti-k(ə-)lē\ *adv* — **ach·ro·mat·ism** \(ˌ)ā-'krō-mə-ˌti-zəm, a-\ *n*

achro·ma·top·sia \ˌā-ˌkrō-mə-'täp-sē-ə\ *n* : a visual defect that is marked by total color blindness in which the colors of the spectrum are seen as tones of white, gray, and black, by poor visual acuity, and by extreme sensitivity to bright light

achro·mia \(ˌ)ā-'krō-mē-ə\ *n* : absence of normal pigmentation esp. in red blood cells and skin

achy \'ā-kē\ *adj* **ach·i·er; ach·i·est** : affected with aches — **ach·i·ness** *n*

achy·lia \(ˌ)ā-'kī-lē-ə\ *n* : ACHYLIA GASTRICA — **achy·lous** \(ˌ)ā-'kī-ləs\ *adj*

achylia gas·tri·ca \-'gas-tri-kə\ *n* **1** : partial or complete absence of gastric juice **2** : ACHLORHYDRIA

¹ac·id \'a-səd\ *adj* **1** : sour, sharp, or biting to the taste **2 a** : of, relating to, or being an acid; *also* : having the reactions or characteristics of an acid ⟨an ∼ solution⟩ **b** *of salts and esters* : derived by partial exchange of replaceable hydrogen ⟨∼ sodium carbonate NaHCO₃⟩ **c** : marked by or resulting from an abnormally high concentration of acid ⟨∼ indigestion⟩ — not used technically

²acid *n* **1** : a sour substance; *specif* : any of various typically water-soluble and sour compounds that in solution are capable of reacting with a base to form a salt, redden litmus, and have a pH less than 7, and that are hydrogen-containing molecules or ions able to give up a proton to a base or are substances able to accept a pair of electrons from a base **2** : LSD

ac·i·dae·mia *chiefly Brit var of* ACIDEMIA

acid–base balance \\'a-səd-'bās-\ *n* : the state of equilibrium between proton donors and proton acceptors in the buffering system of the blood that is maintained at approximately pH 7.35 to 7.45 under normal conditions in arterial blood

ac·i·de·mia \\,a-sə-'dē-mē-ə\ *n* : a condition in which the hydrogen-ion concentration in the blood is increased

acid–fast \\'a-səd-,fast\ *adj* : not easily decolorized by acids (as when stained) — used esp. of bacteria and tissues

acid·ic \ə-'si-dik, a-\ *adj* **1** : acid-forming **2** : ACID

acid·i·fy \-də-,fī\ *vb* **-fied; -fy·ing 1** : to make acid **2** : to convert into an acid — **acid·i·fi·ca·tion** \-,si-də-fə-'kā-shən, a-\ *n* — **acid·i·fi·er** \ə-'si-də-,fī-ər, a-\ *n*

acid·i·ty \ə-'si-də-tē, a-\ *n, pl* **-ties 1** : the quality, state, or degree of being sour or chemically acid **2** : the quality or state of being excessively or abnormally acid : HYPERACIDITY

acid maltase deficiency *n* : POMPE'S DISEASE

acid·o·gen·ic \ə-,si-də-'je-nik, ,a-sə-dō-\ *adj* : acid-forming

[1]**acid·o·phil** \ə-'si-də-,fil, a-\ *also* **acid·o·phile** \-,fīl\ *adj* : ACIDOPHILIC 1

[2]**acidophil** *also* **acidophile** *n* : a substance, tissue, or organism that stains readily with acid stains

acid·o·phil·ic \-'fi-lik\ *adj* **1** : staining readily with acid stains **2** : preferring or thriving in a relatively acid environment 〈~ bacteria〉

ac·i·doph·i·lus \,a-sə-'dä-fə-ləs\ *n* : a lactobacillus (*Lactobacillus acidophilus*) that is added esp. to dairy products (as yogurt and milk) or prepared as a dietary supplement, is part of the normal intestinal and vaginal flora, and is used therapeutically esp. to promote intestinal health; *also* : a preparation containing such bacteria

ac·i·do·sis \,a-sə-'dō-səs\ *n, pl* **-do·ses** \-,sēz\ : an abnormal condition of reduced alkalinity of the blood and tissues marked by sickly sweet breath, headache, nausea and vomiting, and visual disturbances and usu. a result of excessive acid production — compare ALKALOSIS, KETOSIS 1 — **ac·i·dot·ic** \-'dä-tik\ *adj*

acid phosphatase *n* : a phosphatase (as the phosphomonoesterase from the prostate gland) active in acid medium

acid·u·late \ə-'si-jə-,lāt\ *vb* **-lat·ed; -lat·ing** : to make acid or slightly acid — **acid·u·la·tion** \-,si-jə-'lā-shən\ *n*

ac·id·uria \,a-sə-'dur-ē-ə, -'dyur-\ *n* : the condition of having acid in the urine esp. in abnormal amounts — see AMINOACIDURIA

ac·id·uric \,a-sə-'dur-ik, -'dyur-\ *adj* : tolerating a highly acid environment; *also* : ACIDOPHILIC 2

ac·i·nar \'a-sə-nər, -,när\ *adj* : of, relating to, or comprising an acinus 〈pancreatic ~ cells〉

acin·ic \ə-'si-nik\ *adj* : ACINAR

ac·i·nous \'a-sə-nəs, ə-'sī-nəs\ *adj* : consisting of or containing acini

aci·nus \'a-sə-nəs, ə-'sī-\ *n, pl* **aci·ni** \-,nī\ : any of the small sacs that terminate the ducts of some exocrine glands and are lined with secretory cells

Acip·Hex \'as-ə-,feks\ *trademark* — used for a preparation of the sodium salt of rabeprazole

ackee *var of* AKEE

ACL \,ā-(,)sē-'el\ *n* : ANTERIOR CRUCIATE LIGAMENT

ACLS *abbr* advanced cardiac life support

ac·ne \'ak-nē\ *n* : a disorder of the skin caused by inflammation of the skin glands and hair follicles; *specif* : a form found chiefly in adolescents and marked by pimples esp. on the face — **ac·ned** \-nēd\ *adj*

ac·ne·gen·ic \,ak-ni-'je-nik\ *adj* : producing or increasing the severity of acne 〈the ~ effect of some hormones〉

ac·ne·i·form \'ak-nē-ə-,fȯrm, ak-'nē-\ *or* **ac·ne·form** \'ak-nē-,fȯrm\ *adj* : resembling acne 〈an ~ eruption〉

ac·ne ro·sa·cea \,ak-nē-rō-'zā-shē-ə, -shə\ *n, pl* **ac·nae ro·sa·ce·ae** \,ak-nē-rō-'zā-shē-,ē\ : ROSACEA

acne ur·ti·ca·ta \-,ər-tə-'kā-tə\ *n* : an acneiform eruption of the skin characterized by itching papular wheals

acne vul·gar·is \-,vəl-'gar-əs\ *n, pl* **ac·nae vul·gar·es** \-'gar-,ēz\ : a chronic acne involving mainly the face, chest, and shoulders that is common in adolescent humans and various domestic animals and is characterized by the intermittent formation of discrete papular or pustular lesions often resulting in considerable scarring

ACNM *abbr* American College of Nurse-Midwives

acous·tic \ə-'kü-stik\ *or* **acous·ti·cal** \-sti-kəl\ *adj* : of or relating to the sense or organs of hearing, to sound, or to the science of sounds — **acous·ti·cal·ly** \-k(ə-)lē\ *adv*

acoustic meatus *n* : AUDITORY CANAL

acoustic nerve *n* : AUDITORY NERVE

acoustic neuroma *n* : a nonmalignant usu. slow-growing tumor involving the Schwann cells of the vestibular nerve that may be life-threatening if not treated

acoustic tubercle *n* : a pear-shaped prominence on the inferior cerebellar peduncle including the dorsal nucleus of the cochlear nerve

ACP *abbr* American College of Physicians

ac·quain·tance rape \ə-'kwänt-ᵊn(t)s-\ *n* : rape committed by someone known to the victim

ac·quired \ə-'kwīrd\ *adj* **1** : arising in response to the action of the environment on the organism (as in the use or disuse of an organ) — compare GENETIC 2, HEREDITARY **2** : developed after birth — compare CONGENITAL 2, FAMILIAL, HEREDITARY

acquired immune deficiency syndrome *n* : AIDS

acquired immunity *n* : immunity that develops after exposure to a suitable agent (as by an attack of a disease or by injection of antigens) — compare ACTIVE IMMUNITY, NATURAL IMMUNITY, PASSIVE IMMUNITY

acquired immunodeficiency syndrome *n* : AIDS

acr- or **acro-** *comb form* **1** : top : peak : summit ⟨*acro*cephaly⟩ **2** : height ⟨*acro*phobia⟩ **3** : extremity of the body ⟨*acro*cyanosis⟩

ac·rid \'a-krəd\ *adj* : irritatingly sharp and harsh or unpleasantly pungent in taste or odor — **ac·rid·ly** *adv*

ac·ri·dine \'a-krə-ˌdēn\ *n* : a colorless crystalline compound $C_{13}H_9N$ occurring in coal tar and important as the parent compound of dyes and pharmaceuticals

ac·ri·fla·vine \ˌa-krə-'flā-ˌvēn, -vən\ *n* : a yellow acridine dye $C_{14}H_{14}N_3Cl$ obtained by methylation of proflavine as red crystals or usu. in admixture with proflavine as a deep orange powder and used often in the form of its reddish brown hydrochloride as an antiseptic esp. for wounds

ac·ro·cen·tric \ˌa-krō-'sen-trik\ *adj* : having the centromere situated so that one chromosomal arm is much shorter than the other — compare METACENTRIC, TELOCENTRIC — **acrocentric** *n*

ac·ro·ceph·a·lo·syn·dac·ty·ly \-ˌse-fə-(ˌ)lō-sin-'dak-tə-lē\ *n, pl* **-lies** : a congenital syndrome characterized by a peaked head and webbed or fused fingers and toes

ac·ro·ceph·a·ly \ˌa-krō-'se-fə-lē\ *n, pl* **-lies** *also* **-lias** : OXYCEPHALY

ac·ro·chor·don \ˌa-krə-'kór-ˌdän\ *n* : SKIN TAG

ac·ro·cy·a·no·sis \ˌa-krō-ˌsī-ə-'nō-səs\ *n, pl* **-no·ses** \-ˌsēz\ : a disorder of the arterioles of the exposed parts of the hands and feet involving abnormal contraction of the arteriolar walls intensified by exposure to cold and resulting in bluish mottled skin, chilling, and sweating of the affected parts — **ac·ro·cy·a·not·ic** \-'nä-tik\ *adj*

ac·ro·der·ma·ti·tis \ˌa-krō-ˌdər-mə-'tī-təs\ *n* : inflammation of the skin of the extremities

acrodermatitis chron·i·ca atroph·i·cans \ˌkrä-ni-kə-a-ˌträ-fi-ˌkanz\ *n* : a skin condition of the extremities that is a late manifestation of Lyme disease and is characterized by erythematous and edematous lesions which tend to become atrophic giving the skin the appearance of wrinkled tissue paper

acrodermatitis en·tero·path·i·ca \-ˌen-tə-rō-'pa-thi-kə\ *n* : a severe human skin and gastrointestinal disease inherited as a recessive autosomal trait that is characterized by the symptoms of zinc deficiency and clears up when zinc is added to the diet

ac·ro·dyn·ia \ˌa-krō-'di-nē-ə\ *n* : a disease of infants and young children that is an allergic reaction to mercury, is characterized by dusky pink discoloration of hands and feet with local swelling and intense itching, and is accompanied by insomnia, irritability, and sensitivity to light — called also *erythredema, pink disease, Swift's disease* — **ac·ro·dyn·ic** \-'di-nik\ *adj*

¹ac·ro·me·gal·ic \ˌa-krō-mə-'ga-lik\ *adj* : exhibiting acromegaly

²acromegalic *n* : one affected with acromegaly

ac·ro·meg·a·ly \ˌa-krō-'me-gə-lē\ *n, pl* **-lies** : chronic hyperpituitarism that is characterized by a gradual and permanent enlargement of the flat bones (as the lower jaw) and of the hands and feet, abdominal organs, nose, lips, and tongue and that develops after ossification is complete — compare GIGANTISM

acro·mi·al \ə-'krō-mē-əl\ *adj* : of, relating to, or situated near the acromion

acromial process *n* : ACROMION

ac·ro·mi·cria \ˌa-krō-'mi-krē-ə, -'mī-\ *n* : abnormal smallness of the extremities

acromio- *comb form* : acromial and ⟨*acromio*clavicular⟩

acro·mio·cla·vic·u·lar \ə-ˌkrō-mē-(ˌ)ō-klə-'vi-kyə-lər\ *adj* : relating to, being, or affecting the joint connecting the acromion and the clavicle

acro·mi·on \ə-'krō-mē-ˌän, -ən\ *n* : the outer end of the spine of the scapula that protects the glenoid cavity, forms the outer angle of the shoulder, and articulates with the clavicle — called also *acromial process, acromion process*

acro·mi·on·ec·to·my \ə-ˌkrō-mē-ˌän-'ek-tə-mē, -mē-ə-'nek-\ *n, pl* **-mies** : partial or total surgical excision of the acromion

ac·ro·mio·plas·ty \ə-'krō-mē-ō-ˌplas-tē\ *n, pl* **-ties** : surgical removal of the anterior hook of the acromion for the relief of pressure on the rotator cuff

acro·pa·chy \'a-krō-ˌpa-kē, ə-'krä-pə-kē\ *n, pl* **-pa·chies** : OSTEOARTHROPATHY

ac·ro·par·es·the·sia \ˌa-krō-ˌpar-əs-'thē-zhē-ə, -zhə\ *n* : a condition of burning, tingling, or pricking sensations or numbness in the extremities present on awaking and of unknown cause or produced by compression of nerves during sleep

acrop·a·thy \ə-'krä-pə-thē\ *n, pl* **-thies** : a disease affecting the extremities

ac·ro·phobe \'a-krə-ˌfōb\ *n* : a person affected with acrophobia

ac·ro·pho·bia \ˌa-krə-ˈfō-bē-ə\ *n* : abnormal or pathological fear of heights — **ac·ro·pho·bic** \-bik\ *adj*

ac·ro·scle·ro·der·ma \ˌa-krō-ˌskler-ə-ˈdər-mə\ *n* : scleroderma affecting the extremities, face, and chest

ac·ro·scle·ro·sis \ˌa-krō-sklə-ˈrō-səs\ *n, pl* **-ro·ses** \-ˌsēz\ : ACROSCLERODERMA

ac·ro·some \ˈa-krə-ˌsōm\ *n* : an anterior prolongation of a spermatozoon that releases egg-penetrating enzymes — **ac·ro·so·mal** \ˌa-krə-ˈsō-məl\ *adj*

ac·ry·late \ˈak-rə-ˌlāt\ *n* : a salt or ester of acrylic acid

¹**acryl·ic** \ə-ˈkri-lik\ *adj* : of or relating to acrylic acid or its derivatives

²**acrylic** *n* : ACRYLIC RESIN

acrylic acid *n* : a synthetic unsaturated liquid acid $C_3H_4O_2$ that polymerizes readily

acrylic resin *n* : a glassy acrylic thermoplastic used for cast and molded parts (as of dental appliances) or as coatings and adhesives

ACSW *abbr* Academy of Certified Social Workers

ACTH \ˌā-ˌsē-(ˌ)tē-ˈāch\ *n* : a protein hormone of the anterior lobe of the pituitary gland that stimulates the adrenal cortex — called also *adrenocorticotropic hormone*

ac·tin \ˈak-tən\ *n* : a cellular protein found esp. in microfilaments (as those comprising myofibrils) and active in muscular contraction, cellular movement, and maintenance of cell shape — see F-ACTIN, G-ACTIN

actin- *or* **actini-** *or* **actino-** *comb form* **1** : of, utilizing, or caused by actinic radiation (as X-rays) ⟨*actino*therapy⟩ **2** : actinomycete ⟨*actino*mycosis⟩

ac·tin·ic \ak-ˈti-nik\ *adj* : of, relating to, resulting from, or exhibiting chemical changes produced by radiant energy esp. in the visible and ultraviolet parts of the spectrum ⟨∼ keratosis⟩

ac·tin·i·um \ak-ˈti-nē-əm\ *n* : a radioactive trivalent metallic element — symbol *Ac*; see ELEMENT table

ac·ti·no·ba·cil·lo·sis \ˌak-tə-(ˌ)nō-ˌba-sə-ˈlō-səs, ak-ˌti-nō-\ *n, pl* **-lo·ses** \-ˌsēz\ : a disease that affects domestic animals and sometimes humans, resembles actinomycosis, and is caused by a bacterium of the genus *Actinobacillus* (*A. lignieresi*) — see WOODEN TONGUE

ac·ti·no·ba·cil·lus \-bə-ˈsi-ləs\ *n* **1** *cap* : a genus of aerobic gram-negative parasitic bacteria (family Pasteurellaceae) forming filaments resembling streptobacilli — see ACTINOBACILLOSIS **2** *pl* **-li** \-ˌlī, \-ˌlē\ : a bacterium of the genus *Actinobacillus*

ac·ti·no·my·ces \ˌak-tə-(ˌ)nō-ˈmī-ˌsēz, ak-ˌti-nō-\ *n* **1** *cap* : a genus of filamentous or rod-shaped gram-positive bacteria (family Actinomycetaceae) that includes usu. commensal and sometimes pathogenic forms inhabiting mucosal surfaces esp. of the oral cavity — compare ACTINOMYCOSIS **2** *pl* **actinomyces** : a bacterium of the genus *Actinomyces*

ac·ti·no·my·cete \-ˈmī-ˌsēt, -mī-ˈsēt\ *n* : any of an order (Actinomycetales) of filamentous or rod-shaped bacteria (as the actinomyces or streptomyces)

ac·ti·no·my·cin \-ˈmīs-ᵊn\ *n* : any of various red or yellow-red mostly toxic polypeptide antibiotics isolated from soil bacteria (esp. *Streptomyces antibioticus*)

actinomycin D *n* : DACTINOMYCIN

ac·ti·no·my·co·sis \ˌak-tə-nō-ˌmī-ˈkō-səs, ak-ˌti-nō-\ *n, pl* **-co·ses** \-ˌsēz\ : infection with or disease caused by actinomycetes

ac·ti·no·spec·ta·cin \ˌak-tə-(ˌ)nō-ˈspek-tə-sən, ak-ˌti-nō-\ *n* : SPECTINOMYCIN

ac·ti·no·ther·a·py \-ˈther-ə-pē\ *n, pl* **-pies** : application for therapeutic purposes of the chemically active rays of the electromagnetic spectrum (as ultraviolet light or X-rays)

ac·tion \ˈak-shən\ *n* **1** : the process of exerting a force or bringing about an effect that results from the inherent capacity of an agent **2** : a function or the performance of a function of the body (as defecation) or of one of its parts ⟨heart ∼⟩ **3** : an act of will **4** *pl* : BEHAVIOR ⟨aggressive ∼s⟩

action potential *n* : a momentary reversal in the potential difference across a plasma membrane (as of a nerve cell or muscle fiber) that occurs when a cell has been activated by a stimulus — compare RESTING POTENTIAL

ac·ti·vat·ed charcoal *n* : a highly adsorbent fine black odorless tasteless powdered charcoal used in medicine esp. as an antidote in many forms of poisoning and as an antiflatulent

ac·ti·va·tor \ˈak-tə-ˌvā-tər\ *n* **1** : a substance (as a chloride ion) that increases the activity of an enzyme — compare COENZYME **2** : a substance given off by developing tissue that stimulates differentiation of adjacent tissue; *also* : a structure giving off such a stimulant

ac·tive \ˈak-tiv\ *adj* **1** : capable of acting or reacting esp. in some specific way ⟨an ∼ enzyme⟩ **2** : tending to progress or to cause degeneration ⟨∼ tuberculosis⟩ **3** : exhibiting optical activity **4** : requiring the expenditure of energy **5** : producing active immunity ⟨∼ immunization⟩ — **ac·tive·ly** *adv*

active immunity *n* : usu. long-lasting immunity that is acquired through production of antibodies and memory cells within the organism in response to the presence of antigens — compare ACQUIRED IMMUNITY, NATURAL IMMUNITY, PASSIVE IMMUNITY

active site *n* : a region esp. of a biologically active protein (as an enzyme) where catalytic activity takes place and whose shape permits the binding only of a specific reactant molecule

active transport *n* : movement of a chemical substance by the expenditure of energy against a gradient in concentration or electrical potential across a plasma membrane

ac·tiv·i·ty \ak-'ti-və-tē\ *n, pl* **-ties** 1 : natural or normal function ⟨digestive ∼⟩ 2 : the characteristic of acting chemically or of promoting a chemical reaction ⟨the ∼ of a catalyst⟩

ac·to·my·o·sin \ak-tə-'mī-ə-sən\ *n* : a viscous contractile complex of actin and myosin concerned together with ATP in muscular contraction

Ac·to·nel \ak-tə-nel\ *trademark* — used for a preparation of the sodium salt of risedronate

Ac·tos \'ak-ˌtōz\ *trademark* — used for a preparation of the hydrochoride of pioglitazone

act out *vb* : to express (as an impulse or a fantasy) directly in overt behavior without modification to comply with social norms

acu- *comb form* 1 : performed with a needle ⟨*acu*puncture⟩ 2 : applied to selected areas of the body (as in acupuncture) ⟨*acu*pressure⟩

acu·ity \ə-'kyü-ə-tē\ *n, pl* **-ities** : keenness of sense perception ⟨∼ of hearing⟩ — see VISUAL ACUITY

acuminata — see CONDYLOMA ACUMINATUM, VERRUCA ACUMINATA

acuminatum — see CONDYLOMA ACUMINATUM

acu·pres·sure \'a-kyù-ˌpre-shər\ *n* : the application of pressure (as with the fingertips) to the same points on the body stimulated in acupuncture that is used for its therapeutic effects — see SHIATSU — **acu·pres·sur·ist** \-ˌpre-shə-rist\ *n*

acu·punc·ture \-ˌpəŋk-chər\ *n* : an orig. Chinese practice of inserting fine needles through the skin at specific points esp. to cure disease or relieve pain (as in surgery) — **acu·punc·tur·ist** \-chə-rist\ *n*

-acusis *n comb form* : hearing ⟨dipla*cusis*⟩ ⟨hyper*acusis*⟩

acustica — see MACULA ACUSTICA

acuta — see PITYRIASIS LICHENOIDES ET VARIOLIFORMIS ACUTA

acute \ə-'kyüt\ *adj* 1 : sensing or perceiving accurately, clearly, effectively, or sensitively ⟨∼ vision⟩ 2 a : characterized by sharpness or severity ⟨∼ pain⟩ ⟨an ∼ infection⟩ b : having a sudden onset, sharp rise, and short course ⟨an ∼ disease⟩ — compare CHRONIC 2 c : ACUTE CARE ⟨an ∼ hospital⟩ — **acute·ly** *adv* — **acute·ness** *n*

acute abdomen *n* : an acute internal abdominal condition requiring immediate operation

acute care *adj* : providing or concerned with short-term medical care

esp. for serious acute disease or trauma — **acute care** *n*

acute disseminated encephalomyelitis *n* : an acute inflammation of the brain and spinal cord that is thought to be an allergic or immune response following infectious disease or vaccination

acute febrile neutrophilic dermatosis *n* : SWEET'S SYNDROME

acute lymphoblastic leukemia *n* : lymphocytic leukemia that is marked by an abnormal increase in the number of lymphoblasts, that is characterized by rapid onset and progression, and that occurs chiefly during childhood — abbr. *ALL*; compare CHRONIC LYMPHOCYTIC LEUKEMIA

acute lymphocytic leukemia *n* : ACUTE LYMPHOBLASTIC LEUKEMIA

acute myelogenous leukemia *n* : myelogenous leukemia that is marked by an abnormal increase in the number of myeloblasts esp. in bone marrow and blood and that may occur either in childhood or adulthood — abbr. *AML*; called also *acute myeloid leukemia*; compare CHRONIC MYELOGENOUS LEUKEMIA

acute necrotizing ulcerative gingivitis *n* : a periodontal disease that is marked esp. by gray ulceration and necrosis of the gums accompanied by pain, bleeding, and halitosis and that is associated with the proliferation of microorganisms (as *Fusobacterium nucleatum* and *Treponema vincentii*) that are normally part of the oral flora — called also *necrotizing ulcerative gingivitis, trench mouth, Vincent's infection*

acute nonlymphocytic leukemia *n* : any of several forms of mylogenous leukemia marked by an abnormal increase in the number of immature white blood cells that are not of the same lineage as B cells and T cells; esp : ACUTE MYELOGENOUS LEUKEMIA

acute respiratory distress syndrome *n* : respiratory failure in adults or children that results from diffuse injury to the endothelium of the lung (as in sepsis, chest trauma, massive blood transfusion, or pneumonia) and is characterized by pulmonary edema with an abnormally high amount of protein in the edematous fluid and by difficult rapid breathing and hypoxemia — abbr. *ARDS;* called also *adult respiratory distress syndrome*

acy·not·ic \ˌā-ˌsī-ə-'nä-tik\ *adj* : characterized by the absence of cyanosis ⟨∼ patients⟩ ⟨∼ heart disease⟩

acy·clo·vir \ā-'sī-klō-ˌvir\ *n* : a cyclic nucleoside $C_8H_{11}N_5O_3$ used esp. to treat shingles, genital herpes, and chicken pox — see ZOVIRAX

ac·yl \'a-səl, -ˌsēl; 'ā-səl\ *n* : a radical derived usu. from an organic acid by removal of the hydroxyl from all acid groups

AD *abbr* Alzheimer's disease

ADA *abbr* **1** adenosine deaminase **2** American Dental Association **3** American Diabetes Association **4** American Dietetic Association

adac·tyl·ia \ˌā-ˌdak-ˈti-lē-ə\ *n* : congenital lack of fingers or toes

Ad·a·lat \ˈad-ə-ˌlat\ *trademark* — used for a preparation of nifedipine

ad·a·man·ti·no·ma \ˌa-də-ˌmant-ᵊn-ˈō-mə\ *n, pl* **-mas** *also* **-ma·ta** \-mə-tə\ : AMELOBLASTOMA

Ad·am's ap·ple \ˈa-dəmz-ˈa-pəl\ *n* : the projection in the front of the neck that is formed by the thyroid cartilage

ad·ams·ite \ˈa-dəm-ˌzīt\ *n* : a yellow crystalline arsenical $C_{12}H_9AsClN$ used as a respiratory irritant in some forms of tear gas

Adams, Roger (1889–1971), American chemist.

Adams–Stokes syndrome *n* : STOKES-ADAMS SYNDROME

R. Adams — see STOKES-ADAMS SYNDROME

J. Stokes — see CHEYNE-STOKES RESPIRATION

adapt \ə-ˈdapt\ *vb* : to make or become fit often by modification

ad·ap·ta·tion \ˌa-ˌdap-ˈtā-shən\ *n* **1** : the act or process of adapting : the state of being adapted **2** : adjustment to environmental conditions — **adaptive** \ə-ˈdap-tiv\ *adj*

ADD *abbr* : attention deficit disorder

ad·der \ˈa-dər\ *n* **1** : the common venomous European viper of the genus *Vipera* (*V. berus*); *broadly* : a terrestrial viper (family Viperidae) **2** : any of several No. American snakes that are harmless but are popularly believed to be venomous

¹ad·dict \ə-ˈdikt\ *vb* : to cause (a person) to become physiologically dependent upon a substance

²ad·dict \ˈa-(ˌ)dikt\ *n* : one who is addicted to a substance

ad·dic·tion \ə-ˈdik-shən\ *n* : compulsive physiological need for and use of a habit-forming substance (as heroin, nicotine, or alcohol) characterized by tolerance and by well-defined physiological symptoms upon withdrawal; *broadly* : persistent compulsive use of a substance known by the user to be physically, psychologically, or socially harmful — compare HABITUATION — **ad·dic·tive** \-ˈdik-tiv\ *adj*

Ad·dis count \ˈa-dis-ˌkau̇nt\ *n* : a technique for the quantitative determination of cells, casts, and protein in a 12-hour urine sample used in the diagnosis and treatment of kidney disease

Addis, Thomas (1881–1949), American physician.

Ad·di·so·ni·an \ˌa-də-ˈsō-nē-ən, -nyən\ *adj* : of, relating to, or affected with Addison's disease ⟨∼ crisis⟩

Addison, Thomas (1793–1860), English physician.

addisonian anemia *n, often cap 1st A* : PERNICIOUS ANEMIA

Addison's disease *n* : a destructive disease marked by deficient adrenocortical secretion and characterized by extreme weakness, loss of weight, low blood pressure, gastrointestinal disturbances, and brownish pigmentation of the skin and mucous membranes

¹ad·di·tive \ˈa-də-tiv\ *adj* : characterized by, being, or producing effects (as drug responses or gene products) that when the causative factors act together are the sum of their individual effects — **ad·di·tive·ly** *adv* — **ad·di·tiv·i·ty** \ˌa-də-ˈti-və-tē\ *n*

²additive *n* : a substance added to another in relatively small amounts to effect a desired change in properties ⟨food ∼s that improve flavor⟩

ad·duct \ə-ˈdəkt, a-\ *vb* : to draw (as a limb) toward or past the median axis of the body; *also* : to bring together (similar parts) ⟨∼ the fingers⟩ — **ad·duc·tion** \ə-ˈdək-shən, a-\ *n*

ad·duc·tor \-ˈdək-tər\ *n* **1** : any of three powerful triangular muscles that contribute to the adduction of the human thigh: **a** : one arising from the superior ramus of the pubis and inserted into the middle third of the linea aspera — called also *adductor longus* **b** : one arising from the inferior ramus of the pubis and inserted into the iliopectineal line and the upper part of the linea aspera — called also *adductor brevis* **c** : one arising from the inferior ramus of the pubis and the ischium and inserted behind the first two into the linea aspera — called also *adductor magnus* **2** : any of several muscles other than the adductors of the thigh that draw a part toward the median line of the body or toward the axis of an extremity

adductor brev·is \-ˈbre-vəs\ *n* : ADDUCTOR 1b

adductor hal·lu·cis \-ˈhal-yə-sis; -ˈha-lə-səs, -kəs\ *n* : a muscle of the foot that adducts and flexes the big toe and helps to support the arch of the foot — called also *adductor hallucis muscle*

adductor lon·gus \-ˈlȯŋ-gəs\ *n* : ADDUCTOR 1a

adductor mag·nus \-ˈmag-nəs\ *n* : ADDUCTOR 1c

adductor pol·li·cis \-ˈpä-lə-səs, -kəs\ *n* : a muscle of the hand with two heads that adducts the thumb by bringing it toward the palm — called also *adductor pollicis muscle*

adductor tubercle *n* : a tubercle on the proximal part of the medial epicondyle of the femur that is the site of insertion of the adductor magnus

aden- or **adeno-** *comb form* : gland : glandular ⟨*adenitis*⟩ ⟨*adeno*myoma⟩

ad·e·nine \ˈad-ᵊn-ˌēn\ *n* : a purine base $C_5H_5N_5$ that codes hereditary information in the genetic code in DNA and RNA — compare CYTOSINE, GUANINE, THYMINE, URACIL

adenine arabinoside *n* : VIDARABINE
ad·e·ni·tis \ˌad-ᵊn-ˈī-təs\ *n* : inflammation of a gland; *esp* : LYMPHADENITIS
ad·e·no·ac·an·tho·ma \ˌad-ᵊn-(ˌ)ō-ˌa-ˌkan-ˈthō-mə\ *n, pl* **-mas** *also* **-ma·ta** \-mə-tə\ : an adenocarcinoma with epithelial cells differentiated and proliferated into squamous cells
ad·e·no·car·ci·no·ma \-ˌkärs-ᵊn-ˈō-mə\ *n, pl* **-mas** *also* **-ma·ta** \-mə-tə\ : a malignant tumor originating in glandular epithelium — **ad·e·no·car·ci·no·ma·tous** \-mə-təs\ *adj*
ad·e·no·fi·bro·ma \-ˌfī-ˈbrō-mə\ *n, pl* **-mas** *also* **-ma·ta** \-mə-tə\ : a benign tumor of glandular and fibrous tissue
ad·e·no·hy·poph·y·sis \-ˌhī-ˈpä-fə-səs\ *n, pl* **-y·ses** \-ˌsēz\ : the anterior part of the pituitary gland that is derived from the embryonic pharynx and is primarily glandular in nature — called also *anterior lobe*; compare NEUROHYPOPHYSIS — **ad·e·no·hy·poph·y·se·al** \-(ˌ)hī-ˌpä-fə-ˈsē-əl\ *or* **ad·e·no·hy·po·phys·i·al** \-ˌhī-pə-ˈfiz-ē-əl\ *adj*
¹ad·e·noid \ˈad-ᵊn-ˌȯid, ˈad-ˌnȯid\ *adj* **1** : of, like, or relating to glands or glandular tissue; *esp* : like or belonging to lymphoid tissue **2** : of or relating to the adenoids **3 a** : of, relating to, or affected with abnormally enlarged adenoids **b** : characteristic of one affected with abnormally enlarged adenoids ⟨~ facies⟩
²adenoid *n* **1** : an abnormally enlarged mass of lymphoid tissue at the back of the pharynx characteristically obstructing the nasal and ear passages and inducing mouth breathing, a nasal voice, postnasal discharge, and dullness of facial expression — usu. used in pl. **2** : PHARYNGEAL TONSIL
ad·e·noi·dal \ˌad-ᵊn-ˈȯid-ᵊl\ *adj* : exhibiting the characteristics (as snoring, mouth breathing, and a nasal voice) of one affected with abnormally enlarged adenoids : ADENOID — not usu. used technically
ad·e·noid·ec·to·my \ˌad-ᵊn-ˌȯi-ˈdek-tə-mē\ *n, pl* **-mies** : surgical removal of the adenoids
ad·e·noid·itis \ˌad-ᵊn-ˌȯi-ˈdī-təs\ *n* : inflammation of the adenoids
ad·e·no·ma \ˌad-ᵊn-ˈō-mə\ *n, pl* **-mas** *also* **-ma·ta** \-mə-tə\ : a benign tumor of a glandular structure or of glandular origin — **ad·e·no·ma·tous** \-mə-təs\ *adj*
ad·e·no·ma·toid \ˌad-ᵊn-ˈō-mə-ˌtȯid\ *adj* : relating to or resembling an adenoma ⟨an ~ tumor⟩
ad·e·no·ma·to·sis \ˌad-ᵊn-ˌō-mə-ˈtō-səs\ *n, pl* **-to·ses** \-ˌsēz\ : a condition marked by multiple growths consisting of glandular tissue
ad·e·no·my·o·ma \ˌad-ᵊn-ō-(ˌ)mī-ˈō-mə\ *n, pl* **-mas** *also* **-ma·ta** \-mə-tə\ : a benign tumor composed of muscular and glandular elements
ad·e·no·my·o·sis \-ˌmī-ˈō-səs\ *n, pl* **-o·ses** \-ˌsēz\ : endometriosis esp. when

the endometrial tissue invades the myometrium
ad·e·nop·a·thy \ˌad-ᵊn-ˈä-pə-thē\ *n, pl* **-thies** : any disease or enlargement involving glandular tissue; *esp* : one involving lymph nodes
aden·o·sine \ə-ˈden-ə-ˌsēn, -sən\ *n* : a nucleoside $C_{10}H_{13}N_5O_4$ that is a constituent of RNA yielding adenine and ribose on hydrolysis
adenosine deaminase *n* : an enzyme which catalyzes the conversion of adenosine to inosine and whose deficiency causes a form of severe combined immunodeficiency disease as a result of the accumulation of toxic metabolites which inhibit DNA synthesis — abbr. *ADA*
adenosine diphosphate *n* : ADP
adenosine mono·phos·phate \-ˌmä-nə-ˈfäs-ˌfāt, -ˌmō-\ *n* : AMP
adenosine phosphate *n* : any of three phosphates of adenosine: **a** : AMP **b** : ADP **c** : ATP
adenosine 3′,5′-monophosphate \-ˈthrē-ˈfīv-\ *n* : CYCLIC AMP
adenosine tri·phos·pha·tase \-trī-ˈfäs-fə-ˌtās, -ˌtāz\ *n* : ATPASE
adenosine tri·phos·phate \-trī-ˈfäs-ˌfāt\ *n* : ATP
ad·e·no·sis \ˌad-ᵊn-ˈō-səs\ *n, pl* **-no·ses** \-ˌsēz\ : a disease of glandular tissue; *esp* : one involving abnormal proliferation or occurrence of glandular tissue ⟨vaginal ~⟩
S–aden·o·syl·me·thi·o·nine *also* **aden·o·syl·me·thi·o·nine** \(ˌ)es-ə-ˌden-ə-ˌsil-mə-ˈthī-ə-ˌnēn\ *n* : the active form of methionine $C_{15}H_{22}N_6O_5S$ that acts as a methyl group donor (as in the formation of creatine) and is an intermediate in the formation of homocysteine — see SAME
ad·e·not·o·my \ˌad-ᵊn-ˈä-tə-mē\ *n, pl* **-mies** : the operation of dissecting, incising, or removing a gland and esp. the adenoids
ad·e·no·vi·rus \ˌad-ᵊn-ō-ˈvī-rəs\ *n* : any of a family (*Adenoviridae*) of double-stranded DNA viruses that cause infections of the respiratory system, conjunctiva, and gastrointestinal tract and include some capable of inducing malignant tumors in experimental animals — **ad·e·no·vi·ral** \-rəl\ *adj*
ad·e·nyl·ic acid \ˌad-ᵊn-ˈi-lik-\ *n* : AMP
ADH *abbr* antidiuretic hormone
ADHD *abbr* attention-deficit/hyperactivity disorder
ad·here \ad-ˈhir\ *vb* **ad·hered; ad·her·ing 1** : to hold fast or stick by or as if by gluing, suction, grasping, or fusing **2** : to become joined (as in pathological adhesion) — **ad·her·ence** \-ˈhir-ᵊns\ *n*
ad·he·sion \ad-ˈhē-zhən\ *n* **1** : the action or state of adhering; *specif* **2 a** : a sticking together of substances **2 a** : the abnormal union of surfaces normally separate by the formation of new fibrous tissue resulting from an inflammatory process; *also* : the

newly formed uniting tissue ⟨pleural ~s⟩ **b** : the union of wound edges esp. by first intention

¹**ad·he·sive** \-'hē-siv, -ziv\ *adj* **1 a** : tending to adhere or cause adherence **b** : prepared for adhering **2** : characterized by adhesions — **ad·he·sive·ly** *adv*

²**adhesive** *n* **1** : a substance that bonds two materials together by adhering to the surface of each **2** : ADHESIVE TAPE

adhesive capsulitis *n* : FROZEN SHOULDER

adhesive pericarditis *n* : pericarditis in which adhesions form between the two layers of pericardium — see ACCRETIO CORDIS

adhesive tape *n* : tape coated on one side with an adhesive mixture; *esp* : one used for covering wounds

adi·a·do·ko·ki·ne·sis *or* **adi·a·do·cho·ki·ne·sis** \ˌa-dē-ˌa-dō-ˌkō-kə-'nē-səs, ə-ˌdī-ə-ˌdō-(ˌ)kō-, -ki-'nē-\ *n, pl* **-ne·ses** \-ˌsēz\ : inability to make movements exhibiting a rapid change of motion (as in quickly rotating the wrist one way and then the other) due to cerebellar dysfunction — compare DYSDIADOCHOKINESIA

ad·i·ence \'a-dē-əns\ *n* : a tendency to approach or accept a stimulus object or situation — compare ABIENCE — **ad·i·ent** \-ənt\ *adj*

Ad·ie's syndrome \'a-dēz-\ *or* **Ad·ie syndrome** \-dē-\ *n* : a neurologic syndrome that affects esp. women between 20 and 40 and is characterized by an abnormally dilated pupil, absent or diminished light reflexes of the eye, abnormal accommodation, and lack of ankle-jerk and knee-jerk reflexes

    Adie \'ā-dē\, **William John (1886–1935),** British neurologist.

adip- *or* **adipo-** *comb form* : fat : fatty tissue ⟨*adipo*cyte⟩

ad·i·phen·ine \ˌa-di-'fe-ˌnēn\ *n* : an antispasmodic drug administered in the form of its hydrochloride C₂₀H₂₅NO₂·HCl

ad·i·po·cere \'a-də-pə-ˌsir\ *n* : a waxy or unctuous brownish substance consisting chiefly of fatty acids and calcium soaps produced by chemical changes affecting dead body fat and muscle long buried or immersed in moisture

ad·i·po·cyte \'a-də-pə-ˌsīt\ *n* : FAT CELL

ad·i·pose \'a-də-ˌpōs\ *adj* : of or relating to fat; *broadly* : FAT

adipose tissue *n* : connective tissue in which fat is stored and which has the cells distended by droplets of fat

ad·i·pos·i·ty \ˌa-də-'pä-sə-tē\ *n, pl* **-ties** : the quality or state of being fat : OBESITY

ad·i·po·so·gen·i·tal dystrophy \ˌa-də-ˌpō-sō-'je-nət-ᵊl-\ *n* : a combination of obesity, retarded development of the sex glands, and changes in secondary

sex characteristics that results from impaired function or disease of the pituitary gland and hypothalamus — called also *Fröhlich's syndrome*

adiposus — see PANNICULUS ADIPOSUS

adip·sia \ā-'dip-sē-ə, ə-\ *n* : loss of thirst; *also* : abnormal and esp. prolonged abstinence from the intake of fluids

ad·i·tus \'a-də-təs\ *n, pl* **aditus** *or* **ad·i·tus·es** : a passage or opening for entrance

ad·junct \'a-ˌjəŋkt\ *n* : ADJUVANT b

ad·junc·tive \ə-'jəŋk-tiv, a-\ *adj* : involving the medical use of an adjunct ⟨~ therapy⟩ — **ad·junc·tive·ly** *adv*

ad·just \ə-'jəst\ *vb* **1** : to bring about orientation or adaptation of (oneself) **2** : to achieve mental and behavioral balance between one's own needs and the demands of others — **ad·just·ment** \-mənt\ *n*

ad·just·ed *adj* : having achieved an often specified and usu. harmonious relationship with the environment or with other individuals

adjustment disorder *n* : any of a group of psychological disorders characterized by emotional or behavioral symptoms that occur in response to a specific stressor (as divorce or unemployment)

¹**ad·ju·vant** \'a-jə-vənt\ *adj* **1** : serving to aid or contribute **2** : assisting in the prevention, amelioration, or cure of disease ⟨~ chemotherapy following surgery⟩

²**adjuvant** *n* : one that helps or facilitates: as **a** : an ingredient (as in a prescription) that facilitates or modifies the action of the principal ingredient **b** : something (as a drug or method) that enhances the effectiveness of a medical treatment **c** : a substance enhancing the immune response to an antigen

ADL *abbr* activities of daily living

Ad·le·ri·an \ad-'lir-ē-ən, äd-\ *adj* : of, relating to, or being a theory and technique of psychotherapy emphasizing the importance of feelings of inferiority, a will to power, and overcompensation in neurotic processes

    Ad·ler \'äd-lər\, **Alfred (1870–1937),** Austrian psychiatrist.

ad lib \(ˌ)ad-'lib\ *adv* : without restraint or imposed limit : as much or as often as is wanted — often used in writing prescriptions

ad li·bi·tum \ad-'li-bə-təm\ *adv* : AD LIB ⟨rats fed *ad libitum*⟩

ad·min·is·ter \əd-'mi-nə-stər\ *vb* **ad·min·is·tered; ad·min·is·ter·ing** : to give (as medicine) remedially — **ad·min·is·tra·tion** \ad-ˌmi-nə-'strā-shən\ *n*

ad·mit \əd-'mit\ *vb* **ad·mit·ted; ad·mit·ting** : to accept into a hospital as an inpatient

ad·nexa \ad-'nek-sə\ *n pl* : conjoined, subordinate, or associated anatomic parts ⟨the uterine ∼ include the ovaries and fallopian tubes⟩ — **ad-nex-al** \-səl\ *adj*

ad-nex-i-tis \,ad-,nek-'sī-təs\ *n* : inflammation of adnexa

ad-o-les-cence \,ad-ᵊl-'es-ᵊns\ *n* **1** : the state or process of growing up **2** : the period of life from puberty to maturity terminating legally at the age of majority

ad-o-les-cent \-ᵊnt\ *n* : one in the state of adolescence — **adolescent** *adj* — **ad-o-les-cent-ly** *adv*

adop-tive immunotherapy \ə-'däp-tiv-\ *n* : treatment esp. for cancer in which lymphocytes removed from a patient are cultured with interleukin-2 (as to generate lymphokine-activated killer cells or induce proliferation of tumor-infiltrating lymphocytes) and are returned to the patient's body to mediate tumor regression

ADP \,ā-(,)dē-'pē\ *n* : a nucleotide $C_{10}H_{15}N_5O_{10}P_2$ composed of adenosine and two phosphate groups that is formed in living cells as an intermediate between ATP and AMP and that is reversibly converted to ATP for the storing of energy by the addition of a high-energy phosphate group — called also *adenosine diphosphate*

adren- *or* **adreno-** *comb form* **1 a** : adrenal glands ⟨*adreno*cortical⟩ **b** : adrenal and ⟨*adreno*genital⟩ **2** : adrenaline ⟨*adren*ergic⟩

¹**ad-re-nal** \ə-'drēn-ᵊl\ *adj* : of, relating to, or derived from the adrenal glands or their secretion — **ad-re-nal-ly** *adv*

²**adrenal** *n* : ADRENAL GLAND

ad-re-nal-ec-to-my \ə-,drēn-ᵊl-'ek-tə-mē\ *n, pl* **-mies** : surgical removal of one or both adrenal glands

adrenal gland *n* : either of a pair of complex endocrine organs near the anterior medial border of the kidney consisting of a mesodermal cortex that produces glucocorticoid, mineralocorticoid, and androgenic hormones and an ectodermal medulla that produces epinephrine and norepinephrine — called also *adrenal, suprarenal gland*

Adren-a-lin \ə-'dren-ᵊl-ən\ *trademark* — used for a preparation of levorotatory epinephrine

adren-a-line \ə-'dren-ᵊl-ən\ *n* : EPINEPHRINE

ad-ren-er-gic \,a-drə-'nər-jik\ *adj* **1** : liberating or activated by adrenaline or a substance like adrenaline — compare CHOLINERGIC 1, NORADRENERGIC **2** : resembling adrenaline esp. in physiological action — **ad-ren-er-gi-cal-ly** \-ji-k(ə-)lē\ *adv*

ad-re-no-cor-ti-cal \ə-,drē-nō-'kòr-ti-kəl\ *adj* : of, relating to, or derived from the cortex of the adrenal glands

ad-re-no-cor-ti-coid \-,kòid\ *n* : a hormone secreted by the adrenal cortex — **adrenocorticoid** *adj*

ad-re-no-cor-ti-co-ste-roid \-'stir-,òid, -'ster-\ *n* : a steroid (as cortisone or

cortisol) obtained from, resembling, or having physiological effects like those of hormones of the adrenal cortex

ad-re-no-cor-ti-co-tro-pic \-'trō-pik, -'trä-\ *also* **ad-re-no-cor-ti-co-tro-phic** \-'trō-fik, -'trä-\ *adj* : acting on or stimulating the adrenal cortex

adrenocorticotropic hormone *n* : ACTH

ad-re-no-cor-ti-co-tro-pin \-'trō-pən\ *also* **ad-re-no-cor-ti-co-tro-phin** \-fən\ *n* : ACTH

adre-no-gen-i-tal syndrome \ə-,drē-nō-'je-nət-ᵊl-, -,dre-\ *n* : CUSHING'S SYNDROME

adre-no-leu-ko-dys-tro-phy \ə-,drē-nō-'dis-trə-fē\ *n, pl* **-phies** : a rare demyelinating disease of the central nervous system that is inherited as an X-linked recessive trait chiefly affecting males in childhood and that is characterized by progressive blindness, deafness, tonic spasms, and mental deterioration — abbr. *ALD;* called also *Schilder's disease*

adre-no-lyt-ic \ə-,drēn-ᵊl-'i-tik, -,dren-\ *adj* : blocking the release or action of adrenaline at nerve endings

adre-no-med-ul-lary \ə-,drē-nō-'med-ᵊl-,er-ē, -,dre-, -'me-jə-,ler-; -mə-'də-lə-rē\ *adj* : relating to or derived from the medulla of the adrenal glands ⟨∼ extracts⟩

adre-no-re-cep-tor \ə-,drē-nō-ri-'sep-tər, -,dre-\ *n* : an adrenergic receptor

adre-no-ste-rone \ə-,drē-nō-stə-'rōn, -,dre-; ,a-drə-'näs-tə-,\ *n* : a crystalline steroid $C_{19}N_{24}O_3$ obtained from the adrenal cortex and having androgenic activity

Adria-my-cin \,ā-drē-ə-'mīs-ᵊn, ,a-\ *trademark* — used for a preparation of the hydrochloride of doxorubicin

ad-sorb \ad-'sòrb, -'zòrb\ *vb* : to take up and hold by adsorption — **ad-sorb-able** \-'sòr-bə-bəl, -'zòr-\ *adj*

ad-sor-bent \-bənt\ *adj* : having the capacity or tendency to adsorb — **adsorbent** *n*

ad-sorp-tion \ad-'sòrp-shən, -'zòrp-\ *n* : the adhesion in an extremely thin layer of molecules (as of gases) to the surfaces of solid bodies or liquids with which they are in contact — compare ABSORPTION — **ad-sorp-tive** \-'sòrp-tiv, -'zòrp-\ *adj*

adult \ə-'dəlt, 'a-,dəlt\ *n* **1** : one that has arrived at full development or maturity esp. in size, strength, or intellectual capacity **2** : a human male or female after a specific age (as 21) — **adult** *adj* — **adult-hood** \ə-'dəlt-,hùd\ *n*

adul-ter-ate \ə-'dəl-tə-,rāt\ *vb* **-at-ed; -at-ing** : to corrupt, debase, or make impure by the addition of a foreign or inferior substance — **adul-ter-ant** \-rənt\ *n or adj* — **adul-ter-a-tion** \-,rā-shən\ *n*

adult-on-set diabetes *n* : TYPE 2 DIABETES

adult respiratory distress syndrome *n* : ACUTE RESPIRATORY DISTRESS SYNDROME

adult T-cell leukemia *n* : a lymphoproliferative disease that is marked by high counts of malignant T cells and is associated with the retrovirus HTLV-I — called also *adult T-cell leukemia/lymphoma*

Ad·vair Dis·kus \'ad-ˌver-'dis-kəs\ *trademark* — used for a preparation of fluticasone propionate and a salt of salmeterol

ad·vance di·rec·tive \əd-'van(t)s-də-'rek-tiv\ *n* : a legal document (as a living will) signed by a competent person to provide guidance for health-care decisions in the event that the person becomes incompetent to make such decisions

ad·vance·ment \əd-'vans-mənt\ *n* : detachment of a muscle or tendon from its insertion and reattachment (as in the surgical correction of strabismus) at a more advanced point from its insertion ⟨flexor tendon ∼⟩

advancement flap *n* : a flap of tissue stretched and sutured in place to cover a defect at a nearby position

ad·ven·ti·tia \ˌad-vən-'ti-shə, -ven-\ *n* : the outer layer that makes up a tubular organ or structure and esp. a blood vessel, is composed of collagenous and elastic fibers, and is not covered with peritoneum — called also *tunica adventitia* — **ad·ven·ti·tial** \-shəl\ *adj*

ad·ven·ti·tious \-shəs\ *adj* : arising sporadically or in other than the usual location ⟨an ∼ part in embryonic development⟩

Ad·vil \'ad-(ˌ)vil\ *trademark* — used for a preparation of ibuprofen

ady·na·mia \ˌā-dī-'na-mē-ə, ˌa-də-, -'nā-\ *n* : asthenia caused by disease

ady·nam·ic \ˌā-(ˌ)dī-'na-mik, ˌa-də-\ *adj* : characterized by or causing a loss of strength or function ⟨∼ ileus⟩

ae·des \ā-'ē-(ˌ)dēz\ *n* **1** *cap* : a large cosmopolitan genus of mosquitoes that includes vectors of some diseases (as yellow fever and dengue) **2** *pl* **aedes** : any mosquito of the genus *Aedes* — **ae·dine** \-ˌdīn, -ˌdēn\ *adj*

ae·goph·o·ny *chiefly Brit var of* EGOPHONY

aelurophobe, aelurophobia *var of* AILUROPHOBE, AILUROPHOBIA

-aemia *also* **-haemia** *chiefly Brit var of* -EMIA

aer- *or* **aero-** *comb form* **1** : air : atmosphere ⟨aerate⟩ ⟨aerobic⟩ **2** : gas ⟨aerosol⟩ **3** : aviation ⟨aeromedicine⟩

aer·ate \'ar-ˌāt, 'a-ər-\ *vb* **aer·at·ed; aer·at·ing 1** : to supply (the blood) with oxygen by respiration **2** : to supply or impregnate (as a liquid) with air — **aer·a·tion** \ˌar-'ā-shən, ˌa-ər-\ *n*

aero·al·ler·gen \ˌar-ō-'al-ər-jən\ *n* : an allergen carried in the air

aer·obe \'ar-ˌōb, 'a-ər-\ *n* : an organism (as a bacterium) that lives only in the presence of oxygen

aer·o·bic \ˌar-'ō-bik, ˌa-ər-\ *adj* **1** : living, active, or occurring only in the presence of oxygen ⟨∼ respiration⟩ **2** : of, relating to, or induced by aerobes **3 a** : of, relating to, or being activity which increases the body's demand for oxygen thereby resulting in a marked temporary increase in respiration and heart rate ⟨∼ exercise⟩ **b** : relating to, resulting from, or used in aerobics or aerobic activity — **aer·o·bi·cal·ly** \-bi-k(ə-)lē\ *adv*

aer·o·bics \-biks\ *n pl* **1** : a system of physical conditioning involving exercises (as running, walking, swimming, or calisthenics) strenuously performed so as to cause marked temporary increase in respiration and heart rate — used with a sing. or pl. verb **2** : aerobic exercises

aero·bi·ol·o·gy \ˌar-ō-bī-'ä-lə-jē\ *n, pl* **-gies** : the science dealing with the occurrence, transportation, and effects of airborne materials or microorganisms (as viruses or pollen)

aer·odon·tal·gia \ˌar-ō-dän-'tal-jē-ə, -jə\ *n* : toothache resulting from atmospheric decompression

aero·em·bo·lism \-'em-bə-ˌli-zəm\ *n* : decompression sickness caused by rapid ascent to high altitudes and resulting exposure to rapidly lowered air pressure — called also *air bends*

aero·med·i·cine \ˌar-ō-'me-də-sən\ *n* : a branch of medicine that deals with the diseases and disturbances arising from flying and the associated physiological and psychological problems — **aero·med·i·cal** \-'me-di-kəl\ *adj*

aero·oti·tis \ˌar-ə-wō-'tī-təs\ *n* : AERO-OTITIS MEDIA

aero·otitis me·dia \-'mē-dē-ə\ *n* : the traumatic inflammation of the middle ear resulting from differences between atmospheric pressure and pressure in the middle ear

aero·pha·gia \ˌar-ō-'fā-jē-ə, -jə\ *also* **aer·oph·a·gy** \ˌar-'ä-fə-jē, ˌa-ər-\ *n, pl* **-gias** *also* **-gies** : the swallowing of air esp. in hysteria

aero·pho·bia \ˌar-ō-'fō-bē-ə\ *n* : abnormal or excessive fear of drafts or of fresh air — **aero·pho·bic** \-bik\ *adj*

aero·sol \'ar-ə-ˌsäl, -ˌsȯl\ *n* **1** : a suspension of fine solid or liquid particles in gas ⟨smoke is an ∼⟩ **2** : a substance (as a medicine) dispensed from a pressurized container as an aerosol; *also* : the container for this

aero·sol·i·za·tion \ˌar-ə-ˌsä-lə-'zā-shən, -ˌsȯ-\ *n* : dispersal (as of a medicine) in the form of an aerosol — **aero·sol·ize** \'ar-ə-ˌsä-ˌlīz, -ˌsȯ-\ *vb* — **aero·sol·iz·er** *n*

aero·space medicine \'ar-ō-ˌspās-\ *n* : a medical specialty concerned with the health and medical problems of flight personnel both in the earth's atmosphere and in space

aer·oti·tis \ˌar-ō-ˈtī-təs\ *n* : AEROOTITIS MEDIA
Aes·cu·la·pi·an staff \ˌes-kyə-ˈlā-pē-ən-\ *n* : STAFF OF AESCULAPIUS
aetio- *chiefly Brit var of* ETIO-
ae·ti·o·log·ic, ae·ti·ol·o·gy, ae·ti·o·patho·gen·e·sis *chiefly Brit var of* ETIOLOGIC, ETIOLOGY, ETIOPATHOGENESIS
afe·brile \(ˌ)ā-ˈfe-ˌbrīl *also* -ˈfē-\ *adj* : free from fever : not marked by fever
[1]**af·fect** \ˈa-ˌfekt\ *n* : the conscious subjective aspect of an emotion considered apart from bodily changes
[2]**af·fect** \ə-ˈfekt, a-\ *vb* : to produce an effect upon; *esp* : to produce a material influence upon or alteration in
af·fec·tion \ə-ˈfek-shən\ *n* **1** : the action of affecting : the state of being affected **2 a** : a bodily condition **b** : DISEASE, MALADY ⟨a pulmonary ~⟩
af·fec·tive \a-ˈfek-tiv\ *adj* : relating to, arising from, or influencing feelings or emotions : EMOTIONAL ⟨~ symptoms⟩ — **af·fec·tive·ly** *adv* — **af·fec·tiv·i·ty** \ˌa-ˌfek-ˈti-və-tē\ *n*
affective disorder *n* : MOOD DISORDER
[1]**af·fer·ent** \ˈa-fə-rənt, -ˌfer-ənt\ *adj* : bearing or conducting inward; *specif* : conveying impulses toward the central nervous system — compare EFFERENT — **af·fer·ent·ly** *adv*
[2]**afferent** *n* : an afferent anatomical part (as a nerve)
af·fin·i·ty \ə-ˈfin-ət-ē\ *n, pl* **-ties** : an attractive force between substances or particles that causes them to enter into and remain in chemical combination
affinity chromatography *n* : chromatography in which a macromolecule (as a protein) is isolated and purified by passing it in solution through a column treated with a substance having a ligand for which the macromolecule has an affinity
afi·brin·o·gen·emia \ˌā-(ˌ)fī-ˌbri-nə-jə-ˈnē-mē-ə\ *n* : an abnormality of blood clotting caused by usu. congenital absence of fibrinogen in the blood
af·la·tox·in \ˌa-flə-ˈtäk-sən\ *n* : any of several carcinogenic mycotoxins that are produced esp. in stored agricultural crops (as peanuts) by molds (as *Aspergillus flavus*)
AFP *abbr* alpha-fetoprotein
African horse sickness *n* : an often fatal disease esp. of horses, donkeys, and mules that is caused by a reovirus of the genus *Orbivirus* (species *African horse sickness virus*), is endemic in sub-Saharan Africa, is marked by fever, edematous swellings, and internal hemorrhage, and is transmitted esp. by biting flies of the genus *Culicoides*
Af·ri·can·ized bee \ˈa-fri-kə-ˌnīzd-\ *n* : a honeybee that originated in Brazil as an accidental hybrid between an aggressive African subspecies (*Apis mellifera scutellata*) and previously established European honeybees and has spread to Mexico and the southernmost U.S. by breeding with local bees producing populations retaining most of the African bee's traits — called also *Africanized honeybee, killer bee*
African sleeping sickness *n* : SLEEPING SICKNESS 1
African swine fever *n* : highly contagious usu. fatal disease that affects only swine, resembles but is more severe than hog cholera, and is caused by a double-stranded DNA virus (species *African swine fever virus* of the genus *Asfivirus,* family *Asfarviridae*)—called also *swine fever*
African trypanosomiasis *n* : any of several trypanosomiases caused by African trypanosomes; *esp* : SLEEPING SICKNESS 1
af·ter·birth \ˈaf-tər-ˌbərth\ *n* : the placenta and fetal membranes that are expelled after delivery — called also *secundines*
af·ter·care \-ˌkar\ *n* : the care, treatment, help, or supervision given to persons discharged from an institution (as a hospital or prison)
af·ter·ef·fect \ˈaf-tər-i-ˌfekt\ *n* **1** : an effect that follows its cause after an interval **2** : a secondary result esp. in the action of a drug coming on after the subsidence of the first effect
af·ter·im·age \-ˌi-mij\ *n* : a usu. visual sensation occurring after stimulation by its external cause has ceased — called also *aftersensation, aftervision*
af·ter·load \ˈaf-tər-ˌlōd\ *n* : the force against which a ventricle contracts that is contributed to by the vascular resistance esp. of the arteries and by the physical characteristics (as mass and viscosity) of the blood
af·ter·pain \-ˌpān\ *n* : pain that follows its cause only after a distinct interval
af·ter·taste \-ˌtāst\ *n* : persistence of a sensation (as of flavor or an emotion) after the stimulating agent or experience has gone
af·to·sa \af-ˈtō-sə, -zə\ *n* : FOOT-AND-MOUTH DISEASE
Ag *symbol* [Latin *argentum*] silver
aga·lac·tia \ˌā-gə-ˈlak-shē-ə, -shə, -tē-ə\ *n* : the failure of the secretion of milk from any cause other than the normal ending of the lactation period — **aga·lac·tic** \-ˈlak-tik\ *adj*
agam·ma·glob·u·lin·emia \(ˌ)ā-ˌga-mə-ˌglä-byə-lə-ˈnē-mē-ə\ *n* : a pathological condition in which the body forms few or no gamma globulins or antibodies — compare DYSGAMMAGLOBULINEMIA
agan·gli·on·ic \(ˌ)ā-ˌgaŋ-glē-ˈä-nik\ *adj* : lacking ganglia
agar \ˈä-gər\ *n* **1** : a gelatinous colloidal extract of a red alga (as of the genera *Gelidium, Gracilaria,* and *Eucheuma*) used esp. in culture media or as a gelling and stabilizing agent in

foods **2** : a culture medium containing agar

agar–agar \ˌä-gər-ˈä-gər\ *n* : AGAR

aga·rose \ˈä-gə-ˌrōs, ˈä-, -ˌrōz\ *n* : a polysaccharide obtained from agar that is used esp. as a supporting medium in gel electrophoresis

¹age \ˈāj\ *n* **1 a** : the part of life from birth to a given time ⟨a child 10 years of ~⟩ **b** : the time or part of life at which some particular event, qualification, or capacity arises, occurs, or is lost ⟨of reproductive ~⟩ **c** : an advanced stage of life **2** : an individual's development measured in terms of the years requisite for like development of an average individual — see BINET AGE, MENTAL AGE

²age *vb* **aged; ag·ing** *or* **age·ing** : to grow old or cause to grow old

agen·e·sis \(ˌ)ā-ˈje-nə-səs\ *n, pl* **-e·ses** \-ˌsēz\ : lack or failure of development (as of a body part)

agent \ˈā-jənt\ *n* **1** : something that produces or is capable of producing an effect **2** : a chemically, physically, or biologically active principle — see OXIDIZING AGENT, REDUCING AGENT

Agent Orange \-ˈȯr-inj\ *n* : an herbicide widely used as a defoliant in the Vietnam War that is composed of 2,4-D and 2,4,5-T and contains dioxin as a contaminant

age–related macular degeneration *n* : macular degeneration that affects the elderly in either a slowly progressing form marked esp. by the accumulation of yellow deposits in and thinning of the macula lutea or in a rapidly progressing form marked by scarring produced by bleeding and fluid leakage below the macula lutea

age spots *n pl* : benign flat spots evenly covered with darker pigment that occur on sun-exposed skin esp. of persons aged 50 and over — called also *lentigo senilis, liver spots*

ageu·sia \ə-ˈgyü-zē-ə, (ˌ)ā-, -ˈjü-, -sē-\ *n* : the absence or impairment of the sense of taste — **ageu·sic** \-zik, -sik\ *adj*

ag·glu·ti·na·bil·i·ty \ə-ˌglüt-ᵊn-ə-ˈbi-lə-tē\ *n, pl* **-ties** : capacity to be agglutinated — **ag·glu·ti·na·ble** \-ˈglüt-ᵊn-ə-bəl\ *adj*

¹ag·glu·ti·nate \ə-ˈglüt-ᵊn-ˌāt\ *vb* **-nat·ed; -nat·ing** : to undergo or cause to undergo agglutination

²ag·glu·ti·nate \-ᵊn-ət, -ᵊn-ˌāt\ *n* : a clump of agglutinated material

ag·glu·ti·na·tion \ə-ˌglüt-ᵊn-ˈā-shən\ *n* : a reaction in which particles (as red blood cells or bacteria) suspended in a liquid collect into clumps and which occurs esp. as a serological response to a specific antibody — **ag·glu·ti·na·tive** \ə-ˈglüt-ᵊn-ˌā-tiv, -ə-tiv\ *adj*

agglutination test *n* : any of several tests based on the ability of a specific serum to cause agglutination of a suitable system and used in the diagnosis of infections, the identification of microorganisms, and in blood typing — compare WIDAL TEST

ag·glu·ti·nin \ə-ˈglüt-ᵊn-ən\ *n* : a substance (as an antibody) producing agglutination

ag·glu·ti·no·gen \ˌa-glü-ˈti-nə-jən, ə-\ *n* : an antigen whose presence results in the formation of an agglutinin — **ag·glu·ti·no·gen·ic** \-ˌglüt-ᵊn-ə-ˈje-nik\ *adj*

ag·gra·vate \ˈag-rə-ˌvāt\ *vb* **-vat·ed; -vat·ing** **1** : to make worse, more serious, or more severe **2** : to produce inflammation in : IRRITATE

ag·gre·gate \ˈa-gri-ˌgāt\ *vb* **-gat·ed; -gat·ing** : to collect or gather into a mass or whole — **ag·gre·gate** \-gət\ *adj or n* — **ag·gre·ga·tion** \ˌa-gri-ˈgā-shən\ *n*

ag·gres·sion \ə-ˈgre-shən\ *n* : hostile, injurious, or destructive behavior or outlook esp. when caused by frustration

ag·gres·sive \ə-ˈgre-siv\ *adj* **1** : tending toward or exhibiting aggression ⟨~ behavior⟩ **2** : growing, developing, or spreading rapidly ⟨~ bone tumors⟩ **3** : more severe, intensive, or comprehensive than usual esp, in dosage or extent ⟨~ chemotherapy⟩ — **ag·gres·sive·ly** *adv* — **ag·gres·sive·ness** *n* — **ag·gres·siv·i·ty** \ˌa-ˌgre-ˈsi-və-tē\ *n*

agitans — see PARALYSIS AGITANS

agitated depression *n* : a depressive disorder characterized esp. by restlessness, overactivity, and anxiety

ag·i·ta·tion \ˌaj-ə-ˈtā-shən\ *n* : a state of excessive psychomotor activity accompanied by increased tension and irritability — **ag·i·tat·ed** \ˈaj-ə-ˌtāt-əd\ *adj*

agly·cone \a-ˈglī-ˌkōn\ *also* **agly·con** \-ˌkän\ *n* : an organic compound (as a phenol or alcohol) combined with the sugar portion of a glycoside

ag·na·thia \ag-ˈnā-thē-ə, (ˌ)äg-, -ˈna-thē-\ *n* : the congenital complete or partial absence of one or both jaws

ag·no·gen·ic \ˌag-nō-ˈje-nik\ *adj* : of unknown cause ⟨~ metaplasia⟩

ag·no·sia \ag-ˈnō-zhə, -shə\ *n* : loss or diminution of the ability to recognize familiar objects or stimuli usu. as a result of brain damage

-agogue *n comb form* : substance that promotes the secretion or expulsion of ⟨chol*agogue*⟩ ⟨emmena*gogue*⟩

ag·o·nal \ˈa-gən-ᵊl\ *adj* : of, relating to, or associated with agony and esp. the death agony — **ag·o·nal·ly** *adv*

ag·o·nist \ˈa-gə-nist\ *n* **1** : a muscle that on contracting is automatically checked and controlled by the opposing simultaneous contraction of another muscle — called also *agonist muscle, prime mover;* compare ANTAGONIST, SYNERGIST **2** : a chemical substance (as a drug) capable of combining with a receptor on a cell and initiating the same reaction or activity typically produced by the binding of an endogenous substance ⟨binding of adrenergic ∼*s*⟩ — compare ANTAGONIST b

ag·o·ny \'a-gə-nē\ *n, pl* **-nies 1 :** intense pain of mind or body **2 :** the struggle that precedes death

ag·o·ra·pho·bia \ˌa-gə-rə-'fō-bē-ə\ *n* **:** abnormal fear of being helpless in a situation from which escape may be difficult or embarrassing that is characterized initially often by panic or anticipatory anxiety and finally by avoidance of open or public places

¹**ag·o·ra·pho·bic** \-'fō-bik\ *adj* **:** of, relating to, or affected with agoraphobia

²**agoraphobic** *or* **ag·o·ra·phobe** \'a-gə-rə-ˌfōb\ *also* **ag·o·ra·pho·bi·ac** \ˌa-gə-rə-'fō-bē-ˌak\ *n* **:** a person affected with agoraphobia

-agra *n comb form* **:** seizure of pain ⟨pell*agra*⟩ ⟨pod*agra*⟩

agram·ma·tism \(ˌ)ā-'gra-mə-ˌti-zəm\ *n* **:** the pathological inability to use words in grammatical sequence

agran·u·lo·cyte \(ˌ)ā-'gran-yə-lō-ˌsīt\ *n* **:** a leukocyte without cytoplasmic granules — compare GRANULOCYTE

agran·u·lo·cyt·ic angina \ˌā-ˌgran-yə-lō-'si-tik-\ *n* **:** AGRANULOCYTOSIS

agran·u·lo·cy·to·sis \ā-ˌgran-yə-lō-ˌsī-'tō-səs\ *n, pl* **-to·ses** \-ˌsēz\ **:** an acute febrile condition marked by severe depression of the granulocyte-producing bone marrow and by prostration, chills, swollen neck, and sore throat sometimes with local ulceration and believed to be basically a response to the side effects of certain drugs of the coal-tar series (as aminopyrine) — called also *agranulocytic angina, granulocytopenia*

agraph·ia \(ˌ)ā-'gra-fē-ə\ *n* **:** the pathological loss of the ability to write

agraph·ic \-fik\ *adj*

Ag·ry·lin \'ag-rə-lin\ *trademark* — used for a preparation of the hydrochloride of anagrelide

ague \'ā-(ˌ)gyü\ *n* **1 :** a fever (as malaria) marked by paroxysms of chills, fever, and sweating that recur at regular intervals **2 :** a fit of shivering : CHILL

AHA \ā-(ˌ)āch-'ā\ *n* **:** ALPHA HYDROXY ACID

AHA *abbr* **1** American Heart Association **2** American Hospital Association

AHF *abbr* **1** antihemophilic factor **2** [*antihemophilic factor*] factor VIII

AHG *abbr* antihemophilic globulin

AI *abbr* artificial insemination

aid \'ād\ *n* **1 :** the act of helping or treating; *also* **:** the help or treatment given **2 :** an assisting person or group ⟨a laboratory ∼⟩ **3 :** something by which assistance is given : an assisting device; *esp* **:** HEARING AID

AID *abbr* artificial insemination by donor

aide \'ād\ *n* **:** a person who acts as an assistant — see NURSE'S AIDE

AIDS \'ādz\ *n* **:** a disease of the human immune system that is characterized cytologically esp. by reduction in the numbers of CD4-bearing helper T cells to 20 percent or less of normal thereby rendering the subject highly vulnerable to life-threatening conditions (as Pneumocystis carinii pneumonia) and to some that become life-threatening (as Kaposi's sarcoma) and that is caused by infection with HIV commonly transmitted in infected blood esp. during illicit intravenous drug use and in bodily secretions (as semen) during sexual intercourse — called also *acquired immune deficiency syndrome, acquired immunodeficiency syndrome*

AIDS–related complex *n* **:** a group of symptoms (as fever, weight loss, and lymphadenopathy) that is associated with the presence of antibodies to HIV and is followed by the development of AIDS in a certain proportion of cases — abbr. *ARC*

AIDS virus *n* **:** HIV

AIH *abbr* artificial insemination by husband

ail \'āl\ *vb* **1 :** to affect with an unnamed disease or physical or emotional pain or discomfort — used only of unspecified causes **2 :** to become affected with pain or discomfort

ail·ment \'āl-mənt\ *n* **:** a bodily disorder or chronic disease

ai·lu·ro·phobe \ī-'lu̇r-ə-ˌfōb, ā-\ *or* **ae·lu·ro·phobe** \ē-\ *n* **:** a person who hates or fears cats

ai·lu·ro·pho·bia *or* **ae·lu·ro·pho·bia** \-ˌlu̇r-ə-'fō-bē-ə\ *n* **:** abnormal fear of cats

air \'ar\ *n* **:** a mixture of invisible odorless tasteless gases that surrounds the earth, that is composed by volume chiefly of 78 percent nitrogen, 21 percent oxygen, 0.9 percent argon, 0.03 percent carbon dioxide, varying amounts of water vapor, and minute amounts of rare gases (as helium), and that has a pressure at sea level of about 14.7 pounds per square inch

air bends *n pl* **:** AEROEMBOLISM

air·borne \'ar-ˌbȯrn\ *adj* **:** carried or transported by the air ⟨∼ allergens⟩

Air-cast \'ar-ˌkast\ *trademark* — used for a pneumatic brace

air embolism *n* **:** obstruction of the circulation by air that has gained entrance to veins usu. through wounds — compare AEROEMBOLISM

air hunger *n* **:** deep labored breathing at an increased or decreased rate

air sac *n* **:** ALVEOLUS b

air·sick \'ar-ˌsik\ *adj* **:** affected with motion sickness associated with flying — **air·sick·ness** *n*

air·way \-ˌwā\ *n* **:** a passageway for air into or out of the lungs; *specif* **:** a device passed into the trachea by way of the mouth or nose or through an incision to maintain a clear respiratory passageway (as during anesthesia or convulsions)

aka·thi·sia \ˌā-ka-ˈthi-zhē-ə, -zhə, ˌa-, -ˈthē-\ *n* : a condition characterized by uncontrollable motor restlessness

ak·ee *or* **ack·ee** \ˈa-kē, a-ˈkē\ *n* : the fruit of an African tree (*Blighia sapida* of the family Sapindaceae) that has edible flesh when ripe but is poisonous when immature or overripe; *also* : the tree

aki·ne·sia \ˌā-ki-ˈnē-zhē-ə, -zhə\ *n* : loss or impairment of voluntary activity (as of a muscle) — **aki·net·ic** \ˌā-kə-ˈne-tik, -ki-\ *adj*

Al *symbol* aluminum

ala \ˈā-lə\ *n, pl* **alae** \-ˌlē\ : a wing or a winglike anatomic process or part; *esp* : ALA NASI

alaeque — *see* LEVATOR LABII SUPERIORIS ALAEQUE NASI

ala na·si \-ˈnā-ˌsī, -ˌzī\ *n, pl* **alae na·si** \-ˌsī, -ˌzī\ : the expanded outer wall of cartilage on each side of the nose

al·a·nine \ˈa-lə-ˌnēn\ *n* : a simple nonessential crystalline amino acid $C_3H_7NO_2$ formed esp. by the hydrolysis of proteins

alanine aminotransferase *n* : an enzyme which promotes transfer of an amino group from glutamic acid to pyruvic acid and which when present in abnormally high levels in the blood is a diagnostic indication of liver disease — abbr. *ALT*; called also *glutamic pyruvic transaminase*

alar cartilage \ˈā-lər-\ *n* : one of the pair of lower lateral cartilages of the nose

alar ligament *n* : either of a pair of strong rounded fibrous cords of which one arises on each side of the cranial part of the dens, passes obliquely and laterally upward, and inserts on the medial side of a condyle of the occipital bone — called also *check ligament*

alarm reaction *n* : the initial reaction of an organism (as increased hormonal activity) to stress

alas·trim \ˈa-lə-ˌstrim, ˌa-lə-ˈ; ə-ˈlas-trəm\ *n* : VARIOLA MINOR

alba — *see* LINEA ALBA, MATERIA ALBA, PHLEGMASIA ALBA DOLENS

Al·bers–Schön·berg disease \ˈal-bərz-ˈshərn-ˌbərg-, -ˈshön-\ *n* : OSTEOPETROSIS

　Albers–Schönberg, Heinrich Ernst (1865–1921), German radiologist.

albicans, albicantia — *see* CORPUS ALBICANS

albicantes — *see* LINEAE ALBICANTES

al·bi·nism \ˈal-bə-ˌni-zəm, al-ˈbī-\ *n* : the condition of an albino — **al·bi·nis·tic** \ˌal-bə-ˈnis-tik\ *adj*

al·bi·no \al-ˈbī-(ˌ)nō\ *n, pl* **-nos** : an organism exhibiting deficient pigmentation; *esp* : a human being who is congenitally deficient in pigment and usu. has a milky or translucent skin, white or colorless hair, and eyes with pink or blue iris and deep-red pupil — **al·bin·ic** \-ˈbi-nik\ *adj*

al·bi·not·ic \ˌal-bə-ˈnä-tik\ *adj* **1** : of, relating to, or affected with albinism **2** : tending toward albinism

albuginea — *see* TUNICA ALBUGINEA

al·bu·men \al-ˈbyü-mən; ˈal-ˌbyü-, -byə-\ *n* **1** : the white of an egg **2** : ALBUMIN

al·bu·min \al-ˈbyü-mən; ˈal-ˌbyü-, -byə-\ *n* : any of numerous simple heat-coagulable water-soluble proteins that occur in blood plasma or serum, muscle, the whites of eggs, milk, and other animal substances and in many plant tissues and fluids

¹al·bu·min·oid \-mə-ˌnòid\ *adj* : resembling albumin

²albuminoid *n* **1** : PROTEIN 1 **2** : SCLEROPROTEIN

al·bu·min·uria \al-ˌbyü-mə-ˈnùr-ē-ə, -ˈnyùr-\ *n* : the presence of albumin in the urine that is usu. a symptom of disease of the kidneys but sometimes a response to other diseases or physiological disturbances of benign nature — **al·bu·min·uric** \-ˈnùr-ik, -ˈnyùr-\ *adj*

al·bu·te·rol \al-ˈbyü-tə-ˌ ròl\ *n* : a beta-agonist bronchodilator used in the form of its sulfate $(C_{13}H_{21}NO_3)_2 \cdot H_2SO_4$ to treat bronchospasm associated esp. with asthma and chronic obstructive pulmonary disease — called also *salbutamol*; see COMBIVENT, PROVENTIL, VENTOLIN

alcaptonuria *var of* ALKAPTONURIA

al·co·hol \ˈal-kə-ˌhòl\ *n* **1 a** : ethanol esp. when considered as the intoxicating agent in fermented and distilled liquors **b** : drink (as whiskey or beer) containing ethanol **c** : a mixture of ethanol and water that is usu. 95 percent ethanol **2** : any of various compounds that are analogous to ethanol in constitution and that are hydroxyl derivatives of hydrocarbons

alcohol dehydrogenase *n* : any of various dehydrogenases that catalyze reversibly the conversion between an alcohol and an aldehyde or ketone that in humans are zinc-containing dimers found esp. in the liver and gastric mucosa which catalyze the oxidation of an alcohol (as ethanol) to an aldehyde (as acetaldehyde) in the presence of NAD

¹al·co·hol·ic \ˌal-kə-ˈhò-lik, -ˈhä-\ *adj* **1 a** : of, relating to, or caused by alcohol (⟨ hepatitis⟩) **b** : containing alcohol **2** : affected with alcoholism — **al·co·hol·i·cal·ly** \-li-k(ə-)lē\ *adv*

²alcoholic *n* : one affected with alcoholism

al·co·hol·ism \ˈal-kə-ˌhò-ˌli-zəm, -kə-hə-\ *n* **1** : continued excessive or compulsive use of alcoholic drinks **2 a** : poisoning by alcohol **b** : a chronic, progressive, potentially fatal, psychological and nutritional disorder associated with excessive and usu. compulsive drinking of ethanol and characterized by frequent intoxication leading to dependence on or addiction to the substance, impairment of the ability to work and socialize, destructive behaviors (as drunken driving), tissue damage (as cirrhosis of the liver), and severe withdrawal symptoms upon detoxification

ALD *abbr* adrenoleukodystrophy

al·de·hyde \'al-də-ˌhīd\ *n* : ACETALDE- HYDE; *broadly* : any of various highly reactive compounds typified by acetaldehyde and characterized by the group CHO — **al·de·hy·dic** \ˌal-də-'hī-dik\ *adj*

al·do·hex·ose \ˌal-dō-'hek-ˌsōs, -ˌsōz\ *n* : a hexose (as glucose or mannose) of an aldehyde nature

al·dose \'al-ˌdōs, -ˌdōz\ *n* : a sugar containing one aldehyde group per molecule

al·do·ste·rone \al-'däs-tə-ˌrōn; ˌal-dō-'stir-ˌōn, -stə-'rōn\ *n* : a steroid hormone $C_{21}H_{28}O_5$ of the adrenal cortex that functions in the regulation of the salt and water balance of the body

al·do·ste·ron·ism \al-'däs-tə-ˌrō-ˌni-zəm, ˌal-dō-stə-'rō-\ *n* : a condition that is characterized by excessive secretion of aldosterone and typically by loss of body potassium, muscular weakness, and elevated blood pressure — called also *hyperaldosteronism*

al·drin \'ȯl-drən, 'al-\ *n* : an exceedingly poisonous insecticide $C_{12}H_6Cl_6$

K. Alder — see DIELDRIN

alen·dro·nate \ə-'len-drə-ˌnāt\ *n* : a hydrated bisphosphonate sodium salt $C_4H_{12}NNaO_7P_2 \cdot 3H_2O$ used to inhibit bone resorption esp. in the treatment of osteoporosis and Paget's disease of bone — called also *alendronate sodium;* see FOSAMAX

aleu·ke·mia \ˌā-lü-'kē-mē-ə\ *n* : leukemia in which the circulating leukocytes are normal or decreased in number; *esp* : ALEUKEMIC LEUKEMIA

aleu·ke·mic \-'kē-mik\ *adj* : not marked by increase in circulating white blood cells

aleukemic leukemia *n* : leukemia resulting from changes in the tissues forming white blood cells and characterized by a normal or decreased number of white blood cells in the circulating blood — called also *aleukemic myelosis*

Aleve \ə-'lēv\ *trademark* — used for a preparation of the sodium salt of naproxen

Al·ex·an·der technique \ˌal-ig-'zan-dər-\ *n, often cap T* : a technique for positioning and moving the body that is believed to reduce tension

Alexander, Frederick Matthias (1869–1955), Australian elocutionist.

alex·ia \ə-'lek-sē-ə\ *n* : aphasia characterized by loss of ability to read — **alex·ic** \-'lek-sik\ *adj*

alex·in \ə-'lek-sən\ *n* : COMPLEMENT 2 — **alex·in·ic** \ˌa-ˌlek-'si-nik\ *adj*

alex·i·thy·mia \ə-ˌleks-i-'thī-mē-ə\ *n* : inability to express one's feelings

ALG *abbr* antilymphocyte globulin; antilymphocytic globulin

alg- *or* **algo-** *comb form* : pain ⟨*algo*lagnia⟩

al·ga \'al-gə\ *n, pl* **al·gae** \'al-(ˌ)jē\ *also* **algas** : a plant or plantlike organism (as a seaweed) of any of several phyla, divisions, or classes of chiefly aquatic usu. chlorophyll-containing nonvascular organisms — see BROWN ALGA, RED ALGA — **al·gal** \-gəl\ *adj*

al·ge·sia \al-'jē-zē-ə, -'jē-zhə\ *n* : sensitivity to pain — **al·ge·sic** \-'jē-zik, -sik\ *adj*

-al·gia \'al-jə, -jē-ə\ *n comb form* : pain ⟨neur*algia*⟩

al·gi·cide *or* **al·gae·cide** \'al-jə-ˌsīd\ *n* : an agent used to kill algae — **al·gi·cid·al** \ˌal-jə-'sīd-ᵊl\ *adj*

al·gin \'al-jən\ *n* : any of various colloidal substances (as alginic acid) derived from marine brown algae and used esp. as emulsifiers or thickeners

al·gi·nate \'al-jə-ˌnāt\ *n* : a salt of alginic acid

al·gin·ic acid \(ˌ)al-'ji-nik-\ *n* : an insoluble colloidal acid $(C_6H_8O_6)_n$ that is used in making dental preparations and in preparing pharmaceuticals

al·go·gen·ic \ˌal-gō-'je-nik\ *adj* : producing pain

al·go·lag·nia \ˌal-gō-'lag-nē-ə\ *n* : a perversion (as masochism or sadism) in which pleasure and esp. sexual gratification is obtained by inflicting or suffering pain — **al·go·lag·nic** \-nik\ *adj*

al·gor mor·tis \'al-ˌgȯr-'mȯr-təs\ *n* : the gradual cooling of the body following death

ali- *comb form* : wing or winglike part ⟨*ali*sphenoid⟩

alien·ate \'ā-lē-ə-ˌnāt, 'āl-yə-\ *vb* **-at·ed; -at·ing** : to make unfriendly, hostile, or indifferent where attachment formerly existed

alien·ation \ˌā-lē-ə-'nā-shən, ˌāl-yə-\ *n* **1** : a withdrawing or separation of a person or a person's affections from an object or position of former attachment **2** : MENTAL ALIENATION

alien·ist \'ā-lē-ə-nist, 'āl-yə-\ *n* : PSYCHIATRIST

al·i·men·ta·ry \ˌa-lə-'men-tə-rē, -'men-trē\ *adj* : of, concerned with, or relating to nourishment or to the function of nutrition

alimentary canal *n* : DIGESTIVE TRACT

alimentary system *n* : DIGESTIVE SYSTEM

alimentary tract *n* : DIGESTIVE TRACT

al·i·men·ta·tion \ˌa-lə-mən-'tā-shən, -ˌmen-\ *n* : the act or process of affording nutriment or nourishment

al·i·phat·ic \ˌa-lə-'fa-tik\ *adj* : of, relating to, or being an organic compound (as an alkane or alkene) having an open-chain structure

¹al·i·quot \'a-lə-ˌkwät\ *adj* : being an equal fractional part (as of a solution) — **aliquot** *n*

²**aliquot** vb : to divide (as a solution) into equal parts

¹**ali·sphe·noid** \ˌa-lə-'sfē-ˌnȯid, ˌa-\ adj : belonging or relating to or forming the wings of the sphenoid or the pair of bones that fuse with other sphenoidal elements to form the greater wings of the sphenoid in the adult

²**alisphenoid** n : an alisphenoid bone; esp : GREATER WING

alive \ə-'līv\ adj : having life : not dead or inanimate

al·ka·lae·mia chiefly Brit var of ALKALEMIA

al·ka·le·mia \ˌal-kə-'lē-mē-ə\ n : a condition in which the hydrogen ion concentration in the blood is decreased

al·ka·li \'al-kə-ˌlī\ n, pl **-lies** or **-lis** : a substance having marked basic properties — compare BASE

alkali disease n : SELENOSIS

al·ka·line \'al-kə-lən, -ˌlīn\ adj : of, relating to, containing, or having the properties of an alkali or alkali metal : BASIC; esp, of a solution : having a pH of more than 7 — **al·ka·lin·i·ty** \ˌal-kə-'li-nə-tē\ n

alkaline phosphatase n : any of the phosphatases optimally active in alkaline medium and occurring in esp. high concentrations in bone, the liver, the kidneys, and the placenta

al·ka·lin·ize \'al-kə-lə-ˌnīz\ vb **-ized; -iz·ing** : to make alkaline — **al·ka·lin·i·za·tion** \ˌal-kə-ˌli-nə-'zā-shən, -lə-\ n

alkali reserve n : the concentration of one or more basic ions or substances in a fluid medium that buffer its pH by neutralizing acid; esp : the concentration of bicarbonate in the blood

al·ka·lize \'al-kə-ˌlīz\ vb **-lized; -liz·ing** : ALKALINIZE — **al·ka·li·za·tion** \ˌal-kə-lə-'zā-shən\ n

al·ka·liz·er \'al-kə-ˌlī-zər\ n : an alkalinizing agent

al·ka·loid \'al-kə-ˌlȯid\ n : any of numerous usu. colorless, complex, and bitter organic bases (as morphine or caffeine) containing nitrogen and usu. oxygen that occur esp. in seed plants — **al·ka·loi·dal** \ˌal-kə-'lȯid-ᵊl\ adj

al·ka·lo·sis \ˌal-kə-'lō-səs\ n, pl **-lo·ses** \-ˌsēz\ : an abnormal condition of increased alkalinity of the blood and tissues — compare ACIDOSIS, KETOSIS — **al·ka·lot·ic** \ˌal-kə-'lä-tik\ adj

al·kane \'al-ˌkān\ n : any of a series of aliphatic hydrocarbons C_nH_{2n+2} (as methane) in which each carbon is bonded to four other atoms — called also paraffin

al·kap·ton·uria or **al·cap·ton·uria** \(ˌ)al-ˌkap-tə-'nu̇r-ē-ə, -'nyu̇r-\ n : a rare recessive metabolic anomaly marked by inability to complete the degradation of tyrosine and phenylalanine resulting in the presence of homogentisic acid in the urine — **al·kap·ton·uric** or **al·cap·ton·uric** \-'nu̇r-ik, -'nyu̇r-\ n or adj

al·kene \'al-ˌkēn\ n : any of numerous unsaturated hydrocarbons having one

double bond; specif : any of a series of open-chain hydrocarbons C_nH_{2n} (as ethylene)

¹**al·kyl** \'al-kəl\ adj : having a monovalent organic group and esp. one C_nH_{2n+1} (as methyl) derived from an alkane (as methane)

²**alkyl** n : a compound of one or more alkyl groups with a metal

al·kyl·ate \'al-kə-ˌlāt\ vb **-at·ed; -at·ing** : to introduce one or more alkyl groups into (a compound) — **al·kyl·a·tion** \ˌal-kə-'lā-shən\ n

alkylating agent n : a substance that causes replacement of hydrogen by an alkyl group esp. in a biologically important molecule; specif : one with mutagenic activity that inhibits cell division and growth and is used to treat some cancers

ALL abbr acute lymphoblastic leukemia, acute lymphocytic leukemia

all- or **allo-** comb form **1** : other : different \atypical \allergy\ \allopathy\ **2** allo- : isomeric form or variety of (a specified chemical compound) \allopurinol\

al·lan·to·ic \ˌa-lən-'tō-ik, -ˌlan-\ adj : relating to, contained in, or characterized by an allantois

al·lan·to·in \ə-'lan-tə-wən\ n : a crystalline oxidation product $C_4H_6N_4O_3$ of uric acid used to promote healing of local wounds and infections

al·lan·to·is \ə-'lan-tə-wəs\ n, pl **al·lan·to·ides** \ˌa-lən-'tō-ə-ˌdēz, -ˌlan-\ : a vascular fetal membrane that is formed as a pouch from the hindgut and that in placental mammals is intimately associated with the chorion in formation of the placenta

Al·le·gra \ə-'leg-rə, -'lä-grə\ trademark — used for a preparation of the hydrochloride of fexofenadine

al·lele \ə-'lēl\ n **1** : any of the alternative forms of a gene that may occur at a given locus **2** : either of a pair of alternative Mendelian characters (as ability versus inability to taste the chemical phenylthiocarbamide) — **le·lic** \-'lē-lik, -'le-\ adj — **al·lel·ism** \-'lē-ˌli-zəm, -'le-\ n

allelo- comb form : alternative \allelomorph\

al·le·lo·morph \ə-'le-lə-ˌmȯrf, -'lē-\ n : ALLELE — **al·le·lo·mor·phic** \ə-ˌle-lə-'mȯr-fik, -ˌlē-\ adj — **al·le·lo·mor·phism** \ə-'le-lə-ˌmȯr-ˌfi-zəm, -'lē-\ n

al·ler·gen \'a-lər-jən\ n : a substance that induces allergy

al·ler·gen·ic \ˌa-lər-'je-nik\ adj : having the capacity to induce allergy \\~ proteins\ \\~ foods\ — **al·ler·ge·nic·i·ty** \-jə-'ni-sə-tē\ n

al·ler·gic \ə-'lər-jik\ adj **1** : of, relating to, or characterized by allergy \an ~ reaction\ **2** : affected with allergy : subject to an allergic reaction

allergic encephalomyelitis n : encephalomyelitis produced by an allergic response following the introduction of an antigenic substance into the body

al·ler·gic rhinitis *n* : rhinitis caused by exposure to an allergen; *esp* : HAY FEVER

al·ler·gist \-jist\ *n* : a specialist in allergy

al·ler·gol·o·gy \ˌa-lər-ˈjä-lə-jē\ *n, pl* **-gies** : a branch of medicine concerned with allergy

al·ler·gy \ˈa-lər-jē\ *n, pl* **-gies** 1 : altered bodily reactivity (as hypersensitivity) to an antigen in response to a first exposure 2 : exaggerated or pathological reaction (as by sneezing, difficult breathing, itching, or skin rashes) to substances, situations, or physical states that are without comparable effect on the average individual 3 : medical practice concerned with allergies

al·le·thrin \ˈa-lə-thrən\ *n* : a light yellow oily synthetic insecticide $C_{19}H_{26}O_3$

al·le·vi·ate \ə-ˈlē-vē-ˌāt\ *vb* **-at·ed; -at·ing** : to make (as symptoms) less severe or more bearable — **al·le·vi·a·tion** \-ˌlē-vē-ˈā-shən\ *n*

al·le·vi·a·tive \ə-ˈlē-vē-ˌā-tiv\ *adj* : tending to alleviate : PALLIATIVE ⟨a medicine that is ∼ but not curative⟩

al·li·cin \ˈa-lə-sən\ *n* : a liquid compound $C_6H_{10}OS_2$ with a garlic odor and antibacterial properties

allo— see ALL-

al·lo·an·ti·body \ˌa-lō-ˈan-ti-ˌbä-dē\ *n, pl* **-bod·ies** : an antibody produced following introduction of an alloantigen into the system of an individual of a species lacking that particular antigen — called also *isoantibody*

al·lo·an·ti·gen \ˌa-lō-ˈan-tə-jən\ *n* : a genetically determined antigen present in some but not all individuals of a species (as those of a particular blood group) and capable of inducing the production of an alloantibody by individuals which lack it — called also *isoantigen* — **al·lo·an·ti·gen·ic** \-ˌan-tə-ˈje-nik\ *adj*

al·lo·bar·bi·tal \ˌa-lō-ˈbär-bə-ˌtól\ *n* : a white crystalline barbiturate $C_{10}H_{12}N_2O_3$ used as a sedative and hypnotic

al·lo·bar·bi·tone \-ˌtōn\ *n chiefly Brit* : ALLOBARBITAL

al·lo·cor·tex \-ˈkor-ˌteks\ *n* : ARCHIPALLIUM

Al·lo·der·ma·nys·sus \ˌdər-mə-ˈni-səs\ *n* : a genus of bloodsucking mites parasitic on rodents including one (*A. sanguineus*) implicated as a vector of rickettsialpox in humans

al·lo·dyn·ia \ˌal-ə-ˈdin-ē-ə\ *n* : pain resulting from a stimulus (as a light touch of the skin) which would not normally provoke pain; *also* : a condition marked by allodynia

al·lo·ge·ne·ic \ˌa-lō-jə-ˈnē-ik\ *also* **al·lo·gen·ic** \-ˈje-nik\ *adj* : involving, derived from, or being individuals of the same species that are sufficiently unlike genetically to interact antigenically ⟨∼ skin grafts⟩ — compare SYNGENEIC, XENOGENEIC

al·lo·graft \ˈa-lə-ˌgraft\ *n* : a homograft between allogeneic individuals — **allograft** *vb*

al·lo·iso·leu·cine \ˌa-lō-ˌī-sə-ˈlü-ˌsēn\ *n* : either of two stereoisomers of isoleucine of which one is present in bodily fluids of individuals affected with maple syrup urine disease

al·lo·path \ˈa-lə-ˌpath\ *n* : one who practices allopathy

al·lop·a·thy \ə-ˈlä-pə-thē, a-\ *n, pl* **-thies** 1 : a system of medical practice that aims to combat disease by using remedies (as drugs or surgery) which produce effects different from or incompatible with those produced by the disease treated — compare HOMEOPATHY 2 : a system of medical practice making use of all measures that have proved of value in treatment of disease — **al·lo·path·ic** \ˌa-lə-ˈpa-thik\ *adj* — **al·lo·path·i·cal·ly** \-thi-k(ə-)lē\ *adv*

al·lo·pu·ri·nol \ˌa-lō-ˈpyùr-ə-ˌnól, -ˌnōl\ *n* : a drug $C_5H_4N_4O$ used to promote excretion of uric acid esp. in the treatment of gout

all–or–none *adj* : marked either by complete operation or effect or by none at all ⟨∼ response of a nerve cell⟩

all–or–none law *n* : a principle in physiology: in any single nerve or muscle fiber the response to a stimulus above threshold level is maximal and independent of the intensity of the stimulus

all–or–noth·ing *adj* : ALL-OR-NONE

al·lo·ste·ric \ˌa-lō-ˈster-ik, -ˈstir-\ *adj* : of, relating to, or being a change in the shape and activity of a protein (as an enzyme) that results from combination with another substance at a point other than the chemically active site — **al·lo·ste·ri·cal·ly** \-i-k(ə-)lē\ *adv*

al·lo·trans·plant \ˌa-lō-trans-ˈplant\ *vb* : to transplant between genetically different individuals — **al·lo·transplant** \-ˈtrans-ˌ\ *n* — **al·lo·trans·plan·ta·tion** \-ˌtrans-ˌplan-ˈtā-shən\ *n*

al·lo·type \ˈa-lə-ˌtīp\ *n* : an alloantigen that is part of a plasma protein (as an antibody) — compare IDIOTYPE, ISOTYPE — **al·lo·typ·ic** \ˌa-lə-ˈti-pik\ *adj* — **al·lo·typ·i·cal·ly** \-pi-k(ə-)lē\ *adv* — **al·lo·typy** \ˈa-lə-ˌtī-pē\ *n*

al·lox·an \ə-ˈläk-sən\ *n* : a crystalline compound $C_4H_2N_2O_4$ causing diabetes mellitus when injected into experimental animals — called also *mesoxalylurea*

al·loy \ˈa-ˌlói, ə-ˈlói\ *n* : a metal and a nonmetal intimately united usu. by being fused together; *also* : the state of union of the components — **al·loy** \ˈa-ˌlói, ˈa-ˌlói\ *vb*

al·lo·zyme \ˈa-lə-ˌzīm\ *n* : any of the variants of an enzyme that are determined by alleles at a single genetic locus — **al·lo·zy·mic** \ˌa-lə-ˈzī-mik\ *adj*

all–trans–retinoic acid *n* : TRETINOIN

al·lyl \'a-ləl\ *n, often attrib* : an unsaturated radical C_3H_5 compounds of which are found in the oils of garlic and mustard — **al·lyl·ic** \ə-'li-lik, a-\ *adj*

allyl iso·thio·cy·a·nate \-ˌī-sō-ˌthī-ə-'sī-ə-ˌnāt, -nət\ *n* : a colorless pungent irritating liquid ester C_4H_5NS that is the chief constituent of mustard oil used in medicine and is used as a medical counterirritant

N–al·lyl·nor·mor·phine \ˌen-ˌal-əl-ˌnȯr-'mȯr-ˌfēn\ *n* : NALORPHINE

al·oe \'a-(ˌ)lō\ *n* **1** *cap* : a large genus of succulent chiefly southern African plants of the lily family (Liliaceae) **2** : a plant of the genus *Aloe* **3** : the dried juice of the leaves of various aloes used esp. formerly as a purgative and tonic — usu. used in pl. with a sing. verb **4** : ALOE VERA

aloe vera \-'ver-ə, -'vir-\ *n* : an aloe (*Aloe barbadensis* syn *A. vera*) whose leaves furnish a gelatinous emollient extract used esp. in cosmetics and skin creams; *also* : such an extract or a preparation composed primarily of such an extract

al·o·in \'a-lə-wən\ *n* : a bitter yellow crystalline cathartic obtained from the aloe and containing one or more glycosides

al·o·pe·cia \ˌa-lə-'pē-shē-ə, -shə\ *n* : loss of hair, wool, or feathers : BALDNESS — **al·o·pe·cic** \-'pē-sik\ *adj*

alopecia ar·e·a·ta \-ˌar-ē-'ā-tə, -'ä-\ *n* : sudden loss of hair in circumscribed patches with little or no inflammation

¹al·pha \'al-fə\ *n* **1** : the 1st letter of the Greek alphabet — symbol A or α **2** : ALPHA PARTICLE **3** : ALPHA WAVE

²alpha *or* α *adj* **1** : of or relating to one of two or more closely related chemical substances ⟨the *alpha* chain of hemoglobin⟩ — used somewhat arbitrarily to specify ordinal relationship or a particular physical form **2** : closest in position in the structure of an organic molecule to a particular group or atom; *also* : occurring at or having a structure characterized by such a position ⟨α-substitution⟩

al·pha–ad·ren·er·gic \ˌal-fə-ˌa-drə-'nər-jik\ *adj* : of, relating to, or being an alpha-receptor ⟨∼ blocking action⟩

al·pha–ad·re·no·cep·tor \-ə-'drē-nə-ˌsep-tər\ *also* **al·pha–ad·re·no·re·cep·tor** \-ri-ˌsep-tər\ *n* : ALPHA-RECEPTOR

al·pha–ami·no acid *or* **α–ami·no acid** \ə-'mē-nō-\ *n* : any of the more than 20 amino acids that have an amino group in the alpha position with most having the general formula $RCH(NH_2)COOH$, that are synthesized in plant and animal tissues, that are considered the building blocks of proteins from which they can be obtained by hydrolysis, and that play an important role in metabolism, growth, maintenance, and repair of tissue

al·pha–block·er \-ˌbläk-ər\ *n* : any of a group of drugs (as phenoxybenzamine and phentolamine) that combine with and block the activity of an alpha-receptor and are used esp. to treat hypertension

alpha cell *n* : an acidophilic glandular cell (as of the pancreas or the adenohypophysis) — compare BETA CELL

alpha chain disease *n* : IMMUNOPROLIFERATIVE SMALL INTESTINAL DISEASE

alpha–fetoprotein *or* **α–fetoprotein** *n* : a fetal blood protein present abnormally in adults with some forms of cancer (as of the liver) and normally in the amniotic fluid of pregnant women with very low levels tending to be associated with Down syndrome in the fetus and very high levels with neural tube defects (as spina bifida) in which the tube remains open

alpha globulin *n* : any of several globulins of plasma or serum that have at alkaline pH the greatest electrophoretic mobility next to albumin — compare BETA GLOBULIN, GAMMA GLOBULIN

al·pha–he·lix *or* **α–he·lix** \ˌal-fə-'hē-liks\ *n* : the coiled structural arrangement of many proteins consisting of a single chain of amino acids stabilized by hydrogen bonds — compare BETA-SHEET, DOUBLE HELIX — **al·pha–he·li·cal** \-'he-li-kəl, -'hē-\ *adj*

alpha hydroxy acid *n* : a carboxylic acid (as glycolic acid or lactic acid) occurring in natural products (as fruit or yogurt) and used in cosmetics for its exfoliating effect on the surface layer of the skin — called also *AHA*

alpha interferon *n* : an interferon produced by white blood cells that inhibits viral replication, suppresses cell proliferation, and regulates immune response and is used in a form obtained from recombinant DNA to treat various diseases — called also *interferon alpha*

al·pha–ke·to·glu·tar·ic acid *or* **α–ke·toglutaric acid** \-ˌkē-tō-glü-'tar-ik-\ *n* : the alpha keto isomer of ketoglutaric acid formed in various metabolic processes (as the Krebs cycle)

al·pha–lipoprotein *or* **α–lipoprotein** *n* : HDL

al·pha–1–an·ti·tryp·sin \-ˌwən-ˌan-ti-'trip-sən, -ˌtī-\ *n* : a trypsin-inhibiting serum protein whose deficiency is associated with the development of emphysema

alpha particle *n* : a positively charged nuclear particle identical with the nucleus of a helium atom that consists of two protons and two neutrons and is ejected at high speed in certain radioactive transformations

al·pha–re·cep·tor \'al-fə-ri-ˌsep-tər\ *n* : any of a group of receptors that are present on cell surfaces of some effector organs and tissues innervated by the sympathetic nervous system and that mediate certain physiological responses (as vasoconstriction, relaxation of intestinal muscle, and contraction of most smooth muscle) when bound by specific adrenergic agents — compare BETA-RECEPTOR

al·pha–to·coph·er·ol \,al-fə-tō-'kä-fə-,rȯl, -,rōl\ *n* : a tocopherol $C_{29}H_{50}O_2$ with high vitamin E potency

Al·pha·vi·rus \'al-fə-,vī-rəs\ *n* : a genus of togaviruses transmitted by arthropods and esp. mosquitoes and including the Mayaro virus, Semliki Forest virus, Sindbis virus, and the causative agents of chikungunya and equine encephalitis

alpha wave *n* : an electrical rhythm of the brain with a frequency of 8 to 13 cycles per second that is often associated with a state of wakeful relaxation — called also *alpha, alpha rhythm*

al·praz·o·lam \al-'praz-ə-,lam\ *n* : a benzodiazepine tranquilizer $C_{17}H_{13}$-ClN_4 used esp. in the treatment of mild to moderate anxiety — see XANAX

al·pren·o·lol \al-'pre-nə-,lȯl, -,lōl\ *n* : a beta-adrenergic blocking agent that has been used in the form of its hydrochloride $C_{15}H_{23}NO_2$·HCl esp. to treat cardiac arrhythmias

al·pros·ta·dil \al-'präs-tə-dil\ *n* : a prostaglandin $C_{20}H_{34}O_5$ that promotes vasodilation and is used esp. to treat erectile dysfunction — called also *prostaglandin E_1*

ALS *abbr* **1** amyotrophic lateral sclerosis **2** antilymphocyte serum; antilymphocytic serum

al·ser·ox·y·lon \,al-sə-'räk-sə-,län\ *n* : a complex extract from a rauwolfia (*Rauvolfia serpentina*) that has a physiological action resembling but milder than that of reserpine

ALT *abbr* alanine aminotransferase

Al·tace \'al-,tās\ *trademark* — used for a preparation of ramipril

al·te·plase \'al-tə,plās\ *n* : TISSUE PLASMINOGEN ACTIVATOR

al·ter \'ȯl-tər\ *vb* **al·tered; al·ter·ing** : CASTRATE, SPAY

al·ter·ative \'ȯl-tə-,rā-tiv, -rə-\ *n* : a drug used empirically to alter favorably the course of an ailment

altered state of consciousness *n* : any of various states of awareness that deviate from and are usu. clearly demarcated from ordinary waking consciousness

alternans — see PULSUS ALTERNANS

al·ter·nate host \'ȯl-tər-nət-\ *n* : INTERMEDIATE HOST 1

alternating personality *n* : MULTIPLE PERSONALITY DISORDER

al·ter·na·tive \ȯl-'tər-nət-iv\ *adj* : of, relating to, or based on alternative medicine ⟨∼ therapies⟩

alternative medicine *n* : any of various systems of healing or treating disease (as chiropractic, homeopathy, or Ayurveda) not included in the tradi-

tional medical school curricula taught in the U.S. and Britain

altitude sickness *n* : the effects (as nosebleed or nausea) of oxygen deficiency in the blood and tissues developed at high altitudes with reduced atmospheric pressure

al·um \'a-ləm\ *n* : a potassium aluminum sulfate $KAl(SO_4)_2$·$12H_2O$ or an ammonium aluminum sulfate $NH_4Al(SO_4)_2$·$12H_2O$ used esp. as an emetic and as an astringent

alu·mi·na \ə-'lü-mə-nə\ *n* : an oxide of aluminum Al_2O_3 that occurs native as corundum and in hydrated forms and is used in antacids — called also *aluminum oxide*

al·u·min·i·um \,al-yù-'mi-nē-əm\ *chiefly Brit* : ALUMINUM

alu·mi·num \ə-'lü-mə-nəm\ *n, often attrib* : a bluish silver-white malleable ductile light trivalent metallic element — symbol *Al*; see ELEMENT table

aluminum chloride *n* : a deliquescent compound $AlCl_3$ or Al_2Cl_3 that is used as a topical astringent and antiseptic on the skin, and in some deodorants to control sweating

aluminum hydroxide *n* : any of several white gelatinous or crystalline hydrates Al_2O_3·nH_2O of alumina; *esp* : one Al_2O_3·$3H_2O$ or $Al(OH)_3$ used in medicine as an antacid

aluminum oxide *n* : ALUMINA

aluminum sulfate *n* : a colorless salt $Al_2(SO_4)_3$ that is a powerful astringent and is used as a local antiperspirant and in water purification

Al·u·pent \'a-lù-,pent\ *trademark* — used for a preparation of the sulfate of metaproterenol

alvei *pl of* ALVEUS

alve·ol- *or* **alveolo-** *comb form* : alveolus ⟨*alveolectomy*⟩

al·ve·o·lar \al-'vē-ə-lər\ *adj* : of, relating to, resembling, or having alveoli; *esp* : of, relating to, or constituting the part of the jaws where the teeth arise, the air-containing cells of the lungs, or glands with secretory cells about a central space

alveolar arch *n* : the arch of the upper or lower jaw formed by the alveolar processes

alveolar artery *n* : any of several arteries supplying the teeth; *esp* : POSTERIOR SUPERIOR ALVEOLAR ARTERY — compare INFERIOR ALVEOLAR ARTERY

alveolar canals *n pl* : the canals in the jawbones for the passage of the dental nerves and associated vessels

alveolar duct *n* : one of the somewhat enlarged terminal sections of the bronchioles that branch into the terminal alveoli

alveolar nerve — see INFERIOR ALVEOLAR NERVE, SUPERIOR ALVEOLAR NERVE

alveolar process *n* : the bony ridge or raised thickened border on each side of the upper or lower jaw that contains the sockets of the teeth — called also *alveolar ridge*

alveolar vein *n* — see INFERIOR ALVEOLAR VEIN, POSTERIOR SUPERIOR ALVEOLAR VEIN

al·ve·o·lec·to·my \al-ˌvē-ə-ˈlek-tə-mē, ˌal-vē-\ *n, pl* **-mies** : surgical excision of a portion of an alveolar process usu. as an aid in fitting dentures

al·ve·o·li·tis \al-ˌvē-ə-ˈlī-təs, ˌal-vē-\ *n* : inflammation of one or more alveoli esp. of the lung

al·ve·o·lo·plas·ty \al-ˈvē-ə-(ˌ)lō-ˌplas-tē\ *or* **al·veo·plas·ty** \ˈal-vē-ō-\ *n, pl* **-ties** : surgical shaping of the dental alveoli and alveolar processes esp. after extraction of several teeth or in preparation for dentures

al·ve·o·lus \al-ˈvē-ə-ləs\ *n, pl* **-li** \-ˌlī, -(ˌ)lē\ : a small cavity or pit: as **a** : a socket for a tooth **b** : any of the small thin-walled air-containing compartments of the lungs that are typically arranged into saclike clusters into which an alveolar duct terminates and from which respiratory gases are exchanged with the pulmonary capillaries **c** : an acinus of a compound gland **d** : any of the pits in the wall of the stomach into which the glands open

al·ve·us \ˈal-vē-əs\ *n, pl* **al·vei** \-vē-ˌī, -ˌē\ : a thin layer of medullary nerve fibers on the ventricular surface of the hippocampus

Alz·hei·mer's disease \ˈälts-ˌhī-mərz-, ˈalts-\ *also* **Alzheimer disease** *n* : a degenerative brain disease of unknown cause that is the most common form of dementia, that usu. starts in late middle age or in old age, that results in progressive memory loss, impaired thinking, disorientation, and changes in personality and mood, and that is marked histologically by the degeneration of brain neurons esp. in the cerebral cortex and by the presence of neurofibrillary tangles and plaques containing beta-amyloid — abbr. *AD;* called also *Alzheimer's;* compare PRESENILE DEMENTIA

Alzheimer, Alois (1864–1915), German neurologist.

Am *symbol* americium

AMA *abbr* **1** against medical advice **2** American Medical Association

am·a·crine cell \ˈa-mə-ˌkrīn-, (ˌ)ā-ˈma-ˌkrīn-\ *n* : a unipolar nerve cell found in the retina, in the olfactory bulb, and in close connection with the Purkinje cells of the cerebellum

amal·gam \ə-ˈmal-gəm\ *n* : an alloy of mercury with another metal that is solid or liquid at room temperature according to the proportion of mercury present and is used esp. in making tooth cements

am·a·ni·ta \ˌa-mə-ˈnī-tə, -ˈnē-\ *n* **1** *cap* : a genus of widely distributed white-spored basidiomycetous fungi (family

Amanitaceae) that includes some deadly poisonous forms (as the death cap) **2** : a fungus of the genus *Amanita*

am·a·ni·tin \-ˈnit-ᵊn, -ˈnēt-\ *n* : a highly toxic cyclic peptide produced by the death cap that selectively inhibits mammalian RNA polymerase

aman·ta·dine \ə-ˈman-tə-ˌdēn\ *n* : a drug administered orally esp. in the form of its hydrochloride $C_{10}H_{17}N$·HCl to prevent viral infection (as by the virus causing influenza A) and in the treatment of Parkinson's disease — see SYMMETREL

Am·a·ran·thus \ˌa-mə-ˈran-thəs\ *n* : a large genus of coarse herbs (family Amaranthaceae) including some which produce pollen that is an important hay fever allergen

amas·tia \(ˌ)ā-ˈmas-tē-ə\ *n* : the absence or underdevelopment of the mammary glands

am·au·ro·sis \ˌa-mȯ-ˈrō-səs\ *n, pl* **-ro·ses** \-ˌsēz\ : partial or complete loss of sight occurring esp. without an externally perceptible change in the eye — **am·au·rot·ic** \-ˈrä-tik\ *adj*

amaurosis fu·gax \-ˈfü-ˌgaks, -ˈfyü-\ *n* : temporary partial or complete loss of sight esp. from the effects of excessive acceleration (as in flight)

amaurotic idiocy *n* : any of several recessive genetic conditions characterized by the accumulation of lipid-containing cells in the viscera and nervous system, mental retardation, and impaired vision or blindness; *esp* : TAY-SACHS DISEASE

ambi- *prefix* : both ⟨*ambi*valence⟩ ⟨*ambi*sexuality⟩

am·bi·dex·ter·i·ty \ˌam-bi-(ˌ)dek-ˈster-ə-tē\ *n, pl* **-ties** : the quality or state of being ambidextrous

am·bi·dex·trous \ˌam-bi-ˈdek-strəs\ *adj* : using both hands with equal ease — **am·bi·dex·trous·ly** *adv*

Am·bi·en \ˈam-bē-ˌen\ *trademark* — used for a preparation of the tartrate of zolpidem

am·bi·ent \ˈam-bē-ənt\ *adj* : surrounding on all sides ⟨~ air pollution⟩

ambiguus — see NUCLEUS AMBIGUUS

am·bi·sex·u·al \ˌam-bi-ˈsek-shə-wəl\ *adj* : BISEXUAL — **ambisexual** *n* — **am·bi·sex·u·al·i·ty** \-ˌsek-shə-ˈwa-lə-tē\ *n*

am·biv·a·lence \am-ˈbi-və-ləns\ *n* : simultaneous and contradictory attitudes or feelings (as attraction and repulsion) toward an object, person, or action — **am·biv·a·lent** \-lənt\ *adj* — **am·biv·a·lent·ly** *adv*

am·biv·a·len·cy \-lən-sē\ *n, pl* **-cies** : AMBIVALENCE

am·bi·vert \ˈam-bi-ˌvərt\ *n* : a person having characteristics of both extrovert and introvert

ambly- *or* **amblyo-** *comb form* : connected with amblyopia ⟨*amblyo*-scope⟩

Am·bly·om·ma \ˌam-blē-ˈä-mə\ *n* : a genus of ixodid ticks including the lone star tick (*A. americanum*) of the southern U.S. and the African bont tick (*A. hebraeum*)

am·bly·ope \'am-blē-₁ōp\ *n* : an individual affected with amblyopia

am·bly·opia \₁am-blē-'ō-pē-ə\ *n* : dimness of sight esp. in one eye without apparent change in the eye structures — called also *lazy eye, lazy-eye blindness* — **am·bly·opic** \-'ō-pik, -'ä-\ *adj*

am·bly·o·scope \'am-blē-ə-₁skōp\ *n* : an instrument for training amblyopic eyes to function properly

Am·bro·sia \am-'brō-zhə, -zhē-ə\ *n* : a genus of mostly American composite herbs that includes the ragweeds

Am·bu \'am-₁bü\ *trademark* — used for an artificial-respiration device consisting of a bag that is squeezed by hand

am·bu·lance \'am-byə-ləns\ *n* : a vehicle equipped for transporting the injured or sick

am·bu·lant \'am-byə-lənt\ *adj* : walking or in a walking position; *specif* : AMBULATORY ⟨an ~ patient⟩

am·bu·late \-₁lāt\ *vb* **-lat·ed; -lat·ing** : to move from place to place — **am·bu·la·tion** \₁am-byə-'lā-shən\ *n*

am·bu·la·to·ry \'am-byə-lə-₁tōr-ē\ *adj* **1** : of, relating to, or adapted to walking **2 a** : able to walk about and not bedridden ⟨~ patients⟩ **b** : performed on or involving an ambulatory patient or an outpatient ⟨an ~ electrocardiogram⟩ ⟨~ medical care⟩ — **am·bu·la·to·ri·ly** \₁am-byə-lə-'tōr-ə-lē\ *adv*

ameba, amebic, ameboid *var of* AMOEBA, AMOEBIC, AMOEBOID

am·e·bi·a·sis *or* **am·oe·bi·a·sis** \₁a-mi-'bī-ə-səs\ *n, pl* **-a·ses** \-₁sēz\ : infection with or disease caused by amoebas (esp. *Entamoeba histolytica*)

amebic abscess *n* : a specific purulent invasive lesion commonly of the liver caused by parasitic amoebas (esp. *Entamoeba histolytica*)

amebic dysentery *n* : acute human intestinal amebiasis caused by a common amoeba of the genus *Entamoeba* (*E. histolytica*) and marked by dysentery, abdominal pain, and erosion of the intestinal wall

ame·bi·cide *or* **amoe·bi·cide** \ə-'mē-bə-₁sīd\ *n* : a substance used to kill or capable of killing amoebas and esp. parasitic amoebas — **ame·bi·cid·al** *or* **amoe·bi·cid·al** \ə-₁mē-bə-'sīd-ᵊl\ *adj*

ame·bo·cyte *or* **amoe·bo·cyte** \ə-'mē-bə-₁sīt\ *n* : a cell (as a phagocyte) having amoeboid form or movements

amel·a·not·ic \₁ā-₁mē-lə-'nä-tik\ *adj* : containing little or no melanin ⟨~ melanocytes⟩

ame·lia \ə-'mē-lē-ə, (₁)ā-\ *n* : congenital absence of one or more limbs

am·e·lo·blast \'a-mə-lō-₁blast\ *n* : any of a group of columnar cells that produce and deposit enamel on the surface of a developing tooth — **am·e·lo·blas·tic** \₁a-mə-lō-'blas-tik\ *adj*

am·e·lo·blas·to·ma \₁a-mə-lō-blas-'tō-mə\ *n, pl* **-mas** *also* **-ma·ta** \-mə-tə\ : a tumor of the jaw derived from remnants of the embryonic rudiment of tooth enamel — called also *adamantinoma*

am·e·lo·den·tin·al \-'den-₁tēn-ᵊl, -den-'tēn-\ *adj* : of or relating to enamel and dentin

am·e·lo·gen·e·sis \-'je-nə-səs\ *n, pl* **-e·ses** \-₁sēz\ : the process of forming tooth enamel

amelogenesis im·per·fec·ta \-₁im-(₁)pər-'fek-tə\ *n* : faulty development of tooth enamel that is genetically determined

amen·or·rhea \₁ā-₁me-nə-'rē-ə, ₁ä-\ *n* : abnormal absence or suppression of menstruation — **amen·or·rhe·ic** \-'rē-ik\ *adj*

amen·tia \(₁)ā-'men-chē-ə, -chə, (₁)ä-\ *n* : MENTAL RETARDATION; *specif* : a condition of lack of development of intellectual capacity

American cockroach *n* : a free-flying cockroach (*Periplaneta americana*) that is a common domestic pest infesting ships or buildings in the northern hemisphere

American dog tick *n* : a common No. American ixodid tick of the genus *Dermacentor* (*D. variabilis*) esp. of dogs and humans that is an important vector of Rocky Mountain spotted fever and tularemia — called also *dog tick*

am·er·i·ci·um \₁a-mə-'ri-shē-əm, -sē-\ *n* : a radioactive metallic element produced by bombardment of plutonium with high-energy neutrons — symbol *Am*; see ELEMENT table

Ames test \'āmz-\ *n* : a test for identifying potential carcinogens by studying the frequency with which they cause histidine-producing genetic mutants in bacterial colonies of the genus *Salmonella* (*S. typhimurium*) initially lacking the ability to synthesize histidine

Ames, Bruce Nathan (*b* 1928), American biochemist.

ameth·o·caine \ə-'me-thə-₁kān\ *n* : TETRACAINE

ame·thop·ter·in \₁a-mə-'thäp-tə-rən\ *n* : METHOTREXATE

am·e·tro·pia \₁a-mə-'trō-pē-ə\ *n* : an abnormal refractive eye condition (as myopia, hyperopia, or astigmatism) in which images fail to focus upon the retina — **am·e·tro·pic** \-'trō-pik, -'trä-\ *adj*

AMI *abbr* acute myocardial infarction

am·ide \'am-₁īd, -əd\ *n* : an organic compound derived from ammonia or an amine by replacement of an atom of hydrogen with an acyl group

am·i·done \'a-mə-₁dōn\ *n* : METHADONE

amil·o·ride \ə-'mi-lə-₁rīd\ *n* : a diuretic $C_6H_8ClN_7O$ that promotes sodium excretion and potassium retention

amine \ə-'mēn, 'a-₁mēn\ *n* : any of a class of organic compounds derived from ammonia by replacement of one, two, or three hydrogen atoms with alkyl groups

ami·no \ə-'mē-(,)nō\ *adj* : relating to, being, or containing an amine group — often used in combination

amino acid *n* : an amphoteric organic acid containing the amino group NH₂; *esp* : ALPHA-AMINO ACID

ami·no·ac·i·de·mia \ə-,mē-nō-,a-sə-'dē-mē-ə\ *n* : a condition in which the concentration of amino acids in the blood is abnormally increased

ami·no·ac·id·uria \-,a-sə-'dūr-ē-ə, -'dyūr-\ *n* : a condition in which one or more amino acids are excreted in excessive amounts

ami·no·ben·zo·ic acid \ə-,mē-nō-ben-'zō-ik-\ *n* : any of three crystalline derivatives C₇H₇NO₂ of benzoic acid; *esp* : PARA-AMINOBENZOIC ACID

γ-aminobutyric acid *var of* GAMMA-AMINOBUTYRIC ACID

ami·no·glu·teth·i·mide \-glü-'teth-ə-,mīd\ *n* : a glutethimide derivative C₁₃H₁₆N₂O₂ used esp. as an anticonvulsant

ami·no·gly·co·side \-'glī-kə-,sīd\ *n* : any of a group of antibiotics (as streptomycin and neomycin) that inhibit bacterial protein synthesis and are active esp. against gram-negative bacteria

ami·no·pep·ti·dase \ə-,mē-nō-'pep-tə-,dās, -,dāz\ *n* : an enzyme (as one found in the duodenum) that hydrolyzes peptides

am·i·noph·yl·line \,a-mə-'nä-fə-lən\ *n* : a theophylline derivative C₁₆H₂₄N₁₀O₄ used esp. to stimulate the heart in congestive heart failure and to dilate the air passages in respiratory disorders — called also *theophylline ethylenediamine*

β-ami·no·pro·pio·ni·trile \,bā-tə-ə-,mē-nō-,prō-pē-ō-'nī-trəl, -,trīl\ *n* : a potent lathyrogen C₃H₆N₂

am·i·nop·ter·in \,a-mə-'näp-tə-rən\ *n* : a folic acid antagonist C₁₉H₂₀N₈O₅ of glutamic acid that is used as a rodenticide and antileukemic agent

ami·no·py·rine \ə-,mē-nō-'pīr-,ēn\ *n* : a white crystalline compound C₁₃H₁₇N₃O formerly used to relieve pain and fever but now largely abandoned for this purpose because of the occurrence of fatal agranulocytosis as a side effect in some users

ami·no·sal·i·cyl·ic acid \ə-,mē-nō-,sa-lə-'si-lik-\ *n* : any of four isomeric derivatives C₇H₇O₃N of salicylic acid that have a single amino group; *esp* : PARA-AMINOSALICYLIC ACID

ami·no·thi·a·zole \ə-,mē-nō-'thī-ə-,zōl\ *n* : a light yellow crystalline heterocyclic amine C₃H₄N₂S that has been used as a thyroid inhibitor in the treatment of hyperthyroidism

ami·no·trans·fer·ase \-'trans-fə-,rās, -,rāz\ *n* : TRANSAMINASE

ami·o·da·rone \ə-'mē-ō-də-,rōn\ *n* : a drug administered in the form of its hydrochloride C₂₅H₂₉I₂NO₃·HCl to treat ventricular arrhythmias

am·i·trip·ty·line \,a-mə-'trip-tə-,lēn\ *n* : a tricyclic antidepressant drug used in the form of its hydrochloride C₂₀-H₂₃N·HCl to prevent migraines and to treat neuropathic pain and bulimia as well as depression

AML *abbr* acute myelogenous leukemia; acute myeloid leukemia

am·lo·di·pine \am-'lō-də-,pēn\ *n* : a calcium channel blocker administered in the form of its salt C₂₀H₂₅-ClN₂O₅·C₆H₈SO₃H to treat hypertension and angina pectoris — see LOTREL, NORVASC

am·mo·nia \ə-'mō-nyə\ *n* 1 : a pungent colorless gaseous alkaline compound of nitrogen and hydrogen NH₃ that is very soluble in water and can easily be condensed to a liquid by cold and pressure 2 : AMMONIA WATER

am·mo·ni·a·cal \,a-mə-'nī-ə-kəl\ *also* **am·mo·ni·ac** \ə-'mō-nē-,ak\ *adj* : of, relating to, containing, or having the properties of ammonia

ammonia water *n* : a water solution of ammonia — called also *spirit of hartshorn*

am·mo·ni·um \ə-'mō-nē-əm\ *n* : an ion NH₄⁺ derived from ammonia by combination with a hydrogen ion

ammonium carbonate *n* : a carbonate of ammonium; *specif* : the commercial mixture of the bicarbonate and carbamate used esp. in smelling salts

ammonium chloride *n* : a white crystalline volatile salt NH₄Cl that is used in dry cells and as an expectorant — called also *sal ammoniac*

ammonium nitrate *n* : a colorless crystalline salt N₂H₄NO₃ used in veterinary medicine as an expectorant and urinary acidifier

ammonium sulfate *n* : a colorless crystalline salt (NH₄)₂SO₄ used in medicine as a local analgesic

am·ne·sia \am-'nē-zhə\ *n* 1 : loss of memory sometimes including the memory of personal identity due to brain injury, shock, fatigue, repression, or illness or sometimes induced by anesthesia 2 : a gap in one's memory

am·ne·si·ac \am-'nē-zhē-,ak, -zē-\ *also* **am·ne·sic** \-zik, -sik\ *n* : a person affected with amnesia

am·ne·sic \am-'nē-zik, -sik\ *also* **am·ne·si·ac** \-zhē-,ak, -zē-\ *adj* : of or relating to amnesia : affected with or caused by amnesia ⟨an ∼ patient⟩

am·nes·tic \am-'nes-tik\ *adj* : AMNESIC; *also* : causing amnesia ⟨∼ agents⟩

amnii — see LIQUOR AMNII

am·nio \'am-nē-ō\ *n* : AMNIOCENTESIS

amnio- *comb form* : amnion ⟨*amnio*centesis⟩

am·nio·cen·te·sis \,am-nē-ō-(,)sen-'tē-səs\ *n, pl* **-te·ses** \-,sēz\ : the surgical insertion of a hollow needle through the abdominal wall and into the uterus of a pregnant female to obtain amniotic fluid esp. to examine the fetal chromosomes for an abnormality and for the determination of sex

am·ni·og·ra·phy \ˌam-nē-'ä-grə-fē\ *n*, *pl* **-phies** : radiographic visualization of the outlines of the uterine cavity, placenta, and fetus after injection of a radiopaque substance into the amnion

am·ni·on \'am-nē-ˌän, -ən\ *n*, *pl* **am·nions** *or* **am·nia** \-nē-ə\ : a thin membrane forming a closed sac about the embryos of reptiles, birds, and mammals and containing the amniotic fluid

am·nio·scope \'am-nē-ə-ˌskōp\ *n* : an endoscope for observation of the amnion and its contents

am·ni·os·co·py \ˌam-nē-'äs-kə-pē\ *n*, *pl* **-pies** : visual observation of the amnion and its contents by means of an endoscope

am·ni·ote \'am-nē-ˌōt\ *n* : any of a group (Amniota) of vertebrates that undergo embryonic development within an amnion and include the birds, reptiles, and mammals — **amniote** *adj*

am·ni·ot·ic \ˌam-nē-'ä-tik\ *adj* 1 : of or relating to the amnion 2 : characterized by the development of an amnion

amniotic band *n* : strands of amniotic tissue that are formed by premature rupture of the amnion and that become entangled esp. in the extremities of the developing fetus

amniotic band syndrome *n* : the highly variable group of physical abnormalities that can result from the formation of amniotic bands

amniotic cavity *n* : the fluid-filled space between the amnion and the fetus

amniotic fluid *n* : the serous fluid in which the embryo is suspended within the amnion

amniotic sac *n* : AMNION

am·ni·ot·o·my \ˌam-nē-'ä-tə-mē\ *n*, *pl* **-mies** : intentional rupture of the fetal membranes to induce or facilitate labor

amo·bar·bi·tal \ˌa-mō-'bär-bə-ˌtȯl\ *n* : a barbiturate used esp. in the form of its sodium salt $C_{11}H_{17}N_2NaO_3$ as a hypnotic and sedative — called also *amylobarbitone*; see AMYTAL, TUINAL

amo·di·a·quine \ˌa-mə-'dī-ə-ˌkwin, -ˌkwēn\ *or* **amo·di·a·quin** \-ˌkwin\ *n* : a compound derived from quinoline and used in the form of its dihydrochloride $C_{20}H_{22}ClN_3O·2HCl·2H_2O$ as an antimalarial

amoe·ba \ə-'mē-bə\ *n* 1 *cap* : a large genus of naked protozoans with lobed pseudopodia, without permanent organelles or supporting structures, and of wide distribution in fresh and salt water and moist terrestrial environ-

ments 2 *also* ameba *pl* **-bas** *or* **-bae** \-(ˌ)bē\ : a protozoan of the genus *Amoeba*; broadly : an amoeboid protozoan

amoebiasis, amoebicide, amoebocyte *var of* AMEBIASIS, AMEBICIDE, AMEBOCYTE

amoe·bic *also* **ame·bic** \-bik\ *adj* 1 : resembling or relating to an amoeba 2 *usu* amebic : caused by amoebas

amoe·boid *also* **ame·boid** \ə-'mē-ˌbȯid\ *adj* : resembling an amoeba specif. in moving or changing in shape by means of protoplasmic flow

Amoe·bo·tae·nia \ə-ˌmē-(ˌ)bō-'tē-nē-ə\ *n* : a genus of tapeworms (family Dilepididae) parasitic in the intestines of poultry

amor·phous \ə-'mȯr-fəs\ *adj* 1 : having no apparent shape or organization 2 : having no real or apparent crystalline form

amox·a·pine \ə-'mäk-sə-ˌpēn\ *n* : a tricyclic antidepressant drug $C_{17}H_{16}-ClN_3O$

amox·i·cil·lin \ə-ˌmäk-si-'si-lən\ *n* : a semisynthetic penicillin $C_{16}H_{19}N_3O_5S$ derived from ampicillin — see AMOXIL, AUGMENTIN, TRIMOX

Amox·il \ə-'mäk-sil\ *trademark* — used for a preparation of amoxicillin

amox·y·cil·lin \ə-ˌmäk-sē-'si-lən\ *Brit var of* AMOXICILLIN

AMP \ˌā-(ˌ)em-'pē\ *n* : a nucleotide $C_{10}H_{12}N_5O_3H_2PO_4$ that is composed of adenosine and one phosphate group and is reversibly convertible to ADP and ATP in metabolic reactions — called also *adenosine monophosphate*; compare CYCLIC AMP

am·pere \'am-ˌpir, -ˌper\ *n* : a unit of electric current equivalent to a steady current produced by one volt applied across a resistance of one ohm

Am·père \äⁿ-per\, **André Marie (1775–1836)**, French physicist.

am·phet·amine \am-'fe-tə-ˌmēn, -mən\ *n* : a racemic sympathomimetic amine $C_9H_{13}N$ or one of its derivatives (as dextroamphetamine or methamphetamine) frequently abused as a stimulant of the central nervous system but used clinically esp. in the form of its sulfate $C_9H_{13}N·H_2SO_4$ to treat attention deficit disorder and narcolepsy and formerly as a short-term appetite suppressant — see BENZEDRINE

amphi- *or* **amph-** *prefix* : on both sides : of both kinds : both *(amphimixis)*

am·phi·ar·thro·sis \ˌam-fē-(ˌ)är-'thrō-səs\ *n*, *pl* **-thro·ses** \-ˌsēz\ : a slightly movable articulation (as a symphysis or a syndesmosis)

am·phi·bol·ic \ˌam-fə-'bä-lik\ *adj* : having an uncertain or irregular outcome — used of stages in fevers or the critical period of disease when prognosis is uncertain

am·phi·mix·is \ˌam-fə-'mik-səs\ *n*, *pl* **-mix·es** \-ˌsēz\ : the union of gametes in sexual reproduction

am·phi·path·ic \\am-fə-'pa-thik\ *adj* : AMPHIPHILIC — **am·phi·path** \'am-fə-ˌpath\ *n*

am·phi·phil·ic \\am-fə-'fi-lik\ *adj* : of, relating to, consisting of, or being one or more molecules (as of a glycolipid or sphingolipid) in a biological membrane having a polar water-soluble terminal group attached to a water-insoluble hydrocarbon chain — **am·phi·phile** \'am-fə-ˌfil\ *n*

am·phi·stome \'am-fi-ˌstōm\ *n* : any of a suborder (Amphistomata) of digenetic trematodes — compare GASTRODISCOIDES — **amphistome** *adj*

am·phor·ic \am-'fȯr-ik\ *adj* : resembling the sound made by blowing across the mouth of an empty bottle ⟨~ breathing⟩ ⟨~ sounds⟩

am·pho·ter·ic \\am-fə-'ter-ik\ *adj* : capable of reacting chemically either as an acid or as a base

am·pho·ter·i·cin B \\am-fə-'ter-ə-sən-\ *n* : an antifungal antibiotic obtained from a soil actinomycete (*Streptomyces nodosus*) and used esp. to treat systemic fungal infections

am·pi·cil·lin \\am-pə-'si-lən\ *n* : a penicillin $C_{16}H_{19}N_3O_4S$ that is effective against gram-negative and gram-positive bacteria and is used to treat infections of the urinary, respiratory, and intestinal tracts — see PENBRITIN

am·pli·fi·ca·tion \\am-plə-fə-'kā-shən\ *n* 1 : an act, example, or product of amplifying 2 : a usu. massive replication of genetic material and esp. of a gene or DNA sequence (as in a polymerase chain reaction)

am·pli·fy \'am-plə-ˌfī\ *vb* **-fied; -fy·ing** 1 : to make larger or greater (as in amount or intensity) 2 : to cause (a gene or DNA sequence) to undergo amplification

am·pule *or* **am·poule** *also* **am·pul** \'am-ˌpyül, -ˌpül\ *n* 1 : a hermetically sealed small bulbous glass vessel that is used to hold a solution for esp. hypodermic injection 2 : a vial resembling an ampule

am·pul·la \am-'pu̇-lə, 'am-ˌpyü-lə\ *n, pl* **-lae** \-ˌlē\ : a saccular anatomic swelling or pouch: as **a** : the dilatation containing a patch of sensory epithelium at one end of each semicircular canal of the ear **b** : one of the dilatations of the milk-carrying tubules of the mammary glands that serve as reservoirs for milk **c** (1) : the middle portion of the fallopian tube (2) : the distal dilatation of a vas deferens near the opening of the duct leading from the seminal vesicle **d** : a terminal dilatation of the rectum just before it joins the anal canal

ampulla of Va·ter \-'fä-tər\ *n* : a trumpet-mouthed dilatation of the duodenal wall at the opening of the fused pancreatic and common bile ducts — called also *papilla of Vater*

Vater, Abraham (1684–1751), German anatomist.

ampullaris — see CRISTA AMPULLARIS

am·pul·la·ry \am-'pu̇-lə-rē\ *also* **am·pul·lar** \-'pu̇-lər\ *adj* : resembling or relating to an ampulla

am·pu·tate \'am-pyə-ˌtāt\ *vb* **-tat·ed; -tat·ing** : to cut (as a limb) from the body — **am·pu·ta·tion** \\am-pyə-'tā-shən\ *n*

amputation neuroma *n* : NEUROMA 2

am·pu·tee \ˌam-pyə-'tē\ *n* : one that has had a limb amputated

amygdal- *or* **amygdalo-** *comb form* 1 : almond ⟨*amygdalin*⟩ 2 : amygdala ⟨*amygdalectomy*⟩ ⟨*amygdalotomy*⟩

amyg·da·la \ə-'mig-də-lə\ *n, pl* **-lae** \-ˌlē, -ˌlī\ : the one of the four basal ganglia in each cerebral hemisphere that is part of the limbic system and consists of an almond-shaped mass of gray matter in the roof of the lateral ventricle — called also *amygdaloid body, amygdaloid nucleus*

amyg·da·lec·to·my \ə-ˌmig-də-'lek-tə-mē\ *n, pl* **-mies** : surgical removal of the amygdala — **amyg·da·lec·to·mized** \-tə-ˌmīzd\ *adj*

amyg·da·lin \ə-'mig-də-lən\ *n* : a white crystalline cyanogenetic glucoside $C_{20}H_{27}NO_{11}$ found esp. in the seeds of the apricot, peach, and bitter almond

amyg·da·loid \-ˌlȯid\ *adj* 1 : almond-shaped 2 : of, relating to, or affecting an amygdala ⟨~ lesions⟩

amygdaloid body *n* : AMYGDALA

amygdaloid nucleus *n* : AMYGDALA

amyg·da·lot·o·my \ə-ˌmig-də-'lä-tə-mē\ *n, pl* **-mies** : destruction of part of the amygdala (as for the control of epilepsy) esp. by surgical incision

amyl- *or* **amylo-** *comb form* : starch ⟨*amylase*⟩

am·y·lase \'a-mə-ˌlās, -ˌlāz\ *n* : any of a group of enzymes (as amylopsin) that catalyze the hydrolysis of starch and glycogen or their intermediate hydrolysis products

am·yl nitrite \'a-məl-\ *n* : a pale yellow pungent flammable liquid ester $C_5H_{11}NO_2$ that is used chiefly in medicine as a vasodilator esp. in treating angina pectoris and illicitly as an aphrodisiac — called also *isoamyl nitrite;* compare POPPER

am·y·lo·bar·bi·tone \ˌa-mə-lō-'bär-bə-ˌtōn\ *n Brit* : AMOBARBITAL

am·y·loid \'a-mə-ˌlȯid\ *n* : a waxy translucent substance consisting primarily of protein that is deposited in some animal organs and tissue under abnormal conditions (as in Alzheimer's disease) — see BETA-AMYLOID — **amyloid** *adj*

amyloid beta–protein *also* **amyloid β–protein** *n* : BETA-AMYLOID

am·y·loid·osis \ˌa-mə-ˌlȯi-'dō-səs\ *n, pl* **-o·ses** \-ˌsēz\ : a disorder characterized by the deposition of amyloid in organs or tissues of the animal body — see PARAMYLOIDOSIS

amyloid precursor protein *n* : a transmembrane protein from which beta-amyloid is derived by proteolytic cleavage by secretases

am·y·lop·sin \ˌa-mə-'läp-sən\ *n* : the amylase of the pancreatic juice

am·y·lum \'a-mə-ləm\ *n* : STARCH

amyo·to·nia \ˌā-ˌmī-ə-'tō-nē-ə\ *n* : deficiency of muscle tone

amyotonia con·gen·i·ta \-kən-'je-nə-tə\ *n* : a congenital disease of infants characterized by flaccidity of the skeletal muscles

amyo·tro·phia \ˌā-ˌmī-ə-'trō-fē-ə\ *or* **amy·ot·ro·phy** \-ˌmī-'ä-trə-fē\ *n, pl* **-phi·as** *or* **-phies** : atrophy of a muscle — **amyo·tro·phic** \-ˌmī-ə-'trä-fik, -'trō-\ *adj*

amyotrophic lateral sclerosis *n* : a rare fatal progressive degenerative disease that affects pyramidal motor neurons, usu. begins in middle age, and is characterized esp. by increasing and spreading muscular weakness — abbr. *ALS;* called also *Lou Gehrig's disease*

Am·y·tal \'a-mə-ˌtol\ *trademark* — used for a preparation of amobarbital

an- *var of* A-, ANA-

ana \'a-nə\ *adv* : of each an equal quantity — used in prescriptions

ana- *or* **an-** *prefix* : up : upward ⟨*anabolism*⟩

ANA *abbr* **1** American Nurses Association **2** antinuclear antibodies; antinuclear antibody

anabolic steroid *n* : any of a group of usu. synthetic hormones that are derivatives of testosterone, are used medically esp. to promote tissue growth, and are sometimes abused by athletes to increase the size and strength of their muscles and improve endurance

anab·o·lism \ə-'na-bə-ˌli-zəm\ *n* : the constructive part of metabolism concerned esp. with macromolecular synthesis — compare CATABOLISM — **an·a·bol·ic** \ˌa-nə-'bä-lik\ *adj*

an·ac·id·i·ty \ˌa-nə-'si-də-tē\ *n, pl* **-ties** : ACHLORHYDRIA

an·a·clit·ic \ˌa-nə-'kli-tik\ *adj* : of, relating to, or characterized by the direction of love toward an object (as the mother) that satisfies nonsexual needs (as hunger)

anaclitic depression *n* : impaired development of an infant resulting from separation from its mother

anac·ro·tism \ə-'na-krə-ˌti-zəm\ *n* : an abnormality of the blood circulation characterized by a secondary notch in the ascending part of a sphygmographic tracing of the pulse — **an·a·crot·ic** \ˌa-nə-'krä-tik\ *adj*

anae·mia *chiefly Brit var of* ANEMIA

an·aer·obe \'a-nə-ˌrōb, (ˌ)a-'nar-ˌōb\ *n* : an anaerobic organism

an·aer·o·bic \ˌa-nə-'rō-bik, ˌa-ˌnar-'ō-\ *adj* **1 a** : living, active, or occurring in the absence of free oxygen ⟨∼ respiration⟩ **b** : of, relating to, or being activity in which the body incurs an oxygen debt ⟨an ∼ workout⟩ **2** : relating to or induced by anaerobes — **an·aer·o·bi·cal·ly** \-bi-k(ə-)lē\ *adv*

an·aes·the·sia, an·aes·the·si·ol·o·gist, an·aes·the·si·ol·o·gy, an·aes·the·tic, an·aes·the·tist, an·aes·the·tize *chiefly Brit var of* ANESTHESIA, ANESTHESIOLOGIST, ANESTHESIOLOGY, ANESTHETIC, ANESTHETIST, ANESTHETIZE

an·a·gen \'a-nə-ˌjen\ *n* : the active phase of the hair growth cycle preceding telogen

anag·re·lide \ə-'nag-rə-ˌlīd\ *n* : a phosphodiesterase inhibitor administered esp. in the form of its hydrochloride $C_{10}H_7Cl_2N_3O\cdot HCl$ to treat thrombocytosis — see AGRYLIN

anal \'ān-əl\ *adj* **1** : of, relating to, or situated near the anus **2 a** : of, relating to, or characterized by the stage of psychosexual development in psychoanalytic theory during which the child is concerned esp. with its feces **b** : of, relating to, or characterized by personality traits (as parsimony, meticulousness, and ill humor) considered typical of fixation at the anal stage of development — compare GENITAL 3, ORAL 2, PHALLIC 2 — **anal·ly** *adv*

anal *abbr* **1** analysis **2** analytic **3** analyze

anal canal *n* : the terminal section of the rectum

¹an·a·lep·tic \ˌa-nə-'lep-tik\ *adj* : of, relating to, or acting as an analeptic

²analeptic *n* : a restorative agent; *esp* : a drug that acts as a stimulant on the central nervous system

anal eroticism *n* : the experiencing of pleasurable sensations or sexual excitement associated with or symbolic of stimulation of the anus — called also *anal erotism* — **anal erotic** *adj*

an·al·ge·sia \ˌan-əl-'jēzhə, -zhē-ə, -zē-\ *n* : insensibility to pain without loss of consciousness

¹an·al·ge·sic \-'jē-zik, -sik\ *adj* : relating to, characterized by, or producing analgesia

²analgesic *n* : an agent for producing analgesia

an·al·get·ic \-'je-tik\ *n or adj* : ANALGESIC

anal·i·ty \ā-'na-lə-tē\ *n, pl* **-ties** : an anal psychological state, stage, or quality

anal·o·gous \ə-'na-lə-gəs\ *adj* : having similar function but a different structure and origin ⟨∼ organs⟩

an·a·logue *or* **an·a·log** \'an-əl-ˌȯg, -ˌäg\ *n* **1** : an organ similar in function to an organ of another animal or plant but different in structure and origin **2** *usu* **analog** : a chemical compound that is structurally similar to another but differs slightly in composition (as in the replacement of one atom by an atom of a different element or in the presence of a particular functional group)

anal·o·gy \ə-'na-lə-jē\ *n, pl* **-gies** : functional similarity between anatomical parts without similarity of structure and origin — compare HOMOLOGY 1

anal–re·ten·tive \ˈān-ᵊl-ri-ˈten-tiv\ *adj* : exhibiting or typifying personality traits (as frugality and obstinacy) held to be psychological consequences of toilet training — compare ANAL 2b — **anal retentive** *n* — **anal retentiveness** *n*

anal sadism *n* : the cluster of personality traits (as aggressiveness, negativism, destructiveness, and outwardly directed rage) typical of the anal stage of development — **anal–sa·dis·tic** \ˌān-ᵊl-sə-ˈdis-tik\ *adj*

anal sphincter *n* : either of two sphincters controlling the closing of the anus: **a** : an outer sphincter of striated muscle surrounding the anus immediately beneath the skin — called also *external anal sphincter, sphincter ani externus* **b** : an inner sphincter formed by thickening of the circular smooth muscle of the rectum — called also *internal anal sphincter, sphincter ani internus*

anal verge \-ˈvərj\ *n* : the distal margin of the anal canal comprising the muscular rim of the anus

anal·y·sand \ə-ˈna-lə-ˌsand\ *n* : one who is undergoing psychoanalysis

an·a·lyse *Brit var of* ANALYZE

anal·y·sis \ə-ˈna-lə-səs\ *n, pl* **-y·ses** \-ˌsēz\ **1** : separation of a whole into its component parts **2 a** : the identification or separation of ingredients of a substance **b** : a statement of the constituents of a mixture **3** : PSYCHOANALYSIS

an·a·lyst \ˈan-ᵊl-ist\ *n* : PSYCHOANALYST

an·a·lyt·i·cal \ˌan-ᵊl-ˈi-tik\ *or* **an·a·lyt·i·cal** \-ti-kəl\ *adj* **1** : of or relating to analysis; *esp* : separating something into component parts or constituent elements **2** : PSYCHOANALYTIC — **an·a·lyt·i·cal·ly** \-ti-k(ə-)lē\ *adv*

analytic psychology *n* : a modification of psychoanalysis due to C. G. Jung that adds to the concept of the personal unconscious a racial or collective unconscious and advocates that psychotherapy be conducted in terms of the patient's present-day conflicts and maladjustments

an·a·lyze \ˈan-ᵊl-ˌīz\ *vb* **-lyzed; -lyz·ing 1** : to study or determine the nature and relationship of the parts of by analysis; *esp* : to examine by chemical analysis **2** : PSYCHOANALYZE

an·am·ne·sis \ˌa-ˌnam-ˈnē-səs\ *n, pl* **-ne·ses** \-ˌsēz\ **1** : a recalling to mind **2** : a preliminary case history of a medical or psychiatric patient

an·am·nes·tic \-ˈnes-tik\ *adj* **1** : of or relating to anamnesis **2** : of or relating to a secondary response to an immunogenic substance after serum antibodies can no longer be detected in the blood

ana·phase \ˈa-nə-ˌfāz\ *n* : the stage of mitosis and meiosis in which the chromosomes move toward the poles of the spindle — **ana·pha·sic** \ˌa-nə-ˈfā-zik\ *adj*

an·aph·ro·dis·i·ac \-ˈdē-zē-ˌak, -ˈdi-\ *adj* : of, relating to, or causing absence or impairment of sexual desire — **anaphrodisiac** *n*

ana·phy·lac·tic \ˌa-nə-fə-ˈlak-tik\ *adj* : of, relating to, affected by, or causing anaphylaxis or anaphylactic shock — **ana·phy·lac·ti·cal·ly** \-ti-k(ə-)lē\ *adv*

anaphylactic shock *n* : an often severe and sometimes fatal systemic reaction in a susceptible individual upon a second exposure to a specific antigen (as wasp venom or penicillin) after previous sensitization that is characterized esp. by respiratory symptoms, fainting, itching, and hives

ana·phy·lac·toid \ˌa-nə-fə-ˈlak-ˌtoid\ *adj* : resembling anaphylaxis or anaphylactic shock

ana·phy·lax·is \ˌa-nə-fə-ˈlak-səs\ *n, pl* **-lax·es** \-ˌsēz\ **1** : hypersensitivity (as to foreign proteins or drugs) resulting from sensitization following prior contact with the causative agent **2** : ANAPHYLACTIC SHOCK

an·a·pla·sia \ˌa-nə-ˈplā-zhē-ə, -zē-\ *n* : reversion of cells to a more primitive or undifferentiated form

an·a·plas·ma \ˌa-nə-ˈplaz-mə\ *n* **1** *cap* : a genus of bacteria (family Anaplasmataceae) that are found in the red blood cells of ruminants, are transmitted by biting arthropods, and cause anaplasmosis **2** *pl* **-ma·ta** \-mə-tə\ *or* **-mas** : any bacterium of the genus *Anaplasma*

an·a·plas·mo·sis \ˌ-ˌplaz-ˈmō-səs\ *n, pl* **-mo·ses** \-ˌsēz\ : a tick-borne disease of cattle, sheep, and deer caused by a bacterium of the genus *Anaplasma* (*A. marginale*) and characterized esp. by anemia and by jaundice

an·a·plas·tic \ˌa-nə-ˈplas-tik\ *adj* : characterized by, composed of, or being cells which have reverted to a relatively undifferentiated state

an·a·plas·tol·o·gy \ˌ-ˌplas-ˈtä-lə-jē\ *n, pl* **-gies** : a branch of medical technology concerned with the preparation and fitting of prosthetic devices (as artificial eyes and surgical implants) to individual specifications and with the study of the materials from which they are fabricated — **an·a·plas·tol·o·gist** \-jist\ *n*

an·ar·thria \a-ˈnär-thrē-ə\ *n* : inability to articulate remembered words as a result of a brain lesion — compare APHASIA

an·a·sar·ca \ˌa-nə-ˈsär-kə\ *n* : generalized edema with accumulation of serum in the connective tissue

an·a·stal·sis \ˌa-nə-ˈstȯl-səs, -ˈstäl-, -ˈstal-\ *n, pl* **-stal·ses** \-ˌsēz\ : ANTIPERISTALSIS

anas·to·mose \ə-ˈnas-tə-ˌmōz, -ˌmōs\ *vb* **-mosed; -mos·ing** : to connect, join, or communicate by anastomosis

anas·to·mo·sis \ə-ˌnas-tə-'mō-səs, ˌa-nəs-\ *n, pl* **-mo·ses** \-ˌsēz\ **1 a** : a communication between or coalescence of blood vessels **b** : the surgical union of parts and esp. hollow tubular parts **2** : a product of anastomosis; *esp* : a network (as of channels or branches) produced by anastomosis — **anas·to·mot·ic** \-'mä-tik\ *adj*

anas·tro·zole \ə-'nas-trə-ˌzōl\ *n* : a nonsteroidal aromatase inhibitor $C_{17}H_{19}N_5$ that is administered orally to treat breast cancer in postmenopausal women — see ARIMIDEX

anat *abbr* anatomic; anatomical; anatomy

an·a·tom·ic \ˌa-nə-'tä-mik\ *or* **an·a·tom·i·cal** \-mi-kəl\ *adj* **1** : of or relating to anatomy **2** : STRUCTURAL 1 ⟨an ∼ obstruction⟩ — **an·a·tom·i·cal·ly** \-mi-k(ə-)lē\ *adv*

Anatomica — see BASLE NOMINA ANATOMICA, NOMINA ANATOMICA

anatomical dead space *n* : the dead space in that portion of the respiratory system which is external to the alveoli and includes the air-conveying ducts from the nostrils to the terminal bronchioles — compare PHYSIOLOGICAL DEAD SPACE

anatomical position *n* : the normal position of the human body when active

anat·o·mist \ə-'na-tə-mist\ *n* : a specialist in anatomy

anat·o·my \ə-'na-tə-mē\ *n, pl* **-mies** **1** : a branch of morphology that deals with the structure of organisms — compare PHYSIOLOGY 1 **2** : a treatise on anatomic science or art **3** : the art of separating the parts of an organism in order to ascertain their position, relations, structure, and function : DISSECTION **4** : structural makeup esp. of an organism or any of its parts

ana·tox·in \ˌa-nə-'täk-sən\ *n* : TOXOID

anchyl- *or* **anchylo-** — see ANKYL-

anchylose, anchylosis *var of* ANKYLOSE, ANKYLOSIS

an·cil·lary \'an-sə-ˌler-ē\ *adj* : being auxiliary or supplementary

an·co·ne·us \aŋ-'kō-nē-əs\ *n, pl* **-nei** \-nē-ˌī\ : a small triangular extensor muscle that is superficially situated behind and below the elbow joint and that extends the forearm — called also *anconeus muscle*

An·cy·los·to·ma \ˌaŋ-ki-'läs-tə-mə, ˌan-sə-\ *n* : a genus of hookworms (family Ancylostomatidae) that are intestinal parasites of mammals — compare NECATOR

an·cy·lo·stome \aŋ-'ki-lə-ˌstōm, -'si-\ *or* **an·kyl·o·stome** \'ki-\ *n* : any of the genus *Ancylostoma* of hookworms

an·cy·lo·sto·mi·a·sis \ˌaŋ-ki-lō-stə-'mī-ə-səs, ˌan-sə-\ *or* **an·kyl·o·sto·mi·a·sis** \-ki-lō-\ *n, pl* **-a·ses** \-ˌsēz\ : infestation with or disease caused by hookworms; *esp* : a lethargic anemic state due to blood loss through the feeding of hookworms in the small in-

testine — called also *hookworm disease*

andr- *or* **andro-** *comb form* **1** : male ⟨*androgen*⟩ **2** : male and ⟨*androgynous*⟩

an·dro \an-drō\ *n* : ANDROSTENEDIONE

an·dro·gen \an-drə-jən\ *n* : a male sex hormone (as testosterone) — **an·dro·gen·ic** \ˌan-drə-'je-nik\ *adj*

androgenetic alopecia \ˌan-drə-jə-'net-ik-\ *n* : hereditary androgen-dependent hair loss typically characterized by moderate to severe hair loss on the temples and crown in men and diffuse thinning on the crown in women — see MALE-PATTERN BALDNESS

androgen insensitivity syndrome *n* : TESTICULAR FEMINIZATION

an·dro·gen·ize \an-'drä-jə-ˌnīz\ *vb* **-nized; -niz·ing** : to treat or influence with male sex hormone esp. in excessive amounts

an·drog·y·nous \an-'drä-jə-nəs\ *adj* : having the characteristics or nature of both male and female — **an·drog·y·ny** \-nē\ *n*

an·droid \'an-ˌdroid\ *adj* **1** *of the pelvis* : having the angular form and narrow outlet typical of the human male — compare ANTHROPOID, GYNECOID, PLATYPELLOID **2** : relating to or characterized by the distribution of body fat chiefly in the abdominal region ⟨∼ obesity⟩ — compare GYNECOID

an·drol·o·gist \an-'dräl-ə-jəst\ *n* : a specialist in andrology

an·drol·o·gy \an-'dräl-ə-jē\ *n, pl* **-gies** : a branch of medicine concerned with male diseases and esp. with those affecting the reproductive system

an·drom·e·do·tox·in \an-ˌdrä-mə-dō-'täk-sən\ *n* : a toxic compound $C_{31}H_{50}O_{10}$ found in various plants of the heath family (Ericaceae)

an·dro·pause \'an-drə-ˌpöz\ *n* : a gradual and highly variable decline in the production of androgenic hormones and esp. testosterone in the human male together with its associated effects that is held to occur during and after middle age but is often difficult to discriminate from the effects of confounding factors (as chronic illness or stress) that can depress testosterone levels — called also *male climacteric, male menopause, viropause*

an·dro·stene·di·one \ˌan-drə-ˌstēn-'dī-ˌōn, -'stēn-dē-ˌōn\ *n* : a steroid sex hormone $C_{19}H_{26}O_2$ that is secreted by the testis, ovary, and adrenal cortex and is a precursor of testosterone and estrogen

an·dros·ter·one \an-'dräs-tə-ˌrōn\ *n* : an androgenic hormone that is a hydroxy ketone $C_{19}H_{30}O_2$ found in human urine

Anec·tine \ə-'nek-tən\ *trademark* — used for a preparation of succinylcholine

ane·mia \ə-'nē-mē-ə\ *n* **1** : a condition in which the blood is deficient in red blood cells, in hemoglobin, or in total volume — see APLASTIC ANEMIA, HYPERCHROMIC ANEMIA, HYPOCHROMIC ANEMIA, MEGALOBLASTIC ANEMIA, MICROCYTIC ANEMIA, PERNICIOUS ANEMIA, SICKLE-CELL ANEMIA **2** : ISCHEMIA — **ane·mic** \ə-'nē-mik\ *adj* — **ane·mi·cal·ly** \-mi-k(ə-)lē\ *adv*

an·en·ceph·a·lus \ˌan-(ˌ)en-'se-fə-ləs\ *n, pl* **-li** \-ˌlī\ : ANENCEPHALY

an·en·ceph·a·ly \ˌan-(ˌ)en-'se-fə-lē\ *n, pl* **-lies** : congenital absence of all or a major part of the brain — **an·en·ce·phal·ic** \-ˌen-sə-'fa-lik\ *adj or n*

aneph·ric \(ˌ)ā-'ne-frik, (ˌ)ā-\ *adj* : being without functioning kidneys

an·er·gy \'a-(ˌ)nər-jē\ *n, pl* **-gies** : a condition in which the body fails to react to an antigen and esp. one injected under the skin (as in a skin test) — **an·er·gic** \-jik\ *adj*

an·es·the·sia \ˌa-nəs-'thē-zhə\ *n* **1** : loss of sensation esp. to touch usu. resulting from a lesion in the nervous system or from some other abnormality **2** : loss of sensation and usu. of consciousness without loss of vital functions artificially produced by the administration of one or more agents that block the passage of pain impulses along nerve pathways to the brain

an·es·the·si·ol·o·gist \ˌa-nəs-ˌthē-zē-'ä-lə-jist\ *n* : ANESTHETIST; *specif* : a physician specializing in anesthesiology

an·es·the·si·ol·o·gy \-jē\ *n, pl* **-gies** : a branch of medical science dealing with anesthesia and anesthetics

¹an·es·thet·ic \ˌa-nəs-'the-tik\ *adj* **1** : capable of producing anesthesia ⟨~ agents⟩ **2** : of, relating to, or caused by anesthesia ⟨an ~ effect⟩ — **an·es·thet·i·cal·ly** \-ti-k(ə-)lē\ *adv*

²anesthetic *n* : a substance that produces anesthesia

anes·the·tist \ə-'nes-thə-tist\ *n* : one who administers anesthetics — compare ANESTHESIOLOGIST

anes·the·tize \-ˌtīz\ *vb* **-tized; -tiz·ing** : to subject to anesthesia — **anes·the·ti·za·tion** \-ˌnes-thə-tə-'zā-shən\ *n*

an·es·trous \(ˌ)a-'nes-trəs\ *adj* **1** : not exhibiting estrus **2** : of or relating to anestrus

an·es·trus \-trəs\ *n* : the period of sexual quiescence between two periods of sexual activity in cyclically breeding mammals — compare ESTRUS

an·eu·ploid \'an-yù-ˌploid\ *adj* : having or being a chromosome number that is not an exact multiple of the usu. haploid number — **aneuploid** *n* — **an·eu·ploi·dy** \-ˌploi-dē\ *n*

an·eu·rine \'an-yə-ˌrēn, (ˌ)ā-'nyùr-ˌēn\ *n* : THIAMINE

an·eu·rysm *also* **an·eu·rism** \'an-yə-ˌri-zəm\ *n* : an abnormal blood-filled dilatation of a blood vessel and esp. an artery resulting from disease of the vessel wall — **an·eu·rys·mal** *also* **an·eu·ris·mal** \ˌan-yə-'riz-məl\ *adj* — **an·eu·rys·mal·ly** *adv*

ANF *abbr* atrial naturetic factor

angel dust *n* : PHENCYCLIDINE

An·gel·man syndrome \'aŋ-jəl-mən-\ *also* **An·gel·man's syndrome** \-mənz-\ *n* : a genetic disorder characterized by severe mental retardation, seizures, ataxic gait, jerky movements, lack of speech, microcephaly, and frequent smiling and laughter

Angelman, Harry (1915–1996), British pediatrician.

angi- *or* **angio-** *comb form* **1** : blood or lymph vessel ⟨*angioma*⟩ ⟨*angiogenesis*⟩ **2** : blood vessels and ⟨*angiocardiography*⟩

-angia *pl of* -ANGIUM

an·gi·itis \ˌan-jē-'ī-təs\ *n, pl* **-it·i·des** \-'i-tə-ˌdēz\ : VASCULITIS

an·gi·na \an-'jī-nə, 'an-jə-\ *n* : a disease marked by spasmodic attacks of intense suffocative pain: as **a** : a severe inflammatory or ulcerated condition of the mouth or throat ⟨diphtheritic ~⟩ — see LUDWIG'S ANGINA, VINCENT'S ANGINA **b** : ANGINA PECTORIS — **an·gi·nal** \an-'jīn-ᵊl, 'an-jən-\ *adj*

angina pec·to·ris \-'pek-tə-rəs\ *n* : a disease marked by brief paroxysmal attacks of chest pain precipitated by deficient oxygenation of the heart muscles — see UNSTABLE ANGINA; compare CORONARY INSUFFICIENCY, HEART ATTACK, HEART FAILURE 1

an·gi·nose \'an-jə-ˌnōs, an-'jī-\ *or* **gi·nous** \(ˌ)an-'jī-nəs, 'an-jə-\ *adj* : relating to angina or angina pectoris

an·gio·car·dio·gram \ˌan-jē-ō-'kär-dē-ə-ˌgram\ *n* : a radiograph of the heart and its blood vessels prepared by angiocardiography

an·gio·car·di·og·ra·phy \-ˌkär-dē-'ä-grə-fē\ *n, pl* **-phies** : the radiographic visualization of the heart and its blood vessels after injection of a radiopaque substance — **an·gio·car·dio·graph·ic** \-dē-ə-'gra-fik\ *adj*

an·gio·ede·ma \ˌan-jē-ō-i-'dē-mə\ *n, pl* **-mas** *also* **-ma·ta** \-mə-tə\ : an allergic skin disease characterized by patches of circumscribed swelling involving the skin and its subcutaneous layers, the mucous membranes, and sometimes the viscera — called also *angioneurotic edema, giant urticaria, Quincke's disease, Quincke's edema*

an·gio·gen·e·sis \ˌan-jə-ō-sas\ *n, pl* **-e·ses** \-ˌsēz\ : the formation and differentiation of blood vessels

an·gio·gram \'an-jē-ə-ˌgram\ *n* **1** : a radiograph made by angiography **2** : ANGIOGRAPHY

an·gi·og·ra·phy \ˌan-jē-'ä-grə-fē\ *n, pl* **-phies** : the radiographic visualization of the blood vessels after injection of a radiopaque substance — **an·gi·og·ra·pher** \-fər\ *n* — **an·gio·graph·ic** \ˌan-jē-ə-'gra-fik\ *adj* — **an·gio·graph·i·cal·ly** \-fi-k(ə-)lē\ *adv*

an·gio·im·mu·no·blas·tic T–cell lym·phoma \,an-jē-ō-,im-yə-nō-'blas-tik-, -im-,yü-nō-\ *n* : an often fatal non-Hodgkin's lymphoma that involves T cells and is characterized esp. by generalized lymphadenopathy, fever, weight loss, and night sweats — called also *angioimmunoblastic lymphadenopathy, angioimmunoblastic lymphadenopathy with dysproteinemia, immunoblastic lymphadenopathy*

an·gio·ker·a·to·ma \,an-jē-ō-,ker-ə-'tō-mə\ *n, pl* **-mas** *also* **-ma·ta** \-mə-tə\ : a skin disease characterized by small warty elevations or telangiectasias and epidermal thickening

an·gi·ol·o·gy \,an-jē-'ä-lə-jē\ *n, pl* **-gies** : the study of blood vessels and lymphatics

an·gi·o·ma \,an-jē-'ō-mə\ *n, pl* **-mas** *also* **-ma·ta** \-mə-tə\ : a tumor (as a hemangioma) composed chiefly of blood vessels or lymphatic vessels — **an·gi·o·ma·tous** \-mə-təs\ *adj*

an·gi·o·ma·to·sis \,an-jē-(,)ō-mə-'tō-səs\ *n, pl* **-to·ses** \-,sēz\ : a condition characterized by the formation of multiple angiomas

an·gio·neu·rot·ic edema \-nù-,rä-tik, -nyü-\ *n* : ANGIOEDEMA

an·gi·op·a·thy \,an-jē-'ä-pə-thē\ *n, pl* **-thies** : a disease of the blood or lymph vessels

an·gio·plas·ty \'an-jē-ə-,plas-tē\ *n, pl* **-ties** : surgical repair or recanalization of a blood vessel; *esp* : BALLOON ANGIOPLASTY

an·gio·sar·co·ma \,an-jē-ō-sär-'kō-mə\ *n, pl* **-mas** *also* **-ma·ta** \-mə-tə\ : a rare malignant vascular tumor (as of the liver or breast)

an·gio·spasm \'an-jē-ō-,spa-zəm\ *n* : spasmodic contraction of the blood vessels with increase in blood pressure — **an·gio·spas·tic** \,an-jē-ō-'spas-tik\ *adj*

an·gio·ten·sin \,an-jē-ō-'ten-sən\ *n* **1** : either of two forms of a kinin of which one has marked physiological activity and the other is its physiologically inactive precursor; *esp* : ANGIOTENSIN II **2** : a synthetic amide derivative of angiotensin II used to treat some forms of hypotension

an·gio·ten·sin·ase \,an-jē-ō-'ten-sə-,nās, -,nāz\ *n* : any of several enzymes in the blood that hydrolyze angiotensin — called also *hypertensinase*

angiotensin converting enzyme *n* : a proteolytic enzyme that converts angiotensin I to angiotensin II — see ACE INHIBITOR

angiotensin converting enzyme inhibitor *n* : ACE INHIBITOR

an·gio·ten·sin·o·gen \-ten-'si-nə-jən\ *n* : a serum globulin formed by the liver that is cleaved by renin to produce angiotensin I — called also *hypertensinogen*

angiotensin I \-'wən\ *n* : the physiologically inactive form of angiotensin that is composed of 10 amino-acid residues and is a precursor of angiotensin II

angiotensin II \-'tü\ *n* : a protein with vasoconstrictive activity that is composed of eight amino-acid residues and is the physiologically active form of angiotensin

an·gio·to·nin \-'tō-nən\ *n* : ANGIOTENSIN

-angium *n comb form, pl* **-angia** : vessel : receptacle ⟨mes*angium*⟩

an·gle \'aŋ-gəl\ *n* **1** : a corner whether constituting a projecting spur or a partially enclosed space **2** : the figure formed by two lines extending from the same point

an·gle·ber·ry \'aŋ-gəl-,ber-ē\ *n, pl* **-ries** : a papilloma or warty growth of the skin or mucous membranes of cattle and sometimes horses often occurring in great numbers

angle–closure glaucoma *n* : glaucoma in which the drainage channel for the aqueous humor is blocked by the iris — called also *closed-angle glaucoma, narrow-angle glaucoma*; compare OPEN-ANGLE GLAUCOMA

angle of the jaw *n* : GONIAL ANGLE

angle of the mandible *n* : GONIAL ANGLE

ang·strom \'aŋ-strəm\ *n* : a unit of length equal to one ten-billionth of a meter

Ång·ström, Anders Jonas (1814–1874), Swedish astronomer and physicist.

angstrom unit *n* : ANGSTROM

an·gu·lar \'aŋ-gyə-lər\ *adj* **1 a** : having an angle or angles **b** : forming an angle or corner : sharp-cornered **2** : relating to or situated near an anatomical angle; *specif* : relating to or situated near the inner angle of the eye — **an·gu·lar·i·ty** \,aŋ-gyü-'lar-ə-tē\ *n* — **an·gu·lar·ly** *adv*

angular artery *n* : the terminal part of the facial artery that passes up alongside the nose to the inner angle of the orbit

angular gyrus *n* : the cerebral gyrus of the posterior part of the external surface of the parietal lobe that arches over the posterior end of the sulcus between the superior and middle gyri of the temporal lobe — called also *angular convolution*

angularis — see INCISURA ANGULARIS

angular vein *n* : a vein that comprises the first part of the facial vein and runs obliquely down at the side of the upper part of the nose

an·gu·la·tion \,aŋ-gyə-'lā-shən\ *n* : an angular position, formation or shape; *esp* : an abnormal bend or curve in an organ — **an·gu·late** \'aŋ-gyə-,lāt\ *vb*

anguli — see LEVATOR ANGULI ORIS

an·gu·lus \'aŋ-gyə-ləs\ *n, pl* **an·gu·li** \-,lī, -,lē\ : an anatomical angle; *also* : an angular part or relationship

an·he·do·nia \,an-hē-'dō-nē-ə\ *n* : a psychological condition characterized by inability to experience pleasure in acts which normally produce it — compare ANALGESIA — **an·he·don·ic** \-'dä-nik\ *adj*

an·hi·dro·sis *also* **an·hy·dro·sis** \,an-hi-'drō-səs, -hī-\ *n, pl* **-dro·ses** \-,sēz\ : abnormal deficiency or absence of sweating

¹an·hi·drot·ic *also* **an·hy·drot·ic** \-'drä-tik\ *adj* : tending to check sweating

²anhidrotic *also* **anhydrotic** *n* : an anhidrotic agent

anhydr- *or* **anhydro-** *comb form* : lacking water ⟨anhyd*rem*ia⟩

an·hy·drase \an-'hī-,drās, -,drāz\ *n* : an enzyme (as carbonic anhydrase) promoting a specific dehydration reaction and the reverse hydration reaction

an·hy·dre·mia \,an-(,)hī-'drē-mē-ə\ *n* : an abnormal reduction of water in the blood

an·hy·dride \(,)an-'hī-,drīd\ *n* : a compound derived from another by removal of the elements of water

an·hy·dro·hy·droxy·pro·ges·ter·one \an-,hī-drō-,hī-,dräk-sē-prō-'jes-tə-,rōn\ *n* : ETHISTERONE

an·hy·drous \(,)an-'hī-drəs\ *adj* : free from water and esp. water that is chemically combined in a crystalline substance ⟨∼ ammonia⟩

ani *pl of* ANUS

ani — see LEVATOR ANI, PRURITUS ANI

an·ic·ter·ic \,a-(,)nik-'ter-ik\ *adj* : not accompanied or characterized by jaundice ⟨∼ hepatitis⟩

an·i·line \'an-ᵊl-ən\ *n* : an oily liquid poisonous amine $C_6H_5NH_2$ used chiefly in organic synthesis (as of dyes and pharmaceuticals) — **aniline** *adj*

ani·lin·gus \,ā-ni-'lin̄-gəs\ *or* **anil·inc·tus** \-'lin̄k-təs\ *n* : erotic stimulation achieved by contact between mouth and anus

an·i·ma \'a-nə-mə\ *n* : an individual's true inner self that in the analytic psychology of C. G. Jung reflects archetypal ideals of conduct; *also* : an inner feminine part of the male personality — compare ANIMUS, PERSONA

animal heat *n* : BODY HEAT

animal model *n* : an animal similar to humans (as in its physiology) that is used in medical research to obtain results that can be extrapolated to human medicine; *also* : a pathological or physiological condition that occurs in such an animal and is similar to one occurring in humans

animal starch *n* : GLYCOGEN

an·i·mate \'a-nə-mət\ *adj* **1** : possessing or characterized by life **2** : of or relating to animal life as opposed to plant life

an·i·mus \'a-nə-məs\ *n* : an inner masculine part of the female personality in the analytic psychology of C. G. Jung — compare ANIMA

an·ion \'a-,nī-ən\ *n* : the ion in an electrolyzed solution that migrates to the anode; *broadly* : a negatively charged

ion — **an·ion·ic** \,a-(,)nī-'ä-nik\ — **an·ion·i·cal·ly** \-ni-k(ə-)lē\ *adv*

an·irid·ia \,a-,nī-'ri-dē-ə\ *n* : congenital or traumatically induced absence or defect of the iris

anis- *or* **aniso-** *comb form* : unequal ⟨aniseikonia⟩ ⟨anisocytosis⟩

an·i·sa·ki·a·sis \,a-nə-sə-'kī-ə-sis\ *n* : intestinal infection caused by the larvae of a nematode (esp. *Anisakis marina*) and usu. contracted by eating raw fish (as in sushi)

an·is·ei·ko·nia \,a-,nī-,sī-'kō-nē-ə\ *n* : a defect of binocular vision in which the two retinal images of an object differ in size — **an·is·ei·kon·ic** \-'kä-nik\ *adj*

an·iso·co·ria \,a-,nī-sō-'kōr-ē-ə\ *n* : inequality in the size of the pupils of the eyes

an·iso·cy·to·sis \-,sī-'tō-səs\ *n, pl* **-to·ses** \-,sēz\ : variation in size of cells and esp. of the red blood cells (as in pernicious anemia) — **an·iso·cy·tot·ic** \-'tä-tik\ *adj*

an·iso·me·tro·pia \,a-,nī-sə-mə-'trō-pē-ə\ *n* : unequal refractive power in the two eyes — **an·iso·me·tro·pic** \-'trä-pik, -'trō-\ *adj*

an·i·strep·lase \,a-ni-'strep-lās\ *n* : a thrombolytic complex of plasminogen and streptokinase that has been used esp. to treat heart attack — called also APSAC

an·kle \'an̄-kəl\ *n* **1** : the joint between the foot and the leg that constitutes in humans a ginglymus joint between the tibia and fibula above and the talus below — called also *ankle joint* **2** : the region of the ankle joint

an·kle·bone \-,bōn\ *n* : TALUS 1

ankle jerk *n* : a reflex downward movement of the foot produced by a spasmodic contraction of the muscles of the calf in response to sudden extension of the leg or the striking of the Achilles tendon above the heel — called also *Achilles reflex*

ankle joint *n* : ANKLE 1

ankyl- *or* **ankylo-** *also* **anchyl-** *or* **anchylo-** *comb form* : stiffness : immobility ⟨ankylosis⟩

an·ky·lose *also* **an·chy·lose** \'an̄-ki-,lōs, -,lōz\ *vb* **-losed; -los·ing** **1** : to unite or stiffen by ankylosis **2** : to undergo ankylosis

ankylosing spondylitis *n* : rheumatoid arthritis of the spine — called also *Marie-Strümpell disease, rheumatoid spondylitis*

an·ky·lo·sis *also* **an·chy·lo·sis** \,an̄-ki-'lō-səs\ *n, pl* **-lo·ses** \-,sēz\ : stiffness or fixation of a joint by disease or surgery — **an·ky·lot·ic** *also* **an·chy·lot·ic** \-'lä-tik\ *adj*

ankylostome, ankylostomiasis *var of* ANCYLOSTOME, ANCYLOSTOMIASIS

an·la·ge \'än-,lä-gə\ *n, pl* **-gen** \-gən\ *also* **-ges** \-əz\ : the foundation of a subsequent development; *esp* : PRIMORDIUM

an·neal \ə-'nēl\ *vb* **1** : to heat and then cool (double-stranded nucleic acid) in order to separate strands and induce combination at lower temperatures esp. with complementary strands **2** : to be capable of combining with complementary nucleic acid by a process of heating and cooling

an·ne·lid \'an-ᵊl-əd\ *n* : any of a phylum (Annelida) of usu. elongated segmented invertebrates (as earthworms and leeches) — **annelid** *adj*

an·nu·lar \'an-yə-lər\ *adj* : of, relating to, or forming a ring

annulare — see GRANULOMA ANNULARE

annular ligament *n* : a ringlike ligament or band of fibrous tissue encircling a part: as **a** : a strong band of fibers surrounding the head of the radius and retaining it in the radial notch of the ulna **b** : a ring attaching the base of the stapes to the oval window

an·nu·lus *also* **an·u·lus** \'an-yə-ləs\ *n, pl* **-li** \-ₗlī\ *also* **-lus·es** : a ringlike part, structure, or marking; *esp* : any of various ringlike anatomical parts (as the inguinal ring)

annulus fi·bro·sus \-fī-'brō-səs, -fi-\ *n* : a ring of fibrous or fibrocartilaginous tissue (as of an intervertebral disk)

¹ano- *prefix* : upward ⟨*anoopsia*⟩

²ano- *comb form* **1** : anus ⟨*ano*scope⟩ **2** : anus and ⟨*ano*rectal⟩

ano·ci·as·so·ci·a·tion \ə-ₙnō-sē-ə-ₙsō-sē-'ā-shən, a-, -ₙsō-shē-\ *n* : a method of preventing shock and exhaustion incident to surgical operations by preventing communication between the area of operation and the nervous system esp. by means of a local anesthetic or sharp dissection

an·odon·tia \ₐa-nō-'dän-chə, -chē-ə\ *n* : an esp. congenital absence of teeth

¹an·o·dyne \'a-nə-ₙdīn\ *adj* : serving to ease pain

²anodyne *n* : a drug that allays pain

ano·gen·i·tal \ₐā-nō-'je-nə-tᵊl\ *adj* : of, relating to, or involving the genital organs and the anus ⟨an ∼ infection⟩

anom·a·lo·scope \ə-'nä-mə-lə-ₙskōp\ *n* : an optical device designed to test color vision

anom·a·lous \ə-'nä-mə-ləs\ *adj* : deviating from normal; *specif* : having abnormal vision with respect to a particular color but not color-blind

anom·a·ly \ə-'nä-mə-lē\ *n, pl* **-lies** : a deviation from normal esp. of a bodily part

ano·mia \ə-'nä-mē-ə, -'nō-\ *n* : ANOMIC APHASIA

anom·ic \ə-'nä-mik, ā-, -'nō-\ *adj* : relating to or characterized by anomie

anomic aphasia *n* : loss of the power to use or understand words denoting objects

an·o·mie *also* **an·o·my** \'a-nə-mē\ *n* : personal unrest, alienation, and anxiety that comes from a lack of purpose or ideals

an·onych·ia \ₐa-nə-'ni-kē-ə\ *n* : congenital absence of the nails

ano·op·sia \ₐa-nō-'äp-sē-ə\ *or* **an·op·sia** \ə-'näp-\ *n* : upward strabismus

anoph·e·les \ə-'nä-fə-ₗlēz\ *n* **1** *cap* : a genus of mosquitoes that includes all mosquitoes that transmit malaria to humans **2** : any mosquito of the genus *Anopheles* — **anopheles** *adj* — **anoph·e·line** \-ₗlīn\ *adj or n*

an·oph·thal·mia \ₐa-näf-'thal-mē-ə, -äp-\ *n* : congenital absence of the eyes — **an·oph·thal·mic** \-'thal-mik\ *adj*

an·oph·thal·mos \-'thal-məs\ *n* **1** : ANOPHTHALMIA **2** : an individual born without eyes

an·opia \ə-'nō-pē-ə, a-\ *n* : a defect of vision; *esp* : HEMIANOPIA

ano·plas·ty \'ā-nə-ₙplas-tē, 'a-\ *n, pl* **-ties** : a plastic surgery on the anus (as for stricture)

An·op·lo·ceph·a·la \ₐa-nə-(ₗ)plō-'se-fə-lə\ *n* : a genus of taenioid tapeworms including some parasites of horses

anopsia *var of* ANOOPSIA

an·or·chid·ism \ə-'nȯr-ki-ₙdi-zəm, a-\ *n* : congenital absence of one or both testes

ano·rec·tal \ₐā-nō-'rekt-ᵊl, ₐa-nə-\ *adj* : of, relating to, or involving both the anus and rectum ⟨∼ surgery⟩

¹an·o·rec·tic \ₐa-nə-'rek-tik\ *also* **an·o·ret·ic** \-'re-tik\ *adj* **1 a** : lacking appetite **b** : ANOREXIC **2** : causing loss of appetite ⟨∼ drugs⟩

²anorectic *also* **anoretic** *n* **1** : an anorectic agent **2** : ANOREXIC

an·orex·ia \ₐa-nə-'rek-sē-ə, -'rek-shə\ *n* **1** : loss of appetite esp. when prolonged **2** : ANOREXIA NERVOSA

anorexia ner·vo·sa \-(ₗ)nər-'vō-sə, -zə\ *n* : a serious eating disorder primarily of young women in their teens and early twenties that is characterized esp. by a pathological fear of weight gain leading to faulty eating patterns, malnutrition, and usu. excessive weight loss

¹ano·rex·i·ant \ₐa-nə-'rek-sē-ənt, -'rek-shənt\ *n* : a drug that suppresses appetite

²anorexiant *adj* : ANORECTIC 2

¹ano·rex·ic \-'rek-sik\ *adj* **1** : ANORECTIC 1a, 2 **2** : relating to, characteristic of, or affected with anorexia nervosa

²anorexic *n* : a person affected with anorexia nervosa

ano·rex·i·gen·ic \-ₗrek-sə-'je-nik\ *adj* : ANORECTIC 2

an·or·gas·mia \ₐa-nȯr-'gaz-mē-ə\ *n* : sexual dysfunction characterized by failure to achieve orgasm — **an·or·gas·mic** \-mik\ *adj*

ano·scope \'ā-nə-ₙskōp\ *n* : an instrument for facilitating visual examination of the anal canal

ano·sco·py \ā-'näs-kə-pē, ə-, ₗ\ *n, pl* **-pies** : visual examination of the anal canal with an anoscope — **ano·scop·ic** \ₐā-nə-'skä-pik\ *adj*

an·os·mia \a-'näz-mē-ə\ *n* : loss or impairment of the sense of smell — **an·os·mic** \-mik\ *adj*

ano·vag·i·nal \ˌā-nō-'va-jən-ᵊl\ *adj* : connecting the anal canal and the vagina ⟨a congenital ∼ fistula⟩

an·ovu·la·tion \ˌa-ˌnä-vyə-'lā-shən, -ˌnō-\ *n* : failure or absence of ovulation

an·ovu·la·to·ry \(ˌ)a-'nä-vyə-lə-ˌtōr-ē, -'nō\ *adj* 1 : not involving or associated with ovulation ⟨∼ bleeding⟩ 2 : suppressing ovulation ⟨∼ drugs⟩

an·ox·emia \ˌa-ˌnäk-'sē-mē-ə\ *n* : a condition of subnormal oxygenation of the arterial blood — **an·ox·emic** \-mik\ *adj*

an·ox·ia \ə-'näk-sē-ə, a-\ *n* : hypoxia esp. of such severity as to result in permanent damage — **an·ox·ic** \-sik\ *adj*

ANP *abbr* atrial natriuretic peptide

ANS *abbr* autonomic nervous system

an·sa \'an-sə\ *n, pl* **an·sae** \-ˌsē\ : a loop-shaped anatomical structure

ansa cer·vi·ca·lis \-ˌsər-və-'ka-ləs, -'kä-\ *n* : a nerve loop from the upper cervical nerves that accompanies the hypoglossal nerve and innervates the infrahyoid muscles

ansa hy·po·glos·si \-ˌhī-pə-'glä-ˌsī, -'glō-, -(ˌ)sē\ *n* : ANSA CERVICALIS

An·said \'an-sed\ *trademark* — used for a preparation of flurbiprofen

ansa sub·cla·via \-ˌsəb-'klä-vē-ə\ *n* : a nerve loop of sympathetic fibers passing around the subclavian artery

anserinus — see PES ANSERINUS

ant- — see ANTI-

Ant·a·buse \'an-tə-ˌbyüs\ *trademark* — used for a preparation of disulfiram

¹**ant·ac·id** \(ˌ)ant-'a-səd\ *also* **an·ti·ac·id** \ˌan-tē-'a-səd, -ˌtī-\ *adj* : tending to counteract acidity

²**antacid** *also* **antiacid** *n* : an agent (as an alkali or absorbent) that counteracts or neutralizes acidity

an·tag·o·nism \an-'ta-gə-ˌni-zəm\ *n* : opposition in physiological action: **a** : contrariety in the effect of contraction of muscles **b** : interaction of two or more substances such that the action of any one of them on living cells or tissues is lessened — compare SYNERGISM — **an·tag·o·nize** \an-'ta-gə-ˌnīz\ *vb*

an·tag·o·nist \-nist\ *n* : an agent that acts in physiological opposition: as **a** : a muscle that contracts with and limits the action of an agonist with which it is paired — called also *antagonistic muscle*; compare AGONIST 1, SYNERGIST 2 **b** : a chemical substance that opposes the action on the nervous system of a drug or a substance occurring naturally in the body by combining with and blocking its nervous receptor — compare AGONIST 2

an·tag·o·nis·tic \(ˌ)an-ˌta-gə-'nis-tik\ *adj* 1 : characterized by or resulting

from antagonism 2 : relating to or being muscles that are antagonists — **an·tag·o·nis·ti·cal·ly** \-ti-k(ə-)lē\ *adv*

ante- *prefix* 1 : anterior : forward ⟨*ante*hyophysis⟩ 2 **a** : prior to : earlier than ⟨*ante*partum⟩ **b** : in front of ⟨*ante*brachium⟩

an·te·bra·chi·um *or* **an·ti·bra·chi·um** \ˌan-ti-'brā-kē-əm\ *n, pl* **-chia** \-kē-ə\ : the part of the arm or forelimb between the brachium and the carpus : FOREARM

an·te·cu·bi·tal \ˌan-ti-'kyü-bət-ᵊl\ *adj* : of or relating to the inner or front surface of the forearm

antecubital fossa *n* : a triangular cavity of the elbow joint that contains a tendon of the biceps, the median nerve, and the brachial artery

an·te·flex·ion \ˌan-ti-'flek-shən\ *n* : a displacement forward of an organ (as the uterus) so that its axis is bent upon itself

an·te·grade \'an-ti-ˌgrād\ *adj* : ANTEROGRADE 1

an·te·mor·tem \-'mȯr-təm\ *adj* : preceding death

an·te·na·tal \-'nāt-ᵊl\ *adj* : PRENATAL ⟨∼ diagnosis of birth defects⟩ — **an·te·na·tal·ly** *adv*

an·te·par·tum \-'pär-təm\ *adj* : relating to the period before parturition : before childbirth ⟨∼ care⟩

an·te·ri·or \an-'tir-ē-ər\ *adj* 1 : relating to or situated near or toward the head or toward the part in headless animals most nearly corresponding to the head 2 : situated toward the front of the body : VENTRAL — used in human anatomy because of the upright posture of humans — **an·te·ri·or·ly** *adv*

anterior cerebral artery *n* : CEREBRAL ARTERY a

anterior chamber *n* : a space in the eye bounded in front by the cornea and in back by the iris and middle part of the lens — compare POSTERIOR CHAMBER

anterior column *n* : VENTRAL HORN

anterior commissure *n* : a band of nerve fibers crossing from one side of the brain to the other just anterior to the third ventricle

anterior communicating artery *n* : COMMUNICATING ARTERY a

anterior corticospinal tract *n* : VENTRAL CORTICOSPINAL TRACT

anterior cruciate ligament *n* : a cruciate ligament of each knee that attaches the front of the tibia with the back of the femur and functions esp. to prevent hyperextension of the knee and is subject to injury esp. by tearing — called also *ACL*

anterior facial vein *n* : FACIAL VEIN

anterior fontanel *n* : the fontanel occurring at the meeting point of the coronal and sagittal sutures

anterior funiculus *n* : a longitudinal division on each side of the spinal cord comprising white matter between the anterior median fissure and the ventral root — called also *ventral funiculus;* compare LATERAL FUNICULUS, POSTERIOR FUNICULUS

anterior gray column *n* : VENTRAL HORN

anterior horn *n* **1** : VENTRAL HORN **2** : the cornu of the lateral ventricle of each cerebral hemisphere that curves outward and forward into the frontal lobe — compare INFERIOR HORN, POSTERIOR HORN 2

anterior humeral circumflex artery *n* : an artery that branches from the axillary artery in the shoulder, curves around the front of the humerus, and is distributed esp. to the shoulder joint, head of the humerus, biceps brachii, and deltoid muscle — compare POSTERIOR HUMERAL CIRCUMFLEX ARTERY

anterior inferior cerebellar artery *n* : an artery that arises from the basilar artery and divides into branches distributed to the anterior parts of the inferior surface of the cerebellum

anterior inferior iliac spine *n* : a projection on the anterior margin of the ilium that is situated below the anterior superior iliac spine and is separated from it by a notch — called also *anterior inferior spine*

anterior intercostal artery *n* : INTERCOSTAL ARTERY a

anterior jugular vein *n* : JUGULAR VEIN c

anterior lingual gland *n* : either of two mucus-secreting glands of the tip of the tongue

anterior lobe *n* : ADENOHYPOPHYSIS

anterior median fissure *n* : a groove along the anterior midline of the spinal cord that incompletely divides it into symmetrical halves — called also *ventral median fissure*

anterior nasal spine *n* : the nasal spine that is formed by the union of processes of the two premaxillae

anterior pillar of the fauces *n* : PALATOGLOSSAL ARCH

anterior root *n* : VENTRAL ROOT

anterior sacrococcygeal muscle *n* : SACROCOCCYGEUS VENTRALIS

anterior spinal artery *n* : SPINAL ARTERY a

anterior spinothalamic tract *n* : SPINOTHALAMIC TRACT a

anterior superior iliac spine *n* : a projection at the anterior end of the iliac crest — called also *anterior superior spine*

anterior synechia *n* : SYNECHIA a

anterior temporal artery *n* : TEMPORAL ARTERY 3a

anterior tibial artery *n* : TIBIAL ARTERY b

anterior tibial nerve *n* : DEEP PERONEAL NERVE

anterior tibial vein *n* : TIBIAL VEIN b

anterior triangle *n* : a triangular region that is a landmark in the neck and has its apex at the sternum point-

ing downward — compare POSTERIOR TRIANGLE

anterior ulnar recurrent artery *n* : ULNAR RECURRENT ARTERY a

antero- *comb form* : anterior and : extending from front to ⟨*antero*lateral⟩ ⟨*antero*posterior⟩

an·tero·grade \ˈan-tə-(ˌ)rō-ˌgrād\ *adj* **1** : occurring or performed in the normal or forward direction of conduction or flow: as **a** : occurring along nerve cell processes away from the cell body ⟨∼ axonal transport⟩ **b** : occurring in the normal direction or path of blood circulation ⟨restoration of ∼ flow⟩ — compare RETROGRADE 2 **2** : affecting memories of a period immediately following a shock or seizure ⟨∼ amnesia⟩

an·tero·in·fe·ri·or \ˌan-tə-(ˌ)rō-in-ˈfir-ē-ər\ *adj* : located in front and below ⟨the ∼ aspect of the femur⟩ — **an·tero·in·fe·ri·or·ly** *adv*

an·tero·lat·er·al \-ˈla-tə-rəl, -trəl\ *adj* : situated or occurring in front and to the side — **an·tero·lat·er·al·ly** *adv*

an·tero·me·di·al \-ˈmē-dē-əl\ *adj* : located in front and toward the middle

an·tero·pos·te·ri·or \-pō-ˈstir-ē-ər, -pä-\ *adj* : concerned with or extending along a direction or axis from front to back or from anterior to posterior — **an·tero·pos·te·ri·or·ly** *adv*

an·tero·su·pe·ri·or \-sù-ˈpir-ē-ər\ *adj* : located in front and above — **an·tero·su·pe·ri·or·ly** *adv*

an·te·ver·sion \ˌan-ti-ˈvər-zhən, -shən\ *n* : a condition of being anteverted — used esp. of the uterus

an·te·vert \ˈan-ti-ˌvərt, ˌan-ti-ˈ\ *vb* : to displace (a body organ) so that the whole axis is directed farther forward than normal

anth- — see ANTI-

anthelix *var of* ANTIHELIX

¹**an·thel·min·tic** \ˌant-ˌhel-ˈmin-tik, ˌan-ˌthel-\ *also* **an·thel·min·thic** \-ˈmin-thik\ *adj* : expelling or destroying parasitic worms (as tapeworms) esp. of the intestine

²**anthelmintic** *also* **anthelminthic** *n* : an anthelmintic drug

-anthem *or* **-anthema** *n comb form, pl* **-anthems** *or* **-anthemata** : eruption : rash ⟨en*anthem*⟩ ⟨ex*anthema*⟩

anthrac- *or* **anthraco-** *comb form* : carbon : coal ⟨*anthrac*osis⟩

an·thra·co·sil·i·co·sis \ˌan-thrə-(ˌ)kō-ˌsi-lə-ˈkō-səs\ *also* **an·thra·sil·i·co·sis** \ˌan-thrə-ˌsi-\ *n, pl* **-co·ses** \-ˌsēz\ : massive fibrosis of the lungs resulting from inhalation of carbon and quartz dusts and marked by shortness of breath

an·thra·co·sis \ˌan-thrə-ˈkō-səs\ *n, pl* **-co·ses** \-ˌsēz\ : a benign deposition of coal dust within the lungs from inhalation of sooty air — **an·thra·cot·ic** \-ˈkä-tik\ *adj*

an·thra·cy·cline \ˌan-thrə-ˈsī-ˌklēn\ *n* : any of a class of antineoplastic drugs (as doxorubicin) derived from an actinomycete of the genus *Strepto-myces* (esp. *S. peucetius*)

an·thra·lin \\'an-thrǝ-lǝn\ *n* : a yellow-ish brown crystalline compound $C_{14}H_{10}O_3$ used in the treatment of skin diseases (as psoriasis) — called also *dithranol*

an·thrax \\'an-,thraks\ *n, pl* **-thra·ces** \-thrǝ-,sēz\ : an infectious disease of warm-blooded animals (as cattle and sheep) caused by a spore-forming bacterium (*Bacillus anthracis*), trans-missible to humans esp. by the han-dling of infected products (as wool), and characterized by external ulcerat-ing nodules or by lesions in the lungs; *also* : the bacterium causing anthrax

anthrop- *or* **anthropo-** *comb form* : human being ⟨*anthropo*philic⟩

an·thro·poid \\'an-thrǝ-,póid\ *adj, of the pelvis* : having a relatively great an-teroposterior dimension — compare ANDROID, GYNECOID, PLATYPELLOID

an·thro·pom·e·try \,an-thrǝ-'pä-mǝ-trē\ *n, pl* **-tries** : the study of human body measurements esp. on a com-parative basis — **an·thro·po·met·ric** \-pǝ-'me-trik\ *adj*

an·thro·po·phil·ic \,an-thrǝ-(,)pō-'fi-lik\ *also* **an·thro·poph·i·lous** \-'pä-fǝ-lǝs\ *adj* : attracted to humans esp. as a source of food ⟨~ mosquitoes⟩

anti- *or* **ant-** *or* **anth-** *prefix* **1** : oppos-ing in effect or activity ⟨*anti*hista-mine⟩ **2** : serving to prevent, cure, or alleviate ⟨*anti*anxiety⟩

an·ti·abor·tion \,an-tē-ǝ-'bòr-shǝn, -,tī-\ *adj* : opposed to abortion and esp. to the legalization of abortion — **an·ti·abor·tion·ist** \-shǝ-nist\ *n*

antiacid *var of* ANTACID

an·ti·ac·ne \-'ak-nē\ *adj* : alleviating the symptoms of acne ⟨~ creams⟩

an·ti·ag·ing \'āj-iŋ\ *adj* : used or tend-ing to prevent or lessen the effects of aging ⟨~ skin creams⟩

an·ti–AIDS \-'ādz\ *adj* : used to treat or delay the development of AIDS ⟨the ~ drug AZT⟩

¹**an·ti·al·ler·gic** \-ǝ-'lǝr-jik\ *also* **an·ti·al·ler·gen·ic** \-,ǝ-lǝr-'je-nik\ *adj* : tending to relieve or control allergic symptoms

²**antiallergic** *also* **antiallergenic** *n* : an antiallergic agent

an·ti·an·a·phy·lax·is \-,ǝ-nǝ-fǝ-'lak-sǝs\ *n, pl* **-lax·es** \-'lak-,sēz\ : the state of desensitization to an antigen

an·ti·an·dro·gen \-'an-drǝ-jǝn\ *n* : a substance that tends to inhibit the production, activity, or effects of a male sex hormone — **an·ti·an·dro·gen·ic** \-,an-drǝ-'je-nik\ *adj*

an·ti·ane·mic \-ǝ-'nē-mik\ *adj* : effec-tive in or relating to the prevention or correction of anemia

an·ti·an·gi·nal \-an-'jīn-ᵊl, -'an-jǝn-ᵊl\ *adj* : used or tending to prevent or re-lieve angina pectoris ⟨~ drugs⟩

an·ti·an·gio·gen·e·sis \-,an-jē-ō-'jen-ǝ-sǝs\ *n, pl* **-e·ses** \-,sēz\ : the preven-tion or inhibition of angiogenesis — **an·ti·an·gio·gen·ic** \-'jen-ik\ *adj*

an·ti·an·ti·body \,an-tē-'an-ti-,bä-dē, -,tī-\ *n, pl* **-bod·ies** : an antibody with specific immunologic activity against another antibody

an·ti·anx·i·ety \-(,)aŋ-'zī-ǝ-tē\ *adj* : tending to prevent or relieve anxiety

¹**an·ti·ar·rhyth·mic** \-(,)ā-'rith-mik\ *adj* : counteracting or preventing cardiac arrhythmia ⟨an ~ agent⟩

²**antiarrhythmic** *n* : an antiarrhythmic agent

¹**an·ti·ar·thrit·ic** \-är-'thri-tik\ *or* **an·ti·ar·thri·tis** \-'thri-tǝs\ *adj* : tending to relieve or prevent arthritic symptoms

²**antiarthritic** *n* : an antiarthritic agent

an·ti–asth·ma \-'az-mǝ\ *or* **an·ti·asth·ma·tic** \-az-'ma-tik\ *adj* : used to re-lieve the symptoms of asthma

antiasthmatic *n* : an anti-asthma drug

¹**an·ti·bac·te·ri·al** \,an-ti-bak-'tir-ē-ǝl, ,an-,tī\ *adj* : directed or effective against bacteria

²**antibacterial** *n* : an antibacterial agent

an·ti·bi·o·sis \,an-ti-bī-'ō-sǝs, ,an-,tī-; ,an-ti-bē-\ *n, pl* **-o·ses** \-,sēz\ : antago-nistic association between organisms to the detriment of one of them or be-tween one organism and a metabolic product of another

¹**an·ti·bi·ot·ic** \-bī-'ä-tik, -bē-\ *adj* **1** : tending to prevent, inhibit, or de-stroy life **2** : of or relating to antibi-otics or to antibiosis — **an·ti·bi·ot·i·cal·ly** \-ti-k(ǝ-)lē\ *adv*

²**antibiotic** *n* : a substance produced by or a semisynthetic substance derived from a microorganism and able in di-lute solution to inhibit or kill another microorganism

an·ti·body \'an-ti-,bä-dē\ *n, pl* **-bod·ies** : any of a large number of pro-teins of high molecular weight that are produced normally by specialized B cells after stimulation by an antigen and act specifically against the anti-gen in an immune response, that are produced abnormally by some cancer cells, and that typically consist of four subunits including two heavy chains and two light chains — called also *im-munoglobulin*

antibrachium *var of* ANTEBRACHIUM

an·ti·can·cer \,an-ti-'kan-sǝr, ,an-,tī-\ *adj* : used against or tending to arrest cancer ⟨~ drugs⟩ ⟨~ activity⟩

an·ti·car·cin·o·gen \-kär-'si-nǝ-jǝn, -'kärs-ᵊn-ǝ-jen\ *n* : an anticarcino-genic agent

an·ti·car·ci·no·gen·ic \-,kärs-ᵊn-ō-'je-nik\ *adj* : tending to inhibit or prevent the activity of a carcinogen or the de-velopment of carcinoma

an·ti·car·dio·lip·in antibody \-,kärd-ē-ō-'li-pǝn-\ *n* : an antibody that is di-rected against phospholipids and esp. cardiolipin and that is associated with increased risk for recurring arterial and venous thromboses

an·ti·car·ies \,an-ti-'kar-ēz, ,an-,tī-\ *adj* : tending to inhibit the formation of caries

¹an·ti·car·io·gen·ic \-ˌkar-ē-ō-ˈjen-ik\ *adj* : ANTICARIES

an·ti·cho·les·ter·ol \-kə-ˈles-tə-ˌrōl, -ˌrȯl\ *adj* : tending to reduce the level of cholesterol in the blood ⟨∼ drugs⟩

¹an·ti·cho·lin·er·gic \-ˌkō-lə-ˈnər-jik\ *adj* : opposing or blocking the physiological action of acetylcholine

²anticholinergic *n* : a drug having an anticholinergic action

an·ti·cho·lin·es·ter·ase \-ˈnes-tə-ˌrās, -ˌrāz\ *n* : any substance (as neostigmine) that inhibits a cholinesterase by combination with it

an·tic·i·pa·tion \(ˌ)an-ˌti-sə-ˈpā-shən\ *n* **1** : occurrence (as of a symptom) before the normal or expected time **2** : mental attitude that influences a later response — **an·tic·i·pate** \an-ˈti-sə-ˌpāt\ *vb*

an·ti·clot·ting \ˌan-ti-ˈklä-tiŋ, ˌan-ˌtī-\ *adj* : inhibiting the clotting of blood ⟨∼ factors⟩

¹an·ti·co·ag·u·lant \-kō-ˈa-gyə-lənt\ *adj* : of, relating to, or utilizing anticoagulants ⟨∼ therapy⟩

²anticoagulant *n* : a substance that hinders coagulation and esp. coagulation of the blood : BLOOD THINNER

an·ti·co·ag·u·la·tion \-kō-ˌa-gyə-ˈlā-shən\ *n* : the process of hindering the clotting of blood esp. by treatment with an anticoagulant — **an·ti·co·ag·u·late** \-ˈa-gyə-ˌlāt\ *vb* — **an·ti·co·ag·u·la·to·ry** \-lə-ˌtōr-ē\ *adj*

an·ti·co·ag·u·la·tive \-ˈa-gyə-ˌlā-tiv\ *adj* : ANTICOAGULANT ⟨∼ activity⟩

an·ti·co·ag·u·lin \-gyə-lən\ *n* : a substance (as one in snake venom) that retards clotting of vertebrate blood

an·ti·co·don \ˌan-ti-ˈkō-ˌdän\ *n* : a triplet of nucleotide bases in transfer RNA that identifies the amino acid carried and that binds to a complementary codon in messenger RNA during protein synthesis at a ribosome

an·ti·com·ple·ment \-ˈkäm-plə-mənt\ *n* : a substance that interferes with the activity of complement — **an·ti·com·ple·men·ta·ry** \-ˌkäm-plə-ˈmen-tə-rē, -men-trē\ *adj*

¹an·ti·con·vul·sant \-kən-ˈvəl-sənt\ *also* **an·ti·con·vul·sive** \-siv\ *n* : an anticonvulsant drug

²anticonvulsant *also* **anticonvulsive** *adj* : used or tending to control or prevent convulsions (as in epilepsy)

anticus — see SCALENUS ANTICUS, SCALENUS ANTICUS SYNDROME, TIBIALIS ANTICUS

an·ti·dan·druff \-ˈdan-drəf\ *adj* : tending to remove or prevent dandruff ⟨an ∼ shampoo⟩

¹an·ti·de·pres·sant \-di-ˈpres-ᵊnt\ *also* **an·ti·de·pres·sive** \-ˈpre-siv\ *adj* : used or tending to relieve or prevent psychological depression

²antidepressant *also* **antidepressive** *n* : an antidepressant drug — called also *energizer, psychic energizer;* compare TRICYCLIC ANTIDEPRESSANT

¹an·ti·di·a·bet·ic \-ˌdī-ə-ˈbe-tik\ *n* : an antidiabetic drug

²antidiabetic *adj* : tending to relieve diabetes ⟨∼ drugs⟩

¹an·ti·di·ar·rhe·al \-ˌdī-ə-ˈrē-əl\ *adj* : tending to prevent or relieve diarrhea

²antidiarrheal *n* : an antidiarrheal agent

an·ti·di·ure·sis \-ˌdī-yü-ˈrē-səs\ *n, pl* **-ure·ses** \-ˌsēz\ : reduction in or suppression of the excretion of urine

¹an·ti·di·uret·ic \-ˈre-tik\ *adj* : tending to oppose or check excretion of urine

²antidiuretic *n* : an antidiuretic substance

antidiuretic hormone *n* : VASOPRESSIN

an·ti·dote \ˈan-ti-ˌdōt\ *n* : a remedy that counteracts the effects of poison — **an·ti·dot·al** \ˌan-ti-ˈdōt-ᵊl\ *adj* — **an·ti·dot·al·ly** *adv*

an·ti·dro·mic \ˌan-ti-ˈdrä-mik, -ˈdrō-\ *adj* **1** : proceeding or conducting in a direction opposite to the usual one — used esp. of a nerve impulse or fiber ⟨∼ action potentials⟩ **2** : characterized by antidromic conduction ⟨∼ tachycardia⟩ — **an·ti·dro·mi·cal·ly** \-mi-k(ə-)lē\ *adv*

¹an·ti·dys·en·ter·ic \ˌan-ti-ˌdis-ᵊn-ˈter-ik, ˌan-ˌtī-\ *adj* : tending to relieve or prevent dysentery

²antidysenteric *n* : an antidysenteric agent

¹an·ti·emet·ic \-ə-ˈme-tik\ *adj* : used or tending to prevent or check vomiting ⟨∼ drugs⟩

²antiemetic *n* : an antiemetic agent

¹an·ti·ep·i·lep·tic \-ˌe-pə-ˈlep-tik\ *adj* : tending to suppress or prevent epilepsy ⟨∼ treatment⟩

²antiepileptic *n* : an antiepileptic drug

an·ti·es·tro·gen \-ˈes-trə-jən\ *n* : a substance that inhibits the physiological action of an estrogen — **an·ti·es·tro·gen·ic** \-ˌes-trə-ˈje-nik\ *adj*

an·ti·fer·til·i·ty \-(ˌ)fər-ˈti-lə-tē\ *adj* : having the capacity or tending to reduce or destroy fertility : CONTRACEPTIVE ⟨∼ agents⟩

an·ti·fi·bril·la·to·ry \-ˈfi-brə-lə-ˌtōr-ē, -ˈfī-\ *adj* : tending to suppress or prevent cardiac fibrillation

an·ti·fi·bri·no·ly·sin \-ˌfī-brən-ᵊl-ˈīs-ᵊn\ *n* : an antibody that acts specifically against fibrinolysins of hemolytic streptococci and that is used chiefly in some diagnostic tests — called also *antistreptokinase* — **an·ti·fi·bri·no·ly·sis** \-ˈī-səs\ *n* — **an·ti·fi·bri·no·lyt·ic** \-ˈli-tik\ *adj*

¹an·ti·flat·u·lent \-ˈfla-chə-lənt\ *adj* : preventing or relieving flatulence

²antiflatulent *n* : an antiflatulent agent

an·ti·flu \-ˈflü\ *adj* : used to prevent infection by the orthomyxoviruses causing influenza ⟨an ∼ drug⟩

¹an·ti·fun·gal \ˌan-ti-ˈfəŋ-gəl, ˌan-ˌtī-\ *adj* : destroying fungi or inhibiting their growth : FUNGICIDAL, FUNGISTATIC

²**antifungal** *n* : an antifungal agent

an·ti·gen \'an-ti-jən\ *n* : any substance (as an immunogen or a hapten) foreign to the body that evokes an immune response either alone or after forming a complex with a larger molecule (as a protein) and that is capable of binding with a product (as an antibody or T cell) of the immune response — **an·ti·gen·ic** \₁an-ti-'je-nik\ *adj* — **an·ti·gen·i·cal·ly** \-ni-k(ə-)lē\ *adv*

an·ti·gen·emia \₁an-ti-jə-'nē-mē-ə\ *n* : the condition of having an antigen in the blood

antigenic determinant *n* : EPITOPE

an·ti·gen·ic·i·ty \-'ni-sə-tē\ *n, pl* **-ties** : the capacity to act as an antigen

antigen–presenting cell *n* : any of various cells (as a macrophage or a B cell) that take up an antigen and process it into a form recognized by and serving to activate a specific helper T cell

an·ti·glob·u·lin \₁an-ti-'glä-byə-lən, ₁an-₁tī-\ *n* : an antibody that combines with and precipitates globulin

an·ti·go·nad·o·trop·ic \-₁gō-₁na-də-'trä-pik\ *adj* : tending to inhibit the physiological activity of gonadotropic hormones

an·ti·go·nad·o·tro·pin \-'trō-pən\ *n* : an antigonadotropic substance

an·ti·he·lix \-'hē-liks\ *also* **ant·he·lix** \('}ant-\ *n, pl* **-li·ces** \-'he-lə-₁sēz, -'hē-\ *or* **-lix·es** \'hē-lik-səz\ : the curved elevation of cartilage within or in front of the helix

an·ti·he·mo·phil·ic factor \-₁hē-mə-'fi-lik-\ *n* : FACTOR VIII — called also *antihemophilic globulin*

an·ti·hem·or·rhag·ic \-₁he-mə-'ra-jik\ *adj* : tending to prevent or arrest hemorrhage

an·ti·her·pes \-'hər-(₁)pēz\ *adj* : acting against a herpesvirus or the symptoms caused by infection with it ⟨the ∼ drug acyclovir⟩

an·ti·hi·drot·ic \-hi-'drä-tik, -hī-\ *adj* : tending to reduce or prevent sweat secretion

¹**an·ti·his·ta·mine** \-'his-tə-₁mēn, -mən\ *adj* : tending to block or counteract the physiological action of histamine

²**antihistamine** *n* : any of various compounds that oppose the actions of histamine and are used esp. for treating allergic reactions (as hay fever), cold symptoms, and motion sickness

an·ti·his·ta·min·ic \-₁his-tə-'mi-nik\ *adj or n* : ANTIHISTAMINE

an·ti·hor·mone \-'hȯr-₁mōn\ *n* : a substance (as tamoxifen) that blocks the action or inhibits the production of a hormone

an·ti·hu·man \-'hyü-mən\ *adj* : reacting strongly with human antigens ⟨∼ antibodies⟩

an·ti·hy·per·lip·id·emic \-₁hī-pər-₁li-pə-'dē-mik\ *adj* : acting to prevent or counteract the accumulation of lipids in the blood ⟨an ∼ drug⟩

¹**an·ti·hy·per·ten·sive** \-₁hī-pər-'ten-siv\ *also* **an·ti·hy·per·ten·sion** \-₁hī-pər-'ten-chən\ *adj* : used or effective against high blood pressure

²**antihypertensive** *n* : an antihypertensive agent (as a drug)

an·ti·id·io·type \₁an-tī-'i-dē-ə-₁tīp\ *n* : an antibody that treats another antibody as an antigen and suppresses its immunoreactivity — **an·ti·id·io·typ·ic** \-₁i-dē-ə-'ti-pik\ *adj*

¹**an·ti·im·mu·no·glob·u·lin** \₁an-tē-₁i-myə-nō-'glä-byə-lən, ₁an-₁tī-, -₁myü-nō-\ *adj* : acting against specific antibodies ⟨∼ antibodies⟩ ⟨∼ sera⟩

²**anti–immunoglobulin** *n* : an anti-immunoglobulin agent

¹**an·ti·in·fec·tive** \-in-'fek-tiv\ *adj* : used against or tending to counteract or prevent infection ⟨∼ agents⟩

²**anti–infective** *n* : an anti-infective agent

¹**an·ti·in·flam·ma·to·ry** \-in-'fla-mə-₁tōr-ē\ *adj* : counteracting inflammation

²**anti–inflammatory** *n, pl* **-ries** : an anti-inflammatory agent (as a drug)

¹**an·ti·in·su·lin** \-'in-sə-lən\ *adj* : tending to counteract the physiological action of insulin

²**anti–insulin** *n* : an anti-insulin substance

an·ti·ke·to·gen·ic \-'je-nik\ *adj* : tending to prevent or counteract ketosis

an·ti·leu·ke·mic \-lü-'kē-mik\ *also* **an·ti·leu·ke·mia** \-mē-ə\ *adj* : counteracting the effects of leukemia

an·ti·lu·et·ic \-lü-'e-tik\ *n* : ANTISYPHILITIC

an·ti·lym·pho·cyte globulin \-'lim-fə-₁sīt-\ *n* : serum globulin containing antibodies against lymphocytes that is used similarly to antilymphocyte serum

antilymphocyte serum *n* : a serum containing antibodies against lymphocytes that is used for suppressing graft rejection

an·ti·lym·pho·cyt·ic globulin \-₁lim-fə-'si-tik-\ *n* : ANTILYMPHOCYTE GLOBULIN

antilymphocytic serum *n* : ANTILYMPHOCYTE SERUM

¹**an·ti·ma·lar·i·al** \-mə-'ler-ē-əl\ *or* **an·ti·ma·lar·ia** \-ə\ *adj* : serving to prevent, check, or cure malaria

²**antimalarial** *n* : an antimalarial drug

an·ti·man·ic \-'man-ik\ *adj* : counteracting or preventing mania and esp. mania associated with bipolar disorder

an·ti·me·tab·o·lite \-mə-'ta-bə-₁līt\ *n* : a substance (as a sulfa drug) that replaces or inhibits the utilization of a metabolite

¹**an·ti·mi·cro·bi·al** \-mī-₁krō-bē-əl\ *also* **an·ti·mi·cro·bic** \-'krō-bik\ *adj* : destroying or inhibiting the growth of microorganisms and esp. pathogenic microorganisms

²**antimicrobial** *also* **antimicrobic** *n* : an antimicrobial substance

¹**an·ti·mi·tot·ic** \-ˌmī-ˈtä-tik\ *adj* : inhibiting or disrupting mitosis ⟨~ agents⟩

²**antimitotic** *n* : an antimitotic substance

an·ti·mo·ny \ˈan-tə-ˌmō-nē\ *n, pl* **-nies** : a metalloid element that is commonly silvery white, crystalline, and brittle and is used in medicine as a constituent of various antiprotozoal agents (as tartar emetic) — symbol *Sb*; see ELEMENT TABLE

antimonyltartrate — see POTASSIUM ANTIMONYLTARTRATE

antimony potassium tartrate *n* : TARTAR EMETIC

an·ti·mus·ca·rin·ic \-ˌməs-kə-ˈri-nik\ *adj* : inhibiting muscarinic physiological effects ⟨an ~ agent⟩

an·ti·mu·ta·gen·ic \-ˌmyü-tə-ˈje-nik\ *adj* : reducing the rate of mutation

an·ti·my·cin A \ˌan-ti-ˌmīs-ᵊn-ˈā\ *n* : a crystalline antibiotic $C_{28}H_{40}N_2O_9$ used esp. as a fungicide, insecticide, and miticide — called also *antimycin*

an·ti·my·cot·ic \ˌan-ti-mī-ˈkä-tik, ˌan-ˌtī-\ *adj or n* : ANTIFUNGAL

an·ti·nau·sea \-ˈnò-zē-ə, -sē-; -ˈnò-zhə, -shə\ *also* **an·ti·nau·se·ant** \-ˈnò-zē-ənt, -zhē-, -sē-, -shē-\ *adj* : preventing or counteracting nausea ⟨~ drugs⟩

antinauseant *n* : an antinausea agent

¹**an·ti·neo·plas·tic** \-ˌnē-ə-ˈplas-tik\ *adj* : inhibiting or preventing the growth and spread of neoplasms or malignant cells ⟨~ drugs⟩

²**antineoplastic** *n* : an antineoplastic agent

an·ti·neu·rit·ic \-nu̇-ˈri-tik, -nyu̇-\ *adj* : preventing or relieving neuritis

an·ti·no·ci·cep·tive \ˌan-ti-nō-si-ˈsep-tiv, ˌan-ˌtī-\ *adj* : ANALGESIC

an·ti·nu·cle·ar \-ˈnü-klē-ər, -ˈnyü-\ *adj* : being antibodies or autoantibodies that react with components and esp. DNA of cell nuclei and that tend to occur frequently in connective tissue diseases

an·ti·on·co·gene \-ˈäŋ-kō-ˌjēn\ *n* : TUMOR SUPPRESSOR GENE

an·ti·ox·i·dant \-ˈäk-sə-dənt\ *n* : a substance (as beta-carotene or vitamin C) that inhibits oxidation or reactions promoted by oxygen, peroxides, or free radicals — **antioxidant** *adj*

an·ti·par·a·sit·ic \-ˌpar-ə-ˈsi-tik\ *adj* : acting against parasites

an·ti·par·kin·so·nian \-ˌpär-kən-ˈsō-nē-ən, -nyən\ *also* **an·ti·par·kin·son** \-ˈpär-kən-sən\ *adj* : tending to relieve parkinsonism ⟨~ drugs⟩

¹**an·ti·pe·ri·od·ic** \-ˌpir-ē-ˈä-dik\ *adj* : preventing periodic returns of disease

²**antiperiodic** *n* : an antiperiodic agent

an·ti·peri·stal·sis \-ˌper-ə-ˈstol-səs, -ˈstäl-, -ˈstal-\ *n, pl* **-stal·ses** \-ˌsēz\ : reversed peristalsis

an·ti·peri·stal·tic \-tik\ *adj* **1** : opposed to or checking peristaltic motion **2** : relating to antiperistalsis

an·ti·per·spi·rant \-ˈpər-spə-rənt\ *n* : a preparation used to check perspiration

an·ti·phlo·gis·tic \-flə-ˈjis-tik\ *adj or n* : ANTI-INFLAMMATORY

an·ti·phos·pho·lip·id \-ˌfäs-fō-ˈlip-əd\ *adj* : relating to, being, or associated with antibodies (as anticardiolipin antibodies) that act against phospholipids and increase the risk of venous and arterial thromboses and thrombocytopenia ⟨~ syndrome⟩

an·ti·plas·min \-ˈplaz-mən\ *n* : a substance (as an antifibrinolysin) that inhibits the action of plasmin

an·ti·plate·let \-ˈplāt-lət\ *adj* : acting against or destroying blood platelets

an·ti·pneu·mo·coc·cal \-ˌnü-mə-ˈkä-kəl, -ˌnyü-\ *or* **an·ti·pneu·mo·coc·cic** \-ˈkäk-(ˌ)sik\ *or* **an·ti·pneu·mo·coc·cus** \-ˈkä-kəs\ *adj* : destroying or inhibiting pneumococci

an·ti·pro·lif·er·a·tive \-prə-ˈli-fə-ˌrā-tiv\ *adj* : used or tending to inhibit cell growth ⟨~ effects on tumor cells⟩

an·ti·pro·te·ase \-ˈprō-tē-ˌās, -ˌāz\ *n* : a substance that inhibits the enzymatic activity of a protease

an·ti·pro·throm·bin \-(ˌ)prō-ˈthräm-bən\ *n* : a substance that interferes with the conversion of prothrombin to thrombin — compare ANTITHROMBIN, HEPARIN

¹**an·ti·pro·to·zo·al** \-ˌprō-tə-ˈzō-əl\ *adj* : tending to destroy or inhibit the growth of protozoa

²**antiprotozoal** *n* : an antiprotozoal agent

¹**an·ti·pru·rit·ic** \-prü-ˈri-tik\ *adj* : tending to check or relieve itching

²**antipruritic** *n* : an antipruritic agent

an·ti·pseu·do·mo·nal \-ˌsü-də-ˈmōn-ᵊl, -sü-ˈdä-mən-ᵊl\ *adj* : tending to destroy bacteria of the genus *Pseudomonas* ⟨~ activity⟩

¹**an·ti·psy·chot·ic** \-sī-ˈkä-tik\ *adj* : of, being, or involving the use of an antipsychotic ⟨~ drugs⟩

²**antipsychotic** *n* : any of the powerful tranquilizers (as the phenothiazines and butyrophenones) used esp. to treat psychosis and believed to act by blocking dopamine nervous receptors — called also *neuroleptic*

an·ti·py·re·sis \-pī-ˈrē-səs, -ˌsēz\ : treatment of fever by use of antipyretics

¹**an·ti·py·ret·ic** \-pī-ˈre-tik\ *n* : an antipyretic agent — called also *febrifuge*

²**antipyretic** *adj* : preventing, removing, or allaying fever

an·ti·py·rine \-ˈpīr-ˌēn\ *also* **an·ti·py·rin** \-ən\ *n* : an analgesic and antipyretic $C_{11}H_{12}N_2O$ formerly widely used but now largely replaced in oral use by less toxic drugs (as aspirin) — called also *phenazone*

¹**an·ti·ra·chit·ic** \-rə-ˈki-tik\ *adj* : used or tending to prevent the development of rickets ⟨an ~ vitamin⟩

²**antirachitic** *n* : an antirachitic agent

an·ti·re·jec·tion \-ri-ˈjek-shən\ *adj* : used or tending to prevent organ transplant rejection ⟨~ drugs⟩

an·ti·re·sorp·tive \-rē-ˈsȯrp-tiv, -ˈzȯrp-\ *adj* : tending to slow or block the resorption of bone ⟨an ∼ agent⟩

¹**an·ti·ret·ro·vi·ral** \-ˈre-trō-ˌvī-rəl\ *adj* : acting, used, or effective against retroviruses ⟨∼ drugs⟩ ⟨∼ therapy⟩

²**antiretroviral** *n* : an antiretroviral drug

¹**an·ti·rheu·mat·ic** \-rü-ˈma-tik\ *adj* : alleviating or preventing rheumatism

²**antirheumatic** *n* : an antirheumatic agent

an·ti·schis·to·so·mal \-ˌshis-tə-ˈsō-məl\ *adj* : tending to destroy or inhibit the development and reproduction of schistosomes

an·ti·schizo·phren·ic \-ˌskit-sə-ˈfre-nik\ *adj* : tending to relieve or suppress the symptoms of schizophrenia

¹**an·ti·scor·bu·tic** \-skȯr-ˈbyü-tik\ *adj* : counteracting scurvy ⟨the ∼ vitamin is vitamin C⟩

²**antiscorbutic** *n* : a remedy for scurvy

an·ti·se·cre·to·ry \-ˈsē-krə-ˌtōr-ē\ *adj* : tending to inhibit secretion

an·ti·sei·zure \-ˈsē-zhər\ *adj* : preventing or counteracting seizures ⟨∼ drugs⟩

an·ti·sense \ˈan-ˌtī-ˌsens, ˈan-ti-\ *adj* : of, being, relating to, or possessing a sequence of DNA or RNA that is complementary to and pairs with a specific messenger RNA blocking it from being translated into protein and serving to inhibit gene function ⟨∼ RNA⟩ ⟨∼ drug therapy⟩ — compare MISSENSE, NONSENSE

an·ti·sep·sis \ˌan-tə-ˈsep-səs\ *n, pl* **-sep·ses** \-ˌsēz\ : the inhibiting of the growth and multiplication of microorganisms by antiseptic means

¹**an·ti·sep·tic** \ˌan-tə-ˈsep-tik\ *adj* **1 a** : opposing sepsis, putrefaction, or decay; *esp* : preventing or arresting the growth of microorganisms (as on living tissue) **b** : acting or protecting like an antiseptic **2** : relating to or characterized by the use of antiseptics **3** : free of living microorganisms : scrupulously clean : ASEPTIC — **an·ti·sep·ti·cal·ly** \-ti-k(ə-)lē\ *adv*

²**antiseptic** *n* : a substance that checks the growth or action of microorganisms esp. in or on living tissue; *also* : GERMICIDE

an·ti·se·rum \ˈan-ti-ˌsir-əm, ˈan-ˌtī-, -ˌser-\ *n* : a serum containing antibodies — called also *immune serum*

an·ti·so·cial \-ˈsō-shəl\ *adj* : hostile or harmful to organized society: as **a** : being or marked by behavior deviating sharply from the social norm **b** : of, relating to, or characterized by an antisocial personality, the antisocial personality disorder, or behavior typical of either

antisocial personality *n* : a personality exhibiting traits typical of the antisocial personality disorder — called also *psychopathic personality*

antisocial personality disorder *n* : a personality disorder that is characterized by antisocial behavior exhibiting pervasive disregard for and violation of the rights, feelings, and safety of others — called also *psychopathic personality disorder*

¹**an·ti·spas·mod·ic** \-spaz-ˈmä-dik\ *n* : an antispasmodic agent

²**antispasmodic** *adj* : capable of preventing or relieving spasms or convulsions

an·ti·sperm \-ˈspərm\ *adj* : destroying or inactivating sperm ⟨∼ pills⟩

an·ti·strep·to·coc·cal \-ˌstrep-tə-ˈkä-kəl\ *or* **an·ti·strep·to·coc·cic** \-ˈkä-kik, -ˈkäk-sik\ *adj* : tending to destroy or inhibit the growth and reproduction of streptococci ⟨∼ antibodies⟩

an·ti·strep·to·ki·nase \-ˌstrep-tō-ˈkī-ˌnās, -ˌnāz\ *n* : ANTIFIBRINOLYSIN

an·ti·strep·to·ly·sin \-ˌstrep-tə-ˈlīs-ᵊn\ *n* : an antibody against a streptolysin produced by an individual injected with a streptolysin-forming streptococcus

¹**an·ti·syph·i·lit·ic** \-ˌsi-fə-ˈli-tik\ *adj* : effective against syphilis ⟨∼ therapy⟩

²**antisyphilitic** *n* : an antisyphilitic agent

an·ti·throm·bin \-ˈthräm-bən\ *n* : any of a group of substances in blood that inhibit blood clotting by inactivating thrombin — compare ANTIPROTHROMBIN, HEPARIN

an·ti·throm·bo·plas·tin \-ˌthräm-bə-ˈplas-tən\ *n* : an anticoagulant substance that counteracts the effects of thromboplastin

¹**an·ti·throm·bot·ic** \-thräm-ˈbä-tik\ *adj* : used against or tending to prevent thrombosis ⟨∼ agents⟩ ⟨∼ therapy⟩

²**antithrombotic** *n* : an antithrombotic agent

an·ti·thy·roid \-ˈthī-ˌrȯid\ *adj* : able to counteract excessive thyroid activity

an·ti·tox·ic \-ˈtäk-sik\ *adj* **1** : counteracting toxins **2** : being or containing antitoxins ⟨∼ serum⟩

an·ti·tox·in \ˌan-ti-ˈtäk-sən\ *n* : an antibody that is capable of neutralizing the specific toxin (as a specific causative agent of disease) that stimulated its production in the body and is produced in animals for medical purposes by injection of a toxin or toxoid with the resulting serum being used to counteract the toxin in other individuals; *also* : an antiserum containing antitoxins

an·ti·trag·i·cus \ˌan-ti-ˈtra-jə-kəs\ *n, pl* **-i·ci** \-jə-ˌsī, -ˌsē\ : a small muscle arising from the outer part of the antitragus and inserted into the antihelix

an·ti·tra·gus \-ˈtrā-gəs\ *n, pl* **-gi** \-ˌjī, -ˌgī\ : a prominence on the lower posterior portion of the concha of the external ear opposite the tragus

an·ti·try·pano·som·al \-ˌtri-ˌpa-nə-ˈsō-məl\ *or* **an·ti·try·pano·some** \-ˈtri-pa-nə-ˌsōm\ *adj* : TRYPANOCIDAL

an·ti·tryp·sin \ˈan-ti-ˌtrip-sən, ˌan-ˌtī-\ *n* : a substance that inhibits the action of trypsin — see ALPHA-1-ANTITRYPSIN — **an·ti·tryp·tic** \-ˌtrip-tik\ *adj*

an·ti·tu·ber·cu·lous \ˌan-ti-tů-ˈbər-kyə-ləs, ˌan-ˌtī-, -ˈtyü-\ *or* **an·ti·tu·ber·cu·lo·sis** \-ˌbər-kyə-ˈlō-səs\ *also* **an·ti·tu·ber·cu·lar** \-ˈbər-kyə-lər\ *adj* : used or effective against tuberculosis

an·ti·tu·mor \ˈan-ti-ˌtü-mər, ˈan-ˌtī-, -ˌtyü-\ *also* **an·ti·tu·mor·al** \-mə-rəl\ *adj* : ANTICANCER ⟨~ agents⟩

¹**an·ti·tus·sive** \an-ti-ˈtə-siv, ˌan-ˌtī-\ *adj* : tending or having the power to act as a cough suppressant ⟨~ action⟩

²**antitussive** *n* : a cough suppressant

an·ti·ty·phoid \-ˈtī-ˌfóid, -tī-ˈfóid\ *adj* : tending to prevent or cure typhoid

an·ti·ul·cer \-ˈəl-sər\ *adj* : tending to prevent or heal ulcers ⟨~ drugs⟩

an·ti·ven·in \-ˈve-nən\ *n* : an antitoxin to a venom; *also* : an antiserum containing such an antitoxin

An·ti·vert \ˈan-ti-ˌvərt, -ˌtī-\ *trademark* — used for a preparation of the hydrochloride of meclizine

¹**an·ti·vi·ral** \ˌan-ti-ˈvī-rəl, ˌan-ˌtī-\ *also* **an·ti·vi·rus** \-ˈvī-rəs\ *adj* : acting, effective, or directed against viruses

²**antiviral** *n* : an antiviral agent

an·ti·vi·ta·min \ˈan-ti-ˌvī-tə-mən, ˈan-ˌtī-\ *n* : a substance that makes a vitamin metabolically ineffective

antr- *or* **antro-** *comb form* : antrum ⟨*antro*stomy⟩

an·tral \ˈan-trəl\ *adj* : of or relating to an antrum ⟨~ gastritis⟩

an·trec·to·my \an-ˈtrek-tə-mē\ *n, pl* **-mies** : excision of an antrum (as of the stomach or mastoid)

an·tros·to·my \an-ˈträs-tə-mē\ *n, pl* **-mies** : the operation of opening an antrum (as for drainage); *also* : the opening made in such an operation

an·trot·o·my \-ˈträ-tə-mē\ *n, pl* **-mies** : incision of an antrum; *also* : ANTROSTOMY

an·trum \ˈan-trəm\ *n, pl* **an·tra** \-trə\ : a cavity within a bone (as the maxilla) or hollow organ (as the stomach)

antrum of High·more \-ˈhī-ˌmōr\ *n* : MAXILLARY SINUS

Highmore, Nathaniel (1613–1685), British surgeon.

anu·cle·ate \(ˌ)ā-ˈnü-klē-ət, -ˈnyü-\ *also* **anu·cle·at·ed** \-klē-ˌā-təd\ *adj* : lacking a cell nucleus

anulus *var of* ANNULUS

an·uria \ə-ˈnúr-ē-ə, a-, -ˈnyúr-\ *n* : absence of or defective urine excretion — **an·uric** \-ˈnúr-ik, -ˈnyúr-\ *adj*

anus \ˈā-nəs\ *n, pl* **anus·es** *or* **ani** \ˈā-(ˌ)nī\ : the posterior opening of the digestive tract

an·vil \ˈan-vəl, -ˌvil\ *n* : INCUS

anx·i·ety \aŋ-ˈzī-ə-tē\ *n, pl* **-eties** **1 a** : a painful or apprehensive uneasiness of mind usu. over an impending or anticipated ill **b** : a cause of anxiety **2** : an abnormal and overwhelming sense of apprehension and fear often marked by physiological signs (as sweating, tension, and increased pulse), by doubt concerning the reality and nature of the threat, and by

self-doubt about one's capacity to cope with it

anxiety disorder *n* : any of various disorders (as panic disorder, obsessive-compulsive disorder, or generalized anxiety disorder) in which anxiety is a predominant feature — called also *anxiety neurosis, anxiety state*

anxiety reaction *n* : reaction to a feared situation or object in which various manifestations of anxiety are prominent

¹**anx·io·lyt·ic** \ˌaŋ-zē-ō-ˈli-tik, ˌan-sē-\ *n* : a drug that relieves anxiety

²**anxiolytic** *adj* : relieving anxiety

anx·ious \ˈaŋk-shəs\ *adj* **1** : characterized by extreme uneasiness of mind or brooding fear about some contingency **2** : characterized by, resulting from, or causing anxiety

AOB *abbr* alcohol on breath

aort- *or* **aorto-** *comb form* **1** : aorta ⟨*aort*itis⟩ **2** : aortic and ⟨*aorto*coronary⟩

aor·ta \ā-ˈór-tə\ *n, pl* **-tas** *or* **-tae** \-ˌtē\ : the large arterial trunk that carries blood from the heart to be distributed by branch arteries through the body

aor·tic \ā-ˈór-tik\ *also* **aor·tal** \-ˈórt-ᵊl\ *adj* : of, relating to, or affecting an aorta ⟨an ~ aneurysm⟩

aortic arch *n* : ARCH OF THE AORTA

aortic dissection *n* : a pathological splitting of the aortic media

aortic hiatus *n* : an opening in the diaphragm through which the aorta passes

aortic incompetence *n* : AORTIC REGURGITATION

aortic insufficiency *n* : AORTIC REGURGITATION

aor·ti·co·pul·mo·nary \ā-ˌór-tə-kō-ˈpúl-mə-ˌner-ē, -ˈpəl-\ *adj* : relating to or joining the aorta and the pulmonary artery

aor·ti·co·re·nal \-ˈrēn-ᵊl\ *adj* : relating to or situated near the aorta and the kidney

aortic regurgitation *n* : leakage of blood from the aorta back into the left ventricle during diastole because of failure of an aortic valve to close properly — called also *aortic incompetence, aortic insufficiency, Corrigan's disease*

aortic sinus *n* : SINUS OF VALSALVA

aortic stenosis *n* : a condition usu. the result of disease in which the aorta and esp. its orifice is abnormally narrow

aortic valve *n* : the semilunar valve separating the aorta from the left ventricle that prevents blood from flowing back into the left ventricle

aor·ti·tis \ˌā-ór-ˈtī-təs\ *n* : inflammation of the aorta

aor·to·cor·o·nary \ā-ˌór-tō-ˈkór-ə-ˌner-ē, -ˈkär-\ *adj* : of, relating to, or joining the aorta and the coronary arteries ⟨~ bypass surgery⟩

aor·to·fem·o·ral \-ˈfe-mə-rəl\ *adj* : of, relating to, or joining the abdominal aorta and the femoral arteries ⟨an ∼ bypass graft⟩

aor·to·gram \ā-'ȯr-tə-ˌgram\ *n* : an X-ray picture of the aorta made by arteriography

aor·tog·ra·phy \ˌā-ȯr-'tä-grə-fē\ *n, pl* **-phies** : arteriography of the aorta — **aor·to·graph·ic** \(ˌ)ā-ˌȯr-tə-'gra-fik\ *adj*

aor·to·il·i·ac \ˌā-ˌȯr-tō-'i-lē-ˌak\ *adj* : of, relating to, or joining the abdominal aorta and the iliac arteries

aor·to·pul·mo·nary window \ˌā-ˌȯr-tō-'pu̇l-mə-ˌner-ē-, -'pəl-\ *n* : a congenital circulatory defect in which there is direct communication between the aorta and the pulmonary artery — called also *aortopulmonary fenestration*

aor·to·sub·cla·vi·an \-ˌsəb-'klā-vē-ən\ *adj* : relating to or joining the aorta and the subclavian arteries

AOTA *abbr* American Occupational Therapy Association

ap- — see APO-

APAP *abbr* acetaminophen — used esp. when combined with a prescription drug ⟨hydrocodone/APAP⟩

apar·a·lyt·ic \ˌā-ˌpar-ə-'li-tik\ *adj* : not characterized by paralysis

ap·a·thet·ic \ˌa-pə-'the-tik\ *adj* : having or showing little or no feeling or emotion — **ap·a·thet·i·cal·ly** \-ti-k(ə-)lē\ *adv*

ap·a·thy \'a-pə-thē\ *n, pl* **-thies** : lack of feeling or emotion

ap·a·tite \'a-pə-ˌtīt\ *n* : any of a group of calcium phosphate minerals comprising the chief constituent of bones and teeth; *specif* : calcium phosphate fluoride $Ca_5F(PO_4)_3$

APC *abbr* aspirin, phenacetin, and caffeine

¹**ape·ri·ent** \ə-'pir-ē-ənt\ *adj* : gently causing the bowels to move : LAXATIVE

²**aperient** *n* : an aperient agent

ape·ri·od·ic \ˌā-ˌpir-ē-'ä-dik\ *adj* : of irregular occurrence

aperi·stal·sis \ˌā-ˌper-ə-'stȯl-səs, -'stäl-, -'stal-\ *n, pl* **-stal·ses** \-ˌsēz\ : absence of peristalsis

apex \'ā-ˌpeks\ *n, pl* **apex·es** *or* **api·ces** \'ā-pə-ˌsēz\ : a narrowed or pointed end of an anatomical structure: as **a** : the narrow somewhat conical upper part of a lung extending into the root **b** : the lower pointed end of the heart situated in humans opposite the space between the cartilages of the fifth and sixth ribs on the left side **c** : the extremity of the root of a tooth

apex·car·di·og·ra·phy \ˌā-ˌpeks-ˌkär-dē-'ä-grə-fē\ *n, pl* **-phies** : a procedure for measuring the beat in the apex region of the heart by recording movements in the nearby wall of the chest

Ap·gar score \'ap-ˌgär-\ *n* : an index used to evaluate the condition of a newborn infant based on a rating of 0, 1, or 2 for each of the five characteristics of color, heart rate, response to stimulation of the sole of the foot, muscle tone, and respiration with 10 being a perfect score

Apgar, Virginia (1909–1974), American physician.

aph- — see APO-

apha·gia \ə-'fā-jə, a-, -jē-ə\ *n* : loss of the ability to swallow

apha·kia \ə-'fā-kē-ə, a-\ *n* : absence of the crystalline lens of the eye; *also* : the resulting anomalous state of refraction

¹**apha·kic** \ə-'fā-kik, a-\ *adj* : of, relating to, or affected with aphakia

²**aphakic** *n* : an individual who has had the lens of an eye removed

apha·sia \ə-'fā-zhə, -zhē-ə\ *n* : loss or impairment of the power to use or comprehend words usu. resulting from brain damage — see MOTOR APHASIA; compare ANARTHRIA

¹**apha·sic** \ə-'fā-zik\ *adj* : of, relating to, or affected with aphasia

²**aphasic** *or* **apha·si·ac** \ə-'fā-zē-ˌak, -zhē-\ *n* : an individual affected with aphasia

apha·si·ol·o·gy \ə-ˌfā-zē-'ä-lə-jē, -zhē-\ *n, pl* **-gies** : the study of aphasia — **apha·si·ol·o·gist** \-jist\ *n*

aphe·re·sis \ˌā-fə-'rē-səs\ *n, pl* **-re·ses** \-ˌsēz\ : withdrawal of blood from a donor's body, removal of one or more components (as plasma or white blood cells) from the blood, and transfusion of the remaining blood back into the donor — called also *pheresis*; see LEUKAPHERESIS, PLASMAPHERESIS, PLATELETPHERESIS

apho·nia \(ˌ)ā-'fō-nē-ə\ *n* : loss of voice and of all but whispered speech — **apho·nic** \-'fä-nik, -'fō-\ *adj*

aphos·pho·ro·sis \ˌā-ˌfäs-fə-'rō-səs\ *n, pl* **-ro·ses** \-ˌsēz\ : a deficiency disease esp. of cattle caused by inadequate intake of dietary phosphorus

¹**aph·ro·di·si·ac** \ˌa-frə-'dē-zē-ˌak, -'dī-\ *also* **aph·ro·di·si·a·cal** \ˌa-frə-də-'zī-ə-kəl, -'sī-\ *adj* : exciting sexual desire

²**aphrodisiac** *n* : an aphrodisiac agent

aph·tha \'af-thə\ *also* **ap·tha** \'ap-\ *n, pl* **aph·thae** *also* **ap·thae** \-ˌthē\ : a speck, flake, or blister on the mucous membranes (as of the mouth, gastrointestinal tract, or lips) — **aph·thous** \-thəs\ *adj*

aph·thoid \'af-ˌthȯid\ *adj* : resembling thrush ⟨∼ ulcers⟩

aphthous fever *n* : FOOT-AND-MOUTH DISEASE

aphthous stomatitis *n* : a very common disorder of the oral mucosa that is characterized by the formation of canker sores on movable mucous membranes and that has a multiple etiology but is not caused by the virus causing herpes simplex

apic- *or* **apici-** *or* **apico-** *comb form* : apex : tip esp. of an organ ⟨*apicec-tomy*⟩

api·cal \'ā-pi-kəl, 'a-\ *adj* : of, relating to, or situated at an apex — **api·cal·ly** \-k(ə-)lē\ *adv*

apical foramen *n* : the opening of the pulp canal in the root of a tooth

apic·ec·to·my \ˌā-pə-ˈsek-tə-mē\ *n, pl* **-mies** : surgical removal of an anatomical apex (as of the root of a tooth)

apices *pl of* APEX

api·co·ec·to·my \ˌā-pi-(ˌ)kō-ˈek-tə-mē, ˌa-\ *n, pl* **-mies** : excision of the root tip of a tooth

apla·sia \(ˌ)ā-ˈplā-zhə, -zhē-ə, ə-\ *n* : incomplete or faulty development of an organ or part — **aplas·tic** \-ˈplas-tik\ *adj*

aplastic anemia *n* : anemia that is characterized by defective function of the blood-forming organs (as the bone marrow) and is caused by toxic agents (as chemicals or X-rays) or is idiopathic in origin — called also *hypoplastic anemia*

ap·nea \ap-ˈnē-ə, ap-ˈnē-\ *n* 1 : transient cessation of respiration; *esp* : SLEEP APNEA 2 : ASPHYXIA — **ap·ne·ic** \ap-ˈnē-ik\ *adj*

ap·neu·sis \ap-ˈnü-səs, -ˈnyü-\ *n, pl* **ap·neu·ses** \-ˌsēz\ : sustained tonic contraction of the respiratory muscles resulting in prolonged inspiration — **ap·neus·tic** \-ˈnü-stik, -ˈnyü-\ *adj*

ap·noea \ap-ˈnē-ə, ˈap-nē-\ *chiefly Brit var of* APNEA

apo *n* : APOLIPOPROTEIN

apo- *or* **ap-** *or* **aph-** *prefix* : formed from : related to ⟨*apomorphine*⟩

apo·crine \ˈa-pə-krən, -ˌkrīn, -ˌkrēn\ *adj* : producing a fluid secretion by pinching off one end of the secreting cells which then reform and repeat the process ⟨∼ glands⟩; *also* : produced by an apocrine gland — compare ECCRINE, HOLOCRINE, MEROCRINE

apo·en·zyme \ˌa-pō-ˈen-ˌzīm\ *n* : a protein that forms an active enzyme system by combination with a coenzyme and determines the specificity of this system for a substrate

apo·fer·ri·tin \ˌa-pə-ˈfer-ət-ᵊn\ *n* : a colorless crystalline protein capable of storing iron in bodily cells esp. of the liver

apo·li·po·pro·tein \ˌa-pō-ˌlī-pō-ˈprō-ˌtēn, -ˌli-\ *n* : any of the proteins that combine with a lipid to form a lipoprotein and that are now grouped into four classes designated *A*, *B*, *C*, and *E* ⟨∼ B is a major component of LDL⟩

apo·mor·phine \ˌa-pə-ˈmȯr-ˌfēn\ *n* : a morphine derivative that is a dopamine agonist and is injected subcutaneously in the form of its hydrochloride $C_{17}H_{17}NO_2 \cdot HCl \cdot {}^{1}\!/_{2}H_2O$ to treat episodes of immobility associated with advanced Parkinson's disease

apo·neu·ro·sis \ˌa-pə-nu̇-ˈrō-səs, -nyü-\ *n, pl* **-ro·ses** \-ˌsēz\ : any of the broad flat sheets of dense fibrous collagenous connective tissue that cover, invest, and form the terminations and attachments of various muscles — **apo·neu·rot·ic** \-ˈrä-tik\ *adj*

aponeurotica — see GALEA APONEUROTICA

apoph·y·sis \ə-ˈpä-fə-səs\ *n, pl* **-y·ses** \-ˌsēz\ : an expanded or projecting part esp. of an organism — **apoph·y·se·al** \-ˌpä-fə-ˈsē-əl\ *adj*

ap·o·plec·tic \ˌa-pə-ˈplek-tik\ *adj* 1 : of, relating to, or causing stroke 2 : affected with, inclined to, or showing symptoms of stroke — **ap·o·plec·ti·cal·ly** \-ti-k(ə-)lē\ *adv*

ap·o·plexy \ˈa-pə-ˌplek-sē\ *n, pl* **-plex·ies** 1 : STROKE 2 : copious hemorrhage into a cavity or into the substance of an organ ⟨abdominal ∼⟩

apo·pro·tein \ˌa-pə-ˈprō-ˌtēn\ *n* : a protein that combines with a prosthetic group to form a conjugated protein

apo·pto·sis \ˌa-pə-ˈtō-sis\ *n, pl* **-pto·ses** \-ˌsēz\ : a genetically directed process of cell self-destruction that is marked by the fragmentation of nuclear DNA and is a normal physiological process eliminating DNA-damaged, superfluous, or unwanted cells — called also *programmed cell death* — **ap·o·pto·tic** \-ˈtä-tik\ *adj*

apothecaries' measure *n* : a system of liquid units of measure used in compounding medical prescriptions that include the gallon, pint, fluid ounce, fluid dram, and minim

apothecaries' weight *n* : a system of weights used chiefly by pharmacists in compounding medical prescriptions that include the pound of 12 ounces, the dram of 60 grains, and the scruple

apoth·e·cary \ə-ˈpä-thə-ˌker-ē\ *n, pl* **-car·ies** 1 : a person who prepares and sells drugs or compounds for medicinal purposes : DRUGGIST, PHARMACIST 2 : PHARMACY 2a

ap·pa·ra·tus \ˌa-pə-ˈra-təs, -ˈrā-\ *n, pl* **-tus·es** *or* **-tus** : a group of anatomical or cytological parts functioning together — see GOLGI APPARATUS

append- *or* **appendo-** *or* **appendic-** *or* **appendico-** *comb form* : vermiform appendix ⟨*append*ectomy⟩

ap·pend·age \ə-ˈpen-dij\ *n* : a subordinate or derivative body part; *esp* : a limb or analogous part

ap·pen·dec·to·my \ˌa-pən-ˈdek-tə-mē\ *n, pl* **-mies** : surgical removal of the vermiform appendix

ap·pen·di·ce·al \ə-ˌpen-də-ˈsē-əl\ *also* **ap·pen·di·cal** \ə-ˈpen-di-kəl\ *adj* : of, relating to, or involving the vermiform appendix ⟨∼ inflammation⟩

ap·pen·di·cec·to·my \ə-ˌpen-də-ˈsek-tə-mē\ *n, pl* **-mies** *Brit* : APPENDECTOMY

ap·pen·di·ces epi·plo·i·cae \ə-ˈpen-də-ˌsēz-ˌe-pi-ˈploi-sē\ *n pl* : small peritoneal pouches filled with fat that are situated along the large intestine

ap·pen·di·ci·tis \ə-ˌpen-də-ˈsī-təs\ *n* : inflammation of the vermiform appendix

ap·pen·dic·u·lar \ˌa-pən-'di-kyə-lər\ *adj* : of or relating to an appendage: **a** : of or relating to a limb or limbs ⟨the ∼ skeleton⟩ **b** : APPENDICEAL

ap·pen·dix \ə-'pen-diks\ *n, pl* **-dix·es** *or* **-di·ces** \-də-ˌsēz\ : a bodily outgrowth or process; *specif* : VERMIFORM APPENDIX

ap·per·ceive \ˌa-pər-'sēv\ *vb* **-ceived; -ceiv·ing** : to have apperception of

ap·per·cep·tion \ˌa-pər-'sep-shən\ *n* : mental perception; *esp* : the process of understanding something perceived in terms of previous experience — compare ASSIMILATION 3 — **ap·per·cep·tive** \-'sep-tiv\ *adj*

ap·pe·stat \'a-pə-ˌstat\ *n* : the neural center in the brain that regulates appetite and is thought to be in the hypothalamus

ap·pe·tite \'a-pə-ˌtīt\ *n* : any of the instinctive desires necessary to keep up organic life; *esp* : the desire to eat — **ap·pe·ti·tive** \-ˌtī-tiv\ *adj*

ap·pla·na·tion \ˌa-plə-'nā-shən\ *n* : abnormal flattening of a convex surface (as of the cornea of the eye)

applanation tonometer *n* : an ophthalmologic instrument used to determine intraocular pressure by measuring the force necessary to flatten an area of the cornea with a small disk

ap·pli·ance \ə-'plī-əns\ *n* : an instrument or device designed for a particular use ⟨prosthetic ∼s⟩

ap·pli·ca·tion \ˌa-plə-'kā-shən\ *n* **1** : an act of applying **2** : a medicated or protective layer or material

ap·pli·ca·tor \'a-plə-ˌkā-tər\ *n* : one that applies; *specif* : a device for applying a substance (as medicine)

ap·ply \ə-'plī\ *vb* **ap·plied; ap·ply·ing** : to lay or spread on

ap·po·si·tion \ˌa-pə-'zi-shən\ *n* **1** : the placing of things in juxtaposition or proximity; *specif* : deposition of successive layers upon those already present (as in cell walls) — compare ACCRETION **2** : the state of being in juxtaposition or proximity (as in the drawing together of cut edges of tissue in healing) — **ap·pose** \a-'pōz\ *vb* — **ap·po·si·tion·al** \ˌa-pə-'zi-shə-nəl\ *adj*

ap·proach \ə-'prōch\ *n* : the surgical procedure by which access is gained to a bodily part

approach–approach conflict *n* : psychological conflict that results when a choice must be made between two desirable alternatives — compare APPROACH-AVOIDANCE CONFLICT, AVOIDANCE-AVOIDANCE CONFLICT

approach–avoidance conflict *n* : psychological conflict that results when a goal is both desirable and undesirable — compare APPROACH-APPROACH CONFLICT, AVOIDANCE-AVOIDANCE CONFLICT

ap·prox·i·mate \ə-'präk-sə-ˌmāt\ *vb* **-mat·ed; -mat·ing** : to bring together ⟨∼ cut edges of tissue⟩

aprax·ia \(ˌ)ā-'prak-sē-ə\ *n* : loss or impairment of the ability to execute complex coordinated movements without muscular or sensory impairment — **aprac·tic** \-'prak-tik\ *or* **aprax·ic** \-'prak-sik\ *adj*

apro·ti·nin \ā-'prō-tə-nin\ *n* : a polypeptide used for its protease-inhibiting properties esp. in the treatment of pancreatitis — see TRASYLOL

APSAC \'ap-ˌsak\ *n* : ANISTREPLASE

aptha *var of* APHTHA

ap·ti·tude \'ap-tə-ˌtüd, -ˌtyüd\ *n* : a natural or acquired capacity or ability; *esp* : a tendency, capacity, or inclination to learn or understand

aptitude test *n* : a standardized test designed to predict an individual's ability to learn certain skills

apy·rex·ia \ˌā-ˌpī-'rek-sē-ə, ˌa-pə-'rek-\ *n* : absence or intermission of fever

aqua \'a-kwə, 'ä-\ *n, pl* **aquae** \'a-(ˌ)kwē, 'ä-ˌkwī\ *or* **aquas** : WATER; *esp* : an aqueous solution

aq·ue·duct \'a-kwə-ˌdəkt\ *n* : a canal or passage in a part or organ

aqueduct of Syl·vi·us \-'sil-vē-əs\ *n* : a channel connecting the third and fourth ventricles of the brain — called also *cerebral aqueduct*

Du·bois \dü-'bwä, dü-, dyü-\, **Jacques** (*Latin* **Jacobus Sylvius**) (1478–1555), French anatomist.

¹**aque·ous** \'ā-kwē-əs, 'a-\ *adj* **1 a** : of, relating to, or resembling water ⟨an ∼ vapor⟩ **b** : made from, with, or by water ⟨an ∼ solution⟩ **2** : of or relating to the aqueous humor

²**aqueous** *n* : AQUEOUS HUMOR

aqueous flare *n* : FLARE 3

aqueous humor *n* : a transparent fluid occupying the space between the crystalline lens and the cornea of the eye

Ar *symbol* argon

ara–A \ˌar-ə-'ā\ *n* : VIDARABINE

arab·i·nose \ə-'ra-bə-ˌnōs, -ˌnōz\ *n* : a white crystalline sugar $C_5H_{10}O_5$ occurring esp. in vegetable gums

ara·bi·no·side \ˌar-ə-'bi-nə-ˌsīd, ə-'ra-bə-nō-ˌsīd\ *n* : a glycoside that yields arabinose on hydrolysis

ar·a·chi·don·ic acid \ˌar-ə-kə-'dä-nik-\ *n* : a liquid unsaturated fatty acid $C_{20}H_{32}O_2$ that occurs in most animal fats, is a precursor of prostaglandins, and is considered essential in animal nutrition

arachn- *or* **arachno-** *comb form* : spider ⟨*arachno*dactyly⟩

arach·nid \ə-'rak-nəd\ *n* : any of a large class of arthropods (Arachnida) comprising mostly air-breathing invertebrates, including the spiders and scorpions, mites, and ticks, and having a segmented body divided into two regions of which the anterior bears four pairs of legs but no antennae — **arach·nid** *adj*

arach·nid·ism \-nə-ˌdi-zəm\ *n* : poisoning caused by the bite or sting of an arachnid (as a spider, tick, or scorpion); *esp* : a syndrome marked by extreme pain and muscular rigidity due to the bite of a black widow spider

arach·no·dac·ty·ly \ə-ˌrak-nō-ˈdak-tə-lē\ *n, pl* **-lies** : a hereditary condition characterized esp. by excessive length of the fingers and toes

arach·noid \ə-ˈrak-ˌnȯid\ *n* : a thin membrane of the brain and spinal cord that lies between the dura mater and the pia mater — **arachnoid** *also* **arach·noi·dal** \ə-ˌrak-ˈnȯid-ᵊl\ *adj*

arachnoid granulation *n* : any of the small whitish processes that are enlarged villi of the arachnoid membrane of the brain which protrude into the superior sagittal sinus and into depressions in the neighboring bone — called also *arachnoid villus, pacchionian body*

arach·noid·itis \ə-ˌrak-ˌnȯi-ˈdī-təs\ *n* : inflammation of the arachnoid membrane

arach·no·pho·bia \ə-ˌrak-nə-ˈfō-bē-ə\ *n* : pathological fear or loathing of spiders — **arach·no·phobe** \ə-ˈrak-nə-ˌfōb\ *n* — **arach·no·pho·bic** \-ˌrak-nə-ˈfō-bik\ *adj or n*

ar·bor \ˈär-bər\ *n* : a branching anatomical structure resembling a tree

ar·bo·ri·za·tion \ˌär-bə-rə-ˈzā-shən\ *n* : a treelike figure or arrangement of branching parts; *esp* : a treelike part or process (as a dendrite) of a nerve cell

ar·bo·rize \ˈär-bə-ˌrīz\ *vb* **-rized; -riz·ing** : to branch freely and repeatedly

ar·bo·vi·rus \ˌär-bə-ˈvī-rəs\ *n* : any of various RNA viruses (as the causative agents of Japanese B encephalitis, West Nile fever, yellow fever, and dengue) transmitted chiefly by arthropods — **ar·bo·vi·ral** \-rəl\ *adj*

ARC *abbr* 1 AIDS-related complex 2 American Red Cross

ar·cade \är-ˈkād\ *n* 1 : an anatomical structure comprising a series of arches 2 : DENTAL ARCH

arch \ˈärch\ *n* 1 : an anatomical structure that resembles an arch in form or function: as **a** : either of two vaulted portions of the bony structure of the foot that impart elasticity to it **b** : ARCH OF THE AORTA 2 : a fingerprint in which all the ridges run from side to side and make no backward turn

arch- *or* **archi-** *prefix* : primitive : original : primary ⟨*arch*enteron⟩

arch·en·ter·on \är-ˈken-tə-ˌrän, -rən\ *n, pl* **-tera** \-tə-rə\ : the cavity of the gastrula of an embryo forming a primitive gut

ar·che·type \ˈär-ki-ˌtīp\ *n* : an inherited idea or mode of thought in the psychology of C. G. Jung that is derived from the experience of the race and is present in the unconscious of the individual — **ar·che·typ·al** \ˌär-ki-ˈtī-pəl\ *adj*

ar·chi·pal·li·um \ˌär-ki-ˈpa-lē-əm\ *n* : the olfactory part of the cerebral

cortex comprising the hippocampus and part of the parahippocampal gyrus — compare NEOPALLIUM

ar·chi·tec·ton·ics \-tek-ˈtä-niks\ *n sing or pl* : the structural arrangement or makeup of an anatomical part or system — **ar·chi·tec·ton·ic** \-nik\ *adj*

ar·chi·tec·ture \ˈär-kə-ˌtek-chər\ *n* : the basic structural form esp. of a bodily part or of a large molecule — **ar·chi·tec·tur·al** \ˌär-kə-ˈtek-chə-rəl, -ˈtek-shrəl\ *adj* — **ar·chi·tec·tur·al·ly** *adv*

arch of the aorta *n* : the curved transverse part of the aorta that connects the ascending aorta with the descending aorta — called also *aortic arch*

ar·cu·ate \ˈär-kyə-wət, -ˌwāt\ *adj* : curved like a bow

arcuate artery *n* : any of the branches of the interlobar arteries of the kidney that form arches over the base of the pyramids

arcuate ligament — see LATERAL ARCUATE LIGAMENT, MEDIAL ARCUATE LIGAMENT, MEDIAN ARCUATE LIGAMENT

arcuate nucleus *n* : any of several cellular masses in the thalamus, hypothalamus, or medulla oblongata

arcuate popliteal ligament *n* : a triangular ligamentous band in the posterior part of the knee that passes medially downward from the lateral condyle of the femur to the area between the condyles of the tibia and to the head of the fibula — compare OBLIQUE POPLITEAL LIGAMENT

arcuate vein *n* : any of the veins of the kidney that accompany the arcuate arteries, drain blood from the interlobular veins, and empty into the interlobar veins

ar·cus \ˈär-kəs\ *n, pl* **arcus** : an anatomical arch

arcus se·ni·lis \-sə-ˈni-ləs\ *n* : a whitish ring-shaped or bow-shaped deposit in the cornea that frequently occurs in old age

ARDS *abbr* acute respiratory distress syndrome; adult respiratory distress syndrome

ar·ea \ˈar-ē-ə\ *n* : a part of the cerebral cortex having a particular function — see ASSOCIATION AREA, MOTOR AREA, SENSORY AREA

area po·stre·ma \-pōs-ˈtrē-mə, -päs-\ *n* : a tongue-shaped structure in the caudal region of the fourth ventricle of the brain

areata — see ALOPECIA AREATA

arec·o·line \ə-ˈre-kə-ˌlēn\ *n* : a toxic parasympathomimetic alkaloid C_8H_{13}-NO_2 that is used as a veterinary anthelmintic and occurs naturally in betel nuts

are·flex·ia \ˌā-ri-ˈflek-sē-ə\ *n* : absence of reflexes — **are·flex·ic** \-ˈflek-sik\ *adj*

ar·e·na·vi·rus \ˌar-ə-nə-ˈvī-rəs\ *n* 1 *cap* : a genus of single-stranded RNA viruses (family *Arenaviridae*) having dense lipid envelope on the virion covered by club-shaped projections and including the Machupo virus, the Junin virus, and the viruses causing lymphocytic choriomeningitis and Lassa fever **2** : any virus of the genus *Arenavirus* or of the family (*Arenaviridae*) to which it belongs

are·o·la \ə-'rē-ə-lə\ *n, pl* **-lae** \-ˌlē\ *or* **-las 1** : the colored ring around the nipple or around a vesicle or pustule **2** : the portion of the iris that borders the pupil of the eye

are·o·lar \-lər\ *adj* **1** : of, relating to, or like an areola **2** : of, relating to, or consisting of areolar tissue

areolar tissue *n* : fibrous connective tissue having the fibers loosely arranged in a net or meshwork

Ar·gas \'är-gəs, -ˌgas\ *n* : a genus of ticks (family Argasidae) including the fowl ticks (as *A. persicus*)

argent- *or* **argenti-** *or* **argento-** *comb form* : silver 〈*argento*phil〉

ar·gen·taf·fin cell \är-'jen-tə-fən-\ *or* **ar·gen·taf·fine cell** \-fən-, -ˌfēn-\ *n* : any of various specialized epithelial cells of the gastrointestinal tract that stain readily with silver salts

ar·gen·to·phil·ic \ˌär-jen-tə-'fi-lik\ *also* **ar·gen·to·phil** \-'jen-tə-ˌfil\ *or* **ar·gen·to·phile** \-ˌfil\ *adj* : ARGYROPHILIC

ar·gi·nine \'är-jə-ˌnēn\ *n* : a crystalline basic amino acid $C_6H_{14}N_4O_2$ derived from guanidine

arginine vasopressin *n* : vasopressin in which the eighth amino acid residue in its polypeptide chain is an arginine residue — abbr. *AVP*

ar·gon \'är-ˌgän\ *n* : a colorless odorless inert gaseous element — symbol *Ar;* see ELEMENT table

Ar·gyll Rob·ert·son pupil \'är-gīl-'rä-bərt-sən-, är-'gīl-\ *n* : a pupil characteristic of neurosyphilis that fails to react to light but still reacts in accommodation to distance

Robertson, Douglas Argyll (1837–1909), British ophthalmologist.

argyr- *or* **argyro-** *comb form* : silver 〈*argyr*ia〉

ar·gyr·ia \är-'jir-ē-ə\ *n* : permanent dark discoloration of skin caused by overuse of medicinal silver preparations

Ar·gy·rol \'är-jə-ˌról, -ˌról\ *trademark* — used for a silver-protein compound whose aqueous solution is used as a local antiseptic

ar·gyr·o·phil·ic \ˌär-jə-(ˌ)rō-'fi-lik, -rə-\ *also* **ar·gyr·o·phil** \ˌär-jə-(ˌ)rō-ˌfil, -rə-\ *or* **ar·gyr·o·phile** \-ˌfil\ *adj* : having an affinity for silver 〈~ cells〉

ari·bo·fla·vin·osis \ˌā-ˌrī-bə-ˌflā-və-'nō-səs\ *n, pl* **-oses** \-ˌsēz\ : a deficiency disease due to inadequate intake of riboflavin and characterized by sores on the mouth

Ar·i·cept \'ar-ə-ˌsept\ *trademark* — used for a preparation of the hydrochloride of donepezil

Arim·i·dex \ə-'ri-mə-ˌdeks\ *trademark* — used for a preparation of anastrozole

arith·mo·ma·nia \ə-ˌrith-mō-'mā-nē-ə, -nyə\ *n* : a morbid compulsion to count objects

-ar·i·um \'ar-ē-əm\ *n suffix, pl* **-ariums** *or* **-ar·ia** \-ē-ə\ : thing or place belonging to or connected with 〈sani*tarium*〉

arm \'ärm\ *n* **1** : a human upper limb; *esp* : the part between the shoulder and the wrist **2 a** : the forelimb of a vertebrate other than a human being **b** : a limb of an invertebrate animal **c** : any of the usu. two parts of a chromosome lateral to the centromere — **armed** \'ärmd\ *adj*

ar·ma·men·tar·i·um \ˌär-mə-ˌmen-'ter-ē-əm, -mən-\ *n, pl* **-tar·ia** \-ē-ə\ : the equipment and methods used esp. in medicine

arm·pit \'ärm-ˌpit\ *n* : the hollow beneath the junction of the arm and shoulder : AXILLA

Aro·ma·sin \ə-'rō-mə-ˌsin\ *trademark* — used for a preparation of exemestane

aro·ma·tase \ə-'rō-mə-ˌtās, -ˌtāz\ *n* : an enzyme or complex of enzymes that promotes the conversion of an androgen into estrogen

aromatase inhibitor *n* : any of a class of drugs (as anastrozole) that suppress the synthesis of estrogen in the body by inhibiting the action of aromatase and are used to treat breast cancer in postmenopausal women

aro·ma·ther·a·py \ə-ˌrō-mə-'ther-ə-pē\ *n, pl* **-pies** : inhalation or bodily application (as by massage) of fragrant essential oils (as from flowers and fruits) for therapeutic purposes; *broadly* : the use of aroma to enhance a feeling of well-being — **aro·ma·ther·a·pist** \-pist\ *n*

arous·al \ə-'raú-zəl\ *n* : the act of arousing : state of being aroused 〈sexual ~〉; *specif* : responsiveness to stimuli

arouse \ə-'raúz\ *vb* **aroused; arous·ing** : to rouse or stimulate to action or to physiological readiness for activity

ar·rec·tor pi·li muscle \ə-'rek-tər-'pī-ˌlī-, -'pī-lē-\ *n* : one of the small fan-shaped smooth muscles associated with the base of each hair that contract when the body surface is chilled and erect the hairs, compress an oil gland above each muscle, and produce the appearance of goose bumps

¹ar·rest \ə-'rest\ *vb* : to bring to a standstill or state of inactivity

²arrest *n* : the condition of being stopped — see CARDIAC ARREST

ar·rhe·no·blas·to·ma \ə-ˌrē-nō-ˌbla-'stō-mə, ə-ˌrē-ˌnō-\ *n, pl* **-mas** *also* **-ma·ta** \-mə-tə\ : a sometimes malignant tumor of the ovary that by the secretion of male hormone induces development of secondary male characteristics — compare GYNANDRO-BLASTOMA

ar·rhyth·mia \ə-'rith-mē-ə\ n : an alteration in rhythm of the heartbeat either in time or force

ar·rhyth·mic \-mik\ adj **1** : lacking rhythm or regularity **2** : of, relating to, characterized by, or resulting from arrhythmia ⟨∼ death⟩

ARRT abbr **1** American registered respiratory therapist **2** American Registry of Radiologic Technologists

ars- comb form : arsenic ⟨arsine⟩

ar·se·nate \'är-sə-nət, -ˌnāt\ n : a salt or ester of an arsenic acid

¹**ar·se·nic** \-nik\ n **1** : a solid poisonous element that is commonly metallic steel-gray, crystalline, and brittle — symbol As; see ELEMENT table **2** : ARSENIC TRIOXIDE

²**ar·sen·ic** \är-'se-nik\ adj : of, relating to, or containing arsenic esp. with a valence of five

arsenic acid \är-'se-nik-\ n : any of three arsenic-containing acids that are analogous to the phosphoric acids

¹**ar·sen·i·cal** \är-'se-ni-kəl\ adj : of, relating to, containing, or caused by arsenic ⟨∼ poisoning⟩

²**arsenical** n : a compound or preparation containing arsenic

ar·se·nic trioxide \'är-sə-nik-\ n : a poisonous trioxide As_2O_3 or As_4O_6 of arsenic that was formerly used in medicine and dentistry and is now used esp. as an insecticide and weed killer — called also arsenic

ar·sine \är-'sēn, 'är-\ n : a colorless flammable extremely poisonous gas AsH_3 with an odor like garlic

ars·phen·a·mine \ärs-'fe-nə-ˌmēn, -mən\ n : a toxic powder $C_{12}Cl_2H_{14}$-$As_2N_2O_2{\cdot}2H_2O$ formerly used in the treatment esp. of syphilis and yaws — called also salvarsan, six-o-six

ART abbr accredited record technician

ar·te·fact chiefly Brit var of ARTIFACT

ar·te·mis·i·nin \ˌärt-ə-'mis-ēˀn-ən\ n : an antimalarial drug $C_{15}H_{22}O_5$ obtained from the leaves of a Chinese herb (Artemisia annua) or made synthetically

ar·te·ria \är-'tir-ē-ə\ n, pl **-ri·ae** \-ē-ˌē\ : ARTERY

arteri- or **arterio-** comb form **1** : artery ⟨arteriography⟩ **2** : arterial and ⟨arteriovenous⟩

ar·te·ri·al \är-'tir-ē-əl\ adj **1** : of or relating to an artery **2** : relating to or being the bright red blood present in most arteries that has been oxygenated in lungs or gills — compare VENOUS 3 — **ar·te·ri·al·ly** adv

ar·te·rio·gram \är-'tir-ē-ə-ˌgram\ n : a radiograph of an artery made by arteriography

ar·te·ri·og·ra·phy \är-ˌtir-ē-'ä-grə-fē\ n, pl **-phies** : the radiographic visualization of an artery after injection of a radiopaque substance — **ar·te·rio·graph·ic** \-ē-ə-'gra-fik\ adj — **ar·te·rio·graph·i·cal·ly** \-fi-k(ə-)lē\ adv

ar·te·ri·o·la \är-ˌtir-ē-'ō-lə\ n, pl **-lae** \-ˌlē\ : ARTERIOLE

ar·te·ri·ole \är-'tir-ē-ˌōl\ n : any of the small terminal twigs of an artery that ends in capillaries — **ar·te·ri·o·lar** \-ˌtir-ē-'ō-ˌlär, -lər\ adj

ar·te·rio·li·tis \är-ˌtir-ē-ō-'lī-təs\ n : inflammation of the arterioles

ar·te·rio·lu·mi·nal \är-ˌtir-ē-ō-'lü-mən-ˀl\ adj : relating to or being the small vessels that branch from the arterioles of the heart and empty directly into its lumen

ar·te·ri·op·a·thy \är-ˌtir-ē-'ä-pə-thē\ n, pl **-thies** : a disease of the arteries

ar·te·ri·or·rha·phy \är-ˌtir-ē-'ȯr-ə-fē\ n, pl **-phies** : a surgical operation of suturing an artery

ar·te·rio·scle·ro·sis \är-ˌtir-ē-ō-sklə-'rō-səs\ n, pl **-ro·ses** \-ˌsēz\ : a chronic disease characterized by abnormal thickening and hardening of the arterial walls with resulting loss of elasticity — see ATHEROSCLEROSIS

arteriosclerosis ob·lit·e·rans \-ə-'bli-tə-ˌranz\ n : chronic arteriosclerosis marked by occlusion of arteries and esp. those supplying the extremities

ar·te·rio·scle·rot·ic \-'rä-tik\ adj : of, relating to, or affected with arteriosclerosis

²**arteriosclerotic** n : an arteriosclerotic individual

arteriosi — see CONUS ARTERIOSUS

ar·te·rio·si·nu·soi·dal \är-ˌtir-ē-ō-ˌsī-nyə-'sȯid-ˀl, -nə-\ adj : relating to or being the vessels that connect the arterioles and sinusoids of the heart

ar·te·rio·spasm \är-'tir-ē-ō-ˌspa-zəm\ n : spasm of an artery — **ar·te·rio·spas·tic** \-ˌtir-ē-ō-'spas-tik\ adj

arteriosum — see LIGAMENTUM ARTERIOSUM

arteriosus — see CONUS ARTERIOSUS, DUCTUS ARTERIOSUS, PATENT DUCTUS ARTERIOSUS

ar·te·ri·ot·o·my \är-ˌtir-ē-'ä-tə-mē\ n, pl **-mies** : the surgical incision of an artery

ar·te·rio·ve·nous \är-ˌtir-ē-ō-'vē-nəs\ adj : of, relating to, or connecting the arteries and veins ⟨∼ anastomoses⟩

ar·ter·i·tis \ˌär-tə-'rī-təs\ n : arterial inflammation — see GIANT CELL ARTERITIS — **ar·ter·it·ic** \-'ri-tik\ adj

ar·tery \'är-tə-rē\ n, pl **-ter·ies** : any of the tubular branching muscular- and elastic-walled vessels that carry blood from the heart through the body

arthr- or **arthro-** comb form : joint ⟨arthralgia⟩ ⟨arthropathy⟩

ar·thral·gia \är-'thral-jə, -jē-ə\ n : pain in one or more joints — **ar·thral·gic** \-jik\ adj

ar·threc·to·my \är-'threk-tə-mē\ n, pl **-mies** : surgical excision of a joint

¹**ar·thrit·ic** \är-'thri-tik\ adj : of, relating to, or affected with arthritis — **ar·thrit·i·cal·ly** \-ti-k(ə-)lē\ adv

²**arthritic** n : a person affected with arthritis

ar·thri·tis \är-'thrī-təs\ n, pl **-thrit·i·des** \-'thrī-tə-ˌdēz\ : inflammation of joints due to infectious, metabolic, or constitutional causes; *also* : a specific arthritic condition (as gouty arthritis or psoriatic arthritis)

ar·thri·tis de·for·mans \-dē-'fȯr-,manz\ *n* : a chronic arthritis marked by deformation of affected joints

ar·thro·cen·te·sis \,är-(,)thrō-sen-'tē-səs\ *n, pl* **-te·ses** \-,sēz\ : surgical puncture of a joint

ar·thro·de·sis \är-'thrä-də-səs\ *n, pl* **-e·ses** \-,sēz\ : the surgical immobilization of a joint so that the bones grow solidly together : artificial ankylosis

ar·thro·dia \är-'thrō-dē-ə\ *n, pl* **-di·ae** \-dē-,ē\ : GLIDING JOINT

ar·thro·dys·pla·sia \,är-(,)thrō-dis-'plā-zhə, -zhē-ə, -zē-ə\ *n* : abnormal development of a joint

ar·thro·gram \'är-thrō-,gram\ *n* : a radiograph of a joint made by arthrography

ar·throg·ra·phy \är-'thrä-grə-fē\ *n, pl* **-phies** : the radiographic visualization of a joint after the injection of a radiopaque substance — **ar·thro·graph·ic** \,är-thrə-'gra-fik\ *adj*

ar·thro·gry·po·sis \,är-(,)thrō-gri-'pō-səs\ *n* **1** : congenital fixation of a joint in an extended or flexed position **2** : any of a group of congenital conditions characterized by reduced mobility of multiple joints due to contractures causing fixation of the joints in extension or flexion

arthrogryposis mul·ti·plex con·gen·i·ta \-'məl-tə-,pleks-kən-'je-nə-tə\ *n* : ARTHROGRYPOSIS 2

ar·throl·o·gy \är-'thrä-lə-jē\ *n, pl* **-gies** : a science concerned with the study of joints

ar·throp·a·thy \är-'thrä-pə-thē\ *n, pl* **-thies** : a disease of a joint

ar·thro·plas·ty \'är-thrə-,plas-tē\ *n, pl* **-ties** : plastic surgery of a joint : the operative formation or restoration of a joint

ar·thro·pod \'är-thrə-,päd\ *n* : any of a phylum (Arthropoda) of invertebrate animals (as insects, arachnids, and crustaceans) that have a segmented body and jointed appendages and usu. a shell of chitin molted at intervals — **arthropod** *adj* — **ar·throp·o·dan** \är-'thrä-pəd-ᵊn\ *adj*

ar·thro·scope \'är-thrə-,skōp\ *n* : an endoscope inserted through an incision near a joint (as the knee) and used to visually examine, diagnose, and treat the interior of a joint

ar·thros·co·py \är-'thrä-skə-pē\ *n, pl* **-pies** : examination of a joint with an arthroscope; *also* : joint surgery using an arthroscope — **ar·thro·scop·ic** \,är-thrə-'skä-pik\ *adj*

ar·thro·sis \är-'thrō-səs\ *n, pl* **-ses** \-,sēz\ **1** : an articulation or line of juncture between bones **2** : a degenerative disease of a joint

ar·throt·o·my \är-'thrä-tə-mē\ *n, pl* **-mies** : incision into a joint

Ar·thus reaction \'är-thəs-, är-'tēs-\ *n* : a reaction that follows injection of an antigen into an animal in which hypersensitivity has been previously established and that involves infiltrations, edema, sterile abscesses, and in severe cases gangrene — called also *Arthus phenomenon*

Arthus, Nicolas Maurice (1862–1945), French bacteriologist and physiologist.

ar·tic·u·lar \är-'ti-kyə-lər\ *adj* : of or relating to a joint

articular capsule *n* : JOINT CAPSULE

articular cartilage *n* : cartilage that covers the articular surfaces of bones

articular disk *n* : a cartilage interposed between two articular surfaces and partially or completely separating the joint cavity into two compartments

articular process *n* : either of two processes on each side of a vertebra that articulate with adjoining vertebrae: **a** : one on each side of the neural arch that projects upward and articulates with an inferior articular process of the next more cranial vertebra — called also *superior articular process* **b** : one on each side of the neural arch that projects downward and articulates with a superior articular process of the next more caudal vertebra — called also *inferior articular process*

ar·tic·u·late \är-'ti-kyə-,lāt\ *vb* **-lat·ed; -lat·ing 1** : to unite or be united by means of a joint 〈bones that ∼ with each other〉 **2** : to arrange (artificial teeth) on an articulator

ar·tic·u·la·tion \är-,ti-kyə-'lā-shən\ *n* **1** : the action or manner in which the parts come together at a joint **2 a** : a joint between bones or cartilages in the vertebrate skeleton that is immovable when the bones are directly united, slightly movable when they are united by an intervening substance, or more or less freely movable when the articular surfaces are covered with smooth cartilage and surrounded by a joint capsule — see AMPHIARTHROSIS, DIARTHROSIS, SYNARTHROSIS **b** : a movable joint between rigid parts of any animal (as between the segments of an insect appendage) **3 a** (1) : the act of properly arranging artificial teeth (2) : an arrangement of artificial teeth **b** : OCCLUSION 2a

ar·tic·u·la·tor \är-'ti-kyə-,lā-tər\ *n* : an apparatus used in dentistry for obtaining correct articulation of artificial teeth

ar·tic·u·la·to·ry \är-'ti-kyə-lə-,tȯr-ē\ *adj* : of or relating to articulation

ar·ti·fact \'är-tə-,fakt\ *n* **1** : a product of artificial character due to usu. extraneous (as human) agency; *specif* : a product or formation in a microscopic preparation of a fixed tissue or cell that is caused by manipulation or reagents and is not indicative of actual structural relationships **2** : an electrocardiographic and electroencephalographic wave that arises from sources other than the heart or brain — **ar·ti·fac·tu·al** \ˌär-tə-'fak-chə-wəl, -shə-wəl\ *adj*

ar·ti·fi·cial \ˌär-tə-'fi-shəl\ *adj* : humanly contrived often on a natural model ⟨an ∼ limb⟩ — **ar·ti·fi·cial·ly** *adv*

artificial insemination *n* : introduction of semen into part of the female reproductive tract (as the cervical opening, uterus, or fallopian tube) by other than natural means

artificial kidney *n* : an apparatus designed to do the work of the kidney during temporary stoppage of kidney function — called also *hemodialyzer*

artificial respiration *n* : the process of restoring or initiating breathing by forcing air into and out of the lungs to establish the rhythm of inspiration and expiration — see MOUTH-TO-MOUTH

ary·ep·i·glot·tic \ˌar-ē-ˌe-pə-'glä-tik\ *adj* : relating to or linking the arytenoid cartilage and the epiglottis ⟨∼ folds⟩

¹ary·te·noid \ˌar-ə-'tē-ˌnòid, ə-'rit-ʰn-ˌòid\ *adj* **1** : relating to or being either of two small cartilages to which the vocal cords are attached and which are situated at the upper back part of the larynx **2** : relating to or being either of a pair of small muscles or an unpaired muscle of the larynx

²arytenoid *n* : an arytenoid cartilage or muscle

ary·te·noi·dec·to·my \ˌar-ə-ˌtē-ˌnòi-'dek-tə-mē, ə-ˌrit-ʰn-ˌòi-\ *n, pl* **-mies** : surgical excision of an arytenoid cartilage

ary·te·noi·do·pexy \ˌar-ə-tə-'nòi-də-ˌpek-sē, ə-ˌrit-ʰn-'òid-\ *n, pl* **-pex·ies** : surgical fixation of arytenoid muscles or cartilages

As *symbol* arsenic

AS *abbr* **1** aortic stenosis **2** arteriosclerosis

ASA *abbr* [*a*cetyl*s*alicylic *a*cid] aspirin

asa·fet·i·da *or* **asa·foet·i·da** \ˌa-sə-'fi-tə-dē, -'fe-tə-də\ *n* : the fetid gum resin of various Asian plants (genus *Ferula*) of the carrot family (Umbelliferae) that was formerly used in medicine as an antispasmodic and in folk medicine as a general prophylactic against disease

as·bes·tos \as-'bes-təs, az-\ *n* : any of several minerals that readily separate into long flexible fibers, that cause asbestosis and have been implicated as causes of certain cancers, and that have been used esp. formerly as fireproof insulating materials

as·bes·to·sis \ˌas-ˌbes-'tō-səs, ˌaz-\ *n, pl* **-to·ses** \-ˌsēz\ : a pneumoconiosis due to asbestos particles that is marked by fibrosis and scarring of lung tissue

as·ca·ri·a·sis \ˌas-kə-'rī-ə-səs\ *n, pl* **-a·ses** \-ˌsēz\ : infestation with or disease caused by ascarids

as·car·i·cid·al \ə-ˌskar-ə-'sīd-ʰl\ *adj* : capable of destroying ascarids

as·car·i·cide \ə-'skar-ə-ˌsīd\ *n* : an agent destructive of ascarids

as·ca·rid \'as-kə-rəd\ *n* : any of a family (Ascaridae) of nematode worms that are usu. parasitic in the intestines of vertebrates — see ASCARIDIA, ASCARIS — **ascarid** *adj*

As·ca·rid·ia \ˌas-kə-'ri-dē-ə\ *n* : a genus of ascarid nematode worms that include an important intestinal parasite (*A. galli*) of some domestic fowl

as·car·i·di·a·sis \ə-ˌskar-ə-'dī-ə-səs\ *n, pl* **-a·ses** : ASCARIASIS

as·car·i·do·sis \ə-ˌskar-ə-'dō-səs\ *n, pl* **-do·ses** \-ˌsēz\ : ASCARIASIS

as·ca·ris \'as-kə-rəs\ *n* **1** *cap* : a genus of ascarid nematode worms that resemble earthworms in size and superficial appearance and include one (*A. lumbricoides*) parasitic in the human intestine **2** *pl* **as·car·i·des** \ə-'skar-ə-ˌdēz\ : ASCARID

As·ca·rops \'as-kə-ˌräps\ *n* : a genus of nematode worms (family Spiruridae) including a common stomach worm (*A. strongylina*) of swine

as·cend \ə-'send\ *vb* : to move upward: as **a** : to conduct nerve impulses toward or to the brain **b** : to affect the extremities and esp. the lower limbs first and then the central nervous system

ascending aorta *n* : the part of the aorta from its origin to the beginning of the arch

ascending colon *n* : the part of the large intestine that extends from the cecum to the bend on the right side below the liver — compare DESCENDING COLON, TRANSVERSE COLON

ascending lumbar vein *n* : a longitudinal vein on each side that connects the lumbar veins and is frequently the origin of the azygos vein on the right side and of the hemiazygos vein on the left

ascending palatine artery *n* : PALATINE ARTERY 1a

Asch·heim–Zon·dek test \'äsh-ˌhīm-ˌzän-dik-, -'tsän-\ *n* : a test formerly used esp. to determine human pregnancy in its early stages on the basis of the effect of a subcutaneous injection of the patient's urine on the ovaries of an immature female mouse **Asch·heim** \'äsh-ˌhīm\, **Selmor Samuel (1878–1965)**, and **Zon·dek** \'tsòn-ˌdek\, **Bernhard (1891–1966)**, German obstetrician-gynecologists.

Asch·off body \'ä-ˌshòf-\ *n* : one of the tiny lumps in heart muscle typical of rheumatic heart disease; *also* : one of the similar but larger lumps found under the skin esp. in rheumatic fever or polyarthritis — called also *Aschoff nodule* **Aschoff, Karl Albert Ludwig (1866–1942)**, German pathologist.

as·ci·tes \ə-'sī-tēz\ *n, pl* **ascites** : abnormal accumulation of serous fluid in the spaces between tissues and organs in the cavity of the abdomen — **as·cit·ic** \-'si-tik\ adj

as·co·my·cete \ˌas-kō-'mī-ˌsēt, -ˌmī-'sēt\ n : any of a group (as class Ascomycetes or subdivision Ascomycotina) of fungi (as yeasts or molds) with spores formed in asci — **as·co·my·ce·tous** \-ˌmī-'sē-təs\ adj

ascor·bate \ə-'skór-ˌbāt, -bət\ n : a salt of ascorbic acid

ascor·bic acid \ə-'skór-bik-\ n : VITAMIN C

ASCP abbr American Society of Clinical Pathologists

as·cus \'as-kəs\ n, pl **as·ci** \'as-ˌkī, -ˌkē; 'a-ˌsī\ : the membranous oval or tubular spore case of an ascomycete

ASCVD abbr arteriosclerotic cardiovascular disease

-ase n suffix : enzyme ⟨protease⟩

asep·sis \(ˌ)ā-'sep-səs, ə-\ n, pl **asep·ses** \-ˌsēz\ **1** : the condition of being aseptic **2** : the methods of producing or maintaining an aseptic condition

asep·tic \-'sep-tik\ adj **1** : preventing infection ⟨~ techniques⟩ **2** : free or freed from pathogenic microorganisms ⟨an ~ operating room⟩ — **asep·ti·cal·ly** \-ti-k(ə-)lē\ adv

asex·u·al \(ˌ)ā-'sek-shə-wəl\ adj **1** : lacking sex or functional sexual organs **2** : produced without sexual action or differentiation ⟨~ spores⟩ — **asex·u·al·ly** adv

asexual generation n : a generation that reproduces only by asexual processes — used of organisms exhibiting alternation of a sexual and an asexual generation

asexual reproduction n : reproduction (as spore formation, fission, or budding) without union of individuals or gametes

ASHD abbr arteriosclerotic heart disease

Asian flu n : influenza that is caused by a subtype (H2N2) of the orthomyxovirus causing influenza A and that was responsible for about 70,000 deaths in the U.S. in the influenza pandemic of 1957–58 — called also Asian influenza; compare HONG KONG FLU, SPANISH FLU

Asian tiger mosquito n : a black-and-white striped Asian mosquito of the genus Aedes (A. albopictus) that transmits the causative viruses of several diseases (as dengue) and has been introduced into the U.S. — called also tiger mosquito

Asi·at·ic cholera \ˌā-zhē-'a-tik-, -zē-\ n : cholera of Asian origin that is produced by virulent strains of the causative vibrio (Vibrio cholerae)

aso·cial \(ˌ)ā-'sō-shəl\ adj : not social: as **a** : rejecting or lacking the capacity for social interaction **b** : ANTISOCIAL

as·pa·rag·i·nase \ˌas-pə-'ra-jə-ˌnās, -ˌnāz\ n : an enzyme that hydrolyzes asparagine to aspartic acid and ammonia

L-asparaginase — see entry alphabetized in the letter l

as·par·a·gine \ə-'spar-ə-ˌjēn\ n : a white crystalline amino acid $C_4H_8N_2O_3$ that is an amide of aspartic acid

as·par·tame \'as-pər-ˌtām, ə-'spär-\ n : a crystalline compound $C_{14}H_{18}N_2O_5$ that is synthesized from the amino acids phenylalanine and aspartic acid and is used as a low-calorie sweetener — see NUTRASWEET

as·par·tate \-ˌtāt\ n : a salt or ester of aspartic acid

aspartate aminotransferase n : an enzyme that promotes transfer of an amino group from glutamic acid to oxaloacetic acid and that when present in abnormally high levels in the blood is a diagnostic indication of heart attack or liver disease — called also aspartate transaminase, glutamic-oxaloacetic transaminase

as·par·tic acid \ə-'spär-tik-\ n : a crystalline amino acid $C_4H_7NO_4$ that is obtained from many proteins by hydrolysis

as·par·tyl \ə-'spär-təl, a-, -ˌtēl\ n : the bivalent radical –OCCH₂CH(NH₂)CO– of aspartic acid

as·pect \'as-ˌpekt\ n : the part of an object (as an organ) in a particular position

aspera — see LINEA ASPERA

As·per·ger's syndrome \'äs-ˌpər-gərz-\ also **As·per·ger syndrome** \-gər\ n : a developmental disorder resembling autism that is characterized by impaired social interaction, by repetitive patterns of behavior and restricted interests, by normal language and cognitive development, and often by above average performance in a narrow field against a general background of deficient functioning — called also Asperger's disorder

Asperger, Hans (1906–1980), Austrian psychiatrist.

as·per·gil·lin \ˌas-pər-'ji-lən\ n : an antibacterial substance isolated from molds of the genus Aspergillus

as·per·gil·lo·sis \ˌas-pər-(ˌ)ji-'lō-səs\ n, pl **-lo·ses** \-ˌsēz\ : infection with or disease caused (as in poultry) by molds of the genus Aspergillus

as·per·gil·lus \-'ji-ləs\ n **1** cap : a genus of ascomycetous fungi that include many common molds **2** pl **-gil·li** \-'ji-ˌlī, -(ˌ)lē\ : any fungus of the genus Aspergillus

asper·mia \ā-'spər-mē-ə\ n : inability to produce or ejaculate semen — compare AZOOSPERMIA — **asper·mic** \-mik\ adj

as·phyx·ia \as-'fik-sē-ə, əs-\ n : a lack of oxygen or excess of carbon dioxide in the body that is usu. caused by an interruption of breathing and that causes unconsciousness — **as·phyx·i·al** \-sē-əl\ adj

as·phyx·i·ant \-sē-ənt\ n : an agent (as a gas) capable of causing asphyxia

as·phyx·i·ate \-sē-ˌāt\ *vb* **-at·ed; -at·ing** **1** : to cause asphyxia in; *also* : to kill or make unconscious by inadequate oxygen, presence of noxious agents, or other obstruction to normal breathing **2** : to become asphyxiated — **as·phyx·i·a·tion** \-ˌfik-sē-ˈā-shən\ *n* — **as·phyx·i·a·tor** \-ˈfik-sē-ˌā-tər\ *n*

¹as·pi·rate \ˈas-pə-ˌrāt\ *vb* **-rat·ed; -rat·ing** **1** : to draw by suction **2** : to remove (as blood) by aspiration **3** : to take into the lungs by aspiration

²as·pi·rate \-ret\ *n* : material removed by aspiration

as·pi·ra·tion \ˌas-pə-ˈrā-shən\ *n* **1** : the act of breathing and esp. of breathing in **2** : the withdrawal of fluid or friable tissue from the body **3** : the taking of foreign matter into the lungs with the respiratory current — **as·pi·ra·tion·al** \-sh(ə-)nəl\ *adj*

as·pi·ra·tor \ˈas-pə-ˌrā-tər\ *n* : an apparatus for producing suction or moving or collecting materials by suction; *esp* : a hollow tubular instrument connected with a partial vacuum and used to remove fluid or tissue or foreign bodies from the body

as·pi·rin \ˈas-prən, -pə-rən\ *n, pl* **aspirin** *or* **aspirins** **1** : a white crystalline derivative $C_9H_8O_4$ of salicylic acid used for relief of pain and fever **2** : a tablet of aspirin

as·say \ˈaˌsā, aˈsā\ *n* **1** : examination and determination as to characteristics (as weight, measure, or quality) **2** : analysis (as of a drug) to determine the presence, absence, or quantity of one or more components — compare BIOASSAY **3** : a substance to be assayed; *also* : the tabulated result of assaying — **as·say** \aˈsā, ˈaˌsā\ *vb*

as·sim·i·la·ble \ə-ˈsi-mə-lə-bəl\ *adj* : capable of being assimilated

¹as·sim·i·late \ə-ˈsi-mə-ˌlāt\ *vb* **-lat·ed; -lat·ing** **1** : to take in and utilize as nourishment : absorb into the system **2** : to become absorbed or incorporated into the system

²as·sim·i·late \-lət, -ˌlāt\ *n* : something that is assimilated

as·sim·i·la·tion \ə-ˌsi-mə-ˈlā-shən\ *n* **1 a** : an act, process, or instance of assimilating **b** : the state of being assimilated **2** : the incorporation or conversion of nutrients into protoplasm that in animals follows digestion and absorption **3** : the process of receiving new facts or of responding to new situations in conformity with what is already available to consciousness — compare APPERCEPTION

as·sist·ed living \ə-ˌsis-təd-\ *n* : a system of housing and limited care that is designed for senior citizens who need some assistance with daily activities but do not require care in a nursing home

assisted suicide *n* : suicide committed by someone with assistance from another person; *esp* : PHYSICIAN-ASSISTED SUICIDE

as·sist·ive \ə-ˈsis-tiv\ *adj* : providing aid or assistance; *specif* : designed or intended to assist disabled persons

as·so·ci·a·tion \ə-ˌsō-sē-ˈā-shən, -shē-\ *n* **1** : something linked in memory or imagination with a thing or person **2** : the process of forming mental connections or bonds between sensations, ideas, or memories **3** : the aggregation of chemical species to form (as with hydrogen bonds) loosely bound chemical complexes — compare POLYMERIZATION — **as·so·ci·a·tion·al** \-sh(ə-)nəl\ *adj*

association area *n* : an area of the cerebral cortex considered to function in linking and coordinating the sensory and motor areas

association fiber *n* : a nerve fiber connecting different parts of the brain; *esp* : any of the fibers connecting different areas within the cortex of each cerebral hemisphere — compare PROJECTION FIBER

as·so·ci·a·tive \ə-ˈsō-shē-ˌā-tiv, -sē-; -shə-tiv\ *adj* **1** : of or relating to association esp. of ideas or images ⟨a ∼ symbol⟩ **2 a** : dependent on or characterized by association ⟨an ∼ reaction⟩ **b** : acquired by a process of learning ⟨an ∼ reflex⟩

associative learning *n* : a learning process in which discrete ideas and percepts which are experienced together become linked to one another — compare PAIRED-ASSOCIATE LEARNING

associative neuron *n* : INTERNEURON

as·sort·ment \ə-ˈsȯrt-mənt\ — see INDEPENDENT ASSORTMENT

asta·sia \ə-ˈstā-zhə, -zhē-ə\ *n* : muscular incoordination in standing — compare ABASIA — **astat·ic** \ə-ˈsta-tik\ *adj*

as·ta·tine \ˈas-tə-ˌtēn\ *n* : an unstable radioactive halogen element — symbol *At;* see ELEMENT table

as·tem·i·zole \a-ˈste-mə-ˌzōl\ *n* : an antihistamine $C_{28}H_{31}FN_4O$ now withdrawn from use because of its link to ventricular arrythmias and cardiac arrest

as·ter \ˈas-tər\ *n* : a system of microtubules arranged radially about a centriole at either end of the mitotic or meiotic spindle

astere·og·no·sis \(ˌ)ā-ˌster-ē-äg-ˈnō-səs, -ˌstir-\ *n, pl* **-no·ses** \-ˌsēz\ : loss of the ability to recognize the shapes of objects by handling them

as·te·rix·is \ˌas-tə-ˈrik-sis\ *n* : a motor disorder characterized by jerking movements (as of the outstretched hands) and associated with various encephalopathies due esp. to faulty metabolism

asthen- *or* **astheno-** *comb form* : weak ⟨*asthen*opia⟩

as·the·nia \as-ˈthē-nē-ə\ *n* : lack or loss of strength : DEBILITY

as·then·ic \as-'the-nik\ *adj* **1** : of, relating to, or exhibiting asthenia : DEBILITATED **2** : characterized by slender build and slight muscular development : ECTOMORPHIC

as·the·no·pia \,as-thə-'nō-pē-ə\ *n* : weakness or rapid fatigue of the eyes often accompanied by pain and headache — **as·the·no·pic** \-'nä-pik, -'nō-\ *adj*

asth·ma \'az-mə\ *n* : a chronic lung disorder that is marked by recurrent episodes of airway obstruction (as from bronchospasm) manifested by labored breathing accompanied by wheezing and coughing and by a sense of constriction in the chest, and that is triggered by hypersensitivity to various stimuli (as allergens or a rapid change in air temperature)

¹asth·mat·ic \az-'ma-tik\ *adj* : of, relating to, or affected with asthma ⟨an ∼ attack⟩ — **asth·mat·i·cal·ly** \-ti-k(ə-)lē\ *adv*

²asthmatic *n* : a person affected with asthma

asthmaticus — see STATUS ASTHMATICUS

asth·mo·gen·ic \,az-mə-'je-nik\ *adj* : causing asthmatic attacks

¹as·tig·mat·ic \,as-tig-'ma-tik\ *adj* : affected with, relating to, or correcting astigmatism ⟨∼ eyes⟩

²astigmatic *n* : a person affected with astigmatism

astig·ma·tism \ə-'stig-mə-,ti-zəm\ *n* **1** : a defect of an optical system (as a lens) causing rays from a point to fail to meet in a focal point resulting in a blurred and imperfect image **2** : a defect of vision due to astigmatism of the refractive system of the eye and esp. to corneal irregularity — compare EMMETROPIA, MYOPIA

as tol *abbr* as tolerated

astr- or **astro-** *comb form* **1** : star ⟨star-shaped ⟨*astro*cyte⟩ **2** : astrocyte ⟨*astro*blastoma⟩ ⟨*astro*glia⟩

astragal- or **astragalo-** *comb form* : astragalus ⟨*astragal*ectomy⟩

astrag·a·lec·to·my \ə-,stra-gə-'lek-tə-mē\ *n, pl* **-mies** : surgical removal of the astragalus

as·trag·a·lus \ə-'stra-gə-ləs\ *n, pl* **-li** \-,lī, -,lē\ : one of the proximal bones of the tarsus of the higher vertebrates — see TALUS 1

astral ray *n* : one of the thin fibrils that make up the mitotic or meiotic aster

¹as·trin·gent \ə-'strin-jənt\ *adj* : having the property of drawing together the soft organic tissues ⟨∼ cosmetic lotions⟩: **a** : tending to shrink mucous membranes or raw or exposed tissues : checking discharge (as of serum or mucus) : STYPTIC **b** : tending to pucker the tissues of the mouth ⟨∼ fruits⟩ — **as·trin·gen·cy** \-jən-sē\ *n*

²astringent *n* : an astringent agent or substance

as·tro·blas·to·ma \,as-trə-(,)blas-'tō-mə\ *n, pl* **-mas** *also* **-ma·ta** \-mə-tə\ : an astrocytoma of moderate malignancy

as·tro·cyte \'as-trə-,sīt\ *n* : a star-shaped cell; *esp* : any comparatively large much-branched neuroglial cell — **as·tro·cyt·ic** \,as-trə-'si-tik\ *adj*

as·tro·cy·to·ma \,as-trə-sī-'tō-mə\ *n, pl* **-mas** *also* **-ma·ta** \-mə-tə\ : a nerve-tissue tumor composed of astrocytes

as·tro·glia \as-'trä-glē-ə, ,as-trə-'glī-ə\ *n* : glial tissue composed of astrocytes — **as·tro·gli·al** \-əl\ *adj*

asy·lum \ə-'sī-ləm\ *n* : an institution for the relief or care of the destitute or sick and esp. the insane

asym·bo·lia \,ā-(,)sim-'bō-lē-ə\ *n* : loss of the power to understand previously familiar symbols and signs

asym·met·ri·cal \,ā-sə-'me-tri-kəl\ or **asym·met·ric** \-trik\ *adj* **1** : not symmetrical **2** *usu* **assymetric**, *of a carbon atom* : bonded to four different atoms or groups — **asym·met·ri·cal·ly** \-tri-k(ə-)lē\ *adv*

asym·me·try \(,)ā-'si-mə-trē\ *n, pl* **-tries** **1** : lack or absence of symmetry: as **a** : lack of proportion between the parts of a thing; *esp* : want of bilateral symmetry ⟨∼ in the development of the two sides of the brain⟩ **b** : lack of coordination of two parts acting in connection with one another ⟨∼ of convergence of the eyes⟩ **2** : lack of symmetry in spatial arrangement of atoms and groups in a molecule

asymp·tom·at·ic \,ā-,simp-tə-'ma-tik\ *adj* : presenting no symptoms of disease ⟨an ∼ infection⟩ — **asymp·tom·at·i·cal·ly** \-ti-k(ə-)lē\ *adv*

asyn·ap·sis \,ā-sə-'nap-səs\ *n, pl* **-ap·ses** \-,sēz\ : failure of pairing of homologous chromosomes in meiosis

asyn·clit·ism \(,)ā-'sin-klə-,ti-zəm, -'siŋ-\ *n* : presentation of the fetal head during childbirth with the axis oriented obliquely to the axial planes of the pelvis

asy·ner·gia \,ā-sə-'nər-jē-ə, -jə\ or **asyn·er·gy** \(,)ā-'si-nər-jē\ *n, pl* **-gias** or **-gies** : lack of coordination (as of muscles) — **asy·ner·gic** \,ā-sə-'nər-jik\ *adj*

asys·to·le \(,)ā-'sis-tə-(,)lē\ *n* : a condition of weakening or cessation of systole — **asys·tol·ic** \,ā-sis-'tä-lik\ *adj*

At *symbol* astatine

Ata·brine \'a-tə-brən\ *n* : a preparation of quinacrine — formerly a U.S. registered trademark

¹at·a·rac·tic \,a-tə-'rak-tik\ or **at·a·rax·ic** \-'rak-sik\ *adj* : tending to tranquilize ⟨∼ drugs⟩

²ataractic or **ataraxic** *n* : TRANQUILIZER

at·a·rax·ia \,a-tə-'rak-sē-ə\ or **at·a·raxy** \'a-tə-,rak-sē\ *n, pl* **-rax·ias** or **-rax·ies** : calmness untroubled by mental or emotional disturbance

at·a·vism \'a-tə-,vi-zəm\ *n* **1** : recurrence in an organism of a trait or character typical of an ancestral form and usu. due to genetic recombination 2 : an individual or character manifesting atavism : THROWBACK — **at·a·vis·tic** \,a-tə-'vis-tik\ *adj*

atax·ia \ə-'tak-sē-ə, (,)ā-\ *n* : an inability to coordinate voluntary muscular movements that is symptomatic of some nervous disorders — **atax·ic** \-sik\ *adj*

ataxic cerebral palsy *n* : cerebral palsy marked by hypotonic muscles and poor coordination and balance

atel- *or* **atelo-** *comb form* : defective ⟨*atelectasis*⟩

at·el·ec·ta·sis \,at-ə-¹'ek-tə-səs\ *n, pl* **-ta·ses** \-,sēz\ : collapse of the expanded lung; *also* : defective expansion of the pulmonary alveoli at birth — **at·el·ec·tat·ic** \-,ek-'ta-tik\ *adj*

ate·li·o·sis \ə-,te-lē-'ō-səs, -,tē-\ *n, pl* **-o·ses** \-,sēz\ : incomplete development; *esp* : dwarfism associated with anterior pituitary deficiencies and marked by essentially normal intelligence and proportions — compare ACHONDROPLASIA

¹**ate·li·ot·ic** \-ā-tik\ *adj* : of, relating to, or affected with ateliosis

²**ateliotic** *n* : a person affected with ateliosis

aten·o·lol \ə-'te-nə-,lòl, -,lōl\ *n* : a beta-blocker $C_{14}H_{22}N_2O_3$ used to treat hypertension — see TENORMIN

athero- *comb form* : atheroma ⟨*atherogenic*⟩

ath·er·ec·to·my \,a-thə-'rek-tə-mē\ *n, pl* **-mies** : removal of atheromatous plaque from within a blood vessel by utilizing a catheter usu. fitted with a cutting blade or grinding burr

ath·ero·gen·e·sis \,a-thə-rō-'je-nə-səs\ *n, pl* **-e·ses** \-,sēz\ : the formation of atheroma

ath·ero·gen·ic \-'je-nik\ *adj* : relating to or causing atherogenesis ⟨∼ diets⟩ — **ath·ero·ge·nic·i·ty** \-jə-'ni-sə-tē\ *n*

ath·er·o·ma \,a-thə-'rō-mə\ *n, pl* **-mas** *also* **-ma·ta** \-mə-tə\ **1** : fatty degeneration of the inner coat of the arteries **2** : an abnormal fatty deposit in an artery — **ath·er·o·ma·tous** \-'rō-mə-təs\ *adj*

ath·er·o·ma·to·sis \,a-thə-rō-mə-'tō-səs\ *n, pl* **-to·ses** \-,sēz\ : a disease characterized by atheromatous degeneration of the arteries

ath·ero·scle·ro·sis \,a-thə-rō-sklə-'rō-səs\ *n, pl* **-ro·ses** \-,sēz\ : an arteriosclerosis characterized by atheromatous deposits in and fibrosis of the inner layer of the arteries — **ath·ero·scle·rot·ic** \-sklə-'rä-tik\ *adj* — **ath·ero·scle·rot·i·cal·ly** \-i-k(ə-)lē\ *adv*

¹**ath·e·toid** \'a-thə-,tòid\ *adj* : exhibiting or characteristic of athetosis

²**athetoid** *n* : an athetoid individual

athetoid cerebral palsy *n* : cerebral palsy marked by involuntary uncontrolled writhing movements — called also *dyskinetic cerebral palsy*

ath·e·to·sis \,a-thə-'tō-səs\ *n, pl* **-to·ses** \-,sēz\ : a nervous disorder that is marked by continual slow movements esp. of the extremities and is usu. due to a brain lesion

athlete's foot *n* : ringworm of the feet — called also *tinea pedis*

ath·let·ic \ath-'le-tik\ *adj* : characterized by heavy frame, large chest, and powerful muscular development : MESOMORPHIC

athletic supporter *n* : a supporter for the genitals worn by boys and men participating in sports or strenuous activities — called also *jockstrap;* see CUP 1

ath·ro·cyte \'a-thrə-,sīt\ *n* : a cell capable of athrocytosis — **ath·ro·cyt·ic** \,a-thrə-'si-tik\ *adj*

ath·ro·cy·to·sis \,a-thrə-sī-'tō-səs\ *n, pl* **-to·ses** \-,sēz\ : the capacity of some cells (as of the proximal convoluted tubule of the kidney) to pick up foreign material and store it in granular form in the cytoplasm

athy·mic \(,)ā-'thī-mik\ *adj* : lacking a thymus

At·i·van \'at-i-,van\ *trademark* — used for a preparation of lorazepam

At·kins diet \'at-kənz-\ *n* : a weight loss program that emphasizes a diet low in carbohydrates along with little restriction on protein, fat, or total caloric intake

Atkins, Robert Coleman (1930–2003), American cardiologist and nutritionist.

atlant- *or* **atlanto-** *comb form* **1** : atlas ⟨*atlant*al⟩ **2** : atlantal and ⟨*atlanto*occipital⟩

at·lan·tal \-'lant-²l\ *adj* **1** : of or relating to the atlas **2** : ANTERIOR 1, CEPHALIC

at·lan·to·ax·i·al \ət-,lan-tō-'ak-sē-əl, at-\ *adj* : relating to or being anatomical structures that connect the atlas and the axis

at·lan·to·oc·cip·i·tal \-äk-'si-pət-²l\ *adj* : relating to or being structures (as a joint or ligament) joining the atlas and the occipital bone

at·las \'at-ləs\ *n* : the first vertebra of the neck

ATLS *trademark* — used for an instruction course for assessing patient condtion in the case of trauma

at·mo·sphere \'at-mə-,sfir\ *n* **1** : the whole mass of air surrounding the earth **2** : a unit of pressure equal to the pressure of the air at sea level or approximately 14.7 pounds per square inch (101,352 pascals) — **at·mo·spher·ic** \,at-mə-'sfir-ik, -'sfer-\ *adj*

atmospheric pressure *n* : the pressure exerted in every direction at any given point by the weight of the atmosphere

at·om \'a-təm\ *n* : the smallest particle of an element that can exist either alone or in combination — **atom·ic** \ə-'tä-mik\ *adj*

atomic cocktail *n* : a radioactive substance (as iodide of sodium) dissolved in water and administered orally to patients with cancer

atomic number *n* : the number of protons in the nucleus of an element — see ELEMENT table

atomic weight *n* : the average mass of an atom of an element as it occurs in nature — see ELEMENT table

at·om·ize \'a-tə-ˌmīz\ *vb* **-ized; -iz·ing** : to convert to minute particles or to a fine spray — **at·om·i·za·tion** \ˌa-tə-mə-'zā-shən\ *n*

at·om·iz·er \'a-tə-ˌmī-zər\ *n* : an instrument for atomizing usu. a perfume, disinfectant, or medicament

aton·ic \(ˌ)ā-'tä-nik, (ˌ)a-\ *adj* : characterized by atony ⟨an ~ bladder⟩

at·o·ny \'at-ᵊn-ē\ *or* **ato·nia** \(ˌ)ā-'tō-nē-ə\ *n, pl* **-nies** *or* **-ni·as** : lack of physiological tone esp. of a contractile organ

atopic dermatitis *n* : a chronic eczematous skin condition esp. of children marked esp. by intense itching, inflammation, and xerosis and occurring chiefly in those with a personal or familial history of atopy

at·o·py \'a-tə-pē\ *n, pl* **-pies** : a genetic disposition to develop an allergic reaction (as allergic rhinitis, asthma, or atopic dermatitis) and produce elevated levels of IgE upon exposure to an environmental antigen and esp. one inhaled and ingested — **ato·pic** \(ˌ)ā-'tä-pik, -'tō-\ *adj*

ator·va·stat·in \ə-ˌtór-və-'sta-tᵊn\ *n* : a statin that is administered orally in the form of its hydrated calcium salt $(C_{33}H_{34}FN_2O_5)_2Ca·3H_2O$ to lower lipid levels in the blood — see LIPITOR

ATP \ˌā-(ˌ)tē-'pē\ *n* : a phosphorylated nucleotide $C_{10}H_{16}N_5O_{13}P_3$ composed of adenosine and three phosphate groups that supplies energy for many biochemical cellular processes by undergoing enzymatic hydrolysis esp. to ADP — called also *adenosine triphosphate*

ATPase \ˌā-(ˌ)tē-'pē-ˌās, -ˌāz\ *n* : an enzyme that hydrolyzes ATP; *esp* : one that hydrolyzes ATP to ADP and inorganic phosphate — called also *adenosine triphosphatase*

atre·sia \ə-'trē-zhə\ *n* **1** : absence or closure of a natural passage of the body ⟨~ of the small intestine⟩ **2** : absence or disappearance of an anatomical part (as an ovarian follicle) by degeneration — **atret·ic** \ə-'tre-tik\ *adj*

atri- *or* **atrio-** *comb form* **1** : atrium ⟨*atri*al⟩ **2** : atrial and ⟨*atrio*ventricular⟩

atria *pl of* ATRIUM

atri·al \'ā-trē-əl\ *adj* : of, relating to, or affecting an atrium ⟨~ disorders⟩

atrial fibrillation *n* : very rapid uncoordinated contractions of the atria of the heart resulting in a lack of synchronism between heartbeat and pulse beat — called also *auricular fibrillation*

atrial flutter *n* : an irregularity of the heartbeat in which the contractions of the atrium exceed in number those of the ventricle — called also *auricular flutter*

atrial natriuretic peptide *n* : a peptide hormone secreted by the cardiac atria that promotes salt and water excretion and lowers blood pressure — called also *atrial natriuretic factor*

atrial septum *n* : INTERATRIAL SEPTUM

atrich·ia \ā-'tri-kē-ə, ə-\ *n* : congenital or acquired baldness : ALOPECIA

atrio·ven·tric·u·lar \ˌā-trē-(ˌ)ō-ˌven-'tri-kyə-lər\ *adj* **1** : of, relating to, or situated between an atrium and ventricle **2** : of, involving, or being the atrioventricular node

atrioventricular bundle *n* : BUNDLE OF HIS

atrioventricular canal *n* : the canal joining the atrium and ventricle in the tubular embryonic heart

atrioventricular node *n* : a small mass of tissue that is situated in the wall of the right atrium adjacent to the septum between the atria and passes impulses received from the sinoatrial node to the ventricles by way of the bundle of His

atrioventricular valve *n* : a valve between an atrium and ventricle of the heart: **a** : MITRAL VALVE **b** : TRICUSPID VALVE

atri·um \'ā-trē-əm\ *n, pl* **atria** \-trē-ə\ *also* **atri·ums** : an anatomical cavity or passage; *esp* : a chamber of the heart that receives blood from the veins and forces it into a ventricle or ventricles

At·ro·pa \'a-trə-pə\ *n* : a genus of Eurasian and African herbs (as belladonna) of the nightshade family (Solanaceae) that are a source of medicinal alkaloids (as atropine)

atro·phic \(ˌ)ā-'trō-fik, ə-, -'trä-\ *adj* : relating to or characterized by atrophy ⟨an ~ jaw⟩

atrophicans — see ACRODERMATITIS CHRONICA ATROPHICANS

atrophic rhinitis *n* **1** : a disease of swine that is characterized by purulent inflammation of the nasal mucosa, atrophy of the nasal conchae, and abnormal swelling of the face **2** : OZENA

atrophicus — see LICHEN SCLEROSUS ET ATROPHICUS

atrophic vaginitis *n* : inflammation of the vagina with thinning of the epithelial lining that occurs following menopause and is due to a deficiency of estrogen

¹**at·ro·phy** \'a-trə-fē\ *n, pl* **-phies** : decrease in size or wasting away of a body part or tissue; *also* : arrested development or loss of a part or organ incidental to the normal development or life of an animal or plant

²**atrophy** \'a-trə-fē, -ˌfī\ *vb* **-phied; -phy·ing** : to undergo or cause to undergo atrophy

at·ro·pine \'a-trə-ˌpēn\ *n* : a racemic mixture of hyoscyamine usu. obtained from belladonna and related plants (family Solanaceae) and used esp. in the form of its hydrated sulfate ($C_{17}H_{23}NO_3)_2·H_2SO_4·H_2O$ for its anticholinergic effects (as pupil dilation or relief of smooth muscle spasms)

at·ro·pin·ism \ˌrpē-ˌni-zəm\ *n* : poisoning by atropine

at·ro·pin·iza·tion \ˌa-trə-ˌpē-nə-'zā-shən\ *n* : the physiological condition of being under the influence of atropine — **at·ro·pin·ize** \'a-trə-pə-ˌnīz\ *vb*

at·ro·scine \'a-trə-ˌsēn, -ˌsən\ *n* : racemic scopolamine

at·tach·ment \ə-'tach-mənt\ *n* : the physical connection by which one thing is attached to another — **at·tach** \ə-'tach\ *vb*

¹at·tack \ə-'tak\ *vb* : to begin to affect or to act on injuriously

²attack *n* : a fit of sickness; *esp* : an active episode of a chronic or recurrent disease

at·tempt·er \ə-'tem(p)-tər\ *n* : one who attempts suicide

at·tend \ə-'tend\ *vb* : to visit or stay with professionally as a physician or nurse

¹at·tend·ing \ə-'ten-diŋ\ *adj* : serving as a physician or surgeon on the staff of a hospital, regularly visiting and treating patients, and often supervising students, fellows, and the house staff

²attending *n* : an attending physician or surgeon

at·ten·tion \ə-'ten-chən\ *n* **1** : the act or state of attending : the application of the mind to any object of sense or thought **2 a** : an organismic condition of selective awareness or perceptual receptivity **b** : the process of focusing consciousness to produce greater vividness and clarity of certain of its contents relative to others — **at·ten·tion·al** \-'ten-chə-nəl\ *adj*

attention deficit disorder *n* : a syndrome of disordered learning and disruptive behavior that is not caused by any serious underlying physical or mental disorder and that has several subtypes characterized primarily by symptoms of inattention or primarily by symptoms of hyperactivity and impulsive behavior (as speaking out of turn) or by the significant expression of all three — abbr. *ADD*; called also **minimal brain dysfunction**

attention–deficit/hyperactivity disorder *n* : ATTENTION DEFICIT DISORDER

at·ten·u·ate \ə-'ten-yə-ˌwāt\ *vb* **-at·ed; -at·ing** : to reduce the severity of (a disease) or virulence or vitality of (a pathogenic agent) ⟨a procedure to ~ severe diabetes⟩ ⟨*attenuated* bacilli⟩

at·ten·u·a·tion \ə-ˌten-yə-'wā-shən\ *n* : a decrease in the pathogenicity or vitality of a microorganism or in the severity of a disease

at·tic \'a-tik\ *n* : the small upper space of the middle ear — called also *epitympanic recess*

at·ti·co·to·my \ˌa-tə-'kä-tə-mē\ *n, pl* **-mies** : surgical incision of the tympanic attic

at·ti·tude \'a-tə-ˌtüd, -ˌtyüd\ *n* **1** : the arrangement of the parts of the body : POSTURE **2 a** : a mental position with regard to a fact or state **b** : a feeling or emotion toward a fact or state **3** : an organismic state of readiness to respond in a characteristic way to a stimulus (as an object, concept, or situation)

at·ti·tu·di·nal \ˌa-tə-'tüd-ᵊn-əl, -'tyüd-\ *adj* : relating to, based on, or expressive of personal attitudes or feelings

at·tri·tion \ə-'tri-shən\ *n* : the act of rubbing together; *also* : the act of wearing or grinding down by friction ⟨~ of teeth⟩

atyp·ia \(ˌ)ā-'ti-pē-ə\ *n* : ATYPISM

atyp·i·cal \(ˌ)ā-'ti-pi-kəl\ *adj* : not typical : not like the usual or normal type — **atyp·i·cal·ly** \-pi-k(ə-)lē\ *adv*

atypical pneumonia *n* : PRIMARY ATYPICAL PNEUMONIA

atyp·ism \(ˌ)ā-'tī-ˌpi-zəm\ *n* : the condition of being uncharacteristic or lacking uniformity

Au *symbol* [L *aurum*] gold

au·di·ble \'ò-də-bəl\ *adj* : heard or capable of being heard — **au·di·bil·i·ty** \ˌò-də-'bi-lə-tē\ *n* — **au·di·bly** \'ò-də-blē\ *adv*

¹au·dile \'ò-ˌdīl\ *n* : a person whose mental imagery is auditory rather than visual or motor — compare TACTILE, VISUALIZER

²audile *adj* **1** : of or relating to hearing : AUDITORY **2** : of, relating to, or being an audile

audio- *comb form* **1** : hearing ⟨*audiol*ogy⟩ **2** : sound ⟨*audiogenic*⟩

au·dio·gen·ic \ˌò-dē-ō-'je-nik\ *adj* : produced by frequencies corresponding to sound waves — used esp. of epileptoid responses ⟨~ seizures⟩

au·dio·gram \'ò-dē-ō-ˌgram\ *n* : a graphic representation of the relation of vibration frequency and the minimum sound intensity for hearing

au·di·ol·o·gist \ˌò-dē-'ä-lə-jist\ *n* : a specialist in audiology

au·di·ol·o·gy \ˌò-dē-'ä-lə-jē\ *n, pl* **-gies** : a branch of science dealing with hearing; *specif* : therapy of individuals having impaired hearing — **au·di·o·log·i·cal** \-dē-ə-'lä-ji-kəl\ *also* **au·di·o·log·ic** \-dē-ə-'lä-jik\ *adj*

au·di·om·e·ter \ˌò-dē-'ä-mə-tər\ *n* : an instrument used in measuring the acuity of hearing

au·di·om·e·try \ˌò-dē-'ä-mə-trē\ *n, pl* **-tries** : the testing and measurement of hearing acuity for variations in sound intensity and pitch and for tonal purity — **au·dio·met·ric** \-ō-'me-trik\ *adj* — **au·di·om·e·trist** \-'ä-mə-trist\ *n*

au·di·to·ry \'ȯ-də-ˌtōr-ē\ *adj* **1** : of or relating to hearing **2** : attained, experienced, or produced through or as if through hearing ⟨~ images⟩ ⟨~ hallucinations⟩ **3** : marked by great susceptibility to impressions and reactions produced by acoustic stimuli

auditory canal *n* — either of two passages of the ear — called also *acoustic meatus, auditory meatus;* compare EXTERNAL AUDITORY CANAL, INTERNAL AUDITORY CANAL

auditory cortex *n* : a sensory area of the temporal cortex associated with the organ of hearing — called also *auditory area, auditory center*

auditory nerve *n* : either of the eighth pair of cranial nerves connecting the inner ear with the brain, transmitting impulses concerned with hearing and balance, and composed of the cochlear nerve and the vestibular nerve — called also *acoustic nerve, auditory, eighth cranial nerve, vestibulocochlear nerve*

auditory processing disorder *n* : CENTRAL AUDITORY PROCESSING DISORDER

auditory tube *n* : EUSTACHIAN TUBE

Auer·bach's plexus \'aủ-ər-ˌbäks-, -ˌbäks-\ *n* : MYENTERIC PLEXUS

 Auer·bach \'aủ-ər-ˌbäk, -ˌbäk\, **Leopold (1828–1897),** German anatomist.

aug·ment \ȯg-ˈment, 'ȯg-ˌment\ *vb* : to increase in size, amount, degree, or severity — **aug·men·ta·tion** \ˌȯg-mən-ˈtā-shən, -ˌmen-\ *n*

Aug·men·tin \ȯg-ˈmen-tᵊn\ *trademark* — used for a preparation of amoxicillin and the potassium salt of clavulanic acid

aur- *or* **auri-** *comb form* : ear ⟨*aural*⟩

au·ra \'ȯr-ə\ *n, pl* **auras** *also* **au·rae** \-ē\ : a subjective sensation (as of voices or colored lights) experienced before an attack of some disorders (as epilepsy or migraine)

au·ral \'ȯr-əl\ *adj* : of or relating to the ear or to the sense of hearing — **au·ral·ly** *adv*

Au·reo·my·cin \ˌȯr-ē-ō-ˈmī-sən\ *trademark* — used for a preparation of the hydrochloride of chlortetracycline

au·ri·cle \'ȯr-i-kəl\ *n* **1 a** : PINNA **b** : an atrium of the heart **2** : an angular or ear-shaped anatomical lobe or process

au·ric·u·la \ȯ-ˈri-kyủ-lə\ *n, pl* **-lae** \-ˌlē\ : AURICLE; *esp* : AURICULAR APPENDAGE

au·ric·u·lar \ȯ-ˈri-kyủ-lər\ *adj* **1** : of, relating to, or using the ear or the sense of hearing **2** : understood or recognized by the sense of hearing **3** : of or relating to an auricle or auricular appendage ⟨~ fibrillation⟩

auricular appendage *n* : an ear-shaped pouch projecting from each atrium of the heart — called also *auricular appendix*

auricular artery — see POSTERIOR AURICULAR ARTERY

auricular fibrillation *n* : ATRIAL FIBRILLATION

auricular flutter *n* : ATRIAL FLUTTER

au·ric·u·lar·is \ȯ-ˌri-kyủ-ˈlar-əs, -ˈlär-\ *n, pl* **-lar·es** \-ˌēz\ : any of three muscles attached to the cartilage of the external ear that assist in moving the scalp and in some individuals the external ear itself and that consist of one that is anterior, one superior, and one posterior in position — called also respectively *auricularis anterior, auricularis superior, auricularis posterior*

auricular tubercle of Darwin *n* : DARWIN'S TUBERCLE

auricular vein — see POSTERIOR AURICULAR VEIN

auriculo- *comb form* : of or belonging to an auricle of the heart and ⟨*auriculo*ventricular⟩

au·ric·u·lo·tem·po·ral nerve \ȯ-ˌri-kyủ-(ˌ)lō-ˈtem-pə-rəl-\ *n* : the branch of the mandibular nerve that supplies sensory fibers to the skin of the external ear and temporal region and autonomic fibers from the otic ganglion to the parotid gland

au·ric·u·lo·ven·tric·u·lar \-ven-ˈtri-kyủ-lər, -vən-\ *adj* : ATRIOVENTRICULAR

au·ro·thio·glu·cose \ˌȯr-ō-ˌthī-ō-ˈglü-ˌkōs, -ˌkōz\ *n* : GOLD THIOGLUCOSE

aus·cul·ta·tion \ˌȯ-skəl-ˈtā-shən\ *n* : the act of listening to sounds arising within organs (as the lungs or heart) as an aid to diagnosis and treatment — **aus·cul·tate** \'ȯ-skəl-ˌtāt\ *vb* — **aus·cul·ta·to·ry** \ȯ-ˈskəl-tə-ˌtōr-ē\ *adj*

Aus·tra·lia antigen \ȯ-ˈstrāl-yə-\ *also* **Aus·tra·lian antigen** \-yən-\ *n* : HEPATITIS B SURFACE ANTIGEN

aut- *or* **auto-** *comb form* : self : same one ⟨*autism*⟩ **a** : of, by, affecting, from, or for the same individual ⟨*auto*graft⟩ ⟨*auto*transfusion⟩ **b** : arising or produced within the individual and acting or directed toward or against the individual or the individual's own body, tissues, or molecules ⟨*auto*immunity⟩ ⟨*auto*suggestion⟩

au·ta·coid \'ȯ-tə-ˌkȯid\ *n* : a physiologically active substance (as serotonin, bradykinin, or angiotensin) produced by and acting within the body

au·tism \'ȯ-ˌti-zəm\ *n* : a developmental disorder that appears by age three and that is variable in expression but is recognized and diagnosed by impairment of the ability to form normal social relationships, by impairment of the ability to communicate with others, and by stereotyped behavior patterns esp. as exhibited by a preoccupation with repetitive activities of restricted focus rather than with flexible and imaginative ones

¹au·tis·tic \ȯ-ˈtis-tik\ *adj* : of, relating to, or marked by autism ⟨~ behavior⟩

²**autistic** n : a person affected with autism

au·to·ag·glu·ti·na·tion \ˌȯ-tō-ə-ˌglüt-ᵊn-ˈā-shən\ n : agglutination of red blood cells by cold agglutinins in an individual's own serum usu. at lower than body temperature

au·to·ag·glu·ti·nin \ə-ˈglüt-ᵊn-ən\ n : an antibody that agglutinates the red blood cells of the individual producing it — compare COLD AGGLUTININ

Au·to·an·a·lyz·er \ˌȯ-tō-ˈan-ᵊl-ˌī-zər\ trademark — used for an instrument designed for automatic chemical analysis (as of blood glucose level)

au·to·an·ti·body \ˌȯ-(ˌ)tō-ˈan-ti-ˌbä-dē\ n, pl **-bod·ies** : an antibody active against a tissue constituent of the individual producing it

au·to·an·ti·gen \ˌȯ-tō-ˈan-ti-jen\ n : an antigen that is a normal bodily constituent and against which the immune system produces autoantibodies — **au·to·an·ti·gen·ic** \-ˌan-ti-ˈjen-ik\ adj

au·toch·tho·nous \(ˌ)ȯ-ˈtäk-thə-nəs\ adj 1 a : indigenous or endemic to a region 〈∼ malaria〉 b : contracted in the area where reported 2 : originated in that part of the body where found — used chiefly of pathological conditions — **au·toch·tho·nous·ly** adv

au·to·clav·able \ˈȯ-tə-ˌklā-və-bəl\ adj : able to withstand the action of an autoclave — **au·to·clav·abil·i·ty** \ˌȯ-tə-ˌklā-və-ˈbi-lə-tē\ n

au·to·clave \ˈȯ-tō-ˌklāv\ n : an apparatus (as for sterilizing) using superheated steam under pressure — **autoclave** vb

au·to·crine \ˈȯ-tō-ˌkrin\ adj : of, relating to, promoted by, or being a substance secreted by a cell and acting on surface receptors of the same cell 〈∼ growth of cancer〉 — compare PARACRINE

au·to·erot·ism \ˌȯ-tō-ˈer-ə-ˌti-zəm\ or **au·to·erot·i·cism** \-i-ˈrä-tə-ˌsi-zəm\ n 1 : sexual gratification obtained solely through stimulation by oneself of one's own body 2 : sexual feeling arising without known external stimulation — **au·to·erot·ic** \-i-ˈrä-tik\ adj — **au·to·erot·i·cal·ly** \-ti-k(ə-)lē\ adv

au·to·gen·ic \ˌȯ-tə-ˈje-nik\ adj 1 : AUTOGENOUS 2 : of or relating to any of several relaxation techniques that actively involve the patient (as by meditation or biofeedback) in attempts to control physiological variables (as blood pressure)

au·tog·e·nous \ȯ-ˈtä-jə-nəs\ adj 1 : produced independently of external influence or aid : ENDOGENOUS 2 : originating or derived from sources within the same individual 〈an ∼ graft〉 〈∼ vaccine〉

au·to·graft \ˈȯ-tō-ˌgraft\ n : a tissue or organ that is transplanted from one part to another part of the same body — **autograft** vb

au·to·he·mo·ly·sin \ˌȯ-tō-ˌhē-mə-ˈlīs-ᵊn\ n : a hemolysin that acts on the red blood cells of the individual in whose blood it is found

au·to·he·mo·ly·sis \-hi-ˈmä-lə-səs, -ˌhē-mə-ˈlī-səs\ n, pl **-ly·ses** \-ˌsēz\ : hemolysis of red blood cells by factors in the serum of the person from whom the blood is taken

au·to·he·mo·ther·a·py \-ˌhē-mō-ˈther-ə-pē\ n, pl **-pies** : treatment of disease by modification (as by irradiation) of the patient's own blood or by its introduction (as by intramuscular injection) outside the bloodstream

au·to·hyp·no·sis \ˌȯ-tō-hip-ˈnō-səs\ n, pl **-no·ses** \-ˌsēz\ : self-induced and usu. automatic hypnosis — **au·to·hyp·not·ic** \-ˈnä-tik\ adj

au·to·im·mune \-i-ˈmyün\ adj : of, relating to, or caused by antibodies or T cells that attack molecules, cells, or tissues of the organism producing them 〈∼ diseases〉

au·to·im·mu·ni·ty \ˌȯ-tō-i-ˈmyü-nə-tē\ n, pl **-ties** : a condition in which the body produces an immune response against its own tissue constituents — **au·to·im·mu·ni·za·tion** \-ˌi-myə-nə-ˈzā-shən also i-ˌmyü-nə-\ n — **au·to·im·mu·nize** \-ˈi-myə-ˌnīz\ vb

au·to·in·fec·tion \-in-ˈfek-shən\ n : reinfection with larvae produced by parasitic worms already in the body — compare HYPERINFECTION

au·to·in·oc·u·la·tion \-i-ˌnä-kyə-ˈlā-shən\ n 1 : inoculation with vaccine prepared from material from one's own body 2 : spread of infection from one part to other parts of the same body — **au·to·in·oc·u·la·ble** \ˌȯ-tō-i-ˈnä-kyə-lə-bəl\ adj

au·to·ki·ne·sis \ˌȯ-tō-kə-ˈnē-səs, -kī-\ n, pl **-ne·ses** \-ˌsēz\ : spontaneous or voluntary movement

au·tol·o·gous \ȯ-ˈtä-lə-gəs\ adj 1 : derived from the same individual 〈∼ grafts〉 — compare HETEROLOGOUS 1, HOMOLOGOUS 2 : involving one individual as both donor and recipient (as of blood) 〈∼ transfusion〉

au·tol·y·sate \ȯ-ˈtä-lə-ˌsāt, -ˌzāt\ also **au·tol·y·zate** \-ˌzāt\ n : a product of autolysis

au·tol·y·sin \-lə-sən\ n : a substance that produces autolysis

au·tol·y·sis \-lə-səs\ n, pl **-y·ses** \-lə-ˌsēz\ : breakdown of all or part of a cell or tissue by self-produced enzymes — **au·to·lyt·ic** \ˌȯt-ᵊl-ˈi-tik\ adj — **au·to·lyze** \ˈȯt-ᵊl-ˌīz\ vb

au·tom·a·tism \ȯ-ˈtä-mə-ˌti-zəm\ n 1 : an automatic action; esp : any action performed without the doer's intention or awareness 2 : the power or fact of moving or functioning without conscious control either independently of external stimulation (as in the beating of the heart) or more or less directly under the influence of external stimuli (as in the dilating or contracting of the pupil of the eye)

au·to·nom·ic \ˌȯ-tə-ˈnä-mik\ *adj* **1 a** : acting or occurring involuntarily ⟨∼ reflexes⟩ **b** : relating to, affecting, or controlled by the autonomic nervous system ⟨∼ ganglia⟩ **2** : having an effect upon tissue supplied by the autonomic nervous system ⟨∼ drugs⟩ — **au·to·nom·i·cal·ly** \-mi-k(ə-)lē\ *adv*

autonomic nervous system *n* : a part of the vertebrate nervous system that innervates smooth and cardiac muscle and glandular tissues and governs involuntary actions (as secretion, vasoconstriction, or peristalsis) and that consists of the sympathetic nervous system and the parasympathetic nervous system — compare CENTRAL NERVOUS SYSTEM, PERIPHERAL NERVOUS SYSTEM

au·ton·o·my \ȯ-ˈtä-nə-mē\ *n, pl* **-mies 1** : the quality or state of being independent, free, and self-directing **2** : independence from the organism as a whole in the capacity of a part for growth, reactivity, or responsiveness — **au·ton·o·mous** \-məs\ *adj* — **au·ton·o·mous·ly** *adv*

au·to·pro·throm·bin \ˌȯ-tō-prō-ˈthräm-bən\ *n* : any of several blood factors formed in the conversion of prothrombin to thrombin: as **a** : FACTOR VII — called also *autoprothrombin I* **b** : FACTOR IX — called also *autoprothrombin II*

¹au·top·sy \ˈȯ-ˌtäp-sē, -təp-\ *n, pl* **-sies** : an examination of the body after death usu. with such dissection as will expose the vital organs for determining the cause of death or the character and extent of changes produced by disease — called also *necropsy, postmortem, postmortem examination*

²autopsy *vb* **-sied; -sy·ing** : to perform an autopsy on

au·to·ra·dio·gram \ˌȯ-tō-ˈrā-dē-ə-ˌgram\ *n* : AUTORADIOGRAPH

au·to·ra·dio·graph \-ˌgraf\ *n* : an image produced on a photographic film or plate by the radiations from a radioactive substance in an object which is in close contact with the emulsion — called also *radioautogram, radioautograph* — **autoradiograph** *vb* — **au·to·ra·dio·graph·ic** \-ˌrā-dē-ə-ˈgra-fik\ *adj* — **au·to·ra·di·og·ra·phy** \-ˌrā-dē-ˈä-grə-fē\ *n*

au·to·re·ac·tive \ˌȯ-tō-rē-ˈak-tiv\ *adj* : produced by an organism and acting against its own cells or tissues ⟨∼ T cells⟩

au·to·reg·u·la·tion \ˌȯ-tō-ˌre-gyə-ˈlā-shən\ *n* : the maintenance of relative constancy of a physiological process by a bodily part or system under varying conditions; *esp* : the maintenance of a constant supply of blood to an organ in spite of varying arterial pressure — **au·to·reg·u·late** \-ˈre-gyə-ˌlāt\ *vb* — **au·to·reg·u·la·to·ry** \-ˈre-gyə-lə-ˌtōr-ē\ *adj*

au·to·sen·si·ti·za·tion \ˌȯ-tō-ˌsen-sə-tə-ˈzā-shən\ *n* : AUTOIMMUNIZATION

au·to·some \ˈȯ-tə-ˌsōm\ *n* : a chromosome other than a sex chromosome — **au·to·so·mal** \ˌȯ-tə-ˈsō-məl\ *adj* — **au·to·so·mal·ly** *adv*

au·to·sug·ges·tion \-səg-ˈjes-chən, -jesh-\ *n* : an influencing of one's own attitudes, behavior, or physical condition by mental processes other than conscious thought : SELF-HYPNOSIS — **au·to·sug·gest** \-səg-ˈjest\ *vb*

au·to·ther·a·py \ˈȯ-tō-ˌther-ə-pē\ *n, pl* **-pies** : SELF-TREATMENT

au·to·top·ag·no·sia \ˌȯ-tō-ˌtä-pig-ˈnō-zhə\ *n* : loss of the power to recognize or orient a bodily part due to a brain lesion

autotoxicus — see HORROR AUTOTOXICUS

au·to·trans·fu·sion \-trans-ˈfyü-zhən\ *n* : return of autologous blood to the patient's own circulatory system — **au·to·trans·fuse** \-trans-ˈfyüz\ *vb*

au·to·trans·plant \-ˈtrans-ˌplant\ *n* : AUTOGRAFT — **au·to·trans·plant** \-trans-ˈ\ *vb* — **au·to·trans·plan·ta·tion** \-ˌtrans-ˌplan-ˈtā-shən\ *n*

au·to·troph \ˈȯ-tə-ˌtrōf, -ˌträf\ *n* : an autotrophic organism

au·to·tro·phic \ˌȯ-tə-ˈtrō-fik\ *adj* **1** : needing only carbon dioxide or carbonates as a source of carbon and a simple inorganic nitrogen compound for metabolic synthesis **2** : not requiring a specified exogenous factor for normal metabolism — **au·to·tro·phi·cal·ly** \-fi-k(ə-)lē\ *adv* — **au·tot·ro·phy** \ˈȯ-tə-ˌtrō-fē, ȯ-ˈtä-trə-fē\ *n*

au·to·vac·ci·na·tion \ˌȯ-tō-ˌvak-sə-ˈnā-shən\ *n* : vaccination of an individual by material from the individual's own body or with a vaccine prepared from such material

au·tumn cro·cus \ˌȯ-təm-ˈkrō-kəs\ *n* : an herb (*Colchicum autumnale*) of the lily family (Liliaceae) that is the source of medicinal colchicum

¹aux·il·ia·ry \ȯg-ˈzil-yə-rē, -ˈzi-lə-rē, -ˈzil-rē\ *adj* : serving to supplement or assist ⟨∼ springs in a dental appliance⟩

²auxiliary *n* **1** : one who assists or serves another person esp. in dentistry **2** : an organization that assists (as by donations or volunteer services) the work esp. of a hospital

auxo·troph \ˈȯk-sə-ˌtrōf, -ˌträf\ *n* : an auxotrophic strain or individual

auxo·tro·phic \ˌȯk-sə-ˈtrō-fik\ *adj* : requiring a specific growth substance beyond the minimum required for normal metabolism and reproduction of the parental or wild-type strain ⟨∼ mutants of bacteria⟩ — **aux·ot·ro·phy** \ȯk-ˈsä-trə-fē\ *n*

AV *abbr* **1** arteriovenous **2** atrioventricular

Avan·dia \ə-ˌvan-ˈdē-ə\ *trademark* — used for a preparation of the maleate of rosiglitazone

avas·cu·lar \(ˌ)ā-ˈvas-kyə-lər\ *adj* : having few or no blood vessels ⟨∼

tissue⟩ — **avas·cu·lar·i·ty** \-ˌvas-kyə-ˈlar-ə-tē\ n

avascular necrosis n : necrosis of bone tissue due to impaired or disrupted blood supply (as that caused by traumatic injury or disease) resulting in weakened bone that may flatten and collapse — called also *osteonecrosis*

Aven·tyl \ˈä-vən-ˌtil\ trademark — used for a preparation of nortriptyline

aver·sion \ə-ˈvər-zhən, -shən\ n 1 : a feeling of repugnance toward something with a desire to avoid or turn from it 2 : a tendency to extinguish a behavior or to avoid a thing or situation and esp. a usu. pleasurable one because it is or has been associated with a noxious stimulus

aversion therapy n : therapy intended to suppress an undesirable habit or behavior (as smoking or overeating) by associating the habit or behavior with a noxious or punishing stimulus (as an electric shock)

aver·sive \ə-ˈvər-siv, -ziv\ adj : tending to avoid or causing avoidance of a noxious or punishing stimulus ⟨behavior modification by ∼ conditioning⟩ — **aver·sive·ly** adv — **aver·sive·ness** n

avi·an flu \ˈā-vē-ən-\ n : BIRD FLU

avian influenza n : BIRD FLU

avian tuberculosis n : tuberculosis of birds usu. caused by a bacterium of the genus *Mycobacterium* (M. avium); *also* : infection of mammals (as swine) by the same bacterium

avi·din \ˈä-və-din\ n : a protein found in egg white that inactivates biotin by combining with it

avir·u·lent \(ˌ)ā-ˈvir-ə-lənt, -ˈvir-yə-\ adj : not virulent ⟨an ∼ tubercle bacillus⟩

avis — see CALCAR AVIS

avi·ta·min·osis \ˌā-ˌvī-tə-mə-ˈnō-səs\ n, pl -**o·ses** \-ˌsēz\ : disease (as pellagra) resulting from a deficiency of one or more vitamins — called also *hypovitaminosis* — **avi·ta·min·ot·ic** \-mə-ˈnä-tik\ adj

A–V node or **AV node** \ˌā-ˈvē-\ n : ATRIOVENTRICULAR NODE

avoid·ance \ə-ˈvȯid-ᵊns\ n, often attrib : the act or practice of keeping away from or withdrawing from something undesirable; *esp* : an anticipatory response undertaken to avoid a noxious stimulus

avoidance–avoidance conflict n : psychological conflict that results when a choice must be made between two undesirable alternatives — compare APPROACH-APPROACH CONFLICT, APPROACH-AVOIDANCE CONFLICT

avoid·ant \ə-ˈvȯid-ᵊnt\ adj : characterized by turning away or by withdrawal or defensive behavior ⟨an ∼ personality⟩

av·oir·du·pois \ˌa-vər-də-ˈpȯiz, -ˈpwä\ adj : expressed in avoirdupois weight ⟨∼ units⟩ ⟨5 ounces ∼⟩

avoirdupois pound n : POUND b

avoirdupois weight n : a system of weights based on a pound of 16 ounces and an ounce of 437.5 grains (28.350 grams)

AVP abbr arginine vasopressin

avul·sion \ə-ˈvəl-shən\ n : a tearing away of a body part accidentally or surgically — **avulse** \ə-ˈvəls\ vb

avulsion fracture n : the detachment of a bone fragment that results from the pulling away of a ligament, tendon, or joint capsule from its point of attachment on a bone — called also *sprain fracture*

ax- or **axo-** comb form : axon ⟨axodendritic⟩

axe·nic \(ˌ)ā-ˈze-nik, -ˈzē-\ adj : free from other living organisms ⟨an ∼ culture of bacteria⟩ — **axe·ni·cal·ly** \-ni-k(ə-)lē\ adv

ax·i·al \ˈak-sē-əl\ adj 1 : of, relating to, or having the characteristics of an axis 2 : situated around, in the direction of, on, or along an axis

axial skeleton n : the skeleton of the trunk and head

Ax·id \ˈak-sid\ trademark — used for a preparation of nizatidine

ax·il·la \ag-ˈzi-lə, ak-ˈsi-\ n, pl -**lae** \-(ˌ)lē, -ˌlī\ or -**las** : the cavity beneath the junction of the arm or anterior appendage and shoulder or pectoral girdle containing the axillary artery and vein, a part of the brachial plexus of nerves, many lymph nodes, and fat and areolar tissue; *esp* : ARMPIT

ax·il·lary \ˈak-sə-ˌler-ē\ adj : of, relating to, or located near the axilla ⟨∼ lymph nodes⟩

axillary artery n : the part of the main artery of the arm that lies in the axilla and that is continuous with the subclavian artery above and the brachial artery below

axillary nerve n : a large nerve arising from the posterior cord of the brachial plexus and supplying the deltoid and teres minor muscles and the skin of the shoulder

axillary node n : any of the lymph nodes of the axilla

axillary vein n : the large vein passing through the axilla continuous with the basilic vein below and the subclavian vein above

ax·is \ˈak-səs\ n, pl **ax·es** \-ˌsēz\ 1 a : a straight line about which a body or a geometric figure rotates or may be thought of as rotating b : a straight line with respect to which a body, organ, or figure is symmetrical 2 a : the second vertebra of the neck of the higher vertebrates that is prolonged anteriorly within the foramen of the first vertebra and united with the dens which serves as a pivot for the atlas and head to turn upon — called also *epistropheus* b : any of various central, fundamental, or axial parts ⟨the cerebrospinal ∼⟩ ⟨the skeletal ∼⟩ c : AXILLA

axis cylinder *n* : AXON; *esp* : the axon of a myelinated neuron

axo·ax·o·nal \,ak-sō-'ak-sən-ᵊl, -,ak-'sän-, -'sōn-\ *or* **axo·ax·on·ic** \-ak-'sä-nik\ *adj* : relating to or being a synapse between an axon of one neuron and an axon of another

axo·den·drit·ic \,ak-sō-den-'dri-tik\ *adj* : relating to or being a nerve synapse between an axon of one neuron and a dendrite of another

axo·lem·ma \'ak-sə-,le-mə\ *n* : the plasma membrane of an axon

ax·on \'ak-,sän\ *also* **ax·one** \-,sōn\ *n* : a usu. long and single nerve-cell process that usu. conducts impulses away from the cell body — **ax·o·nal** \'ak-sən-ᵊl; ak-'sän-, -'sōn-\ *adj*

ax·on·o·tme·sis \,ak-sə-nət-'mē-səs\, *n, pl* **-me·ses** \-,sēz\ : axonal nerve damage that does not completely sever the surrounding endoneurial sheath so that regeneration can take place

axo·plasm \'ak-sə-,pla-zəm\ *n* : the protoplasm of an axon — **axo·plas·mic** \,ak-sə-'plaz-mik\ *adj*

axo·so·mat·ic \,ak-sō-sō-'ma-tik\ *adj* : relating to or being a nerve synapse between the cell body of one neuron and an axon of another

Ayer·za's disease \ə-'yer-zəz-\ *n* : a complex of symptoms marked esp. by cyanosis, dyspnea, polycythemia, and sclerosis of the pulmonary artery

Ayerza, Abel (1861–1918), Argentinean physician.

Ay·ur·ve·da \,ī-yər-'vā-də\ *n* : the traditional system of medicine of India that seeks to treat and integrate body, mind, and spirit using a holistic approach that emphasizes diet, herbal remedies, exercise, meditation, breathing, and physical therapy — **Ay·ur·ve·dic** \-dik\ *adj*

Ayurvedic medicine *n* : AYURVEDA

az- *or* **azo-** *comb form* : containing nitrogen esp. as an azo group ⟨*azo*sulfamide⟩

aza·ci·ti·dine \,a-zə-'si-tə-,den, -'sī-\ *or* **5-aza·cy·ti·dine** \'fīv-\ *also* **azacytidine** *n* : an antineoplastic cytidine analog $C_8H_{12}N_4O_5$ that is administered by subcutaneous injection in the treatment of myelodysplastic syndrome

aza·thi·o·prine \,a-zə-'thī-ə-,prēn\ *n* : a purine antimetabolite $C_9H_7N_7O_2S$ that is used esp. as an immunosuppressant — see IMURAN

az·i·do·thy·mi·dine \,a-zi-dō-'thī-mə-,dēn\ *n* : AZT

azith·ro·my·cin \ə-,zith-rō-'mī-sᵊn\ *n* : a semisynthetic macrolide antibiotic $C_{38}H_{72}N_2O_{12}$ that is derived from erythromycin and is used esp. as an antibacterial agent — see ZITHROMAX

Az·ma·cort \'az-mə-,kȯrt\ *trademark* — used for a preparation of triamcinolone

azo \'ā-(,)zō, 'a-\ *adj* : relating to, containing, or being the group N=N united at both ends to carbon

azo dye *n* : any of numerous dyes containing azo groups

azo·osper·mia \,ā-,zō-ə-'spər-mē-ə, ə-,zō-\ *n* : absence of spermatozoa from the seminal fluid — compare ASPERMIA — **azo·osper·mic** \-'spər-mik\ *adj*

azo·sul·fa·mide \,ā-zō-'səl-fə-,mīd\ *n* : a dark red crystalline azo compound $C_{18}H_{14}N_4Na_2O_{10}S_3$ of the sulfa class having antibacterial effect similar to that of sulfanilamide — called also *prontosil*

azot- *or* **azoto-** *comb form* : nitrogen : nitrogenous substance ⟨*azot*uria⟩

azo·te·mia \,ā-zō-'tē-mē-ə\ *n* : an excess of nitrogenous bodies in the blood as a result of kidney insufficiency — compare UREMIA — **azo·te·mic** \-'tē-mik\ *adj*

azo·tu·ria \,ā-zō-'tùr-ē-ə, -'tyùr-\ *n* : an abnormal condition of horses characterized by an excess of urea or other nitrogenous substances in the urine and by muscle damage esp. to the hindquarters

AZT \,ā-(,)zē-'tē\ *n* : an antiviral drug $C_{10}H_{13}N_5O_4$ that inhibits replication of some retroviruses (as HIV) and is used to treat AIDS — called also *azidothymidine, ZDV, zidovudine;* see RETROVIR

az·tre·o·nam \,az-'trē-ō-,nam\ *n* : a synthetic monobactam antibiotic $C_{13}H_{17}N_5O_8S_2$ used esp. against gramnegative bacteria

azygo- *comb form* : azygos ⟨*azygo*graphy⟩

azy·gog·ra·phy \,ā-zī-'gä-grə-fē\ *n, pl* **-phies** : radiographic visualization of the azygos system of veins after injection of a radiopaque medium

¹**azy·gos** \ā-'zī-gəs\ *n* : an azygos anatomical part

²**azy·gos** *also* **azy·gous** \(,)ā-'zī-gəs\ *adj* : not being one of a pair ⟨the ∼ muscle of the uvula⟩

azygos vein *n* : any of a system of three veins which drain the thoracic wall and much of the abdominal wall and which form a collateral circulation when either the inferior or superior vena cava is obstructed; *esp* : a vein that receives blood from the right half of the thoracic and abdominal walls, ascends along the right side of the vertebral column, and empties into the superior vena cava — compare ACCESSORY HEMIAZYGOS VEIN, HEMIAZYGOS VEIN

B

b *abbr* bicuspid

B \'bē\ *n* : the one of the four ABO blood groups characterized by the presence of antigens designated by the letter B and by the presence of antibodies against the antigens present in the A blood group

B *symbol* boron

Ba *symbol* barium

ba·be·sia \bə-'bē-zhə, -zhē-ə\ *n* **1** *cap* : a genus of sporozoans (family Babesiidae) parasitic in mammalian red blood cells and transmitted by the bite of a tick **2** : any sporozoan of the genus *Babesia* or sometimes the family (Babesiidae) to which it belongs — called also *piroplasm*

Babès, Victor (1854–1926), Romanian bacteriologist.

babe·si·a·sis \ˌba-bə-'sī-ə-səs\ *n, pl* **-a·ses** \-ˌsēz\ : BABESIOSIS

ba·be·si·o·sis \ˌba-bə-'sī-ə-səs, bə-ˌbē-zē-'ō-səs\ *n, or* **-oses** \-ˌsēz\ : infection with or disease caused by babesias — called also *babesiasis*

Ba·bin·ski reflex \bə-'bin-skē-\ *also* **Ba·bin·ski's reflex** \-skēz-\ *n* : a reflex movement in which when the sole is tickled the great toe turns upward instead of downward and which is normal in infancy but indicates damage to the central nervous system (as in the pyramidal tracts) when occurring later in life — called also *Babinski sign, Babinski's sign*; compare PLANTAR REFLEX

Babinski, Joseph–François–Felix (1857–1932), French neurologist.

ba·by \'bā-bē\ *n, pl* **babies** : an extremely young child or animal; *esp* : INFANT

baby talk *n* **1** : the imperfect speech or modified forms used by small children learning to talk **2** : the consciously imperfect or altered speech often used by adults in speaking to small children

baby tooth *n* : MILK TOOTH

bacill- *or* **bacilli-** *or* **bacillo-** *comb form* : bacillus ⟨*bacillosis*⟩

ba·cil·lary \'ba-sə-ˌler-ē, bə-'si-lə-rē\ *also* **ba·cil·lar** \bə-'si-lər, 'ba-sə-lər\ *adj* **1** : shaped like a rod; *also* : consisting of small rods **2** : of, relating to, or caused by bacilli ⟨~ meningitis⟩

bacillary angiomatosis *n* : a disease esp. of the skin that occurs in immunocompromised individuals, is characterized by reddish elevated lesions, and is caused by either of two bacteria of the genus *Bartonella* (*B. henselae* and *B. quintana*) — called also *epithelioid angiomatosis*

ba·cille Calmette–Guérin \ba-'sēl-\ *n* : BACILLUS CALMETTE-GUÉRIN

bac·il·le·mia \ˌba-sə-'lē-mē-ə\ *n* : BACTEREMIA

bac·il·lo·sis \ˌba-sə-'lō-səs\ *n, pl* **-lo·ses** \-ˌsēz\ : infection with bacilli

bac·il·lu·ria \ˌba-sə-'lur-ē-ə, -'lyur-\ *n* : the passage of bacilli with the urine — **bac·il·lu·ric** \-ik\ *adj*

ba·cil·lus \bə-'si-ləs\ *n, pl* **-li** \-ˌlī *also* -lē\ **1 a** *cap* : a genus of aerobic rod-shaped gram-positive bacteria (family Bacillaceae) that include many saprophytes and some parasites (as *B. anthracis* of anthrax) **b** : any bacterium of the genus *Bacillus*; *broadly* : a straight rod-shaped bacterium **2** : BACTERIUM; *esp* : a disease-producing bacterium

bacillus Cal·mette–Gué·rin \-ˌkal-'met-(ˌ)gā-'raⁿ, -'ran\ *n* : an attenuated strain of tubercle bacillus developed by repeated culture on a medium containing bile and used in preparation of tuberculosis vaccines — compare BCG VACCINE

Calmette, Albert Léon Charles (1863–1933), French bacteriologist, and **Guérin, Camille (1872–1961),** French veterinarian.

bac·i·tra·cin \ˌba-sə-'trās-ᵒn\ *n* : a polypeptide antibiotic isolated from a bacillus (*Bacillus subtilis* or *B. licheniformis*) and usu. used topically esp. against gram-positive bacteria

Tracy \'trā-sē\, **Margaret,** American hospital patient.

back \'bak\ *n* **1 a** : the rear part of the human body esp. from the neck to the end of the spine **b** : the corresponding part of a lower animal (as a quadruped) **c** : SPINAL COLUMN **2** : the part of the upper surface of the tongue behind the front and lying opposite the soft palate when the tongue is at rest

back·ache \'bak-ˌāk\ *n* : a pain in the lower back

back·board \'bak-ˌbȯrd\ *n* : a stiff board on which an injured person and esp. one with neck or spinal injuries is placed and immobilized in order to prevent further injury during transport

back·bone \-ˌbōn\ *n* **1** : SPINAL COLUMN, SPINE **2** : the longest chain of atoms or groups of atoms in a usu. long molecule (as a protein)

¹back·cross \'bak-ˌkrȯs\ *vb* : to cross (a first-generation hybrid) with one of the parental types

²backcross *n* : a mating that involves backcrossing; *also* : an individual produced by backcrossing

back·ing \'ba-kiŋ\ *n* : the metal portion of a dental crown, bridge, or similar structure to which a porcelain or plastic tooth facing is attached

back·rest \'bak-ˌrest\ *n* : a rest for the back

back·side \-'sīd\ *n* : BUTTOCKS — often used in pl.

bac·lo·fen \'ba-klō-ˌfen\ *n* : a gamma= aminobutyric acid analog $C_{10}H_{12}ClNO_2$ used as a relaxant of skeletal muscle esp. in treating spasticity (as in multiple sclerosis)

bact *abbr* **1** bacteria; bacterial **2** bacteriological; bacteriology **3** bacterium

bacter- *or* **bacteri-** *or* **bacterio-** *comb form* : bacteria : bacterial ⟨*bacteriolysis*⟩

bac·ter·emia \ˌbak-tə-'rē-mē-ə\ *n* : the usu. transient presence of bacteria in the blood — **bac·ter·emic** \-mik\ *adj*

¹**bacteria** *pl of* BACTERIUM

²**bacteria** *n* : BACTERIUM — not usu. used technically

bac·te·ri·al \bak-'tir-ē-əl\ *adj* : of, relating to, or caused by bacteria ⟨a ~ chromosome⟩ ⟨~ infection⟩ — **bac·te·ri·al·ly** *adv*

bacterial vag·i·no·sis \-ˌva-jə-'nō-səs\ *n* : vaginitis that is marked by a grayish vaginal discharge usu. of foul odor and that is associated with the presence of a bacterium esp. of the genus *Gardnerella* (*G. vaginalis* syn. *Haemophilus vaginalis*) — abbr. *BV;* called also *nonspecific vaginitis*

bac·te·ri·cid·al \bak-ˌtir-ə-'sīd-ᵊl\ *also* **bac·te·ri·o·cid·al** \-ˌtir-ē-ə-'sīd-\ *adj* : destroying bacteria — **bac·te·ri·cid·al·ly** *adv* — **bac·te·ri·cide** \-'tir-ə-ˌsīd\ *n*

bac·te·ri·cid·in \bak-ˌtir-ə-'sīd-ᵊn\ *or* **bac·te·ri·o·cid·in** \-ˌtir-ē-ə-'sīd-\ *n* : a bactericidal antibody

bac·ter·in \'bak-tə-rən\ *n* : a suspension of killed or attenuated bacteria for use as a vaccine

bac·te·rio·cin \bak-'tir-ē-ə-sən\ *n* : an antibiotic (as colicin) produced by bacteria

bac·te·ri·ol·o·gist \(ˌ)bak-ˌtir-ē-'ä-lə-jist\ *n* : a specialist in bacteriology

bac·te·ri·ol·o·gy \(ˌ)bak-ˌtir-ē-'ä-lə-jē\ *n, pl* **-gies 1** : a science that deals with bacteria and their relations to medicine, industry, and agriculture **2** : bacterial life and phenomena — **bac·te·ri·o·log·ic** \bak-ˌtir-ē-ə-'lä-jik\ *or* **bac·te·ri·o·log·i·cal** \-'lä-ji-kəl\ *adj* — **bac·te·ri·o·log·i·cal·ly** \-ji-k(ə-)lē\ *adv*

bac·te·ri·o·ly·sin \bak-ˌtir-ē-ə-'lī-sᵊn\ *n* : an antibody that acts to destroy a bacterium

bac·te·ri·ol·y·sis \(ˌ)bak-ˌtir-ē-'ä-lə-səs\ *n, pl* **-y·ses** \-ˌsēz\ : destruction or dissolution of bacterial cells — **bac·te·ri·o·lyt·ic** \bak-ˌtir-ē-ə-'li-tik\ *adj*

bac·te·rio·phage \bak-'tir-ē-ə-ˌfāj, -ˌfäzh\ *n* : a virus that infects bacteria — called also *phage*

bacteriophage lambda *n* : PHAGE LAMBDA

bac·te·rio·sta·sis \bak-ˌtir-ē-ō-'stā-səs\ *n, pl* **-sta·ses** \-ˌsēz\ : inhibition of the growth of bacteria without destruction

bac·te·rio·stat \-'tir-ē-ō-ˌstat\ *also* **bac·te·rio·stat·ic** \-ˌtir-ē-ō-'sta-tik\ *n* : an agent that causes bacteriostasis

bac·te·rio·stat·ic \-ˌtir-ē-ō-'sta-tik\ *adj* : causing bacteriostasis ⟨a ~ agent⟩ — **bac·te·rio·stat·i·cal·ly** \-ti-k(ə-)lē\ *adv*

bac·te·ri·um \bak-'tir-ē-əm\ *n, pl* **-ria** \-ē-ə\ : any of a domain (Bacteria) of prokaryotic round, spiral, or rod= shaped single-celled microorganisms that are often aggregated into colonies or motile by means of flagella, that live in soil, water, organic matter, or the bodies of plants and animals, and that are usu. autotrophic, saprophytic, or parasitic in nutrition, and that are noted for their biochemical effects and pathogenicity; *broadly* : PROKARYOTE

bac·te·ri·uria \bak-ˌtir-ē-'ur-ē-ə, -'yur-\ *n* : the presence of bacteria in the urine — **bac·te·ri·uric** \-ik\ *adj*

bac·te·roi·des \-'roi-(ˌ)dēz\ *n* **1** *cap* : a genus of gram-negative anaerobic bacteria (family Bacteroidaceae) that have rounded ends and occur usu. in the normal intestinal flora **2** *pl* **-roides** : a bacterium of the genus *Bacteroides* or of a closely related genus

Bac·trim \'bak-trim\ *trademark* — used for a preparation of sulfamethoxazole and trimethoprim

Bac·tro·ban \'bak-trō-ˌban\ *trademark* — used for a preparation of mupirocin

bad cholesterol *n* : LDL

¹**bag** \'bag\ *n* **1** : a pouched or pendulous bodily part or organ; *esp* : UDDER **2** : a puffy or sagging protuberance of flabby skin ⟨~s under the eyes⟩

²**bag** *vb* **bagged; bag·ging** : to ventilate the lungs of (a patient) using a hand-squeezed bag attached to a face mask

ba·gasse \bə-'gas\ *n* : plant residue (as of sugarcane or grapes) left after a product (as juice) has been extracted

bag·as·so·sis \ˌba-gə-'sō-səs\ *n, pl* **-so·ses** \-ˌsēz\ : an industrial disease characterized by cough, difficult breathing, chills, fever, and prolonged weakness and caused by the inhalation of the dust of bagasse — called also *bagasse disease*

bag of waters *n* : the double-walled fluid-filled sac that encloses and protects the fetus in the mother's womb and that breaks releasing its fluid during the birth process

Bain·bridge reflex \'bān-(ˌ)brij-\ *n* : a homeostatic reflex mechanism that causes acceleration of heartbeat following the stimulation of local muscle spindles when blood pressure in the venae cavae and right atrium is increased

Bainbridge, Francis Arthur (1874–1921), British physiologist.

Ba·ker's cyst \'bā-kərz-\ *n* : a swelling behind the knee that is composed of a membrane-lined sac filled with synovial fluid and is associated with certain joint disorders (as arthritis)

Baker, William Morrant (1839–1896), British surgeon.

bak·er's itch \ˌbā-kərz-\ *n* : GROCER'S ITCH

bak·ing soda \'bā-kiŋ-\ *n* : SODIUM BICARBONATE

BAL \ˌbē-(ˌ)ā-'el\ *n* : DIMERCAPROL

balan- *or* **balano-** *comb form* : glans penis ⟨*balan*itis⟩ ⟨*balano*posthitis⟩

bal·ance \'ba-ləns\ *n* 1 : an instrument for weighing 2 : mental and emotional steadiness 3 : the relation in physiology between the intake of a particular nutrient and its excretion — see NITROGEN BALANCE, WATER BALANCE

bal·anced \-lənst\ *adj* 1 : having the physiologically active elements mutually counteracting ⟨a ~ solution⟩ 2 *of a diet or ration* : furnishing all needed nutrients in the amount, form, and proportions needed to support healthy growth and productivity

bal·a·ni·tis \ˌba-lə-'nī-təs\ *n* : inflammation of the glans penis

bal·a·no·pos·thi·tis \ˌba-lə-(ˌ)nō-päs-'thī-təs\ *n* : inflammation of the glans penis and of the foreskin

bal·an·ti·di·a·sis \ˌba-lən-tə-'dī-ə-səs, bə-ˌlan-\ *also* **bal·an·tid·i·o·sis** \ˌba-lən-ˌti-dē-'ō-səs\ *n, pl* **-a·ses** *also* **-o·ses** \-ˌsēz\ : infection with or disease caused by protozoans of the genus *Balantidium*

bal·an·tid·i·um \ˌba-lən-'ti-dē-əm\ *n* 1 *cap* : a genus of large parasitic ciliate protozoans (order Heterotricha) including one (*B. coli*) that infests the intestines of some mammals and esp. swine and may cause a chronic ulcerative dysentery in humans 2 *pl* **-ia** \-dē-ə\ : a protozoan of the genus *Balantidium* — **ba·lan·tid·i·al** \-dē-əl\ *adj*

bald \'bȯld\ *adj* : lacking all or a significant part of the hair on the head or sometimes on other parts of the body — **bald** *vb*

bald·ness *n* : the state of being bald — see MALE-PATTERN BALDNESS

Bal·kan frame \'bȯl-kən-\ *n* : a frame employed in the treatment of fractured bones of the leg or arm that provides overhead weights and pulleys for suspension, traction, and continuous extension of the splinted fractured limb

ball \'bȯl\ *n* 1 : a roundish protuberant part of the body: as **a** : the rounded eminence by which the base of the thumb is continuous with the palm of the hand **b** : the rounded broad part of the sole of the human foot between toes and arch and on which the main weight of the leg first rests in normal walking 2 : EYEBALL 3 *often vulgar* : TESTIS

ball–and–socket joint *n* : an articulation (as the hip joint) in which the rounded head of one bone fits into a cuplike cavity of the other and admits movement in any direction — called also *enarthrosis*

bal·lism \'ba-ˌli-zəm\ *or* **bal·lis·mus** \bə-'liz-məs\ *n, pl* **-lisms** *or* **-lis·mus·es** : the abnormal swinging jerking movements sometimes seen in chorea

bal·lis·to·car·dio·gram \bə-ˌlis-tō-'kär-dē-ə-ˌgram\ *n* : the record made by a ballistocardiograph

bal·lis·to·car·dio·graph \-ˌgraf\ *n* : a device for measuring the amount of blood passing through the heart in a specified time by recording the recoil movements of the body that result from contraction of the heart muscle in ejecting blood from the ventricles — **bal·lis·to·car·dio·graph·ic** \-ˌkär-dē-ə-'gra-fik\ *adj* — **bal·lis·to·car·di·og·ra·phy** \-ē-'ä-grə-fē\ *n*

¹bal·loon \bə-'lün\ *n* : a nonporous bag of tough light material that can be inflated (as in a bodily cavity) with air or gas

²balloon *vb* : to inflate, swell, or puff out like a balloon

balloon angioplasty *n* : dilation of an obstructed artherosclerotic artery by the passage of a balloon catheter through the vessel to the area of disease where inflation of the catheter's tip compresses the plaque against the vessel wall

balloon catheter *n* : a catheter that has two lumens and an inflatable tip which can be expanded by the passage of gas, water, or a radiopaque medium through one of the lumens and that is used esp. to measure blood pressure in a blood vessel or to expand a partly closed or obstructed bodily passage or tube (as a coronary artery) — called also *balloon-tipped catheter*; see PERCUTANEOUS TRANSLUMINAL ANGIOPLASTY

bal·lotte·ment \bə-'lät-mənt\ *n* : a sharp upward pushing against the uterine wall with a finger inserted into the vagina for diagnosing pregnancy by feeling the return impact of the displaced fetus; *also* : a similar procedure for detecting a floating kidney

balm \'bäm, 'bälm, 'bȧm\ *n* 1 : an aromatic preparation (as a healing ointment) 2 : a soothing restorative agency

balne- *or* **balneo-** *comb form* : bath : bathing ⟨*balneo*therapy⟩

bal·ne·ol·o·gy \ˌbal-nē-'ä-lə-jē\ *n, pl* **-gies** : the science of the therapeutic use of baths

bal·neo·ther·a·py \ˌbal-nē-ō-'ther-ə-pē\ *n, pl* **-pies** : the treatment of disease by baths

bal·sam \'bȯl-səm\ *n* 1 : any of several resinous substances used esp. in medicine 2 : BALM 2 — **bal·sam·ic** \bȯl-'sa-mik\ *adj*

balsam of Pe·ru \-pə-'rü\ *n* : a balsam from a tropical American leguminous tree (*Myroxylon pereirae*) used esp. as an irritant and to promote wound healing — called also *Peru balsam, Peruvian balsam*

balsam of To·lu \-tə-'lü\ *n* : a balsam from a tropical American leguminous tree (*Myroxylon balsamum*) used esp. as an expectorant and as a flavoring for cough syrups — called also *tolu, tolu balsam*

bam·boo spine \(ˌ)bam-'bü-\ *n* : a spinal column in the advanced stage of ankylosing spondylitis esp. as observed in an X-ray with ossified layers at the margins of the vertebrae giving the whole an appearance of a stick of bamboo

Ban·croft·i·an filariasis \'ban-ˌkröf-tē-ən-, 'baŋ-\ *or* **Ban·croft's filariasis** \-ˌkröfts-\ *n* : filariasis caused by a slender white filaria of the genus *Wuchereria* (*W. bancrofti*) that is transmitted in larval form by mosquitoes, lives in lymph vessels and lymphoid tissues, and often causes elephantiasis by blocking lymphatic drainage

Ban·croft \'ban-ˌkröft, 'baŋ-\, **Joseph** (1836–1894), British physician.

band \'band\ *n* 1 : a thin flat encircling strip esp. for binding: as **a** : a strip of cloth used to protect a newborn baby's navel — called also *belly-band* **b** : a thin flat strip of metal that encircles a tooth ⟨orthodontic ∼*s*⟩ 2 : a strip separated by some characteristic color or texture or considered apart from what is adjacent: as **a** : a line or streak of differentiated cells **b** : one of the alternating dark and light segments of skeletal muscle fibers **c** : a strip of abnormal tissue either congenital or acquired; *esp* : a strip of connective tissue that causes obstruction of the bowel

¹band·age \'ban-dij\ *n* : a strip of fabric used to cover a wound, hold a dressing in place, immobilize an injured part, or apply pressure — see CAPELINE, ESMARCH BANDAGE, PRESSURE BANDAGE, SPICA, VELPEAU BANDAGE

²bandage *vb* **ban·daged; ban·dag·ing** : to bind, dress, or cover with a bandage

Band–Aid \'ban-ˌdād\ *trademark* — used for a small adhesive strip with a gauze pad for covering minor wounds

band form *n* : a young neutrophil in the stage of development following a metamyelocyte and having an elongated nucleus that has not yet become lobed as in a mature neutrophil — called also *band cell, stab cell*

band keratopathy *n* : calcium deposition in Bowman's membrane and the stroma of the cornea that appears as an opaque gray streak and occurs in hypercalcemia and various chronic inflammatory conditions of the eye

bane·ber·ry \'bān-ˌber-ē, -bə-rē, -brē\ *n, pl* **-ber·ries** : the acrid poisonous berry of any plant of a genus (*Actaea*) of the buttercup family (Ranunculaceae); *also* : one of these plants

bang *var of* BHANG

Bang's disease \'baŋz-\ *n* : BRUCELLOSIS; *specif* : contagious abortion of cattle caused by a bacterium of the genus *Brucella* (*B. abortus*) — called also *Bang's*

Bang \'bȧŋ\, **Bernhard Lauritz Frederik** (1848–1932), Danish veterinarian.

bank \'baŋk\ *n* : a depot for the collection and storage of a biological product of human origin for medical use ⟨a sperm ∼⟩ — see BLOOD BANK

Ban·ti's disease \'bän-tēz-\ *n* : a disorder characterized by congestion and great enlargement of the spleen usu. accompanied by anemia, leukopenia, and cirrhosis of the liver — called also *Banti's syndrome*

Ban·ti \'bän-tē\, **Guido** (1852–1925), Italian physician.

¹bar \'bär\ *n, often attrib* 1 : a piece of metal that connects parts of a removable partial denture 2 : a straight stripe, band, or line much longer than it is wide 3 : the space in front of the molar teeth of a horse in which the bit is placed

²bar *vb* **barred; bar·ring** : to cut free and ligate (a vein in a horse's leg) above and below the site of a projected operative procedure

³bar *n* : a unit of pressure equal to 100,000 pascals

bar- *or* **baro-** *comb form* : weight : pressure ⟨*bari*atrics⟩ ⟨*baro*trauma⟩

Bá·rá·ny chair \bə-'rän-(y)ē-ˌcha(ə)r, -ˌche(ə)r\ *n* : a chair used esp. for demonstrating the effects of circular motion (as on airplane pilots)

Bá·rá·ny \'bá-ˌränʸ\, **Robert** (1876–1936), Austrian otologist.

barb \'bärb\ *n, slang* : BARBITURATE

barbae — see SYCOSIS BARBAE

bar·ber's itch \ˌbär-bərz-\ *n* : ringworm of the face and neck

bar·bi·tal \'bär-bə-ˌtȯl\ *n* : a crystalline barbituate C₈H₁₂N₂O₃ formerly used as a sedative and hypnotic often in the form of its soluble sodium salt — see VERONAL

bar·bi·tone \'bär-bə-ˌtōn\ *n, Brit* : BARBITAL

bar·bi·tu·rate \bär-'bi-chə-rət\ *n* 1 : a salt or ester of barbituric acid 2 : any of various derivatives of barbituric acid (as phenobarbital) used esp. as sedatives, hypnotics, and antispasmodics

bar·bi·tu·ric acid \ˌbär-bə-ˈtür-ik, -ˈtyu̇r-\ *n* : a synthetic crystalline acid C₄H₄N₂O₃ that is a derivative of pyrimidine; *also* : any of its acid derivatives of which some are used as hypnotics

bar·bi·tur·ism \ˌbär-ˈbi-chə-ˌri-zəm, ˈbär-bi-\ *n* : a condition characterized by deleterious effects on the mind or body by excess use of barbiturates

barefoot doctor *n* : an auxiliary medical worker trained to provide health care in rural areas of China

bar·ia·tri·cian \ˌbar-ē-ə-ˈtri-shən\ *n* : a specialist in bariatrics

bar·iat·rics \ˌbar-ē-ˈa-triks\ *n* : a branch of medicine that deals with the treatment of obesity — **bar·i·at·ric** \-trik\ *adj*

bar·i·to·sis \ˌbar-ə-ˈtō-səs\ *n, pl* **-to·ses** \-ˌsēz\ : pneumoconiosis caused by inhalation of dust composed of barium or its compounds

bar·i·um \ˈbar-ē-əm\ *n* : a silver-white malleable toxic bivalent metallic element — symbol *Ba;* see ELEMENT table

barium chloride *n* : a water-soluble toxic salt BaCl₂·2H₂O used as a reagent in analysis and as a cardiac stimulant

barium enema *n* : a suspension of barium sulfate injected into the lower bowel to render it radiopaque, usu. followed by injection of air to inflate the bowel and increase definition, and used in the radiographic diagnosis of intestinal lesions

barium meal *n* : a solution of barium sulfate that is swallowed by a patient to facilitate fluoroscopic or radiographic diagnosis

barium sulfate *n* : a colorless crystalline insoluble salt BaSO₄ used medically chiefly as a radiopaque substance

Bar·low's disease \ˈbär-ˌlōz-\ *n* : IN-FANTILE SCURVY

Barlow, Sir Thomas (1845–1945), British physician.

Barlow's syndrome *n* : MITRAL VALUE PROLAPSE

Barlow, John Brereton (*b* 1924), South African cardiologist.

baro- — see BAR-

baro·re·cep·tor \ˌbar-ō-ri-ˈsep-tər\ *also* **baro·cep·tor** \-ō-ˈsep-\ *n* : a sensory nerve ending esp. in the walls of large arteries (as the carotid sinus) that is sensitive to changes in blood pressure — called also *pressoreceptor*

baro·re·flex \ˈbar-ō-ˌrē-fleks\ *n* : the reflex mechanism by which baroreceptors regulate blood pressure — called also *baroreceptor reflex*

baro·trau·ma \-ˈtrau̇-mə, -ˈtrȯ-\ *n, pl* **-mas** *also* **-ma·ta** \-mə-tə\ : injury of a part or organ as a result of changes in barometric pressure; *specif* : AERO= OTITIS MEDIA

Barr body \ˈbär-\ *n* : a densely staining inactivated condensed X chromosome that is present in each somatic cell of most female mammals and is used as a test of genetic femaleness (as in a fetus or an athlete) — called also *sex chromatin*

Barr, Murray Llewellyn (1908–1995), Canadian anatomist.

bar·rel chest \ˈbar-əl-\ *n* : the enlarged chest with a rounded cross section and fixed horizontal position of the ribs that occurs in chronic pulmonary emphysema

bar·ren \ˈbar-ən\ *adj* : incapable of producing offspring — used esp. of females or matings — **bar·ren·ness** \-ən-nəs\ *n*

Bar·rett's esophagus \ˈbar-its-\ *n* : metaplasia of the lower esophagus that occurs especially as a result of chronic gastroesophageal reflux and is associated with an increased risk for esophageal carcinoma — called also *Barrett's epithelium*

Barrett, Norman Rupert (1903–1979), British surgeon.

bar·ri·er \ˈbar-ē-ər\ *n* : a material object or set of objects that separates, demarcates, or serves as a barricade — see BLOOD-BRAIN BARRIER, PLACENTAL BARRIER

bar·tho·lin·itis \ˌbär-ˌtō-lə-ˈnī-təs\ *n, pl* **-lin·ites** \-ˌtēz\ : inflammation of the Bartholin's glands

Bar·tho·lin's gland \ˈbärt-ᵊl-ənz-, ˈbärthə-lənz-\ *n* : either of two oval racemose glands lying one to each side of the lower part of the vagina and secreting a lubricating mucus — called also *gland of Bartholin, greater vestibular gland;* compare COWPER'S GLAND

Bar·tho·lin \ˈbär-ˈtü-lin\, **Caspar Thomeson** (1655–1738), Danish anatomist.

bar·ton·el·la \ˌbärt-ᵊn-ˈe-lə\ *n* 1 *cap* : a genus of gram-negative bacteria (family Bartonellaceae) that include the causative agent (*B. bacilliformis*) of bartonellosis 2 : any bacterium of the genus *Bartonella*

Bar·ton \ˈbär-ˌtōn\, **Alberto L.** (1874–1950), Peruvian physician.

bar·ton·el·lo·sis \ˌbärt-ᵊn-ˌe-ˈlō-səs\ *n, pl* **-lo·ses** \-ˌsēz\ : a disease that occurs in So. America, is characterized by severe anemia and high fever followed by an eruption like warts on the skin, and is caused by a bacterium of the genus *Bartonella* (*B. bacilliformis*) that invades the red blood cells and is transmitted by sand flies (genus *Phlebotomus*) — called also *Carrión's disease*

Bart·er's syndrome \ˈbär-tərz-\ *n* : a kidney disorder that usu. first appears during childhood and is characterized esp. by hypokalemia, aldosteronism, hyperreninemia, and juxtaglomerular cell hyperplasia

Bartter, Frederic Crosby (1914–1983), American physiologist.

ba·sal \ˈbā-səl, -zəl\ *adj* 1 : relating to, situated at, or forming the base 2 : of, relating to, or essential for maintaining the fundamental vital activities of an organism (as respiration, heartbeat, or excretion) (∼ diet) 3 : serving as or serving to induce an initial comatose or unconscious state that forms a basis for further anesthetization (∼ anesthesia) — **ba·sal·ly** *adv*

basal cell *n* : one of the innermost cells of the deeper epidermis of the skin

basal–cell carcinoma *n* : a skin cancer derived from and preserving the form of the basal cells of the skin

basale — see STRATUM BASALE

basal ganglion *n* : any of four deeply placed masses of gray matter within each cerebral hemisphere comprising the caudate nucleus, the lentiform nucleus, the amygdala, and the claustrum — usu. used in pl.; called also *basal nucleus*

basalia — see STRATUM BASALE

basalis — see DECIDUA BASALIS

basal lamina *n* 1 : the part of the gray matter of the embryonic neural tube from which the motor nerve roots arise 2 : a thin extracellular layer chiefly of collagen, proteoglycans, and glycoproteins (as laminin) that lies adjacent to the basal surface of epithelial cells or surrounds individual muscle, fat, and Schwann cells and that separates these cells from underlying or surrounding connective tissue or adjacent cells — compare RETICULAR LAMINA

basal metabolic rate *n* : the rate at which heat is given off by an organism at complete rest

basal metabolism *n* : the turnover of energy in a fasting and resting organism using energy solely to maintain vital cellular activity, respiration, and circulation as measured by the basal metabolic rate

basal nucleus *n* : BASAL GANGLION

basal plate *n* : an underlying structure: as **a** : the ventral portion of the neural tube **b** : the part of the decidua of a placental mammal that is intimately fused with the placenta

base \'bās\ *n, pl* **bas·es** \'bā-səz\ 1 : that portion of a bodily organ or part by which it is attached to another more central structure of the organism ⟨the ~ of the thumb⟩ 2 **a** : the usu. inactive ingredient of a preparation serving as the vehicle for the active medicinal preparation **b** : the chief active ingredient of a preparation — called also *basis* 3 **a** : any of various typically water-soluble and bitter tasting compounds that in solution have a pH greater than 7, are capable of reacting with an acid to form a salt, and are molecules or ions able to take up a proton from an acid or are substances able to give up a pair of electrons to an acid — compare ALKALI **b** : any of the five purine or pyrimidine bases of DNA and RNA that include cytosine, guanine, adenine, thymine, and uracil — **based** \'bāst\ *adj*

Ba·se·dow's disease \'bä-zə-,dōz-\ *n* : GRAVES' DISEASE

    Basedow \'bä-zə-,dō\, **Karl Adolph von** (1799–1854), German physician.

base·line \'bās-,līn\ *n* : a set of critical observations or data used for comparison or a control

base·ment membrane \'bā-smənt-\ *n* 1 : a thin supporting layer that separates a layer of epithelial cells from the underlying lamina propria and is composed of the basal lamina and reticular lamina 2 : BASAL LAMINA 2

base pair *n* : one of the pairs of nucleotide bases on complementary strands of nucleic acid that consist of a purine on one strand joined to a pyrimidine on the other strand by hydrogen bonds and that include adenine linked to thymine in DNA or to uracil in RNA and guanine linked to cytosine in both DNA and RNA

base pairing *n* : the pairing of purine and pyrimidine bases linked by hydrogen bonds in two complementary strands of DNA

base·plate \'bās-,plāt\ *n* 1 : the portion of an artificial denture in contact with the jaw 2 : the sheet of plastic material used in the making of trial denture plates

base unit *n* : one of a set of simple units in a system of measurement from which other units may be derived

basi- *also* **baso-** *comb form* 1 : of or belonging to the base or lower part of ⟨*basi*cranial⟩ 2 : chemical base ⟨*baso*philic⟩

ba·sic \'bā-sik, -zik\ *adj* 1 : of, relating to, or forming the base or essence 2 **a** : of, relating to, containing, or having the character of a base **b** : having an alkaline reaction

ba·si·cra·ni·al \,bā-si-'krā-nē-əl\ *adj* : of or relating to the base of the skull

ba·sid·io·my·cete \bə-,si-dē-ō-'mī-,sēt\ *n* : any of a large class (Basidiomycetes) or subdivision (Basidiomycotina) of higher fungi that include rusts (order Uredinales), smuts (order Ustilaginales), and numerous edible forms (as many mushrooms) — **ba·sid·io·my·ce·tous** \-mī-'sē-təs\ *adj*

bas·i·lar \'ba-zə-lər, -sə- *also* 'bā-\ *adj* : of, relating to, or situated at the base ⟨~ fractures of the skull⟩

basilar artery *n* : an unpaired artery that is formed by the union of the two vertebral arteries, runs forward within the skull just under the pons, divides into the two posterior cerebral arteries, and supplies the pons, cerebellum, posterior part of the cerebrum, and the inner ear

basilar membrane *n* : a membrane that extends from the margin of the bony shelf of the cochlea to the outer wall and that supports the organ of Corti

basilar process *n* : an anterior median projection of the occipital bone in front of the foramen magnum articulating in front with the body of the sphenoid by the basilar suture

basilic vein *n* : a vein of the upper arm lying along the inner border of the biceps muscle, draining the whole limb, and opening into the axillary vein

¹ba·si·oc·cip·i·tal \,bā-sē-äk-'sip-ət-³l\ *adj* : relating to or being a bone in the base of the cranium immediately in front of the foramen magnum that is represented in humans by the basilar process of the occipital bone

²**basioccipital** *n* : the basioccipital bone

ba·si·on \'bā-sē-ˌän, -zē-\ *n* : the midpoint of the anterior margin of the foramen magnum

ba·sis \'bā-səs\ *n, pl* **ba·ses** \-ˌsēz\ 1 : any of various anatomical parts that function as a foundation 2 : BASE 2b

ba·si·sphe·noid \ˌbā-səs-'fē-ˌnóid\ *also* **ba·si·sphe·noi·dal** \-səs-fi-'nóid-ᵊl\ *adj* : relating to or being the part of the base of the cranium that lies between the basioccipital and the presphenoid bones and that usu. ossifies separately and becomes a part of the sphenoid bone only in the adult — **basisphenoid** *n*

basket cell *n* : any of the cells in the molecular layer of the cerebellum whose axons pass inward and end in a basketlike network around the Purkinje cells

Basle Nom·i·na An·a·tom·i·ca \'bä-zəl-'nä-mə-nə-ˌa-nə-'tä-mi-kə\ *n* : the anatomical nomenclature adopted at the 1895 meeting of the German Anatomical Society at Basel, Switzerland, and superseded by the Nomina Anatomica in 1955 — *abbr.* BNA

baso- — see BASI-

ba·so·phil \'bā-sə-ˌfil, -zə-\ *or* **ba·so·phile** \-ˌfil\ *n* : a basophilic substance or structure; *esp* : a white blood cell with basophilic granules that is similar in function to a mast cell

ba·so·phil·ia \ˌbā-sə-'fi-lē-ə, -zə-\ *n* 1 : tendency to stain with basic dyes 2 : an abnormal condition in which some tissue element has increased basophilia

ba·so·phil·ic \-'fi-lik\ *also* **ba·so·phil** \'bā-sə-ˌfil, -zə-\ *or* **ba·so·phile** \-ˌfil\ *adj* : staining readily with or being a basic stain

basophilism — see PITUITARY BASOPHILISM

bath \'bath, 'bàth\ *n, pl* **baths** \'bathz, 'baths, 'bàthz, 'bàths\ 1 : a washing or soaking (as in water) of all or part of the body — see MUD BATH, SITZ BATH 2 : water used for bathing 3 : SPA 1 — usu. used in pl.

bathe \'bāth\ *vb* **bathed; bath·ing** 1 : to wash in a liquid (as water) 2 : to apply water or a liquid medicament to

ba·tra·cho·tox·in \bə-ˌtra-kə-'täk-sən, ˌba-trə-kō-\ *n* : a very powerful steroid venom $C_{31}H_{42}N_2O_6$ extracted from the skin of a So. American frog (*Phyllobates aurotaenia*)

Bat·ten disease \'ba-tᵊn-\ *n* : a fatal lipofuscinosis that is inherited as an autosomal recessive trait and has an onset between five and eight or nine years of age

Batten, Frederick Eustace (1865–1918), British neurologist and pediatrician.

battered child syndrome *n* : the complex of physical injuries (as fractures, hematomas, and contusions) that results from gross abuse (as by a parent) of a young child

battered woman syndrome *also* **battered woman's syndrome** *n* : the highly variable symptom complex of physical and psychological injuries exhibited by a woman repeatedly abused esp. physically by her mate — called also *battered wife syndrome, battered women's syndrome*

bat·tery \'ba-tə-rē\ *n, pl* **-ter·ies** : a group or series of tests; *esp* : a group of intelligence or personality tests given to a subject as an aid in psychological analysis

battle fatigue *n* : COMBAT FATIGUE — **bat·tle-fa·tigued** *adj*

Bau·hin's valve \'bō-ˌanz-, bō-'aⁿz-\ *n* : ILEOCECAL VALVE

Bauhin, Gaspard *or* **Caspar (1560–1624),** Swiss anatomist and botanist.

BBB *abbr* 1 blood-brain barrier 2 bundle branch block

BC *abbr* board-certified

B cell *n* : any of the lymphocytes that have antigen-binding antibody molecules on the surface, that comprise the antibody-secreting plasma cells when mature, and that in mammals differentiate in the bone marrow — called also *B lymphocyte;* compare T CELL

BCG *abbr* bacillus Calmette-Guérin

BCG vaccine \ˌbē-(ˌ)sē-'jē-\ *n* : a vaccine prepared from a living attenuated strain of tubercle bacilli and used to vaccinate human beings against tuberculosis

A. L. C. Calmette and **C. Guérin** — see BACILLUS CALMETTE-GUÉRIN

BCLS *abbr* basic cardiac life support

BCNU \ˌbē-(ˌ)sē-(ˌ)en-'yü\ *n* : CARMUSTINE

B complex *n* : VITAMIN B COMPLEX

b.d. *abbr* [Latin *bis die*] twice a day — used in writing prescriptions

B–DNA \'bē-ˌdē-ˌen-'ā\ *n* : the typical form of double helix DNA in which the chains twist up and to the right around the front of the axis of the helix — compare Z-DNA

Be *symbol* beryllium

BE *abbr* board-eligible

bead·ing \'bē-diŋ\ *n* : the beadlike nodules occurring in rickets at the junction of the ribs with their cartilages — called also *rachitic rosary*

bear down *vb* : to contract the abdominal muscles and the diaphragm during childbirth

¹**beat** \'bēt\ *vb* **beat; beat·en** \'bēt-ᵊn\ *or* **beat; beat·ing** : PULSATE, THROB

²**beat** *n* : a single stroke or pulsation (as of the heart) ⟨cardiac ∼s⟩ — see EXTRASYSTOLE

Beau's lines \'bōz-\ *n pl* : transverse grooves or ridges on the nail plate that are temporary and usu. occur after a severe illness

Beau \bō\, **Joseph-Honoré-Simon (1806–1865),** French physician.

Beck Depression Inventory \'bek-\ *n* : a standardized psychiatric questionnaire that is used in the diagnosis of depression

Beck, Aaron Temkin (*b* 1921), American psychiatrist.

Beck·er muscular dystrophy \'bekər-\ *or* **Beck·er's muscular dystrophy** \-kərz\ *n* : a less severe form of Duchenne muscular dystrophy with later onset and slower progression of the disease that is inherited as an X⁼ linked recessive trait and is characterized by dystrophin of deficient or abnormal molecular weight

Becker, P. E., 20th-century German human geneticist.

Beck·with-Wie·de·mann syndrome \'bek-wəth-'wē-də-mən-\ *n* : an inherited disease that is characterized by macroglossia, umbilical hernia, hypoglycemia, abnormal enlargement of the viscera, and increased risk of Wilms' tumor and rhabdomyosarcoma

Beckwith, John Bruce (*b* 1933), American pathologist.

bec·lo·meth·a·sone \,be-klō-'me-thə-,zōn, -,sōn\ *n* : a steroid anti-inflammatory drug administered in the form of its dipropionate $C_{28}H_{37}ClO_7$ as an inhalant to treat asthma and as a nasal spray to treat rhinitis — see BECONASE

Bec·on·ase \'bek-ə-,nās, -,nāz\ *trademark* — used for a preparation of the dipropionate of beclomethasone

bed \'bed\ *n* 1 **a** : a piece of furniture on or in which one may lie and sleep — see HOSPITAL BED **b** : the equipment and services needed to care for one hospitalized patient 2 : a layer of specialized or altered tissue esp. when separating dissimilar structures — see NAIL BED, VASCULAR BED

bed·bug \'bed-,bəg\ *n* : a wingless bloodsucking bug (*Cimex lectularius*) sometimes infesting houses and esp. beds and feeding on human blood — called also *chinch*

bed·pan \'bed-,pan\ *n* : a shallow vessel used by a bedridden person for urination or defecation

bed rest *n* : confinement of a sick person to bed

bed·rid·den \'bed-,rid-ᵊn\ *also* **bed·rid** \-,rid\ *adj* : confined to bed (as by illness)

¹bed·side \'bed-,sīd\ *n* : a place beside a bed esp. of a bedridden person

²bedside *adj* 1 : of, relating to, or conducted at the bedside of a bedridden patient ⟨a ~ diagnosis⟩ 2 : suitable for a bedridden person

bedside manner *n* : the manner that a physician assumes toward patients

bed·so·nia \bed-'sō-nē-ə\ *n, pl* **-ni·ae** \-nē-ē, -,ī\ : CHLAMYDIA 2a

Bed·son \'bed-sᵊn\, **Sir Samuel Phillips** (1886–1969), English bacteriologist.

bed·sore \'bed-,sōr\ *n* : an ulceration of tissue deprived of adequate blood sup-

ply by prolonged pressure — called also *decubitus, decubitus ulcer, pressure sore;* compare PRESSURE POINT 1

bed–wet·ting \-,we-tiŋ\ *n* : enuresis esp. when occurring in bed during sleep — **bed–wet·ter** \-,we-tər\ *n*

bee \'bē\ *n* : HONEYBEE; *broadly* : any of numerous hymenopterous insects (superfamily Apoidea) that differ from the related wasps esp. in the heavier hairier body and in having sucking as well as chewing mouthparts — see AFRICANIZED BEE

beef measles *n, sing or pl* : the infestation of beef muscle by cysticerci of the beef tapeworm which make oval white vesicles giving a measly appearance to beef

beef tapeworm *n* : a tapeworm of the genus *Taenia* (*T. saginata*) that infests the human intestine as an adult, has a cysticercus larva that develops in cattle, and is contracted through ingestion of the larva in raw or rare beef

bees·wax \'bēz-,waks\ *n* 1 : WAX 1 2 : YELLOW WAX

be·hav·ior \bi-'hā-vyər\ *n* 1 : the manner of conducting oneself 2 **a** : anything that an organism does involving action and response to stimulation **b** : the response of an individual, group, or species to its environment — **be·hav·ior·al** \-vyə-rəl\ *adj* — **be·hav·ior·al·ly** *adv*

behavioral science *n* : a science (as psychology or sociology) that deals with human action and seeks to generalize about human behavior in society — **behavioral scientist** *n*

be·hav·ior·ism \bi-'hā-vyə-,ri-zəm\ *n* : a school of psychology that takes the objective evidence of behavior (as measured responses to stimuli) as the only concern of its research and the only basis of its theory without reference to conscious experience — **be·hav·ior·ist** \-rist\ *n or adj* — **be·hav·ior·is·tic** \-,hā-vyə-'ris-tik\ *adj*

behavior modification *also* **behavioral modification** *n* : psychotherapy that is concerned with the treatment of observable behaviors rather than underlying psychological processes and emphasizes the substitution of desirable responses and behavior patterns for undesirable ones — called also *behavior therapy;* compare COGNITIVE THERAPY

behavior therapist *or* **behavioral therapist** *n* : a specialist in behavior modification

behavior therapy *or* **behavioral therapy** *n* : BEHAVIOR MODIFICATION

be·hav·iour, be·hav·iour·ism *chiefly Brit var of* BEHAVIOR, BEHAVIORISM

Beh·cet's syndrome \bə-'chets-\ *n* : a group of symptoms of unknown etiology that occur esp. in young men and include esp. ulcerative lesions of the mouth and genitalia and inflammation of the eye (as uveitis and iridocyclitis) — called also *Behcet's disease*

Behçet, Hulusi (1889–1948), Turkish dermatologist.

bej·el \'be-jəl\ *n* : a disease that is endemic chiefly in children of dry hot regions of northern Africa, Asia, and the Middle East, is marked by bone and skin lesions, and is caused by a spirochete of the genus *Treponema* (*T. endemicum*) closely related to the causative agent of syphilis — called also *endemic syphilis*

¹**belch** \'belch\ *vb* : to expel gas from the stomach suddenly : ERUCT

²**belch** *n* : an act or instance of belching : ERUCTATION

bel·la·don·na \ˌbe-lə-'dä-nə\ *n* **1** : an Old World poisonous plant of the genus *Atropa* (*A. belladonna*) having a root and leaves that yield atropine — called also *deadly nightshade* **2** : a medicinal preparation (as atropine) extracted from the belladonna and containing anticholinergic alkaloids

bel·lows \'be-(ˌ)lōz\ *n sing or pl* : LUNGS

Bell's palsy *n* : paralysis of the facial nerve producing distortion on one side of the face

Bell, Sir Charles (1774–1842), British anatomist.

bel·ly \'be-lē\ *n, pl* **bellies 1 a** : ABDOMEN 1a **b** : the undersurface of an animal's body **c** : the stomach and its adjuncts **2** : the enlarged fleshy body of a muscle

bel·ly·ache \'be-lē-ˌāk\ *n* : pain in the abdomen and esp. in the stomach : STOMACHACHE

bel·ly·band \-ˌband\ *n* : a band around or across the belly; *esp* : BAND 1a

belly button *n* : the human navel

be·me·gride \'be-mə-ˌgrīd, 'bē-\ *n* : an analeptic drug $C_{18}H_{13}NO_2$ used esp. to counteract the effects of barbiturates

Ben·a·dryl \'be-nə-ˌdril\ *trademark* — used for a preparation of the hydrochloride of diphenhydramine

ben·a·ze·pril \bən-'ā-zə-pril\ *n* : an ACE inhibitor used in the form of its hydrochloride $C_{24}H_{28}N_2O_5 \cdot HCl$ for the treatment of hypertension — see LOTENSIN, LOTREL

Bence–Jones protein \'bens-'jōnz-\ *n* : a polypeptide composed of one or two antibody light chains that is found esp. in the urine of persons affected with multiple myeloma

Bence–Jones, Henry (1814–1873), British physician.

Ben·der Gestalt test \ˌben-dər-\ *n* : a test in which the subject copies geometric figures and which is used esp. to assess organic brain damage and degree of nervous system maturation

Bender, Lauretta (1897–1987), American psychiatrist.

bends \'bendz\ *n sing or pl* : the painful manifestations (as joint pain) of decompression sickness; *also* : DECOMPRESSION SICKNESS — usu. used with *the* ⟨a case of the ∼⟩

Ben·e·dict's solution \'be-nə-ˌdikts-\ *n* : a blue solution that contains sodium carbonate, sodium citrate, and copper sulfate $CuSO_4$ and is used to test for reducing sugars in Benedict's test

Ben·e·dict \'be-nə-ˌdikt\, **Stanley Rossiter** (1884–1936), American chemist.

Benedict's test *n* : a test for the presence of a reducing sugar (as in urine) by heating the solution to be tested with Benedict's solution which yields a red, yellow, or orange precipitate upon warming with a reducing sugar (as glucose or maltose)

Ben–Gay \ˌben-'gā\ *trademark* — used for a preparation of methyl salicylate and menthol

be·nign \bi-'nīn\ *adj* **1** : of a mild type or character that does not threaten health or life ⟨∼ malaria⟩ ⟨a ∼ tumor⟩ — compare MALIGNANT 1 **2** : having a good prognosis : responding favorably to treatment ⟨a ∼ psychosis⟩ — **be·nig·ni·ty** \bi-'nig-nə-tē\ *n*

benign intracranial hypertension *n* : PSEUDOTUMOR CEREBRI

benign prostatic hyperplasia *n* : adenomatous hyperplasia of the periurethral part of the prostate gland that occurs esp. in men over 50 years old and that tends to obstruct urination by constricting the urethra — abbr. *BPH*; called also *benign prostatic hypertrophy*

ben·ny \'be-nē\ *n, pl* **bennies** *slang* : a tablet of amphetamine taken as a stimulant

benz- *or* **benzo-** *comb form* **1** : related to benzene or benzoic acid ⟨*benz*oate⟩ **2** : containing a benzene ring fused on one side to one side of another ring ⟨*benz*imidazole⟩

benz·al·ko·ni·um chloride \ˌben-zal-'kō-nē-əm-\ *n* : a white or yellowish white mixture of chloride salts used as an antiseptic and germicide — see ZEPHIRAN

ben·za·thine penicillin G \'ben-zə-ˌthēn-, -thən-\ *n* : PENICILLIN G BENZATHINE

Ben·ze·drine \'ben-zə-ˌdrēn\ *n* : a preparation of the sulfate of amphetamine $(C_9H_{13}N)_2 \cdot H_2SO_4$ formerly used in medicine — formerly a U.S. registered trademark

ben·zene \'ben-ˌzēn, ben-'\ *n* : a colorless volatile flammable toxic liquid aromatic hydrocarbon C_6H_6 used in organic synthesis, as a solvent, and as a motor fuel

benzene hexa·chlor·ide \-ˌhek-sə-'klōr-ˌīd\ *n* : a compound $C_6H_6Cl_6$ occurring in several stereoisomeric forms : BHC; *esp* : GAMMA BENZENE HEXACHLORIDE — see LINDANE

benzene ring *n* : a ring of six carbon atoms linked by alternate single and double bonds in a plane symmetrical hexagon that occurs in benzene and related compounds

ben·zes·trol \ben-'zes-₁tról, -₁tról\ n : a crystalline estrogenic compound $C_{20}H_{26}O_2$

ben·zi·dine \'ben-zə-₁dēn\ n : a crystalline base $C_{12}H_{12}N_2$ used esp. in making dyes and in a test for blood

benzidine test n : a test for blood (as in feces) based on its production of a blue color in a solution containing benzidine

benzilate — see QUINUCLIDINYL BENZILATE

benz·imid·azole \₁ben-₁zi-mə-'da-₁zōl, ₁ben-zə-'mi-də-₁zōl\ n : a crystalline base $C_7H_6N_2$ used esp. to inhibit the growth of various viruses, parasitic worms, and fungi; also : one of its derivatives

benzo– — see BENZ-

ben·zo[a]·py·rene \₁ben-zō-₁ā-'pīr-₁ēn, -zō-₁al-fə-, -pī-'rēn\ also 3,4-**benz·py·rene** \-benz-'pīr-₁ēn, -₁benz-pī-'rēn\ n : the yellow crystalline highly carcinogenic isomer of the benzopyrene mixture that is formed esp. in the burning of cigarettes, coal, and gasoline

ben·zo·ate \'ben-zə-₁wāt\ n : a salt or ester of benzoic acid

ben·zo·caine \'ben-zə-₁kān\ n : a crystalline ester $C_9H_{11}NO_2$ used as a local anesthetic — called also *ethyl aminobenzoate*

ben·zo·di·az·e·pine \₁ben-zō-dī-'a-zə-₁pēn\ n : any of a group of aromatic lipophilic amines (as diazepam and chlordiazepoxide) used esp. as tranquilizers

ben·zo·ic acid \ben-₁zō-ik-\ n : a white crystalline acid $C_6H_6O_2$ used as a preservative of foods and in medicine

ben·zo·in \'ben-zə-wən, -₁wēn; -₁zóin\ n 1 : a yellowish balsamic resin from trees (genus *Styrax* of the family Styracaceae) of southeastern Asia used esp. as an expectorant and topically to relieve skin irritations 2 : a white crystalline hydroxy ketone $C_{14}H_{12}O_2$

ben·zo·mor·phan \₁ben-zō-'mór-₁fan\ n : any of a group of synthetic compounds including some potent analgesics (as phenazocine or pentazocine)

ben·zo·phe·none \₁ben-zō-fi-'nōn, -'fē-₁nōn\ n : a colorless crystalline ketone $C_{13}H_{10}O$ used in sunscreens

ben·zo·py·rene \₁ben-zō-'pīr-₁ēn, -₁pī-'rēn\ or **benz·py·rene** \benz-'pīr-₁ēn, ₁benz-pī-'rēn\ n : a mixture of two isomeric hydrocarbons $C_{20}H_{12}$ of which one is highly carcinogenic — see BENZO[A]PYRENE

ben·zo·yl peroxide \'ben-zə-₁wil-, -₁zóil-\ n : a white crystalline compound $C_{14}H_{10}O_4$ used in medicine esp. in the treatment of acne

benz·pyr·in·i·um bromide \₁benz-pə-'ri-nē-əm-\ n : a cholinergic agent $C_{15}H_{17}BrN_2O_2$ that has actions similar to those of neostigmine — called also *benzpyrinium*

benz·tro·pine \benz-'trō-₁pēn, -pən\ n : a parasympatholytic drug used in

the form of its mesylate $C_{21}H_{25}NO$-CH_4O_3S esp. in the treatment of Parkinson's disease

ben·zyl benzoate \'ben-₁zēl-, -zəl-\ n : a colorless oily ester $C_{14}H_{12}O_2$ used esp. as a scabicide

ben·zyl·pen·i·cil·lin \₁ben-₁zēl-(₁)pe-nə-'si-lən, -zəl-\ n : PENICILLIN G

beri·beri \₁ber-ē-'ber-ē\ n : a deficiency disease marked by inflammatory or degenerative changes of the nerves, digestive system, and heart and caused by a lack of or inability to assimilate thiamine

berke·li·um \'bər-klē-əm\ n : a radioactive metallic element — symbol *Bk*; see ELEMENT table

ber·lock dermatitis \'bər-₁läk-\ n : a brownish discoloration of the skin that develops on exposure to sunlight after the use of perfume containing certain essential oils

Ber·tin's column \ber-'ta^nz-\ n : RENAL COLUMN

  Ber·tin \ber-ta^n\, **Exupère Joseph (1712–1781),** French anatomist.

be·ryl·li·o·sis \bə-₁ri-lē-'ō-səs\ also **ber·yl·lo·sis** \ber-ə-'lō-\ n, pl **-li·o·ses** \-₁sēz\; or **-lo·ses** \-₁sēz\ : poisoning resulting from exposure to fumes and dusts of beryllium compounds or alloys and occurring chiefly as an acute pneumonitis or as a granulomatosis involving the lungs

be·ryl·li·um \bə-'ri-lē-əm\ n : a steel-gray light strong brittle toxic bivalent metallic element — symbol *Be*; see ELEMENT table

bes·ti·al·i·ty \bes-chē-'a-lə-tē, ₁bēs-\ n, pl **-ties** : sexual relations between a human being and a lower animal

¹be·ta \'bā-tə\ n 1 : the second letter of the Greek alphabet — B or β 2 : BETA PARTICLE 3 : BETA WAVE

²beta or **β-** adj 1 : of or relating to one of two or more closely related chemical substances ⟨the *beta* chain of hemoglobin⟩ — used somewhat arbitrarily to specify ordinal relationship or a particular physical form 2 : second in a position in the structure of an organic molecule from a particular group or atom; also : occurring at or having a structure characterized by such a position ⟨β-substitution⟩ 3 : producing a zone of decolorization when grown on blood media — used of some hemolytic streptococci or of the hemolysis they cause

be·ta–ad·ren·er·gic \-₁a-drə-'nər-jik\ adj : of, relating to, or being a beta-receptor ⟨∼ blocking action⟩

beta–adrenergic receptor n : BETA-RECEPTOR

be·ta–ad·re·no·cep·tor \-ə-'drē-nə-₁sep-tər\ also **be·ta–ad·re·no·re·cep·tor** \-ri-₁sep-tər\ n : BETA-RECEPTOR

be·ta–ag·o·nist \-'a-gə-nəst\ n : any of various drugs (as albuterol or terbutaline) that combine with and activate a beta-receptor

be·ta–am·y·loid also **β–amyloid** \-'a-mə-ˌlȯid\ n : an amyloid that is derived from amyloid precursor protein and is the primary component of plaques characteristic of Alzheimer's disease — called also *amyloid beta-protein, beta-amyloid protein*

be·ta–block·ade \-blä-'kād\ n : blockade of beta-receptor activity

be·ta–block·er \-'blä-kər\ n : any of a group of drugs (as propranolol) that combine with and block the activity of a beta-receptor to decrease the heart rate and force of contractions and lower high blood pressure and that are used esp. to treat hypertension, angina pectoris, and ventricular and supraventricular arrhythmias

be·ta–block·ing \-'blä-kiŋ\ adj : blocking or relating to the blocking of beta-receptor activity ⟨~ drugs⟩

be·ta–car·o·tene or **β–carotene** \-'kar-ə-ˌtēn\ n : an isomer of carotene that is found in dark green and dark yellow vegetables and fruits

beta cell n : any of various secretory cells distinguished by their basophilic staining characters: as **a** : a pituitary basophil **b** : an insulin-secreting cell of the islets of Langerhans — compare ALPHA CELL

Be·ta·dine \'bā-tə-ˌdīn\ trademark — used for a preparation of povidone-iodine

be·ta–en·dor·phin or **β–endorphin** \ˌbā-tə-en-'dȯr-fən\ n : an endorphin of the pituitary gland with much greater analgesic potency than morphine — see BETA-LIPOTROPIN

beta globin also **β–globin** \-'glō-bən\ n : the chain of hemoglobin that is designated beta and that when deficient or defective causes various anemias (as beta-thalassemia or sickle-cell anemia)

beta globulin n : any of several globulins of plasma or serum that have at alkaline pH electrophoretic mobilities intermediate between those of the alpha globulins and gamma globulins

beta hemolysis n : a sharply defined clear colorless zone of hemolysis surrounding colonies of certain streptococci on blood agar plates — **be·ta–he·mo·lyt·ic** \ˌbā-tə-ˌhē-mə-'li-tik\ adj

be·ta·ine \'bē-tə-ˌēn\ n : an ammonium salt C₅H₁₁NO₂ that is used to treat homocystinuria and is also used in the form of its hydrochloride C₅H₁₁NO₂·HCl as a source of hydrochloric acid esp. to treat hypochlorhydria

beta interferon n : an interferon that is produced esp. by fibroblasts, possesses antiviral activity, and is used in a form obtained from recombinant DNA esp. in the treatment of multiple sclerosis

be·ta–lac·tam or **β–lactam** \ˌbā-tə-'lak-ˌtam\ n : any of a large class of antibiotics (as the penicillins and cephalosporins) with a lactam ring

be·ta–lac·ta·mase or **β–lactamase** \-'lak-tə-ˌmās, -ˌmāz\ n : an enzyme found esp. in staphylococcal bacteria that inactivates penicillins by hydrolyzing them — called also *penicillinase*

beta–lipoprotein or **β–lipoprotein** n : LDL

be·ta–li·po·tro·pin \ˌbā-tə-ˌli-pə-'trō-pən, -ˌlī-\ n : a lipotropin of the anterior pituitary that contains beta-endorphin as the terminal sequence of 31 amino acids in its polypeptide chain

be·ta·meth·a·sone \ˌbā-tə-'me-thə-ˌzōn, -ˌsōn\ n : a potent glucocorticoid C₂₂H₂₉FO₅ that is isomeric with dexamethasone and has potent anti-inflammatory activity

beta particle n : a high-speed electron emitted from the nucleus of an atom during radioactive decay

be·ta–pleat·ed sheet \-'plē-təd\ n : BETA-SHEET

beta ray n **1** : BETA PARTICLE **2** : a stream of beta particles — called also *beta radiation*

be·ta–re·cep·tor \ˌbā-tə-ri-'sep-tər\ n : any of a group of receptors that are present on cell surfaces of some effector organs and tissues innervated by the sympathetic nervous system and that mediate certain physiological responses (as vasodilation, relaxation of bronchial and uterine smooth muscle, and increased heart rate) when bound by specific adrenergic agents — called also *beta-adrenergic receptor, beta-adrenoceptor*; compare ALPHA-RECEPTOR

beta rhythm n : BETA WAVE

be·ta–sheet \-ˌshēt\ n : the structural arrangement of many proteins in which two or more short regions of the polypeptide chain align adjacently and are stabilized by hydrogen bonds into sheets with a pleated appearance — called also *beta-pleated sheet*; compare ALPHA-HELIX

be·ta–si·tos·ter·ol also **β–sitosterol** \-sī-'täs-tə-ˌrȯl, -ˌrōl\ n : a sterol widespread in plant products (as wheat germ, soybeans, and corn oil) that is used in dietary supplements and is held to lower cholesterol levels and relieve symptoms of benign prostatic hyperplasia

be·ta–thalassemia or **β–thalassemia** n : thalassemia in which the hemoglobin chain designated beta is affected and which comprises Cooley's anemia in the homozygous condition and thalassemia minor in the heterozygous condition

beta wave n : an electrical rhythm of the brain with a frequency of 13 to 30 cycles per second that is associated with normal conscious waking experience — called also *beta, beta rhythm*

be·tel nut \'bē-tᵊl-\ n : the astringent seed of an Asian palm (*Areca catechu*) that is a source of arecoline

be·tha·ne·chol \bə-'thā-nə-ˌkȯl, -'tha-, -ˌkōl\ *n* : a parasympathomimetic agent administered in the form of its chloride $C_7H_{17}ClN_2O_2$ and used esp. to treat gastric and urinary retention — see URECHOLINE

be·tween-brain \bi-'twēn-ˌbrān\ *n* : DIENCEPHALON

Betz cell \'bets-\ *n* : a very large pyramidal nerve cell of the motor area of the cerebral cortex

Betz, Vladimir Aleksandrovich (1834–1894), Russian anatomist.

Bex·tra \'bek-strə\ *trademark* — used for a preparation of valdecoxib

be·zoar \'bē-ˌzȯr\ *n* : any of various calculi found in the gastrointestinal organs esp. of ruminants — called also *bezoar stone*

BFP *abbr* biologic false-positive

BGH *abbr* bovine growth hormone

Bh *symbol* bohrium

BHA \ˌbē-(ˌ)āch-'ā\ *n* : a phenolic antioxidant $C_{11}H_{16}O_2$ used esp. to preserve fats and oils in food — called also *butylated hydroxyanisole*

bhang *also* **bang** \'bäŋ, 'bȯŋ, 'baŋ\ *n* **1 a** : HEMP 1 **b** : the leaves and flowering tops of uncultivated hemp : CANNABIS — compare MARIJUANA **2** : an intoxicant product obtained from bhang — compare HASHISH

BHC \ˌbē-(ˌ)āch-'sē\ *n* **1** : BENZENE HEXACHLORIDE **2** : LINDANE

BHT \ˌbē-(ˌ)āch-'tē\ *n* : a phenolic antioxidant $C_{15}H_{24}O$ used esp. to preserve fats and oils in food, cosmetics, and pharmaceuticals — called also *butylated hydroxytoluene*

Bi *symbol* bismuth

¹bi- *prefix* **1 a** : two ⟨*bi*lateral⟩ **b** : into two parts ⟨*bi*furcate⟩ **2** : twice : doubly : on both sides ⟨*bi*convex⟩ **3** : between, involving, or affecting two (specified) symmetrical parts ⟨*bi*labial⟩ **4 a** : containing one (specified) constituent in double the proportion of the other constituent or in double the ordinary proportion ⟨*bi*carbonate⟩ **b** : DI- ⟨*bi*phenyl⟩

²bi- *or* **bio-** *comb form* : life : living organisms or tissue ⟨*bio*chemistry⟩

bi·ar·tic·u·lar \ˌbī-är-'tik-yə-lər\ *adj* : of or relating to two joints

bib·li·o·ther·a·py \ˌbi-blē-ō-'ther-ə-pē\ *n, pl* **-pies** : the use of selected reading materials as therapeutic adjuvants in medicine and in psychiatry; *also* : guidance in the solution of personal problems through directed reading — **bib·li·o·ther·a·peu·tic** \-ther-ə-'pyütik\ *adj* — **bib·li·o·ther·a·pist** \-'therə-pist\ *n*

bi·carb \'bī-ˌkärb, bī-'\ *n* : SODIUM BICARBONATE

bi·car·bon·ate \(ˌ)bī-'kär-bə-ˌnāt, -nət\ *n* : an acid carbonate

bicarbonate of soda *n* : SODIUM BICARBONATE

bi·ceps \'bī-ˌseps\ *n, pl* **biceps** *also* **bicepses** : a muscle having two heads: as **a** : the large flexor muscle of the

front of the upper arm **b** : the large flexor muscle of the back of the upper leg

biceps bra·chii \-'brā-kē-ˌē, -ˌī\ *n* : BICEPS a

biceps fe·mo·ris \-'fē-mə-rəs, -'fe-\ *n* : BICEPS b

biceps flex·or cu·bi·ti \-'flek-ˌsȯr-'kyü-bə-ˌtī, -tē\ *n* : BICEPS a

bi·chlo·ride of mercury \(ˌ)bī-'klȯrˌīd-\ *n* : MERCURIC CHLORIDE

bi·cip·i·tal \(ˌ)bī-'si-pət-ᵊl\ *adj* **1** *of muscles* : having two heads or origins **2** : of or relating to a biceps muscle

bicipital aponeurosis *n* : an aponeurosis given off from the tendon of the biceps of the arm and continuous with the deep fascia of the forearm

bicipital groove *n* : a furrow on the upper part of the humerus occupied by the long head of the biceps — called also *intertubercular groove*

bicipital tuberosity *n* : the rough eminence which is on the anterior inner aspect of the neck of the radius and into which the tendon of the biceps is inserted

bi·con·cave \ˌbī-(ˌ)kän-'kāv, (ˌ)bī-'kän-ˌ\ *adj* : concave on both sides — **bi·con·cav·i·ty** \ˌbī-(ˌ)kän-'ka-və-tē\ *n*

bi·con·vex \ˌbī-(ˌ)kän-'veks, (ˌ)bī-'kän-ˌ, ˌbī-kən-'\ *adj* : convex on both sides — **bi·con·vex·i·ty** \ˌbī-kən-'vek-sə-tē, -(ˌ)kän-\ *n*

bi·cor·nu·ate \(ˌ)bī-'kȯrn-yə-ˌwāt, -wət\ *or* **bi·cor·nate** \-'kȯr-ˌnāt, -nət\ *adj* : having two horns or horn-shaped processes ⟨a ~ uterus⟩

bi·cu·cul·line \bī-'kü-kyə-ˌlēn, -lən\ *n* : a convulsant alkaloid $C_{20}H_{17}NO_6$ obtained from plants (family Fumariaceae) and having the capacity to antagonize the action of gammaaminobutyric acid

¹bi·cus·pid \(ˌ)bī-'kəs-pəd\ *adj* : having or ending in two points ⟨~ teeth⟩

²bicuspid *n* : either of the two doublepointed teeth that are situated between the canines and the molars on each side of each jaw : PREMOLAR

bicuspid valve *n* : MITRAL VALVE

bi·cy·clic \bī-'sī-klik, -'si-\ *adj* : containing two usu. fused rings in the structure of a molecule

bid *abbr* [Latin *bis in die*] twice a day — used in writing prescriptions

bi·det \bi-'dā\ *n* : a bathroom fixture used esp. for bathing the external genitals and the anal region

bi·di·rec·tion·al \ˌbī-də-'rek-sh(ə-)nəl, -dī-\ *adj* : involving, moving, or taking place in two usu. opposite directions ⟨~ flow⟩ — **bi·di·rec·tion·al·ly** *adv*

bi·fid \'bī-ˌfid, -fəd\ *adj* : divided into two equal lobes or parts by a median cleft ⟨repair of a ~ digit⟩

bifida — see SPINA BIFIDA, SPINA BIFIDA OCCULTA

¹bi·fo·cal \(ˌ)bī-'fō-kəl\ *adj* **1** : having two focal lengths **2** : having one part that corrects for near vision and one for distant vision ⟨a ~ eyeglass lens⟩

²**bifocal** *n* **1** : a bifocal glass or lens **2** **bifocals** *pl* : eyeglasses with bifocal lenses

bi·func·tion·al \ˌbī-ˈfəŋk-sh(ə-)nəl\ *adj* : having two functions ⟨∼ neurons⟩

bi·fur·cate \ˈbī-(ˌ)fər-ˌkāt, bī-ˈfər-\ *vb* **-cat·ed; -cat·ing** : to divide into two branches or parts — **bi·fur·cate** \(ˌ)bī-ˈfər-kət, -ˌkāt; ˈbī-(ˌ)fər-ˌkāt\ *or* **bi·fur·cat·ed** \-ˌkā-təd\ *adj* — **bi·fur·ca·tion** \ˌbī-(ˌ)fər-ˈkā-shən\ *n*

bi·gem·i·ny \bī-ˈje-mə-nē\ *n, pl* **-nies** : the state of having a pulse characterized by two beats close together with a pause following each pair of beats — **bi·gem·i·nal** \-nəl\ *adj*

big·head \ˈbig-ˌhed\ *n* : any of several diseases of animals: as **a** : equine osteoporosis **b** : an acute photosensitization of sheep and goats that follows the ingestion of various plants

big toe *n* : the innermost and largest digit of the foot — called also *great toe*

bi·gua·nide \(ˌ)bī-ˈgwä-ˌnīd, -nəd\ *n* : any of a group of hypoglycemia-inducing drugs (as metformin) used esp. in the treatment of diabetes — see PROGUANIL

bi·ki·ni incision \bə-ˈkē-nē-\ *n* : PFANNENSTIEL'S INCISION

bi·la·bi·al \(ˌ)bī-ˈlā-bē-əl\ *adj* : of or relating to both lips

bi·lat·er·al \(ˌ)bī-ˈla-tə-rəl, -ˈla-trəl\ *adj* **1** : of, relating to, or affecting the right and left sides of the body or the right and left members of paired organs ⟨∼ nephrectomy⟩ **2** : having bilateral symmetry — **bi·lat·er·al·i·ty** \(ˌ)bī-ˌla-tə-ˈra-lə-tē\ *n* — **bi·lat·er·al·ly** *adv*

bilateral symmetry *n* : symmetry in which similar anatomical parts are arranged on opposite sides of a median axis so that one and only one plane can divide the individual into essentially identical halves

bi·lay·er \ˈbī-ˌlā-ər\ *n* : a film or membrane with two molecular layers — **bilayer** *adj*

bile \ˈbīl\ *n* : a yellow or greenish viscid alkaline fluid secreted by the liver and passed into the duodenum where it aids esp. in the emulsification and absorption of fats

bile acid *n* : any of several steroid acids (as cholic acid) that occur in bile usu. in the form of sodium salts conjugated with glycine or taurine

bile duct *n* : a duct by which bile passes from the liver or gallbladder to the duodenum

bile fluke *n* : CHINESE LIVER FLUKE

bile pigment *n* : any of several coloring matters (as bilirubin) in bile

bile salt *n* **1** : a salt of bile acid **2 bile salts** *pl* : a dry mixture of the salts of the gall of the ox used as a liver stimulant and as a laxative

bil·har·zia \bil-ˈhär-zē-ə, -ˈhärt-sē-\ *n* **1** : SCHISTOSOME **2** : SCHISTOSOMIASIS — **bil·har·zi·al** \-zē-əl, -sē-\ *adj*

Bil·harz \ˈbil-ˌhärts\, **Theodor Maximillian (1825–1862)**, German anatomist and helminthologist.

bil·har·zi·a·sis \ˌbil-ˌhär-ˈzī-ə-səs, -ˌhärt-ˈsī-\ *n, pl* **-a·ses** \ˌsēz\ : SCHISTOSOMIASIS

bili- *comb form* **1** : bile ⟨*bili*ary⟩ **2** : derived from bile ⟨*bili*rubin⟩

bil·i·ary \ˈbi-lē-ˌer-ē\ *adj* **1** : of, relating to, or conveying bile **2** : affecting the bile-conveying structures

biliary atresia *n* : absence or underdevelopment of the bile ducts and esp. the extrahepatic bile ducts

biliary cirrhosis *n* : cirrhosis of the liver due to inflammation or obstruction of the bile ducts resulting in the accumulation of bile in and functional impairment of the liver

biliary dyskinesia *n* : pain or discomfort in the epigastric region resulting from spasm esp. of the sphincter of Oddi following cholecystectomy

biliary fever *n* : piroplasmosis esp. of dogs and horses

biliary tree *n* : the bile ducts and gallbladder

bil·ious \ˈbil-yəs\ *adj* **1** : of or relating to bile **2** : marked by or affected with disordered liver function and esp. excessive secretion of bile — **bil·ious·ness** *n*

bil·i·ru·bin \ˌbi-li-ˈrü-bən, ˈbi-li-ˌ\ *n* : a reddish yellow pigment $C_{33}H_{36}N_4O_6$ that occurs esp. in bile and in blood and causes jaundice if accumulated in excess

bil·i·ru·bi·nae·mia \ˌbi-li-ˌrü-bə-ˈnē-mē-ə\ *chiefly Brit var of* BILIRUBINEMIA

bil·i·ru·bi·ne·mia \-ˈnē-mē-ə\ *n* : HYPERBILIRUBINEMIA

bil·i·ru·bi·nu·ria \-ˈnùr-ē-ə, -nyùr-\ *n* : excretion of bilirubin in the urine

bil·i·ver·din \ˌbi-li-ˈvərd-ᵊn, ˈbi-li-ˌ\ *n* : a green pigment $C_{33}H_{34}N_4O_6$ that occurs in bile and is an intermediate in the degradation of hemoglobin heme groups to bilirubin

bi·lobed \(ˌ)bī-ˈlōbd\ *adj* : divided into two lobes ⟨a ∼ organ⟩

Bil·tri·cide \ˈbil-trə-ˌsīd\ *trademark* — used for a preparation of praziquantel

bi·man·u·al \(ˌ)bī-ˈman-yə-wəl\ *adj* : done with or requiring the use of both hands ⟨a ∼ pelvic examination⟩

bin- *comb form* : two : two by two : two at a time ⟨*bin*aural⟩

bi·na·ry \ˈbī-nə-rē\ *adj* **1** : compounded or consisting of or marked by two things or parts **2** : composed of two chemical elements, an element and a radical that acts as an element, or two such radicals

binary fission *n* : reproduction of a cell by division into two approximately equal parts

bin·au·ral \(ˌ)bī-ˈnòr-əl, (ˌ)bi-\ *adj* : of, relating to, or involving two or both ears — **bin·au·ral·ly** *adv*

bind \ˈbīnd\ *vb* **bound** \ˈbaùnd\; **binding** **1** : to wrap up (an injury) with a cloth : BANDAGE 2 : to take up and hold usu. by chemical forces : combine with ⟨cellulose ∼*s* water⟩ 3 : to combine or be taken up esp. by chemical action ⟨an antibody *bound* to a specific antigen⟩ 4 : to make costive : CONSTIPATE

bind·er \'bīn-dər\ *n* 1 : a broad bandage applied (as about the chest) for support 2 : a substance (as glucose or acacia) used in pharmacy to hold together the ingredients of a compressed tablet

Bi·net age \bē-'nā-, bi-\ *n* : mental age as determined by the Binet-Simon scale

Bi·net \bē-nā\, **Alfred (1857–1911),** French psychologist, and **Si·mon** \sē-mōⁿ\, **Théodore (1873–1961),** French physician.

Bi·net–Si·mon scale \bi-'nā-sē-'mōⁿ-\ *n* : an intelligence test consisting orig. of tasks graded from the level of the average 3-year-old to that of the average 12-year-old but later extended in range — called also *Binet-Simon test, Binet test;* see STANFORD-BINET TEST

¹**binge** \'binj\ *n* : an act of excessive or compulsive consumption esp. of food or alcoholic beverages

²**binge** *vb* **binged; binge·ing** or **bing·ing** : to go on a binge — **bing·er** \'bin-jər\ *n*

binge eating disorder *n* : an eating disorder characterized by recurring episodes of excessive food consumption accompanied by a sense of lack of control but without intervening periods of compensatory behavior (as self-induced vomiting or purging by laxatives)

bin·oc·u·lar \bī-'nä-kyə-lər, bə-\ *adj* : of, relating to, using, or adapted to the use of both eyes ⟨a ∼ infection⟩ ⟨∼ vision⟩ — **bin·oc·u·lar·ly** *adv*

bi·no·mi·al \bī-'nō-mē-əl\ *n* : a biological species name consisting of two terms — **binomial** *adj*

binomial nomenclature *n* : a system of nomenclature in which each species of animal or plant receives a name of two terms of which the first identifies the genus to which it belongs and the second the species itself

bin·ovu·lar \(,)bī-'nä-vyə-lər, -'nō-\ *adj* : BIOVULAR ⟨∼ twinning⟩

bi·nu·cle·ate \(,)bī-'nü-klē-ət, -'nyü-\ also **bi·nu·cle·at·ed** \-klē-,ā-təd\ *adj* : having two nuclei ⟨∼ lymphocytes⟩

bio- — see BI-

bio·ac·cu·mu·la·tion \bī-(,)ō-ə-,kyü-myə-'lā-shən\ *n* : the accumulation of a substance (as a pesticide) in a living organism

bio·ac·tive \,bī-ō-'ak-tiv\ *adj* : having an effect on a living organism — **bio·ac·tiv·i·ty** \-ak-'ti-və-tē\ *n*

bio·as·say \,bī-(,)ō-'a-,sā, -a-'sā\ *n* : determination of the relative strength of a substance (as a drug) by comparing its effect on a test organism with that of a standard preparation — **bio·as·say** \-a-'sā, -'a-,sā\ *vb*

bio·avail·abil·i·ty \,bī-(,)ō-ə-,vā-lə-'bi-lə-tē\ *n, pl* **-ties** : the degree and rate at which a substance (as a drug) is absorbed into a living system or is made available at the site of physiological activity — **bio·avail·able** \-'vā-lə-bəl\ *adj*

bio·cat·a·lyst \,bī-ō-'kat-ᵊl-əst\ *n* : ENZYME

bio·chem·i·cal \,bī-ō-'ke-mi-kəl\ *adj* 1 : of or relating to biochemistry 2 : characterized by, produced by, or involving chemical reactions in living organisms ⟨∼ processes⟩ — **bio·chemical** *n* — **bio·chem·i·cal·ly** \-k(ə-)lē\ *adv*

bio·chem·is·try \,bī-ō-'ke-mə-strē\ *n, pl* **-tries** 1 : chemistry that deals with the chemical compounds and processes occurring in organisms 2 : the chemical characteristics and reactions of a particular living organism or biological substance ⟨a change in the patient's ∼⟩ — **bio·chem·ist** \-'ke-mist\ *n*

bio·chip \'bī-ō-,chip\ *n* : MICROARRAY

bio·cide \'bī-ə-,sīd\ *n* : a substance (as glutaraldehyde) that is destructive to many different organisms — **bio·cid·al** \,bī-ə-'sīd-ᵊl\ *adj*

bio·com·pat·i·bil·i·ty \,bī-ō-kəm-,pa-tə-'bi-lə-tē\ *n, pl* **-ties** : the condition of being compatible with living tissue or a living system by not being toxic or injurious and not causing immunological rejection — **bio·com·pat·i·ble** \-kəm-'pa-tə-bəl\ *adj*

bio·de·grad·able \,bī-ō-di-'grā-də-bəl\ *adj* : capable of being broken down esp. into innocuous products by the action of living things (as microorganisms) — **bio·de·grad·abil·i·ty** \-,grā-də-'bi-lə-tē\ *n* — **bio·deg·ra·da·tion** \-,de-grə-'dā-shən\ *n* — **bio·de·grade** \-di-'grād\ *vb*

bio·elec·tri·cal \-i-'lek-tri-kəl\ also **bio·elec·tric** \-'trik\ *adj* : of or relating to electric phenomena in living organisms ⟨human cortical ∼ activity⟩ — **bio·elec·tric·i·ty** \-,lek-'tri-sə-tē\ *n*

bio·elec·tron·ics \-i-(,)lek-'trä-niks\ *n* 1 : a branch of science that deals with electronic control of physiological function 2 : a branch of science that deals with the role of electron transfer in biological processes — **bio·elec·tron·ic** \-'nik\ *adj*

bio·en·er·get·ics \,e-nər-'je-tiks\ *n* : a system of therapy that combines breathing and body exercises, psychological therapy, and the free expression of impulses and emotions and that is held to increase well-being by releasing blocked physical and psychic energy — **bio·en·er·get·ic** \-'tik\ *adj*

bio·en·gi·neer·ing \,en-jə-'nir-in\ *n* 1 : biological or medical application of engineering principles or engineering equipment — called also *biomedical* *engineering* 2 : the application of biological techniques (as genetic recombination) to create modified versions of organisms (as crops); *esp* : GENETIC ENGINEERING — **bio·en·gi·neer** \-'nir\ *n or vb*

bio·equiv·a·lence \-i-'kwi-və-ləns\ *n* : the property wherein two drugs with identical active ingredients or two different dosage forms (as tablet and oral suspension) of the same drug possess similar bioavailability and produce the same effect at the site of physiological activity — **bio·equiv·a·lent** \-lənt\ *adj*

bio·equiv·a·len·cy \-lən-sē\ *n, pl* **-cies** : BIOEQUIVALENCE

bio·eth·i·cist \-'e-thə-sist\ *n* : an expert in bioethics

bio·eth·ics \-'e-thiks\ *n* : the discipline dealing with the ethical implications of biological research and applications esp. in medicine — **bio·ethic** \-'thik\ *n* — **bio·ethical** \-'thi-kəl\ *adj*

bio·feed·back \-'fēd-,bak\ *n* : the technique of making unconscious or involuntary bodily processes (as heartbeat or brain waves) perceptible to the senses (as by the use of an oscilloscope) in order to manipulate them by conscious mental control

bio·film \'bī-ō-,film\ *n* : a thin usu. resistant layer of microorganisms (as bacteria) that form on and coat various surfaces (as of catheters)

bio·fla·vo·noid \-'flā-və-,nòid\ *n* : any of various biologically active flavonoids (as quercetin) derived from plants and found esp. in fruits and vegetables

bio·gen·ic \-'je-nik\ *adj* : produced by living organisms ⟨∼ amines⟩

bio·haz·ard \'bī-ō-,ha-zərd\ *n* : a biological agent or condition that constitutes a hazard to humans or the environment; *also* : a hazard posed by such an agent or condition — **bio·haz·ard·ous** \,bī-ō-'ha-zər-dəs\ *adj*

bio·iden·ti·cal \,bī-ō-ī-'den-ti-kəl\ *adj* : possessing identical molecular structure esp. in relation to an endogenously produced substance ⟨∼ estrogens⟩

bio·in·for·mat·ics \,bī-ō-,in-fər-'ma-tiks\ *n* : the collection, classification, storage, and analysis of biochemical and biological information using computers esp. as applied in molecular genetics and genomics — **bio·in·for·mat·ic** \-tik\ *adj*

biol *abbr* biologic; biological; biologist; biology

bi·o·log·ic \,bī-ə-'lä-jik\ *or* **bi·o·log·i·cal** \-ji-kəl\ *n* : a biological product (as a globulin or antigen) used in the prevention or treatment of disease

biological *also* **biologic** *adj* 1 : of or relating to biology or to life and living processes 2 : used in or produced by applied biology 3 : related by direct genetic relationship rather than by adoption or marriage ⟨∼ parents⟩ — **bi·o·log·i·cal·ly** \-ji-k(ə-)lē\ *adv*

biological clock *n* : an inherent timing mechanism in a living system (as a cell) that is inferred to exist in order to explain various cyclical behaviors and physiological processes

biological control *n* 1 : reduction in numbers or elimination of pest organisms by interference with their ecology 2 : an agent used in biological control

biological half–life *or* **biologic half–life** *n* : the time that a living body requires to eliminate one half the quantity of an administered substance (as a radioisotope) through its normal channels of elimination

biological warfare *n* : warfare involving the use of biological weapons; *also* : warfare involving the use of herbicides

biological weapon *n* : a harmful biological agent (as a pathogenic microorganism) used as a weapon to cause death or disease

biologic false–positive *n* : a positive serological reaction for syphilis given by blood of a person who does not have syphilis

bi·ol·o·gist \bī-'ä-lə-jist\ *n* : a specialist in biology

bi·ol·o·gy \bī-'ä-lə-jē\ *n, pl* **-gies** 1 : a branch of science that deals with living organisms and vital processes 2 : the laws and phenomena relating to an organism or group

bio·mark·er \'bī-ō-,mär-kər\ *n* : a biological or biologically derived indicator (as a metabolite in the body) of a process, event, or condition (as disease or exposure to a toxin)

bio·ma·te·ri·al \,bī-ō-mə-'tir-ē-əl\ *n* : material that is suitable for introduction into living tissue esp. as part of a medical device (as an artificial heart valve or joint)

bio·me·chan·ics \,bī-ō-mi-'ka-niks\ *n sing or pl* : the mechanics of biological and esp. muscular activity; *also* : the scientific study of this — **bio·me·chan·i·cal** \-ni-kəl\ *adj*

bio·med·i·cal \-'me-di-kəl\ *adj* 1 : of or relating to biomedicine ⟨∼ studies⟩ 2 : of, relating to, or involving biological, medical, and physical science — **bio·med·i·cal·ly** \-k(ə-)lē\ *adv*

biomedical engineering *n* : BIOENGINEERING 1 — **biomedical engineer** *n*

bio·med·i·cine \-'me-də-sən\ *n* : medicine based on the application of the principles of the natural sciences and esp. biology and biochemistry

bio·met·rics \-'me-triks\ *n sing or pl* : BIOMETRY

bi·om·e·try \bī-'ä-mə-trē\ *n, pl* **-tries** : the statistical analysis of biological observations and phenomena — **bio·met·ric** \,bī-ō-'me-trik\ *or* **bio·met·ri·cal** \-tri-kəl\ *adj* — **bio·me·tri·cian** \-me-'tri-shən\ *n*

bio·mi·cro·scope \bī-ō-'mī-krə-ˌskōp\ n : a binocular microscope used for examination of the anterior part of the eye

bio·mi·cros·co·py \-mī-'kräs-kə-pē\ n, pl **-pies** : the microscopic examination and study of living cells and tissues; specif : examination of the living eye with the biomicroscope

bio·mol·e·cule \ˌbī-ō-'mä-li-ˌkyül\ n : an organic molecule and esp. a macromolecule (as a protein or nucleic acid) in living organisms — **bio·mo·lec·u·lar** \-mə-'le-kyə-lər\ adj

bi·on·ic \bī-'ä-nik\ adj **1** : of or relating to bionics **2** : having normal biological capability or performance enhanced by or as if by electronic or electrically actuated mechanical devices

bi·on·ics \bī-'ä-niks\ n sing or pl : a science concerned with the application of data about the functioning of biological systems to the solution of engineering problems

bio·phar·ma·ceu·ti·cal \ˌbī-ō-ˌfär-mə-'sü-ti-kəl\ adj : of or relating to biopharmaceutics or biopharmaceuticals

biopharmaceutical n : a pharmaceutical derived from biological sources and esp. one produced by biotechnology

bio·phar·ma·ceu·tics \ˌbī-ō-ˌfär-mə-'sü-tiks\ n : the study of the relationships between the physical and chemical properties, dosage, and form of administration of a drug and its activity in the living body

bio·phys·i·cist \-'fi-zə-sist\ n : a specialist in biophysics

bio·phys·ics \ˌbī-ō-'fi-ziks\ n : a branch of science concerned with the application of physical principles and methods to biological problems — **bio·phys·i·cal** \-zi-kəl\ adj

bio·poly·mer \ˌbī-ō-'pä-lə-mər\ n : a polymeric substance (as a protein or polysaccharide) formed in a biological system

bio·pros·the·sis \-präs-'thē-səs\ n, pl **-the·ses** \-ˌsēz\ : a prosthesis (as a porcine heart valve) consisting of an animal part or containing animal tissue — **bio·pros·thet·ic** \-präs-'thet-ik\ adj

bi·op·sy \'bī-ˌäp-sē\ n, pl **-sies** : the removal and examination of tissue, cells, or fluids from the living body — **biopsy** vb

bio·psy·chol·o·gy \ˌbī-ō-sī-'kä-lə-jē\ n, pl **-gies** : PSYCHOBIOLOGY — **bio·psy·cho·log·i·cal** \-ˌsī-kə-'lä-ji-kəl\ adj — **bio·psy·chol·o·gist** \-sī-'kä-lə-jist\ n

bio·psy·cho·so·cial \-ˌsī-kō-'sō-shəl\ adj : of, relating to, or concerned with the biological, psychological, and social aspects of disease

bio·re·ac·tor \-rē-'ak-tər\ n : a device or apparatus in which living organisms and esp. bacteria synthesize useful substances (as interferon) or break down harmful ones (as in sewage)

bio·rhythm \'bī-ō-ˌri-thəm\ n : an innately determined rhythmic biological process or function (as sleep behavior); also : an innate rhythmic determiner of such a process or function — **bio·rhyth·mic** \ˌbī-ō-'rith-mik\ adj

bio·safe·ty \'bī-ō-ˌsāf-tē\ n, pl **-ties** : safety with respect to the effects of biological research on humans and the environment

bio·sci·ence \'bī-ō-ˌsī-əns\ n : BIOLOGY; also : LIFE SCIENCE — **bio·sci·en·tist** \ˌbī-ō-'sī-ən-tist\ n

bio·sen·sor \'bī-ō-ˌsen-ˌsòr, -sər\ n : a device and esp. one consisting of a biological component (as an enzyme or bacterium) that aids in the detection of a target substance

-bi·o·sis \(ˌ)bī-'ō-səs, bē-\ n comb form, pl **-bi·o·ses** \-ˌsēz\ : mode of life ⟨para*biosis*⟩ ⟨sym*biosis*⟩

bio·sta·tis·tics \ˌbī-ō-stə-'tis-tiks\ n : statistical processes and methods applied to the analysis of biological phenomena — **bio·stat·is·ti·cian** \-ˌsta-tə-'sti-shən\ n

bio·syn·the·sis \ˌbī-ō-'sin-thə-səs\ n, pl **-the·ses** : production of a chemical compound by a living organism — **bio·syn·the·size** \-'sin-thə-ˌsīz\ vb — **bio·syn·thet·ic** \-sin-'the-tik\ adj — **bio·syn·thet·i·cal·ly** \-ti-k(ə-)lē\ adv

bio·tech \'bī-ō-ˌtek\ n : BIOTECHNOLOGY 1

bio·tech·ni·cal \ˌbī-ō-'tek-ni-kəl\ adj : of or relating to biotechnology

bio·tech·nol·o·gy \ˌbī-ō-tek-'nä-lə-jē\ n, pl **-gies** **1** : the manipulation (as through genetic engineering) of living organisms or their components to produce useful usu. commercial products (as novel pharmaceuticals); also : any of various applications of biological science used in such manipulation **2** : ERGONOMICS 1 — **bio·tech·no·log·i·cal** \-ˌtek-nə-'lä-ji-kəl\ adj — **bio·tech·no·log·i·cal·ly** \-k(ə-)lē\ adv — **bio·tech·nol·o·gist** \-tek-'nä-lə-jəst\ n

bio·te·lem·e·try \-tə-'le-mə-trē\ n, pl **-tries** : remote detection and measurement of a human or animal condition, activity, or function (as heartbeat or body temperature) — **bio·tel·e·met·ric** \-ˌte-lə-'me-trik\ adj

bi·ot·ic \bī-'ä-tik\ adj : of or relating to life; esp : caused or produced by living beings

-bi·ot·ic \bī-'ä-tik\ adj comb form **1** : relating to life ⟨anti*biotic*⟩ **2** : having a (specified) mode of life ⟨necro*biotic*⟩

bi·o·tin \'bī-ə-tən\ n : a colorless crystalline growth vitamin $C_{10}H_{16}N_2O_3S$ of the vitamin B complex found esp. in yeast, liver, and egg yolk — called also *vitamin H*

bio·tox·in \'bī-ō-ˌtäk-sən\ n : a toxic substance of biological origin

bio·trans·for·ma·tion \'bī-ō-ˌtrans-fər-'mā-shən, -ˌfȯr-\ n : the transformation of chemical compounds within a living system

bi·ovu·lar \(ˌ)bī-'ä-vyə-lər, -'ō-\ adj, of fraternal twins : derived from two ova

bi·pa·ri·etal \ˌbī-pə-'rī-ət-ᵊl\ adj : of or relating to the parietal bones; specif : being a measurement between the most distant opposite points of the two parietal bones

bi·ped \'bī-ˌped\ n : a two-footed animal — **biped** or **bi·ped·al** \(ˌ)bī-'ped-ᵊl\ adj

bi·pen·nate \(ˌ)bī-'pe-ˌnāt\ adj : resembling a feather barbed on both sides — used of muscles

bi·pen·ni·form \ˌ'pe-ni-ˌfȯrm\ adj : BIPENNATE

bi·per·i·den \bī-'per-ə-dən\ n : a white crystalline muscle relaxant $C_{21}H_{29}NO$ used esp. to reduce the symptoms (as tremors and muscle rigidity) associated with Parkinson's disease

bi·phe·nyl \(ˌ)bī-'fen-ᵊl, -'fēn-\ n : a white crystalline hydrocarbon C_6H_5-C_6H_5

bi·po·lar \(ˌ)bī-'pō-lər\ adj 1 : involving or being electrodes or leads attached to two different bodily sites (as the arms and legs) for recording the difference in electrical potential between the two sites 2 of a neuron : having an efferent and an afferent process 3 : being, characteristic of, or affected with a bipolar disorder ⟨∼ depression⟩ — compare UNIPOLAR 2

bipolar disorder n : any of several mood disorders characterized usu. by alternating episodes of depression and mania or by episodes of depression alternating with mild nonpsychotic excitement — called also bipolar affective disorder, bipolar illness, manic depression, manic-depressive illness, manic-depressive psychosis

bird flu n : influenza of birds caused esp. by strains of a subtype (H5N1) of the orthomyxovirus causing influenza A that may mutate and be passed to humans causing mild to fatally severe respiratory illness and that in wild birds often cause a fulminant and highly contagious fatal systemic illness — called also avian flu, avian influenza, fowl plague

bird louse n : BITING LOUSE

¹**birth** \'bərth\ n, often attrib 1 : the emergence of a new individual from the body of its parent 2 : the act or process of bringing forth young from the womb — **birth** vb

²**birth** adj : BIOLOGICAL 3

birth canal n : the channel formed by the cervix, vagina, and vulva through which the fetus passes during birth

birth certificate n : a copy of an official record of a person's date and place of birth and parentage

birth control n 1 : control of the number of children born esp. by preventing or lessening the frequency of conception : CONTRACEPTION 2 : contraceptive devices or preparations

birth control pill n : any of various preparations that usu. contain progestogen and an estrogen, are taken orally esp. on a daily basis, and act as contraceptives typically by preventing ovulation — called also oral contraceptive, oral contraceptive pill

birth defect n : a physical or biochemical defect (as cleft palate, phenylketonuria, or Down syndrome) that is present at birth and may be inherited or environmentally induced

birthing center n : a facility usu. staffed by nurse-midwives that provides a less institutionalized setting than a hospital for women who wish to deliver by natural childbirth

birthing room n : a comfortably furnished hospital room where both labor and delivery take place and in which the baby usu. remains during the hospital stay

birth·mark \'bərth-ˌmärk\ n : an unusual mark or blemish on the skin at birth : NEVUS — **birthmark** vb

birth pang n : one of the regularly recurrent pains that are characteristic of childbirth — usu. used in pl.

birth·rate \'bərth-ˌrāt\ n : the ratio between births and individuals in a specified population and time often expressed as number of live births per hundred or per thousand population per year — called also natality

birth trauma n : physical injury (as cephalhematoma, facial paralysis, or clavicular fracture) sustained by an infant in the process of birth

bis·a·co·dyl \ˌbi-sə-'kō-(ˌ)dil\ n : a white crystalline laxative $C_{22}H_{19}NO_4$ used orally or as a suppository

¹**bi·sex·u·al** \(ˌ)bī-'sek-shə-wəl\ adj 1 a : possessing characters of both sexes : HERMAPHRODITIC b : of, relating to, or characterized by a tendency to direct sexual desire toward individuals of both sexes 2 : of, relating to, or involving two sexes — **bi·sex·u·al·i·ty** \ˌbī-ˌsek-shə-'wa-lə-tē\ n — **bi·sex·u·al·ly** adv

²**bisexual** n : a bisexual individual

bis·hy·droxy·cou·ma·rin \ˌbis-(ˌ)hī-ˌdräk-sē-'kü-mə-rən\ n : DICUMAROL

bis·muth \'biz-məth\ n : a brittle grayish white chiefly trivalent metallic element — symbol Bi; see ELEMENT table

bismuth sub·car·bon·ate \-ˌsəb-'kär-bə-ˌnāt, -nət\ n : a white or pale yellowish white powder used chiefly in treating gastrointestinal disorders, topically as a protective in lotions and ointments, and in cosmetics

bismuth sub·ni·trate \-ˌsəb-'nī-ˌtrāt\ n : a white powder $Bi_5O(OH)_9(NO_3)_4$ that is used in medicine similarly to bismuth subcarbonate

bismuth sub·sa·lic·y·late \-ˌsəb-sə-'li-sə-ˌlāt\ n : an antidiarrheal drug

$C_7H_5BiO_4$ also used to relieve heartburn, indigestion, and nausea — see PEPTO-BISMOL

bis·phos·pho·nate \bis-'fäs-fə-,nāt\ *n* : any of a group of drugs (as alendronate) that are potent inhibitors of osteoclast-mediated bone resorption

bis·tou·ry \'bis-tə-rē\ *n, pl* **-ries** : a small slender straight or curved surgical knife with a sharp or blunt point

bi·sul·fate \bī-'səl-,fāt\ *n* : an acid sulfate

bi·tar·trate \bī-'tär-,trāt\ *n* : an acid tartrate

¹bite \'bīt\ *vb* **bit** \'bit\; **bit·ten** \'bit-ᵊn\ *also* **bit**; **bit·ing** **1** : to seize esp. with teeth or jaws so as to enter, grip, or wound **2** : to wound, pierce, or sting esp. with a fang or a proboscis

²bite *n* **1** : the act or manner of biting; *esp* : OCCLUSION 2a **2** : a wound made by biting

bite block *n* : a device used in dentistry for recording the spatial relation of the jaws esp. in respect to the occlusion of the teeth

bi·tem·po·ral \(,)bī-'tem-pə-rəl\ *adj* : relating to, involving, or joining the two temporal bones or the areas that they occupy

bite plane *n* : a removable dental appliance used to cover the occlusal surfaces of the teeth so that they cannot be brought into contact

bite plate *n* : a removable usu. plastic dental appliance used in orthodontics and prosthodontics: as **a** : a U-shaped device worn in the upper or lower jaw and used esp. to reposition that jaw or prevent bruxism **b** : RETAINER 2

bite-wing \'bīt-,wiŋ\ *n* : dental X-ray film designed to show the crowns of the upper and lower teeth simultaneously

biting fly *n* : a dipteran fly (as a mosquito or horsefly) having mouthparts adapted for piercing and biting

biting louse *n* : any of numerous wingless insects (order Mallophaga) parasitic esp. on birds — called also *bird louse*

biting midge *n* : any of a large family (Ceratopogonidae) of tiny dipteran flies of which some are vectors of filarial worms

Bi·tot's spots \bē-'tō-\ *n* : shiny pearly spots of triangular shape occurring on the conjunctiva in severe vitamin A deficiency esp. in children

Bi·tot \bē-'tō\, **Pierre A.** (1822–1888), French physician.

bit·ter \'bi-tər\ *adj* : being or inducing the one of the four basic taste sensations that is peculiarly acrid, astringent, or disagreeable — compare SALT, SOUR, SWEET — **bit·ter·ness** *n*

bitter almond *n* : an almond with a bitter taste that contains amygdalin; *also* : a tree (*Prunus dulcis amara*) of the rose family (Rosaceae) producing bitter almonds

bi·uret \,bī-yə-'ret\ *n* : a white crystalline compound $N_3H_5C_2O_2$ formed by heating urea

biuret reaction *n* : a reaction that is shown by biuret, proteins, and most peptides on treatment in alkaline solution with copper sulfate and that results in a violet color

biuret test *n* : a test esp. for proteins using the biuret reaction

¹bi·va·lent \(,)bī-'vā-lᵊnt\ *adj* **1** : having two combining sites ⟨a ~ antibody⟩ **2** : associated in pairs in synapsis **3** : conferring immunity to two diseases or two serotypes ⟨a ~ vaccine⟩

²bivalent *n* : a pair of synaptic chromosomes

bi·valve \'bī-,valv\ *vb* **bi·valved**; **bi·valv·ing** : to split (a cast) along one or two sides (as to relieve pressure)

Bk *symbol* berkelium

BK *abbr* below knee

black–and–blue \,blak-ᵊn-'blü\ *adj* : darkly discolored from blood effused by bruising

black box *adj* : being or containing a warning of a serious or life-threatening side effect (as stroke, muscle damage, or suicidal tendencies) that is highlighted by a black border ⟨a *black box* warning on the drug's label⟩

black death *n, often cap B&D* **1** : PLAGUE 2 **2** : a severe epidemic of plague and esp. bubonic plague that occurred in Asia and Europe in the 14th century

black disease *n* : a fatal toxemia of sheep associated with simultaneous infection by liver flukes (*Fasciola hepatica*) and an anaerobic toxin-producing clostridium (*Clostridium novyi*) and characterized by liver necrosis and subcutaneous hemorrhage

black eye *n* : a discoloration of the skin around the eye from bruising

black·fly \'blak-,flī\ *n, pl* **-flies** : any of a family (Simuliidae) and esp. genus *Simulium* of bloodsucking dipteran flies

black hairy tongue *n* : a dark furry or hairy discoloration of the tongue that is due to hyperplasia of the filiform papillae usu. with an overgrowth of microorganisms — called also *black-tongue*

black·head \'blak-,hed\ *n* **1** : a small plug of sebum blocking the duct of a sebaceous gland esp. on the face — compare MILIUM **2** : a destructive disease of turkeys and related birds caused by a protozoan of the genus *Histomonas* (*H. meleagridis*)

black henbane *n* : HENBANE

black·leg \'blak-,leg\ *n* : a usu. fatal toxemia esp. of young cattle caused by toxins produced by an anaerobic soil bacterium of the genus *Clostridium* (*C. chauvoei* syn. *C. feseri*)

black-legged tick *n* : either of two ixodid ticks: **a** : DEER TICK **b** : a tick

(*Ixodes pacificus*) of the western U.S. and British Columbia that is the vector of several diseases (as Lyme disease)

black lung *n* : pneumoconiosis caused by habitual inhalation of coal dust — called also *black lung disease*

black·out \'blak-,aut\ *n* : a transient dulling or loss of vision, consciousness, or memory (as from temporary impairment of cerebral circulation or an alcoholic binge) — compare GRAYOUT, REDOUT — **black out** *vb*

black quarter *n* : BLACKLEG

black rat *n* : a rat of the genus *Rattus* (*R. rattus*) that has been the chief vector of bubonic plague

black·tongue \'blak-,tͻng\ *n* **1** : BLACK HAIRY TONGUE **2** : a disease of dogs that is caused by a deficient diet and that is identical with pellagra in humans

black·wa·ter \'blak-,wȯ-tər, -,wä-\ *n* : any of several diseases (as blackwater fever or Texas fever) characterized by dark-colored urine

blackwater fever *n* : a rare febrile complication of repeated malarial attacks that is marked by destruction of blood cells with hemoglobinuria and extensive kidney damage

black widow *n* : a venomous New World spider of the genus *Latrodectus* (*L. mactans*) the female of which is black with an hourglass-shaped red mark on the abdominal underside

blad·der \'bla-dər\ *n* **1** : a membranous sac in animals that serves as the receptacle of a liquid or contains gas; *esp* : URINARY BLADDER **2** : a vesicle or pouch forming part of an animal body (the ~ of a tapeworm larva)

bladder worm *n* : CYSTICERCUS

blade \'blād\ *n* **1** : a broad flat body part (as the shoulder blade) **2** : the flat portion of the tongue immediately behind the tip; *also* : this portion together with the tip **3** : a flat working and esp. cutting part of an implement (as a scalpel)

blain \'blān\ *n* : an inflammatory swelling or sore

Bla·lock–Taus·sig operation \'blā-,läk-'tau̇-sig-\ *n* : surgical correction of the tetralogy of Fallot — called also *blue-baby operation*

Blalock, Alfred (1899–1964), and Taussig, Helen B. (1898–1986), American physicians.

blast \'blast\ *n* : BLAST CELL

blast- *or* **blasto-** *comb form* : bud : budding : germ (*blasto*disc) (*blas*tula)

-blast \,blast\ *n comb form* : formative unit esp. of living matter : germ : cell layer (epi*blast*)

blast cell *n* : an immature cell; *esp* : a usu. large blood cell precursor that is in the earliest stage of development in which it is recognizably committed to development along a particular cell lineage

blast crisis *n* : the terminal stage of chronic myelogenous leukemia that is marked by a significant increase in the proportion of blast cells — called also *blastic crisis*

blas·te·ma \bla-'stē-mə\ *n, pl* **-mas** *also* **-ma·ta** \-mə-tə\ : a mass of living substance capable of growth and differentiation

-blas·tic \'blas-tik\ *adj comb form* : sprouting or germinating (in a specified way) (hemocyto*blastic*) : having (such or so many) sprouts, buds, or germ layers (meso*blastic*)

blas·to·coel *or* **blas·to·coele** \'blas-tə-,sēl\ *n* : the cavity of a blastula — **blas·to·coe·lic** \,blas-tə-'sē-lik\ *adj*

blas·to·cyst \'blas-tə-,sist\ *n* : the modified blastula of a placental mammal

blas·to·derm \-,dərm\ *n* : a blastodisc after completion of cleavage and formation of the blastocoel

blas·to·der·mic vesicle \,blas-tə-'dər-mik-\ *n* : BLASTOCYST

blas·to·disc *or* **blas·to·disk** \'blas-tə-,disk\ *n* : the embryo-forming portion of an egg with discoidal cleavage usu. appearing as a small disc on the upper surface of the yolk mass

blas·to·gen·e·sis \,blas-tə-'je-nə-səs\ *n, pl* **-e·ses** \-,sēz\ : the transformation of lymphocytes into larger cells capable of undergoing mitosis — **blas·to·gen·ic** \-'je-nik\ *adj*

blas·to·mere \'blas-tə-,mir\ *n* : a cell produced during cleavage of a fertilized egg — called also *cleavage cell*

Blas·to·my·ces \,blas-tə-'mī-,sēz\ *n* : a genus of yeastlike fungi that contains the causative agent (*B. dermatitidis*) of North American blastomycosis

blas·to·my·cin \-'mīs-ᵊn\ *n* : a preparation of growth products of the causative agent of North American blastomycosis that is used esp. to test for this disease

blas·to·my·co·sis \-,mī-'kō-səs\ *n, pl* **-co·ses** \-,sēz\ : either of two infectious diseases caused by yeastlike fungi — see NORTH AMERICAN BLASTOMYCOSIS, SOUTH AMERICAN BLASTOMYCOSIS — **blas·to·my·cot·ic** \-'kä-tik\ *adj*

blas·to·pore \'blas-tə-,pō(ə)r, -,pȯ(ə)r\ *n* : the opening of the archenteron

blas·tu·la \'blas-chə-lə\ *n, pl* **-las** *or* **-lae** \-,lē\ : an early metazoan embryo typically having the form of a hollow fluid-filled rounded cavity bounded by a single layer of cells — compare GASTRULA, MORULA — **blas·tu·lar** \-lər\ *adj* — **blas·tu·la·tion** \,blas-chə-'lā-shən\ *n*

Blat·ta \'bla-tə\ *n* : a genus (family Blattidae) of cockroaches including the common oriental cockroach (*B. orientalis*) that infests dwellings in most parts of the world

Blat·tel·la \bla-'te-lə\ *n* : a genus of cockroaches including the German cockroach

83

bleb \'bleb\ n 1 : a small blister — compare BULLA 2 2 : a vesicular outpocketing of a plasma or nuclear membrane

¹**bleed** \'blēd\ vb **bled** \'bled\; **bleeding** 1 : to emit or lose blood 2 : to escape by oozing or flowing (as from a wound); also : to remove or draw blood from

²**bleed** n : the escape of blood from vessels : HEMORRHAGE

bleed·er \'blē-dər\ n 1 : BLOODLETTER 2 : HEMOPHILIAC 3 : a large blood vessel (as one cut during surgery) that is losing blood 4 : a horse that has experienced exercise-induced pulmonary hemorrhage

bleed·ing n : an act, instance, or result of being bled or the process by which something is bled: as a : the escape of blood from vessels : HEMORRHAGE b : PHLEBOTOMY

bleeding time n : a period of time of usu. about two and a half minutes during which a small wound (as a pinprick) continues to bleed

blem·ish \'ble-mish\ n : a mark of physical deformity or injury; esp : any small mark on the skin (as a pimple)

blen·nor·rha·gia \,ble-nə-'rā-jē-ə, -jə\ n 1 : BLENNORRHEA 2 : GONORRHEA

blennorrhagica — see KERATOSIS BLENNORRHAGICA

blennorrhagicum — see KERATODERMA BLENNORRHAGICUM

blen·nor·rhea \,ble-nə-'rē-ə\ n : an excessive secretion and discharge of mucus — **blen·nor·rheal** \-'rē-əl\ adj

blen·nor·rhoea chiefly Brit var of BLENNORRHEA

bleo·my·cin \,blē-ə-'mīs-ᵊn\ n : a mixture of glycoprotein antibiotics derived from a streptomyces (Streptomyces verticillus) and used in the form of the sulfates as an antineoplastic agent

blephar- or **blepharo-** comb form : eyelid ⟨blepharospasm⟩

bleph·a·ri·tis \-'rī-təs\ n, pl **-rit·i·des** \-'ri-tə-,dēz\ : inflammation esp. of the margins of the eyelids

bleph·a·ro·con·junc·ti·vi·tis \,ble-fə-(,)rō-kən-,jəŋk-tə-'vī-təs\ n : inflammation of the eyelid and conjunctiva

bleph·a·ro·plas·ty \'ble-fə-rō-,plas-tē\ n, pl **-ties** : plastic surgery on an eyelid esp. to remove fatty or excess tissue

bleph·a·rop·to·sis \,ble-fə-rəp-'tō-səs\ n, pl **-to·ses** \-,sēz\ : a drooping or abnormal relaxation of the upper eyelid

bleph·a·ro·spasm \'ble-fə-rō-,spa-zəm, -rə-\ n : spasmodic winking from involuntary contraction of the orbicularis oculi muscle of the eyelids

bleph·a·rot·o·my \,ble-fə-'rä-tə-mē\ n, pl **-mies** : surgical incision of an eyelid

blind \'blīnd\ adj 1 a : lacking or deficient in sight; esp : having less than ¹/₁₀ of normal vision in the more efficient eye when refractive defects are fully corrected by lenses b : of or relating to sightless persons ⟨~ care⟩ 2 : made or done without sight of certain objects or knowledge of certain facts that could serve for guidance or cause bias ⟨a ~ test⟩ — see DOUBLE-BLIND, SINGLE-BLIND 3 : having but one opening or outlet ⟨the cecum is a ~ pouch⟩ — **blind** vb — **blind·ly** adv — **blind·ness** n

blind gut n : the cecum of the large intestine

blind spot n : the point in the retina where the optic nerve enters that is devoid of rods and cones and is insensitive to light — called also optic disk

blind stag·gers \-'sta-gərz\ n sing or pl : a severe form of selenosis characterized esp. by impairment of vision and an unsteady gait; also : a similar condition not caused by selenium poisoning

blink \'bliŋk\ vb 1 : to close and open the eye involuntarily 2 : to remove (as tears) from the eye by blinking — **blink** n

blis·ter \'blis-tər\ n 1 : a fluid-filled elevation of the epidermis 2 : an agent that causes blistering — **blister** vb — **blis·tery** \-tə-rē\ adj

¹**bloat** \'blōt\ vb : to make or become turgid: a : to produce edema in b : to cause or result in accumulation of gas in the digestive tract of c : to cause abdominal distension in

²**bloat** n 1 : a flatulent digestive disturbance of domestic animals and esp. cattle 2 : a condition of large dogs marked by distension and usu. life-threatening rotation of the stomach

¹**block** \'bläk\ n, often attrib 1 : interruption of normal physiological function of a tissue or organ; esp : HEART BLOCK 2 a : BLOCK ANESTHESIA b : NERVE BLOCK 1 3 : interruption of a train of thought by competing thoughts or psychological suppression

²**block** vb 1 : to prevent normal functioning of (a bodily element) 2 : to experience or exhibit psychological blocking or blockage 3 : to obstruct the effect of

block·ade \blä-'kād\ n 1 : interruption of normal physiological function (as transmission of nerve impulses) of a tissue or organ 2 : inhibition of a physiologically active substance (as a hormone) — **blockade** vb

block·age \'blä-kij\ n 1 : the action of blocking or the state of being blocked 2 : internal resistance to understanding a communicated idea, to learning new material, or to adopting a new mode of response because of existing habitual ways of thinking, perceiving, and acting — compare BLOCKING

block anesthesia n : local anesthesia (as by injection) produced by interruption of the flow of impulses along a nerve trunk — compare REGIONAL ANESTHESIA

block·er \'blä-kər\ *n* : one that blocks — see ALPHA-BLOCKER, BETA-BLOCKER, CALCIUM CHANNEL BLOCKER

block·ing \'blä-kiŋ\ *n* : interruption of a trend of associative thought by the arousal of an opposing trend or through the welling up into consciousness of a complex of unpleasant ideas — compare BLOCKAGE 2

blocking antibody *n* : an antibody that combines with an antigen without visible reaction but prevents another antibody from later combining with or producing its usual effect on that antigen

blood \'bləd\ *n, often attrib* **1** : the fluid that circulates in the heart, arteries, capillaries, and veins of a vertebrate animal carrying nourishment and oxygen to and bringing away waste products from all parts of the body **2** : a fluid of an invertebrate comparable to blood

blood bank *n* : a place for storage of or an institution storing blood or plasma; *also* : blood so stored

blood banking *n* : the activity of administering or working in a blood bank

blood–borne \-ˌbȯrn\ *adj* : carried or transmitted by the blood

blood–brain barrier *n* : a barrier created by the modification of brain capillaries (as by reduction in fenestration and formation of tight cell-to-cell contacts) that prevents many substances from leaving the blood and crossing the capillary walls into the brain tissues — abbr. *BBB*

blood cell *n* : a cell or platelet normally present in blood — see RED BLOOD CELL, WHITE BLOOD CELL

blood clot *n* : CLOT

blood count *n* : the determination of the blood cells in a definite volume of blood; *also* : the number of cells so determined — see COMPLETE BLOOD COUNT, DIFFERENTIAL BLOOD COUNT

blood doping *n* : a technique for temporarily improving athletic performance in which oxygen-carrying red blood cells previously withdrawn from an athlete are injected back just before an event

blood fluke *n* : SCHISTOSOME

blood gas *n* : dissolved carbon dioxide and oxygen in blood typically expressed in terms of partial pressure; *also* : a test of usu. arterial blood to measure the partial pressures and concentrations of carbon dioxide and oxygen along with the pH and bicarbonate level

blood group *n* : one of the classes (as A, B, AB, or O) into which individual vertebrates and esp. human beings or their blood can be separated on the basis of the presence or absence of specific antigens in the blood — called also *blood type*

blood grouping *n* : BLOOD TYPING

blood·less \'bləd-ləs\ *adj* : free from or lacking blood ⟨a ∼ surgical field⟩

blood·let·ter \'bləd-ˌle-tər\ *n* : a practitioner of phlebotomy

blood·let·ting \-ˌle-tiŋ\ *n* : PHLEBOTOMY

blood·mo·bile \-mō-ˌbēl\ *n* : a motor vehicle staffed and equipped for collecting blood from donors

blood packing *n* : BLOOD DOPING

blood plasma *n* : the pale yellow fluid portion of whole blood that consists of water and its dissolved constituents including proteins (as albumin, fibrinogen, and globulins), electrolytes (as sodium and chloride), sugars (as glucose), lipids (as cholesterol and triglycerides), metabolic waste products (as urea), amino acids, hormones, and vitamins

blood platelet *n* : PLATELET

blood poisoning *n* : SEPTICEMIA

blood pressure *n* : pressure exerted by the blood upon the walls of the blood vessels and esp. arteries, usu. measured on the radial artery by means of a sphygmomanometer, and expressed in millimeters of mercury either as a fraction having as numerator the maximum pressure that follows systole of the left ventricle of the heart and as denominator the minimum pressure that accompanies cardiac diastole or as a whole number representing the first value only ⟨a *blood pressure* of 120/80⟩ ⟨a *blood pressure* of 120⟩ — abbr. *BP*

blood serum *n* : SERUM a(1)

blood·shot \'bləd-ˌshät\ *adj, of an eye* : inflamed to redness

blood·stain \-ˌstān\ *n* : a discoloration caused by blood — **blood·stained** \-ˌstānd\ *adj*

blood·stream \-ˌstrēm\ *n* : the flowing blood in a circulatory system

blood·suck·er \-ˌsə-kər\ *n* : an animal that sucks blood; *esp* : LEECH — **blood·suck·ing** \-kiŋ\ *adj*

blood sugar *n* : the glucose in the blood; *also* : its concentration (as in milligrams per 100 milliliters)

blood test *n* : a test of the blood (as a serological test for syphilis)

blood thinner *n* : a drug used to prevent the formation of blood clots by hindering coagulation of the blood

blood type *n* : BLOOD GROUP

blood typ·ing \-ˌtī-piŋ\ *n* : the action or process of determining an individual's blood group

blood vessel *n* : any of the vessels through which blood circulates in the body

blood·worm \'bləd-ˌwərm\ *n* : any of several nematode worms of the genus *Strongylus* that are parasitic in the large intestine of horses — called also *palisade worm, red worm*

bloody \'blə-dē\ *adj* **blood·i·er; -est 1 a** : containing or made up of blood **b** : of or contained in the blood **2 a**

: smeared or stained with blood **b** : dripping blood : BLEEDING ⟨a ~ nose⟩

blot \'blät\ *n* : a sheet usu. of a cellulose derivative that contains spots of immobilized macromolecules (as of DNA, RNA, or protein) or their fragments and that is used to identify specific components of the spots by applying a suitable molecular probe (as a complementary nucleic acid or a radioactively labeled antibody) — see NORTHERN BLOT, SOUTHERN BLOT, WESTERN BLOT — **blot** *vb*

blotch \'bläch\ *n* : a discolored patch on the skin ⟨a face covered with ~es⟩ — **blotch** *vb* — **blotchy** \'blä-chē\ *adj*

blow·fish \'blō-ˌfish\ *n* : PUFFER FISH

blow·fly \-ˌflī\ *n, pl* **-flies** : any of a family (Calliphoridae) of dipteran flies (as a bluebottle or screwworm)

BLS *abbr* basic life support

blue baby *n* : an infant with a bluish tint usu. from a congenital heart defect marked by mingling of venous and arterial blood

blue–baby operation *n* : BLALOCK-TAUSSIG OPERATION

blue bag *n* : gangrenous mastitis of sheep

blue·bot·tle \'blü-ˌbät-ᵊl\ *n* : any of several blowflies (genus *Calliphora*) that have an irridescent blue body or abdomen

blue·comb \'blü-ˌkōm\ *n* : an acute infectious disease of domestic turkeys that is caused by a virus of the genus *Coronavirus* (species *Turkey coronavirus*)

blue heaven *n, slang* : amobarbital or its sodium derivative in a blue tablet or capsule

blue mold *n* : any of various fungi of the genus *Penicillium* that produce blue or blue-green surface growth

blue nevus *n* : a small blue or bluish black spot on the skin that is sharply circumscribed, rounded, and flat or slightly raised and is usu. benign but often mistaken for a melanoma

blues \'blüz\ *n sing or pl* : low spirits : MELANCHOLY

blue·tongue \'blü-ˌtəŋ\ *n* : a virus disease esp. of sheep marked by hyperemia, cyanosis, and by swelling and sloughing of the mucous membranes esp. about the mouth and tongue and caused by a reovirus of the genus *Orbivirus* (species *Bluetongue virus*)

blunt dissection *n* : surgical separation of tissue layers by means of an instrument without a cutting edge or by the fingers

blunt trauma *n* : an injury caused by a blunt object or collision with a blunt surface (as in a car accident)

B lym·pho·cyte \'bē-ˈlim-fə-ˌsīt\ *n* : B CELL

BM *abbr* **1** Bachelor of Medicine **2** bowel movement

BMD *abbr* bone mineral density

BMI *abbr* body mass index

BMR *abbr* basal metabolic rate

BMT *abbr* bone marrow transplant; bone marrow transplantation

BNA *abbr* Basle Nomina Anatomica

BO *abbr* body odor

board \'bōrd\ *n* **1** : a group of persons having supervisory, managerial, investigative, or advisory powers ⟨medical licensing ~s⟩ ⟨a ~ of health⟩ **2** : an examination given by an examining board — often used in pl.

board–certified *adj* : being a physician who has graduated from medical school, completed residency, trained under supervision in a specialty, and passed a qualifying exam given by a medical specialty board — abbr. *BC*

board–eligible *adj* : being a physician who has graduated from medical school, completed residency, trained under supervision in a specialty, and is eligible to take a qualifying exam given by a medical specialty board — abbr. *BE*

Bo·dan·sky unit \bə-ˈdan-skē-, -ˈdän-\ *n* : a unit that is used as a measure of phosphatase concentration (as in the blood) esp. in the diagnosis of various pathological conditions and that has a normal value for the blood averaging about 7 for children and about 4 for adults

Bodansky, Aaron (1887–1960), American biochemist.

bod·i·ly \'bäd-ᵊl-ē\ *adj* : of or relating to the body ⟨~ organs⟩

body \'bä-dē\ *n, pl* **bod·ies** **1 a** (1) : the material part or nature of a human being (2) : a dead organism : CORPSE **b** : a human being **2 a** : the main part of a plant or animal body esp. as distinguished from limbs and head : TRUNK **b** : the main part of an organ (as the uterus)

body bag *n* : a large zippered bag in which a human corpse is placed esp. for transportation

body build \-ˌbild\ *n* : the distinctive physical makeup of a human being

body cavity *n* : a cavity within an animal body; *specif* : COELOM

body clock *n* : the internal mechanisms that schedule bodily functions and activities — not usu. used technically

body dysmorphic disorder *n* : pathological preoccupation with an imagined or slight physical defect of one's body — called also *body dysmorphia*

body heat *n* : heat produced in the body of a living animal by metabolic and physical activity — called also *animal heat*

body image *n* : a subjective picture of one's own physical appearance established both by self-observation and by noting the reactions of others

body louse *n* : a louse feeding primarily on the body; *esp* : a sucking louse of the genus *Pediculus* (*P. humanus humanus* syn. *P. h. corporis*) feeding on the human body and living in clothing — called also *cootie*

body mass index *n* : a measure of body fat that is the ratio of the weight of the body in kilograms to the square of its height in meters ⟨a *body mass index* in adults of 25 to 29.9 is considered an indication of overweight, and 30 or more an indication of obesity⟩ — abbr. *BMI*

body odor *n* : an unpleasant odor from a perspiring or unclean person

body ringworm *n* : TINEA CORPORIS

body stalk *n* : the mesodermal cord that contains the umbilical vessels and that connects a fetus with its chorion

body·work \-,wərk\ *n* : therapeutic touching or manipulation of the body by using specialized techniques

Boeck's sarcoid \'beks-\ *n* : SARCOIDOSIS

   Boeck \'bek\, **Caesar Peter Moeller** (1845–1917), Norwegian dermatologist.

Bohr effect \'bōr-\ *n* : the decrease in oxygen affinity of a respiratory pigment (as hemoglobin) in response to decreased blood pH resulting from increased carbon dioxide concentration
   Bohr, Christian (1855–1911), Danish physiologist.

bohr·i·um \'bōr-ē-əm\ *n* : a short-lived radioactive element that is artificially produced — symbol *Bh*; see ELEMENT table

boil \'bȯil\ *n* : a localized swelling and inflammation of the skin resulting from usu. bacterial infection of a hair follicle and adjacent tissue, having a hard central core, and forming pus — called also *furuncle*

boiling point *n* : the temperature at which a liquid boils

bo·lus \'bō-ləs\ *n* **1** : a rounded mass: as **a** : a large pill **b** : a soft mass of chewed food **2 a** : a dose of a substance (as a drug) given intravenously **b** : a large dose of a substance given by injection for the purpose of rapidly achieving the needed therapeutic concentration in the bloodstream

bombé — see IRIS BOMBÉ

bom·be·sin \'bäm-bə-sin\ *n* : a polypeptide that is found in the brain and gastrointestinal tract and has been shown experimentally to cause the secretion of various substances (as gastrin and cholecystokinin) and to inhibit intestinal motility

bond \'bänd\ *n* : an attractive force that holds together atoms, ions, or groups of atoms in a molecule or crystal — usu. represented in formulas by a line or dot — **bond** *vb*

bond·ing *n* **1** : the formation of a close personal relationship (as between a mother and child) esp. through frequent or constant association — see MALE BONDING **2** : a dental technique in which a material and esp. plastic or porcelain is attached to

a tooth surface to correct minor defects (as chipped or discolored teeth) esp. for cosmetic purposes

bone \'bōn\ *n, often attrib* **1** : one of the hard parts of the skeleton of a vertebrate ⟨the ∼s of the arm⟩ **2** : the hard largely calcareous connective tissue of which the adult skeleton of most vertebrates is chiefly composed ⟨cancellous ∼⟩ ⟨compact ∼⟩ — compare CARTILAGE 1

bone marrow *n* : a soft highly vascular modified connective tissue that occupies the cavities and cancellous part of most bones and occurs in two forms: **a** : one that is whitish or yellowish, consists chiefly of fat cells, and is found esp. in the cavities of long bones — called also *yellow marrow* **b** : one that is reddish, consists of little fat, is the chief site of red blood cell and blood granulocyte formation, and occurs in the normal adult in cancellous tissue esp. of certain flat bones — called also *red marrow*

bont tick \'bänt-\ *n* : a southern African tick of the genus *Amblyomma* (*A. hebraeum*) that attacks livestock, birds, and sometimes humans and transmits heartwater of sheep, goats, and cattle; *broadly* : any African tick of the genus *Amblyomma*

bony *also* **bon·ey** \'bō-nē\ *adj* **bon·i·er; -est** : consisting of or resembling bone ⟨∼ prominences of the skull⟩

bony labyrinth *n* : the cavity in the petrous portion of the temporal bone that contains the membranous labyrinth of the inner ear and is divided into the vestibule, cochlea, and semicircular canals — called also *osseous labyrinth*

Bo·oph·i·lus \bō-'ä-fə-ləs\ *n* : a genus of ticks several of which are pests esp. of cattle and vectors of disease — see CATTLE TICK

boost·er \'bü-stər\ *n* : a substance that increases the effectiveness of a medicament; *esp* : BOOSTER SHOT

booster shot *n* : a supplementary dose of an immunizing agent — called also *booster, booster dose*

bo·rac·ic acid \bə-'ra-sik-\ *n* : BORIC ACID

bor·bo·ryg·mus \,bȯr-bə-'rig-məs\ *n, pl* **-mi** \-,mī\ : a rumbling sound made by the movement of gas in the intestine — **bor·bo·ryg·mic** \-mik\ *adj*

bor·der·line \'bȯr-dər-,līn\ *adj* **1** : being in an intermediate position or state : not fully classifiable as one thing or its opposite; *esp* : not quite up to what is usual, standard, or expected ⟨∼ intelligence⟩ **2** : exhibiting typical but not altogether conclusive symptoms ⟨a ∼ diabetic⟩ **3** : of, relating to, being, or exhibiting a behavior pattern typical of or suggestive of borderline personality disorder

borderline personality disorder *n* : a disordered behavior pattern with onset by early adulthood that is characterized by multiple types of psychological instability and impulsiveness

Bor·de·tel·la \ˌbȯr-də-ˈte-lə\ *n* : a genus of bacteria comprising minute and very short gram-negative strictly aerobic coccuslike bacilli and including the causative agent (*B. pertussis*) of whooping cough

J.–J.–B.–V. Bordet — see BORDET= GENGOU BACILLUS

Bor·det–Gen·gou bacillus \bȯr-ˈdā-zhäⁿ-ˈgü-\ *n* : a small ovoid bacillus of the genus *Bordetella* (*B. pertussis*) that is the causative agent of whooping cough

Bordet, Jules–Jean–Baptiste–Vincent (1870–1961), Belgian bacteriologist, and Gengou, Octave (1875–1957), French bacteriologist.

bore \ˈbȯr\ *n* : the internal diameter of a tube (as a hypodermic needle or catheter)

bo·ric acid \ˈbȯr-ik-\ *n* : a white crystalline acid H_3BO_3 used esp. as a weak antiseptic — called also *boracic acid*

Born·holm disease \ˈbȯrn-ˌhōlm-\ *n* : EPIDEMIC PLEURODYNIA

bo·ron \ˈbȯr-ˌän\ *n* : a trivalent metalloid element found in nature only in combination — symbol *B;* see ELEMENT table

bor·re·lia \bə-ˈre-lē-ə, -ˈrē-\ *n* 1 *cap* : a genus of small spirochetes (family Spirochaetaceae) that are parasites of humans and warm-blooded animals and include the causative agents of relapsing fever in Africa (*B. duttoni*) and Lyme disease in the U.S. (*B. burgdorferi*) 2 : a spirochete of the genus *Borrelia*

bor·rel·i·o·sis \bə-ˌre-lē-ˈō-səs\ *n, pl* -o·ses \-ˌsēz\ : infection with or disease caused by a spirochete of the genus *Borrelia; specif* : LYME DISEASE

bos·se·lat·ed \ˈbä-sə-ˌlä-təd, ˈbō-\ *adj* : marked or covered with protuberances 〈a ~ tumor〉

bot *also* **bott** \ˈbät\ *n* : the larva of a botfly; *esp* : one infesting the horse

bo·tan·i·cal \bə-ˈta-ni-kəl\ *n* : a vegetable drug esp. in the crude state

bot·fly \ˈbät-ˌflī\ *n, pl* -**flies** : any of various stout dipteran flies (family Oestridae) with larvae parasitic in cavities or tissues of various mammals including humans

Bo·tox \ˈbō-ˌtäks\ *trademark* — used for a preparation of botulinum toxin type A

bot·ry·oid \ˈbä-trē-ˌȯid\ *adj* : having the form of a bunch of grapes 〈~ sarcoma〉

botryoides — see SARCOMA BOTRYOIDES

bot·ry·o·my·co·sis \ˌbä-trē-(ˌ)ō-mī-ˈkō-səs\ *n, pl* -co·ses \-ˌsēz\ : a bacterial infection of domestic animals and humans marked by the formation of usu. superficial vascular granulomatous masses, associated esp. with wounds, and sometimes followed by

metastatic visceral tumors — **bot·ry·o·my·cot·ic** \-ˈkä-tik\ *adj*

bot·tle \ˈbät-ᵊl\ *n, often attrib* : liquid food usu. consisting of milk and supplements that is fed from a bottle (as to an infant) in place of mother's milk

bottle baby *n* : a baby that is chiefly or wholly bottle-fed as contrasted with a baby that is chiefly or wholly breast= fed

bot·tle–feed \ˈbät-ᵊl-ˌfēd\ *vb* -**fed**; -**feed·ing** : to feed (an infant) from a nursing bottle rather than by breast= feeding

bottle jaw *n* : a pendulous edematous condition of the tissues under the lower jaw in cattle and sheep resulting from infestation with bloodsucking gastrointestinal parasites (as of the genus *Haemonchus*)

bot·u·lin \ˈbä-chə-lən\ *n* : BOTULINUM TOXIN

bot·u·li·num \ˌbä-chə-ˈlī-nəm\ *also* **bot·u·li·nus** \-nəs\ *n* : a spore-forming bacterium of the genus *Clostridium* (*C. botulinum*) that secretes botulinum toxin — **bo·tu·li·nal** \-ˈlīn-ᵊl\ *adj*

botulinum toxin *also* **botulinus toxin** *n* : a very powerful bacterial neurotoxin that acts primarily on the parasympathetic nervous system, is produced by botulinum, and causes botulism — called also *botulin*

botulinum toxin A *n* : a purified botulinum toxin used by injection esp. to treat strabismus, blepharospasm, spasmodic torticollis, and severe axillary hyperhidrosis and to minimize wrinkles — see BOTOX

bot·u·lism \ˈbä-chə-ˌli-zəm\ *n* : acute food poisoning caused by botulinum toxin produced in food by a bacterium of the genus *Clostridium* (*C. botulinum*) and characterized by muscle weakness and paralysis, disturbances of vision, swallowing, and speech, and a high mortality rate

Bou·chard's node \bü-ˈshärz\ *n* : a bony enlargement of the middle joint of a finger that is commonly associated with osteoarthritis — compare HEBERDEN'S NODE

Bouchard, Charles Jacques (1837–1915), French pathologist.

bou·gie \ˈbü-ˌzhē, -ˌjē\ *n* 1 : a tapering cylindrical instrument for introduction into a tubular passage of the body 2 : SUPPOSITORY

bou·gie·nage *or* **bou·gi·nage** \ˌbü-zhē-ˈnäzh\ *n* : the dilation of a tubular cavity (as a constricted esophagus) with a bougie

-boulia — see -BULIA

bound \ˈbaůnd\ *adj* 1 : made costive : CONSTIPATED 2 : held in chemical or physical combination

bou·ton \bü-ˈtōⁿ\ *n* : a terminal club= shaped enlargement of a nerve fiber at a synapse with another neuron

bou·ton·neuse fever \ˌbü-tȯ-ˈnüz-, -ˈnœz-\ *n* : a disease of the Mediterranean area that is characterized by headache, pain in muscles and joints, and an eruption over the body and is caused by a tick-borne rickettsia (*Rickettsia conorii*) — called also *fièvre boutonneuse, Marseilles fever*; see TICK-BITE FEVER

Bo·vic·o·la \bō-'vi-kə-lə\ *n* : a genus of biting lice (order Mallophaga) including several that infest the hair of domestic mammals

bo·vine \'bō-ˌvīn, -ˌvēn\ *n* : an ox (genus *Bos*) or a closely related animal — **bovine** *adj*

bovine growth hormone *n* : the naturally occurring growth hormone of bovines or a recombinant version that stimulates milk production — abbr. *BGH*

bovine mastitis *n* : inflammation of the udder of a cow resulting from injury or more commonly from bacterial infection

bovine spongiform encephalopathy *n* : a fatal prion disease of cattle that affects the nervous system, resembles or is identical to scrapie of sheep and goats, and is prob. transmitted by infected tissue in food — abbr. *BSE*; called also *mad cow disease*

bovine viral diarrhea *n* : an infectious disease of cattle that may range from a subclinical or mild infection to a severe illness marked chiefly by fever, diarrhea, anorexia, and ulceration esp. of the mouth and is caused by two flaviviruses of the genus *Pestivirus* (species *Bovine viral diarrhea virus 1* and *Bovine viral diarrhea virus 2*) — called also *bovine virus diarrhea*; see MUCOSAL DISEASE

bovinum — see COR BOVINUM

bow \'bō\ *n* : a frame for the lenses of eyeglasses; *also* : the curved sidepiece of the frame passing over the ear

bow·el \'baül\ *n* : INTESTINE, GUT; *also* : one of the divisions of the intestines — usu. used in pl. except in medical use ⟨move your ~s⟩ ⟨surgery of the involved ~⟩

bowel worm *n* : a common strongylid nematode worm of the genus *Chabertia* (*C. ovina*) infesting the colon of sheep and feeding on blood and tissue

bow·en·oid papulosis \'bō-ə-ˌnȯid-\ *n* : a condition associated with certain human papillomaviruses (genus *Alphapapillomavirus*) and marked by pigmented papules in the anogenital area which usu. follow a benign course

J. T. Bowen — see BOWEN'S DISEASE

Bow·en's disease \'bō-ənz-\ *n* : a precancerous lesion of the skin or mucous membranes characterized by small solid elevations covered by thickened horny tissue

Bow·en \'bō-ən\, **John Templeton** (1857–1941), American dermatologist.

bow·leg \'bō-ˌleg\ *n* : a leg bowed outward at or below the knee — called also *genu varum*

bow-legged \'bō-ˌle-gəd, -ˌlegd\ *adj* : having bowlegs

Bow·man's capsule \'bō-mənz-\ *n* : a thin membranous double-walled capsule surrounding the glomerulus of a vertebrate nephron — called also *capsule of Bowman, glomerular capsule*

Bow·man \'bō-mən\, **Sir William** (1816–1892), British ophthalmologist, anatomist, and physiologist.

Bowman's gland *n* : OLFACTORY GLAND

Bowman's membrane *n* : the thin outer layer of the substantia propria of the cornea immediately underlying the epithelium

box·ing \'bäk-siŋ\ *n* : construction of the base of a dental cast by building up the walls of an impression while preserving important landmarks

box jellyfish *n* : SEA WASP

bp *abbr* base pair

BP *abbr* blood pressure

BPH *abbr* benign prostatic hyperplasia

BPharm *abbr* bachelor of pharmacy

Br *symbol* bromine

¹**brace** \'brās\ *n, pl* **brac·es** 1 : an appliance that gives support to movable parts (as a joint), to weak muscles, or to strained ligaments (as of the lower back) 2 **braces** *pl* : an orthodontic appliance usu. of metallic wire that is used esp. to exert pressure to straighten misaligned teeth and that is not removable by the patient

²**brace** *vb* **braced; brac·ing** : to furnish or support with a brace

brachi- or **brachio-** *comb form* 1 : arm ⟨*brachio*radialis⟩ 2 : brachial and ⟨*brachio*cephalic artery⟩

bra·chi·al \'brā-kē-əl\ *adj* : of or relating to the arm

brachial artery *n* : the chief artery of the upper arm that is a direct continuation of the axillary artery and divides into the radial and ulnar arteries just below the elbow — see DEEP BRACHIAL ARTERY

bra·chi·a·lis \ˌbrā-kē-'a-ləs, -'ā-, -'ä-\ *n* : a flexor that lies in front of the lower part of the humerus whence it arises and is inserted into the ulna

brachial plexus *n* : a complex network of nerves that is formed chiefly by the lower four cervical nerves and the first thoracic nerve and supplies nerves to the chest, shoulder, and arm

brachial vein *n* : one of a pair of veins accompanying the brachial artery and uniting with each other and with the basilic vein to form the axillary vein

brachii — see BICEPS BRACHII, TRICEPS BRACHII

bra·chio·ce·phal·ic artery \ˌbrā-kē-(ˌ)ō-sə-'fa-lik-\ *n* : a short artery that arises from the arch of the aorta and divides into the carotid and subclavian arteries of the right side — called also *innominate artery*

brachiocephalicus — see TRUNCUS BRACHIOCEPHALICUS

brachiocephalic vein *n* : either of two large veins that occur one on each side of the neck, receive blood from the head and neck, are formed by the union of the internal jugular and the subclavian veins, and unite to form the superior vena cava — called also *innominate vein*

bra·chio·ra·di·alis \ˌbrā-kē-ō-ˌrā-dē-ˈa-ləs, -ˈā-, -ˈä-\ *n, pl* **-ales** \-ˌlēz\ : a flexor of the radial side of the forearm arising from the lateral supracondylar ridge of the humerus and inserted into the styloid process of the radius

bra·chi·um \ˈbrā-kē-əm\ *n, pl* **-chia** \-kē-ə\ : the upper segment of the arm extending from the shoulder to the elbow

brachium con·junc·ti·vum \-ˌkän-(ˌ)jəŋk-ˈtī-vəm\ *n* : CEREBELLAR PEDUNCLE a

brachium pon·tis \-ˈpän-təs\ *n* : CEREBELLAR PEDUNCLE b

brachy- *comb form* : short ⟨*brachy*cephalic⟩ ⟨*brachy*dactylous⟩

brachy·ce·phal·ic \ˌbra-ki-sə-ˈfa-lik\ *adj* : short-headed or broad-headed with a cephalic index of over 80 — **brachy·ceph·a·ly** \-ˈse-fə-lē\ *n*

brachy·dac·ty·lous \ˌbra-ki-ˈdak-tə-ləs\ *adj* : having abnormally short digits — **brachy·dac·ty·ly** \-lē\ *n*

brachy·ther·a·py \-ˈther-ə-pē\ *n, pl* **-pies** : radiotherapy in which the source of radiation is placed (as by implantation) in or close to the area being treated

Brad·ford frame \ˈbrad-fərd-\ *n* : a frame used to support a patient with disease or fractures of the spine, hip, or pelvis

Bradford, Edward Hickling (1848–1926), American orthopedist.

brady- *comb form* : slow ⟨*brady*cardia⟩

bra·dy·car·dia \ˌbrā-di-ˈkär-dē-ə *also* ˌbra-\ *n* : relatively slow heart action whether physiological or pathological — compare TACHYCARDIA

bra·dy·ki·ne·sia \-kī-ˈnē-zhē-ə, -zhə, -zē-ə\ *n* : extreme slowness of movements and reflexes (as in catatonic schizophrenia)

bra·dy·ki·nin \-ˈkī-nən\ *n* : a kinin that is formed locally in injured tissue, acts in vasodilation of small arterioles, and is considered to play a part in inflammatory processes

bra·dy·pnea \ˌbrā-dəp-ˈnē-ə, ˌbra-\ *n* : abnormally slow breathing

bra·dy·pnoea *chiefly Brit var of* BRADYPNEA

braille \ˈbrāl\ *n, often cap* : a system of writing for the blind that uses characters made up of raised dots — **braille** *vb*

Braille \ˈbrī, ˈbrāl\, Louis (1809–1852), French inventor and teacher.

brain \ˈbrān\ *n* : the portion of the vertebrate central nervous system enclosed in the skull and continuous with the spinal cord through the foramen magnum that is composed of neurons and supporting and nutritive structures (as glia) and that integrates sensory information from inside and outside the body in controlling autonomic function (as heartbeat and respiration), in coordinating and directing correlated motor responses, and in the process of learning

brain attack *n* : STROKE

brain·case \-ˌkās\ *n* : the part of the skull that encloses the brain — see CRANIUM

brain death *n* : final cessation of activity in the central nervous system esp. as indicated by a flat electroencephalogram for a predetermined length of time — **brain–dead** *adj*

brain stem *n* : the part of the brain composed of the midbrain, pons, and medulla oblongata and connecting the spinal cord with the forebrain and cerebrum

brain vesicle *n* : any of the divisions into which the developing embryonic brain of vertebrates is marked off by incomplete transverse constrictions

brain·wash·ing \ˈbrān-ˌwȯ-shiŋ, -ˌwä-\ *n* : a forcible indoctrination to induce someone to give up basic political, social, or religious beliefs and attitudes and to accept contrasting regimented ideas — **brain·wash** *vb*

brain wave *n* **1** : rhythmic fluctuations of voltage between parts of the brain resulting in the flow of an electric current **2** : a current produced by brain waves — compare ALPHA WAVE, BETA WAVE

bran \ˈbran\ *n* : the edible broken seed coats of cereal grain separated from the flour or meal by sifting

branch \ˈbranch\ *n* : something that extends from or enters into a main body or source ⟨a ~ of an artery⟩ — **branch** *vb* — **branched** \ˈbrancht\ *adj*

bran·chi·al \ˈbran-kē-əl\ *adj* : of or relating to the parts of the body derived from the embryonic branchial arches and clefts

branchial arch *n* : one of a series of bony or cartilaginous arches that develop in the walls of the mouth cavity and pharynx of a vertebrate embryo and correspond to the gill arches of fishes and amphibians — called also *pharyngeal arch, visceral arch*

branchial cleft *n* : one of the open or potentially open clefts that occur on each side of the neck region of a vertebrate embryo between the branchial arches and correspond to the gill slits of fishes and amphibians — called also *pharyngeal cleft*

brash \ˈbrash\ *n* : WATER BRASH

Brax·ton–Hicks contractions \ˈbrakstən-ˈhiks-\ *n, pl* : relatively painless nonrhythmic contractions of the uterus that occur during pregnancy

with increasing frequency over time but are not associated with labor
Hicks, John Braxton (1823–1897), British gynecologist.

braxy \'brak-sē\ *n, pl* **brax·ies** : a malignant edema of sheep that involves gastrointestinal invasion by a bacterium of the genus *Clostridium* (*C. septicum*)

BRCA \,bē-,är-,sē-'ā\ *n* : either of two tumor suppressor genes that in mutated form tend to be associated with an increased risk of certain cancers and esp. breast and ovarian cancers

¹**break** \'brāk\ *vb* **broke** \'brōk\; **broken** \'brō-kən\; **break·ing** **1 a** : to snap into pieces : FRACTURE ⟨∼ a bone⟩ **b** : to fracture the bone of (a bodily part) ⟨the blow *broke* her arm⟩ **c** : to dislocate or dislocate and fracture a bone of (the neck or back) **2 a** : to cause an open wound in : RUPTURE ⟨∼ the skin⟩ **b** : to rupture the surface of and permit flowing out or effusing ⟨∼ an artery⟩ **3** : to fail in health or strength — often used with *down* **4** : to suffer complete or marked loss of resistance, composure, resolution, morale, or command of a situation — often used with *down*

²**break** *n* **1** : an act or action of breaking : FRACTURE **2** : a condition produced by breaking ⟨the ∼ in his leg⟩

break·bone fever \'brāk-,bōn-\ *n* : DENGUE

¹**break·down** \'brāk-,daùn\ *n* **1** : a failure to function **2** : a physical, mental, or nervous collapse **3** : the process of decomposing ⟨∼ of food during digestion⟩ — **break down** *vb*

²**breakdown** *adj* : obtained or resulting from disintegration or decomposition of a substance

break out *vb* **1** : to become affected with a skin eruption **2** of a disease : to manifest itself by skin eruptions **3** : to become covered with ⟨*break out* in a sweat⟩

break·through bleeding \,brāk-,thrü-\ *n* : an abnormal flow of blood from the uterus that occurs between menstrual periods esp. due to irregular sloughing of the endometrium in women on contraceptive hormones

breast \'brest\ *n* **1** : either of the pair of mammary glands extending from the front of the chest in pubescent and adult females; *also* : either of the analogous but rudimentary organs of the male chest esp. when enlarged **2** : the fore or ventral part of the body between the neck and the abdomen

breast·bone \'brest-,bōn\ *n* : STERNUM

breast–feed \'brest-,fēd\ *vb* : to feed (an infant) from a mother's breast rather than from a nursing bottle

breast lift *n* : plastic surgery to elevate and often reshape a sagging breast — called also *mastopexy*

breath \'breth\ *n* **1 a** : the faculty of breathing **b** : an act or an instance of breathing or inhaling ⟨recovering her

∼ after the race⟩ **2 a** : air inhaled and exhaled in breathing ⟨bad ∼⟩ **b** : something (as moisture on a cold surface) produced by breath or breathing — **out of breath** : breathing very rapidly (as from strenuous exercise)

Breath·a·ly·zer \'bre-thə-,lī-zər\ *trademark* — used for a device that is used to determine the alcohol content of a breath sample

breathe \'brēth\ *vb* **breathed; breathing** **1** : to draw air into and expel it from the lungs : RESPIRE; *broadly* : to take in oxygen and give out carbon dioxide through natural processes **2** : to inhale and exhale freely

breath·er \'brē-thər\ *n* : one that breathes usu. in a specified way — see MOUTH BREATHER

breathing tube *n* : ENDOTRACHEAL TUBE

breath·less \'breth-ləs\ *adj* **1** : panting or gasping for breath **2** : suffering from dyspnea

breech \'brēch\ *n* **1** : the hind end of the body : BUTTOCKS **2** : BREECH PRESENTATION; *also* : a fetus that is presented at the uterine cervix buttocks or legs first

breech delivery *n* : delivery of a fetus by breech presentation — called also *breech birth*

breech presentation *n* : presentation of the fetus in which the buttocks or legs are the first parts to appear at the uterine cervix

breg·ma \'breg-mə\ *n, pl* **-ma·ta** \-mə-tə\ : the point of junction of the coronal and sagittal sutures of the skull — **breg·mat·ic** \breg-'ma-tik\ *adj*

bre·tyl·i·um \brə-'ti-lē-əm\ *n* : an antiarrhythmic drug administered in the form of its tosylate $C_{18}H_{24}BrNO_3S$ in the treatment of ventricular fibrillation and tachycardia and formerly used as an antihypertensive

brevis — see ABDUCTOR POLLICIS BREVIS, ADDUCTOR BREVIS, EXTENSOR CARPI RADIALIS BREVIS, EXTENSOR DIGITORUM BREVIS, EXTENSOR HALLUCIS BREVIS, EXTENSOR POLLICIS BREVIS, FLEXOR DIGITI MINIMI BREVIS, FLEXOR DIGITORUM BREVIS, FLEXOR HALLUCIS BREVIS, FLEXOR POLLICIS BREVIS, PALMARIS BREVIS, PERONEUS BREVIS

brewer's yeast *n* : the dried pulverized cells of a yeast of the genus *Saccharomyces* (*S. cerevisiae*) used as a source of B-complex vitamins

bridge \'brij\ *n* **1 a** : the upper bony part of the nose **b** : the curved part of a pair of glasses that rests upon this part of the nose **2 a** : PONS **b** : a strand of protoplasm extending between two cells **c** : a partial denture held in place by anchorage to adjacent teeth

bridge·work \-,wərk\ *n* : dental bridges; *also* : prosthodontics concerned with their construction

bright·ness \'brīt-nəs\ *n* : the one of the three psychological dimensions of color perception by which visual stimuli are ordered continuously from light to dark and which is correlated with light intensity — compare HUE, SATURATION

Bright's disease \'brīts-\ *n* : any of several kidney diseases marked esp. by albumin in the urine

Bright \'brīt\, **Richard** (1789–1858), British internist and pathologist.

Brill's disease \'brilz-\ *n* : an acute infectious disease milder than epidemic typhus but caused by the same rickettsia

Brill \'bril\, **Nathan Edwin** (1860–1925), American physician.

bring up *vb* : VOMIT

British an·ti·lew·is·ite \-ˌan-tē-'lü-ə-ˌsīt, -ˌan-ˌtī-\ *n* : DIMERCAPROL

W. L. Lewis — see LEWISITE

brit·tle \'brit-ºl\ *adj* : affected with or being a form of type 1 diabetes characterized by large and unpredictable fluctuations in blood glucose level ⟨∼ diabetes⟩

broach \'brōch\ *n* : a fine tapered flexible instrument used in dentistry to remove dental pulp and to dress a root canal

broad bean *n* : the large flat edible seed of an Old World upright vetch (*Vicia faba*); *also* : the plant itself — called also *fava bean;* see FAVISM

broad ligament *n* : either of the two lateral ligaments of the uterus composed of a double sheet of peritoneum and bearing the ovary supended from the dorsal surface

broad–spectrum *adj* : effective against a wide range of organisms (as insects or bacteria) ⟨∼ antibiotics⟩ — compare NARROW-SPECTRUM

Bro·ca's aphasia \'brō-ˌkäz-\ *n* : MOTOR APHASIA

Bro·ca \brō-'kä\, **Pierre–Paul** (1824–1880), French surgeon and anthropologist.

Broca's area *n* : a brain center associated with the motor control of speech and usu. located in the left but sometimes in the right inferior frontal gyrus — called also *Broca's convolution, Broca's convolution of Broca*

Brod·mann area \'bräd-mən-\ *or* **Brod·mann's area** \-mənz-\ *n* : one of the several structurally distinguishable and presumably functionally distinct regions into which the cortex of each cerebral hemisphere can be divided

Brod·mann \'brōt-ˌmän, 'bräd-mən\, **Korbinian** (1868–1918), German neurologist.

broke *past of* BREAK

bro·ken \'brō-kən\ *adj* : having undergone or been subjected to fracture

broken wind *n* : HEAVES 1 — **bro·ken–wind·ed** \-'wind-əd\ *adj*

brom– *or* **bromo–** *comb form* **1** : bromine ⟨*bromide*⟩ **2** *now usu*

bromo– : containing bromine in place of hydrogen — in names of organic compounds ⟨*bromouracil*⟩

bro·me·lain *also* **bro·me·lin** \'brō-mə-lən\ *n* : a protease obtained from the juice of the pineapple (*Ananas comosus* of the family Bromeliaceae)

bro·mide \'brō-ˌmīd\ *n* **1** : a binary compound of bromine with another element or a radical including some (as potassium bromide) used as sedatives **2** : a dose of bromide taken usu. as a sedative

brom·hi·dro·sis \ˌbrō-mə-'drō-səs *also* ˌbrō-hə-\ *also* **bro·mi·dro·sis** \ˌbrō-mə-\ *n, pl* **-dro·ses** \-ˌsēz\ : foul-smelling sweat

bro·mine \'brō-ˌmēn\ *n* : a nonmetallic element that is normally a red corrosive toxic liquid — symbol *Br*; see ELEMENT table

bro·mism \'brō-ˌmi-zəm\ *n* : an abnormal state due to excessive or prolonged use of bromides

bro·mo \'brō-(ˌ)mō\ *n, pl* **bromos** : a dose of a proprietary effervescent mixture used as a headache remedy, sedative, and antacid; *also* : such a proprietary preparation

bro·mo·crip·tine \ˌbrō-mō-'krip-ˌtēn\ *n* : a polypeptide alkaloid $C_{32}H_{40}$-BrN_5O_5 that is a derivative of ergot and mimics the activity of dopamine in selectively inhibiting prolactin secretion

bro·mo·de·oxy·ur·i·dine \ˌbrō-mō-ˌdē-ˌäk-sē-'yùr-ə-ˌdēn, -dən\ *or* **5–bro·mo·de·oxy·ur·i·dine** \'fīv-\ *n* : a mutagenic analog $C_9H_{11}O_5NBr$ of thymidine that induces chromosomal breakage esp. in heterochromatic regions — abbr. *BUdR*

bro·mo·der·ma \'brō-mə-ˌdər-mə\ *n* : a skin eruption caused in susceptible persons by the use of bromides

bro·mo·ura·cil \ˌbrō-mō-'yùr-ə-ˌsil, -səl\ *n* : a mutagenic uracil derivative $C_4H_3N_2O_2Br$ that is an analog of thymine and pairs readily with adenine and sometimes with guanine

brom·phen·ir·a·mine \ˌbrōm-fen-'ir-ə-ˌmēn\ *n* : an H_1 antagonist used in the form of its maleate $C_{16}H_{19}BrN_2$-$C_4H_4O_4$ esp. to treat allergies and the common cold

bronch– *or* **broncho–** *comb form* : bronchial tube : bronchial ⟨*bronchitis*⟩

bronchi *pl of* BRONCHUS

bronchi– *or* **bronchio–** *comb form* : bronchial tubes ⟨*bronchi*ectasis⟩

bron·chi·al \'brän-kē-əl\ *adj* : of or relating to the bronchi or their ramifications in the lungs — **bron·chi·al·ly** *adv*

bronchial artery *n* : any branch of the descending aorta or first intercostal artery that accompanies the bronchi

bronchial asthma *n* : asthma resulting from spasmodic contraction of bronchial muscles

bronchial pneumonia *n* : BRONCHOPNEUMONIA

bronchial tree *n* : the bronchi together with their branches

bronchial tube *n* : a primary bronchus; *also* : any of its branches

bronchial vein *n* : any vein accompanying the bronchi and their branches and emptying into the azygos and superior intercostal veins

bron·chi·ec·ta·sis \,brän-kē-'ek-tə-səs\ *also* **bron·chi·ec·ta·sia** \-ek-'tā-zhə, -zhē-ə\ *n, pl* **-ta·ses** \-,sēz\ *also* **-ta·sias** \-zhəz, -zhē-əz\ : a chronic inflammatory or degenerative condition of one or more bronchi or bronchioles marked by dilatation and loss of elasticity of the walls — **bron·chi·ec·tat·ic** \-ek-'ta-tik\ *adj*

bron·chio·gen·ic \,brän-kē-ō-'je-nik\ *adj* : BRONCHOGENIC

bron·chi·ole \'brän-kē-,ōl\ *n* : a minute thin-walled branch of a bronchus — **bron·chi·o·lar** \,brän-kē-'ō-lər\ *adj*

bron·chi·ol·itis \,brän-kē-ō-'lī-təs\ *n* : inflammation of the bronchioles

bronchiolitis ob·lit·er·ans \-ə-'bli-tə-,ranz\ *n* : a pathological process producing obstruction of the bronchioles due to inflammation and fibrosis

bron·chi·o·lus \brän-'kī-ə-ləs\ *n, pl* **-o·li** \-,lī\ : BRONCHIOLE

bron·chi·tis \brän-'kī-təs, brän-\ *n* : acute or chronic inflammation of the bronchial tubes; *also* : a disease marked by this — **bron·chit·ic** \-'ki-tik\ *adj*

broncho- — see BRONCH-

bron·cho·al·ve·o·lar \,brän-kō-al-'vē-ə-lər\ *adj* : of, relating to, or involving the bronchioles and alveoli of the lungs ⟨~ lavage⟩

bron·cho·con·stric·tion \-kən-'strik-shən\ *n* : constriction of the bronchial air passages — **bron·cho·con·stric·tive** \-tiv\ *adj*

bron·cho·con·stric·tor \-'strik-tər\ *adj* : causing or involving bronchoconstriction — **bronchoconstrictor** *n*

bron·cho·di·la·ta·tion \-,dī-lə-'tā-shən, -,dī-\ *n* : BRONCHODILATION

bron·cho·di·la·tion \-dī-'lā-shən\ *n* : expansion of the bronchial air passages

bron·cho·di·la·tor \-dī-'lā-tər, -dī-,lā-\ *also* **bron·cho·di·la·to·ry** \-dī-'lā-tə-rē\ *adj* : causing or involving bronchodilation ⟨~ activity⟩ ⟨~ drugs⟩ — **bronchodilator** *n*

bron·cho·gen·ic \,brän-kə-'je-nik\ *adj* : of, relating to, or arising in or by way of the air passages of the lungs ⟨~ carcinoma⟩

bron·cho·gram \'brän-kə-,gram, -kō-\ *n* : a radiograph of the bronchial tree after injection of a radiopaque substance

bron·chog·ra·phy \brän-'kä-grə-fē, brän-\ *n, pl* **-phies** : the radiographic visualization of the bronchi and their branches after injection of a radiopaque substance — **bron·cho·graph·ic** \,brän-kə-'gra-fik\ *adj*

bron·choph·o·ny \brän-'kä-fə-nē\ *n, pl* **-nies** : the sound of the voice heard through the stethoscope over a healthy bronchus and over other portions of the chest in cases of consolidation of the lung tissue — compare PECTORILOQUY

bron·cho·plas·ty \'brän-kə-,plas-tē\ *n, pl* **-ties** : surgical repair of a bronchial defect

bron·cho·pleu·ral \,brän-kō-'plùr-əl\ *adj* : joining a bronchus and the pleural cavity ⟨a ~ fistula⟩

bron·cho·pneu·mo·nia \,brän-(,)kō-nü-'mō-nyə, -nyü-\ *n* : pneumonia involving many relatively small areas of lung tissue — called also *bronchial pneumonia* — **bron·cho·pneu·mon·ic** \-'mä-nik\ *adj*

bron·cho·pul·mo·nary \,brän-kō-'pùl-mə-,ner-ē, -'pəl-\ *adj* : of, relating to, or affecting the bronchi and the lungs

bronchopulmonary dysplasia *n* : a chronic lung condition that is caused by tissue damage to the lungs and usu. occurs in immature infants who have received mechanical ventilation and supplemental oxygen as treatment for respiratory distress syndrome

bron·cho·scope \'brän-kə-,skōp\ *n* : a usu. flexible endoscope for inspecting or passing instruments into the bronchi — **bron·cho·scop·ic** \,brän-kə-'skä-pik\ *adj* — **bron·chos·co·pist** \brän-'käs-kə-pist\ *n* — **bron·chos·co·py** \brän-'käs-kə-pē\ *n*

bron·cho·spasm \'brän-kə-,spa-zəm\ *n* : constriction of the air passages of the lung (as in asthma) by spasmodic contraction of the bronchial muscles — **bron·cho·spas·tic** \,brän-kə-'spas-tik\ *adj*

bron·cho·spi·rom·e·try \,brän-kō-spī-'rä-mə-trē\ *n, pl* **-tries** : independent measurement of the vital capacity of each lung by means of a spirometer in direct continuity with one of the primary bronchi — **bron·cho·spi·rom·e·ter** \-'rä-mə-tər\ *n*

bron·cho·ste·no·sis \,brän-kō-stə-'nō-səs\ *n, pl* **-no·ses** \-,sēz\ : stenosis of a bronchus

bron·chus \'brän-kəs\ *n, pl* **bron·chi** \'brän-,kī, -,kē\ : either of the two primary divisions of the trachea that lead respectively into the right and the left lung; *broadly* : BRONCHIAL TUBE

broth \'bròth\ *n, pl* **broths** \'bròths, 'bròthz\ **1** : liquid in which meat or sometimes vegetable food has been cooked **2** : a fluid culture medium

brow \'braù\ *n* **1** : EYEBROW **2** : either of the lateral prominences of the forehead **3** : FOREHEAD

brown alga *n* : any of a major taxonomic group (Phaeophyta) of variable mostly marine algae with chlorophyll masked by brown pigment

brown dog tick *n* : a widely distributed reddish brown tick of the genus *Rhipicephalus* (*R. sanguineus*) that occurs esp. on dogs and that transmits canine babesiosis

brown fat *n* : a mammalian heat-producing tissue occurring esp. in human newborn infants — called also *brown adipose tissue*

brown lung disease *n* : BYSSINOSIS

brown rat *n* : a common domestic rat of the genus *Rattus* (*R. norvegicus*) that has been introduced worldwide — called also *Norway rat*

brown recluse spider *n* : a venomous spider of the genus *Loxosceles* (*L. reclusa*) esp. of the southern and central U.S. that produces a dangerous cytotoxin — called also *brown recluse*

brown snake *n* : any of several Australian venomous elapid snakes (genus *Pseudonaja* syn. *Demansia*); *esp* : a widely distributed brownish or blackish snake (*P. textilis*)

brow·ridge \'braů-ˌrij\ *n* : SUPERCILIARY RIDGE

BRP *abbr* bathroom privileges

bru·cel·la \brü-'se-lə\ *n* **1** *cap* : a genus of nonmotile capsulated bacteria (family Brucellaceae) that cause disease in humans and domestic animals **2** *pl* **-cel·lae** \-ˈse-(ˌ)lē\ *or* **-cel·las** : any bacterium of the genus *Brucella*
　Bruce \'brüs\, **Sir David** (1855–1931),　British bacteriologist.

bru·cel·lo·sis \ˌbrü-sə-'lō-səs\ *n, pl* **-lo·ses** \-ˌsēz\ : a disease caused by bacteria of the genus *Brucella*: **a** : a disease of humans caused by any of four organisms (*Brucella melitensis* of goats, *B. suis* of hogs, *B. abortus* of cattle, and *B. canis* of dogs), characterized esp. by weakness, fatigue, night sweats, chills, remittent fever, and generalized aches and pains, and acquired through direct contact with infected animals or animal products or from the consumption of milk, dairy products, or meat from infected animals — called also *Malta fever, undulant fever* **b** : CONTAGIOUS ABORTION

bru·cine \'brü-ˌsēn\ *n* : a poisonous alkaloid $C_{23}H_{26}N_2O_4$ found with strychnine in nux vomica
　Bruce \'brüs\, **James** (1730–1794), British explorer.

Brud·zin·ski sign \brü-'jin-skē-, brüd-'zin-\ *or* **Brud·zin·ski's sign** \-skēz-\ *n* : any of several symptoms of meningeal irritation occurring esp. in meningitis: as **a** : flexion of the lower limbs induced by passive flexion of the head on the chest **b** : flexion of one lower limb following passive flexion of the other
　Brudzinski, Josef (1874–1917), Polish physician.

¹bruise \'brüz\ *vb* **bruised; bruis·ing 1** : to inflict a bruise on : CONTUSE **2** : WOUND, INJURE; *esp* : to inflict psychological hurt on **3** : to become bruised

²bruise *n* **1** : an injury transmitted through unbroken skin to underlying tissue causing rupture of small blood vessels and escape of blood into the tissue with resulting discoloration : CONTUSION **2** : an injury esp. to the feelings

bruit \'brü-ē\ *n* : any of several generally abnormal sounds heard on auscultation

Brun·ner's gland \'brů-nərz-\ *n* : any of the compound racemose glands in the submucous layer of the duodenum that secrete alkaline mucus and a potent proteolytic enzyme — called also *gland of Brunner*
　Brun·ner \'brů-nər\, **Johann Conrad** (1653–1727), Swiss anatomist.

brush border *n* : a stria of microvilli on the plasma membrane of an epithelial cell (as in a kidney tubule) that is specialized for absorption

brux·ism \'brək-ˌsi-zəm\ *n* : the habit of unconsciously gritting or grinding the teeth esp. in situations of stress or during sleep

BS *abbr* **1** bowel sounds **2** breath sounds

BSE *abbr* bovine spongiform encephalopathy

BSN *abbr* bachelor of science in nursing

BST *abbr* blood serological test

bu·bo \'bü-(ˌ)bō, 'byü-\ *n, pl* **buboes** : an inflammatory swelling of a lymph node esp. in the groin — **bu·bon·ic** \bü-'bä-nik, byü-\ *adj*

bubonic plague *n* : plague caused by a bacterium of the genus *Yersinia* (*Y. pestis* syn. *Pasteurella pestis*) and characterized esp. by the formation of buboes — compare PNEUMONIC PLAGUE

buc·cal \'bə-kəl\ *adj* **1** : of, relating to, near, involving, or supplying a cheek ⟨the ∼ surface of a tooth⟩ **2** : of, relating to, involving, or lying in the mouth — **buc·cal·ly** *adv*

buccal gland *n* : any of the small racemose mucous glands in the mucous membrane lining the cheeks

buc·ci·na·tor \'bək-sə-ˌnā-tər\ *n* : a thin broad muscle forming the wall of the cheek and serving to compress the cheek against the teeth — called also *buccinator muscle*

bucco- *comb form* : buccal and ⟨*buccolingual*⟩

buc·co·lin·gual \ˌbə-kō-'liŋ-gwəl, -gyə-wəl\ *adj* **1** : relating to or affecting the cheek and the tongue **2** : of or relating to the buccal and lingual aspects of a tooth ⟨the ∼ width of a molar⟩ — **buc·co·lin·gual·ly** *adv*

buc·co·pha·ryn·ge·al \-ˌfar-ən-'jē-əl, -fə-'rin-jəl, -jē-əl\ *adj* : relating to or near the cheek and the pharynx

buck·thorn \'bək-ˌthȯrn\ *n* : any of a genus (*Rhamnus* of the family Rhamnaceae) of shrubs and trees some of which yield purgative principles in their bark or sap

buck·tooth \-'tüth\ *n, pl* **buck·teeth** : a large projecting front tooth — **buck·toothed** \-'tütht\ *adj*

¹**bud** \'bəd\ *n* **1 a** : an asexual reproductive structure **b** : a primordium having potentialities for growth and development into a definitive structure ⟨an embryonic limb ∼⟩ **2** : an anatomical structure (as a tactile corpuscle) resembling a bud

²**bud** *vb* **bud·ded; bud·ding** : to reproduce asexually esp. by the pinching off of a small part of the parent

bu·des·o·nide \ˌbyü-'de-sō-ˌnīd\ *n* : an anti-inflammatory glucocorticoid $C_{25}H_{34}O_6$ used to treat rhinitis

BUdR *abbr* bromodeoxyuridine

Buer·ger's disease \'bər-gərz-, 'bur-\ *n* : thromboangiitis of the small arteries and veins of the extremities and esp. the feet resulting in occlusion, ischemia, and gangrene — called also *thromboangiitis obliterans*

Buer·ger \'bər-gər, 'bur-\, **Leo (1879–1943),** American pathologist.

¹**buff·er** \'bə-fər\ *n* : a substance or mixture of substances (as bicarbonates) that in solution tends to stabilize the hydrogen-ion concentration by neutralizing within limits both acids and bases

²**buffer** *vb* : to treat (as a solution or its acidity) with a buffer; *also* : to prepare (aspirin) with an antacid

buffy coat \'bə-fē-\ *n* : the superficial layer of yellowish or buff coagulated plasma from which the red corpuscles have settled out in slowly coagulated blood

bu·fo·ten·ine \ˌbyü-fə-'te-ˌnēn, -nən\ *or* **bu·fo·ten·in** \-nən\ *n* : a toxic hallucinogenic alkaloid $C_{12}H_{16}N_2O$ that is obtained esp. from poisonous secretions of toads (order Anura and esp. family Bufonidae) and from some mushrooms and has hypertensive and vasoconstrictor activity

bug \'bəg\ *n* **1 a** : an insect or other creeping or crawling invertebrate animal (as a spider) — not used technically **b** : any of several insects (as the bedbug or cockroach) commonly considered obnoxious **c** : any of an order (Hemiptera and esp. its suborder Heteroptera) of insects that have sucking mouthparts and forewings thickened at the base and that lack a pupal stage between the immature stages and the adult — called also *true bug* **2 a** : a disease-producing microorganism and esp. a germ **b** : a disease caused by such microorganisms; *esp* : any of various respiratory conditions (as influenza) of viral origin

building–related illness *n* : a clinically diagnosable disease or condition (as Legionnaires' disease or an allergic reaction) caused by a microorganism or substance demonstrably present in a building

bulb \'bəlb\ *n* **1** : a rounded dilation or expansion of something cylindrical ⟨the ∼ of a thermometer⟩; *esp* : a rounded or pear-shaped enlargement on a small base ⟨the ∼ of an eyedropper⟩ **2** : a rounded part: as **a** : a rounded enlargement of one end of a part — see BULB OF THE PENIS, BULB OF THE VESTIBULE, END BULB, OLFACTORY BULB **b** : MEDULLA OBLONGATA; *broadly* : the hindbrain exclusive of the cerebellum

bulb- *or* **bulbo-** *comb form* **1** : bulb ⟨*bulbar*⟩ **2** : bulbar and ⟨*bulbospinal*⟩

bul·bar \'bəl-bər, -ˌbär\ *adj* : of or relating to a bulb; *specif* : involving the medulla oblongata

bulbar paralysis *n* : destruction of nerve centers of the medulla oblongata and paralysis of the parts innervated from the medulla with interruption of their functions (as swallowing or speech)

bulbi — see PHTHISIS BULBI

bul·bo·cav·er·no·sus \ˌbəl-(ˌ)bō-ˌkavər-'nō-səs\ *n, pl* **-no·si** \-ˌsī\ : a muscle that in the male surrounds and compresses the bulb of the penis and the bulbar portion of the urethra and in the female serves to compress the vagina — see SPHINCTER VAGINAE

bulb of the penis *n* : the proximal expanded part of the corpus cavernosum of the male urethra

bulb of the vestibule *n* : a structure in the female vulva that is homologous to the bulb of the penis and the adjoining corpus spongiosum in the male and that consists of an elongated mass of erectile tissue on each side of the vaginal opening united anteriorly to the contralateral mass by a narrow median band passing along the lower surface of the clitoris

bul·bo·spi·nal \ˌbəl-bō-'spīn-ᵊl\ *adj* : of, relating to, or connecting the medulla oblongata and the spinal cord

bul·bo·spon·gio·sus muscle \ˌbəl-(ˌ)bō-ˌspən-jē-'ō-səs-\ *n* : BULBOCAVERNOSUS

bul·bo·ure·thral gland \-yú-'rē-thrəl\ *n* : COWPER'S GLAND

bul·bous \'bəl-bəs\ *adj* : resembling a bulb esp. in roundness or the gross enlargement of a part

bul·bus \'bəl-bəs\ *n, pl* **bul·bi** \-ˌbī, -ˌbē\ : a bulb-shaped anatomical part

-bulia *also* **-boulia** *n comb form* : condition of having (such) will ⟨*abulia*⟩

-bulic *adj comb form* : of, relating to, or characterized by a (specified) state of will ⟨*abulic*⟩

bu·lim·a·rex·ia \ˌbü-ˌli-mə-'rek-sē-ə, ˌbyü-, -ˌlē-\ *n* : BULIMIA 2 — **bu·lim·a·rex·ic** \-sik\ *n or adj*

bu·lim·ia \bü-'li-mē-ə, byü-, -'lē-\ *n* **1** : an abnormal and constant craving for food **2** : a serious eating disorder that occurs chiefly in females, is characterized by compulsive overeating usu. followed by self-induced vomiting or laxative or diuretic abuse, and is often accompanied by guilt and depression

bulimia ner·vo·sa \-(ˌ)nər-ˈvō-sə, -zə\ *n* : BULIMIA 2

¹**bu·lim·ic** \-ˈmik\ *adj* : of, relating to, or affected with bulimia ⟨∼ patients⟩

²**bulimic** *n* : a person affected with bulimia

bulk \ˈbəlk\ *n* : material (as indigestible fibrous residues of food) that forms a mass in the intestine; *esp* : FIBER 2

bul·la \ˈbu̇-lə\ *n, pl* **bul·lae** \ˈbu̇-ˌlē, -ˌlī\ **1** : a hollow thin-walled rounded bony prominence **2** : a large vesicle or blister — compare BLEB

bull·nose \ˈbu̇l-ˌnōz\ *n* : a necrobacillosis arising in facial wounds of swine

bullosa — see EPIDERMOLYSIS BULLOSA

bul·lous \ˈbu̇-ləs\ *adj* : resembling or characterized by bullae : VESICULAR

bullous pemphigoid *n* : a chronic skin disease affecting esp. elderly persons that is characterized by the formation of numerous hard blisters over a widespread area

bu·met·a·nide \byü-ˈme-tə-ˌnīd\ *n* : a diuretic $C_{17}H_{20}N_2O_5S$ used in the treatment of edema — see BUMEX

Bu·mex \ˈbyü-ˌmeks\ *trademark* — used for a preparation of bumetanide

BUN \ˌbē-(ˌ)yü-ˈen\ *n* : the concentration of nitrogen in the form of urea in the blood

bun·dle \ˈbənd-ᵊl\ *n* : a small band of mostly parallel fibers (as of nerve or muscle) : FASCICULUS, TRACT

bundle branch *n* : either of the parts of the bundle of His passing respectively to the right and left ventricles

bundle branch block *n* : heart block due to a lesion in one of the bundle branches

bundle of His \-ˈhis\ *n* : a slender bundle of modified cardiac muscle that passes from the atrioventricular node in the right atrium to the right and left ventricles by way of the septum and that maintains the normal sequence of the heartbeat — called also *atrioventricular bundle, His bundle*
  His, Wilhelm (1863–1934), German physician.

bun·ga·ro·tox·in \ˈbəŋ-gə-rō-ˌtäk-sən\ *n* : a potent neurotoxin obtained from the venom of an Asian elapid snake (genus *Bungarus*)

bun·ion \ˈbən-yən\ *n* : an inflamed swelling of the small fluid-filled sac on the first joint of the big toe accompanied by enlargement and protrusion of the joint

bun·io·nec·to·my \ˌbən-yə-ˈnek-tə-mē\ *n, pl* **-mies** : surgical excision of a bunion

Bu·nos·to·mum \byü-ˈnäs-tə-məm\ *n* : a genus of nematode worms including the hookworms of sheep and cattle

bun·ya·vi·rus \ˈbən-yə-ˌvī-rəs\ *n* : any of a family (*Bunyaviridae*) of usu.

spherical or pleomorphic single-stranded RNA viruses that are usu. transmitted by the bite of an arthropod (as a mosquito) or in the bodily secretions of rodents and that include the causative agents of Rift Valley fever, sandfly fever, and some forms of encephalitis (as La Crosse encephalitis) and hemorrhagic fever

Bunyavirus *n, syn of* ORTHOBUNYAVIRUS

buph·thal·mos \büf-ˈthal-məs, byüf-, ˌbəf-, -ˌmäs\ *also* **buph·thal·mia** \-mē-ə\ *n, pl* **-mos·es** *also* **-mias** : marked enlargement of the eye that is usu. congenital and attended by symptoms of glaucoma

bu·piv·a·caine \byü-ˈpi-və-ˌkān\ *n* : a local anesthetic $C_{18}H_{28}N_2O$ that is like lidocaine in its action but is longer acting

bu·pre·nor·phine \ˌbyü-prə-ˈnȯr-ˌfēn\ *n* : a narcotic analgesic that is used in the form of its hydrochloride $C_{29}H_{41}NO_4·HCl$ intravenously or intramuscularly to treat moderate to severe pain and sublingually to treat opioid dependence

bu·pro·pi·on \byü-ˈprō-pē-ˌän\ *n* : a drug used in the form of its hydrochloride $C_{13}H_{18}ClNO·HCl$ as an antidepressant and as an aid to stop smoking — see WELLBUTRIN, ZYBAN

bur \ˈbər\ *n* **1** *usu* **burr** : a small surgical cutting tool (as for making an opening in bone) **2** : a bit used on a dental drill

bur·den \ˈbər-dən\ *n* : LOAD 1

Burk·hol·de·ria \ˌbərk-hōl-ˈder-ē-ə\ *n* : a genus of bacteria (family Burkholderiacea) formerly placed in the genus *Pseudomonas* and including the causative agents of glanders (*B. mallei*) and melioidosis (*B. pseudomallei*)
  Burkholder, Walter Hagemeyer (1891–1983), American botanist.

Bur·kitt's lymphoma \ˈbər-kəts-\ *also* **Burkitt lymphoma** \-kət-\ *n* : a non-Hodgkin's lymphoma of B cell origin that occurs esp. in children of central Africa and is associated with Epstein-Barr virus
  Bur·kitt \ˈbər-kət\, **Denis Parsons** (1911–1993), British surgeon.

Burkitt's tumor *also* **Burkitt tumor** *n* : BURKITT'S LYMPHOMA

¹**burn** \ˈbərn\ *vb* **burned** \ˈbərnd, ˈbərnt\ *or* **burnt** \ˈbərnt\; **burn·ing 1** : to produce or undergo discomfort or pain ⟨iodine ∼s so⟩; *also* : to injure or damage by exposure to fire, heat, or radiation ⟨∼ed his hand⟩ **2** : to receive sunburn ⟨she ∼s easily⟩

²**burn** *n* **1** : bodily injury resulting from exposure to heat, caustics, electricity, or some radiations, marked by varying degrees of skin destruction and hyperemia often with the formation of watery blisters and in severe cases by charring of the tissues, and classified according to the extent and

degree of the injury — see FIRST=
DEGREE BURN, SECOND-DEGREE
BURN, THIRD-DEGREE BURN **2** : an
abrasion having the appearance of a
burn ⟨friction ~s⟩ **3** : a burning sensation

burn center *also* **burns center** *n* : a
specialized facility usu. affiliated with
a hospital that provides advanced
care and treatment for patients with
severe burn

burn·er \'bər-nər\ *n* : STINGER 2

¹**burn·ing** \'bər-niŋ\ *adj* **1** : affecting
with or as if with heat ⟨a ~ fever⟩ **2**
: resembling that produced by a burn
⟨a ~ sensation⟩

²**burning** *n* : a sensation of being on fire
or excessively heated ⟨gastric ~⟩

burning mouth syndrome *n* : a
chronic burning sensation of the oral
mucous membranes esp. of the
tongue that chiefly affects postmenopausal women and is of unknown cause

burn·out \'bərn-‚aút\ *n* **1 a** : exhaustion of physical or emotional strength
usu. as a result of prolonged stress or
frustration **b** : a person affected with
burnout **2** : a person showing the effects of drug abuse

Bu·row's solution \'bü-(‚)rōz-\ *n* : a
solution of the acetate of aluminum
used as an antiseptic and astringent
   Bu·row \'bü-(‚)rō\, **Karl August von
(1809–1874)**, German military surgeon and anatomist.

¹**burp** \'bərp\ *n* : BELCH

²**burp** *vb* **1** : BELCH 2 **2** : to help (a baby)
expel gas from the stomach esp. by
patting or rubbing the back

burr *var of* BUR

bur·row \'bər-(‚)ō\ *n* : a passage or
gallery formed in or under the skin by
the wandering of a parasite (as the
mite of scabies) — **burrow** *vb*

bur·sa \'bər-sə\ *n, pl* **bur·sas** \-səz\ *or*
bur·sae \-‚sē, -‚sī\ : a bodily pouch or
sac: as **a** : a small serous sac between
a tendon and a bone **b** : BURSA OF
FABRICIUS — **bur·sal** \-səl\ *adj*

bursa of Fa·bri·cius \-fə-'bri-shəs,
-shē-əs\ *n* : a blind glandular sac that
opens into the cloaca of birds and
functions in B cell production
   **Fabricius, Johann Christian (1745–
1808)**, Danish entomologist.

bur·si·tis \(‚)bər-'sīt-əs\ *n* : inflamma-
tion of a bursa (as of the shoulder or
elbow)

bush·mas·ter \'büsh-‚mas-tər\ *n* : a
tropical American pit viper (*Lachesis
mutus*)

Bu·Spar \'byü-‚spär\ *trademark* —
used for a preparation of the hydrochloride of buspirone

bu·spi·rone \byü-'spī-‚rōn\ *n* : a mild
antianxiety tranquilizer that is used in
the form of its hydrochloride C_{21}-
$H_{31}N_5O_2 \cdot HCl$ and does not induce significant tolerance or psychological
dependence — see BUSPAR

bu·sul·fan \byü-'səl-fən\ *n* : an antineoplastic agent $C_6H_{14}O_6S_2$ used in
the treatment of chronic myelogenous leukemia — see MYLERAN

bu·ta·bar·bi·tal \‚byü-tə-'bär-bə-‚tal\ *n*
: a synthetic barbiturate used esp. in
the form of its sodium salt $C_{10}H_{15}N_2$-
NaO_3 as a sedative and hypnotic

bu·ta·caine \'byü-tə-‚kān\ *n* : a local
anesthetic that is applied in the form
of its sulfate $(C_{18}H_{30}N_2O_2)_2 \cdot H_2SO_4$ to
mucous membranes

Bu·ta·zol·i·din \‚byü-tə-'zä-lə-dən\ *n*
: a preparation of phenylbutazone —
formerly a U.S. registered trademark

bute \'byüt\ *n* : PHENYLBUTAZONE

bu·tor·pha·nol \byü-'tór-fə-‚nól\ *n* : a
synthetic opioid drug used esp. in
the form of its tartrate $C_{21}H_{29}NO_2$-
$C_4H_6O_6$ as nasal spray or by injection esp. for the relief of pain — see
STADOL

butoxide — see PIPERONYL BUTOXIDE

¹**but·ter·fly** \'bə-tər-‚flī\ *n, pl* **-flies 1** *pl*
: a feeling of hollowness or queasiness
caused esp. by emotional or nervous
tension or anxious anticipation **2** : a
bandage with wing-shaped extensions

²**butterfly** *adj* : being, relating to, or affecting the area of the face including
both cheeks connected by a band
across the nose ⟨the typical ~ lesion
of lupus erythematosus⟩

butterfly needle *n* : a short needle that
has plastic tabs on either side which
aid esp. in manipulating and stabiliz-
ing the needle during insertion

but·tock \'bə-tək\ *n* **1** : the back of a
hip that forms one of the fleshy parts
on which a person sits **2 buttocks** *pl*
: the seat of the body; *also* : the corresponding part of a quadruped : RUMP

but·ton \'bət-ᵊn\ *n* : something that resembles a small knob or disk: as **a**
: the terminal segment of a rattlesnake's rattle **b** : COTYLEDON 1

bu·tyl·at·ed hy·droxy·an·i·sole \'byü-tə-
‚lā-təd-‚hī-‚dräk-sē-'a-nə-‚sōl\ *n*
: BHA

butylated hy·droxy·tol·u·ene \-(‚)hī-
‚dräk-sē-'täl-yə-‚wēn\ *n* : BHT

bu·tyl nitrite \'byüt-ᵊl-\ *n* : a colorless
pungent liquid $C_4H_9NO_2$ inhaled illicitly for its stimulating effects which
are similar to those of amyl nitrite —
called also *isobutyl nitrite*; compare
POPPER

bu·tyr·ic acid \byü-'tir-ik-\ *n* : either
of two isomeric fatty acids $C_4H_8O_2$;
esp : one of unpleasant odor found in
rancid butter and in perspiration

bu·ty·ro·phe·none \‚byü-tə-(‚)rō-fə-
'nōn\ *n* : any of a class of antipsychotic drugs (as haloperidol) used
esp. in the treatment of schizophrenia

BV *abbr* bacterial vaginosis

B vitamin *n* : any vitamin of the vitamin B complex

Bx *abbr* [by analogy with *Rx*] biopsy

by·pass \'bī-‚pas\ *n* : a surgically established shunt; *also* : a surgical procedure for the establishment of a

shunt — see CORONARY BYPASS, GAS-
TRIC BYPASS, JEJUNOILEAL BYPASS —
bypass vb

bys·si·no·sis \ˌbi-sə-'nō-səs\ n, pl **-no-
ses** \-ˌsēz\ : an occupational respiratory disease associated with inhalation of cotton, flax, or hemp dust and
characterized initially by chest tightness, shortness of breath, and cough,
and eventually by irreversible lung
disease — called also *brown lung,
brown lung disease*

BZ \ˌbē-'zē\ n : a gas $C_{21}H_{23}NO_3$ that
when breathed produces incapacitat-
ing physical and mental effects —
called also *quinuclidinyl benzilate*

C

c abbr 1 canine 2 centimeter 3 curie
4 or **c** [Latin *cum*] with — used in
writing prescriptions

C abbr 1 Celsius 2 centigrade 3 cervical — used esp. with a number from
1 to 7 to indicate a vertebra or segment of the spinal cord 4 cocaine 5
[Latin *congius*] gallon 6 cytosine

C symbol carbon

Ca symbol calcium

CA abbr chronological age

CABG \'ka-bij\ abbr coronary artery
bypass graft

cacao butter var of COCOA BUTTER

ca·chec·tic \ka-'kek-tik, ka-\ adj : relating to or affected by cachexia

ca·chet \ka-'shā\ n : a medicinal preparation for swallowing consisting
of a case usu. of rice-flour paste containing an unpleasant-tasting medicine

ca·chex·ia \kə-'kek-sē-ə, ka-\ n : general physical wasting and malnutrition usu. associated with chronic
disease

cac·o·dyl·ic acid \ˌka-kə-'di-lik-\ n : a
toxic crystalline compound of arsenic
$C_2H_7AsO_2$ used esp. as an herbicide

ca·cos·mia \kə-'käs-mē-ə, ka-ˌ-'käz-\
n : a hallucination of a disagreeable
odor

CAD abbr coronary artery disease

ca·dav·er \kə-'da-vər\ n : a dead body;
specif : one intended for dissection —
ca·dav·er·ic \-və-rik\ adj

ca·dav·er·ous \kə-'da-və-rəs\ adj 1 : of
or relating to a corpse 2 of a complexion : being pallid or livid like a corpse

cade oil n : JUNIPER TAR

cad·mi·um \'kad-mē-əm\ n : a bluish
white malleable ductile toxic bivalent
metallic element — symbol Cd; see
ELEMENT table

cadmium sulfide n : a yellow-brown
poisonous salt CdS used esp. in the
treatment of seborrheic dermatitis of
the scalp

ca·du·ceus \kə-'dü-sē-əs, -'dyü-, -shəs\
n, pl **-cei** \-sē-ˌī\ : a medical insignia
bearing a representation of a staff
with two entwined snakes and two
wings at the top — compare STAFF OF
AESCULAPIUS

caec- or **caeci-** or **caeco-** chiefly Brit
var of CEC-

cae·cal, cae·cum chiefly Brit var of CE-
CAL, CECUM

cae·sar·e·an also **caesarian** var of CE-
SAREAN

cae·si·um chiefly Brit var of CESIUM

ca·fé au lait spot \ka-'fā-ō-'lā-\ n : any
of the medium brown spots usu. on
the trunk, pelvis, and creases of the
elbow and knees that are often numerous in neurofibromatosis — usu.
used in pl.

caf·feine \ka-'fēn, 'ka-ˌ\ n : a bitter alkaloid $C_8H_{10}N_4O_2$ found esp. in coffee
and tea and used medicinally as a
stimulant and diuretic — **caf·fein·ic**
\ka-'fē-nik\ adj

caf·fein·ism \-ˌni-zəm\ n : a morbid
condition caused by caffeine (as from
excessive consumption of coffee)

-caine n comb form : synthetic alkaloid
anesthetic ⟨*procaine*⟩ ⟨lido*caine*⟩

cais·son disease \'kā-ˌsän-, 'käs-ᵊn-\
n : DECOMPRESSION SICKNESS

caj·e·put·ol or **caj·u·put·ol** \'ka-jə-pə-
ˌtol, -ˌtōl\ n : EUCALYPTOL

caked breast \'kākt-\ n : a localized
hardening in one or more segments of
a lactating breast caused by accumulation of blood in dilated veins and
milk in obstructed ducts

cal abbr small calorie

Cal abbr large calorie

Cal·a·bar swelling \'ka-lə-ˌbär-\ n : a
transient subcutaneous swelling marking the migratory course through the
tissues of the adult filarial eye worm of
the genus *Loa* (*L. loa*)

cal·a·mine \'ka-lə-ˌmīn, -mən\ n : a
mixture of zinc oxide or zinc carbonate with a small amount of ferric oxide that is used in lotions, liniments,
and ointments

Cal·an \'ka-ˌlän\ trademark — used
for a preparation of the hydrochloride of verapamil

cal·ca·ne·al \kal-'kā-nē-əl\ adj 1 : relating to the heel 2 : relating to the
calcaneus

calcaneal tendon n : ACHILLES TEN-
DON

calcaneo- comb form : calcaneal and
⟨*calcaneo*cuboid⟩

cal·ca·neo·cu·boid \(ˌ)kal-ˌkā-nē-ō-
'kyü-ˌbȯid\ adj : of or relating to the
calcaneus and the cuboid bone

calcaneonavicular — see PLANTAR CALCANEONAVICULAR LIGAMENT

cal·ca·ne·um \kal-'kā-nē-əm\ n, pl **-nea** \-nē-ə\ : CALCANEUS

cal·ca·ne·us \-nē-əs\ n, pl **-nei** \-nē-ˌī\ : a tarsal bone that in humans is the large bone of the heel — called also *heel bone, os calcis*

cal·car \'kal-ˌkär\ n, pl **cal·car·ia** \kal-'kar-ē-ə\ : a small anatomical prominence or projection

calcar avis \-'ā-vəs, -'ä-\ n, pl **calcaria avi·um** \-vē-əm\ : a curved ridge on the medial wall of the posterior horn of each lateral ventricle of the brain opposite the calcarine sulcus

cal·car·e·ous \kal-'kar-ē-əs\ adj : resembling, consisting of, or containing calcium carbonate; *also* : containing calcium

cal·ca·rine sulcus \'kal-kə-ˌrīn-\ n : a sulcus in the mesial surface of the occipital lobe of the cerebrum — called also *calcarine fissure*

cal·cif·er·ol \kal-'sif-ə-ˌról, -ˌról\ n : an alcohol $C_{28}H_{43}OH$ usu. prepared by irradiation of ergosterol and used as a dietary supplement in nutrition and medicinally esp. in the control of rickets — called also *ergocalciferol, viosterol, vitamin D, vitamin D₂*; see DRISDOL

cal·cif·ic \kal-'si-fik\ adj : involving or caused by calcification ⟨∼ lesions⟩

cal·ci·fi·ca·tion \ˌkal-sə-fə-'kā-shən\ n **1** : impregnation with calcareous matter: as **a** : deposition of calcium salts within the matrix of cartilage often as the preliminary step in the formation of bone **b** : abnormal deposition of calcium salts within tissue **2** : a calcified structure or part — **cal·ci·fy** \'kal-sə-ˌfī\ vb

cal·ci·no·sis \ˌkal-sə-'nō-səs\ n, pl **-no·ses** \-ˌsēz\ : the abnormal deposition of calcium salts in a part or tissue of the body

calcis — see OS CALCIS

cal·ci·to·nin \ˌkal-sə-'tō-nən\ n : a polypeptide hormone esp. from the thyroid gland that tends to lower the level of calcium in the blood plasma — called also *thyrocalcitonin*

cal·ci·tri·ol \ˌkal-sə-'trī-ˌól, -ˌól\ n : a physiologically active metabolic derivative $C_{27}H_{44}O_3$ of cholecalciferol that is synthesized in the liver and kidney and stimulates the intestinal absorption of calcium — called also *1,25-dihydroxycholecalciferol*

cal·ci·um \'kal-sē-əm\ n, often attrib : a silver-white bivalent metal that is an essential constituent of most plants and animals — symbol *Ca*; see ELEMENT table

calcium blocker n : CALCIUM CHANNEL BLOCKER

calcium carbonate n : a calcium salt $CaCO_3$ that is found in limestone, chalk, and bones and that is used in pharmaceuticals as an antacid and to supplement bodily calcium stores

calcium channel blocker n : any of a class of drugs (as verapamil) that prevent or slow the influx of calcium ions into smooth muscle cells esp. of the heart and that are used to treat some forms of angina pectoris and some cardiac arrhythmias — called also *calcium blocker*

calcium chloride n : a white salt $CaCl_2$ used in medicine as a source of calcium and as a diuretic

calcium gluconate n : a white powdery salt $C_{12}H_{22}CaO_{14}$ used to supplement bodily calcium stores

calcium hydroxide n : a strong alkali $Ca(OH)_2$ — see SODA LIME

calcium lactate n : a white crystalline salt $C_6H_{10}CaO_6 \cdot 5H_2O$ used chiefly in medicine as a source of calcium and in foods (as in baking powder)

calcium levulinate n : a white powdery salt $C_{10}H_{14}CaO_6 \cdot H_2O$ used in medicine as a source of calcium

calcium oxalate n : an insoluble crystalline salt $CaC_2O_4 \cdot H_2O$ that is sometimes excreted in urine or retained in the form of urinary calculi

calcium pantothenate n : a white powdery salt $C_{18}H_{32}CaN_2O_{10}$ made synthetically and used as a source of pantothenic acid

calcium phosphate n : any of various phosphates of calcium: as **a** : the phosphate $CaHPO_4$ used in pharmaceutical preparations and animal feeds **b** : a naturally occurring phosphate $Ca_5(F,Cl,OH,\frac{1}{2}CO_3)(PO_4)_3$ that contains other elements or radicals and is the chief constituent of bones and teeth

calcium propionate n : a mold-inhibiting salt $C_6H_{10}CaO_4$ used chiefly as a food preservative

calcium stearate n : a white powder consisting essentially of calcium salts of stearic acid and palmitic acid and used as a conditioning agent in food and pharmaceuticals

calcium sulfate n : a white calcium salt $CaSO_4$ used esp. as a diluent in tablets and in plaster of paris

cal·co·sphe·rite \ˌkal-kō-'sfir-ˌīt\ n : a granular or laminated deposit of calcium salts in the body

cal·cu·lo·sis \ˌkal-kyə-'lō-səs\ n, pl **-lo·ses** \-ˌsēz\ : the formation of or the condition of having a calculus or calculi

cal·cu·lous \'kal-kyə-ləs\ adj : caused or characterized by a calculus or calculi ⟨∼ disease⟩

cal·cu·lus \-ləs\ n, pl **-li** \-ˌlī, -ˌlē\; also **-lus·es 1** : a concretion usu. of mineral salts around organic material found esp. in hollow organs or ducts **2** : a concretion on teeth : TARTAR

Cald·well-Luc operation \'kóld-ˌwel-'lük-, 'käld-, -'lᵫk-\ n : a surgical procedure used esp. for clearing a blocked or infected maxillary sinus that involves entering the sinus through the mouth by way of an inci-

sion into the canine fossa above a canine tooth, cleaning the sinus, and creating a new and enlarged opening for drainage through the nose
Caldwell, George Walter (1866–1946), American surgeon.
Luc \lük\, **Henri** (1855–1925), French laryngologist.

calf \'kaf, 'kàf\ *n, pl* **calves** \'kavz, 'kàvz\ : the fleshy back part of the leg below the knee

calf bone *n* : FIBULA

calf diphtheria *n* : an infectious disease of the mouth and pharynx of calves and young cattle associated with the presence of large numbers of a bacterium of the genus *Fusobacterium* (*F. necrophorum*) and commonly resulting in pneumonia and generalized septicemia if untreated

cal·i·ber \'ka-lə-bər\ *n* : the diameter of a round body; *esp* : the internal diameter of a hollow cylinder

cal·i·bre *chiefly Brit var of* CALIBER

caliceal *var of* CALYCEAL

cal·i·ci·vi·rus \kə-'li-sə-,vī-rəs\ *n* : any of a family (*Caliciviridae*) of single-stranded RNA viruses that include the Norwalk virus and the causative virus of vesicular exanthema — see HEPATITIS E

cal·i·for·ni·um \,ka-lə-'fȯr-nē-əm\ *n* : an artificially prepared radioactive element — symbol *Cf*; see ELEMENT table

cal·i·per \'ka-lə-pər\ *n* : any of various measuring instruments having two usu. adjustable arms, legs, or jaws used esp. to measure diameter or thickness — usu. used in pl.

cal·is·then·ics \,ka-ləs-'the-niks\ *n sing or pl* **1** : systematic rhythmic bodily exercises performed usu. without apparatus **2** *usu sing* : the art or practice of calisthenics — **cal·is·then·ic** \-nik\ *adj*

calix *var of* CALYX

cal·li·per *chiefly Brit var of* CALIPER

cal·lis·then·ics *Brit var of* CALISTHENICS

cal·lo·sal \ka-'lō-səl\ *adj* : of, relating to, or being the corpus callosum

cal·los·i·ty \ka-'lä-sə-tē\ *n, pl* **-ties** : the quality or state of being callous; *esp* : marked or abnormal hardness and thickness (as of the skin)

callosum — see CORPUS CALLOSUM

cal·lous \'ka-ləs\ *adj* **1** : being hardened and thickened **2** : having calluses

cal·loused *or* **cal·lused** \'ka-ləst\ *adj* : CALLOUS 2 〈~ hands〉

cal·lus \'ka-ləs\ *n* **1** : a thickening of or a hard thickened area on skin **2** : a mass of exudate and connective tissue that forms around a break in a bone and is converted into bone in the healing of the break

calm·ant \'kä-mənt, 'kälm-\ *n* : SEDATIVE

calm·ative \'kä-mə-tiv, 'käl-mə-\ *n or adj* : SEDATIVE

cal·mod·u·lin \kal-'mä-jə-lən\ *n* : a calcium-binding protein that regulates cellular metabolic processes (as muscle-fiber contraction) by modifying the activity of specific calcium-dependent enzymes

cal·o·mel \'ka-lə-məl, -,mel\ *n* : a white tasteless compound Hg₂Cl₂ used esp. as a fungicide and insecticide and formerly in medicine as a purgative — called also *mercurous chloride*

cal·or \'ka-,lȯr\ *n* : bodily heat that is a sign of inflammation

calori- *comb form* : heat 〈*calori*genic〉 〈*calori*meter〉

ca·lo·ric \kə-'lȯr-ik, -'lär-; 'ka-lə-rik\ *adj* **1** : of or relating to heat **2** : of or relating to calories — **ca·lo·ri·cal·ly** \kə-'lȯr-i-k(ə-)lē, -'lär-\ *adv*

cal·o·rie *also* **cal·o·ry** \'ka-lə-rē\ *n, pl* **-ries** **1 a** : the amount of heat required at a pressure of one atmosphere to raise the temperature of one gram of water one degree Celsius that is equal to about 4.19 joules — abbr. *cal*; called also *gram calorie, small calorie* **b** : the amount of heat required to raise the temperature of one kilogram of water one degree Celsius that is equal to 1000 gram calories — abbr. *Cal*; called also *kilocalorie, kilogram calorie, large calorie* **2 a** : a unit equivalent to the large calorie expressing heat-producing or energy-producing value in food when oxidized in the body **b** : an amount of food having an energy-producing value of one large calorie

cal·o·rif·ic \,ka-lə-'ri-fik\ *adj* **1** : CALORIC **2** : of or relating to the production of heat

ca·lo·ri·gen·ic \kə-,lȯr-ə-'je-nik, -,lär-; ,ka-lə-rə-\ *adj* : generating heat or energy 〈~ foodstuffs〉

cal·o·rim·e·ter \,ka-lə-'ri-mə-tər\ *n* : any of several apparatuses for measuring quantities of absorbed or evolved heat or for determining specific heats — **ca·lo·ri·met·ric** \,ka-lə-rə-'me-trik; kə-,lȯr-ə-, -,lär-\ *adj* — **ca·lo·ri·met·ri·cal·ly** \-tri-k(ə-)lē\ *adv* — **cal·o·rim·e·try** \,ka-lə-'ri-mə-trē\ *n*

cal·va \'kal-və\, *n, pl* **calvas** *or* **cal·vae** \-,vē, -,vī\ : the upper part of the human cranium

cal·var·ia \kal-'var-ē-ə\ *n, pl* **-i·ae** \-ē-,ē, -ē-,ī\ : CALVARIUM

cal·var·i·um \-ē-əm\ *n, pl* **-ia** \-ē-ə\ : an incomplete skull; *esp* : the portion of a skull including the braincase and excluding the lower jaw or lower jaw and facial portion — **cal·var·i·al** \-ē-əl\ *adj*

calves *pl of* CALF

cal·vi·ti·es \kal-'vi-shē-,ēz, -(,)shēz\ *n, pl* **calvities** : the condition of being bald : BALDNESS

calx \'kalks\ *n, pl* **cal·ces** \'kal-,sēz\

ca·ly·ce·al *or* **ca·li·ce·al** \,ka-lə-'sē-əl, ,kā-\ *adj* : of or relating to a calyx

calyces *pl of* CALYX

Ca·lym·ma·to·bac·te·ri·um \kə-ˌli-mə-tō-bak-ˈtir-ē-əm\ n : a genus of pleomorphic nonmotile bacteria (family Brucellaceae) including only the causative agent (*C. granulomatis*) of granuloma inguinale — see DONOVAN BODY

ca·lyx also **ca·lix** \ˈkā-liks, ˈka-\ n, pl **ca·lyx·es** or **ca·ly·ces** \ˈkā-lə-ˌsēz, ˈka-\ : a cuplike division of the renal pelvis surrounding one or more renal papillae

CAM abbr complementary and alternative medicine

cam·i·sole \ˈka-mə-ˌsōl\ n : a long-sleeved straitjacket

cAMP abbr cyclic AMP

cam·phor \ˈkam-fər\ n : a gummy volatile aromatic crystalline compound $C_{10}H_{16}O$ that is obtained esp. from the wood and bark of an evergreen tree (*Cinnamomum camphora*) of the laurel family (Lauraceae) and is used esp. as a liniment and mild topical analgesic and as an insect repellent

cam·phor·at·ed \ˈkam-fə-ˌrā-təd\ adj : impregnated or treated with camphor

cam·phor·ic acid \kam-ˈfȯr-ik-, -ˈfär-\ n : the dextrorotatory form of a white crystalline acid $C_{10}H_{16}O_2$ that is used in pharmaceuticals

cam·pim·e·ter \kam-ˈpi-mə-tər\ n : an instrument for testing indirect or peripheral visual perception of form and color — **cam·pim·e·try** \-trē\ n

camp·to·cor·mia \ˌkam-tə-ˈkȯr-mē-ə\ n : an hysterical condition marked by forward bending of the trunk and sometimes accompanied by lumbar pain

camp·to·dac·ty·ly \ˌkam-tə-ˈdak-tə-lē\ n, pl **-lies** : permanent flexion of one or more finger joints

camp·to·the·cin \ˌkamp-tə-ˈthē-sən\ n : an alkaloid $C_{20}H_{16}N_2O_4$ from the wood of a Chinese tree (*Camptotheca acuminata* of the family Nyssaceae) that has shown some antileukemic and antitumor activity; also : a semisynthetic or synthetic derivative of this

cam·py·lo·bac·ter \ˈkam-pə-lō-ˌbak-tər\ n 1 cap : a genus of slender spirally curved rod bacteria (family Spirillaceae) including some forms pathogenic for domestic animals or humans — HELICOBACTER 2 : any bacterium of the genus *Campylobacter*

ca·nal \kə-ˈnal\ n : a tubular anatomical passage or channel : DUCT

can·a·lic·u·lus \ˌkan-ᵊl-ˈi-kyə-ləs\ n, pl **-li** \-ˌlī, -ˌlē\ : a minute canal in a bodily structure — **can·a·lic·u·lar** \-lər\ adj

ca·na·lis \kə-ˈna-ləs, -ˈnä-\ n, pl **ca·na·les** \-ˈna-(ˌ)lēz, -ˈnä-(ˌ)lās\ : CANAL

can·a·li·za·tion \ˌkan-ᵊl-ə-ˈzā-shən\ n 1 : surgical formation of holes or canals for drainage without tubes 2 : natural formation of new channels in tissue (as formation of new blood vessels through a blood clot) 3 : establishment of new pathways in the

central nervous system by repeated passage of nerve impulses

can·a·lize \ˈkan-ᵊl-ˌīz\ vb **-lized; -lizing** 1 : to drain (a wound) by forming channels without the use of tubes 2 : to develop new channels (as new capillaries in a blood clot)

canal of Schlemm \-ˈshlem\ n : a circular canal lying in the substance of the sclerocorneal junction of the eye and draining the aqueous humor from the anterior chamber into the veins draining the eyeball — called also *Schlemm's canal, sinus venosus sclerae*

  Schlemm, Friedrich S. (1795–1858), German anatomist.

Can·a·van disease \ˈka-nə-ˌvan\ also **Can·a·van's disease** \-ˌvanz-\ n : a rare usu. fatal demyelinating disease of infancy that is caused by an enzyme deficiency that is inherited as an autosomal recessive trait and that typically affects individuals of eastern European Jewish ancestry

  Canavan, Myrtelle May (1879–1953), American pathologist.

can·cel·lous \ˈkan-ˈse-ləs, ˈkan-sə-\ adj : having a porous structure made up of intersecting plates and bars that form small cavities or cells ⟨∼ bone⟩ — compare COMPACT

can·cer \ˈkan-sər\ n 1 : a malignant tumor of potentially unlimited growth that expands locally by invasion and systemicaly by metastasis 2 : an abnormal state marked by a cancer — **can·cer·ous** \-sə-rəs\ adj

cancer eye n : a malignant squamous cell epithelioma of cattle that originates in the mucous membranes of the eye

can·cer·i·ci·dal or **can·cer·o·ci·dal** \ˌkan-sə-rə-ˈsīd-ᵊl\ adj : destructive of cancer cells

can·cer·i·za·tion \-ˌzā-shən\ n : transformation into cancer or from a normal to a cancerous state

can·cer·o·gen·ic \-ˈje-nik, -rō-\ or **can·cer·i·gen·ic** \-rə-\ adj : CARCINOGENIC

can·cer·ol·o·gy \ˌkan-sə-ˈrä-lə-jē\ n, pl **-gies** : the study of cancer — **can·cer·ol·o·gist** \-jist\ n

can·cer·pho·bia \ˌkan-sər-ˈfō-bē-ə\ or **can·cer·o·pho·bia** \-sər-ō-ˈfō-\ n : an abnormal dread of cancer

can·crum oris \ˌkaŋ-krəm-ˈōr-əs, -ˈär-\ n, pl **can·cra oris** \-krə-\ : noma of the oral tissues — called also *gangrenous stomatitis*

can·de·la \kan-ˈdel-ə, -ˈde-\ n : a unit of luminous intensity in the International System of Units — called also *candle*

can·di·ci·din \ˌkan-də-ˈsīd-ᵊn\ n : an antibiotic obtained from a streptomyces (*Streptomyces griseus*) and active against some fungi of the genus *Candida*

can·di·da \ˈkan-də-də\ n 1 cap : a genus of parasitic fungi that resemble yeasts, occur esp. in the mouth, vagina, and intestinal tract where they are usu. benign but can become pathogenic, and have been grouped with the imperfect fungi but are now often placed with the ascomycetes **2** : any fungus of the genus *Candida*; *esp* : one (*C. albicans*) causing thrush — **can·di·dal** \-dəd-ᵊl\ *adj*

can·di·di·a·sis \ˌkan-də-ˈdī-ə-səs\ *n, pl* **-a·ses** \-ˌsēz\ : infection with or disease caused by a fungus of the genus *Candida* — called also *monilia, moniliasis*

can·dle \ˈkand-ᵊl\ *n* **1** : a medicated candle or lozenge used for fumigation **2** : CANDELA

candy striper *n* : a volunteer nurse's aide

ca·nic·o·la fever \kə-ˈni-kə-lə-\ *n* : an acute disease of humans and dogs characterized by gastroenteritis and mild jaundice and caused by a spirochete of the genus *Leptospira* (*L. canicola*)

¹ca·nine \ˈkā-ˌnīn\ *n* **1** : a conical pointed tooth; *esp* : one situated between the lateral incisor and the first premolar **2** : a canine mammal : DOG

²canine *adj* : of or relating to dogs or to the family (Canidae) to which they belong

canine distemper *n* : DISTEMPER a

canine fossa *n* : a depression external to and somewhat above the prominence on the surface of the superior maxillary bone caused by the socket of the canine tooth

ca·ni·nus \kā-ˈnī-nəs, kə-\ *n, pl* **ca·ni·ni** \-ˈnī-ˌnī\ : LEVATOR ANGULI ORIS

ca·ni·ti·es \kə-ˈni-shē-ˌēz\ *n* : grayness or whiteness of the hair

can·ker \ˈkaŋ-kər\ *n* **1 a** : an erosive or spreading sore : CANKER SORE **2 a** : a chronic inflammation of the ear in dogs, cats, or rabbits; *esp* : a localized form of mange **b** : a chronic and progressive inflammation of the hooves of horses resulting in softening and destruction of the horny layers — **can·kered** \-kərd\ *adj*

canker sore *n* : a painful shallow ulceration of the oral mucous membranes that has a grayish-white base surrounded by a reddish inflamed area and is characteristic of aphthous stomatitis

can·na·bi·noid \ˈka-nə-bə-ˌnȯid, kə-ˈna-\ *n* : any of various chemical constituents (as THC) of cannabis or marijuana

can·na·bis \ˈka-nə-bəs\ *n* **1 a** *cap* : a genus of annual herbs (family Moraceae) that have leaves with three to seven elongate leaflets and pistillate flowers in spikes along the leafy erect stems and that include the hemp (*C. sativa*) **b** : HEMP 1 **2** : any of the preparations (as marijuana or hashish) or chemicals (as THC) that are derived from the hemp and are psychoactive

cannabis in·di·ca \-ˈin-di-kə\ *n, pl* **can·na·bes in·di·cae** \ˈka-nə-ˌbēz-ˈin-də-ˌsē, -ˌbäs-ˈin-di-ˌkī\ : cannabis of a variety obtained in India

can·na·bism \ˈka-nə-ˌbi-zəm\ *n* **1** : habituation to the use of cannabis **2** : chronic poisoning from excessive smoking or chewing of cannabis

can·ni·bal \ˈka-nə-bəl\ *n* : one that eats the flesh of its own kind — **cannibal** *adj*

can·ni·bal·ism \-bə-ˌli-zəm\ *n* **1** : the usu. ritualistic eating of human flesh by a human being **2** : the eating of the flesh or the eggs of any animal by its own kind

can·non \ˈka-nən\ *n* : the part of the leg in which the cannon bone is found

cannon bone *n* : a bone in hoofed mammals that supports the leg from the hock joint to the fetlock

can·nu·la *also* **can·u·la** \ˈkan-yə-lə\ *n, pl* **-las** *or* **-lae** \-ˌlē, -ˌlī\ : a small tube for insertion into a body cavity, duct, or vessel

can·nu·late \-ˌlāt\ *vb* **-lat·ed; -lat·ing** : to insert a cannula into — **can·nu·la·tion** \ˌkan-yə-ˈlā-shən\ *n*

can·nu·lize \ˈkan-yə-ˌlīz\ *vb* **-lized; -liz·ing** : CANNULATE — **can·nu·li·za·tion** \ˌkan-yə-lə-ˈzā-shən\ *n*

ca·no·la \kə-ˈnō-lə\ *n* **1** : a rape plant (*Brassica napus*) of the mustard family of an improved variety with seeds that are low in erucic acid and are the source of canola oil **2** : CANOLA OIL

canola oil *n* : an edible vegetable oil obtained from the seeds of canola that is high in monounsaturated fatty acids

can·thar·i·din \kan-ˈthar-əd-ᵊn\ *n* : a bitter crystalline compound $C_{10}H_{12}O_4$ that is the active blister-producing ingredient of cantharides

can·thar·is \ˈkan-thə-rəs\ *n, pl* **can·thar·i·des** \kan-ˈthar-ə-ˌdēz\ **1** : SPANISH FLY 1 **2** *cantharides* : a preparation of dried beetles and esp. Spanish flies that contains cantharidin and is used in medicine as a blister-producing agent and formerly as an aphrodisiac — used with a sing. or pl. verb; called also *Spanish fly*

can·tha·xan·thin \ˌkan-thə-ˈzan-ˌthin\ *n* : a carotenoid $C_{40}H_{52}O_2$ used esp. as a color additive in food

can·thus \ˈkan-thəs\ *n, pl* **can·thi** \ˈkan-ˌthī, -ˌthē\ : either of the angles formed by the meeting of the upper and lower eyelids

¹cap \ˈkap\ *n, often attrib* **1** : something that serves as a cover or protection esp. for a tip, knob, or end (as of a tooth) **2** : PATELLA, KNEECAP **3** *Brit* : CERVICAL CAP

²cap *vb* **capped; cap·ping 1** : to invest (a student nurse) with a cap as an indication of completion of a probationary period of study **2** : to cover (a diseased or exposed part of a tooth) with a protective substance

cap *abbr* capsule

ca·pac·i·ta·tion \kə-ˌpa-sə-'tā-shən\ n : the change undergone by sperm in the female reproductive tract that enables them to penetrate and fertilize an egg — **ca·pac·i·tate** \-ˌtāt\ vb

ca·pac·i·ty \kə-'pa-sə-tē, -'pas-tē\ n, pl **-ties 1** : a measure of content : VOLUME — see VITAL CAPACITY **2** : legal qualification, competency, power, or fitness

cap·e·line \'ka-pə-ˌlēn, -lən\ n : a cup-shaped bandage for the head, the shoulder, or the stump of an amputated limb

cap·il·lar·ia \ˌka-pə-'lar-ē-ə\ n 1 cap : a genus of slender white nematode worms (family Trichuridae) that include serious pathogens of the digestive tract of fowls and some tissue and organ parasites of mammals including one (C. hepatica) which is common in rodents and occas. invades the human liver sometimes with fatal results **2** : a nematode worm of the genus Capillaria — **cap·il·lar·id** \-'lar-əd, kə-'pi-lə-rəd\ n

ca·pil·la·ri·a·sis \kə-ˌpi-lə-'rī-ə-səs\ also **cap·il·lar·i·o·sis** \ˌka-pə-ˌler-ē-'ō-səs\ n, pl **-a·ses** \-'rī-ə-ˌsēz\ also **-o·ses** \-'ō-ˌsēz\ : infestation with or disease caused by nematode worms of the genus Capillaria

cap·il·lar·o·scope \ˌka-pə-'lar-ə-ˌskōp\ n : a microscope that permits visual examination of the living capillaries in nail beds, skin, and conjunctiva — **cap·il·la·ros·co·py** \ˌka-pə-lə-'räs-kə-pē\ n

¹cap·il·lary \'ka-pə-ˌler-ē\ adj **1 a** : resembling a hair esp. in slender elongated form **b** : having a very small bore ⟨a ~ tube⟩ **2** : of or relating to capillaries

²capillary n, pl **-lar·ies 1** : a minute thin-walled vessel of the body; esp : any of the smallest blood vessels connecting arterioles with venules and forming networks throughout the body **2** : a capillary tube

capillary bed n : the whole system of capillaries of a body, part, or organ

capita pl of CAPUT

¹cap·i·tate \'ka-pə-ˌtāt\ adj : abruptly enlarged and globe-shaped

²capitate n : the largest bone of the wrist that is situated between the hamate and the trapezoid in the distal row of carpal bones and that articulates with the third metacarpal

cap·i·tat·ed \'ka-pə-ˌtā-təd\ adj : of, relating to, participating in, or being a health-care system in which a medical provider is given a set fee per patient (as by an HMO) regardless of treatment required

cap·i·ta·tion \ˌka-pə-'tā-shən\ n **1** : a fixed per capita medical payment made periodically to a medical service provider (as a physician) by a managed care group (as in an HMO) in return for medical care provided to enroll individuals **2** : a capitated health-care system

cap·i·ta·tum \ˌka-pə-'tā-təm, -'tä-\ n, pl **cap·i·ta·ta** \-tə\ : CAPITATE

cap·i·tel·lum \ˌka-pə-'te-ləm\ n, pl **-tel·la** \-lə\ : a knoblike protuberance esp. at the end of a bone (as the humerus)

capitis — see LONGISSIMUS CAPITIS, LONGUS CAPITIS, OBLIQUUS CAPITIS INFERIOR, OBLIQUUS CAPITIS SUPERIOR, PEDICULOSIS CAPITIS, RECTUS CAPITIS POSTERIOR MAJOR, RECTUS CAPITIS POSTERIOR MINOR, SEMISPINALIS CAPITIS, SPINALIS CAPITIS, SPLENIUS CAPITIS, TINEA CAPITIS

ca·pit·u·lum \kə-'pi-chə-ləm\ n, pl **-la** \-lə\ : a rounded protuberance of an anatomical part — **ca·pit·u·lar** \-lər, -ˌlär\ adj

Cap·lets \'ka-pləts\ trademark — used for capsule-shaped medicinal tablets

-capnia n comb form : carbon dioxide in the blood ⟨hypercapnia⟩

cap·no·gram \'kap-nō-ˌgram\ n : the waveform tracing produced by a capnograph

cap·no·graph \'kap-nō-ˌgraf\ n : a monitoring device that measures the concentration of carbon dioxide in exhaled air and displays a numerical readout and waveform tracing — **cap·no·graph·ic** \ˌkap-nō-'gra-fik\ adj — **cap·nog·ra·phy** \kap-'nä-grə-fē\ n

cap·nom·e·ter \kap-'nä-mə-tər\ n : a monitoring device that measures and numerically displays the concentration of carbon dioxide in exhaled air — **cap·nom·e·try** \-trē\ n

Cap·o·ten \'ka-pō-ˌten\ trademark — used for a preparation of captopril

cap·re·o·my·cin \ˌka-prē-ō-'mīs-ᵊn\ n : an antibiotic obtained from a bacterium of the genus Streptomyces (S. capreolus) that is used to treat tuberculosis

ca·pro·ic acid \kə-ˌprō-ik-\ n : a liquid fatty acid $C_6H_{12}O_2$ that is found as a glyceryl ester in fats and oils and is used in pharmaceuticals and flavors

cap·ry·late \'ka-prə-ˌlāt\ n : a salt or ester of caprylic acid — see SODIUM CAPRYLATE

ca·pryl·ic acid \kə-'pri-lik-\ n : a fatty acid $C_8H_{16}O_2$ of rancid odor occurring in fats and oils

cap·sa·i·cin \kap-'sā-ə-sən\ n : a colorless irritant substance $C_{18}H_{27}NO_3$ obtained from various capsicums and used in topical creams for its analgesic properties

cap·si·cum \'kap-si-kəm\ n **1** : any of a genus (Capsicum) of tropical plants of the nightshade family (Solanaceae) that are widely cultivated for their many-seeded usu. fleshy-walled berries **2** : the dried ripe fruit of some capsicums (as C. frutescens) used as a gastric and intestinal stimulant

cap·sid \'kap-səd\ n : the protein shell of a virus particle that surrounds its nucleic acid

cap·so·mer \'kap-sə-mər\ or **cap·so·mere** \'kap-sə-ˌmir\ n : one of the subunits making up a viral capsid

capsul- or **capsuli-** or **capsulo-** comb form : capsule ⟨capsulitis⟩

cap·su·la \'kap-sə-lə\ n, pl **cap·su·lae** \-lē, -lī\ : CAPSULE

cap·su·lar \'kap-sə-lər\ adj : of, relating to, affecting, or resembling a capsule

capsular contracture n : shrinking and tightening of the mass of scar tissue around a breast implant that may result in pain and in unnatural firmness and distortion of the breast

capsularis — see DECIDUA CAPSULARIS

cap·su·lat·ed \-,lā-təd\ also **cap·su·late** \-,lāt, -lət\ adj : enclosed in a capsule

cap·su·la·tion \,kap-sə-'lā-shən\ n : enclosure in a capsule

cap·sule \'kap-səl, -(,)sül\ n **1 a** : a membrane or saclike structure enclosing a part or organ ⟨the ∼ of the kidney⟩ **b** : either of two layers or laminae of white matter in the cerebrum: **(1)** : a layer that consists largely of fibers passing to and from the cerebral cortex and that lies internal to the lentiform nucleus — called also *internal capsule* **(2)** : one that lies between the lentiform nucleus and the claustrum — called also *external capsule* **2** : a shell usu. of gelatin for packaging something (as a drug or vitamins); also : a usu. medicinal or nutritional preparation for oral use consisting of the shell and its contents **3** : a viscous or gelatinous often polysaccharide envelope surrounding certain microscopic organisms (as the pneumococcus)

cap·su·lec·to·my \,kap-sə-'lek-tə-mē\ n, pl **-mies** : excision of a capsule (as of a joint, kidney, or lens)

capsule of Bow·man \'bō-mən\ n : BOWMAN'S CAPSULE

capsule of Te·non \-tə-'nōⁿ\ n : TENON'S CAPSULE

cap·su·li·tis \,kap-sə-'lī-təs\ n : inflammation of a capsule (as that of the crystalline lens)

cap·su·lor·rha·phy \,kap-sə-'lȯr-ə-fē\ n, pl **-phies** : suture of a cut or wounded capsule (as of the knee joint)

cap·su·lot·o·my \-'lä-tə-mē\ n, pl **-mies** : incision of a capsule esp. of the crystalline lens (as in cataract surgery)

cap·to·pril \'kap-tə-,pril\ n : an antihypertensive drug $C_9H_{15}NO_3S$ that is an ACE inhibitor — see CAPOTEN

ca·put \'kä-,pût, -pət; 'ka-pət\ n, pl **ca·pi·ta** \'kä-pə-,tä, 'ka-pə-tə\ **1** : a knoblike protuberance (as of a bone or muscle) **2** : CAPUT SUCCEDANEUM

caput suc·ce·da·ne·um \-,sək-sə-'dā-nē-əm\ n, pl **capita suc·ce·da·nea** \-ə\ : an edematous swelling formed upon the presenting part of the scalp of a newborn infant as a result of trauma sustained during delivery

Car·a·fate \'kar-ə-,fāt\ trademark — used for a preparation of sucralfate

ca·ra·te \kə-'rä-tē\ n : PINTA

carb \'kärb\ or **car·bo** \'kär-,bō\ n : CARBOHYDRATE; also : a high-carbohydrate food — usu. used in pl.

car·ba·chol \'kär-bə-,kȯl, -,kōl\ n : a synthetic parasympathomimetic drug $C_6H_{15}ClN_2O_2$ that is used in veterinary medicine and topically to treat glaucoma

car·ba·mate \'kär-bə-,māt, kär-'ba-,māt\ n : a salt or ester of carbamic acid — see URETHANE

car·ba·maz·e·pine \,kär-bə-'ma-zə-,pēn\ n : a tricyclic anticonvulsant and analgesic $C_{15}H_{12}N_2O$ used in the treatment of trigeminal neuralgia and epilepsy — see TEGRETOL

car·bam·ic acid \,kär-'ba-mik-\ n : an acid CH_3NO_2 known in the form of salts and esters

carb·ami·no·he·mo·glo·bin \,kär-bə-,mē-(,)nō-'hē-mə-,glō-bən\ n : CARBHEMOGLOBIN

car·bar·sone \kär-'bär-,sōn\ n : a white powder $C_7H_9N_2O_4As$ used esp. in treating intestinal amebiasis

car·ba·zole \'kär-bə-,zōl\ n : a crystalline slightly basic cyclic compound $C_{12}H_9N$ used in testing for carbohydrates (as sugars)

car·ben·i·cil·lin \,kär-,be-nə-'si-lən\ n : a broad-spectrum semisynthetic penicillin $C_{17}H_{18}N_2O_6S$ that is used esp. against gram-negative bacteria (as pseudomonas)

carb·he·mo·glo·bin \(,)kärb-'hē-mə-,glō-bən\ or **car·bo·hemo·glo·bin** \,kär-bō-\ n : a compound of hemoglobin with carbon dioxide

carbo var of CARB

car·bo·hy·drase \,kär-bō-'hī-,drās, -bə-, -,drāz\ n : any of a group of enzymes (as amylase) that promote hydrolysis or synthesis of a carbohydrate (as a disaccharide)

car·bo·hy·drate \-,drāt, -drət\ n : any of various neutral compounds of carbon, hydrogen, and oxygen (as sugars, starches, and celluloses) most of which are formed by green plants and which constitute a major class of animal foods

car·bol·fuch·sin paint \'kär-(,)bäl-'fyük-sən-, -(,)bȯl-\ n : a solution containing boric acid, phenol, resorcinol, and fuchsin in acetone, alcohol, and water that is applied externally in the treatment of fungal infections of the skin — called also *Castellani's paint*

car·bol·ic \kär-'bä-lik\ n : PHENOL 1

carbolic acid n : PHENOL 1

car·bo–load \'kär-,bō-'lōd\ vb : to consume a large amount of carbohydrates through food intake usu. in order to improve performance in an upcoming athletic event (as a marathon)

car·bo·my·cin \ˌkär-bə-ˈmīs-ᵊn\ *n* : a colorless crystalline basic macrolide antibiotic $C_{42}H_{67}NO_{16}$ produced by a bacterium of the genus *Streptomyces* (*S. halstedii*) and active esp. in inhibiting the growth of gram-positive bacteria

car·bon \ˈkär-bən\ *n, often attrib* : a nonmetallic element found native (as in diamonds and graphite) or as a constituent of coal, petroleum, asphalt, limestone, and organic compounds or obtained artificially (as in activated charcoal) — symbol *C;* see ELEMENT table

car·bon·ate \ˈkär-bə-ˌnāt, -nət\ *n* : a salt or ester of carbonic acid

carbon dioxide *n* : a heavy colorless gas CO_2 that does not support combustion, dissolves in water to form carbonic acid and is formed esp. in animal respiration and in the decay or combustion of animal and vegetable matter

carbon 14 *n* : a heavy radioactive isotope of carbon of mass number 14 used esp. in tracer studies

car·bon·ic \kär-ˈbä-nik-\ *n* : a weak acid H_2CO_3 known only in solution that reacts with bases to form carbonates

carbonic anhydrase *n* : a zinc-containing enzyme that occurs in living tissues (as red blood cells) and aids carbon-dioxide transport from the tissues and its release from the blood in the lungs by catalyzing the reversible hydration of carbon dioxide to carbonic acid

carbon monoxide *n* : a colorless odorless very toxic gas CO that is formed as a product of the incomplete combustion of carbon

carbon tetrachloride *n* : a colorless nonflammable toxic carcinogenic liquid CCl_4 that has an odor resembling that of chloroform and is used as a solvent and a refrigerant

car·bo·plat·in \ˈkär-bō-ˌpla-tᵊn\ *n* : a platinum-containing antineoplastic drug $C_6H_{12}N_2O_4$Pt that is an analog of cisplatin with somewhat reduced toxicity and that is used in the treatment of various cancers

car·boxy·he·mo·glo·bin \ˌkär-ˌbäk-sē-ˈhē-mə-ˌglō-bən\ *n* : a very stable combination of hemoglobin and carbon monoxide formed in the blood when carbon monoxide is inhaled with resulting loss of ability of the blood to combine with oxygen

car·box·yl \kär-ˈbäk-səl\ *n* : a monovalent group —COOH typical of organic acids — called also *carboxyl group* — **car·box·yl·ic** \ˌkär-(ˌ)bäk-ˈsil-ik\ *adj*

car·box·yl·ase \kär-ˈbäk-sə-ˌlās, -ˌlāz\ *n* : an enzyme that catalyzes decarboxylation or carboxylation

car·box·yl·ate \-ˌlāt, -lət\ *n* : a salt or ester of a carboxylic acid — **car·box·yl·ate** \-ˌlāt\ *vb* — **car·box·yl·ation** \(ˌ)kär-ˌbäk-sə-ˈlā-shen\ *n*

carboxylic acid *n* : an organic acid (as an acetic acid) containing one or more carboxyl groups

car·boxy·meth·yl·cel·lu·lose \(ˌ)kär-ˌbäk-sē-ˌme-thəl-ˈsel-yə-ˌlōs, -ˌlōz\ *n* : a derivative of cellulose used in the form of its sodium salt is used as a bulk laxative in medicine

car·boxy·pep·ti·dase \-ˈpep-tə-ˌdās, -ˌdāz\ *n* : an enzyme that hydrolyzes peptides and esp. polypeptides by splitting off sequentially the amino acids at the end of the peptide chain which contain free carboxyl groups

car·bun·cle \ˈkär-ˌbəŋ-kəl\ *n* : a painful local purulent inflammation of the skin and deeper tissues with multiple openings for the discharge of pus and usu. necrosis and sloughing of dead tissue — **car·bun·cu·lar** \kär-ˈbəŋ-kyə-lər\ *adj*

car·bun·cu·lo·sis \kär-ˌbəŋ-kyə-ˈlō-səs\ *n, pl* **-lo·ses** \-ˌsēz\ : a condition marked by the formation of many carbuncles simultaneously or in rapid succession

carcin- *or* **carcino-** *comb form* : tumor : cancer ⟨*carcino*genic⟩

car·ci·no·em·bry·on·ic antigen \ˌkärs-ᵊn-ō-ˌem-brē-ˈä-nik-\ *n* : a glycoprotein present in fetal gut tissues during the first two trimesters of pregnancy and in peripheral blood of patients with some forms of cancer (as of the digestive system) — abbr. *CEA*

car·cin·o·gen \kär-ˈsi-nə-jən, ˈkärs-ᵊn-ə-ˌjen\ *n* : a substance or agent causing cancer

car·ci·no·gen·e·sis \ˌkärs-ᵊn-ō-ˈje-nə-səs\ *n, pl* **-e·ses** \-ˌsēz\ : the production of cancer

car·ci·no·gen·ic \ˌkärs-ᵊn-ō-ˈje-nik\ *adj* : producing or tending to produce cancer ⟨~ compounds⟩ — **car·ci·no·gen·i·cal·ly** \-ni-k(ə-)lē\ *adv* — **car·ci·no·ge·nic·i·ty** \-jə-ˈni-sə-tē\ *n*

car·ci·noid \ˈkärs-ᵊn-ˌóid\ *n* : a benign or malignant tumor arising esp. from the mucosa of the gastrointestinal tract (as in the stomach or appendix)

carcinoid syndrome *n* : a syndrome that is caused by vasoactive substances secreted by carcinoid tumors and is characterized by flushing, cyanosis, abdominal cramps, diarrhea, and valvular heart disease

car·ci·no·ma \ˌkärs-ᵊn-ˈō-mə\ *n, pl* **-mas** *also* **-ma·ta** \-mə-tə\ : a malignant tumor of epithelial origin — compare SARCOMA — **car·ci·no·ma·tous** \-mə-təs\ *adj*

carcinoma in situ *n* : carcinoma in the stage of development when the cancer cells are still within their site of origin (as the mouth or uterine cervix)

car·ci·no·ma·to·sis \-ˌō-mə-ˈtō-səs\ *n, pl* **-to·ses** \-ˌsēz\ : a condition in which multiple carcinomas develop simultaneously usu. after dissemination from a primary source

car·ci·no·sar·co·ma \ˈkärs-ᵊn-ō-(ˌ)sär-ˈkō-mə\ *n, pl* **-mas** *also* **-ma·ta** \-mə-tə\ : a malignant tumor combining elements of carcinoma and sarcoma

cardi- *or* **cardio-** *comb form* : heart : cardiac : cardiac and ⟨*cardio*gram⟩

car·dia \ˈkär-dē-ə\ *n, pl* **car·di·ae** \-ˌē\ *or* **cardias 1** : the opening of the esophagus into the stomach **2** : the part of the stomach adjoining the cardia

¹**-car·dia** \ˈkär-dē-ə\ *n comb form* : heart action or location (of a specified type) ⟨tachy*cardia*⟩

²**-cardia** *pl of* -CARDIUM

¹**car·di·ac** \ˈkär-dē-ˌak\ *adj* **1 a** : of, relating to, situated near, or acting on the heart **b** : of or relating to the cardia of the stomach **2** : of, relating to, or affected with heart disease

²**cardiac** *n* : a person with heart disease

cardiac arrest *n* : abrupt temporary or permanent cessation of the heartbeat (as from ventricular fibrillation or asystole) — called also *sudden cardiac arrest*

cardiac asthma *n* : asthma due to heart disease (as heart failure) that occurs in paroxysms usu. at night and is characterized by difficult wheezing respiration, pallor, and anxiety — called also *paroxysmal dyspnea*

cardiac cycle *n* : the complete sequence of events in the heart from the beginning of one beat to the beginning of the following beat : a complete heartbeat including systole and diastole

cardiac failure *n* : HEART FAILURE

cardiac gland *n* : any of the branched tubular mucus-secreting glands of the cardia of the stomach; *also* : one of the similar glands of the esophagus

cardiac muscle *n* : the principal muscle tissue of the vertebrate heart that is made up of elongated striated fibers joined at usu. branched ends by intercalated disks and that is synchronized to function in contraction esp. by electrical signals of extrinsic origin passing through gap junctions in the intercalated disks — compare SMOOTH MUSCLE, STRIATED MUSCLE

cardiac nerve *n* : any of the three nerves connecting the cervical ganglia of the sympathetic nervous system with the cardiac plexus

cardiac neurosis *n* : NEUROCIRCULATORY ASTHENIA

cardiac output *n* : the volume of blood ejected from the left side of the heart in one minute — called also *minute volume*

cardiac plexus *n* : a nerve plexus of the autonomic nervous system supplying the heart and neighboring structures and situated near the heart and the arch and ascending part of the aorta

cardiac reserve *n* : the difference between the rate at which a heart pumps blood at a particular time and its maximum capacity for pumping blood

cardiac sphincter *n* : the somewhat thickened muscular ring surrounding the opening between the esophagus and the stomach

cardiac tamponade *n* : mechanical compression of the heart by large amounts of fluid or blood within the pericardial space that limits the normal range of motion and function of the heart

cardiac valve *n* : HEART VALVE

cardiac vein *n* : any of the veins returning the blood from the tissues of the heart that open into the right atrium either directly or through the coronary sinus

car·di·al·gia \ˌkär-dē-ˈal-jə, -jē-ə\ *n* **1** : HEARTBURN **2** : pain in the heart

car·di·ec·to·my \ˌkär-dē-ˈek-tə-mē\ *n, pl* **-mies** : excision of the cardiac portion of the stomach

cardinal vein *n* : any of four longitudinal veins of the vertebrate embryo running anteriorly and posteriorly along each side of the spinal column with the pair on each side meeting at and discharging blood to the heart through a large venous sinus — called also *cardinal sinus, Cuvierian vein*

¹**car·dio** \ˈkär-dē-ō\ *adj* : CARDIOVASCULAR 2 ⟨∼ exercises⟩

²**cardio** *n* : cardiovascular exercise

cardio- — see CARDI-

car·dio·ac·cel·er·a·tor \ˌkär-dē-(ˌ)ō-ik-ˈse-lə-ˌrā-tər, -ak-\ *adj* : speeding up the action of the heart — **car·dio·ac·cel·er·a·tion** \-ˌse-lə-ˈrā-shən\ *n*

car·dio·ac·tive \-ˈak-tiv\ *adj* : having an influence on the heart ⟨∼ drugs⟩

car·dio·cir·cu·la·to·ry \ˈsər-kyə-lə-ˌtōr-ē\ *adj* : of or relating to the heart and circulatory system ⟨∼ failure⟩

car·dio·dy·nam·ics \-dī-ˈna-miks\ *n sing or pl* : the dynamics of the heart's action in pumping blood — **car·dio·dy·nam·ic** \-mik\ *adj*

car·dio·gen·ic \-ˈje-nik\ *adj* : originating in the heart : caused by a cardiac condition ⟨∼ pulmonary edema⟩

cardiogenic shock *n* : shock resulting from failure of the heart to pump an adequate amount of blood as a result of heart disease and esp. heart attack

car·dio·gram \ˈkär-dē-ə-ˌgram\ *n* : the curve or tracing made by a cardiograph

car·dio·graph \-ˌgraf\ *n* : an instrument that registers graphically movements of the heart — **car·dio·graph·ic** \ˌkär-dē-ə-ˈgra-fik\ *adj* — **car·di·og·ra·phy** \ˌkär-dē-ˈä-grə-fē\ *n*

car·dio·in·hib·i·to·ry \ˌkär-dē-(ˌ)ō-in-ˈhi-bə-ˌtōr-ē\ *adj* : interfering with or slowing the normal sequence of events in the cardiac cycle ⟨the ∼ center of the medulla⟩

car·dio·lip·in \ˌkär-dē-ō-ˈli-pən\ *n* : a phospholipid used in combination with lecithin and cholesterol as an antigen in diagnostic blood tests for syphilis

car·di·ol·o·gy \ˌkär-dē-'ä-lə-jē\ *n, pl* **-gies** : the study of the heart and its action and diseases — **car·di·o·log·i·cal** \-ə-'lä-ji-kəl\ *adj* — **car·di·ol·o·gist** \-'ä-lə-jist\ *n*

car·dio·meg·a·ly \ˌkär-dē-ō-'me-gə-lē\ *n, pl* **-lies** : enlargement of the heart

car·dio·my·op·a·thy \ˌkär-dē-ō-(ˌ)mī-'ä-pə-thē\ *n, pl* **-thies** : any structural or functional disease of heart muscle that is marked esp. by enlargement of the heart, by hypertrophy of cardiac muscle, or by rigidity and loss of flexibility of the heart walls and that may be idiopathic or attributable to a specific cause (as heart valve disease, untreated high blood pressure, or viral infection)

car·di·op·a·thy \ˌkär-dē-'ä-pə-thē\ *n, pl* **-thies** : any disease of the heart

car·dio·plas·ty \'kär-dē-ō-ˌplas-tē\ *n, pl* **-ties** : plastic surgery performed on the gastric cardiac sphincter

car·dio·ple·gia \ˌkär-dē-ō-'plē-jə, -jē-ə\ *n* : temporary cardiac arrest induced (as by drugs) during heart surgery — **car·dio·ple·gic** \-jik\ *adj*

car·dio·pro·tec·tive \ˌkär-dē-ō-prə-'tek-tiv\ *adj* : serving to protect the heart ⟨~ effects of ACE inhibitors⟩

car·dio·pul·mo·nary \ˌkär-dē-ō-'pùl-mə-ˌner-ē, -'pəl-\ *adj* : of or relating to the heart and lungs ⟨a ~ bypass⟩

cardiopulmonary resuscitation *n* : a procedure designed to restore normal breathing after cardiac arrest that includes the clearance of air passages to the lungs, the mouth-to-mouth method of artificial respiration, and heart massage by the exertion of pressure on the chest — abbr. *CPR*

car·dio·re·nal \-'rēn-ᵊl\ *adj* : of or relating to the heart and the kidneys

car·dio·re·spi·ra·to·ry \ˌkär-dē-ō-'res-pə-rə-ˌtōr-ē, -ri'spī-rə-\ *adj* : of or relating to the heart and the respiratory system : CARDIOPULMONARY

car·dio·scle·ro·sis \ˌkär-dē-(ˌ)ō-sklə-'rō-səs\ *n, pl* **-ro·ses** \-ˌsēz\ : induration of the heart caused by formation of fibrous tissue in the cardiac muscle

car·dio·spasm \'kär-dē-ō-ˌspa-zəm\ *n* : failure of the cardiac sphincter to relax during swallowing with resultant esophageal obstruction — compare ACHALASIA

car·dio·ta·chom·e·ter \ˌkär-dē-(ˌ)ō-ta-'kä-mə-tər\ *n* : a device for prolonged graphic recording of the heartbeat

car·dio·tho·rac·ic \-thə-'ra-sik\ *adj* : relating to, involving, or specializing in the heart and chest ⟨~ surgery⟩

car·di·ot·o·my \ˌkär-dē-'ä-tə-mē\ *n, pl* **-mies** 1 : surgical incision of the heart 2 : surgical incision of the stomach cardia

¹car·dio·ton·ic \ˌkär-dē-ō-'tä-nik\ *adj* : tending to increase the tonus of heart muscle ⟨~ steroids⟩

²cardiotonic *n* : a cardiotonic substance

car·dio·tox·ic \-'täk-sik\ *adj* : having a toxic effect on the heart — **car·dio·tox·ic·i·ty** \-täk-'si-sə-tē\ *n*

¹car·dio·vas·cu·lar \-'vas-kyə-lər\ *adj* 1 : of, relating to, or involving the heart and blood vessels ⟨~ disease⟩ 2 : used, designed, or performed to cause a temporary increase in heart rate ⟨a ~ workout⟩

²cardiovascular *n* : a substance (as a drug) that affects the heart or blood vessels

car·dio·ver·sion \-'vər-zhən, -shən\ *n* : application of an electric shock in order to restore normal heartbeat

car·dio·ver·ter \ˌkär-dē-ō-ˌvər-tər\ *n* : a device for the administration of an electric shock in cardioversion

car·di·tis \kär-'dī-təs\ *n, pl* **car·dit·i·des** \-'di-tə-ˌdēz\ : inflammation of the heart muscle : MYOCARDITIS

-car·di·um \'kär-dē-əm\ *n comb form, pl* **-car·dia** \-ē-ə\ : heart ⟨epi*cardium*⟩

Car·di·zem \'kär-də-ˌzem\ *trademark* — used for a preparation of the hydrochloride of diltiazem

Car·du·ra \kär-'dùr-ə\ *trademark* — used for a preparation of the mesylate of doxazosin

care \'ker, 'kar\ *n* : responsibility for or attention to health, well-being, and safety — see ACUTE CARE, HEALTH CARE, INTENSIVE CARE, PRIMARY CARE, TERTIARY CARE — **care** *vb*

care·giv·er \-ˌgi-vər\ *n* : a person who provides direct care (as for children, elderly people, or the chronically ill) — **care·giv·ing** \-ˌgi-viŋ\ *n*

car·ies \'kar-ēz, 'ker-\ *n, pl* **caries** : a progressive destruction of bone or tooth; *esp* : tooth decay

ca·ri·na \kə-'rī-nə, -'rē-\ *n, pl* **carinas** *or* **ca·ri·nae** \'rī-ˌnē, -'rē-ˌnī\ : any of various keel-shaped anatomical structures, ridges, or processes

carinii — see PNEUMOCYSTIS CARINII PNEUMONIA

cario- *comb form* : caries ⟨*cario*genic⟩

car·io·gen·ic \ˌkar-ē-ō-'je-nik\ *adj* : producing or promoting the development of tooth decay ⟨~ foods⟩

car·io·stat·ic \-'sta-tik\ *adj* : tending to inhibit the formation of dental caries

car·i·ous \'kar-ē-əs, 'ker-\ *adj* : affected with caries ⟨~ teeth⟩

ca·ri·so·pro·dol \kə-ˌrī-sə-'prō-ˌdòl, -zə-, -ˌdōl\ *n* : a drug $C_{12}H_{24}N_2O_4$ related to meprobamate that is used to relax muscle and relieve pain

¹car·min·a·tive \kär-'mi-nə-tiv, 'kär-mə-ˌnā-\ *adj* : expelling gas from the stomach or intestines so as to relieve flatulence or abdominal pain or distension

²carminative *n* : a carminative agent

car·mus·tine \'kär-mə-ˌstēn\ *n* : a nitrosourea $C_5H_9Cl_2N_3O_2$ used as an antineoplastic drug (as in the treatment of brain tumors) — called also *BCNU*

car·ni·tine \'kär-nə-ˌtēn\ n : a quaternary ammonium compound $C_7H_{15}NO_3$ present esp. in muscle and involved in the transfer of fatty acids across mitochondrial membranes

car·o·ten·ae·mia *chiefly Brit var of* CAROTENEMIA

car·o·tene \'kar-ə-ˌtēn\ n : any of several orange or red hydrocarbon pigments (as $C_{40}H_{56}$) that occur in plants and in the fatty tissues of plant-eating animals and are convertible to vitamin A — see BETA-CAROTENE

car·o·ten·emia \ˌkar-ə-tə-'nē-mē-ə\ n : a yellowing of the skin resembling jaundice that is associated with increased levels of carotene in the blood

ca·rot·enoid \kə-'rät-ᵊn-ˌoid\ n : any of various usu. yellow to red pigments (as carotenes) found widely in plants and animals — **carotenoid** adj

caroticum — see GLOMUS CAROTICUM

ca·rot·id \kə-'rä-təd\ adj : of, situated near, or involving a carotid artery

carotid artery n : either of the two main arteries that supply blood to the head of which the left in humans arises from the arch of the aorta and the right by bifurcation of the brachiocephalic artery — called also *carotid;* see COMMON CAROTID ARTERY, EXTERNAL CAROTID ARTERY, INTERNAL CAROTID ARTERY

carotid body n : a small body of vascular tissue that adjoins the carotid sinus, functions as a chemoreceptor sensitive to change in the oxygen content of blood, and mediates reflex changes in respiratory activity — called also *carotid gland, glomus caroticum*

carotid canal n : the canal by which the internal carotid artery enters the skull — called also *carotid foramen*

carotid plexus n : a network of nerves of the sympathetic nervous system surrounding the internal carotid artery

carotid sinus n : a small but richly innervated arterial enlargement that is located near the point in the neck where the common carotid artery divides into the internal and the external carotid arteries and that functions in the regulation of heart rate and blood pressure

carp- *or* **carpo-** *comb form* **1** : carpus ⟨*carp*ectomy⟩ **2** : carpal and ⟨*carp*ometacarpal⟩

¹car·pal \'kär-pəl\ adj : relating to the carpus

²carpal n : a carpal element : CARPALE

car·pa·le \kär-'pa-(ˌ)lē, -'pä-, -'pä-\ n, pl **-lia** \-lē-ə\ : a carpal bone; esp : one of the distal series articulating with the metacarpals

carpal tunnel n : a passage between the flexor retinaculum of the hand and the carpal bones that is sometimes a site of compression of the median nerve

carpal tunnel syndrome n : a condition caused by compression of the median nerve in the carpal tunnel and characterized esp. by weakness, pain, and disturbances of sensation in the hand and fingers

car·pec·to·my \ˌkär-'pek-tə-mē\ n, pl **-mies** : excision of a carpal bone

carpi — see EXTENSOR CARPI RADIALIS BREVIS, EXTENSOR CARPI RADIALIS LONGUS, EXTENSOR CARPI ULNARIS, FLEXOR CARPI RADIALIS, FLEXOR CARPI ULNARIS

carpo- — see CARP-

car·po·meta·car·pal \ˌkär-pō-'me-tə-ˌkär-pəl\ adj : relating to, situated between, or joining a carpus and metacarpus ⟨a ∼ joint⟩

car·po·ped·al spasm \ˌkär-pə-'ped-ᵊl-, -'pēd-\ n : a spasmodic contraction of the muscles of the hands and feet or esp. of the wrists and ankles (as that occurring in alkalosis and tetany)

car·pus \'kär-pəs\ n, pl **car·pi** \-ˌpī, -ˌpē\ **1** : WRIST **2** : the group of bones supporting the wrist comprising in humans a proximal row which contains the scaphoid, lunate, triquetrum, and pisiform that articulate with the radius and a distal row which contains the trapezium, trapezoid, capitate, and hamate that articulate with the metacarpals

car·riage \'kar-ij\ n : the condition of harboring a pathogen within the body

car·ri·er \'kar-ē-ər\ n **1 a** : a person, animal, or plant that harbors and transmits the causative agent of an infectious disease; esp : one that carries the causative agent systemically but is asymptomatic or immune to it ⟨a ∼ of typhoid fever⟩ — compare RESERVOIR 2, VECTOR 1 **b** : an individual possessing a specified gene and capable of transmitting it to offspring but not expressing or only weakly expressing its phenotype; esp : one that is heterozygous for a recessive factor **2** : a vehicle serving esp. as a diluent (as for a drug)

Car·ri·ón's disease \ˌkar-ē-'ònz-\ n : BARTONELLOSIS

Carrión, Daniel A. (1850–1885), Peruvian medical student.

car·ry \'kar-ē\ vb **1** : to harbor (a pathogen) within the body **2** : to possess a specified gene; specif : to possess one copy of a specified recessive gene and be capable of transmitting it to offspring

car·sick \'kär-ˌsik\ adj : affected with motion sickness esp. in an automobile — **car sickness** n

car·ti·lage \'kärt-ᵊl-ij, 'kärt-lij\ n **1** : a usu. translucent somewhat elastic tissue that composes most of the skeleton of vertebrate embryos and except for a small number of structures (as some joints, respiratory passages, and the external ear) is replaced by bone during ossification in the higher vertebrates **2** : a part or structure composed of cartilage

car·ti·lag·i·nous \ˌkärt-ᵊl-ˈa-jə-nəs\ adj : composed of, relating to, or resembling cartilage

car·un·cle \ˈkar-ən-kəl, kə-ˈrəŋ-\ n : a small fleshy growth; specif : a reddish growth situated at the urethral meatus in women and causing pain and bleeding — see LACRIMAL CARUNCLE

ca·run·cu·la \kə-ˈrəŋ-kyə-lə\ n, pl **-lae** \-ˌlē, -ˌlī\ : CARUNCLE

cary- or **caryo-** — see KARY-

ca·san·thra·nol \kə-ˈsan-thrə-ˌnȯl\ n : a cathartic mixture of glycosides extracted from cascara sagrada — see PERI-COLACE

cas·cade \(ˌ)kas-ˈkād\ n : a molecular, biochemical, or physiological process occurring in a succession of stages each of which is closely related to or depends on the output of the previous stage ⟨an enzymatic ∼⟩ ⟨a ∼ of immunologic reactions⟩

cas·cara sa·gra·da \kas-ˈkar-ə-sə-ˈgräd-ə, -ˈkär-; ˈkas-kə-rə-\ n : the dried bark of a buckthorn (Rhamnus purshiana) of the Pacific coast of the U.S. that is used as a mild laxative — called also cascara

case \ˈkās\ n **1** : the circumstances and situation of a particular person or group **2** : an instance of disease or injury ⟨10 ∼s of pneumonia⟩ **b** : PATIENT 1

ca·se·ation \ˌkā-sē-ˈā-shən\ n : necrosis with conversion of damaged tissue into a soft cheesy substance — **ca·se·ate** \ˈkā-sē-ˌāt\ vb

case·book \ˈkās-ˌbuk\ n : a book containing medical records of illustrative cases that is used for reference and instruction

case history n : a record of an individual's personal or family history and environment for use in analysis or instructive illustration

ca·sein \kā-ˈsēn, ˈkā-sē-ən\ n : any of several phosphoproteins of milk

case·load \ˈkās-ˌlōd\ n : the number of cases handled (as by a clinic) in a particular period

caseosa — see VERNIX CASEOSA

ca·se·ous \ˈkā-sē-əs\ adj : marked by caseation

caseous lymphadenitis n : a chronic infectious disease of sheep and goats characterized by caseation of the lymph glands and occas. of parts of the lungs, liver, spleen, and kidneys that is caused by a bacterium of the genus Corynebacterium (C. pseudotuberculosis) — called also pseudotuberculosis

case·work \ˈkās-ˌwərk\ n : social work involving direct consideration of the problems, needs, and adjustments of the individual case (as a person or family in need of psychiatric aid) — **case·work·er** \-ˌwər-kər\ n

cas·sette also **ca·sette** \kə-ˈset, ka-\ n : a lightproof magazine for holding the intensifying screens and film in X-ray photography

cast \ˈkast\ n **1** : a slight strabismus : a rigid casing (as of fiberglass or of gauze impregnated with plaster of paris) used for immobilizing a usu. diseased or broken part **3** : a mass of plastic matter formed in cavities of diseased organs (as the kidneys) and discharged from the body

Cas·tel·la·ni's paint \ˌkas-tə-ˈlä-nēz-\ n : CARBOLFUCHSIN PAINT

Cas·tel·la·ni \ˌkas-tə-ˈlä-nē, Aldo (1878–1971), Italian physician.

cas·tor bean \ˈkas-tər-\ n : the very poisonous seed of the castor-oil plant; also : CASTOR-OIL PLANT

castor oil n : a pale viscous fatty oil from castor beans used esp. as a cathartic

castor–oil plant n : a tropical Old World herb (Ricinus communis) of the spurge family (Euphorbiaceae) widely grown as an ornamental or for its oil-rich castor beans that are a source of castor oil

¹cas·trate \ˈkas-ˌtrāt\ vb **cas·trat·ed; cas·trat·ing 1 a** : to deprive of the testes : GELD **b** : to deprive of the ovaries : SPAY **2** : to render impotent or deprive of vitality esp. by psychological means — **cas·trat·er** or **cas·tra·tor** \-ˈtrā-tər\ n — **cas·tra·tion** \kas-ˈtrā-shən\ n

²castrate n : a castrated individual

castration complex n : a child's fear or delusion of genital injury at the hands of the parent of the same sex as punishment for unconscious guilt over oedipal strivings; broadly : the often unconscious fear or feeling of bodily injury or loss of power at the hands of authority

ca·su·al·ty \ˈka-zhəl-tē, ˈka-zhə-wəl-\ n, pl **-ties 1** : a serious or fatal accident **2** : a military person lost through death, wounds, injury, sickness, internment, or capture or through being missing in action **3 a** : injury or death from accident **b** : one injured or killed (as by accident)

ca·su·is·tic \ˌka-zhə-ˈwis-tik\ adj : of or based on the study of actual cases or case histories

cat \ˈkat\ n, often attrib **1** : a carnivorous mammal (Felis catus) long domesticated and kept as a pet or for catching rats and mice **2** : any of a family (Felidae) of mammals including the domestic cat, lion, tiger, leopard, cougar, and their relatives

CAT abbr computed axial tomography; computerized axial tomography

cata- or **cat-** or **cath-** prefix : down ⟨catamnesis⟩ ⟨cataplexy⟩

ca·tab·o·lism \kə-ˈta-bə-ˌli-zəm\ n : destructive metabolism involving the release of energy and resulting in the breakdown of complex materials within the organism — compare ANABOLISM — **cat·a·bol·ic** \ˌka-tə-ˈbä-lik\ adj — **cat·a·bol·i·cal·ly** \-li-k(ə-)lē\ adv

ca·tab·o·lite \-ˌlīt\ *n* : a product of catabolism

ca·tab·o·lize \-ˌlīz\ *vb* **-lized; -liz·ing** : to subject to or undergo catabolism

cat·a·lase \'kat-ᵊl-ˌās, -ˌāz\ *n* : an enzyme that consists of a protein complex with hematin groups and catalyzes the decomposition of hydrogen peroxide into water and oxygen

cat·a·lep·sy \'kat-ᵊl-ˌep-sē\ *n, pl* **-sies** : a trancelike state of consciousness (as that occurring in catatonic schizophrenia) that is marked by a loss of voluntary motion and a fixed posture in which the limbs remain in whatever position they are placed — compare WAXY FLEXIBILITY

¹**cat·a·lep·tic** \ˌkat-ᵊl-'ep-tik\ *adj* : of, having the characteristics of, or affected with catalepsy ⟨a ~ state⟩

²**cataleptic** *n* : one affected with catalepsy

ca·tal·y·sis \kə-'ta-lə-səs\ *n, pl* **-y·ses** \-ˌsēz\ : a change and esp. increase in the rate of a chemical reaction induced by a catalyst — **cat·a·lyt·ic** \ˌkat-ᵊl-'it-ik\ *adj* — **cat·a·lyt·i·cal·ly** \-ti-k(ə-)lē\ *adv*

cat·a·lyst \'ka-tᵊl-əst\ *n* : a substance (as an enzyme) that enables a chemical reaction to proceed at a usu. faster rate or under different conditions (as at a lower temperature) than otherwise possible

cat·a·lyze \'kat-ᵊl-ˌīz\ *vb* **-lyzed; -lyz·ing** : to bring about the catalysis of (a chemical reaction) — **cat·a·lyz·er** *n*

cata·me·nia \ˌka-tə-'mē-nē-ə\ *n pl* : MENSES — **cata·me·ni·al** \-nē-əl\ *adj*

cat·am·ne·sis \ˌkat-ˌam-'nē-səs\ *n, pl* **-ne·ses** \-ˌsēz\ : the follow-up medical history of a patient — **cat·am·nes·tic** \-'nes-tik\ *adj*

cat·a·plasm \'ka-tə-ˌpla-zəm\ *n* : POULTICE

cat·a·plexy \'ka-tə-ˌplek-sē\ *n, pl* **-plex·ies** \-ˌsēz\ : sudden loss of muscle power with retention of clear consciousness following a strong emotional stimulus (as fright, anger, or shock)

cat·a·ract \'ka-tə-ˌrakt\ *n* : a clouding of the lens of the eye or its surrounding transparent membrane that obstructs the passage of light

cat·a·ract·ous \'ka-tə-ˌrak-təs\ *adj* : of, relating to, or affected with an eye cataract

ca·tarrh \kə-'tär\ *n* : inflammation of a mucous membrane in humans or animals; *esp* : one chronically affecting the human nose and air passages — **ca·tarrh·al** \-əl\ *adj*

catarrhal fever *n* : MALIGNANT CATARRHAL FEVER

cata·to·nia \ˌka-tə-'tō-nē-ə\ *n* : a marked psychomotor disturbance that may involve stupor or mutism, negativism, rigidity, purposeless excitement, echolalia, echopraxia, and inappropriate or bizarre posturing and is associated with various medical conditions (as schizophrenia and mood disorders)

¹**cata·ton·ic** \ˌka-tə-'tä-nik\ *adj* : of, relating to, marked by, or affected with catatonia ⟨~ schizophrenia⟩ — **cata·ton·i·cal·ly** \-ni-k(ə-)lē\ *adv*

²**catatonic** *n* : a catatonic person

catch·ment area \'kach-mənt-\ *n* : the geographical area served by an institution

cat cry syndrome *n* : CRI DU CHAT SYNDROME

cat distemper *n* : PANLEUKOPENIA

cat·e·chol·amine \ˌka-tə-'kō-lə-ˌmēn, -'kô-\ *n* : any of various amines (as epinephrine, norepinephrine, and dopamine) that function as hormones or neurotransmitters or both

cat·e·chol·amin·er·gic \-ˌkō-lə-mē-'nər-jik\ *adj* : involving, liberating, or mediated by catecholamine ⟨~ transmission in the nervous system⟩

cat fever *n* : PANLEUKOPENIA

cat flea *n* : a common flea of the genus *Ctenocephalides* (*C. felis*) that breeds chiefly on cats, dogs, and rats

cat·gut \'kat-ˌgət\ *n* : a tough cord made usu. from sheep intestines and used esp. for sutures in closing wounds

cath \'kath\ *vb* : to insert a catheter into : subject to catheterization

cath *abbr* **1** cathartic **2** catheter; catheterization

cath- — see CATA-

ca·thar·sis \kə-'thär-səs\ *n, pl* **ca·thar·ses** \-ˌsēz\ **1** : PURGATION **2** : elimination of a complex by bringing it to consciousness and affording it expression — compare ABREACTION

¹**ca·thar·tic** \kə-'thär-tik\ *adj* : of, relating to, or producing catharsis

²**cathartic** *n* : a cathartic medicine : PURGATIVE

ca·thect \kə-'thekt\ *vb* : to invest with mental or emotional energy

ca·thec·tic \kə-'thek-tik, ka-\ *adj* : of, relating to, or invested with mental or emotional energy

cath·e·ter \'ka-thə-tər, 'kath-tər\ *n* : a tubular medical device for insertion into canals, vessels, passageways, or body cavities for diagnostic or therapeutic purposes (as to permit injection or withdrawal of fluids or to keep a passage open)

cath·e·ter·i·za·tion \ˌka-thə-tə-rə-'zā-shən, ˌkath-tə-rə-\ *n* : the use of or insertion of a catheter (as in or into the bladder, trachea, or heart) — **cath·e·ter·ize** \'ka-thə-tə-ˌrīz, 'kath-tə-\ *vb*

cath·e·ter·ized *adj* : obtained by catheterization ⟨~ urine specimens⟩

ca·thex·is \kə-'thek-səs, ka-\ *n, pl* **ca·thex·es** \-ˌsēz\ **1** : investment of mental or emotional energy in a person, object, or idea **2** : libidinal energy that is either invested or being invested

cath·ode–ray oscilloscope \'ka-ˌthōd-\ *n* : OSCILLOSCOPE

cathode–ray tube *n* : a vacuum tube in which a beam of electrons is projected on a fluorescent screen to produce a luminous spot

cat·ion \'kat-ˌī-ən, 'ka-(ˌ)tī-ən\ *n* : the ion in an electrolyte that migrates to the cathode; *also* : a positively charged ion — **cat·ion·ic** \ˌkat-(ˌ)ī-'ä-nik, ˌka-(ˌ)tī-\ *adj* — **cat·ion·i·cal·ly** *adv*

cat louse *n* : a biting louse (*Felicola subrostratus* of the family Trichodectidae) common on cats esp. in warm regions

CAT scan \'kat-\ *n* : a sectional view of the body constructed by computed tomography — **CAT scanning** *n*

CAT scanner *n* : a medical instrument consisting of integrated X-ray and computing equipment and used for computed tomography

cat scratch disease *n* : an illness that is characterized by chills, slight fever, and swelling of the lymph glands and is caused by a gram-negative bacterium of the genus *Bartonella* (*B. henselae* syn. *Rochalimaea henselae*) transmitted esp. by a cat scratch — called also *cat scratch fever*

cat tapeworm *n* : a common tapeworm of the genus *Taenia* (*T. taeniaeformis*) of cats who ingest cysticercus-infected livers of various rodents

cattle grub *n* : either of two warble flies of the genus *Hypoderma* esp. in the larval stage: **a** : COMMON CATTLE GRUB **b** : NORTHERN CATTLE GRUB

cattle louse *n* : a louse infesting cattle — see LONG-NOSED CATTLE LOUSE, SHORT-NOSED CATTLE LOUSE

cattle tick *n* : either of two ixodid ticks of the genus *Boophilus* (*B. annulatus* and *B. microplus*) that infest cattle and transmit the protozoan that causes Texas fever

cau·dad \'kȯ-ˌdad\ *adv* : toward the tail or posterior end

cau·da equi·na \ˌkau̇-də-ē-'kwē-nə, 'kȯ-də-, -'kwī-\ *n, pl* **caudae equi·nae** \ˌkau̇-ˌdī-ē-'kwē-ˌnī, 'kȯ-ˌdē-ē-'kwī-ˌnē\ : the roots of the upper sacral nerves that extend beyond the termination of the spinal cord at the first lumbar vertebra in the form of a bundle of filaments within the spinal canal resembling a horse's tail

cau·dal \'kȯd-ᵊl\ *adj* 1 : of, relating to, or being a tail 2 : situated in or directed toward the hind part of the body — **cau·dal·ly** *adv*

caudal anesthesia *n* : loss of pain sensation below the umbilicus produced by injection of an anesthetic into the caudal portion of the spinal canal — called also *caudal analgesia*

caudate lobe \'kȯ-ˌdāt-\ *n* : a lobe of the liver bounded on the right by the inferior vena cava, on the left by the fissure of the ductus venosus, and connected with the right lobe by a narrow prolongation

caudate nucleus *n* : the one of the four basal ganglia in each cerebral hemisphere that comprises a mass of gray matter in the corpus striatum, forms part of the floor of the lateral ventricle, and is separated from the lentiform nucleus by the internal capsule — called also *caudate*

caul \'kȯl\ *n* 1 : GREATER OMENTUM 2 : the inner embryonic membrane of higher vertebrates esp. when covering the head at birth

cauliflower ear *n* : an ear deformed from injury and excessive growth of reparative tissue

cau·sal·gia \kȯ-'zal-jə, -'sal-, -jē-ə\ *n* : a constant usu. burning pain resulting from injury to a peripheral nerve — **cau·sal·gic** \-jik\ *adj*

¹caus·tic \'kȯ-stik\ *adj* : capable of destroying or eating away organic tissue and esp. animal tissue by chemical action

²caustic *n* : a caustic agent: as **a** : a substance that burns or destroys organic tissue by chemical action : ESCHAROTIC **b** : a strong corrosive alkali (as sodium hydroxide)

cau·ter·ize \'kȯ-tə-ˌrīz\ *vb* **-ized; -iz·ing** : to sear with a cautery or caustic — **cau·ter·i·za·tion** \ˌkȯ-tə-rə-'zā-shən\ *n*

cau·tery \'kȯ-tə-rē\ *n, pl* **-ter·ies** 1 : the act or effect of cauterizing : CAUTERIZATION 2 : an agent (as a hot iron or caustic) used to burn, sear, or destroy tissue

¹ca·va \'kā-və, 'kä-\ *n, pl* **ca·vae** \'kä-ˌvē, -ˌvī; 'kä-ˌvē\ : VENA CAVA — **ca·val** \-vəl\ *adj*

²cava *pl of* CAVUM

cavernosum, cavernosa — see CORPUS CAVERNOSUM

cav·ern·ous \'ka-vər-nəs\ *adj* 1 : having caverns or cavities 2 *of tissue* : composed largely of vascular sinuses and capable of dilating with blood to bring about the erection of a body part

cavernous sinus *n* : either of a pair of large venous sinuses situated in a groove at the side of the body of the sphenoid bone in the cranial cavity and opening behind into the petrosal sinuses

cav·i·tary \'ka-və-ˌter-ē\ *adj* : of, relating to, or characterized by bodily cavitation (< lesions)

cav·i·ta·tion \ˌka-və-'tā-shən\ *n* 1 : the formation of cavities in an organ or tissue esp. in disease 2 : a cavity formed by cavitation — **cav·i·tate** \'ka-və-ˌtāt\ *vb*

cav·i·ty \'ka-və-tē\ *n, pl* **-ties** 1 : an unfilled space within a mass 2 : an area of decay in a tooth : CARIES

ca·vum \'kä-vəm, 'kā-\ *n, pl* **ca·va** \-və\ : an anatomical recess or hollow

cavus — see PES CAVUS

Cb *symbol* columbium

CB *abbr* [Latin *Chirurgiae Baccalaureus*] bachelor of surgery

CBC *abbr* complete blood count

CBW *abbr* chemical and biological warfare

cc *abbr* cubic centimeter

CC *abbr* **1** chief complaint **2** current complaint

CCK *abbr* cholecystokinin

CCU *abbr* **1** cardiac care unit **2** coronary care unit **3** critical care unit

Cd *symbol* cadmium

CD *abbr* cluster of differentiation — used with an integer to denote any of numerous antigenic proteins on the surface of leukocytes (as T cells or B cells); see CD8, CD4

CDC *abbr* Centers for Disease Control and Prevention

CD8 \ˌsē-(ˌ)dē-'āt\ *n, often attrib* : a glycoprotein found esp. on the surface of cytotoxic T cells that usu. functions to facilitate recognition by cytotoxic T cell receptors of antigens complexed with molecules of a class that are found on the surface of most nucleated cells and are the product of genes of the major histocompatibility complex

CD4 \ˌsē-(ˌ)dē-'fōr\ *n, often attrib* : a large glycoprotein that is found esp. on the surface of helper T cells, that is the receptor for HIV, and that usu. functions to facilitate recognition by helper T cells of antigens complexed with molecules of a class that are found on the surface of antigen‑presenting cells and are the product of genes of the major histocompatibility complex

cDNA \ˌsē-ˌdē-(ˌ)en-'ā\ *n* : a DNA that is complementary to a given RNA which serves as a template for synthesis of the DNA in the presence of a reverse transcriptase — called also **complementary DNA**

Ce *symbol* cerium

CEA *abbr* carcinoembryonic antigen

cec- *or* **ceci-** *or* **ceco-** *comb form* : cecum ⟨*cecitis*⟩ ⟨*cecostomy*⟩

ce·cal \'sē-kəl\ *adj* : of or like a cecum — **ce·cal·ly** *adv*

ce·ci·tis \sē-'sīt-əs\ *n* : inflammation of the cecum

Ce·clor \'sē-klȯr\ *trademark* — used for a preparation of cefaclor

ce·co·pexy \'sē-kə-ˌpek-sē\ *n, pl* **-pex·ies** : a surgical operation to fix the cecum to the abdominal wall

ce·cos·to·my \sē-'käs-tə-mē\ *n, pl* **-mies** : the surgical formation of an opening into the cecum to serve as an artificial anus

ce·cum \'sē-kəm\ *n, pl* **ce·ca** \-kə\ : the blind pouch at the beginning of the large intestine into which the ileum opens from one side and which is continuous with the colon

cef·a·clor \'se-fə-klȯr\ *n* : a semisynthetic cephalosporin antibiotic $C_{15}H_{14}ClN_3O_4S \cdot H_2O$ that is administered orally to treat bacterial infections of the skin and of the respiratory and urinary tracts — see CECLOR

ce·faz·o·lin \si-'fa-zə-lən\ *n* : a semisynthetic cephalosporin antibiotic administered parenterally in the form of its sodium salt $C_{14}H_{13}N_8NaO_4S_3$

ce·fix·ime \ˌse-'fiks-ˌēm\ *n* : a semisynthetic cephalosporin antibiotic $C_{16}H_{15}N_5O_7S_2$ administered orally

ce·fo·tax·ime \ˌse-fə-'tak-ˌsēm\ *n* : a semisynthetic cephalosporin antibiotic that is administered parenterally in the form of its sodium salt $C_{16}H_{16}$‑ $N_5NaO_7S_2$

ce·fox·i·tin \si-'fäk-sə-tən\ *n* : a semisynthetic cephamycin antibiotic administered parenterally in the form of its sodium salt $C_{16}H_{16}N_3NaO_7S_2$

cef·taz·i·dime \sef-'taz-ə-ˌdēm\ *n* : a semisynthetic cephalosporin antibiotic that is administered parenterally in the form of its hydrate $C_{22}H_{22}N_6O_7S_2 \cdot 5H_2O$

Cef·tin \'sef-tin\ *trademark* — used for a preparation of an ester of cefuroxime

cef·tri·ax·one \ˌsef-ˌtrī-'ak-ˌsōn\ *n* : semisynthetic cephalosporin antibiotic that is administered parenterally in the form of its hydrated disodium salt $C_{18}H_{16}N_8Na_2O_7S_3 \cdot 3\frac{1}{2}H_2O$

ce·fur·ox·ime \si-'fyu̇r-ə-ˌzēm\ *n* : a semisynthetic cephalosporin antibiotic that is administered parenterally in the form of its sodium salt $C_{16}H_{15}N_4NaO_8S$ or orally as an ester derivative $C_{20}H_{22}N_4O_{10}S$ — see CEFTIN

-cele *n comb form* : tumor : hernia ⟨*cystocele*⟩

-cele — see -COELE

Cel·e·brex \'se-lə-ˌbreks\ *trademark* — used for a preparation of celecoxib

cel·e·cox·ib \ˌse-lə-'käk-sib\ *n* : an NSAID $C_{17}H_{14}F_3N_3O_2S$ that is a COX-2 inhibitor administered orally esp. to relieve the pain and inflammation of osteoarthritis and rheumatoid arthritis — see CELEBREX

Ce·lexa \sə-'lek-sə\ *trademark* — used for a preparation of the hydrobromide of citalopram

celi- *or* **celio-** *comb form* : belly : abdomen ⟨*celioscopy*⟩ ⟨*celiotomy*⟩

¹**ce·li·ac** \'sē-lē-ˌak\ *adj* **1** : of or relating to the abdominal cavity **2** : belonging to or prescribed for celiac disease ⟨the ∼ syndrome⟩ ⟨a ∼ diet⟩

²**celiac** *n* : a celiac part (as a nerve)

celiac artery *n* : a short thick artery arising from the aorta just below the diaphragm and dividing almost immediately into the gastric, hepatic, and splenic arteries — called also *celiac axis, truncus celiacus*

celiac disease *n* : a chronic hereditary intestinal disorder in which an inability to absorb the gliadin portion of gluten results in the gliadin triggering an immune response that damages the intestinal mucosa — called also *celiac sprue, gluten-sensitive enteropathy, nontropical sprue, sprue*

celiac ganglion *n* : either of a pair of collateral sympathetic ganglia that are the largest of the autonomic nervous system and lie one on each side of the celiac artery near the adrenal gland on the same side

celiac plexus *n* : a nerve plexus that is situated in the abdomen behind the stomach and in front of the aorta and the crura of the diaphragm, surrounds the celiac artery and the root of the superior mesenteric artery, contains several ganglia of which the most important are the celiac ganglia, and distributes nerve fibers to all the abdominal viscera — called also *solar plexus*

celiac sprue *n* : CELIAC DISEASE

celiacus — see TRUNCUS CELIACUS

ce·li·os·co·py \ˌsē-lē-'äs-kə-pē\ *n, pl* **-pies** : examination of the abdominal cavity by surgical insertion of an endoscope through the abdominal wall

ce·li·ot·o·my \ˌsē-lē-'ä-tə-mē\ *n, pl* **-mies** : surgical incision of the abdomen

cell \'sel\ *n* : a small usu. microscopic mass of protoplasm bounded externally by a semipermeable membrane, usu. including one or more nuclei and various nonliving products, capable alone or interacting with other cells of performing all the fundamental functions of life, and forming the smallest structural unit of living matter capable of functioning independently

cell body *n* : the nucleus-containing central part of a neuron exclusive of its axons and dendrites that is the major structural element of the gray matter of the brain and spinal cord, the ganglia, and the retina — called also *perikaryon, soma*

cell count *n* : a count of cells esp. of the blood or other body fluid in a standard volume (as a cubic millimeter)

cell cycle *n* : the complete series of events from one cell division to the next — see G₁ PHASE, G₂ PHASE, M PHASE, S PHASE

cell division *n* : the process by which cells multiply involving both nuclear and cytoplasmic division — compare MEIOSIS, MITOSIS

celled \'seld\ *adj* : having (such or so many) cells — used in combination ⟨single-*celled* organisms⟩

cell line *n* : a cell culture selected for uniformity from a cell population derived from a usu. homogeneous tissue source (as an organ) ⟨a *cell line* derived from a malignant tumor⟩

cell-me·di·at·ed \'sel-'mē-dē-ˌā-təd\ *adj* : relating to or being the part of immunity or the immune response that is mediated primarily by T cells and esp. cytotoxic T cells rather than by antibodies secreted by B cells ⟨∼ immunity⟩ — compare HUMORAL 2

cell membrane *n* **1** : a membrane of a cell; *esp* : PLASMA MEMBRANE **2** : CELL WALL

cell of Ley·dig \-'lī-dig\ *n* : LEYDIG CELL

cell sap *n* **1** : the liquid contents of a plant cell vacuole **2** : CYTOSOL

cell theory *n* : a theory in biology that includes one or both of the statements that the cell is the fundamental structural and functional unit of living matter and that the organism is composed of autonomous cells with its properties being the sum of those of its cells

cel·lu·lar \'sel-yə-lər\ *adj* **1** : of, relating to, or consisting of cells **2** : CELL-MEDIATED ⟨∼ immunity⟩ — **cel·lu·lar·i·ty** \ˌsel-yə-'lar-ə-tē\ *n*

cellular respiration *n* : any of various energy-yielding oxidative reactions in living matter that typically involve transfer of oxygen and production of carbon dioxide and water as end products

cel·lu·lite \'sel-yə-ˌlīt, -ˌlēt\ *n* : deposits of subcutaneous fat within fibrous connective tissue (as in the thighs, hips, and buttocks) that give a puckered and dimpled appearance to the skin surface

cel·lu·li·tis \ˌsel-yə-'lī-təs\ *n* : diffuse and esp. subcutaneous inflammation of connective tissue

cel·lu·lose \'sel-yə-ˌlōs, -ˌlōz\ *n* : a polysaccharide ($C_6H_{10}O_5)_x$ of glucose units that constitutes the chief part of the cell walls of plants — **cel·lu·los·ic** \ˌsel-yə-'lō-sik, -zik\ *adj*

cellulose acetate phthal·ate \-'ta-ˌlāt\ *n* : a derivative of cellulose used as a coating for enteric tablets

cell wall *n* : the usu. rigid nonliving permeable wall that surrounds the plasma membrane and encloses and supports the cells of most plants, bacteria, fungi, and algae

Cel·si·us \'sel-sē-əs, -shəs\ *adj* : relating to or having a scale for measuring temperature on which the interval between the triple point and the boiling point of water is divided into 99.99 degrees with 0.01° being the triple point and 100.00° the boiling point — abbr. *C*; compare CENTIGRADE

Celsius, Anders (1701–1744), Swedish astronomer.

ce·ment \si-'ment\ *n* **1** : CEMENTUM **2** : a plastic composition made esp. of zinc or silica for filling dental cavities

ce·men·ta·tion \ˌsē-ˌmen-'tā-shən\ *n* : the act or process of attaching (as a dental restoration to a natural tooth) by means of cement

ce·men·ti·cle \si-'men-ti-kəl\ *n* : a calcified body formed in the periodontal ligament of a tooth

ce·men·to·enam·el \si-ˌmen-tō-i-'na-məl\ *adj* : of, relating to, or joining the cementum and enamel of a tooth

ce·men·to·ma \ˌsē-ˌmen-'tō-mə\ *n, pl* **-mas** *also* **-ma·ta** \-mə-tə\ : a tumor resembling cementum in structure

ce·men·tum \si-ˈmen-təm\ n : a specialized external bony layer covering the dentin of the part of a tooth normally within the gum — called also *cement*; compare DENTIN, ENAMEL

cen·sor \ˈsen-sər\ n : a hypothetical psychic agency that represses unacceptable notions before they reach consciousness — **cen·so·ri·al** \sen-ˈsōr-ē-əl\ adj

cen·sor·ship \ˈsen-sər-ˌship\ n : exclusion from consciousness by the psychic censor

cen·ter \ˈsen-tər\ n : a group of nerve cells having a common function — called also *nerve center*

cen·te·sis \sen-ˈtē-səs\ n, pl **cen·te·ses** \-ˌsēz\ : surgical puncture (as of a tumor or membrane) — usu. used in compounds ⟨para*centesis*⟩

cen·ti·grade \ˈsen-tə-ˌgrād, ˈsän-\ adj : relating to, conforming to, or having a thermometer scale on which the interval between the freezing and boiling points of water is divided into 100 degrees with 0° representing the freezing point and 100° the boiling point ⟨10° ∼⟩ — abbr. C; compare CELSIUS

cen·ti·gram \-ˌgram\ n : a unit of mass and weight equal to ¹/₁₀₀ gram

cen·ti·li·ter \-ˌlē-tər\ n : a unit of liquid capacity equal to ¹/₁₀₀ liter

cen·ti·me·ter \-ˌmē-tər\ n : a unit of length equal to ¹/₁₀₀ meter

centimeter–gram–second adj : CGS

cen·ti·pede \ˈsen-tə-ˌpēd\ n : any of a class (Chilopoda) of long flattened many-segmented predaceous arthropods with each segment bearing one pair of legs of which the foremost pair is modified into poison fangs

centra pl of CENTRUM

cen·tral \ˈsen-trəl\ adj **1** : of or concerning the centrum of a vertebra **2 a** : of, relating to, or comprising the brain and spinal cord **b** : originating within or caused by factors originating in the central nervous system ⟨∼ precocious puberty⟩ **3** : affecting or involving the trunk of the body and esp. the abdomen ⟨∼ adiposity⟩ — **cen·tral·ly** adv

central artery n : a branch of the ophthalmic artery or the lacrimal artery that enters the substance of the optic nerve and supplies the nerve

central artery of the retina n : a branch of the ophthalmic artery that passes to the retina in the middle of the optic nerve and branches to form the arterioles of the retina — called also *central retinal artery*

central auditory processing disorder n : a disorder that is marked by a deficit in the way the brain receives, differentiates, analyzes, and interprets auditory information (as speech) and that is not attributable to impairments in peripheral hearing or intellect

central canal n : a minute canal running through the gray matter of the whole length of the spinal cord and continuous anteriorly with the ventricles of the brain

central deafness n : hearing loss or impairment resulting from defects in the central nervous system (as in the auditory cortex) rather than in the ear itself or the auditory nerve — compare CONDUCTION DEAFNESS, NERVE DEAFNESS

central diabetes insipidus n : diabetes insipidus caused by insufficient production of vasopressin and resulting from damage to the pituitary gland or hypothalamus

centralis — see FOVEA CENTRALIS

central line n : an IV line that is inserted into a large vein (as the superior vena cava) typically in the neck or near the heart for therapeutic or diagnostic purposes

central lobe n : INSULA

central nervous system n : the part of the nervous system which in vertebrates consists of the brain and spinal cord, to which sensory impulses are transmitted and from which motor impulses pass out, and which supervises and coordinates the activity of the entire nervous system — compare AUTONOMIC NERVOUS SYSTEM, PERIPHERAL NERVOUS SYSTEM

central pontine myelinolysis n : demyelination that occurs in the pons and is associated with malnutrition, alcoholism, liver disease, or hyponatremia

central retinal artery n : CENTRAL ARTERY OF THE RETINA

central retinal vein n : CENTRAL VEIN OF THE RETINA

central sulcus n : the sulcus separating the frontal lobe of the cerebral cortex from the parietal lobe — called also *fissure of Rolando*, *Rolandic fissure*

central tendon n : a 3-lobed aponeurosis located near the central portion of the diaphragm caudal to the pericardium and composed of intersecting planes of collagenous fibers

central vein n : any of the veins in the lobules of the liver that occur one in each lobule running from the apex to the base, receive blood from the sinusoids, and empty into the sublobular veins — called also *intralobular vein*

central vein of the retina n : a vein that is formed by union of the veins draining the retina, passes with the central artery of the retina in the optic nerve, and empties into the superior ophthalmic vein — called also *central retinal vein*

central venous pressure n : the venous pressure of the right atrium of the heart obtained by inserting a catheter into the median cubital vein and advancing it to the right atrium through the superior vena cava — abbr. CVP

cen·tre *chiefly Brit var of* CENTER

cen·tric \'sen-trik\ *adj* **1** : of or relating to a nerve center **2** *of dental occlusion* : involving spatial relationships such that all teeth of both jaws meet in a normal manner and forces exerted by the lower on the upper jaw are perfectly distributed in the dental arch

cen·trif·u·gal \sen-'tri-fyə-gəl, -fi-\ *adj* : passing outward (as from a nerve center to a muscle or gland) : EFFERENT — **cen·trif·u·gal·ly** *adv*

cen·tri·fu·ga·tion \sen-trə-fyü-'gā-shən\ *n* : the process of centrifuging

¹cen·tri·fuge \'sen-trə-ˌfyüj\ *n* : a machine using centrifugal force for separating substances of different densities, for removing moisture, or for simulating gravitational effects

²centrifuge *vb* **-fuged; -fug·ing** : to subject to centrifugal action esp. in a centrifuge

cen·tri·lob·u·lar \ˌsen-trə-'lä-byə-lər\ *adj* : relating to or affecting the center of a lobule ⟨∼ necrosis in the liver⟩; *also* : affecting the central parts of the lobules containing clusters of branching functional and anatomical units of the lung ⟨∼ emphysema⟩

cen·tri·ole \'sen-trē-ˌōl\ *n* : one of a pair of cellular organelles that occur esp. in animals, are adjacent to the nucleus, function in the formation of the spindle apparatus during cell division, and consist of a cylinder with nine microtubules arranged peripherally in a circle

cen·trip·e·tal \sen-'tri-pət-əl\ *adj* : passing inward (as from a sense organ to the brain or spinal cord) : AFFERENT — **cen·trip·e·tal·ly** *adv*

cen·tro·mere \'sen-trə-ˌmir\ *n* : the point or region on a chromosome to which the spindle attaches during mitosis and meiosis — called also *kinetochore* — **cen·tro·mer·ic** \ˌsen-trə-'mer-ik, -'mir-\ *adj*

cen·tro·some \'sen-trə-ˌsōm\ *n* : the centriole-containing region of clear cytoplasm adjacent to the cell nucleus

cen·trum \'sen-trəm\ *n, pl* **centrums** *or* **cen·tra** \-trə\ **1** : the center esp. of an anatomical part **2** : the body of a vertebra ventral to the neural arch

Cen·tru·roi·des \ˌsen-trə-'rói-(ˌ)dēz\ *n* : a genus of scorpions containing the only U.S. forms dangerous to humans

cephal- *or* **cephalo-** *comb form* **1** : head ⟨*cephal*algia⟩ ⟨*cephalo*metry⟩ **2** : cephalic and ⟨*cephalo*pelvic⟩

ceph·a·lad \'se-fə-ˌlad\ *adv* : toward the head or anterior end of the body

ceph·a·lal·gia \ˌse-fə-'lal-jə, -jē-ə\ *n* : HEADACHE

ceph·a·lex·in \ˌse-fə-'lek-sən\ *n* : a semisynthetic cephalosporin $C_{16}H_{17}N_3O_4S$ with a spectrum of antibiotic activity similar to the penicillins that is often administered in the form of its hydrochloride $C_{16}H_{17}N_3O_4S·HCl$

ce·phal·gia \se-'fal-jə, -jē-ə\ *n* : HEADACHE

ceph·al·he·ma·to·ma \ˌse-fəl-ˌhē-mə-'tō-mə\ *n, pl* **-mas** *also* **-ma·ta** \-mə-tə\ : a usu. benign swelling formed from a hemorrhage beneath the periosteum of the skull and occurring esp. over one or both of the parietal bones in newborn infants as a result of trauma sustained during delivery

-cephali *pl of* -CEPHALUS

ce·phal·ic \sə-'fa-lik\ *adj* **1** : of or relating to the head **2** : directed toward or situated on or in or near the head — **ce·phal·i·cal·ly** \-li-k(ə-)lē\ *adv*

cephalic flexure *n* : the middle of the three anterior flexures of an embryo in which the front part of the brain bends downward in an angle of 90 degrees

cephalic index *n* : the ratio multiplied by 100 of the maximum breadth of the head to its maximum length — compare CRANIAL INDEX

cephalic vein *n* : any of various superficial veins of the arm; *specif* : a large vein of the upper arm lying along the outer edge of the biceps muscle and emptying into the axillary vein

ceph·a·lin \'ke-fə-lən, 'se-\ *n* : PHOSPHATIDYLETHANOLAMINE

cephalo- — see CEPHAL-

ceph·a·lo·cau·dal \ˌse-fə-lō-'kòd-əl\ *adj* : proceeding or occurring in the long axis of the body esp. in the direction from head to tail — **ceph·a·lo·cau·dal·ly** *adv*

ceph·a·lom·e·ter \ˌse-fə-'lä-mə-tər\ *n* : an instrument for measuring the head

ceph·a·lom·e·try \ˌse-fə-'lä-mə-trē\ *n, pl* **-tries** : the science of measuring the head in living individuals — **ceph·a·lo·met·ric** \ˌse-fə-lō-'me-trik\ *adj*

ceph·a·lo·pel·vic disproportion \ˌse-fə-lō-'pel-vik-\ *n* : a condition in which a maternal pelvis is small in relation to the size of the fetal head

ceph·a·lor·i·dine \ˌse-fə-'lòr-ə-ˌdēn, -'lär-\ *n* : a semisynthetic broad-spectrum antibiotic $C_{19}H_{17}N_3O_4S_2$ derived from cephalosporin

ceph·a·lo·spo·rin \ˌse-fə-lə-'spòr-ən\ *n* : any of several beta-lactam antibiotics produced by an imperfect fungus (genus *Acremonium*) or made semisynthetically

ceph·a·lo·thin \'se-fə-lə-(ˌ)thin\ *n* : a semisynthetic broad-spectrum antibiotic $C_{16}H_{15}N_2NaO_6S_2$ that is an analog of a cephalosporin and is effective against penicillin-resistant staphylococci

ceph·a·lo·tho·ra·cop·a·gus \ˌse-fə-lō-ˌthòr-ə-'kä-pə-gəs\ *n, pl* **-a·gi** \-ˌgī, -ˌgē\ : teratological twin fetuses joined at the head, neck, and thorax

-cephalus *n comb form, pl* **-cephali** : cephalic abnormality (of a specified type) ⟨hydro*cephalus*⟩

ceph·a·my·cin \ˌse-fə-'mī-sᵊn\ *n* : any of several beta-lactam antibiotics produced by various bacteria of the genus *Streptomyces*

cer·amide \'sir-ə-ˌmīd\ *n* : any of a group of lipids formed by linking a fatty acid to sphingosine and found widely but in small amounts in plant and animal tissue

cer·amide·tri·hexo·si·dase \ˌsir-ə-ˌmīd-ˌtrī-ˌhek-sə-'sī-ˌdās, -ˌdāz\ *n* : an enzyme that breaks down ceramide-trihexoside and is deficient in individuals affected with Fabry's disease

cer·amide·tri·hexo·side \-(ˌ)trī-'hek-sə-ˌsīd\ *n* : a lipid that accumulates in body tissues of individuals affected with Fabry's disease

ce·rate \'sir-ˌāt\ *n* : an unctuous preparation for external use consisting of wax or resin mixed with oil, lard, and medicinal ingredients

cer·a·to·hy·al \ˌser-ə-(ˌ)tō-'hī-əl\ *or* **cer·a·to·hy·oid** \-'hī-ˌoid\ *n* : the smaller inner projection of the two lateral projections on each side of the human hyoid bone — called also *lesser cornu;* compare THYROHYAL

cer·car·ia \(ˌ)sər-'kar-ē-ə, -'ker-\ *n, pl* **-i·ae** \-ē-ˌē\ : a usu. tadpole-shaped larval trematode worm that develops in a molluscan host from a redia — **cer·car·i·al** \-əl\ *adj*

cer·clage \ser-'kläzh, (ˌ)sər-\ *n* : any of several procedures for increasing tissue resistance in a functionally incompetent uterine cervix that usu. involve reinforcement with an inert substance esp. in the form of sutures near the internal opening

ce·rea flex·i·bil·i·tas \ˌsir-ē-ə-ˌflek-sə-'bi-lə-ˌtas, -ˌtäs\ *n* : the capacity (as in catalepsy) to maintain the limbs or other bodily parts in whatever position they have been placed

cerebell- *or* **cerebelli-** *or* **cerebello-** *comb form* : cerebellum ⟨*cerebell*itis⟩

cerebella *pl of* CEREBELLUM

cer·e·bel·lar \ˌser-ə-'be-lər\ *adj* 1 : of, relating to, or affecting the cerebellum ⟨∼ neurons⟩ 2 : caused by disease of the cerebellum ⟨∼ ataxia⟩

cerebellar artery *n* : any of several branches of the basilar and vertebral arteries that supply the cerebellum

cerebellaris — see PEDUNCULUS CEREBELLARIS INFERIOR, PEDUNCULUS CEREBELLARIS MEDIUS, PEDUNCULUS CEREBELLARIS SUPERIOR

cerebellar peduncle *n* : any of three large bands of nerve fibers that join each hemisphere of the cerebellum with the parts of the brain below and in front: **a** : one connecting the cerebellum with the midbrain — called also *brachium conjunctivum, pedunculus cerebellaris superior, superior cerebellar peduncle* **b** : one connecting the cerebellum with the pons — called also *brachium pontis, middle cerebellar peduncle, middle peduncle, pedunculus cerebellaris medius* **c** : one that connects the cerebellum with the medulla oblongata and the spinal cord — called also *inferior cere-*

bellar peduncle, pedunculus cerebellaris inferior, restiform body

cerebelli — see FALX CEREBELLI, TENTORIUM CEREBELLI

cer·e·bel·li·tis \ˌser-ə-bə-'lī-təs, -be-\ *n* : inflammation of the cerebellum

cer·e·bel·lo·pon·tine angle \ˌser-ə-ˌbe-lō-ˌpän-ˌtēn-, -ˌtīn-\ *n* : a region of the brain at the junction of the pons and cerebellum that is a frequent site of tumor formation

cer·e·bel·lum \ˌser-ə-'be-ləm\ *n, pl* **-bellums** *or* **-bel·la** \-lə\ : a large dorsally projecting part of the brain concerned esp. with the coordination of muscles and the maintenance of bodily equilibrium, situated between the brain stem and the back of the cerebrum and formed in humans of two lateral lobes and a median lobe

cerebr- *or* **cerebro-** *comb form* 1 : brain : cerebrum ⟨*cerebr*ation⟩ 2 : cerebral and ⟨*cerebro*spinal⟩

cerebra *pl of* CEREBRUM

ce·re·bral \sə-'rē-brəl, 'ser-ə-\ *adj* 1 : of or relating to the brain or the intellect 2 : of, relating to, or being the cerebrum ⟨∼ blood flow⟩

cerebral accident *n* : STROKE

cerebral aqueduct *n* : AQUEDUCT OF SYLVIUS

cerebral artery *n* : any of the arteries supplying the cerebral cortex: **a** : an artery that arises from the internal carotid artery, forms the anterior portion of the circle of Willis where it is linked to the artery on the opposite side by the anterior communicating artery, and passes on to supply the medial surfaces of the cerebrum — called also *anterior cerebral artery* **b** : an artery that arises from the internal carotid artery, passes along the lateral fissure, and supplies the lateral surfaces of the cerebral cortex — called also *middle cerebral artery* **c** : an artery that arises by the terminal forking of the basilar artery where it forms the posterior portion of the circle of Willis and passes on to supply the lower surfaces of the temporal and occipital lobes — called also *posterior cerebral artery*

cerebral cortex *n* : the convoluted surface layer of gray matter of the cerebrum that functions chiefly in coordination of sensory and motor information — called also *pallium;* see NEOCORTEX

cerebral dominance *n* : dominance in development and functioning of one of the cerebral hemispheres

cerebral edema *n* : the accumulation of fluid in and resultant swelling of the brain (as that caused by trauma, a tumor, lack of oxygen at high altitudes, or exposure to a toxin)

cerebral hemisphere *n* : either of the two hollow convoluted lateral halves of the cerebrum

cerebral hemorrhage n : bleeding from a ruptured blood vessel in the brain and esp. in the cerebrum

cerebral palsy n : a disability resulting from damage to the brain before, during, or shortly after birth and outwardly manifested by muscular incoordination and speech disturbances — see ATAXIC CEREBRAL PALSY, ATHETOID CEREBRAL PALSY, SPASTIC CEREBRAL PALSY — **cerebral palsied** adj

cerebral peduncle n : either of two large bundles of nerve fibers passing from the pons forward and outward to form the main connection between the cerebral hemispheres and the spinal cord

cerebral vein n : any of various veins that drain the surface and inner tissues of the cerebral hemispheres — see GALEN'S VEIN, GREAT CEREBRAL VEIN

cer·e·brate \'ser-ə-ˌbrāt\ vb **-brat·ed; -brat·ing** : to use the mind — **cer·e·bra·tion** \ˌser-ə-'brā-shən\ n

cerebri — see CRURA CEREBRI, FALX CEREBRI, HYPOPHYSIS CEREBRI, PSEUDOTUMOR CEREBRI

cerebro- — see CEREBR-

ce·re·bro·side \sə-'rē-brə-ˌsīd, 'ser-ə-\ n : any of various lipids composed of ceramide and a monosaccharide and found esp. in the myelin sheath of nerves

ce·re·bro·spi·nal \sə-ˌrē-brō-'spīn-ᵊl, ˌser-ə-\ adj : of or relating to the brain and spinal cord or to these together with the cranial and spinal nerves that innervate voluntary muscles

cerebrospinal fluid n : a liquid that is comparable to serum but contains less dissolved material, that is secreted from the blood into the lateral ventricles of the brain, and that serves chiefly to maintain uniform pressure within the brain and spinal cord — called also spinal fluid

cerebrospinal meningitis n : inflammation of the meninges of both brain and spinal cord; specif : an infectious epidemic and often fatal meningitis caused by the meningococcus — called also cerebrospinal fever

ce·re·bro·vas·cu·lar \sə-ˌrē-brō-'vas-kyə-lər, ˌser-ə-\ adj : of or involving the cerebrum and the blood vessels supplying it (∼ disease)

cerebrovascular accident n : STROKE

ce·re·brum \sə-'rē-brəm, 'ser-ə-\ n, pl **-brums** or **-bra** \-brə\ : the expanded anterior portion of the brain that overlies the rest of the brain, consists of cerebral hemispheres and connecting structures, and is considered to be the seat of conscious mental processes : TELENCEPHALON

cer·e·sin \'ser-ə-sən\ n : a white or yellow hard mineral wax

ce·ri·um \'sir-ē-əm\ n : a malleable ductile metallic element — symbol Ce; see ELEMENT table

ce·roid \'sir-ˌoid\ n : a yellow to brown pigment found esp. in the liver in cirrhosis

cert abbr certificate; certification; certified; certify

cer·ti·fy \'sər-tə-ˌfī\ vb **-fied; -fy·ing** 1 : to attest officially to the insanity of 2 : to designate as having met the requirements to practice medicine or a particular medical specialty — **cer·ti·fi·able** \ˌsər-tə-'fī-ə-bəl\ adj — **cer·ti·fi·ably** \-blē\ adv — **cer·ti·fi·ca·tion** \-fə-'kā-shən\ n

cerulea — see PHLEGMASIA CERULEA DOLENS

ceruleus, cerulei — see LOCUS COERULEUS

ce·ru·lo·plas·min \sə-ˌrü-lō-'plaz-mən\ n : a blue copper-binding serum oxidase that appears to catalyze the conversion of ferrous iron in tissues to ferric iron and is deficient in Wilson's disease

ce·ru·men \sə-'rü-mən\ n : EARWAX

ce·ru·mi·nous gland \sə-'rü-mə-nəs-\ n : one of the modified sweat glands of the ear that produce earwax

cervic- or **cervici-** or **cervico-** comb form 1 : neck : cervix of an organ ⟨cervicitis⟩ 2 : cervical and ⟨cervicothoracic⟩ ⟨cervicovaginal⟩

cer·vi·cal \'sər-vi-kəl\ adj : of or relating to a neck or cervix ⟨∼ cancer⟩

cervical canal n : the passage through the cervix uteri

cervical cap n : a usu. rubber or plastic contraceptive device in the form of a thimble-shaped molded cap that fits snugly over the uterine cervix and blocks sperm from entering the uterus — called also Dutch cap

cervical flexure n : a ventral bend in the neural tube of the embryo marking the point of transition from brain to spinal cord

cervical ganglion n : any of three sympathetic ganglia on each side of the neck

cervicalis — see ANSA CERVICALIS

cervical nerve n : one of the spinal nerves of the cervical region of which there are eight on each side in most mammals including humans

cervical plexus n : a plexus formed by the anterior divisions of the four upper cervical nerves

cervical plug n : a mass of tenacious secretion by glands of the uterine cervix present during pregnancy and tending to close the uterine orifice

cervical rib n : a supernumerary rib sometimes found in the neck above the usual first rib

cervical vertebra n : any of the seven vertebrae of the neck

cer·vi·cec·to·my \ˌsər-və-'sek-tə-mē\ n, pl **-mies** : surgical excision of the uterine cervix — called also trachelectomy

cervici- or **cervico-** — see CERVIC-

cervicis — see ILIOCOSTALIS CERVICIS, LONGISSIMUS CERVICIS, SEMI-

SPINALIS CERVICIS, SPINALIS CERVI-
CIS, SPLENIUS CERVICIS, TRANSVER-
SALIS CERVICIS

cer·vi·ci·tis \ˌsər-və-ˈsī-təs\ n : inflammation of the uterine cervix

cer·vi·co·fa·cial \ˌsər-və-kō-ˈfā-shəl\
adj : of, relating to, or affecting the
neck and upper part of the face ⟨∼ actinomycosis⟩

cervicofacial nerve \ˌsər-və-(ˌ)kō-ˈfā-
shəl-\ n : a branch of the facial nerve
supplying the lower part of the face
and upper part of the neck

cer·vi·co·tho·rac·ic \ˌsər-vi-(ˌ)kō-thə-
ˈra-sik, -thó-\ adj : of or relating to the
neck and thorax

cer·vi·co·vag·i·nal \-ˈva-jən-ᵊl\ adj : of
or relating to the uterine cervix and
the vagina ⟨∼ flora⟩ ⟨∼ carcinoma⟩

cer·vix \ˈsər-viks\ n, pl **cer·vi·ces** \-və-
ˌsēz, ˌsər-ˈvī-(ˌ)sēz\ or **cervixes 1**
: NECK 1a; esp : the back part of the
neck **2** : a constricted portion of an
organ or part: as **a** : the narrow lower
or outer end of the uterus **b** : on the constricted cementoenamel junction on a
tooth

cervix ute·ri \-ˈyü-tə-ˌrī\ n : CERVIX 2a

¹**ce·sar·e·an** or **cae·sar·e·an** also **ce·
sar·i·an** or **cae·sar·i·an** \si-ˈzar-ē-ən\
adj : of, relating to, or being a cesarean section ⟨a ∼ birth⟩

²**cesarean** or **caesarean** also **cesarian**
or **caesarian** n : CESAREAN SECTION
  Cae·sar \ˈsē-zər\, Gaius Julius
  (100–44 BC), Roman general and
  statesman.

cesarean section n : surgical incision
of the walls of the abdomen and
uterus for delivery of offspring

ce·si·um \ˈsē-zē-əm\ n : a silver-white
soft ductile element — symbol Cs; see
ELEMENT TABLE

ces·tode \ˈses-ˌtōd\ n : TAPEWORM —
cestode adj

ce·tir·i·zine \se-ˈtir-ə-ˌzēn\ n : an H₁
antagonist administered orally in the
form of its dihydrochloride C₂₁H₂₅-
ClN₂O₃·2HCl to treat allergic rhinitis
and chronic hives — see ZYRTEC

cet·ri·mide \ˈse-trə-ˌmīd\ n : a mixture
of bromides of ammonium used esp.
as a detergent and antiseptic

ce·tyl alcohol \ˈsēt-ᵊl-\ n : a waxy crystalline alcohol C₁₆H₃₄O used in pharmaceutical and cosmetic preparations

ce·tyl·py·ri·din·i·um chloride \ˌsēt-ᵊl-
ˌpī-rə-ˈdi-nē-əm-\ n : a white powder
consisting of a quaternary ammonium salt C₂₁H₃₈ClN·H₂O and used as
a detergent and antiseptic

Cf symbol californium

CF abbr cystic fibrosis

CFS abbr chronic fatigue syndrome

CG abbr chorionic gonadotropin

cgs adj, often cap C&G&S : of, relating
to, or being a system of units based on
the centimeter as the unit of length,
the gram as the unit of mass, and the
second as the unit of time

Cha·ber·tia \shə-ˈbər-tē-ə, -ˈbər-\ n : a
genus of strongylid nematode worms
including one (C. ovina) that infests

the colon esp. of sheep and causes a
bloody diarrhea
  Cha·bert \shá-ˈber\, Philibert
  (1737–1814), French veterinarian.

chafe \ˈchāf\ n : injury caused by friction — **chafe** vb

Cha·gas' disease \ˈshä-gəs-, -gə-səz-\
n : a tropical American disease that is
caused by a trypanosome (Trypanosoma cruzi) transmitted by
blood-sucking insects of the genus
Triatoma, that has an acute form primarily affecting children and marked
esp. by chagoma, fever, edema, enlargement of the spleen, liver, and
lymph nodes, and that also has a
chronic form which may or may not
follow an acute episode and is
marked esp. by cardiac and gastrointestinal complications
  Chagas, Carlos Ribeiro Justiniano
  (1879–1934), Brazilian physician.

cha·go·ma \shə-ˈgō-mə\ n, pl **-mas** or
-ma·ta \-tə\ : a swelling resembling a
tumor that appears at the site of infection in Chagas' disease

chain \ˈchān\ n : a number of atoms or
chemical groups connected by chemical bonds ⟨a carbon ∼⟩

κ–chain var of KAPPA CHAIN

chain reflex n : a series of responses
each serving as a stimulus that evokes
the next response

chair·side \ˈchar-ˌsīd\ adj : relating to,
performed in the vicinity of, or assisting in the work done on a patient in a
dentist's chair ⟨a dental ∼ assistant⟩

chair time n : the time that a dental
patient spends in the dentist's chair

cha·la·sia \kə-ˈlā-zhə, ka-\ n : the relaxation of a ring of muscle (as the
cardiac sphincter of the esophagus)
surrounding a bodily opening

cha·la·zion \kə-ˈlā-zē-ən, -ˌän\ n, pl
-zia \-zē-ə\ : a small circumscribed tumor of the eyelid formed by retention
of secretions of the meibomian gland

chal·i·co·sis \ˌka-li-ˈkō-səs\ n, pl **-co·
ses** \-ˌsēz\ : a pulmonary disorder occurring among stone cutters that is
caused by inhalation of stone dust

chalk \ˈchók\ n : a soft limestone
sometimes used medicinally as a
source of calcium carbonate — see
PRECIPITATED CHALK, PREPARED
CHALK — **chalky** \ˈchó-kē\ adj

chal·lenge \ˈcha-lənj\ n : the process
of provoking or testing physiological
activity by exposure to a specific substance; esp : a test of immunity by exposure to an antigen after immunization against it — **challenge** vb

chal·lenged adj : having a physical or
mental disability or deficiency

cha·lone \ˈkā-ˌlōn, ˈka-\ n : a substance (as a glycoprotein) that inhibits
mitosis in the specific tissue which secretes it

cham·ber \ˈchām-bər\ n : an enclosed
space within the body of an animal —
see ANTERIOR CHAMBER, POSTERIOR
CHAMBER, VITREOUS CHAMBER

chamber pot *n* : a bedroom vessel for urination and defecation

chan·cre \'shaŋ-kər\ *n* : a primary sore or ulcer at the site of entry of a pathogen (as in tularemia); *esp* : the initial lesion of syphilis

chan·croid \'shaŋ-ˌkrȯid\ *n* : a venereal disease caused by a bacterium of the genus *Haemophilus* (*H. ducreyi*) and characterized by chancres that unlike those of syphilis lack firm indurated margins — called also *soft chancre;* see DUCREY'S BACILLUS

change of life *n* 1 : MENOPAUSE 1a(2) 2 : ANDROPAUSE

chan·nel \'chan-ᵊl\ *n* 1 : a usu. tubular enclosed passage 2 : a passage created in a selectively permeable membrane by a conformational change in membrane proteins; *also* : the proteins of such a passage — see ION CHANNEL

chap \'chap\ *n* : a crack in or a sore roughening of the skin caused by exposure to wind or cold — **chap** *vb*

Chap Stick \'chap-ˌstik\ *trademark* — used for a lip balm in stick form

char·ac·ter \'kar-ik-tər\ *n* 1 : one of the attributes or features that make up and distinguish the individual 2 : the detectable expression of the action of a gene or group of genes 3 : the complex of mental and ethical traits marking and often individualizing a person, group, or nation

¹char·ac·ter·is·tic \ˌkar-ik-tə-'ris-tik\ *adj* : serving to reveal and distinguish the individual character — **char·ac·ter·is·ti·cal·ly** \-ti-k(ə-)lē\ *adv*

²characteristic *n* : a distinguishing trait, quality, or property

cha·ras \'chär-əs\ *n* : HASHISH

char·coal \'chär-ˌkōl\ *n* : a dark or black porous carbon prepared from vegetable or animal substances — see ACTIVATED CHARCOAL

Char·cot–Ley·den crystals \ˌshär-ˌkō-'lī-dᵊn-\ *n pl* : minute colorless crystals that occur in various pathological discharges and esp. in the sputum following an asthmatic attack and that are thought to be formed by the disintegration of eosinophils

Char·cot \shär-'kō\, Jean–Martin (1825–1893), French neurologist.
Leyden, Ernst Viktor von (1832–1910), German physician.

Char·cot–Ma·rie–Tooth disease \(ˌ)shär-'kō-mə-'rē-'tüth-\ *n* : PERONEAL MUSCULAR ATROPHY

P. Marie — see MARIE-STRÜMPELL DISEASE
Tooth, Howard Henry (1856–1925), British physician.

Char·cot's joint \(ˌ)shär-'kōz-\ or **Char·cot joint** \-'kō\ *n* : a degenerative condition affecting one or more joints that is marked by joint instability and hypermobility and results from peripheral nerve damage (as that associated with diabetes mellitus

and tabes dorsalis) — called also *Charcot's disease*

charge \'chärj\ *n* 1 : a plaster or ointment used on a domestic animal 2 : CATHEXIS 2

charge nurse *n* : a nurse who is in charge of a health-care unit (as a hospital ward, emergency room, or nursing home)

char·la·tan \'shär-lə-tən\ *n* : QUACK

char·ley horse \'chär-lē-ˌhȯrs\ *n* : a muscular pain, cramping, or stiffness esp. of the quadriceps that results from a strain or bruise

chart \'chärt\ *n* : a record of medical information for a patient

CHD *abbr* coronary heart disease

check·bite \'chek-ˌbīt\ *n* 1 a : an act of biting into a sheet of material (as wax) to record the relation between the opposing surfaces of upper and lower teeth b : the record obtained 2 : the material for checkbites

check ligament *n* 1 : ALAR LIGAMENT 2 : either of two expansions of the sheaths of rectus muscles of the eye each of which prob. restrains the activity of the muscle with which it is associated

check·up \'chek-ˌəp\ *n* : EXAMINATION; *esp* : a general physical examination

Che·diak–Hi·ga·shi syndrome \shäd-'yäk-hē-'gä-shē\ *n* : a genetic disorder inherited as an autosomal recessive trait and characterized by partial albinism, abnormal granules in the white blood cells, and marked susceptibility to bacterial infections

Che·diak \shäd-'yäk\, Moises (*fl* 1952), French physician.
Hi·ga·shi \hē-'gä-shē\, Ototaka (*fl* 1954), Japanese physician.

cheek \'chēk\ *n* 1 : the fleshy side of the face below the eye and above and to the side of the mouth; *broadly* : the lateral aspect of the head 2 : BUTTOCK 1

cheek·bone \'chēk-ˌbōn\ *n* : the prominence below the eye that is formed by the zygomatic bone; *also* : ZYGOMATIC BONE

cheek tooth *n* : any of the molar or premolar teeth

cheese skipper *n* : the larva of a dipteran fly (*Piophila casei*) that lives in cheese and cured meats and is a cause of intestinal myiasis

cheesy \'chē-zē\ *adj* **chees·i·er; -est** : resembling cheese in consistency ⟨∼ lesions⟩ ⟨a ∼ discharge⟩

cheil- or cheilo- also chil- or chilo- *comb form* : lip ⟨*cheil*itis⟩ ⟨*cheilo*plasty⟩

cheil·i·tis \kī-'lī-təs\ *n* : inflammation of the lip

chei·lo·plas·ty \'kī-lō-ˌplas-tē\ *n, pl* **-ties** : plastic surgery to repair lip defects

cheil·os·chi·sis \kī-'läs-kə-səs\ *n, pl* **-chi·ses** \-ˌsēz\ : CLEFT LIP

chei·lo·sis \kī-ˈlō-səs\ *n, pl* **-lo·ses** \-ˌsēz\ : an abnormal condition of the lips characterized by scaling of the surface and by the formation of fissures in the corners of the mouth

cheir- *or* **cheiro-** — see CHIR-

chei·ro·pom·pho·lyx \ˌkī-rō-ˈpäm-fə-ˌliks\ *n* : a skin disease characterized by itching vesicles or blebs occurring in groups on the hands or feet

che·late \ˈkē-ˌlāt\ *n* : a compound having a ring structure that usu. contains a metal ion held by coordinate bonds — **chelate** *adj or vb* — **che·la·tion** \kē-ˈlā-shən\ *n*

che·lat·ing agent \ˈkē-ˌlā-tin-\ *n* : CHELATOR

che·la·tion therapy \kē-ˈlā-shən-\ : the use of a chelator (as EDTA) to bind with a metal in the body to form a chelate so that the metal loses its toxic effect or physiological activity

che·la·tor \ˈkē-ˌlā-tər\ *n* : any of various compounds that combine with metals to form chelates and that include some used medically in the treatment of metal poisoning (as by lead)

chem *abbr* chemical; chemist; chemistry

chem- *or* **chemo-** *also* **chemi-** *comb form* : chemical : chemistry ⟨*chemo-therapy*⟩

¹**chem·i·cal** \ˈke-mi-kəl\ *adj* **1** : of, relating to, used in, or produced by chemistry **2** : acting or operated or produced by chemicals — **chem·i·cal·ly** \-mi-k(ə-)lē\ *adv*

²**chemical** *n* **1** : a substance obtained by a chemical process or used for producing a chemical effect **2** : DRUG 2

chemical dependence *n* : addiction to or dependence on drugs — **chemically dependent** *adv*

chemical dependency *n* : CHEMICAL DEPENDENCE

chemical peel *n* : a cosmetic procedure for the removal of facial blemishes and wrinkles involving the application of a caustic chemical and esp. an acid to the skin

chemical warfare *n* : warfare using incendiary mixtures, smokes, or irritant, burning, poisonous, or asphyxiating gases

chem·ist \ˈke-məst\ *n* **1** : one trained in chemistry **2** *Brit* : PHARMACIST

chem·is·try \ˈke-mə-strē\ *n, pl* **-tries 1** : a science that deals with the composition, structure, and properties of substances and of the transformations that they undergo **2 a** : the composition and chemical properties of a substance ⟨the ∼ of hemoglobin⟩ **b** : chemical processes and phenomena (as of an organism) ⟨blood ∼⟩

chemist's shop *n, Brit* : a place where medicines are sold

chemo \ˈkē-mō\ *n* : CHEMOTHERAPY

chemo- — see CHEM-

che·mo·dec·to·ma \ˌkē-mō-ˈdek-tə-mə, ˌke-\ *n, pl* **-mas** *also* **-ma·ta** \-mə-tə\ : a tumor that affects tissue (as of the carotid body) populated with chemoreceptors

che·mo·nu·cle·ol·y·sis \-ˌnü-klē-ˈä-lə-səs, -ˌnyü-\ *n, pl* **-y·ses** \-ˌsēz\ : treatment of a slipped disk by the injection of chymopapain to dissolve the displaced nucleus pulposus

che·mo·pal·li·dec·to·my \-ˌpa-lə-ˈdek-tə-mē\ *n, pl* **-mies** : destruction of the globus pallidus by the injection of a chemical agent (as ethyl alcohol) esp. for the relief of parkinsonian tremors

che·mo·pre·ven·tion \-pri-ˈven-chən\ *n* : the use of chemical agents to prevent the development of cancer — **che·mo·pre·ven·tive** \-tiv\ *adj*

che·mo·pro·phy·lax·is \-ˌprō-fə-ˈlak-səs, -ˌprä-\ *n, pl* **-lax·es** \-ˌsēz\ : prevention of infectious disease by the use of chemical agents — **che·mo·pro·phy·lac·tic** \-ˈlak-tik\ *adj*

che·mo·ra·di·a·tion \-ˌrā-dē-ˈā-shən\ *n* : CHEMORADIOTHERAPY

che·mo·ra·dio·ther·a·py \-ˌrā-dē-ō-ˈther-ə-pē\ *n* : treatment that combines chemotherapy and radiotherapy

che·mo·re·cep·tion \-ri-ˈsep-shən\ *n* : the physiological reception of chemical stimuli — **che·mo·re·cep·tive** \-tiv\ *adj*

che·mo·re·cep·tor \-ri-ˈsep-tər\ *n* : a sense organ (as a taste bud) responding to chemical stimuli

che·mo·re·flex \ˌkē-mō-ˈrē-ˌfleks *also* ˌke-\ *n* : a physiological reflex initiated by a chemical stimulus or in a chemoreceptor — **chemoreflex** *adj*

che·mo·re·sis·tance \-ri-ˈzis-təns\ *n* : the quality or state of being resistant to a chemical (as a drug) — **che·mo·re·sis·tant** \-tənt\ *adj*

che·mo·sen·si·tiv·i·ty \-ˌsen-sə-ˈti-və-tē\ *n, pl* **-ties** : susceptibility to the action of a chemical agent (as a therapeutic drug) ⟨∼ of cancer cells⟩ — **che·mo·sen·si·tive** \ˈsen-sə-tiv\ *adj*

che·mo·sis \kə-ˈmō-səs\ *n, pl* **-mo·ses** \-ˌsēz\ : swelling of the conjunctival tissue around the cornea

che·mo·sur·gery \ˌkē-mō-ˈsər-jə-rē\ *n, pl* **-ger·ies** : removal by chemical means of diseased or unwanted tissue — **che·mo·sur·gi·cal** \-ˈsər-ji-kəl\ *adj*

che·mo·tac·tic \-ˈtak-tik\ *adj* : involving, inducing, or exhibiting chemotaxis — **che·mo·tac·ti·cal·ly** \-ti-k(ə-)lē\ *adv*

che·mo·tax·is \-ˈtak-səs\ *n, pl* **-tax·es** \-ˌsēz\ : orientation or movement of an organism or cell in relation to chemical agents

¹**che·mo·ther·a·peu·tic** \-ˌther-ə-ˈpyü-tik\ *adj* : of, relating to, or used in chemotherapy — **che·mo·ther·a·peu·ti·cal·ly** \-ti-k(ə-)lē\ *adv*

²**chemotherapeutic** *n* : an agent used in chemotherapy

che·mo·ther·a·py \-ˈther-ə-pē\ *n, pl* **-pies** : the use of chemical agents in the treatment or control of disease or mental disorder — **che·mo·ther·a·pist** \-pist\ *n*

che·mot·ic \ki-ˈmä-tik\ *adj* : marked by or affected with chemosis

che·mot·ro·pism \ki-ˈmä-trə-ˌpi-zəm, ke-\ *n* : orientation of cells or organisms in relation to chemical stimuli

che·no·de·ox·y·cho·lic acid \ˌkē-(ˌ)nō-ˌdē-ˌäk-si-ˈkō-lik-, -ˈkä-\ *n* : a bile acid $C_{24}H_{40}O_4$ that facilitates fat absorption and cholesterol excretion

che·no·di·ol \ˌkē-nō-ˈdī-ˌól, -ˌōl\ *n* : CHENODEOXYCHOLIC ACID

cher·ub·ism \ˈcher-ù-ˌbi-zəm\ *n* : a hereditary condition characterized by swelling of the jawbones and esp. in young children by a characteristic facies marked by protuberant cheeks and upturned eyes

chest \ˈchest\ *n* **1** : MEDICINE CHEST **2** : the part of the body enclosed by the ribs and sternum

chest·nut \ˈches-(ˌ)nət\ *n* : a callosity on the inner side of the leg of the horse

chesty \ˈches-tē\ *adj* : of, relating to, or affected with disease of the chest — not used technically

Cheyne–Stokes respiration \ˈchān-ˈstōks-\ *n* : cyclic breathing marked by a gradual increase in the rapidity of respiration followed by a gradual decrease and total cessation for from 5 to 50 seconds and found esp. in advanced kidney and heart disease, asthma, and increased intracranial pressure — called also *Cheyne-Stokes breathing*

    Cheyne \ˈchān, ˈchā-nē\, **John (1777–1836)**, British physician.

    Stokes \ˈstóks\, **William (1804–1878)**, British physician.

CHF *abbr* congestive heart failure

Chi·ari–From·mel syndrome \kē-ˈär-ē-ˈfró-məl-, -ˈfrä-\ *n* : a condition usu. occurring postpartum and characterized by amenorrhea, galactorrhea, obesity, and atrophy of the uterus and ovaries

    Chiari, Johann Baptist (1817–1854), German surgeon.

    Frommel, Richard Julius Ernst (1854–1912), German gynecologist.

chi·asm \ˈkī-ˌa-zəm, ˈkē-\ *n* : CHIASMA 1

chi·as·ma \kī-ˈaz-mə, kē-\ *n, pl* **chi·as·ma·ta** \-mə-tə\ **1** : an anatomical intersection or decussation — see OPTIC CHIASMA **2** : a cross-shaped configuration of paired chromatids visible in the diplotene of meiotic prophase and considered the cytological equivalent of genetic crossing-over — **chi·as·mat·ic** \ˌkī-əz-ˈma-tik, kē-\ *adj*

chiasmatic groove *n* : a narrow transverse groove that lies near the front of the superior surface of the body of the sphenoid bone, is continuous with the optic foramen, and houses the optic chiasma

chicken mite *n* : a small mite of the genus *Dermanyssus* (*D. gallinae*) that infests poultry esp. in warm regions

chicken pox *n* : an acute contagious disease esp. of children that is marked by low-grade fever and formation of vesicles and is caused by a herpesvirus of the genus *Varicellovirus* (species *Human herpesvirus 3*) — called also *varicella*; — see SHINGLES

chief cell *n* **1** : one of the cells that line the lumen of the fundic glands of the stomach; *esp* : a small cell with granular cytoplasm that secretes pepsin — compare PARIETAL CELL **2** : one of the secretory cells of the parathyroid glands

chig·ger \ˈchi-gər, ˈji-\ *n* **1** : CHIGOE 1 **2** : a 6-legged mite larva (family Trombiculidae) that sucks the blood and causes intense irritation

chi·goe \ˈchi-(ˌ)gō, ˈchē-\ *n* **1** : a tropical flea belonging to the genus *Tunga* (*T. penetrans*) of which the fertile female causes great discomfort by burrowing under the skin — called also *chigger, sand flea* **2** : CHIGGER 2

chi kung *also* **ch'i kung** \ˈchē-ˈkùŋ\ *n, often cap C&K* : QIGONG

chik·un·gun·ya \ˌchi-kən-ˈgùn-yə\ *n* : a febrile disease that resembles dengue, occurs esp. in parts of Africa, India, and southeastern Asia, and is caused by a togavirus of the genus *Alphavirus* (species *Chikungunya virus*) transmitted by mosquitoes esp. of the genus *Aedes* — called also *chikungunya fever*

chil– *or* **chilo–** — see CHEIL-

chil·blain \ˈchil-ˌblān\ *n* : an inflammatory swelling or sore caused by exposure (as of the feet or hands) to cold — called also *pernio*

child \ˈchīld\ *n, pl* **chil·dren** \ˈchil-drən, -dərn\ **1** : an unborn or recently born person **2** : a young person esp. between infancy and youth — **with child** : PREGNANT

child·bear·ing \ˈchīld-ˌbar-iŋ\ *n* : the act of bringing forth children : PARTURITION — **childbearing** *adj*

child·bed \-ˌbed\ *n* : the condition of a woman in childbirth

childbed fever *n* : PUERPERAL FEVER

child·birth \-ˌbərth\ *n* : PARTURITION

child guidance *n* : the clinical study and treatment of the behavioral and emotional problems of children by a staff of specialists usu. comprising a physician or psychiatrist, a clinical psychologist, and a psychiatric social worker

child·hood \ˈchīld-ˌhùd\ *n* : the state or period of being a child

child psychiatry *n* : psychiatry applied to the treatment of children

child psychology *n* : the study of the psychological characteristics of infants and children and the application of general psychological principles to infancy and childhood

¹chill \ˈchil\ *n* **1** : a sensation of cold accompanied by shivering **2** : a disagreeable sensation of coldness

²**chill** vb **1 a** : to make or become cold **b** : to shiver or quake with or as if with cold **2** : to become affected with a chill

chill factor n : WINDCHILL

chi·me·ra or **chi·mae·ra** \kī-'mir-ə, kə-\ n : an individual, organ, or part consisting of tissues of diverse genetic constitution — **chi·me·ric** \-'mir-ik, -'mer-\ adj — **chi·me·rism** \-'mir-,i-zəm, kə-; 'kī-mə-,ri-\ n

chin \'chin\ n : the lower portion of the face lying below the lower lip and including the prominence of the lower jaw — called also *mentum* — **chin·less** \-ləs\ adj

chin·bone \'chin-,bōn\ n : JAW 1b; esp : the median anterior part of the bone of the lower jaw

chinch \'chinch\ n : BEDBUG

Chi·na white \'chī-nə-'(h)wīt\ n, often cap W, slang **1** : a pure potent form of heroin originating in southeastern Asia **2** : an illicit analog of the analgesic fentanyl that resembles heroin in its physical appearance and physiological effects

Chinese liver fluke n : a common and destructive Asian liver fluke of the genus *Clonorchis* (*C. sinensis*) that esp. in eastern and southeastern Asia is a serious human parasite invading the liver following consumption of raw infected fish and causing clonorchiasis

Chinese restaurant syndrome n : a group of symptoms (as chest pain, headache, and facial flushing) that is held to affect susceptible persons eating food and esp. Chinese food heavily seasoned with monosodium glutamate

chin–blow·er \'chip-,blō-ər\ n : a dental instrument usu. consisting of a rubber bulb with a long metal tube that is used to blow drilling debris from a cavity being prepared for filling

chir- or **chiro-** also **cheir-** or **cheiro-** comb form : hand ⟨chiropractic⟩

chi·rop·o·dy \kə-'rä-pə-dē, shə-, kī-\ n, pl **-dies** : PODIATRY — **chi·ro·po·di·al** \,kī-rə-'pō-dē-əl\ adj — **chi·rop·o·dist** \kə-'rä-pə-dist, shə-, kī-\ n

chi·ro·prac·tic \'kī-rə-,prak-tik\ n : a system of therapy which holds that disease results from a lack of normal nerve function and which employs manipulation and specific adjustment of body structures (as the spinal column) — **chiropractic** adj — **chi·ro·prac·tor** \-tər\ n

chis·el \'chi-zəl\ n : a metal tool with a cutting edge at the end of a blade; esp : one used in dentistry

chi·tin \'kīt-ᵊn\ n : a horny polysaccharide that forms part of the hard outer integument esp. of insects, arachnids, and crustaceans — **chi·tin·ous** \'kīt-ᵊn-əs\ adj

chla·myd·ia \klə-'mi-dē-ə\ n **1** cap : a genus of coccoid to spherical gram-negative intracellular bacteria (family Chlamydiaceae) including one (*C. trachomatis*) that causes or is associated with various diseases of the eye and genitourinary tract including trachoma, lymphogranuloma venereum, cervicitis, and some forms of nongonococcal urethritis **2** pl **-iae** also **-ias a** : a bacterium of the genus *Chlamydia* **b** : an infection or disease caused by chlamydiae — **chla·myd·ial** \-əl\ adj

chlo·as·ma \klō-'az-mə\ n, pl **-ma·ta** \-mə-tə\ : irregular brownish or blackish spots esp. on the face that occur sometimes in pregnancy and in disorders of or functional changes in the uterus and ovaries

chlor- or **chloro-** comb form **1** : green ⟨*chlor*osis⟩ **2** : chlorine : containing or caused by chlorine ⟨*chlor*acne⟩

chloracetophenone var of CHLORO-ACETOPHENONE

chlor·ac·ne \(,)klȯr-'ak-nē\ n : a skin eruption resembling acne and resulting from exposure to chlorine or its compounds

chlo·ral \'klȯr-əl\ n : CHLORAL HYDRATE

chloral hydrate n : a bitter white crystalline drug $C_2H_3Cl_3O_2$ used as a hypnotic and sedative

chlo·ral·ose \'klȯr-ə-,lōs, -,lōz\ n : a bitter crystalline compound C_8H_{11}-Cl_3O_6 used esp. to anesthetize animals — **chlo·ral·osed** \-,lōst, -,lōzd\ adj

chlo·ram·bu·cil \klȯr-'am-byə-,sil\ n : an anticancer drug $C_{14}H_{19}Cl_2NO_2$ used esp. to treat leukemias, multiple myeloma, and some lymphomas

chlo·ra·mine \'klȯr-ə-,mēn\ n : any of various organic compounds containing nitrogen and chlorine; esp : CHLORAMINE-T

chloramine–T \-'tē\ n : a white or faintly yellow crystalline compound $C_7H_7ClNNaO_2S\cdot3H_2O$ used as an antiseptic (as in treating wounds)

chlor·am·phen·i·col \,klȯr-,am-'fe-ni-kȯl, -,kōl\ n : a broad-spectrum antibiotic $C_{11}H_{12}Cl_2N_2O_5$ isolated from cultures of a soil actinomycete of the genus *Streptomyces* (*S. venezuelae*) or prepared synthetically — see CHLOROMYCETIN

chlor·bu·tol \'klȯr-byə-,tȯl\ n, chiefly Brit : CHLOROBUTANOL

chlor·cy·cli·zine \klȯr-'sī-klə-,zēn\ n : a cyclic antihistamine administered in the form of its hydrochloride $C_{18}H_{21}ClN_2\cdot HCl$

chlor·dane \'klȯr-,dān\ n : a viscous volatile liquid insecticide $C_{10}H_6Cl_8$ formerly used in the U.S.

chlor·di·az·epox·ide \,klȯr-dī-,a-zə-'päk-,sīd\ n : a benzodiazepine structurally and pharmacologically related to diazepam and used in the form of its hydrochloride $C_{16}H_{14}ClN_3O\cdot HCl$ esp. as a tranquilizer and to treat the withdrawal symptoms of alcoholism — see LIBRIUM

chlor·hex·i·dine \klōr-'hek-sə-ˌdīn, -ˌdēn\ n : an antibacterial compound $C_{22}H_{30}Cl_2N_{10}$ used as a local antiseptic (as in mouthwash) and disinfectant esp. in the form of its hydrochloride, gluconate, or acetate

chlo·ride \'klōr-ˌīd\ n : a compound of chlorine with another element or radical; *esp* : a salt or ester of hydrochloric acid

chloride shift n : the passage of chloride ions from the plasma into the red blood cells when carbon dioxide enters the plasma from the tissues and their return to the plasma when the carbon dioxide is discharged in the lungs that is a major factor both in maintenance of blood pH and in transport of carbon dioxide

chlo·ri·nate \'klōr-ə-ˌnāt\ vb -nat·ed; -nat·ing : to treat or cause to combine with chlorine or a chlorine compound — **chlo·ri·na·tion** \ˌklōr-ə-'nā-shən\ n

chlo·rine \'klōr-ˌēn, -ən\ n : a halogen element that is isolated as a heavy greenish yellow gas of pungent odor and is used esp. as a bleach, oxidizing agent, and disinfectant in water purification — symbol *Cl;* see ELEMENT table

chlor·mer·o·drin \klōr-'mer-ə-drən\ n : a mercurial compound $C_5H_{11}ClHg$-N_2O_2 formerly used esp. as a diuretic

chloro- — see CHLOR-

chlo·ro·ace·to·phe·none \ˌklōr-ō-ˌa-sə-(ˌ)tō-fə-'nōn, -ə-ˌsē-\ *or* **chlor·ace·to·phe·none** \ˌklōr-ˌa-, ˌklōr-ə-ˌsē\ n : a chlorine-containing compound C_8H_7ClO used esp. as a tear gas

chlo·ro·az·o·din \ˌklōr-ō-'a-zəd-³n\ n : a yellow crystalline compound $C_2H_4Cl_2N_6$ used in solution as a surgical antiseptic

chlo·ro·bu·ta·nol \-'byüt-³n-ˌòl, -'òl\ n : a white crystalline alcohol $C_4H_7Cl_3O$ that is used as a local anesthetic, sedative, and preservative (as for hypodermic solutions)

chlo·ro·cre·sol \-'krē-ˌsòl, -ˌsōl\ n : a chlorine derivative C_7H_7ClO of cresol used as an antiseptic and preservative

¹**chlo·ro·form** \'klōr-ə-ˌfòrm\ n : a colorless volatile heavy toxic liquid $CHCl_3$ with an ether odor used esp. as a solvent — called also *trichloromethane*

²**chloroform** vb : to treat with chloroform esp. so as to produce anesthesia or death

chlo·ro·gua·nide \ˌklōr-ō-'gwä-ˌnīd, -nəd\ n : PROGUANIL

chlo·ro·leu·ke·mia \-lü-'kē-mē-ə\ n : CHLOROMA

chlo·ro·ma \klə-'rō-mə\ n, pl -mas *also* -ma·ta \-mə-tə\ : a leukemic condition marked by the formation of usu. green-colored tumors composed of myeloid tissue; *also* : one of these tumors

Chlo·ro·my·ce·tin \ˌklōr-ō-mī-'sēt-³n\ *trademark* — used for chloramphenicol

chlo·ro·phyll \'klōr-ə-ˌfil, -fəl\ n 1 : the green photosynthetic coloring matter of plants 2 : a waxy green chlorophyll-containing substance extracted from green plants and used as a coloring agent or deodorant

chlo·ro·pic·rin \ˌklōr-ə-'pik-rən\ n : a heavy colorless liquid CCl_3NO_2 that causes tears and vomiting and is used esp. as a soil fumigant

chlo·ro·pro·caine \ˌklōr-ō-'prō-ˌkān\ n : a local anesthetic administered by injection in the form of its hydrochloride $C_{13}H_{19}ClN_2O_2$·HCl — see NESACAINE

chlo·ro·quine \'klōr-ə-ˌkwēn\ n : an antimalarial drug administered in the form of its diphosphate $C_{18}H_{26}$-ClN_3·$2H_3PO_4$ or hydrochloride $C_{18}H_{26}ClN_3$·HCl

chlo·ro·sis \klə-'rō-səs\ n, pl -ro·ses \-ˌsēz\ : an iron-deficiency anemia esp. of adolescent girls that may impart a greenish tint to the skin — called also *greensickness* — **chlo·rot·ic** \-'rä-tik\ adj

chlo·ro·thi·a·zide \ˌklōr-ə-'thī-ə-ˌzīd, -zəd\ n : a thiazide diuretic $C_7H_6ClN_3O_4S_2$ that is taken orally or is administered in the form of its sodium salt $C_7H_5ClN_3NaO_4S_2$ by intravenous injection esp. in the treatment of edema and hypertension — see DIURIL

chlo·ro·tri·an·i·sene \-ˌtrī-'a-nə-ˌsēn\ n : a synthetic estrogen $C_{23}H_{21}ClO_3$ used esp. formerly to treat menopausal symptoms

chlor·phen·e·sin carbamate \(ˌ)klōr-'fe-nə-sin-\ n : a drug $C_{10}H_{12}ClNO_4$ used as a skeletal muscle relaxant

chlor·phen·ir·amine \(ˌ)klōr-fen-'ir-ə-ˌmēn\ n : an antihistamine that is usu. administered in the form of its maleate $C_{16}H_{19}ClN_2$·$C_4H_4O_4$

chlor·prom·a·zine \klōr-'prä-mə-ˌzēn\ n : a phenothiazine derivative that has antipsychotic, sedative, and antiemetic properties and is used in the form of its hydrochloride $C_{17}H_{19}$-ClN_2S·HCl esp. to manage the symptoms of psychotic disorders (as in schizophrenia) — see LARGACTIL, THORAZINE

chlor·prop·amide \-'prä-pə-ˌmīd, -'prō-\ n : a sulfonylurea drug $C_{10}H_{13}ClN_2O_3S$ used orally to reduce blood sugar in the treatment of type 2 diabetes

chlor·tet·ra·cy·cline \ˌklōr-ˌte-trə-'sī-ˌklēn\ n : a yellow crystalline broad-spectrum antibiotic $C_{22}H_{23}ClN_2O_8$ produced by a soil actinomycete of the genus *Streptomyces* (*S. aureofaciens*) and sometimes used in animal feeds to stimulate growth — see AUREOMYCIN

chlor·thal·i·done \klōr-'tha-lə-ˌdōn\ n : a diuretic sulfonamide $C_{14}H_{11}$-ClN_2O_4S used esp. in the treatment of edema and hypertension — see HYGROTON

cho·a·na \'kō-ə-nə\ *n, pl* **-nae** \-,nē\ : either of the pair of posterior apertures of the nasal cavity that open into the nasopharynx — called also *posterior naris* — **cho·a·nal** \-nəl\ *adj*

Cho·a·no·tae·nia \,kō-ə-(,)nō-'tē-nē-ə\ *n* : a genus of tapeworms including one (*C. infundibulum*) which is an intestinal parasite of birds

¹choke \'chōk\ *vb* **choked; chok·ing 1** : to keep from breathing in a normal way by compressing or obstructing the windpipe or by poisoning or adulterating available air **2** : to have the windpipe blocked entirely or partly

²choke *n* **1** : the act of choking **2 chokes** *pl* : decompression sickness when marked by suffocation — used with *the*

choked disk *n* : PAPILLEDEMA

chol- *or* **chole-** *or* **cholo-** *comb form* : bile : gall ⟨*cholate*⟩ ⟨*cholo*rrhea⟩

cho·lae·mia *chiefly Brit var of* CHOLEMIA

cho·la·gogue \'kä-lə-,gäg, 'kō-\ *n* : an agent that promotes an increased flow of bile — **cho·la·gog·ic** \,kä-lə-'gä-jik, ,kō-\ *adj*

chol·an·gio·car·ci·no·ma \kə-,lan-jē-ə-,kär-sⁿ-'ō-mə\ *n* : a usu. slow-growing malignant tumor of the bile duct that arises from biliary epithelium and is typically an adenocarcinoma

chol·an·gio·gram \kə-'lan-jē-ə-,gram, kō-\ *n* : a radiograph of the bile ducts made after the ingestion or injection of a radiopaque substance

chol·an·gi·og·ra·phy \kə-,lan-jē-'ä-grə-fē, (,)kō-\ *n, pl* **-phies** : radiographic visualization of the bile ducts after ingestion or injection of a radiopaque substance — **chol·an·gio·graph·ic** \-jē-ə-'gra-fik\ *adj*

chol·an·gi·o·li·tis \-ə-'lī-təs, (,)kō-\ *n, pl* **-lit·i·des** \-'li-tə-,dēz\ : inflammation of bile capillaries — **chol·an·gi·o·lit·ic** \-'li-tik\ *adj*

cholangiopancreatography — see ENDOSCOPIC RETROGRADE CHOLANGIOPANCREATOGRAPHY

chol·an·gi·tis \,kō-,lan-'jī-təs\ *n, pl* **-git·i·des** \-'ji-tə-,dēz\ : inflammation of one or more bile ducts

cho·late \'kō-,lāt\ *n* : a salt or ester of cholic acid

cho·le·cal·cif·er·ol \,kō-lə-(,)kal-'si-fə-,rol, -,rōl\ *n* : a sterol $C_{27}H_{43}OH$ that is a natural form of vitamin D found esp. in fish, egg yolks, and fish-liver oils and is formed in the skin on exposure to sunlight or ultraviolet rays — called also *vitamin D, vitamin D₃*

cho·le·cys·tec·to·my \,kō-lə-(,)sis-'tek-tə-mē\ *n, pl* **-mies** : surgical excision of the gallbladder — **cho·le·cys·tec·to·mized** \-,mīzd\ *adj*

cho·le·cys·ti·tis \-(,)sis-'tī-təs\ *n, pl* **-tit·i·des** \-'ti-tə-,dēz\ : inflammation of the gallbladder

cho·le·cys·to·en·ter·os·to·my \-,sis-tō-,en-tə-'räs-tə-mē\ *n, pl* **-mies** : surgical union of and creation of a passage between the gallbladder and the intestine

cho·le·cys·to·gram \-'sis-tə-,gram\ *n* : a radiograph of the gallbladder made after ingestion or injection of a radiopaque substance

cho·le·cys·tog·ra·phy \-(,)sis-'tä-grə-fē\ *n, pl* **-phies** : the radiographic visualization of the gallbladder after ingestion or injection of a radiopaque substance — **cho·le·cys·to·graph·ic** \-,sis-tə-'gra-fik\ *adj*

cho·le·cys·to·ki·net·ic \-,sis-tə-kə-'ne-tik, -kī-\ *adj* : tending to cause the gallbladder to contract and discharge bile

cho·le·cys·to·ki·nin \-,sis-tə-'kī-nən\ *n* : a hormone secreted esp. by the duodenal mucosa that regulates the emptying of the gallbladder and secretion of enzymes by the pancreas and that has been found in the brain — called also *cholecystokinin-pancreozymin, pancreozymin*

cho·le·cys·tor·rha·phy \-(,)sis-'tor-ə-fē\ *n, pl* **-phies** : repair of the gallbladder by suturing

cho·le·cys·tos·to·my \-(,)sis-'täs-tə-mē\ *n, pl* **-mies** : surgical incision of the gallbladder usu. to effect drainage

cho·le·cys·tot·o·my \-'tä-tə-mē\ *n, pl* **-mies** : surgical incision of the gallbladder esp. for exploration or to remove a gallstone

cho·le·doch·al \'kō-lə-,dä-kəl, kə-'le-də-kəl\ *adj* : relating to, being, or occurring in the common bile duct

cho·le·do·chi·tis \kə-,le-də-'kī-təs, ,kō-lə-\ *n* : inflammation of the common bile duct

cho·led·o·cho·je·ju·nos·to·my \kə-,le-də-(,)kō-ji-(,)jü-'näs-tə-mē\ *n, pl* **-mies** : surgical creation of a passage uniting the common bile duct and the jejunum

cho·led·o·cho·li·thi·a·sis \-li-'thī-ə-səs\ *n, pl* **-a·ses** \-,sēz\ : a condition marked by presence of calculi in the gallbladder and common bile duct

cho·led·o·cho·li·thot·o·my \-li-'thä-tə-mē\ *n, pl* **-mies** : surgical incision of the common bile duct for removal of a gallstone

cho·led·o·chor·rha·phy \kə-,le-də-'kōr-ə-fē\ *n, pl* **-ra·phies** : surgical union of the separated ends of the common bile duct by suturing

cho·led·o·chos·to·my \-'käs-tə-mē\ *n, pl* **-mies** : surgical incision of the common bile duct usu. to effect drainage

cho·led·o·chot·o·my \-'kä-tə-mē\ *n, pl* **-mies** : surgical incision of the common bile duct

cho·led·o·chus \kə-'le-də-kəs\ *n, pl* **-o·chi** \-,kī, -,kē\ : COMMON BILE DUCT

cho·le·glo·bin \'kō-lə-,glō-bən, 'kä-\ *n* : a green pigment that occurs in bile and is formed by breakdown of hemoglobin

cho·le·lith \'kō-li-ˌlith, 'kä-\ *n* : GALLSTONE

cho·le·li·thi·a·sis \ˌkō-li-li-'thī-ə-səs\ *n, pl* **-a·ses** \-ˌsēz\ : production of gallstones; *also* : the resulting abnormal condition

cho·le·mia \kō-'lē-mē-ə\ *n* : the presence of excess bile in the blood usu. indicative of liver disease — **cho·le·mic** \-mik\ *adj*

cho·le·poi·e·sis \ˌkō-lə-ˌpȯi-'ē-səs, ˌkä-\ *n, pl* **-e·ses** \-ˌsēz\ : production of bile — **cho·le·poi·et·ic** \-'e-tik\ *adj*

chol·era \'kä-lə-rə\ *n* : any of several diseases of humans and domestic animals usu. marked by severe gastrointestinal symptoms: as **a** : an acute diarrheal disease caused by an enterotoxin produced by a comma-shaped gram-negative bacillus of the genus *Vibrio* (*V. cholerae* syn. *V. comma*) when it is present in large numbers in the proximal part of the human small intestine — see ASIATIC CHOLERA **b** : FOWL CHOLERA **c** : HOG CHOLERA — **chol·e·ra·ic** \ˌkä-lə-'rā-ik\ *adj*

cholera mor·bus \-'mȯr-bəs\ *n* : a gastrointestinal disturbance characterized by abdominal pain, diarrhea, and sometimes vomiting — not used technically

cho·le·re·sis \ˌkō-lə-'rē-səs, ˌkä-\ *n, pl* **-re·ses** \-ˌsēz\ : the flow of bile from the liver esp. when increased above a previous or normal level

¹**cho·le·ret·ic** \ˌkō-lə-'re-tik, ˌkä-\ *adj* : promoting bile secretion by the liver (⁓ action of bile salts)

²**choleretic** *n* : a choleretic agent

cho·le·scin·tig·ra·phy \ˌkō-lə-sin-'ti-grə-fē\ *n, pl* **-phies** : scintigraphy of the biliary system

cho·le·sta·sis \ˌkō-lə-'stā-səs, ˌkä-\ *n, pl* **-sta·ses** \-'stā-ˌsēz\ : a checking or failure of bile flow — **cho·le·stat·ic** \-'sta-tik\ *adj*

cho·les·te·a·to·ma \kə-ˌles-tē-ə-'tō-mə, ˌkō-lə-ˌstē-, ˌkä-lə-\ *n, pl* **-mas** *also* **-ma·ta** \-mə-tə\ **1** : an epidermoid cyst usu. in the brain appearing as a compact shiny flaky mass **2** : a tumor usu. growing in a confined space (as the middle ear) and frequently constituting a sequel to chronic otitis media — **cho·les·te·a·to·ma·tous** \-mə-təs\ *adj*

cho·les·ter·ol \kə-'les-tə-ˌrōl, -ˌrȯl\ *n* : a steroid alcohol $C_{27}H_{45}OH$ present in animal cells and body fluids that regulates membrane fluidity, functions as a precursor molecule in various metabolic pathways, and as a constituent of LDL may cause arteriosclerosis — **cho·les·ter·ic** \kə-'les-tə-rik, ˌkō-lə-'ster-ik, ˌkä-\ *adj*

cho·les·ter·ol·ae·mia *also* **cho·les·te·rae·mia** *chiefly Brit var of* CHOLESTEROLEMIA

cho·les·ter·ol·emia \kə-ˌles-tə-rə-'lē-mē-ə\ *also* **cho·les·ter·emia** \-'rē-mē-ə\ *n* : the presence of cholesterol in the blood

cho·les·ter·ol·osis \kə-ˌles-tə-rə-'lō-səs\ *or* **cho·les·ter·o·sis** \kə-ˌles-tə-'rō-səs\ *n, pl* **-oses** \-ˌsēz\ : abnormal deposition of cholesterol (as in blood vessels or the gallbladder)

cho·le·styr·amine \kō-'les-tir-ə-ˌmēn\ *n* : a strongly basic synthetic resin used esp. to lower cholesterol levels

cho·lic acid \'kō-lik-\ *n* : a crystalline bile acid $C_{24}H_{40}O_5$

cho·line \'kō-ˌlēn\ *n* : a basic compound $C_5H_{15}NO_2$ that is found in various foods (as egg yolks and legumes) or is synthesized in the liver, is a precursor of acetylcholine, and is essential to liver function

choline ace·tyl·trans·fer·ase \-ə-ˌsē-tᵊl-'trans-fər-ˌās\ *n* : an enzyme that catalyzes the synthesis of acetylcholine from acetyl coenzyme A and choline

cho·lin·er·gic \ˌkō-lə-'nər-jik\ *adj* **1** *of autonomic nerve fibers* : liberating, activated by, or involving acetylcholine — compare ADRENERGIC 1, NORADRENERGIC **2** : resembling acetylcholine esp. in physiologic action — **cho·lin·er·gi·cal·ly** \-ji-k(ə-)lē\ *adv*

cho·lin·es·ter·ase \ˌkō-lə-'nes-tə-ˌrās, -ˌrāz\ *n* **1** : ACETYLCHOLINESTERASE **2** : an enzyme that hydrolyzes choline esters and that is found esp. in blood plasma — called also *pseudocholinesterase*

¹**cho·li·no·lyt·ic** \ˌkō-lə-nō-'li-tik\ *adj* : interfering with the action of acetylcholine or cholinergic agents

²**cholinolytic** *n* : a cholinolytic substance

¹**cho·li·no·mi·met·ic** \ˌkō-lə-nō-mə-'me-tik, ˌkä-, -mī-\ *adj* : resembling acetylcholine or simulating its physiologic action

²**cholinomimetic** *n* : a cholinomimetic substance

cholo- — see CHOL-

cho·lor·rhea \ˌkä-lə-'rē-ə, ˌkō-\ *n* : excessive secretion of bile

cho·lor·rhoea *chiefly Brit var of* CHOLORRHEA

chol·uria \kō-'lùr-ē-ə, kōl-'yùr-\ *n* : presence of bile in urine

chondr- *or* **chondri-** *or* **chondro-** *comb form* : cartilage ⟨*chondro*clast⟩

chon·dral \'kän-drəl\ *adj* : of or relating to cartilage

chon·dri·tis \kän-'drī-təs\ *n* : inflammation of cartilage

chon·dro·blast \'kän-drə-ˌblast, -drō-\ *n* : a cell that produces cartilage — **chon·dro·blas·tic** \ˌkän-drə-'blas-tik, -drō-\ *adj*

chon·dro·clast \'kän-drə-ˌklast, -drō-\ *n* : a cell that absorbs cartilage

chon·dro·cos·tal \ˌkän-drə-'käst-ᵊl, -drō-\ *adj* : of or relating to the costal cartilages and the ribs

chon·dro·cyte \'kän-drə-ˌsīt, -drō-\ *n* : a cartilage cell

chon·dro·dys·pla·sia \ˌkän-drə-dis-'plā-zhə, -drō-, -zhē-ə\ *n* : a hereditary skeletal disorder characterized by the formation of exostoses at the epiphyses and resulting in arrested development and deformity — called also *dyschondroplasia*

chon·dro·dys·tro·phia \-dis-'trō-fē-ə\ *n* : ACHONDROPLASIA

chon·dro·dys·tro·phy \-'dis-trə-fē\ *n, pl* **-phies** : ACHONDROPLASIA — **chon·dro·dys·tro·phic** \-dis-'trō-fik\ *adj*

chon·dro·gen·e·sis \-'je-nə-səs\ *n, pl* **-e·ses** \-,sēz\ : the development of cartilage — **chon·dro·gen·ic** \-'je-nik\ *adj*

chon·droid \'kän-,dròid\ *adj* : resembling cartilage

chon·droi·tin \kän-'dròit-ᵊn, -'dròi-ət-ᵊn\ *n* : any of several glycosaminoglycans occurring in sulfated form in various tissues (as cartilage and tendons)

chon·drol·o·gy \kän-'drä-lə-jē\ *n, pl* **-gies** : a branch of anatomy concerned with cartilage

chon·dro·ma \kän-'drō-mə\ *n, pl* **-mas** \-məz\ *also* **-ma·ta** \-mə-tə\ : a benign tumor containing the structural elements of cartilage — **chon·dro·ma·tous** \(')kän-'drä-mə-təs, -'drō-\ *adj*

chon·dro·ma·la·cia \,kän-drō-mə-'lā-shə, -shē-ə\ *n* : abnormal softness of cartilage

chondromalacia patellae *n* : pain over the front of the knee with softening of the articular cartilage of the patella

chon·dro·os·teo·dys·tro·phy \-,äs-tē-ō-'dis-trə-fē\ *n, pl* **-phies** : any of several mucopolysaccharidoses (as Hurler's syndrome) characterized esp. by disorders of bone and cartilage

chon·dro·phyte \'kän-drō,fit\ *n* : an outgrowth or spur of cartilage

chon·dro·sar·co·ma \,kän-drō-sär-'kō-mə\ *n, pl* **-mas** *also* **-ma·ta** \-mə-tə\ : a sarcoma containing cartilage cells

chon·dro·ster·nal \,kän-drō-'stərn-ᵊl\ *adj* : of or relating to the costal cartilages and sternum

Cho·part's joint \(,)shō-'pärz-\ *n* : the tarsal joint that comprises the talonavicular and calcaneocuboid articulations

    Cho·part \shō-pár\, **François (1743–1795)**, French surgeon.

chor·da ten·din·ea \'kòr-də-,ten-'di-nē-ə\ *n, pl* **chor·dae ten·din·e·ae** \-nē-,ē\ : any of the delicate tendinous cords that are attached to the edges of the atrioventricular valves of the heart and to the papillary muscles and serve to prevent the valves from being pushed into the atrium during the ventricular contraction

chorda tym·pa·ni \-'tim-pə-,nī\ *n* : a branch of the facial nerve that traverses the middle ear cavity and the infratemporal fossa and supplies autonomic fibers to the sublingual and submandibular glands and sensory fibers to the anterior part of the tongue

chor·dee \'kòr-,dē, -,dā, ,kòr-'\ *n* : painful erection of the penis often with a downward curvature that may be present in a congenital condition (as hypospadias) or accompany gonorrhea

chor·do·ma \kòr-'dō-mə\ *n, pl* **-mas** *also* **-ma·ta** \-mə-tə\ : a malignant tumor that is derived from remnants of the embryonic notochord and occurs along the spine

chordotomy *var of* CORDOTOMY

cho·rea \kə-'rē-ə\ *n* : any of various nervous disorders of infectious or organic origin marked by spasmodic movements of the limbs and facial muscles and by incoordination — called also *Saint Vitus' dance*; see HUNTINGTON'S DISEASE, SYDENHAM'S CHOREA — **cho·re·at·ic** \,kòr-ē-'a-tik\ *adj* — **cho·re·ic** \kə-'rē-ik\ *adj*

cho·re·i·form \kə-'rē-ə-,fòrm\ *adj* : resembling chorea ⟨~ convulsions⟩

cho·reo·ath·e·to·sis \,-ə-thə-'tō-səs\ *n, pl* **-to·ses** \-,sēz\ : a nervous disturbance marked by the involuntary movements characteristic of chorea and athetosis

cho·rio·al·lan·to·is \,kòr-ē-ō-ə-'lan-tə-wəs\ *n, pl* **-to·ides** \-,ō-,a-lən-'tō-ə-,dēz, -,lan-\ : a vascular fetal membrane composed of the fused chorion and adjacent wall of the allantois — called also *chorioallantoic membrane* — **cho·rio·al·lan·to·ic** \-,a-lən-'tō-ik\ *adj*

cho·rio·am·ni·o·ni·tis \,-am-nē-ō-'nī-təs\ *n* : inflammation of the fetal membranes

cho·rio·cap·il·lar·is \,-ka-pə-'lar-əs\ *n* : the inner of the two vascular layers of the choroid of the eye that is composed largely of capillaries

cho·rio·car·ci·no·ma \,-kärs-ᵊn-'ō-mə\ *n, pl* **-mas** *also* **-ma·ta** \-mə-tə\ : a malignant tumor derived from trophoblastic tissue that develops typically in the uterus following pregnancy, miscarriage, or abortion esp. when associated with a hydatidiform mole or rarely in the testes or ovaries chiefly as a component of a mixed germ-cell tumor

cho·rio·ep·i·the·li·o·ma \,-,e-pə-,thē-lē-'ō-mə\ *n, pl* **-mas** *also* **-ma·ta** \-mə-tə\ : CHORIOCARCINOMA

cho·ri·o·ma \,kòr-ē-'ō-mə\ *n, pl* **-mas** *or* **-ma·ta** \-mə-tə\ : a tumor formed of chorionic tissue

cho·rio·men·in·gi·tis \,-,me-nən-'jī-təs\ *n, pl* **-git·i·des** \-'ji-tə-,dēz\ : cerebral meningitis; *specif* : LYMPHOCYTIC CHORIOMENINGITIS

cho·ri·on \'kòr-ē-,än\ *n* : the highly vascular outer embryonic membrane that is associated with the allantois in the formation of the placenta

cho·ri·on·ep·i·the·li·o·ma \,kòr-ē-,ä-,ne·pə-,thē-lē-'ō-mə\ *n, pl* **-mas** *also* **-ma·ta** \-mə-tə\ : CHORIOCARCINOMA

chorion fron·do·sum \-frən-'dō-səm\ *n* : the part of the chorion that has persistent villi and that with the decidua basalis forms the placenta — see CHORIONIC VILLUS SAMPLING

cho·ri·on·ic \ˌkōr-ē-'ä-nik\ *adj* **1** : of, relating to, or being part of the chorion ⟨∼ villi⟩ **2** : secreted or produced by chorionic or a related tissue (as in the placenta or a choriocarcinoma)

chorionic so·ma·to·mam·mo·tro·pin \-ˌsō-mə-tə-ˌma-mə-'trō-pᵊn\ *n* : PLACENTAL LACTOGEN

chorionic villus sampling *also* **chorionic villi sampling** *n* : biopsy of the chorion frondosum through the abdominal wall or by way of the vagina and uterine cervix at 10 to 12 weeks of gestation to obtain fetal cells for the prenatal diagnosis of chromosomal abnormalities — abbr. *CVS*

Cho·ri·op·tes \ˌkōr-ē-'äp-ˌtēz\ *n* : a genus of small parasitic mites infesting domestic animals — **cho·ri·op·tic** \-'äp-tik\ *adj*

chorioptic mange *n* : mange caused by mites of the genus *Chorioptes* that usu. attack only the surface of the skin — compare DEMODECTIC MANGE, SARCOPTIC MANGE

cho·rio·ret·i·nal \ˌkōr-ē-ō-'ret-ᵊn-əl\ *adj* : of, relating to, or affecting the choroid and the retina of the eye

cho·rio·ret·i·ni·tis \-ˌret-ᵊn-'ī-təs\ *also* **cho·roi·do·ret·i·ni·tis** \kə-ˌrȯi-dō-\ *n, pl* **-nit·i·des** \-'i-tə-ˌdēz\ : inflammation of the retina and choroid of the eye

cho·roid \'kōr-ˌȯid\ *n* : a vascular membrane containing large branched pigment cells that lies between the retina and the sclera of the eye — called also *choroid coat* — **choroid** or **cho·roi·dal** \kə-'rȯid-ᵊl\ *adj*

choroidea — see TELA CHOROIDEA

cho·roi·de·re·mia \ˌkōr-ˌȯi-də-'rē-mē-ə\ *n* : progressive degeneration of the choroid that is an X-linked trait chiefly affecting males and that is characterized by night blindness, constriction of the visual field, and eventual blindness

cho·roid·i·tis \ˌkōr-ˌȯi-'dī-təs\ *also* **cho·ri·oid·i·tis** \ˌkōr-ē-ȯi-\ *n* : inflammation of the choroid of the eye

cho·roi·do·iri·tis \kə-ˌrȯi-dō-ī-'rī-təs\ *n* : inflammation of the choroid and the iris of the eye

cho·roid·op·a·thy \ˌkōr-ˌȯi-'dä-pə-thē\ *n, pl* **-thies** : a diseased condition affecting the choroid of the eye

choroid plexus *n* : a highly vascular portion of the pia mater that projects into the ventricles of the brain and secretes cerebrospinal fluid

Christ·mas disease \'kris-məs-\ *n* : a hereditary sex-linked hemorrhagic disease involving absence of a coagulation factor in the blood and failure of the clotting mechanism — called also *hemophilia B;* compare HEMOPHILIA

Christmas, Stephen, British child patient.

Christmas factor *n* : FACTOR IX

chrom·aes·the·sia *chiefly Brit var of* CHROMESTHESIA

chro·maf·fin \'krō-mə-fən\ *adj* : staining deeply with chromium salts

chro·maf·fi·no·ma \ˌkrō-mə-fə-'nō-mə, krō-ˌma-\ *n, pl* **-mas** *also* **-ma·ta** \-mə-tə\ : a tumor containing chromaffin cells; *esp* : PHEOCHROMOCYTOMA

chro·ma·phil \'krō-mə-ˌfil\ *adj* : CHROMAFFIN ⟨∼ tissue⟩

chromat- or **chromato-** *comb form* **1** : color ⟨*chromatid*⟩ **2** : chromatin ⟨*chromatolysis*⟩

chro·mat·ic \krō-'ma-tik\ *adj* **1** : of, relating to, or characterized by color or color phenomena or sensations ⟨∼ stimuli⟩ **2** : capable of being colored by staining agents ⟨∼ substances⟩

chromatic vision *n* **1** : normal color vision in which the colors of the spectrum are distinguished and evaluated **2** : CHROMATOPSIA

chro·ma·tid \'krō-mə-təd\ *n* : one of the usu. paired and parallel strands of a duplicated chromosome joined by a single centromere — see CHROMONEMA

chro·ma·tin \'krō-mə-tən\ *n* : a complex of a nucleic acid with basic proteins (as histone) in eukaryotic cells that is usu. dispersed in the interphase nucleus and condensed into chromosomes in mitosis and meiosis — **chro·ma·tin·ic** \ˌkrō-mə-'ti-nik\ *adj*

chro·ma·tism \'krō-mə-ˌti-zəm\ *n* : CHROMESTHESIA

chromato- — see CHROMAT-

chro·mato·gram \krō-'ma-tə-ˌgram, krə-\ *n* **1** : the pattern formed on the adsorbent medium by the layers of components separated by chromatography **2** : a time-based graphic record of a chromatographic separation

chro·mato·graph \krō-'ma-tə-ˌgraf, krə-\ *n* : an instrument for producing chromatograms — **chromatograph** *vb*

chro·ma·tog·ra·phy \ˌkrō-mə-'tä-grə-fē\ *n, pl* **-phies** : a process in which a chemical mixture carried by a liquid or gas is separated into components as a result of differential distribution of the solutes as they flow around or over a stationary liquid or solid phase — **chro·mato·graph·ic** \krō-ˌma-tə-'gra-fik, krə-\ *adj* — **chro·mato·graph·i·cal·ly** \-fi-k(ə-)lē\ *adv*

chro·ma·tol·y·sis \ˌkrō-mə-'tä-lə-səs\ *n, pl* **-y·ses** \-ˌsēz\ : the dissolution and breaking up of chromophil material (as chromatin) of a cell — **chro·mato·lyt·ic** \krō-ˌmat-ᵊl-'i-tik, krə-\ *adj*

chro·ma·to·phore \krō-'ma-tə-ˌfōr, krə-\ *n* : a pigment-bearing cell esp. in the skin

chro·ma·top·sia \ˌkrō-mə-'täp-sē-ə\ *n* : a disturbance of vision which is sometimes caused by drugs and in which colorless objects appear colored

chro·ma·to·sis \ˌkrō-mə-'tō-səs\ *n, pl* **-to·ses** \-ˌsēz\ : PIGMENTATION; *specif* : deposit of pigment in a normally unpigmented area or excessive pigmentation in a normally pigmented area

chrom·es·the·sia \ˌkrō-mes-'thē-zhə, -zhē-ə\ *n* : synesthesia in which color is perceived in response to stimuli (as words or numbers) that contain no element of color — called also *chromatism*

chro·mid·i·al substance \krō-'mi-dē-əl-\ *n* : NISSL SUBSTANCE

chro·mi·dro·sis \ˌkrō-mə-'drō-səs\ *also* **chrom·hi·dro·sis** \ˌkrōm-(h)ə-\ *n, pl* **-dro·ses** \-ˌsēz\ : secretion of colored sweat

chro·mi·um \'krō-mē-əm\ *n* : a blue-white metallic element found naturally only in combination — symbol *Cr;* see ELEMENT table

chromium picolinate *n* : a biologically active chromium salt $C_{18}H_{12}CrN_3O_6$ that is used as a dietary supplement

chro·mo·blas·to·my·co·sis \ˌkrō-mə-ˌblas-tə-ˌmī-'kō-səs\ *n, pl* **-co·ses** \-ˌsēz\ : a skin disease that is caused by any of several pigmented fungi (esp. genera *Phialophora, Cladosporium,* and *Fonsecaea*) and is marked by the formation of warty colored nodules usu. on the legs — called also *chromomycosis*

¹**chro·mo·mere** \'krō-mə-ˌmir\ *n* : the highly refractile portion of a blood platelet — compare HYALOMERE

²**chromomere** *n* : one of the small bead-shaped and heavily staining concentrations of chromatin that are linearly arranged along the chromosome — **chro·mo·mer·ic** \ˌkrō-mə-'mer-ik, -'mir-\ *adj*

chro·mo·my·co·sis \ˌkrō-mə-ˌmī-'kō-səs\ *n, pl* **-co·ses** \-ˌsēz\ : CHROMOBLASTOMYCOSIS

chro·mo·ne·ma \ˌkrō-mə-'nē-mə\ *n, pl* **-ne·ma·ta** \-'nē-mə-tə\ : the coiled filamentous core of a chromatid — **chro·mo·ne·mat·ic** \-ni-'ma-tik\ *adj*

¹**chro·mo·phobe** \'krō-mə-ˌfōb\ *adj* : not readily absorbing stains : difficult to stain ⟨∼ tumors⟩

²**chromophobe** *n* : a chromophobe cell esp. of the pituitary gland

chro·mo·pro·tein \ˌkrō-mə-'prō-ˌtēn\ *n* : any of various proteins (as hemoglobins or carotenoids) having a pigment as a prosthetic group

chro·mo·some \'krō-mə-ˌsōm, -ˌzōm\ *n* : any of the rod-shaped or thread-like DNA-containing structures of cellular organisms that are located in the nucleus of eukaryotes, are usu. ring-shaped in prokaryotes (as bacteria), and contain most or all of the genes of the organism; *also* : the genetic material of a virus — **chro·mo·som·al** \ˌkrō-mə-'sō-məl, -'zō-\ *adj* — **chro·mo·som·al·ly** *adv*

chromosome complement *n* : the entire group of chromosomes in a nucleus

chromosome number *n* : the usu. constant number of chromosomes characteristic of a particular kind of animal or plant

chron·ax·ie *or* **chron·axy** \'krō-ˌnak-sē, 'krä-\ *n, pl* **-ax·ies** : the minimum time required for excitation of a structure (as a nerve cell) by a constant electric current of twice the threshold voltage

¹**chron·ic** \'krä-nik\ *also* **chron·i·cal** \-ni-kəl\ *adj* **1 a** : marked by long duration, by frequent recurrence over a long time, and often by slowly progressing seriousness : not acute ⟨∼ indigestion⟩ **b** : suffering from a disease or ailment of long duration or frequent recurrence ⟨a ∼ arthritic⟩ **2 a** : having a slow progressive course of indefinite duration — used esp. of degenerative invasive diseases, some infections, psychoses, and inflammations ⟨∼ heart disease⟩ ⟨∼ arthritis⟩; compare ACUTE 2b **b** : infected with a disease-causing agent (as a virus) and remaining infectious over a long period of time but not necessarily expressing symptoms ⟨∼ carriers⟩ — **chron·i·cal·ly** \-ni-k(ə-)lē\ *adv* — **chro·nic·i·ty** \krä-'ni-sə-tē, krō-\ *n*

²**chronic** *n* : one that suffers from a chronic disease

chronica — see ACRODERMATITIS CHRONICA ATROPHICANS

chronic alcoholism *n* : ALCOHOLISM 2b

chronic care *adj* : providing or concerned with long-term medical care lasting usu. more than 90 days esp. for individuals with chronic physical or mental impairment — **chronic care** *n*

chronic fatigue syndrome *n* : a disorder of uncertain cause that is characterized by persistent profound fatigue usu. accompanied by impairment in short-term memory or concentration, sore throat, tender lymph nodes, muscle or joint pain, and headache unrelated to any preexisting medical condition and that typically has an onset at about 30 years of age — abbr. *CFS;* called also *myalgic encephalomyelitis*

chronic granulocytic leukemia *n* : CHRONIC MYELOGENOUS LEUKEMIA

chronic granulomatous disease *n* : either of two diseases that are inherited as X-linked and autosomal traits, are characterized by recurrent infections which lead to granuloma formation at infection sites (as the skin or lungs), and result from a defect in the ability of white blood cells to destroy bacteria and fungi

chronic lymphocytic leukemia *n* : lymphocytic leukemia that is marked by an abnormal increase in the number of mature lymphocytes and esp. B cells, that is characterized by slow onset and progression, and that occurs esp. in older adults — abbr. *CLL;* compare ACUTE LYMPHOCYTIC LEUKEMIA

chronic myelogenous leukemia *n* : myelogenous leukemia that is marked by an abnormal increase in granulocytes esp. in bone marrow and blood, occurs esp. in adults, and is associated with the presence of the Philadelphia chromosome — abbr. *CML;* called also *chronic myeloid leukemia, chronic granulocytic leukemia;* compare ACUTE MYELOGENOUS LEUKEMIA

chronic obstructive pulmonary disease *n* : pulmonary disease (as emphysema or chronic bronchitis) that is characterized by chronic typically irreversible airway obstruction resulting in a slowed rate of exhalation — abbr. *COPD*

chronicum — see ERYTHEMA CHRONICUM MIGRANS

chronicus — see LICHEN SIMPLEX CHRONICUS

chronic venous insufficiency *n* : inability of the veins of the legs to return blood to the heart that is chiefly due to absence of or damage to venous valves (as from deep vein thrombosis or phlebitis) resulting in the pooling of blood in the lower legs and that is marked by edema, pain, reddened or discolored skin, varicose veins, eczema, and ulceration of the legs — called also *postphlebitic syndrome*

chro·no·bi·ol·o·gy \ˌkrä-nə-bī-ˈä-lə-jē, ˌkrō-\ *n, pl* **-gies** : the study of biological rhythms — **chro·no·bi·o·log·ic** \-ˌbī-ə-ˈlä-jik\ *or* **chro·no·bi·o·log·i·cal** \-ji-kəl\ *adj* — **chro·no·bi·ol·o·gist** \-bī-ˈä-lə-jist\ *n*

chro·no·log·i·cal age \ˌkrän-ᵊl-ˈä-ji-kəl-, ˌkrōn-\ *n* : the age of a person as measured from birth to a given date — compare ACHIEVEMENT AGE

chro·no·ther·a·py \ˌkrä-nə-ˈther-ə-pē, ˌkrō-\ *n, pl* **-pies** : treatment of a sleep disorder (as insomnia) by changing sleeping and waking times in an attempt to reset the patient's biological clock

chro·no·trop·ic \-ˈträ-pik\ *adj* : influencing the rate esp. of the heartbeat

chro·not·ro·pism \krə-ˈnä-trə-ˌpi-zəm\ *n* : interference with the rate of the heartbeat

chrys·a·ro·bin \ˌkri-sə-ˈrō-bən\ *n* : a brownish to orange-yellow powder that is obtained from the wood of a Brazilian leguminous tree (*Andira araroba*) and is used to treat skin diseases

chrys·i·a·sis \krə-ˈsī-ə-səs\ *n, pl* **-a·ses** \-ˌsēz\ : an ash-gray or mauve pigmentation of the skin due to deposition of gold in the tissues

Chrys·ops \ˈkri-ˌsäps\ *n* : a genus of small horseflies (family Tabanidae)

that includes the deerflies and mango flies

chryso·ther·a·py \ˌkri-sə-ˈther-ə-pē\ *n, pl* **-pies** : treatment (as of arthritis) by injection of gold salts

Churg–Strauss syndrome \ˈchərg-ˈstrau̇s-\ *n* : granulomatosis that typically affects the lungs but may involve other organs or tissues, is accompanied by vasculitis, eosinophilia, and asthma, and is sometimes considered to be a variant form of polyarteritis nodosa

    Churg, Jacob (*b* **1910**), and **Strauss, Lotte (1913–1985),** American pathologists.

Chvos·tek's sign \ˈvȯs-ˌteks-, ˈkvȯs-\ *or* **Chvos·tek sign** \-ˌtek-\ *n* : a twitch of the facial muscles following gentle tapping over the facial nerve in front of the ear that indicates hyperirritability of the facial nerve

    Chvostek, Franz (1835–1884), Austrian surgeon.

chyl- *or* **chyli-** *or* **chylo-** *comb form* : chyle ⟨*chyluria*⟩ ⟨*chylothorax*⟩

chyle \ˈkīl\ *n* : lymph that is milky from emulsified fats, is characteristically present in the lacteals, and is most apparent during intestinal absorption of fats

chyli — see CISTERNA CHYLI

-chylia *n comb form* : condition of having (such) chyle ⟨*achylia*⟩

chy·lo·mi·cron \ˌkī-lō-ˈmī-ˌkrän\ *n* : a lipoprotein rich in triglyceride and common in the blood during fat digestion and assimilation

chy·lo·mi·cro·nae·mia *chiefly Brit var of* CHYLOMICRONEMIA

chy·lo·mi·cro·ne·mia \-ˌmī-krə-ˈnē-mē-ə\ *n* : an excessive number of chylomicrons in the blood

chy·lo·tho·rax \-ˈthȯr-ˌaks\ *n, pl* **-rax·es** *or* **-ra·ces** \-ˈthȯr-ə-ˌsēz\ : an effusion of chyle or chylous fluid into the thoracic cavity

chy·lous \ˈkī-ləs\ *adj* : consisting of or like chyle ⟨~ ascites⟩

chy·lu·ria \kī-ˈlu̇r-ē-ə, kīl-ˈyu̇r-\ *n* : the presence of chyle in the urine as a result of organic disease (as of the kidney) or of mechanical lymphatic esp. parasitic obstruction

chyme \ˈkīm\ *n* : the semifluid mass of partly digested food expelled by the stomach into the duodenum — **chy·mous** \ˈkī-məs\ *adj*

chy·mo·pa·pa·in \ˌkī-mō-pə-ˈpā-ən, -ˈpī-ən\ *n* : a proteolytic enzyme from the latex of the papaya that is used in meat tenderizer and has been used medically in chemonucleolysis

chy·mo·tryp·sin \ˌkī-mō-ˈtrip-sən\ *n* : a protease that hydrolyzes peptide bonds and is formed in the intestine from chymotrypsinogen — **chy·mo·tryp·tic** \-ˈtrip-tik\ *adj*

chy·mo·tryp·sin·o·gen \-ˌtrip-ˈsi-nə-jən\ *n* : a zymogen that is secreted by the pancreas and is converted by trypsin to chymotrypsin

Ci·al·is \sē-'a-ləs\ *trademark* — used for a preparation of tadalafil

cic·a·trix \'si-kə-ˌtriks, sə-'kā-triks\ *n, pl* **cic·a·tri·ces** \ˌsi-kə-'trī-(ˌ)sēz, sə-'kā-trə-ˌsēz\ : a scar resulting from formation and contraction of fibrous tissue in a flesh wound — **cic·a·tri·cial** \ˌsi-kə-'tri-shəl\ *adj*

cic·a·tri·zant \ˌsi-kə-'trīz-°nt\ *adj* : promoting the healing of a wound or the formation of a cicatrix

cic·a·tri·za·tion \ˌsi-kə-trə-'zā-shən\ *n* : scar formation at the site of a healing wound — **cic·a·trize** \'si-kə-ˌtrīz\ *vb*

CICU *abbr* coronary intensive care unit

cic·u·tox·in \ˌsi-kyə-'täk-sən, 'si-kyə-ˌ\ *n* : an amorphous poisonous principle $C_{19}H_{26}O_3$ in water hemlock, spotted cowbane, and related plants

cigarette drain *n* : a cigarette-shaped gauze wick enclosed in rubber dam tissue or rubber tubing for draining wounds — called also *Penrose drain*

ci·gua·tera \ˌsē-gwə-'ter-ə, ˌsi-\ *n* : poisoning caused by the ingestion of various normally edible tropical fish in whose flesh a toxic substance has accumulated

ci·gua·tox·in \'sē-gwə-ˌtäk-sən,'si-\ *n* : a potent neurotoxin that is produced by a marine dinoflagellate (*Gambierdiscus toxicus*) and causes ciguatera poisoning in those who eat fish in which toxic levels of it have become concentrated; *also* : any of several related neurotoxins causing ciguatera

cilia *pl of* CILIUM

ciliaris — see ORBICULARIS CILIARIS, ZONULA CILIARIS

cil·i·ary \'si-lē-ˌer-ē\ *adj* **1** : of or relating to cilia **2** : of, relating to, or being the annular suspension of the lens of the eye

ciliary artery *n* : any of several arteries that arise from the ophthalmic artery or its branches and supply various parts of the eye — see LONG POSTERIOR CILIARY ARTERY, SHORT POSTERIOR CILIARY ARTERY

ciliary body *n* : an annular structure on the inner surface of the anterior wall of the eyeball composed largely of the ciliary muscle and bearing the ciliary processes

ciliary ganglion *n* : a small autonomic ganglion on the nasociliary branch of the ophthalmic nerve receiving preganglionic fibers from the oculomotor nerve and sending postganglionic fibers to the ciliary muscle and to the sphincter pupillae

ciliary muscle *n* : a circular band of smooth muscle fibers situated in the ciliary body and serving as the chief agent in accommodation when it contracts by drawing the ciliary processes centripetally and relaxing the suspensory ligament of the lens so that the lens is permitted to become more convex

ciliary nerve — see LONG CILIARY NERVE, SHORT CILIARY NERVE

ciliary process *n* : any of the vascular folds on the inner surface of the ciliary body that give attachment to the suspensory ligament of the lens

ciliary ring *n* : ORBICULUS CILIARIS

cil·i·ate \'si-lē-ət, -ˌāt\ *n* : any of a phylum or subphylum (Ciliophora) of ciliated protozoans

cil·i·at·ed \'si-lē-ˌā-təd\ *or* **ciliate** *adj* : provided with cilia

cil·io·ret·i·nal \ˌsi-lē-ō-'ret-°n-əl\ *adj* : of, relating to, or supplying the part of the eye including the ciliary body and the retina

cil·i·um \'si-lē-əm\ *n, pl* **cil·ia** \-ə\ **1** : EYELASH **2** : a minute short hairlike process often forming part of a fringe; *esp* : one of a cell that serves esp. in free unicellular organisms to produce locomotion or in higher forms a current of fluid

ci·met·i·dine \sī-'me-tə-ˌdēn\ *n* : an H_2 antagonist $C_{10}H_{16}N_6S$ that is used to inhibit gastric acid secretion in conditions in which such secretion produces duodenal or gastric ulcers or erosive lesions — see TAGAMET

ci·mex \'sī-ˌmeks\ *n* **1** *pl* **ci·mi·ces** \'sī-mə-ˌsēz, 'si-\ : BEDBUG **2** *cap* : a genus of bloodsucking bugs (family Cimicidae) that includes the common bedbug

cin- *or* **cino-** — see KIN-

cin·cho·caine \'siŋ-kə-ˌkān, 'sin-\ *chiefly Brit* : DIBUCAINE

cin·cho·na \siŋ-'kō-nə, sin-'chō-\ *n* : the dried bark of any of several trees (genus *Cinchona* of the family Rubiaceae and esp. *C. ledgeriana* and *C. succirubra*) containing alkaloids (as quinine) used esp. formerly as a specific in malaria, an antipyretic in other fevers, and a tonic and stomachic — called also *cinchona bark*

Chin·chón \chin-'chōn\, **Countess of (Doña Francisca Henríquez de Ribera)**, Spanish noblewoman.

cin·cho·nism \'siŋ-kə-ˌni-zəm, 'sin-chə-\ *n* : a disorder due to excessive or prolonged use of cinchona or its alkaloids and marked by temporary deafness, ringing in the ears, headache, dizziness, and rash

cine·an·gio·car·di·og·ra·phy \ˌsi-nē-ˌan-jē-ō-ˌkär-dē-'ä-grə-fē\ *n, pl* **-phies** : motion-picture photography of a fluoroscopic screen recording passage of a contrasting medium through the chambers of the heart and large blood vessels — **cine·an·gio·car·dio·graph·ic** \-ˌkär-dē-ə-'gra-fik\ *adj*

cine·an·gi·og·ra·phy \-ˌan-jē-'ä-grə-fē\ *n, pl* **-phies** : motion-picture photography of a fluorescent screen recording passage of a contrasting medium through the blood vessels — **cine·an·gio·graph·ic** \-jē-ə-'gra-fik\ *adj*

cine·flu·o·rog·ra·phy \-ˌflùr-'ä-grə-fē\ *n, pl* **-phies** : the process of making motion pictures of images of objects by means of X-rays with the aid of a fluorescent screen (as for revealing the motions of organs in the body) — compare CINERADIOGRAPHY — **cine-flu-o-ro-graph-ic** \-ˌflür-ə-'gra-fik\ *adj*

cin-e-ole \'si-nē-ˌōl\ *n* : EUCALYPTOL

cin-e-plas-ty \'si-nə-ˌplas-tē\ *also* **ki-ne-plas-ty** \'ki-nə-, 'ki-\ *n, pl* **-ties 1** : surgical fitting of a lever to a muscle in an amputation stump to facilitate the operation of an artificial hand **2** : surgical isolation of a loop of muscle of chest or arm, covering it with skin, and attaching to it a prosthetic device to be operated by contraction of the muscle in the loop — **cin-e-plas-tic** \ˌsi-nə-'plas-tik\ *also* **ki-ne-plas-tic** \ˌki-nə-, ˌkī-\ *adj*

cine-ra-di-og-ra-phy \ˌsi-nē-ˌrā-dē-'ä-grə-fē\ *n, pl* **-phies** : the process of making radiographs of moving objects (as the heart or joints) in sufficiently rapid sequence so that the radiographs or copies made from them may be projected as motion pictures — compare CINEFLUOROGRAPHY — **cine-ra-dio-graph-ic** \-ˌrā-dē-ō-'gra-fik\ *adj*

ci-ne-rea \sə-'nir-ē-ə\ *n* : the gray matter of nerve tissue

cinereum — see TUBER CINEREUM

cine-roent-gen-og-ra-phy \ˌsi-nē-ˌrent-gən-'ä-grə-fē\ *n, pl* **-phies** : CINERADIOGRAPHY

cin-gu-late gyrus \'siŋ-gyə-lət-, -ˌlāt-\ *n* : a medial gyrus of each cerebral hemisphere that partly surrounds the corpus callosum

cin-gu-lot-o-my \ˌsiŋ-gyə-'lä-tə-mē\ *n, pl* **-mies** : surgical destruction of all or part (as the cingulum) of the cingulate gyrus

cin-gu-lum \'siŋ-gyə-ləm\ *n, pl* **cin-gu-la** \-lə\ **1** : a ridge about the base of the crown of a tooth **2** : a tract of association fibers lying within the cingulate gyrus and connecting the callosal and hippocampal convolutions of the brain

cin-na-mon \'si-nə-mən\ *n, often attrib* **1** : any of several Asian trees (genus *Cinnamomum*) of the laurel family (Lauraceae) **2** : an aromatic spice prepared from the dried inner bark of a cinnamon (esp. *C. zeylanicum*); *also* : the bark

cino- — see KIN-

Cip-ro \'si-prō\ *trademark* — used for a preparation of ciprofloxacin

cip-ro-flox-a-cin \ˌsip-rə-'fläk-sə-sən\ *n* : a fluoroquinolone $C_{17}H_{18}FN_3O_3$ that is often administered in the form of its hydrochloride $C_{17}H_{18}FN_3O_3$·HCl and is effective esp. against gram-negative bacteria — see CIPRO

cir-ca-di-an \(ˌ)sər-'kā-dē-ən, -'kā-; ˌsər-kə-'dī-ən, -'dē-\ *adj* : being, having, characterized by, or occurring in approximately 24-hour periods or cycles (as of biological activity or function) ⟨~ rhythms in behavior⟩

cir-ci-nate \'sərs-ᵊn-ˌāt\ *adj, of lesions* : having a sharply circumscribed and somewhat circular margin

circle of Wil-lis \-'wi-ləs\ *n* : a complete ring of arteries at the base of the brain that is formed by the cerebral and communicating arteries and is a site of aneurysms

Willis, Thomas (1621–1675), British physician.

circling disease *n* : listeriosis of sheep or cattle

cir-cu-lar \'sər-kyə-lər\ *adj* : MANIC-DEPRESSIVE; *esp* : BIPOLAR 3

circulares — see PLICAE CIRCULARES

circular sinus *n* : a circular venous channel around the pituitary gland formed by the cavernous and intercavernous sinuses

cir-cu-late \'sər-kyə-ˌlāt\ *vb* **-lat-ed; -lat-ing** : to flow or be propelled naturally through a closed system of channels (as blood vessels)

circulating nurse *n* : a registered nurse who makes preparations for an operation and continually monitors patient and staff during its course and who works outside the sterile field in which the operation takes place

cir-cu-la-tion \ˌsər-kyə-'lā-shən\ *n* : the movement of blood through the vessels of the body that is induced by the pumping action of the heart and serves to distribute nutrients and oxygen to and remove waste products from all parts of the body — see PULMONARY CIRCULATION, SYSTEMIC CIRCULATION

cir-cu-la-to-ry \'sər-kyə-lə-ˌtōr-ē\ *adj* : of or relating to circulation or the circulatory system ⟨~ failure⟩

circulatory system *n* : the system of blood, blood vessels, lymphatics, and heart concerned with the circulation of blood and lymph

cir-cu-lus \'sər-kyə-ləs\ *n, pl* **-li** \-ˌlī\ : an anatomical circle or ring esp. of veins or arteries

cir-cum-cise \'sər-kəm-ˌsīz\ *vb* **-cised; -cis-ing** : to cut off the foreskin of (a male) or the clitoris of (a female) — **cir-cum-cis-er** *n*

cir-cum-ci-sion \ˌsər-kəm-'si-zhən\ *n* **1 a** : the act of circumcising; *esp* : the cutting off of the foreskin of males that is practiced as a religious rite by Jews and Muslims and as a sanitary measure in modern surgery **b** : FEMALE GENITAL MUTILATION **2** : the condition of being circumcised

cir-cum-cor-ne-al injection \ˌsir-kəm-'kȯr-nē-əl-\ *n* : enlargement of the ciliary and conjunctival blood vessels near the margin of the cornea with reduction in size peripherally

cir-cum-duc-tion \ˌsər-kəm-'dək-shən\ *n* : movement of a limb or extremity so that the distal end describes a circle while the proximal end remains fixed — **cir-cum-duct** \-'dəkt\ *vb*

cir·cum·flex \'sər-kəm-ˌfleks\ *adj, of nerves and blood vessels* : bending around

circumflex artery *n* : any of several paired curving arteries: as **a** : either of two arteries that branch from the deep femoral artery or from the femoral artery itself: (1) : LATERAL FEMORAL CIRCUMFLEX ARTERY (2) : MEDIAL FEMORAL CIRCUMFLEX ARTERY **b** : either of two branches of the axillary artery that wind around the neck of the humerus: (1) : ANTERIOR HUMERAL CIRCUMFLEX ARTERY (2) : POSTERIOR HUMERAL CIRCUMFLEX ARTERY **c** : CIRCUMFLEX ILIAC ARTERY **d** : a branch of the subscapular artery supplying the muscles of the shoulder

circumflex iliac artery *n* : either of two arteries arching anteriorly near the inguinal ligament: **a** : an artery lying internal to the iliac crest and arising from the external iliac artery **b** : a more superficially located artery that is a branch of the femoral artery

circumflex nerve *n* : AXILLARY NERVE

cir·cum·oral \ˌsər-kəm-ˈōr-əl, -ˈär-\ *adj* : surrounding the mouth 〈~ pallor〉

cir·cum·scribed \'sər-kəm-ˌskrībd\ *adj* : confined to a limited area 〈~ patches of hair loss〉

cir·cum·stan·ti·al·i·ty \ˌsər-kəm-ˌstan-chē-ˈa-lə-tē\ *n, pl* **-ties** : a conversational pattern (as in some manic states) exhibiting excessive attention to irrelevant and digressive details

cir·cum·val·late \ˌsər-kəm-ˈva-ˌlāt, -lət\ *adj* : enclosed by a ridge of tissue

circumvallate papilla *n* : any of the usu. 8 to 12 large papillae near the back of the tongue each of which is surrounded with a marginal sulcus and supplied with taste buds responsive esp. to bitter flavors — called also *vallate papilla*

cir·rho·sis \sə-ˈrō-səs\ *n, pl* **-rho·ses** \-ˌsēz\ : widespread disruption of normal liver structure by fibrosis and the formation of regenerative nodules that is caused by any of various chronic progressive conditions affecting the liver (as long-term alcohol abuse or hepatitis) — see BILIARY CIRRHOSIS

¹**cir·rhot·ic** \sə-ˈrä-tik\ *adj* : of, relating to, caused by, or affected with cirrhosis 〈~ degeneration〉 〈a ~ liver〉

²**cirrhotic** *n* : an individual affected with cirrhosis

cirs- *or* **cirso-** *comb form* : swollen vein : varix 〈cirsoid〉

cir·soid \'sər-ˌsȯid\ *adj* : resembling a dilated tortuous vein 〈~ aneurysms〉

CIS *abbr* carcinoma in situ

cis·plat·in \'sis-ˈplat-ᵊn\ *n* : a platinum-containing antineoplastic drug $Cl_2H_6N_2Pt$ used esp. as a palliative therapy in testicular and ovarian tumors and in advanced bladder cancer — see PLATINOL

cis–platinum \-ˈplat-ᵊn-əm\ *n* : CISPLATIN

13–cis–retinoic acid *n* : ISOTRETINOIN

cis·ter·na \sis-ˈtər-nə\ *n, pl* **-nae** \-ˌnē\ : a fluid-containing sac or cavity in an organism: as **a** : CISTERNA MAGNA **b** : CISTERNA CHYLI

cisterna chy·li \-ˈkī-ˌlī\ *n, pl* **cisternae chyli** : a dilated lymph channel usu. opposite the first and second lumbar vertebrae and marking the beginning of the thoracic duct

cis·ter·nal \(ˌ)sis-ˈtərn-ᵊl\ *adj* : of or relating to a cisterna and esp. the cisterna magna — **cis·ter·nal·ly** *adv*

cisterna mag·na \-ˈmag-nə\ *n, pl* **cisternae mag·nae** \-ˌnē\ : a large subarachnoid space between the caudal part of the cerebellum and the medulla oblongata

cis·ter·nog·ra·phy \ˌsis-(ˌ)tər-ˈnä-grə-fē\ *n, pl* **-phies** : radiographic visualization of the subarachnoid spaces containing cerebrospinal fluid following injection of an opaque contrast medium

cis·tron \'sis-ˌträn\ *n* : a segment of DNA that is equivalent to a gene and that specifies a single functional unit (as a protein or enzyme) — **cis·tron·ic** \sis-ˈträ-nik\ *adj*

ci·tal·o·pram \sī-ˈta-lə-ˌpram\ *n* : a drug that functions as an SSRI and is administered orally in the form of its hydrobromide $C_{20}H_{21}FN_2O·HBr$ to treat depression and anxiety — see CELEXA

cit·rate \'si-ˌtrāt\ *n* : a salt or ester of citric acid

cit·rat·ed \'si-ˌtrā-təd\ *adj* : treated with a citrate esp. of sodium or potassium to prevent coagulation 〈~ blood〉

cit·ric acid \'si-trik-\ *n* : a sour organic acid $C_6H_8O_7$ occurring in cellular metabolism, obtained esp. from lemon and lime juices or by fermentation of sugars, and used as a flavoring

citric acid cycle *n* : KREBS CYCLE

ci·tri·nin \si-ˈtrī-nən\ *n* : a toxic antibiotic $C_{13}H_{14}O_5$ that is produced esp. by two molds of the genus *Penicillium* (*P. citrinum*) and the genus *Aspergillus* (*A. niveus*) and is effective against some gram-positive bacteria

ci·trov·o·rum factor \sə-ˈträ-və-rəm-\ *n* : LEUCOVORIN

cit·rul·line \'si-trə-ˌlēn; si-ˈtrə-ˌlēn, -lən\ *n* : a crystalline amino acid $C_6H_{13}N_3O_3$ formed esp. as an intermediate in the conversion of ornithine to arginine in the living system

cit·rul·lin·ae·mia *chiefly Brit var of* CITRULLINEMIA

cit·rul·lin·emia \ˌsi-trə-lə-ˈnē-mē-ə, si-ˌtrə-lə-ˈnē-\ *n* : an inherited disorder of amino acid metabolism marked by excess amounts of citrulline in the blood, urine, and cerebrospinal fluid and ammonia intoxication

cit·rus \'si-trəs\ *n, often attrib* : any of a group of trees and shrubs (*Citrus* and related genera) of the rue family (Rutaceae) grown in warm regions for their edible fruit (as the orange or lemon); *also* : the fruit

CJD *abbr* Creutzfeldt-Jakob disease

CK *abbr* creatine kinase

cl *abbr* centiliter

Cl *symbol* chlorine

CLA *abbr* certified laboratory assistant

clair·voy·ance \klar-'vȯi-əns, kler-\ : the power or faculty of discerning objects or matters not present to the senses — **clair·voy·ant** \-ənt\ *adj or n*

clam·my \'kla-mē\ *adj* **clam·mi·er; -est** : being moist and sticky ⟨~ hands⟩

clamp \'klamp\ *n* : any of various instruments or appliances having parts brought together for holding or compressing something; *esp* : an instrument used to hold, compress, or crush vessels and hollow organs and to aid in surgical excision of parts ⟨an arterial ~⟩ — **clamp** *vb*

clang association *n* : word association based on similar sound rather than meaning

clap \'klap\ *n* : GONORRHEA — often used with *the*

Clar·i·nex \'klar-ə-,neks\ *trademark* — used for a preparation of desloratadine

cla·rith·ro·my·cin \klə-,rith-rə-'mī-sᵊn\ *n* : a semisynthetic macrolide antibiotic $C_{38}H_{69}NO_{13}$ used esp. in the treatment of various respiratory tract infections

Clar·i·tin \'klar-ə-,tin\ *trademark* — used for a preparation of loratadine

clasp \'klasp\ *n* : a device designed to encircle a tooth to hold a denture in place

class \'klas\ *n* : a major category in biological taxonomy ranking above the order and below the phylum

clas·sic \'kla-sik\ *or* **clas·si·cal** \-si-kəl\ *adj* : standard or recognized esp. because of great frequency or consistency of occurrence ⟨the ~ symptoms of a disease⟩

classical conditioning *n* : conditioning in which the conditioned stimulus (as the sound of a bell) is paired with and precedes the unconditioned stimulus (as the sight of food) until the conditioned stimulus alone is sufficient to elicit the response (as salivation in a dog) — compare OPERANT CONDITIONING

clau·di·ca·tion \,klȯ-də-'kā-shən\ *n* : the quality or state of being lame 2 : INTERMITTENT CLAUDICATION

claus·tro·phobe \'klȯ-strə-,fōb\ *n* : one affected with claustrophobia

claus·tro·pho·bia \,klȯ-strə-'fō-bē-ə\ *n* : abnormal dread of being in closed or narrow spaces

¹claus·tro·pho·bic \,klȯ-strə-'fō-bik\ *adj* 1 : suffering from or inclined to claustrophobia 2 : inducing or suggesting claustrophobia — **claus·tro·pho·bi·cal·ly** \-bi-k(ə-)lē\ *adv*

²claustrophobic *n* : CLAUSTROPHOBE

claus·trum \'klȯ-strəm, 'klaů-\ *n, pl* **claus·tra** \-strə\ : the one of the four basal ganglia in each cerebral hemisphere that consists of a thin lamina of gray matter between the lentiform nucleus and the insula

clav·i·cle \'kla-vi-kəl\ *n* : a bone of the pectoral girdle that links the scapula and sternum, is situated just above the first rib on either side of the neck, and has the form of a narrow elongated S — called also *collarbone* — **cla·vic·u·lar** \kla-'vi-kyə-lər, klə-\ *adj*

clavicular notch *n* : a notch on each side of the upper part of the manubrium that is the site of articulation with a clavicle

cla·vi·cu·lec·to·my \kla-,vi-kyə-'lek-tə-mē, klə-\ *n, pl* **-mies** : surgical removal of all or part of a clavicle

clav·u·lan·ic acid \,klav-yə-,la-nik-\ *n* : a beta-lactam antibiotic $C_8H_9NO_5$ produced by a bacterium of the genus *Streptomyces* (*S. clavuligerus*) — see AUGMENTIN

cla·vus \'klā-vəs, 'klä-\ *n, pl* **cla·vi** \'klā-,vī, 'klä-,vē\ : CORN

claw foot *n* : a deformity of the foot characterized by an exaggerated curvature of the longitudinal arch

claw hand *n* : a deformity of the hand characterized by extreme extension of the wrist and the first phalanges and extreme flexion of the other phalanges

claw toe *n* : HAMMERTOE

¹clean \'klēn\ *adj* **1 a** : free from dirt or pollution **b** : free from disease or infectious agents **2** : free from drug addiction

²clean *vb* **1** : to brush (the teeth) with a cleanser (as a dentifrice) **2** : to perform dental prophylaxis on (the teeth)

¹clear \'klir\ *adj* **1** *of the skin or complexion* : good in texture and color and without blemish or discoloration **2** : free from abnormal sounds on auscultation

²clear *vb* : to rid (the throat) of phlegm or of something that makes the voice indistinct or husky

clear·ance \'klir-əns\ *n* : the volume of blood or plasma that could be freed of a specified constituent in a specified time (usu. one minute) by excretion of the constituent into the urine through the kidneys — called also *renal clearance*

cleav·age \'klē-vij\ *n* **1** : the series of synchronized mitotic cell divisions of the fertilized egg that results in the formation of the blastomeres and changes the single-celled zygote into a multicellular embryo; *also* : one of these cell divisions **2** : the splitting of a molecule into simpler molecules — **cleave** \'klēv\ *vb*

cleavage cell *n* : BLASTOMERE

cleft \'kleft\ *n* **1** : a usu. abnormal fissure or opening esp. when resulting from failure of parts to fuse during embryonic development **2 a** : a V-shaped indented formation : a hollow between ridges or protuberances **3** : SYNAPTIC CLEFT

cleft lip *n* : a birth defect characterized by one or more clefts in the upper lip resulting from failure of the embryonic parts of the lip to unite — called also *cheiloschisis*

cleft palate *n* : congenital fissure of the roof of the mouth produced by failure of the two maxillae to unite during embryonic development and often associated with cleft lip

cleid- *or* **cleido-** *comb form* : clavicular : clavicular and ⟨*cleido*cranial⟩

clei·do·cra·ni·al dysostosis \,klī-dō-'krā-nē-əl-\ *n* : a rare condition inherited as an autosomal dominant trait and characterized esp. by partial or complete absence of the clavicles, defective ossification of the skull, and faulty occlusion due to missing, misplaced, or supernumerary teeth

clem·as·tine \'kle-mə-,stēn\ *n* : an antihistamine administered in the form of its fumarate $C_{21}H_{26}ClNO·C_4H_4O_4$

cle·oid \'klē-,ȯid\ *n* : a dental excavator with a claw-shaped working point

clerk \'klǝrk\ *n* : a third- or fourth-year medical student undergoing clinical training in a clerkship — **clerk** *vb*

clerk·ship \'klǝrk-,ship\ *n* : a course of clinical medical training in a specialty that usu. lasts a minimum of several weeks and takes place during the third or fourth year of medical school

click \'klik\ *n* : a short sharp sound heard in auscultation and associated with various heart abnormalities

cli·mac·ter·ic \klī-'mak-tə-rik, ,klī-,mak-'ter-ik\ *n* **1** : MENOPAUSE 1a(2) **2** : ANDROPAUSE — **climacteric** *adj*

cli·mac·te·ri·um \,klī-,mak-'tir-ē-əm\ *n, pl* **-ria** \-ē-ə\ : the bodily and mental involutional changes accompanying the transition from middle life to old age; *specif* : menopause and the bodily and psychological changes that accompany it

cli·mac·tic \klī-'mak-tik\ *adj* : of, relating to, or constituting a climax

cli·ma·to·ther·a·py \,klī-mə-tō-'ther-ə-pē\ *n, pl* **-pies** : treatment of disease by means of residence in a suitable climate

cli·max \'klī-,maks\ *n* **1** : the highest or most intense point **2** : ORGASM **3 a** : MENOPAUSE 1a(2) **b** : ANDROPAUSE

clin *abbr* clinical

clin·da·my·cin \,klin-də-'mī-sən\ *n* : an antibiotic $C_{18}H_{33}ClN_2O_5S$ derived from and used similarly to lincomycin

clin·ic \'kli-nik\ *n* **1 a** : a session or class of medical instruction in a hospital held at the bedside of patients serving as case studies **b** : a group of selected patients presented with discussion before doctors for purposes of instruction **2 a** : an institution connected with a hospital or medical school where diagnosis and treatment are made available to outpatients **b** : a form of group practice in which several physicians (as specialists) work in cooperative association

clin·i·cal \'kli-ni-kəl\ *adj* : of, relating to, or conducted in or as if in a clinic: as **a** : involving or concerned with the direct observation of living patients ⟨a full-time ~ practice⟩ **b** : of, relating to, based on, or characterized by observable or diagnosable symptoms of disease ⟨~ tuberculosis⟩ ⟨the ~ presentation of Lyme disease⟩ **c** : applying objective or standardized methods (as interviews and personality tests) to the description, evaluation, and modification of human behavior ⟨~ psychology⟩ — **clin·i·cal·ly** \-k(ə-)lē\ *adv*

clinical crown *n* : the part of a tooth that projects above the gums

clinical depression *n* : depression of sufficient severity to be brought to the attention of a physician and to require treatment; *specif* : MAJOR DEPRESSIVE DISORDER

clinical thermometer *n* : a thermometer for measuring body temperature that has a constriction in the tube above the bulb preventing movement of the column of liquid downward once it has reached its maxium temperature so that it continues to indicate the maximum temperature until the liquid is shaken back down into the bulb — called also *fever thermometer*

clinical trial *n* : a scientifically controlled study of the safety and effectiveness of a therapeutic agent (as a drug or vaccine) using consenting human subjects

cli·ni·cian \kli-'ni-shən\ *n* : one qualified in the clinical practice of medicine, psychiatry, or psychology

clinico- *comb form* : clinical : clinical and ⟨*clinico*pathologic⟩

clin·i·co·path·o·log·ic \,kli-ni-(,)kō-,pa-thə-'lä-jik\ *or* **clin·i·co·path·o·log·i·cal** \-'lä-ji-kəl\ *adj* : relating to or concerned both with the signs and symptoms directly observable by the physician and with the results of laboratory examination ⟨a ~ study of the patient⟩ — **clin·i·co·path·o·log·i·cal·ly** \-ji-k(ə-)lē\ *adv*

cli·no·dac·ty·ly \,klī-nō-'dak-tə-lē\ *n, pl* **-ty·lies** : a deformity of the hand marked by deviation or deflection of the fingers

cli·noid process \'klī-,nȯid-\ *n* : any of several processes of the sphenoid bone

clip \'klip\ *n* : a device used to arrest bleeding from vessels or tissues during operations

clitorid- *or* **clitorido-** *comb form* : clitoris ⟨*clitorid*ectomy⟩

clit·o·ri·dec·to·my \ˌkli-tə-rə-'dek-tə-mē\ *also* **clit·o·rec·to·my** \-'rek-tə-mē\ *n, pl* **-mies** : excision of all or part of the clitoris

clitoridis — see PREPUTIUM CLITORIDIS

cli·to·ris \'kli-tə-rəs, kli-'tòr-əs\ *n, pl* **cli·to·ri·des** \kli-'tòr-ə-ˌdēz\ : a small erectile organ at the anterior or ventral part of the vulva homologous to the penis — **cli·to·ral** \'kli-tə-rəl\ *also* **cli·tor·ic** \kli-'tòr-ik, -'tär-\ *adj*

cli·vus \'klī-vəs\ *n, pl* **cli·vi** \-ˌvī\ : the smooth sloping surface on the upper posterior part of the body of the sphenoid bone supporting the pons and the basilar artery

CLL *abbr* chronic lymphocytic leukemia

clo·a·ca \klō-'ā-kə\ *n, pl* **-acae** \-ˌkē, -ˌsē\ **1** : the terminal part of the embryonic hindgut of a mammal before it divides into rectum, bladder, and genital precursors **2** : a passage in a bone leading to a cavity containing a sequestrum — **clo·a·cal** \-kəl\ *adj*

cloacal membrane *n* : a plate of fused embryonic ectoderm and endoderm closing the fetal anus

clo·a·ci·tis \ˌklō-ə-'sī-təs\ *n* : a chronic inflammatory process of the cloaca of the domestic chicken — called also *vent gleet*

clo·be·ta·sol \klō-'bā-tə-ˌsòl\ *n* : a potent synthetic corticosteroid that is used topically in the form of its propionate $C_{25}H_{32}ClFO_5$ esp. to treat inflammatory skin conditions

clock \'kläk\ *n* : BIOLOGICAL CLOCK

clo·faz·i·mine \klō-'faz-ə-ˌmēn\ *n* : a reddish brown powdered dye $C_{27}H_{22}Cl_2N_4$ that is used esp. to treat lepromatous leprosy

clo·fi·brate \klō-'fī-ˌbrāt, -'fi-\ *n* : a synthetic drug $C_{12}H_{15}ClO_3$ used esp. to lower abnormally high concentrations of fats and cholesterol in the blood

Clo·mid \'klō-mid\ *trademark* — used for a preparation of the citrate of clomiphene

clo·mi·phene \'klä-mə-ˌfēn, 'klō-\ *n* : a synthetic drug used in the form of its citrate $C_{26}H_{28}ClNO·C_6H_8O_7$ to induce ovulation

clo·mip·ra·mine \klō-'mi-prə-ˌmēn\ *n* : a tricyclic antidepressant used in the form of its hydrochloride $C_{19}H_{23}-ClN_2·HCl$ to treat obsessive-compulsive disorder

clo·naz·e·pam \(ˌ)klō-'na-zə-ˌpam\ *n* : a benzodiazepine $C_{15}H_{10}ClN_3O_3$ used esp. as an anticonvulsant in the treatment of epilepsy

clone \'klōn\ *n* **1** : the aggregate of genetically identical cells or organisms asexually produced by a single progenitor cell or organism **2** : an individual grown from a single somatic cell or cell nucleus and genetically identical to it **3** : a group of replicas of all or part of a macromolecule and

esp. DNA — **clon·al** \'klōn-ᵊl\ *adj* — **clon·al·ly** *adv* — **clone** *vb*

clon·ic \'klä-nik\ *adj* : exhibiting, relating to, or involving clonus ⟨~ contraction⟩ ⟨~ spasm⟩ — **clo·nic·i·ty** \klō-'ni-sə-tē, klä-\ *n*

clo·ni·dine \'klä-nə-ˌdēn, 'klō-, -ˌdin\ *n* : an antihypertensive drug used in the form of its hydrochloride $C_9H_9-Cl_2N_3·HCl$ esp. to treat essential hypertension, to prevent migraine headache, and to diminish opiate withdrawal symptoms

clo·nor·chi·a·sis \ˌklō-nòr-'kī-ə-səs\ *n, pl* **-a·ses** \-ˌsēz\ : infestation with or disease caused by the Chinese liver fluke (*Clonorchis sinensis*) that invades bile ducts of the liver after ingestion in uncooked fish and when present in numbers causes severe systemic reactions including edema, liver enlargement, and diarrhea

Clo·nor·chis \klō-'nòr-kəs\ *n* : a genus of trematode worms (family Opisthorchiidae) that includes the Chinese liver fluke (*C. sinensis*)

clo·nus \'klō-nəs\ *n* : a series of alternating contractions and partial relaxations of a muscle that in some nervous diseases occurs in the form of convulsive spasms — compare TONUS 2

clo·pid·o·grel \klō-'pi-də-ˌgrel\ *n* : an antithrombotic agent that is administered in the form of its bisulfate $C_{16}H_{16}ClNO_2S·H_2SO_4$ and inhibits ADP-induced aggregation of platelets — see PLAVIX

clor·az·e·pate \ˌklòr-'a-zə-ˌpāt\ *n* : a benzodiazepine $C_{16}H_{10}ClN_2O_3·KOH$ taken orally to treat anxiety, partial seizures, and acute alcohol withdrawal — called also *clorazepate dipotassium*; see TRANXENE

closed \'klōzd\ *adj* **1** : covered by unbroken skin ⟨a ~ fracture⟩ **2** : not discharging pathogenic organisms to the outside ⟨a case of ~ tuberculosis⟩ — compare OPEN 1c

closed-angle glaucoma *n* : ANGLE-CLOSURE GLAUCOMA

closed reduction *n* : the reduction of a displaced part (as a fractured bone) by manipulation without incision — compare OPEN REDUCTION

clos·trid·i·um \kläs-'tri-dē-əm\ *n* **1** *cap* : a genus of saprophytic mostly anaerobic bacteria (family Bacillaceae) that are commonly found in soil and in the intestinal tracts of humans and animals and that include important pathogens — see BLACK-LEG, BOTULISM, GAS GANGRENE, TETANUS BACILLUS; compare LIMBERNECK **2** *pl* **clos·trid·ia** \-dē-ə\ **a** : any bacterium of the genus *Clostridium* **b** : a spindle-shaped or ovoid bacterial cell; *esp* : one swollen at the center by an endospore — **clos·trid·i·al** \-dē-əl\ *adj*

clo·sure \'klō-zhər\ *n* **1 a** : an act of closing up or condition of being closed up **b** : a drawing together of edges or parts to form a united integument **2** : the perception of incomplete figures or situations as though complete by ignoring the missing parts or by compensating for them by projection based on past experience **3** : an often comforting or satisfying sense of finality

¹**clot** \'klät\ *n* : a coagulated mass produced by clotting of blood

²**clot** *vb* **clot·ted; clot·ting** : to undergo a sequence of reactions that results in conversion of fluid blood into a coagulum and that involves shedding of blood, release of thromboplastin, inactivation of heparin, conversion of prothrombin to thrombin, interaction of thrombin with fibrinogen to form an insoluble fibrin network, and contraction of the network to squeeze out excess fluid : COAGULATE

clot–bust·er \'klät-ˌbəs-tər\ *n* : a drug (as streptokinase or tissue plasminogen activator) used to dissolve blood clots — **clot–bust·ing** \-tiŋ\ *adj*

clot retraction *n* : the process by which a blood clot becomes smaller and draws the edges of a broken blood vessel together and which involves the shortening of fibrin threads and the squeezing out of excess serum

clo·tri·ma·zole \klō-'trī-mə-ˌzōl, -ˌzōl\ *n* : an antifungal agent $C_{22}H_{17}ClN_2$ used to treat candida infections, tinea, and ringworm — see LOTRIMIN

clotting factor *n* : any of several plasma components (as fibrinogen, prothrombin, and thromboplastin) that are involved in the clotting of blood — see FACTOR VIII, PLASMA THROMBOPLASTIN ANTECEDENT, TRANSGLUTAMINASE; compare FACTOR V, FACTOR VII, FACTOR IX, FACTOR X, FACTOR XII, FACTOR XIII

clove oil \'klōv-\ *n* : a colorless to pale yellow essential oil that is obtained from the dried aromatic flower buds of a tropical tree (*Syzygium aromaticum*) of the myrtle family (Myrtaceae) and is a source of eugenol, has a powerful germicidal action, and is used topically to relieve toothache

cloverleaf skull *n* : a birth defect in which some or all of the usu. separate bones of the skull have grown together resulting in a 3-lobed skull with associated deformities of the features and skeleton

clox·a·cil·lin \ˌkläk-sə-'si-lən\ *n* : a semisynthetic oral penicillin $C_{19}H_{17}-ClN_3NaO_5S$ effective esp. against staphylococci which secrete beta-lactamase — see TEGOPEN

clo·za·pine \'klō-zə-ˌpēn\ *n* : an antipsychotic drug $C_{18}H_{19}ClN_4$ with serious side effects that is used in the management of severe schizophrenia — see CLOZARIL

Clo·za·ril \'klō-zə-ril\ *trademark* — used for a preparation of clozapine

clubbed \'kləbd\ *adj* **1** : having a bulbous enlargement of the tip with convex overhanging nail ⟨a ∼ finger⟩ **2** : affected with clubfoot — **club·bing** \'klə-biŋ\ *n*

club·foot \'kləb-ˌfůt\ *n, pl* **club·feet** \-ˌfēt\ **1** : any of numerous congenital deformities of the foot in which it is twisted out of position or shape — called also *talipes*; compare TALIPES EQUINOVARUS, TALIPES EQUINUS, TALIPES VALGUS, TALIPES VARUS **2** : a foot affected with clubfoot — **club·foot·ed** \-ˌfů-təd\ *adj*

club·hand \ˌhand\ *n* **1** : a congenital deformity in which the hand is short and distorted **2** : a hand affected with clubhand

clump \'kləmp\ *n* : a clustered mass of particles (as cells) — compare AGGLUTINATION — **clump** *vb*

clus·ter \'klə-stər\ *n* : a larger than expected number of cases of disease occurring in a particular locality, group of people, or period of time

cluster headache *n* : a headache that is characterized by severe unilateral pain in the eye or temple, affects primarily men, and tends to recur in a series of attacks

clut·ter·ing \'klə-tə-riŋ\ *n* : a speech defect in which phonetic units are dropped, condensed, or otherwise distorted as a result of overly rapid agitated utterance

Clut·ton's joints \'klət-ᵊnz-\ *n pl* : symmetrical hydrarthrosis esp. of the knees or elbows that occurs in congenital syphilis

  Clut·ton \'klət-ᵊn\, **Henry Hugh (1850–1909)**, British surgeon.

cly·sis \'klī-səs\ *n, pl* **cly·ses** \-ˌsēz\ : the introduction of large amounts of fluid into the body usu. by parenteral injection to replace that lost (as from hemorrhage or in dysentery or burns), to provide nutrients, or to maintain blood pressure — see HYPODERMOCLYSIS, PROCTOCLYSIS

clys·ter \'klis-tər\ *n* : ENEMA

cm *abbr* centimeter

Cm *symbol* curium

CMA *abbr* certified medical assistant

CMHC *abbr* Community Mental Health Center

CML *abbr* chronic myelogenous leukemia; chronic myeloid leukemia

CMV *abbr* cytomegalovirus

CNA *abbr* certified nurse's aid

cne·mi·al \'nē-mē-əl\ *adj* : relating to the shin or shinbone

cne·mis \'nē-məs\ *n, pl* **cnem·i·des** \'ne-mə-ˌdēz\ : SHIN, TIBIA

cni·dar·i·an \nī-'dar-ē-ən\ *n* : COELENTERATE — **cnidarian** *adj*

CNM *abbr* certified nurse-midwife

CNS *abbr* central nervous system

Co *symbol* cobalt

c/o *abbr* complains of

co·ad·min·is·tra·tion \ˌkō-əd-ˌmi-nə-'strā-shən\ *n* : the administration of two or more drugs together — **co·ad·min·is·ter** \-'mi-nə-stər\ *vb*

co·ag·u·lant \kō-'a-gyə-lənt\ *n* : something that produces coagulation

co·ag·u·lase \kō-'a-gyə-ˌlās, -ˌlāz\ *n* : any of several enzymes that cause coagulation (as of blood)

¹**co·ag·u·late** \kō-'a-gyə-ˌlāt\ *vb* **-lat·ed; -lat·ing 1** : to become or cause to become viscous or thickened into a coherent mass : CLOT **2** : to subject to coagulation — **co·ag·u·la·bil·i·ty** \kō-ˌa-gyə-lə-'bi-lə-tē\ *n* — **co·ag·u·la·ble** \-'a-gyə-lə-bəl\ *adj*

²**co·ag·u·late** \-lət, -ˌlāt\ *n* : COAGULUM

co·ag·u·la·tion \kō-ˌa-gyə-'lā-shən\ *n* **1 a** : a change to a viscous, jellylike, or solid state; *esp* : a change from a liquid to a thickened curdlike state not by evaporation but by chemical reaction **b** : the process by which such change of state takes place consisting of the alteration of a soluble substance (as protein) into an insoluble form or of the flocculation or separation of colloidal or suspended matter **2** : a substance or body formed by coagulation : COAGULUM **3** : disruption of tissue by physical means (as by application of an electric current) so that denaturation and clumping of protein occur

coagulation time *n* : the time required by shed blood to clot that is a measure of the normality of the blood

co·ag·u·lop·a·thy \kō-ˌa-gyə-'lä-pə-thē\ *n, pl* **-thies** : a disease or condition affecting the blood's ability to coagulate

co·ag·u·lum \kō-'a-gyə-ləm\ *n, pl* **-u·la** \-lə\ *or* **-u·lums** : a coagulated mass or substance : CLOT

coal tar *n* : tar obtained by distillation of bituminous coal and used in the treatment of some skin diseases by direct local application to the skin

co·apt \kō-'apt\ *vb* : to close or fasten together : cause to adhere — **co·ap·ta·tion** \(ˌ)kō-ˌap-'tā-shən\ *n*

co·arct \kō-'ärkt\ *vb* : to cause (the aorta) to become narrow or (the heart) to constrict

co·arc·ta·tion \(ˌ)kō-ˌärk-'tā-shən\ *n* : a stricture or narrowing esp. of a canal or vessel (as the aorta)

coarse \'kōrs\ *adj* **1** : visible to the naked eye or by means of a compound microscope **2** *of a tremor* : of wide excursion **3** : harsh, raucous, or rough in tone — used of some sounds heard in auscultation in pathological states of the chest (∼ rales)

coat \'kōt\ *n* **1** : the external growth on an animal **2** : a layer of one substance covering or lining another; *esp* : one covering or lining an organ

coat·ed \'kō-təd\ *adj, of the tongue* : covered with a whitish or yellowish deposit of desquamated cells, bacteria, and debris

Coats's disease \'kōts, 'kōt-səz-\ *n* : a chronic inflammatory disease of the eye that is characterized by white or yellow areas around the optic disk due to edematous accumulation under the retina and that leads to destruction of the macula and to blindness

Coats \'kōts\, **George (1876–1915)**, British ophthalmologist.

co·bal·a·min \kō-'ba-lə-mən\ *n* : VITAMIN B₁₂

co·balt \'kō-ˌbȯlt\ *n* : a tough lustrous silver-white magnetic metallic element — symbol *Co*; see ELEMENT table

cobalt 60 *n* : a heavy radioactive isotope of cobalt having the mass number 60 and used as a source of gamma rays esp. in place of radium (as in the treatment of cancer and in radiography) — called also *radiocobalt*

co·bra \'kō-brə\ *n* **1** : any of several venomous Asian and African elapid snakes (genera *Naja* and *Ophiophagus*) **2** : RINGHALS **3** : MAMBA

COC *abbr* combination oral contraceptive; combined oral contraceptive

co·ca \'kō-kə\ *n* **1** : any of several So. American shrubs (genus *Erythroxylon* of the family Erythroxylaceae); *esp* : one (*E. coca*) that is the primary source of cocaine **2** : dried leaves of a coca (as *Erythroxylon coca*) containing alkaloids including cocaine

co·caine \kō-'kān, 'kō-\ *n* : a bitter crystalline alkaloid $C_{17}H_{21}NO_4$ obtained from coca leaves that is used medically esp. in the form of its hydrochloride $C_{17}H_{21}NO_4 \cdot HCl$ as a topical anesthetic and illicitly for its euphoric effects and that may result in a compulsive psychological need

co·cain·ize \kō-'kā-ˌnīz\ *vb* **-ized; -izing** : to treat or anesthetize with cocaine — **co·cain·i·za·tion** \-ˌkā-nə-'zā-shən\ *n*

co·car·cin·o·gen \ˌkō-kär-'si-nə-jən, kō-'kärs-ᵊn-ə-jen\ *n* : an agent that aggravates the carcinogenic effects of another substance — **co·car·cin·o·gen·ic** \ˌkō-ˌkärs-ᵊn-ō-'je-nik\ *adj*

coc·cal \'kä-kəl\ *adj* : of or relating to a coccus

cocci *pl of* COCCUS

coc·cid·ia \käk-'si-dē-ə\ *n pl* : sporozoans of an order (Coccidia) parasitic in the digestive epithelium of vertebrates and including several forms of economic importance — compare CRYPTOSPORIDIUM, EIMERIA, ISOSPORA — **coc·cid·i·an** \-dē-ən\ *adj or n*

Coc·cid·i·oi·des \käk-ˌsi-dē-'ȯi-ˌdēz\ *n* : a genus of imperfect fungi including one (*C. immitis*) causing coccidioidomycosis

coc·cid·i·oi·din \-'ȯid-ᵊn, -'ȯi-ˌdin\ *n* : an antigen prepared from a fungus of the genus *Coccidioides* (*C. immitis*) and used to detect skin sensitivity to and, by inference, infection with this organism

coc·cid·i·oi·do·my·co·sis \-ˌȯi-dō-(ˌ)mī-kō-səs\ *n, pl* **-co·ses** \-ˌsēz\ : a disease of humans and domestic animals caused by a fungus of the genus *Coccidioides* (*C. immitis*) and marked esp. by fever and localized pulmonary symptoms — called also *San Joaquin fever, San Joaquin valley fever, valley fever*

coc·cid·io·my·co·sis \(ˌ)käk-ˌsi-dē-ō-(ˌ)mī-ˈkō-səs\ *n, pl* **-co·ses** \-ˌsēz\ : COCCIDIOIDOMYCOSIS

coc·cid·i·o·sis \(ˌ)käk-ˌsi-dē-ˈō-səs\ *n, pl* **-o·ses** \-ˌsēz\ : infestation with or disease caused by coccidia

coc·cid·io·stat \(ˌ)käk-ˈsi-dē-ō-ˌstat\ *n* : a chemical agent added to animal feed (as for poultry) that serves to retard the life cycle or reduce the population of a pathogenic coccidium to the point that disease is minimized and the host develops immunity

coc·co·ba·cil·lus \ˌkä-(ˌ)kō-bə-ˈsi-ləs\ *n, pl* **-li** \-ˌlī, -ˌlē\ : a very short bacillus esp. of the genus *Pasteurella* — **coc·co·ba·cil·la·ry** \-ˈba-sə-ˌler-ē, -bə-ˈsi-lə-rē\ *adj*

coc·coid \ˈkä-ˌkȯid\ *adj* : of, related to, or resembling a coccus — **coccoid** *n*

coc·cus \ˈkä-kəs\ *n, pl* **coc·ci** \ˈkä-ˌkī,-ˌkē; ˈkäk-ˌsī, -ˌsē\ : a spherical bacterium

coccyg- *or* **coccygo-** *comb form* : coccyx ⟨*coccyg*ectomy⟩

coc·cy·geal \käk-ˈsi-jəl, -jē-əl\ *adj* : of, relating to, or affecting the coccyx

coccygeal body *n* : GLOMUS COCCYGEUM

coccygeal gland *n* : GLOMUS COCCYGEUM

coccygeal nerve *n* : either of the 31st or lowest pair of spinal nerves

coc·cy·gec·to·my \ˌkäk-sə-ˈjek-tə-mē\ *n, pl* **-mies** : the surgical removal of the coccyx

coccygeum — see GLOMUS COCCYGEUM

coc·cyg·e·us \käk-ˈsi-jē-əs\ *n, pl* **coc·cyg·ei** \-jē-ˌī\ : a muscle arising from the ischium and sacrospinous ligament and inserted into the coccyx and sacrum — called also *coccygeus muscle, ischiococcygeus*

coc·cy·go·dyn·ia \ˌkäk-sə-(ˌ)gō-ˈdi-nē-ə\ *n* : pain in the coccyx and adjacent regions

coc·cyx \ˈkäk-siks\ *n, pl* **coc·cy·ges** \-sə-ˌjēz\ *also* **coc·cyx·es** \-sik-səz\ : a small bone that articulates with the sacrum and that usu. consists of four fused vertebrae which form the terminus of the spinal column

co·chlea \ˈkō-klē-ə, ˈkä-\ *n, pl* **co·chle·as** *or* **co·chle·ae** \-ē, -ˌī\ : a division of the bony labyrinth of the inner ear coiled into the form of a snail shell and consisting of a spiral canal in the petrous part of the temporal bone in which lies a smaller membranous spiral passage that communicates with the saccule at the base of the spiral, ends blindly near its apex,

and contains the organ of Corti — **co·chle·ar** \-ər\ *adj*

cochlear canal *n* : COCHLEAR DUCT

cochlear duct *n* : the spirally arranged canal in the bony canal of the cochlea that contains the organ of Corti, is triangular in cross section, and is bounded by the vestibular membrane above, by the periosteum lined wall of the cochlea laterally, and by the basilar membrane below — called also *cochlear canal, scala media*

cochlear implant *n* : an electronic prosthetic device that enables individuals with sensorineural hearing loss to recognize some sounds and consists of an external microphone and speech processor and one or more electrodes implanted in the cochlea — **cochlear implantation** *n*

cochlear microphonic *n* : an electrical potential arising in the cochlea when the mechanical energy of a sound stimulus is transformed to electrical energy as the action potential of the transmitting nerve — called also *microphonic*

cochlear nerve *n* : a branch of the auditory nerve that arises in the spiral ganglion of the cochlea and conducts sensory stimuli from the organ of hearing to the brain — called also *cochlear, cochlear branch, cochlear division*

cochlear nucleus *n* : the nucleus of the cochlear nerve situated in the caudal part of the pons and consisting of dorsal and ventral parts which are continuous and lie on the dorsal and lateral aspects of the inferior cerebellar peduncle

co·chleo·ves·tib·u·lar \ˌkō-klē-(ˌ)ō-ve-ˈsti-byə-lər, ˌkä-\ *adj* : relating to or affecting the cochlea and vestibule of the ear ⟨∼ disorders⟩

Coch·lio·my·ia \ˌkä-klē-ə-ˈmī-ə\ *n* : a genus of No. American blowflies that includes the screwworms (*C. hominivorax* and *C. macellaria*)

Cock·ayne syndrome \kä-ˈkān-\ *n* : a rare disease that is inherited as an autosomal recessive trait, is marked esp. by growth and developmental failure, photosensitivity, and premature aging, and that is either present at birth or has an onset during infancy or childhood — called also *Cockayne's syndrome*

Cockayne, Edward Alfred (1880–1956), British physician.

cock·roach \ˈkäk-ˌrōch\ *n* : any of an order or suborder (Blattodea syn. Blattaria) of chiefly nocturnal insects including some that are domestic pests — see BLATTA, BLATTELLA

cock·tail \ˈkäk-ˌtāl\ *n* : a mixture of agents usu. in solution that is taken or used esp. for medical treatment or diagnosis

cocoa butter *or* **cacao butter** *n* : a pale vegetable fat obtained from cacao beans that is used in the manufacture of chocolate candy, in cosmetics as an emollient, and in pharmacy for making suppositories — called also *theobroma oil*

co·con·scious \(ˌ)kō-ˈkän-chəs\ *n* : mental processes outside the main stream of consciousness but sometimes available to it — **coconscious** *adj*

co·con·scious·ness *n* : COCONSCIOUS

¹**code** \ˈkōd\ *n* **1** : GENETIC CODE **2** : CODE BLUE

²**code** *vb* **cod·ed; cod·ing 1** : to specify the genetic code ⟨a gene that ∼s for a protein⟩ **2** : to experience cardiac arrest or respiratory failure ⟨the patient *coded* a second time⟩

code blue *n, often cap C&B* : a declaration of or a state of medical emergency and call for medical personnel and equipment for attempt to resuscitate a patient esp. when in cardiac arrest or respiratory distress or failure; *also* : the attempt to resuscitate the patient

co·deine \ˈkō-ˌdēn, ˈkō-dē-ən\ *n* : a morphine derivative that is found in opium, is weaker in action than morphine, and is used esp. in the form of its sulfate $(C_{18}H_{21}NO_3)_2 \cdot H_2SO_4$ or phosphate $C_{18}H_{21}NO_3 \cdot H_3PO_4$ esp. as an analgesic and an antitussive

co·de·pen·dence \ˌkō-di-ˈpen-dəns\ *n* : CODEPENDENCY

co·de·pen·den·cy \-dən-sē\ *n, pl* **-cies** : a psychological condition or a relationship in which a person is controlled or manipulated by another who is affected with a pathological condition (as an addiction); *broadly* : dependence on the needs of or control by another

¹**co·de·pen·dent** \-dənt\ *n* : a codependent person

²**codependent** *adj* : participating in or exhibiting codependency

co·dex \ˈkō-ˌdeks\ *n, pl* **co·di·ces** \ˈkō-də-ˌsēz, ˈkä-\ : an official or standard collection of drug formulas and descriptions

cod–liver oil *n* : a pale yellow fatty oil obtained from the liver of the cod (*Gadus morhua* of the family Gadidae) and related fishes and used in medicine chiefly as a source of vitamins A and D

co·dom·i·nant \(ˌ)kō-ˈdä-mə-nənt\ *adj* : being fully expressed in the heterozygous condition — **codominant** *n*

co·don \ˈkō-ˌdän\ *n* : a specific sequence of three consecutive nucleotides that is part of the genetic code and that specifies a particular amino acid in a protein or starts or stops protein synthesis — called also *triplet*

co·ef·fi·cient \ˌkō-ə-ˈfi-shənt\ *n* : a number that serves as a measure of some property or characteristic (as of a substance, device, or process)

-coele *or* **-coel** *also* **-cele** *n comb form* : cavity : chamber ⟨blasto*coel*⟩

coe·len·ter·ate \si-ˈlen-tə-ˌrāt, -rət\ *n* : any of a phylum (Cnidaria syn. Coelenterata) of invertebrate animals including the jellyfishes, corals, and sea anemones and having bodies with similar parts regularly arranged around a central axis — called also *cnidarian* — **coelenterate** *adj*

coeli- *or* **coelio-** *chiefly Brit var of* CELI-

coe·li·ac, coe·li·os·co·py, coe·li·ot·o·my *chiefly Brit var of* CELIAC, CELIOSCOPY, CELIOTOMY

coe·lom \ˈsē-ləm\ *n, pl* **coeloms** *or* **coe·lo·ma·ta** \si-ˈlō-mə-tə\ : the usu. epithelium-lined body cavity between the body wall and digestive tract of metazoans above the lower worms — **coe·lo·mate** \ˈsē-lə-ˌmāt\ *adj or n* — **coe·lo·mic** \si-ˈlä-mik, -ˈlō-\ *adj*

coe·nu·ro·sis \ˌsēn-yə-ˈrō-səs, ˌsen-\ *or* **coe·nu·ri·a·sis** \-ˈrī-ə-səs\ *n, pl* **-o·ses** \-ˌsēz\ *or* **-a·ses** \-ˌsēz\ : infestation with or disease caused by coenuri

coe·nu·rus \sə-ˈnur-əs, sē-, -ˈnyur-\ *n, pl* **coe·nu·ri** \-ˈnùr-ˌī, -ˈnyùr-\ : a complex tapeworm larva growing interstitially in vertebrate tissues and consisting of a large fluid-filled sac from the inner wall of which numerous scolices develop — see GID, MULTICEPS

co·en·zyme \(ˌ)kō-ˈen-ˌzīm\ *n* : a thermostable nonprotein compound that forms the active portion of an enzyme system after combination with an apoenzyme — compare ACTIVATOR 1 — **co·en·zy·mat·ic** \-ˌen-zə-ˈma-tik, -(ˌ)zī-\ *adj* — **co·en·zy·mat·i·cal·ly** \-ti-k(ə-)lē\ *adv*

coenzyme A *n* : a coenzyme $C_{21}H_{36}N_7O_{16}P_3S$ that occurs in all living cells and is essential to the metabolism of carbohydrates, fats, and some amino acids

coenzyme Q *n* : UBIQUINONE

coenzyme Q10 *n* : a ubiquinone $C_{59}H_{90}O_4$ of humans and most other mammals that possesses antioxidant properties

coeruleus, coerulei — see LOCUS COERULEUS

co·fac·tor \ˈkō-ˌfak-tər\ *n* **1** : a substance that acts with another substance to bring about certain effects; *esp* : COENZYME **2** : something (as a diet or virus) that acts with or aids another factor in causing disease

cogener *var of* CONGENER

Cog·gins test \ˈkä-gənz-\ *n* : a serological immunodiffusion test for the diagnosis of equine infectious anemia esp. in horses by the presence of antibodies to the causative virus — called also *Coggins* — **Coggins test** *vb*
Coggins, Leroy (*b* 1932), American veterinary virologist.

Cog·nex \ˈkäg-ˌneks\ *trademark* — used for a preparation of the hydrochloride of tacrine

cog·ni·tion \käg-ˈni-shən\ *n* : cognitive mental processes; *also* : a product of these processes

cog·ni·tive \'käg-nə-tiv\ *adj* : of, relating to, or being conscious intellectual activity (as thinking, reasoning, remembering, imagining, or learning words) — **cog·ni·tive·ly** *adv*

cognitive behavioral therapy *also* **cognitive behavior therapy** *n* : COGNITIVE THERAPY

cognitive dissonance *n* : psychological conflict resulting from simultaneously held incongruous beliefs and attitudes

cognitive psychology *n* : a branch of psychology concerned with cognition esp. with respect to the internal events occurring between sensory stimulation and the overt expression of behavior — compare BEHAVIORISM — **cognitive psychologist** *n*

cognitive science *n* : an interdisciplinary science that draws on many fields (as psychology, artificial intelligence, linguistics, and philosophy) in developing theories about human perception, thinking, and learning — **cognitive scientist** *n*

cognitive therapy *n* : psychotherapy esp. for depression that emphasizes the substitution of desirable patterns of thinking for maladaptive or faulty ones — compare BEHAVIOR MODIFICATION

co·he·sion \kō-'hē-zhən\ *n* **1** : the act or process of sticking together tightly **2** : the molecular attraction by which the particles of a body are united throughout the mass — **co·he·sive** \kō-'hē-siv, -ziv\ *adj* — **co·he·sive·ly** *adv* — **co·he·sive·ness** *n*

co·hort \'kō-,hȯrt\ *n* : a group of individuals having a statistical factor (as age or risk) in common

co·in·fec·tion \,kō-in-'fek-shən\ *n* : concurrent infection of a cell or organism with two microorganisms — **co·in·fect** \-'fekt\ *vb*

coin lesion *n* : a round well-circumscribed nodule in a lung that is seen in an X-ray photograph as a shadow the size and shape of a coin

coital exanthema *n* : EQUINE COITAL EXANTHEMA

co·ition \kō-'i-shən\ *n* : COITUS — **co·ition·al** \-'ish-nəl, -'i-shən-ᵊl\ *adj*

co·itus \'kō-ə-təs, kō-'ē-; 'kȯi-təs\ *n* : physical union of male and female genitalia accompanied by rhythmic movements : SEXUAL INTERCOURSE **1** — compare ORGASM — **co·ital** \-ət-ᵊl, -ēt-ᵊl\ *adj* — **co·ital·ly** \-ᵊl-ē\ *adv*

coitus in·ter·rup·tus \-,in-tə-'rəp-təs\ *n* : coitus in which the penis is withdrawn prior to ejaculation to prevent the deposit of sperm in the vagina

coitus res·er·va·tus \-,re-zər-'vä-təs\ *n* : prolonged coitus in which ejaculation of sperm is deliberately withheld

col- *or* **coli-** *or* **colo-** *comb form* **1** : colon ⟨*colitis*⟩ **2** : colon bacillus ⟨*coli*form⟩

cola *pl of* COLON

col·chi·cine \'käl-chə-,sēn, 'käl-kə-\ *n* : a poisonous alkaloid $C_{22}H_{25}NO_6$ that inhibits mitosis, is extracted from the corms or seeds of the autumn crocus, and is used in the treatment of gout and acute attacks of gouty arthritis

col·chi·cum \-kəm\ *n* : the dried corm or dried ripe seeds of the autumn crocus containing the alkaloid colchicine

¹cold \'kōld\ *adj* **1 a** : having or being a temperature that is noticeably lower than body temperature and esp. that is uncomfortable for humans **b** : having a relatively low temperature or one that is lower than normal or expected **c** : receptive to the sensation of coldness : stimulated by cold **2** : marked by the loss of normal body heat ⟨~ hands⟩ **3** : DEAD **4** : exhibiting little or no radioactivity — **cold·ness** *n*

²cold *n* **1** : bodily sensation produced by loss or lack of heat **2** : a bodily disorder popularly associated with chilling: **a** *in humans* : COMMON COLD **b** *in domestic animals* : CORYZA

COLD *abbr* chronic obstructive lung disease

cold agglutinin *n* : any of several agglutinins sometimes present in the blood (as of patients with primary atypical pneumonia) that at low temperatures agglutinate compatible as well as incompatible red blood cells, including the patient's own — compare AUTOAGGLUTININ

cold–blood·ed \'kōld-'blə-dəd\ *adj* : having a body temperature not internally regulated but approximating that of the environment : POIKILOTHERMIC — **cold–blood·ed·ness** *n*

cold cream *n* : a soothing and cleansing cosmetic basically consisting of a perfumed emulsion of a bland vegetable oil or heavy mineral oil

cold pack *n* : a sheet or blanket wrung out of cold water, wrapped around the patient's body, and covered with dry blankets — compare HOT PACK

cold sore *n* : a vesicular lesion that typically occurs in or around the mouth, that initially causes pain, burning, or itching before bursting and crusting over, and that is caused by a herpes simplex virus — called also *fever blister*

cold sweat *n* : perspiration accompanied by feelings of chill or cold and usu. induced by or accompanied by dread, fear, or shock

cold turkey *n* : abrupt complete cessation of the use of an addictive drug; *also* : the symptoms experienced by one undergoing withdrawal from a drug — **cold turkey** *adv or adj*

col·ec·to·my \kə-'lek-tə-mē, kō-\ *n, pl* **-mies** : excision of a portion or all of the colon

co·les·ti·pol \kə-'les-tə-,pȯl\ *n* : a strongly basic resin with an affinity for bile acids that is used in the form of its hydrochloride to treat hypercholesterolemia and disorders associated with the accumulation of bile acids

co·li \'kō-ˌlī\ adj : of or relating to bacteria normally inhabiting the intestine or colon and esp. to species of the genus *Escherichia* (as *E. coli*) — **coli** comb form — see COL-

co·li·ba·cil·lo·sis \ˌkō-lə-ˌba-sə-'lō-səs\ n, pl **-lo·ses** \-ˌsēz\ : infection with or disease caused by colon bacilli (esp. *E. coli*)

¹**col·ic** \'kä-lik\ n 1 : an attack of acute abdominal pain localized in a hollow organ and often caused by spasm, obstruction, or twisting 2 : a condition marked by recurrent episodes of prolonged and uncontrollable crying in an otherwise healthy infant that is of unknown cause and usu. subsides after three to four months of age

²**colic** adj : of or relating to colic : COLICKY ⟨~ crying⟩

³**co·lic** \'kō-lik, 'kä-\ adj : of or relating to the colon

colic artery n : any of three arteries that branch from the mesenteric arteries and supply the large intestine

co·li·cin \'kō-lə-sən\ also **co·li·cine** \-ˌsēn\ n : any of various antibacterial proteins that are produced by strains of intestinal bacteria (as *E. coli*) and that often act to inhibit macromolecular synthesis in related strains

col·icky \'kä-li-kē\ adj 1 : relating to or associated with colic ⟨~ pain⟩ 2 : suffering from colic ⟨~ babies⟩

col·i·form \'kō-lə-ˌfȯrm, 'kä-\ adj : of, relating to, or being gram-negative rod-shaped bacteria (as *E. coli*) normally present in the intestine — **coliform** n

co·li·phage \'kō-lə-ˌfāj, -ˌfäzh\ n : a bacteriophage active against colon bacilli

co·lis·tin \kə-'lis-tən, kō-\ n : a polymyxin produced by a bacterium of the genus *Bacillus* (*B. polymyxa* var. *colistinus*)

co·li·tis \kō-'lī-təs, kə-\ n : inflammation of the colon — see ULCERATIVE COLITIS

colla pl of COLLUM

col·la·gen \'kä-lə-jən\ n : an insoluble fibrous protein of vertebrates that is the chief constituent of the fibrils of connective tissue (as in skin and tendons) and of the organic substance of bones and yields gelatin and glue on prolonged heating with water — **col·lag·e·nous** \kə-'la-jə-nəs\ adj

col·la·ge·nase \kə-'la-jə-ˌnās, 'kä-lə-, -ˌnāz\ n : any of a group of proteolytic enzymes that decompose collagen and gelatin

collagen disease n : CONNECTIVE TISSUE DISEASE

col·la·gen·o·lyt·ic \ˌkä-lə-jə-nə-'li-tik, -je-\ adj : relating to or having the capacity to break down collagen

col·la·ge·no·sis \ˌkä-lə-jə-'nō-səs\ n, pl **-no·ses** \-ˌsēz\ : CONNECTIVE TISSUE DISEASE

collagen vascular disease n : CONNECTIVE TISSUE DISEASE

¹**col·lapse** \kə-'laps\ vb **col·lapsed; col·laps·ing** 1 : to fall or shrink together abruptly and completely : fall into a jumbled or flattened mass through the force of external pressure ⟨a blood vessel that *collapsed*⟩ 2 : to break down in vital energy, stamina, or self-control through exhaustion or disease; esp : to fall helpless or unconscious — **col·laps·ibil·i·ty** \-ˌlap-sə-'bi-lə-tē\ n — **col·laps·ible** \-'lap-sə-bəl\ adj

²**collapse** n 1 : a breakdown in vital energy, strength, or stamina : complete sudden enervation 2 : a state of extreme prostration and physical depression resulting from circulatory failure, great loss of body fluids, or heart disease and occurring terminally in diseases such as cholera, typhoid fever, and pneumonia 3 : an airless state of a lung of spontaneous origin or induced surgically — see ATELECTASIS 4 : an abnormal falling together of the walls of an organ

col·lar \'kä-lər\ n : a protective or supportive device (as a brace or cast) worn around the neck

col·lar·bone \'kä-lər-ˌbōn\ n : CLAVICLE

¹**col·lat·er·al** \kə-'la-tə-rəl, -trəl\ adj 1 : relating to or being branches of a bodily part ⟨~ sprouting of nerves⟩ 2 : relating to or being part of the collateral circulation ⟨~ blood flow⟩

²**collateral** n 1 : a branch esp. of a blood vessel, nerve, or the axon of a nerve cell 2 : a bodily part that is lateral in position

collateral circulation n : circulation of blood established through enlargement of minor vessels and anastomosis of vessels with those of adjacent parts when a major vein or artery is functionally impaired (as by obstruction); also : the modified vessels through which such circulation occurs

collateral ligament n : any of various ligaments on one or the other side of a hinge joint (as the knee, elbow, or the joints between the phalanges of the toes and fingers): as **a** : LATERAL COLLATERAL LIGAMENT **b** : MEDIAL COLLATERAL LIGAMENT

collateral sulcus n : a sulcus of the tentorial surface of the cerebrum lying below and external to the calcarine sulcus and causing an elevation on the floor of the lateral ventricle between the hippocampi — called also *collateral fissure*

collecting tubule n : a nonsecretory tubule that receives urine from several nephrons and discharges it into the pelvis of the kidney — called also *collecting duct*

collective unconscious *n* : the genetically determined part of the unconscious that esp. in the psychoanalytic theory of C. G. Jung occurs in all the members of a people or race

Col·les' fracture \'kä-ləs-, -,lēz-\ *n* : a fracture of the lower end of the radius with backward displacement of the lower fragment and radial deviation of the hand at the wrist that produces a characteristic deformity — compare SMITH FRACTURE

Col·les \'kä-ləs\, **Abraham (1773–1843),** British surgeon.

col·lic·u·lus \kə-'li-kyə-ləs\ *n, pl* **-u·li** \-,lī, -,lē\ : an anatomical prominence; *esp* : any of the four prominences constituting the corpora quadrigemina — see INFERIOR COLLICULUS, SUPERIOR COLLICULUS

col·li·ma·tor \'kä-lə-,mā-tər\ *n* : a device for obtaining a beam of radiation (as X-rays) of limited cross section

col·li·qua·tion \,kä-lə-'kwā-zhən, -shən\ *n* : the breakdown and liquefaction of tissue — **col·li·qua·tive** \'kä-li-,kwā-tiv, kə-'li-kwə-\ *adj*

col·lo·di·on \kə-'lō-dē-ən\ *n* : a viscous solution of pyroxylin used as a coating for wounds

col·loid \'kä-,lȯid\ *n* **1** : a gelatinous or mucinous substance found in tissues in disease or normally (as in the thyroid) **2 a** : a substance that consists of particles dispersed throughout another substance which are too small for resolution with an ordinary light microscope but are incapable of passing through a semipermeable membrane **b** : a mixture (as smoke) consisting of a colloid together with the medium in which it is dispersed — **col·loi·dal** \kə-'lȯid-ᵊl, kä-\ *adj* — **col·loi·dal·ly** *adv*

col·lum \'kä-ləm\ *n, pl* **col·la** \-lə\ : an anatomical neck or neckline part or process

col·lu·to·ri·um \,kä-lə-'tōr-ē-əm\ *n, pl* **-to·ria** \-ē-ə\ : MOUTHWASH

col·lyr·i·um \kə-'lir-ē-əm\ *n, pl* **-ia** \-ē-ə\ *or* **-i·ums** : an eye lotion : EYEWASH

colo- — see COL-

col·o·bo·ma \,kä-lə-'bō-mə\ *n, pl* **-mas** *also* **-ma·ta** \-mə-tə\ : a fissure of the eye usu. of congenital origin

co·lon \'kō-lən\ *n, pl* **colons** *or* **co·la** \-lə\ : the part of the large intestine that extends from the cecum to the rectum

colon bacillus *n* : any of several bacilli esp. of the genus *Escherichia* that are normally commensal in vertebrate intestines; esp : E. COLI

¹co·lon·ic \kō-'lä-nik, kə-\ *adj* : of or relating to the colon

²colonic *n* : ENEMA — see HIGH COLONIC

colonic irrigation *n* : ENEMA

col·o·nize \'kä-lə-,nīz\ *vb* **-nized; -niz·ing** : to establish a colony in or on — **col·o·ni·za·tion** \,kä-lə-nə-'zā-shən\ *n*

co·lon·o·scope \kō-'lä-nə-,skōp\ *n* : a flexible endoscope for inspecting and passing instruments into the colon (as to obtain tissue for biopsy)

co·lo·nos·co·py \,kō-lə-'näs-kə-pē, ,kä-\ *n, pl* **-pies** : endoscopic examination of the colon — **co·lon·o·scop·ic** \kō-,lä-nə-'skä-pik\ *adj*

col·o·ny \'kä-lə-nē\ *n, pl* **-nies** : a circumscribed mass of microorganisms usu. growing in or on a solid medium

colony–stimulating factor *n* : any of several glycoproteins that promote the differentiation of stem cells esp. into blood granulocytes and macrophages and that stimulate their proliferation into colonies in culture

co·lo·proc·tos·to·my \,kō-lə-,präk-'täs-tə-mē, ,kä-\ *n, pl* **-mies** : surgical formation of an artificial passage between the colon and the rectum

col·or \'kə-lər\ *n, often attrib* **1 a** : a phenomenon of light (as red, brown, pink, or gray) or visual perception that enables one to differentiate otherwise identical objects **b** : the aspect of objects and light sources that may be described in terms of hue, lightness, and saturation for objects and hue, brightness, and saturation for light sources **c** : a hue as contrasted with black, white, or gray **2** : complexion tint; *esp* : the tint characteristic of good health

Colorado tick fever *n* : a mild disease of the western U.S. and western Canada that is characterized by the absence of a rash, intermittent fever, malaise, headaches, and myalgia and is caused by a reovirus (species *Colorado tick fever virus* of the genus *Coltivirus*) transmitted by the Rocky Mountain wood tick

col·or–blind \-,blīnd\ *adj* : affected with partial or total inability to distinguish one or more chromatic colors — **color blindness** *n*

co·lo·rec·tal \,kō-lə-'rekt-ᵊl, ,kä-\ *adj* : relating to or affecting the colon and the rectum ⟨∼ cancer⟩ ⟨∼ surgery⟩

col·or·im·e·ter \,kə-lə-'ri-mə-tər\ *n* : any of various instruments used to objectively determine the color of a solution — **col·or·i·met·ric** \,kə-lə-rə-'me-trik\ *adj* — **col·or·i·met·ri·cal·ly** \-tri-k(ə-)lē\ *adv* — **col·or·im·e·try** \,kə-lə-'ri-mə-trē\ *n*

color index *n* : a figure that represents the ratio of the amount of hemoglobin to the number of red cells in a given volume of blood and that is a measure of the normality of the hemoglobin content of the individual cells

color vision *n* : perception of and ability to distinguish colors

co·los·to·mize \kə-'läs-tə-,mīz\ *vb* **-mized; -miz·ing** : to perform a colostomy on

co·los·to·my \kə-'läs-tə-mē\ *n, pl* **-mies** : surgical formation of an artificial anus by connecting the colon to an opening in the abdominal wall

col·os·to·my bag *n* : a container kept constantly in position to receive feces discharged through a colostomy

co·los·trum \kə-'läs-trəm\ *n* : milk secreted for a few days after parturition and characterized by high protein and antibody content — **co·los·tral** \-trəl\ *adj*

col·our *chiefly Brit var of* COLOR

colp- *or* **colpo-** *comb form* : vagina ⟨*colpi*tis⟩ ⟨*colpo*scope⟩

col·pec·to·my \käl-'pek-tə-mē\ *n, pl* **-to·mies** : partial or complete surgical excision of the vagina — called also *vaginectomy*

col·pi·tis \käl-'pī-təs\ *n* : VAGINITIS 1

col·po·cen·te·sis \ˌkäl-(ˌ)pō-sen-'tē-səs\ *n, pl* **-te·ses** \-ˌsēz\ : surgical puncture of the vagina

col·po·clei·sis \ˌkäl-pō-'klī-səs\ *n, pl* **-clei·ses** \-ˌsēz\ : the suturing of posterior and anterior walls of the vagina to prevent uterine prolapse

col·po·per·i·ne·or·rha·phy \ˌkäl-pō-ˌper-ə-(ˌ)nē-'ȯr-ə-fē\ *n, pl* **-phies** : the suturing of an injury to the vagina and the perineum

col·po·pexy \'käl-pə-ˌpek-sē\ *n, pl* **-pex·ies** : fixation of the vagina by suturing it to the adjacent abdominal wall

col·por·rha·phy \käl-'pȯr-ə-fē\ *n, pl* **-phies** : surgical repair of the vaginal wall

-colpos *n comb form* : vaginal disorder (of a specified type) ⟨hemato*colpos*⟩

col·po·scope \'käl-pə-ˌskōp\ *n* : an instrument designed to facilitate visual inspection of the vagina — **col·po·scop·ic** \ˌkäl-pə-'skä-pik\ *adj* — **col·po·scop·i·cal·ly** \-pi-k(ə-)lē\ *adv* — **col·pos·co·py** \käl-'päs-kə-pē\ *n*

col·pot·o·my \käl-'pä-tə-mē\ *n, pl* **-mies** : surgical incision of the vagina

co·lum·bi·um \kə-'ləm-bē-əm\ *n* : NIOBIUM

col·u·mel·la \ˌkä-lə-'me-lə, ˌkäl-yə-\ *n, pl* **-mel·lae** \-'me-(ˌ)lē, -ˌlī\ : any of various anatomical parts likened to a column: **a** : the bony central axis of the cochlea **b** : the lower part of the nasal septum — **col·u·mel·lar** \-lər\ *adj*

col·umn \'kä-ləm\ *n* : a longitudinal subdivision of the spinal cord that resembles a column or pillar: as **a** : any of the principal longitudinal subdivisions of gray matter or white matter in each lateral half of the spinal cord — see DORSAL HORN, GRAY COLUMN, LATERAL COLUMN 1, VENTRAL HORN; compare FUNICULUS a **b** : any of a number of smaller bundles of spinal nerve fibers : FASCICULUS

co·lum·nar \kə-'ləm-nər\ *adj* : of, relating to, being, or composed of tall narrow somewhat cylindrical epithelial cells ⟨~ epithelium⟩

column chromatography *n* : chromatography in which the substances to be separated are introduced onto the top of a column packed with an adsorbent (as silica gel or alumina), pass through the column at different rates that depend on the affinity of each substance for the adsorbent and for the solvent or solvent mixture, and are usu. collected in solution as they pass from the column at different times — compare GAS CHROMATOGRAPHY, PAPER CHROMATOGRAPHY, THIN-LAYER CHROMATOGRAPHY

column of Ber·tin \-ber-'taⁿ\ *n* : RENAL COLUMN

E. J. Bertin — see BERTIN'S COLUMN

column of Bur·dach \-'bər-dək, -'bu̇r-, -ˌdäk\ *n* : FASCICULUS CUNEATUS

Bur·dach \'bu̇r-ˌdäk\, **Karl Friedrich (1776–1847),** German anatomist.

co·ma \'kō-mə\ *n* : a state of profound unconsciousness caused by disease, injury, or poison

co·ma·tose \'kō-mə-ˌtōs, 'kä-\ *adj* : of, resembling, or affected with coma ⟨a ~ patient⟩ ⟨a ~ condition⟩

combat fatigue *n* : a post-traumatic stress disorder occurring under wartime conditions (as combat) that cause intense stress — called also *battle fatigue, shell shock, war neurosis*

combination therapy *n* : the use of two or more therapies and esp. drugs to treat a disease or condition

Com·bi·vent \'käm-bə-ˌvent\ *trademark* — used for a preparation of ipratropium bromide and the sulfate of albuterol

com·e·do \'kä-mə-ˌdō\ *n, pl* **com·e·do·nes** \ˌkä-mə-'dō-(ˌ)nēz\ : BLACKHEAD 1

com·e·do·car·ci·no·ma \ˌkä-mə-ˌdō-ˌkärs-ʰn-'ō-mə\ *n, pl* **-mas** *also* **-ma·ta** \-mə-tə\ : a breast cancer that arises in the larger ducts and is characterized by slow growth, late metastasis, and the accumulation of solid plugs of atypical and degenerating cells in the ducts

com·e·do·gen·ic \ˌkä-mə-də-'je-nik\ *adj* : tending to clog pores esp. by the formation of blackheads ⟨~ cosmetics⟩

come to *vb* : to recover consciousness

comitans — see VENA COMITANS

com·men·sal·ism \kə-'men-sə-ˌli-zəm\ *n* : a relation between two kinds of organisms in which one obtains food or other benefits from the other without damaging or benefiting it — **com·men·sal** \-səl\ *adj or n* — **com·men·sal·ly** *adv*

com·mi·nut·ed \ˌkä-mə-'nü-təd, -'nyü-\ *adj* : being a fracture in which the bone is splintered or crushed into numerous pieces

com·mis·su·ra \ˌkä-mə-'shu̇r-ə\ *n, pl* **-rae** \-'shu̇r-ē\ : COMMISSURE

com·mis·sure \'kä-mə-ˌshu̇r\ *n* **1** : a point or line of union or junction between two anatomical parts (as the lips at their angles or adjacent heart valves) **2** : a connecting band of nerve tissue in the brain or spinal cord — see ANTERIOR COMMISSURE, CORPUS CALLOSUM, GRAY COMMISSURE, HABENULAR COMMISSURE, HIPPOCAMPAL COMMISSURE, POSTERIOR COMMISSURE — com·mis·su·ral \ˌkä-mə-ˈshùr-əl\ adj

com·mis·sur·ot·o·my \ˌkä-mə-ˌshùr-ˈä-tə-mē, -shə-ˈrä-\ n, pl -mies : the operation of cutting through a band of muscle or nerve fibers; specif : separation of the flaps of a mitral valve to relieve mitral stenosis : VALVULOTOMY

com·mit \kə-ˈmit\ vb com·mit·ted; com·mit·ting : to place in a prison or mental institution — com·mit·ment \kə-ˈmit-mənt\ n — com·mit·ta·ble \-ˈmi-tə-bəl\ adj

com·mon \ˈkä-mən\ adj : formed of or dividing into two or more branches ⟨the ∼ facial vein⟩ ⟨∼ iliac vessels⟩

common bile duct n : the duct formed by the union of the hepatic and cystic ducts and opening into the duodenum

common carotid artery n : the part of either carotid artery between its point of origin and its division into the internal and external carotid arteries — called also common carotid

common cattle grub n : a cattle grub of the genus Hypoderma (H. lineatum) whose larva is particularly destructive to cattle

common cold n : an acute contagious disease of the upper respiratory tract that is marked by inflammation of the mucous membranes of the nose, throat, eyes, and eustachian tubes with a watery but purulent discharge and is caused by any of several viruses (as a rhinovirus or an adenovirus)

common iliac artery n : ILIAC ARTERY 1

common iliac vein n : ILIAC VEIN a

common interosseous artery n : a short thick artery that arises from the ulnar artery near the proximal end of the radius and that divides into anterior and posterior branches which pass down the forearm toward the wrist

common peroneal nerve n : the smaller of the branches into which the sciatic nerve divides passing outward and downward from the popliteal space and to the neck of the fibula where it divides into the deep peroneal nerve and the superficial peroneal nerve — called also lateral popliteal nerve, peroneal nerve

com·mo·tio \kə-ˈmō-shē-ō\ n : CONCUSSION

commotio cor·dis \-ˈkòr-dəs\ n : concussion of the heart that is caused by a blow to the chest over the region of the heart by a blunt object which does not penetrate the body and that usu. results in ventricular fibrillation leading to sudden cardiac death if treatment by defibrillation is not immediately given

com·mu·ni·ca·ble \kə-ˈmyü-ni-kə-bəl\ adj : capable of being transmitted from person to person, animal to animal, animal to human, or human to animal : TRANSMISSIBLE — com·mu·ni·ca·bil·i·ty \-ˌmyü-ni-kə-ˈbi-lə-tē\ n

communicable disease n : an infectious disease transmissible (as from person to person) by direct contact with an affected individual or the individual's discharges or by indirect means (as by a vector) — compare CONTAGIOUS DISEASE

communicans — see RAMUS COMMUNICANS, WHITE RAMUS COMMUNICANS

communicantes — see RAMUS COMMUNICANS

com·mu·ni·cate \kə-ˈmyü-nə-ˌkāt\ vb -cat·ed; -cat·ing : to cause to pass from one to another ⟨some diseases are easily communicated⟩

communicating artery n : any of three arteries in the brain that form parts of the circle of Willis: a : one connecting the anterior cerebral arteries — called also anterior communicating artery b : either of two arteries that occur one on each side of the circle of Willis and connect an internal carotid artery with a posterior cerebral artery — called also posterior communicating artery

com·mu·ni·ca·tion \kə-ˌmyü-nə-ˈkā-shən\ n 1 : the act or process of transmitting information (as about ideas, attitudes, emotions, or objective behavior) 2 : information communicated 3 : a connection between bodily parts ⟨an artificial ∼ between the esophagus and the stomach⟩

communis — see EXTENSOR DIGITORUM COMMUNIS

co·mor·bid \kō-ˈmòr-bəd\ adj : existing simultaneously with and usu. independently of another medical condition ⟨bipolar disorder with ∼ substance abuse⟩

co·mor·bid·i·ty \ˌkō-mòr-ˈbi-də-tē\ n 1 : a comorbid condition 2 : the occurrence of comorbid conditions : occurrence as a comorbid condition

com·pact \kəm-ˈpakt, käm-, ˈkäm-ˌ\ adj : having a dense structure without small cavities or cells ⟨∼ bone⟩ — compare CANCELLOUS

compacta — see PARS COMPACTA

compactum — see STRATUM COMPACTUM

com·par·a·tive \kəm-ˈpar-ə-tiv\ adj : characterized by the systematic comparison of phenomena and esp. of likenesses and dissimilarities ⟨∼ anatomy⟩

com·part·ment syndrome \kəm-ˈpärt-mənt-\ n : a painful condition resulting from the expansion or overgrowth of enclosed tissue (as of a leg muscle) within its anatomical enclosure (as a muscular sheath) producing pressure that interferes with circulation and adversely affects the function and health of the tissue itself — called also *com·part·men·tal syndrome* \kəm-ˌpärt-'men-tᵊl-\

com·pat·i·ble \kəm-'pa-tə-bəl\ *adj* **1** : capable of existing together in a satisfactory relationship (as marriage) **2** : capable of being used in transfusion or grafting without immunological reaction (as agglutination or tissue rejection) **3** *of medications* : capable of being administered jointly without interacting to produce deleterious effects or impairing their respective actions — **com·pat·i·bil·i·ty** \-ˌpa-tə-'bi-lə-tē\ *n*

Com·pa·zine \'käm-pə-ˌzēn\ *trademark* — used for a preparation of prochlorperazine

com·pen·sate \'käm-pən-ˌsāt, -ˌpen-\ *vb* **-sat·ed; -sat·ing 1** : to subject to or remedy by physiological compensation **2** : to undergo or engage in psychological or physiological compensation

com·pen·sat·ed *adj* : buffered so that there is no change in the pH of the blood ⟨∼ acidosis⟩ — compare UNCOMPENSATED

com·pen·sa·tion \ˌkäm-pən-'sā-shən, -ˌpen-\ *n* **1** : correction of an organic defect by excessive development or by increased functioning of another organ or unimpaired parts of the same organ ⟨cardiac ∼⟩ — see DECOMPENSATION **2** : a psychological mechanism by which feelings of inferiority, frustration, or failure in one field are counterbalanced by achievement in another

com·pen·sa·to·ry \kəm-'pen-sə-ˌtōr-ē\ *adj* : making up for a loss; *esp* : serving as psychological or physiological compensation

com·pe·tence \'käm-pə-təns\ *n* : the quality or state of being functionally adequate ⟨immune system ∼⟩

com·pe·ten·cy \-tən-sē\ *n, pl* **-cies** : COMPETENCE

com·pe·tent \'käm-pə-tənt\ *adj* : having the capacity to function or develop in a particular way

com·pet·i·tive \kəm-'pe-tə-tiv\ *adj* : depending for effectiveness on the relative concentration of two or more substances ⟨∼ protein binding⟩

com·plain \kəm-'plān\ *vb* : to speak of one's illness or symptoms

com·plaint \kəm-'plānt\ *n* : a bodily ailment or disease

com·ple·ment \'käm-plə-mənt\ *n* **1** : a group or set (as of chromosomes) that is typical of the complete organism or one of its parts — see CHROMOSOME COMPLEMENT **2** : the thermolabile group of proteins in normal blood serum and plasma that in combination with antibodies causes the destruction esp. of particulate antigens

com·ple·men·tar·i·ty \ˌkäm-plə-(ˌ)men-'tar-ə-tē, -mən-\ *n, pl* **-ties** : correspondence in reverse of part of one molecule to part of another: as **a**

: the arrangement of chemical groups and electric charges that enables a combining group of an antibody to combine with a specific determinant group of an antigen or hapten **b** : the correspondence between strands or nucleotides of DNA or sometimes RNA that permits their precise pairing

com·ple·men·ta·ry \ˌkäm-plə-'men-tə-rē, -trē\ *adj* : characterized by molecular complementarity; *esp* : characterized by the capacity for precise pairing of purine and pyrimidine bases between strands of DNA and sometimes RNA such that the structure of one strand determines the other — **com·ple·men·ta·ri·ly** \-'men-trə-lē, -(ˌ)men-'ter-ə-lē, -'men-tə-rə-lē\ *adv* — **com·ple·men·ta·ri·ness** \-'men-tə-rē-nəs, -'men-trē-\ *n*

complementary DNA *n* : cDNA

complementary medicine *n* : any of the practices (as acupuncture) of alternative medicine accepted and utilized by mainstream medical practitioners; *also* : ALTERNATIVE MEDICINE

complement fixation *n* : the process of binding serum complement to the product formed by the union of an antibody and the antigen for which it is specific

complement fixation test *n* : a diagnostic test for the presence of a particular antibody in the serum of a patient that involves inactivation of the complement in the serum, addition of measured amounts of the antigen for which the antibody is specific and of foreign complement, and detection of the presence or absence of complement fixation by the addition of a suitable indicator system — see WASSERMAN TEST

com·plete \kəm-'plēt\ *adj* **1** *of insect metamorphosis* : having a pupal stage intercalated between the motile immature stages and the adult — compare INCOMPLETE 1 **2** *of a bone fracture* : characterized by a break passing entirely across the bone — compare INCOMPLETE 2

complete blood count *n* : a blood count that includes separate counts for red and white blood cells — called also *complete blood cell count;* compare DIFFERENTIAL BLOOD COUNT

¹com·plex \käm-'pleks, kəm-, 'käm-ˌ\ *adj* **1** : formed by the union of simpler chemical substances ⟨∼ proteins⟩

²com·plex \'käm-ˌpleks\ *n* **1** : a group of repressed memories, desires, and ideas that exert a dominant influence on the personality and behavior ⟨a guilt ∼⟩ — see CASTRATION COMPLEX, ELECTRA COMPLEX, INFERIORITY COMPLEX, OEDIPUS COMPLEX, PERSECUTION COMPLEX, SUPERIORITY COMPLEX **2** : a group of chromosomes arranged or behaving in a particular way — see GENE COMPLEX **3** : a chemical association of two or more species (as ions or molecules) joined usu. by weak electrostatic bonds rather than covalent bonds **4** : the sum of the factors (as symptoms and lesions) characterizing a disease ⟨primary tuberculous ∼⟩

³**com·plex** \käm-ˈpleks, kəm-ˈ, ˈkäm-ˌ\ *vb* : to form or cause to form into a complex ⟨RNA ∼ed with protein⟩

com·plex·ion \kəm-ˈplek-shən\ *n* : the hue or appearance of the skin and esp. of the face ⟨a dark ∼⟩ — **com·plex·ioned** \-shənd\ *adj*

com·plex·us \kəm-ˈplek-səs, käm-\ *n* : SEMISPINALIS CAPITIS — called also *complexus muscle*

com·pli·ance \kəm-ˈplī-əns\ *n* **1** : the ability or process of yielding to changes in pressure without disruption of structure or function ⟨pulmonary ∼⟩ **2** : the process of complying with a regimen of treatment

com·pli·cate \ˈkäm-plə-ˌkāt\ *vb* **-cat·ed; -cat·ing** : to cause to be more complex or severe ⟨a virus disease *complicated* by bacterial infection⟩

com·pli·cat·ed *adj of a bone fracture* : characterized by injury to nearby parts

com·pli·ca·tion \ˌkäm-plə-ˈkā-shən\ *n* : a secondary disease or condition that develops in the course of a primary disease or condition and arises either as a result of it or from independent causes

com·pos men·tis \ˌkäm-pəs-ˈmen-təs\ *adj* : of sound mind, memory, and understanding

¹**com·pound** \käm-ˈpaůnd, kəm-ˈ, ˈkäm-ˌ\ *vb* : to form by combining parts ⟨∼ a medicine⟩

²**com·pound** \ˈkäm-ˌpaůnd, käm-ˈ,kəm-ˈ\ *adj* : composed of or resulting from union of separate elements, ingredients, or parts ⟨∼ glands⟩

³**com·pound** \ˈkäm-ˌpaůnd\ *n* : something formed by a union of elements or parts; *specif* : a distinct substance formed by chemical union of two or more ingredients in definite proportion by weight

compound benzoin tincture *n* : FRIAR'S BALSAM

compound fracture *n* : a bone fracture resulting in an open wound through which bone fragments usu. protrude — compare SIMPLE FRACTURE

compound microscope *n* : a microscope consisting of an objective and an eyepiece mounted in a telescoping tube

¹**com·press** \kəm-ˈpres\ *vb* : to press or squeeze together ⟨a ∼ed nerve⟩

²**com·press** \ˈkäm-ˌpres\ *n* **1** : a covering consisting usu. of a folded cloth that is applied and held firmly by the aid of a bandage over a wound dressing to prevent oozing **2** : a folded wet or dry cloth applied firmly to a part (as to allay inflammation)

compressed–air illness *n* : DECOMPRESSION SICKNESS

com·pres·sion \kəm-ˈpre-shən\ *n* : the act, process, or result of compressing esp. when involving a compressing force on a bodily part ⟨∼ of a nerve⟩

compression fracture *n* : fracture (as of a vertebra) caused by compression of one bone against another

¹**com·pro·mise** \ˈkäm-prə-ˌmīz\ *vb* **-mised; -mis·ing** : to cause the impairment of ⟨a *compromised* immune system⟩

²**compromise** *n* : the condition of having been compromised : IMPAIRMENT ⟨cardiovascular ∼⟩

com·pul·sion \kəm-ˈpəl-shən\ *n* : an irresistible persistent impulse to perform an act (as excessive hand washing); *also* : the act itself — compare OBSESSION, PHOBIA

¹**com·pul·sive** \-siv\ *adj* : of, relating to, caused by, or suggestive of psychological compulsion or obsession ⟨repetitive and ∼ behavior⟩ ⟨a ∼ gambler⟩ — **com·pul·sive·ly** *adv* — **com·pul·sive·ness** *n* — **com·pul·siv·i·ty** \ˌkäm-ˌpəl-ˈsi-və-tē, kəm-\ *n*

²**compulsive** *n* : one who is subject to a psychological compulsion

com·put·ed axial tomography \kəm-ˈpyü-təd-\ *n* : COMPUTED TOMOGRAPHY — abbr. CAT

computed tomographic *adj* : using, produced by, or obtained by computed tomography

computed tomography *n* : radiography in which a three-dimensional image of a body structure is constructed by computer from a series of plane cross-sectional images made along an axis — abbr. CT

com·pu·ter·ized axial tomography \kəm-ˈpyü-tə-ˌrīzd-\ *n* : COMPUTED TOMOGRAPHY — abbr. CAT

computerized tomography *n* : COMPUTED TOMOGRAPHY — abbr. CT

co·na·tion \kō-ˈnā-shən\ *n* : an inclination (as an instinct or a craving) to act purposefully : IMPULSE **2** — **co·na·tive** \ˈkō-nə-tiv, -ˌnā-; ˈkä-\ *adj*

conc *abbr* concentrated; concentration

con·ca·nav·a·lin \ˌkän-kə-ˈna-və-lən\ *n* : either of two crystalline globulins occurring esp. in the seeds of a tropical American leguminous plant (*Canavalia ensiformis*); *esp* : one that is a potent hemagglutinin

con·ceive \kən-ˈsēv\ *vb* **con·ceived; con·ceiv·ing** : to become pregnant

con·cen·trate \ˈkän-sən-ˌtrāt, -ˌsen-\ *vb* **-trat·ed; -trat·ing** **1 a** : to bring or direct toward a common center or objective **b** : to accumulate in bodily tissues ⟨fish ∼ mercury⟩ **2** : to make less dilute **3** : to fix one's powers, efforts, or attention on one thing

con·cen·tra·tion \ˌkän-sən-ˈtrā-shən, -ˌsen-\ *n* **1** : the act or action of concentrating: as **a** : a directing of the attention or of the mental faculties toward a single object **b** : an increasing of strength (as of a solute) by partial or total removal of diluents **2** : a crude active principle of a vegetable esp. for pharmaceutical use in the form of a powder or resin **3** : the relative content of a component (as dissolved or dispersed material) of a solution, mixture, or dispersion that may be expressed in percentage by weight or by volume, in parts per million, or in grams per liter

Con·cer·ta \kän-'ser-tə\ *trademark* — used for a preparation of the hydrochloride of methylphenidate

con·cep·tion \kən-'sep-shən\ *n* **1 a** : the process of becoming pregnant involving fertilization or implantation or both **b** : EMBRYO, FETUS **2 a** : the capacity, function, or process of forming or understanding ideas or abstractions or their symbols **b** : a general idea

con·cep·tive \kən-'sep-tiv\ *adj* : capable of or relating to conception

con·cep·tus \kən-'sep-təs\ *n* : a fertilized egg, embryo, or fetus

conch \'käŋk, 'känch\ *n, pl* **conchs** \'käŋks, 'köŋks\ *or* **conch·es** \'kän-chəz\ : CONCHA 1

con·cha \'käŋ-kə, 'köŋ-\ *n, pl* **con·chae** \-ˌkē, -ˌkī\ **1** : the largest and deepest concavity of the external ear **2** : NASAL CONCHA — **con·chal** \-kəl\ *adj*

con·cor·dant \kən-'körd-ʾnt\ *adj, of twins* : similar with respect to one or more particular characters — compare DISCORDANT — **con·cor·dance** \-ʾn(t)s\ *n*

con·cre·ment \'käŋ-krə-mənt, 'kän-\ *n* : CONCRETION

con·cre·tion \kän-'krē-shən, kən-\ *n* : a hard usu. inorganic mass (as a bezoar or tophus) formed in a living body

con·cuss \kən-'kəs\ *vb* : to affect with concussion

con·cus·sion \kən-'kə-shən\ *n* **1** : a hard blow or collision **2** : a condition resulting from the effects of a hard blow; *esp* : a jarring injury of the brain resulting in disturbance of cerebral function — **con·cus·sive** \-'kə-siv\ *adj*

con·den·sa·tion \ˌkän-ˌden-'sā-shən, -dən-\ *n* **1** : the act or process of condensing: as **a** : a chemical reaction involving union between molecules often with elimination of a simple molecule (as water) **b** : the conversion of a substance (as water) from the vapor state to a denser liquid or solid state **2** : representation of several apparently discrete ideas by a single symbol esp. in dreams \<an abnormal hardening of an organ or tissue \<connective tissue ~*s*\>

con·dense \kən-'dens\ *vb* **con·densed; con·dens·ing** : to make denser or more compact; *esp* : to subject to or undergo condensation — **condensed** *adj*

¹con·di·tion \kən-'di-shən\ *n* **1** : something essential to the appearance or occurrence of something else; *esp* : an environmental requirement **2 a** : a usu. defective state of health \<a serious heart ~\> **b** : a state of physical fitness

²condition *vb* **con·di·tioned; con·di·tion·ing** : to cause to undergo a change so that an act or response previously associated with one stimulus becomes associated with another — **con·di·tion·able** \-'di-sh(ə-)nə-bəl\ *adj*

con·di·tion·al \kən-'dish-nəl, -'di-shən-ᵊl\ *adj* **1** : CONDITIONED \<~ reflex\> **2** : eliciting a conditional response \<a ~ stimulus\> — **con·di·tion·al·ly** \-'dish-nə-lē, -'di-shən-ᵊl-ē\ *adv*

con·di·tioned *adj* : determined or established by conditioning

con·dom \'kän-dəm\ *n* **1** : a sheath commonly of rubber worn over the penis (as to prevent conception or venereal infection during sexual intercourse) — called also **sheath** \ **2** : a device inserted into the vagina that is similar in form and function to a condom

con·duct \kən-'dəkt, 'kän-ˌdəkt\ *vb* **1** : to act as a medium for conveying **2** : to have the quality of transmitting something — **con·duc·tance** \kən-'dək-təns\ *n*

con·duc·tion \kən-'dək-shən\ *n* **1** : transmission through or by means of something (as a conductor) **2** : the transmission of excitation through living tissue and esp. nervous tissue

conduction deafness *n* : hearing loss or impairment resulting from interference with the transmission of sound waves to the organ of Corti — called also *conductive deafness, transmission deafness;* compare CENTRAL DEAFNESS, NERVE DEAFNESS

con·duc·tive \-'dək-tiv\ *adj* **1** : having the power to conduct **2** : caused by failure in the mechanisms for sound transmission in the external or middle ear \<~ hearing loss\> — **con·duc·tiv·i·ty** \ˌkän-ˌdək-'ti-və-tē, kən-\ *n*

con·duc·tor \kən-'dək-tər\ *n* **1** : a material or object capable of transmitting electricity, heat or sound **2** : a bodily part (as a nerve fiber) that transmits excitation

condyl- *or* **condylo-** *comb form* : joint : condyle \<*condyl*ectomy\>

con·dy·lar·thro·sis \ˌkän-də-lär-'thrō-səs\ *n, pl* **-thro·ses** \-ˌsēz\ : articulation by means of a condyle

con·dyle \'kän-ˌdīl, 'känd-ᵊl\ *n* : an articular prominence of a bone — used chiefly of such as occur in pairs resembling a pair of knuckles (as those of the occipital bone for articulation with the atlas, those at the distal end of the humerus and femur, and those of the lower jaw); see LATERAL

CONDYLE, MEDIAL CONDYLE — **con-dy-lar** \'kän-də-lər\ *adj* — **con-dy-loid** \'kän-də-ˌlȯid\ *adj*

con-dy-lec-to-my \ˌkän-dī-'lek-tə-mē, ˌkänd-ᵊl-'ek-\ *n, pl* **-mies** : surgical removal of a condyle

con-dy-loid joint \'kän-də-ˌlȯid\ *n* : an articulation in which an ovoid head is received into an elliptical cavity permitting all movements except axial rotation

condyloid process *n* : the rounded process by which the ramus of the mandible articulates with the temporal bone

con-dy-lo-ma \ˌkän-də-'lō-mə\ *n, pl* **-ma-ta** \-mə-tə\ *also* **-mas** : GENITAL WART — **con-dy-lo-ma-tous** \-mə-təs\ *adj*

condyloma acu-mi-na-tum \-ə-ˌkyü-mə-'nā-təm\ *n, pl* **condylomata acu-mi-na-ta** \-'nā-tə\ : GENITAL WART

condyloma la-tum \-'lä-təm\ *n, pl* **condylomata la-ta** \-tə\ : a highly infectious flattened often hypertrophic papule of secondary syphilis that forms in moist areas of skin and at mucocutaneous junctions

cone \'kōn\ *n* **1** : any of the conical photosensitive receptor cells of the retina that function in color vision — compare ROD 1 **2** : any of a family (Conidae) of tropical marine gastropod mollusks that include a few highly poisonous forms **3** : a cusp of a tooth esp. in the upper jaw

cone-nose \'kōn-ˌnōz\ *n* : any of various large bloodsucking bugs esp. of the genus *Triatoma* including some capable of inflicting painful bites — called also *kissing bug*

con-fab-u-la-tion \kən-ˌfa-byə-'lā-shən, ˌkän-\ *n* : a filling in of gaps in memory by unconstrained fabrication — **con-fab-u-late** \kən-'fa-byə-ˌlāt\ *vb*

con-fec-tion \kən-'fek-shən\ *n* : a medicinal preparation usu. made with sugar, syrup, or honey — called also *electuary*

con-fine \kən-'fīn\ *vb* **con-fined; con-fin-ing** : to keep from leaving accustomed quarters (as one's room or bed) under pressure of infirmity, childbirth, or detention

con-fined \kən-'fīnd\ *adj* : undergoing childbirth

con-fine-ment \kən-'fīn-mənt\ *n* : an act of confining : the state of being confined; *esp* : LYING-IN

con-flict \'kän-ˌflikt\ *n* : mental struggle resulting from incompatible or opposing needs, drives, wishes, or external or internal demands — **con-flict-ful** \'kän-ˌflikt-fəl\ *adj* — **con-flic-tu-al** \kän-'flik-chə-wəl, kən-\ *adj*

con-flict-ed \kən-'flik-təd\ *adj* : having or expressing emotional conflict 〈~ about one's sexual identity〉

con-flu-ence of sinuses \'kän-ˌflü-ənts-, kən-'flü-\ *n* : the junction of several of the sinuses of the dura mater in the internal occipital region — called also *confluence of the sinuses*

con-flu-ent \'kän-ˌflü-ənt, kən-'\ *adj* **1** : flowing or coming together; *also* : run together 〈~ pustules〉 **2** : characterized by confluent lesions 〈~ smallpox〉 — compare DISCRETE

con-for-ma-tion \ˌkän-(ˌ)fȯr-'mā-shən, -fər-\ *n* : any of the spatial arrangements of a molecule that can be obtained by rotation of the atoms about a single bond — **con-for-ma-tion-al** \-shnəl, -shən-ᵊl\ *adj* — **con-for-ma-tion-al-ly** *adv*

con-form-er \kən-'fȯr-mər\ *n* : a mold (as of plastic) used to prevent collapse or closing of a cavity, vessel, or opening during surgical repair

con-fu-sion \kən-'fyü-zhən\ *n* : disturbance of consciousness characterized by inability to engage in orderly thought or by lack of power to distinguish, choose, or act decisively — **con-fused** \-'fyüzd\ *adj* — **con-fu-sion-al** \-zhnəl, -zhən-ᵊl\ *adj*

con-geal \kən-'jēl\ *vb* **1** : to change from a fluid to a solid state by or as if by cold **2** : to make viscid or curdled : COAGULATE

con-ge-ner \'kän-jə-nər, kən-'jē-\ *also* **co-ge-ner** \'kō-jē-nər\ *n* **1** : a member of the same taxonomic genus as another plant or animal **2** : a chemical substance related to another — **con-ge-ner-ic** \ˌkän-jə-'ner-ik\ *adj*

congenita — see AMYOTONIA CONGENITA, ARTHROGRYPOSIS MULTIPLEX CONGENITA, MYOTONIA CONGENITA, OSTEOGENESIS IMPERFECTA CONGENITA

con-gen-i-tal \kän-'je-nət-ᵊl\ *adj* **1** : existing at or dating from birth 〈~ deafness〉 **2** : acquired during development in the uterus and not through heredity 〈~ syphilis〉 — compare ACQUIRED 2, FAMILIAL, HEREDITARY — **con-gen-i-tal-ly** *adv*

congenital megacolon *n* : HIRSCHSPRUNG'S DISEASE

con-gest-ed \kən-'jes-təd\ *adj* : containing an excessive accumulation of blood or mucus 〈~ lungs〉

con-ges-tion \kən-'jes-chən, -'jesh-\ *n* : an excessive accumulation esp. of blood or mucus 〈nasal ~〉 〈vascular ~〉 — **con-ges-tive** \-'jes-tiv\ *adj*

congestive heart failure *n* : heart failure in which the heart is unable to maintain adequate circulation of blood in the tissues of the body or to pump out the venous blood returned to it by the venous circulation

con-glu-ti-nate \kən-'glüt-ᵊn-ˌāt, kän-\ *vb* **-nat-ed; -nat-ing** : to unite or become united by or as if by a glutinous substance 〈blood platelets ~ in blood clotting〉 — **con-glu-ti-na-tion** \-ˌglüt-ᵊn-'ā-shən\ *n*

Congo red \'kän-(ˌ)gō-\ *n* : an azo dye $C_{32}H_{22}N_6Na_2O_6S_2$ used in a number of diagnostic tests and esp. for the detection of amyloidosis

congress • conscious sedation

148

con·gress \'käŋ-grəs, -rəs\ n : COITUS

coni pl of CONUS

con·iza·tion \ˌkō-nə-'zā-shən, ˌkä-\ n : the electrosurgical excision of a cone of tissue from a diseased uterine cervix

con·joined \kən-'jȯind\ adj : of, relating to, or being conjoined twins

conjoined twins n pl : twins that are physically united at some part or parts of their bodies at birth

con·ju·ga·ta \ˌkän-jə-'gā-tə\ n, pl **-ga·tae** \-ˌgä-ˌtē\ : CONJUGATE DIAMETER

¹**con·ju·gate** \'kän-ji-gət, -jə-ˌgāt\ adj 1 : functioning or operating simultaneously as if joined 2 of an acid or base : related by the difference of a proton — **con·ju·gate·ly** adv

²**con·ju·gate** \-jə-ˌgāt\ vb **-gat·ed; -gat·ing** 1 : to unite (as with the elimination of water) so that the product is easily broken down (as by hydrolysis) into the original compounds 2 : to pair and fuse in conjugation 3 : to pair in synapsis

³**con·ju·gate** \-ji-gət, -jə-ˌgāt\ n : a chemical compound formed by the union of two compounds or united with another compound — **con·ju·gat·ed** \'kän-jə-ˌgā-təd\ adj

conjugated estrogen n : a mixture of estrogens and esp. of estrone and equilin for oral administration in the form of the sodium salts of their sulfate esters — usu. used in pl. with a sing. or pl. verb; see PREMARIN, PREMPRO

conjugate diameter n : the anteroposterior diameter of the human pelvis measured from the sacral promontory to the pubic symphysis — called also conjugata, true conjugate

conjugated protein n : a compound of a protein with a nonprotein ⟨hemoglobin is a conjugated protein of heme and globin⟩

conjugate vaccine n : a vaccine containing bacterial capsular polysaccharide joined to a protein to enhance immunogenicity; esp : one that is used to immunize infants and children against invasive disease caused by Hib bacteria

con·ju·ga·tion \ˌkän-jə-'gā-shən\ n 1 : the act of conjugating : the state of being conjugated 2 a : temporary cytoplasmic union with exchange of nuclear material that is the usual sexual process in ciliated protozoans b : the one-way transfer of DNA between bacteria in cellular contact — **con·ju·ga·tion·al** \-shnəl, -shən-ᵊl\ adj

con·junc·ti·va \ˌkän-jəŋk-'tī-və, kən-\ n, pl **-vas** or **-vae** \-ˌ(ˌ)vē\ : the mucous membrane that lines the inner surface of the eyelids and is continued over the foreeyeball — **con·junc·ti·val** \-vəl\ adj

con·junc·ti·vi·tis \kən-ˌjəŋk-ti-'vī-təs\ n : inflammation of the conjunctiva

con·junc·ti·vo·plas·ty \kən-'jəŋk-ti-(ˌ)vō-ˌplas-tē\ n, pl **-plas·ties** : plastic repair of a defect in the conjunctiva

con·junc·ti·vo·rhi·nos·to·my \kən-jəŋk-ti-(ˌ)vō-ˌrī-'näs-tə-mē\ n, pl **-mies** : surgical creation of a passage through the conjunctiva to the nasal cavity

conjunctivum — see BRACHIUM CONJUNCTIVUM

connective tissue n : a tissue of mesodermal origin that consists of various cells (as fibroblasts and macrophages) and interlacing protein fibers (as of collagen) embedded in a chiefly carbohydrate ground substance, that supports, ensheathes, and binds together other tissues, and that includes loose and dense forms (as adipose tissue, tendons, ligaments, and aponeuroses) and specialized forms (as cartilage and bone)

connective tissue disease n : any of various diseases or abnormal states (as rheumatoid arthritis, systemic lupus erythematosus, polyarteritis nodosa, scleroderma, and dermatomyositis) characterized by inflammatory or degenerative changes in connective tissue — called also collagen disease, collagenolysis, collagen vascular disease

con·nec·tor \kə-'nek-tər\ n : a part of a partial denture which joins its components

conniventes — see VALVULAE CONNIVENTES

Conn's syndrome \'känz-\ n : PRIMARY ALDOSTERONISM
  Conn, Jerome W. (1907–1994), American physician.

con·san·guine \kän-'saŋ-gwən, kən-\ adj : CONSANGUINEOUS

con·san·guin·e·ous \ˌkän-ˌsan-'gwi-nē-əs, -ˌsaŋ-\ adj : of the same blood or origin; specif : relating to or involving persons (as first cousins) that are relatively closely related ⟨∼ marriages⟩ — **con·san·guin·i·ty** \-nə-tē\ n

con·science \'kän-chəns\ n : the part of the superego in psychoanalysis that transmits commands and admonitions to the ego

¹**con·scious** \'kän-chəs\ adj 1 : capable of or marked by thought, will, design, or perception : relating to, being, or being part of consciousness ⟨the ∼ mind⟩ 2 : having mental faculties undulled by sleep, faintness, or stupor — **con·scious·ly** adv

²**conscious** n : CONSCIOUSNESS 3

con·scious·ness \-nəs\ n 1 : the totality in psychology of sensations, perceptions, ideas, attitudes, and feelings of which an individual or a group is aware at any given time or within a given time span 2 : waking life (as that to which one returns after sleep, trance, or fever) in which one's normal mental powers are present 3 : the upper part of mental life of which the person is aware as contrasted with unconscious processes

conscious sedation n : an induced state of sedation characterized by a minimally depressed consciousness such that the patient is able to continuously and independently maintain a patent airway, retain protective reflexes, and remain responsive to verbal commands and physical stimulation — compare DEEP SEDATION

con·sen·su·al \kən-'sen-chə-wəl\ adj **1** : existing or made by mutual consent ⟨∼ sexual behavior⟩ **2** : relating to or being the constrictive pupillary response of an eye that is covered when the other eye is exposed to light — **con·sen·su·al·ly** adv

con·ser·va·tive \kən-'sər-və-tiv\ adj : designed to preserve parts or restore or preserve function ⟨∼ surgery⟩ — compare AGGRESSIVE 2, RADICAL — **con·ser·va·tive·ly** adv

con·serve \kən-'sərv\ vb **con·served; con·serv·ing** : to maintain (a quantity) constant during a process of chemical, physical, or evolutionary change

con·sol·i·da·tion \kən-ˌsä-lə-'dā-shən\ n : the process by which an infected lung passes from an aerated collapsible condition to one of airless solid consistency through the accumulation of exudate in the alveoli and adjoining ducts; *also* : tissue that has undergone consolidation

con·spe·cif·ic \ˌkän-spi-'si-fik\ adj : of the same species — **conspecific** n

constant region n : the part of the polypeptide chain of a light or heavy chain of an antibody that ends in a free carboxyl group –COOH and that is relatively constant in its sequence of amino-acid residues from one antibody to another — called also *constant domain;* compare VARIABLE REGION

con·stel·la·tion \ˌkän-stə-'lā-shən\ n : a set of ideas, conditions, symptoms, or traits that fall into or appear to fall into a pattern

con·sti·pa·tion \ˌkän-stə-'pā-shən\ n : abnormally delayed or infrequent passage of usu. dry hardened feces — **con·sti·pate** \'kän-stə-ˌpāt\ vb — **con·sti·pat·ed** \-ˌpā-təd\ adj

con·sti·tu·tion \ˌkän-stə-'tü-shən, -'tyü-\ n : the physical makeup of the individual comprising inherited qualities modified by environment — **con·sti·tu·tion·al** \-shnəl, -shən-ᵊl\ adj

con·sti·tu·tion·al \-shnəl, -shən-ᵊl\ n : a walk taken for one's health

con·strict \kən-'strikt\ vb **1** : to make narrow or draw together **2** : to subject (as a body part) to compression ⟨∼ a nerve⟩ — **con·stric·tion** \-'strik-shən\ n — **con·stric·tive** \-'strik-tiv\ adj

con·stric·tor \-'strik-tər\ n : a muscle that contracts a cavity or orifice or compresses an organ — see INFERIOR CONSTRICTOR, MIDDLE CONSTRICTOR, SUPERIOR CONSTRICTOR

constrictor pha·ryn·gis inferior \-fə-'rin-jəs-\ n : INFERIOR CONSTRICTOR

constrictor pharyngis me·di·us \-'mē-dē-əs\ n : MIDDLE CONSTRICTOR

constrictor pharyngis superior n : SUPERIOR CONSTRICTOR

con·struct \'kän-ˌstrəkt\ n : something constructed esp. by mental synthesis ⟨form a ∼ of a physical object⟩

con·sult \kən-'səlt\ vb : to ask the advice or opinion of ⟨∼ a doctor⟩

con·sul·tant \kən-'səlt-ᵊnt\ n : one (as a physician, surgeon, or psychologist) called in for professional advice or services

con·sul·ta·tion \ˌkän-səl-'tā-shən\ n : a deliberation between physicians on a case or its treatment — **con·sul·ta·tive** \kən-'səl-tə-tiv, 'kän-səl-ˌtā-tiv\ adj

con·sult·ing \kən-'səl-tiŋ\ adj **1** : serving as a consultant ⟨a ∼ physician⟩ **2** : of or relating to consultation or a consultant ⟨a ∼ room⟩

con·sum·ma·to·ry \kən-'sə-mə-ˌtōr-ē\ adj : of, relating to, or being a response or act (as eating or copulating) that terminates a period of usu. goal-directed behavior

con·sump·tion \kən-'səmp-shən\ n **1** : a progressive wasting away of the body esp. from pulmonary tuberculosis **2** : TUBERCULOSIS

¹con·sump·tive \-'səmp-tiv\ adj : of, relating to, or affected with consumption ⟨a ∼ cough⟩

²consumptive n : a person affected with consumption

¹con·tact \'kän-ˌtakt\ n **1** : union or junction of body surfaces ⟨sexual ∼⟩ **2** : direct experience through the senses **3** : CONTACT LENS

²contact adj : caused or transmitted by direct or indirect contact (as with an allergen or a contagious disease)

contact lens n : a thin lens designed to fit over the cornea and usu. worn to correct defects in vision

con·ta·gion \kən-'tā-jən\ n **1** : the transmission of a disease by direct or indirect contact **2** : CONTAGIOUS DISEASE **3** : a disease-producing agent (as a virus)

contagiosa — see IMPETIGO CONTAGIOSA, MOLLUSCUM CONTAGIOSUM

contagiosum — see MOLLUSCUM CONTAGIOSUM

con·ta·gious \-jəs\ adj **1** : communicable by contact — compare INFECTIOUS 2 **2** : bearing contagion **3** : used for contagious diseases ⟨a ∼ ward⟩ — **con·ta·gious·ly** adv — **con·ta·gious·ness** n

contagious abortion n **1** : brucellosis in domestic animals characterized by abortion; *esp* : a disease affecting esp. cattle that is caused by a brucella (*Brucella abortus*) contracted by ingestion, by copulation, or possibly by wound infection **2** : any of several contagious or infectious diseases of domestic animals marked by abortion (as vibrionic abortion of sheep) — called also *infectious abortion*

contagious disease n : an infectious disease communicable by contact with one who has it, with a bodily discharge of such a patient, or with an object touched by such a patient or by bodily discharges — compare COMMUNICABLE DISEASE

con·ta·gium \kən-'tā-jəm, -jē-əm\ n, pl **-gia** \-jə, -jē-ə\ : a virus or living organism capable of causing a communicable disease

con·tam·i·nant \kən-'ta-mə-nənt\ n : something that contaminates

con·tam·i·nate \kən-'ta-mə-ˌnāt\ vb **-nat·ed; -nat·ing 1** : to soil, stain, or infect by contact or association ⟨bacteria *contaminated* the wound⟩ **2** : to make unfit for use by the introduction of unwholesome or undesirable elements ⟨water *contaminated* by sewage⟩ — **con·tam·i·na·tion** \kən-ˌta-mə-'nā-shən\ n

con·tent \'kän-ˌtent\ n : the subject matter or symbolic significance of something — see LATENT CONTENT, MANIFEST CONTENT

con·ti·nence \'känt-ᵊn-əns\ n **1** : self-restraint in refraining from sexual intercourse **2** : the ability to retain a bodily discharge voluntarily ⟨fecal ~⟩ — **con·ti·nent** \-ənt\ adj — **con·ti·nent·ly** adv

continuous positive airway pressure n : a technique of assisting breathing by maintaining the air pressure in the lungs and air passages constant and above atmospheric pressure throughout the breathing cycle — abbr. *CPAP*

con·tra·cep·tion \ˌkän-trə-'sep-shən\ n : deliberate prevention of conception or impregnation — **con·tra·cep·tive** \-'sep-tiv\ adj or n

contraceptive pill n : BIRTH CONTROL PILL

con·tract \kən-'trakt, 'kän-ˌtrakt\ vb **1** : to become affected with ⟨~ pneumonia⟩ **2** : to draw together so as to become diminished in size **3** of a muscle or muscle fiber : to undergo contraction; esp : to shorten and thicken

con·trac·tile \kən-'trakt-ᵊl, -'trak-ˌtīl\ adj : having or concerned with the power or property of contracting

con·trac·til·i·ty \ˌkän-ˌtrak-'ti-lə-tē\ n, pl **-ties** : the capability or quality of shrinking or contracting; esp : the power of muscle fibers of shortening into a more compact form

con·trac·tion \kən-'trak-shən\ n **1** : the action or process of contracting : the state of being contracted **2** : the action of a functioning muscle or muscle fiber in which force is generated accompanied esp. by shortening and thickening of the muscle or muscle fiber or sometimes by its lengthening; esp : the shortening and thickening of a functioning muscle or muscle fiber **3** : one of usu. a series of rhythmic tightening actions of the uterine muscles (as during labor)

con·trac·tor \'kän-ˌtrak-tər, kən-'\ n : something (as a muscle) that contracts or shortens

con·trac·ture \kən-'trak-chər\ n : a permanent shortening (as of muscle, tendon, or scar tissue) producing deformity or distortion — see DUPUYTREN'S CONTRACTURE

con·tra·in·di·ca·tion \ˌkän-trə-ˌin-də-'kā-shən\ n : something (as a symptom or condition) that makes a particular treatment or procedure inadvisable — **con·tra·in·di·cate** \-'in-də-ˌkāt\ vb

con·tra·lat·er·al \-'la-tə-rəl, -'la-trəl\ adj : occurring on, affecting, or acting in conjunction with a part on the opposite side of the body — compare IPSILATERAL

contrast bath n : a therapeutic immersion of a part of the body (as an extremity) alternately in hot and cold water

contrast medium n : a substance comparatively opaque to X-rays that is introduced into the body to contrast an internal part with its surrounding tissue in radiographic visualization — called also *contrast agent, contrast material*

con·tre·coup \'kōn-trə-ˌkü, 'kän-\ n : injury (as when the brain strikes the skull) occurring on the side of an organ opposite to the side on which a blow or impact is received — compare COUP

¹**con·trol** \kən-'trōl\ vb **con·trolled; con·trol·ling 1** : to incorporate suitable controls in ⟨a *controlled* experiment⟩ **2** : to reduce the incidence or severity of esp. to innocuous levels ⟨~ outbreaks of cholera⟩

²**control** n **1** : an act or instance of controlling something ⟨~ of acute intermittent porphyria⟩ **2** : one that is used in controlling something: as **a** : an experiment in which the subjects are treated as in a parallel experiment except for omission of the procedure or agent under test and which is used as a standard of comparison in judging experimental effects — called also *control experiment* **b** : one (as an organism) that is part of a control

con·trolled \kən-'trōld\ adj : regulated by law with regard to possession and use ⟨~ drugs⟩

controlled hypotension n : low blood pressure induced and maintained to reduce blood loss or to provide a bloodless field during surgery

con·tu·sion \kən-'tü-zhən, -'tyü-\ n : injury to tissue usu. without laceration : BRUISE 1 — **con·tuse** \-'tüz, -'tyüz\ vb

co·nus \'kō-nəs\ n, pl **co·ni** \-ˌnī, -ˌ(ˌ)nē\ : CONUS ARTERIOSUS

co·nus ar·te·ri·o·sus \'kō-nəs-är-ˌtir-ē-'ō-səs\ n, pl **co·ni ar·te·ri·o·si** \-ˌnī-är-ˌtir-ē-'ō-ˌsī, -ˌ(ˌ)nē-\ : a conical prolongation of the right ventricle from which the pulmonary arteries emerge

conus med·ul·lar·is \-ˌmed-ᵊl-ˈer-əs, -ˌme-jə-ˈler-\ n : a tapering lower part of the spinal cord at the level of the first lumbar segment

con·va·les·cence \ˌkän-və-ˈles-ᵊns\ n 1 : gradual recovery of health and strength after disease 2 : the time between the subsidence of a disease and complete restoration to health — **con·va·lesce** \ˌkän-və-ˈles\ vb

¹con·va·les·cent \ˌkän-və-ˈles-ᵊnt\ adj 1 : recovering from sickness or debility : partially restored to health or strength 2 : of, for, or relating to convalescence or convalescents ⟨a ∼ ward⟩

²convalescent n : one recovering from sickness

convalescent home n : an institution for the care of convalescing patients

con·ver·gence \kən-ˈvər-jəns\ n 1 : movement of the two eyes so coordinated that the images of a single point fall on corresponding points of the two retinas 2 : overlapping synaptic innervation of a single cell by more than one nerve fiber — compare DIVERGENCE 2 — **con·verge** \-ˈvərj\ vb — **con·ver·gent** \-ˈvər-jənt\ adj

convergent thinking n : thinking that weighs alternatives within an existing construct or model in solving a problem or answering a question to find one best solution and that is measured by IQ tests — compare DIVERGENT THINKING

con·ver·sion \kən-ˈvər-zhən, -shən\ n : the transformation of an unconscious mental conflict into a symbolically equivalent bodily symptom

conversion disorder n : a psychoneurosis in which bodily symptoms (as paralysis of the limbs) appear without physical basis — called also conversion hysteria, conversion reaction

con·vo·lut·ed \ˈkän-və-ˌlü-təd\ adj : folded in curved or tortuous windings; specif : having convolutions

convoluted tubule n 1 : PROXIMAL CONVOLUTED TUBULE 2 : DISTAL CONVOLUTED TUBULE

con·vo·lu·tion \ˌkän-və-ˈlü-shən\ n : any of the irregular ridges on the surface of the brain and esp. of the cerebrum — called also gyrus; compare SULCUS

convolution of Broca n : BROCA'S AREA

¹con·vul·sant \kən-ˈvəl-sənt\ adj : causing convulsions : CONVULSIVE

²convulsant n : an agent and esp. a drug that causes convulsions

con·vulse \kən-ˈvəls\ vb **con·vulsed; con·vuls·ing** 1 : to shake or agitate violently; esp : to shake or cause to shake with or as if with irregular spasms 2 : to become affected with convulsions

con·vul·sion \kən-ˈvəl-shən\ n 1 : an abnormal violent and involuntary contraction or series of contractions of the muscles — often used in pl. 2 : SEIZURE 1 — **con·vul·sive** \-siv\ adj — **con·vul·sive·ly** adv

convulsive therapy n : SHOCK THERAPY

Coo·ley's anemia \ˈkü-lēz-\ n : a severe thalassemic anemia that is associated with the presence of microcytes, enlargement of the liver and spleen, increase in the erythroid bone marrow, and jaundice and that occurs esp. in children of Mediterranean parents — called also thalassemia major

    Cooley, Thomas Benton (1871–1945), American pediatrician.

Coo·mas·sie blue \kü-ˈma-sē-, -ˈmä-\ n : a bright blue acid dye used as a biological stain esp. for proteins in gel electrophoresis

Coombs test \ˈkümz-\ n : an agglutination test used to detect proteins and esp. antibodies on the surface of red blood cells

    Coombs, Robert Royston Amos (b 1921), British immunologist.

Coo·pe·ria \kü-ˈpir-ē-ə\ n : a genus of small reddish brown nematode worms (family Trichostrongylidae) including several infesting the small intestine of sheep, goats, and cattle

    Curtice, Cooper (1856–1939), American veterinarian.

coordinate bond n : a covalent bond that consists of a pair of electrons supplied by only one of the two atoms it joins

co·or·di·na·tion \(ˌ)kō-ˌórd-ᵊn-ˈā-shən\ n 1 : the act or action of bringing into a common action, movement, or condition 2 : the harmonious functioning of parts (as muscle and nerves) for most effective results — **co·or·di·nate** \kō-ˈórd-ᵊn-ˌāt\ vb — **co·or·di·nat·ed** \-ˌā-təd\ adj

coo·tie \ˈkü-tē\ n : BODY LOUSE

co·pay \ˈkō-ˈpā\ n : CO-PAYMENT

co·pay·ment \(ˌ)kō-ˈpā-mənt\ n : a relatively small fixed fee that a health insurer (as an HMO) requires the patient to pay upon incurring a medical expense (as for a routine office visit, surgical procedure, or prescription drug) covered by the health insurer

COPD abbr chronic obstructive pulmonary disease

cope \ˈkōp\ vb **coped; cop·ing** : to deal with and attempt to overcome problems and difficulties — usu. used with with ⟨helping children ∼ with grief⟩

COPE abbr chronic obstructive pulmonary emphysema

cop·per \ˈkä-pər\ n, often attrib : a common reddish metallic element that is ductile and malleable — symbol Cu; see ELEMENT table

cop·per·head \ˈkä-pər-ˌhed\ n : a pit viper (Agkistrodon contortrix) of the eastern and central U.S. that usu. has a copper-colored head and often a reddish-brown hourglass pattern on the body and is capable of inflicting a very painful but rarely fatal bite

copper sulfate *n* : a sulfate of copper that is most familiar in its blue hydrous crystalline form $CuSO_4 \cdot 5H_2O$, is used as an algicide and fungicide, and formerly used in solution as an emetic

copr- *or* **copro-** *comb form* **1** : dung : feces ⟨*copro*phagy⟩ **2** : obscenity ⟨*copro*lalia⟩

cop·ro·an·ti·body \ˌkä-prō-ˈan-ti-ˌbä-dē\ *n, pl* **-bod·ies** : an antibody whose presence in the intestinal tract can be demonstrated by examination of an extract of the feces

cop·ro·la·lia \ˌkä-prə-ˈlā-lē-ə\ *n* **1** : obsessive or uncontrollable use of obscene language **2** : the use of obscene language as sexual gratification — **cop·ro·la·lic** \-ˈla-lik\ *adj*

cop·ro·pha·gia \ˌkä-prə-ˈfā-jə, -jē-ə\ *n* : COPROPHAGY

co·proph·a·gy \kə-ˈpräf-ə-jē\ *n, pl* **-gies** : the eating of feces that is normal behavior among many esp. young animals — **co·proph·a·gous** \-gəs\ *adj*

cop·ro·phil·ia \ˌkä-prə-ˈfi-lē-ə\ *n* : marked interest in excrement; *esp* : the use of feces or filth for sexual excitement — **cop·ro·phil·i·ac** \-ˌak\ *n*

cop·ro·por·phy·rin \ˌkä-prə-ˈpȯr-fə-rən\ *n* : any of four isomeric porphyrins $C_{36}H_{38}N_4O_8$ of which types I and III are found in feces and urine esp. in certain pathological conditions

cop·u·late \ˈkä-pyə-ˌlāt\ *vb* **-lat·ed; -lat·ing** : to engage in sexual intercourse — **cop·u·la·tion** \ˌkä-pyə-ˈlā-shən\ *n* — **cop·u·la·to·ry** \ˈkä-pyə-lə-ˌtȯr-ē\ *adj*

coraco- *comb form* : coracoid and ⟨*coraco*humeral⟩

cor·a·co·acro·mi·al \ˌkȯr-ə-(ˌ)kō-ə-ˈkrō-mē-əl\ *adj* : relating to or connecting the acromion and the coracoid process

cor·a·co·bra·chi·a·lis \ˌkȯr-ə-(ˌ)kō-ˌbrā-kē-ˈā-ləs\ *n, pl* **-a·les** \-ˌlēz\ : a muscle extending between the coracoid process and the middle of the medial surface of the humerus — called also *coracobrachialis muscle*

cor·a·co·cla·vic·u·lar ligament \-klə-ˌvi-kyə-lər-, -kla-\ : a ligament that joins the clavicle and the coracoid process of the scapula

cor·a·co·hu·mer·al \-ˈhyü-mə-rəl\ *adj* : relating to or connecting the coracoid process and the humerus

¹cor·a·coid \ˈkȯr-ə-ˌkȯid, ˈkär-\ *adj* : of, relating to, or being a process of the scapula in most mammals or a well-developed cartilage bone of many lower vertebrates that extends from the scapula to or toward the sternum

²coracoid *n* : a coracoid bone or process

coracoid process *n* : a process of the scapula in most mammals representing the remnant of the coracoid bone

of lower vertebrates that has become fused with the scapula and in humans is situated on its superior border and serves for the attachment of various muscles

coral snake \ˈkȯr-əl-, ˈkär-\ *n* : any of several venomous chiefly tropical New World elapid snakes of the genus *Micrurus* that are brilliantly banded in red, black, and yellow or white and include two (*M. fulvius* and *M. euryxanthus*) ranging northward into the southern U.S.

cor bo·vi·num \ˈkȯr-bō-ˈvī-nəm\ *n* : a greatly enlarged heart

cord \ˈkȯrd\ *n* : a slender flexible anatomical structure (as a nerve) — see SPERMATIC CORD, SPINAL CORD, UMBILICAL CORD, VOCAL CORD 1

cord blood *n* : blood from the umbilical cord of a fetus or newborn

cor·dec·to·my \kȯr-ˈdek-tə-mē\ *n, pl* **-mies** : surgical removal of one or more vocal cords

cordia pulmonalia *pl of* COR PULMONALE

cordis — see ACCRETIO CORDIS, VENAE CORDIS MINIMAE

cor·do·cen·te·sis \ˌkȯr-dō-sen-ˈtē-səs\ *n* : the withdrawal of a sample of fetal blood from the umbilical cord by transabdominal insertion of a needle guided by ultrasound

cor·dot·o·my *or* **chor·dot·o·my** \kȯr-ˈdä-tə-mē\ *n, pl* **-mies** : surgical division of a tract of the spinal cord for relief of severe intractable pain

core \ˈkȯr\ *n* : the central part of a body, mass, or part

core biopsy *n* : a biopsy in which a cylindrical sample of tissue is obtained (as from a kidney or breast) by a hollow needle

co·re·pres·sor \ˌkō-ri-ˈpres-ər\ *n* : a substance that activates a particular genetic repressor by combining with it

core temperature *n* : the temperature deep within a living body (as in the viscera)

Co·ri cycle \ˈkȯr-ē-\ *n* : the cycle in carbohydrate metabolism consisting of the conversion of glycogen to lactic acid in muscle, diffusion of the lactic acid into the bloodstream which carries it to the liver where it is converted into glycogen, and the breakdown of liver glycogen to glucose which is transported to muscle by the bloodstream and reconverted into glycogen

Cori, Carl Ferdinand (1896–1984) and **Gerty Theresa (1896–1957)**, American biochemists.

co·ri·um \ˈkȯr-ē-əm\ *n, pl* **co·ria** \-ē-ə\ : DERMIS

corn \ˈkȯrn\ *n* : a local hardening and thickening of epidermis (as on a toe)

corne- *or* **corneo-** *comb form* : cornea : corneal and ⟨*corneo*scleral⟩

cor·nea \ˈkȯr-nē-ə\ *n* : the transparent part of the coat of the eyeball that covers the iris and pupil and admits light to the interior — **cor·ne·al** \-əl\ adj

cor·neo·scler·al \ˌkȯr-nē-ə-'skler-əl\ adj : of, relating to, or affecting both the cornea and the sclera

cor·ner \'kȯ(r)-nər\ n : CORNER TOOTH

corner tooth n : one of the third or outer pair of incisor teeth of each jaw of a horse — compare DIVIDER, NIPPER

cor·ne·um \'kȯr-nē-əm\ n, pl **cor·nea** \-nē-ə\ : STRATUM CORNEUM

cor·nic·u·late cartilage \kȯr-'ni-kyə-lət-\ n : either of two small nodules of yellow elastic cartilage articulating with the apex of the arytenoid

cor·ni·fi·ca·tion \ˌkȯr-nə-fə-'kā-shən\ n 1 : conversion into horn or a horny substance or tissue : KERATINIZATION 2 : the cytological changes that occur in the vaginal epithelium esp. of rodents in response to stimulation by estrogen — **cor·ni·fy** \'kȯr-nə-fī\ vb

corn oil n : a yellow fatty oil obtained from the germ of Indian corn kernels

cor·nu \'kȯr-(ˌ)nü, -(ˌ)nyü\ n, pl **cor·nua** \-nü-ə, -ˌnyü-\ : a horn-shaped anatomical structure (as either of the lateral divisions of a bicornuate uterus or one of the lateral processes of the hyoid bone) — **cor·nu·al** \-nü-əl, -nyü-\ adj

co·ro·na \kə-'rō-nə\ n : the upper portion of a bodily part

co·ro·nal \'kȯr-ən-ᵊl, 'kär-; kə-'rōn-\ adj 1 : of, relating to, or being a corona 2 : lying in the direction of the coronal suture 3 : of or relating to the frontal plane that passes through the long axis of the body

coronal suture n : a suture extending across the skull between the parietal and frontal bones — called also *frontoparietal suture*

co·ro·na ra·di·a·ta \kə-'rō-nə-ˌrā-dē-'ä-tə, -'ä-\ n, pl **co·ro·nae ra·di·a·tae** \-(ˌ)nē-ˌrā-dē-'ā-(ˌ)tē, -'ä-\ 1 : the zone of small follicular cells immediately surrounding the ovum in the graafian follicle and accompanying the ovum on its discharge from the follicle 2 : a large mass of myelinated nerve fibers radiating from the internal capsule to the cerebral cortex

¹**cor·o·nary** \'kȯr-ə-ˌner-ē, 'kär-\ adj 1 : of, relating to, affecting, or being the coronary arteries or veins of the heart ⟨∼ sclerosis⟩; broadly : of or relating to the heart 2 : of, relating to, or affected with coronary artery disease ⟨a ∼ care unit⟩

²**coronary** n, pl **-nar·ies** 1 a : CORONARY ARTERY b : CORONARY VEIN 2 : CORONARY THROMBOSIS; broadly : HEART ATTACK

coronary artery n : either of two arteries that arise one from the left and one from the right side of the aorta immediately above the semilunar valves and supply the tissues of the heart itself

coronary artery disease n : a condition and esp. one caused by atherosclerosis that reduces the blood flow through the coronary arteries to the heart muscle and typically results in chest pain or heart damage — called also *coronary disease, coronary heart disease*

coronary band n : a thickened band of extremely vascular tissue that lies at the upper border of the wall of the hoof of the horse and related animals and that plays an important part in the secretion of the horny walls — called also *coronary cushion*

coronary bypass n : a surgical bypass operation performed to shunt blood around an obstruction in a coronary artery that usu. involves grafting one end of a segment of vein (as of the saphenous vein) removed from another part of the body into the aorta and the other end into the coronary artery beyond the obstructed area to allow for increased blood flow — called also *coronary artery bypass*

coronary disease n : CORONARY ARTERY DISEASE

coronary failure n : heart failure in which the heart muscle is deprived of the blood necessary to meet its functional needs as a result of narrowing or blocking of one or more of the coronary arteries — compare CONGESTIVE HEART FAILURE

coronary heart disease n : CORONARY ARTERY DISEASE

coronary insufficiency n : cardiac insufficiency of relatively mild degree — compare ANGINA PECTORIS, HEART ATTACK, HEART FAILURE 1

coronary ligament n 1 : the folds of peritoneum connecting the posterior surface of the liver and the diaphragm 2 : a part of the joint capsule of the knee connecting each meniscus with the margin of the head of the tibia

coronary occlusion n : the partial or complete blocking (as by a thrombus or by sclerosis) of a coronary artery

coronary plexus n : one of two nerve plexuses that are extensions of the cardiac plexus along the coronary arteries

coronary sinus n : a venous channel that is derived from the sinus venosus, is continuous with the largest of the cardiac veins, receives most of the blood from the walls of the heart, and empties into the right atrium

coronary thrombosis n : the blocking of a coronary artery of the heart by a thrombus

coronary vein n 1 a : any of several veins that drain the tissues of the heart and empty into the coronary sinus b : CARDIAC VEIN — not used technically 2 : a vein draining the lesser curvature of the stomach and emptying into the portal vein

co·ro·na·vi·rus \kə-'rō-nə-ˌvī-rəs\ *n* **1** *cap* : a genus of single-stranded RNA viruses (family *Coronaviridae*) that infect birds and many mammals including humans and that include the causative agents of bluecomb, feline infectious peritonitis, and SARS **2** : any virus of the genus *Coronavirus* or of the family (*Coronaviridae*) to which it belongs

cor·o·ner \'kȯr-ə-nər, 'kär-\ *n* : a usu. elected public officer who is typically not required to have specific medical qualifications and whose principal duty is to inquire by an inquest into the cause of any death which there is reason to suppose is not due to natural causes — see MEDICAL EXAMINER 1

cor·o·net \ˌkȯr-ə-'net, ˌkär-\ *n* : the lower part of a horse's pastern where the horn terminates in skin

cor·o·noid·ec·to·my \ˌkȯr-ə-ˌnȯi-'dek-tə-mē\ *n, pl* **-mies** : surgical removal of the mandibular coronoid process

cor·o·noid fossa \'kȯr-ə-ˌnȯid-\ *n* : a depression of the humerus into which the coronoid process fits when the arm is flexed — compare OLECRANON FOSSA

coronoid process *n* **1** : the anterior process of the superior border of the ramus of the mandible **2** : a flared process of the lower anterior part of the upper articular surface of the ulna fitting into the coronoid fossa when the arm is flexed

cor·po·ra *pl of* CORPUS

cor·po·ral \'kȯr-pə-rəl, -prəl\ *adj* : of, relating to, or affecting the body ⟨~ punishment⟩

cor·po·ra quad·ri·gem·i·na \ˌkȯr-pə-rə-ˌkwä-drə-'je-mə-nə, ˌkȯr-prə-\ *n pl* : two pairs of colliculi on the dorsal surface of the midbrain composed of white matter externally and gray matter within, the superior pair containing correlation centers for optic reflexes and the inferior pair containing correlation centers for auditory reflexes

cor·po·re·al \kȯr-'pȯr-ē-əl\ *adj* : having, consisting of, or relating to a physical material body

corporis — see PEDICULOSIS CORPORIS, TINEA CORPORIS

corpse \'kȯrps\ *n* : a dead body esp. of a human being

corps·man \'kȯr-mən, 'kȯrz-\ *n, pl* **corps·men** \-mən\ : a military enlisted person trained to give first aid and minor medical treatment

cor pul·mo·na·le \ˌkȯr-ˌpu̇l-mə-'nä-lē, -ˌpäl-, -'na-\ *n, pl* **cor·dia pul·mo·na·lia** \'kȯr-dē-ə-ˌpu̇l-mə-'nä-lē-ə, -ˌpäl-, -'na-\ : disease of the heart characterized by hypertrophy and dilatation of the right ventricle and secondary to disease of the lungs or their blood vessels

cor·pus \'kȯr-pəs\ *n, pl* **cor·po·ra** \-pə-rə, -prə\ **1** : the human or animal body esp. when dead **2** : the main

part or body of a bodily structure or organ

corpus al·bi·cans \-'al-bə-ˌkanz\ *n, pl* **corpora al·bi·can·tia** \-ˌal-bə-'kan-chē-ə\ **1** : MAMMILLARY BODY **2** : the white fibrous scar that remains in the ovary after resorption of the corpus luteum and replaces a discharged graafian follicle

corpus cal·lo·sum \-ka-'lō-səm\ *n, pl* **corpora cal·lo·sa** \-sə\ : the great band of commissural fibers uniting the cerebral hemispheres

corpus ca·ver·no·sum \-ˌka-vər-'nō-səm\ *n, pl* **corpora ca·ver·no·sa** \-sə\ : a mass of erectile tissue with large interspaces capable of being distended with blood; *esp* : one of those that form the bulk of the body of the penis or of the clitoris

cor·pus·cle \'kȯr-(ˌ)pə-səl\ *n* **1** : a living cell; *esp* : one (as a red or white blood cell or a cell in cartilage or bone) not aggregated into continuous tissues **2** : any of various small circumscribed multicellular bodies — usu. used with a qualifying term ⟨Malpighian ~s⟩ — **cor·pus·cu·lar** \kȯr-'pəs-kyə-lər\ *adj*

corpuscle of Krause *n* : KRAUSE'S CORPUSCLE

corpus he·mor·rhag·i·cum \-ˌhe-mə-'ra-ji-kəm\ *n* : a ruptured graafian follicle containing a blood clot that is absorbed as the cells lining the follicle form the corpus luteum

corpus lu·te·um \-'lü-tē-əm, -lü-'tē-əm\ *n, pl* **corpora lu·tea** \-ə\ : a yellowish mass of progesterone-secreting endocrine tissue that consists of pale secretory cells derived from granulosa cells, that forms immediately after ovulation from the ruptured graafian follicle in the mammalian ovary, and that regresses rather quickly if the ovum is not fertilized but persists throughout the ensuing pregnancy if it is fertilized

corpus spon·gi·o·sum \-ˌspən-jē-'ō-səm, -ˌspän-\ *n* : the median longitudinal column of erectile tissue of the penis that contains the urethra and is ventral to the two corpora cavernosa

corpus stri·a·tum \-ˌstrī-'ā-təm\ *n, pl* **corpora stri·a·ta** \-'ā-tə\ : either of a pair of masses of nerve tissue which lie beneath and external to the anterior cornua of the lateral ventricles of the brain and form part of their floor and each of which contains a caudate nucleus and a lentiform nucleus separated by sheets of white matter to give the mass a striated appearance in section

corpus ute·ri \-'yü-tə-ˌrī\ *n* : the main body of the uterus above the constriction behind the cervix and below the openings of the fallopian tubes

¹cor·rec·tive \kə-'rek-tiv\ *adj* : intended to correct ⟨~ lenses⟩ ⟨~ surgery⟩ — **cor·rec·tive·ly** *adv*

²**corrective** *n* : a medication that removes undesirable or unpleasant side effects of other medication

corresponding points *n pl* : points on the retinas of the two eyes which when simultaneously stimulated normally produce a single visual impression

Cor·ri·gan's disease \'kor-i-gənz-\ *n* : AORTIC REGURGITATION

Cor·ri·gan \'kor-i-gən\, **Sir Dominic John** (1802–1880), British pathologist.

Corrigan's pulse *or* **Corrigan pulse** *n* : a pulse characterized by a sharp rise to full expansion followed by immediate collapse that is seen in aortic insufficiency — called also *water-hammer pulse*

cor·rode \kə-'rōd\ *vb* **cor·rod·ed; cor·rod·ing** : to eat or be eaten away gradually (as by chemical action) — **cor·ro·sion** \kə-'rō-zhən\ *n*

¹**cor·ro·sive** \-'rō-siv, -ziv\ *adj* : tending or having the power to corrode ⟨~ acids⟩ — **cor·ro·sive·ness** *n*

²**corrosive** *n* : a substance that corrodes : CAUSTIC

corrosive sublimate *n* : MERCURIC CHLORIDE

cor·ru·ga·tor \'kor-ə-ˌgā-tər\ *n* : a muscle that contracts the skin into wrinkles; *esp* : one that draws the eyebrows together and wrinkles the brow in frowning

cor·tex \'kor-ˌteks\ *n, pl* **cor·ti·ces** \'kor-tə-ˌsēz\ *or* **cor·tex·es** : the outer or superficial part of an organ or body structure (as the kidney, adrenal gland, or a hair); *esp* : CEREBRAL CORTEX

cor·ti·cal \'kor-ti-kəl\ *adj* 1 : of, relating to, or consisting of cortex ⟨~ tissue⟩ 2 : involving or resulting from the action or condition of the cerebral cortex ⟨~ blindness⟩ — **cor·ti·cal·ly** *adv*

cortico- *comb form* 1 : cortex ⟨*cortico*tropic⟩ 2 : cortical and ⟨*cortico*spinal⟩

cor·ti·co·ad·re·nal \ˌkor-ti-kō-ə-'drēn-ᵊl\ *adj* : of or relating to the cortex of the adrenal gland ⟨~ insufficiency⟩

cor·ti·co·bul·bar \-'bəl-bər, -ˌbär\ *adj* : relating to or connecting the cerebral cortex and the medulla oblongata

cor·ti·coid \'kor-ti-ˌkoid\ *n* : CORTICOSTEROID — **corticoid** *adj*

cor·ti·co·pon·tine \ˌkor-ti-kō-'pän-ˌtīn\ *adj* : relating to or connecting the cerebral cortex and the pons

cor·ti·co·pon·to·cer·e·bel·lar \-ˌpän-tō-ˌser-ə-'be-lər\ *adj* : of, relating to, or being a tract of nerve fibers or a path for nervous impulses that passes from the cerebral cortex through the internal capsule to the pons to the white matter and cortex of the cerebellum

cor·ti·co·spi·nal \-'spīn-ᵊl\ *adj* : of or relating to the cerebral cortex and

spinal cord or to the corticospinal tract

corticospinal tract *n* : any of four columns of motor fibers of which two run on each side of the spinal cord and which are continuations of the pyramids of the medulla oblongata: **a** : LATERAL CORTICOSPINAL TRACT **b** : VENTRAL CORTICOSPINAL TRACT

cor·ti·co·ste·roid \ˌkor-ti-kō-'stir-ˌoid, -'ster-\ *n* : any of various adrenal-cortex steroids (as corticosterone, cortisone, and aldosterone) that are divided on the basis of their major biological activity into glucocorticoids and mineralocorticoids

cor·ti·co·ste·rone \ˌkor-tə-'käs-tə-ˌrōn, -kō-stə-'; ˌkor-ti-kō-'stir-ˌōn, -'ster-\ *n* : a colorless crystalline corticosteroid $C_{21}H_{30}O_4$ of the adrenal cortex that is important in protein and carbohydrate metabolism

cor·ti·co·tro·pic \ˌkor-ti-kō-'trō-pik\ *also* **cor·ti·co·tro·phic** \-fik\ *adj* : influencing or stimulating the adrenal cortex ⟨~ cells⟩

cor·ti·co·tro·pin \-'trō-pən\ *also* **cor·ti·co·tro·phin** \-fən\ *n* : ACTH; *also* : a preparation of ACTH that is used esp. in the treatment of rheumatoid arthritis and rheumatic fever

corticotropin–releasing factor *also* **corticotrophin–releasing factor** *n* : a substance secreted by the median eminence of the hypothalamus that regulates the release of ACTH by the anterior lobe of the pituitary gland

corticotropin–releasing hormone *also* **corticotrophin–releasing hormone** *n* : CORTICOTROPIN-RELEASING FACTOR

cor·tin \'kort-ᵊn\ *n* : the active principle of the adrenal cortex now known to consist of several hormones

cor·ti·sol \'kor-tə-ˌsȯl, -ˌzȯl, -ˌsōl, -ˌzōl\ *n* : a glucocorticoid $C_{21}H_{30}O_5$ produced by the adrenal cortex upon stimulation by ACTH that mediates various metabolic processes (as gluconeogenesis), has anti-inflammatory and immunosuppressive properties, and whose levels in the blood may become elevated in response to physical or psychological stress — called also *hydrocortisone*

cor·ti·sone \-ˌsōn, -ˌzōn\ *n* : a glucocorticoid $C_{21}H_{28}O_5$ that is produced naturally in small amounts by the adrenal cortex and is used in the form of its synthetic acetate $C_{23}H_{30}O_6$ esp. as replacement therapy for deficient adrenocortical secretion and as an anti-inflammatory agent (as for rheumatoid arthritis) — compare 11-DEHYDROCORTICOSTERONE

cory·ne·bac·te·ri·um \ˌkor-ə-(ˌ)nē-bak-'tir-ē-əm\ *n* 1 *cap* : a large genus of usu. gram-positive nonmotile bacteria that occur as irregular or branching rods and include a number of important parasites — see DIPH-

THERIA **2** *pl* **-ria** \-ē-ə\ : any bacterium of the genus *Corynebacterium*

co·ry·ne·form \kə-'ri-nə-ˌfȯrm\ *adj* : being or resembling bacteria of the genus *Corynebacterium*

co·ry·za \kə-'rī-zə\ *n* : an acute inflammatory contagious disease involving the upper respiratory tract: **a** : COMMON COLD **b** : any of several diseases of domestic animals characterized by inflammation of and discharge from the mucous membranes of the upper respiratory tract, sinuses, and eyes; *esp* : INFECTIOUS CORYZA — **co·ry·zal** \-zəl\ *adj*

cos·me·ceu·ti·cal \ˌkäz-mə-'sü-ti-kəl\ *n* : a preparation (as of benzoyl peroxide or retinol) that possesses both cosmetic and pharmaceutical properties

cos·me·sis \käz-'mē-səs\ *n, pl* **-me·ses** \-ˌsēz\ **1** : preservation, restoration, or enhancement of physical appearance **2** : the outer aesthetic covering (as of silicone) of a limb prosthesis

¹cos·met·ic \käz-'me-tik\ *n* : a cosmetic preparation for external use

²cosmetic *adj* **1** : of, relating to, or making for beauty esp. of the complexion ⟨~ salves⟩ **2** : correcting defects esp. of the face ⟨~ surgery⟩ — **cos·met·i·cal·ly** *adv*

cos·mid \'käz-məd\ *n* : a plasmid into which a short nucleotide sequence of a bacteriophage has been inserted to create a vector capable of cloning large segments of DNA

cost- *or* **costi-** *or* **costo-** *comb form* : rib : costal and ⟨*costochondral*⟩

cos·ta \'käs-tə\ *n, pl* **cos·tae** \-(ˌ)tē, -ˌtī\ : RIB

cos·tal \'käst-ᵊl\ *adj* : of, relating to, involving, or situated near a rib

costal breathing *n* : inspiration and expiration produced chiefly by movements of the ribs

costal cartilage *n* : any of the cartilages that connect the distal ends of the ribs with the sternum and by their elasticity permit movement of the chest in respiration

costarum — see LEVATORES COSTARUM

cos·tive \'käs-tiv, 'kȯs-\ *adj* **1** : affected with constipation **2** : causing constipation — **cos·tive·ness** *n*

cos·to·cer·vi·cal trunk \ˌkäs-tə-'sər-və-kəl, -tō-\ *n* : a branch of the subclavian artery that divides to supply the first or first two intercostal spaces and the deep structures of the neck — see INTERCOSTAL ARTERY b

cos·to·chon·dral \-'kän-drəl\ *adj* : relating to or joining a rib and costal cartilage ⟨a ~ junction⟩

cos·to·chon·dri·tis \-ˌkän-'drī-təs\ *n* : TIETZE'S SYNDROME

cos·to·di·a·phrag·mat·ic \ˌkäs-tə-ˌdī-ə-fra-'ma-tik, ˌkäs-tō-, -frag-, -ˌfrag-\ *adj* : relating to or involving the ribs and diaphragm

cos·to·phren·ic \ˌkäs-tə-'fre-nik, -tō-\ *adj* : of or relating to the ribs and the diaphragm

cos·to·trans·verse \ˌkäs-tə-trans-'vərs, -tō-, -tranz-, -'trans-ˌ, -'tranz-\ *adj* : relating to or connecting a rib and the transverse process of a vertebra ⟨a ~ joint⟩

cos·to·trans·ver·sec·to·my \-ˌtrans-(ˌ)vər-'sek-tə-mē, -ˌtranz-\ *n, pl* **-mies** : surgical excision of part of a rib and the transverse process of the adjoining vertebra

cos·to·ver·te·bral \-(ˌ)vər-'tē-brəl, -'vər-tə-brəl\ *adj* : of or relating to a rib and its adjoining vertebra ⟨~ pain⟩

¹cot \'kät\ *n* : a protective cover for a finger — called also *fingerstall*

²cot *n* : a wheeled stretcher for hospital, mortuary, or ambulance service

COTA *abbr* certified occupational therapy assistant

cot death *n chiefly Brit* : SUDDEN INFANT DEATH SYNDROME

co·throm·bo·plas·tin \(ˌ)kō-ˌthräm-bō-'plas-tən\ *n* : FACTOR VII

co·tin·ine \'kō-tᵊn-ˌēn, -ˌin\ *n* : an alkaloid $C_{10}H_{12}N_2O$ that is the principal metabolite of nicotine and is widely used as an indicator of recent exposure to nicotine

co–tri·mox·a·zole \ˌkō-ˌtrī-'mäk-sə-ˌzōl\ *n* : a bactericidal combination of trimethoprim and sulfamethoxazole in the ratio of one to five used esp. for chronic urinary tract infections

cot·ton·mouth \'kät-ᵊn-ˌmaůth\ *n* : WATER MOCCASIN

cottonmouth moccasin *n* : WATER MOCCASIN

cot·y·le·don \ˌkät-ᵊl-'ēd-ᵊn\ *n* : a lobule of a mammalian placenta — **cot·y·le·don·ary** \-'ēd-ᵊn-ˌer-ē\ *adj*

¹couch \'kaůch\ *vb* : to treat (a cataract or a person who has a cataract) by displacing the lens of the eye into the vitreous humor

²couch *n* : an article of furniture used (as by a patient undergoing psychoanalysis) for sitting or reclining — **on the couch** : receiving psychiatric treatment

¹cough \'kȯf\ *vb* **1** : to expel air from the lungs suddenly with a sharp short noise usu. in a series of efforts **2** : to expel by coughing — often used with *up* ⟨~ up mucus⟩

²cough *n* **1** : a condition marked by repeated frequent coughing ⟨he has a bad ~⟩ **2** : a sudden sharp-sounding expulsion of air from the lungs acting as a protective mechanism to clear the air passages or as a symptom of pulmonary disturbance

cough drop *n* : a lozenge used to relieve coughing

cough syrup *n* : any of various sweet usu. medicated liquids used to relieve coughing

cou·lomb \'kü-ˌläm, -ˌlōm, kü-'\ *n* : the practical mks unit of electric charge equal to the quantity of electricity transferred by a current of one ampere in one second

Coulomb, Charles–Augustin de (1736–1806), French physicist.

Cou·ma·din \'kü-mə-dən\ *trademark* — used for a preparation of the sodium salt of warfarin

cou·ma·phos \'kü-mə-ˌfäs\ *n* : an organophosphorus systemic insecticide $C_{14}H_{16}ClO_5PS$ administered esp. to cattle and poultry as a feed additive

cou·ma·rin \'kü-mə-rən\ *n* : a toxic white crystalline lactone $C_9H_6O_2$ found in plants or made synthetically and used as the parent compound in anticoagulant agents (as warfarin); *also* : a derivative of this compound

coun·sel·ing \'kaùn-s(ə-)liŋ\ *n* : professional guidance of the individual by utilizing psychological methods

coun·sel·or *or* **coun·sel·lor** \'kaùn-s(ə-)lər\ *n* : a person engaged in counseling

¹**count** \'kaùnt\ *vb* : to indicate or name by units or groups so as to find the total number of units involved

²**count** *n* : the total number of individual things in a given unit or sample (as of blood) obtained by counting all or a subsample of them

¹**count·er** \'kaùn-tər\ *n* : a level surface over which transactions are conducted or food is served or on which goods are displayed or work is conducted — **over the counter** : without a prescription ⟨drugs available *over the counter*⟩

²**counter** *n* : a device for indicating a number or amount — see GEIGER COUNTER

coun·ter·act \ˌkaùn-tər-'akt\ *vb* : to make ineffective or restrain or neutralize the usu. ill effects of by an opposite force — **coun·ter·ac·tion** \-'ak-shən\ *n*

coun·ter·con·di·tion·ing \-kən-'di-shə-niŋ\ *n* : conditioning in order to replace an undesirable response (as fear) to a stimulus (as an engagement in public speaking) by a favorable one

coun·ter·cur·rent \ˌkaùn-tər-'kər-ənt, -'kə-rənt\ *adj* **1** : flowing in an opposite direction **2** : involving flow of materials in opposite directions

coun·ter·elec·tro·pho·re·sis \-i-ˌlek-trō-fə-'rē-səs\ *n, pl* **-re·ses** \-ˌsēz\ : an electrophoretic method of testing blood esp. for hepatitis antigens

coun·ter·im·mu·no·elec·tro·pho·re·sis \-ˌimyə-nō-i-ˌlek-trō-fə-'rē-səs\ *n, pl* **-re·ses** : COUNTERELECTROPHORESIS

coun·ter·ir·ri·tant \-'ir-ə-tənt\ *n* : an agent applied locally to produce superficial inflammation with the object of reducing inflammation in deeper adjacent structures — **counterirritant** *adj*

coun·ter·ir·ri·ta·tion \-ˌtā-shən\ *n* : the reaction produced by treatment with a counterirritant; *also* : the treatment itself

coun·ter·pho·bic \-ˌfō-bik\ *adj* : relating to or characterized by a preference for or the seeking out of a situation that is feared ⟨∼ reaction patterns⟩

coun·ter·pul·sa·tion \-ˌpəl-ˌsā-shən\ *n* : a technique for reducing the work load on the heart by lowering systemic blood pressure just before or during expulsion of blood from the ventricle and by raising blood pressure during diastole — see INTRA-AORTIC BALLOON COUNTERPULSATION

coun·ter·shock \-ˌshäk\ *n* : therapeutic electric shock applied to a heart for the purpose of altering a disturbed rhythm

coun·ter·stain \-ˌstān\ *n* : a stain used to color parts of a microscopy specimen not affected by another stain; *esp* : a cytoplasmic stain used to contrast with or enhance a nuclear stain — **counterstain** *vb*

coun·ter·trac·tion \'kaùn-tər-ˌtrak-shən\ *n* : a traction opposed to another traction used in reducing fractures

coun·ter·trans·fer·ence \ˌkaùn-tər-trans-'fər-əns, -'trans-(ˌ)\ *n* **1** : psychological transference esp. by a psychotherapist during the course of treatment; *esp* : the psychotherapist's reactions to the patient's transference **2** : the complex of feelings of a psychotherapist toward the patient

coup \'kü\ *n* : injury occurring on the side of an organ (as the brain) on which a blow or impact is received — compare CONTRECOUP

cou·pling \'kə-pliŋ, -pə-liŋ\ *n* : the joining of or the part of the body that joins the hindquarters to the forequarters of a quadruped

course \'kōrs\ *n* **1** : the series of events or stages comprising a natural process **2** : a series of doses or medications administered over a designated period

court plaster \'kōrt-\ *n* : an adhesive plaster esp. of silk coated with isinglass and glycerin

cou·vade \kü-'väd\ *n* **1** : a custom in some cultures in which when a child is born the father takes to bed as if bearing the child **2** : COUVADE SYNDROME

couvade syndrome *n* : a phenomenon in which a male experiences symptoms of pregnancy (as nausea or weight gain) during the time his partner or another woman he is particularly close to is pregnant

Cou·ve·laire uterus \ˌkü-və-'ler-\ *n* : a pregnant uterus in which the placenta has detached prematurely with extravasation of blood into the uterine musculature

Couvelaire, Alexandre (1873–1948), French obstetrician.

co·va·lent bond \(ˌ)kō-ˈvā-lənt-\ *n* : a chemical bond formed between atoms by the sharing of electrons

cover glass *n* : a piece of very thin glass or plastic used to cover material on a microscope slide

cov·er·slip \'kə-vər-ˌslip\ *n* : COVER GLASS

Cow·dria \'kaú-drē-ə\ *n* : a genus of small pleomorphic intracellular rickettsial bacteria known chiefly from ticks but including the causative organism (*C. ruminantium*) of heartwater of ruminants

Cow·dry \'kaú-drē\, **Edmund Vincent (1888–1975),** American anatomist.

cow·hage *also* **cow·age** \'kaú-ij\ *n* : a tropical leguminous woody vine (*Mucuna pruriens*) with crooked pods covered with barbed hairs that cause severe itching; *also* : these hairs formerly used as a vermifuge

Cow·per's gland \'kaú-pərz-, 'kü-, 'kú-\ *n* : either of two small glands of which one lies on each side of the male urethra below the prostate gland and discharges a secretion into the semen — called also *bulbourethral gland;* compare BARTHOLIN'S GLAND

Cow·per \'kaú-pər, 'kü-, 'kú-\, **William (1666–1709),** British anatomist.

cow·pox \'kaú-ˌpäks\ *n* : a mild eruptive disease of the cow that is caused by a poxvirus of the genus *Orthopoxvirus* (species *Cowpox virus*) and that when communicated to humans protects against smallpox — called also *variola vaccinia*

cox \'käks\ *n* : CYCLOOXYGENASE

cox- *or* **coxo-** *comb form* : hip : thigh : of the hip and ⟨*coxo*femoral⟩

coxa \'käk-sə\ *n, pl* **cox·ae** \-ˌsē, -ˌsī\ : HIP JOINT, HIP

coxa vara \'käk-sə-'var-ə\ *n* : a deformed hip joint in which the neck of the femur is bent downward

Cox·i·el·la \ˌkäk-sē-'e-lə\ *n* : a genus of small pleomorphic rickettsial bacteria occurring intercellularly in ticks and intracellularly in the cytoplasm of vertebrates and including the causative organism (*C. burnetii*) of Q fever

Cox \'käks\, **Herald Rea** (*b* 1907), American bacteriologist.

coxo·fem·o·ral \ˌkäk-sō-'fe-mə-rəl\ *adj* : of or relating to the hip and thigh

COX–1 \'käks-'wən\ *n* : the isoform of cyclooxygenase that is expressed in most tissues of the body and is not involved in producing the pain and inflammation of arthritis

cox·sack·ie·vi·rus \ˌ(ˌ)käk-ˌsa-kē-'vī-rəs\ *n* : any of numerous serotypes of three picornaviruses of the genus *Enterovirus* (species *Human enterovirus A, Human enterovirus B,* and *Human enterovirus C*) associated with human diseases (as meningitis, herpangina, or epidemic pleurodynia)

COX–2 \'käks-'tü\ *n* **1** : the isoform of cyclooxygenase that is expressed esp. in the brain and kidneys and at sites of inflammation **2** : COX-2 INHIBITOR

cox–2 inhibitor *n* : any of a class of NSAID drugs (as celecoxib) that selectively block the isoform COX-2 but not the isoform COX-1 of cyclooxygenase and that are intended to relieve the pain and inflammation of arthritis while minimizing gastrointestinal side effects — called also *COX-2 blocker*

Co·zaar \'kō-ˌzär\ *trademark* — used for a preparation of the potassium salt of losartan

CP *abbr* cerebral palsy

CPAP *abbr* continuous positive airway pressure

CPB *abbr* competitive protein binding

C–pep·tide \'sē-'pep-ˌtīd\ *n* : a protein fragment 35 amino-acid residues long produced by enzymatic cleavage of proinsulin in the formation of insulin

CPK *abbr* creatine phosphokinase

CPR *abbr* cardiopulmonary resuscitation

Cr *symbol* chromium

CR *abbr* conditioned response

crab louse *n, pl* **crab lice** : a sucking louse of the genus *Phthirius* (*P. pubis*) infesting the pubic region of the human body — called also *pubic louse*

crabs \'krabz\ *n pl* : infestation with crab lice

crack \'krak\ *n, often attrib* : a potent form of cocaine that is obtained by treating the hydrochloride of cocaine with sodium bicarbonate to create small chips used illicitly usu. for smoking

crack baby *n* : an infant born physiologically addicted to crack as a result of continued exposure to the drug in the mother's womb

cra·dle \'krād-ºl\ *n* : a frame to keep the bedding from contact with an injured part of the body

cradle cap *n* : a seborrheic condition in infants that usu. affects the scalp and is characterized by greasy gray or dark brown adherent scaly crusts

¹cramp \'kramp\ *n* **1** : a painful involuntary spasmodic contraction of a muscle ⟨a ~ in the leg⟩ **2** : a temporary paralysis of muscles from overuse — see WRITER'S CRAMP **3 a** : sharp abdominal pain — usu. used in pl. **b** : persistent and often intense though dull lower abdominal pain associated with dysmenorrhea — usu. used in pl.

²cramp *vb* : to affect with or be affected with a cramp or cramps

crani- *or* **cranio-** *comb form* **1** : cranium ⟨*cranio*synostosis⟩ **2** : cranial and ⟨*cranio*sacral⟩

-crania *n comb form* : condition of the skull or head ⟨hemi*crania*⟩

cra·ni·ad \'krā-nē-ˌad\ *adv* : toward the head or anterior end

cra·ni·al \'krā-nē-əl\ *adj* **1** : of or relating to the skull or cranium **2** : CEPHALIC — **cra·ni·al·ly** *adv*

cranial arteritis *n* : GIANT CELL ARTERITIS

cra·ni·al fossa *n* : any of the three large depressions in the posterior, middle, and anterior aspects of the floor of the cranial cavity

cranial index *n* : the ratio multiplied by 100 of the maximum breadth of the bare skull to its maximum length from front to back — compare CEPHALIC INDEX

cranial nerve *n* : any of the 12 paired nerves that arise from the lower surface of the brain with one of each pair on each side and pass through openings in the skull to the periphery of the body — see ABDUCENS NERVE, ACCESSORY NERVE, AUDITORY NERVE, FACIAL NERVE, GLOSSOPHARYNGEAL NERVE, HYPOGLOSSAL NERVE, OCULOMOTOR NERVE, OLFACTORY NERVE, OPTIC NERVE, TRIGEMINAL NERVE, TROCHLEAR NERVE, VAGUS NERVE

cra·ni·ec·to·my \ˌkrā-nē-ˈek-tə-mē\ *n, pl* **-mies** : the surgical removal of a portion of the skull

cra·nio·ce·re·bral \ˌkrā-nē-ō-sə-ˈrē-brəl, -ˈser-ə-\ *adj* : involving both cranium and brain ⟨~ injury⟩

cra·nio·fa·cial \ˌkrā-nē-ō-ˈfā-shəl\ *adj* : of, relating to, or involving both the cranium and the face

craniofacial dysostosis *n* : CROUZON SYNDROME

cra·ni·ol·o·gy \ˌkrā-nē-ˈä-lə-jē\ *n, pl* **-gies** : a science dealing with variations in size, shape, and proportions of skulls among human races

cra·ni·om·e·try \-ˈä-mə-trē\ *n, pl* **-tries** : a science dealing with cranial measurement

cra·ni·op·a·gus \ˌkrā-nē-ˈä-pə-gəs\ *n, pl* **-a·gi** \-pə-ˌjē, -ˌjī\ : a pair of twins joined at the heads

cra·nio·pha·ryn·ge·al \ˌkrā-nē-ō-fa-ˈrən-jē-əl, -fə-ˈrin-jəl, -jē-əl\ *adj* : relating to or connecting the cavity of the skull and the pharynx

cra·nio·pha·ryn·gi·o·ma \-ˌfar-ən-jē-ˈō-mə, -fə-ˌrin-jē-ˈō-mə\ *n, pl* **-mas** *also* **-ma·ta** \-mə-tə\ : a tumor of the brain near the pituitary gland that develops esp. in children or young adults from epithelium derived from the embryonic craniopharyngeal canal and that is often associated with increased intracranial pressure

cra·nio·plas·ty \ˈkrā-nē-ˌō-ˌplas-tē\ *n, pl* **-ties** : the surgical correction of skull defects

cra·nio·ra·chis·chi·sis \ˌkrā-nē-ō-rə-ˈkis-kə-səs\ *n, pl* **-chi·ses** \-ˌsēz\ : a congenital fissure of the skull and spine

cra·nio·sa·cral \ˌkrā-nē-ō-ˈsa-krəl, -ˈsā-\ *adj* **1** : of or relating to the cranium and the sacrum **2** : PARASYMPATHETIC

cra·ni·os·chi·sis \ˌkrā-nē-ˈäs-kə-səs\ *n, pl* **-chi·ses** \-ˌsēz\ : a congenital fissure of the skull

cra·nio·ste·no·sis \ˌkrā-nē-ō-stə-ˈnō-səs\ *n, pl* **-no·ses** \-ˌsēz\ : malformation of the skull caused by premature closure of the cranial sutures

cra·nio·syn·os·to·sis \-ˌsi-ˌnäs-ˈtō-səs\ *n, pl* **-to·ses** \-ˌsēz\ *or* **-to·sis·es** : premature fusion of the sutures of the skull

cra·ni·o·ta·bes \ˌkrā-nē-ə-ˈtā-(ˌ)bēz\ *n, pl* **craniotabes** : a thinning and softening of the infantile skull in spots usu. due to rickets or syphilis

cra·ni·ot·o·my \ˌkrā-nē-ˈä-tə-mē\ *n, pl* **-mies 1** : the operation of cutting or crushing the fetal head to effect delivery **2** : surgical opening of the skull

cra·ni·um \ˈkrā-nē-əm\ *n, pl* **-ni·ums** *or* **-nia** \-nē-ə\ : SKULL; *specif* : BRAINCASE

crank \ˈkrank\ *n* : CRYSTAL 2

cra·ter \ˈkrā-tər\ *n* : an eroded lesion of a wall or surface ⟨ulcer ~s⟩

cra·ter·i·za·tion \ˌkrā-tər-ə-ˈzā-shən\ *n* : surgical excision of a crater-shaped piece of bone

craz·ing \ˈkrāz-iŋ\ *n* : the formation of minute cracks (as in acrylic resin teeth) usu. attributed to shrinkage or to moisture

cra·zy \ˈkrā-zē\ *adj* **craz·i·er; -est** : MAD, INSANE — **cra·zi·ly** \-zə-lē\ *adv* — **cra·zi·ness** \-zē-nəs\ *n*

crazy bone *n* : FUNNY BONE

CRD *abbr* chronic respiratory disease

C–re·ac·tive protein \ˈsē-rē-ˈak-tiv-\ *n* : a protein produced by the liver that is normally present in trace amounts in the blood serum but is elevated during episodes of acute inflammation

cream \ˈkrēm\ *n* **1** : the yellowish part of milk containing from 18 to about 40 percent butterfat **2** : something having the consistency of cream; *esp* : a usu. emulsified medicinal or cosmetic preparation — **creamy** \ˈkrē-mē\ *adj*

crease \ˈkrēs\ *n* : a line or mark made by or as if by folding a pliable substance (as the skin) — **crease** *vb*

cre·a·tine \ˈkrē-ə-ˌtēn, -ət-ᵊn\ *n* : a nitrogenous substance $C_4H_9N_3O_2$ found esp. in vertebrate muscles either free or as phosphocreatine

creatine kinase *n* : any of three isoenzymes found esp. in skeletal and myocardial muscle and the brain that catalyze the transfer of a high-energy phosphate group from phosphocreatine to ADP with the formation of ATP and creatine and typically occur in elevated levels in the blood following injury to brain or muscle tissue

creatine phosphate *n* : PHOSPHOCREATINE

creatine phosphokinase *n* : CREATINE KINASE

cre·at·i·nine \krē-ˈat-ᵊn-ˌēn, -ᵊn-ən\ *n* : a white crystalline strongly basic compound $C_4H_7N_3O$ formed from creatine and found esp. in muscle, blood, and urine

cre·a·tin·uria \ˌkrē-ə-tə-ˈnuṙ-ə, -ˈnyuṙ-\ *n* : the presence of creatine in urine; *esp* : an increased or abnormal amount in the urine

creeping eruption *n* : a human skin disorder that is characterized by a red line of eruption which fades at one end as it progresses at the other and that is usu. caused by insect or worm larvae and esp. those of the dog hookworm burrowing in the deeper layers of the skin — called also *larval migrans, larva migrans*

creeps \ˈkrēps\ *n pl* : a deficiency disease esp. of sheep and cattle associated with an abnormal dietary calcium-phosphorus ratio

cre·mas·ter \krē-ˈmas-tər, krə-\ *n* : a thin muscle consisting of loops of fibers derived from the internal oblique muscle and descending upon the spermatic cord to surround and suspend the testicle — called also *cremaster muscle* — **cre·mas·ter·ic** \ˌkrē-mə-ˈster-ik\ *adj*

crème \ˈkrem, ˈkrēm\ *n, pl* **crèmes** \ˈkrem, ˈkremz, ˈkrēmz\ : CREAM 2

cre·nat·ed \ˈkrē-ˌnā-təd\ *also* **cre·nate** \-ˌnāt\ *adj* : having the margin or surface cut into rounded scallops ⟨∼ red blood cells⟩

cre·na·tion \kri-ˈnā-shən\ *n* : shrinkage of red blood cells resulting in crenated margins

cre·o·sote \ˈkrē-ə-ˌsōt\ *n* **1** : an oily liquid mixture of phenolic compounds obtained by the distillation of wood tar and used esp. as a disinfectant and as an expectorant in chronic bronchitis **2** : a brownish oily liquid consisting chiefly of aromatic hydrocarbons obtained by distillation of coal tar and used esp. as a wood preservative

crep·i·tant rale \ˈkre-pə-tənt-\ *n* : a peculiar crackling sound audible with inspiration in pneumonia and other lung diseases

crep·i·ta·tion \ˌkre-pə-ˈtā-shən\ *n* : a grating or crackling sound or sensation (as that produced by the fractured ends of a bone moving against each other) ⟨∼ in the arthritic knee⟩

crep·i·tus \ˈkre-pə-təs\ *n, pl* **crepitus** : CREPITATION

crescent of Gian·nuz·zi *or* **crescent of Gia·nuz·zi** \-jə-ˈnüt-sē\ *n* : DEMILUNE

G. Giannuzzi — see DEMILUNE OF GIANNUZZI

cre·sol \ˈkrē-ˌsȯl, -ˌsōl\ *n* : any of three poisonous colorless crystalline or liquid isomeric phenols C_7H_8O that are used as disinfectants, in making phenolic resins, and in organic synthesis — see METACRESOL

crest \ˈkrest\ *n* : a ridge esp. on a bone ⟨the ∼ of the tibia⟩ — see OCCIPITAL CREST

Cres·tor \ˈkre-ˌstȯr\ *trademark* — used for the calcium salt of rosuvastatin

cre·tin \ˈkrēt-ᵊn\ *n, often offensive* : one affected with cretinism — **cre·tin·ous** \-ᵊn-əs\ *adj*

cre·tin·ism \-ˈtē-ˌni-zəm\ *n* : a usu. congenital abnormal condition marked by physical stunting and mental retardation and caused by severe thyroid deficiency

Creutz·feldt–Ja·kob disease *also* **Creutz·feld–Ja·cob disease** \ˈkrȯits-ˌfelt-ˈyä-(ˌ)kōb-, -(ˌ)kȯp-\ *n* : a rare progressive fatal prion disease marked by development of porous brain tissue, premature dementia in middle age, and gradual loss of muscular coordination — abbr. *CJD;* called also *Jakob-Creutzfeldt disease;* see VARIANT CREUTZFELDT-JAKOB DISEASE

Creutzfeldt, Hans Gerhard (1885–1964), and Jakob, Alfons Maria (1884–1931), German psychiatrists.

crev·ice \ˈkre-vəs\ *n* : a narrow fissure or cleft — see GINGIVAL CREVICE

cre·vic·u·lar \kri-ˈvi-kyə-lər\ *adj* : of, relating to, or involving a crevice and esp. the gingival crevice

crib·bing \ˈkri-biŋ\ *n* : a vice of horses in which they grasp a solid object (as a stall door) with their teeth and gulp air

crib biting *n* : CRIBBING

crib death *n* : SUDDEN INFANT DEATH SYNDROME

crib·ri·form plate \ˈkri-brə-ˌfȯrm-\ *n* **1** : the horizontal plate of the ethmoid bone perforated with numerous foramina for the passage of the olfactory nerve filaments from the nasal cavity — called also *lamina cribrosa* **2** : LAMINA DURA

cribrosa — see LAMINA CRIBROSA

crick \ˈkrik\ *n* : a painful spasmodic condition of muscles (as of the neck or back) — **crick** *vb*

crico- *comb form* **1** : cricoid cartilage and ⟨cricothyroid⟩ **2** : of the cricoid cartilage and ⟨crico·pharyngeal⟩

cri·co·ar·y·te·noid \ˌkrī-kō-ˌar-ə-ˈtē-ˌnȯid, -kō-ə-ˈrit-ᵊn-ˌȯid\ *n* **1** : a muscle of the larynx that arises from the upper margin of the arch of the cricoid cartilage, inserts into the front of the process of the arytenoid cartilage, and helps to narrow the opening of the vocal cords — called also *lateral cricoarytenoid* **2** : a muscle of the larynx that arises from the posterior surface of the lamina of the cricoid cartilage, inserts into the posterior of the process of the arytenoid cartilage, and widens the opening of the vocal cords — called also *posterior cricoarytenoid*

cri·coid cartilage \ˈkrī-ˌkȯid-\ *n* : a cartilage of the larynx which articulates with the lower cornua of the thyroid cartilage and with which the arytenoid cartilages articulate — called also *cricoid*

cri·co·pha·ryn·geal \ˌkrī-kō-ˌfar-ən-ˈjē-əl, -fə-ˈrin-jəl, -jē-əl\ *adj* : of or relating to the cricoid cartilage and the pharynx

¹**cri·co·thy·roid** \-'thī-ˌroid\ *adj* : relating to or connecting the cricoid cartilage and the thyroid cartilage

²**cricothyroid** *n* : a triangular muscle of the larynx that is attached to the cricoid and thyroid cartilages and is the principal tensor of the vocal cords — called also *cricothyroid muscle*

cri·co·thy·roi·de·us \ˌkrī-kō-thī-'roi-dē-əs\ *n, pl* **-dei** \-dē-ˌī\ : CRICOTHYROID

cricothyroid membrane *n* : a membrane of yellow elastic tissue that is attached below to the cricoid cartilage, in front to the thyroid cartilage, and in back to the arytenoid cartilages and that forms the vocal ligaments with its thickened upper margins

cri·co·thy·roi·dot·o·my \ˌkrī-kō-ˌthī-ˌroi-'dä-tə-mē\ *n, pl* **-mies** : tracheotomy by incision through the skin and cricothyroid membrane esp. as an emergency procedure for relief of an obstructed airway

cri du chat syndrome \ˌkrē-dù-'shä-, -də-\ *n* : an inherited condition characterized by a mewing cry, mental retardation, physical anomalies, and the absence of part of a chromosome — called also *cat cry syndrome*

¹**crip·ple** \'kri-pəl\ *n, sometimes offensive* : a lame or partly disabled individual

²**cripple** *vb* **crip·pled**; **crip·pling** \-p(ə-)liŋ\ : to deprive of the use of a limb and esp. a leg ⟨*crippled* by arthritis⟩

crip·pler \-p(ə-)lər\ *n* : a disease that results in crippling

cri·sis \'krī-səs\ *n, pl* **cri·ses** \-ˌsēz\ **1** : the turning point for better or worse in an acute disease or fever; *esp* : a sudden turn for the better (as sudden abatement in severity of symptoms or abrupt drop in temperature) — compare LYSIS 1 **2** : a paroxysmal attack of pain, distress, or disordered function ⟨tabetic ∼⟩ ⟨cardiac ∼⟩ **3** : an emotionally significant event or radical change of status in a person's life **4** : a psychological or social condition characterized by unusual instability caused by excessive stress and either endangering or felt to endanger the continuity of an individual or group; *esp* : such a social condition requiring the transformation of cultural patterns and values

crisis center *n* : a facility run usu. by nonprofessionals who counsel those who telephone for help in a personal crisis

cris·ta \'kris-tə\ *n, pl* **cris·tae** \-ˌtē, -ˌtī\ **1** : one of the areas of specialized sensory epithelium in the ampullae of the semicircular canals of the ear serving as end organs for the vestibular sense **2** : an elevation of the surface of a bone for the attachment of a muscle or tendon **3** : any of the inwardly pro-

jecting folds of the inner membrane of a mitochondrion

crista amp·ul·lar·is \-ˌam-p(y)ù-'lar-əs\ *n* : CRISTA 1

crista gal·li \-'ga-lē, -'gȯ-\ *n* : an upright process on the anterior portion of the cribriform plate to which the anterior part of the falx cerebri is attached

crit·i·cal \'kri-ti-kəl\ *adj* **1** : relating to, indicating, or being the stage of a disease at which an abrupt change for better or worse may be anticipated with reasonable certainty ⟨the ∼ phase of a fever⟩ **2** : being or relating to an illness or condition involving danger of death ⟨a ∼ care⟩ ⟨a ∼ head injury⟩ — **crit·i·cal·ly** \-k(ə-)lē\ *adv*

Crix·i·van \'krik-sə-ˌvan\ *trademark* — used for a preparation of the sulfate of indinavir

CRNA *abbr* certified registered nurse anesthetist

crock \'kräk\ *n, slang* : a complaining medical patient whose illness is largely imaginary or psychosomatic

Crohn's disease \'krōnz-\ *also* **Crohn disease** \'krōn-\ *n* : chronic ileitis that typically involves the distal portion of the ileum, often spreads to the colon, and is characterized by diarrhea, cramping, and loss of appetite and weight with local abscesses and scarring — called also *regional enteritis, regional ileitis*

   Crohn \'krōn\, **Burrill Bernard** (1884–1983), American physician.

cromoglycate — see SODIUM CROMOGLYCATE

cro·mo·lyn sodium \'krō-mə-lən-\ *n* : a drug $C_{23}H_{14}Na_2O_{11}$ that inhibits the release of histamine from mast cells and is used usu. as an inhalant to prevent the onset of bronchial asthma attacks — called also *cromolyn, disodium cromoglycate, sodium cromoglycate;* see INTAL

¹**cross** \'krȯs\ *n* **1** : an act of crossing dissimilar individuals or kind **2** : a crossbred individual or kind

²**cross** *vb* : to interbreed or cause (an animal or plant) to interbreed with one of a different kind : HYBRIDIZE

³**cross** *adj* : CROSSBRED, HYBRID

cross·bred \'krȯs-'bred\ *adj* : produced by crossbreeding : HYBRID — **cross·bred** \-ˌbred\ *n*

¹**cross·breed** \'krȯs-ˌbrēd, -'brēd\ *vb* **-bred** \-ˌbred, -'bred\; **-breed·ing** : HYBRIDIZE, CROSS; *esp* : to cross (two varieties or breeds) within the same species

²**cross·breed** \-ˌbrēd\ *n* : HYBRID

cross·bridge \'krȯs-ˌbrij\ *n* : the globular head of a myosin molecule that projects from a myosin filament in muscle and in the sliding filament hypothesis of muscle contraction is held to attach temporarily to an adjacent actin filament and draw it into the A band of a sarcomere between the myosin filaments

crossed \'krȯst\ *adj* : forming a decussation ⟨a ~ tract of nerve fibers⟩

cross-eye \'krȯs-ˌī\ *n* **1** : strabismus in which the eye turns inward toward the nose — called also *esotropia*; compare WALLEYE 2a **2 cross-eyes** \-ˈīz\ *pl* : eyes affected with cross-eye — **cross-eyed** \-ˈīd\ *adj*

cross-ing-over \ˌkrȯ-siŋ-ˈō-vər\ *n* : an interchange of genes or segments between homologous chromosomes

cross-link \'krȯs-ˌliŋk\ *n* : a crosswise connecting part (as an atom) that connects parallel chains in a complex chemical molecule (as a protein) — **cross-link** *vb*

cross-match-ing \'krȯs-ˈma-chiŋ\ or **cross-match** \-ˈmach\ *n* : the testing of the compatibility of the bloods of a transfusion donor and a recipient by mixing the serum of each with the red cells of the other to determine the absence of agglutination reactions — **crossmatch** *vb*

¹cross-over \'krȯs-ˌō-vər\ *n* **1** : an instance or product of genetic crossing-over **2** : a crossover interchange in an experiment

²crossover *adj* : involving or using interchange of the control group and the experimental group during the course of an experiment

cross-re-ac-tion \ˌkrȯs-rē-ˈak-shən\ *n* : reaction of one antigen with antibodies developed against another antigen — **cross-re-act** \-ˈakt\ *vb* — **cross-re-ac-tive** \-rē-ˈak-tiv\ *adj* — **cross-re-ac-tiv-i-ty** \-(ˌ)rē-ˌak-ˈti-və-tē\ *n*

cross section *n* : a cutting or piece of something cut off at right angles to an axis; *also* : a representation of such a cutting — **cross-sec-tion-al** \ˌkrȯs-ˈsek-shə-nəl\ *adj*

cross-tol-er-ance \'krȯs-ˈtä-lə-rəns\ *n* : tolerance or resistance to a drug that develops through continued use of another drug with similar pharmacological action

cro-ta-lar-ia \ˌkrō-tə-ˈlar-ē-ə, ˌkrä-\ *n* **1** *cap* : a large genus of usu. tropical and subtropical leguminous plants including some containing toxic alkaloids esp. in the seeds that are poisonous to farm animals and humans **2** : any plant of the genus *Crotalaria* — called also *rattlebox*

Cro-ta-lus \'krōt-ᵊl-əs, 'krät-\ *n* : a genus of American pit vipers including many of the rattlesnakes

crotch \'kräch\ *n* : an angle formed by the parting of two legs, branches, or members

-crotic *adj comb form* : having (such) a heartbeat or pulse ⟨dicrotic⟩

-crotism *n comb form* : condition of having (such) a heartbeat or pulse ⟨dicrotism⟩

Cro-ton bug \'krōt-ᵊn-\ *n* : GERMAN COCKROACH

cro-ton oil \'krōt-ᵊn-\ *n* : a viscid acrid oil from an Asian plant (*Croton tiglium* of the family Euphorbiaceae) that was formerly used as a cathartic but is now used esp. in pharmacological experiments as an irritant

croup \'krüp\ *n* : inflammation, edema, and subsequent obstruction of the larynx, trachea, and bronchi esp. of infants and young children that is typically caused by a parainfluenza virus and is marked by episodes of difficult breathing and low-pitched cough resembling the bark of a seal — **croup-ous** \'krü-pəs\ *adj* — **croupy** \-pē\ *adj*

Crou-zon syndrome \krü-ˈzän-\ *also* **Crou-zon's syndrome** \-ˈzänz-\ *n* : a craniofacial disorder that is inherited as an autosomal dominant trait and is characterized by malformation of the skull due to premature ossification and closure of the sutures — called also *craniofacial dysostosis, Crouzon's disease*

Crouzon, Octave (1874–1938), French neurologist.

¹crown \'kraun\ *n* **1** : the topmost part of the skull or head **2** : the part of a tooth external to the gum or an artificial substitute for this

²crown *vb* **1** : to put an artificial crown on (a tooth) **2** *in childbirth* : to appear at the vaginal opening — used of the first part (as the crown of the head) of the infant to appear

crow's-foot \'krōz-ˌfut\ *n, pl* **crow's-feet** \-ˌfēt\ : a wrinkle extending from the outer corner of the eye — usu. used in pl.

CRT \ˌsē-(ˌ)är-ˈtē\ *n, pl* **CRTs** *or* **CRT's** : CATHODE-RAY TUBE; *also* : a display device incorporating a cathode-ray tube

CRTT *abbr* certified respiratory therapy technician

cru-ci-ate \'krü-shē-ˌāt\ *adj* : shaped like a cross

cruciate ligament *n* : any of several more or less cross-shaped ligaments: as **a** : either of two ligaments in the knee joint which cross each other from femur to tibia: (1) : ANTERIOR CRUCIATE LIGAMENT (2) : POSTERIOR CRUCIATE LIGAMENT **b** : a complex ligament made up of the transverse ligament of the atlas and vertical fibrocartilage extending from the dens to the border of the foramen magnum

crude protein *n* : the approximate amount of protein in foods that is calculated from the determined nitrogen content and that may contain an appreciable error if the nitrogen is derived from nonprotein material or from a protein of unusual composition

cru-ra *pl of* CRUS

cru-ra ce-re-bri \ˌkrur-ə-ˈser-ə-ˌbrī, -ˈker-ə-ˌbrē\ *n pl* : CRUS 2c

crura for-ni-cis \-ˈfȯr-nə-ˌsis, -ə-ˌkis\ *n pl* : CRUS 2e

cru-ral \'krur-əl\ *adj* : of or relating to the thigh or leg; *specif* : FEMORAL

cruris — see TINEA CRURIS

crus \'krüs, 'krəs\ *n, pl* **cru·ra** \'krür-ə\ **1** : the lower or hind limb esp. between the knee and the ankle or tarsus : SHANK **2** : any of various anatomical parts likened to a leg or to a pair of legs: as **a** : either of the diverging proximal ends of the corpora cavernosa **b** : the tendinous attachments of the diaphragm to the bodies of the lumbar vertebrae forming the sides of the aortic opening — often used in pl. **c** *pl* : the peduncles of the cerebrum — called also *crura cerebri* **d** *pl* : the peduncles of the cerebellum **e** *pl* : the posterior pillars of the fornix — called also *crura fornicis* **f** (1) : a long bony process of the incus that articulates with the stapes; *also* : a shorter one projecting from the body of the incus perpendicular to this (2) : either of the two bony processes forming the sides of the arch of the stapes

crush syndrome *n* : the physical responses to severe crushing injury of muscle tissue involving esp. shock and partial or complete renal failure; *also* : the renal failure associated with such responses

crust \'krəst\ *n* **1** : SCAB 2 **2** : an encrusting deposit of serum, cellular debris, and bacteria present over or about lesions in some skin diseases (as impetigo or eczema) — **crust** *vb*

crutch \'krəch\ *n* **1** : a support typically fitting under the armpit for use as an aid in walking **2** : the crotch esp. of an animal

cry- *or* **cryo-** *comb form* : cold : freezing ⟨*cryo*surgery⟩

cryo·bi·ol·o·gy \ˌkrī-ō-bī-'ä-lə-jē\ *n, pl* **-gies** : the study of the effects of extremely low temperature on living organisms and cells — **cryo·bi·o·log·i·cal** \-ˌbī-ə-'lä-ji-kəl\ *adj* — **cryo·bi·ol·o·gist** \ˌkrī-ō-bī-'ä-lə-jist\ *n*

cryo·cau·tery \-'kò-tə-rē\ *n, pl* **-ter·ies** : destruction of tissue by use of extreme cold

cryo·ex·trac·tion \-ik-'strak-shən\ *n* : extraction of a cataract through use of a cryoprobe whose refrigerated tip adheres to and freezes tissue of the lens permitting its removal

cryo·ex·trac·tor \-ik-'strak-tər, -'ek-ˌ\ *n* : a cryoprobe used for removal of cataracts

cryo·fi·brin·o·gen \-fī-'bri-nə-jən\ *n* : fibrinogen that precipitates upon cooling to 4°C (39°F) and redissolves at 37°C (98.6°F)

cryo·gen·ic \ˌkrī-ə-'je-nik\ *adj* **1 a** : of or relating to the production of very low temperatures **b** : being or relating to very low temperatures **2** : requiring or involving the use of a cryogenic temperature ⟨~ surgery⟩ — **cryo·gen·i·cal·ly** \-ni-k(ə-)lē\ *adv*

cryo·gen·ics \-niks\ *n* : a branch of physics that deals with the production and effects of very low temperatures

cryo·glob·u·lin \ˌkrī-ō-'glä-byə-lən\ *n* : any of several proteins similar to gamma globulins (as in molecular weight) that precipitate usu. in the cold from blood serum esp. in pathological conditions (as multiple myeloma)

cryo·glob·u·lin·emia \-ˌglä-byə-lə-'nē-mē-ə\ *n* : the condition of having abnormal quantities of cryoglobulins in the blood

cry·on·ics \krī-'ä-niks\ *n* : the practice of freezing the body of a person who has died from a disease in hopes of restoring life at some future time when a cure for the disease has been developed — **cry·on·ic** \-nik\ *adj*

cryo·pexy \'krī-ə-ˌpek-sē\ *n, pl* **-pex·ies** : cryosurgery for fixation of the retina in retinal detachment or for repair of a retinal tear or hole

cryo·pre·cip·i·tate \ˌkrī-ō-prə-'si-pə-tət, -ˌtāt\ *n* : a precipitate that is formed by cooling a solution — **cryo·pre·cip·i·ta·tion** \-ˌsi-pə-'tā-shən\ *n*

cryo·pres·er·va·tion \-ˌpre-zər-'vā-shən\ *n* : preservation (as of sperm or eggs) by subjection to extremely low temperatures — **cryo·pre·serve** \-pri-'zərv\ *vb*

cryo·probe \'krī-ə-ˌprōb\ *n* : a blunt chilled instrument used to freeze tissues in cryosurgery

cryo·pro·tec·tive \ˌkrī-ō-prə-'tek-tiv\ *adj* : serving to protect against the deleterious effects of subjection to freezing temperatures ⟨a ~ agent⟩ — **cryo·pro·tec·tant** \-tənt\ *n* or *adj*

cryo·stat \'krī-ə-ˌstat\ *n* : an apparatus for maintaining a constant low temperature esp. below 0°C; *esp* : one containing a microtome for obtaining sections of frozen tissue — **cryo·stat·ic** \ˌkrī-ə-'sta-tik\ *adj*

cryo·sur·gery \ˌkrī-ō-'sərj-rē, -'sər-jə-rē\ *n, pl* **-ger·ies** : surgery in which diseased or abnormal tissue (as a tumor or wart) is destroyed or removed by freezing (as by the use of liquid nitrogen) — **cryo·sur·geon** \-'sər-jən\ *n* — **cryo·sur·gi·cal** \-'sər-ji-kəl\ *adj*

cryo·ther·a·py \-'ther-ə-pē\ *n, pl* **-pies** : the therapeutic use of cold; *esp* : CRYOSURGERY

crypt \'kript\ *n* **1** : an anatomical pit or depression **2** : a simple tubular gland (as a crypt of Lieberkühn)

crypt- *or* **crypto-** *comb form* : hidden : covered ⟨*crypto*genic⟩

crypt·ec·to·my \krip-'tek-tə-mē\ *n, pl* **-mies** : surgical removal or destruction of a crypt

cryp·tic \'krip-tik\ *adj* : not recognized ⟨a ~ infection⟩

cryp·ti·tis \krip-'tī-təs\ *n* : inflammation of a crypt (as an anal crypt)

cryp·to·coc·co·sis \ˌkrip-tə-(ˌ)kä-'kō-səs\ *n, pl* **-co·ses** \-(ˌ)sēz\ : an infectious disease that is caused by a fungus of the genus *Cryptococcus* (*C. neoformans*) and is characterized by the production of nodular lesions or abscesses in the subcutaneous tissues, joints, and esp. the lungs, brain, and meninges — called also *torulosis*

cryp·to·coc·cus \-'kä-kəs\ n 1 cap : a genus of imperfect fungi that resemble yeasts and include a number of saprophytes and a few serious pathogens 2 pl **-coc·ci** \-'käk-ˌsī, -ˌsē; -'kä-ˌkī, -ˌkē\ : any fungus of the genus *Cryptococcus* — **cryp·to·coc·cal** \-'kä-kəl\ adj

crypt of Lie·ber·kühn \-'lē-bər-ˌkün, -ˌkyün, -ˌkün-\ n : any of the tubular glands of the intestinal mucous membrane — called also *intestinal gland*
    Lieberkühn, Johannes Nathanael (1711–1756), German anatomist.

crypt of Mor·ga·gni \-mȯr-'gän-yē\ n : any of the pouched cavities of the rectal mucosa immediately above the anorectal junction, intervening between vertical folds of the rectal mucosa
    Morgagni, Giovanni Battista (1682–1771), Italian anatomist and pathologist.

cryp·to·ge·net·ic \ˌkrip-tō-jə-'ne-tik\ adj : CRYPTOGENIC

cryp·to·gen·ic \ˌkrip-tə-'je-nik\ adj : of obscure or unknown origin

crypt·or·chid \krip-'tȯr-kəd\ n : one affected with cryptorchidism — compare MONORCHID — **cryptorchid** adj

crypt·or·chi·dism \-kə-ˌdi-zəm\ also **crypt·or·chism** \-ˌki-zəm\ n : a condition in which one or both testes fail to descend normally — compare MONORCHIDISM

cryp·to·spo·rid·i·o·sis \ˌkrip-tō-spȯr-ˌi-dē-'ō-səs\ n, pl **-o·ses** \-ˌsēz\ : a disease caused by cryptosporidia

cryp·to·spo·rid·i·um \ˌkrip-tō-spȯr-'i-dē-əm\ n 1 cap : a genus of coccidian protozoans parasitic in the gut of many vertebrates including humans and sometimes causing diarrhea esp. in individuals who are immunocompromised (as in AIDS) 2 pl **-rid·ia** \-dē-ə\ : any protozoan of the genus *Cryptosporidium*

cryp·to·xan·thin \ˌkrip-tə-'zan-thən\ n : a carotenoid alcohol $C_{40}H_{55}OH$ that occurs in many plants, in blood serum, and in some animal products (as butter and egg yolk) and that is a precursor of vitamin A

cryp·to·zo·ite \-'zō-ˌīt\ n : a malaria parasite that develops in tissue cells and gives rise to the forms that invade blood cells — compare METACRYPTOZOITE

crys·tal \'krist-ᵊl\ n 1 : a body that is formed by the solidification of a chemical element, a compound, or a mixture and has a regularly repeating internal arrangement of its atoms and often external plane faces 2 : ICE; *broadly* : methamphetamine in any form when used illicitly — **crystal** adj — **crys·tal·line** \'kris-tə-lən, -ˌlīn, -ˌlēn\ adj

crys·tal·lin \'kris-tə-lən\ n : either of two globulins in the crystalline lens

crystallina — see MILIARIA CRYSTALLINA

crystalline lens n : the lens of the eye

crys·tal·lize also **crys·tal·ize** \'kris-tə-ˌlīz\ vb **-lized** also **-ized**; **-liz·ing** also **-iz·ing** : to cause to form crystals or assume crystalline form — **crys·tal·liz·able** \ˌkris-tə-'lī-zə-bəl\ adj — **crys·tal·li·za·tion** \ˌkris-tə-lə-'zā-shən\ n

crys·tal·lu·ria \ˌkris-tə-'lùr-ē-ə, -təl-'yùr-\ n : the presence of crystals in the urine indicating renal irritation

crystal meth n : ICE — called also *crystal methamphetamine*

cs abbr conditioned stimulus

Cs symbol cesium

CS \ˌsē-'es\ n : a potent lacrimatory and nausea-producing gas $C_{10}H_5ClN_2$ used in riot control and chemical warfare

C–sec·tion \'sē-ˌsek-shən\ n : CESAREAN SECTION

CSF \ˌsē-(ˌ)es-'ef\ n : COLONY-STIMULATING FACTOR

CSF abbr cerebrospinal fluid

CT abbr computed tomography; computerized tomography

CTD abbr cumulative trauma disorder

Cteno·ce·phal·i·des \ˌte-nō-sə-'fa-lə-ˌdēz\ n : a genus of fleas (family Pulicidae) including the dog flea (C. canis) and cat flea (C. felis)

CTL \ˌsē-(ˌ)tē-'el\ n : CYTOTOXIC T LYMPHOCYTE

CTS abbr carpal tunnel syndrome

CT scan \'sē-ˌtē-\ n : CAT SCAN — **CT scanning** n

CT scanner n : CAT SCANNER

Cu symbol copper

¹cu·bi·tal \'kyü-bət-ᵊl\ adj : of or relating to a cubitus

²cubital n : CUBITUS

cubiti — see BICEPS FLEXOR CUBITI

cu·bi·tus \'kyü-bə-təs\ n, pl **cu·bi·ti** \-ˌtī\ 1 : FOREARM, ANTEBRACHIUM 2 : ULNA

cubitus valgus n : a condition of the arm in which the forearm deviates away from the midline of the body when extended

cubitus varus n : a condition of the arm in which the forearm deviates toward the midline of the body when extended

¹cu·boid \'kyü-ˌbȯid\ adj 1 : relating to or being the cuboid ⟨the ~ bone⟩ 2 : shaped approximately like a cube

²cuboid n : the outermost bone in the distal row of tarsal bones of the foot that supports the fourth and fifth metatarsals

cu·boi·dal \kyü-'bȯid-ᵊl\ adj 1 : CUBOID 2 : composed of nearly cubical elements ⟨~ epithelium⟩

cud \'kəd\ n : food brought up into the mouth by a ruminating animal from its first stomach to be chewed again

cue \'kyü\ n : a minor stimulus acting as an indication of the nature of the perceived object or situation

cuff \'kəf\ *n* **1** : an inflatable band that is wrapped around an extremity to control the flow of blood through the part when recording blood pressure with a sphygmomanometer **2** : an anatomical structure shaped like a cuff; *esp* : ROTATOR CUFF

cuffed \'kəft\ *adj* : provided with an often inflatable encircling part ⟨a ∼ endotracheal tube⟩

cui·rass \kwi-'ras, kyū-\ *n* **1** : a plaster cast for the trunk and neck **2** : a respirator that covers the chest or the chest and abdomen and provides artificial respiration by means of an electric pump

cul–de–sac \ˌkəl-di-'sak, ˌkül-\ *n, pl* **culs–de–sac** *same or* ˌkəlz-, ˌkülz-\ *also* **cul–de–sacs** \-'saks\ **1** : a blind diverticulum or pouch; *also* : the closed end of such a pouch **2** : POUCH OF DOUGLAS

cul–de–sac of Douglas *n* : POUCH OF DOUGLAS

culdo– *comb form* : pouch of Douglas ⟨*culdoscopy*⟩

cul·do·cen·te·sis \ˌkəl-dō-ˌsen-'tē-səs, ˌkül-\ *n, pl* **-te·ses** \-ˌsēz\ : removal of material from the pouch of Douglas by means of puncture of the vaginal wall

cul·dos·co·py \ˌkəl-'däs-kə-pē, ˌkül-\ *n, pl* **-pies** : a technique for endoscopic visualization and minor operative procedures on the female pelvic organs in which the instrument is introduced through a puncture in the wall of the pouch of Douglas — **cul·do·scop·ic** \ˌkəl-də-'skä-pik, ˌkül-\ *adj*

cul·dot·o·my \ˌkəl-'dä-tə-mē, ˌkül-\ *n, pl* **-mies** : surgical incision of the pouch of Douglas

cu·lex \'kyü-ˌleks\ *n* **1** *cap* : a large cosmopolitan genus of mosquitoes (family Culicidae) that includes the common house mosquito (*C. pipiens*) of Europe and No. America, a widespread tropical mosquito (*C. quinquefasciatus* syn. *C. fatigans*) which transmits some filarial worms parasitic in humans, and other mosquitoes which act as vectors of viral encephalitides **2** : a mosquito of the genus *Culex* — **cu·li·cine** \'kyü-lə-ˌsīn\ *adj or n*

cu·li·cide \'kyü-lə-ˌsīd\ *n* : an insecticide that destroys mosquitoes

Cu·li·coi·des \ˌkyü-lə-'kòi-ˌdēz\ *n* : a genus of bloodsucking midges (family Ceratopogonidae) of which some are intermediate hosts of filarial parasites

cul·men \'kəl-mən\ *n* : a lobe of the cerebellum lying in the superior vermis just in front of the primary fissure

cul·ti·vate \'kəl-tə-ˌvāt\ *vb* **-vat·ed; -vat·ing** : CULTURE 1

cul·ti·va·tion \ˌkəl-tə-'vā-shən\ *n* : CULTURE 2

¹cul·ture \'kəl-chər\ *n* **1 a** : the integrated pattern of human behavior that includes thought, speech, action, and artifacts and depends upon the human capacity for learning and transmitting knowledge to succeeding generations **b** : the customary beliefs, social forms, and material traits of a racial, religious, or social group **2 a** : the act or process of growing living material (as bacteria or viruses) in prepared nutrient media **b** : a product of cultivation in nutrient media — **cul·tur·al** \'kəl-chə-rəl\ *adj* — **cul·tur·al·ly** *adv*

²culture *vb* **cul·tured; cul·tur·ing 1** : to grow (as microorganisms or tissues) in a prepared medium **2** : to start a culture from; *also* : to make a culture of ⟨∼ milk⟩

culture shock *n* : a sense of confusion and uncertainty sometimes with feelings of anxiety that may affect people exposed to an alien culture or environment without adequate preparation

cu·mu·la·tive \'kyü-myə-lə-tiv, -ˌlā-\ *adj* : increasing in effect by successive doses (as of a drug or poison) — **cu·mu·la·tive·ly** *adv*

cumulative trauma disorder *n* : REPETITIVE STRAIN INJURY

cu·mu·lus \'kyü-myə-ləs\ *n, pl* **cu·mu·li** \-ˌlī, -ˌlē\ : the projecting mass of granulosa cells that bears the developing ovum in a graafian follicle — called also *discus proligerus*

cumulus ooph·o·rus \-ō-'ä-fə-rəs\ *n* : CUMULUS

cu·ne·ate fasciculus \'kyü-nē-ˌāt-, -ət-\ *n, pl* **cuneate fasciculi** : FASCICULUS CUNEATUS

cuneate nucleus *n* : NUCLEUS CUNEATUS

cuneatus — see FASCICULUS CUNEATUS, NUCLEUS CUNEATUS

¹cu·ne·i·form \kyü-'nē-ə-ˌfòrm, 'kyü-; 'kyü-nə-\ *adj* **1** : of, relating to, or being a cuneiform bone or cartilage **2** *of a human skull* : wedge-shaped as viewed from above

²cuneiform *n* : a cuneiform bone or cartilage

cuneiform bone *n* **1** : any of three small bones of the tarsus situated between the navicular and the first three metatarsals: **a** : one on the medial side of the foot that is just proximal to the first metatarsal bone and is the largest of the three bones — called also *medial cuneiform, medial cuneiform bone* **b** : one that is situated between the other two bones proximal to the second metatarsal bone and is the smallest of the three bones — called also *intermediate cuneiform, intermediate cuneiform bone* **c** : one that is situated proximal to the third metatarsal bone and that lies between the intermediate cuneiform bone and the cuboid — called also *lateral cuneiform bone* **2** : TRIQUETRAL BONE

cuneiform cartilage *n* : either of a pair of rods of yellow elastic cartilage of which each lies on one side of the larynx in an aryepiglottic fold just below the arytenoid cartilage

cu·ne·us \'kyü-nē-əs\ *n, pl* **cu·nei** \-nē-ˌī\ : a convolution of the mesial surface of the occipital lobe of the brain above the calcarine sulcus that forms a part of the visual cortex

cun·ni·lin·gus \ˌkə-ni-'liŋ-gəs\ *also* **cun·ni·linc·tus** \-'liŋk-təs\ *n* : oral stimulation of the vulva or clitoris

¹**cup** \'kəp\ *n* **1** : an athletic supporter reinforced for providing extra protection to the wearer in certain strenuous sports (as hockey or football) **2** : a cap of metal or plastic shaped like the femoral head and used in plastic reconstruction of the hip joint

²**cup** *vb* **cupped; cup·ping 1** : to treat by cupping **2** : to undergo or perform cupping

cup·ping *n* : a technique formerly employed for drawing blood to the surface of the body by application of a glass vessel from which air had been evacuated by heat to form a partial vacuum

cu·pu·la \'kyü-pyü-lə, -pü-\ *n, pl* **cu·pu·lae** \-ˌlē\ **1** : the bony apex of the cochlea **2** : the peak of the pleural sac covering the apex of the lung

cur·able \'kyúr-ə-bəl\ *adj* : capable of being cured

cu·ra·re *also* **cu·ra·ri** \kyù-'rär-ē, kú-\ *n* : a dried aqueous extract esp. of a vine (as *Strychnos toxifera* of the family Loganiaceae or *Chondodendron tomentosum* of the family Menispermaceae) that produces muscle relaxation and is used in arrow poisons by So. American Indians — compare TUBOCURARINE

cu·ra·ri·form \kyù-'rär-ə-ˌfòrm, kú-\ *adj* : producing or characterized by the muscular relaxation typical of curare ⟨∼ drugs⟩

cu·ra·rize \-'rär-ˌīz\ *vb* **-rized; -riz·ing** : to treat with curare — **cu·ra·ri·za·tion** \-ˌrär-ə-'zā-shən\ *n*

cu·ra·tive \'kyúr-ə-tiv\ *adj* : relating to or used in the cure of diseases — **curative** *n* — **cu·ra·tive·ly** *adv*

curb \'kərb\ *n* : a swelling on the back of the hind leg of a horse just behind the lowest part of the hock joint that is due to strain or rupture of the ligament and generally causes lameness

¹**cure** \'kyúr\ *n* **1** : recovery from a disease ⟨his ∼ was complete⟩; *also* : remission of signs or symptoms of a disease esp. during a prolonged period of observation ⟨a clinical ∼⟩ **2** : a drug, treatment, regimen, or other agency that cures a disease **3** : a course or period of treatment; *esp* : one designed to interrupt an addiction or compulsive habit or to improve general health **4** : SPA

²**cure** *vb* **cured; cur·ing 1 a** : to make or become healthy, sound, or normal again ⟨∼ a patient of his illness⟩ **b** : to bring about recovery from ⟨∼ a disease⟩ **2** : to take a cure (as at a spa) — **cur·er** *n*

cu·ret·tage \ˌkyúr-ə-'täzh\ *n* : a surgical scraping or cleaning by means of a curette

¹**cu·rette** *also* **cu·ret** \kyù-'ret\ *n* : a surgical instrument that has a scoop, loop, or ring at its tip and is used in performing curettage

²**curette** *also* **curet** *vb* **cu·rett·ed; cu·rett·ing** : to perform curettage on — **cu·rette·ment** \kyù-'ret-mənt\ *n*

cu·rie \'kyúr-(ˌ)ē, kyù-'rē\ *n* **1** : a unit quantity of any radioactive nuclide in which 3.7×10^{10} disintegrations occur per second **2** : a unit of radioactivity equal to 3.7×10^{10} disintegrations per second

Curie, Pierre (1859–1906) and **Marie Slodowska (1867–1934),** French chemists and physicists.

cu·ri·um \'kyúr-ē-əm\ *n* : a metallic radioactive trivalent element produced artificially — symbol *Cm;* see ELEMENT table

Curl·ing's ulcer \'kər-liŋz-\ *n* : acute gastroduodenal ulceration following severe skin burns

Curling, Thomas Blizard (1811–1888), British surgeon.

cur·rent \'kər-ənt\ *n* : a flow of electric charge; *also* : the rate of such flow

cur·va·ture \'kər-və-ˌchúr, -chər, -ˌtyúr\ *n* **1** : an abnormal curving (as of the spine) — see KYPHOSIS, SCOLIOSIS **2** : a curved surface of an organ (as the stomach) — see GREATER CURVATURE, LESSER CURVATURE

cush·ing·oid \'kú-shiŋ-ˌóid\ *adj, often cap* : resembling Cushing's disease esp. in facies or habitus

Cushing's disease \'kú-shiŋz-\ *n* : Cushing's syndrome esp. when caused by excessive production of ACTH by the pituitary gland

Cushing, Harvey Williams (1869–1939), American neurosurgeon.

Cushing's syndrome *n* : an abnormal bodily condition that is caused by excess corticosteroids and esp. cortisol usu. from adrenal or pituitary hyperfunction and is characterized esp. by obesity, hypertension, muscular weakness, and easy bruising — called *also adrenogenital syndrome*

cush·ion \'kú-shən\ *n* **1** : a bodily part resembling a pad **2** : a medical procedure or drug that eases discomfort without necessarily affecting the basic condition of the patient

cusp \'kəsp\ *n* **1** : a point on the grinding surface of a tooth **2** : a fold or flap of a cardiac valve — **cus·pal** \'kəs-pəl\ *adj*

cusp·id \'kəs-pəd\ *n* : a canine tooth

cus·pi·date \'kəs-pə-ˌdāt\ *adj* : having a cusp : terminating in a point

cus·to·di·al \ˌkəs-'tō-dē-əl\ *adj* **1** : relating to, providing, or being protective care or services for basic needs ⟨∼ care⟩ **2** : having sole or primary custody of a child ⟨∼ parents⟩

¹**cut** \'kət\ *vb* **cut; cut·ting 1 a :** to penetrate with or as if with an edged instrument **b :** to cut or operate on in surgery: as **(1) :** to subject (a domestic animal) to castration **(2) :** to perform lithotomy on **c :** to experience the emergence of (a tooth) through the gum **2 :** to function as or in the manner of an edged tool ⟨a knife that ∼s well⟩ **3 :** to subject to trimming or paring ⟨∼ one's nails⟩

²**cut** *n* **1 a :** an opening made with an edged instrument **b :** a wound made by something sharp **2 :** a stroke or blow with the edge of a sharp implement (as a knife)

cu·ta·ne·ous \kyu̇-'tā-nē-əs\ *adj :* of, relating to, or affecting the skin ⟨a ∼ infection⟩ — **cu·ta·ne·ous·ly** *adv*

cutaneous T–cell lymphoma *n :* any of several non-Hodgkin's lymphomas (as mycosis fungoides or Sezary syndrome) that are marked by clusters of malignant helper T cells in the epidermis causing skin lesions and eruptions which typically progress to tumors and may spread to lymph nodes and internal organs

cut·down \'kət-ˌdau̇n\ *n :* incision of a superficial blood vessel (as a vein) to facilitate insertion of a catheter (as for administration of fluids)

Cu·te·re·bra \ˌkyü-tə-'rē-brə, kyü-'ter-ə-brə\ *n :* a genus of botflies (family Cuterebridae) with larvae that form tumors under the skin of small mammals (as rodents and rabbits)

cu·ti·cle \'kyü-ti-kəl\ *n* **1 a :** the outermost layer of integument composed of epidermis **b :** the outermost membranous layer of a hair consisting of cornified epithelial cells **2 :** dead or horny epidermis (as that surrounding the base and sides of a fingernail or toenail) — **cu·tic·u·lar** \kyü-'ti-kyə-lər\ *adj*

cu·ti·re·ac·tion \ˌkyü-ti-rē-'ak-shən, 'kyü-ti-rē-ˌ\ *n :* a local inflammatory reaction of the skin that occurs in certain infectious diseases following the application to or injection into the skin of a preparation of organisms producing the disease

cu·tis \'kyü-təs\ *n, pl* **cu·tes** \-ˌtēz\ *or* **cu·tis·es :** DERMIS

Cu·vie·ri·an vein \(ˌ)kyü-'vir-ē-ən-, ˌkyü-vē-'ir-\ *n :* CARDINAL VEIN

Cu·vier \'kü-vē-ˌā, 'kyü-; kūē-'vyā\, **Georges** *(orig.* **Jean–Léopold–Nicolas–Frédéric)** **(1769–1832),** French naturalist.

CVA *abbr* cerebrovascular accident
CVD *abbr* cardiovascular disease
CVP *abbr* central venous pressure
CVS *abbr* chorionic villus sampling

cyan- *or* **cyano-** *comb form* **1 :** blue ⟨cyanosis⟩ **2 :** cyanide ⟨cyanogenetic⟩

cy·a·nide \'sī-ə-ˌnīd, -nəd\ *n :* any of several compounds (as potassium cyanide) that contain the monovalent group –CN, react with and inactivate respiratory enzymes, and are rapidly lethal producing drowsiness, tachycardia, coma, and finally death

cy·a·no·ac·ry·late \ˌsī-ə-nō-'a-krə-ˌlāt, sī-ˌa-nō-\ *n :* any of several liquid acrylate monomers used as adhesives in medicine on living tissue to close wounds in surgery

cy·a·no·co·bal·a·min \-kō-'ba-lə-mən\ *also* **cy·a·no·co·bal·a·mine** \-ˌmēn\ *n* : VITAMIN B₁₂

cy·a·no·ge·net·ic \ˌsī-ə-nō-jə-'ne-tik, sī-ˌa-nō-\ *or* **cy·a·no·gen·ic** \-'je-nik\ *adj :* capable of producing cyanide (as hydrogen cyanide) ⟨a ∼ glucoside⟩ — **cy·a·no·gen·e·sis** \-'je-nə-səs\ *n*

cy·a·no·met·he·mo·glo·bin \ˌsī-ə-ˌnō-(ˌ)met-'hē-mə-ˌglō-bən\ *or* **cy·an·met·he·mo·glo·bin** \ˌsī-ˌan-(ˌ)met-, ˌsī-ən-\ *n :* a bright red crystalline compound formed by the action of hydrogen cyanide on methemoglobin or on oxyhemoglobin at body temperature

cy·a·nosed \'sī-ə-ˌnōst, -ˌnōzd\ *adj :* affected with cyanosis

cy·a·no·sis \ˌsī-ə-'nō-səs\ *n, pl* **-no·ses** \-ˌsēz\ : a bluish or purplish discoloration (as of skin) due to deficient oxygenation of the blood — **cy·a·not·ic** \-'nä-tik\ *adj*

cycl- *or* **cyclo-** *comb form* **1 :** ciliary body (of the eye) ⟨cyclitis⟩ ⟨cyclodialysis⟩ **2 :** containing a ring of atoms — in names of organic compounds ⟨cyclohexane⟩

cy·cla·mate \'sī-klə-ˌmāt, -mət\ *n :* an artificially prepared salt of sodium or calcium used esp. formerly as a sweetener but now largely discontinued because of the possibly harmful effects of its metabolic breakdown product cyclohexylamine

cy·clan·de·late \sī-'kland-ᵊl-ˌāt\ *n :* an antispasmodic drug C₁₇H₂₄O₃ used esp. as a vasodilator in the treatment of diseased arteries

cy·claz·o·cine \sī-'kla-zə-ˌsēn, -sən\ *n :* an analgesic drug C₁₈H₂₅NO that inhibits the effect of morphine and related addictive drugs and is used in the treatment of drug addiction

¹**cy·cle** \'sī-kəl\ *n :* a recurring series of events: as **a (1) :** a series of stages through which an organism tends to pass once in a fixed order; *also :* a series of stages through which a population of organisms tends to pass more or less together — see LIFE CYCLE **(2)** : a series of physiological, biochemical, or psychological stages that recur in the same individual — see CARDIAC CYCLE, MENSTRUAL CYCLE, KREBS CYCLE **b :** one complete performance of a vibration, electric oscillation, current alternation, or other periodic process — **cy·clic** \'sī-klik, 'si-\ *or* **cy·cli·cal** \'sī-kli-kəl, 'si-\ *adj* — **cy·cli·cal·ly** *also* **cy·clic·ly** *adv*

²**cycle** *vb* **cy·cled; cy·cling :** to undergo the estrous cycle

cy·clec·to·my \sī-'klek-tə-mē, si-\ *n, pl* **-mies** : surgical removal of part of the ciliary muscle or body

cyclic adenosine monophosphate *n* : CYCLIC AMP

cyclic AMP *n* : a cyclic mononucleotide of adenosine that is formed from ATP and is responsible for the intracellular mediation of hormonal effects on various cellular processes — abbr. *cAMP*

cyclic GMP \-jē-(ˌ)em-'pē\ *n* : a cyclic mononucleotide of guanosine that acts similarly to cyclic AMP as a second messenger in response to hormones

cyclic guanosine monophosphate *n* : CYCLIC GMP

cy·clic·i·ty \sī-'kli-sə-tē, si-\ *n, pl* **-ties** : the quality or state of being cyclic

cy·clin \'sī-klən, 'si-\ *n* : any of a group of proteins active in controlling the cell cycle and in initiating DNA synthesis

cy·cli·tis \sə-'klī-təs, sī-\ *n* : inflammation of the ciliary body

cy·cli·zine \'sī-klə-ˌzēn\ *n* : an antiemetic drug used esp. in the form of its hydrochloride $C_{18}H_{22}N_2$·HCl in the treatment of motion sickness — see MAREZINE

cyclo- — see CYCL-

cy·clo·ben·za·prine \ˌsī-klō-'ben-zə-ˌprēn\ *n* : a skeletal muscle relaxant used in the form of its hydrochloride $C_{20}H_{21}N$·HCl to relieve muscle spasms and pain

cy·clo·di·al·y·sis \ˌsī-klō-dī-'a-lə-səs\ *n, pl* **-y·ses** \-ˌsēz\ : surgical detachment of the ciliary body from the sclera to reduce tension in the eyeball in some cases of glaucoma

cy·clo·di·a·ther·my \-'dī-ə-ˌthər-mē\ *n, pl* **-mies** : partial or complete destruction of the ciliary body by diathermy to relieve some conditions (as glaucoma) characterized by increased tension within the eyeball

Cy·clo·gyl \'sī-klō-ˌgil\ *trademark* — used for a preparation of the hydrochloride of cyclopentolate

cy·clo·hex·ane \ˌsī-klō-'hek-ˌsān\ *n* : a pungent saturated hydrocarbon C_6H_{12} found in petroleum or made synthetically

cy·clo·hex·yl·a·mine \-hek-'si-lə-ˌmēn\ *n* : a colorless liquid amine $C_6H_{11}NH_2$ of cyclohexane that is believed to be harmful as a metabolic breakdown product of cyclamate

¹**cy·cloid** \'sī-ˌklȯid\ *n* : a cycloid individual

²**cycloid** *adj* : relating to, having, or being a personality characterized by alternating high and low moods — compare CYCLOTHYMIC

cy·clo·ox·y·gen·ase \ˌsī-klō-'äk-si-jə-ˌnās, -äk-'si-jə-, -ˌnāz\ *n* : an enzyme that catalyzes the conversion of arachidonic acid to prostaglandins, inactivated by aspirin and other NSAIDS, and has two isoforms — see COX-1, COX-2

cy·clo·pen·to·late \ˌsī-klō-'pen-tə-ˌlāt, ˌsi-\ *n* : an anticholinergic drug used esp. in the form of its hydrochloride $C_{17}H_{25}NO_3$·HCl to dilate the pupil of the eye for ophthalmologic examination — see CYCLOGYL

cy·clo·phos·pha·mide \-'fäs-fə-ˌmīd\ *n* : an immunosuppressive and antineoplastic drug $C_7H_{15}Cl_2N_2O_2P$ used in the treatment of lymphomas and some leukemias — see CYTOXAN

cy·clo·pia \sī-'klō-pē-ə\ *n* : a developmental anomaly characterized by the presence of a single median eye

cy·clo·ple·gia \ˌsī-klō-'plē-jə, -jē-ə\ *n* : paralysis of the ciliary muscle of the eye

¹**cy·clo·ple·gic** \-'plē-jik\ *adj* : producing, involving, or characterized by cycloplegia ⟨∼ agents⟩ ⟨∼ refraction⟩

²**cycloplegic** *n* : a cycloplegic agent

cy·clo·pro·pane \-'prō-ˌpān\ *n* : a flammable gaseous saturated cyclic hydrocarbon C_3H_6 sometimes used as a general anesthetic

cy·clops \'sī-ˌkläps\ *n, pl* **cy·clo·pes** \sī-'klō-(ˌ)pēz\ : an individual or fetus abnormal in having a single eye or the usual two orbits fused

cy·clo·ser·ine \ˌsī-klō-'ser-ˌēn, ˌsi-\ *n* : a broad-spectrum antibiotic $C_3H_6N_2O_2$ produced by an actinomycete of the genus *Streptomyces* (*S. orchidaceus*) and used esp. in the treatment of tuberculosis

cy·clo·spo·ra \ˌsī-klō-'spȯr-ə\ *n* **1** *cap* : a genus of coccidian protozoans including one (*C. cayetanensis*) causing diarrhea in humans **2** : a protozoan of the genus *Cyclospora*

cy·clo·spo·ri·a·sis \ˌsī-klō-spə-'rī-ə-səs\ *n, pl* **-a·ses** \-ˌsēz\ : infection with or disease caused by a cyclospora

cy·clo·spor·in \ˌsī-klō-'spȯr-ᵊn\ *n* : any of a group of polypeptides obtained as metabolites from various imperfect fungi (as *Tolypocladium inflatum* syn. *Trichoderma polysporum*); *esp* : CYCLOSPORINE

cyclosporin A *n* : CYCLOSPORINE

cy·clo·spo·rine \ˌsī-klə-'spȯr-ᵊn, -ˌēn\ *n* : a cyclosporin $C_{62}H_{111}N_{11}O_{12}$ used as an immunosuppressive drug esp. to prevent rejection of transplanted organs

cy·clo·thyme \'sī-klə-ˌthīm\ *n* : a cyclothymic individual

cy·clo·thy·mia \ˌsī-klə-'thī-mē-ə\ *n* : cyclothymic mood disorder

¹**cy·clo·thy·mic** \-'thī-mik\ *adj* : relating to, having, or being a mood disorder characterized by alternating short episodes of depression and hypomania in a form less severe than that of bipolar disorder — compare CYCLOID

²**cyclothymic** *n* : a cyclothymic individual

cy·clo·tome \'sī-klə-ˌtōm\ *n* : a knife used in cyclotomy

cy·clot·o·my \sī-'klä-tə-mē\ *n, pl* **-mies** : incision or division of the ciliary body

cy·clo·tro·pia \ˌsī-klə-ˈtrō-pē-ə\ n : squint in which the eye rolls outward or inward around its front-to-back axis

cy·e·sis \sī-ˈē-səs\ n, pl **cy·e·ses** \-ˌsēz\ : PREGNANCY

cyl·in·droid \ˈsil-ən-ˌdròid, sə-ˈlin-\ n : a spurious or mucous urinary cast that resembles a hyaline cast but has one tapered, stringy, twisted end

cyl·in·dro·ma \ˌsil-ən-ˈdrō-mə\ n, pl **-mas** also **-ma·ta** \mə-tə\ : a tumor characterized by cylindrical masses consisting of epithelial cells and hyalinized stroma: **a** : a malignant tumor esp. of the respiratory tract or salivary glands **b** : a benign tumor of the skin and esp. the scalp

cyl·in·dru·ria \ˌsil-ən-ˈdrùr-ē-ə\ n : the presence of casts in the urine

cy·no·mol·gus monkey \ˌsī-nə-ˈmäl-gəs-\ n : a macaque (Macaca fascicularis syn. M. cynomolgus) of southeastern Asia, Borneo, and the Philippines that is often used in medical research

cy·no·pho·bia \-ˈfō-bē-ə\ n : a morbid fear of dogs

cy·pro·hep·ta·dine \ˌsī-prō-ˈhep-tə-ˌdēn\ n : a drug $C_{21}H_{21}N$ that acts antagonistically to histamine and serotonin and is used esp. in the treatment of asthma

cy·prot·er·one \sī-ˈprä-tə-ˌrōn\ n : a synthetic steroid used in the form of its acetate $C_{24}H_{29}ClO_4$ to inhibit androgenic secretions (as testosterone)

cyst \ˈsist\ n **1** : a closed sac having a distinct membrane and developing abnormally in a body cavity or structure **2** : a body resembling a cyst: **a** : a capsule formed about a minute organism going into a resting or spore stage; also : this capsule with its contents **b** : a resistant cover about a parasite produced by the parasite or the host — compare HYDATID 2a

cyst- or cysti- or cysto- comb form **1** : bladder 〈cystitis〉 〈cystoplasty〉 **2** : cyst 〈cystogastrostomy〉

-cyst \ˌsist\ n comb form : bladder : sac 〈blastocyst〉

cyst·ad·e·no·ma \ˌsis-ˌtad-ᵊn-ˈō-mə\ n, pl **-mas** also **-ma·ta** \mə-tə\ : an adenoma marked by a cystic structure — **cyst·ad·e·no·ma·tous** \-mə-təs\ adj

cys·te·amine \sis-ˈtē-ə-mən\ n : a cysteine derivative used in the form of its bitartrate $C_2H_7NS·C_4H_6O_6$ to treat cystinosis and esp. formerly as an antidote for acetaminophen overdose

cys·tec·to·my \sis-ˈtek-tə-mē\ n, pl **-mies** **1** : the surgical excision of a cyst 〈ovarian ∼〉 **2** : the removal of all or a portion of the urinary bladder

cys·teine \ˈsis-tə-ˌēn\ n : a sulfur-containing amino acid $C_3H_7NO_2S$ occurring in many proteins and glutathione and readily oxidizable to cystine

cysti- — see CYST-

cys·tic \ˈsis-tik\ adj **1** : relating to, composed of, or containing cysts 〈a ∼ tumor〉 **2** : of or relating to the urinary bladder or the gallbladder **3** : enclosed in a cyst 〈a ∼ worm larva〉

cystica — see OSTEITIS FIBROSA CYSTICA, OSTEITIS FIBROSA CYSTICA GENERALISTA

cystic duct n : the duct from the gallbladder that unites with the hepatic duct to form the common bile duct

cys·ti·cer·coid \ˌsis-tə-ˈsər-ˌkòid\ n : a tapeworm larva having an invaginated scolex and solid hind part

cys·ti·cer·co·sis \-(ˌ)sər-ˈkō-səs\ n, pl **-co·ses** \-ˌsēz\ : infestation with or disease caused by cysticerci

cys·ti·cer·cus \-ˈsər-kəs\ n, pl **-cer·ci** \-ˈsər-ˌsī, -ˌkī\ : a tapeworm larva that consists of a fluid-filled sac containing an invaginated scolex, is situated in the tissues of an intermediate host, and is capable of developing into an adult tapeworm when eaten by a suitable definitive host — called also bladder worm, measle — **cys·ti·cer·cal** \-ˈsər-kəl\ adj

cystic fibrosis n : a common hereditary disease esp. in Caucasian populations that appears usu. in early childhood, is inherited as an autosomal recessive trait, involves functional disorder of the exocrine glands, and is marked esp. by faulty digestion due to a deficiency of pancreatic enzymes, by difficulty in breathing due to mucus accumulation in airways, and by excessive loss of salt in the sweat — called also fibrocystic disease of the pancreas, mucoviscidosis

cys·tine \ˈsis-ˌtēn\ n : a crystalline amino acid $C_6H_{12}N_2O_4S_2$ that is widespread in proteins (as keratins) and is a major metabolic sulfur source

cys·ti·no·sis \ˌsis-tə-ˈnō-səs\ n, pl **-no·ses** \-ˌsēz\ : a recessive autosomally inherited disease characterized esp. by cystinuria and deposits of cystine throughout the body — **cys·ti·not·ic** \-ˈnä-tik\ adj

cys·ti·nu·ria \ˌsis-tə-ˈnùr-ē-ə, -ˈnyùr-\ n : a metabolic defect characterized by excretion of excessive amounts of cystine in the urine and sometimes by the formation of stones in an urinary tract and inherited as an autosomal recessive trait — **cys·tin·uric** \-ˈnùr-ik, -ˈnyùr-\ adj

cys·ti·tis \sis-ˈtī-təs\ n, pl **cys·tit·i·des** \-ˈti-tə-ˌdēz\ : inflammation of the urinary bladder — **cys·tit·ic** \(ˈ)sis-ˈti-tik\ adj

cysto- — see CYST-

cys·to·cele \ˈsis-tə-ˌsēl\ n : hernia of a bladder and esp. the urinary bladder : vesical hernia

cys·to·gas·tros·to·my \ˌsis-tō-(ˌ)gas-ˈträs-tə-mē\ n, pl **-mies** : creation of a surgical opening between the stomach and a nearby cyst for drainage

cys·to·gram \ˈsis-tə-ˌgram\ n : a radiograph made by cystography

cys·tog·ra·phy \sis-ˈtä-grə-fē\ n, pl **-phies** : X-ray photography of the urinary bladder after injection of a contrast medium — **cys·to·graph·ic** \-tə-'gra-fik\ *adj*

cys·toid \'sis-,tȯid\ *adj* : resembling a bladder

cys·to·lith \'sis-tə-,lith\ *n* : a urinary calculus

cys·to·li·thi·a·sis \,sis-tō-li-'thī-ə-səs\ *n, pl* **-a·ses** \-,sēz\ : the presence of calculi in the urinary bladder

cys·to·li·thot·o·my \-li-'thä-tə-mē\ *n, pl* **-mies** : surgical removal of a calculus from the urinary bladder

cys·tom·e·ter \sis-'tä-mə-tər\ *n* : an instrument designed to measure pressure within the urinary bladder in relation to its capacity — **cys·to·met·ric** \,sis-tə-'me-trik\ *adj* — **cys·tom·e·try** \sis-'tä-mə-trē\ *n*

cys·to·met·ro·gram \,sis-tə-'me-trə-,gram, -'mē-\ *n* : a graphic recording of a cystometric measurement

cys·to·me·trog·ra·phy \-mə-'trä-grə-fē\ *n, pl* **-phies** : the process of making a cystometrogram

cys·to·plas·ty \'sis-tə-,plas-tē\ *n, pl* **-ties** : a plastic surgery on the urinary bladder

cys·to·py·eli·tis \,sis-tə-,pī-ə-'lī-təs\ *n* : inflammation of the urinary bladder and of the pelvis of one or both kidneys

cys·tor·rha·phy \sis-'tȯr-ə-fē\ *n, pl* **-phies** : suture of a wound, injury, or rupture in the urinary bladder

cys·to·sar·co·ma phyl·lo·des \,sis-tō-sär-'kō-mə-fi-'lō-,dēz\ *n* : a slow-growing tumor of the breast that resembles a fibroadenoma

cys·to·scope \'sis-tə-,skōp\ *n* : a rigid endoscope for inspecting and passing instruments into the urethra and bladder — **cys·to·scop·ic** \,sis-tə-'skä-pik\ *adj* — **cys·tos·co·pist** \sis-'täs-kə-pist\ *n*

cys·tos·co·py \sis-'täs-kə-pē\ *n, pl* **-pies** : the use of a cystoscope to examine the bladder

cys·tos·to·my \sis-'täs-tə-mē\ *n, pl* **-mies** : formation of an opening into the urinary bladder by surgical incision

cys·tot·o·my \sis-'tä-tə-mē\ *n, pl* **-mies** : surgical incision of the urinary bladder

cys·to·ure·ter·itis \,sis-tō-,yùr-ə-tə-'rī-təs\ *n* : combined inflammation of the urinary bladder and ureters

cys·to·ure·thro·cele \,sis-tō-yù-'rē-thrə-,sēl\ *n* : herniation of the neck of the female bladder and associated urethra into the vagina

cys·to·ure·thro·gram \-yù-'rē-thrə-,gram\ *n* : an X-ray photograph of the urinary bladder and urethra made after injection of these organs with a contrast medium — **cys·to·ure·throg·ra·phy** \-,yùr-i-'thrä-grə-fē\ *n*

cys·to·ure·thro·scope \,sis-tō-yù-'rē-thrə-,skōp\ *n* : an instrument used for the examination of the posterior urethra and bladder — **cys·to·ure·thros·co·py** \-,yùr-i-'thräs-kə-pē\ *n*

cyt- *or* **cyto-** *comb form* **1** : cell ⟨*cytol*ogy⟩ **2** : cytoplasm ⟨*cyto*kinesis⟩

cyt·ar·a·bine \sī-'tar-ə-,bēn\ *n* : CYTOSINE ARABINOSIDE

-cyte \,sīt\ *n comb form* : cell ⟨leuko*cyte*⟩

cy·ti·dine \'sī-tə-,dēn\ *n* : a nucleoside containing cytosine

cy·to·ar·chi·tec·ton·ics \,sī-tō-,är-kə-(,)tek-'tä-niks\ *n sing or pl* : CYTOARCHITECTURE — **cy·to·ar·chi·tec·ton·ic** \-nik\ *adj*

cy·to·ar·chi·tec·ture \,sī-tō-'är-kə-,tek-chər\ *n* : the cellular makeup of a bodily tissue or structure — **cy·to·ar·chi·tec·tur·al** \-,är-kə-'tek-chə-rəl\ *adj* — **cy·to·ar·chi·tec·tur·al·ly** *adv*

cy·to·chem·is·try \-'ke-mə-strē\ *n, pl* **-tries** **1** : microscopic biochemistry **2** : the chemistry of cells — **cy·to·chem·i·cal** \-'ke-mi-kəl\ *adj* — **cy·to·chem·i·cal·ly** \-mi-k(ə-)lē\ *adv* — **cy·to·chem·ist** \-'ke-mist\ *n*

cy·to·chrome \'sī-tə-,krōm\ *n* : any of several intracellular hemoprotein respiratory pigments that are enzymes functioning in electron transport as carriers of electrons

cytochrome c *n, often italicized third c* : the most abundant and stable of the cytochromes

cytochrome oxidase *n* : an iron-porphyrin enzyme important in cell respiration because of its ability to catalyze the oxidation of reduced cytochrome c in the presence of oxygen

cy·to·cid·al \,sī-tə-'sīd-ᵊl\ *adj* : killing or tending to kill individual cells ⟨∼ RNA viruses⟩

cy·to·di·ag·no·sis \,sī-tō-,dī-ig-'nō-səs, -əg-\ *n, pl* **-no·ses** \-,sēz\ : diagnosis based upon the examination of cells found in the tissues or fluids of the body — **cy·to·di·ag·nos·tic** \-'näs-tik\ *adj*

cy·to·dif·fer·en·ti·a·tion \,sī-tō-,di-fə-,ren-chē-'ā-shən\ *n* : the development of specialized cells (as muscle, blood, or nerve cells) from undifferentiated precursors

cy·to·ge·net·ics \-jə-'ne-tiks\ *n sing or pl* : a branch of biology that deals with the study of heredity and variation by the methods of both cytology and genetics — **cy·to·ge·net·ic** \-jə-'ne-tik\ *or* **cy·to·ge·net·i·cal** \-ti-kəl\ *adj* — **cy·to·ge·net·i·cal·ly** \-ti-k(ə-)lē\ *adv* — **cy·to·ge·net·i·cist** \-'ne-tə-sist\ *n*

cy·toid body \'sī-,tȯid-\ *n* : one of the white globular masses resembling cells that are found in the retina in some abnormal conditions

cy·to·ker·a·tin \,sī-tō-'ker-ə-t³n\ *n* : any of a class of fibrous proteins that are intermediate filaments present usu. in pairs chiefly in epithelial cells and that are sometimes used as markers to identify malignancies of epithelial origin

cy·to·kine \'sī-tə-,kīn\ *n* : any of a class of immunoregulatory substances (as lymphokines) that are secreted by cells of the immune system

cy·to·ki·ne·sis \ˌsī-tō-kə-ˈnē-səs, -kī-\ *n, pl* **-ne·ses** \-ˌsēz\ **1** : the cytoplasmic changes accompanying mitosis **2** : cleavage of the cytoplasm into daughter cells following nuclear division — compare KARYOKINESIS — **cy·to·ki·net·ic** \-ˈne-tik\ *adj*

cytol *abbr* cytological; cytology

cy·tol·o·gy \sī-ˈtä-lə-jē\ *n, pl* **-gies 1** : a branch of biology dealing with the structure, function, multiplication, pathology, and life history of cells **2** : the cytological aspects of a process or structure — **cy·to·log·i·cal** \ˌsīt-ᵊl-ˈä-ji-kəl\ *or* **cy·to·log·ic** \-ˈä-jik\ *adj* — **cy·to·log·i·cal·ly** \-ji-k(ə-)lē\ *adv* — **cy·tol·o·gist** \sī-ˈtä-lə-jist\ *n*

cy·to·ly·sin \ˌsīt-ᵊl-ˈīs-ᵊn\ *n* : a substance (as an antibody that lyses bacteria) producing cytolysis

cy·tol·y·sis \sī-ˈtä-lə-səs\ *n, pl* **-y·ses** \-ˌsēz\ : the usu. pathologic dissolution or disintegration of cells — **cy·to·lyt·ic** \ˌsīt-ᵊl-ˈi-tik\ *adj*

cytolytic T cell *n* : CYTOTOXIC T CELL

cytolytic T lymphocyte *n* : CYTOTOXIC T CELL

cy·to·meg·al·ic \ˌsī-tō-mi-ˈga-lik\ *adj* : characterized by or causing the formation of enlarged cells

cytomegalic inclusion disease *n* : a severe disease esp. of newborns that is caused by a cytomegalovirus and usu. affects the salivary glands, brain, kidneys, liver, and lungs — called also *inclusion disease*

cy·to·meg·a·lo·vi·rus \ˌsī-tə-ˌme-gə-lō-ˈvī-rəs\ *n* : a herpesvirus (species *Human herpesvirus 5* of the genus *Cytomegalovirus*) that causes cellular enlargement and formation of eosinophilic inclusion bodies esp. in the nucleus and that acts as an opportunistic infectious agent in immunosuppressed conditions (as AIDS)

cy·tom·e·ter \sī-ˈtä-mə-tər\ *n* : an apparatus for counting and measuring cells

cy·tom·e·try \sī-ˈtä-mə-trē\ *n, pl* **-tries** : a technical specialty concerned with the counting of cells and esp. blood cells — see FLOW CYTOMETRY — **cy·to·met·ric** \ˌsī-tə-ˈme-trik\ *adj*

cy·to·mor·phol·o·gy \ˌsī-tə-mȯr-ˈfä-lə-jē\ *n, pl* **-gies** : the morphology of cells — **cy·to·mor·pho·log·i·cal** \-ˌmȯr-fə-ˈlä-ji-kəl\ *adj*

cy·to·path·ic \ˌsī-tə-ˈpa-thik\ *adj* : of, relating to, characterized by, or producing pathological changes in cells

cy·to·patho·gen·ic \-ˌpa-thə-ˈje-nik\ *adj* : causing or involving pathological changes in cells — **cy·to·patho·ge·nic·i·ty** \-jə-ˈni-sə-tē\ *n*

cy·to·pa·thol·o·gy \-pə-ˈthä-lə-jē, -pa-\ *n, pl* **-gies** : a branch of pathology that deals with manifestations of disease at the cellular level — **cy·to·patho·log·ic** \-ˌpa-thə-ˈlä-jik\ *also* **cy·to·patho·log·i·cal** \-ji-kəl\ *adj* — **cy·to·pa·thol·o·gist** \-pə-ˈthä-lə-jist, -pa-\ *n*

cy·to·pe·nia \-ˈpē-nē-ə\ *n* : a deficiency of cellular elements of the blood; *esp* : deficiency of a specific element (as granulocytes in granulocytopenia) — **cy·to·pe·nic** \-ˈpē-nik\ *adj*

cy·to·phil·ic \ˌsī-tə-ˈfi-lik\ *adj* : having an affinity for cells

cy·to·pho·tom·e·ter \ˌsī-tō-fō-ˈtä-mə-tər\ *n* : a photometer for use in cytophotometry

cy·to·pho·tom·e·try \-(ˌ)fō-ˈtä-mə-trē\ *n, pl* **-tries** : photometry applied to the study of the cell or its constituents — **cy·to·pho·to·met·ric** \-ˌfō-tə-ˈme-trik\ *adj* — **cy·to·pho·to·met·ri·cal·ly** \-tri-k(ə-)lē\ *adv*

cy·to·phys·i·ol·o·gy \ˌsī-tō-ˌfi-zē-ˈä-lə-jē\ *n, pl* **-gies** : the physiology of cells — **cy·to·phys·i·o·log·i·cal** \-zē-ə-ˈlä-ji-kəl\ *adj*

cy·to·pi·pette \ˌsī-tō-pī-ˈpet\ *n* : a pipette with a bulb that contains a fluid which is released into the vagina and then sucked back with a sample of cells for a vaginal smear

cy·to·plasm \ˈsī-tə-ˌpla-zəm\ *n* : the organized complex of inorganic and organic substances external to the nuclear membrane of a cell and including the cytosol and membrane-bound organelles (as mitochondria) — **cy·to·plas·mic** \ˌsī-tə-ˈplaz-mik\ *adj* — **cy·to·plas·mi·cal·ly** \-mi-k(ə-)lē\ *adv*

cy·to·sine \ˈsī-tə-ˌsēn\ *n* : a pyrimidine base $C_4H_5N_3O$ that codes genetic information in the polynucleotide chain of DNA or RNA — compare ADENINE, GUANINE, THYMINE, URACIL

cytosine arabinoside *n* : a cytotoxic antineoplastic agent $C_9H_{13}N_3O_5$ that is a synthetic isomer of the naturally occurring nucleoside of cytosine and arabinose and is used esp. in the treatment of acute myelogenous leukemia in adults

cy·to·skel·e·ton \ˌsī-tō-ˈske-lə-ᵊn\ *n* : the network of protein filaments and microtubules in the cytoplasm that controls cell shape, maintains intracellular organization, and is involved in cell movement — **cy·to·skel·e·tal** \-ᵊl\ *adj*

cy·to·sol \ˈsī-tə-ˌsäl, -ˌsȯl\ *n* : the fluid portion of the cytoplasm exclusive of organelles and membranes — called also *hyaloplasm, ground substance* — **cy·to·sol·ic** \ˌsī-tə-ˈsä-lik, -ˈsȯ-\ *adj*

¹cy·to·stat·ic \ˌsī-tə-ˈsta-tik\ *adj* : tending to retard cellular activity and multiplication (~ treatment of tumors) — **cy·to·stat·i·cal·ly** \-ti-k(ə-)lē\ *adv*

²cytostatic *n* : a cytostatic agent

cy·to·tech·ni·cian \ˌsī-tō-(ˌ)tek-ˈni-shən\ *n* : CYTOTECHNOLOGIST

cy·to·tech·nol·o·gist \-ˈnä-lə-jist\ *n* : a medical technician trained in cytotechnology

cy·to·tech·nol·o·gy \-ˈnä-lə-jē\ *n, pl* **-gies** : a specialty in medical technology concerned with the identification of cells and cellular abnormalities (as in cancer)

cy·to·tox·ic \ˌsī-tə-ˈtäk-sik\ *adj* : toxic to cells ⟨∼ lymphocytes⟩ ⟨∼ drugs⟩ — **cy·to·tox·ic·i·ty** \-(ˌ)täk-ˈsi-sə-tē\ *n*

cytotoxic T cell *n* : a T cell that usu. bears CD8 molecular markers on its surface and that functions in cell-mediated immunity by destroying a cell (as one infected with a virus) having a specific antigenic molecule on its surface — called also *CTL, cytolytic T cell, cytolytic T lymphocyte, killer T cell, killer T lymphocyte;* compare HELPER T CELL, SUPPRESSOR T CELL

cy·to·tox·in \-ˈtäk-sən\ *n* : a substance (as a toxin or antibody) having a toxic effect on cells

cy·to·tro·pho·blast \ˌsī-tə-ˈtrō-fə-ˌblast\ *n* : the inner cellular layer of the trophoblast of an embryonic placenta-forming mammal that gives rise to the plasmodial syncytiotrophoblast covering the placental villi — **cy·to·tro·pho·blas·tic** \-ˌtrō-fə-ˈblas-tik\ *adj*

Cy·tox·an \sī-ˈtäk-sən\ *trademark* — used for a preparation of cyclophosphamide

d *abbr* **1** died **2** diopter **3** disease

d- \ˈdē, ˈdē\ *prefix* **1** : dextrorotatory — usu. printed in italic ⟨*d*-tartaric acid⟩ **2** : having a similar configuration at a selected carbon atom to the configuration of dextrorotatory glyceraldehyde — usu. printed as a small capital ⟨D-fructose⟩

2,4-D — see entry alphabetized as TWO,FOUR-D in the letter *t*

da·car·ba·zine \dä-ˈkär-bə-ˌzēn\ *n* : an antineoplastic agent $C_6H_{10}N_6O$ used to treat esp. metastatic malignant melanoma, tumors of adult soft tissue, and Hodgkin's disease

dacry- *or* **dacryo-** *comb form* : lacrimal ⟨*dacryo*cystitis⟩

dac·ryo·ad·e·nec·to·my \ˌda-krē-(ˌ)ō-ˌad-ᵊn-ˈek-tə-mē\ *n, pl* **-mies** : excision of a lacrimal gland

dac·ryo·cyst \ˈda-krē-ə-ˌsist\ *n* : LACRIMAL SAC

dac·ryo·cys·tec·to·my \ˌda-krē-(ˌ)ō-sis-ˈtek-tə-mē\ *n, pl* **-mies** : excision of a lacrimal sac

dac·ryo·cys·ti·tis \-sis-ˈtī-təs\ *n* : inflammation of the lacrimal sac

dac·ryo·cys·tog·ra·phy \-sis-ˈtä-grə-fē\ *n, pl* **-phies** : radiographic visualization of the lacrimal sacs and associated structures after injection of a contrast medium

dac·ryo·cys·to·rhi·nos·to·my \-ˌsis-tə-ˌrī-ˈnäs-tə-mē\ *n, pl* **-mies** : surgical creation of a passage for drainage between the lacrimal sac and the nasal cavity

dac·ryo·cys·tos·to·my \-sis-ˈtäs-tə-mē\ *n, pl* **-mies** : an operation on a lacrimal sac to form a new opening (as for drainage)

dac·ryo·cys·tot·o·my \-sis-ˈtä-tə-mē\ *n, pl* **-mies** : incision (as for drainage) of a lacrimal sac

dac·ryo·lith \ˈda-krē-ə-ˌlith\ *n* : a concretion formed in a lacrimal passage

dac·ryo·ste·no·sis \ˌda-krē-(ˌ)ō-sti-ˈnō-səs\ *n, pl* **-o·ses** \-ˌsēz\ : a narrowing of the lacrimal duct

dac·ti·no·my·cin \ˌdak-tə-nō-ˈmīs-ᵊn\ *n* : a toxic antineoplastic drug $C_{62}H_{86}N_{12}O_{16}$ of the actinomycin group — called also *actinomycin D*

dactyl- *or* **dactylo-** *comb form* : finger : toe : digit ⟨*dactylo*logy⟩

-dac·tyl·ia *n comb form* : -DACTYLY ⟨*adactylia*⟩

-dac·tyl·ism *n comb form* : -DACTYLY ⟨oligo*dactylism*⟩

dac·ty·lol·o·gy \ˌdak-tə-ˈlä-lə-jē\ *n, pl* **-gies** : FINGER SPELLING

-dac·ty·lous *adj comb form* : having (such or so many) fingers or toes ⟨brachy*dactylous*⟩

-dac·ty·ly *n comb form, pl* **-lies** : condition of having (such or so many) fingers or toes ⟨poly*dactyly*⟩

dag·ga \ˈda-gə, ˈdä-\ *n chiefly SoAfr* : MARIJUANA

DAH *abbr* disordered action of the heart

Dal·mane \ˈdal-ˌmān\ *trademark* — used for a preparation of flurazepam hydrochloride

Dal·ton·ism \ˈdȯlt-ᵊn-ˌi-zəm\ *n* : red-green color blindness occurring as a recessive sex-linked genetic trait; *broadly* : any form of color blindness

Dalton, John (1766–1844), British chemist and physicist.

1dam \ˈdam\ *n* : a female parent — used esp. of a domestic animal

2dam *n* : RUBBER DAM — see DENTAL DAM

3dam *abbr* dekameter

damp \ˈdamp\ *n* : a noxious or stifling gas or vapor; *esp* : one occurring in coal mines — usu. used in pl.; see BLACK DAMP, FIREDAMP

da·na·zol \ˈdä-nə-ˌzȯl, ˈda-, -ˌzōl\ *n* : a synthetic androgenic derivative $C_{22}H_{27}NO_2$ of ethisterone that suppresses hormone secretion by the adenohypophysis and used esp. in the treatment of endometriosis

D&C *n* : DILATION AND CURETTAGE

D&E *n* : DILATION AND EVACUATION

dan·der \'dan-dər\ *n* : DANDRUFF; *specif* : minute scales from hair, feathers, or skin that may act as allergens

dan·druff \'dan-drəf\ *n* : scaly white or grayish flakes of dead skin cells esp. of the scalp; *also* : the condition marked by excessive shedding of such flakes and usu. accompanied by itching — **dan·druffy** \-drə-fē\ *adj*

dan·dy fever \'dan-dē-\ *n* : DENGUE

Dane particle \'dān-\ *n* : a spherical particle found in the serum in hepatitis B that is the virion of the causative virus

Dane, David Maurice Surrey (1923–1998), British pathologist.

dap·sone \'dap-,sōn, -,zōn\ *n* : an antimicrobial agent $C_{12}H_{12}N_2O_2S$ used esp. against leprosy and dermatitis herpetiformis — called also *diaminodiphenyl sulfone*

Da·rier's disease \dar-'yāz-\ *n* : a genetically determined skin condition characterized by patches of keratotic papules — called also *keratosis follicularis*

Da·rier \dàr-'yā\, **Jean Ferdinand (1856–1938)**, French dermatologist.

dark adaptation *n* : the phenomena including dilation of the pupil, increase in retinal sensitivity, shift of the region of maximum luminosity toward the blue, and regeneration of rhodopsin by which the eye adapts to conditions of reduced illumination — compare LIGHT ADAPTATION — **dark–adapted** *adj*

dark field *n* : the dark area that serves as the background for objects viewed in an ultramicroscope — **dark–field** *adj*

dark–field microscope *n* : ULTRAMICROSCOPE — **dark–field microscopy** *n*

darm·stadt·i·um \,därm-'sta-tē-əm\ *n* : a short-lived radioactive element that is artificially produced — symbol *Ds*; see ELEMENT table

dar·tos \'där-,täs, -,təs\ *n* : a thin layer of vascular contractile tissue that contains smooth muscle fibers but no fat and is situated beneath the skin of the scrotum or beneath that of the labia majora

Dar·vo·cet–N \'där-vō-,set-'en\ *trademark* — used for a preparation of the napsylate of propoxyphene in combination with acetaminophen

Dar·von \'där-,vän\ *trademark* — used for a preparation of the hydrochloride of propoxyphene

Dar·win·ism \'där-wə-,ni-zəm\ *n* : a theory of the origin and perpetuation of new species of animals and plants that offspring of a given organism vary, that natural selection favors the survival of some of these variations over others, that new species may have arisen from the same ancestors — **Dar·win·ist** \-nist\ *n or adj*

Dar·win \'där-wən\, **Charles Robert (1809–1882)**, British naturalist.

Darwin's tubercle *n* : the slight projection occas. present on the edge of the external human ear and assumed by some scientists to represent the pointed part of the ear of quadrupeds — called also *auricular tubercle of Darwin*

DASH \'dash\ *n* [*dietary approaches to stop hypertension*] : a diet that is designed to lower blood pressure and emphasizes the consumption of fruit, vegetables, grains, and low-fat or non-fat dairy products

da·ta \'dā-tə, 'da-, 'dä-\ *n sing or pl* : factual information (as measurements or statistics) used as a basis for reasoning, discussion, or calculation

date rape *n* : rape committed by the victim's date; *broadly* : ACQUAINTANCE RAPE

date rape drug *n* : a drug (as GHB) given surreptitiously (as in a drink) to induce an unconscious or sedated state in a potential date rape victim

da·tu·ra \də-'tùr-ə, -'tyùr-\ *n* 1 *cap* : a genus of strong-scented herbs, shrubs, and trees (family Solanaceae) related to the potato and tomato and including some used as sources of medicinal alkaloids (as stramonium from jimsonweed) or in folk rites or illicitly for their poisonous, narcotic, or hallucinogenic properties 2 : any plant of the genus *Datura*

dau *abbr* daughter

¹**daugh·ter** \'dó-tər\ *n* 1 a : a human female having the relation of child to a parent b : a female offspring of an animal 2 : an atomic species that is the immediate product of the radioactive decay of a given element

²**daughter** *adj* 1 : having the characteristics or relationship of a daughter 2 : belonging to the first generation of offspring, organelles, or molecules produced by reproduction, division, or replication ⟨a ~ cell⟩ ⟨~ chromosomes⟩ ⟨~ DNA molecules⟩

dau·no·my·cin \,dó-nə-'mīs-ᵊn, ,daú-\ *n* : DAUNORUBICIN

dau·no·ru·bi·cin \-'rü-bə-sən\ *n* : an antibiotic that is a nitrogenous glycoside used in the form of its hydrochloride $C_{27}H_{29}NO_{10} \cdot HCl$ esp. in the treatment of some leukemias

dawn phenomenon *n* : a rise in the level of glucose in the blood plasma that occurs in early morning before breakfast and that may progress to hyperglycemia in diabetics — compare SOMOGYI EFFECT

day·dream \'dā-,drēm\ *n* : a visionary creation of the imagination experienced while awake; *esp* : a gratifying reverie usu. of wish fulfillment — **daydream** *vb* — **day·dream·er** *n*

day·mare \'dā-,mar\ *n* : a nightmarish fantasy experienced while awake

day nursery *n* : a public center for the care and training of young children

Day·pro *trademark* — used for a preparation of oxaprozin

Db *symbol* dubnium

DBCP \ˌdē-(ˌ)bē-(ˌ)sē-ˈpē\ *n* : an agricultural pesticide C₃H₅Br₂Cl that is a suspected carcinogen and cause of sterility in human males — called also *dibromochloropropane*

DBP *abbr* diastolic blood pressure

DC *abbr* doctor of chiropractic

DCIS *abbr* ductal carcinoma in situ

DD *abbr* developmentally disabled

DDAVP \ˌdē-ˌdē-ˌā-ˌvē-ˈpē\ *trademark* — used for a preparation of the acetate of desmopressin

ddC \ˌdē-(ˌ)dē-ˈsē\ *n, often all cap* : a synthetic nucleoside analog C₉H₁₃-N₃O₃ that inhibits replication of retroviruses and is used in the treatment of advanced HIV infection — called also *dideoxycytidine, zalcitabine*

DDD \ˈdē\ *n* : an insecticide C₁₄H₁₀Cl₄ closely related chemically and similar in properties to DDT

DDE \ˈē\ *n* : a persistent organochlorine C₁₅H₈Cl₄ that is produced by the metabolic breakdown of DDT

ddl \ˈī\ *n, often all cap* : a synthetic nucleoside analog C₁₀H₁₂N₄O₃ having properties and uses similar to those of ddC — called also *didanosine, dideoxyinosine;* see VIDEX

DDS *abbr* doctor of dental surgery

DDT \ˌdē-(ˌ)dē-ˈtē\ *n* : a colorless odorless water-insoluble crystalline insecticide C₁₄H₉Cl₅ that tends to accumulate in ecosystems and has toxic effects on many vertebrates

DDVP \ˌdē-(ˌ)dē-(ˌ)vē-ˈpē\ *n* : DICHLORVOS

¹**dead** \ˈded\ *adj* **1** : deprived of life : having died **2** : lacking power to move, feel, or respond : NUMB

²**dead** *n, pl* **dead** : one that is dead — usu. used collectively

dead·ly \ˈded-lē\ *adj* **dead·li·er; -est** : likely to cause or capable of causing death ⟨a ~ disease⟩ ⟨a ~ poison⟩ — **dead·li·ness** \-nəs\ *n*

deadly nightshade *n* : BELLADONNA 1

dead space *n* **1** : space in the respiratory system in which air does not undergo significant gaseous exchange — see ANATOMICAL DEAD SPACE, PHYSIOLOGICAL DEAD SPACE **2** : a space (as that in the chest following excision of a lung) left in the body as the result of a surgical procedure

deaf \ˈdef\ *adj* : lacking or deficient in the sense of hearing — **deaf·ness** *n*

deaf–aid \ˈdef-ˌād\ *n, chiefly Brit* : HEARING AID

deaf·en \ˈde-fən\ *vb* **deaf·ened; deaf·en·ing 1** : to make deaf **2** : to cause deafness or stun one with noise — **deaf·en·ing·ly** \-f(ə-)niŋ-lē\ *adv*

de·af·fer·en·ta·tion \ˌdē-ˌa-fə-ˌren-ˈtā-shən\ *n* : the freeing of a motor nerve from sensory components by severing the dorsal root central to the dorsal ganglion

¹**deaf–mute** \ˈdef-ˈmyüt\ *adj, often offensive* : lacking the sense of hearing and the ability to speak — **deaf–mute·ness** *n, sometimes offensive* — **deaf–mut·ism** \-ˈmyü-ˌti-zəm\ *n, sometimes offensive*

²**deaf–mute** *n, often offensive* : a deaf person who cannot speak

de·am·i·nase \(ˌ)dē-ˈa-mə-ˌnās, -ˌnāz\ *also* **des·am·i·nase** \(ˌ)des-\ *n* : an enzyme that hydrolyzes amino compounds (as amino acids) with removal of the amino group

de·am·i·nate \-ˌnāt\ *vb* **-nat·ed -nat·ing** : to remove the amino group from (a compound) — **de·am·i·na·tion** \(ˌ)dē-ˌa-mə-ˈnā-shən\ *n*

de·a·nol \ˈdē-ə-ˌnȯl\ *n* : DMAE

death \ˈdeth\ *n* **1** : the irreversible cessation of all vital functions esp. as indicated by permanent stoppage of the heart, respiration, and brain activity : the end of life — see BRAIN DEATH **2** : the cause or occasion of loss of life ⟨drinking was the ~ of him⟩ **3** : the state of being dead

death·bed \ˈdeth-ˌbed\ *n* **1** : the bed in which a person dies **2** : the last hours of life — **on one's deathbed** : near the point of death

death cap *n* : a very poisonous mushroom of the genus *Amanita* (*A. phalloides*) of deciduous woods of No. America and Europe that varies in color from pure white to olive or yellow and has a prominent cup at the base of the stem — called also *death cup;* see THIOCTIC ACID

death instinct *n* : an innate and unconscious tendency toward self-destruction postulated in psychoanalytic theory to explain aggressive and destructive behavior not satisfactorily explained by the pleasure principle — called also *Thanatos;* compare EROS

death rate *n* : the ratio of deaths to number of individuals in a population usu. expressed as number of deaths per hundred or per thousand population for a given time

death rattle *n* : a rattling or gurgling sound produced by air passing through mucus in the lungs and air passages of a dying person

death wish *n* : the conscious or unconscious desire for the death of another or of oneself

de·bil·i·tate \di-ˈbi-lə-ˌtāt\ *vb* **-tat·ed; -tat·ing** : to impair the strength of ⟨a body *debilitated* by disease⟩ — **de·bil·i·ta·tion** \-ˌbi-lə-ˈtā-shən\ *n*

de·bil·i·ty \di-ˈbi-lə-tē\ *n, pl* **-ties** : the quality or state of being weak, feeble, or infirm; *esp* : physical weakness

de·bride·ment \di-ˈbrēd-mənt, dā-, -ˌmänt, -ˌmäⁿ\ *n* : the usu. surgical removal of lacerated, devitalized, or contaminated tissue — **de·bride** \də-ˈbrēd, dā-\ *vb*

de·bris \də-'brē, dā-', 'dā-ˌ\ *n, pl* **debris** : organic waste from dead or damaged tissue

de·bris·o·quin \di-'bri-sō-ˌkwin\ *or* **de·bris·o·quine** \-ˌkwīn\ *n* : an antihypertensive drug used esp. in the form of its sulfate $(C_{10}H_{13}N_3)_2 \cdot H_2SO_4$

de·bulk \dē-'bəlk\ *vb* : to remove all or most of the substance of (a tumor or lesion)

dec *abbr* deceased

Dec·a·dron \'de-kə-ˌdrän\ *trademark* — used for a preparation of dexamethasone

de·cal·ci·fi·ca·tion \(ˌ)dē-ˌkal-sə-fə-'kā-shən\ *n* : the removal or loss of calcium or calcium compounds (as from bones) — **de·cal·ci·fy** \-'kal-sə-ˌfī\ *vb*

deca·me·tho·ni·um \ˌde-kə-mə-'thō-nē-əm\ *n* : a synthetic ion used in the form of either its bromide $C_{16}H_{38}Br_2N_2$ or iodide salts $C_{16}H_{38}I_2N_2$ as a skeletal muscle relaxant

de·cap·i·tate \di-'ka-pə-ˌtāt\ *vb* **-tat·ed; -tat·ing** : to cut off the head of — **de·cap·i·ta·tion** \-ˌka-pə-'tā-shən\ *n*

de·cap·su·late \(ˌ)dē-'kap-sə-ˌlāt\ *vb* **-lat·ed; -lat·ing** : to remove the capsule from (∼ a kidney) — **de·cap·su·la·tion** \-ˌkap-sə-'lā-shən\ *n*

de·car·box·yl·ase \ˌdē-kär-'bäk-sə-ˌlās, -ˌlāz\ *n* : any of a group of enzymes that accelerate decarboxylation esp. of amino acids

de·car·box·yl·ate \-sə-ˌlāt\ *vb* **-lat·ed; -lat·ing** : to remove carboxyl from — **de·car·box·yl·a·tion** \-ˌbäk-sə-'lā-shən\ *n*

de·cay \di-'kā\ *n* **1 a** : ROT 1; *specif* : aerobic decomposition of proteins chiefly by bacteria **b** : the product of decay **2 a** : spontaneous decrease in the number of radioactive atoms in radioactive material **b** : spontaneous disintegration (as of an atom or a nuclear particle) — **decay** *vb*

de·ceased \di-'sēst\ *adj* : no longer living; *esp* : recently dead — used of persons

deceased *n, pl* **deceased** : a dead person

de·cer·e·brate \(ˌ)dē-'ser-ə-brət, -ˌbrāt; ˌdē-sə-'rē-brət\ *adj* : having the cerebrum removed or made inactive; *also* : characteristic of decerebration (∼ rigidity)

de·cer·e·bra·tion \(ˌ)dē-ˌser-ə-'brā-shən\ *n* : loss of cerebral function (as from disease or surgical cutting of the brain stem); *also* : removal of the cerebrum (as by surgery) — **de·cer·e·brate** \(ˌ)dē-'ser-ə-ˌbrāt\ *vb*

deci·bel \'de-sə-ˌbel, -bəl\ *n* : a unit for expressing the relative intensity of sounds on a scale from zero for the average least perceptible sound to about 130 for the average pain level

de·cid·ua \di-'si-jə-wə\ *n, pl* **-uae** \-ˌwē\ **1** : the part of the mucous membrane lining the uterus that in higher placental mammals undergoes special modifications in preparation for and during pregnancy and is cast off at parturition, being made up in the human of a part lining the uterus, a part enveloping the embryo, and a part participating with the chorion in the formation of the placenta — see DECIDUA BASALIS, DECIDUA CAPSULARIS, DECIDUA PARIETALIS **2** : the mucous membrane of the uterus cast off in the ordinary process of menstruation — **de·cid·u·al** \-wəl\ *adj*

decidua ba·sa·lis \-bə-'sä-ləs\ *n* : the part of the endometrium in the pregnant human female that participates with the chorion in the formation of the placenta

decidua cap·su·lar·is \-ˌkap-sə-'lar-əs\ *n* : the part of the decidua in the pregnant human female that envelops the embryo

decidua pa·ri·etal·is \-pə-ˌrī-ə-'ta-ləs\ *n* : the part of the decidua in the pregnant human female lining the uterus

decidua pla·cen·tal·is \-ˌplā-sən-'ta-ləs, -sen-\ *n* : DECIDUA BASALIS

decidua re·flexa \-ri-'flek-sə\ *n* : DECIDUA CAPSULARIS

decidua ser·o·ti·na \-ˌser-ə-'tē-nə, -'tī-\ *n* : DECIDUA BASALIS

de·cid·u·ate \di-'si-jə-wət\ *adj* : having the fetal and maternal tissues firmly interlocked so that a layer of maternal tissue is torn away at parturition and forms a part of the afterbirth

decidua ve·ra \-'vir-ə, -'ver-\ *n* : DECIDUA PARIETALIS

de·cid·u·oma \di-ˌsi-jə-'wō-mə\ *n, pl* **-ma·ta** \-mə-tə\ *also* **-mas** **1** : a mass of tissue formed in the uterus following pregnancy that contains remnants of chorionic or decidual tissue **2** : decidual tissue induced in the uterus (as by trauma) in the absence of pregnancy

de·cid·u·ous \di-'si-jə-wəs\ *adj* **1** : falling off or shed at a certain stage in the life cycle **2** : having deciduous parts (a ∼ dentition)

deciduous tooth *n* : MILK TOOTH

deci·gram \'de-sə-ˌgram\ *n* : a metric unit of mass and weight equal to $\frac{1}{10}$ gram

deci·li·ter \'de-sə-ˌlē-tər\ *n* : a metric unit of capacity equal to $\frac{1}{10}$ liter

deci·me·ter \'de-sə-ˌmē-tər\ *n* : a metric unit of length equal to $\frac{1}{10}$ meter

de·clar·a·tive \di-'klar-ə-tiv\ *adj* : being or comprising memory characterized by the conscious recall of facts and events — compare PROCEDURAL

de·claw \(ˌ)dē-'klȯ\ *vb* : to remove the claws of (a cat) usu. with the nail matrix and all or part of the last bone of the toe

de·cline \di-'klīn, 'dē-ˌklīn\ *n* **1** : a gradual physical or mental sinking and wasting away **2** : the period during which the end of life is approaching **3** : a wasting disease; *esp* : pulmonary tuberculosis — **de·cline** \di-'klīn\ *vb*

de·clive \di-'klīv\ *n* : a part of the monticulus of the cerebellum that is dorsal to the culmen

de·clot \(,)dē-'klät\ *vb* **de·clot·ted; de·clot·ting** : to remove blood clots from

de·coc·tion \di-'käk-shən\ *n* **1** : the act or process of boiling usu. in water so as to extract the flavor or active principle — compare INFUSION 2a **2** : an extract or liquid preparation obtained by decoction esp. of a medicinal plant — **de·coct** \-'käkt\ *vb*

de·col·or·ize \(,)dē-'kəl-ə-,rīz\ *vb* **-or·ized; -or·iz·ing** : to remove color from — **de·col·or·iza·tion** \-,kə-lə-rə-'zā-shən\ *n*

de·com·pen·sa·tion \(,)dē-,käm-pən-'sā-shən, -pen-\ *n* : loss of physiological compensation or psychological balance; *esp* : inability of the heart to maintain adequate circulation — **de·com·pen·sate** \-'käm-pən-,sāt, -,pen-\ *vb* — **de·com·pen·sa·to·ry** \dē-kəm-'pen-sə-,tōr-ē\ *adj*

de·com·pose \,dē-kəm-'pōz\ *vb* **-posed; -pos·ing 1** : to separate into constituent parts or elements or into simpler compounds **2** : to undergo chemical breakdown : DECAY, ROT — **de·com·pos·able** \-'pō-zə-bəl\ *adj* — **de·com·po·si·tion** \(,)dē-,käm-pə-'zi-shən\ *n*

de·com·pres·sion \,dē-kəm-'pre-shən\ *n* **1 a** : the decrease of ambient air pressure experienced in an air lock on return to atmospheric pressure after a period of breathing compressed air (as in a diving apparatus or caisson) or experienced in ascent to a great altitude without a pressure suit or pressurized cabin **b** : the decrease of water pressure experienced by a diver when ascending rapidly **2** : an operation or technique used to relieve pressure upon an organ (as in fractures of the skull or spine) or within a hollow organ (as in intestinal obstruction) — **de·com·press** \-'pres\ *vb*

decompression chamber *n* **1** : a chamber in which excessive pressure can be reduced gradually to atmospheric pressure **2** : a chamber in which an individual can be gradually subjected to decreased atmospheric pressure (as in simulating conditions at high altitudes)

decompression sickness *n* : a sometimes fatal disorder that is marked by neuralgic pains and paralysis, distress in breathing, and often collapse and that is caused by the release of gas bubbles (as of nitrogen) in tissue upon too rapid decrease in air pressure after a stay in a compressed atmosphere — called also *bends, decompression illness, caisson disease;* see AEROEMBOLISM

de·com·pres·sive \,dē-kəm-'pre-siv\ *adj* : tending to relieve or reduce pressure ⟨∼ lumbar laminectomy⟩

de·con·di·tion \,dē-kən-'di-shən\ *vb* **1** : to cause to lose physical fitness **2**

: to cause extinction of (a conditioned response)

de·con·di·tion·ing \-'di-shə-niŋ\ *n* : a decrease in the responsiveness of heart muscle that sometimes occurs after long periods of weightlessness and may be marked by decrease in blood volume and pooling of the blood in the legs upon return to normal conditions

¹**de·con·ges·tant** \,dē-kən-'jes-tənt\ *n* : an agent that relieves congestion (as of mucous membranes)

²**decongestant** *adj* : relieving or tending to relieve congestion

de·con·ges·tion \-'jes-chən\ *n* : the process of relieving congestion — **de·con·ges·tive** \-'jes-tiv\ *adj*

de·con·tam·i·nate \,dē-kən-'ta-mə-,nāt\ *vb* **-nat·ed; -nat·ing** : to rid of contamination (as radioactive material) — **de·con·tam·i·na·tion** \-,ta-mə-'nā-shən\ *n*

¹**de·cor·ti·cate** \(,)dē-'kȯr-tə-,kāt\ *vb* **-cat·ed; -cat·ing** : to remove all or part of the cortex from (as the brain)

²**de·cor·ti·cate** \-,kāt, -kət\ *adj* : lacking a cortex and esp. the cerebral cortex

de·cor·ti·ca·tion \-,kȯr-ti-'kā-shən\ *n* : the surgical removal of the cortex of an organ, an enveloping membrane, or a constrictive fibrinous covering ⟨the ∼ of a lung⟩

de·cu·bi·tal \di-'kyü-bət-ᵊl\ *adj* **1** : relating to or resulting from lying down ⟨a ∼ sore⟩ **2** : relating to or resembling a decubitus

de·cu·bi·tus \-bə-təs\ *n, pl* **-bi·ti** \-,tī, -,tē\ **1** : a position assumed in lying down ⟨the dorsal ∼⟩ **2 a** : ULCER **b** : BEDSORE **3** : prolonged lying down (as in bed)

decubitus ulcer *n* : BEDSORE

de·cus·sa·tion \,dē-(,)kə-'sā-shən\ *n* : the action of intersecting or crossing (as of nerve fibers) esp. in the form of an X — see DECUSSATION OF PYRAMIDS **2 a** : a band of nerve fibers that connects unlike centers on opposite sides of the nervous system **b** : a crossed tract of nerve fibers passing between centers on opposite sides of the central nervous system : COMMISSURE — **de·cus·sate** \'de-kə-,sāt, di-'kə-,sāt\ *vb*

decussation of pyramids *n* : the crossing of the fibers of the corticospinal tracts from one side of the central nervous system to the other near the junction of the medulla and the spinal cord

de·dif·fer·en·ti·a·tion \(,)dē-,di-fə-,ren-chē-'ā-shən\ *n* : reversion of specialized structures (as cells) to a more generalized or primitive condition often as a preliminary to major change — **de·dif·fer·en·ti·ate** \-'ren-chē-,āt\ *vb*

deep \'dēp\ *adj* **1** : extending well inward from an outer surface ⟨a ∼ gash⟩ **b** (1) : not located superficially within the body or one of its parts ⟨∼

veins⟩ (2) : resulting from or involving stimulation of deep structures ⟨~ pain⟩ ⟨~ reflexes⟩ **2** : being below the level of the conscious ⟨~ neuroses⟩ — **deep·ly** *adv*

deep brachial artery *n* : the largest branch of the brachial artery in the upper part of the arm

deep external pudendal artery *n* : EXTERNAL PUDENDAL ARTERY b

deep facial vein *n* : a tributary of the facial vein draining part of the pterygoid plexus and nearby structures

deep fascia *n* : a firm fascia that ensheathes and binds together muscles and other internal structures — compare SUPERFICIAL FASCIA

deep femoral artery *n* : the large deep branch of the femoral artery formed where it divides about two inches (five centimeters) below the inguinal ligament

deep inguinal ring *n* : the internal opening of the inguinal canal — called also *internal inguinal ring*; compare SUPERFICIAL INGUINAL RING, INGUINAL RING

deep palmar arch *n* : PALMAR ARCH a

deep peroneal nerve *n* : a nerve that arises as a branch of the common peroneal nerve and that innervates or gives off branches innervating the muscles of the anterior part of the leg, the extensor digitorum brevis of the foot, and the skin between the big toe and the second toe — compare SUPERFICIAL PERONEAL NERVE

deep petrosal nerve *n* : a sympathetic nerve that originates in the carotid plexus, passes through the cartilage of the Eustachian tube, joins with the greater petrosal nerve to form the Vidian nerve, and as part of this nerve is distributed to the mucous membranes of the nasal cavity and palate

deep sedation *n* : an induced state of sedation characterized by depressed consciousness such that the patient is unable to continuously and independently maintain a patent airway and experiences a partial loss of protective reflexes and ability to respond to verbal commands or physical stimulation — compare CONSCIOUS SEDATION

deep temporal artery *n* : TEMPORAL ARTERY I

deep temporal nerve *n* : either of two motor branches of the mandibular nerve on each side of the body that are distributed to the temporalis

deep temporal vein *n* : TEMPORAL VEIN b

deep vein thrombosis *n* : a condition marked by the formation of a thrombus within a deep vein (as of the leg or pelvis) that may be asymptomatic or be accompanied by symptoms (as swelling and pain) and that is potentially life threatening if dislodgment of the thrombus results in pulmonary embolism — abbr. *DVT*

deer·fly \'dir-ˌflī\ *n* : any of numerous small horseflies esp. of the genus *Chrysops* that include important vectors of tularemia

deer tick *n* : a tick of the genus *Ixodes* (*I. scapularis* syn. *I. dammini*) that transmits the bacterium causing Lyme disease

deet \'dēt\ *n, often all cap* : a colorless oily liquid insect and tick repellent $C_{12}H_{17}NO$

def·e·cate \'de-fi-ˌkāt\ *vb* **-cat·ed; -cat·ing 1** : to discharge from the anus **2** : to discharge feces from the bowels — **def·e·ca·tion** \ˌde-fi-'kā-shən\ *n*

de·fect \'dē-ˌfekt, di-'\ *n* : a lack or deficiency of something necessary for adequacy in form or function

¹**de·fec·tive** \di-'fek-tiv\ *adj* : falling below the norm in structure or in mental or physical function ⟨~ eyesight⟩ — **de·fec·tive·ness** \-nəs\ *n*

²**defective** *n* : a person who is subnormal physically or mentally

de·fem·i·nize \(ˌ)dē-'fe-mə-ˌnīz\ *vb* **-nized; -niz·ing** : to divest of feminine qualities or physical characteristics : MASCULINIZE — **de·fem·i·ni·za·tion** \-ˌfe-mə-nə-'zā-shən\ *n*

de·fense \di-'fens\ *n* : a means or method of protecting the physical or functional integrity of body or mind ⟨a ~ against anxiety⟩

defense mechanism *n* : an often unconscious mental process (as repression, projection, or sublimation) that makes possible compromise solutions to personal problems

de·fen·sive \di-'fen-siv, 'dē-ˌ\ *adj* **1** : serving to defend or protect (as the ego) **2** : devoted to resisting or preventing aggression or attack ⟨~ behavior⟩ — **de·fen·sive·ly** *adv* — **de·fen·sive·ness** *n*

defensive medicine *n* : the practice of ordering medical tests, procedures, or consultations of doubtful clinical value in order to protect the prescribing physician from malpractice suits

deferens — see DUCTUS DEFERENS, VAS DEFERENS

deferentes — see DUCTUS DEFERENS

deferentia — see VAS DEFERENS

de·fer·ox·amine \ˌdē-fə-'räk-sə-ˌmēn\ *n* : a chelator that is used in the form of its mesylate $C_{25}H_{48}N_6O_8 \cdot CH_4O_3S$ as an antidote to iron poisoning or overload

de·fer·ves·cence \ˌdē-(ˌ)fər-'ves-ᵊns, ˌde-fər-\ *n* : the subsidence of a fever

de·fi·bril·la·tion \(ˌ)dē-ˌfi-brə-'lā-shən, -ˌfī-\ *n* : restoration of the rhythm of a fibrillating heart — **de·fi·bril·late** \(ˈ)dē-'fi-brə-ˌlāt, -'fī-\ *vb*

de·fi·bril·la·tor \-'fi-brə-ˌlā-tər, -'fī-\ *n* : an electronic device used to defibrillate a heart by applying an electric shock to it

de·fi·brin·ate \-'fi-brə-ˌnāt, -'fī-\ *vb* **-at·ed; -at·ing** : to remove fibrin from (blood) — de·fi·brin·ation \-ˌfī-brə-ˈnā-shən, -ˌfī-\ n

de·fi·cien·cy \di-ˈfi-shən-sē\ n, pl -cies 1 : a shortage of substances (as vitamins) necessary to health 2 : DELETION

deficiency anemia n : NUTRITIONAL ANEMIA

deficiency disease n : a disease (as scurvy) caused by a lack of essential dietary elements and esp. a vitamin or mineral

¹de·fi·cient \di-ˈfi-shənt\ adj 1 : lacking in some necessary quality or element ⟨a ∼ diet⟩ 2 : not up to a normal standard or complement ⟨∼ strength⟩

²deficient n : one that is deficient

de·fi·cit \ˈde-fə-sət\ n : a deficiency of a substance ⟨a potassium ∼⟩; also : a lack or impairment of a functional capacity ⟨cognitive ∼s⟩

de·fin·i·tive \di-ˈfi-nə-tiv\ adj : fully differentiated or developed

definitive host n : the host in which the sexual reproduction of a parasite takes place — compare INTERMEDIATE HOST 1

de·flo·ra·tion \ˌde-flə-ˈrā-shən, ˌdē-\ n : rupture of the hymen — de·flo·rate \ˈde-flə-ˌrāt, ˈdē-\ vb

de·flu·vi·um \dē-ˈflü-vē-əm\ n : the pathological loss of a part (as hair or nails)

de·fo·cus \ˌdē-ˈfō-kəs\ vb de·fo·cused; de·fo·cus·ing : to cause to be out of focus ⟨∼ed his eye⟩ ⟨a ∼ed image⟩

deformans — see ARTHRITIS DEFORMANS, DYSTONIA MUSCULORUM DEFORMANS, OSTEITIS DEFORMANS

de·formed \di-ˈfórmd, dē-\ adj : misshapen esp. in body or limbs

de·for·mi·ty \di-ˈfòr-mə-tē\ n, pl -ties 1 : the state of being deformed 2 : a physical blemish or distortion

deg abbr degree

de·gen·er·a·cy \di-ˈje-nə-rə-sē\ n, pl -cies 1 : sexual perversion 2 : the coding of an amino acid by more than one codon of the genetic code

¹de·gen·er·ate \-rət\ adj 1 a : having deteriorated progressively (as in the process of evolution) esp. through loss of structure and function b : having sunk to a lower and usu. corrupt and vicious state 2 : having more than one codon representing an amino acid; also : being such a codon

²degenerate n : one that is degenerate

de·gen·er·a·tion \di-ˌje-nə-ˈrā-shən, ˌdē-\ n 1 : progressive deterioration of physical characters from a level representing the norm of earlier generations or forms 2 : deterioration of a tissue or an organ in which its function is diminished or its structure impaired — de·gen·er·ate \-ˈje-nə-ˌrāt\ vb — de·gen·er·a·tive \di-ˈje-nə-ˌrā-tiv, -rə-\ adj

degenerative arthritis n : OSTEOARTHRITIS

degenerative disease n : a disease (as arteriosclerosis or osteoarthritis) characterized by progressive degenerative changes in tissue

degenerative joint disease n : OSTEOARTHRITIS

de·germ \(ˌ)dē-ˈjərm\ vb : to remove germs from (as the skin)

de·glu·ti·tion \ˌdē-ˌglü-ˈti-shən, ˌde-\ n : the act, power, or process of swallowing

deg·ra·da·tion \ˌde-grə-ˈdā-shən\ n : change of a chemical compound to a less complex compound — deg·ra·da·tive \ˈde-grə-ˌdā-tiv\ adj

de·grade \di-ˈgrād\ vb 1 : to reduce the complexity of (a chemical compound) by splitting off one or more groups or larger components : DECOMPOSE 2 : to undergo chemical degradation — de·grad·able \-ˈgrā-də-bəl\ adj

de·gran·u·la·tion \(ˌ)dē-ˌgran-yə-ˈlā-shən\ n : the process by which cytoplasmic granules (as of mast cells) release their contents — de·gran·u·late \-ˈgran-yə-ˌlāt\ vb

de·gree \di-ˈgrē\ n 1 : a measure of damage to tissue caused by injury or disease — see FIRST-DEGREE BURN, SECOND-DEGREE BURN, THIRD-DEGREE BURN 2 : one of the divisions or intervals marked on a scale of a measuring instrument; specif : any of various units for measuring temperature

de·his·cence \di-ˈhis-ᵊns\ n : the parting of the sutured lips of a surgical wound — de·hisce \-ˈhis\ vb

de·hu·mid·i·fy \ˌdē-hyü-ˈmi-də-ˌfī, ˌdē-yü-\ vb -fied; -fy·ing : to remove moisture from (as air) — de·hu·mid·i·fi·ca·tion \-ˌmi-də-fə-ˈkā-shən\ n — de·hu·mid·i·fi·er \-ˈmi-də-ˌfī-ər\ n

de·hy·drate \(ˌ)dē-ˈhī-ˌdrāt\ vb -drat·ed; -drat·ing 1 : to remove bound water or hydrogen and oxygen from (a chemical compound) in the proportion in which they form water 2 : to remove water from (as foods) 3 : to lose water or body fluids — de·hy·dra·tor \-ˌdrā-tər\ n

de·hy·dra·tion \ˌdē-hī-ˈdrā-shən\ n : the process of dehydrating; esp : an abnormal depletion of body fluids

de·hy·dro·ascor·bic acid \(ˌ)dē-ˌhī-drō-ə-ˈskòr-bik-\ n : a crystalline oxidation product $C_6H_6O_6$ of vitamin C

7–de·hy·dro·cho·les·ter·ol \ˈse-vən-(ˌ)dē-ˌhī-drō-kə-ˈles-tə-ˌról, -ˌrōl\ n : a crystalline steroid alcohol $C_{27}H_{44}OH$ that occurs (as in the skin) in humans and that yields vitamin D_3 on irradiation with ultraviolet light

24–dehydrocholesterol \ˌtwen-tē-ˈfòr-\ n : DESMOSTEROL

de·hy·dro·cho·lic acid \(ˈ)dē-ˌhī-drə-ˌkō-lik-\ n : a colorless crystalline acid $C_{24}H_{34}O_5$ used often in the form of its sodium salt $C_{24}H_{33}NaO_5$ esp. as a laxative and choleretic

11–de·hy·dro·cor·ti·co·ste·rone \ˌi-ˈle-vən-(ˌ)dē-ˌhī-drō-ˌkòr-tə-ˈkäs-tə-ˌrōn,

-ˌkō-stə-ˈrōn, -kō-ˈstir-ˌōn\ *n* : a steroid $C_{21}H_{28}O_4$ extracted from the adrenal cortex and also made synthetically — compare CORTISONE

de·hy·dro·epi·an·dros·ter·one \(ˌ)dē-ˌhī-drō-ˌe-pē-an-ˈdräs-tə-ˌrōn\ *n* : an androgenic ketosteroid $C_{19}H_{28}O_2$ that is secreted by the adrenal cortex and is an intermediate in the biosynthesis of testosterone — abbr. *DHA, DHEA*

de·hy·dro·ge·nase \dē-(ˌ)hī-ˈdrä-jə-ˌnās, -ˈhī-drə-jə-, -ˌnāz\ *n* : an enzyme that accelerates the removal of hydrogen from metabolites and its transfer to other substances — see ALCOHOL DEHYDROGENASE

de·hy·dro·ge·nate \dē-(ˌ)hī-ˈdrä-jə-ˌnāt, -ˈhī-drə-jə-\ *vb* -**nat·ed; -nat·ing** : to remove hydrogen from — **de·hy·dro·ge·na·tion** \dē-(ˌ)hī-ˌdrä-jə-ˈnā-shən, -ˌhī-drə-jə-\ *n*

de·hy·dro·ge·nize \(ˌ)dē-ˈhī-drə-jə-ˌnīz\ *vb* -**ized; -iz·ing** : DEHYDROGENATE

de·in·sti·tu·tion·al·ize \(ˌ)dē-ˌin-stə-ˈtü-shə-nə-lə-ˈzā-shən, -ˈtyü-\ : the release of institutionalized individuals from institutional care (as in a psychiatric hospital) to care in the community — **de·in·sti·tu·tion·al·ize** \-ˈtü-shə-nə-ˌlīz, -ˈtyü-\ *vb*

de·ion·ize \(ˌ)dē-ˈī-ə-ˌnīz\ *vb* -**ized; -iz·ing** : to remove ions from ⟨∼ water⟩ — **de·ion·iza·tion** \-ˌī-ə-nə-ˈzā-shən\ *n* — **de·ion·iz·er** \-ˈī-ə-ˌnī-zər\ *n*

Dei·ters' nucleus \ˈdī-tərz-\ *n* : LATERAL VESTIBULAR NUCLEUS

dé·jà vu \ˌdā-ˌzhä-ˈvü\ *n* : PARAMNESIA b

delayed hypersensitivity *n* : hypersensitivity (as in a tuberculin test) in which the typical symptoms of inflammation and induration appear in an individual previously exposed to an antigen after an interval of 12 to 48 hours following a subsequent exposure

delayed-stress disorder *n* : POSTTRAUMATIC STRESS DISORDER

delayed-stress syndrome *n* : POSTTRAUMATIC STRESS DISORDER

de·lead \(ˌ)dē-ˈled\ *vb* : to remove lead from ⟨∼ a chemical⟩

del·e·te·ri·ous \ˌde-lə-ˈtir-ē-əs\ *adj* : harmful often in a subtle or an unexpected way ⟨∼ genes⟩

de·le·tion \di-ˈlē-shən\ *n* **1** : the absence of a section of genetic material from a gene or chromosome **2** : the mutational process that results in a deletion

de·lin·quen·cy \di-ˈliŋ-kwən-sē, -ˈlin-\ *n, pl* -**cies** : conduct that is out of accord with accepted behavior or the law; *esp* : JUVENILE DELINQUENCY

¹de·lin·quent \-kwənt\ *n* : a delinquent person; *specif* : one whose behavior has been labeled juvenile delinquency

²delinquent *adj* **1** : offending by neglect or violation of duty or of law **2** : of, relating to, or characteristic of delinquents : marked by delinquency ⟨∼ behavior⟩ — **de·lin·quent·ly** *adv*

de·lir·i·um \di-ˈlir-ē-əm\ *n* : a mental disturbance characterized by confusion, disordered speech, and hallucinations — **de·lir·i·ous** \-ē-əs\ *adj* — **de·lir·i·ous·ly** *adv*

delirium tre·mens \-ˈtrē-mənz, -ˈtre-\ *n* : a violent delirium with tremors that is induced by excessive and prolonged use of alcoholic liquors — called also *d.t.'s* \ˈdē-ˈtēz\

de·liv·er \di-ˈli-vər\ *vb* **de·liv·ered; de·liv·er·ing 1 a** : to assist (a parturient female) in giving birth ⟨she was ∼*ed* of a fine boy⟩ **b** : to aid in the birth of ⟨∼ a child with forceps⟩ **2** : to give birth to ⟨she ∼*ed* a healthy girl⟩

de·liv·ery \di-ˈli-və-rē\ *n, pl* -**er·ies** : the act of giving birth : the expulsion or extraction of a fetus and its membranes : PARTURITION **2** : the procedure of assisting birth of the fetus and expulsion of the placenta by manual, instrumental, or surgical means

delivery room *n* : a hospital room esp. equipped for the delivery of pregnant women

de·louse \(ˌ)dē-ˈlaus, -ˈlaúz\ *vb* **de·loused; de·lous·ing** : to remove lice from

del·phin·i·um \del-ˈfin-ē-əm\ *n* **1** *cap* : a genus of perennial herbs of the buttercup family (Ranunculaceae) having showy flowers and including several esp. of the western U.S. that are toxic to grazing animals and fowl. cattle **2** : any plant of the genus *Delphinium*

delt \ˈdelt\ *n* : DELTOID — usu. used in pl.

¹del·ta \ˈdel-tə\ *n* **1** : the fourth letter of the Greek alphabet — symbol Δ or δ **2** : DELTA WAVE

²delta or δ- *adj* : of or relating to one of four or more closely related chemical substances ⟨the *delta* chain of fetal hemoglobin⟩ — used somewhat arbitrarily to specify ordinal relationship or a particular physical form

delta agent *n* : HEPATITIS D VIRUS

delta hepatitis *n* : HEPATITIS D

delta-9-tet·ra·hy·dro·can·nab·i·nol \ˈdel-tə-ˈnīn-ˌte-trə-ˌhī-drə-kə-ˈna-bə-ˌnȯl, -ˌnōl\ *n* : THC a

delta-9-THC \-ˌtē-ˌāch-ˈsē\ *n* : THC a

delta virus *n* : HEPATITIS D VIRUS

delta wave *n* : a high amplitude electrical rhythm of the brain with a frequency of less than 6 cycles per second that occurs esp. in deep sleep, in infancy, and in many diseased conditions of the brain — called also *delta, delta rhythm*

¹del·toid \ˈdel-ˌtȯid\ *n* : a large triangular muscle that covers the shoulder joint, serves to raise the arm laterally, arises from the upper anterior part of the outer third of the clavicle and from the acromion and spine of the scapula, and is inserted into the outer side of the middle of the shaft of the humerus — called also *deltoid muscle;* see DELTOID TUBEROSITY

²deltoid *adj* : relating to, associated with, or supplying the deltoid

del·toi·de·us \del-'tȯi-dē-əs\ *n, pl* **-dei** \-dē-ˌē, -ˌī\ : DELTOID

deltoid ligament *n* : a strong radiating ligament of the inner aspect of the ankle that binds the base of the tibia to the bones of the foot

deltoid tuberosity *n* : a rough triangular bump on the outer side of the middle of the humerus that is the site of insertion of the deltoid

delts \'delts\ *pl of* DELT

de·lude \di-'lüd\ *vb* **de·lud·ed; de·lud·ing** : to mislead the mind or judgment of

de·lu·sion \di-'lü-zhən\ *n* **1 a** : the act of deluding : the state of being deluded **b** : an abnormal mental state characterized by the occurrence of psychotic delusions **2** : a false belief regarding the self or persons or objects outside the self that persists despite the facts and occurs in some psychotic states — **de·lu·sion·al** \di-'lü-zhən-ᵊl\ *adj*

delusion of reference *n* : IDEA OF REFERENCE

de·mas·cu·lin·ize \(ˌ)dē-'mas-kyə-lə-ˌnīz, di-\ *vb* **-ized; -iz·ing** : to remove the masculine character or qualities of — **de·mas·cu·lin·iza·tion** \-ˌmas-kyə-lə-nə-'zā-shən, -ˌni-\ *n*

dem·e·car·i·um \ˌde-mi-'kar-ē-əm, -'ker-\ *n* : a long-acting cholinesterase-inhibiting ammonium compound that is used as the bromide $C_{32}H_{52}Br_2N_4O_4$ in an ophthalmic solution esp. in the treatment of glaucoma and esotropia

de·mec·lo·cy·cline \ˌde-mə-klō-'sī-ˌklēn\ *n* : a broad-spectrum tetracycline antibiotic produced by an actinomycete of the genus *Streptomyces* (*S. aureofaciens*) and used esp. in the form of its hydrochloride $C_{21}H_{21}ClN_2O_8 \cdot HCl$

de·ment·ed \di-'men-təd\ *adj* **1** : MAD, INSANE **2** : suffering from or exhibiting cognitive dementia — **de·ment·ed·ly** *adv* — **de·ment·ed·ness** *n*

de·men·tia \di-'men-chə\ *n* : a usu. progressive condition (as Alzheimer's disease) marked by the development of multiple cognitive deficits (as memory impairment, aphasia, and inability to plan and initiate complex behavior) — **de·men·tial** \-chəl\ *adj*

dementia par·a·lyt·i·ca \-ˌpar-ə-'li-ti-kə\ *n, pl* **de·men·ti·ae par·a·lyt·i·cae** \di-'men-chē-ˌē,-par-ə-'li-ti-ˌsē\ : GENERAL PARESIS

dementia prae·cox \-'prē-ˌkäks\ *n* : SCHIZOPHRENIA

dementia pu·gi·lis·ti·ca \-ˌpyü-jə-'lis-stə-kə\ *n* : a neurological disorder affecting boxers that is caused by cumulative cerebral injuries and is characterized esp. by impaired cognitive functioning and parkinsonism

de·ment·ing \di-'men-tiŋ\ *adj* : causing or characterized by dementia

Dem·er·ol \'de-mə-ˌrȯl, -ˌrōl\ *trademark* — used for meperidine

demi·lune \'de-mē-ˌlün\ *n* : one of the small crescentic groups of granular deeply staining zymogen-secreting cells lying between the clearer mucus-producing cells and the basement membrane in the alveoli of mixed salivary glands — called also *crescent of Giannuzzi*

demilune of Gian·nuz·zi *also* **demilune of Gia·nuz·zi** \-jä-'nüt-sē\ *n* : DEMILUNE

   Giannuzzi, Giuseppe (1839–1876), Italian anatomist.

de·min·er·al·iza·tion \(ˌ)dē-ˌmi-nə-rə-lə-'zā-shən\ *n* **1** : loss of mineral (as salts of calcium) from the body esp. in disease **2** : the process of removing mineral matter or salts (as from water) — **de·min·er·al·ize** \-'mi-nə-rə-ˌlīz\ *vb*

dem·o·dec·tic mange \ˌde-mə-'dek-tik-\ *n* : mange caused by mites of the genus *Demodex* that burrow in the hair follicles esp. of dogs — compare CHORIOPTIC MANGE, SARCOPTIC MANGE

de·mo·dex \'de-mə-ˌdeks, 'dē-\ *n* **1** *cap* : a genus (family Demodicidae) of minute mites that live in the hair follicles esp. about the face of humans and various furred mammals and in the latter often cause demodectic mange **2** : any mite of the genus *Demodex* : FOLLICLE MITE

dem·o·di·co·sis \ˌde-mō-də-'kō-səs\ *n, pl* **-co·ses** \-ˌsēz\ : DEMODECTIC MANGE

de·mog·ra·phy \di-'mä-grə-fē\ *n, pl* **-phies** : the statistical study of human populations esp. with reference to size and density, distribution, and vital statistics — **de·mog·ra·pher** \-fər\ *n* — **de·mo·graph·ic** \ˌde-mə-'gra-fik, ˌdē-\ *adj* — **de·mo·graph·i·cal·ly** \-fi-k(ə-)lē\ *adv*

¹de·mul·cent \di-'məl-sᵊnt\ *adj* : tending to soothe or soften

²demulcent *n* : a usu. mucilaginous or oily substance that can soothe or protect an abraded mucous membrane

de·my·elin·at·ing \(ˌ)dē-'mī-ə-lə-ˌnā-tiŋ\ *adj* : causing or characterized by the loss or destruction of myelin

de·my·elin·ation \-ˌmī-ə-lə-'nā-shən\ *n* : the state resulting from the loss or destruction of myelin; *also* : the process of such loss or destruction

de·my·elin·iza·tion \-lə-nə-'zā-shən\ *n* : DEMYELINATION

de·na·tur·ant \(ˌ)dē-'nā-chər-ənt\ *n* : a denaturing agent

de·na·ture \-'nā-chər\ *vb* **de·na·tured; de·na·tur·ing** **1** : to make (alcohol) unfit for drinking (as by adding an obnoxious substance) without impairing usefulness for other purposes **2** : to modify the molecular structure of (as a protein or DNA) esp. by heat, acid, alkali, or ultraviolet radiation so as to destroy or diminish some of the original properties and esp. the specific biological activity — **de·na·tur·ation** \-ˌnā-chə-ˈrā-shən\ n

den·drite \ˈdren-ˌdrīt\ n : any of the usu. branching protoplasmic processes that conduct impulses toward the body of a nerve cell — **den·drit·ic** \den-ˈdri-tik\ adj

dendritic cell n : any of various antigen-presenting cells with long irregular processes

den·dro·den·drit·ic \ˌden-drō-ˌden-ˈdri-tik\ adj : relating to or being a nerve synapse between a dendrite of one cell and a dendrite of another

de·ner·vate \ˈdē-(ˌ)nər-ˌvāt\ vb -vat·ed; -vat·ing : to deprive of a nerve supply (as by cutting a nerve) — **de·ner·va·tion** \ˌdē-(ˌ)nər-ˈvā-shən\ n

den·gue \ˈden-gē, -ˌgā\ n : an acute infectious disease that is characterized by headache, severe joint pain, and a rash and that is caused by a virus of the genus *Flavivirus* (species *Dengue virus*) transmitted by mosquitoes of the genus *Aedes* — called also *breakbone fever, dandy fever, dengue fever*

dengue hemorrhagic fever n : dengue marked by hemorrhagic symptoms (as hemorrhagic lesions of the skin and thrombocytopenia) — called also *hemorrhagic dengue*

de·ni·al \di-ˈnī-əl\ n : a psychological defense mechanism in which confrontation with a personal problem or with reality is avoided by denying the existence of the problem or reality

den·i·da·tion \ˌden-ə-ˈdā-shən\ n : the sloughing of the endometrium of the uterus esp. during menstruation

de·ni·trog·e·nate \(ˌ)dē-ˌnī-ˈträ-jə-ˌnāt\ vb -nat·ed; -nat·ing : to reduce the stored nitrogen in the body by forced breathing of pure oxygen for a period of time esp. as a measure designed to prevent development of decompression sickness — **de·ni·trog·e·na·tion** \-ˌträ-jə-ˈnā-shən\ n

dens \ˈdenz\ n, pl **den·tes** \ˈden-ˌtēz\ : a toothlike process that projects from the anterior end of the centrum of the axis in the spinal column and serves as a pivot on which the atlas rotates — called also *odontoid process*

densa — see MACULA DENSA

den·si·tom·e·ter \ˌden-sə-ˈtä-mə-tər\ n : an instrument for determining optical, photographic, or mass density ⟨an X-ray bone ~⟩ — **den·si·to·met·ric** \ˌden-sə-tə-ˈme-trik\ adj — **den·si·tom·e·try** \ˌden-sə-ˈtä-mə-trē\ n

den·si·ty \ˈden-sə-tē\ n, pl -ties 1 : the quantity per unit volume, unit area, or unit length: as **a** : the mass of a substance per unit volume **b** : the distribution of a quantity (as mass, electricity, or energy) per unit usu. of space **c** : the average number of individuals or units per space unit 2 : the degree of opacity of a translucent medium

dent- or **denti-** or **dento-** comb form 1 : tooth : teeth ⟨*dental*⟩ 2 : dental and ⟨*dento*facial⟩

den·tal \ˈdent-ᵊl\ adj 1 : relating to, specializing in, or used in dentistry 2 : relating to or used on the teeth ⟨~ paste⟩ — **den·tal·ly** adv

dental arch n : the curve of the row of teeth in each jaw — called also *arcade*

dental dam n : a rubber dam used in dentistry

dental floss n : a thread used to clean between the teeth

dental formula n : an abridged expression for the number and kind of teeth of mammals in which the kind of teeth are represented by *i* (incisor), *c* (canine), *pm* (premolar) or *b* (bicuspid), and *m* (molar) and the number in each jaw is written like a fraction with the figures above the horizontal line showing the number in the upper jaw and those below the number in the lower jaw and with a dash separating the figures representing the teeth on each side of the jaw ⟨the *dental formula* of a human adult is

$$i\,\frac{2\text{-}2}{2\text{-}2},\ c\,\frac{1\text{-}1}{1\text{-}1},\ b \text{ or } pm\,\frac{2\text{-}2}{2\text{-}2},$$

$$m\,\frac{3\text{-}3}{3\text{-}3} = 32\rangle$$

dental hygienist n : one who assists a dentist esp. in cleaning teeth

dental lamina n : a linear zone of epithelial cells of the covering of each embryonic jaw that gives rise to the enamel organs of the teeth — called also *dental ridge*

dental nerve — see INFERIOR ALVEOLAR NERVE

dental papilla n : the mass of mesenchyme that gives rise to the dentin and the pulp of the tooth

dental plate n : DENTURE 2

dental pulp n : the highly vascular sensitive tissue occupying the central cavity of a tooth

dental surgeon n : DENTIST; esp : one engaging in oral surgery

dental technician n : a technician who makes dental appliances

den·tate \ˈden-ˌtāt\ adj : having teeth or pointed conical projections ⟨the ~ border of the retina⟩

dentate gyrus n : a narrow strip of cortex associated with the hippocampal sulcus that continues forward to the uncus

dentate nucleus n : a large laminar nucleus of gray matter forming an incomplete capsule within the white matter of each cerebellar hemisphere

dentes pl of DENS

denti- — see DENT-

den·ti·cle \ˈden-ti-kəl\ n : PULP STONE

den·tic·u·late ligament \den-ˈti-kyə-lət-\ n : a band of fibrous pia mater extending along the spinal cord on each side between the dorsal and ventral roots

den·ti·frice \'den-tə-frəs\ n : a powder, paste, or liquid for cleaning the teeth

den·tig·er·ous cyst \den-'ti-jə-rəs-\ n : an epithelial cyst containing fluid and one or more imperfect teeth

den·tin \'dent-ᵊn\ or **den·tine** \'den-ₜtēn, den-'tēn\ n : a calcareous material similar to bone but harder and denser that composes the principal mass of a tooth and is formed by the odontoblasts — compare CEMENTUM, ENAMEL — **den·tin·al** \'dent-ᵊn-əl; 'den-ₜtēn-ᵊl, den-'\ adj

dentinal tubule n : one of the minute parallel tubules of the dentin of a tooth that communicate with the dental pulp

den·tino·enam·el \den-ₜtē-nō-i-'na-məl\ adj : relating to or connecting the dentin and enamel of a tooth ⟨the ∼ junction⟩

den·tino·gen·e·sis \den-ₜtē-nə-'je-nə-səs\ n, pl **-e·ses** \-ₜsēz\ : the formation of dentin

dentinogenesis im·per·fec·ta \-ₜim-pər-'fek-tə\ n : a disorder of tooth development inherited as an autosomal dominant trait and characterized by relatively soft enamel that makes the teeth abnormally vulnerable to fracture, abrasion, and wear

den·tist \'den-tist\ n : a licensed practitioner who is skilled in the prevention, diagnosis, and treatment of diseases, injuries, and malformations of the teeth, jaws, and mouth and who makes and inserts false teeth — **den·tist·ry** \'den-tə-strē\ n

den·ti·tion \den-'ti-shən\ n 1 : the development and cutting of teeth 2 : the character of a set of teeth esp. with regard to their number, kind, and arrangement 3 : TEETH

dento- — see DENT-

den·to·al·ve·o·lar \den-tō-al-'vē-ə-lər\ adj : of, relating to, or involving the teeth and their sockets ⟨∼ structures⟩

den·to·fa·cial \den-tə-'fā-shəl\ adj : of or relating to the dentition and face

den·to·gin·gi·val \den-tō-'jin-jə-vəl\ adj : of, relating to, or connecting the teeth and the gums ⟨the ∼ junction⟩

den·tu·lous \'den-chə-ləs\ adj : having teeth

den·ture \'den-chər\ n 1 : a set of teeth 2 : an artificial replacement for one or more teeth; esp : a set of false teeth

den·tur·ist \-chə-rist\ n : a dental technician who makes, fits, and repairs dentures directly for the public

de·nu·da·tion \dē-nü-'dā-shən, ₍de-, -nyü-\ n : the act or process of removing surface layers (as of skin) or an outer covering (as of myelin); also : the condition that results from this — **de·nude** \di-'nüd, -'nyüd\ vb

¹**de·odor·ant** \dē-'ō-də-rənt\ adj : destroying or masking offensive odors

²**deodorant** n : any of various preparations or solutions (as a soap or disinfectant) that destroy or mask unpleasant odors; esp : a cosmetic that neutralizes perspiration odors

de·odor·ize \dē-'ō-də-ₜrīz\ vb **-ized; -iz·ing** : to eliminate or prevent the offensive odor of — **de·odor·iza·tion** \-ₜō-də-rə-'zā-shən\ n — **de·odor·iz·er** n

de·oxy \₍₎dē-'äk-sē\ also **des·oxy** \₍₎dez-\ adj : containing less oxygen per molecule than the compound from which it is derived — usu. used in combination ⟨*deoxy*ribonucleic acid⟩

de·oxy·cho·late \₍₎dē-ₜäk-sē-'kō-ₜlāt\ n : a salt or ester of deoxycholic acid

de·oxy·cho·lic acid \-'kō-lik-\ n : a crystalline acid $C_{24}H_{40}O_4$ found esp. in bile

deoxycorticosterone var of DESOXYCORTICOSTERONE

de·oxy·cor·tone chiefly Brit var of DESOXYCORTONE

de·ox·y·gen·ate \₍₎dē-'äk-si-jə-ₜnāt, ₍₎dē-äk-'si-jə-\ vb **-at·ed; -at·ing** : to remove oxygen from — **de·ox·y·gen·ation** \-ₜäk-si-jə-'nā-shən, ₍₎dē-äk-ₜsi-jə-\ n

de·ox·y·gen·at·ed adj : having the hemoglobin in the reduced state

de·oxy·ri·bo·nu·cle·ase \₍₎dē-'äk-si-ₜrī-bō-'nü-klē-ₜās, -'nyü-, -ₜāz\ n : an enzyme that hydrolyzes DNA to nucleotides — called also DNase

de·oxy·ri·bo·nu·cle·ic acid \₍₎dē-ₜäk-si-ₜrī-bō-nü-'klē-ik-, -nyü-, -'klā-\ also **des·oxy·ri·bo·nu·cle·ic acid** \₍₎des-\ n : DNA

de·oxy·ri·bo·nu·cle·o·tide \-'nü-klē-ə-ₜtīd, -'nyü-\ n : a nucleotide that contains deoxyribose and is a constituent of DNA

de·oxy·ri·bose \₍₎dē-ₜäk-si-'rī-ₜbōs, -ₜbōz\ n : a pentose sugar $C_5H_{10}O_4$ that is a structural element of DNA

Dep·a·kene \'de-pə-ₜkēn\ trademark — used for a preparation of valproic acid

Dep·a·kote \'de-pə-ₜkōt\ trademark — used for a preparation of divalproex sodium

de·pen·dence \di-'pen-dəns\ n 1 : the quality or state of being dependent upon or unduly subject to the influence of another 2 a : drug addiction b : HABITUATION 2b

de·pen·den·cy \-dən-sē\ n, pl **-cies** : DEPENDENCE

de·pen·dent \di-'pen-dənt\ adj 1 : unable to exist, sustain oneself, or act appropriately or normally without the assistance or direction of another 2 : affected with a drug dependence 3 a : occurring under the influence of gravity ⟨∼ drainage⟩ b : affecting the lower part of the body and esp. the legs ⟨∼ edema⟩ — **de·pen·dent·ly** adv

dependent lividity n : LIVOR MORTIS

de·per·son·al·iza·tion \(ˌ)dē-ˌpər-sə-nə-lə-lə-ˈzā-shən\ n : the act or process of causing or the state resulting from loss of the sense of personal identity; *esp* : a psychopathological syndrome characterized by loss of identity and feelings of unreality or strangeness about one's own behavior — **de·per·son·al·ize** \(ˈ)dē-ˈpər-sə-nə-ˌlīz\ vb

de·phos·phor·y·la·tion \(ˌ)dē-ˌfäs-ˌfôr-ə-ˈlā-shən\ n : the process of removing phosphate groups from an organic compound (as ATP) by hydrolysis; *also* : the resulting state — **de·phos·phor·y·late** \-ˈfäs-ˈfôr-ə-ˌlāt\ vb

de·pig·men·ta·tion \(ˌ)dē-ˌpig-mən-ˈtā-shən, -ˌmen-\ n : loss of normal pigmentation — **de·pig·ment·ed** \-ˈpig-mən-təd, -ˌmen-\ adj — **de·pig·ment·ing** \-tiŋ\ adj

dep·i·la·tion \ˌde-pə-ˈlā-shən\ n : the removal of hair, wool, or bristles by chemical or mechanical methods — **dep·i·late** \ˈde-pə-ˌlāt\ vb

[1]**de·pil·a·to·ry** \di-ˈpi-lə-ˌtōr-ē\ adj : having the power to remove hair

[2]**depilatory** n : a cosmetic for the temporary removal of undesired hair

de·plete \di-ˈplēt\ vb **de·plet·ed; de·plet·ing** : to empty of a principal substance ⟨tissues *depleted* of vitamins⟩

de·ple·tion \di-ˈplē-shən\ n : the act or process of depleting or the state of being depleted: as **a** : the reduction or loss of blood, body fluids, chemical constituents, or stored materials from the body (as by hemorrhage or malnutrition) **b** : a debilitated state caused by excessive loss of body fluids or other constituents

de·po·lar·iza·tion \(ˌ)dē-ˌpō-lə-rə-ˈzā-shən\ n : loss of polarization; *esp* : loss of the difference in charge between the inside and outside of the plasma membrane of a muscle or nerve cell due to a change in permeability and migration of sodium ions to the interior — **de·po·lar·ize** \-ˈpō-lə-ˌrīz\ vb

Depo-Pro·vera \ˈde-pō-prō-ˈver-ə\ *trademark* — used for a preparation of medroxyprogesterone acetate

de·pos·it \də-ˈpä-zət\ n : matter laid down or accumulated by a normal or abnormal process — **deposit** vb

[1]**de·pot** \-ˈdē-(ˌ)pō, ˈdē-\ n : a bodily location where a substance is stored usu. for later utilization ⟨fat ∼s⟩

[2]**depot** adj : being in storage ⟨∼ fat⟩; *also* : acting over a prolonged period ⟨∼ insulin⟩

dep·re·nyl \ˈdep-rə-ˌnil\ n : a monoamine oxidase inhibitor $C_{13}H_{17}N$; *esp* : SELEGILINE

de·press \di-ˈpres\ vb **1** : to diminish the activity, strength, or yield of **2** : to lower in spirit or mood

[1]**de·pres·sant** \-ᵊnt\ adj : tending to depress; *esp* : lowering or tending to lower functional or vital activity ⟨a drug with a ∼ effect on heart rate⟩

[2]**depressant** n : one that depresses;

specif : an agent that reduces bodily functional activity or an instinctive desire (as appetite)

de·pressed \di-ˈprest\ adj **1** : low in spirits; *specif* : affected by psychological depression ⟨a severely ∼ patient⟩ **2** : having the central part lower than the margin ⟨a ∼ pustule⟩

depressed fracture n : a fracture esp. of the skull in which the fragment is depressed below the normal surface

de·pres·sion \di-ˈpre-shən\ n **1** : a displacement downward or inward ⟨∼ of the jaw⟩ **2** : an act of depressing or a state of being depressed: as **a** (1) : a state of feeling sad (2) : a mood disorder marked esp. by sadness, inactivity, difficulty with thinking and concentration, a significant increase or decrease in appetite and time spent sleeping, feelings of dejection and hopelessness, and sometimes suicidal thoughts or an attempt to commit suicide **b** : a reduction in functional activity, amount, quality, or force ⟨∼ of autonomic function⟩

[1]**de·pres·sive** \di-ˈpre-siv\ adj **1** : tending to depress **2** : of, relating to, marked by, or affected by psychological depression ⟨∼ symptoms⟩

[2]**depressive** n : one who is affected with or prone to psychological depression

depressive disorder n : any of several mood disorders and esp. dysthymia and major depressive disorder that are characterized by prolonged or recurring symptoms of psychological depression without manic episodes

de·pres·sor \di-ˈpre-sər\ n : one that depresses: as **a** : a muscle that draws down a part — compare LEVATOR **b** : a device for pressing a part down or aside — see TONGUE DEPRESSOR **c** : a nerve or nerve fiber that decreases the activity or the tone of the organ or part it innervates

depressor sep·ti \-ˈsep-ˌtī\ n : a small muscle of each side of the upper lip that is inserted into the nasal septum and wing of the nose on each side and constricts the nasal opening by drawing the wing downward

de·pri·va·tion \ˌde-prə-ˈvā-shən, ˌdē-ˌprī-\ n : the act or process of removing or the condition resulting from removal of something normally present and usu. essential for mental or physical well-being ⟨sleep ∼⟩ ⟨sensory ∼⟩ — **de·prive** \di-ˈprīv\ vb

de·pro·gram \(ˌ)dē-ˈprō-ˌgram\ vb -grammed *also* -gramed; -gramming *also* -gram·ing : to dissuade or try to dissuade from strongly held convictions (as of a religious nature) or a firmly established or innate behavior pattern

de·pro·tein·ate \(ˌ)dē-ˈprō-ˌtē-ˌnāt, -ˈprō-tē-ə-ˌnāt\ vb -at·ed; -at·ing : DEPROTEINIZE — **de·pro·tein·ation** \(ˌ)dē-ˌprō-ˌtē-ˈnā-shən, -ˌprō-tē-ə-\ n

de·pro·tein·i·za·tion \(ₗ)dē-ₗprō-ₗtē-nə-ˈzā-shən, -ₗprō-tē-ə-nə-\ *n* : the process of removing protein

de·pro·tein·ize \(ₗ)dē-ˈprō-ₗtē-ₗnīz, -ˈprō-tē-ə-ₗnīz\ *vb* **-ized; -iz·ing** : to subject to deproteinization

depth \ˈdepth\ *n, pl* **depths 1** : the distance between upper and lower or between dorsal and ventral points of a body **2** : the quality of a state of consciousness, a bodily state, or a physiological function of being intense or complete ⟨the ~ of anesthesia⟩

depth perception *n* : the ability to judge the distance of objects and the spatial relationship of objects at different distances

depth psychology *n* : PSYCHOANALYSIS; *also* : psychology concerned esp. with the unconscious mind

de·Quer·vain's disease \də-(ₗ)kər-ˈvāⁿz-\ *n* : inflammation of tendons and their sheaths at the styloid process of the radius that often causes pain in the thumb side of the wrist
   Quer·vain \ker-ˈvaⁿ\, **Fritz de (1868–1940)**, Swiss physician.

de·range·ment \di-ˈrānj-mənt\ *n* **1** : a disturbance of normal bodily functioning or operation **2** : INSANITY — **de·range** \di-ˈrānj\ *vb*

de·re·al·iza·tion \(ₗ)dē-ₗrē-ə-lə-ˈzā-shən\ *n* : a feeling of altered reality that occurs often in schizophrenia and in some drug reactions

de·re·press \ₗdē-ri-ˈpres\ *vb* : to activate (a gene or enzyme) by releasing from a blocked state — **de·re·pres·sion** \-ˈpre-shən\ *n*

¹de·riv·a·tive \di-ˈri-və-tiv\ *adj* **1** : formed by derivation **2** : made up of or marked by derived elements

²derivative *n* **1** : something that is obtained from, grows out of, or results from an earlier or more fundamental state or condition **2** : a chemical substance related structurally to another substance and theoretically derivable from it **b** : a substance that can be made from another substance

de·rive \di-ˈrīv\ *vb* **de·rived; de·riv·ing** : to take, receive, or obtain, esp. from a specified source; *specif* : to obtain (a chemical substance) actually or theoretically from a parent substance — **der·i·va·tion** \ₗder-ə-ˈvā-shən\ *n*

derm- *or* **derma-** *or* **dermo-** *comb form* : skin ⟨*dermal*⟩ ⟨*dermo*pathy⟩

-derm \ₗdərm\ *n comb form* : covering ⟨ecto*derm*⟩

-der·ma \ˈdər-mə\ *n comb form, pl* **-dermas** *or* **-der·ma·ta** \-mə-tə\ : skin or skin ailment of a (specified) type ⟨sclero*derma*⟩

derm·abra·sion \ₗdər-mə-ˈbrā-zhən\ *n* : surgical removal of skin blemishes or imperfections (as scars or tattoos) by abrasion

Der·ma·cen·tor \ˈdər-mə-ₗsen-tər\ *n* : a large widely distributed genus of ornate ixodid ticks including several vectors of important diseases (as Rocky Mountain spotted fever)

der·mal \ˈdər-məl\ *adj* **1** : of or relating to skin and esp. to the dermis : CUTANEOUS **2** : EPIDERMAL

Der·ma·nys·sus \ₗdər-mə-ˈni-səs\ *n* : a genus (family Dermanyssidae) of blood-sucking mites that are parasitic on birds — see CHICKEN MITE

dermat- *or* **dermato-** *comb form* : skin ⟨*dermat*itis⟩ ⟨*dermato*logy⟩

der·ma·ti·tis \ₗdər-mə-ˈtī-təs\ *n, pl* **-ti·tis·es** *or* **-tit·i·des** \-ˈti-tə-ₗdēz\ : inflammation of the skin — **der·ma·tit·ic** \-ˈti-tik\ *adj*

dermatitis her·pe·ti·for·mis \-ₗhər-pə-tə-ˈfōr-məs\ *n* : chronic dermatitis characterized by eruption of itching papules, vesicles, and lesions resembling hives typically in clusters

Der·ma·to·bia \ₗdər-mə-ˈtō-bē-ə\ *n* : a genus of botflies including one (*D. hominis*) whose larvae live under the skin of domestic mammals and sometimes of humans in tropical America

der·ma·to·fi·bro·ma \ₗdər-mə-tō-fī-ˈbrō-mə\ *n, pl* **-mas** *also* **-ma·ta** \-mə-tə\ : a benign chiefly fibroblastic nodule of the skin found esp. on the extremities of adults

der·ma·to·fi·bro·sar·co·ma \-ₗfī-brō-sär-ˈkō-mə\ *n, pl* **-mas** *also* **-ma·ta** \-mə-tə\ : a fibrosarcoma affecting the skin

dermatofibrosarcoma pro·tu·ber·ans \-prō-ˈtü-bə-rənz, -ˈtyü-\ *n* : a dermal fibroblastic tumor composed of firm nodular masses that usu. do not metastasize

der·ma·to·glyph·ics \ₗdər-mə-tə-ˈgli-fiks\ *n* **1** : skin patterns; *esp* : patterns of the specialized skin of the inferior surfaces of the hands and feet **2** : the science of the study of skin patterns — **der·ma·to·glyph·ic** \-fik\ *adj*

der·ma·to·graph·ia \-ˈgra-fē-ə\ *n* : DERMOGRAPHISM

der·ma·to·graph·ism \-ˈgra-ₗfi-zəm\ *n* : DERMOGRAPHISM

der·ma·to·log·ic \ₗdər-mət-ᵊl-ˈä-jik\ *or* **der·ma·to·log·i·cal** \-ji-kəl\ *adj* : of or relating to dermatology

der·ma·to·log·i·cal \-ji-kəl\ *n* : a medicinal agent for application to the skin

der·ma·tol·o·gy \ₗdər-mə-ˈtä-lə-jē\ *n, pl* **-gies** : a branch of medicine dealing with the skin, its structure, functions, and diseases — **der·ma·tol·o·gist** \-mə-ˈtä-lə-jist\ *n*

der·ma·tome \ˈdər-mə-ₗtōm\ *n* **1** : an instrument for cutting skin for use in grafting **2** : the lateral wall of a somite from which the dermis is produced — **der·ma·to·mal** \ₗdər-mə-ˈtō-məl\ *or* **der·ma·to·mic** \-ˈtō-mik\ *adj*

der·ma·to·my·co·sis \ₗdər-mə-tō-ₗmī-ˈkō-səs, (ₗ)dər-mə-\ *n, pl* **-co·ses** \-ₗsēz\ : a disease (as ringworm) of the skin caused by infection with a fungus

der·ma·to·my·o·si·tis \-ₗmī-ə-ˈsī-təs\ *n,*

pl **-si·tis·es** *or* **-sit·i·des** \-'si-tə-ˌdēz\
: polymyositis that is accompanied by
involvement of the skin and that is
marked esp. by reddish erythematous
eruptions, by periorbital edema, and
by violet-colored erythema of the eyelids and region over the upper eyelids

der·ma·to·pa·thol·o·gy \ˌdər-ˌma-tə-pə-'thä-lə-jē, -pa-\ *n, pl* **-gies** : pathology of the
skin — **der·ma·to·pa·thol·o·gist**
\-jist\ *n*

Der·ma·toph·a·goi·des \ˌdər-mə-ˌtä-fə-'goi-(ˌ)dēz\ *n* : a genus of mites
(family Pyroglyphidae) including sev-
eral that scavenge shed flakes of human skin and dander and cause
allergy — see HOUSE-DUST MITE

der·ma·to·phyte \(ˌ)dər-'ma-tə-ˌfīt, 'dər-mə-tə-\ *n* : a fungus parasitic
upon the skin or skin derivatives (as
hair or nails) — compare DERMATO-
MYCOSIS — **der·ma·to·phy·tic** \(ˌ)dər-ˌma-tə-'fi-tik, ˌdər-mə-\ *adj*

der·ma·to·phy·tid \(ˌ)dər-'ma-tə-'fī-təd, ˌdər-mə-\ *n* : a skin eruption asso-
ciated with a fungus infection; *esp*
: one considered to be due to allergic
reaction

der·ma·to·phy·to·sis \-fī-'tō-səs\ *n, pl*
-to·ses \-ˌsēz\ : a disease (as athlete's
foot) of the skin or skin derivatives
that is caused by a dermatophyte

der·ma·to·plas·ty \(ˌ)dər-'ma-tə-ˌplas-tē, 'dər-mə-\ *n, pl* **-ties** : plastic sur-
gery of the skin

der·ma·to·sis \ˌdər-mə-'tō-səs\ *n, pl*
-to·ses \-ˌsēz\ : a disease of the skin

-der·ma·tous \dər-mə-təs\ *adj comb
form* : having a (specified) type of skin
⟨sclero*dermatous*⟩

-der·mia \'dər-mē-ə\ *n comb form*
: skin or skin ailment of a (specified)
type ⟨kerato*dermia*⟩

der·mis \'dər-məs\ *n* : the sensitive
vascular inner mesodermic layer of
the skin — called also *corium, cutis*

-der·mis \dər-məs\ *n comb form*
: layer of skin or tissue ⟨epi*dermis*⟩

der·mo- — see DERM-

der·mo·graph·ia \ˌdər-mə-'gra-fē-ə\ *n*
: DERMOGRAPHISM

der·mog·ra·phism \(ˌ)dər-'mä-grə-ˌfi-zəm\ *n* : a condition in which pressure
or friction on the skin gives rise to a
transient raised usu. reddish mark so
that a line traced on the skin becomes
visible — called also *dermatographia,
dermatographism*

der·moid \'dər-ˌmóid\ *also* **der·moi·dal** \(ˌ)dər-'móid-əl\ *adj* **1** : made up
of cutaneous elements and esp. ecto-
dermal derivatives ⟨a ∼ tumor⟩ **2**
: resembling skin

dermoid cyst *n* : a cystic tumor often
of the ovary that contains skin and
skin derivatives (as hair or teeth) —
called also *dermoid*

der·mo·ne·crot·ic \ˌdər-mō-ni-'krä-tik\ *adj* : relating to or causing necrosis of the skin ⟨a ∼ toxin⟩

der·mop·a·thy \(ˌ)dər-'mä-pə-thē\ *n, pl*
-thies : a disease of the skin

DES \ˌdē-(ˌ)ē-'es\ *n* : DIETHYLSTIL-
BESTROL

desaminase *var of* DEAMINASE

des·ce·met·o·cele \ˌde-sə-'me-tə-ˌsēl\
n : protrusion of Descemet's membrane through the cornea

Des·ce·met's membrane \ˌde-sə-'māz-, ˌdes-'māz-\ *n* : a transparent
highly elastic apparently structureless
membrane that covers the inner surface of the cornea and is lined with
endothelium — called also *membrane
of Descemet, posterior elastic lamina*

Des·ce·met \des-'mā\, **Jean (1732–1810)**, French physician.

descending *adj* **1** : moving or directed downward **2** : being a nerve,
nerve fiber, or nerve tract that carries
nerve impulses in a direction away
from the central nervous system : EF-
FERENT, MOTOR

descending aorta *n* : the part of the
aorta from the arch to its bifurcation
into the two common iliac arteries
that passes downward in the thoracic
and abdominal cavities

descending colon *n* : the part of the
large intestine on the left side that extends from the bend below the spleen
to the sigmoid colon — compare
ASCENDING COLON, TRANSVERSE
COLON

de·scen·sus \di-'sen-səs\ *n* : the
process of descending or prolapsing

de·sen·si·tize \(ˌ)dē-'sen-sə-ˌtīz\ *vb*
-tized; -tiz·ing **1** : to make a (sensitized or hypersensitive individual) insensitive or nonreactive to a
sensitizing agent **2** : to extinguish an
emotional response (as of fear or anxiety) to stimuli which formerly induced it : make emotionally
insensitive — **de·sen·si·ti·za·tion**
\-ˌsen-sə-tə-'zā-shən\ *n*

de·sen·si·tiz·er \-'sen-sə-ˌtī-zər\ *n* : a
desensitizing agent; *esp* : a drug that
reduces sensitivity to pain

de·ser·pi·dine \di-'sər-pə-ˌdēn\ *n* : an
alkaloid $C_{32}H_{38}N_2O_9$ that is obtained
from a plant of the genus *Rauwolfia*
(*R. canescens*) and is used esp. as an
antihypertensive

de·sex \(ˌ)dē-'seks\ *vb* : CASTRATE,
SPAY

¹**des·ic·cant** \'de-si-kənt\ *adj* : tending
to dry or desiccate

²**desiccant** *n* : a drying agent (as calcium chloride)

des·ic·cate \'de-si-ˌkāt\ *vb* **-cat·ed;
-cat·ing** : to dry up or cause to dry up
: deprive or exhaust of moisture; *esp*
: to dry thoroughly

des·ic·ca·tion \ˌde-si-'kā-shən\ *n* : the
act or process of desiccating or the
state of being or becoming desiccated;
esp : a complete or nearly complete
deprivation of moisture or of water
not chemically combined : DEHYDRA-
TION

designer drug *n* **1** : a synthetic version of a controlled substance (as
heroin) that is produced with a

slightly altered molecular structure to avoid classification as an illicit drug **2** : a synthetic drug created (as by genetic engineering) to treat a particular medical condition

de·si·pra·mine \ˌde-zə-'pra-mən, də-'zi-prə-ˌmēn\ *n* : a tricyclic antidepressant administered in the form of its hydrochloride $C_{18}H_{22}N_2 \cdot HCl$ esp. in the treatment of endogenous depressions (as bipolar disorder) — see NORPRAMIN, PERTOFRANE

-de·sis \də-səs\ *n comb form, pl* **-de·ses** \-ˌsēz\ : binding or fixation 〈*arthrodesis*〉

des·lo·rat·a·dine \ˌdez-lə-'ra-tə-ˌdēn, -ˌdin\ *n* : a long-acting H_1 antagonist $C_{19}H_{19}ClN_2$ that is used to treat seasonal and perennial allergic rhinitis and chronic hives — see CLARINEX

desm- *or* **desmo-** *comb form* : connective tissue 〈*desmo*plasia〉

des·meth·yl·imip·ra·mine \ˌdes-ˌme-thəl-im-'i-prə-ˌmēn\ *n* : DESIPRAMINE

des·moid \'dez-ˌmȯid\ *n* : a dense benign connective-tissue tumor

des·mo·pla·sia \ˌdez-mə-'plā-zhə, -zhē-ə\ *n* : formation of fibrous connective tissue by proliferation of fibroblasts

des·mo·plas·tic \-'plas-tik\ *adj* : characterized by the formation of fibrous tissue 〈~ fibromas〉

des·mo·pres·sin \ˌdes-mō-'pre-s⁹n\ *n* : a synthetic hormone that is used in the form of its hydrated acetate salt $C_{46}H_{64}N_{14}O_{12}S_2 \cdot C_2H_4O_2 \cdot 3H_2O$ for its antidiuretic effect and for its effect of increasing certain clotting factors — see DDAVP

des·mo·some \'dez-mə-ˌsōm\ *n* : a specialized local thickening of the plasma membrane of an epithelial cell that serves to anchor contiguous cells together — **des·mo·som·al** \-ˌsō-məl\ *adj*

des·mos·ter·ol \dez-'mä-stə-ˌrȯl, -ˌrōl\ *n* : a precursor $C_{27}H_{43}OH$ of cholesterol that tends to accumulate in blood serum when cholesterol synthesis is inhibited — called also *24-dehydrocholesterol*

deso·ges·trel \ˌdes-ə-'jes-trɪl\ *n* : a synthetic progestogen $C_{22}H_{30}O$ used in birth control pills in combination with ethinyl estradiol

desoxy *var of* DEOXY

desoxyribonucleic acid *var of* DEOXYRIBONUCLEIC ACID

des·oxy·cor·ti·co·ste·rone \(ˌ)dez-ˌäk-si-ˌkȯr-ti-'käs-tə-ˌrōn, -ˌkō-stə-'rōn\ *or* **de·oxy·cor·ti·co·ste·rone** \(ˌ)dē-\ *n* : a steroid hormone $C_{21}H_{30}O_3$ of the adrenal cortex

des·oxy·cor·tone \(ˌ)dez-ˌäk-si-'kȯr-ˌtōn\ *n* : DESOXYCORTICOSTERONE

des·qua·mate \'des-kwə-ˌmāt\ *vb* **-mat·ed; -mat·ing** : to peel off in the form of scales : scale off 〈*desquamated* epithelial cells〉 — **des·qua·ma·tion** \ˌdes-kwə-'mā-shən\ *n*

des·qua·ma·tive \'des-kwə-ˌmā-tiv, di-'skwa-mə-\ *adj*

destroying angel *n* : any of several very poisonous white mushrooms of the genus *Amanita* (as *A. verna* or *A. virosa*); *also* : a death cap (*A. phalloides*) whether white or colored

detached retina *n* : RETINAL DETACHMENT

detachment of the retina *n* : RETINAL DETACHMENT

detail man *n* : a representative of a drug manufacturer who introduces new drugs esp. to physicians and pharmacists — called also *detailer*

¹**de·ter·gent** \di-'tər-jənt\ *adj* : having a cleansing action

²**detergent** *n* : a cleansing agent (as a soap)

de·te·ri·o·rate \di-'tir-ē-ə-ˌrāt\ *vb* **-rat·ed; -rat·ing** : to become impaired in quality, functioning, or condition : DEGENERATE — **de·te·ri·o·ra·tion** \di-ˌtir-ē-ə-'rā-shən\ *n*

de·ter·mi·nant \di-'tər-mə-nənt\ *n* **1** : GENE **2** : EPITOPE

de·ter·mi·nate \di-'tər-mə-nət\ *adj* : relating to, being, or undergoing determinate cleavage 〈a ~ egg〉

determinate cleavage *n* : cleavage of an egg in which each division irreversibly separates portions of the zygote with specific potencies for further development — compare INDETERMINATE CLEAVAGE

de·ter·min·er \-'tər-mə-nər\ *n* : GENE

de·tick \(ˌ)dē-'tik\ *vb* : to remove ticks from 〈~ dogs〉

¹**de·tox** \(ˌ)dē-'täks\ *vb* : DETOXIFY 2

²**de·tox** \'dē-ˌtäks\ *n, often attrib* **1** : detoxification from an intoxicating or addictive substance 〈a ~ clinic〉 **2** : a detox program or facility

de·tox·i·cant \(ˌ)dē-'täk-si-kənt\ *n* : a detoxicating agent

de·tox·i·cate \-'täk-sə-ˌkāt\ *vb* **-cat·ed; -cat·ing** : DETOXIFY — **de·tox·i·ca·tion** \-ˌtäk-sə-'kā-shən\ *n*

de·tox·i·fy \-'täk-sə-ˌfī\ *vb* **-fied; -fy·ing** **1 a** : to remove a poison or toxin or the effect of such from **b** : to render (a harmful substance) harmless **2** : to free (as a drug user or an alcoholic) from an intoxicating or an addictive substance in the body or from dependence on or addiction to such a substance — **de·tox·i·fi·ca·tion** \-ˌtäk-sə-fə-'kā-shən\ *n*

de·tru·sor \di-'trü-zər, -sər\ *n* : the outer largely longitudinally arranged musculature of the bladder wall — called also *detrusor muscle*

detrusor uri·nae \-yə-'rī-(ˌ)nē\ *n* : the external longitudinal musculature of the urinary bladder

de·tu·mes·cence \ˌdē-tü-'mes-⁹ns, -tyü-\ *n* : subsidence or diminution of swelling or erection — **de·tu·mes·cent** \-⁹nt\ *adj*

deu·ter·anom·a·lous \ˌdü-tə-rə-'nä-mə-ləs, ˌdyü-\ *adj* : exhibiting partial loss of green color vision so that an increased intensity of this color is required in a mixture of red and green to match a given yellow

deu·ter·anom·a·ly \,-mə-lē\ *n, pl* **-lies** : the condition of being deuteranomalous — compare PROTANOMALY, TRICHROMATISM

deu·ter·an·ope \'dü-tə-rə-,nōp, 'dyü-\ *n* : an individual affected with deuteranopia

deu·ter·an·opia \,dü-tə-rə-'nō-pē-ə, ,dyü-\ *n* : color blindness marked by usu. complete loss of ability to distinguish colors — **deu·ter·an·opic** \-'nō-pik, -'nä-\ *adj*

deux — see FOLIE À DEUX

de·vas·cu·lar·iza·tion \(,)dē-,vas-kyə-lə-rə-'zā-shən\ *n* : loss of the blood supply to a bodily part due to destruction or obstruction of blood vessels — **de·vas·cu·lar·ized** \-'vas-kyə-lə-,rīzd\ *adj*

de·vel·op \di-'ve-ləp\ *vb* **1 a** : to make active or promote the growth of ⟨∼ed her muscles by weight lifting⟩ **b** : to go through a process of natural growth, differentiation, or evolution by successive stages **2** : to become infected or affected by ⟨∼ed tuberculosis⟩ **3** : to acquire secondary sex characteristics

de·vel·op·ment \di-'ve-ləp-mənt\ *n* **1** : the action or process of developing: as **a** : the process of growth and differentiation by which the potentialities of a zygote, spore, or embryo are realized **b** : the gradual advance through evolutionary stages : EVOLUTION **2** : the state of being developed — **de·vel·op·men·tal** \-,ve-ləp-'ment-ᵊl\ *adj* — **de·vel·op·men·tal·ly** *adv*

developmentally disabled *adj* : having a physical or mental disability (as mental retardation) that impedes, limits, or prevents normal development — abbr. *DD* — **developmental disability** *n*

developmental quotient *n* : a number expressing the development of a child determined by dividing the age of the group into which test scores place the child by the child's chronological age and multiplying by 100

de·vi·ance \'dē-vē-əns\ *n* : deviant quality, state, or behavior

1de·vi·ant \-ənt\ *adj* : deviating esp. from some accepted norm : characterized by deviation (as from a standard of conduct) ⟨socially ∼ behavior⟩

2deviant *n* : something that deviates from a norm; *esp* : a person who differs markedly (as in social adjustment or sexual behavior) from what is considered normal for a group

1de·vi·ate \'dē-vē-ət, -vē-,āt\ *adj* : characterized by or given to significant departure from the behavioral norms of a particular society

2deviate *n* : one that deviates from a norm; *esp* : a person who differs markedly from a group norm

de·vi·at·ed septum \,dē-vē-,ā-təd-\ *n* : deviation of the nasal septum from its normal position that results from a developmental abnormality or trauma

de·vi·a·tion \,dē-vē-'ā-shən\ *n* : an act or instance of diverging (as in growth or behavior) from an established way or in a new direction

de·vi·tal·iza·tion \(,)dē-,vīt-ᵊl-ə-'zā-shən\ *n* : destruction and usu. removal of the pulp from a tooth — **de·vi·tal·ize** \-'vīt-ᵊl-,īz\ *vb*

dew·claw \'dü-,klò, 'dyü-\ *n* : a vestigial digit not reaching to the ground on the foot of a mammal; *also* : a claw or hoof terminating such a digit — **dew·clawed** \-,klòd\ *adj*

dew·lap \-,lap\ *n* : loose skin hanging under the neck esp. of a bovine animal — **dew·lapped** \-,lapt\ *adj*

de·worm \(,)dē-'wərm\ *vb* : to rid (as a dog) of worms : WORM

de·worm·er \-'wər-mər\ *n* : WORMER

dex \'deks\ *n* : the sulfate of dextroamphetamine

DEXA *abbr* dual-energy X-ray absorptiometry

dexa·meth·a·sone \,dek-sə-'me-thə-,sōn, -,zōn\ *n* : a synthetic glucocorticoid $C_{22}H_{29}FO_5$ also used in the form of its acetate $C_{24}H_{31}FO_6$ or sodium phosphate $C_{22}H_{28}FNa_2O_8P$ esp. as an anti-inflammatory and antiallergic agent — see DECADRON

Dex·e·drine \'dek-sə-,drēn, -drən\ *trademark* — used for a preparation of the sulfate of dextroamphetamine

dex·fen·flur·amine \,deks-'fen-flùr-ə-,mēn\ *n* : the dextrorotatory form of fenfluramine formerly used in the form of its hydrochloride to treat obesity but no longer used due to its association with heart disease affecting the heart valves — see FEN-PHEN

dex·ies \'dek-sēz\ *n pl, slang* : tablets or capsules of the sulfate of dextroamphetamine

dextr- or **dextro-** *comb form* **1** : right : on or toward the right ⟨*dextro*cardia⟩ **2** *usu* **dextro-** : dextrorotatory ⟨*dextro*amphetamine⟩

1dex·tral \'dek-strəl\ *adj* : of or relating to the right; *esp* : RIGHT-HANDED — **dex·tral·ly** *adv*

2dextral *n* : a person exhibiting dominance of the right hand and eye

dex·tral·i·ty \dek-'stra-lə-tē\ *n, pl* **-ties** : the quality or state of having the right side or some parts (as the hand or eye) different from and usu. more efficient than the left or corresponding part; *also* : RIGHT-HANDEDNESS

dex·tran \'dek-,stran, -strən\ *n* : any of numerous biopolymers $(C_6H_{10}O_5)_n$ of variable molecular weight that are produced by bacteria (genus *Leuconostoc*), are found in dental plaque, and are used esp. after suitable chemical modification as blood plasma substitutes and as pharmaceutical agents

dex·tran·ase \-strə-ˌnās, -ˌnāz\ *n* : a hydrolase that prevents tooth decay by breaking down dextran and eliminating plaque

dex·trin \ˈdek-strən\ *n* : any of various soluble gummy polysaccharides $(C_6H_{10}O_5)_x$ obtained from starch by the action of heat, acids, or enzymes

dex·tro \ˈdek-(ˌ)strō\ *adj* : DEXTRORO-TATORY

dex·tro·am·phet·amine \ˌdek-(ˌ)strō-am-ˈfe-tə-ˌmēn, -mən\ *n* : a drug consisting of dextrorotatory amphetamine that is usu. administered as the sulfate $(C_9H_{13}N)_2 \cdot H_2SO_4$, is a strong stimulant of the central nervous system, is a common drug of abuse, and is used medicinally esp. in the treatment of narcolepsy and attention deficit disorder — see DEXEDRINE

dex·tro·car·dia \ˌdek-strō-ˈkär-dē-ə\ *n* : an abnormal condition in which the heart is situated on the right side and the great blood vessels of the right and left sides are reversed — **dex·tro·car·di·al** \-dē-əl\ *adj*

dex·tro·me·thor·phan \ˌdek-strō-mi-ˈthȯr-ˌfan\ *n* : a nonaddictive cough suppressant that is widely used esp. in the form of its hydrobromide $C_{18}H_{25}NO \cdot HBr$ in over-the-counter cough and cold preparations

dex·tro·pro·poxy·phene \ˌdek-strə-prō-ˈpäk-sə-ˌfēn\ *n* : PROPOXYPHENE

dex·tro·ro·ta·to·ry \-ˈrō-tə-ˌtȯr-ē\ *also* **dex·tro·ro·ta·ry** \-ˈrō-tə-rē\ *adj* : turning clockwise or toward the right; *esp* : rotating the plane of polarization of light toward the right ⟨∼ crystals⟩ — compare LEVOROTATORY

dex·trose \ˈdek-ˌstrōs, -ˌstrōz\ *n* : dextrorotatory glucose — called also *grape sugar*

d4T \ˌdē-ˌfȯr-ˈtē\ *n* : a synthetic antiretroviral nucleoside $C_{10}H_{12}N_2O_4$ that is an analog of thymidine and is used orally in the treatment of HIV infection — called also *stavudine*

DFP \ˌdē-(ˌ)ef-ˈpē\ *n* : ISOFLUROPHATE

DHA *abbr* 1 dehydroepiandrosterone 2 dihydroxyacetone 3 docosahexaenoic acid

DHEA *abbr* dehydroepiandrosterone

DHPG \ˌdē-(ˌ)āch-(ˌ)pē-ˈjē\ *n* : GANCICLOVIR

DHT *abbr* dihydrotestosterone

di- *comb form* 1 : twice : twofold : double ⟨*dizygotic*⟩ 2 : containing two atoms, radicals, or groups ⟨*dioxide*⟩

Diaβeta *trademark* — used for a preparation of glyburide

di·a·be·tes \ˌdī-ə-ˈbē-tēz, -təs\ *n, pl* **diabetes** : any of various abnormal conditions characterized by the secretion and excretion of excessive amounts of urine; *esp* : DIABETES MELLITUS

diabetes in·sip·i·dus \-in-ˈsi-pə-dəs\ *n* : a disorder that is caused by insufficient secretion of vasopressin by the pituitary gland or by a failure of the

kidneys to respond to circulating vasopressin and that is characterized by intense thirst and by the excretion of large amounts of urine — see CENTRAL DIABETES INSIPIDUS, NEPHROGENIC DIABETES INSIPIDUS

diabetes mel·li·tus \-ˈme-lə-təs\ *n* : a variable disorder of carbohydrate metabolism caused by a combination of hereditary and environmental factors and usu. characterized by inadequate secretion or utilization of insulin, by excessive urine production, by excessive amounts of sugar in the blood and urine, and by thirst, hunger, and loss of weight — see TYPE 1 DIABETES, TYPE 2 DIABETES

¹**di·a·bet·ic** \ˌdī-ə-ˈbe-tik\ *adj* 1 : of or relating to diabetes or diabetics 2 : affected with diabetes 3 : occurring in or caused by diabetes ⟨∼ coma⟩ 4 : suitable for diabetics ⟨∼ food⟩

²**diabetic** *n* : a person affected with diabetes

diabeticorum — see NECROBIOSIS LIPOIDICA DIABETICORUM

di·a·be·to·gen·ic \ˌdī-ə-ˌbē-tə-ˈje-nik\ *adj* : producing diabetes ⟨∼ drugs⟩

di·a·be·tol·o·gist \ˌdī-ə-bə-ˈtä-lə-jist\ *n* : a specialist in diabetes

di·a·ce·tic acid \ˌdī-ə-ˌsēt-ik-\ *n* : ACETOACETIC ACID

di·ace·tyl·mor·phine \ˌdī-ə-ˌsēt-əl-ˈmȯr-ˌfēn, dī-ˌa-sət-əl-\ *n* : HEROIN

di·ag·nose \ˈdī-ig-ˌnōs, -ˌnōz, ˌdī-ig-ˈ, -əg-\ *vb* **-nosed; -nos·ing** 1 : to recognize (as a disease) by signs and symptoms 2 : to diagnose a disease or condition in ⟨*diagnosed* the patient⟩ — **di·ag·nos·able** *also* **di·ag·nose·able** \ˌdī-ig-ˈnō-sə-bəl, -əg-, -zə-\ *adj*

di·ag·no·sis \ˌdī-ig-ˈnō-səs, -əg-\ *n, pl* **-no·ses** \-ˌsēz\ 1 : the art or act of identifying a disease from its signs and symptoms 2 : the decision reached by diagnosis

diagnosis related group *n* : DRG

¹**di·ag·nos·tic** \-ˈnäs-tik\ *also* **di·ag·nos·ti·cal** \-ti-kəl\ *adj* 1 : of, relating to, or used in diagnosis 2 : using the methods of or yielding a diagnosis — **di·ag·nos·ti·cal·ly** \-ti-k(ə-)lē\ *adv*

²**diagnostic** *n* : the art or practice of diagnosis — often used in pl.

di·ag·nos·ti·cian \-(ˌ)näs-ˈti-shən\ *n* : a specialist in medical diagnostics

di·a·ki·ne·sis \ˌdī-ə-kə-ˈnē-səs, -(ˌ)kī-\ *n, pl* **-ne·ses** \-ˌsēz\ : the final stage of the meiotic prophase marked by contraction of each chromosome pair — **di·a·ki·net·ic** \-ˈne-tik\ *adj*

di·al·y·sance \dī-ˈa-lə-səns\ *n* : blood volume in milliliters per unit time cleared of a substance by dialysis

di·al·y·sate \dī-ˈa-lə-ˌzāt, -ˌsāt\ *also* **di·al·y·zate** \-ˌzāt\ *n* 1 : the material that passes through the membrane in dialysis 2 : the liquid into which material passes by way of the membrane in dialysis

di·al·y·sis \dī-ˈa-lə-səs\ *n, pl* **-y·ses** \-ˌsēz\ 1 : the separation of substances in solution by means of their unequal diffusion through semipermeable membranes; *esp* : such a separation of colloids from soluble substances **2** : either of two medical procedures to remove wastes or toxins from the blood and adjust fluid and electrolyte imbalances by utilizing rates at which substances diffuse through a semipermeable membrane: **a** : the process of removing blood from an artery (as of a kidney patient), purifying it by dialysis, adding vital substances and returning it to a vein — called also *hemodialysis* **b** : a procedure performed in the peritoneal cavity in which the peritoneum acts as the semipermeable membrane — called also *peritoneal dialysis* — **di·a·lyt·ic** \ˌdī-ə-ˈli-tik\ *adj*

dialysis dementia *n* : a neurological syndrome that occurs in some long-term dialysis patients, is associated with aluminum intoxication (as from aluminum-containing compounds in the dialysis fluid), and is marked esp. by motor and speech disturbance (as dysarthria and myoclonus), progressive dementia, and seizures

di·a·lyze \ˈdī-ə-ˌlīz\ *vb* **-lyzed; -lyz·ing** **1** : to subject to or undergo dialysis **2** : to separate or obtain by dialysis — **di·a·lyz·abil·i·ty** \ˌdī-ə-ˌlī-zə-ˈbi-lə-tē\ *n* — **di·a·lyz·able** \-ˈlī-zə-bəl\ *adj*

di·a·lyz·er \-ˌlī-zər\ *n* : an apparatus in which dialysis is carried out consisting essentially of one or more containers for liquids separated into compartments by membranes

di·am·e·ter \dī-ˈa-mə-tər\ *n* **1** : a unit of magnification of a magnifying device equal to the number of times the linear dimensions of the object are increased **2** : one of the maximal breadths of a part of the body ⟨the transverse ~ of the inlet of the pelvis⟩

di·ami·no·di·phe·nyl sul·fone \ˌdī-ə-ˌmē-(ˌ)nō-ˌdī-ˈfen-ᵊl-ˈsəl-ˌfōn, -ˈfēn-\ *n* : DAPSONE

di·a·mond·back rattlesnake \ˈdī-mənd-ˌbak-, ˈdī-ə-\ *n* : either of two large and deadly rattlesnakes of the genus *Crotalus* (*C. adamanteus* of the southeastern U.S. and *C. atrox* of the south central and southwestern U.S. and Mexico) — called also *diamondback, diamondback rattler*

dia·mor·phine \ˌdī-ə-ˈmȯr-ˌfēn\ *n* : HEROIN

di·a·pe·de·sis \ˌdī-ə-pə-ˈdē-səs\ *n, pl* **-de·ses** \-ˌsēz\ : the passage of blood cells through capillary walls into the tissues — **di·a·pe·det·ic** \-ˈde-tik\ *adj*

¹di·a·per \ˈdī-pər, ˈdī-ə-\ *n* : a basic garment esp. for infants consisting of a folded cloth or other absorbent material drawn up between the legs and fastened about the waist

²diaper *vb* **di·a·pered; di·a·per·ing** : to put on or change the diaper of (an infant)

diaper rash *n* : skin irritation of the diaper-covered area and usu. the buttocks of an infant esp. from exposure to feces and urinary ammonia

di·a·pho·re·sis \ˌdī-ə-fə-ˈrē-səs, (ˌ)dī-ˌa-fə-\ *n, pl* **-re·ses** \-ˌsēz\ : PERSPIRATION; *esp* : profuse perspiration artificially induced

¹di·a·pho·ret·ic \-ˈre-tik\ *adj* **1** : having the power to increase sweating **2** : perspiring profusely : SWEATY

²diaphoretic *n* : an agent capable of inducing sweating

di·a·phragm \ˈdī-ə-ˌfram\ *n* **1** : a body partition of muscle and connective tissue; *specif* : the partition separating the chest and abdominal cavities in mammals — compare PELVIC DIAPHRAGM, UROGENITAL DIAPHRAGM **2** : a device that limits the aperture of a lens or optical system **3** : a molded cap usu. of thin rubber fitted over the uterine cervix to act as a mechanical contraceptive barrier

di·a·phrag·ma sel·lae \ˌdī-ə-ˈfrag-mə-ˈse-ˌlī, -ˌlē\ *n, pl* : a small horizontal fold of the dura mater that roofs over the sella turcica and is pierced by a small opening for the infundibulum

di·a·phrag·mat·ic \ˌdī-ə-frə-ˈma-tik, -ˌfrag-\ *adj* : of, involving, or resembling a diaphragm ⟨~ hernia⟩

di·aph·y·se·al \ˌdī-ˌa-fə-ˈsē-əl, -ˈzē-\ *or* **di·a·phys·i·al** \ˌdī-ə-ˈfi-zē-əl\ *adj* : of, relating to, or involving a diaphysis

di·a·phy·sec·to·my \ˌdī-ə-fə-ˈzek-tə-mē, -ˈsek-\ *n, pl* **-mies** : surgical excision of all or part of a diaphysis (as of the femur)

di·aph·y·sis \dī-ˈa-fə-səs\ *n, pl* **-y·ses** \-ˌsēz\ : the shaft of a long bone — compare EPIPHYSIS 1

di·ar·rhea \ˌdī-ə-ˈrē-ə\ *n* : abnormally frequent intestinal evacuations with more or less fluid stools

di·ar·rhe·al \-ˈrē-əl\ *adj* : DIARRHEIC

di·ar·rhe·ic \-ˈrē-ik\ *adj* : of or relating to diarrhea

di·ar·rhet·ic \-ˈre-tik\ *adj* : DIARRHEIC

di·ar·rhoea, di·ar·rhoe·al, di·ar·rhoe·ic, di·ar·rhoet·ic *chiefly Brit var of* DIARRHEA, DIARRHEAL, DIARRHEIC, DIARRHEIC

di·ar·thro·sis \ˌdī-är-ˈthrō-səs\ *n, pl* **-thro·ses** \-ˌsēz\ **1** : articulation that permits free movement **2** : a freely movable joint — called also *synovial joint* — **di·ar·thro·di·al** \ˌdī-ˌär-ˈthrō-dē-əl\ *adj*

di·a·stase \ˈdī-ə-ˌstās, -ˌstāz\ *n* **1** : AMYLASE; *esp* : a mixture of amylases from malt **2** : ENZYME

di·as·ta·sis \dī-ˈas-tə-səs\ *n, pl* **-ta·ses** \-ˌsēz\ **1** : an abnormal separation of parts normally joined together **2** : the rest phase of cardiac diastole occurring between filling of the ventricle and the start of atrial contraction

di·a·stat·ic \ˌdī-ə-ˈsta-tik\ *adj* : relating to or having the properties of diastase; *esp* : converting starch into sugar di·a·ste·ma \ˌdī-ə-ˈstē-mə\ n, pl -mas or -ma·ta \-mə-tə\ : a space between teeth in a jaw

di·a·ste·ma·to·my·e·lia \ˌdī-ə-ˌstē-mə-tō-mī-ˈē-lē-ə, -ˌste-\ n : congenital division of all or part of the spinal cord

di·as·to·le \dī-ˈas-tə-(ˌ)lē\ n : the passive rhythmical expansion or dilation of the cavities of the heart during which they fill with blood — compare SYSTOLE — di·a·stol·ic \ˌdī-ə-ˈstä-lik\ adj

diastolic blood pressure n : the lowest arterial blood pressure of a cardiac cycle occurring during diastole of the heart — called also diastolic pressure; compare SYSTOLIC BLOOD PRESSURE

di·a·stroph·ic dwarfism \ˌdī-ə-ˈsträ-fik-\ n : an inherited dysplasia affecting bones and joints and characterized esp. by clubfoot, deformities of the digits of the hand, malformed pinnae, and cleft palate

dia·ther·my \ˈdī-ə-ˌthər-mē\ n, pl -mies : the generation of heat in tissue by electric currents for medical or surgical purposes — see ELECTROCOAGULATION — dia·ther·mic \ˌdī-ə-ˈthər-mik\ adj

di·ath·e·sis \dī-ˈa-thə-səs\ n, pl -e·ses \-ˌsēz\ : a constitutional predisposition toward a particular state or condition and esp. one that is abnormal or diseased

dia·tri·zo·ate \ˌdī-ə-ˌtrī-ˈzō-ˌāt\ n : either of two salts of the acid $C_{11}H_9I_3N_2O_4$ administered in solution as a radiopaque medium for various forms of radiographic diagnosis — see HYPAQUE

di·az·e·pam \dī-ˈa-zə-ˌpam\ n : a synthetic tranquilizer $C_{16}H_{13}ClN_2O$ used esp. to relieve anxiety and tension and as a muscle relaxant — see VALIUM

Di·az·i·non \ˌdī-ˈa-zə-ˌnän\ trademark — used for an organophosphate insecticide $C_{12}H_{21}N_2O_3PS$ that is a cholinesterase inhibitor dangerous to humans if ingested

di·az·ox·ide \ˌdī-ˌa-ˈzäk-ˌsīd\ n : a drug $C_8H_7ClN_2O_2S$ used in the treatment of hypoglycemia and in the emergency treatment of hypertension

di·benz·an·thra·cene or 1,2:5,6-di·benz·an·thra·cene \(ˌ)wən-ˌtü-ˌfiv-ˌsiks-\dī-ˌben-ˈzan-thrə-ˌsēn\ n : a carcinogenic cyclic hydrocarbon $C_{22}H_{14}$ found in trace amounts in coal tar

di·ben·zo·fu·ran \ˈdī-ˌben-zō-ˈfyü-ˌran, -fyə-ˈran\ n : a highly toxic chemical compound $C_{12}H_8O$ that is used in chemical synthesis and as an insecticide and is a hazardous pollutant in its chlorinated form

di·bro·mo·chlo·ro·pro·pane \(ˌ)dī-ˌbrō-mō-ˌklōr-ō-ˈprō-ˌpān\ n : DBCP

di·bu·caine \ˈdī-byü-ˌkān, ˈdī-ˌ\ n : a local anesthetic $C_{20}H_{29}N_3O_2$ used for temporary relief of pain and itching esp. from burns, sunburn, insect bites, or hemorrhoids — called also cinchocaine

dibucaine number n : a number expressing the percentage by which cholinesterase activity in a serum sample is inhibited by dibucaine

DIC abbr disseminated intravascular coagulation

di·cen·tric \(ˌ)dī-ˈsen-trik\ adj : having two centromeres ⟨a ~ chromosome⟩ — dicentric n

dich- or dicho- comb form : apart : separate ⟨dichotic⟩

di·chlo·ra·mine-T \ˌdī-ˌklōr-ə-ˌmēn-ˈtē\ n : a yellow crystalline compound $C_7H_7Cl_2NO_2S$ used esp. formerly as an antiseptic

p–dichlorobenzene var of PARADICHLOROBENZENE

2,4–di·chlo·ro·phen·oxy·ace·tic acid also di·chlo·ro·phen·oxy·ace·tic acid \(ˌ)tü-ˌfōr-ˌ)dī-ˌklōr-ō-(ˌ)fē-ˌnäk-sē-ə-ˈsē-tik-\ n : 2,4-D

di·chlor·vos \(ˌ)dī-ˈklōr-ˌväs, -vəs\ n : an organophosphorus insecticide and anthelmintic $C_4H_7Cl_2O_4P$ used esp. in veterinary medicine — called also DDVP

dich·ot·ic \(ˌ)dī-ˈkō-tik\ adj : relating to or involving the presentation of a stimulus to one ear that differs in some respect (as pitch, loudness, frequency, or energy) from a stimulus presented to the other ear ⟨~ listening⟩ — dich·oti·cal·ly \-ti-k(ə-)lē\ adv

di·chot·o·my \dī-ˈkä-tə-mē\ n, pl -mies : a division or forking into branches; esp : repeated bifurcation — di·chot·o·mous \dī-ˈkä-tə-məs\ adj

di·chro·mat \ˈdī-krō-ˌmat, (ˌ)dī-ˈ\ n : one affected with dichromatism

di·chro·ma·tism \dī-ˈkrō-mə-ˌti-zəm\ n : partial color blindness in which only two colors are perceptible — di·chro·mat·ic \ˌdī-krō-ˈma-tik\ adj

Dick test \ˈdik-\ n : a test to determine susceptibility or immunity to scarlet fever by an injection of scarlet fever toxin

Dick, George Frederick (1881–1967) and Gladys Henry (1881–1963), American physicians.

di·clo·fe·nac \dī-ˈklō-fə-ˌnak\ n : a nonsteroidal anti-inflammatory drug used in the form of its sodium salt $C_{14}H_{10}Cl_2NNaO_2$ or potassium salt $C_{14}H_{10}Cl_2KNaO_2$ esp. to treat the symptoms of rheumatoid arthritis, osteoarthritis, and ankylosing spondylitis — see VOLTAREN

di·clox·a·cil·lin \(ˌ)dī-ˌkläk-sə-ˈsi-lən\ n : a semisynthetic penicillin used in the form of its sodium salt $C_{19}H_{16}Cl_2N_3NaO_5S\cdot H_2O$ esp. against beta-lactamase producing staphylococci

di·cou·ma·rin \(ˌ)dī-ˈkü-mə-rən\ n : DICUMAROL

Di·cro·coe·li·um \ˌdī-krə-ˈsē-lē-əm\ n : a genus (family Dicrocoeliidae) of small digenetic trematodes infesting the livers of ruminants or occas. other

mammals including humans — see
LANCET FLUKE

di·crot·ic \(ˌ)dī-ˈkrä-tik\ *adj* **1** *of the pulse* : having a double beat (as in certain febrile states in which the heart is overactive and the arterial walls are lacking in tone) — compare MONO-CROTIC **2** : being or relating to the second part of the arterial pulse occurring during diastole of the heart or of an arterial pressure recording made during the same period — **di·cro·tism** \ˈdī-krə-ˌti-zəm\ *n*

dicrotic notch *n* : a secondary upstroke in the descending part of a pulse tracing corresponding to the transient increase in aortic pressure upon closure of the aortic valve

Dic·ty·o·cau·lus \ˌdik-tē-ə-ˈkȯ-ləs\ *n* : a genus (family Metastrongylidae) of small slender lungworms infesting mammals (as ruminants) and often causing severe respiratory symptoms

dic·tyo·some \ˈdik-tē-ə-ˌsōm\ *n* : any of the membranous or vesicular structures making up the Golgi apparatus

di·cu·ma·rol *also* **di·cou·ma·rol** \dī-ˈkü-mə-ˌról, -ˈkyü-, -ˌröl\ *n* : an anticoagulant $C_{19}H_{12}O_6$ that acts similarly to warfarin and is used esp. in preventing and treating thromboembolic disease

di·cy·clo·mine \(ˌ)dī-ˈsī-klə-ˌmēn, -ˈsi-\ *n* : an anticholinergic drug used in the form of its hydrochloride $C_{19}H_{35}NO_2 \cdot HCl$ for its antispasmodic effect on smooth muscle in gastrointestinal functional disorders

di·dan·o·sine \dī-ˈda-nə-ˌsēn\ *n* : DDI

di·de·oxy·cy·ti·dine \ˌdī-(ˌ)dē-ˌäk-sē-ˈsi-tə-dēn, -ˈsī-\ *n* : DDC

di·de·oxy·ino·sine \-ˈi-nə-ˌsēn, -ˈī-, -ˌsən\ *n* : DDI

die \ˈdī\ *vb* **died; dy·ing** \ˈdī-iŋ\ **1** : to suffer total and irreversible loss of the bodily attributes and functions that constitute life **2** : to suffer or face the pains of death

diel·drin \ˈdēl-drən\ *n* : a white crystalline persistent chlorinated hydrocarbon insecticide $C_{12}H_8Cl_6O$

Diels \ˈdēls\, **Otto Paul Hermann (1876–1954),** and **Al·der** \ˈȯl-dər\, **Kurt (1902–1958),** German chemists.

di·en·ceph·a·lon \ˌdī-ən-ˈse-fə-ˌlän, -ˌdī-(ˌ)en-, -lən\ *n* : the posterior subdivision of the forebrain — called also *betweenbrain* — **di·en·ce·phal·ic** \-sə-ˈfa-lik\ *adj*

die·ner \ˈdē-nər\ *n* : a laboratory helper esp. in a medical school

di·en·es·trol \ˌdī-ə-ˈnes-ˌtról, -ˌtrōl\ *n* : a white crystalline estrogenic compound $C_{18}H_{18}O_2$ structurally related to diethylstilbestrol and used topically to treat atrophic vaginitis and kraurosis vulvae

di·en·oes·trol \ˌdī-ə-ˈnēs-ˌtról, -ˌtrōl\ *chiefly Brit var of* DIENESTROL

Di·ent·amoe·ba \ˌdī-ˌen-tə-ˈmē-bə\ *n* : a genus of amoebic protozoans par-

asitic in the intestines of humans and monkeys that include one (*D. fragilis*) known to cause abdominal pain, anorexia, and loose stools in humans

di·es·trus \(ˌ)dī-ˈes-trəs\ *n* : a period of sexual quiescence that intervenes between two periods of estrus — **di·es·trous** \-trəs\ *adj*

¹di·et \ˈdī-ət\ *n* **1** : food and drink regularly provided or consumed **2** : habitual nourishment **3** : the kind and amount of food prescribed for a person or animal for a special reason **4** : a regimen of eating and drinking sparingly so as to reduce one's weight

²diet *vb* : to eat or cause to eat less or according to a prescribed rule

³diet *adj* : reduced in calories ⟨a ∼ soft drink⟩

¹di·etary \ˈdī-ə-ˌter-ē\ *n, pl* **di·etar·ies** : the kinds and amounts of food available to or eaten by an individual, group, or population

²dietary *adj* : of or relating to a diet or to the rules of a diet ⟨∼ habits⟩ — **di·etari·ly** \ˌdī-ə-ˈter-ə-lē\ *adv*

dietary fiber *n* : FIBER 2

Dietary Reference Intake *n* : a set of guidelines for the daily intake of nutrients (as vitamins, protein, and fats) and other food components (as fiber) — abbr. *DRI*

dietary supplement *n* : a product taken orally that contains one or more ingredients that are intended to supplement one's diet and are not considered food

di·et·er \ˈdī-ə-tər\ *n* : one that diets; *esp* : a person that consumes a reduced allowance of food in order to lose weight

di·etet·ic \ˌdī-ə-ˈte-tik\ *adj* **1** : of or relating to diet **2** : adapted (as by the elimination of salt or sugar) for use in special diets — **di·etet·i·cal·ly** \-ti-k(ə-)lē\ *adv*

di·etet·ics \-ˈte-tiks\ *n, sing or pl* : the science or art of applying the principles of nutrition to feeding

diethylamide — see LYSERGIC ACID DIETHYLAMIDE

di·eth·yl·car·bam·azine \ˌdī-ˌe-thəl-kär-ˈba-mə-ˌzēn, -zən\ *n* : an anthelmintic derived from piperazine and administered in the form of its crystalline citrate $C_{10}H_{21}N_3O \cdot C_6H_8O_7$ esp. to control filariasis in humans and roundworms in dogs and cats

di·eth·yl ether \(ˌ)dī-ˈe-thəl-\ *n* : ETHER 1

di·eth·yl·pro·pi·on \(ˌ)dī-ˌe-thəl-ˈprō-pē-ˌän\ *n* : a sympathomimetic amine related structurally to amphetamine and used esp. in the form of its hydrochloride $C_{13}H_{19}NO \cdot HCl$ as an appetite suppressant to promote weight loss — see TENUATE

di·eth·yl·stil·bes·trol \-stil-ˈbes-ˌtról, -ˌtrōl\ *n* : a colorless crystalline synthetic compound $C_{18}H_{20}O_2$ used as a potent estrogen but contraindicated in pregnancy for its tendency to cause cancer or birth defects in offspring — called also *DES, stilbestrol*

di·eth·yl·stil·boes·trol \-ˈbēs-ˌtrȯl, -ˌtrōl\ *chiefly Brit var of* DIETHYLSTILBESTROL

di·e·ti·tian *or* **di·e·ti·cian** \ˌdī-ə-ˈti-shən\ *n* : a specialist in dietetics

Dietl's crisis \ˈdēt-ᵊlz-\ *n* : an attack of violent pain in the kidney region accompanied by chills, nausea, vomiting, and collapse that is caused by the formation of kinks in the ureter and is usu. associated with a floating kidney

Dietl \ˈdēt-ᵊl\, **Josef** (1804–1878), Polish physician.

diet pill *n* : a pill and esp. one containing amphetamine prescribed esp. formerly to promote weight loss by increasing metabolism or depressing appetite

differential blood count *n* : a blood count which includes separate counts for each kind of white blood cell — compare COMPLETE BLOOD COUNT

differential cell count *n* : a count of cells that includes a separate count for each type of cell; *esp* : DIFFERENTIAL BLOOD COUNT

differential diagnosis *n* : the distinguishing of a disease or condition from others presenting similar symptoms

dif·fer·en·ti·ate \ˌdif-ə-ˈren-chē-ˌāt\ *vb* **-at·ed; -at·ing** **1 a** : to constitute a difference that distinguishes **2 a** : to cause differentiation of in the course of development **b** : to undergo differentiation **3** : to sense, recognize, or give expression to a difference (as in stimuli) **4** : to cause differentiation in (a specimen for microscopic examination) by staining

dif·fer·en·ti·a·tion \-ˌren-chē-ˈā-shən\ *n* **1 a** : the act or process of differentiating **b** : the enhancement of microscopically visible differences between tissue or cell parts by partial selective decolorization or removal of excess stain **2 a** : modification of different parts of the body for performance of particular functions **b** : the sum of the developmental processes whereby apparently unspecialized cells, tissues, and structures attain their adult form and function

differently abled *adj* : DISABLED, CHALLENGED

dif·flu·ent \ˈdi-(ˌ)flü-ənt\ *adj* : soft like mush ⟨a ~ spleen⟩

dif·fu·sate \di-ˈfyü-ˌzāt\ *n* : DIALYSATE

¹**dif·fuse** \di-ˈfyüs\ *adj* : not concentrated or localized ⟨~ sclerosis⟩

²**dif·fuse** \di-ˈfyüz\ *vb* **dif·fused; dif·fus·ing** **1** : to subject to or undergo diffusion **2** : to break up and distribute (incident light) by reflection (as from a rough surface) — **dif·fus·ible** \di-ˈfyü-zə-bəl\ *adj* — **dif·fus·ibil·i·ty** \-ˌfyü-zə-ˈbi-lə-tē\ *n*

dif·fu·sion \di-ˈfyü-zhən\ *n* **1** : the process whereby particles of liquids,

gases, or solids intermingle as the result of their spontaneous movement caused by thermal agitation and in dissolved substances move from a region of higher to one of lower concentration **2 a** : reflection of light by a rough reflecting surface **b** : transmission of light through a translucent material — **dif·fu·sion·al** \-ˈfyü-zhə-nəl\ *adj*

Di·flu·can \dī-ˈflük-ˌän\ *trademark* — used for a preparation of fluconazole

di·flu·ni·sal \(ˌ)dī-ˈflü-nə-ˌsal\ *n* : a nonsteroidal anti-inflammatory drug $C_{13}H_8F_2O_3$ related to aspirin that is used to relieve mild to moderately severe pain — see DOLOBID

di·gas·tric muscle \(ˌ)dī-ˈgas-trik-\ *n* : either of a pair of muscles that extend from the anterior inferior margin of the mandible to the temporal bone and serve to depress the lower jaw and raise the hyoid bone esp. during swallowing — called also *digastric*

di·gas·tri·cus \-tri-kəs\ *n* : DIGASTRIC MUSCLE

di·ge·net·ic \ˌdī-jə-ˈne-tik\ *adj* : of or relating to a subclass (Digenea) of trematode worms in which sexual reproduction as an internal parasite of a vertebrate alternates with asexual reproduction in a mollusk and which include a number of parasites (as the Chinese liver fluke) of humans

Di·George syndrome \də-ˈjȯrj-\ *also* **Di·George's syndrome** \-ˈjȯr-jəz-\ *n* : a rare congenital disease that is characterized esp. by absent or underdeveloped thymus and parathyroid glands, heart defects, immunodeficiency, hypocalcemia, and characteristic facial features (as wide-set eyes and small jaws)

Di George, Angelo Mario (*b* 1921), American endocrinologist and pediatrician.

¹**di·gest** \ˈdī-ˌjest\ *n* : a product of digestion

²**di·gest** \dī-ˈjest, də-\ *vb* **1** : to convert (food) into absorbable form **2 a** : to soften, decompose, or break down by heat and moisture or chemicals **b** : to extract soluble ingredients from by warming with a liquid — **di·ges·ter** \-ˈjes-tər\ *n*

di·ges·tant \-ˈjes-tənt\ *n* : a substance that digests or aids in digestion

di·gest·ibil·i·ty \-ˌjes-tə-ˈbi-lə-tē\ *n, pl* **-ties** **1** : the fitness of something for digestion **2** : the percentage of a foodstuff taken into the digestive tract that is absorbed into the body

di·gest·ible \-ˈjes-tə-bəl\ *adj* : capable of being digested

di·ges·tion \-ˈjes-chən\ *n* : the action, process, or power of digesting; *esp* : the process of making food absorbable by mechanically and enzymatically breaking it down into simpler chemical compounds in the digestive tract

¹**di·ges·tive** \-'jes-tiv\ n 1 : something that aids digestion esp. of food 2 : a substance which promotes suppuration

²**digestive** adj 1 : relating to or functioning in digestion ⟨~ processes⟩ 2 : having the power to cause or promote digestion ⟨~ enzymes⟩

digestive gland n : a gland secreting digestive enzymes

digestive system n : the bodily system concerned with the ingestion, digestion, and absorption of food and the discharge of residual wastes and consisting of the digestive tract and accessory glands (as the salivary glands and the pancreas) that secrete digestive enzymes — called also *alimentary system*

digestive tract n : the tubular passage typically extending from mouth to anus or cloaca that functions in digestion and absorption of food and elimination of residual waste and that in most mammals includes the mouth, pharynx, esophagus, stomach, intestine, and anus — called also *alimentary canal, alimentary tract*

dig·i·lan·id \₁di-jə-'la-nəd\ or **dig·i·lan·ide** \-₁nīd, -nəd\ n : LANATOSIDE

digilanid A or **digilanide A** n : LANATOSIDE a

digilanid B or **digilanide B** n : LANATOSIDE b

digilanid C or **digilanide C** n : LANATOSIDE c

dig·it \'di-jət\ n : any of the divisions (as a finger or toe) in which the limbs of amphibians and all higher vertebrates terminate and which in humans are five in number on each limb

dig·i·tal \'di-jət-ᵊl\ adj 1 : of, relating to, or supplying one or more fingers or toes ⟨a ~ branch of an artery⟩ 2 : done with a finger ⟨a ~ rectal examination⟩ — **dig·i·tal·ly** adv

dig·i·tal·in \₁di-jə-'ta-lən, -'tä-\ n : a white crystalline steroid glycoside $C_{36}H_{56}O_{14}$ obtained from seeds esp. of a common European foxglove (*Digitalis purpurea*) 2 : a mixture of the glycosides of digitalis leaves or seeds

dig·i·tal·is \-ləs\ n 1 a cap : a genus of Eurasian herbs (family Scrophulariaceae) that have stalks of showy bell-shaped flowers b : FOXGLOVE 2 : the dried leaf of a common European foxglove (*D. purpurea*) that contains physiologically active glycosides, that is a powerful cardiac stimulant and a diuretic, and that is used in standardized powdered form esp. in the treatment of congestive heart failure and in the management of atrial fibrillation, atrial flutter, and paroxysmal tachycardia of the atria; *broadly* : any of various glycosides (as digoxin or digitoxin) that are constituents of digitalis or are derived from a related foxglove (*D. lanata*)

dig·i·ta·li·za·tion \₁di-jət-ᵊl-ə-'zā-shən\ n : the administration of digitalis (as

in heart disease) until the desired physiological adjustment is attained; *also* : the bodily state so produced — **dig·i·ta·lize** \'di-jət-ᵊl-₁īz\ vb

digital nerve n 1 : any of several branches of the median nerve and the ulnar nerve supplying the fingers and thumb 2 : any of several branches of the medial plantar nerve supplying the toes

Dig·i·tek \'di-jə-₁tek\ *trademark* — used for a preparation of digoxin

digiti — see ABDUCTOR DIGITI MINIMI, EXTENSOR DIGITI MINIMI, EXTENSOR DIGITI QUINTI PROPRIUS, FLEXOR DIGITI MINIMI BREVIS, OPPONENS DIGITI MINIMI

digitorum — see EXTENSOR DIGITORUM BREVIS, EXTENSOR DIGITORUM COMMUNIS, EXTENSOR DIGITORUM LONGUS, FLEXOR DIGITORUM BREVIS, FLEXOR DIGITORUM LONGUS, FLEXOR DIGITORUM PROFUNDUS, FLEXOR DIGITORUM SUPERFICIALIS

dig·i·tox·in \₁di-jə-'täk-sən\ n : a poisonous glycoside $C_{41}H_{64}O_{13}$ that is the most active constituent of digitalis; *also* : a mixture of digitalis glycosides consisting chiefly of digitoxin

di·glyc·er·ide \dī-'gli-sə-₁rīd\ n : an ester of glycerol that contains two ester groups and involves one or two acids

di·gox·in \di-'jäk-sən, -'gäk-\ n : a poisonous cardiotonic glycoside $C_{41}H_{64}O_{14}$ obtained from the leaves of a foxglove (*Digitalis lanata*) and used similarly to digitalis — see DIGITEK, LANOXIN

di·hy·dro·chlo·ride \(₁)dī-₁hī-drə-'klȯr-₁īd\ n : a chemical compound with two molecules of hydrochloric acid

di·hy·dro·co·de·inone \-kō-'dē-ə-₁nōn\ n : HYDROCODONE

di·hy·dro·er·got·a·mine \-₁hī-drō-₁ər-'gä-tə-₁mēn\ n : a hydrogenated derivative of ergotamine that is used in the form of its mesylate $C_{33}H_{37}N_5O_5 \cdot CH_4O_3S$ in the treatment of migraine

di·hy·dro·fo·late reductase \-'fō-₁lāt\ n : an enzyme that is essential for DNA and protein synthesis

di·hy·dro·mor·phi·none \-'mȯr-fə-₁nōn\ n : HYDROMORPHONE

di·hy·dro·strep·to·my·cin \-₁strep-tə-'mīs-ᵊn\ n : a toxic antibiotic $C_{21}H_{41}N_7O_{12}$ formerly used but abandoned because of its tendency to impair hearing

di·hy·dro·tachy·ste·rol \-₁ta-ki-'ster-₁ȯl, -'stir-, -₁ȯl\ n : an alcohol $C_{28}H_{45}OH$ used in the treatment of hypocalcemia

di·hy·dro·tes·tos·ter·one \-te-'stäs-tə-₁rōn\ n : a biologically active metabolite $C_{19}H_{30}O_2$ of testosterone having similar androgenic activity — abbr. *DHT*

di·hy·dro·the·elin \-'thē-ə-lən\ n : ESTRADIOL

di·hy·droxy·ac·e·tone \₁dī-hī-₁dräk-sē-'a-sə-₁tōn\ n : a glyceraldehyde isomer

$C_3H_6O_3$ that is used esp. to stain the skin to simulate a tan

1,25-di·hy·droxy·cho·le·cal·cif·er·ol \ˌwən-ˌtwen-tē-ˌfīv-ˌdī-hī-ˌdräk-sē-ˌkō-lə-(ˌ)kal-ˈsi-fə-ˌról, -ˌról\ n : CALCITRIOL

di·hy·droxy·phe·nyl·al·a·nine \ˌdī-hī-ˌdräk-sē-ˌfen-ᵊl-ˈa-lə-ˌnēn, -ˌfēn-\ n **1** or **3,4–dihydroxyphenylalanine** \ˌthrē-ˌfór-\ : DOPA **2** or L–**3,4–dihydroxyphenylalanine** \ˌel-\ or L–**dihydroxyphenylalanine** : L-DOPA

di·io·do·hy·droxy·quin \ˌdī-ˌī-ə-ˌdō-hī-ˈdräk-si-kwən\ n : IODOQUINOL

di·io·do·hy·droxy·quin·o·line \-hī-ˌdräk-si-ˈkwin-ᵊl-ˌēn\ n : IODOQUINOL

di·io·do·ty·ro·sine \-ˈti-rə-ˌsēn\ n : a compound $C_9H_9I_2NO_3$ of tyrosine and iodine that is produced in the thyroid gland from monoiodotyrosine and that combines with monoiodotyrosine to form triiodothyronine

di·iso·pro·pyl   flu·o·ro·phos·phate \ˌdī-ˌī-sə-ˈprō-pəl-ˌflúr-ō-ˈfäs-ˌfāt\ n : ISOFLUROPHATE

di·lac·er·a·tion \ˌdī-ˌla-sə-ˈrā-shən\ n : injury (as partial fracture) to a developing tooth that results in a curve in the long axis as development continues — **di·lac·er·at·ed** \(ˌ)dī-ˈla-sə-ˌrā-təd\ adj

Di·lan·tin \dī-ˈlant-ᵊn, də-\ trademark — used for a preparation of phenytoin

di·la·ta·tion \ˌdi-lə-ˈtā-shən, ˌdī-, ˌdī-\ n **1** : the condition of being stretched beyond normal dimensions esp. as a result of overwork or disease or of abnormal relaxation **2** : DILATION 2

di·la·ta·tor \ˈdi-lə-ˌtā-tər, ˈdī-\ n : DILATOR b

di·late \dī-ˈlāt, ˈdī-\ vb **di·lat·ed; di·lat·ing 1** : to enlarge, stretch, or cause to expand **2** : to become expanded or swollen

di·la·tion \dī-ˈlā-shən\ n **1** : the state of being dilated : DILATATION **2** : the action of stretching or enlarging an organ or part of the body

dilation and curettage n : a medical procedure in which the uterine cervix is dilated and a curette is inserted into the uterus to scrape away the endometrium (as for the diagnosis or treatment of abnormal bleeding or for surgical abortion during the early part of the second trimester of pregnancy) — called also *D&C*

dilation and evacuation n : a surgical abortion that is typically performed midway during the second trimester of pregnancy and in which the uterine cervix is dilated and fetal tissue is removed using surgical instruments (as a forceps and curette) and suction — called also *D&E*

dilation and extraction n : a surgical abortion that is typically performed during the third trimester or later part of the second trimester of pregnancy and in which the uterine cervix is dilated and death of the fetus is in-

duced after it has passed partway through the birth canal — called also *D&X, partial-birth abortion*

di·la·tor \(ˌ)dī-ˈlā-tər, də-\ n : one that dilates: as **a** : an instrument for expanding a tube, duct, or cavity ⟨a urethral $\sim$⟩ **b** : a muscle that dilates a part **c** : a drug (as a vasodilator) causing dilation

Di·lau·did \(ˌ)dī-ˈló-did\ trademark — used for a preparation of hydromorphone

dil·do \ˈdil-(ˌ)dō\ n, pl **dildos** also **dil·does** : an object resembling a penis used for sexual stimulation

dil·ti·a·zem \dil-ˈtī-ə-(ˌ)zem\ n : a calcium channel blocker used esp. in the form of its hydrochloride $C_{22}H_{26}$-$N_2O_4S \cdot HCl$ as a coronary vasodilator — see CARDIZEM

¹dil·u·ent \ˈdil-yə-wənt\ n : a diluting agent (as the vehicle in a medicinal preparation)

²diluent adj : making thinner or less concentrated by admixture

¹di·lute \dī-ˈlüt, də-\ vb **di·lut·ed; di·lut·ing** : to make thinner or more liquid by admixture — **di·lut·er** also **di·lut·or** \-ˈlü·tər\ n

²dilute adj : of relatively low strength or concentration

di·lu·tion \dī-ˈlü-shən, də-\ n **1** : the action of diluting : the state of being diluted **2** : something (as a solution) that is diluted

di·men·hy·dri·nate \ˌdī-ˌmen-ˈhī-drə-ˌnāt\ n : an antihistamine $C_{24}H_{28}$-ClN_5O_3 used esp. to prevent nausea (as in motion sickness)

di·mer \ˈdī-mər\ n : a polymer formed from two molecules of a monomer — **di·mer·ic** \(ˌ)dī-ˈmer-ik\ adj

di·mer·cap·rol \ˌdī-(ˌ)mər-ˈka-ˌpról, -ˌpról\ n : a colorless viscous oily compound $C_3H_8OS_2$ with an offensive odor used in treating arsenic, mercury, and gold poisoning — called also BAL, British anti-lewisite

di·meth·yl·ami·no·eth·a·nol \(ˌ)dī-ˈme-thə-lə-ˌmē-nō-ˈe-thə-ˌnól, -nōl\ n : DMAE

di·meth·yl·ni·tros·amine \(ˌ)dī-ˌme-thəl-(ˌ)nī-ˈtrō-sə-ˌmēn\ n : a carcinogenic nitrosamine $C_2H_6N_2O$ that occurs esp. in tobacco smoke — called also nitrosodimethylamine

dimethyl sul·fox·ide \-səl-ˈfäk-sīd\ n : an anti-inflammatory agent $(CH_3)_2SO$ used in the treatment of interstitial cystitis — called also DMSO

di·meth·yl·tryp·ta·mine \-ˈtrip-tə-ˌmēn\ n : a hallucinogenic drug $C_{12}H_{16}N_2$ that is chemically similar to but shorter acting than psilocybin — called also DMT

dim·ple \ˈdim-pəl\ n : a slight natural indentation or hollow in the surface of some part of the human body (as on a cheek or the chin) — **dimple** vb

dinitrate — see ISOSORBIDE DINITRATE

di·ni·tro·phe·nol \ˌdī-ˌnī-trō-ˈfē-ˌnól,

-fi-\\ *n* : any of six isomeric compounds $C_6H_4N_2O_5$ some of whose derivatives are pesticides; *esp* : a highly toxic compound formerly used in weight control

di·no·fla·gel·late \\ˌdī-nō-ˈfla-jə-lət, -ˌlāt, -flə-ˈje-lət\\ *n* : any of an order (Dinoflagellata) of chiefly marine planktonic plantlike unicellular flagellates of which some cause red tide

Di·oc·to·phy·ma \\ˌdī-ˌäk-tə-ˈfī-mə\\ *n* : a genus (family Dioctophymidae) of nematode worms including a single species (*D. renale*) which is a destructive parasite of the kidney of dogs, minks, and sometimes humans

di·oes·trus *chiefly Brit var of* DIESTRUS

di·op·ter \\dī-ˈäp-tər, ˈdī-ˌäp-\\ *n* : a unit of measurement of the refractive power of a lens equal to the reciprocal of the focal length in meters

di·op·tric \\(ˌ)dī-ˈäp-trik\\ *adj* **1** : producing or serving in refraction of a beam of light : REFRACTIVE; *specif* : assisting vision by refracting and focusing light **2** : produced by means of refraction

Di·o·van \\ˈdī-ə-ˌvan\\ *trademark* — uesd for a preparation of valsartan

di·ox·ide \\(ˌ)dī-ˈäk-ˌsīd\\ *n* : an oxide (as carbon dioxide) containing two atoms of oxygen in a molecule

di·ox·in \\(ˌ)dī-ˈäk-sən\\ *n* : any of several persistent toxic hydrocarbons that occur esp. as by-products of various industrial processes and waste incineration; *esp* : TCDD — see AGENT ORANGE

di·oxy·ben·zone \\(ˌ)dī-ˌäk-sē-ˈben-ˌzōn, -ben-ˈ\\ *n* : a sunscreen $C_{14}H_{12}O_4$ that absorbs throughout the ultraviolet spectrum

dip \\ˈdip\\ *n* : a liquid preparation of an insecticide or parasiticide for the dipping of animals ⟨a sheep ∼⟩ — **dip** *vb*

di·pep·ti·dase \\dī-ˈpep-tə-ˌdās, -ˌdāz\\ *n* : any of various enzymes that hydrolyze dipeptides but not polypeptides

di·pep·tide \\(ˌ)dī-ˈpep-ˌtīd\\ *n* : a peptide that yields two molecules of amino acid on hydrolysis

di·pha·sic \\(ˌ)dī-ˈfā-zik\\ *adj* : having two phases: as **a** : exhibiting a stage of stimulation followed by a stage of depression or vice versa ⟨the ∼ action of certain drugs⟩ **b** : relating to or being a record of a nerve impulse that is negative and positive — compare MONOPHASIC 1, POLYPHASIC 1

di·phen·hy·dra·mine \\ˌdī-ˌfen-ˈhī-drə-ˌmēn\\ *n* : an antihistamine used esp. in the form of its hydrochloride $C_{17}H_{21}NO \cdot HCl$ to treat allergy symptoms and motion sickness and to induce sleep — see BENADRYL

di·phen·oxy·late \\ˌdī-ˌfen-ˈäk-sə-ˌlāt\\ *n* : an antidiarrheal agent used in the form of its hydrochloride $C_{30}H_{32}N_2O_2 \cdot HCl$ in combination with the sulfate of atropine — see LOMOTIL

di·phe·nyl·hy·dan·to·in \\(ˌ)dī-ˌfen-əl-hī-ˈdan-tə-wən, -ˌfēn-\\ *n* : PHENYTOIN

di·phos·phate \\(ˌ)dī-ˈfäs-ˌfāt\\ *n* : a phosphate containing two phosphate groups

2,3–di·phos·pho·glyc·er·ate *also* **di·phos·pho·glyc·er·ate** \\(ˌ)tü-ˌthrē-)dī-ˌfäs-fō-ˈgli-sə-ˌrāt\\ *n* : a phosphate that occurs in human red blood cells and facilitates release of oxygen by decreasing the oxygen affinity of hemoglobin

di·phos·pho·pyr·i·dine nucleotide \\-ˌpir-ə-ˌdēn-\\ *n* : NAD

diph·the·ria \\dif-ˈthir-ē-ə, dip-\\ *n* : an acute febrile contagious disease marked by the formation of a false membrane esp. in the throat and caused by a bacterium of the genus *Corynebacterium* (*C. diphtheriae*) which produces a toxin causing inflammation of the heart and nervous system — **diph·the·ri·al** \\-ē-əl\\ *adj*

diph·the·rit·ic \\ˌdif-thə-ˈri-tik, ˌdip-\\ *adj* : relating to, produced in, or affected with diphtheria; *also* : resembling diphtheria esp. in the formation of a false membrane ⟨∼ dysentery⟩

1diph·the·roid \\ˈdif-thə-ˌrȯid\\ *adj* : resembling diphtheria

2diphtheroid *n* : a bacterium (esp. genus *Corynebacterium*) that resembles the bacterium of diphtheria but does not produce diphtheria toxin

di·phyl·lo·both·ri·a·sis \\(ˌ)dī-ˌfi-lō-bä-ˈthrī-ə-səs\\ *n, pl* **-a·ses** \\-ˌsēz\\ : infestation with or disease caused by the fish tapeworm

Di·phyl·lo·both·ri·um \\-ˈbä-thrē-əm\\ *n* : a genus of tapeworms (family Diphyllobothriidae) that includes the fish tapeworm (*D. latum*) of humans

dipl- *or* **diplo-** *comb form* : double : twofold ⟨*diplo*coccus⟩ ⟨*diplo*pia⟩

dip·la·cu·sis \\ˌdi-plə-ˈkyü-səs\\ *n, pl* **-cu·ses** \\-ˌsēz\\ : the hearing of a single tone as if it were two tones of different pitch

di·ple·gia \\dī-ˈplē-jə, -jē-ə\\ *n* : paralysis of corresponding parts (as the legs) on both sides of the body

dip·lo·coc·cus \\ˌdi-plō-ˈkä-kəs\\ *n, pl* **-coc·ci** \\-ˈkä-ˌkī, -kē; ˈkäk-ˌsī, -sē\\ : any of various encapsulated bacteria (as the pneumococcus) that usu. occur in pairs and that were formerly grouped in a single taxon (genus *Diplococcus*) but are now all assigned to other genera — **dip·lo·coc·cal** \\-kəl\\ *adj*

dip·loe \\ˈdi-plə-ˌwē\\ *n* : cancellous bony tissue between the external and internal layers of the skull — **di·plo·ic** \\də-ˈplō-ik, dī-\\ *adj*

diploic vein *n* : any of several veins situated in channels in the diploe

1dip·loid \\ˈdi-ˌplȯid\\ *adj* : having the basic chromosome number doubled — **dip·loi·dy** \\-ˌplȯi-dē\\ *n*

2diploid *n* : a single cell, individual, or generation characterized by the diploid chromosome number

dip·lo·mate \'di-plə-ˌmāt\ *n* : a physician qualified to practice in a medical specialty by advanced training and experience in the specialty followed by passing an intensive examination by a national board of senior specialists

dip·lo·pia \di-'plō-pē-ə\ *n* : a disorder of vision in which two images of a single object are seen (as from unequal action of the eye muscles) — called also *double vision* — **dip·lo·pic** \-'plō-pik, -'plä-\ *adj*

dip·lo·tene \'di-plə-ˌtēn\ *n* : a stage of meiotic prophase which follows the pachytene and during which the paired homologous chromosomes begin to separate and chiasmata become visible — **diplotene** *adj*

di·pole \'dī-ˌpōl\ *n* 1 : a pair of equal and opposite electric charges or magnetic poles of opposite sign separated by a small distance 2 : a body or system (as a molecule) having such charges — **di·po·lar** \-ˌpō-lər, -'pō-\ *adj*

di·po·tas·si·um \ˌdī-pə-'ta-sē-əm\ *adj* : containing two atoms of potassium in a molecule

di·pro·pi·o·nate \(ˌ)dī-'prō-pē-ə-ˌnāt\ *n* : an ester containing two propionate groups

dip·so·ma·nia \ˌdip-sə-'mā-nē-ə, -nyə\ *n* : an uncontrollable craving for alcoholic liquors — **dip·so·ma·ni·ac** \-nē-ˌak\ *n* — **dip·so·ma·ni·a·cal** \ˌdip-sō-mə-'nī-ə-kəl\ *adj*

dip·stick \'dip-ˌstik\ *n* : a chemically sensitive strip of paper used to identify one or more constituents (as glucose or protein) of urine by immersion

dip·ter·an \'dip-tə-rən\ *adj* : of, relating to, or being a fly (sense 2a) — **dipteran** *n* — **dip·ter·ous** \-rəs\ *adj*

Di·py·lid·i·um \ˌdī-pī-'li-dē-əm, -pə-\ *n* : a genus of taenioid tapeworms including the dog tapeworm (*D. caninum*)

di·pyr·i·dam·ole \(ˌ)dī-ˌpir-ə-'da-ˌmōl, -ˌmōl\ *n* : a drug $C_{24}H_{40}N_8O_4$ used as a coronary vasodilator — see PERSANTINE

di·rec·tive \də-'rek-tiv, dī-\ *adj* : of or relating to psychotherapy in which the therapist introduces information, content, or attitudes not previously expressed by the client

di·rec·tor \də-'rek-tər, dī-\ *n* : an instrument grooved to guide and limit the motion of a surgical knife

direct pyramidal tract *n* : VENTRAL CORTICOSPINAL TRACT

Di·ro·fi·lar·ia \ˌdī-rō-(ˌ)fī-'lar-ē-ə\ *n* : a genus (family Dipetalonematidae) of filarial worms that includes the heartworm (*D. immitis*) — **di·ro·fi·lar·i·al** \-ē-əl\ *adj*

di·ro·fil·a·ri·a·sis \-ˌfi-lə-'rī-ə-səs\ *n*, *pl* **-a·ses** \-ˌsēz\ : infestation with filarial worms of the genus *Dirofilaria* and esp. with the heartworm (*D. immitis*)

dirty \'dər-tē\ *adj* **dirt·i·er**; **-est** : contaminated with infecting organisms

dis·abil·i·ty \ˌdi-sə-'bi-lə-tē\ *n*, *pl* **-ties** 1 : the condition of being disabled 2 : inability to pursue an occupation because of physical or mental impairment

dis·able \di-'sā-bəl, -'zā-\ *vb* **dis·abled**; **dis·abling** : to deprive of a mental or physical capacity

dis·abled *adj* : incapacitated by illness, injury, or wounds; *broadly* : physically or mentally impaired

dis·able·ment \-mənt\ *n* : the act of becoming disabled to the extent that full wages cannot be earned; *also* : the state of being so disabled

di·sac·cha·ri·dase \(ˌ)dī-'sa-kə-rə-ˌdās, -ˌdāz\ *n* : an enzyme (as maltase) that hydrolyzes disaccharides

di·sac·cha·ride \(ˌ)dī-'sa-kə-ˌrīd\ *n* : any of a class of sugars (as sucrose) that on hydrolysis yields two monosaccharide molecules

dis·ar·tic·u·la·tion \ˌdi-sär-ˌti-kyə-'lā-shən\ *n* : separation or amputation of a body part at a joint ⟨~ of the shoulder⟩ — **dis·ar·tic·u·late** \-'ti-kyə-ˌlāt\ *vb*

disc, discectomy *var of* DISK, DISKECTOMY

disc- *or* **disci-** *or* **disco-** *comb form* : disk ⟨*disci*form⟩

¹**dis·charge** \dis-'chärj, 'dis-\ *vb* **discharged**; **dis·charg·ing** 1 : to release from confinement, custody, or care ⟨~ a patient from the hospital⟩ 2 a : to give outlet to or emit ⟨a boil *discharging* pus⟩ b : to release or give expression to (as a pent-up emotion)

²**dis·charge** \'dis-ˌchärj, dis-'\ *n* 1 : the act of relieving of something ⟨~ of a repressed impulse⟩ 2 : release from confinement, custody, or care 3 : something that is emitted or evacuated ⟨a purulent ~⟩

disci *pl of* DISCUS

dis·ci·form \'di-sə-ˌfȯrm\ *adj* : round or oval in shape

dis·cis·sion \də-'si-shən, -zhən\ *n* : an incision (as in treating cataract) of the capsule of the lens of the eye

dis·clos·ing \dis-'klō-ziŋ\ *adj* : being or using an agent (as a tablet or liquid) that contains a usu. red dye that adheres to and stains dental plaque

discogram, discography *var of* DISKOGRAM, DISKOGRAPHY

¹**dis·coid** \'dis-ˌkȯid\ *adj* 1 : resembling a disk : being flat and circular 2 : characterized by macules ⟨~ lupus erythematosus⟩

²**discoid** *n* : an instrument with a disk-shaped blade used in dentistry for carving

dis·coi·dal \dis-'kȯid-ᵊl\ *adj* : of, resembling, or producing a disk; *esp* : having the villi restricted to one or more disklike areas

dis·cop·a·thy \dis-'kä-pə-thē\ *n*, *pl* **-thies** : any disease affecting an intervertebral disk

dis·cor·dant \dis-'kȯrd-ᵊnt\ *adj, of twins* : dissimilar with respect to one or more particular characters — compare CONCORDANT — **dis·cor·dance** \-ᵊns\ *n*

dis·crete \dis-'krēt, 'dis-,\ *adj* : characterized by distinct unconnected lesions ⟨∼ smallpox⟩ — compare CONFLUENT 2

dis·crim·i·nate \dis-'kri-mə-,nāt\ *vb* **-nat·ed; -nat·ing** : to respond selectively to (a stimulus)

dis·crim·i·na·tion \dis-,kri-mə-'nā-shən\ *n* : the process by which two stimuli differing in some aspect are responded to differently

dis·cus \'dis-kəs\ *n, pl* **dis·ci** \-,kī, -kē\ : any of various rounded and flattened anatomical structures

discus pro·lig·er·us \-prō-'li-jə-rəs\ *n* : CUMULUS

dis·ease \di-'zēz\ *n* : an impairment of the normal state of the living body or one of its parts that interrupts or modifies the performance of the vital functions and is a response to environmental factors (as malnutrition), to specific infective agents (as viruses), to inherent defects of the organism (as genetic anomalies), or to combinations of these factors : SICKNESS, ILLNESS — **dis·eased** \-'zēzd\ *adj*

dis·equi·lib·ri·um \(,)di-,sē-kwə-'li-brē-əm, -,se-\ *n, pl* **-ri·ums** *or* **-ria** : loss or lack of equilibrium

disfunction *var of* DYSFUNCTION

dis·har·mo·ny \(,)di-'här-mə-nē\ *n, pl* **-nies** : lack of harmony — see OCCLUSAL DISHARMONY

dis·in·fect \dis-ᵊn-'fekt\ *vb* : to free from infection esp. by destroying harmful microorganisms — **dis·in·fec·tion** \-'fek-shən\ *n*

¹**dis·in·fec·tant** \-'fek-tənt\ *n* : a chemical that destroys vegetative forms of harmful microorganisms (as bacteria and fungi) esp. on inanimate objects but that may be less effective in destroying spores

²**disinfectant** *adj* : serving or tending to disinfect : suitable for use in disinfecting

dis·in·fest \dis-ᵊn-'fest\ *vb* : to rid of small animal pests (as insects or rodents) — **dis·in·fes·ta·tion** \(,)dis-,in-,fes-'tā-shən\ *n*

dis·in·fes·tant \dis-ᵊn-'fes-tənt\ *n* : a disinfesting agent

dis·in·hib·it \dis-in-'hi-bət\ *vb* : to cause the loss or reduction of an inhibition ⟨∼ of a reflex⟩ — **dis·in·hi·bi·tion** \(,)dis-,in-hə-'bi-shən, -,si-nə-\ *n*

dis·in·hib·i·to·ry \-in-'hi-bə-,tōr-ē\ *adj* : tending to overcome psychological inhibition ⟨∼ drugs⟩

dis·in·ter \dis-in-'tər\ *vb* : to take out of the grave or tomb — **dis·in·ter·ment** \-mənt\ *n*

dis·junc·tion \dis-'jəŋk-shən\ *n* : the separation of chromosomes or chromatids during anaphase of mitosis or meiosis

disk *or* **disc** \'disk\ *n* : any of various rounded or flattened anatomical structures: as **a** : a mammalian blood cell **b** : BLIND SPOT **c** : INTERVERTEBRAL DISK — see SLIPPED DISK

disk·ec·to·my *also* **disc·ec·to·my** \'kek-tə-mē\ *n, pl* **-mies** : surgical removal of an intervertebral disk

disk·o·gram *also* **disc·o·gram** \'dis-kə-,gram\ *n* : a radiograph of an intervertebral disk made after injection of a radiopaque substance

dis·kog·ra·phy *also* **dis·cog·ra·phy** \dis-'kä-grə-fē\ *n, pl* **-phies** : the process of making a diskogram

dis·lo·cate \'dis-lō-,kāt, -lə-; (,)dis-'lō-,kāt\ *vb* **-cat·ed; -cat·ing** : to put (a body part) out of order by displacing a bone from its normal connections with another bone ⟨he *dislocated* his shoulder⟩; *also* : to displace (a bone) from normal connections with another bone ⟨the humerus was *dislocated* in the fall⟩

dis·lo·ca·tion \dis-(,)lō-'kā-shən, -lə-\ *n* : displacement of one or more bones at a joint : LUXATION

dismutase — see SUPEROXIDE DISMUTASE

di·so·di·um \(,)dī-'sō-dē-əm\ *adj* : containing two atoms of sodium in a molecule

disodium cromoglycate *n* : CROMOLYN SODIUM

disodium ed·e·tate \-'e-də-,tāt\ *n* : a disodium salt $C_{10}H_{14}N_2Na_2O_8·2H_2O$ of EDTA that has an affinity for calcium and is used to treat hypercalcemia and pathological calcification

di·so·mic \dī-'sō-mik\ *adj* : having one or more chromosomes present in two copies ⟨the ∼ state is normal in humans⟩ — **di·so·my** \-mē\ *n*

di·so·pyr·a·mide \dī-(,)sō-'pir-ə-,mīd\ *n* : a cardiac depressant used in the form of its phosphate $C_{21}H_{29}N_3O$·H_3PO_4 to treat life-threatening ventricular arrhythmias

¹**dis·or·der** \(,)di-'sȯr-dər, -'zȯr-\ *vb* **dis·or·dered; dis·or·der·ing** : to disturb the regular or normal functions of

²**disorder** *n* : an abnormal physical or mental condition : AILMENT

dis·or·dered *adj* **1** : not functioning in a normal orderly healthy way ⟨∼ bodily functions⟩ **2** : mentally unbalanced

dis·or·ga·ni·za·tion \(,)di-,sȯr-gə-nə-'zā-shən\ *n* : psychopathological inconsistency in personality, mental functions, or overt behavior — **dis·or·ga·nize** \(,)di-'sȯr-gə-,nīz\ *vb*

dis·ori·ent \(,)di-'sȯr-ē-,ent\ *vb* : to produce a state of disorientation in : DISORIENTATE

dis·ori·en·ta·tion \(,)di-,sȯr-ē-ən-'tā-shən, -,en-\ *n* : a usu. transient state of confusion esp. as to time, place, or identity often as a result of disease or drugs — **dis·ori·en·tate** \-'sōr-ē-ən-ˌtāt, -en-\ *vb*

dis·par·i·ty \di-'spar-ə-tē\ *n, pl* **-ties** : the state of being different or dissimilar (as in the sensory information received) — see RETINAL DISPARITY

dis·pen·sa·ry \di-'spen-sə-rē\ *n, pl* **-ries** : a place where medicine or medical or dental treatment is dispensed

dis·pen·sa·to·ry \di-'spen-sə-ˌtōr-ē\ *n, pl* **-ries** **1** : a book or medicinal formulary containing a systematic description of the drugs and preparations used in medicine **2** : DISPENSARY

dis·pense \di-'spens\ *vb* **dis·pensed; dis·pens·ing** **1** : to put up (a prescription or medicine) **2** : to prepare and distribute (medication) — **dis·pen·sa·tion** \ˌdis-pən-'sā-shən, -pen-\ *n*

dispensing optician *n, Brit* : a person qualified and licensed to fit and supply eyeglasses

dis·place·ment \di-'splā-smənt\ *n* **1** : the act or process of removing something from its usual or proper place or the state resulting from this : DISLOCATION ⟨the ~ of a knee joint⟩ **2** : the quantity in which or the degree to which something is displaced **3 a** : the direction of an emotion or impulse away from its original object (as an idea or person) to something that is more acceptable **b** : SUBLIMATION **c** : the substitution of another form of behavior for what is usual or expected esp. when the usual response is nonadaptive — **dis·place** \-'splās\ *vb*

dis·pro·por·tion \ˌdis-prə-'pōr-shən\ *n* : absence of symmetry or the proper dimensional relationship — see CEPHALOPELVIC DISPROPORTION

dis·rup·tive \dis-'rəp-tiv\ *adj* : characterized by psychologically disorganized behavior ⟨a confused and ~ patient in the manic phase⟩

dissecans — see OSTEOCHONDRITIS DISSECANS

dis·sect \di-'sekt, dī-; 'dī-ˌ\ *vb* **1** : to cut so as to separate into pieces or to expose the several parts of (as an animal or a cadaver) for scientific examination; *specif* : to separate or follow along natural lines of cleavage (as through connective tissue) **2** : to make a medical dissection — **dis·sec·tor** \-'sek-tər, -ˌsek-\ *n*

dis·sec·tion \di-'sek-shən, dī-; 'dī-ˌ\ *n* **1** : the act or process of dissecting or separating: as **a** : the surgical removal along natural lines of cleavage of tissues which are or might become diseased **b** : the digital separation of tissues (as in heart-valve operations) **c** : a pathological splitting or separation of tissue — see AORTIC DISSECTION **2 a** : something (as a part or the whole of an animal) that has been dissected **b** : an anatomical specimen prepared in this way

dis·sem·i·nat·ed \di-'se-mə-ˌnā-təd\ *adj* : widely dispersed in a tissue, organ, or the entire body — see ACUTE DISSEMINATED ENCEPHALOMYELITIS — **dis·sem·i·na·tion** \-ˌse-mə-'nā-shən\ *n*

disseminated intravascular coagulation *n* : an acute or chronic thrombotic and hemorrhagic disorder that arises secondary to various disease states (as acute promyelocytic leukemia, abruptio placentae, or major trauma) and is marked by uncontrolled systemic coagulation resulting in thrombosis which in acute cases typically leads to generalized bleeding due to depletion of clotting factors and increased fibrinolysis — abbr. *DIC*

dis·so·ci·a·tion \(ˌ)di-ˌsō-sē-'ā-shən, -shē-\ *n* **1** : the process by which a chemical combination breaks up into simpler constituents **2** : the separation of whole segments of the personality (as in multiple personality disorder) or of discrete mental processes (as in the schizophrenias) from the mainstream of consciousness or of behavior — **dis·so·ci·ate** \-'sō-sē-ˌāt, -shē-\ *vb* — **dis·so·cia·tive** \(ˌ)di-'sō-shē-ˌā-tiv, -sē-, -shə-tiv\ *adj*

dissociative identity disorder *n* : MULTIPLE PERSONALITY DISORDER

dis·so·lu·tion \ˌdi-sə-'lü-shən\ *n* : the act or process of dissolving

dis·solve \di-'zälv, -'zȯlv\ *vb* **dis·solved; dis·solv·ing** **1** : to pass or cause to pass into solution **2** : to cause to melt or liquefy **3** : to become fluid — **dis·solv·er** *n*

dis·so·nance \'di-sə-nəns\ *n* : inconsistency between the beliefs one holds or between one's actions and one's beliefs — see COGNITIVE DISSONANCE

dist- — see DISTO-

dis·tal \'dist-ᵊl\ *adj* **1** : situated away from the point of attachment or origin or a central point: as **a** : located away from the center of the body ⟨the ~ end of a bone⟩ — compare PROXIMAL 1a **b** : located away from the mesial plane of the body — compare MESIAL 2 **c** : of, relating to, or being the surface of a tooth that is next to the following tooth counting from the middle of the front of the upper or lower jaw or that faces the back of the mouth in the case of the last tooth on each side — compare MESIAL 3, PROXIMAL 1b **2** : physical or social rather than sensory — compare PROXIMAL 2 — **dis·tal·ly** *adv*

distal convoluted tubule *n* : the convoluted portion of the nephron lying between the loop of Henle and the nonsecretory part of the nephron and concerned esp. with the concentration of urine — called also *convoluted tubule, distal tubule*

distalis — see PARS DISTALIS

distal radioulnar joint *n* : a pivot joint

between the lower end of the ulna and the ulnar notch on the lower end of the radius that permits rotation of the distal end of the radius around the longitudinal axis of the ulna — called also *inferior radioulnar joint*

dis·tem·per \dis-'tem-pər\ *n* : a disordered or abnormal bodily state esp. of quadruped mammals: as **a** : a highly contagious virus disease esp. of dogs that is marked by fever, leukopenia, and respiratory, gastrointestinal, and neurological symptoms and that is caused by a paramyxovirus of the genus *Morbillivirus* (species *Canine distemper virus*) — called also *canine distemper* **b** : STRANGLES **c** : PANLEUKOPENIA

dis·tend \di-'stend\ *vb* : to enlarge or stretch out (as from internal pressure)

dis·ten·si·ble \-'sten-sə-bəl\ *adj* : capable of being distended, extended, or dilated ⟨∼ blood vessels⟩ — **dis·ten·si·bil·i·ty** \-,sten-sə-'bi-lə-tē\ *n*

dis·ten·sion *or* **dis·ten·tion** \di-'stenchən\ *n* : the act of distending esp. the state of being distended esp. unduly or abnormally

disto- *also* **dist-** *or* **disti-** *comb form* : distal ⟨*disto*buccal⟩

dis·to·buc·cal \dis-tō-'bə-kəl\ *adj* : relating to or located on the distal and buccal surfaces of a molar or premolar — **dis·to·buc·cal·ly** *adv*

dis·to·lin·gual \-'liŋ-gwel, -gyə-wəl\ *adj* : relating to or situated on the distal and lingual surfaces of a tooth

dis·to·ma·to·sis \,dī-,stō-mə-'tō-səs\ *n, pl* **-to·ses** \-,sēz\ : infestation with or disease (as liver rot) caused by digenetic trematode worms

dis·to·mi·a·sis \,dī-stō-'mī-ə-səs\ *n, pl* **-a·ses** \-,sēz\ : DISTOMATOSIS

dis·tor·tion \di-'stor-shən\ *n* **1** : the censorship of unacceptable unconscious impulses so that they are unrecognizable to the ego in the manifest content of a dream **2** : a lack of correspondence of size or intensity in an image resulting from defects in an optical system

dis·tract·i·bil·i·ty \di-,strak-tə-'bi-lə-tē\ *n, pl* **-ties** : a condition in which the attention of the mind is easily distracted by small and irrelevant stimuli — **dis·tract·ible** \-'strak-tə-bəl\ *adj*

dis·trac·tion \di-'strak-shən\ *n* **1 a** : diversion of the attention **b** : mental derangement **2** : excessive separation (as from improper traction) of fracture fragments — **dis·tract** \di-'strakt\ *vb*

dis·tress \di-'stres\ *n* : pain or suffering affecting the body, a bodily part, or the mind ⟨gastric ∼⟩ ⟨respiratory ∼⟩

dis·tri·bu·tion \dis-trə-'byü-shən\ *n* : the pattern of branching and termination of a ramifying anatomical structure (as a nerve or artery)

district nurse *n, Brit* : a qualified nurse who is employed by a local authority to visit and treat patients in their own homes — compare VISITING NURSE

dis·turbed \di-'stərbd\ *adj* : showing symptoms of emotional illness or mental disorder ⟨∼ children⟩ — **dis·tur·bance** \-'stər-bəns\ *n*

di·sul·fi·ram \dī-'səl-fə-,ram\ *n* : a compound $C_{10}H_{20}N_2S_4$ that causes a severe physiological reaction to alcohol and is used esp. in the treatment of alcoholism — called also *tetraethylthiuram disulfide;* see ANTABUSE

di·sul·phi·ram *chiefly Brit var of* DISULFIRAM

di·thra·nol \'dī-thrə-,nōl, 'di-, -,nōl\ *n, chiefly Brit* : ANTHRALIN

di·ure·sis \,dī-yə-'rē-səs\ *n, pl* **di·ure·ses** \-,sēz\ : an increased excretion of urine

¹di·uret·ic \,dī-yə-'re-tik\ *adj* : tending to increase the excretion of urine — **di·uret·i·cal·ly** \-ti-k(ə-)lē\ *adv*

²diuretic *n* : an agent that increases the excretion of urine

Di·ur·il \'dī-yùr-il\ *trademark* — used for a preparation of chlorothiazide

di·ur·nal \dī-'ərn-ᵊl\ *adj* **1** : having a daily cycle ⟨∼ rhythms⟩ **2** : of, relating to, or occurring in the daytime ⟨∼ activity⟩ — **di·ur·nal·ly** *adv*

di·val·pro·ex sodium \dī-'val-prō-eks-\ *n* : a combination of valproate and valproic acid that is used esp. to treat manic episodes of bipolar disorder and absence seizures of epilepsy — called also *divalproex;* see DEPAKOTE

di·ver·gence \də-'vər-jəns, dī-\ *n* **1** : a drawing apart **2** : dissemination of the effect of activity of a single nerve cell through multiple synaptic connections — compare CONVERGENCE 2 — **di·verge** \-'vərj\ *vb* — **di·ver·gent** \-'vər-jənt\ *adj*

divergent thinking *n* : creative thinking that may follow many lines of thought and tends to generate new and original solutions to problems — compare CONVERGENT THINKING

diverticula *pl of* DIVERTICULUM

di·ver·tic·u·lar \,dī-vər-'ti-kyə-lər\ *adj* : consisting of or resembling a diverticulum

diverticular disease *n* : a disorder characterized by diverticulosis or diverticulitis

di·ver·tic·u·lec·to·my \,dī-vər-,ti-kyə-'lek-tə-mē\ *n, pl* **-mies** : the surgical removal of a diverticulum

di·ver·tic·u·li·tis \-'lī-təs\ *n* : inflammation or infection of a diverticulum of the colon that is marked by abdominal pain or tenderness often accompanied by fever, chills, and cramping

di·ver·tic·u·lop·exy \-'lä-pək-sē\ *n, pl* **-ex·ies** : surgical obliteration or fixation of a diverticulum

di·ver·tic·u·lo·sis \-'lō-səs\ *n, pl* **-lo·ses** \-,sēz\ : an intestinal disorder characterized by the presence of many diverticula in the colon that is typically symptomless but may be marked by symptoms (as bleeding or constipation)

di·ver·tic·u·lum \ˌdī-vər-'ti-kyə-ləm\ *n, pl* **-la** \-lə\ **1** : an abnormal pouch or sac opening from a hollow organ (as the colon or bladder) **2** : a blind tube or sac branching off from a cavity or canal of the body

di·vide \də-'vīd\ *vb* **di·vid·ed; di·vid·ing 1** : to separate into two or more parts ⟨~ a nerve surgically⟩ **2** : to undergo replication, multiplication, fission, or separation into parts ⟨actively *dividing* cells⟩

di·vid·er \də-'vī-dər\ *n* : the second incisor tooth of a horse situated between the center and corner incisors on each side — compare NIPPER

di·vi·sion \də-'vi-zhən\ *n* **1** : the act or process of dividing : the state of being divided — see CELL DIVISION **2** : a group of organisms forming part of a larger group; *specif* : a primary category of the plant kingdom that is typically equivalent to a phylum — **di·vi·sion·al** \-'vi-zhə-nəl\ *adj*

di·zy·got·ic \ˌdī-zī-'gä-tik\ *also* **di·zy·gous** \(ˌ)dī-'zī-gəs\ *adj, of twins* : FRATERNAL

diz·zi·ness \'di-zē-nəs\ *n* : the condition of being dizzy; *esp* : a sensation of unsteadiness accompanied by a feeling of movement within the head

diz·zy \'di-zē\ *adj* **diz·zi·er; -est** : having a whirling sensation in the head with a tendency to fall **2** : mentally confused — **diz·zi·ly** \'di-zə-lē\ *adv*

DJD *abbr* degenerative joint disease

DM *abbr* **1** diabetes mellitus **2** diastolic murmur **3** myotonic dystrophy

DMAE \ˌdē-ˌem-ˌā-'ē\ *n* : a choline analog C₄H₁₁NO used esp. as a dietary supplement and skin toner — called also *deanol, dimethylaminoethanol*

DMD *abbr* [Latin *dentariae medicinae doctor*] **1** doctor of dental medicine **2** Duchenne muscular dystrophy; Duchenne's muscular dystrophy

DMF *abbr* decayed, missing, and filled teeth

DMSO \ˌdē-(ˌ)em-(ˌ)es-'ō\ *n* : DIMETHYL SULFOXIDE

DMT \ˌdē-(ˌ)em-'tē\ *n* : DIMETHYLTRYPTAMINE

DNA \ˌdē-(ˌ)en-'ā\ *n* : any of various nucleic acids that are usu. the molecular basis of heredity, are localized esp. in cell nuclei, and are constructed of a double helix held together by hydrogen bonds between purine and pyrimidine bases which project inward from two chains containing alternate links of deoxyribose and phosphate — called also *deoxyribonucleic acid;* see RECOMBINANT DNA

DNA fingerprint *n* : the base-pair pattern in an individual's DNA obtained by DNA fingerprinting — called also *genetic fingerprint*

DNA fingerprinting *n* : a technique

that involves extracting and identifying the base-pair pattern of an individual's DNA — called also *DNA typing, genetic fingerprinting*

DNA methylation *n* : the enzymatically controlled methylation of a nucleotide base (as cytosine) in a molecule of DNA that plays a role in suppressing gene expression

DNA polymerase *n* : any of several polymerases that promote replication or repair of DNA usu. using single-stranded DNA as a template

DNAR *abbr* do not attempt resuscitation

DN·ase \(ˌ)dē-'en-ˌās, -ˌāz\ *also* **DNA-ase** \(ˌ)dē-ˌen-'ā-ˌās, -ˌāz\ *n* : DEOXYRIBONUCLEASE

DNA virus *n* : a virus whose genome consists of DNA

DNR *abbr* do not resuscitate

DO *abbr* doctor of osteopathy

DOA *abbr* dead on arrival

DOB *abbr* date of birth

do·bu·ta·mine \dō-'byü-tə-ˌmēn\ *n* : a drug administered intravenously in the form of its hydrochloride C₁₈H₂₃NO₃·HCl esp. to increase cardiac output and lower wedge pressure in heart failure and after cardiopulmonary bypass surgery

doc \'däk\ *n* : DOCTOR — used chiefly as a familiar term of address

do·ce·tax·el \ˌdō-sə-'tak-səl\ *n* : a semisynthetic antineoplastic drug C₄₃H₅₃NO₁₄·3H₂O derived from the needles of a European yew tree (*Taxus baccata*) — see TAXOTERE

do·co·sa·hex·a·e·no·ic acid \ˌdō-kō-sə-ˌhek-sə-ˌē-ˌnō-ik-\ *n* : an omega-3 fatty acid C₂₂H₃₂O₂ found esp. in fish of cold waters — abbr *DHA*

¹doc·tor \'däk-tər\ *n* **1 a** : a person who has earned one of the highest academic degrees (as a PhD) conferred by a university **b** : a person awarded an honorary doctorate by a college or university **2** : a person skilled or specializing in healing arts; *esp* : one (as a physician, dentist, or veterinarian) who holds an advanced degree and is licensed to practice

²doctor *vb* **doc·tored; doc·tor·ing 1 a** : to give medical treatment to **b** : to practice medicine **2** : CASTRATE, SPAY

doc·u·sate \'dä-kyü-ˌsāt\ *n* : any of several laxative salts and esp. the sodium salt C₂₀H₃₇NaO₇S used to soften stools — see PERI-COLACE

dog \'dȯg\ *n, often attrib* : a highly variable carnivorous domesticated mammal (*Canis familiaris*); *broadly* : any member of the family (Canidae) to which the dog belongs

dog flea *n* : a flea of the genus *Ctenocephalides* (*C. canis*) that feeds chiefly on dogs and cats

dog tapeworm *n* : a tapeworm of the genus *Dipylidium* (*D. caninum*) occurring in dogs and cats and sometimes in humans

dog tick *n* : AMERICAN DOG TICK

dolens — see PHLEGMASIA ALBA DOLENS, PHLEGMASIA CERULEA DOLENS

dolicho- *comb form* : long ⟨*dolicho*cephalic⟩

dol·i·cho·ce·phal·ic \ˌdä-li-kō-sə-ˈfa-lik\ *adj* : having a relatively long head with a cephalic index of less than 75 — **dol·i·cho·ceph·a·ly** \-ˈse-fə-lē\ *n*

Do·lo·bid \ˈdō-lə-ˌbid\ *trademark* — used for a preparation of diflunisal

do·lor \ˈdō-lər, ˈdä-\ *n* : mental suffering or anguish

DOM \ˌdē-(ˌ)ō-ˈem\ *n* : STP

do·main \dō-ˈmān\ *n* **1** : any of the three-dimensional subunits of a protein that together make up its tertiary structure **2** : the highest taxonomic category in biological classification ranking above the kingdom

dome \ˈdōm\ *n* : a rounded-arch element in the wave tracing in an electroencephalogram

do·mi·cil·i·ary \ˌdä-mə-ˈsi-lē-ˌer-ē, ˌdō-\ *adj* **1** : provided or attended in the home rather than in an institution ⟨∼ midwifery⟩ **2** : providing, constituting, or provided by an institution for chronically ill or permanently disabled persons requiring minimal medical attention ⟨∼ care⟩

dom·i·nance \ˈdä-mə-nəns\ *n* : the fact or state of being dominant: as **a** : the property of one of a pair of alleles or traits that suppresses expression of the other in the heterozygous condition **b** : functional asymmetry between a pair of bodily structures (as the right and left hands)

¹dom·i·nant \-nənt\ *adj* **1** : exerting forcefulness or having dominance in a social hierarchy **2** : being the one of a pair of bodily structures that is the more effective or predominant in action ⟨the ∼ eye⟩ **3** : of, relating to, or exerting genetic dominance — **dom·i·nant·ly** *adv*

²dominant *n* **1** : a dominant genetic character or factor **2** : a dominant individual in a social hierarchy

DOMS *abbr* delayed onset muscle soreness

do·nee \dō-ˈnē\ *n* : a recipient of biological material (as blood or a graft)

don·ep·e·zil \dä-ˈne-pə-zil\ *n* : a drug used in the form of its hydrochloride $C_{24}H_{29}NO_3 \cdot HCl$ in the palliative treatment of mild to moderate dementia — see ARICEPT

Don Juan·ism \ˈdän-ˈhwä-ˌni-zəm, -ˈwä-\ *n, pl* Don Juanisms : male sexual promiscuity : SATYRIASIS

do·nor \ˈdō-nər, -ˌnȯr\ *n* **1** : one used as a source of biological material (as blood or an organ) **2** : a compound capable of giving up a part (as an atom) for combination with an acceptor

Don·o·van body \ˈdä-nə-vən-, ˈdə-\ *n* : an encapsulated gram-negative bacterium of the genus *Calymmatobacterium* (*C. granulomatis*) that is the causative agent of granuloma inguinale — compare LEISHMAN-DONOVAN BODY

C. Donovan — see LEISHMAN-DONOVAN BODY

do·pa \ˈdō-pə, -(ˌ)pä\ *n* : an amino acid $C_9H_{11}NO_4$ that in the levorotatory form is found in the broad bean and is used in the treatment of Parkinson's disease

L–dopa — see entry alphabetized in the letter *l*

do·pa·mine \ˈdō-pə-ˌmēn\ *n* : a monoamine $C_8H_{11}NO_2$ that is a decarboxylated form of dopa and occurs esp. as a neurotransmitter in the brain and as an intermediate in the biosynthesis of epinephrine — see INTROPIN

do·pa·mi·ner·gic \ˌdō-pə-ˌmē-ˈnər-jik\ *adj* : liberating, activated by, or involving dopamine or related substances ⟨∼ activity⟩ ⟨∼ neurons⟩

dope \ˈdōp\ *n* **1** : a preparation of an illicit, habit-forming, or narcotic drug (as heroin or marijuana) **2** : a preparation given to a racehorse to help or hinder its performance — **dope** *vb*

Dopp·ler \ˈdä-plər\ *adj* **1** : of, relating to, or utilizing a shift in frequency in accordance with the Doppler effect **2** : of, relating to, using, or produced by Doppler ultrasound ⟨∼ images⟩ ⟨∼ echocardiography⟩

Doppler, Christian Johann (1803–1853), Austrian physicist and mathematician.

Doppler effect *n* : a change in the frequency with which waves (as sound or light) from a given source reach an observer when the source and the observer are in motion with respect to each other so that the frequency increases or decreases according to the speed at which the distance is decreasing or increasing

Doppler ultrasound *n* : ultrasound that utilizes the Doppler effect to measure movement or flow in the body and esp. blood flow — called also *Doppler ultrasonography*

dors- — see DORSO-

dorsa *pl of* DORSUM

¹dor·sal \ˈdȯr-səl\ *adj* **1** : being or located near, on, or toward the upper surface of an animal (as a quadruped) opposite the lower or ventral surface **2** : being or located near, on, or toward the back or posterior part of the human body — **dor·sal·ly** \-sə-lē\ *adv*

²dorsal *n* : a dorsally located part; *esp* : a thoracic vertebra

dorsal horn *n* : a longitudinal subdivision of gray matter in the dorsal part of each lateral half of the spinal cord that receives terminals from some afferent fibers of the dorsal roots of the spinal nerves — called also *dorsal column, posterior column, posterior gray column, posterior horn*; compare LATERAL COLUMN 1, VENTRAL HORN

dorsal interosseus *n* **1** : any of four small muscles of the hand that act to draw the fingers away from the long axis of the middle finger, flex the fingers at the metacarpophalangeal joints, and extend their distal two phalanges 2 : any of four small muscles of the foot that act to draw the toes away from the long axis of the second toe, flex their proximal phalanges, and extend the distal phalanges

dorsalis — see INTEROSSEUS DORSALIS, SACROCOCCYGEUS DORSALIS, TABES DORSALIS

dorsalis pe·dis \dȯr-'sa-ləs-'pe-dəs, -'sä-, -'sä-, -'pē-\ n : an artery of the upper surface of the foot that is a direct continuation of the anterior tibial artery — called also *dorsalis pedis artery*

dorsal lip n : the margin of the fold of blastula wall that delineates the dorsal limit of the blastopore

dorsal mesogastrium n : MESOGASTRIUM 2

dorsal root n : the one of the two roots of a spinal nerve that passes posteriorly to the spinal cord separating the posterior and lateral funiculi and that consists of sensory fibers — called also *posterior root;* compare VENTRAL ROOT

dorsal root ganglion n : SPINAL GANGLION

dorsal spinocerebellar tract n : SPINOCEREBELLAR TRACT a

dorsi — see ILIOCOSTALIS DORSI, LATISSIMUS DORSI, LONGISSIMUS DORSI

dor·si·flex·ion \ˌdȯr-sə-'flek-shən\ n : flexion in a dorsal direction; *esp* : flexion of the foot in an upward direction — compare PLANTAR FLEXION — **dor·si·flex** \'dȯr-sə-ˌfleks\ vb

dor·si·flex·or \'dȯr-sə-ˌflek-sər\ n : a muscle causing flexion in a dorsal direction

dorso- or **dorsi-** also **dors-** comb form 1 : dorsal ⟨dorsiflexion⟩ 2 : dorsal and ⟨dorsolateral⟩

dor·so·lat·er·al \ˌdȯr-sō-'la-tə-rəl, -'la-trəl\ adj : of, relating to, or involving both the back and the sides ⟨the ~ prefrontal cortex⟩ — **dor·so·lat·er·al·ly** adv

dorsolateral tract n : a slender column of white matter between the dorsal gray column and the periphery of the spinal cord — called also *tract of Lissauer*

dor·so·lum·bar \ˌdȯr-sō-'ləm-bər\ adj : of or involving structures in the region occupied by the dorsal and lumbar vertebrae ⟨the ~ spine⟩

dor·so·me·di·al \-'mē-dē-əl\ adj : located toward the back and near the midline ⟨the ~ hypothalamus⟩

dor·so·ven·tral \-'ven-trəl\ adj : relating to, involving, or extending along the axis joining the dorsal and ventral sides — **dor·so·ven·tral·ly** adv

dor·sum \'dȯr-səm\ n, pl **dor·sa** \-sə\ 1 : the upper surface of an appendage or part 2 : BACK; *esp* : the entire dorsal surface of an animal

dos·age \'dō-sij\ n 1 a : the addition of an ingredient or the application of an agent in a measured dose b : the presence and relative representation or strength of a factor or agent (as a gene) 2 a : DOSE 1 b (1) : the giving of a dose (2) : regulation or determination of doses

¹dose \'dōs\ n 1 a : the measured quantity of a therapeutic agent to be taken at one time b : the quantity of radiation administered or absorbed 2 : a gonorrheal infection

²dose vb **dosed; dos·ing** 1 : to divide (as a medicine) into doses 2 : to give a dose to; *esp* : to give medicine to 3 : to take medicine 4 : to treat with an application or agent

dose–response adj : of, relating to, or graphing the pattern of physiological response to varied dosage (as of a drug or toxic substance)

do·sim·e·ter \dō-'si-mə-tər\ n : a device for measuring doses of radiations (as X-rays) — **do·si·met·ric** \ˌdō-sə-'me-trik\ adj — **do·sim·e·try** \dō-'si-mə-trē\ n

double bind n : a psychological predicament in which a person receives from a single source conflicting messages that allow no appropriate response to be made

dou·ble–blind \ˌdə-bəl-'blīnd\ adj : of, relating to, or being an experimental procedure in which neither the subjects nor the experimenters know which subjects are in the test and control groups during the actual course of the experiments — compare OPEN-LABEL, SINGLE-BLIND

double bond n : a chemical bond in which two pairs of electrons are shared by two atoms in a molecule and which is usu. represented in chemical formulas by two lines

double chin n : a fleshy or fatty fold under the chin — **dou·ble–chinned** \-'chind\ adj

double helix n : the structural arrangement of DNA in space that consists of paired polynucleotide strands stabilized by chemical bonds between the chains linking purine and pyrimidine bases — compare ALPHA-HELIX, WATSON-CRICK MODEL — **dou·ble–he·li·cal** \-'he-li-kəl, -'hē-\ adj

dou·ble–joint·ed \ˌdə-bəl-'jȯin-təd\ adj : having a joint that permits an exceptional degree of freedom of motion of the parts joined

double pneumonia n : pneumonia affecting both lungs

double vision n : DIPLOPIA

douche \'düsh\ n 1 a : a jet or current of liquid (as a cleansing solution) directed against or into a bodily part or cavity (as the vagina) b : an act of cleansing with a douche 2 : a device for giving douches — **douche** vb

Doug·las bag \'də-gləs-\ n : an inflatable bag used to collect expired air for the determination of oxygen consumption and basal metabolic rate
  Douglas, Claude Gordon (1882–1963), British physiologist.

Douglas's cul–de–sac \'də-glə-saz-\ n : POUCH OF DOUGLAS

Douglas's pouch n : POUCH OF DOUGLAS

dou·la \'dü-lə\ n : a woman experienced in childbirth who provides advice, information, emotional support, and physical comfort to a mother before, during, and just after childbirth

douloureux — see TIC DOULOUREUX

dow·a·ger's hump \'dau̇-i-jərz-\ n : an abnormal outward curvature of the upper back with round shoulders and stooped posture caused esp. by bone loss and anterior compression of the vertebrae in osteoporosis

down·er \'dau̇-nər\ n : a depressant drug; esp : BARBITURATE

down·stream \'dau̇n-'strēm\ adv or adj : in the same direction along a molecule of DNA or RNA as that in which transcription and translation take place and toward the end having a hydroxyl group attached to the position labeled 3' in the terminal nucleotide — compare UPSTREAM

Down syndrome \'dau̇n-\ or **Down's syndrome** \'dau̇nz-\ n : a congenital condition characterized esp. by moderate to severe mental retardation, upward slanting eyes usu. with epicanthic folds, a broad short skull, broad hands with short fingers, decreased muscle tone, and by trisomy of the human chromosome numbered 21 — called also *Down's, trisomy 21*
  Down \'dau̇n\, John Langdon Haydon (1828–1896), British physician.

dox·a·zo·sin \däk-'sā-zō-sin\ n : an alpha-blocker used in the form of its mesylate $C_{23}H_{25}N_5O_5·CH_4O_3S$ to relieve urethral obstruction in benign prostatic hyperplasia and to treat hypertension — see CARDURA

dox·e·pin \'däk-sə-,pin, -pən\ n : a tricyclic antidepressant administered as the hydrochloride $C_9H_{21}NO·HCl$ — see SINEQUAN

doxo·ru·bi·cin \,däk-sə-'rü-bə-sən\ n : an antibiotic with broad antitumor activity that is obtained from a bacterium of the genus *Streptomyces* (*S. peucetius*) and is used in the form of its hydrochloride $C_{27}H_{29}NO_{11}·HCl$ — see ADRIAMYCIN

doxy·cy·cline \,däk-sə-'sī-,klēn\ n : a broad-spectrum tetracycline antibiotic $C_{22}H_{24}N_2O_8$ with potent antibacterial activity that is often taken orally by travelers as a prophylactic against diarrhea — see VIBRAMYCIN

dox·yl·amine \däk-'si-lə-,mēn, -mən\ n : an antihistamine usu. used in the form of its succinate $C_{17}H_{22}N_2O·C_4H_6O_4$

DP abbr doctor of podiatry

DPH abbr 1 department of public health 2 doctor of public health

DPM abbr doctor of podiatric medicine

DPT abbr diphtheria-pertussis-tetanus (vaccine)

dr abbr dram

Dr abbr doctor

drac·on·ti·a·sis \,dra-,kän-'tī-ə-səs\ n, pl **-a·ses** \-,sēz\ : DRACUNCULIASIS

dra·cun·cu·li·a·sis \drə-,kən-kyə-'lī-ə-səs\ n, pl **-a·ses** \-,sēz\ : infestation with or disease caused by the guinea worm — called also *guinea worm disease*

dra·cun·cu·lo·sis \-'lō-səs\ n, pl **-lo·ses** \-,sēz\ : DRACUNCULIASIS

Dra·cun·cu·lus \drə-'kən-kyə-ləs\ n : a genus (family Dracunculidae) of greatly elongated nematode worms including the guinea worm

draft \'draft, 'draft\ n 1 : a portion (as of medicine) poured out or mixed for drinking : DOSE 2 : a current of air in a closed-in space — **drafty** \'draf-tē, 'draf-\ adj

¹drain \'drān\ vb 1 : to draw off (liquid) gradually or completely ⟨∼ pus from an abscess⟩ 2 : to carry away or give passage to a bodily fluid or a discharge from ⟨∼ an abscess⟩

²drain n : a tube or cylinder usu. of absorbent material for drainage of a wound — see CIGARETTE DRAIN

drain·age \'drā-nij\ n : the act or process of drawing off fluids from a cavity or wound by means of suction or gravity

Draize test \'drāz-\ n : a test that is used as a criterion for harmfulness of chemicals to the human eye and that involves dropping the test substance into one eye of rabbits without anesthesia with the other eye used as a control — called also *Draize eye test*
  Draize, John H. (1900–1992), American pharmacologist.

dram \'dram\ n 1 : either of two units of weight: **a** : an avoirdupois unit equal to 1.772 grams or 27.344 grains **b** : a unit of apothecaries' weight equal to 3.888 grams or 60 grains 2 : FLUID DRAM

Dram·amine \'dra-mə-,mēn\ trademark — used for a preparation of dimenhydrinate

drape n : a sterile covering used in an operating room — usu. used in pl. — **drape** vb

dras·tic \'dras-tik\ adj : acting rapidly or violently — used chiefly of purgatives — **dras·ti·cal·ly** \-ti-k(ə-)lē\ adv

draught chiefly Brit var of DRAFT

draw \'drȯ\ vb **drew** \'drü\; **drawn** \'drȯn\; **draw·ing** 1 : INHALE 2 **a** : to localize or cause to move toward a surface — used in the phrase *draw to a head* ⟨using a poultice to ∼ inflammation to a head⟩ **b** : to cause local congestion : induce blood or other body fluid to localize at a particular point

draw·sheet \'drȯ-ˌshēt\ *n* : a narrow sheet used chiefly in hospitals and stretched across the bed lengthwise often over a rubber sheet underneath the patient's trunk

DRE *abbr* digital rectal exam; digital rectal examination

dream \'drēm\ *n, often attrib* : a series of thoughts, images, or emotions occurring during sleep and esp. during REM sleep — **dream** *vb*

¹**drench** \'drench\ *n* : a poisonous or medicinal drink; *specif* : a large dose of medicine mixed with liquid and put down the throat of an animal

²**drench** *vb* : to administer a drench to (an animal)

dress \'dres\ *vb* : to apply dressings or medicaments to

dress·ing *n* : a covering (as of ointment or gauze) applied to a lesion

Dress·ler's syndrome \'dre-slərz-\ *n* : pericarditis after heart attack or open-heart surgery that is often recurrent and is typically accompanied by fever, chest pain, and pericardial and pleural effusions

Dressler, William (1890–1969), American cardiologist.

DRG \ˌdē-(ˌ)är-'jē\ *n* : any of the payment categories that are used to classify patients and esp. Medicare patients for the purpose of reimbursing hospitals for each case in a given category with a fixed fee regardless of the actual costs incurred — called also *diagnosis related group*

DRI *abbr* Dietary Reference Intake

drier *comparative of* DRY

driest *superlative of* DRY

drift \'drift\ *n* **1** : movement of a tooth in the dental arch **2** : GENETIC DRIFT — **drift** *vb*

drill *n* : an instrument with an edged or pointed end for making holes in hard substances (as teeth) by revolving — **drill** *vb*

Drink·er respirator \'driŋ-kər-\ *n* : IRON LUNG

Drinker, Philip (1894–1972), American industrial hygienist.

drip \'drip\ *n* **1 a** : a falling in drops — see POSTNASAL DRIP **b** : liquid that falls, overflows, or is extruded in drops **2** : a device for the administration of a fluid at a slow rate esp. into a vein; *also* : a material so administered ⟨a glucose ∼⟩ — see GRAVITY DRIP — **drip** *vb*

Dris·dol \'dris-ˌdȯl, -ˌdōl\ *trademark* — used for a preparation of calciferol

drive \'drīv\ *n* : an urgent, basic, or instinctual need : a motivating physiological condition of the organism ⟨a sexual ∼⟩

dro·nab·i·nol \ˌdrō-'na-bə-ˌnȯl\ *n* : a synthetic delta-9-tetrahydrocannabinol used to control nausea caused by chemotherapy and to stimulate appetite in cases of AIDS-induced anorexia — see MARINOL

drool \'drül\ *vb* **1** : to secrete saliva in

anticipation of food **2** : to let saliva or some other substance flow from the mouth — **drool** *n*

¹**drop** \'dräp\ *n* **1 a** : the quantity of fluid that falls in one spherical mass **b drops** *pl* : a dose of medicine measured by drops ⟨eye ∼s⟩ **2** : the smallest practical unit of liquid measure that varies in size according to the specific gravity and viscosity of the liquid and to the conditions under which it is formed

²**drop** *vb* **dropped; drop·ping 1** : to fall in drops **2** *of an animal* : to give birth to ⟨lambs *dropped* in June⟩ **3** : to take (a drug) orally ⟨∼ acid⟩

dro·per·i·dol \drō-'per-ə-ˌdȯl\ *n* : a butyrophenone tranquilizer $C_{22}H_{22}$-FN_3O_2 used esp. as a sedative, antiemetic, and antipsychotic

drop foot *n* : FOOT DROP

drop·let \'dräp-lət\ *n* : a tiny drop (as of a liquid)

droplet infection *n* : infection transmitted by airborne droplets of saliva or sputum containing infectious organisms

drop·per \'drä-pər\ *n* : a short glass tube fitted with a rubber bulb and used to measure liquids by drops — called also *eyedropper, medicine dropper* — **drop·per·ful** \-ˌfu̇l\ *n*

drop·si·cal \'dräp-si-kəl\ *adj* : relating to or affected with edema

drop·sy \'dräp-sē\ *n, pl* **drop·sies** : EDEMA

dros·pir·e·none \drō-'spir-ə-ˌnōn\ *n* : a synthetic progestogen $C_{24}H_{30}O_3$ that is an analog of spironolactone and is used in birth control pills in combination with ethinyl estradiol

drown \'drau̇n\ *vb* **drowned** \'drau̇nd\; **drown·ing** \'drau̇-niŋ\ **1** : to suffocate in water or some other liquid **2** : to suffocate because of excess of body fluid that interferes with the passage of oxygen from the lungs to the body tissues (as in pulmonary edema)

DrPH *abbr* doctor of public health

¹**drug** \'drəg\ *n* **1 a** : a substance used as a medication or in the preparation of medication **b** *according to the Food, Drug, and Cosmetic Act* (1) : a substance recognized in an official pharmacopoeia or formulary (2) : a substance intended for use in the diagnosis, cure, mitigation, treatment, or prevention of disease (3) : a substance other than food intended to affect the structure or function of the body (4) : a substance intended for use as a component of a medicine but not a device or a component, part, or accessory of a device **2** : something and often an illicit substance that causes addiction, habituation, or a marked change in consciousness

²**drug** *vb* **drugged; drug·ging 1** : to affect with a drug; *esp* : to stupefy by a narcotic drug **2** : to administer a drug to **3** : to take drugs for narcotic effect

drug·gist \'drə-gist\ *n* : one who sells or dispenses drugs and medicines; use **a** : PHARMACIST **b** : a person who owns or manages a drugstore

drug·mak·er \'drəg-ˌmā-kər\ *n* : one that manufactures pharmaceuticals

drug·store \-ˌstȯr\ *n* : a retail store where medicines and miscellaneous articles (as food, cosmetics, and film) are sold — called also *pharmacy*

drum \'drəm\ *n* : TYMPANIC MEMBRANE

drum·head \-ˌhed\ *n* : TYMPANIC MEMBRANE

drum·stick \-ˌstik\ *n* : a small projection from the cell nucleus that occurs in a small percentage of the polymorphonuclear leukocytes in the normal human female

druse \'drüz, 'drü-zə\ *n, pl* **dru·sen** \'drü-zən\ : one of the small yellowish deposits of cellular debris that accumulate between the pigmented epithelial layer of the retina and the inner collagenous layer of the choroid

dry \'drī\ *adj* **dri·er** \'drī-ər\; **dri·est** \-əst\ **1** : marked by the absence or scantiness of secretions, effusions, or other forms of moisture **2** *of a cough* : not accompanied by the raising of mucus or phlegm

dry eye *n* : a condition associated with inadequate tear production and marked by redness of the conjunctiva and by itching and burning of the eye — called also *dry eye syndrome, keratoconjunctivitis sicca*

dry gangrene *n* : gangrene that develops in the presence of arterial obstruction, is sharply localized, and is characterized by dryness of the dead tissue which is distinguishable from adjacent tissue by a line of inflammation

dry mouth *n* : XEROSTOMIA

dry out *vb* : to undergo an extended period of withdrawal from alcohol or drug use esp. at a special clinic : DETOXIFY

dry socket *n* : a tooth socket in which after tooth extraction a blood clot fails to form or disintegrates without undergoing organization; *also* : a condition that is marked by the occurrence of such a socket or sockets and that is usu. accompanied by neuralgic pain but without suppuration

Ds *symbol* darmstadtium

DSC *abbr* doctor of surgical chiropody

DTP *abbr* diphtheria, tetanus, pertussis (vaccine)

d.t.'s \ˌdē-'tēz\ *n, pl often cap* **D&T** : DELIRIUM TREMENS

dual–energy X–ray absorptiometry *n* : absorptiometry in which the density or mass of a material (as bone) is measured by comparing the material's absorption of X-rays of two different energies and which is used esp. for determining the mineral content of bone — abbr. *DEXA, DXA*

DUB *abbr* dysfunctional uterine bleeding

dub·ni·um \'düb-nē-əm\ *n* : a short-lived radioactive element that is artificially produced — symbol *Db;* see ELEMENT table

Du·chenne \dü-'shen, də-\ *also* **Du·chenne's** \-'shenz\ *adj* : relating to or being Duchenne muscular dystrophy
　　Du·chenne \dǖ-'shen\, **Guillaume–Benjamin–Amand** (1806–1875), French neurologist.

Duchenne dystrophy *also* **Duchenne's dystrophy** *n* : DUCHENNE MUSCULAR DYSTROPHY

Duchenne muscular dystrophy *also* **Duchenne's muscular dystrophy** *n* : a severe progressive form of muscular dystrophy of males that appears in early childhood, affects the muscles of the legs before those of the arms, is inherited as an X-linked recessive trait, is characterized by complete absence of the protein dystrophin, and usu. has a fatal outcome by age 20 — abbr. *DMD;* see BECKER MUSCULAR DYSTROPHY

Du·crey's bacillus \dü-'krāz-\ *n* : a gram-negative bacillus of the genus *Haemophilus* (*H. ducreyi*) that is the causative agent of chancroid
　　Du·crey \dü-'krā\, **Augusto** (1860–1940), Italian dermatologist.

duct \'dəkt\ *n* : a bodily tube or vessel esp. when carrying the secretion of a gland

duc·tal \'dək-tᵊl\ *adj* : of or belonging to a duct : made up of ducts

ductal carcinoma in situ *n* : any of a histologically variable group of precancerous or early carcinomas of the lactiferous ducts that have the potential of becoming invasive and spreading to other tissues — abbr. *DCIS*

duc·tion \'dək-shən\ *n* : a turning or rotating movement of the eye

duct·less \'dəkt-ləs\ *adj* : being without a duct

ductless gland *n* : ENDOCRINE GLAND

duct of Bel·li·ni \-be-'lē-nē\ *n* : any of the large excretory ducts of the uriniferous tubules of the kidney that open on the free surface of the papillae
　　Bellini, Lorenzo (1643–1704), Italian anatomist and physiologist.

duct of Gart·ner \-'gärt-nər\ *n* : GARTNER'S DUCT

duct of Ri·vi·nus \-rə-'vē-nəs\ *n* : any of several small inconstant efferent ducts of the sublingual gland
　　Rivinus, Augustus Quirinus (1652–1723), German anatomist and botanist.

duct of San·to·ri·ni \-ˌsan-tə-'rē-nē, -ˌsän-\ *n* : ACCESSORY PANCREATIC DUCT
　　Santorini, Giovanni Domenico (1681–1737), Italian anatomist.

duct of Wir·sung \-'vir-(₁)zùŋ, -zəŋ\ *n* : PANCREATIC DUCT a

Wirsung, Johann Georg (1600–1643), German anatomist.

duct·ule \'dək-(₁)tyül\ *n* : a small duct

duc·tu·li ef·fe·ren·tes \'dək-tyù-₁lī-₁ef-ə-'ren-(₁)tēz, -tù-, -(₁)lē-\ *n pl* : a group of ducts that convey sperm from the testis to the epididymis

duc·tu·lus \'dək-tyù-ləs, -tù-\ *n, pl* **-li** \-₁lī, -(₁)lē\ : DUCTULE

duc·tus \'dək-təs\ *n, pl* **ductus** : DUCT

ductus ar·te·ri·o·sus \-är-₁tir-ē-'ō-səs\ *n* : a short broad vessel in the fetus that connects the pulmonary artery with the aorta and conducts most of the blood directly from the right ventricle to the aorta bypassing the lungs

ductus de·fer·ens \-'de-fə-₁renz, -rənz\ *n, pl* **ductus de·fer·en·tes** \-₁de-fə-'ren-tēz\ : VAS DEFERENS

ductus re·uni·ens \-rē-'yü-nē-₁enz, -'ü-\ *n* : a passage in the ear that connects the cochlea and the saccule

ductus ve·no·sus \-vi-'nō-səs\ *n* : a vein passing through the liver and connecting the left umbilical vein with the inferior vena cava of the fetus, losing its circulatory function after birth, and persisting as the ligamentum venosum of the liver

Duf·fy \'də-fē\ *adj* : relating to, characteristic of, or being a system of blood groups determined by the presence or absence of any of several antigens in red blood cells ⟨~ blood typing⟩

Duffy, Richard (1906–1956), British hemophiliac.

Dührs·sen's incisions \'dǖr-sənz-\ *n pl* : a set of three incisions in the cervix of the uterus to facilitate delivery if dilation is inadequate

Dührs·sen \'dǖr-sən\, Alfred (1862–1933), German obstetrician-gynecologist.

dull \'dəl\ *adj* **1** : mentally slow or stupid **2** : slow in perception or sensibility **3** : lacking sharpness or edge or point ⟨a ~ scalpel⟩ **4** : lacking in force, intensity, or acuteness ⟨a ~ pain⟩ — **dull** *vb* — **dull·ness** *or* **dul·ness** \'dəl-nəs\ *n* — **dul·ly** *adv*

dumb \'dəm\ *adj, often offensive* : lacking the ability to speak

dumb rabies *n* : PARALYTIC RABIES

dum·dum fever \'dəm-₁dəm-\ *n* : KALA-AZAR

¹dum·my \'də-mē\ *n, pl* **dummies** : PLACEBO

²dummy *adj* : being a placebo ⟨a ~ pill⟩

dump·ing syndrome \'dəm-piŋ-\ *n* : a condition characterized by weakness, dizziness, flushing and warmth, nausea, and palpitation immediately after or shortly after eating and produced by abnormally rapid emptying of the stomach esp. in persons who have had part of the stomach removed

duoden- *or* **duodeno-** *comb form* **1** : duodenum ⟨*duoden*itis⟩ **2** : duodenal and ⟨*duodeno*jejunal⟩

du·o·de·nal ulcer \₁dü-ə-'dēn-°l-, ₁dyü-; dù-'äd-°n-əl-, dyù-\ *n* : a peptic ulcer situated in the duodenum

du·o·de·ni·tis \dù-₁äd-°n-'ī-təs, dyù-\ *n* : inflammation of the duodenum

du·o·de·no·cho·led·o·chot·o·my \dù-₁äd-°n-ō-kə-₁le-də-'kä-tə-mē, dyù-\ *n, pl* **-mies** : choledochotomy performed by approach through the duodenum by incision

du·o·de·nog·ra·phy \dù-₁äd-°n-'ä-grə-fē, dyù-\ *n, pl* **-phies** : radiographic visualization of the duodenum with a contrast medium

du·o·de·no·je·ju·nal \dù-₁äd-°n-ō-ji-'jün-°l, dyù-\ *adj* : of, relating to, or joining the duodenum and the jejunum

du·o·de·no·je·ju·nos·to·my \-ji-jü-'näs-tə-mē\ *n, pl* **-mies** : a surgical operation that joins part of the duodenum and the jejunum with creation of an artificial opening between them

du·o·de·not·o·my \dù-₁äd-°n-'ä-tə-mē, dyù-\ *n, pl* **-mies** : incision of the duodenum

du·o·de·num \₁dü-ə-'dē-nəm, ₁dyü-; dù-'äd-°n-əm, dyù-\ *n, pl* **-de·na** \-°n-ə, -'ēn-ə\ *or* **-de·nums** : the first, shortest, and widest part of the small intestine that in humans is about 10 inches (25 centimeters) long and that extends from the pylorus to the undersurface of the liver where it descends for a variable distance and receives the bile and pancreatic ducts and then bends to the left and finally upward to join the jejunum near the second lumbar vertebra — **du·o·de·nal** \-'dēn-°l, -°n-əl\ *adj*

du·plex \'dü-₁pleks, 'dyü-\ *n* : a molecule having two complementary polynucleotide strands of DNA or of RNA — **duplex** *adj*

du·pli·cate \'dü-pli-₁kāt, 'dyü-\ *vb* **-cat·ed; -cat·ing** : to become duplicate : REPLICATE

du·pli·ca·tion \₁dü-pli-'kā-shən, ₁dyü-\ *n* **1** : the act or process of duplicating : the quality or state of being duplicated **2** : a part of a chromosome in which the genetic material is repeated; *also* : the process of forming a duplication

Du·puy·tren's contracture \də-₁pwē-'trä°z-, -'pwē-trənz-\ *n* : a condition marked by fibrosis with shortening and thickening of the palmar aponeurosis resulting in flexion contracture of the fingers into the palm of the hand

Du·puy·tren \də-pwē-'trä°\, Guillaume (1777–1835), French surgeon.

dura — see LAMINA DURA

du·ral \'dùr-əl, 'dyùr-\ *adj* : of or relating to the dura mater

dural sinus *n* : SINUS OF THE DURA MATER

du·ra ma·ter \'dùr-ə-₁mä-tər, 'dyùr-, -₁mä-\ *n* : the tough fibrous membrane lined with endothelium on the inner surface that envelops the brain and spinal cord external to the arachnoid and pia mater, that in the cranium closely lines the bone and contains numerous blood vessels and venous sinuses, and that in the spinal cord is separated from the bone by a considerable space and contains no venous sinuses — called also *dura*

dust cell *n* : a pulmonary macrophage that takes up and eliminates foreign particles introduced into the lung alveoli with inspired air

dust·ing powder \'dəs-tiŋ-\ *n* : a powder used on the skin or on wounds esp. for allaying irritation or absorbing moisture

dust mite *n* : any of various mites (esp. family Pyroglyphidae) commonly found in dust; *esp* : HOUSE-DUST MITE

Dutch cap *n* : CERVICAL CAP

DV *abbr* daily value

DVM *abbr* doctor of veterinary medicine

DVT *abbr* deep vein thrombosis

¹**dwarf** \'dworf\ *n, pl* **dwarfs** \'dworfs\ *also* **dwarves** \'dworvz\ *often attrib* **1** : a person of unusually small stature; *esp* : one whose bodily proportions are abnormal **2** : an animal much below normal size

²**dwarf** *vb* : to restrict the growth of

dwarf·ism \'dwor-ˌfi-zəm\ *n* : the condition of stunted growth

Dx *abbr* diagnosis

DXA *abbr* dual-energy X-ray absorptiometry

Dy *symbol* dysprosium

dy·ad \'dī-ˌad, -əd\ *n* : a meiotic chromosome after separation of the two homologous members of a tetrad

Dy·a·zide \'dī-ə-ˌzīd\ *trademark* — used for a preparation of hydrochlorothiazide and triamterene

dy·dro·ges·ter·one \ˌdī-drō-'jes-tə-ˌrōn\ *n* : a synthetic progestational agent $C_{21}H_{28}O_2$ — called also *isopregnenone*

dying *pres part of* DIE

-dynamia *n comb form* : strength : condition of having (such) strength ⟨adynamia⟩

dy·nam·ic \dī-'na-mik\ *also* **dy·nam·i·cal** \-mi-kəl\ *adj* **1 a** : of or relating to physical force or energy **b** : of or relating to dynamics **2** : FUNCTIONAL 1b ⟨a ~ disease⟩ — **dy·nam·i·cal·ly** \-mi-k(ə-)lē\ *adv*

dy·nam·ics \dī-'na-miks\ *n sing or pl* **1** : a branch of mechanics that deals with forces and their relation primarily to the motion but sometimes also to the equilibrium of bodies **2** : PSYCHODYNAMICS **3** : the pattern of change or growth of an object or phenomenon ⟨personality ~⟩

dy·na·mom·e·ter \ˌdī-nə-'mä-mə-tər\ *n* : an instrument for measuring the force of muscular contraction esp. of the hand

dyne \'dīn\ *n* : the unit of force in the

cgs system equal to the force that would give a free mass of one gram an acceleration of one centimeter per second per second

dy·nein \'dī-ˌnēn, -ˌnē-ən\ *n* : an ATPase that regulates the movement of cellular organelles and structures (as cilia and chromosomes) by controlling the motion of microtubules

dy·nor·phin \dī-'nor-fən\ *n* : any of a group of potent opioid peptides found in the mammalian central nervous system

dy·phyl·line \dī-'fi-ˌlēn\ *n* : a theophylline derivative $C_{10}H_{14}N_4O_4$ used as a diuretic and for its bronchodilator and peripheral vasodilator effects

dys- *prefix* **1** : abnormal ⟨*dys*plasia⟩ **2** : difficult ⟨*dys*pnea⟩ **3** : impaired ⟨*dys*function⟩

dys·aes·the·sia *chiefly Brit var of* DYSESTHESIA

dys·ar·thria \dis-'är-thrē-ə\ *n* : difficulty in articulating words due to disease of the central nervous system — compare DYSPHASIA — **dys·ar·thric** \-thrik\ *adj*

dys·ar·thro·sis \ˌdis-ˌär-'thrō-səs\ *n, pl* **-thro·ses** \-ˌsēz\ **1** : a condition of reduced joint motion due to deformity, dislocation, or disease **2** : DYSARTHRIA

dys·au·to·no·mia \ˌdis-ˌȯ-tə-'nō-mē-ə\ *n* : a disorder of the autonomic nervous system that causes disturbances in all or some autonomic functions and may result from the course of a disease (as diabetes) or from injury or poisoning; *esp* : FAMILIAL DYSAUTONOMIA — **dys·au·to·nom·ic** \-'nä-mik\ *adj*

dys·ba·rism \'dis-bə-ˌri-zəm\ *n* : the complex of symptoms (as the bends or headache) that accompanies exposure to excessively low or rapidly changing environmental air pressure

dys·cal·cu·lia \ˌdis-ˌkal-'kyü-lē-ə\ *n* : impairment of mathematical ability due to an organic condition of the brain

dys·che·zia \dis-'kē-zē-ə, -'ke-, -zhə, -zhē-ə\ *n* : constipation associated with a defective reflex for defecation

dys·chon·dro·pla·sia \ˌdis-ˌkän-drō-'plā-zhə, -zhē-ə\ *n* : CHONDRODYSPLASIA

dys·cra·sia \dis-'krā-zhə, -zhē-ə\ *n* : an abnormal condition of the body; *esp* : an imbalance of components of the blood

dys·di·ad·o·cho·ki·ne·sia *or* **dys·di·ad·o·ko·ki·ne·sia** \ˌdis-ˌdī-ˌa-də-ˌkō-kī-'nē-zhə, -zhē-ə\ *n* : impairment of the ability to make movements exhibiting a rapid change of motion that is caused by cerebellar dysfunction — compare ADIADOKOKINESIS

dys·en·ter·ic \ˌdis-ᵊn-'ter-ik\ *adj* : of or relating to dysentery

dys·en·tery \'dis-ᵊn-ˌter-ē\ *n, pl* **-ter·ies** **1** : a disease characterized by severe diarrhea with passage of mucus and blood and usu. caused by infection **2** : DIARRHEA

dys·es·the·sia \ˌdis-es-ˈthē-zh(ē)ə, -zhē-ə\ *n* : impairment of sensitivity esp. to touch — **dys·es·thet·ic** \-ˈthet-ik\ *adj*

dys·func·tion *also* **dis·func·tion** \(ˈ)dis-ˈfəŋk-shən\ *n* : impaired or abnormal functioning (as of an organ of the body) — **dys·func·tion·al** \-shnəl, -shən-ᵊl\ *adj* — **dys·func·tion·ing** \-shə-niŋ\ *n*

dysfunctional uterine bleeding *n* : abnormal uterine bleeding that is not associated with a physical lesion (as a tumor), inflammation, or pregnancy — abbr. *DUB*

dys·gam·ma·glob·u·li·ne·mia \ˌdis-ˌga-mə-ˌglä-byə-lə-ˈnē-mē-ə\ *n* : a disorder involving abnormality in structure or frequency of gamma globulins — compare AGAMMAGLOBULINEMIA

dys·gen·e·sis \(ˌ)dis-ˈje-nə-səs\ *n, pl* **-e·ses** \-ˌsēz\ : defective development esp. of the gonads (as in Klinefelter's syndrome or Turner's syndrome)

dys·ger·mi·no·ma \ˌdis-ˌjər-mə-ˈnō-mə\ *n, pl* **-mas** *also* **-ma·ta** \-mə-tə\ : a germinoma of the ovary

dys·geu·sia \(ˌ)dis-ˈgü-zē-ə, -ˈgyü-, -zhə, -zhē-ə\ *n* : dysfunction of the sense of taste

dys·graph·ia \(ˌ)dis-ˈgra-fē-ə\ *n* : impairment of the ability to write caused by brain damage

dys·hi·dro·sis \ˌdis-ˌhī-ˈdrō-səs, -hə-\ *n, pl* **-dro·ses** \-ˌsēz\ : POMPHOLYX

dys·kary·o·sis \ˌdis-ˌkar-ē-ˈō-səs\ *n, pl* **-o·ses** \-ˌsēz\ *or* **-o·sis·es** : abnormality esp. of exfoliated cells (as from the uterine cervix) that affects the nucleus but not the cytoplasm

dys·ker·a·to·sis \ˌdis-ˌker-ə-ˈtō-səs\ *n, pl* **-to·ses** \-ˌsēz\ : faulty development of the epidermis with abnormal keratinization — **dys·ker·a·tot·ic** \-ˈtä-tik\ *adj*

dys·ki·ne·sia \ˌdis-kə-ˈnē-zhə, -kī-, -zhē-ə\ *n* : impairment of voluntary movements resulting in fragmented or jerky motions (as in Parkinson's disease) — see TARDIVE DYSKINESIA — **dys·ki·net·ic** \-ˈne-tik\ *adj*

dyskinetic cerebral palsy *n* : ATHETOID CEREBRAL PALSY

dys·lec·tic \dis-ˈlek-tik\ *adj or n* : DYSLEXIC

dys·lex·ia \dis-ˈlek-sē-ə\ *n* : a variable often familial learning disability involving difficulties in acquiring and processing language that is typically manifested by a lack of proficiency in reading, spelling, and writing

¹**dys·lex·ic** \-ˈlek-sik\ *adj* : affected with dyslexia

²**dyslexic** *n* : a dyslexic person

dys·lip·id·emia \dis-ˌli-pə-ˈdē-mē-ə\ *n* : a condition marked by abnormal concentrations of lipids or lipoproteins in the blood — **dys·lip·id·emic** \-mik\ *adj*

dys·men·or·rhea \(ˌ)dis-ˌme-nə-ˈrē-ə\ *n* : painful menstruation — **dys·men·or·rhe·ic** \-ˈrē-ik\ *adj*

dys·met·ria \dis-ˈme-trē-ə\ *n* : impaired ability to estimate distance in muscular action

dys·mor·phia \-ˈmȯr-fē-ə\ *n* **1** : DYSMORPHISM **2** : BODY DYSMORPHIC DISORDER — **dys·mor·phic** \-fik\ *adj*

dys·mor·phism \-ˈmȯr-ˌfi-zəm\ *n* : an anatomical malformation

dys·mor·phol·o·gy \-mȯr-ˈfä-lə-jē\ *n* : a branch of clinical medicine concerned with human teratology — **dys·mor·phol·o·gist** \-jist\ *n*

dys·os·mia \di-ˈsäz-mē-ə, -ˈsäs-\ *n* : dysfunction of the sense of smell

dys·os·to·sis \ˌdi-ˌsäs-ˈtō-səs\ *n, pl* **-ses** \-ˌsēz\ : defective formation of bone — **dys·os·tot·ic** \-ˈtä-tik\ *adj*

dys·pa·reu·nia \ˌdis-pə-ˈrü-nē-ə, -nyə\ *n* : difficult or painful sexual intercourse

dys·pep·sia \dis-ˈpep-shə, -sē-ə\ *n* : INDIGESTION

¹**dys·pep·tic** \-ˈpep-tik\ *adj* : relating to or having dyspepsia

²**dyspeptic** *n* : a person having dyspepsia

dys·pha·gia \dis-ˈfā-jə, -jē-ə\ *n* : difficulty in swallowing — **dys·phag·ic** \-ˈfa-jik\ *adj*

dys·pha·sia \dis-ˈfā-zhə, -zhē-ə\ *n* : loss of or deficiency in the power to use or understand language as a result of injury to or disease of the brain — compare DYSARTHRIA

¹**dys·pha·sic** \-ˈfā-zik\ *adj* : relating to or affected with dysphasia

²**dysphasic** *n* : a dysphasic person

dys·pho·nia \dis-ˈfō-nē-ə\ *n* : defective use of the voice

dys·pho·ria \dis-ˈfōr-ē-ə\ *n* : a state of feeling unwell or unhappy — compare EUPHORIA — **dys·phor·ic** \-ˈfȯr-ik, -ˈfär-\ *adj*

dys·pla·sia \dis-ˈplā-zhə, -zhē-ə\ *n* : abnormal growth or development (as of organs or cells); *broadly* : abnormal anatomic structure due to such growth — **dys·plas·tic** \-ˈplas-tik\ *adj*

dys·pnea \ˈdis-nē-ə, ˈdisp-\ *n* : difficult or labored respiration — compare EUPNEA — **dys·pne·ic** \-nē-ik\ *adj*

dys·pnoea *chiefly Brit var of* DYSPNEA

dys·prax·ia \dis-ˈprak-sē-ə, -ˈprak-shə, -shē-ə\ *n* : impairment of the ability to perform coordinated movements — **dys·prax·ic** \-sik\ *adj*

dys·pro·si·um \dis-ˈprō-zē-əm, -zhəm, -zhē-əm\ *n* : an element that forms highly magnetic compounds — symbol *Dy*; see ELEMENT table

dys·pro·tein·ae·mia *chiefly Brit var of* DYSPROTEINEMIA

dys·pro·tein·emia \ˌdis-ˌprōt-ᵊn-ˈē-mē-ə, -ˌprō-ˌtē-ˈnē-, -ˌprōt-ē-ə-ˈnē-\ *n* : any abnormality of the protein content of the blood — **dys·pro·tein·emic** \-mik\ *adj*

dys·ra·phism \dis-ˈrā-ˌfi-zəm\ *n* : incomplete fusion of parts; *esp* : defective closure of the neural tube ⟨spinal ∼⟩

dys·reg·u·la·tion \ˌdis-ˌre-gyə-'lā-shən\ *n* : impairment of regulatory mechanisms (as those governing metabolism or organ function) — **dys·reg·u·lat·ed** \-'re-gyə-ˌlā-təd\ *adj*

dys·rhyth·mia \dis-'rith-mē-ə\ *n* 1 : an abnormal rhythm; *esp* : a disordered rhythm exhibited in a record of electrical activity of the brain or heart 2 : JET LAG — **dys·rhyth·mic** \-mik\ *adj*

dys·syn·er·gia \ˌdis-sə-'nər-jə, -jē-ə\ *n* : DYSKINESIA — **dys·syn·er·gic** \-'nər-jik\ *adj*

dys·thy·mia \dis-'thī-mē-ə\ *n* : a mood disorder characterized by chronic mildly depressed or irritable mood often accompanied by other symptoms (as eating and sleeping disturbances, and poor self-esteem) — **dys·thy·mic** \-mik\ *adj or n*

dysthymic disorder *n* : DYSTHYMIA

dys·to·cia \dis-'tō-shə, -shē-ə\ *or* **dys·to·kia** \-'tō-kē-ə\ *n* : slow or difficult labor or delivery

dys·to·nia mus·cu·lo·rum de·for·mans \-ˌməs-kyə-'lȯr-əm-di-'fȯr-ˌmanz\ *n* : a

rare inherited neurological disorder characterized by progressive muscular spasticity causing severe involuntary contortions esp. of the trunk and limbs — called also *torsion dystonia*

dys·tro·phic \dis-'trō-fik\ *adj* 1 : relating to or caused by faulty nutrition 2 : relating to or affected with a dystrophy ⟨∼ muscles⟩ 3 a : occurring at sites of damaged or necrotic tissue ⟨∼ calcification⟩ b : characterized by disordered growth ⟨∼ nails⟩

dystrophica — see MYOTONIA DYSTROPHICA

dystrophic epidermolysis bullosa *n* : any of several inherited forms of epidermolysis bullosa that are marked esp. by blister formation between the basement membrane and lamina propria

dys·tro·phin \'dis-trə-ˌfin\ *n* : a protein that is absent in Duchenne muscular dystrophy and deficient or of abnormal molecular weight in Becker muscular dystrophy

dys·tro·phy \'dis-trə-fē\ *n, pl* **-phies** 1 : a condition produced by faulty nutrition 2 : any myogenic atrophy; *esp* : MUSCULAR DYSTROPHY

dys·uria \dis-'yūr-ē-ə\ *n* : difficult or painful discharge of urine — **dys·uric** \-'yūr-ik\ *adj*

E

e- *prefix* : missing : absent ⟨edentulous⟩

EAE *abbr* experimental allergic encephalomyelitis

ear \'ir\ *n* 1 : the vertebrate organ of hearing and equilibrium consisting in most mammals of a sound-collecting outer ear separated from a sound-transmitting middle ear that in turn is separated from a sensory inner ear by membranous fenestrae 2 a : the external ear of humans and most mammals b : a human earlobe — **eared** \'ird\ *adj*

ear·ache \'ir-ˌāk\ *n* : an ache or pain in the ear — called also *otalgia*

ear·drum \-ˌdrəm\ *n* : TYMPANIC MEMBRANE

ear·lobe \'ir-ˌlōb\ *n* : the pendent part of the ear esp. of humans

ear mange *n* : canker of the ear esp. in cats and dogs that is caused by mites; *esp* : OTODECTIC MANGE

ear mite *n* : any of various mites attacking the ears of mammals

ear·mold \'ir-ˌmōld\ *n* : a device that fits within the outer ear, is connected by way of a tube to a hearing aid worn behind the ear, and serves esp. to channel the amplified sound from the hearing aid to the ear canal

ear pick *n* : a device for removing wax or foreign bodies from the ear

ear·piece \'ir-ˌpēs\ *n* 1 : a part of an instrument (as a stethoscope) that is inserted into the outer opening of the ear 2 : one of the two sidepieces that support eyeglasses by passing over or behind the ears

ear·plug \-ˌpləg\ *n* : a device of pliable material for insertion into the outer opening of the ear (as to keep out water or deaden sound)

ear tick *n* : any of several ticks infesting the ears of mammals; *esp* : SPINOSE EAR TICK

ear·wax \'ir-ˌwaks\ *n* : the yellow waxy secretion from the glands of the external ear — called also *cerumen*

east coast fever *n* : an acute fatal febrile disease of cattle that occurs in Africa and is caused by a protozoan of the genus *Theileria* (*T. parva*) transmitted by ticks esp. of the genera *Rhipicephalus* and *Hyalomma*

eastern equine encephalitis *n* : EQUINE ENCEPHALITIS a

eastern equine encephalomyelitis *n* : EQUINE ENCEPHALITIS a

eating disorder *n* : any of several psychological disorders (as anorexia nervosa or bulimia) characterized by serious disturbances of eating behavior

Ea·ton agent \'ēt-ᵊn-\ n : a bacterium of the genus *Mycoplasma* (*M. pneumoniae*) that is the causative agent of primary atypical pneumonia.

Eaton, Monroe Davis (*b* 1904), American microbiologist.

Eaton–Lambert syndrome n : LAMBERT-EATON SYNDROME

Ebo·la \i-'bō-lə, ē-\ n 1 : EBOLA VIRUS 2 : the hemorrhagic fever caused by the Ebola virus — called also *Ebola fever*

Ebola virus n : any of several filoviruses (esp. species *Zaire ebolavirus* of the genus *Ebolavirus*) of African origin that cause an often fatal hemorrhagic fever

eb·ur·nat·ed \'e-bər-ˌnā-təd, 'ē-\ adj : hard and dense like ivory 〈~ cartilage〉 〈~ bone〉 — **eb·ur·na·tion** \ˌe-bər-'nā-shən, ˌē-\ n

EBV abbr Epstein-Barr virus

EB virus \ˌē-'bē-\ n : EPSTEIN-BARR VIRUS

ec- prefix : out of : outside of : outside 〈*eccrine*〉

eccentric hypertrophy n : hypertrophy of the wall of a hollow organ and esp. the heart with dilatation of its cavity

ec·chon·dro·ma \ˌe-kən-'drō-mə\ n, pl **-ma·ta** \-mə-tə\ also **-mas** : a cartilaginous tumor projecting from bone or cartilage

ec·chy·mo·sis \ˌe-kə-'mō-səs\ n, pl **-mo·ses** \-ˌsēz\ : the escape of blood into the tissues from ruptured blood vessels marked by a livid black-and-blue or purple spot or area; also : the discoloration so caused — **ec·chy·mosed** \'e-kə-ˌmōzd, -ˌmōst\ adj — **ec·chy·mot·ic** \-'mä-tik\ adj

ec·crine \'e-krən, -ˌkrīn, -ˌkrēn\ adj : of, relating to, having, or being eccrine glands — compare APOCRINE, HOLOCRINE, MEROCRINE

eccrine gland n : any of the rather small sweat glands that produce a fluid secretion without removing cytoplasm from the secreting cells and that are restricted to the human skin — called also *eccrine sweat gland*

ECG abbr electrocardiogram

Echid·noph·a·ga \ˌek-(ˌ)id-'nä-fə-gə\ n : a genus of fleas (family Pulicidae) including the sticktight flea (*E. gallinacea*

ech·i·na·cea \ˌe-ki-'nā-sē-ə, -shə\ n : the dried root or other part of any of three herbs (*Echinacea angustifolia*, *E. pallida*, and *E. purpurea*) that are used chiefly in dietary supplements and herbal remedies and that are held to stimulate the immune system; also : any of these herbs

echi·no·coc·co·sis \i-ˌkī-nə-kä-'kō-səs\ n, pl **-co·ses** \-ˌsēz\ : infestation with or disease caused by a tapeworm of the genus *Echinococcus*; esp : HYDATID DISEASE

echi·no·coc·cus \-nə-'kä-kəs\ n 1 cap : a genus of taeniid tapeworms (as *E. granulosus* and *E. multilocularis*) that alternate a minute adult living in a harmless commensal in the intestine of dogs and other carnivores with a hydatid larva invading tissues esp. of the liver of mammals (as cattle, sheep, swine, and humans) and acting as a serious often fatal pathogen — see HYDATID DISEASE 2 pl **-coc·ci** \-'kä-ˌkī, -ˌkē; -'käk-ˌsī, -ˌsē\ : any tapeworm of the genus *Echinococcus*; also : HYDATID 1

echo abbr — echocardiogram; echocardiography

echo·car·dio·gram \ˌe-kō-'kär-dē-ə-ˌgram\ n : a visual record made by echocardiography; also : the procedure for producing such a record

echo·car·di·og·ra·phy \ˌ-ˌkär-dē-'ä-grə-fē\ n, pl **-phies** : the use of ultrasound to examine and measure the structure and functioning of the heart and to diagnose abnormalities and disease — **echo·car·dio·graph·er** \-grə-fər\ n — **echo·car·dio·graph·ic** \-dē-ə-'gra-fik\ adj

echo·en·ceph·a·lo·gram \ˌe-kō-in-'se-fə-lə-ˌgram\ n : a visual record obtained by echoencephalography

echo·en·ceph·a·log·ra·phy \-in-ˌse-fə-'lä-grə-fē\ n, pl **-phies** : the use of ultrasound to examine and measure internal structures (as the ventricles) of the skull and to diagnose abnormalities and disease — **echo·en·ceph·a·lo·graph·ic** \-fə-lə-'gra-fik\ adj

echo·gen·ic \ˌe-kə-'je-nik\ adj : reflecting ultrasound waves — **echo·ge·nic·i·ty** \-jə-'ni-sə-tē\ n

echo·gram \'e-kō-ˌgram\ n : SONOGRAM

echo·graph \-ˌgraf\ n : an instrument used for echography

echog·ra·phy \i-'kä-grə-fē\ n, pl **-phies** : ULTRASOUND 2 — **echo·graph·ic** \ˌe-kō-'gra-fik\ adj — **echo·graph·i·cal·ly** \-fi-k(ə-)lē\ adv

echo·la·lia \ˌe-kō-'lā-lē-ə\ n : the often pathological repetition of what is said by other people as if echoing them — **echo·lal·ic** \-'la-lik\ adj

echo·prax·ia \ˌe-kō-'prak-sē-ə\ n : pathological repetition of the actions of other people as if echoing them

echo·thi·o·phate iodide \'thī-ə-ˌfāt-\ n : a long-acting anticholinesterase $C_9H_{23}INO_3PS$ used esp. to reduce intraocular pressure in the treatment of glaucoma — called also *echothiophate*

echo·vi·rus \'e-kō-ˌvī-rəs\ n : any of numerous serotypes of a picornavirus of the genus *Enterovirus* (species *Human enterovirus B*) that are found in the gastrointestinal tract and are sometimes associated with respiratory ailments and meningitis

ec·lamp·sia \i-'klamp-sē-ə, e-\ n : a convulsive state : an attack of convulsions: as **a** : convulsions or coma late in pregnancy in an individual affected with preeclampsia **b** : a condition comparable to milk fever of cows occurring in domestic animals (as dogs and cats) — **ec·lamp·tic** \-tik\ *adj*

E. coli \ˌē-ˈkō-ˌlī\ *n, pl* **E. coli** *also* **E. colis** : a straight rod-shaped gramnegative bacterium (*Escherichia coli* of the family Enterobacteriaceae) occurring in various strains that may live as harmless inhabitants of the human lower intestine or may produce a toxin causing intestinal illness marked esp. by diarrhea

ecol·o·gy \i-ˈkä-lə-jē, e-\ *n, pl* **-gies 1** : a branch of science concerned with the interrelationship of organisms and their environments **2** : the totality or pattern of relations between organisms and their environment **3** : HUMAN ECOLOGY — **eco·log·i·cal** \ˌē-kə-ˈlä-ji-kəl, ˌe-\ *also* **eco·log·ic** \-jik\ *adj* — **eco·log·i·cal·ly** \-ji-k(ə-)lē\ *adv* — **ecol·o·gist** \i-ˈkä-lə-jist, e-\ *n*

eco·sys·tem \ˈē-kō-ˌsis-təm, ˈe-\ *n* : the complex of a community and its environment functioning as an ecological unit in nature

écra·seur \ˌā-krä-ˈzər, ˌē-\ *n* : a surgical instrument used to encircle and sever a projecting mass of tissue

ec·sta·sy \ˈek-stə-sē\ *n, pl* **-sies 1** : a trance state in which intense absorption is accompanied by loss of sense perception and voluntary control **2** *often cap* : a synthetic amphetamine analog $C_{11}H_{15}NO_2$ used illicitly for its mood-enhancing and hallucinogenic properties — called also *methylene dioxymethamphetamine, MDMA* — **ec·stat·ic** \ek-ˈsta-tik\ *adj*

ECT *abbr* electroconvulsive therapy

ec·ta·sia \ek-ˈtā-zhē-ə, -zhə\ *n* : the expansion of a hollow or tubular organ — **ec·tat·ic** \ek-ˈta-tik\ *adj*

ec·ta·sis \ek-tə-səs\ *n, pl* **-ta·ses** \-ˌsēz\ : ECTASIA

ec·thy·ma \ek-ˈthī-mə\ *n* **1** : a cutaneous eruption marked by large flat pustules that have a hardened base surrounded by inflammation and occur esp. on the lower legs **2** : sore mouth of sheep — **ec·thy·ma·tous** \ek-ˈthī-mə-təs, -ˈthī-\ *adj*

ecto- *also* **ect-** *comb form* : outside : external ⟨*ectoderm*⟩

ec·to·derm \-ˌdərm\ *n* **1** : the outermost of the three primary germ layers of an embryo **2** : a tissue (as neural tissue) derived from ectoderm — **ec·to·der·mal** \ˌek-tə-ˈdər-məl\ *adj*

ec·to·en·zyme \ˌek-tō-ˈen-ˌzīm\ *n* : an enzyme acting outside the cell

ec·to·mor·phic \ˌek-tə-ˈmȯr-fik\ *adj* : having a light lean body build — compare ENDOMORPHIC, MESOMORPHIC — **ec·to·morph** \ˈek-tə-ˌmȯrf\ *n* — **ec·to·mor·phy** \ˈek-tə-ˌmȯr-fē\ *n*

-ec·to·my \ˈek-tə-mē\ *n comb form, pl* **-ec·to·mies** : surgical removal ⟨append*ectomy*⟩

ec·to·par·a·site \ˌek-tō-ˈpar-ə-ˌsīt\ *n* : a parasite that lives on the exterior of its host — compare ENDOPARASITE — **ec·to·par·a·sit·ic** \-ˌpar-ə-ˈsi-tik\ *adj*

ec·to·pia \ek-ˈtō-pē-ə\ *n* : an abnormal congenital or acquired position of an organ or part ⟨∼ of the heart⟩

ec·top·ic \ek-ˈtä-pik\ *adj* **1** : occurring in an abnormal position ⟨an ∼ kidney⟩ **2** : originating in an area of the heart other than the sinoatrial node ⟨∼ beats⟩; *also* : initiating ectopic heartbeats ⟨an ∼ pacemaker⟩ — **ec·top·i·cal·ly** \-pi-k(ə-)lē\ *adv*

ectopic pregnancy *n* : gestation elsewhere than in the uterus (as in a fallopian tube or in the peritoneal cavity) — called also *ectopic gestation, extrauterine pregnancy*

ec·to·pla·cen·ta \ˌek-tō-plə-ˈsen-tə\ *n* : TROPHOBLAST — **ec·to·pla·cen·tal** \-ˈsent-ᵊl\ *adj*

ec·to·plasm \ˈek-tə-ˌpla-zəm\ *n* : the outer relatively rigid granule-free layer of the cytoplasm — compare ENDOPLASM

ec·to·py \ˈek-tə-pē\ *n, pl* **-pies** : ECTOPIA

ectro- *comb form* : congenitally absent — usu. indicating absence of a particular part or part ⟨*ectro*dactyly⟩

ec·tro·dac·ty·ly \-ˈdak-tə-lē\ *n, pl* **-lies** : congenital complete or partial absence of one or more digits

ec·tro·me·lia \ˌek-trō-ˈmē-lē-ə\ *n* **1** : congenital absence or imperfection of one or more limbs **2** : MOUSEPOX

ec·tro·pi·on \ek-ˈtrō-pē-ˌän, -ən\ *n* : an abnormal turning out of a part (as an eyelid)

ec·ze·ma \ig-ˈzē-mə, ˈeg-zə-mə, ˈek-sə-\ *n* : an inflammatory condition of the skin characterized by redness, itching, and oozing vesicular lesions which become scaly, crusted, or hardened — **ec·zem·a·tous** \ig-ˈze-mə-təs\ *adj*

ec·ze·ma·toid \ig-ˈzē-mə-ˌtȯid, -ˈze-\ *adj* : resembling eczema

ED *abbr* **1** effective dose **2** emergency department **3** erectile dysfunction

EDB *abbr* ethylene dibromide

ede·ma \i-ˈdē-mə\ *n, pl* **-mas** *also* **-ma·ta** \-mə-tə\ : an abnormal excess accumulation of serous fluid in connective tissue or in a serous cavity — called also *dropsy* — **edem·a·tous** \-ˈde-mə-təs\ *adj*

eden·tu·lous \(ˌ)ē-ˈden-chə-ləs\ *adj* : TOOTHLESS ⟨an ∼ upper jaw⟩

edetate — see DISODIUM EDETATE

Ed·ing·er–West·phal nucleus \ˌe-diŋ-ər-ˈwest-ˌfäl-, -ˌfȯl-\ *n* : the lateral portion of the group of nerve cells lying ventral to the aqueduct of Sylvius which give rise to autonomic fibers of the oculomotor nerve

Ed·ing·er \ˈe-diŋ-ər\, **Ludwig** (1855–1918), German neurologist.

West·phal \ˈwest-ˌfäl, -ˌfȯl\, **Carl Friedrich Otto** (1833–1890), German neurologist.

EDR *abbr* electrodermal response

ed·ro·pho·ni·um \ˌe-drə-ˈfō-nē-əm\ *n* : an anticholinesterase $C_{10}H_{16}ClNO$ used esp. to stimulate skeletal muscle and in the diagnosis of myasthenia gravis — called also *edrophonium chloride;* see TENSILON

EDTA \ˌē-(ˌ)dē-(ˌ)tē-ˈā\ *n* : a white crystalline acid $C_{10}H_{16}N_2O_8$ used in medicine as an anticoagulant and as a chelator in the treatment of lead poisoning — called also *ethylenediaminetetraacetic acid*

ed·u·ca·ble \ˈe-jə-kə-bəl\ *adj* : affected with mild mental retardation and capable of developing academic, social, and occupational skills within the capabilities of one with a mental age between 9 and 12 years — compare TRAINABLE

Ed·wards syndrome \ˈed-wərdz-\ *n* : TRISOMY 18

Edwards, John Hilton (b 1928), British geneticist.

EEE *abbr* eastern equine encephalitis; eastern equine encephalomyelitis

EEG *abbr* electroencephalogram; electroencephalograph

EENT *abbr* eye, ear, nose, and throat

ef·face·ment \i-ˈfās-mənt, e-\ *n* : obliteration of the uterine cervix by shortening and softening during labor so that only the external orifice remains — **ef·face** \-ˈfās\ *vb*

ef·fect \i-ˈfekt\ *n* : something that is produced by an agent or cause

ef·fec·tive \i-ˈfek-tiv\ *adj* : producing a decided, decisive, claimed, or desired effect — **ef·fec·tive·ness** *n*

ef·fec·tor \i-ˈfek-tər, -ˌtȯr\ *n* **1** : a bodily organ (as a gland or muscle) that becomes active in response to stimulation **2** : a substance (as an inducer or corepressor) that activates, controls, or inactivates a process or action (as protein synthesis)

¹ef·fer·ent \ˈe-fə-rənt; ˈe-ˌfer-ənt, ˈē-fer-\ *adj* : conducting outward from a part or organ; *specif* : conveying nervous impulses to an effector ⟨∼ neurons⟩ — compare AFFERENT

²efferent *n* : an efferent part (as a blood vessel or nerve fiber)

efferentes — see DUCTULI EFFERENTES

efferentia — see VASA EFFERENTIA

Ef·fex·or \ə-ˈfek-ˌsȯr\ *trademark* — used for a preparation of the hydrochloride of venlafaxine

ef·fleu·rage \ˌe-flə-ˈräzh, -(ˌ)flü-\ *n* : a light stroking movement used in massage

effort syndrome *n* : NEUROCIRCULATORY ASTHENIA

ef·fuse \i-ˈfyüs, e-\ *adj* : spread out flat without definite form

ef·fu·sion \i-ˈfyü-zhən, e-\ *n* **1** : the escape of a fluid from anatomical vessels by rupture or exudation **2** : the fluid that escapes by extravasation — see PLEURAL EFFUSION

eges·tion \i-ˈjes-chən\ *n* : the act or process of discharging undigested or waste material from a cell or organism; *specif* : DEFECATION — **egest** \i-ˈjest\ *vb*

EGF *abbr* epidermal growth factor

egg \ˈeg, ˈāg\ *n* **1** : the hard-shelled reproductive body produced by a bird and esp. by the common domestic chicken (*Gallus gallus*) **2** : an animal reproductive body consisting of an ovum together with its nutritive and protective envelopes and having the capacity to develop into a new individual capable of independent existence **3** : OVUM

egg cell *n* : OVUM

ego \ˈē-(ˌ)gō\ *n, pl* **egos** **1** : the self esp. as contrasted with another self or the world **2** : the one of the three divisions of the psyche in psychoanalytic theory that serves as the organized conscious mediator between the person and reality esp. by functioning both in the perception of and adaptation to reality — compare ¹ID, SUPEREGO

¹ego·cen·tric \ˌē-gō-ˈsen-trik\ *adj* **1** : limited in outlook or concern to one's own activities or needs **2** : being self-centered or selfish — **ego·cen·tri·cal·ly** \-tri-k(ə-)lē\ *adv* — **ego·cen·tric·i·ty** \ˌē-gō-(ˌ)sen-ˈtris-ət-ē, -sən-\ *n* — **ego·cen·trism** \-ˈsen-ˌtri-zəm\ *n*

²egocentric *n* : an egocentric person

ego–defense *n* : DEFENSE MECHANISM

ego–dys·ton·ic \-dis-ˈtä-nik\ *adj* : incompatible with or unacceptable to the ego — compare EGO-SYNTONIC

ego ideal *n* : the positive standards, ideals, and ambitions that according to psychoanalytic theory are assimilated from the superego

ego–involvement *n* : an involvement of one's self-esteem in the performance of a task or in an object — **ego–involve** *vb*

ego·ism \ˈē-gə-ˌwi-zəm\ *n* **1 a** : a doctrine that individual self-interest is the actual motive of all conscious action **b** : a doctrine that individual self-interest is the valid end of all actions **2** : excessive concern for oneself without exaggerated feelings of self-importance — compare EGOTISM — **ego·ist** \-wist\ *n* — **ego·is·tic** \ˌē-gə-ˈwis-tik\ *also* **ego·is·ti·cal** \-ti-kəl\ *adj* — **ego·is·ti·cal·ly** \-ti-k(ə-)lē\ *adv*

ego·ma·nia \ˌē-gō-ˈmā-nē-ə, -nyə\ *n* : the quality or state of being extremely egocentric — **ego·ma·ni·ac** \-nē-ˌak\ *n* — **ego·ma·ni·a·cal** \-mə-ˈnī-ə-kəl\ *adj* — **ego·ma·ni·a·cal·ly** \-k(ə-)lē\ *adv*

egoph·o·ny \ē-ˈgä-fə-nē\ *n, pl* **-nies** : a modification of the voice resembling bleating heard on auscultation of the chest in some diseases (as in pleurisy with effusion)

ego–syn·ton·ic \ˌē-gō-sin-ˈtä-nik\ *adj* : compatible with or acceptable to the ego — compare EGO-DYSTONIC

ego·tism \ˈē-gə-ˌti-zəm\ *n* : an exaggerated sense of self-importance — compare EGOISM 2 — **ego·tist** \-tist\ *n* — **ego·tis·tic** \ˌē-gə-ˈtis-tik\ *or* **ego·tis·ti·cal** \-ˈtis-ti-kəl\ *adj* — **ego·tis·ti·cal·ly** \-ˈtis-ti-k(ə-)lē\ *adv*

Eh·lers–Dan·los syndrome \ˈā-lərz-ˈdan-(ˌ)läs\ *n* : a rare inherited disorder of connective tissue characterized esp. by extremely flexible joints, elastic skin, and excessive bruising
Ehlers \ˈā-(ˌ)lerz\, **Edvard L.** (1863–1937), Danish dermatologist.
Dan·los \däⁿ-lō\, **Henri–Alexandre** (1844–1912), French dermatologist.

Ehr·lich·ia \er-ˈli-kē-ə\ *n* : a genus of gram-negative nonmotile rickettsial bacteria that are intracellular parasites infecting esp. circulating white blood cells (as monocytes and granulocytes), that are transmitted chiefly by tick bites, and that are pathogens of animals and humans
Ehr·lich \ˈār-ˌlik\, **Paul** (1854–1915), German chemist and bacteriologist.

ehrlichiosis *n* : infection with or a disease caused by rickettsial bacteria of the genus *Ehrlichia*

EIA *abbr* **1** enzyme immunoassay **2** equine infectious anemia **3** exercise-induced asthma

ei·co·sa·noid \ī-ˈkō-sə-ˌnòid\ *n* : any of a class of compounds (as the prostaglandins and leukotrienes) derived from polyunsaturated fatty acids and involved in cellular activity

ei·co·sa·pen·ta·e·no·ic acid \ˌī-kō-sə-ˌpen-tə-ē-ˌnō-ik-\ *n* : an omega-3 fatty acid $C_{20}H_{30}O_2$ found especially in fish oils — abbr. *EPA*

ei·det·ic \ī-ˈde-tik\ *adj* : marked by or involving extraordinarily accurate and vivid recall esp. of visual images — **ei·det·i·cal·ly** \-ti-k(ə-)lē\ *adv*

eighth cranial nerve *n* : AUDITORY NERVE

eighth nerve *n* : AUDITORY NERVE

ei·ko·nom·e·ter \ˌī-kə-ˈnä-mə-tər\ *n* : a device to detect aniseikonia or to test stereoscopic vision

Ei·me·ria \ī-ˈmir-ē-ə\ *n* : a genus of coccidian protozoans that invade the visceral epithelia and esp. the intestinal wall of many vertebrates and include serious pathogens
Eimer \ˈī-mər\, **Theodor Gustav Heinrich** (1843–1898), German zoologist.

ein·stei·ni·um \īn-ˈstī-nē-əm\ *n* : a radioactive element produced artificially — symbol *Es;* see ELEMENT table
Einstein \ˈīn-ˌstīn, -ˌshtīn\, **Albert** (1879–1955), German physicist.

Ei·sen·meng·er complex \ˈī-zən-ˌmeng-ər-\ *or* **Ei·sen·meng·er's complex** \-ərz-\ *n* : the combination of a congenital defect in the septum between the ventricles of the heart with its early complications (as left to right blood flow through the defect and increased blood pressure in the pulmonary arteries)

Eisenmenger, Victor (1864–1932), German physician.

Eisenmenger syndrome *or* **Eisenmenger's syndrome** *n* : the septal defect of Eisenmenger's complex with its later complications (as right to left blood flow through the septal defect and marked hypertrophy of the right ventricle) that are essentially surgically irreversible

¹ejac·u·late \i-ˈja-kyə-ˌlāt\ *vb* **-lat·ed; -lat·ing** : to eject from a living body; *specif* : to eject (semen) in orgasm — **ejac·u·la·tor** \-ˌlā-tər\ *n*

²ejac·u·late \-lət\ *n* : the semen released by one ejaculation

ejac·u·la·tion \i-ˌja-kyə-ˈlā-shən\ *n* : the act or process of ejaculating; *specif* : the sudden or spontaneous discharging of a fluid (as semen in orgasm) from a duct — see PREMATURE EJACULATION

ejac·u·la·tio prae·cox \-ˈlā-shē-ō-ˈprē-ˌkäks\ *n* : PREMATURE EJACULATION

ejac·u·la·to·ry \i-ˈja-kyə-lə-ˌtōr-ē\ *adj* : associated with or concerned in physiological ejaculation ⟨~ vessels⟩

ejaculatory duct *n* : either of the paired ducts in the human male that are formed by the junction of the duct from the seminal vesicle with the vas deferens, pass through the prostate, and open into or close to the prostatic utricle

ejection fraction *n* : the ratio of the volume of blood the heart empties during systole to the volume of blood in the heart at the end of diastole expressed as a percentage usu. between 50 and 80 percent

ejec·tor \i-ˈjek-tər\ *n* : something that ejects — see SALIVA EJECTOR

EKG \ˌē-(ˌ)kā-ˈjē\ *n* **1** : ELECTROCARDIOGRAM **2** : ELECTROCARDIOGRAPH

el·a·pid \ˈe-lə-pəd\ *n* : any of a family (Elapidae) of venomous snakes with hollow fangs that include the cobras and mambas, the coral snakes of the New World, and the majority of Australian snakes — **elapid** *adj*

elast- *or* **elasto-** *comb form* : elasticity ⟨*elasto*sis⟩

elas·tase \i-ˈlas-ˌtās, -ˌtāz\ *n* : an enzyme esp. of pancreatic juice that digests elastin

¹elas·tic \i-ˈlas-tik\ *adj* : capable of being easily stretched or expanded and resuming former shape — **elas·ti·cal·ly** \-ti-k(ə-)lē\ *adv* — **elas·tic·i·ty** \i-ˌlas-ˈtis-ə-tē\ *n*

²elastic *n* **1 a** : easily stretched rubber usu. prepared in cords, strings, or bands **b** : a band of elastic used esp. in orthodontics; *also* : one placed around a tooth at the gum line in effecting its nonsurgical removal **2 a** : an elastic fabric usu. made of yarns containing rubber **b** : something made from this fabric

elastic cartilage *n* : a yellowish flexible cartilage having the matrix infiltrated in all directions by a network of elastic fibers and occurring chiefly in the external ear, eustachian tube, and some cartilages of the larynx and epiglottis

elastic fiber *n* : a thick very elastic smooth yellowish anastomosing fiber of connective tissue that contains elastin

elastic stocking *n* : a stocking woven or knitted with an elastic material and used (as in the treatment of varicose veins) to provide support for the leg

elastic tissue *n* : tissue consisting chiefly of elastic fibers that is found esp. in some ligaments and tendons

elasticum — see PSEUDOXANTHOMA ELASTICUM

elas·tin \i-ˈlas-tən\ *n* : a protein that is similar to collagen and is the chief constituent of elastic fibers

elas·to·sis \i-ˌlas-ˈtō-səs\ *n, pl* **-to·ses** \-ˌsēz\ : a condition marked by loss of elasticity of the skin in elderly people due to degeneration of connective tissue

El·a·vil \ˈe-lə-ˌvil\ *trademark* — used for a preparation of amitriptyline

el·bow \ˈel-ˌbō\ *n* : the joint between the human forearm and the upper arm that supports the outer curve of the arm when bent — called also *elbow joint*

el·der·care \ˈel-dər-ˌker\ *n* : the care of older persons and esp. the care of an older parent by a son or daughter

elec·tive \i-ˈlek-tiv\ *adj* : beneficial to the patient but not essential for survival ⟨∼ vascular surgery⟩

elective mutism *n* : SELECTIVE MUTISM

Elec·tra complex \i-ˈlek-trə-\ *n* : the Oedipus complex when it occurs in a female

electrical potential *or* **electric potential** *n* : the potential energy measured in volts of a unit of positive charge in an electric field

electric eel *n* : a large eel-shaped fish (*Electrophorus electricus* of the family Electrophoridae) of the Orinoco and Amazon basins capable of delivering a severe shock of electricity

electric ray *n* : any of various round-bodied short-tailed rays (family Torpedinidae) of warm seas capable of delivering a shock of electricity

electric shock *n* **1** : SHOCK 3 **2** : ELECTROCONVULSIVE THERAPY

electric shock therapy *n* : ELECTROCONVULSIVE THERAPY

electric shock treatment *n* : ELECTROCONVULSIVE THERAPY

elec·tro·car·dio·gram \-ˈkär-dē-ə-ˌgram\ *n* : the tracing made by an electrocardiograph; *also* : the procedure for producing an electrocardiogram

elec·tro·car·dio·graph \-ˌgraf\ *n* : an instrument for recording the changes of electrical potential occurring during the heartbeat used esp. in diagnosing abnormalities of heart action —

elec·tro·car·dio·graph·ic \-ˌkär-dē-ə-ˈgra-fik\ *adj* — **elec·tro·car·dio·graph·i·cal·ly** \-fi-k(ə-)lē\ *adv* — **elec·tro·car·di·og·ra·phy** \-dē-ˈä-grə-fē\ *n*

elec·tro·cau·tery \-ˈkȯ-tə-rē\ *n, pl* **-ter·ies 1** : a cautery operated by an electric current **2** : the cauterization of tissue by means of an electrocautery

elec·tro·co·ag·u·la·tion \-kō-ˌa-gyə-ˈlā-shən\ *n* : the surgical coagulation of tissue by diathermy — **elec·tro·co·ag·u·late** \-kō-ˈa-gyə-ˌlāt\ *vb*

elec·tro·con·vul·sive \i-ˌlek-trō-kən-ˈvəl-siv\ *adj* : of, relating to, or involving a convulsive response to a shock of electricity

electroconvulsive therapy *n* : the treatment of mental disorder and esp. depression by the application of electric current to the head of a usu. anesthetized patient that induces unconsciousness and convulsive seizures in the brain — abbr. *ECT;* called also *electric shock, electric shock therapy, electroshock therapy*

elec·tro·cor·ti·cal \-ˈkȯr-ti-kəl\ *adj* : of, relating to, or being electrical activity occurring in the cerebral cortex

elec·tro·cor·ti·co·gram \-ˈkȯr-ti-kə-ˌgram\ *n* : an electroencephalogram made with the electrodes in direct contact with the brain

elec·tro·cor·ti·cog·ra·phy \-ˌkȯr-ti-ˈkä-grə-fē\ *n, pl* **-phies** : the process of recording electrical activity in the brain by placing electrodes in direct contact with the cerebral cortex — **elec·tro·cor·ti·co·graph·ic** \-kə-ˈgra-fik\ *adj* — **elec·tro·cor·ti·co·graph·i·cal·ly** \-fi-k(ə-)lē\ *adv*

elec·troc·u·lo·gram \i-ˌlek-ˈträ-kyə-lə-ˌgram\ *n* : a recording of the moving eye

elec·tro·cute \i-ˈlek-trə-ˌkyüt\ *vb* **-cut·ed; -cut·ing 1** : to execute (a criminal) by electricity **2** : to kill by a shock of electricity — **elec·tro·cu·tion** \-ˌlek-trə-ˈkyü-shən\ *n*

elec·trode \i-ˈlek-ˌtrōd\ *n* : a conductor used to establish electrical contact with a nonmetallic part of a circuit

elec·tro·der·mal \i-ˌlek-trō-ˈdər-məl\ *adj* : of or relating to electrical activity in or electrical properties of the skin

elec·tro·des·ic·ca·tion \-ˌde-si-ˈkā-shən\ *n* : the drying of tissue by a high-frequency electric current applied with a needle-shaped electrode — called also *fulguration* — **elec·tro·des·ic·cate** \-ˈde-si-ˌkāt\ *vb*

elec·tro·di·ag·no·sis \-ˌdī-ig-ˈnō-səs\ *n, pl* **-no·ses** \-ˌsēz\ : diagnosis based on electrodiagnostic methods

elec·tro·di·ag·nos·tic \-ˌdī-ig-ˈnäs-tik\ *adj* : involving or obtained by the recording of responses to electrical stimulation or of spontaneous electrical activity (as in electromyography) for purposes of diagnosing a pathological condition — **elec·tro·di·ag·nos·ti·cal·ly** \-ti-k(ə-)lē\ *adv*

elec·tro·di·al·y·sis \i-ˌlek-trō-dī-'a-lə-səs\ *n, pl* **-y·ses** \-ˌsēz\ : dialysis accelerated by an electromotive force applied to electrodes adjacent to the membranes — **elec·tro·di·a·lyt·ic** \-ˌdī-ə-'li-tik\ *adj*

elec·tro·en·ceph·a·lo·gram \-in-'se-fə-lə-ˌgram\ *n* : the tracing of brain waves made by an electroencephalograph

elec·tro·en·ceph·a·lo·graph \-ˌgraf\ *n* : an apparatus for detecting and recording brain waves — called also *encephalograph* — **elec·tro·en·ceph·a·lo·graph·ic** \-ˌse-fə-lə-'gra-fik\ *adj* — **elec·tro·en·ceph·a·lo·graph·i·cal·ly** \-fi-k(ə-)lē\ *adv* — **elec·tro·en·ceph·a·log·ra·phy** \-'lä-grə-fē\ *n*

elec·tro·en·ceph·a·log·ra·pher \-in-ˌse-fə-'lä-grə-fər\ *n* : a person who specializes in electroencephalography

elec·tro·gen·ic \-'je-nik\ *adj* : of or relating to the production of electrical activity in living tissue — **elec·tro·gen·e·sis** \i-ˌlek-trə-'je-nə-səs\ *n*

elec·tro·gram \i-'lek-trə-ˌgram\ *n* : a tracing of the electrical potentials of a tissue (as the brain or heart) made by means of electrodes placed directly in the tissue instead of on the surface of the body

elec·tro·graph·ic \i-ˌlek-trə-'gra-fik\ *adj* : relating to, involving, or produced by the use of electrodes implanted directly in living tissue \<~ stimulation of the brain\> — **elec·tro·graph·i·cal·ly** \-fi-k(ə-)lē\ *adv*

elec·tro·ky·mo·graph \-'kī-mə-ˌgraf\ *n* : an instrument for recording graphically the motion of the heart as seen in silhouette on a fluoroscopic screen — **elec·tro·ky·mog·ra·phy** \-kī-'mä-grə-fē\ *n*

elec·trol·o·gist \i-ˌlek-'trä-lə-jist\ *n* : a person who removes hair by means of an electric current applied to the body with a needle-shaped electrode

elec·trol·y·sis \i-ˌlek-'trä-lə-səs\ *n, pl* **-y·ses** \-ˌsēz\ **1 a** : the producing of chemical changes by passage of an electric current through an electrolyte **b** : subjection to this action **2** : the destruction of hair roots by an electrologist using an electric current

elec·tro·lyte \i-'lek-trə-ˌlīt\ *n* **1** : a nonmetallic electric conductor in which current is carried by the movement of ions **2 a** : a substance (as an acid or salt) that when dissolved in a suitable solvent (as water) or when fused becomes an ionic conductor **b** : any of the ions (as of sodium, potassium, or calcium) that in a biological fluid regulate or affect most metabolic processes (as the flow of nutrients into and waste products out of cells)

elec·tro·lyt·ic \i-ˌlek-trə-'li-tik\ *adj* : of or relating to electrolysis or an electrolyte; *also* : involving or produced by electrolysis — **elec·tro·lyt·i·cal·ly** \-ti-k(ə-)lē\ *adv*

elec·tro·mag·net·ic \-mag-'ne-tik\ *adj* : of, relating to, or produced by electromagnetism

electromagnetic field *n* : a field (as around a high voltage power line) that possesses a definite amount of electromagnetic energy

electromagnetic radiation *n* : a series of electromagnetic waves

electromagnetic spectrum *n* : the entire range of wavelengths or frequencies of electromagnetic radiation extending from gamma rays to the longest radio waves

electromagnetic wave *n* : one of the waves propagated by simultaneous periodic variations of electric and magnetic field intensity and including radio waves, infrared, visible light, ultraviolet, X-rays, and gamma rays

elec·tro·mag·ne·tism \i-ˌlek-trō-'mag-nə-ˌti-zəm\ *n* **1** : magnetism developed by a current of electricity **2** : physics dealing with the relations between electricity and magnetism

elec·tro·mo·tive force \i-ˌlek-trō-'mō-tiv-, -trə-\ *n* : something that moves or tends to move electricity : the amount of energy derived from an electrical source per unit quantity of electricity passing through the source (as a cell or generator)

elec·tro·myo·gram \i-ˌlek-trō-'mī-ə-ˌgram\ *n* : a tracing made with an electromyograph

elec·tro·myo·graph \-ˌgraf\ *n* : an instrument that converts the electrical activity associated with functioning skeletal muscle into a visual record or into sound and has been used to diagnose neuromuscular disorders and in biofeedback training — **elec·tro·myo·graph·ic** \-ˌmī-ə-'gra-fik\ *adj* — **elec·tro·myo·graph·i·cal·ly** \-fi-k(ə-)lē\ *adv* — **elec·tro·my·og·ra·phy** \-mī-'ä-grə-fē\ *n*

elec·tron \i-'lek-ˌträn\ *n* : an elementary particle consisting of a charge of negative electricity equal to about 1.602×10^{-19} coulomb and having a mass when at rest of about 9.109534×10^{-28} gram

elec·tro·nar·co·sis \i-ˌlek-trō-när-'kō-səs\ *n, pl* **-co·ses** \-ˌsēz\ : unconsciousness induced by passing a weak electric current through the brain

elec·tron·ic \i-ˌlek-'trä-nik\ *adj* : of or relating to electrons or electronics — **elec·tron·i·cal·ly** \-ni-k(ə-)lē\ *adv*

elec·tron·ics \i-ˌlek-'trä-niks\ *n* **1** : the physics of electrons and electronic devices **2** : electronic devices or equipment

electron micrograph *n* : a micrograph made with an electron microscope

electron microscope *n* : an electron-optical instrument in which a beam of electrons is used to produce an enlarged image of a minute object — **electron microscopist** *n* — **electron microscopy** *n*

electron transport *n* : the sequential

transfer of electrons esp. by cytochromes in cellular respiration from an oxidizable substrate to molecular oxygen by a series of oxidation-reduction reactions

elec·tro·nys·tag·mog·ra·phy \i-ˌlek-trō-ˌnis-ˌtag-ˈmä-grə-fē\ *n, pl* **-phies** : the use of electrooculography to study nystagmus — **elec·tro·nys·tag·mo·graph·ic** \-(ˌ)nis-ˌtag-mə-ˈgra-fik\ *adj*

elec·tro·oc·u·lo·gram \-ˈä-kyə-lə-ˌgram\ *n* : a record of the standing voltage between the front and back of the eye that is correlated with eyeball movement (as in REM sleep) and obtained by electrodes suitably placed on the skin near the eye

elec·tro·oc·u·log·ra·phy \-ˌä-kyə-ˈlä-grə-fē\ *n, pl* **-phies** : the preparation and study of electrooculograms — **elec·tro·oc·u·lo·graph·ic** \-lə-ˈgra-fik\ *adj*

elec·tro·phe·ro·gram \-trə-ˈfir-ə-ˌgram, -ˈfer-\ *n* : ELECTROPHORETOGRAM

elec·tro·pho·re·sis \-trə-fə-ˈrē-səs\ *n, pl* **-re·ses** \-ˌsēz\ : the movement of suspended particles through a fluid or gel under the action of an electromotive force applied to electrodes in contact with the suspension — **elec·tro·pho·rese** \-ˈrēs, -ˈrēz\ *vb* — **elec·tro·pho·ret·ic** \-ˈre-tik\ *adj* — **elec·tro·pho·ret·i·cal·ly** \-ti-k(ə-)lē\ *adv*

elec·tro·pho·reto·gram \-fə-ˈre-tə-ˌgram\ *n* : a record that consists of the separated components of a mixture (as of proteins) produced by electrophoresis in a supporting medium

elec·tro·phren·ic \i-ˌlek-trə-ˈfre-nik\ *adj* : relating to or induced by electrical stimulation of the phrenic nerve

elec·tro·phys·i·ol·o·gy \i-ˌlek-trō-ˌfi-zē-ˈä-lə-jē\ *n, pl* **-gies** **1** : physiology that is concerned with the electrical aspects of physiological phenomena **2** : electrical phenomena associated with a physiological process (as the function of a body or bodily part) — **elec·tro·phys·i·o·log·i·cal** \-ə-lä-ji-kəl\ *also* **elec·tro·phys·i·o·log·ic** \-jik\ *adj* — **elec·tro·phys·i·o·log·i·cal·ly** \-ji-k(ə-)lē\ *adv* — **elec·tro·phys·i·ol·o·gist** \-ˈä-lə-jist\ *n*

elec·tro·re·sec·tion \-rē-ˈsek-shən\ *n* : resection by electrosurgical means

elec·tro·ret·i·no·gram \-ˈret-ⁿn-ə-ˌgram\ *n* : a graphic record of electrical activity of the retina

elec·tro·ret·i·no·graph \-ˌgraf\ *n* : an instrument for recording electrical activity in the retina — **elec·tro·ret·i·no·graph·ic** \-ˌret-ⁿn-ə-ˈgra-fik\ *adj* — **elec·tro·ret·i·nog·ra·phy** \-ⁿn-ˈä-grə-fē\ *n*

elec·tro·shock \i-ˈlek-trō-ˌshäk\ *n* **1** : SHOCK 3 **2** : ELECTROCONVULSIVE THERAPY

electroshock therapy *n* : ELECTROCONVULSIVE THERAPY

elec·tro·sleep \-ˌslēp\ *n* : profound relaxation or a state of unconsciousness induced by the passage of a very low

voltage electric current through the brain

elec·tro·stat·ic \i-ˌlek-trə-ˈsta-tik\ *adj* : of or relating to stationary electric charges or to the study of the forces of attraction and repulsion acting between such charges

elec·tro·stim·u·la·tion \i-ˌlek-trō-ˌstim-yə-ˈlā-shən\ *n* : shocks of electricity administered in nonconvulsive doses

elec·tro·sur·gery \-ˈsər-jə-rē\ *n, pl* **-ger·ies** : surgery by means of diathermy — **elec·tro·sur·gi·cal** \-ji-kəl\ *adj*

elec·tro·ther·a·py \-ˈther-ə-pē\ *n, pl* **-pies** : treatment of disease by means of electricity (as in diathermy)

elec·tro·tome \i-ˈlek-trə-ˌtōm\ *n* : an electric cutting instrument used in electrosurgery

elec·tro·ton·ic \i-ˌlek-trə-ˈtä-nik\ *adj* **1** : of, induced by, relating to, or constituting electrotonus ⟨the ∼ condition of a nerve⟩ **2** : of, relating to, or being the spread of electrical activity through living tissue or cells in the absence of repeated action potentials — **elec·tro·ton·i·cal·ly** \-ni-k(ə-)lē\ *adv*

elec·trot·o·nus \i-ˌlek-ˈträt-ⁿn-əs\ *n* : the altered sensitivity of a nerve when a constant current of electricity passes through any part of it

elec·tu·ary \i-ˈlek-chə-ˌwer-ē\ *n, pl* **-ar·ies** : CONFECTION; *esp* : a medicated paste prepared with a sweet (as honey) and used in veterinary practice

el·e·doi·sin \ˌe-lə-ˈdòis-ⁿn\ *n* : a small protein $C_{54}H_{85}N_{13}O_{15}S$ from the salivary glands of several octopuses (genus *Eledone*) that is a powerful vasodilator and hypotensive agent

el·e·ment \ˈe-lə-mənt\ *n* **1** : any of more than 100 fundamental substances that consist of atoms of only one kind and that singly or in combination constitute all matter **2** : one of the basic constituent units (as a cell or fiber) of a tissue

el·e·men·tal \ˌe-lə-ˈment-ⁿl\ *adj* : of, relating to, or being an element; *specif* : existing as an uncombined chemical element

elementary body *n* : an infectious particle of any of several microorganisms; *esp* : a chlamydial cell of an extracellular infectious form that attaches to receptors on the membrane of the host cell and is taken up by endocytosis — compare RETICULATE BODY

elementary particle *n* : any of the subatomic units of matter and energy (as the electron, neutrino, proton, or photon) that do not appear to be made up of other smaller particles

el·e·phan·ti·a·sis \ˌe-lə-fən-ˈtī-ə-səs, -ˌfan-\ *n, pl* **-a·ses** \-ˌsēz\ : enlargement and thickening of tissues; *specif* : the enormous enlargement of a limb or the scrotum caused by obstruction of lymphatics by filarial worms of the genus *Wuchereria* (*W. bancrofti*) or a related genus (*Brugia malayi*)

CHEMICAL ELEMENTS

ELEMENT NAME	SYMBOL & ATOMIC NUMBER	ATOMIC WEIGHT[1]	ELEMENT NAME	SYMBOL & ATOMIC NUMBER	ATOMIC WEIGHT[1]
actinium	(Ac = 89)	227.0277	meitnerium	(Mt = 109)	(268)
aluminum	(Al = 13)	26.98154	mendelevium	(Md = 101)	(258)
americium	(Am = 95)	(243)	mercury	(Hg = 80)	200.59
antimony	(Sb = 51)	121.760	molybdenum	(Mo = 42)	95.94
argon	(Ar = 18)	39.948	neodymium	(Nd = 60)	144.24
arsenic	(As = 33)	74.92160	neon	(Ne = 10)	20.180
astatine	(At = 85)	(210)	neptunium	(Np = 93)	(237)
barium	(Ba = 56)	137.33	nickel	(Ni = 28)	58.6934
berkelium	(Bk = 97)	(247)	niobium	(Nb = 41)	92.90638
beryllium	(Be = 4)	9.012182	nitrogen	(N = 7)	14.0067
bismuth	(Bi = 83)	208.98038	nobelium	(No = 102)	(259)
bohrium	(Bh = 107)	(264)	osmium	(Os = 76)	190.23
boron	(B = 5)	10.81	oxygen	(O = 8)	15.9994
bromine	(Br = 35)	79.904	palladium	(Pd = 46)	106.42
cadmium	(Cd = 48)	112.41	phosphorus	(P = 15)	30.973761
calcium	(Ca = 20)	40.078	platinum	(Pt = 78)	195.078
californium	(Cf = 98)	(251)	plutonium	(Pu = 94)	(244)
carbon	(C = 6)	12.011	polonium	(Po = 84)	(209)
cerium	(Ce = 58)	140.116	potassium	(K = 19)	39.0983
cesium	(Cs = 55)	132.90545	praseodymium	(Pr = 59)	140.90765
chlorine	(Cl = 17)	35.453	promethium	(Pm = 61)	(145)
chromium	(Cr = 24)	51.996	protactinium	(Pa = 91)	(231)
cobalt	(Co = 27)	58.93320	radium	(Ra = 88)	(226)
copper	(Cu = 29)	63.546	radon	(Rn = 86)	(222)
curium	(Cm = 96)	(247)	rhenium	(Re = 75)	186.207
darmstadtium	(Ds = 110)	(269)	rhodium	(Rh = 45)	102.90550
dubnium	(Db = 105)	(262)	rubidium	(Rb = 37)	85.4678
dysprosium	(Dy = 66)	162.50	ruthenium	(Ru = 44)	101.07
einsteinium	(Es = 99)	(252)	rutherfordium	(Rf = 104)	(261)
erbium	(Er = 68)	167.259	samarium	(Sm = 62)	150.36
europium	(Eu = 63)	151.964	scandium	(Sc = 21)	44.95591
fermium	(Fm = 100)	(257)	seaborgium	(Sg = 106)	(266)
fluorine	(F = 9)	18.998403	selenium	(Se = 34)	78.96
francium	(Fr = 87)	(223)	silicon	(Si = 14)	28.0855
gadolinium	(Gd = 64)	157.25	silver	(Ag = 47)	107.8682
gallium	(Ga = 31)	69.723	sodium	(Na = 11)	22.989770
germanium	(Ge = 32)	72.64	strontium	(Sr = 38)	87.62
gold	(Au = 79)	196.96655	sulfur	(S = 16)	32.07
hafnium	(Hf = 72)	178.49	tantalum	(Ta = 73)	180.9479
hassium	(Hs = 108)	(277)	technetium	(Tc = 43)	(98)
helium	(He = 2)	4.002602	tellurium	(Te = 52)	127.60
holmium	(Ho = 67)	164.93032	terbium	(Tb = 65)	158.92534
hydrogen	(H = 1)	1.0079	thallium	(Tl = 81)	204.3833
indium	(In = 49)	114.818	thorium	(Th = 90)	232.0381
iodine	(I = 53)	126.90447	thulium	(Tm = 69)	168.93421
iridium	(Ir = 77)	192.217	tin	(Sn = 50)	118.71
iron	(Fe = 26)	55.845	titanium	(Ti = 22)	47.867
krypton	(Kr = 36)	83.80	tungsten	(W = 74)	183.84
lanthanum	(La = 57)	138.9055	uranium	(U = 92)	(238)
lawrencium	(Lr = 103)	(262)	vanadium	(V = 23)	50.9415
lead	(Pb = 82)	207.2	xenon	(Xe = 54)	131.29
lithium	(Li = 3)	6.941	ytterbium	(Yb = 70)	173.04
lutetium	(Lu = 71)	174.967	yttrium	(Y = 39)	88.90585
magnesium	(Mg = 12)	24.305	zinc	(Zn = 30)	65.39
manganese	(Mn = 25)	54.93805	zirconium	(Zr = 40)	91.224

[1]Weights are based on the naturally occurring isotope compositions and scaled to $^{12}C = 12$. For elements lacking stable isotopes, the mass number of the most stable nuclide is shown in parentheses.

el·e·vat·ed \'e-lə-ˌvā-təd\ *adj* : increased esp. abnormally ⟨an ∼ pulse rate⟩ ⟨∼ temperature⟩

el·e·va·tion \ˌe-lə-'vā-shən\ *n* **1** : a swelling esp. on the skin **2** : a usu. abnormal increase (as in degree or amount) ⟨an ∼ of temperature⟩

el·e·va·tor \'e-lə-ˌvā-tər\ *n* **1** : a dental instrument that is used for removing teeth or the roots of teeth which cannot be gripped with a forceps **2** : a surgical instrument for raising a depressed part (as a bone) or for separating contiguous parts

eleventh cranial nerve *n* : ACCESSORY NERVE

elim·i·nate \i'li-mə-ˌnāt\ *vb* **-nat·ed; -nat·ing** : to expel (as waste) from the living body

elim·i·na·tion \i-ˌli-mə-'nā-shən\ *n* **1** : the act of discharging or excreting waste products or foreign substances from the body **2** **eliminations** *pl* : bodily discharges (as urine and feces)

ELISA \ē-'li-sə, -zə\ *n* : ENZYME= LINKED IMMUNOSORBENT ASSAY

elix·ir \i-'lik-sər\ *n* : a sweetened liquid usu. containing alcohol that is used in medication either for its medicinal ingredients or as a flavoring

Eliz·a·be·than collar \i-ˌli-zə-'bē-thən-\ *n* : a broad circle of stiff material (as plastic) placed about the neck of a cat or dog to prevent it from licking or biting an injured part

el·lip·to·cyte \i-'lip-tə-ˌsīt\ *n* : an elliptical red blood cell

el·lip·to·cy·to·sis \i-ˌlip-tə-ˌsī-'tō-səs\ *n, pl* **-to·ses** \-ˌsēz\ : a human hereditary trait manifested by the presence in the blood of red blood cells which are oval in shape with rounded ends

el·u·ant *or* **el·u·ent** \'el-yə-wənt\ *n* : a solvent used in eluting

el·u·ate \'el-yə-wət, -ˌwāt\ *n* : the washings obtained by eluting

elute \ē-'lüt\ *vb* **elut·ed; elut·ing** : to wash out or extract; *specif* : to remove (adsorbed material) from an adsorbent by means of a solvent

EM *abbr* **1** electromagnetic **2** electron microscope; electron microscopy **3** emergency medicine

ema·ci·ate \i-'mā-shē-ˌāt\ *vb* **-at·ed; -at·ing** **1** : to cause to lose flesh so as to become very thin **2** : to waste away physically — **ema·ci·a·tion** \-ˌmā-shē-'ā-shən, -sē-\ *n*

emas·cu·late \i-'mas-kyə-ˌlāt\ *vb* **-lat·ed; -lat·ing** : to deprive of virility or procreative power : CASTRATE — **emas·cu·la·tion** \-ˌmas-kyə-'lā-shən\ *n*

emas·cu·la·tor \i-'mas-kyə-ˌlā-tər\ *n* : an instrument often with a broad surface and a cutting edge used in castrating livestock

em·balm \im-'bäm, -'bälm\ *vb* : to treat (a dead body) so as to protect from decay — **em·balm·er** *n*

em·bar·rass \im-'bar-əs\ *vb* : to impair the activity of (a bodily function) or the function of (a bodily part)

em·bar·rass·ment \im-'bar-əs-mənt\ *n* : difficulty in functioning as a result of disease ⟨respiratory ∼⟩

em·bed *also* **im·bed** \im-'bed\ *vb* **em·bed·ded** *also* **im·bed·ded; em·bed·ding** *also* **im·bed·ding** : to prepare (a microscopy specimen) for sectioning by infiltrating with and enclosing in a supporting substance — **em·bed·ment** \-'bed-mənt\ *n*

embol- *comb form* : embolus ⟨*embol*ectomy⟩

em·bo·lec·to·my \ˌem-bə-'lek-tə-mē\ *n, pl* **-mies** : surgical removal of an embolus

emboli *pl of* EMBOLUS

em·bol·ic \em-'bä-lik, im-\ *adj* : of or relating to an embolus or embolism

em·bo·lism \'em-bə-ˌli-zəm\ *n* **1** : the sudden obstruction of a blood vessel by an embolus **2** : EMBOLUS

em·bo·li·za·tion \ˌem-bə-lə-'zā-shən\ *n* **1** : the process by which or state in which a blood vessel or organ is obstructed by the lodgment of a material mass (as an embolus) ⟨pulmonary ∼⟩ ⟨∼ of a thrombus⟩ **2** : an operation in which pellets are introduced into the circulatory system in order to induce embolization in specific abnormal blood vessels

em·bo·lize \'em-bə-ˌlīz\ *vb* **-lized; -liz·ing** **1** *of an embolus* : to lodge in and obstruct (as a blood vessel or organ) **2** : to break up into emboli or become an embolus

em·bo·lo·ther·a·py \ˌem-bə-lō-'ther-ə-pē\ *n* : the intentional blockage of an artery with an object (as a balloon inserted by a catheter) to control or prevent hemorrhaging

em·bo·lus \'em-bə-ləs\ *n, pl* **-li** \-ˌlī\ : an abnormal particle (as an air bubble) circulating in the blood — compare THROMBUS

em·bra·sure \im-'brā-zhər\ *n* : the sloped valley between adjacent teeth

em·bro·ca·tion \ˌem-brə-'kā-shən\ *n* : LINIMENT

embry- *or* **embryo-** *comb form* : embryo ⟨*embryo*ma⟩

em·bryo \'em-brē-ˌō\ *n, pl* **em·bry·os** : an animal in the early stages of growth and differentiation that are characterized by cleavage, the laying down of fundamental tissues, and the formation of primitive organs and organ systems; *esp* : the developing human individual from the time of implantation to the end of the eighth week after conception — compare FETUS

em·bryo·gen·e·sis \ˌem-brē-ō-'je-nə-səs\ *n, pl* **-e·ses** \-ˌsēz\ : the formation and development of the embryo — **em·bryo·ge·net·ic** \-jə-'ne-tik\ *adj*

em·bry·og·e·ny \ˌem-brē-'ä-jə-nē\ *n, pl* **-nies** : EMBRYOGENESIS — **em·bryo·gen·ic** \-brē-ō-'je-nik\ *adj*

em·bry·ol·o·gist \ˌem-brē-'ä-lə-jist\ *n* : a specialist in embryology

em·bry·ol·o·gy \-jē\ *n, pl* **-gies** **1** : a

branch of biology dealing with embryos and their development **2** : the features and phenomena exhibited in the formation and development of an embryo — **em·bry·o·log·i·cal** \-brē-ə-ˈlä-ji-kəl\ *also* **em·bry·o·log·ic** \-jik\ *adj* — **em·bry·o·log·i·cal·ly** \-ji-k(ə-)lē\ *adv*

em·bry·o·ma \ˌem-brē-ˈō-mə\ *n, pl* **-mas** *also* **-ma·ta** \-mə-tə\ : a tumor derived from embryonic structures : TERATOMA

embryon- *or* **embryoni-** *comb form* : embryo ⟨*embryonic*⟩

em·bry·o·nal \em-ˈbrī-ən-ᵊl\ *adj* : EMBRYONIC 1

embryonal carcinoma *n* : a highly malignant cancer of the testis

em·bry·o·nate \ˈem-brē-ə-ˌnāt\ *vb* **-nat·ed; -nat·ing** *of an egg or zygote* : to produce or differentiate into an embryo

em·bry·o·nat·ed *adj* : having an embryo

em·bry·on·ic \ˌem-brē-ˈä-nik\ *adj* **1** : of or relating to an embryo **2** : being in an early stage of development — **em·bry·on·i·cal·ly** \-ni-k(ə-)lē\ *adv*

embryonic disk *or* **embryonic disc** *n* **1 a** : BLASTODISC **b** : BLASTODERM **2** : the part of the inner cell mass of a blastocyst from which the embryo of a placental mammal develops

embryonic membrane *n* : a structure (as the amnion) that derives from the fertilized ovum but does not form a part of the embryo

em·bry·op·a·thy \ˌem-brē-ˈä-pə-thē\ *n, pl* **-thies** : a developmental abnormality of an embryo or fetus esp. when caused by a disease (as German measles or mumps) in the mother

em·bryo·tox·ic·i·ty \ˌem-brē-ō-ˌtäk-ˈsi-sə-tē\ *n, pl* **-ties** : the state of being toxic to embryos — **em·bryo·tox·ic** \-ˈtäk-sik\ *adj*

embryo transfer *n* : a procedure used esp. in animal breeding in which an embryo from a superovulated female is removed and reimplanted in the uterus of another female — called also *embryo transplant*

emer·gence \i-ˈmər-jəns\ *n* : a recovering of consciousness (as from anesthesia)

emer·gen·cy \i-ˈmər-jən-sē\ *n, pl* **-cies** : an unforeseen combination of circumstances or the resulting state that calls for immediate action: as **a** : a sudden bodily alteration (as a ruptured appendix) such as is likely to require immediate medical attention **b** : a usu. distressing event or condition that can often be anticipated or prepared for but seldom exactly foreseen

emergency medical technician *n* : EMT

emergency medicine *n* : a medical specialty concerned with the care and treatment of acutely ill or injured patients who need immediate medical attention

emergency room *n* : a hospital room or area staffed and equipped for the reception and treatment of persons with conditions (as illness or trauma) requiring immediate medical care

emer·gent \i-ˈmər-jənt\ *adj* : calling for prompt or urgent action

eme·sis \ˈe-mə-səs, i-ˈmē-\ *n, pl* **eme·ses** \-ˌsēz\ : VOMITING

¹**emet·ic** \i-ˈme-tik\ *n* : an agent that induces vomiting

²**emetic** *adj* : having the capacity to induce vomiting

em·e·tine \ˈe-mə-ˌtēn\ *n* : an amorphous alkaloid $C_{29}H_{40}N_2O_4$ extracted from ipecac root and used as an emetic and expectorant

EMF *abbr* **1** electromagnetic field **2** electromotive force

EMG *abbr* electromyogram; electromyograph; electromyography

-emia \ˈē-mē-ə\ *or* **-he·mia** \ˈhē-\ *n comb form* **1** : condition of having (such) blood ⟨leuk*emia*⟩ ⟨septic*emia*⟩ **2** : condition of having (a specified thing) in the blood ⟨ur*emia*⟩

Em·i·nase \ˈe-mi-ˌnās, -ˌnāz\ *trademark* — used for a preparation of anistreplase

em·i·nence \ˈe-mə-nəns\ *n* : a protuberance or projection on a bodily part and esp. a bone

emissary vein *n* : any of the veins that pass through apertures in the skull and connect the venous sinuses of the dura mater with veins external to the skull

emis·sion \ē-ˈmi-shən\ *n* **1** : a discharge of fluid from a living body; *esp* : EJACULATE — see NOCTURNAL EMISSION **2** : substances and esp. pollutants discharged into the air (as by a smokestack or an automobile engine)

em·men·a·gogue \ə-ˈme-nə-ˌgäg, e-\ *n* : an agent that promotes the menstrual discharge

em·me·tro·pia \ˌe-mə-ˈtrō-pē-ə\ *n* : the normal refractive condition of the eye in which with accommodation relaxed parallel rays of light are all brought accurately to a focus upon the retina — compare ASTIGMATISM, MYOPIA — **em·me·trop·ic** \-ˈträ-pik, -ˈtrō-\ *adj*

¹**emol·lient** \i-ˈmäl-yənt\ *adj* : making soft or supple; *also* : soothing esp. to the skin or mucous membrane

²**emollient** *n* : an emollient agent

emo·tion \i-ˈmō-shən\ *n* : a conscious mental reaction (as anger or fear) subjectively experienced as strong feeling usu. directed toward a specific object and typically accompanied by physiological and behavioral changes in the body — **emo·tion·al** \-shə-nəl\ *adj* — **emo·tion·al·i·ty** \-ˌmō-shə-ˈna-lə-tē\ *n* — **emo·tion·al·ly** *adv*

em·pa·thy \ˈem-pə-thē\ *n, pl* **-thies** : the action of understanding, being aware of, being sensitive to, and vicariously experiencing the feelings, thoughts, and experience of another of either the past or present without having the feelings, thoughts, and experience fully communicated in an objectively explicit manner; *also* : the capacity for empathy — **em·path·ic** \em-ˈpa-thik, im-\ *adj* — **em·path·i·cal·ly** *adv* — **em·pa·thize** \ˈem-pə-ˌthīz\ *vb*

em·phy·se·ma \ˌem-fə-ˈzē-mə, -ˈsē-\ *n* : a condition characterized by air-filled expansions like blisters in interstitial or subcutaneous tissues; *specif* : a condition of the lung that is marked by distension and eventual rupture of the alveoli with progressive loss of pulmonary elasticity, that is accompanied by shortness of breath with or without cough, and that may lead to impairment of heart action — **em·phy·se·ma·tous** \-ˈze-mə-təs, -ˈse-, -ˈzē-, -ˈsē-\ *adj* — **em·phy·se·mic** \-ˈzē-mik, -ˈsē-\ *adj*

em·pir·ic \im-ˈpir-ik, em-\ *n* : EMPIRICIST

em·pir·i·cal \-i-kəl\ *or* **em·pir·ic** \-ik\ *adj* **1** : originating in or based on observation or experiment **2** : capable of being verified or disproved by observation or experiment ⟨∼ laws⟩ — **em·pir·i·cal·ly** \-i-k(ə-)lē\ *adv*

empirical formula *n* : a chemical formula showing the simplest ratio of elements in a compound rather than the total number of atoms in the molecule ⟨CH_2O is the *empirical formula* for glucose⟩

em·pir·i·cism \im-ˈpir-ə-ˌsi-zəm, em-\ *n* **1 a** : a former school of medical practice founded on experience without the aid of science or theory **b** : QUACKERY **2** : the practice of relying on observation and experiment esp. in the natural sciences

em·pir·i·cist \-sist\ *n* : one who relies on observation and experiment

empty sella syndrome *n* : a condition in which the subarachnoid space extends into the sella turcica causing it to become filled with cerebrospinal fluid and the pituitary gland is compressed but usu. functions normally

em·py·ema \ˌem-ˌpī-ˈē-mə\ *n, pl* **-ema·ta** \-mə-tə\ *also* **-emas** : the presence of pus in a bodily cavity (as the pleural cavity) — called also *pyothorax* — **em·py·emic** \-mik\ *adj*

EMS *abbr* **1** emergency medical service; emergency medical services **2** eosinophilia-myalgia syndrome

EMT \ˌē-(ˌ)em-ˈtē\ *n* : a specially trained medical technician licensed to provide basic emergency services (as cardiopulmonary resuscitation) before and during transportation to a hospital — called also *emergency medical technician;* compare PARAMEDIC 2

emul·si·fi·er \i-ˈməl-sə-ˌfī-ər\ *n* : a surface-active agent (as a soap) promoting the formation and stabilization of an emulsion

emul·si·fy \-ˌfī\ *vb* **-fied; -fy·ing** : to disperse (as an oil) in an emulsion; *also* : to convert (two or more mutually insoluble liquids) into an emulsion — **emul·si·fi·ca·tion** \-ˌməl-sə-fə-ˈkā-shən\ *n*

emul·sion \i-ˈməl-shən\ *n* **1 a** : a mixture of mutually insoluble liquids in which one is dispersed throughout the other usu. in droplets of larger than colloidal size **b** : the state of such a mixture **2** : SUSPENSION 2

en·abler \i-ˈnā-b(ə-)lər\ *n* : one who enables another to persist in self-destructive behavior (as substance abuse) by providing excuses or by helping that individual avoid the consequences of such behavior

enal·a·pril \e-ˈna-lə-ˌpril\ *n* : an antihypertensive drug that is an ACE inhibitor administered orally in the form of its maleate $C_{20}H_{28}N_2O_5 \cdot C_4H_4O_4$ — see VASOTEC

enal·a·pril·at \e-ˈna-lə-ˌpri-lət\ *n* : the metabolically active form $C_{18}H_{24}N_2O_5 \cdot 2H_2O$ of enalapril administered intravenously — see VASOTEC

enam·el \in-ˈa-məl\ *n* : the hard calcareous substance that forms a thin layer partly covering the teeth and consists of minute prisms secreted by ameloblasts, arranged at right angles to the surface, and bound together by a cement substance — compare CEMENTUM, DENTIN

enamel organ *n* : an ectodermal ingrowth from the dental lamina that encloses the anterior part of the developing dental papilla and the cells of the inner enamel layer adjacent to the papilla and differentiates into columnar ameloblasts which lay down the enamel rods of the tooth

enamel rod *n* : one of the elongated prismatic bodies making up the enamel of a tooth — called also *enamel prism*

enanthate — see TESTOSTERONE ENANTHATE

en·an·them \i-ˈnan-thəm\ *or* **en·an·the·ma** \ˌen-ˌan-ˈthē-mə\ *n, pl* **-thems** *or* **-the·ma·ta** \-mə-tə\ : an eruption on a mucous surface

en·an·tio·mer \i-ˈnan-tē-ə-mər\ *n* : either of a pair of chemical compounds whose molecular structures have a mirror-image relationship to each other — **en·an·tio·mer·ic** \-ˌnan-tē-ə-ˈmer-ik\ *adj* — **en·an·tio·mer·i·cal·ly** \-i-k(ə-)lē\ *adv*

en·an·tio·morph \i-ˈnan-tē-ə-ˌmȯrf\ *n* : ENANTIOMER

en·ar·thro·sis \ˌe-ˌnär-ˈthrō-səs\ *n, pl* **-thro·ses** \-ˌsēz\ : BALL-AND-SOCKET JOINT

en·cap·su·late \in-ˈkap-sə-ˌlāt\ *vb* **-lat·ed; -lat·ing** : to encase or become encased in or as if in a capsule — **en·cap·su·la·tion** \-ˌkap-sə-ˈlā-shən\ *n*

en·cap·su·lat·ed *adj* : surrounded by a gelatinous or membranous envelope

en·ceinte \äⁿ-ˈsant\ *adj* : PREGNANT

encephal- *or* **encephalo-** *comb form*

1 : brain 〈*encephal*itis〉 〈*encephalo*cele〉 **2** : of, relating to, or affecting the brain and 〈*encephalo*myelitis〉
-encephali *pl of* -ENCEPHALUS

en·ceph·a·li·tis \in-ˌse-fə-ˈlī-təs\ *n, pl* -lit·i·des \-ˈli-tə-ˌdēz\ : inflammation of the brain — en·ceph·a·lit·ic \-ˈli-tik\ *adj*

encephalitis le·thar·gi·ca \-li-ˈthär-ji-kə, -le-\ *n* : epidemic virus encephalitis in which somnolence is marked

en·ceph·a·lit·o·gen \in-ˌse-fə-ˈli-tə-jən, -ˌjen\ *n* : an encephalitogenic agent (as a virus)

en·ceph·a·lit·o·gen·ic \in-ˌse-fə-ˌli-tə-ˈje-nik\ *adj* : tending to cause encephalitis 〈an ∼ strain of a virus〉

en·ceph·a·lo·cele \in-ˈse-fə-lō-ˌsēl\ *n* : hernia of the brain that is either congenital or due to trauma

en·ceph·a·lo·gram \in-ˈse-fə-lə-ˌgram\ *n* : an X-ray picture of the brain made by encephalography

en·ceph·a·lo·graph \-ˌgraf\ *n* **1** : ENCEPHALOGRAM **2** : ELECTROENCEPHALOGRAPH

en·ceph·a·log·ra·phy \in-ˌse-fə-ˈlä-grə-fē\ *n, pl* -phies : radiography of the brain after the cerebrospinal fluid has been replaced by a gas (as air) — en·ceph·a·lo·graph·ic \-lə-ˈgra-fik\ *adj* — en·ceph·a·lo·graph·i·cal·ly \-fi-k(ə)lē\ *adv*

en·ceph·a·lo·ma·la·cia \in-ˌse-fə-lō-mə-ˈlā-shē-ə, -shə\ *n* : softening of the brain due to degenerative changes in nervous tissue

en·ceph·a·lo·my·eli·tis \in-ˌse-fə-lō-ˌmī-ə-ˈlī-təs\ *n, pl* -elit·i·des \-ˈli-tə-ˌdēz\ : concurrent inflammation of the brain and spinal cord — see ACUTE DISSEMINATED ENCEPHALOMYELITIS, ALLERGIC ENCEPHALOMYELITIS, EQUINE ENCEPHALOMYELITIS — en·ceph·a·lo·my·elit·ic \-ə-ˈli-tik\ *adj*

en·ceph·a·lo·my·elop·a·thy \-ˌmī-ə-ˈlä-pə-thē\ *n, pl* -thies : any disease that affects the brain and spinal cord

en·ceph·a·lo·myo·car·di·tis \-ˌmī-ə-ˌkär-ˈdī-təs\ *n* : an acute febrile virus disease that is caused by a picornavirus (genus *Cardiovirus*) and is marked by degeneration and inflammation of skeletal and cardiac muscle and lesions of the central nervous system

en·ceph·a·lop·a·thy \in-ˌse-fə-ˈlä-pə-thē\ *n, pl* -thies : a disease of the brain; *esp* : one involving alterations of brain structure — en·ceph·a·lo·path·ic \-lə-ˈpa-thik\ *adj*

-en·ceph·a·lus \in-ˈse-fə-ləs\ *n comb form, pl* -en·ceph·a·li \-ˌlī, -ˌlē\ : fetus having (such) a brain 〈inien*cephalus*〉 **2** : condition of having (such) a brain 〈hydr*encephalus*〉

-en·ceph·a·ly \in-ˈse-fə-lē\ *n comb form, pl* -en·ceph·a·lies \in-ˈse-fə-lēz\ : condition of having (such) a brain 〈micr*encephaly*〉

en·chon·dral \(ˌ)en-ˈkän-drəl, (ˌ)en-\ *adj* : ENDOCHONDRAL

en·chon·dro·ma \ˌen-ˌkän-ˈdrō-mə, ˌen-\ *n, pl* -mas *also* -ma·ta \-mə-tə\ : a tumor consisting of cartilaginous tissue; *esp* : one arising where cartilage does not normally exist

en·code \in-ˈkōd, en-\ *vb* : to specify the genetic code for

en·co·pre·sis \ˌen-ˌkä-ˈprē-səs, -kə-\ *n, pl* -re·ses \-ˌsēz\ : involuntary passage of feces

encounter group *n* : a usu. unstructured group that seeks to develop the capacity of the individual to express feelings and to form emotional ties by unrestrained confrontation of individuals — compare T-GROUP

encrustation *var of* INCRUSTATION

en·cyst \in-ˈsist, en-\ *vb* : to enclose in or become enclosed in a cyst 〈an ∼*ed* tumor〉 — en·cyst·ment *n*

end- *or* endo- *comb form* **1** : within : inside 〈*end*aural〉 〈*endo*skeleton〉 **2** : taking in 〈*endo*cytosis〉

end·ar·ter·ec·to·my \ˌen-ˌdär-tə-ˈrek-tə-mē\ *n, pl* -mies : surgical removal of the inner layer of an artery when thickened and atheromatous or occluded (as by intimal plaques)

end·ar·te·ri·tis \ˌen-ˌdär-tə-ˈrī-təs\ *n* : inflammation of the intima of one or more arteries

endarteritis ob·lit·er·ans \-ə-ˈbli-tə-ˌranz, -ˌranz\ *n* : endarteritis in which the intimal tissue plugs the lumen of an affected artery — called also *obliterating endarteritis*

end artery *n* : a terminal artery (as a coronary artery) supplying all or most of the blood to a body part

end·au·ral \(ˌ)en-ˈdȯr-əl\ *adj* : performed or applied within the ear

end·brain \ˈend-ˌbrān\ *n* : TELENCEPHALON

end brush *n* : END PLATE

end bud *n* : TAIL BUD

end bulb *n* : a bulbous termination of a sensory nerve fiber (as in the skin)

end·di·a·stol·ic \ˌen-ˌdī-ə-ˈstä-lik\ *adj* : relating to or occurring in the moment immediately preceding contraction of the heart 〈∼ pressure〉

¹en·dem·ic \en-ˈde-mik, en-\ *adj* : restricted or peculiar to a locality or region 〈∼ diseases〉 — compare EPIDEMIC 1, SPORADIC — en·dem·i·cal·ly \-mi-k(ə-)lē\ *adv*

²endemic *n* **1** : an endemic disease or an instance of its occurrence **2** : an endemic organism

en·de·mic·i·ty \ˌen-ˌde-ˈmi-sə-tē, -də-\ *n, pl* -ties : the quality or state of being endemic

endemic syphilis *n* : BEJEL

endemic typhus *n* : MURINE TYPHUS

en·de·mism \ˈen-də-ˌmi-zəm\ *n* : ENDEMICITY

end foot *n, pl* end feet : BOUTON

endo- — see END-

en·do·ab·dom·i·nal \,en-dō-ab-'dä-mən-ᵊl\ *adj* : relating to or occurring in the interior of the abdomen

en·do·an·eu·rys·mor·rha·phy \,en-dō-,an-yə-,riz-'mòr-ə-fē\ *n, pl* **-phies** : a surgical treatment of aneurysm that involves opening its sac and collapsing, folding, and suturing its walls

en·do·bron·chi·al \,en-dō-'bräŋ-kē-əl\ *adj* : located within a bronchus ⟨~ tuberculosis⟩ — **en·do·bron·chi·al·ly** *adv*

en·do·car·di·al \-'kär-dē-əl\ *adj* **1** : situated within the heart **2** : of or relating to the endocardium ⟨~ biopsy⟩

endocardial fibroelastosis *n* : a condition usu. associated with congestive heart failure and enlargement of the heart that is characterized by conversion of the endocardium to fibroelastic tissue

en·do·car·di·tis \-,kär-'dī-təs\ *n* : inflammation of the lining of the heart and its valves

en·do·car·di·um \-'kär-dē-əm\ *n, pl* **-dia** \-dē-ə\ : a thin serous membrane lining the cavities of the heart

en·do·cer·vi·cal \'sər-vi-kəl\ *adj* : of, relating to, or affecting the endocervix

en·do·cer·vi·ci·tis \-,sər-və-'sī-təs\ *n* : inflammation of the lining of the uterine cervix

en·do·cer·vix \-'sər-viks\ *n, pl* **-vi·ces** \-və-,sēz\ : the epithelial and glandular lining of the uterine cervix

en·do·chon·dral \,en-də-'kän-drəl\ *adj* : relating to, formed by, or being ossification that takes place from centers arising in cartilage and involves deposition of lime salts in the cartilage matrix followed by secondary absorption and replacement by true bony tissue

¹en·do·crine \'en-də-krən,   ,-krīn, -,krēn\ *adj* **1** : secreting internally; *specif* : producing secretions that are distributed in the body by way of the bloodstream ⟨an ~ system⟩ **2** : of, relating to, affecting, or resembling an endocrine gland or secretion

²endocrine *n* **1** : HORMONE **2** : ENDOCRINE GLAND

endocrine gland *n* : a gland (as the thyroid or the pituitary) that produces an endocrine secretion — called also *ductless gland, gland of internal secretion*

endocrine system *n* : the glands and parts of glands that produce endocrine secretions, help to integrate and control bodily metabolic activity, and include esp. the pituitary, thyroid, parathyroids, adrenals, islets of Langerhans, ovaries, and testes

endocrine therapy *n* : HORMONE THERAPY b

en·do·cri·no·log·ic \,en-də-,krin-ᵊl-'ä-jik, -,krīn-, -,krēn-\ *or* **en·do·cri·no·log·i·cal** \-ji-kəl\ *adj* : involving or relating to the endocrine glands or secretions or to endocrinology

en·do·cri·nol·o·gy \,en-də-kri-'nä-lə-jē, -,krī-\ *n, pl* **-gies** : a science dealing with the endocrine glands — **en·do·cri·nol·o·gist** \-jist\ *n*

en·do·cri·nop·a·thy \-krə-'nä-pə-thē, -,krī-, -,krē-\ *n, pl* **-thies** : a disease marked by dysfunction of an endocrine gland — **en·do·crin·o·path·ic** \-,kri-nə-'pa-thik, -,krī-, -,krē-\ *adj*

en·do·cyt·ic \-'si-tik\ *adj* : of or relating to endocytosis — ENDOCYTOTIC

en·do·cy·to·sis \-sī-'tō-səs\ *n, pl* **-to·ses** \-,sēz\ : incorporation of substances into a cell by phagocytosis or pinocytosis — **en·do·cy·tose** \-'sī-,tōs, -,tōz\ *vb* — **en·do·cy·tot·ic** \-sī-'tä-tik\ *adj*

en·do·derm \'en-də-,dərm\ *n* : the innermost of the three primary germ layers of an embryo that is the source of the epithelium of the digestive tract and its derivatives and of the lower respiratory tract; *also* : a tissue that is derived from this germ layer — **en·do·der·mal** \,en-də-'dər-məl\ *adj*

en·do·don·tia \,en-də-'dän-chē-ə, -chə\ *n* : ENDODONTICS

en·do·don·tics \-'dän-tiks\ *n* : a branch of dentistry concerned with diseases of the pulp — **en·do·don·tic** \-tik\ *adj* — **end·odon·ti·cal·ly** \-ti-k(ə-)lē\ *adv* — **en·do·don·tist** \-tist\ *n* : a specialist in endodontics

en·do·en·zyme \,en-dō-'en-,zīm\ *n* : an enzyme that functions inside the cell — compare EXOENZYME

en·dog·e·nous \en-'dä-jə-nəs\ *also* **en·do·gen·ic** \,en-də-'je-nik\ *adj* **1** : caused by factors within the body or mind or arising from internal structural or functional causes ⟨~ malnutrition⟩ ⟨~ depression⟩ **2** : relating to or produced by metabolic synthesis in the body ⟨~ opioids⟩ — compare EXOGENOUS — **en·dog·e·nous·ly** *adv*

en·do·lymph \'en-də-,limf\ *n* : the watery fluid in the membranous labyrinth of the ear — **en·do·lym·phat·ic** \,en-də-lim-'fa·tik\ *adj*

en·do·me·ninx \,en-də-'mē-niŋs, -'me-\ *n, pl* **-nin·ges** \-mə-'nin-(,)jēz\ : the layer of embryonic mesoderm from which the arachnoid coat and pia mater of the brain develop

en·do·me·tri·al \,en-də-'mē-trē-əl\ *adj* : of, belonging to, or consisting of endometrium

en·do·me·tri·o·ma \-,mē-trē-'ō-mə\ *n, pl* **-mas** *also* **-ma·ta** \-mə-tə\ **1** : a tumor containing endometrial tissue **2** : ENDOMETRIOSIS — used chiefly of isolated foci of endometrium outside the uterus

en·do·me·tri·o·sis \,en-dō-,mē-trē-'ō-səs\ *n, pl* **-oses** \-,sēz\ : the presence and growth of functioning endometrial tissue in places other than the uterus that often results in severe pain and infertility — see ADENOMYOSIS — **en·do·me·tri·ot·ic** \-'ä-tik\ *adj*

en·do·me·tri·tis \-mə-'trī-təs\ *n* : inflammation of the endometrium

en·do·me·tri·um \-'mē-trē-əm\ *n, pl* **-tria** \-trē-ə\ : the mucous membrane lining the uterus

en·do·morph \'en-də-ˌmȯrf\ *n* : an endomorphic individual

en·do·mor·phic \ˌen-də-'mȯr-fik\ *adj* : having a heavy rounded body build often with a marked tendency to become overweight — compare ECTOMORPHIC, MESOMORPHIC — **en·do·mor·phy** \'en-də-ˌmȯr-fē\ *n*

en·do·myo·car·di·al \ˌen-dō-ˌmī-ə-'kär-dē-əl\ *adj* : of, relating to, or affecting the endocardium and the myocardium ⟨∼ fibrosis⟩ — **en·do·myo·car·di·um** \-dē-əm\ *n*

en·do·my·si·um \ˌen-də-'mi-zē-əm, -zhē-əm, -zhəm\ *n, pl* **-sia** \-zē-ə, -zhē-ə, -zhə\ : the delicate connective tissue surrounding the individual muscular fibers — compare EPIMYSIUM — **en·do·my·si·al** \-zē-əl, -zhē-əl, -zhəl\ *adj*

en·do·neu·ri·um \ˌen-dō-'nu̇r-ē-əm, -'nyu̇r-\ *n, pl* **-ria** \-ē-ə\ : the delicate connective tissue network holding together the individual fibers of a nerve trunk — **en·do·neu·ri·al** \-ē-əl\ *adj*

en·do·nu·cle·ase \-'nü-klē-ˌās, -'nyü-, -ˌāz\ *n* : an enzyme that breaks down a nucleotide chain into two or more shorter chains by breaking the internal phosphodiester bonds — compare EXONUCLEASE

en·do·nu·cleo·lyt·ic \-ˌnü-klē-ō-'li-tik, -ˌnyü-\ *adj* : breaking a nucleotide chain into two parts at an internal point ⟨∼ nicks⟩

en·do·para·site \-'par-ə-ˌsīt\ *n* : a parasite that lives in the internal organs or tissues of its host — compare ECTOPARASITE — **en·do·para·sit·ic** \-ˌpar-ə-'si-tik\ *adj* — **en·do·para·sit·ism** \-'par-ə-ˌsī-ˌti-zəm, -sə-\ *n*

en·do·pep·ti·dase \-'pep-tə-ˌdās, -ˌdāz\ *n* : any of a group of enzymes that hydrolyze peptide bonds within the long chains of protein molecules — PROTEASE — compare EXOPEPTIDASE

en·do·per·ox·ide \-pə-'räk-ˌsīd\ *n* : any of various biosynthetic intermediates in the formation of prostaglandins

en·do·phle·bi·tis \ˌen-dō-fli-'bī-təs\ *n, pl* **-bi·tis·es** *or* **-bit·i·des** \-'bi-tə-ˌdēz\ : inflammation of the intima of a vein

en·doph·thal·mi·tis \ˌen-ˌdäf-thal-'mī-təs\ *n* : inflammation that affects the interior of the eyeball

en·do·phyt·ic \ˌen-dō-'fi-tik\ *adj* : tending to grow inward into tissues in fingerlike projections from a superficial site of origin — used of tumors; compare EXOPHYTIC

en·do·plasm \'en-də-ˌpla-zəm\ *n* : the inner relatively fluid part of the cytoplasm — compare ECTOPLASM — **en·do·plas·mic** \ˌen-də-'plaz-mik\ *adj*

endoplasmic reticulum *n* : a system of interconnected vesicular and lamellar cytoplasmic membranes that functions esp. in the transport of materials within the cell and that is studded with ribosomes in some places

en·do·pros·the·sis \ˌen-dō-präs-'thē-səs\ *n, pl* **-the·ses** \-ˌsēz\ : an artificial device to replace a missing bodily part that is placed inside the body

end organ *n* : a structure forming the peripheral end of a path of nerve conduction and consisting of an effector or a receptor with its associated nerve terminations

en·dor·phin \en-'dȯr-fən\ *n* : any of a group of endogenous peptides (as enkephalin and dynorphin) that are found esp. in the brain and produce some of the same effects (as pain relief) as those of opiates; *specif* : BETA-ENDORPHIN

β-endorphin *var of* BETA-ENDORPHIN

en·do·scope \'en-də-ˌskōp\ *n* : an illuminated usu. fiber-optic flexible or rigid tubular instrument for visualizing the interior of a hollow organ (as the bladder or esophagus) and that typically has one or more channels to enable passage of instruments (as forceps or scissors) — **en·dos·co·py** \en-'däs-kə-pē\ *n*

en·do·scop·ic \ˌen-də-'skä-pik\ *adj* : of, relating to, or performed by means of an endoscope or endoscopy — **en·do·scop·i·cal·ly** \-pi-k(ə-)lē\ *adv*

endoscopic retrograde chol·an·gio·pan·cre·atog·ra·phy \-kə-ˌlan-jē-ə-ˌpaṇ-krē-ə-'täg-rə-fē\ *n* : radiographic visualization of the pancreatic and biliary ducts by means of endoscopic injection of a contrast medium through the ampulla of Vater

en·dos·co·pist \en-'däs-kə-pist\ *n* : a person trained in the use of the endoscope

en·do·skel·e·ton \ˌen-dō-'skel-ət-ᵊn\ *n* : an internal skeleton or supporting framework in an animal — **en·do·skel·e·tal** \-ət-ᵊl\ *adj*

en·do·spore \-ˌspȯr\ *n* : an asexual spore developed within the cell esp. in bacteria

en·do·stat·in \ˌen-də-'sta-tᵊn\ *n* : a polypeptide that is found esp. in epithelial basement membrane and inhibits angiogenesis, tumor growth, and endothelial cell proliferation

end·os·te·al \en-'däs-tē-əl\ *adj* **1** : of or relating to the endosteum **2** : located within bone or cartilage — **end·os·te·al·ly** *adv*

end·os·te·um \-'däs-tē-əm\ *n, pl* **-tea** \-ə\ : the layer of vascular connective tissue lining the medullary cavities of bone

endotheli- *or* **endothelio-** *comb form* : endothelium ⟨endothelioma⟩

en·do·the·li·al \ˌen-də-'thē-lē-əl\ *adj* : of, relating to, or produced from endothelium

en·do·the·lin \ˌen-dō-'thē-lin\ *n* : any of several polypeptides that play a role in regulating vasomotor activity, cell proliferation, and the production of hormones, and that have been implicated in the development of vascular disease

en·do·the·li·o·ma \-ˌthē-lē-ˈō-mə\ *n, pl* **-mas** *also* **-ma·ta** \-mə-tə\ : a tumor developing from endothelial tissue

en·do·the·li·um \ˌen-də-ˈthē-lē-əm\ *n, pl* **-lia** \-ə\ : an epithelium of mesoblastic origin composed of a single layer of thin flattened cells that lines internal body cavities (as the serous cavities or the interior of the heart)

en·do·tox·emia \ˌen-dō-täk-ˈsē-mē-ə\ *n* : the presence of endotoxins in the blood

en·do·tox·in \ˌen-dō-ˈtäk-sən\ *n* : a toxin of internal origin; *specif* : a poisonous substance present in bacteria but separable from the cell body only on its disintegration — compare EXO-TOXIN — **en·do·tox·ic** \-sik\ *adj*

en·do·tra·che·al \-ˈtrā-kē-əl\ *adj* **1** : placed within the trachea **2** : applied or effected through the trachea ⟨∼ anesthesia⟩ ⟨∼ intubation⟩

endotracheal tube *n* : a tube inserted (as through the nose or mouth) into the trachea to maintain an unobstructed passageway esp. to deliver oxygen or anesthesia to the lungs — called also *breathing tube*

end plate *n* : a complex terminal arborization of the axon of a motor neuron that contacts with a muscle fiber — called also *end brush*

end–stage \ˈend-ˌstāj\ *adj* : being or occurring in the final stages of a terminal disease or condition ⟨∼ liver failure⟩

end–stage renal disease *n* : the final stage of kidney failure that is marked by the complete or nearly complete irreversible loss of renal function — called also *end-stage kidney disease, end-stage kidney failure, end-stage renal failure*

end–tid·al \ˈend-ˌtī-dᵊl\ *adj* : of or relating to the last portion of expired tidal air ⟨∼ carbon dioxide concentrations⟩

en·e·ma \ˈe-nə-mə\ *n, pl* **enemas** *also* **ene·ma·ta** \ˌe-nə-ˈmä-tə, ˈe-nə-mə-tə\ : the injection of liquid into the intestine by way of the anus (as for cleansing); *also* : the liquid so injected

en·er·get·ics \-tiks\ *n* : the total energy relations and transformations of a physical, chemical, or biological system

en·er·giz·er \ˈe-nər-ˌjī-zər\ *n* : ANTIDEPRESSANT

en·er·gy \ˈe-nər-jē\ *n, pl* **-gies 1** : PSYCHIC ENERGY **2** : the capacity for doing work

en·er·vate \ˈe-nər-ˌvāt\ *vb* **-vat·ed; -vat·ing** : to lessen the vitality or strength of — **en·er·va·tion** \ˌe-nər-ˈvā-shən\ *n*

en·flur·ane \en-ˈflu̇r-ˌān\ *n* : a liquid inhalational general anesthetic $C_3H_2ClF_5O$ prepared from methanol

en·gage·ment \in-ˈgāj-mənt\ *n* : the phase of parturition in which the fetal head passes into the cavity of the true pelvis

en·gi·neer \ˌen-jə-ˈnir\ *vb* : to modify or produce by genetic engineering

en·gorge \in-ˈgȯrj\ *vb* **en·gorged; en·gorg·ing 1** : to fill with blood to the point of congestion ⟨the gastric mucosa was greatly *engorged*⟩ **2** : to suck blood to the limit of body capacity ⟨a tick *engorging* on its host⟩ — **en·gorge·ment** *n*

en·graft \in-ˈgraft\ *vb* : GRAFT — **en·graft·ment** *n*

en·gram *also* **en·gramme** \ˈen-ˌgram\ *n* : a \hypothetical change in neural tissue postulated in order to account for persistence of memory — called also *memory trace*

en·hanc·er \in-ˈhan-sər, en-\ *n* : a nucleotide sequence that increases the rate of genetic transcription by increasing the activity of the nearest promoter on the same DNA molecule

en·keph·a·lin \in-ˈke-fə-lən, -(ˌ)lin\ *n* : either of two pentapeptide endorphins: **a** : LEUCINE-ENKEPHALIN **b** : METHIONINE-ENKEPHALIN

en·keph·a·lin·er·gic \-ˌke-fə-lə-ˈnər-jik\ *adj* : liberating or activated by enkephalins ⟨∼ neurons⟩

eno·lase \ˈē-nə-ˌlās, -ˌlāz\ *n* : an enzyme that is found esp. in muscle and is important in the metabolism of carbohydrates

en·oph·thal·mos \ˌe-ˌnäf-ˈthal-məs, -ˌnäp-, -ˌmäs\ *also* **en·oph·thal·mus** \-məs\ *n* : a sinking of the eyeball into the orbital cavity

en·os·to·sis \ˌe-ˌnäs-ˈtō-səs\ *n, pl* **-to·ses** \-ˌsēz\ : a bony tumor arising within a bone

Eno·vid \e-ˈnō-vid\ *n* : a preparation of norethynodrel and mestranol — formerly a U.S. registered trademark

en·sheathe \in-ˈshēth\ *vb* : to cover with or as if with a sheath

ensiform cartilage *n* : XIPHOID PROCESS

ensiform process *n* : XIPHOID PROCESS

ENT *abbr* ear, nose, and throat

ent- *or* **ento-** *comb form* : inner : within ⟨*ent*optic⟩ ⟨*ento*derm⟩

ent·am·e·bi·a·sis *or* **ent·am·oe·bi·a·sis** \ˌen-ˌta-mi-ˈbī-ə-səs, -ˌtä-\ *n, pl* **-a·ses** \-ˌsēz\ : infection with or disease caused by an entamoeba

ent·amoe·ba \ˌen-tə-ˈmē-bə\ *n* **1** *cap* : a genus of amoeboid protozoans (order Amoebida) that are parasitic in the vertebrate digestive tract and esp. in the intestines and that include the causative agent (*E. histolytica*) of amebic dysentery **2** *also* **ent·ame·ba** *pl* **-bas** *or* **-bae** \-bē\ : any protozoan of the genus *Entamoeba* — **ent·amoe·bic** *also* **ent·ame·bic** \-bik\ *adj*

enter- *or* **entero-** *comb form* **1** : intestine ⟨*enter*itis⟩ **2** : intestinal and ⟨*entero*hepatic⟩

en·ter·al \'en-tə-rəl\ *adj* : ENTERIC — **en·ter·al·ly** *adv*

en·ter·ec·to·my \ˌen-tə-'rek-tə-mē\ *n, pl* **-mies** : the surgical removal of a portion of the intestine

en·ter·ic \en-'ter-ik, in-\ *adj* **1** : of, relating to, or affecting the intestines ⟨∼ diseases⟩; *broadly* : ALIMENTARY **2** : being or possessing a coating designed to pass through the stomach unaltered and disintegrate in the intestines ⟨∼ aspirin⟩

enteric fever *n* : TYPHOID FEVER; *also* : PARATYPHOID

entericus — see SUCCUS ENTERICUS

en·ter·i·tis \ˌen-tə-'rī-təs\ *n, pl* **en·ter·it·i·des** \-'ri-tə-ˌdēz\ *or* **en·ter·i·tis·es** **1** : inflammation of the intestines and esp. of the human ileum **2** : a disease of domestic animals (as panleukopenia of cats) marked by enteritis and diarrhea

En·tero·bac·ter \'en-tə-rō-ˌbak-tər\ *n* : a genus of enterobacteria that are widely distributed in nature (as in feces, soil, or water) and include some that may be pathogenic

en·tero·bac·te·ri·um \ˌen-tə-rō-bak-'tir-ē-əm\ *n, pl* **-ria** \-ē-ə\ : any of a family (Enterobacteriaceae) of gram-negative rod-shaped bacteria (as E. coli or salmonella) that ferment glucose and include some serious pathogens — **en·tero·bac·te·ri·al** \-ē-əl\ *adj*

en·tero·bi·a·sis \-'bī-ə-səs\ *n, pl* **-a·ses** \-ˌsēz\ : infestation with or disease caused by pinworms of the genus *Enterobius* that occurs esp. in children

En·te·ro·bi·us \ˌen-tə-'rō-bē-əs\ *n* : a genus of small nematode worms (family Oxyuridae) that includes the common pinworm (*E. vermicularis*) of the human intestine

en·ter·o·cele \'en-tə-rō-ˌsēl\ *n* : a hernia containing a portion of the intestines

en·tero·chro·maf·fin \ˌen-tə-rō-'krō-mə-fən\ *adj* : of, relating to, or being epithelial cells of the intestinal mucosa that stain esp. with chromium salts and usu. contain serotonin

en·tero·coc·cus \ˌen-tə-rō-'kä-kəs\ *n* **1** *cap* : a genus of gram-positive bacteria that resemble streptococci and were formerly classified with them **2** *pl* **-coc·ci** \-'käk-ˌsī, -ˌsē; -'käk-ˌkī, -ˌkē\ : any bacterium of the genus *Enterococcus*; *esp* : one (*E. faecalis*) normally present in the intestine — **en·tero·coc·cal** \-'kä-kəl\ *adj*

en·tero·co·li·tis \ˌen-tə-rō-kə-'lī-təs\ *n* : enteritis affecting both the large and small intestine

en·tero·en·ter·os·to·my \-ˌen-tə-'räs-tə-mē\ *n, pl* **-mies** : surgical anastomosis of two parts of the intestine with creation of an opening between them

en·tero·gas·tric reflex \-ˌgas-trik-\ *n* : reflex inhibition of the emptying of the stomach's contents through the

pylorus that occurs when the duodenum is stimulated by the presence of irritants, is overloaded, or is obstructed

en·tero·gas·trone \-'gas-ˌtrōn\ *n* : a hormone that is held to be produced by the duodenal mucosa and to inhibit gastric motility and secretion — compare UROGASTRONE

en·tero·he·pat·ic \-hi-'pa-tik\ *adj* : of or involving the intestine and the liver

en·tero·hep·a·ti·tis \-ˌhe-pə-'tī-təs\ *n* : BLACKHEAD 2

en·tero·ki·nase \-'kī-ˌnās, -ˌnāz\ *n* : an enzyme that activates trypsinogen by converting it to trypsin

en·ter·o·lith \'en-tə-rō-ˌlith\ *n* : a calculus occurring in the intestine

enteropathica — see ACRODERMATITIS ENTEROPATHICA

en·tero·patho·gen·ic \ˌen-tə-rō-ˌpa-thə-'je-nik\ *adj* : tending to produce disease in the intestinal tract ⟨∼ bacteria⟩ — **en·tero·patho·gen** \-'pa-thə-jən\

en·ter·op·a·thy \ˌen-tə-'rä-pə-thē\ *n, pl* **-thies** : a disease of the intestinal tract

en·ter·os·to·my \ˌen-tə-'räs-tə-mē\ *n, pl* **-mies** : a surgical formation of an opening into the intestine through the abdominal wall — **en·ter·os·to·mal** \-tə-məl\ *adj*

en·ter·ot·o·my \ˌen-tə-'rä-tə-mē\ *n, pl* **-mies** : incision into the intestines

en·tero·tox·emia \ˌen-tə-rō-ˌtäk-'sē-mē-ə\ *n* : a disease (as pulpy kidney disease of lambs) attributed to absorption of a toxin from the intestine — called also *overeating disease*

en·tero·toxi·gen·ic \-ˌtäk-sə-'je-nik\ *adj* : producing enterotoxin

en·tero·tox·in \-'täk-sən\ *n* : a toxin that is produced by microorganisms (as some staphylococci) and causes gastrointestinal symptoms

en·tero·vi·rus \-'vī-rəs\ *n* **1** *cap* : a genus of picornaviruses that typically occur in the gastrointestinal tract but may infect other tissues (as nerve and muscle) and that include the poliovirus, coxsackieviruses, and echoviruses **2** : any virus of the genus *Enterovirus* — **en·tero·vi·ral** \-rəl\ *adj*

ento- — see ENT-

en·to·derm \'en-tə-ˌdərm\ *n* : ENDODERM

en·to·mo·pho·bia \ˌen-tə-mō-'fō-bē-ə\ *n* : fear of insects

ent·op·tic \(ˌ)en-'täp-tik\ *adj* : lying or originating within the eyeball — used esp. of visual sensations due to the shadows of retinal blood vessels or of opaque particles in the vitreous body falling upon the retina

en·to·rhi·nal \ˌen-tə-'rī-nᵊl\ *adj* : of, relating to, or being the part of the cerebral cortex in the medial temporal lobe that serves as the main cortical input to the hippocampus

en·trap·ment \in-'trap-mənt\ *n* : chronic compression of a peripheral nerve (as the median nerve or ulnar nerve) usu. between ligamentous and bony surfaces that is marked by pain, numbness, tingling, or weakness

en·tro·pi·on \en-'trō-pē-ˌän, -ən\ *n* : the inversion or turning inward of the border of the eyelid against the eyeball

¹**enu·cle·ate** \(ˌ)ē-'nü-klē-ˌāt, -'nyü-\ *vb* **-at·ed; -at·ing 1** : to deprive of a nucleus **2** : to remove without cutting into ⟨~ the eyeball⟩ — **enu·cle·ation** \(ˌ)ē-ˌnü-klē-'ā-shən, -ˌnyü-\ *n*

²**enu·cle·ate** \-klē-ət, -ˌāt\ *adj* : lacking a nucleus ⟨~ cells⟩

en·ure·sis \ˌen-yu̇-'rē-səs\ *n, pl* **-ure·ses** \-ˌsēz\ : an involuntary discharge of urine : incontinence of urine — **en·uret·ic** \-'re-tik\ *adj or n*

en·ve·lope \'en-və-ˌlōp, 'än-\ *n* : a natural enclosing covering (as a membrane or integument)

en·ven·om·ation \in-ˌve-nə-'mā-shən\ *n* : an act or instance of impregnating with a venom (as of a snake or spider); *also* : ENVENOMIZATION — **en·ven·om·ate** \-'ve-nə-ˌmāt\ *vb*

en·ven·om·iza·tion \-mə-'zā-shən\ *n* : a poisoning caused by a bite or sting

en·vi·ron·ment \in-'vī-rən-mənt, -'vī-ərn-\ *n* **1** : the complex of physical, chemical, and biotic factors (as climate, soil, and living things) that act upon an organism or an ecological community and ultimately determine its form and survival **2** : the aggregate of social and cultural conditions that influence the life of an individual or community — **en·vi·ron·men·tal** \-ˌvī-rən-'ment-ᵊl, -ˌvī-ərn-\ *adj* — **en·vi·ron·men·tal·ly** *adv*

¹**en·zo·ot·ic** \ˌen-zə-'wä-tik\ *adj, of animal diseases* : peculiar to or constantly present in a locality — **en·zo·ot·i·cal·ly** \-ti-k(ə-)lē\ *adv*

²**enzootic** *n* : an enzootic disease

en·zy·mat·ic \ˌen-zə-'ma-tik\ *also* **en·zy·mic** \en-'zī-mik\ *adj* : of, relating to, or produced by an enzyme — **en·zy·mat·i·cal·ly** \-ti-k(ə-)lē\ *also* **en·zy·mi·cal·ly** \en-'zī-mi-k(ə-)lē\ *adv*

en·zyme \'en-ˌzīm\ *n* : any of numerous complex proteins that are produced by living cells and catalyze specific biochemical reactions at body temperatures

enzyme immunoassay *n* : an immunoassay (as an enzyme-linked immunosorbent assay) in which an enzyme bound to an antigen or antibody functions as a label — abbr. *EIA*

enzyme–linked immunosorbent assay *n* : a quantitative in vitro test for an antibody or antigen in which the test material is adsorbed on a surface and exposed to a complex of an enzyme linked to an antibody specific for the antigen or an enzyme linked to an anti-immunoglobulin specific for the antibody followed by reaction of the enzyme with a substrate to yield a colored product correspon-

ding to the concentration of the test material — called also *ELISA*

en·zy·mol·o·gy \ˌen-ˌzī-'mä-lə-jē, -zə-\ *n, pl* **-gies** : a branch of biochemistry dealing with enzymes, their nature, activity, and significance — **en·zy·mo·log·i·cal** \-mə-'lä-ji-kəl\ *adj* — **en·zy·mol·o·gist** \-ˌzī-'mä-lə-jist\ *n*

EOG *abbr* electrooculogram

eon·ism \'ē-ə-ˌni-zəm\ *n* : TRANSVESTISM

   Éon de Beau·mont \ā-ōⁿ-də-bō-mōⁿ\, **Charles (1728–1810),** French chevalier and adventurer.

eo·sin \'ē-ə-sən\ *also* **eo·sine** \-sən, -ˌsēn\ *n* : a red fluorescent dye $C_{20}H_8Br_4O_5$; *also* : its red to brown sodium or potassium salt used esp. as a biological stain

eo·sin·o·pe·nia \ˌē-ə-ˌsi-nə-'pē-nē-ə, -nyə\ *n* : an abnormal decrease in the number of eosinophils in the blood — **eo·sin·o·pe·nic** \-'pē-nik\ *adj*

¹**eo·sin·o·phil** \ˌē-ə-'si-nə-ˌfil\ *also* **eo·sin·o·phile** \-ˌfīl\ *adj* : EOSINOPHILIC 1

²**eosinophil** *also* **eosinophile** *n* : a white blood cell or other granulocyte with cytoplasmic inclusions readily stained by eosin

eo·sin·o·phil·ia \ˌē-ə-ˌsi-nə-'fi-lē-ə\ *n* : abnormal increase in the number of eosinophils in the blood that is characteristic of allergic states and various parasitic infections

eosinophilia–myalgia syndrome *n* : eosinophilia with severe myalgia that occurred esp. in 1989 and 1990 in individuals who made extensive use of L-tryptophan containing a toxic contaminant — abbr. *EMS*; called also *eosinophilia-myalgia*

eo·sin·o·phil·ic \-ˌsi-nə-'fi-lik\ *adj* **1** : staining readily with eosin **2** : of, relating to, or characterized by eosinophilia

eosinophilic granuloma *n* : a disease of adolescents and young adults marked by the formation of granulomas in bone and the presence in them of macrophages and eosinophilic cells with secondary deposition of cholesterol

ep— see EPI-

EPA *abbr* eicosapentaenoic acid

ep·ar·te·ri·al \ˌe-pär-'tir-ē-əl\ *adj* : situated above an artery; *specif* : of or relating to the first branch of the right bronchus

ependym- *or* **ependymo-** *comb form* : ependyma ⟨*ependymitis*⟩

ep·en·dy·ma \e-'pen-də-mə\ *n* : an epithelial membrane lining the ventricles of the brain and the canal of the spinal cord — **ep·en·dy·mal** \(ˌ)e-'pen-də-məl\ *adj*

ep·en·dy·mi·tis \ˌe-ˌpen-də-'mī-təs\ *n, pl* **-mit·i·des** \-'mi-tə-ˌdēz\ : inflammation of the ependyma

ep·en·dy·mo·ma \(ˌ)e-ˌpen-də-'mō-mə\ *n, pl* **-mas** *also* **-ma·ta** \-mə-tə\ : a glioma arising in or near the ependyma

ep·eryth·ro·zo·on \ˌe-pə-ˌrith-rə-ˈzō-ˌän\ *n* **1** *cap* : a genus of bacteria (family Anaplasmataceae) comprising blood parasites of vertebrates **2** *pl* **-zoa** \-ˈzō-ə\ : a bacterium of the genus *Eperythrozoon*

ep·eryth·ro·zo·on·o·sis \-ˌzō-ə-ˈnō-səs\ *n, pl* **-o·ses** \-ˌsēz\ : infection with or disease caused by bacteria of the genus *Eperythrozoon*

ephed·ra \i-ˈfe-drə, ˈe-fə-drə\ *n* **1 a** *cap* : a genus of shrubs (family Gnetaceae) of dry regions including some (esp. *E. sinica*) that are a source of ephedrine — see MA HUANG **b** : any plant of the genus *Ephedra* **2** : an extract of ma huang containing ephedrine and related alkaloids and used as a dietary supplement

ephed·rine \i-ˈfe-drən\ *n* : a crystalline alkaloid $C_{10}H_{15}NO$ extracted from a Chinese ephedra (*Ephedra sinica*) or synthesized that has the physiological action of epinephrine and is usu. used in the form of its hydrochloride or sulfate as a bronchodilator, nasal decongestant, and vasopressor — see PSEUDOEPHEDRINE

ephe·lis \i-ˈfē-ləs\ *n, pl* **-li·des** \-ˈfē-lə-ˌdēz, -ˈfe-\ : FRECKLE

ephem·er·al \i-ˈfe-mə-rəl\ *adj* : lasting a very short time

epi- *or* **ep-** *prefix* : upon ⟨*epicranial*⟩ : besides ⟨*epiphenomenon*⟩ : attached to ⟨*epididymis*⟩ : outer ⟨*epiblast*⟩

epi·an·dros·ter·one \ˌe-pē-ˌan-ˈdräs-tə-ˌrōn\ *n* : an androsterone derivative $C_{19}H_{30}O_2$ that occurs in normal human urine

epi·blast \ˈe-pə-ˌblast\ *n* : the outer layer of the blastoderm : ECTODERM — **epi·blas·tic** \ˌe-pə-ˈblas-tik\ *adj*

epi·can·thic fold \ˌe-pə-ˈkan-thik-\ *n* : a prolongation of a fold of the skin of the upper eyelid over the inner angle or both angles of the eye — called also *epicanthal fold*

epi·can·thus \-ˈkan-thəs\ *n* : EPICANTHIC FOLD

epi·car·di·um \ˌe-pi-ˈkär-dē-əm\ *n, pl* **-dia** \-ə\ : the visceral part of the pericardium that closely envelops the heart — called also *visceral pericardium;* compare PARIETAL PERICARDIUM — **epi·car·di·al** \-dē-əl\ *adj*

epi·con·dyle \ˌe-pi-ˈkän-ˌdīl, -dəl\ *n* : any of several prominences on the distal part of a long bone serving for the attachment of muscles and ligaments: **a** : one on the outer aspect of the distal part of the humerus or proximal to the lateral condyle of the femur — called also *lateral epicondyle* **b** : a larger and more prominent one on the inner aspect of the distal part of the humerus or proximal to the medial condyle of the femur — called also *medial epicondyle;* see EPITROCHLEA — **epi·con·dy·lar** \-də-lər\ *adj*

epi·con·dy·li·tis \-ˌkän-ˌdī-ˈlī-təs, -də-\ *n* : inflammation of an epicondyle or of adjacent tissues — compare TENNIS ELBOW

epi·cra·ni·al \-ˈkrā-nē-əl\ *adj* : situated on the cranium

epicranial aponeurosis *n* : GALEA APONEUROTICA

epi·cra·ni·um \-ˈkrā-nē-əm\ *n, pl* **-nia** \-nē-ə\ : the structures covering the vertebrate cranium

epi·cra·ni·us \ˌe-pə-ˈkrā-nē-əs\ *n, pl* **-cra·nii** \-nē-ˌī\ : OCCIPITOFRONTALIS

ep·i·crit·ic \ˌe-pə-ˈkri-tik\ *adj* : of, relating to, being, or mediating cutaneous sensory reception that is marked by accurate discrimination between small degrees of sensation — compare PROTOPATHIC

¹ep·i·dem·ic \ˌe-pə-ˈde-mik\ *also* **ep·i·dem·i·cal** \-mi-kəl\ *adj* **1** : affecting or tending to affect in an atypically large number of individuals within a population, community, or region at the same time ⟨typhoid was ∼⟩ — compare ENDEMIC, SPORADIC **2** : of, relating to, or constituting an epidemic — **ep·i·dem·i·cal·ly** \-mi-k(ə-)lē\ *adv*

²epidemic *n* : an outbreak of epidemic disease

epidemic hemorrhagic fever *n* : KOREAN HEMORRHAGIC FEVER

ep·i·de·mic·i·ty \ˌe-pə-ˌde-ˈmi-sə-tē, -də-\ *n, pl* **-ties** : the quality or state of being epidemic; *specif* : the relative ability to spread from one host to others ⟨∼ of typhoid bacteria⟩

epidemic keratoconjunctivitis *n* : an infectious often epidemic disease that is caused by an adenovirus of the genus *Mastadenovirus* (esp. species *Human adenovirus B* and *Human adenovirus D*) and is marked by pain, by redness and swelling of the conjunctiva, by edema of the tissues around the eye, and by tenderness of the adjacent lymph nodes

epidemic parotitis *n* : MUMPS

epidemic pleurodynia *n* : an acute epidemic form of pleurisy characterized by sudden onset with fever, headache, and acute diaphragmatic pain and caused by various coxsackieviruses (esp. serotypes of species *Human enterovirus B* of the genus *Enterovirus*)

epidemic typhus *n* : TYPHUS a

ep·i·de·mi·ol·o·gist \ˌe-pə-ˌdē-mē-ˈä-lə-jist, -ˌde-\ *n* : a specialist in epidemiology

ep·i·de·mi·ol·o·gy \-jē\ *n, pl* **-gies 1** : a branch of medical science that deals with the incidence, distribution, and control of disease in a population **2** : the sum of the factors controlling the presence or absence of a disease or pathogen — **ep·i·de·mi·o·log·i·cal** \-ə-ˈläj-i-kəl\ *also* **ep·i·de·mi·o·log·ic** \-jik\ *adj* — **ep·i·de·mi·o·log·i·cal·ly** \-ji-k(ə-)lē\ *adv*

epiderm- *or* **epidermo-** *comb form* : epidermis ⟨*epidermitis*⟩

ep·i·derm \'e-pə-ˌdərm\ *n* : EPIDERMIS
epi·der·mal \ˌe-pə-'dər-məl\ *adj* : of, relating to, or arising from the epidermis
epidermal growth factor *n* : a polypeptide hormone that stimulates cell proliferation esp. of epithelial cells by binding to receptor proteins on the cell surface — abbr. *EGF*
epidermal necrolysis *n* : TOXIC EPIDERMAL NECROLYSIS
epi·der·mic \ˌe-pə-'dər-mik\ *adj* : EPIDERMAL
epi·der·mis \-məs\ *n* : the outer epithelial layer of the external integument of the animal body that is derived from the embryonic epiblast; *specif* : the outer nonsensitive and nonvascular layer of the skin that overlies the dermis
epi·der·mi·tis \-(ˌ)dər-'mī-təs\ *n, pl* **-mi·tis·es** *or* **-mit·i·des** \-'mi-tə-ˌdēz\ : inflammation of the epidermis
epidermo- — see EPIDERM-
epi·der·moid \-'dər-ˌmȯid\ *adj* : resembling epidermis or epidermal cells : made up of elements like those of epidermis ⟨~ cancer of the lung⟩
epidermoid cyst *n* : a cystic tumor containing epidermal or similar tissue — called also *epidermoid;* see CHOLESTEATOMA
ep·i·der·mol·y·sis \ˌep-ə-(ˌ)dər-'mä-lə-səs\ *n, pl* **-y·ses** \-ˌsēz\ : a state of detachment or loosening of the epidermis
epidermolysis bul·lo·sa \-bə-'lō-sə\ *n* : any of a group of inherited disorders (as dystrophic epidermolysis bullosa and junctional epidermolysis bullosa) of variable severity marked esp. by the formation of large fluid-filled blisters which develop chiefly in response to minor mechanical trauma
epidermolysis bullosa ac·qui·si·ta \-ˌa-kwə-'sī-tə\ *n* : an autoimmune skin disorder similar to epidermolysis bullosa that occurs in adults and is usu. associated with another disorder (as Crohn's disease or diabetes)
epidermolysis bullosa sim·plex \-'sim-ˌpleks\ *n* : any of several forms of epidermolysis bullosa that are marked by blister formation within the epidermis sometimes accompanied by thickening of the skin and that are chiefly inherited as an autosomal dominant trait
Ep·i·der·moph·y·ton \-(ˌ)dər-'mä-fə-ˌtän\ *n* : a genus of fungi that comprises dermatophytes causing disease (as athlete's foot and tinea cruris), that now usu. includes a single species (*E. floccosums* syns. *E. inguinale* and *E. cruris*), and that is sometimes considered a synonym of *Trichophyton*
ep·i·der·moph·y·to·sis \-ˌmä-fə-'tō-səs\ *n, pl* **-to·ses** \-ˌsēz\ : a disease (as athlete's foot) of the skin or nails caused by a dermatophyte
epididym- *or* **epididymo-** *comb form* **1** : epididymis ⟨*epididym*ectomy⟩ **2** : epididymis and ⟨*epididymo*-orchitis⟩

ep·i·did·y·mec·to·my \-ˌdi-də-'mek-tə-mē\ *n, pl* **-mies** : excision of the epididymis
ep·i·did·y·mis \-'di-də-məs\ *n, pl* **-mi·des** \-mə-ˌdēz\ : a system of ductules that emerges posteriorly from the testis, holds sperm during maturation, and forms a tangled mass before uniting into a single coiled duct which comprises the highly convoluted body and tail of the system and is continuous with the vas deferens — see VASA EFFERENTIA — **ep·i·did·y·mal** \-məl\ *adj*
ep·i·did·y·mi·tis \-ˌdi-də-'mī-təs\ *n* : inflammation of the epididymis
ep·i·did·y·mo-or·chi·tis \-ˌdi-də-ˌmō-ȯr-'kī-təs\ *n* : combined inflammation of the epididymis and testis
ep·i·did·y·mo·vas·os·to·my \-va-'säs-tə-mē\ *n, pl* **-mies** : surgical severing of the vas deferens with anastomosis of the distal part to the epididymis esp. to circumvent an obstruction
¹**epi·du·ral** \ˌep-i-'dúr-əl, -'dyúr-\ *adj* : situated upon or administered or placed outside the dura mater — **epi·du·ral·ly** *adv*
²**epidural** *n* : an injection of an anesthetic to produce epidural anesthesia
epidural anesthesia *n* : anesthesia produced by injection of a local anesthetic into the peridural space of the spinal cord beneath the ligamentum flavum — called also *peridural anesthesia*
epi·gas·tric \ˌe-pə-'gas-trik\ *adj* **1** : lying upon or over the stomach **2 a** : of or relating to the anterior walls of the abdomen ⟨~ veins⟩ **b** : of or relating to the abdominal region lying between the hypochondriac regions and above the umbilical region
epigastric artery *n* : any of the three arteries supplying the anterior walls of the abdomen
epi·gas·tri·um \ˌe-pə-'gas-trē-əm\ *n, pl* **-tria** \-trē-ə\ : the epigastric region
epi·glot·tic \ˌe-pə-'glä-tik\ *or* **epi·glot·tal** \-'glät-ᵊl\ *adj* : of, relating to, or produced with the aid of the epiglottis
epi·glot·ti·dec·to·my \-ˌglä-tə-'dek-tə-mē\ *n, pl* **-mies** : excision of all or part of the epiglottis
epi·glot·tis \-'glä-təs\ *n* : a thin lamella of yellow elastic cartilage that ordinarily projects upward behind the tongue and just in front of the glottis and that with the arytenoid cartilages serves to cover the glottis during the act of swallowing
epi·glot·ti·tis \-ˌglä-'tī-təs\ *n* : inflammation of the epiglottis
epi·ker·a·to·pha·kia \ˌe-pə-ˌker-ə-tə-'fā-kē-ə\ *n* : the grafting of human corneal tissue to a recipient in order to correct a refractive defect (as nearsightedness or astigmatism)
ep·i·la·tion \-'lā-shən\ *n* : the loss or removal of hair
ep·i·lep·sy \'e-pə-ˌlep-sē\ *n, pl* **-sies** : any of various disorders marked by

abnormal electrical discharges in the brain and typically manifested by sudden brief episodes of altered or diminished consciousness, involuntary movements, or convulsions — see GRAND MAL; PETIT MAL; FOCAL EPILEPSY; JACKSONIAN EPILEPSY; MYOCLONIC EPILEPSY; TEMPORAL LOBE EPILEPSY

epilept- or **epilepti-** or **epilepto-** comb form : epilepsy ⟨epileptiform⟩

ep·i·lep·tic \ˌe-pə-ˈlep-tik\ adj : relating to, affected with, or having the characteristics of epilepsy — **epileptic** n — **ep·i·lep·ti·cal·ly** \-ti-k(ə-)lē\ adv

epilepticus — see STATUS EPILEPTICUS

ep·i·lep·ti·form \-ˈlep-tə-ˌfȯrm\ adj : resembling that of epilepsy ⟨an ∼ seizure⟩

ep·i·lep·to·gen·ic \-ˌlep-tə-ˈjen-ik\ adj : inducing or tending to induce epilepsy ⟨an ∼ drug⟩

ep·i·lep·toid \-ˈlep-ˌtȯid\ adj **1** : EPILEPTIFORM **2** : exhibiting symptoms resembling those of epilepsy

epi·loia \ˌe-pə-ˈlȯi-ə\ n : TUBEROUS SCLEROSIS

epi·my·si·um \ˌe-pə-ˈmizh-ē-əm, -zē-\ n, pl **-sia** \-zhē-ə, -zē-ə\ : the external connective-tissue sheath of a muscle — compare ENDOMYSIUM

epi·neph·rine also **epi·neph·rin** \ˌe-pə-ˈne-frən\ n : a crystalline sympathomimetic hormone $C_9H_{13}NO_3$ that is the principal blood-pressure-raising hormone secreted by the adrenal medulla, is prepared from adrenal extracts or made synthetically, and is used medicinally esp. as a heart stimulant, as a vasoconstrictor (as to treat life-threatening allergic reactions and to prolong the effects of local anesthetics), and as a bronchodilator — called also *adrenaline*

¹epi·neu·ral \ˌe-pə-ˈnu̇r-əl, -ˈnyu̇r-\ adj : arising from the neural arch of a vertebra

²epineural n : a spine or process arising from the neural arch of a vertebra

epi·neu·ri·um \ˌe-pə-ˈnu̇r-ē-əm, -ˈnyu̇r-\ n : the external connective-tissue sheath of a nerve trunk

epi·phe·nom·e·non \ˌe-pi-fə-ˈnä-mə-ˌnän, -nən\ n : an accidental or accessory event or process occurring in the course of a disease but not necessarily related to that disease

epiph·o·ra \i-ˈpi-fə-rə\ n : a watering of the eyes due to excessive secretion of tears or to obstruction of the lacrimal passages

epiph·y·se·al \i-ˌpi-fə-ˈsē-əl\ also **epi·phys·i·al** \ˌe-pə-ˈfiz-ē-əl\ adj : of or relating to an epiphysis

epiphyseal line n : the line marking the site of the epiphyseal plate

epiphyseal plate n : the cartilage that contains an epiphysis, unites it with the shaft, and is the site of longitudinal growth of the bone — called also *epiphyseal cartilage*

epiph·y·si·od·e·sis \i-ˌpi-fə-sē-ˈä-də-səs, ˌe-pə-ˌfi-zē-\ n, pl **-e·ses** \-ˌsēz\ : the surgical reattachment of a separated epiphysis to the shaft of its bone

epiph·y·sis \i-ˈpi-fə-səs\ n, pl **-y·ses** \-ˌsēz\ **1** : a part or process of a bone that ossifies separately and later becomes ankylosed to the main part of the bone; esp : an end of a long bone — compare DIAPHYSIS **2** : PINEAL GLAND

epiph·y·si·tis \i-ˌpi-fə-ˈsī-təs\ n : inflammation of an epiphysis

epi·plo·ec·to·my \ˌe-pə-plō-ˈek-tə-mē\ n, pl **-mies** : OMENTECTOMY

ep·i·plo·ic \ˌe-pə-ˈplō-ik\ adj : of or associated with an omentum : OMENTAL

epiploicae — see APPENDICES EPIPLOICAE

epiploic foramen n : the only opening between the omental bursa and the general peritoneal sac — called also *foramen of Winslow*

ep·i·plo·on \ˌe-pə-ˈplō-ˌän\ n, pl **-ploa** \-ˈplō-ə\ : OMENTUM; specif : GREATER OMENTUM

epi·pter·ic \ˌep-ip-ˈter-ik\ adj : relating to or being a small Wormian bone sometimes present in the human skull between the parietal and the greater wing of the sphenoid

epi·sclera \ˌe-pə-ˈskler-ə\ n : the layer of connective tissue between the conjunctiva and the sclera of the eye

epi·scler·al \-ˈskler-əl\ adj **1** : situated upon the sclerotic coat of the eye **2** : of or relating to the episclera

epi·scle·ri·tis \-sklə-ˈrī-təs\ n : inflammation of the superficial layers of the sclera

episio- comb form **1** : vulva ⟨*episio*tomy⟩ **2** : vulva and ⟨*episio*perineorrhaphy⟩

epi·sio·per·i·ne·or·rha·phy \i-ˌpi-zē-ō-ˌper-ə-nē-ˈȯr-ə-fē, -ˌpē-\ n, pl **-phies** : surgical repair of the vulva and perineum by suturing

epi·si·or·rha·phy \-zē-ˈȯr-ə-fē\ n, pl **-phies** : surgical repair of injury to the vulva by suturing

epi·si·ot·o·my \i-ˌpi-zē-ˈä-tə-mē, -ˌpē-\ n, pl **-mies** : surgical enlargement of the vulval orifice for obstetrical purposes during parturition

ep·i·sode \ˈe-pə-ˌsōd, -ˌzōd\ n : an event that is distinctive and separate although part of a larger series; esp : an occurrence of a usu. recurrent pathological abnormal condition — **ep·i·sod·ic** \ˌe-pə-ˈsä-dik, -ˈzä-\ adj — **ep·i·sod·i·cal·ly** \-di-k(ə-)lē\ adv

epi·some \ˈe-pə-ˌsōm, -ˌzōm\ n : a genetic determinant (as the DNA of some bacteriophages) that can replicate either autonomously in bacterial cytoplasm or as an integral part of their chromosomes — compare PLASMID — **epi·som·al** \ˌe-pə-ˈsō-məl, -ˈzō-\ adj — **epi·som·al·ly** \-mə-lē\ adv

ep·i·spa·di·as \ˌe-pə-ˈspā-dē-əs\ n : a

congenital defect in which the urethra opens upon the upper surface of the penis

epis·ta·sis \i-'pis-tə-səs\ *n, pl* **-ta·ses** \-,sēz\ **1 a** : suppression of a secretion or discharge **b** : a scum on the surface of urine **2** : suppression of the effect of a gene by a nonallelic gene — **epi·stat·ic** \,e-pə-'sta-tik\ *adj*

ep·i·stax·is \,e-pə-'stak-səs\ *n, pl* **-stax·es** \-,sēz\ : NOSEBLEED

ep·i·stro·phe·us \,e-pə-'strō-fē-əs\ *n* : AXIS 2a

epi·thal·a·mus \,e-pə-'tha-lə-məs\ *n, pl* **-mi** \-,mī\ : a dorsal segment of the diencephalon containing the habenula and the pineal gland

epithel- *or* **epitheli-** *or* **epithelio-** *comb form* : epithelium ⟨*epithelioma*⟩

epi·the·li·al \,e-pə-'thē-lē-əl\ *adj* : of or relating to epithelium ⟨~ cells⟩

epi·the·li·oid \-'thē-lē-,ȯid\ *adj* : resembling epithelium

epithelioid angiomatosis *n* : BACILLARY ANGIOMATOSIS

epi·the·li·o·ma \,thē-lē-'ō-mə\ *n, pl* **-mas** *also* **-ma·ta** \-mə-tə\ : a tumor derived from epithelial tissue

epi·the·li·um \,e-pə-'thē-lē-əm\ *n, pl* **-lia** \-lē-ə\ : a membranous cellular tissue that covers a free surface or lines a tube or cavity of an animal body and serves esp. to enclose and protect the other parts of the body, to produce secretions and excretions, and to function in assimilation

epi·the·li·za·tion \,e-pə-,thē-lə-'zā-shən\ *or* **epi·the·li·al·i·za·tion** \-,thē-lē-ə-lə-\ *n* : the process of becoming covered with or converted to epithelium — **epi·the·lize** \,e-pə-'thē-,līz\ *or* **epi·the·li·al·ize** \-'thē-lē-ə-,līz\ *vb*

epi·thet \'e-pə-,thet, -,thət\ *n* : the part of a scientific name identifying the species, variety, or other subunit within a genus — see SPECIFIC EPITHET

epi·tope \'e-pə-,tōp\ *n* : a molecular region on the surface of an antigen capable of eliciting an immune response and of combining with the specific antibody produced by such a response — called also *determinant, antigenic determinant*

epi·troch·lea \,e-pi-'trä-klē-ə\ *n* : the medial epicondyle at the distal end of the humerus — **epi·troch·le·ar** \-klē-ər\ *adj*

epi·tym·pan·ic \-tim-'pa-nik\ *adj* : situated above the tympanic membrane

epitympanic recess *n* : ATTIC

epi·tym·pa·num \-'tim-pə-nəm\ *n* : the upper portion of the middle ear — compare HYPOTYMPANUM

Ep·i·vir \'e-pə-,vir\ *trademark* — used for a preparation of lamivudine

epi·zo·ot·ic \,e-pə-zō-'wä-tik\ *n* : an outbreak of disease affecting many animals of one kind at the same time; *also* : the disease itself — **epizootic** *adj*

epizootic lymphangitis *n* : a chronic

contagious inflammation chiefly affecting the superficial lymphatics and lymph nodes of horses, mules, and donkeys and caused by a fungus of the genus *Histoplasma* (*H. farciminosum*)

epi·zo·ot·i·ol·o·gy \,e-pə-zō-,wä-tē-'ä-lə-jē\ *also* **epi·zo·ot·ol·o·gy** \-,zō-ə-'tä-lə-jē\ *n, pl* **-gies** **1** : a science that deals with the character, ecology, and causes of outbreaks of animal diseases **2** : the sum of the factors controlling the occurrence of a disease or pathogen of animals — **epi·zo·oti·o·log·i·cal** \-zō-,wō-tē-ə-'lä-ji-kəl, -,wä-\ *also* **epi·zo·oti·o·log·ic** \-jik\ *adj*

EPO *abbr* erythropoietin

Ep·o·gen \'e-pə-jən\ *trademark* — used for a preparation of erythropoietin

ep·o·nych·i·um \,e-pə-'ni-kē-əm\ *n* : the horny band of epidermis that extends over the proximal edge of a nail : CUTICLE

ep·onym \'e-pə-,nim\ *n* **1** : the person for whom something (as a disease) is or is believed to be named **2** : a name (as of a drug or a disease) based on or derived from the name of a person — **epon·y·mous** \i-'pä-nə-məs, e-\ *adj*

ep·ooph·o·ron \,e-pō-'ä-fə-,rän\ *n* : a rudimentary organ homologous with the male epididymis that lies in the broad ligament of the uterus — called also *organ of Rosenmüller, parovarium*

Ep·som salt \'ep-səm-\ *n* : EPSOM SALTS

Epsom salts *n* : a bitter white crystalline salt $MgSO_4 \cdot 7H_2O$ that is a hydrated magnesium sulfate with cathartic properties

Ep·stein–Barr virus \'ep-,stīn-'bär-\ *n* : a herpesvirus (species *Human herpesvirus 4* of the genus *Lymphocryptovirus*) that causes infectious mononucleosis and is associated with Burkitt's lymphoma and nasopharyngeal carcinoma — abbr. *EBV;* called also *EB virus*

Epstein, Michael Anthony (*b* 1921), **and Barr, Yvonne M.** (*b* 1932), British virologists.

Ep·stein's pearls \'ep-,stīnz-, -,stēnz-\ *n pl* : temporary small white cysts that occur along the midline of the hard palate of many newborn infants

Epstein, Alois (1849–1918), Czech pediatrician.

epu·lis \ə-'pyü-ləs\ *n, pl* **epu·li·des** \-lə-,dēz\ : a tumor or tumorous growth of the gum

Equa·nil \'e-kwə-,nil\ *trademark* — used for a preparation of meprobamate

equa·tion·al \i-'kwā-zhə-nəl\ *adj* : dividing into two equal parts — used esp. of the mitotic cell division usu. following reduction in meiosis — **equa·tion·al·ly** *adv*

equa·tor \i-'kwā-tər, 'ē-,\ *n* **1** : a circle dividing the surface of a body into two usu. equal and symmetrical parts esp. at the place of greatest width ⟨the ~ of the lens of the eye⟩ 2 : EQUA-TORIAL PLANE — **equa·to·ri·al** \ˌē-kwə-ˈtōr-ē-əl, ˌe-\ *adj*

equatorial plane *n* : the plane perpendicular to the spindle of a dividing cell and midway between the poles

equatorial plate *n* 1 : METAPHASE PLATE 2 : EQUATORIAL PLANE

equi·an·al·ge·sic \ˌē-kwi-ˌan-ᵊl-ˈjē-zik, ˌe-, -sik\ *adj* : producing the same degree of analgesia

equi·len·in \ē-ˈkwe-lə-nən, ə-ˈkwi-lə-nən\ *n* : a weakly estrogenic steroid hormone $C_{18}H_{18}O_2$ obtained from the urine of pregnant mares

equi·lib·ri·um \ˌē-kwə-ˈli-brē-əm, ˌe-\ *n, pl* **-ri·ums** *or* **-ria** \-brē-ə\ 1 : a state of balance between opposing forces or actions that is either static (as in a body acted on by forces whose resultant is zero) or dynamic (as in a reversible chemical reaction when the velocities in both directions are equal) 2 : a state of intellectual or emotional balance

eq·ui·lin \ˈe-kwə-lən\ *n* : an estrogenic steroid $C_{18}H_{20}O_2$ obtained from the urine of pregnant mares

equina — see CAUDA EQUINA

equine \ˈē-ˌkwīn, ˈe-\ *n* : any of a family (Equidae) of hoofed mammals that include the horses, asses and zebras; *esp* : HORSE — **equine** *adj*

equine babesiosis *n* : EQUINE PIROPLASMOSIS

equine coital exanthema *n* : a highly contagious disease of horses that is caused by a herpesvirus of the genus *Varicellovirus* (species *Equid herpesvirus 3*) transmitted chiefly by copulation — called also *coital exanthema*

equine encephalitis *n* : any of three virus diseases chiefly of equines and humans in various parts of No. and So. America that are transmitted esp. by mosquitoes, are characterized in humans by flulike symptoms which often progress to encephalitis and sometimes to coma and death, and are caused by three togaviruses of the genus *Alphavirus* (species *Eastern equine encephalitis virus*, *Western equine encephalitis virus*, and *Venezuelan equine encephalitis virus*): **a** : one that occurs in the eastern U.S. and Canada — called also *eastern equine encephalitis*, *eastern equine encephalomyelitis* **b** : one that occurs in the western U.S. and Canada — called also *western equine encephalitis*, *western equine encephalomyelitis* **c** : one that occurs from northern So. America to Mexico — called also *Venezuelan equine encephalitis*, *Venezuelan equine encephalomyelitis*

equine encephalomyelitis *n* : EQUINE ENCEPHALITIS

equine infectious anemia *n* : a serious sometimes fatal disease of horses that is caused by a retrovirus of the genus *Lentivirus* (species *Equine infectious anemia virus*) and is marked by intermittent fever, depression, weakness, edema and anemia — called also *swamp fever*

equine piroplasmosis *n* : a tick-borne disease that affects horses and related equines, is caused by two protozoans of the genus *Babesia* (*B. caballi* and *B. equi*), and is characterized esp. by fever, anemia, weakness, and icterus — called also *equine babesiosis*

equinovarus — see TALIPES EQUINOVARUS

equinus — see TALIPES EQUINUS

equi·po·tent \ˌē-kwə-ˈpōt-ᵊnt, ˌe-\ *adj* : having equal effects or capacities

Er *symbol* erbium

ER *abbr* emergency room

er·bi·um \ˈər-bē-əm\ *n* : a metallic element that occurs with yttrium — symbol *Er;* see ELEMENT table

Erb's palsy \ˈerbz-, ˈerps-\ *n* : paralysis affecting the muscles of the upper arm and shoulder that is caused by an injury during birth to the upper part of the brachial plexus

Erb, Wilhelm Heinrich (1840–1921), German neurologist.

erect \i ˈrekt\ *adj* 1 : standing up or out from the body ⟨~ hairs⟩ 2 : being in a state of physiological erection

erec·tile \i-ˈrekt-ᵊl, -ˈrek-ˌtīl\ *adj* : capable of being raised to an erect position; *esp* : CAVERNOUS 2 — **erec·til·i·ty** \-ˌrek-ˈti-lə-tē\ *n*

erectile dysfunction *n* : chronic inability to achieve or maintain an erection satisfactory for sexual intercourse : IMPOTENCE 2 — abbr. *ED*

erec·tion \i-ˈrek-shən\ *n* 1 : the state marked by firm turgid form and erect position of a previously flaccid bodily part containing cavernous tissue when that tissue becomes dilated with blood 2 : an occurrence of erection in the penis or clitoris

erec·tor \i-ˈrek-tər\ *n* : a muscle that raises or keeps a part erect

erector spi·nae \-ˈspī-ˌnē\ *n* : SACROSPINALIS

erep·sin \i-ˈrep-sən\ *n* : a proteolytic fraction obtained esp. from the intestinal juice

er·e·thism \ˈer-ə-ˌthi-zəm\ *n* : abnormal irritability or responsiveness to stimulation

erg \ˈərg\ *n* : a cgs unit of work equal to the work done by a force of one dyne acting through a distance of one centimeter

ERG *abbr* electroretinogram

erg- *or* **ergo-** *comb form* : work ⟨*ergo*meter⟩

-er·gic \ˈər-jik\ *adj comb form* 1 : allergic ⟨hyper*ergic*⟩ 2 : exhibiting or stimulating activity esp. of (such) a neurotransmitter substance ⟨adren*ergic*⟩ ⟨dopamin*ergic*⟩

ergo- *comb form* : ergot ⟨*ergo*sterol⟩

er·go·cal·cif·er·ol \ˌər-(ˌ)gō-kal-ˈsi-fə-ˌrȯl, -ˌrōl\ *n* : CALCIFEROL

er·go·loid mes·y·lates \'ər-gə-ˌlȯid-\ *n sing or pl* : a combination of equal amounts of three ergot alkaloids used with varying success in the treatment of cognitive decline and dementia esp. in elderly patients — see HYDERGINE

er·gom·e·ter \(ˌ)ər-'gä-mə-tər\ *n* : an apparatus for measuring the work performed (as by a person exercising); *also* : an exercise machine equipped with an ergometer — **er·go·met·ric** \ˌər-gə-'me-trik\ *adj*

er·go·met·rine \ˌər-gə-'me-ˌtrēn, -trən\ *n* : ERGONOVINE

er·go·nom·ics \ˌər-gə-'nä-miks\ *n sing or pl* : an applied science concerned with designing and arranging things people use so that the people and things interact most efficiently and safely — called also *biotechnology, human engineering, human factors, human factors engineering* **2** : the design characteristics of an object resulting esp. from the application of the science of ergonomics — **er·go·nom·ic** \-ik\ *adj* — **er·go·nom·i·cal·ly** \-mi-k(ə-)lē\ *adv* — **er·gon·o·mist** \(ˌ)ər-'gä-nə-mist\ *n*

er·go·no·vine \ˌər-gə-'nō-ˌvēn, -vən\ *n* : an alkaloid $C_{19}H_{23}N_3O_2$ that is derived from ergot and is used esp. in the form of its maleate $C_{19}H_{23}N_3O_2 \cdot C_4H_4O_4$ to prevent or treat postpartum bleeding

er·gos·ter·ol \ˌər-'gäs-tə-ˌrȯl, -ˌrōl\ *n* : a steroid alcohol $C_{28}H_{44}O$ that occurs esp. in yeast, molds, and ergot and is converted by ultraviolet irradiation ultimately into vitamin D_2

er·got \'ər-gət, -ˌgät\ *n* **1** : the black or dark purple sclerotium of fungi of an ascomycetous genus (*Claviceps*); *also* : any fungus of this genus **2 a** : the dried sclerotial bodies of an ergot fungus grown on rye and containing several ergot alkaloids **b** : ERGOT ALKALOID

ergot alkaloid *n* : any of a group of alkaloids found in ergot or produced synthetically that include some (as ergonovine and ergotamine) noted esp. for their contractile effect on smooth muscle (as of the uterus or blood vessels)

er·got·a·mine \(ˌ)ər-'gä-tə-ˌmēn\ *n* : an alkaloid that is derived from ergot and is used chiefly in the form of its tartrate $(C_{33}H_{35}N_5O_5)_2 \cdot C_4H_6O_6$ esp. in treating migraine

er·got·ism \'ər-gə-ˌti-zəm\ *n* : a toxic condition produced by eating grain, grain products (as rye bread), or grasses infected with ergot fungus or by chronic excessive use of an ergot drug

er·got·ized \-ˌtīzd\ *adj* : infected with ergot; *also* : poisoned by ergot

erigens, erigentes — see NERVUS ERIGENS

eri·o·dic·ty·on \ˌer-ē-ə-'dik-tē-ˌän\ *n* : the dried leaves of yerba santa used as a flavoring in medicine

erode \i-'rōd\ *vb* **erod·ed; erod·ing 1** : to eat into or away by slow destruction of substance ⟨acids that ~ the teeth⟩ ⟨bone *eroded* by cancer⟩ **2** : to remove with an abrasive

erog·e·nous \i-'rä-jə-nəs\ *adj* **1** : producing sexual excitement or libidinal gratification when stimulated : sexually sensitive **2** : of, relating to, or arousing sexual feelings — **er·o·ge·ne·ity** \ˌer-ə-jə-'nē-ə-tē\ *n*

Eros \'er-ˌäs, 'ir-\ *n* : the sum of life-preserving instincts that are manifested as impulses to gratify basic needs (as sex), as sublimated impulses motivated by the same needs, and as impulses to protect and preserve the body and mind — compare DEATH INSTINCT

ero·sion \i-'rō-zhən\ *n* **1 a** : the superficial destruction of a surface area of tissue (as mucous membrane) by inflammation, ulceration, or trauma ⟨~ of the uterine cervix⟩ **b** : progressive loss of the hard substance of a tooth **2** : an instance or product of erosion — **ero·sive** \i-'rō-siv, -ziv\ *adj*

erot·ic \i-'rä-tik\ *also* **erot·i·cal** \i-'rä-ti-kəl\ *adj* **1** : of, devoted to, or tending to arouse sexual love or desire **2** : strongly marked or affected by sexual desire — **erot·i·cal·ly** \-ti-k(ə-)lē\ *adv*

erot·i·cism \i-'rä-tə-ˌsi-zəm\ *n* **1** : a state of sexual arousal or anticipation **2** : insistent sexual impulse or desire

erot·i·cize \-ˌsīz\ *vb* **-cized; -ciz·ing** : to make erotic — **erot·i·ci·za·tion** \-ˌrä-tə-sə-'zā-shən\ *n*

er·o·tism \'er-ə-ˌti-zəm\ *n* : EROTICISM

er·o·tize \'er-ə-ˌtīz\ *vb* **-tized; -tiz·ing** : to invest with erotic significance or sexual feeling — **er·o·ti·za·tion** \ˌer-ə-tə-'zā-shən\ *n*

eroto- *comb form* : sexual desire ⟨*eroto*mania⟩

ero·to·gen·ic \i-ˌrō-tə-'je-nik, -ˌrä-\ *adj* : EROGENOUS

ero·to·ma·nia \-'mā-nē-ə\ *n* **1** : excessive sexual desire **2** : a psychological disorder marked by the delusional belief that one is the object of another person's love or sexual desire

ero·to·ma·ni·ac \-'mā-nē-ˌak\ *n* : one affected with erotomania

ero·to·pho·bia \-'fō-bē-ə\ *n* : a morbid aversion to sexual love or desire

ERT *abbr* estrogen replacement therapy

eru·cic acid \i-'rük-sik-\ *n* : a crystalline fatty acid $C_{22}H_{42}O_2$ found in the form of its glycerides esp. in an oil obtained from the seeds of the rape plant (*Brassica napus* of the mustard family)

eruct \i-'rəkt\ *vb* : BELCH

eruc·ta·tion \i-ˌrək-'tā-shən, ˌē-\ *n* : an act or instance of belching

erupt \i-'rəpt\ *vb* **1** *of a tooth* : to emerge through the gum **2** : to break out (as with a skin eruption) — **erup·tive** \-'rəp-tiv\ *adj*

erup·tion \i-'rəp-shən\ *n* **1** : an act,

process, or instance of erupting; *specif* : the breaking out of an exanthem or enanthem on the skin or mucous membrane (as in measles) **2** : something produced by an act or process of erupting: as **a** : the condition of the skin or mucous membrane caused by erupting **b** : one of the lesions (as a pustule) constituting this condition

er·y·sip·e·las \er-ə-'si-pə-ləs, ir-\ *n* 1 : an acute febrile disease that is associated with intense often vesicular and edematous local inflammation of the skin and subcutaneous tissues and that is caused by a hemolytic streptococcus **2** : SWINE ERYSIPELAS — used esp. when the disease affects hosts other than swine

er·y·sip·e·loid \er-ə-'si-pə-ˌlȯid, ir-\ *n* : an acute dermatitis resembling erysipelas that is caused by the bacterium of the genus *Erysipelothrix* (*E. rhusiopathiae*) that causes swine erysipelas, is typically marked by usu. painful reddish purple lesions esp. on the hands, and that is contracted by direct contact with infected animal flesh — **erysipeloid** *adj*

er·y·sip·e·lo·thrix \er-ə-'si-pə-lō-ˌthriks\ *n* **1** *cap* : a genus of gram-positive, rod-shaped bacteria (family Erysipelotrichaceae) including one (*E. rhusiopathiae*) that is the causative agent of swine erysipelas, an arthritis of lambs, and human erysipeloid **2** : a bacterium of the genus *Erysipelothrix*

er·y·the·ma \er-ə-'thē-mə\ *n* : abnormal redness of the skin due to capillary congestion (as in inflammation) — **er·y·the·mal** \-məl\ *adj*

erythema chron·i·cum mi·grans \-'krä-nə-kəm-'mī-grənz\ *n* : ERYTHEMA MIGRANS

erythema in·fec·ti·o·sum \-in-ˌfek-shē-'ō-səm\ *n* : FIFTH DISEASE

erythema mi·grans \-'mī-grənz\ *n* : a spreading annular erythematous skin lesion that is an early symptom of Lyme disease and that develops at the site of the bite of a tick (as the deer tick) infected with the causative spirochete

erythema mul·ti·for·me \-ˌməl-tə-'fȯr-mē\ *n* : a skin disease characterized by papular or vesicular lesions and reddening or discoloration of the skin often in concentric zones about the lesions

erythema no·do·sum \-nō-'dō-səm\ *n* : a skin condition characterized by small tender reddened nodules under the skin (as over the shin bones) often accompanied by fever and transitory arthritic pains

erythematosus — see LUPUS ERYTHEMATOSUS, LUPUS ERYTHEMATOSUS CELL, PEMPHIGUS ERYTHEMATOSUS, SYSTEMIC LUPUS ERYTHEMATOSUS

er·y·them·a·tous \er-ə-'the-mə-təs, -'thē-\ *adj* : relating to or marked by erythema

er·y·thor·bate \er-ə-'thȯr-ˌbāt\ *n* : a salt of erythorbic acid that is used in foods as an antioxidant

er·y·thor·bic acid \er-ə-'thȯr-bik-\ *n* : a stereoisomer of vitamin C

erythr- *or* **erythro-** *comb form* **1** : red ⟨*erythrocyte*⟩ **2** : erythrocyte ⟨*erythroid*⟩

er·y·thrae·mia *chiefly Brit var of* ERYTHREMIA

er·y·thras·ma \er-ə-'thraz-mə\ *n* : a chronic contagious dermatitis that affects warm moist areas of the body (as the armpit and groin) and is caused by a bacterium of the genus *Corynebacterium* (*C. minutissimum*)

eryth·re·de·ma \i-ˌri-thrə-'dē-mə\ *n* : ACRODYNIA

er·y·thre·mia \er-ə-'thrē-mē-ə\ *n* : POLYCYTHEMIA VERA

er·y·thrism \'er-ə-ˌthri-zəm\ *n* : a condition marked by exceptional prevalence of red pigmentation (as in skin or hair) — **er·y·thris·tic** \er-ə-'thris-tik\ *also* **er·y·thris·mal** \-'thriz-məl\ *adj*

eryth·ri·tyl tet·ra·ni·trate \i-'ri-thrə-ˌtil ˌte-trə-'nī-ˌtrāt\ *n* : a vasodilator $C_4H_{10}N_4O_{12}$ used to prevent angina pectoris — called also *erythritol tetranitrate*

erythro- — see ERYTHR-

eryth·ro·blast \i-'ri-thrə-ˌblast\ *n* : a polychromatic nucleated cell of red marrow that synthesizes hemoglobin and that is an intermediate in the initial stage of red blood cell formation; *broadly* : a cell ancestral to red blood cells — compare NORMOBLAST — **eryth·ro·blas·tic** \-ˌri-thrə-'blas-tik\ *adj*

eryth·ro·blas·to·pe·nia \i-ˌri-thrə-ˌblas-tə-'pē-nē-ə\ *n* : a deficiency in bone-marrow erythroblasts

eryth·ro·blas·to·sis \-ˌblas-'tō-səs\ *n, pl* **-to·ses** \-ˌsēz\ : abnormal presence of erythroblasts in the circulating blood; *esp* : ERYTHROBLASTOSIS FETALIS

erythroblastosis fe·ta·lis \-fi-'ta-ləs\ *n* : a hemolytic disease of the fetus and newborn that is characterized by an increase in circulating erythroblasts and by jaundice and that occurs when the system of an Rh-negative mother produces antibodies to an antigen in the blood of an Rh-positive fetus — called also *hemolytic disease of the newborn, Rh disease*

eryth·ro·blas·tot·ic \i-ˌri-thrə-blas-'tä-tik\ *adj* : of, relating to, or affected by erythroblastosis ⟨an ~ infant⟩

eryth·ro·cyte \i-'ri-thrə-ˌsīt\ *n* : RED BLOOD CELL — **eryth·ro·cyt·ic** \-ˌri-thrə-'si-tik\ *adj*

eryth·ro·cy·to·pe·nia \i-ˌri-thrə-ˌsī-tə-'pē-nē-ə\ *n* : deficiency of red blood cells

eryth·ro·cy·tor·rhex·is \-'rek-səs\ *n, pl* **-rhex·es** \-'rek-ˌsēz\ : rupture of a red blood cell

eryth·ro·cy·to·sis \i-ˌri-thrə-ˌsī-'tō-səs\

n, *pl* **-to·ses** \-'tō-,sēz\ : an increase in the number of circulating red blood cells esp. resulting from a known stimulus (as hypoxia)

eryth·ro·der·ma \-'dər-mə\ *n, pl* **-mas** \-məz\ *or* **-ma·ta** \-mə-tə\ : ERYTHEMA

eryth·ro·der·mia \-'dər-mē-ə\ *n* : ERYTHEMA

eryth·ro·gen·ic \-'je-nik\ *adj* 1 : producing red blood cells : ERYTHROPOIETIC 2 : inducing reddening of the skin

ery·throid \i-'ri-,thròid, 'er-ə-\ *adj* : relating to erythrocytes or their precursors

eryth·ro·leu·ke·mia \i-,ri-thrə-lü-'kē-mē-ə\ *n* : a malignant disorder that is marked by proliferation of erythroblastic and myeloblastic tissue and in later stages by leukemia — **eryth·ro·leu·ke·mic** \-mik\ *adj*

eryth·ro·mel·al·gia \-mə-'lal-jə\ *n* : a state of excessive dilation of the superficial blood vessels usu. of the feet accompanied by hyperemia, increased skin temperature, and burning pain

eryth·ro·my·cin \i-,ri-thrə-'mīs-³n\ *n* : a broad-spectrum antibiotic $C_{37}H_{67}NO_{13}$ produced by a bacterium of the genus *Streptomyces* (*S. erythreus*), resembling penicillin in antibacterial activity, and effective also against amoebas, treponemata, and pinworms — see ILOSONE, ILOTYCIN

eryth·ro·phago·cy·to·sis \i-'ri-thrə-,fa-gə-sə-'tō-səs, -,sī-\ *n, pl* **-to·ses** \-'tō-,sēz\ : phagocytosis of red blood cells esp. by macrophages

eryth·ro·pla·sia \-'plā-zhə, -zhē-ə\ *n* : a reddened patch with a velvety surface on the oral or genital mucosa that is considered to be a precancerous lesion

eryth·ro·poi·e·sis \-,ri-thrō-pòi-'ē-səs\ *n, pl* **-e·ses** \-,sēz\ : the production of red blood cells (as from the bone marrow) — **eryth·ro·poi·et·ic** \-'e-tik\ *adj*

erythropoietic protoporphyria *n* : a rare porphyria usu. appearing in young children and marked by excessive protoporphyrin in red blood cells, blood plasma, and feces and by skin lesions resulting from photosensitivity

eryth·ro·poi·e·tin \-'pòi-ət-³n\ *n* : a hormonal substance that is formed esp. in the kidney and stimulates red blood cell formation — abbr. *EPO*; see EPOGEN

eryth·ro·sine \i-'ri-thrə-sən, -,sēn\ *also* **eryth·ro·sin** \-sən\ *n* : a brick-red powdered xanthene dye $C_{20}H_6I_4Na_2O_5$ that is used as a biological stain and in dentistry as an agent to disclose plaque on teeth — called also *erythrosine sodium*

Es *symbol* einsteinium

ESB *abbr* electrical stimulation of the brain

es·cape \i-'skāp\ *n* 1 : evasion of something undesirable ⟨~ from pain and suffering⟩ 2 : distraction or relief from routine or reality; *esp* : mental distraction or relief by flight into idealizing fantasy or fiction — **escape** *vb* — **escape** *adj*

escape mechanism *n* : a mode of behavior or thinking adopted to evade unpleasant facts or responsibilities : DEFENSE MECHANISM

es·cap·ism \i-'skā-,pi-zəm\ *n* : habitual diversion of the mind to purely imaginative activity or entertainment as an escape from reality or routine — **es·cap·ist** \-pist\ *adj or n*

es·char \'es-,kär\ *n* : a scab formed esp. after a burn

¹es·cha·rot·ic \,es-kə-'rä-tik\ *adj* : producing an eschar

²escharotic *n* : an escharotic agent (as a drug)

Esch·e·rich·ia \,e-shə-'ri-kē-ə\ *n* : a genus of aerobic gram-negative rod-shaped bacteria (family Enterobacteriaceae) that include occas. pathogenic forms (as some strains of *E. coli*) normally present in the human intestine and other forms which typically occur in soil and water

Esch·e·rich \'e-shə-rik\, **Theodor** **(1857–1911),** German pediatrician.

es·ci·tal·o·pram \,e-sə-'ta-lə-,pram\ *n* : a drug that functions as an SSRI and is administered orally in the form of its oxalate $C_{20}H_{21}FN_2O \cdot C_2H_2O_4$ to treat depression and anxiety — see LEXAPRO

es·cutch·eon \i-'skə-chən\ *n* : the configuration of adult pubic hair

es·er·ine \'e-sə-,rēn\ *n* : PHYSOSTIGMINE

Es·march bandage \'es-,märk, 'ez-\ *or* **Es·march's bandage** \-,märks-\ *n* : a tight rubber bandage for driving the blood out of a limb

Esmarch, Johannes Friedrich August von (1823–1908), German surgeon.

eso- *prefix* : inner ⟨*eso*tropia⟩

es·omep·ra·zole \,e-sō-'me-prə-,zōl\ *n* : an isomer of omeprazole that is administered in the form of its magnesium salt $(C_{17}H_{18}N_3O_3S)_2Mg$ esp. in the treatment of erosive esophagitis, gastroesophageal reflux disease, and duodenal ulcer — see NEXIUM

esophag- *or* **esophago-** *comb form* 1 : esophagus ⟨*esophag*ectomy⟩ ⟨*esophago*plasty⟩ 2 : esophagus and ⟨*esophago*gastrectomy⟩

esoph·a·ge·al \i-,sä-fə-'jē-əl\ *adj* : of or relating to the esophagus

esophageal artery *n* : any of several arteries that arise from the front of the aorta, anastomose along the esophagus, and terminate by anastomosis with adjacent arteries

esophageal gland *n* : one of the racemose glands in the walls of the esophagus that in humans are small and serve principally to lubricate the food

esoph·a·ge·al hia·tus *n* : the aperture in the diaphragm that gives passage to the esophagus — see HIATAL HERNIA

esophageal plexus *n* : a nerve plexus formed by the branches of the vagus nerve which surround and supply the esophagus

esophageal speech *n* : a method of speaking which is used by individuals whose larynx has been removed and in which phonation is achieved by expelling swallowed air from the esophagus

esoph·a·gec·to·my \i-₁sä-fə-'jek-tə-mē\ *n, pl* **-mies** : excision of part of the esophagus

esophagi *pl of* ESOPHAGUS

esoph·a·gi·tis \i-₁sä-fə-'jī-təs, -'gī, (₁)ē-\ *n* : inflammation of the esophagus

esophago- — see ESOPHAG-

esoph·a·go·gas·trec·to·my \i-₁sä-fə-gō-₁gas-'trek-tə-mē\ *n, pl* **-mies** : excision of part of the esophagus (esp. the lower third) and the stomach

esoph·a·go·gas·tric \-'gas-trik\ *adj* : of, relating to, involving, or affecting the esophagus and the stomach

esoph·a·go·gas·tros·co·py \-₁gas-'träs-kə-pē\ *n, pl* **-pies** : examination of the interior of the esophagus and stomach by means of an endoscope

esoph·a·go·gas·tros·to·my \-₁gas-'träs-tə-mē\ *n, pl* **-mies** : the surgical formation of an artificial communication between the esophagus and the stomach

esoph·a·go·je·ju·nos·to·my \-₁je-jə-'näs-tə-mē\ *n, pl* **-mies** : the surgical formation of an artificial communication between the esophagus and the jejunum

esoph·a·go·my·ot·o·my \-mī-'ä-tə-mē\ *n, pl* **-mies** : incision through the musculature of the esophagus and esp. the distal part (as for the relief of esophageal achalasia)

esoph·a·go·plas·ty \i-'sä-fə-gə-₁plas-tē\ *n, pl* **-ties** : plastic surgery for the repair or reconstruction of the esophagus

esoph·a·go·scope \-₁skōp\ *n* : an endoscope for inspecting the interior of the esophagus

esoph·a·gos·co·py \i-₁sä-fə-'gäs-kə-pē\ *n, pl* **-pies** : examination of the esophagus by means of an esophagoscope — **esoph·a·go·scop·ic** \i-₁sä-fə-gə-'skä-pik\ *adj*

esophagostomiasis *var of* OE-SOPHAGOSTOMIASIS

esoph·a·gos·to·my \i-₁sä-fə-'gäs-tə-mē\ *n, pl* **-mies** : surgical creation of an artificial opening into the esophagus

esoph·a·got·o·my \-'gä-tə-mē\ *n, pl* **-mies** : incision of the esophagus (as for the removal of an obstruction or the relief of esophageal achalasia)

esoph·a·gus \i-'sä-fə-gəs\ *n, pl* **-gi** \-₁gī, -₁jī\ : a muscular tube that in adult humans is about nine inches (23

centimeters) long and passes from the pharynx down the neck between the trachea and the spinal column and behind the left bronchus where it pierces the diaphragm slightly to the left of the middle line and joins the cardiac end of the stomach

es·o·pho·ria \₁e-sə-'fōr-ē-ə, *sometimes* ₁ē-\ *n* : squint in which the eyes tend to turn inward toward the nose

es·o·tro·pia \₁e-sə-'trō-pē-ə, ₁ē-\ *n* : CROSS-EYE 1 — **es·o·trop·ic** \-'trä-pik\ *adj*

ESP \₁ē-(₁)es-'pē\ *n* : EXTRASENSORY PERCEPTION

es·pun·dia \is-'pün-dē-ə, -'pün-\ *n* : mucocutaneous leishmaniasis of the mouth, pharynx, and nose that is prevalent in Central and So. America — compare UTA

ESR *abbr* erythrocyte sedimentation rate

ESRD *abbr* end-stage renal disease

es·sen·tial \i-'sen-chəl\ *adj* **1** : being a substance that is not synthesized by the body in a quantity sufficient for normal health and growth and that must be obtained from the diet ⟨∼ fatty acids⟩ — compare NONESSEN-TIAL **2** : having no obvious or known cause : IDIOPATHIC ⟨∼ disease⟩

essential amino acid *n* : any of various alpha-amino acids that are required for normal health and growth, are either not manufactured in the body or manufactured in insufficient quantities, are usu. supplied by dietary protein, and in humans include histidine, isoleucine, leucine, lysine, methionine, phenylalanine, threonine, tryptophan, and valine

essential hypertension *n* : a common form of hypertension that occurs in the absence of any evident cause, is marked by elevated peripheral vascular resistance, and has multiple risk factors (as family history of hypertension, obesity, and sedentary lifestyle) — called also *idiopathic hypertension, primary hypertension;* see MALIGNANT HYPERTENSION

essential oil *n* : any of a large class of volatile oils of vegetable origin that give plants their characteristic odors and are used esp. in perfumes, flavorings, and pharmaceutical preparations — called also *volatile oil*

essential thrombocythemia *n* : THROMBOCYTHEMIA

essential tremor *n* : a common disorder of movement characterized by uncontrolled trembling of the hands and often involuntary nodding of the head and tremulousness of the voice

EST *abbr* electroshock therapy

es·ter \'es-tər\ *n* : any of a class of often fragrant compounds that can be represented by the formula RCOOR′ and that are usu. formed by the reaction between an acid and an alcohol usu. with elimination of water

es·ter·ase \'es-tə-ˌrās, -ˌrāz\ *n* : an enzyme that accelerates the hydrolysis or synthesis of esters

es·ter·i·fy \e-'ster-ə-ˌfī\ *vb* **-fied; -fy·ing** : to convert into an ester — **es·ter·i·fi·ca·tion** \e-ˌster-ə-fə-'kā-shən\ *n*

estr- *or* **estro-** *comb form* : estrus ⟨*estrogen*⟩

Es·trace \'e-ˌstrās\ *trademark* — used for a preparation of estradiol

Es·tra·derm \'e-strə-dərm\ *trademark* — used for a preparation of estradiol

es·tra·di·ol \ˌes-trə-'dī-ˌȯl, -ˌōl\ *n* : a natural estrogenic hormone $C_{18}H_{24}O_2$ secreted chiefly by the ovaries that is the most potent of the naturally occurring estrogens and is administered in its natural or semisynthetic esterified form esp. to treat menopausal symptoms — called also *dihydrotheelin*; see ESTRACE, ESTRADERM

es·tral cycle \'es-trəl-\ *n* : ESTROUS CYCLE

es·trin \'es-trən\ *n* : an estrogenic hormone; *esp* : ESTRONE

es·tri·ol \'es-ˌtrī-ˌȯl, e-'strī-, -ˌōl\ *n* : a relatively weak natural estrogenic hormone $C_{18}H_{24}O_3$ that is found in the body chiefly as a metabolite of estradiol, is the main estrogen secreted by the placenta during pregnancy, and is the estrogen typically found in the urine of pregnant women

estro- — see ESTR-

es·tro·gen \'es-trə-jən\ *n* : any of various natural steroids (as estradiol) that are formed from androgen precursors, are secreted chiefly by the ovaries, placenta, adipose tissue, and testes, and stimulate the development of female secondary sex characteristics and promote the growth and maintenance of the female reproductive system; *also* : any of various synthetic or semisynthetic steroids (as ethinyl estradiol) that mimic the physiological effect of natural estrogens

es·tro·gen·ic \ˌes-trə-'je-nik\ *adj* 1 : promoting estrus 2 : of, relating to, caused by, or being an estrogen — **es·tro·gen·i·cal·ly** \-ni-k(ə-)lē\ *adv* — **es·tro·gen·ic·i·ty** \-jə-'ni-sə-tē\ *n*

estrogen replacement therapy *n* : the administration of estrogen esp. to treat menopausal symptoms and prevent postmenopausal osteoporosis — abbr. ERT

es·trone \'es-ˌtrōn\ *n* : a natural estrogenic hormone that is a ketone $C_{18}H_{22}O_2$ found in the body chiefly as a metabolite of estradiol, is also secreted esp. by the ovaries, and is used to treat various conditions relating to estrogen deficiency (as ovarian failure and menopausal symptoms)

es·trous \'es-trəs\ *adj* 1 : of, relating to, or characteristic of estrus 2 : being in heat

estrous cycle *n* : the correlated phenomena of the endocrine and generative systems of a female mammal from the beginning of one period of

estrus to the beginning of the next — called also *estral cycle, estrus cycle*

es·tru·al \'es-trə-wəl\ *adj* : ESTROUS

es·trus \'es-trəs\ *n* : a regularly recurrent state of sexual excitability during which the female of most mammals will accept the male and is capable of conceiving : HEAT; *also* : a single occurrence of this state

es·zo·pic·lone \ˌes-zō-'pi-ˌklōn\ *n* : a sedative and hypnotic drug $C_{17}H_{17}ClN_6O_3$ used to treat insomnia — see LUNESTA

eth·a·cryn·ic acid \ˌe-thə-'kri-nik-\ *n* : a potent synthetic diuretic $C_{13}H_{12}Cl_2O_4$ used esp. to treat edema

eth·am·bu·tol \e-'tham-byü-ˌtȯl, -ˌtōl\ *n* : a synthetic drug used in the form of its dihydrochloride $C_{10}H_{24}N_2O_2\cdot2HCl$ esp. in the treatment of tuberculosis — see MYAMBUTOL

etha·mi·van \e-'thа-mə-ˌvan, ˌe-thə-'mī-vən\ *n* : a central nervous stimulant $C_{12}H_{17}NO_3$ used esp. formerly as a respiratory stimulant

eth·a·nol \'e-thə-ˌnȯl, -ˌnōl\ *n* : a colorless volatile flammable liquid C_2H_5OH that is the intoxicating agent in liquors and is also used as a solvent — called also *ethyl alcohol, grain alcohol;* see ALCOHOL 1

eth·chlor·vy·nol \eth-'klȯr-və-ˌnȯl, -ˌnōl\ *n* : a hypnotic and sedative drug C_7H_9ClO used esp. to treat insomnia — see PLACIDYL

eth·ene \'e-ˌthēn\ *n* : ETHYLENE

ether \'ē-thər\ *n* 1 : a light volatile flammable liquid $C_4H_{10}O$ used esp. formerly as an anesthetic — called also *diethyl ether, ethyl ether* 2 : any of various organic compounds characterized by an oxygen atom attached to two carbon atoms

ether·ize \'ē-thə-ˌrīz\ *vb* **-ized; -iz·ing** : to treat or anesthetize with ether

¹**eth·i·cal** \'e-thi-kəl\ *also* **eth·ic** \-thik\ *adj* 1 : conforming to accepted professional standards of conduct 2 *of a drug* : restricted to sale only on a doctor's prescription — **eth·i·cal·ly** \-thi-k(ə-)lē\ *adv*

²**ethical** *n* : an ethical drug

eth·ics \'e-thiks\ *n sing or pl* : the principles of conduct governing an individual or a group ⟨medical ∼⟩

ethid·i·um bromide \e-'thi-dē-əm-\ *n* : a biological dye $C_{21}H_{20}BrN_3$ that is used esp. to stain nucleic acids

ethi·nyl estradiol *or* **ethy·nyl·es·tra·di·ol** \'e-thə-nil-ˌes-trə-'dī-ˌȯl, -ˌōl\ *n* : a potent synthetic estrogen $C_{20}H_{24}O_2$ used in combination (as with norgestrel or norethindrone) as a birth control pill or alone in the treatment of menopausal symptoms or female hypogonadism or in the palliative treatment of prostate or breast cancer — see ORTHO EVRA, ORTHO-NOVUM, ORTHO TRI-CYCLEN, YASMIN

eth·i·on·amide \ˌe-thē-'ä-nə-ˌmīd\ *n* : a compound $C_8H_{10}N_2S$ used against mycobacteria (as in tuberculosis)

ethi·o·nine \e-ˈthī-ə-ˌnēn\ n : an amino acid $C_6H_{13}NO_2S$ that is biologically antagonistic to methionine

ethis·ter·one \i-ˈthis-tə-ˌrōn\ n : a synthetic female sex hormone $C_{21}H_{28}O_2$ administered in cases of progesterone deficiency — called also *anhydrohydroxyprogesterone*

ethmo- comb form : ethmoid and ⟨*ethmomaxillary*⟩

¹**eth·moid** \ˈeth-ˌmȯid\ or **eth·moi·dal** \eth-ˈmȯid-ᵊl\ adj : of, relating to, adjoining, or being one or more bones of the walls and septum of the nasal cavity

²**ethmoid** n : ETHMOID BONE

ethmoidal air cells n pl : the cavities in the lateral masses of the ethmoid bone that communicate with the nasal cavity

ethmoid bone n : a light spongy cubical bone forming much of the walls of the nasal cavity and part of those of the orbits

eth·moid·ec·to·my \ˌeth-ˌmȯi-ˈdek-tə-mē\ n, pl -mies : excision of all or some of the ethmoidal air cells or part of the ethmoid bone

eth·moid·itis \-ˈdī-təs\ n : inflammation of the ethmoid bone or its sinuses

ethmoid sinus also **ethmoidal sinus** n : either of two sinuses each of which is situated in a lateral part of the ethmoid bone alongside the nose and consists of ethmoidal air cells

eth·mo·max·il·lary \ˌeth-(ˌ)mō-ˈmak-sə-ˌler-ē\ adj : of or relating to the ethmoid and maxillary bones

eth·no·med·i·cine \ˌeth-nō-ˈme-də-sən\ n : the comparative study of how different cultures view disease and how they treat or prevent it; also : the medical beliefs and practices of indigenous cultures — **eth·no·med·i·cal** \-ˈme-di-kəl\ adj

etho·sux·i·mide \ˌe-(ˌ)thō-ˈsək-sə-ˌmīd, -ˌməd\ n : an anticonvulsant drug $C_7H_{11}NO_2$ used to treat epilepsy

eth·o·to·in \ˌe-thə-ˈtō-ən\ n : an anticonvulsant drug $C_{11}H_{12}N_2O_2$ used to treat epilepsy — see PEGANONE

ethyl alcohol \ˈe-thəl-\ n : ETHANOL

ethyl aminobenzoate n : BENZOCAINE

ethyl bromide n : a volatile liquid compound C_2H_5Br used as an inhalation anesthetic

ethyl carbamate n : URETHANE

ethyl chloride n : a pungent flammable gaseous or volatile liquid C_2H_5Cl used esp. as a topical anesthetic

eth·yl·ene \ˈe-thə-ˌlēn\ n : a colorless flammable gaseous unsaturated hydrocarbon C_2H_4 used in medicine as a general inhalation anesthetic and occurring in plants where it functions esp. as a natural growth regulator that promotes the ripening of fruit — called also *ethene*

ethylene bromide n : ETHYLENE DIBROMIDE

eth·yl·ene·di·amine \ˌe-thə-ˌlēn-ˈdī-ə-ˌmēn, -ˌdī-ˈa-mən\ n : a colorless volatile liquid base $C_2H_8N_2$ used in medicine to stabilize aminophylline when used in injections

eth·yl·ene·di·amine·tetra·ac·e·tate \ˌe-thə-ˌlēn-ˌdī-ə-ˌmēn-ˌte-trə-ˈa-sə-ˌtāt, -ˌdī-ˌa-mən-\ n : a salt of EDTA

eth·yl·ene·di·amine·tetra·ace·tic acid \-ə-ˈsē-tik-\ n : EDTA

ethylene di·bro·mide \-dī-ˈbrō-ˌmīd\ n : a colorless toxic liquid compound $C_2H_4Br_2$ that has been shown by experiments with laboratory animals to be strongly carcinogenic and that was formerly used in the U.S. as an agricultural pesticide — abbr. *EDB*; called also *ethylene bromide*

ethylene glycol n : a thick liquid alcohol $C_2H_6O_2$ used esp. as an antifreeze

ethylene oxide n : a colorless flammable toxic gaseous or liquid compound C_2H_4O used in fumigation and sterilization (as of medical instruments)

eth·yl·es·tren·ol \ˌe-thəl-ˈes-trə-ˌnȯl, -ˌnōl\ n : an anabolic steroid $C_{20}H_{32}O$ having androgenic activity — see MAXIBOLIN

ethyl ether n : ETHER 1

eth·yl·mor·phine \ˌe-thəl-ˈmȯr-ˌfēn\ n : a synthetic toxic alkaloid used esp. in the form of its hydrochloride $C_{19}H_{23}NO_3$·HCl similarly to morphine and codeine

eth·y·no·di·ol diacetate \ˌe-thi-nō-ˈdī-ˌōl, -ˌȯl-\ n : a synthetic progestogen $C_{24}H_{32}O_4$ used esp. in birth control pills usu. in combination with an estrogen

ethynylestradiol var of ETHINYL ESTRADIOL

et·i·dro·nate \ˌē-tə-ˈdrō-ˌnāt, ˌe-\ n : a white disodium bisphosphonate salt $C_2H_6Na_2O_7P_2$ that inhibits the formation, growth, and dissolution of hydroxyapatite crystals — called also *etidronate disodium*

etio- comb form : cause ⟨*etiologic*⟩

etio·chol·an·ol·one \ˌē-tē-ō-ˌkō-ˈla-nə-ˌlōn, ˌe-\ n : a testosterone metabolite $C_{19}H_{30}O_2$ that occurs in urine

eti·o·log·ic \ˌē-tē-ə-ˈlä-jik\ or **eti·o·log·i·cal** \-ji-kəl\ adj 1 : of, relating to, or based on etiology ⟨~ investigations⟩ 2 : causing or contributing to the cause of a disease or condition — **eti·o·log·i·cal·ly** \-ji-k(ə-)lē\ adv

eti·ol·o·gy \ˌē-tē-ˈä-lə-jē\ n, pl -gies 1 : the cause or causes of a disease or abnormal condition 2 : a branch of medical science dealing with the causes and origin of diseases

etio·patho·gen·e·sis \ˌē-tē-ō-ˌpa-thə-ˈje-nə-səs, ˌe-\ n, pl -e·ses \-ˌsēz\ : the cause and development of a disease or abnormal condition

eto·po·side \ˌē-tə-ˈpō-ˌsīd, ˌe-\ n : a drug $C_{29}H_{32}O_{13}$ used to treat various neoplastic diseases (as carcinoma of the lungs, acute myelogenous leukemia, and Ewing's sarcoma)

etor·phine \ē-ˈtȯr-ˌfēn, i-\ n : a synthetic narcotic drug $C_{25}H_{33}NO_4$ related to morphine but with more potent analgesic properties

etret·i·nate \i-'tre-t^n-ˌāt\ n : a retinoid drug $C_{23}H_{30}O_3$ used esp. to treat severe recalcitrant psoriasis

eu- comb form **1** : good : normal ⟨*eu*thyroid⟩ **2** : true ⟨*eu*globulin⟩

Eu symbol europium

eu·ca·lyp·tol also **eu·ca·lyp·tole** \ˌyü-kə-'lip-ˌtöl, -ˌtöl\ n : a liquid $C_{10}H_{18}O$ with an odor of camphor that occurs in many essential oils (as of eucalyptus) and is used esp. as an expectorant — called also *cajeputol, cineole*

eu·ca·lyp·tus oil \ˌyü-kə-'lip-təs-\ n : any of various essential oils obtained from the leaves of an Australian tree (genus *Eucalyptus* and esp. *E. globulus*) of the myrtle family (Myrtaceae) and used in pharmaceutical preparations (as antiseptics or cough drops)

euc·at·ro·pine \yü-'ka-trə-ˌpēn\ n : a synthetic alkaloid used in the form of its white crystalline hydrochloride $C_{17}H_{25}NO_3 \cdot HCl$ as a mydriatic

eu·chro·ma·tin \(ˌ)yü-'krō-mə-tən\ n : the genetically active portion of chromatin that is largely composed of genes — **eu·chro·mat·ic** \ˌyü-krō-'ma-tik\ adj

eu·gen·ics \yü-'je-niks\ n : a science that deals with the improvement (as by control of human mating) of hereditary qualities of a race or breed — **eu·gen·ic** \-nik\ adj — **eu·gen·i·cist** \-nə-sist\ n — **eu·gen·i·cal·ly** adv

eu·ge·nol \'yü-jə-ˌnól, -ˌnôl\ n : an aromatic liquid phenol $C_{10}H_{12}O_2$ found esp. in clove oil and used in dentistry as an analgesic

eu·glob·u·lin \yü-'glä-byə-lən\ n : a simple protein that does not dissolve in pure water

eu·gly·ce·mia \ˌyü-glī-'sē-mē-ə\ n : a normal level of sugar in the blood

eu·kary·ote also **eu·cary·ote** \(ˌ)yü-'kar-ē-ˌōt, -ē-ət\ n : an organism composed of one or more cells containing visibly evident nuclei and organelles — compare PROKARYOTE — **eu·kary·ot·ic** also **eu·cary·ot·ic** \-ˌkar-ē-'ä-tik\ adj

eu·nuch \'yü-nək, -nik\ n : a man or boy deprived of the testes or external genitals — **eu·nuch·ism** \-nə-ˌki-zəm, -ni-\ n

¹**eu·nuch·oid** \'yü-nə-ˌkóid\ adj : of, relating to, or characterized by eunuchoidism : resembling a eunuch

²**eunuchoid** n : a sexually deficient individual; esp : one lacking in sexual differentiation and tending toward the intersex state

eu·nuch·oid·ism \'yü-nə-ˌkói-ˌdi-zəm\ n : a state suggestive of that of a eunuch in being marked by deficiency of sexual development, by persistence of prepubertal characteristics, and often by the presence of characteristics typical of the opposite sex

eu·pep·sia \yü-'pep-shə, -sē-ə\ n : good digestion — **eu·pep·tic** \-'pep-tik\ adj

eu·phen·ics \yü-'fe-niks\ n : the therapeutic techniques and procedures for ameliorating deleterious phenotypic effects of a genetic defect esp. without altering the genotype of the individual — **eu·phen·ic** \-nik\ adj

eu·pho·ria \yü-'fór-ē-ə\ n : a feeling of well-being or elation; esp : one that is groundless, disproportionate to its cause, or inappropriate to one's life situation — compare DYSPHORIA — **eu·phor·ic** \-'fór-ik, -'fär-\ adj — **eu·phor·i·cal·ly** \-i-k(ə-)lē\ adv

¹**eu·pho·ri·ant** \yü-'fór-ē-ənt\ n : a drug that tends to induce euphoria

²**euphoriant** adj : tending to induce euphoria ⟨a ∼ drug⟩

eu·phor·i·gen·ic \yü-ˌfór-ə-'je-nik\ adj : tending to cause euphoria

eup·nea \yüp-'nē-ə\ n : normal respiration — compare DYSPNEA — **eup·ne·ic** \-'nē-ik\ adj

eup·noea chiefly Brit var of EUPNEA

eu·ro·pi·um \yü-'rō-pē-əm\ n : a bivalent and trivalent metallic element — symbol *Eu*; see ELEMENT table

-e·us \ē-əs\ n comb form, pl **-ei** \ē-ˌī\ also **-e·us·es** \ē-ə-səz\ : muscle that constitutes, has the form of, or joins a (specified) part, thing, or structure ⟨glut*eus*⟩ ⟨rhomboid*eus*⟩

eu·sta·chian tube \yü-'stā-shən-, -shē-ən-, -kē-ən-\ n, often cap E : a bony and cartilaginous tube connecting the middle ear with the nasopharynx and equalizing air pressure on both sides of the tympanic membrane — called also *auditory tube, pharyngotympanic tube*

Eu·sta·chio \äü-'stäk-yō\, **Bartolomeo** (ca 1520–1574), Italian anatomist.

eu·tha·na·sia \ˌyü-thə-'nā-zhə, -zhē-ə\ n : the act or practice of killing hopelessly sick or injured individuals (as persons or domestic animals) in a relatively painless way for reasons of mercy; also : the act or practice of allowing a hopelessly sick or injured patient to die by taking less than complete medical measures to prolong life — called also *mercy killing*

eu·than·a·tize \'yü-thə-ˌnīz\ also **eu·than·a·tize** \yü-'tha-nə-ˌtīz\ vb **-nized** also **-tized; -niz·ing** also **-tiz·ing** : to subject to euthanasia

eu·then·ics \yü-'the-niks\ n sing or pl : a science that deals with development of human well-being by improvement of living conditions — **eu·the·nist** \yü-'the-nist, 'yü-thə-\ n

eu·thy·roid \(ˌ)yü-'thī-ˌróid\ adj : characterized by normal thyroid function — **eu·thy·roid·ism** \-ˌrói-ˌdi-zəm\ n

evac·u·ant \i-'va-kyə-wənt\ n : an emetic, diuretic, or purgative agent — **evacuant** adj

evac·u·ate \i-'va-kyə-ˌwāt\ vb **-at·ed; -at·ing 1** : to remove the contents of

⟨∼ an abscess⟩ **2** : to discharge (as urine or feces) from the body as waste : VOID — **evac·u·a·tive** \-ˌwā-tiv\ adj

evac·u·a·tion \i-ˌva-kyə-ˈwā-shən\ n **1** : the act or process of evacuating **2** : something evacuated or discharged

evag·i·na·tion \i-ˌva-jə-ˈnā-shən\ n **1** : a process of turning outward or inside out ⟨∼ of a cell membrane⟩ **2** : a part or structure that is produced by evagination — called also *outpocketing, outpouching* — **evag·i·nate** \i-ˈva-jə-ˌnāt\ vb

ev·a·nes·cent \ˌe-və-ˈnes-ᵊnt\ adj : tending to disappear quickly : of relatively short duration ⟨an ∼ rash⟩

Ev·ans blue \ˈe-vənz-\ n : a dye $C_{34}H_{24}N_6Na_4O_{14}S_4$ that on injection into the bloodstream combines with serum albumin and is used to determine blood volume colorimetrically

Evans, Herbert McLean (1882–1971), American anatomist and physiologist.

event \i-ˈvent\ n : an adverse or damaging medical occurrence ⟨a heart attack or other cardiac ∼⟩

even·tra·tion \ˌē-ˌven-ˈtrā-shən\ n : protrusion of abdominal organs through the abdominal wall

ever·sion \i-ˈvər-zhən, -shən\ n **1** : the act of turning inside out : the state of being turned inside out ⟨∼ of the eyelid⟩ **2** : the condition (as of the foot) of being turned or rotated outward — compare INVERSION 1b

evert \i-ˈvərt\ vb : to turn outward ⟨∼ the foot⟩; also : to turn inside out

evis·cer·ate \i-ˈvi-sə-ˌrāt\ vb **-at·ed; -at·ing 1 a** : to remove the viscera of **b** : to remove an organ from (a patient) or the contents of (an organ) **2** : to protrude through a surgical incision or suffer protrusion of a part through an incision — **evis·cer·a·tion** \-ˌvi-sə-ˈrā-shən\ n

Evis·ta \ē-ˈvi-stə\ trademark — used for a preparation of raloxifene

evo·ca·tion \ˌē-vō-ˈkā-shən, ˌe-\ n : INDUCTION 2b

evo·ca·tor \ˈē-vō-ˌkā-tər, ˈe-\ n : the specific chemical constituent responsible for the physiological effects of an organizer

evoked potential \ē-ˈvōkt-\ n : an electrical response esp. in the cerebral cortex as recorded following stimulation of a peripheral sense receptor

evo·lu·tion \ˌe-və-ˈlü-shən, ˌē-\ n **1** : a process of change in a certain direction **2 a** : the historical development of a biological group (as a race or species) : PHYLOGENY **b** : a theory that the various types of animals and plants have their origin in other preexisting types and that the distinguishable differences are due to modifications in successive generations — **evo·lu·tion·ari·ly** \-shə-ˌner-ə-lē\ adv — **evo·lu·tion·ary** \-shə-ˌner-ē\ adj — **evo·lu·tio·nist** \-shə-nist\ n

evolve \i-ˈvälv, -ˈvȯlv\ vb **evolved; evolv·ing** : to produce or develop by natural evolutionary processes

evul·sion \i-ˈvəl-shən\ n : the act of extracting forcibly : EXTRACTION ⟨∼ of a tooth⟩ — **evulse** \i-ˈvəls\ vb

ewe–neck \ˈyü-ˈnek\ n : a thin neck with a concave arch occurring as a defect in dogs and horses — **ewe–necked** \-ˈnekt\ adj

Ew·ing's sarcoma \ˈyü-iŋz-\ n : a malignant bone tumor esp. of a long bone or the pelvis — called also *Ewing's tumor*

Ewing, James (1866–1943), American pathologist.

ex- — see EXO-

ex·ac·er·bate \ig-ˈza-sər-ˌbāt\ vb **-bat·ed; -bat·ing** : to cause (a disease or its symptoms) to become more severe — **ex·ac·er·ba·tion** \-ˌza-sər-ˈbā-shən\ n

ex·al·ta·tion \ˌeg-ˌzȯl-ˈtā-shən, ˌek-ˌsȯl-\ n **1** : marked or excessive intensification of a mental state or of the activity of a bodily part or function **2** : an abnormal sense of personal well-being, power, or importance : a delusional euphoria

ex·am \ig-ˈzam\ n : EXAMINATION

ex·am·i·na·tion \ig-ˌza-mə-ˈnā-shən\ n : the act or process of inspecting or testing for evidence of disease or abnormality — see PHYSICAL EXAMINATION — **ex·am·ine** \ig-ˈza-mən\ vb

ex·am·in·ee \ig-ˌza-mə-ˈnē\ n : a person who is examined

ex·am·in·er \ig-ˈza-mə-nər\ n : one that examines — see MEDICAL EXAMINER

ex·an·them \eg-ˈzan-thəm, ˈek-ˌsan-ˌthem\ or **ex·an·the·ma** \ˌeg-ˌzan-ˈthē-mə\ n, pl **-thems** also **-them·a·ta** \ˌeg-ˌzan-ˈthe-mə-tə\ or **-themas** : an eruptive disease (as measles) with a symptomatic eruption — **ex·an·them·a·tous** \ˌeg-ˌzan-ˈthe-mə-təs\ or **ex·an·the·mat·ic** \-ˌzan-thə-ˈma-tik\ adj

exanthema su·bi·tum or **exanthem subitum** \-sə-ˈbī-təm\ n : ROSEOLA INFANTUM

ex·ca·va·tion \ˌek-skə-ˈvā-shən\ n **1** : the action or process of forming or undergoing formation of a cavity or hole **2** : a cavity formed by or as if by cutting, digging, or scooping — **ex·ca·vate** \ˈek-skə-ˌvāt\ vb

ex·ca·va·tor \ˈek-skə-ˌvā-tər\ n : an instrument used to open bodily cavities (as in the teeth) or remove material from them

excavatum — see PECTUS EXCAVATUM

ex·ce·men·to·sis \ˌeks-si-ˌmen-ˈtō-səs\ n, pl **-to·ses** \-ˌsēz\ or **-to·sis·es** : abnormal outgrowth of the cementum of the root of a tooth

ex·change transfusion \iks-ˈchānj-\ n : simultaneous withdrawal of the recipient's blood and transfusion with the donor's blood esp. in the treatment of erythroblastosis

ex·ci·mer la·ser \'ek-si-ˌmər-\ *n* : a laser that uses a compound of a halogen and a noble gas to generate radiation usu. in the ultraviolet region of the spectrum — called also *excimer*

ex·cip·i·ent \ik-'si-pē-ənt\ *n* : a usu. inert substance (as starch) that forms a vehicle (as for a drug)

ex·ci·sion \ik-'si-zhən\ *n* : surgical removal or resection (as of a diseased part) — **ex·cise** \-'sīz\ *vb* — **ex·ci·sion·al** \-'si-zhə-nəl\ *adj*

ex·cit·able \ik-'sī-tə-bəl\ *adj, of living tissue or an organism* : capable of being activated by and reacting to stimuli : exhibiting irritability — **ex·cit·abil·i·ty** \-ˌsī-tə-'bi-lə-tē\ *n*

ex·ci·tant \ik-'sīt-ᵊnt, 'ek-sə-tənt\ *n* : an agent that arouses or augments physiological activity (as of the nervous system) — **excitant** *adj*

ex·ci·ta·tion \ˌek-ˌsī-'tā-shən, -sə-\ *n* : EXCITATION: as **a** : the disturbed or altered condition resulting from arousal of activity (as by neural or electrical stimulation) in an individual organ or tissue **b** : the arousing of such activity

ex·cit·a·to·ry \ik-'sī-tə-ˌtōr-ē\ *adj* **1** : tending to induce excitation (as of a neuron) **2** : exhibiting, resulting from, related to, or produced by excitement or excitation

ex·cite \ik-'sīt\ *vb* **ex·cit·ed; ex·cit·ing** : to increase the activity of (as a living organism) : STIMULATE

ex·cite·ment \-'sīt-mənt\ *n* **1** : the act of exciting **2** : the state of being excited: as **a** : aroused, augmented, or abnormal activity of an organism or functioning of an organ or part **b** : extreme motor hyperactivity (as in catatonic schizophrenia or bipolar disorder)

ex·ci·to·tox·ic \ik-ˌsī-tə-'täk-sik\ *adj* : being, involving, or resulting from the action of an agent that binds to a nerve cell receptor, stimulates the cell, and damages it or causes its death ⟨∼ neuronal death⟩ — **ex·ci·to·tox·ic·i·ty** \-ˌ(ˌ)täk-'si-sə-tē\ *n*

ex·ci·to·tox·in \ik-'sī-tə-ˌtäk-sən\ *n* : an excitotoxic agent

ex·co·ri·a·tion \(ˌ)ek-ˌskōr-ē-'ā-shən\ *n* **1** : the act of abrading or wearing off the skin **2** : a raw irritated lesion (as of the skin or a mucosal surface) — **ex·co·ri·ate** \ek-'skōr-ē-ˌāt\ *vb*

ex·cre·ment \'ek-skrə-mənt\ *n* : waste matter discharged from the body; *esp* : waste (as feces) discharged from the digestive tract — **ex·cre·men·tal** \ˌek-skrə-'ment-ᵊl\ *adj*

ex·cres·cence \ik-'skres-ᵊns\ *n* : an outgrowth or enlargement: as **a** : a natural and normal appendage or development **b** : an abnormal outgrowth — **ex·cres·cent** \ik-'skres-ᵊnt\ *adj*

ex·cre·ta \ik-'skrē-tə\ *n pl* : waste matter eliminated or separated from an organism — compare EXCRETION 2 — **ex·cre·tal** \-'skrē-təl\ *adj*

ex·crete \ik-'skrēt\ *vb* **ex·cret·ed; ex·cret·ing** : to separate and eliminate or discharge (waste) from the blood or tissues or from the active protoplasm

ex·cret·er \-'skrē-tər\ *n* : one that excretes something and esp. an atypical bodily product (as a pathogenic microorganism)

ex·cre·tion \ik-'skrē-shən\ *n* **1** : the act or process of excreting **2 a** : something excreted; *esp* : a metabolic waste product (as urea or carbon dioxide) that is eliminated from the body and is distinguished from waste materials (as feces) that are merely passed into or through the digestive tract without being incorporated into the body proper **b** : waste material (as feces) discharged from the body : EXCREMENT — not used technically

ex·cre·to·ry \'ek-skrə-ˌtōr-ē\ *adj* : of, relating to, or functioning in excretion ⟨∼ ducts⟩

ex·cur·sion \ik-'skər-zhən\ *n* **1** : a movement outward and back or from a mean position or axis **2** : one complete movement of expansion and contraction of the lungs and their membranes (as in breathing)

ex·cyst \eks-'sist\ *vb* : to emerge from a cyst — **ex·cys·ta·tion** \ˌeks-ˌsis-'tā-shən\ *n* — **ex·cyst·ment** \eks-'sist-mənt\ *n*

exe·mes·tane \ek-sə-'mes-ˌtān\ *n* : a steroidal aromatase inhibitor $C_{20}H_{24}O_2$ that is administered orally to treat breast cancer in postmenopausal women — see AROMASIN

ex·en·ter·a·tion \ig-ˌzen-tə-'rā-shən\ *n* : surgical removal of the contents of a bodily cavity (as the orbit or pelvis) — **ex·en·ter·ate** \ig-'zen-tə-ˌrāt\ *vb*

ex·er·cise \'ek-sər-ˌsīz\ *n* **1** : regular or repeated use of a faculty or bodily organ **2** : bodily exertion for the sake of developing and maintaining physical fitness — **exercise** *vb*

ex·er·cis·er \'ek-sər-ˌsī-zər\ *n* **1** : one that exercises **2** : an apparatus for use in physical exercise

Ex·er·cy·cle \'ek-sər-ˌsī-kəl\ *trademark* — used for a stationary bicycle

ex·er·e·sis \ig-'zer-ə-səs\ *n, pl* **-e·ses** \-ˌsēz\ : surgical removal of a part or organ (as a nerve)

ex·er·tion·al \ig-'zər-shə-nəl\ *adj* : precipitated by physical exertion but usu. relieved by rest ⟨∼ dyspnea⟩

ex·flag·el·la·tion \(ˌ)eks-ˌfla-jə-'lā-shən\ *n* : the formation of microgametes in sporozoans (as the malaria parasite) by extrusion of nuclear material into peripheral processes resembling flagella

ex·fo·li·ant \(ˌ)eks-'fō-lē-ənt\ *n* : a mechanical or chemical agent (as an abrasive skin wash or salicylic acid) that is applied to the skin to remove dead cells from the surface — called also *exfoliator*

ex·fo·li·ate \(ˌ)eks-ˈfō-lē-ˌāt\ *vb* **-at·ed; -at·ing 1 :** to cast or come off in scales or laminae **2 :** to remove the surface of in scales or laminae **3 :** to shed (teeth) by exfoliation

ex·fo·li·a·tion \(ˌ)eks-ˌfō-lē-ˈā-shən\ *n* **:** the action or process of exfoliating: as **a :** the peeling of the horny layer of the skin **b :** the shedding of surface components **c :** the shedding of a superficial layer of bone or of a tooth or part of a tooth — **ex·fo·li·a·tive** \eks-ˈfō-lē-ˌā-tiv\ *adj*

exfoliative cytology *n* **:** the study of cells shed from body surfaces esp. for determining the presence or absence of a cancerous condition

ex·fo·li·a·tor \(ˌ)eks-ˈfō-lē-ˌā-tər\ **:** EXFOLIANT

ex·ha·la·tion \eks-hə-ˈlā-shən, ˌek-sə-\ *n* **1 :** the action of forcing air out of the lungs **2 :** something (as the breath) that is exhaled or given off — **ex·hale** \eks-ˈhāl, ek-ˈsāl\ *vb*

ex·haust \ig-ˈzȯst\ *vb* **1 a :** to draw off or let out completely **b :** to empty by drawing off the contents; *specif* **:** to create a vacuum in **2 a :** to use up **:** consume completely **b :** to tire extremely or completely **3 :** to extract completely with a solvent

ex·haus·tion \ig-ˈzȯs-chən\ *n* **1 :** the act or process of exhausting **:** the state of being exhausted **2 :** neurosis following overstrain or overexertion esp. in military combat

ex·hi·bi·tion·ism \ˌek-sə-ˈbi-shə-ˌni-zəm\ *n* **1 a :** a perversion marked by a tendency to indecent exposure **b :** an act of such exposure **2 :** the act or practice of behaving so as to attract attention to oneself — **ex·hi·bi·tion·ist** \-nist\ *n* — **ex·hi·bi·tion·is·tic** \-ˌbish-ə-ˈnis-tik\ *also* **exhibitionist** *adj*

ex·hume \ig-ˈzüm, igz-ˈyüm; iks-ˈhyüm, -ˈyüm\ *vb* **ex·humed; ex·hum·ing :** DISINTER — **ex·hu·ma·tion** \ˌeks-hyü-ˈmā-shən, ˌeks-yü-; ˌegz-yü-, ˌeg-zü-\ *n*

ex·i·tus \ˈek-sə-təs\ *n, pl* **exitus :** DEATH; *esp* **:** fatal termination of a disease

exo- *or* **ex-** *comb form* **:** outside **:** outer 〈*exoenzyme*〉

exo·crine \ˈek-sə-krən, -ˌkrīn, -ˌkrēn\ *adj* **:** producing, being, or relating to a secretion that is released outside its source 〈∼ insufficiency〉

exocrine gland *n* **:** a gland (as a salivary gland) that releases a secretion external to or at the surface of an organ by means of a canal or duct — called also *gland of external secretion*

exo·cri·nol·o·gy \ˌek-sə-kri-ˈnä-lə-jē, -ˌkrī-, -ˌkrē-\ *n, pl* **-gies :** the study of external secretions (as pheromones) that serve an integrative function

exo·cy·to·sis \ˌek-sō-sī-ˈtō-səs\ *n, pl* **-to·ses** \-ˌsēz\ **:** the release of cellular substances (as secretory products) contained in cell vesicles by fusion of the vesicular membrane with the plasma membrane and subsequent release of the contents to the exterior of the cell — **exo·cy·tot·ic** \-ˈtä-tik\ *adj*

ex·odon·tia \ˌek-sō-ˈdän-chə, -chē-ə\ *n* **:** a branch of dentistry that deals with the extraction of teeth — **ex·odon·tist** \-ˈdän-tist\ *n*

exo·en·zyme \ˌek-sō-ˈen-ˌzīm\ *n* **:** an extracellular enzyme

exo·eryth·ro·cyt·ic \ˌek-sō-i-ˌri-thrə-ˈsi-tik\ *adj* **:** occurring outside the red blood cells — used of stages of malaria parasites

ex·og·e·nous \ek-ˈsä-jə-nəs\ *also* **ex·o·gen·ic** \ˌek-sō-ˈje-nik\ *adj* **1 :** growing from or on the outside **2 :** caused by factors (as food or a traumatic event) or an agent (as a disease-producing organism) from outside the organism or system 〈∼ obesity〉 **3 :** introduced from or produced outside the organism or system; *specif* **:** not synthesized within the organism or system — compare ENDOGENOUS — **ex·og·e·nous·ly** *adv*

ex·om·pha·los \ek-ˈsäm-fə-ləs\ *n* **:** UMBILICAL HERNIA; *also* **:** OMPHALOCELE

ex·on \ˈek-ˌsän\ *n* **:** a polynucleotide sequence in a nucleic acid that codes information for protein synthesis and that is copied and spliced together with other such sequences to form messenger RNA — compare INTRON — **ex·on·ic** \ek-ˈsä-nik\ *adj*

exo·nu·cle·ase \ˌek-sō-ˈnü-klē-ˌās, -ˈnyü-, -ˌāz\ *n* **:** an enzyme that breaks down a nucleic acid by removing nucleotides one by one from the end of a chain — compare ENDONUCLEASE

exo·nu·cleo·lyt·ic \ˌek-sō-ˌnü-klē-ə-ˈli-tik, -ˌnyü-\ *adj* **:** breaking a nucleotide chain into two parts at a point adjacent to one of its ends

exo·pep·ti·dase \-ˈpep-tə-ˌdās, -ˌdāz\ *n* **:** any of a group of enzymes that hydrolyze peptide bonds formed by the terminal amino acids of peptide chains **:** PEPTIDASE — compare ENDOPEPTIDASE

ex·o·pho·ria \ˌek-sə-ˈfōr-ē-ə\ *n* **:** latent strabismus in which the visual axes tend outward toward the temple — compare HETEROPHORIA

ex·oph·thal·mia \ˌek-ˌsäf-ˈthal-mē-ə\ *n* **:** EXOPHTHALMOS

ex·oph·thal·mic goiter \ˌek-säf-ˈthal-mik-\ *n* **:** GRAVES' DISEASE

ex·oph·thal·mos *also* **ex·oph·thal·mus** \ˌek-säf-ˈthal-məs, -səf-\ *n* **:** abnormal protrusion of the eyeball — **exophthalmic** *adj*

exo·phyt·ic \ˌek-sō-ˈfi-tik\ *adj* **:** tending to grow outward beyond the surface epithelium from which it originates — used of tumors; compare ENDOPHYTIC

ex·os·tec·to·my \ˌek-(ˌ)säs-ˈtek-tə-mē\ *n, pl* **-mies :** excision of an exostosis

ex·os·to·sis \ˌek-(ˌ)säs-ˈtō-səs\ *n, pl*

-to·ses \-ˌsēz\ : a spur or bony outgrowth from a bone or the root of a tooth — **ex·os·tot·ic** \-ˈtä-tik\ *adj*

exo·tox·in \ˌek-sō-ˈtäk-sən\ *n* : a soluble poisonous substance produced during growth of a microorganism and released into the surrounding medium — compare ENDOTOXIN

exo·tro·pia \ˌek-sə-ˈtrō-pē-ə\ *n* : WALL-EYE 2a

ex·pand·er \ik-ˈspan-dər\ *n* : any of several colloidal substances (as dextran) of high molecular weight used as a blood or plasma substitute for increasing the blood volume — called also *extender*

ex·pect \ik-ˈspekt\ *vb* : to be pregnant : await the birth of one's child — used in progressive tenses ⟨she's ∼*ing* next month⟩

ex·pec·tan·cy \-ˈspek-tən-sē\ *n, pl* **-cies** : the expected amount (as of the number of years of life) based on statistical probability — see LIFE EXPECTANCY

ex·pec·tant \-ˈspek-tənt\ *adj* : expecting the birth of a child ⟨∼ mothers⟩

ex·pec·to·rant \ik-ˈspek-tə-rənt\ *n* : an agent that promotes the discharge or expulsion of mucus from the respiratory tract; *broadly* : ANTITUSSIVE — **expectorant** *adj*

ex·pec·to·rate \-ˌrāt\ *vb* **-rat·ed; -rat·ing** 1 : to eject matter from the throat or lungs by coughing or hawking and spitting 2 : SPIT

ex·pec·to·ra·tion \ik-ˌspek-tə-ˈrā-shən\ *n* 1 : the act or an instance of expectorating 2 : expectorated matter

ex·per·i·ment \ik-ˈsper-ə-mənt, -ˈspir-\ *n* 1 : a procedure carried out under controlled conditions in order to discover an unknown effect or law, to test or establish a hypothesis, or to illustrate a known law 2 : the process of testing — **experiment** *vb* — **ex·per·i·men·ta·tion** \ik-ˌsper-ə-mən-ˈtā-shən, -ˌspir-, -ˌmen-\ *n* — **experiment·er** \-ˈsper-ə-ˌmen-tər, -ˈspir-\ *n*

ex·per·i·men·tal \ik-ˌsper-ə-ˈment-ᵊl, -ˌspir-\ *adj* 1 : of, relating to, or based on experience or experiment 2 : founded on or derived from experiment 3 *of a disease* : intentionally produced esp. in laboratory animals for the purpose of study ⟨∼ diabetes⟩ — **ex·per·i·men·tal·ly** *adv*

experimental allergic encephalomyelitis *n* : an inflammatory autoimmune disease that has been induced in laboratory animals and esp. mice and is used as an animal model in studying multiple sclerosis in humans — abbr *EAE*; called also *experimental autoimmune encephalomyelitis*

ex·pi·ra·tion \ˌek-spə-ˈrā-shən\ *n* 1 a : the act or process of releasing air from the lungs through the nose or mouth b : the escape of carbon dioxide from the body protoplasm (as through the blood and lungs or by diffusion) 2 : something produced by breathing out

ex·pi·ra·to·ry \ik-ˈspī-rə-ˌtōr-ē, ek-; ˈek-spə-rə-\ *adj* : of, relating to, or employed in the expiration of air from the lungs ⟨∼ muscles⟩

expiratory reserve volume *n* : the additional amount of air that can be expired from the lungs by determined effort after normal expiration — compare INSPIRATORY RESERVE VOLUME

ex·pire \ik-ˈspīr, ek-\ *vb* **ex·pired; ex·pir·ing** 1 : to breathe one's last breath : DIE 2 a : to breathe out from or as if from the lungs b : to emit breath

ex·plant \ˈek-ˌsplant\ *n* : living tissue removed from an organism and placed in a medium for tissue culture — **ex·plant** \(ˌ)ek-ˈsplant\ *vb* — **ex·plan·ta·tion** \ˌek-ˌsplan-ˈtā-shən\ *n*

ex·plor·ato·ry \ik-ˈsplōr-ə-ˌtōr-ē\ *adj* : of, relating to, or being exploration ⟨∼ surgery⟩

ex·plore \ik-ˈsplōr\ *vb* **ex·plored; ex·plor·ing** : to examine (as by surgery) esp. for diagnostic purposes — **ex·plo·ra·tion** \ˌek-splə-ˈrā-shən\ *n*

ex·plor·er \ik-ˈsplōr-ər\ *n* : an instrument for exploring cavities esp. in teeth : PROBE 1

ex·pose \ik-ˈspōz\ *vb* **ex·posed; ex·pos·ing** 1 : to subject to risk from a harmful action or condition ⟨children *exposed* to measles⟩ 2 : to lay open to view: as a : to engage in indecent exposore of (oneself) b : to reveal (a bodily part) esp. by dissection

ex·po·sure \ik-ˈspō-zhər\ *n* 1 : the fact or condition of being exposed: as a : the condition of being unprotected esp. from severe weather b : the condition of being subject to some detrimental effect or harmful condition ⟨∼ to bronchial irritants⟩ ⟨∼ to the flu⟩ 2 : the act or an instance of exposing — see INDECENT EXPOSURE

exposure therapy *n* : psychotherapy that involves repeated real, visualized, or simulated exposure to or confrontation with a feared situation or object or a traumatic event or memory in order to achieve habituation and that is used esp. in the treatment of post-traumatic stress disorder, anxiety disorder, or phobias

ex·press \ik-ˈspres, ek-\ *vb* 1 : to make known or exhibit by an expression 2 : to force out by pressure ⟨∼ breast milk by electric pump⟩ 3 : to cause (a gene) to manifest its effects in the phenotype

ex·pres·sion \ik-ˈspre-shən\ *n* 1 a : something that manifests, represents, reflects, embodies, or symbolizes something else ⟨the first clinical ∼ of a disease⟩ b (1) : the detectable effect of a gene; *also* : the sum of the processes (as transcription and translation) by which a gene is manifested in the phenotype (2) : EXPRESSIVITY

2 : facial aspect or vocal intonation as indicative of feeling

ex·pres·siv·i·ty \ˌek-ˌspre-ˈsi-və-tē\ *n, pl* **-ties** : the relative capacity of a gene to affect the phenotype — compare PENETRANCE

ex·pul·sive \ik-ˈspəl-siv\ *adj* : serving to expel (∼ efforts during labor)

ex·qui·site \ik-ˈskwi-zət\ *adj* : existing in an extreme degree : ACUTE (∼ pain) — **ex·qui·site·ly** \-lē\ *adv*

ex·san·gui·na·tion \(ˌ)eks-ˌsaŋ-gwə-ˈnā-shən\ *n* : the action or process of draining or losing blood — **ex·san·gui·nate** \eks-ˈsaŋ-gwə-ˌnāt\ *vb*

ex·sic·co·sis \ˌek-si-ˈkō-səs\ *n, pl* **-co·ses** \-ˌsēz\ : insufficient intake of fluids; *also* : the resulting condition of bodily dehydration

ex·stro·phy \ˈek-strə-fē\ *n, pl* **-phies** : eversion of a part or organ; *specif* : a congenital malformation of the bladder in which the normally internal mucosa of the organ lies exposed on the abdominal wall

ex·tend \ik-ˈstend\ *vb* : to straighten out (as an arm or leg)

extended family *n* : a family that includes in one household near relatives in addition to a nuclear family

ex·tend·er \ik-ˈsten-dər\ *n* **1** : a substance added to a product esp. in the capacity of a diluent, adulterant, or modifier **2** : EXPANDER

ex·ten·si·bil·i·ty \ik-ˌsten-sə-ˈbi-lə-tē\ *n, pl* **-ties** : the capability of being stretched (∼ of muscle) — **ex·ten·si·ble** \ik-ˈsten-sə-bəl\ *adj*

ex·ten·sion \ik-ˈsten-chən\ *n* **1** : the stretching of a fractured or dislocated limb so as to restore it to its natural position **2** : an unbending movement around a joint in a limb (as the knee or elbow) that increases the angle between the bones of the limb at the joint — compare FLEXION 1

ex·ten·sor \ik-ˈsten-sər, -ˌsȯr\ *n* : a muscle serving to extend a bodily part (as a limb) — called also *extensor muscle;* compare FLEXOR

extensor car·pi ra·di·al·is brev·is \-ˈkär-ˌpī-ˌrā-dē-ˈä-ləs-ˈbre-vəs, -ˈkär-ˌpē-\ *n* : a short muscle on the radial side of the back of the forearm that extends and may abduct the hand

extensor carpi radialis lon·gus \-ˈlȯŋ-gəs\ *n* : a long muscle on the radial side of the back of the forearm that extends and abducts the hand

extensor carpi ul·nar·is \-ˌəl-ˈnar-əs\ *n* : a muscle on the ulnar side of the back of the forearm that extends and adducts the hand

extensor dig·i·ti min·i·mi \-ˈdi-jə-ˌtī-ˈmi-nə-ˌmī, -ˈdi-jə-ˌtē-ˈmi-nə-ˌmē\ *n* : a slender muscle on the medial side of the extensor digitorum communis that extends the little finger

extensor digiti quin·ti pro·pri·us \-ˈkwin-ˌtī-ˈprō-prē-əs, -ˈkwin-ˌtē-\ *n* : EXTENSOR DIGITI MINIMI

extensor dig·i·to·rum brev·is \-ˌdi-jə-

ˈtȯr-əm-ˈbre-vəs *n* : a muscle on the dorsum of the foot that extends the toes

extensor digitorum com·mu·nis \-kə-ˈmyü-nəs, -ˈkä-myə-\ *n* : a muscle on the back of the forearm that extends the fingers and wrist

extensor digitorum lon·gus \-ˈlȯŋ-gəs\ *n* : a pennate muscle on the lateral part of the front of the leg that extends the four small toes and dorsally flexes and pronates the foot

extensor hal·lu·cis brev·is \-ˈha-lü-səs-ˈbre-vəs, -lyü-, -ˈha-lə-kəs-\ *n* : the part of the extensor digitorum brevis that extends the big toe

extensor hallucis lon·gus \-ˈlȯŋ-gəs\ *n* : a long thin muscle situated on the shin that extends the big toe and dorsiflexes and supinates the foot

extensor in·di·cis \-ˈin-də-səs, -də-kəs\ *n* : a thin muscle that arises from the ulna in the more distal part of the forearm and extends the index finger

extensor indicis pro·pri·us \-ˈprō-prē-əs\ *n* : EXTENSOR INDICIS

extensor pol·li·cis brev·is \-ˈpä-lə-səs-ˈbre-vəs, -lə-kəs-\ *n* : a muscle that arises from the dorsal surface of the radius, extends the first phalanx of the thumb, and abducts the hand

extensor pollicis lon·gus \-ˈlȯŋ-gəs\ *n* : a muscle that arises dorsolaterally from the middle part of the ulna, extends the second phalanx of the thumb, and abducts the hand

extensor ret·i·nac·u·lum \-ˌret-ᵊn-ˈa-kyə-ləm\ *n* **1** : either of two fibrous bands of fascia crossing the front of the ankle: **a** : a lower band that is attached laterally to the superior aspect of the calcaneus and passes medially to divide in the shape of a Y and that passes over or both over and under the tendons of the extensor muscles at the ankle — called also *inferior extensor retinaculum* **b** : an upper band passing over and binding down the tendons of the tibialis anterior, extensor hallucis longus, extensor digitorum longus, and peroneus tertius just above the ankle joint — called also *superior extensor retinaculum, transverse crural ligament* **2** : a fibrous band of fascia crossing the back of the wrist and binding down the tendons of the extensor muscles

ex·te·ri·or·ize \ek-ˈstir-ē-ə-ˌrīz\ *vb* **-ized; -iz·ing** **1** : EXTERNALIZE **2** : to bring out of the body (as for surgery) (the section of perforated colon was *exteriorized*) — **ex·te·ri·or·iza·tion** \-ˌstir-ē-ə-rə-ˈzā-shən\ *n*

ex·tern *also* **ex·terne** \ˈek-ˌstərn\ *n* : a nonresident doctor or medical student at a hospital — **ex·tern·ship** \-ˌship\ *n*

externa — see MUSCULARIS EXTERNA, OTITIS EXTERNA, THECA EXTERNA

ex·ter·nal \ek-ˈstərn-ᵊl\ *adj* **1** : capable of being perceived outwardly : BODILY (∼ signs of a disease) **2 a** : situated at, on, or near the outside ⟨an ∼ muscle⟩ **b** : directed toward the outside : having an outside object ⟨∼ perception⟩ **c** : used by applying to the outside ⟨an ∼ lotion⟩ **3 a** (1) : situated near or toward the surface of the body; *also* : situated away from the mesial plane ⟨the ∼ condyle of the humerus⟩ (2) : arising or acting from outside : having an outside origin ⟨∼ stimuli⟩ **b** : of, relating to, or consisting of something outside the mind : having existence independent of the mind ⟨∼ reality⟩ — **ex·ter·nal·ly** *adv*

external anal sphincter *n* : ANAL SPHINCTER a

external auditory canal *n* : the auditory canal leading from the opening of the external ear to the eardrum — called also *external acoustic meatus, external auditory meatus*

external capsule *n* : CAPSULE 1b (2)

external carotid artery *n* : the outer branch of the carotid artery that supplies the face, tongue, and external parts of the head — called also *external carotid*

external ear *n* : the parts of the ear that are external to the eardrum; *also* : PINNA

external iliac artery *n* : ILIAC ARTERY 2

external iliac node *n* : any of the lymph nodes grouped around the external iliac artery and the external iliac vein — compare INTERNAL ILIAC NODE

external iliac vein *n* : ILIAC VEIN b

external inguinal ring *n* : SUPERFICIAL INGUINAL RING

external intercostal muscle *n* : INTERCOSTAL MUSCLE a — called also *external intercostal*

ex·ter·nal·ize \ek-'stern-ᵊl-ˌīz\ *vb* **-ized; -iz·ing 1 a** : to transform from a mental image into an apparently real object (as in hallucinations) : attribute (a mental image) to external causation **b** : to invent an explanation for by attributing to causes outside the self : RATIONALIZE, PROJECT **2** : to direct outward socially ⟨*externalized* anger⟩ — **ex·ter·nal·iza·tion** \-ˌstern-ᵊl-ə-'zā-shən\ *n*

external jugular vein *n* : JUGULAR VEIN b — called also *external jugular*

external malleolus *n* : MALLEOLUS a

external maxillary artery *n* : FACIAL ARTERY

external oblique *n* : OBLIQUE a 1

external occipital crest *n* : OCCIPITAL CREST a

external occipital protuberance *n* : OCCIPITAL PROTUBERANCE a

external pterygoid muscle *n* : PTERYGOID MUSCLE a

external pudendal artery *n* : either of two branches of the femoral artery: **a** : one that is distributed to the skin of the lower abdomen, to the penis and scrotum in the male, and to one of the labia majora in the female — called

also *superficial external pudendal artery* **b** : one that follows a deeper course, that is distributed to the medial aspect of the thigh, to the skin of the scrotum and perineum in the male, and to one of the labia majora in the female — called also *deep external pudendal artery*

external respiration *n* : exchange of gases between the external environment and the lungs or between the alveoli of the lungs and the blood — compare INTERNAL RESPIRATION

externe *var of* EXTERN

externus — see OBLIQUUS EXTERNUS ABDOMINIS, OBTURATOR EXTERNUS, SPHINCTER ANI EXTERNUS

ex·tero·cep·tive \ˌek-stə-rō-'sep-tiv\ *adj* : activated by, relating to, or giving stimuli received by an organism from outside

ex·tero·cep·tor \-'sep-tər\ *n* : a sense receptor (as of touch, smell, vision, or hearing) excited by exteroceptive stimuli — compare INTEROCEPTOR

ex·tinc·tion \ik-'stiŋk-shən\ *n* : the process of eliminating or reducing a conditioned response by not reinforcing it

ex·tin·guish \ik-'stiŋ-gwish\ *vb* : to cause extinction of (a conditioned response)

ex·tir·pa·tion \ˌek-stər-'pā-shən\ *n* : complete excision or surgical destruction of a body part — **ex·tir·pate** \'ek-stər-ˌpāt\ *vb*

extra- *prefix* : outside : beyond ⟨*extra*uterine⟩

ex·tra·cap·su·lar \ˌek-strə-'kap-sə-lər, -syü-lər\ *adj* **1** : situated outside a capsule **2** *of a cataract operation* : involving removal of the front part of the capsule and the central part of the lens — compare INTRACAPSULAR 2

ex·tra·cel·lu·lar \-'sel-yə-lər\ *adj* : situated or occurring outside a cell or the cells of the body ⟨∼ digestion⟩ ⟨∼ enzymes⟩ — **ex·tra·cel·lu·lar·ly** *adv*

ex·tra·chro·mo·som·al \-ˌkrō-mə-'sō-məl, -'zō-\ *adj* : situated or controlled by factors outside the chromosome ⟨∼ inheritance⟩ ⟨∼ DNA⟩

ex·tra·cor·po·re·al \-kōr-'pōr-ē-əl\ *adj* : occurring or based outside the living body ⟨heart surgery employing ∼ circulation⟩ — **ex·tra·cor·po·re·al·ly** *adv*

ex·tra·cra·ni·al \-'krā-nē-əl\ *adj* : situated or occurring outside the cranium

¹ex·tract \ik-'strakt\ *vb* **1** : to pull or take out forcibly ⟨∼*ed* a wisdom tooth⟩ **2** : to separate the medicinally-active components of a plant or animal tissue by the use of solvents — **ex·trac·tion** \-'strak-shən\ *n*

²ex·tract \'ek-ˌstrakt\ *n* : something prepared by extracting; *esp* : a medicinally-active pharmaceutical solution

¹ex·trac·tive \ik-'strak-tiv, 'ek-ˌ\ *adj* : of, relating to, or involving the process of extracting

²extractive *n* : EXTRACT

ex·tra·du·ral \ˌek-strə-ˈd(y)ür-əl, -dyür-\ *adj* : situated or occurring outside the dura mater but within the skull ⟨an ∼ hemorrhage⟩

ex·tra·em·bry·on·ic \-ˌem-brē-ˈä-nik\ *adj* : situated outside the embryo proper; *esp* : developed from the zygote but not part of the embryo ⟨∼ membranes⟩

extraembryonic coelom *n* : the space between the chorion and amnion which in early stages is continuous with the coelom of the embryo proper

ex·tra·fu·sal \ˌek-strə-ˈfyü-zəl\ *adj* : situated outside a striated muscle spindle ⟨∼ muscle fibers⟩ — compare INTRAFUSAL

ex·tra·gen·i·tal \-ˈje-nə-t⁹l\ *adj* : situated or originating outside the genital region or organs

ex·tra·he·pat·ic \-hi-ˈpa-tik\ *adj* : situated or originating outside the liver

ex·tra·in·tes·ti·nal \-in-ˈtes-tə-nəl\ *adj* : situated or occurring outside the intestines ⟨∼ infections⟩

ex·tra·mac·u·lar \-ˈma-kyə-lər\ *adj* : relating to or being the part of the retina other than the macula lutea

ex·tra·med·ul·lary \-ˈmed-⁹l-ˌer-ē, -ˈme-jə-ˌler-ē, -mə-ˈdə-lə-rē\ *adj* 1 : situated or occurring outside the spinal cord or the medulla oblongata 2 : located or taking place outside the bone marrow

ex·tra·mi·to·chon·dri·al \-ˌmī-tə-ˈkän-drē-əl\ *adj* : situated or occurring in the cell outside the mitochondria

ex·tra·nu·cle·ar \-ˈnü-klē-ər, -ˈnyü-\ *adj* : situated in or affecting the parts of a cell external to the nucleus : CYTOPLASMIC

ex·tra·oc·u·lar muscle \-ˈä-kyə-lər-\ *n* : any of six small voluntary muscles that pass between the eyeball and the orbit and control the movement of the eyeball in relation to the orbit

ex·tra·oral \-ˈōr-əl, -ˈär-\ *adj* : situated or occurring outside the mouth

ex·tra·per·i·to·ne·al \-ˌper-ət-⁹n-ˈē-əl\ *adj* : located or taking place outside the peritoneal cavity ⟨∼ spaces⟩

ex·tra·pi·tu·itary \-pə-ˈtü-ə-ˌter-ē, -ˈtyü-\ *adj* : situated or arising outside the pituitary gland ⟨∼ tissue⟩

ex·tra·pla·cen·tal \-plə-ˈsent-⁹l\ *adj* : being outside of or independent of the placenta

ex·tra·pul·mo·nary \-ˈpùl-mə-ˌner-ē, -ˈpəl-\ *adj* : situated or occurring outside the lungs ⟨∼ tuberculosis⟩

ex·tra·py·ra·mi·dal \-pə-ˈra-məd-⁹l, -ˌpir-ə-ˈmid-⁹l\ *adj* : situated outside of and esp. involving descending nerve tracts other than the pyramidal tracts ⟨∼ brain lesions⟩

ex·tra·re·nal \-ˈrēn-⁹l\ *adj* : situated or occurring outside the kidneys

ex·tra·ret·i·nal \-ˈre-tə-nəl\ *adj* : situated or occurring outside the retina

ex·tra·sen·so·ry \ˌek-strə-ˈsen-sə-rē\ *adj* : residing beyond or outside the ordinary senses

extrasensory perception *n* : perception (as in telepathy, clairvoyance, and precognition) that involves awareness of information about events external to the self not gained through the senses and not deducible from previous experience — called also *ESP*

ex·tra·sys·to·le \-ˈsis-tə-(ˌ)lē\ *n* : a prematurely occurring beat of one of the chambers of the heart that leads to momentary arrhythmia but leaves the fundamental rhythm unchanged — called also *premature beat* — **ex·tra·sys·tol·ic** \-sis-ˈtä-lik\ *adj*

ex·tra·uter·ine \-ˈyü-tə-rən, -ˌrīn\ *adj* : situated or occurring outside the uterus

extrauterine pregnancy *n* : ECTOPIC PREGNANCY

ex·trav·a·sate \ik-ˈstra-və-ˌsāt, -ˌzāt\ *vb* **-sat·ed; -sat·ing** : to force out, cause to escape, or pass by infiltration or effusion from a proper vessel or channel (as a blood vessel) into surrounding tissue

ex·trav·a·sa·tion \ik-ˌstra-və-ˈzā-shən, -ˈsā-\ *n* 1 : the action of extravasating 2 a : an extravasated fluid (as blood) ⟨∼s from the nose and mouth⟩ b : a deposit formed by extravasation

ex·tra·vas·cu·lar \ˌek-strə-ˈvas-kyə-lər\ *adj* : not occurring or contained in body vessels ⟨∼ pulmonary fluid⟩ — **ex·tra·vas·cu·lar·ly** *adv*

ex·tra·ven·tric·u·lar \-ven-ˈtri-kyə-lər, -vən-\ *adj* : located or taking place outside a ventricle ⟨∼ lesions⟩

extraversion, extravert *var of* EXTROVERSION, EXTROVERT

ex·trem·i·ty \ik-ˈstre-mə-tē\ *n, pl* **-ties** 1 : the farthest or most remote part, section, or point 2 : a limb of the body; *esp* : a hand or foot

ex·trin·sic \ek-ˈstrin-zik, -sik\ *adj* 1 : originating or due to causes or factors from or on the outside of a body, organ, or part 2 : originating outside a part and acting on the part as a whole — used esp. of certain muscles; compare INTRINSIC 2 — **ex·trin·si·cal·ly** \-zi-k(ə-)lē, -si-\ *adv*

extrinsic factor *n* : VITAMIN B₁₂

extro- *prefix* : outside : outward ⟨*extro*vert⟩ — compare INTRO-

ex·tro·ver·sion *or* **ex·tra·ver·sion** \ˌek-strə-ˈvər-zhən, -shən\ *n* : the act, state, or habit of being predominantly concerned with and obtaining gratification from what is outside the self — compare INTROVERSION

ex·tro·vert *also* **ex·tra·vert** \ˈek-strə-ˌvort\ *n* : one whose personality is characterized by extroversion; *broadly* : a gregarious and unreserved person — compare INTROVERT — **ex·tro·vert** *also* **ex·tra·vert** *adj* — **ex·tro·vert·ed** *also* **ex·tra·vert·ed** \-ˌvər-təd\ *adj*

ex·trude \ik-ˈstrüd\ *vb* **ex·trud·ed; ex·trud·ing** : to force, press, or push out; *also* : to become extruded ⟨blood *ex-*

truding through arteries⟩ — **ex·tru·sion** \ik-'strü-zhən\ *n*

ex·tu·ba·tion \ek-,stü-'bā-shən, -,styü-\ *n* : the removal of a tube esp. from the larynx after intubation — **ex·tu·bate** \ek-'stü-,bāt, -'styü-, 'ek-,stü-, -,styü-\ *vb*

ex·u·ber·ant \ig-'zü-bə-rənt\ *adj* : characterized by extreme proliferation ⟨~ granulation tissue⟩

ex·u·date \'ek-sù-,dāt, -syù-, -shù-\ *n* : exuded matter; *esp* : the material composed of serum, fibrin, and white blood cells that escapes from blood vessels into a superficial lesion or area of inflammation

ex·u·da·tion \,ek-sù-'dā-shən, -syù-, -shù-\ *n* **1** : the process of exuding **2** : EXUDATE — **ex·u·da·tive** \ig-'zü-də-tiv; 'ek-sù-,dā-tiv, -syù-, -shù-\ *adj*

ex·ude \ig-'züd\ *vb* **ex·ud·ed; ex·ud·ing** **1** : to ooze or cause to ooze out **2** : to undergo diffusion

eye \'ī\ *n* **1 a** : a nearly spherical hollow organ that is lined with a sensitive retina, is lodged in a bony orbit in the skull, is the vertebrate organ of sight, and is normally paired **2** : all the visible structures within and surrounding the orbit and including eyelids, eyelashes, and eyebrows **3** : the faculty of seeing with eyes

eye·ball \'ī-,bȯl\ *n* : the more or less globular capsule of the vertebrate eye formed by the sclera and cornea together with their contained structures

eye bank *n* : a storage place for human corneas from the newly dead for transplanting to the eyes of those blind through corneal defects

eye·brow \'ī-,braù\ *n* : the ridge over the eye or hair growing on it — called also *brow*

eye chart *n* : a chart that is read at a fixed distance for purposes of testing sight; *esp* : one with rows of letters or objects of decreasing size

eye contact *n* : visual contact with another person's eyes

eye·cup \'ī-,kəp\ *n* **1** : a small oval cup with a rim curved to fit the orbit of the eye used for applying liquid remedies to the eyes **2** : OPTIC CUP

eyed \'īd\ *adj* : having an eye or eyes esp. of a specified kind or number — often used in combination ⟨a blue-*eyed* patient⟩

eyed·ness \'īd-nəs\ *n* : preference for the use of one eye instead of the other

eye doctor *n* : a specialist (as an optometrist or ophthalmologist) in the examination, treatment, or care of the eyes

eye·drop·per \'ī-,drä-pər\ *n* : DROPPER

eye·drops \'ī-,dräps\ *n pl* : a medicated solution for the eyes that is applied in drops — **eye·drop** \-,dräp\ *adj*

eye·glass \'ī-,glas\ *n* **1 a** : a lens worn to aid vision; *specif* : MONOCLE **b eye·glass·es** *pl* : GLASSES, SPECTACLES **2** : EYECUP 1

eye gnat *n* : any of several small dipteran flies (genus *Hippelates* of the family Chloropidae and esp. *H. pusio*) including some that are held to be vectors of pinkeye and yaws — called also *eye fly*

eye·ground \'ī-,graùnd\ *n* : the fundus of the eye; *esp* : the retina as viewed through an ophthalmoscope

eye·lash \'ī-,lash\ *n* **1** : the fringe of hair edging the eyelid — usu. used in pl. **2** : a single hair of the eyelashes

eye·lid \'ī-,lid\ *n* : either of the movable lids of skin and muscle that can be closed over the eyeball — called also *palpebra*

eye·sight \'ī-,sīt\ *n* : SIGHT 2

eye socket *n* : ORBIT

eye·strain \'ī-,strān\ *n* : weariness or a strained state of the eye

eye·tooth \'ī-,tüth\ *n, pl* **eye·teeth** \-,tēth\ : a canine tooth of the upper jaw

eye·wash \'ī-,wȯsh, -,wäsh\ *n* : an eye lotion

eye·wear \'ī-,war, -,wer\ *n* : corrective or protective devices (as glasses or contact lenses) for the eyes

eye worm *n* **1** : either of two slender nematode worms of the genus *Oxyspirura* (*O. mansoni* and *O. petrowi*) living beneath the nictitating membrane of the eyes of birds and esp. chickens **2** : any member of the nematode genus *Thelazia* living in the tear duct and beneath the eyelid of dogs, cats, sheep, humans, and other mammals and sometimes causing blindness **3** : an African filarial worm of the genus *Loa* (*L. loa*) that migrates through the eyeball and subcutaneous tissues of humans — compare CALABAR SWELLING

ezet·i·mibe \e-'ze-tə-,mib\ *n* : a drug $C_{24}H_{21}F_2NO_3$ that lowers the amount of cholesterol in the blood by selectively inhibiting its absorption in the intestine — see VYTORIN, ZETIA

f *symbol* focal length
F *abbr* Fahrenheit
F *symbol* fluorine
fab \'fab\ *n* : a fragment of an antibody

that contains one antigen-binding site, one complete light chain, and part of one heavy chain — called also *Fab fragment*

fab·ri·ca·tion \ˌfa-bri-ˈkā-shən\ *n* : CONFABULATION

Fa·bry's disease \ˈfä-brēz-\ *n* : a disorder of lipid metabolism that is inherited as an X-linked recessive trait and is characterized by skin lesions esp. on the lower trunk, severe pain in the extremities, corneal opacities, and vascular disease affecting the kidneys, heart, or brain

  Fabry, Johannes (1860–1930), German dermatologist.

FACC *abbr* Fellow of the American College of Cardiology

FACD *abbr* Fellow of the American College of Dentists

face \ˈfās\ *n, often attrib* : the front part of the head including the chin, mouth, nose, cheeks, eyes, and usu. the forehead

face·bow \ˈfās-ˌbō\ *n* : a device used in dentistry to determine the positional relationships of the maxillae to the temporomandibular joints of a patient

face fly *n* : a European fly of the genus *Musca* (*M. autumnalis*) that is widely established in No. America and causes distress in livestock by clustering about the face

face–lift \ˈfās-ˌlift\ *n* : plastic surgery on the face and neck to remove defects and imperfections (as wrinkles) typical of aging — called also *rhytidectomy* — **face–lift** *vb*

face–lifting \-ˌlif-tin\ *n* : FACE-LIFT

fac·et \ˈfa-sət\ *n* : a smooth flat or nearly flat circumscribed anatomical surface (as of a bone) — **fac·et·ed** or **fac·et·ted** \ˈfa-sə-təd\ *adj*

fac·et·ec·to·my \ˌfa-sə-ˈtek-tə-mē\ *n, pl* **-mies** : excision of a facet esp. of a vertebra

¹**fa·cial** \ˈfā-shəl\ *adj* **1** : of, relating to, or affecting the face (~ neuralgia) **2** : concerned with or used in improving the appearance of the face **3** : relating to or being the buccal and labial surface of a tooth — **fa·cial·ly** \-shə-lē\ *adv*

²**facial** *n* : a treatment to improve the appearance of the face

facial artery *n* : an artery that arises from the external carotid artery and gives off branches supplying the neck and face — called also *external maxillary artery;* compare MAXILLARY ARTERY

facial bone *n* : any of the 14 bones of the facial region of the human skull that do not take part in forming the braincase

facial canal *n* : a passage in the petrous part of the temporal bone that transmits various branches of the facial nerve

facial colliculus *n* : a medial eminence on the floor of the fourth ventricle of the brain produced by the nucleus of the abducens nerve and the flexure of the facial nerve around it

facial nerve *n* : either of the seventh

pair of cranial nerves that supply motor fibers esp. to the muscles of the face and jaw and sensory and parasympathetic fibers to the tongue, palate, and fauces — called also *seventh cranial nerve, seventh nerve*

facial vein *n* : a vein that arises as the angular vein, drains the superficial structures of the face, and empties into the internal jugular vein — called also *anterior facial vein;* see DEEP FACIAL VEIN, POSTERIOR FACIAL VEIN

-fa·cient \ˈfā-shənt\ *adj comb form* : making : causing 〈aborti*facient*〉

fa·cies \ˈfā-ˌshēz, -shē-ˌēz\ *n, pl* **facies 1** : an appearance and expression of the face characteristic of a particular condition esp. when abnormal 〈adenoid ~〉 **2** : an anatomical surface

fa·cil·i·ta·tion \fə-ˌsi-lə-ˈtā-shən\ *n* **1** : the lowering of the threshold for reflex conduction along a particular neural pathway **2** : the increasing of the ease or intensity of a response by repeated stimulation — **fa·cil·i·tate** \-ˈsi-lə-ˌtāt\ *vb* — **fa·cil·i·ta·to·ry** \-ˈsi-lə-tə-ˌtōr-ē\ *adj*

fac·ing \ˈfā-sin\ *n* : a front of porcelain or plastic used in dental crowns and bridgework to face the metal replacement and simulate the natural tooth

facio- *comb form* : facial and 〈*facio*scapulohumeral〉

fa·cio·scap·u·lo·hu·mer·al \ˌfā-shē-ō-ˌska-pyə-lō-ˈhyü-mə-rəl\ *adj* : relating to or affecting the muscles of the face, scapula, and arm

FACOG *abbr* Fellow of the American College of Obstetricians and Gynecologists

FACP *abbr* Fellow of the American College of Physicians

FACR *abbr* Fellow of the American College of Radiology

FACS *abbr* Fellow of the American College of Surgeons

F–ac·tin \ˈef-ˌak-tən\ *n* : a fibrous actin polymerized in the form of a double helix that is produced in the presence of a metal cation (as of calcium) and ATP — compare G-ACTIN

fac·ti·tious \fak-ˈti-shəs\ *adj* : not produced by natural means

fac·tor \ˈfak-tər\ *n* **1 a** : something that actively contributes to the production of a result **b** : a substance that functions in or promotes the function of a particular physiological process or bodily system **2** : GENE — **fac·to·ri·al** \fak-ˈtōr-ē-əl\ *adj*

factor VIII \-ˈāt\ *n* : a glycoprotein clotting factor of blood plasma that is essential for blood clotting and is absent or inactive in hemophilia — called also *antihemophilic factor, thromboplastinogen*

factor XI \-ˈle-vən\ *n* : PLASMA THROMBOPLASTIN ANTECEDENT

factor V \-ˈfīv\ *n* : a globulin clotting factor that occurs in inactive form in blood plasma and that in its active form is one of the factors accelerating the formation of thrombin from prothrombin in the clotting of blood — called also *accelerator globulin, labile factor, proaccelerin*

factor IX \-'nīn\ *n* : a clotting factor whose absence is associated with Christmas disease — called also *autoprothrombin II, Christmas factor*

factor VII \-'se-vən\ *n* : a clotting factor formed in the kidney under the influence of vitamin K that may be deficient due to a hereditary disorder or to a vitamin K deficiency — called also *autoprothrombin I, cothromboplastin, proconvertin, stable factor*

factor X \-'ten\ *n* : a clotting factor that is converted to a proteolytic enzyme which converts prothrombin to thrombin in a reaction dependent on calcium ions and other clotting factors — called also *Stuart-Prower factor*

factor XIII \-,thərt-'tēn\ *n* : a clotting factor that causes monomeric fibrin to polymerize and become stable and insoluble — called also *fibrinase;* see TRANSGLUTAMINASE

factor XII \-'twelv\ *n* : a clotting factor that facilitates blood coagulation but whose deficiency tends not to promote hemorrhage — called also *Hageman factor*

facts of life *n pl* : the fundamental physiological processes and behavior involved in sex and reproduction

fac·ul·ta·tive \'fa-kəl-,tā-tiv\ *adj* **1** : taking place under some conditions but not under others ⟨∼ parasitism⟩ **2** : exhibiting an indicated lifestyle under some environmental conditions but not under others ⟨∼ anaerobes⟩ — **fac·ul·ta·tive·ly** *adv*

FAD \,ef-(,)ā-'dē\ *n* : FLAVIN ADENINE DINUCLEOTIDE

fae·cal, fae·ca·lith, fae·cal·oid, fae·ces *chiefly Brit var of* FECAL, FECALITH, FECALOID, FECES

fag·o·py·rism \,fa-gō-'pī-,ri-zəm\ *n* : a photosensitization esp. of swine and sheep that is due to eating large quantities of buckwheat (esp. *Fagopyrum esculentum* of the family Polygonaceae)

Fahr·en·heit \'far-ən-,hīt\ *adj* : relating or conforming to a thermometric scale on which under standard atmospheric pressure the boiling point of water is at 212 degrees above the zero of the scale and the freezing point is at 32 degrees above zero — *abbr.* F

Fahrenheit, Daniel Gabriel (1686–1736), German physicist.

fail \'fāl\ *vb* **1** : to weaken or lose strength **2** : to stop functioning normally ⟨the patient's heart ∼ed⟩

fail·ure \'fāl-yər\ *n* : a state of inability to perform a vital function ⟨respiratory ∼⟩ — see HEART FAILURE

¹faint \'fānt\ *adj* : weak, dizzy, and likely to faint — **faint·ness** \-nəs\ *n*

²faint *vb* : to lose consciousness because of a temporary decrease in the blood supply to the brain

³faint *n* : the physiological action of fainting; *also* : the resulting condition : SYNCOPE

faith healing *n* : a method of treating diseases by prayer and exercise of faith in God — **faith healer** *n*

falces *pl of* FALX

falciform ligament *n* : an anteroposterior fold of peritoneum attached to the under surface of the diaphragm and sheath of the rectus muscle and along a line on the anterior and upper surfaces of the liver extending back from the notch on the anterior margin

fal·cip·a·rum malaria \fal-'si-pə-rəm-, fôl-\ *n* : severe malaria caused by a parasite of the genus *Plasmodium* (*P. falciparum*) and marked by irregular recurrence of paroxysms and usu. prolonged or continuous fever — called also *malignant malaria, malignant tertian malaria;* compare VIVAX MALARIA

fallen arch *n* : FLATFOOT

falling sickness *n* : EPILEPSY

fal·lo·pian tube \fə-'lō-pē-ən-\ *n, often cap F* : either of the pair of tubes that carry the eggs from the ovary to the uterus — called also *uterine tube*

Fal·lop·pio \fäl-'lòp-yō\ *or* **Fal·lop·pia** \-'lòp-yä\, **Gabriele** (*Latin* **Gabriel Fal·lo·pi·us** \fə-'lō-pē-əs\) **(1523–1562),** Italian anatomist.

Fallot's tetralogy \(,)fa-'lōz-\ *n* : TETRALOGY OF FALLOT

fall·out \'fò-,laut\ *n* **1** : the often radioactive particles stirred up by or resulting from a nuclear explosion and descending through the atmosphere; *also* : other polluting particles (as volcanic ash) descending likewise **2** : descent (as of fallout) through the atmosphere

¹false \'fòls\ *adj* **fals·er; fals·est** **1** : not corresponding to truth or reality **2** : artificially made ⟨a set of ∼ teeth⟩

false joint *n* : PSEUDARTHROSIS

false labor *n* : pains resembling those of normal labor but occurring at irregular intervals and without dilation of the cervix

false membrane *n* : a fibrinous deposit with enmeshed necrotic cells formed esp. in croup and diphtheria — called also *pseudomembrane*

false mo·rel \-mò-'rel\ *n* : any fungus of the genus *Gyromitra*

false–negative *adj* : relating to or being an individual or a test result that is erroneously classified in a negative category (as of diagnosis) because of imperfect testing methods or procedures — compare FALSE-POSITIVE — **false negative** *n*

false neurotransmitter *n* : a biological amine that can be stored in presynaptic vesicles but that has little or no effect on postsynaptic receptors when released into the synaptic cleft — called also *false transmitter*

false pelvis *n* : the upper broader portion of the pelvic cavity — called also *false pelvic cavity*; compare TRUE PELVIS

false–positive *adj* : relating to or being an individual or a test result that is erroneously classified in a positive category (as of diagnosis) because of imperfect testing methods or procedures — compare FALSE-NEGATIVE — **false positive** *n*

false pregnancy *n* : PSEUDOCYESIS, PSEUDOPREGNANCY

false rib *n* : a rib whose cartilages unite indirectly or not at all with the sternum — compare FLOATING RIB

false vocal cords *n pl* : the upper pair of vocal cords that are not directly concerned with speech production — called also *superior vocal cords, ventricular folds*

falx \\`falks, `fólks\\, *pl* **fal·ces** \\`fal-ˌsēz, `fól-\\ : a sickle-shaped part or structure: as **a** : FALX CEREBRI **b** : FALX CEREBELLI

falx ce·re·bel·li \\-ˌser-ə-`be-ˌlī\\ *n* : the smaller of the two folds of dura mater separating the hemispheres of the brain that lies between the lateral lobes of the cerebellum

falx cer·e·bri \\-`ser-ə-ˌbrī\\ *n* : the larger of the two folds of dura mater separating the hemispheres of the cerebral brain that lies between the cerebral hemispheres and contains the sagittal sinuses

FAMA *abbr* Fellow of the American Medical Association

fam·ci·clo·vir \\ˌfam-`sī-klō-ˌvir\\ *n* : a precursor $C_{14}H_{19}N_5O_4$ of penciclovir that is administered orally esp. to treat shingles and herpes genitalis — see FAMVIR

fa·mil·ial \\fə-`mil-yəl\\ *adj* : tending to occur in more members of a family than expected by chance alone ⟨a ∼ disorder⟩ — compare ACQUIRED 2, CONGENITAL 2, HEREDITARY

familial adenomatous polyposis *n* : a disease of the large intestine that is inherited as an autosomal dominant trait and is marked by the formation esp. in the colon and rectum of numerous adenomatous polyps which typically become malignant if left untreated — abbr. *FAP;* called also *familial polyposis*

familial dysautonomia *n* : a disorder of the autonomic nervous system that is inherited as an autosomal recessive trait, typically affects individuals of eastern European Jewish ancestry, and is characterized esp. by lack of tears, difficulty in swallowing, orthostatic hypotension, poor thermoregulation, episodic vomiting, excessive sweating, and sensory deficits (as of pain)

familial hypercholesterolemia *n* : a disorder of lipid metabolism that is inherited as an autosomal dominant trait and is marked by elevated levels of LDL in the blood plasma resulting esp. in xanthomas, atherosclerosis, and an increased risk of heart attack and coronary artery disease

familial polyposis *n* : any of several inherited diseases (as Gardner's syndrome) that are characterized esp. by the formation of polyps in the gastrointestinal tract; *esp* : FAMILIAL ADENOMATOUS POLYPOSIS

fam·i·ly \\`fam-lē, `fa-mə-\\ *n, pl* **-lies 1** : the basic unit in society traditionally consisting of two parents rearing their children; *also* : any of various social units differing from but regarded as equivalent to the traditional family ⟨a single-parent ∼⟩ **2** : a group of related plants or animals forming a category ranking above a genus and below an order and usu. comprising several to many genera — **family** *adj*

family doctor *n* **1** : a doctor regularly consulted by a family **2** : FAMILY PHYSICIAN

family physician *n* **1** : FAMILY DOCTOR 1 **2** : a doctor specialized in family practice

family planning *n* : planning intended to determine the number and spacing of one's children through effective methods of birth control

family practice *n* : a medical practice or specialty which provides continuing general medical care for the individual and family — called also *family medicine*

family practitioner *n* **1** : FAMILY DOCTOR 1 **2** : FAMILY PHYSICIAN 2

fa·mo·ti·dine \\fə-`mō-tə-ˌdīn\\ *n* : an H_2 antagonist $C_8H_{15}N_7O_2S_3$ used to inhibit gastric acid secretion (as in the treatment of gastric and duodenal ulcers and gastroesophageal reflux disease) — see PEPCID

Fam·vir \\`fam-ˌvir\\ *trademark* — used for a preparation of famciclovir

Fan·co·ni's anemia \\fän-`kō-nēz-, fan-\\ *n* : aplastic anemia that is inherited as an autosomal recessive trait and is characterized by progressive pancytopenia, hypoplastic bone marrow, skeletal anomalies (as short stature), microcephaly, hypogonadism, and a predisposition to leukemia

Fanconi, Guido (1892–1979), Swiss pediatrician.

Fanconi syndrome *also* **Fanconi's syndrome** *n* : a disorder of reabsorption in the proximal convoluted tubules of the kidney marked esp. by the presence of glucose, amino acids, and phosphates in the urine

fang \\`faŋ\\ *n*  **1** : a long sharp tooth: as  **a** : one by which an animal's prey is seized and held or torn  **b** : one of the long hollow or grooved and often erectile teeth of a venomous snake  **2** : the root of a tooth or one of the processes or prongs into which a root divides — **fanged** \\`faŋd\\ *adj*

fan·go \'faŋ-(ˌ)gō, 'fäŋ-\ *n* : a clay mud from hot springs at Battaglio, Italy, that is applied externally in the therapeutic treatment of certain medical conditions (as rheumatism)

fan·ta·size \'fan-tə-ˌsīz\ *vb* **-sized; -siz·ing 1** : to indulge in fantasy **2** : to portray in the mind by fantasy

¹**fan·ta·sy** *also* **phan·ta·sy** \'fan-tə-sē, -zē\ *n, pl* **-sies** : the power or process of creating esp. unrealistic or improbable mental images in response to psychological need; *also* : a mental image or a series of mental images (as a daydream) so created

²**fantasy** *also* **phantasy** *vb* **-sied; -sy·ing** : FANTASIZE

FAP *abbr* familial adenomatous polyposis

FAPA *abbr* Fellow of the American Psychological Association

fa·rad·ic \fə-'ra-dik, far-'a-\ *also* **far·a·da·ic** \far-ə-'dā-ik\ *adj* : of or relating to an asymmetric alternating current of electricity ⟨∼ muscle stimulation⟩

Far·a·day \'far-ə-ˌdā\, **Michael** (1791–1867), British physicist and chemist.

far·a·dism \'far-ə-ˌdi-zəm\ *n* : the application of a faradic current of electricity (as for therapeutic purposes)

far·cy \'fär-sē\ *n, pl* **far·cies** : GLANDERS; *esp* : cutaneous glanders

farmer's lung *n* : an acute pulmonary disorder that is characterized by sudden onset, fever, cough, expectoration, and breathlessness and that results from the inhalation of dust from moldy hay or straw

far point *n* : the point farthest from the eye at which an object is accurately focused on the retina when the accommodation is completely relaxed — compare NEAR POINT

far·sight·ed \'fär-ˌsī-təd\ *adj* **1** : seeing or able to see to a great distance **2** : affected with hyperopia — **far·sight·ed·ly** *adv*

far·sight·ed·ness *n* **1** : the quality or state of being farsighted **2** : HYPEROPIA

FAS *abbr* fetal alcohol syndrome

fasc *abbr* fasciculus

fas·cia \'fa-shə, 'fā-, -shē-ə\ *n, pl* **-ci·ae** \-shē-ˌē\ *or* **-cias** : a sheet of connective tissue (as an aponeurosis) covering or binding together body structures; *also* : tissue occurring in such a sheet — see DEEP FASCIA, SUPERFICIAL FASCIA — **fas·cial** \-shəl, -shē-əl\ *adj*

fasciae — see TENSOR FASCIAE LATAE

fascia la·ta \-'lä-tə, -'lā-\ *n, pl* **fasciae la·tae** \-'lä-tē, -'lā-\ : the deep fascia that forms a complete sheath for the thigh

fas·ci·cle \'fa-si-kəl\ *n* : a small bundle; *esp* : FASCICULUS

fasciculata — see ZONA FASCICULATA

fas·cic·u·la·tion \fə-ˌsi-kyə-'lā-shən, fa-\ *n* : muscular twitching involving the simultaneous contraction of contiguous groups of muscle fibers

fas·cic·u·lus \fə-'si-kyə-ləs, fa-\ *n, pl* **-li** \-ˌlī\ : a slender bundle of fibers: **a** : a bundle of skeletal muscle cells bound together by fasciae and forming one of the constituent elements of a muscle **b** : a bundle of nerve fibers that follow the same course but do not necessarily have like functional connections **c** : TRACT 2

fasciculus cu·ne·atus \-ˌkyü-nē-'ā-təs\ *n* : either of a pair of nerve tracts of the posterior funiculus of the spinal cord that are situated on opposite sides of the posterior median septum lateral to the fasciculus gracilis and that carry nerve fibers from the upper part of the body — called also *column of Burdach, cuneate fasciculus*

fasciculus grac·i·lis \-'gra-sə-ləs\ *n* : either of a pair of nerve tracts of the posterior funiculus of the spinal cord that carry nerve fibers from the lower part of the body — called also *gracile fasciculus*

fas·ci·ec·to·my \ˌfa-shē-'ek-tə-mē, -sē-\ *n, pl* **-mies** : surgical excision of strips of fascia

fas·ci·i·tis \ˌfa-shē-'ī-təs, -sē-\ *also* **fas·ci·tis** \fa-'shī-təs, -'sī-\ *n* : inflammation of a fascia

Fas·ci·o·la \fa-'sē-ə-lə, -'sī-\ *n* : a genus of digenetic trematode worms (family Fasciolidae) including common liver flukes of various mammals

fas·ci·o·li·a·sis \fə-ˌsē-ə-'lī-ə-səs, -ˌsī-\ *n, pl* **-a·ses** \-ˌsēz\ : infestation with or disease caused by liver flukes of the genus *Fasciola* (*F. hepatica* or *F. gigantica*)

fas·ci·o·li·cide \fə-'sē-ə-lə-ˌsīd, fa-\ *n* : an agent that destroys liver flukes of the genus *Fasciola*

Fas·ci·o·loi·des \ˌfa-ˌsē-ə-'lói-(ˌ)dēz, -ˌsī-\ *n* : a genus of trematode worms (family Fasciolidae) including the giant liver flukes of ruminant mammals

fas·ci·o·lop·si·a·sis \-ˌläp-'sī-ə-səs\ *n, pl* **-a·ses** \-ˌsēz\ : infestation with or disease caused by an intestinal fluke of the genus *Fasciolopsis* (*F. buski*)

Fas·ci·o·lop·sis \-'läp-səs\ *n* : a genus of trematode worms (family Fasciolidae) that includes an intestinal parasite (*F. buski*) esp. of humans and swine in much of eastern Asia

fas·ci·ot·o·my \ˌfa-shē-'ä-tə-mē\ *n, pl* **-mies** : surgical incision of a fascia

¹**fast** \'fast\ *adj* : resistant to change (as from destructive action) — used chiefly of organisms and in combination with the agent resisted ⟨acid-*fast* bacteria⟩

²**fast** *vb* **1 a** : to abstain from food **b** : to eat sparingly or abstain from some foods **2** : to deny food to ⟨the patient was ∼ed before treatment⟩

³**fast** *n* **1** : the practice of fasting **2** : a time of fasting

fas·tig·ial nucleus \fa-'sti-jē-əl-\ *n* : a nucleus lying near the midline in the roof of the fourth ventricle of the brain

fas·tig·i·um \fa-'sti-jē-əm\ *n* : the period at which the symptoms of a disease are most pronounced

fast·ing \'fas-tiŋ\ *adj* : of or taken from a fasting subject ⟨~ blood sugar levels⟩; *also* : occurring from or caused by fasting ⟨~ hyperglycemia⟩

fast-twitch \'fast-ˌtwich\ *adj* : of, relating to, or being muscle fiber that contracts quickly esp. during brief high-intensity physical activity requiring strength — compare SLOW-TWITCH

¹fat \'fat\ *adj* **fat·ter; fat·test** : fleshy with superfluous flabby tissue that is not muscle : OBESE — **fat·ness** *n*

²fat *n* **1** : animal tissue consisting chiefly of cells distended with greasy or oily matter — see BROWN FAT **2 a** : oily or greasy matter making up the bulk of adipose tissue **b** : any of numerous compounds of carbon, hydrogen, and oxygen that are glycerides of fatty acids, are the chief constituents of plant and animal fat, are a major class of energy-rich food, and are soluble in organic solvents but not in water **c** : a solid or semisolid fat as distinguished from an oil **3** : the condition of fatness : OBESITY

fa·tal \'fāt-ᵊl\ *adj* : causing death — **fa·tal·ly** *adv*

fatal familial insomnia *n* : a rare fatal prion disease that is inherited as an autosomal dominant trait, that is marked by progressive neurodegenerative changes esp. in the thalamus, and that tends to follow a clinical course exhibiting disturbances of the sleep cycle, intractable insomnia, motor disturbances (as ataxia and myoclonus), dysautonomia, dementia, coma, stupor, and death

fa·tal·i·ty \fā-'ta-lə-tē, fə-\ *n, pl* **-ties** **1** : the quality or state of causing death or destruction : DEADLINESS **2 a** : death resulting from a disaster **b** : one who suffers from such a death

fat cell *n* : a fat-containing cell of adipose tissue — called also *adipocyte*

fat de·pot \-'de-(ˌ)pō, -'dē-\ *n* : ADIPOSE TISSUE

fat farm *n* : a health spa that specializes in weight reduction

father figure *n* : one often of particular power or influence who serves as an emotional substitute for a father

father image *n* : an idealization of one's father often projected onto someone to whom one looks for guidance and protection

fa·ti·ga·bil·i·ty *also* **fa·ti·gua·bil·i·ty** \fə-ˌtē-gə-'bil-lə-tē, ˌfa-ti-\ *n, pl* **-ties** : susceptibility to fatigue

fa·tigue \fə-'tēg\ *n* **1** : weariness or exhaustion from labor, exertion, or stress **2** : the temporary loss of power to respond induced in a sensory receptor or motor end organ by continued stimulation — **fatigue** *vb*

fat pad *n* : a flattened mass of fatty tissue

fat-sol·u·ble \'fat-ˌsäl-yə-bəl\ *adj* : soluble in fats or fat solvents

fat·ty \'fa-tē\ *adj* **fat·ti·er; -est** **1 a** : unduly stout **b** : marked by an abnormal deposit of fat **2** : derived from or chemically related to fat — **fat·ti·ness** *n*

fatty acid *n* **1** : any of numerous saturated acids $C_nH_{2n+1}COOH$ (as acetic acid) containing a single carboxyl group and including many that occur naturally usu. in the form of esters in fats, waxes, and essential oils **2** : any of the saturated or unsaturated acids (as palmitic acid) with a single carboxyl group and usu. an even number of carbon atoms that occur naturally in the form of glycerides in fats and fatty oils

fatty degeneration *n* : a process of tissue degeneration marked by the deposition of fat globules in the cells — called also *steatosis*

fatty infiltration *n* : infiltration of the tissue of an organ with excess amounts of fat

fatty liver *n* **1** : an abnormal condition of the liver that is characterized by excess lipid accumulation in the hepatocytes and is caused esp. by injury, malnutrition, or hepatotoxins **2** : a liver affected with fatty liver

fatty oil *n* : a fat that is liquid at ordinary temperatures — called also *fixed oil*

fau·ces \'fo-ˌsēz\ *n sing or pl* : the narrow passage from the mouth to the pharynx situated between the soft palate and the base of the tongue — called also *isthmus of the fauces* — **fau·cial** \'fo-shəl\ *adj*

fau·na \'fon-ə, 'fän-\ *n, pl* **faunas** *also* **fau·nae** \-ˌē, -ˌī\ : animal life; *esp* : the animals characteristic of a region, period, or special environment — compare FLORA 1 — **fau·nal** \-ᵊl\ *adj* — **fau·nal·ly** \-ᵊl-ē\ *adv*

fava bean \'fä-və-\ *n* : BROAD BEAN

fa·vism \'fä-ˌvi-zəm, 'fā-\ *n* : a condition esp. of males of Mediterranean descent that is marked by the development of hemolytic anemia upon consumption of broad beans or inhalation of broad bean pollen and is caused by a usu. inherited deficiency of glucose-6-phosphate

fa·vus \'fā-vəs\ *n* : a contagious skin disease of humans and many domestic animals and fowls that is caused by a fungus (as *Trichophyton schoenleinii*) — **fa·vic** \-vik\ *adj*

FDA *abbr* Food and Drug Administration

Fe *symbol* iron

febri- *comb form* : fever ⟨febrifuge⟩

feb·ri·fuge \'fe-brə-ˌfyüj\ *n or adj* : ANTIPYRETIC

fe·brile \'fe-ˌbrīl, 'fē-\ *adj* : marked or caused by fever : FEVERISH

fe·cal \'fē-kəl\ *adj* : of, relating to, or constituting feces — **fe·cal·ly** *adv*

fe·ca·lith \'fē-kə-ˌlith\ *n* : a concretion of dry compact feces formed in the intestine or vermiform appendix

fe·cal·oid \-kə-ˌlȯid\ *adj* : resembling dung

fe·ces \'fē-(ˌ)sēz\ *n pl* : bodily waste discharged through the anus : EXCREMENT

Fech·ner's law \'fek-nərz-, 'fek-\ *n* : WEBER-FECHNER LAW

fec·u·lent \'fe-kyə-lənt\ *adj* : foul with impurities : FECAL

fe·cund \'fe-kənd, 'fē-\ *adj* **1** : characterized by having produced many offspring **2** : capable of producing : not sterile or barren — **fe·cun·di·ty** \fi-'kən-də-tē, fe-\ *n*

fe·cun·date \'fe-kən-ˌdāt, 'fē-\ *vb* **-dat·ed; -dat·ing** : IMPREGNATE — **fe·cun·da·tion** \ˌfe-kən-'dā-shən, ˌfē-\ *n*

feed·back \'fēd-ˌbak\ *n* **1** : the partial reversion of the effects of a process to its source or to a preceding stage **2** : the return to a point of origin of evaluative or corrective information about an action or process; *also* : the information so transmitted

feedback inhibition *n* : inhibition of an enzyme controlling an early stage of a series of biochemical reactions by the end product when it reaches a critical concentration

fee-for-service *n, often attrib* : separate payment to a health-care provider for each medical service rendered to a patient ⟨a ∼ health plan⟩

feel·ing \'fē-liŋ\ *n* **1** : the one of the basic physical senses of which the skin contains the chief end organs and of which the sensations of touch and temperature are characteristic : TOUCH; *also* : a sensation experienced through this sense **2** : an emotional state or reaction **3** : the overall quality of one's awareness as measured along a pleasantness-unpleasantness continuum

fee splitting *n* : payment by a medical specialist (as a surgeon) of a part of the specialist's fee to the physician who made the referral — **fee splitter** *n*

feet *pl of* FOOT

Feh·ling's solution \'fā-liŋz-\ *or* **Fehling solution** \-liŋ-\ *n* : a blue solution of Rochelle salt and copper sulfate used as an oxidizing agent in a test for sugars and aldehydes in which the precipitation of a red oxide of copper indicates a positive result

Fehling, Hermann von (1812–1885), German chemist.

fel·ba·mate \'fel-bə-ˌmāt\ *n* : an anticonvulsant drug $C_{11}H_{14}N_2O_4$ used to treat severe epilepsy or epilepsy that is unresponsive to other drugs

Fel·den·krais \'fel-dən-ˌkrīs\ *trademark* — used for a system of aided body movements intended to increase bodily awareness and ease tension

fe·line \'fē-ˌlīn\ *adj* : of, relating to, or affecting cats or the cat family (Felidae) — **feline** *n*

feline distemper *n* : PANLEUKOPENIA

feline enteritis *n* : PANLEUKOPENIA

feline infectious anemia *n* : a widespread contagious disease of cats characterized by weakness, lethargy, loss of appetite, and hemolytic anemia and caused by a bacterial parasite of red blood cells belonging to the genus *Haemobartonella* (*H. felis*)

feline infectious peritonitis *n* : an almost invariably fatal infectious disease of cats caused by a virus of the genus *Coronavirus* (species *Feline coronavirus*) and characterized by fever, weight and appetite loss, and ascites with a thick yellow fluid

feline leukemia *n* : a disease of cats caused by the feline leukemia virus, characterized by leukemia and lymphoma, and often resulting in death

feline leukemia virus *n* : a retrovirus (species *Feline leukemia virus* of the genus *Gammaretrovirus*) that is widespread in cat populations, is usu. transmitted by direct contact, and is associated with or causes malignant lymphoma, feline leukemia, anemia, glomerulonephritis, and immunosuppression — abbr. *FeLV*

feline panleukopenia *n* : PANLEUKOPENIA

feline pneumonitis *n* : an infectious disease of the eyes and upper respiratory tract of cats that is caused by a bacterium of the genus *Chlamydia* (*C. psittaci*) and is characterized esp. by conjunctivitis and rhinitis

fel·late \'fe-ˌlāt, fə-'lāt\ *vb* **fel·lat·ed; fel·lat·ing** : to perform fellatio on someone — **fel·la·tor** \-ˌla-tər, -'lā-\ *n*

fel·la·tio \fə-'lā-shē-ˌō, fe-, -'lā-tē-\ *also* **fel·la·tion** \-'lā-shən\ *n, pl* **-tios** *also* **-tions** : oral stimulation of the penis

fellea — see VESICA FELLEA

fel·low \'fe-(ˌ)lō\ *n* : a young physician who has completed training as an intern and resident and is granted a stipend and position allowing further study or research in a specialty

fe·lo·di·pine \fə-'lō-də-ˌpēn\ *n* : a calcium channel blocker $C_{18}H_{19}Cl_2NO_4$ used esp. in the treatment of hypertension

fel·on \'fe-lən\ *n* : WHITLOW

Fel·ty's syndrome \'fel-tēz-\ *n* : a condition characterized esp. by rheumatoid arthritis, neutropenia, and splenomegaly

Felty, Augustus Roi (1895–1964), American physician.

FeLV *abbr* feline leukemia virus

fe·male \'fē-ˌmāl\ *n* : an individual that bears young or produces eggs as distinguished from one that produces sperm; *esp* : a woman or girl as distinguished from a man or boy — **female** *adj* — **fe·male·ness** *n*

female genital mutilation *n* : clitoridectomy esp. as a cultural rite sometimes with removal of the labia that is now outlawed in many nations including the U.S. — abbr. *FGM;* called also *female circumcision*

female hormone *n* : a sex hormone (as an estrogen) primarily produced and functioning in the female

Fem·a·ra \'fe-mə-rə\ *trademark* — used for a preparation of letrozole

fem·i·nize \'fe-mə-ˌnīz\ *vb* **-nized; -niz·ing** : to cause (a male or castrate) to take on feminine characters (as by implantation of ovaries or administration of estrogenic substances) — **fem·i·ni·za·tion** \ˌfe-mə-nə-'zā-shən\ *n*

femora *pl of* FEMUR

fem·o·ral \'fe-mə-rəl\ *adj* : of or relating to the femur or thigh

femoral artery *n* : the chief artery of the thigh that lies in the anterior part of the thigh — see DEEP FEMORAL ARTERY

femoral canal *n* : the space that is situated between the femoral vein and the inner wall of the femoral sheath

femoral nerve *n* : the largest branch of the lumbar plexus that supplies extensor muscles of the thigh and skin areas on the front of the thigh and medial surface of the leg and foot and that sends articular branches to the hip and knee joints

femoral ring *n* : the oval upper opening of the femoral canal often the seat of a hernia

femoral sheath *n* : the fascial sheath investing the femoral vessels

femoral triangle *n* : an area in the upper anterior part of the thigh bounded by the inguinal ligament, the sartorius, and the adductor longus — called also *femoral trigone, Scarpa's triangle*

femoral vein *n* : the chief vein of the thigh that is a continuation of the popliteal vein and continues above the inguinal ligament as the external iliac vein

femoris — see BICEPS FEMORIS, PROFUNDA FEMORIS, PROFUNDA FEMORIS ARTERY, QUADRATUS FEMORIS, QUADRICEPS FEMORIS, RECTUS FEMORIS

femoro- *comb form* : femoral and ⟨*femoro*popliteal⟩

fem·o·ro·pop·li·te·al \ˌfe-mə-rō-ˌpä-plə-'tē-əl, -pä-'pli-tē-əl\ *adj* : of, relating to, or connecting the femoral and popliteal arteries ⟨a ~ bypass⟩

fe·mur \'fē-mər\ *n, pl* **fe·murs** *or* **fem·o·ra** \'fe-mə-rə\ : the proximal bone of the hind or lower limb that is the longest and largest bone in the human body, extends from the hip to the knee, articulates above with the acetabulum, and articulates with the tibia below by a pair of condyles — called also *thigh bone*

fe·nes·tra \fə-'nes-trə\ *n, pl* **-trae** \-ˌtrē, -ˌtrī\ **1** : a small anatomical opening (as in a bone): as **a** : OVAL WINDOW **b** : ROUND WINDOW **2 a** : a small opening cut in bone : WINDOW 2 **b** : a

small opening in a surgical instrument — **fe·nes·tral** \-trəl\ *adj*

fenestra coch·le·ae \-'kä-klē-ˌē, -'kō-klē-ˌī\ *n* : ROUND WINDOW

fenestra oval·is \-ˌō-'vä-ləs\ *n* : OVAL WINDOW

fenestra ro·tun·da \-ˌrō-'tən-də\ *n* : ROUND WINDOW

fen·es·trat·ed \'fe-nə-ˌstrā-təd\ *adj* : having one or more openings or pores ⟨~ blood capillaries⟩

fen·es·tra·tion \ˌfe-nə-'strā-shən\ *n* **1 a** : a natural or surgically created opening in a surface **b** : the presence of such openings **2** : the operation of cutting an opening in the bony labyrinth between the inner ear and tympanum to replace natural fenestrae that are not functional

fenestra ves·ti·bu·li \-ves-'ti-byə-ˌlī\ *n* : OVAL WINDOW

fen·flur·amine \ˌfen-'flùr-ə-ˌmēn\ *n* : an anorectic amphetamine derivative $C_{12}H_{16}F_3N$ formerly used in the form of its hydrochloride to treat obesity but no longer used due to its association with heart valve disease — see DEXFENFLURAMINE, FENPHEN

fen·o·fi·brate \ˌfe-nō-'fī-ˌbrāt\ *n* : a hypolipidemic agent $C_{20}H_{21}ClO_4$ used to treat hypercholesterolemia and hypertriglyceridemia — see TRICOR

fen·o·pro·fen \ˌfe-nə-'prō-fən\ *n* : an anti-inflammatory analgesic used in the form of its hydrated calcium salt $C_{30}H_{26}CaO_6 \cdot 2H_2O$ esp. to treat arthritis

fen–phen \'fen-ˌfen\ *n* : a former diet drug combination of phentermine with either fenfluramine or dexfenfluramine — called also *phen-fen*

fen·ta·nyl \'fent-ᵊn-ˌil\ *n* : a synthetic opioid narcotic analgesic $C_{22}H_{28}N_2O$ with pharmacological action similar to morphine that is administered esp. in the form of its citrate $C_{22}H_{28}N_2O \cdot C_6H_8O_7$

fer·ment \'fər-ˌment, (ˌ)fər-'\ *n* : ENZYME; *also* : FERMENTATION

fer·men·ta·tion \ˌfər-mən-'tā-shən, -ˌmen-\ *n* : an enzymatically controlled anaerobic breakdown of an energy-rich compound (as a carbohydrate to carbon dioxide and alcohol); *broadly* : an enzymatically controlled transformation of an organic compound — **fer·ment** \(ˌ)fər-'ment\ *vb* — **fer·men·ta·tive** \(ˌ)fər-'men-tə-tiv\ *adj*

fer·mi·um \'fer-mē-əm, 'fər-\ *n* : a radioactive metallic element artificially produced — symbol *Fm;* see ELEMENT table

fer·ric \'fer-ik\ *adj* **1** : of, relating to, or containing iron **2** : being or containing iron usu. with a valence of three

ferric chloride *n* : a salt $FeCl_3$ that is used in medicine in a water solution or tincture usu. as an astringent or styptic

ferric oxide n : the red or black oxide of iron Fe$_2$O$_3$

ferric py·ro·phos·phate \-ˌpī-rō-ˈfäs-ˌfāt\ n : a green or yellowish green salt Fe$_4$(P$_2$O$_7$)$_3$·nH$_2$O that is used as a source of iron esp. to fortify food

fer·ri·he·mo·glo·bin \ˌfer-ˌī-ˈhē-mə-ˌglō-bən, ˌfer-i-\ n : METHEMOGLOBIN

fer·ri·tin \ˈfer-ət-ᵊn\ n : a crystalline iron-containing protein that functions in the storage of iron and is found esp. in the liver and spleen

fer·rous \ˈfer-əs\ adj 1 : of, relating to, or containing iron 2 : being or containing iron with a valence of two

ferrous fumarate n : a reddish orange to red-brown powder C$_4$H$_2$FeO$_4$ used orally to treat iron-deficiency anemia

ferrous gluconate n : a yellowish gray or pale greenish yellow powder or granules C$_{12}$H$_{22}$FeO$_{14}$ used as a hematinic in the treatment of iron-deficiency anemia

ferrous sulfate n : an astringent iron salt obtained usu. in pale green crystalline form FeSO$_4$·7H$_2$O and used in medicine chiefly for treating iron-deficiency anemia

fer·tile \ˈfərt-ᵊl, ˈfər-ˌtīl\ adj 1 : capable of growing or developing ⟨a ~ egg⟩ 2 : developing spores or spore-bearing organs 3 a : capable of breeding or reproducing b of an estrous cycle : marked by the production of one or more viable eggs

fer·til·i·ty \(ˌ)fər-ˈti-lə-tē\ n, pl **-ties** 1 : the quality or state of being fertile 2 : the birthrate of a population — compare MORTALITY 2b

fer·til·iza·tion \ˌfərt-ᵊl-ə-ˈzā-shən\ n : an act or process of making fertile; specif : the process of union of two gametes whereby the somatic chromosome number is restored and the development of a new individual is initiated — **fer·til·ize** \ˈfərt-ᵊl-ˌīz\ vb

fertilization membrane n : a resistant membranous layer in eggs of many animals that forms following fertilization by the thickening and separation of the vitelline membrane from the cell surface and that prevents multiple fertilization

fes·cue foot \ˈfes-(ˌ)kyü-\ n : a disease of the feet of cattle resembling ergotism that is associated with feeding on fescue grass (genus *Festuca* and esp. *F. elatior* syn. *F. arundinacea*)

¹**fes·ter** \ˈfes-tər\ n : a suppurating sore : PUSTULE

²**fester** vb **fes·tered**; **fes·ter·ing** : to generate pus

fes·ti·nat·ing \ˈfes-tə-ˌnā-tin\ adj : being a walking gait (as in Parkinson's disease) characterized by involuntary acceleration — **fes·ti·na·tion** \ˌfes-tə-ˈnā-shən\ n

fe·tal \ˈfēt-ᵊl\ adj : of, relating to, or being a fetus

fetal alcohol syndrome n : a highly variable group of birth defects including mental retardation, deficient growth, central nervous system dysfunction, and malformations of the skull and face that tend to occur in the offspring of women who consume large amounts of alcohol during pregnancy — abbr. *FAS*

fetal hemoglobin n : hemoglobin that consists of two alpha chains and two gamma chains and that predominates in the blood of a newborn and persists in increased proportions in some forms of anemia (as thalassemia) — called also *hemoglobin F*

fetalis — see ERYTHROBLASTOSIS FETALIS, HYDROPS FETALIS

fetal position n : a position (as of a sleeping person) in which the body lies curled up on one side with the arms and legs drawn up toward the chest and the head bowed forward and which is assumed in some forms of psychological regression

feti- — see FETO-

fe·ti·cide \ˈfē-tə-ˌsīd\ n : the action or process of causing the death of a fetus

fe·tish also **fe·tich** \ˈfe-tish, ˈfē-\ n : an object or bodily part whose real or fantasized presence is psychologically necessary for sexual gratification and that is an object of fixation to the extent that it may interfere with complete sexual expression

fe·tish·ism also **fe·tich·ism** \-ti-ˌshi-zəm\ n : the pathological displacement of erotic interest and satisfaction to a fetish — **fe·tish·ist** \-shist\ n — **fe·tish·is·tic** \ˌfe-ti-ˈshis-tik also \-ˈtē-\ adj — **fe·tish·is·ti·cal·ly** \-ti-k(ə-)lē\ adv

fet·lock \ˈfet-ˌläk\ n 1 a : a projection bearing a tuft of hair on the back of the leg above the hoof of a horse or similar animal b : the tuft of hair itself 2 : the joint of the limb at the fetlock

feto- or **feti-** comb form : fetus ⟨feticide⟩

fe·tol·o·gist \fē-ˈtä-lə-jist\ n : a specialist in fetology

fe·tol·o·gy \fē-ˈtä-lə-jē\ n, pl **-gies** : a branch of medical science concerned with the study and treatment of the fetus in the uterus

fe·to·pro·tein \ˌfē-tō-ˈprō-ˌtēn, -tē-ən\ n : any of several fetal antigens present in the adult in some abnormal conditions; esp : ALPHA-FETOPROTEIN

fe·tor he·pat·i·cus \ˈfē-tər-hi-ˈpa-ti-kəs, -ˌtor'-\ n : a characteristically disagreeable odor to the breath that is a sign of liver failure

fe·to·scope \ˈfē-tə-ˌskōp\ n 1 : an endoscope for visual examination of the pregnant uterus 2 : a stethoscope for listening to the fetal heartbeat

fe·tos·co·py \fē-ˈtäs-kə-pē\ n, pl **-pies** : examination of the pregnant uterus by means of a fetoscope

fe·to·tox·ic \ˌfē-tə-ˈtäk-sik\ adj : toxic to fetuses — **fe·to·tox·i·ci·ty** \-täk-ˈsi-sə-tē\ n

fe·tus \ˈfē-təs\ n, pl **fe·tus·es** : an unborn or unhatched vertebrate esp. after attaining the basic structural plan of its kind; *specif* : a developing human from usu. two months after conception to birth — compare EMBRYO

Feul·gen reaction \'fȯil-gən\ *n* : the development of a purple color by DNA in a microscopic preparation stained with a modified Schiff's reagent

Feulgen, Robert Joachim (1884–1955), German biochemist.

¹fe·ver \'fē-vər\ *n* **1** : a rise of body temperature above the normal **2** : an abnormal bodily state characterized by increased production of heat, accelerated heart action and pulse, and systemic debility with weakness, loss of appetite, and thirst **3** : any of various diseases of which fever is a prominent symptom — **fe·ver·ish** \-və-rish\ *adj*

²fever *vb* **fe·vered; fe·ver·ing** : to affect with or be in a fever

fever blister *n* : COLD SORE

fever therapy *n* : a treatment of disease by fever induced by various artificial means

fever thermometer *n* : CLINICAL THERMOMETER

fex·o·fen·a·dine \,fek-sō-'fe-nə-,dēn\ *n* : an H₁ antagonist administered orally in the form of its hydrochloride $C_{32}H_{39}NO_4 \cdot HCl$ to relieve symptoms of seasonal allergic rhinitis — see ALLEGRA

FFA *abbr* free fatty acids

FGF *abbr* fibroblast growth factor

FGM *abbr* female genital mutilation

fi·ber \'fī-bər\ *n* **1 a** : a strand of nerve tissue : AXON, DENDRITE **b** : one of the filaments composing most of the intercellular matrix of connective tissue **c** : one of the elongated contractile cells of muscle tissue **2** : indigestible material in food that stimulates the intestine to peristalsis — called also *bulk, dietary fiber, roughage*

fiber of Mül·ler \-'myü-lər, -'mə-\ *n* : any of the glial fibers that extend through the entire thickness of the retina — called also *Müller cell, sustentacular fiber of Müller*

H. Müller — see MÜLLER CELL

fiber optics *n pl* **1** : thin transparent fibers of glass or plastic that transmit light throughout their length by internal reflections; *also* : a bundle of such fibers used in an instrument (as an endoscope) **2** : the technique of the use of fiber optics — used with a sing. verb — **fi·ber-op·tic** *adj*

fi·ber·scope \'fī-bər-,skōp\ *n* : a flexible endoscope that utilizes fiber optics to transmit light and is used for visual examination of inaccessible areas (as the stomach)

fiber tract *n* : TRACT 2

fibr- *or* **fibro-** *comb form* **1** : fiber : fibrous tissue ⟨*fibro*genesis⟩ **2** : fibrous and ⟨*fibro*elastic⟩

fi·bre *chiefly Brit var of* FIBER

fi·bril \'fī-brəl, 'fi-\ *n* : a small filament or fiber: as **a** : one of the fine threads into which a striated muscle fiber can be longitudinally split **b** : NEUROFIBRIL

fi·bril·la \fī-'bri-lə, fi-; 'fī-bri-lə, 'fi-\ *n*, *pl* **fi·bril·lae** \-,lē\ : FIBRIL

fi·bril·lar \'fī-brə-lər, 'fī-; fī-'bri-, fi-\ *adj* **1** : of or like fibrils or fibers ⟨a ~ network⟩ **2** : of or exhibiting fibrillation ⟨~ twitchings⟩

fi·bril·lary \'fī-brə-,ler-ē, 'fi-; fī-'bri-lə-rē, fi-\ *adj* **1** : of or relating to fibrils or fibers **2** : of, relating to, or marked by fibrillation ⟨~ chorea⟩

fi·bril·la·tion \,fi-brə-'lā-shən, ,fī-\ *n* **1** : an act or process of forming fibers or fibrils **2 a** : a muscular twitching involving individual muscle fibers acting without coordination **b** : very rapid irregular contractions of the muscle fibers of the heart resulting in a lack of synchronism between heartbeat and pulse — **fi·bril·late** \'fī-brə-,lāt, 'fi-\ *vb*

fi·bril·lin \'fī-brə-lin, 'fi-\ *n* : a large extracellular glycoprotein of connective tissue that is a structural component of microfibrils associated esp. with elastin

fi·bril·lo·gen·e·sis \,fi-brə-lō-'je-nə-səs, ,fī-\ *n*, *pl* **-e·ses** \-,sēz\ : the development of fibrils

fi·brin \'fī-brən\ *n* : a white insoluble fibrous protein formed from fibrinogen by the action of thrombin esp. in the clotting of blood

fi·brin·ase \-brə-,nās, -,nāz\ *n* : FACTOR XIII

fi·brin·o·gen \fī-'bri-nə-jən\ *n* : a plasma protein that is produced in the liver and is converted into fibrin during blood clot formation

fi·brin·o·gen·o·pe·nia \(,)fī-,bri-nə-,jenə-'pē-nē-ə, -nyə\ *n* : a deficiency of fibrin or fibrinogen or both in the blood

fi·bri·noid \'fi-brə-,nȯid, 'fī-\ *n*, *often attrib* : a homogeneous material that resembles fibrin and is formed in the walls of blood vessels and in connective tissue in some pathological conditions and normally in the placenta

fi·bri·no·ly·sin \,fī-brən-ᵊl-'īs-ᵊn\ *n* : any of several proteolytic enzymes that promote the dissolution of blood clots; *esp* : PLASMIN

fi·bri·no·ly·sis \-'fī-səs, -brə-'nä-lə-səs\ *n*, *pl* **-ly·ses** \-,sēz\ : the usu. enzymatic breakdown of fibrin — **fi·bri·no·lyt·ic** \-brən-ᵊl-'i-tik\ *adj*

fi·bri·no·pe·nia \,fī-brə-nō-'pē-nē-ə, -nyə\ *n* : FIBRINOGENOPENIA

fi·bri·no·pep·tide \-'pep-,tīd\ *n* : any of the polypeptides that are cleaved from fibrinogen by thrombin during blood clot formation

fi·bri·no·pur·u·lent \-'pyur-yə-lənt, -ə-lənt\ *adj* : containing, characterized by, or exuding fibrin and pus

fi·bri·nous \'fi-brə-nəs, 'fī-\ *adj* : marked by the presence of fibrin

fibro- — see FIBR-

fi·bro·ad·e·no·ma \ˌfī-(ˌ)brō-ˌad-ᵊn-'ō-mə\ *n*, *pl* **-mas** *also* **-ma·ta** \-mə-tə\ : adenoma with a large amount of fibrous tissue

fi·bro·blast \'fī-brə-ˌblast, 'fi-\ *n* : a connective-tissue cell of mesenchymal origin that secretes proteins and esp. molecular collagen from which the extracellular fibrillar matrix of connective tissue forms — **fi·bro·blas·tic** \ˌfī-brə-'blas-tik, ˌfi-\ *adj*

fibroblast growth factor *n* : any of several protein growth factors that stimulate the proliferation esp. of endothelial cells and that promote angiogenesis — abbr. *FGF*

fi·bro·car·ti·lage \ˌfī-(ˌ)brō-'kärt-ᵊl-ij\ *n* : cartilage in which the matrix except immediately about the cells is largely composed of fibers like those of ordinary connective tissue; *also* : a structure or part composed of such cartilage — **fi·bro·car·ti·lag·i·nous** \-ˌkärt-ᵊl-'a-jə-nəs\ *adj*

fi·bro·cys·tic \ˌfī-brə-'sis-tik, ˌfi-\ *adj* : characterized by the presence or development of fibrous tissue and cysts

fibrocystic disease of the pancreas *n* : CYSTIC FIBROSIS

fi·bro·cyte \'fī-brə-ˌsīt, 'fi-\ *n* : FIBROBLAST; *specif* : a spindle-shaped cell of fibrous tissue

fi·bro·elas·tic \ˌfī-(ˌ)brō-i-'las-tik\ *adj* : consisting of both fibrous and elastic elements ⟨~ tissue⟩

fi·bro·elas·to·sis \-ˌlas-'tō-səs\ *n*, *pl* **-to·ses** \-ˌsēz\ : a condition of the body or one of its organs characterized by proliferation of fibroelastic tissue — see ENDOCARDIAL FIBROELASTOSIS

fi·bro·gen·e·sis \ˌfī-brə-'je-nə-səs\ *n*, *pl* **-e·ses** \-ˌsēz\ : the development or proliferation of fibers or fibrous tissue

fi·bro·gen·ic \-'je-nik\ *adj* : promoting the development of fibers

¹fi·broid \'fī-ˌbròid, 'fi-\ *adj* : resembling, forming, or consisting of fibrous tissue

²fibroid *n* : a benign tumor esp. of the uterine wall that consists of fibrous and muscular tissue

fi·bro·ma \fī-'brō-mə\ *n*, *pl* **-mas** *also* **-ma·ta** \-tə\ : a benign tumor consisting mainly of fibrous tissue — **fi·bro·ma·tous** \-təs\ *adj*

fi·bro·ma·toid \fī-'brō-mə-ˌtòid\ *adj* : resembling a fibroma

fi·bro·ma·to·sis \(ˌ)fī-ˌbrō-mə-'tō-səs\ *n*, *pl* **-to·ses** \-ˌsēz\ : a condition marked by the presence of or a tendency to develop multiple fibromas

fi·bro·my·al·gia \-ˌmī-'al-jə, -jē-ə\ *n* : a chronic disorder characterized by widespread pain, tenderness, and stiffness of muscles and associated connective tissue structures that is typically accompanied by fatigue, headache, and sleep disturbances — called also *fibromyalgia syndrome, fibromyositis*

fi·bro·my·o·ma \-ˌmī-'ō-mə\ *n*, *pl* **-mas** *also* **-ma·ta** \-mə-tə\ : a mixed tumor containing both fibrous and muscle tissue — **fi·bro·my·o·ma·tous** \-mə-təs\ *adj*

fi·bro·my·o·si·tis \-ˌmī-ə-'sī-təs\ *n* : FIBROMYALGIA

fi·bro·myx·o·ma \-mik-'sō-mə\ *n*, *pl* **-mas** *also* **-ma·ta** \-mə-tə\ : a myxoma containing fibrous tissue

fi·bro·nec·tin \ˌfī-brə-'nek-tən\ *n* : any of a group of glycoproteins of cell surfaces, blood plasma, and connective tissue that promote cellular adhesion and migration

fi·bro·pla·sia \ˌfī-brə-'plā-zhə, -zhē-ə\ *n* : the process of forming fibrous tissue — **fi·bro·plas·tic** \-'plas-tik\ *adj*

fibrosa — see OSTEITIS FIBROSA, OSTEITIS FIBROSA CYSTICA, OSTEITIS FIBROSA CYSTICA GENERALISTA, OSTEODYSTROPHIA FIBROSA

fi·bro·sar·co·ma \-sär-'kō-mə\ *n*, *pl* **-mas** *also* **-ma·ta** \-mə-tə\ : a sarcoma of relatively low malignancy consisting chiefly of spindle-shaped cells that tend to form collagenous fibrils

fi·brose \'fī-ˌbrōs\ *vb* **-brosed; -bros·ing** : to form fibrous tissue

fi·bro·se·rous \ˌfī-brō-'sir-əs\ *adj* : composed of a serous membrane supported by a firm layer of fibrous tissue

fi·bro·sis \fī-'brō-səs\ *n*, *pl* **-bro·ses** \-ˌsēz\ : a condition marked by increase of interstitial fibrous tissue : fibrous degeneration — **fi·brot·ic** \-'brä-tik\ *adj*

fi·bro·si·tis \ˌfī-brə-'sī-təs\ *n* : a rheumatic disorder of fibrous tissue : FIBROMYALGIA — **fi·bro·sit·ic** \-'sit-ik\ *adj*

fibrosus — see ANNULUS FIBROSUS

fi·brous \'fī-brəs\ *adj* **1** : containing, consisting of, or resembling fibers **2** : characterized by fibrosis

fibrous ankylosis *n* : ankylosis due to the growth of fibrous tissue

fib·u·la \'fi-byə-lə\ *n*, *pl* **-lae** \-lē, -ˌlī\ *or* **-las** : the outer or postaxial and usu. the smaller of the two bones of the hind or lower limb below the knee that is the slenderest bone of the human body in proportion to its length and articulates above with the external tuberosity of the tibia and below with the talus — called also *calf bone* — **fib·u·lar** \-lər\ *adj*

fibular collateral ligament *n* : LATERAL COLLATERAL LIGAMENT

Fick principle \'fik-\ *n* : a generalization in physiology which states that blood flow is proportional to the difference in concentration of a substance (as oxygen) in the blood as it enters and leaves an organ and which is used to determine cardiac output — called also *Fick method*

Fick, Adolf Eugen (1829–1901), German physiologist.

FICS *abbr* Fellow of the International College of Surgeons

field \'fēld\ *n* **1** : a complex of forces that serve as causative agents in human behavior **2** : a region of embryonic tissue potentially capable of a particular type of differentiation **3 a** : an area that is perceived or under observation **b** : the site of a surgical operation

field hospital *n* : a military organization of medical personnel with equipment for establishing a temporary hospital in the field

field of vision *n* : VISUAL FIELD

fièvre bou·ton·neuse \'fyev-rə-,bü-tȯ-'nœz\ *n* : BOUTONNEUSE FEVER

fifth cranial nerve *n* : TRIGEMINAL NERVE

fifth disease *n* : an acute eruptive disease esp. of children that is caused by a parvovirus (species *Human parvovirus B19* of the genus *Erythrovirus*), is first manifested by a blotchy red rash on the cheeks followed by a maculopapular rash on the extremities, and is usu. accompanied by fever and malaise — called also *erythema infectiosum*

fifth nerve *n* : TRIGEMINAL NERVE

figure–ground \'fi-gyər-'graȯnd\ *adj* : relating to or being the relationships between the parts of a perceptual field which is perceived as divided into a part consisting of figures having form and standing out from the part comprising the background and being relatively formless

fil·a·ment \'fi-lə-mənt\ *n* : a single thread or a thin flexible threadlike object, process, or appendage; *esp* : an elongated thin series of cells attached one to another (as of some bacteria) — **fil·a·men·tous** \,fi-lə-'men-təs\ *adj*

fi·lar·ia \fə-'lar-ē-ə\ *n, pl* **fi·lar·i·ae** \-ē-,ē, -,ī\ : any of numerous slender filamentous nematodes that as adults are parasites in the blood or tissues and as larvae usu. develop in biting insects and that include forms causing elephantiasis, loaiasis, and onchocerciasis in humans and heartworm in dogs — **fi·lar·i·al** \-ē-əl\ *adj* — **fi·lar·i·id** \-ē-əd\ *adj or n*

fi·lar·i·a·sis \,fi-lə-'rī-ə-səs\ *n, pl* **-a·ses** \-,sēz\ : infestation with or disease caused by filariae

fi·lar·i·cide \fə-'lar-ə-,sīd\ *n* : an agent that is destructive to filariae — **fi·lar·i·cid·al** \-,lar-ə-'sīd-ᵊl\ *adj*

fi·lar·i·form \-ə-,fȯrm\ *adj, of a larval nematode* : resembling a filaria esp. in having a slender elongated form and in possessing a delicate capillary esophagus

fil·gras·tim \fil-'gras-təm\ *n* : a recombinant version of granulocyte colony-stimulating factor that is administered by injection esp. to stimulate production of neutrophils following chemotherapy — see NEUPOGEN

fili- *or* **filo-** *comb form* : thread ⟨*filiform*⟩

fil·ial generation \'fi-lē-əl-, 'fil-yəl-\ *n* : a generation in a breeding experiment that is successive to a parental generation — see F₁ GENERATION, F₂ GENERATION

fi·li·form \'fi-lə-,fȯrm, 'fī-\ *n* : an extremely slender bougie

filiform papilla *n* : any of numerous minute pointed papillae on the tongue

fil·i·pin \'fi-lə-pin\ *n* : an antifungal antibiotic $C_{35}H_{58}O_{11}$ produced by a bacterium of the genus *Streptomyces* (*S. filipinensis*)

fill \'fil\ *vb* **1** : to repair the cavities of (teeth) **2** : to supply as directed ⟨~ a prescription⟩

fil·let \'fi-lət\ *n* : a band of anatomical fibers; *specif* : LEMNISCUS

fill·ing \'fi-liŋ\ *n* **1** : material (as amalgam) used to fill a cavity in a tooth **2** : simple sporadic lymphangitis of the leg of a horse commonly due to overfeeding and insufficient exercise

film \'film\ *n* **1 a** : a thin skin or membranous covering **b** : an abnormal growth on or in the eye **2** : an exceedingly thin layer : LAMINA

film badge *n* : a small pack of sensitive photographic film worn as a badge for indicating exposure to radiation

filo- — see FILI-

fi·lo·vi·rus \'fi-lō-,vī-rəs\ *n* : any of a family (*Filoviridae*) of single-stranded chiefly filamentous RNA viruses that infect vertebrates and include the Ebola viruses and the Marburg virus

fil·ter \'fil-tər\ *n* **1** : a porous article or mass (as of paper) through which a gas or liquid is passed to separate out matter in suspension **2** : an apparatus containing a filter medium — **filter** *vb*

fil·ter·able \'fil-tə-rə-bəl\ *also* **fil·tra·ble** \-trə-bəl\ *adj* : capable of being filtered or of passing through a filter — **fil·ter·abil·i·ty** \,fil-tə-rə-'bi-lə-tē\ *n*

filterable virus *n* : any of the infectious agents that pass through a fine filter (as of unglazed porcelain) with the filtrate and remain virulent and that include the viruses and various other groups (as the mycoplasmas and rickettsiae) which were orig. considered viruses before their cellular nature was established

filter paper *n* : porous paper used esp. for filtering

fil·trate \'fil-,trāt\ *n* : fluid that has passed through a filter

fil·tra·tion \fil-'trā-shən\ *n* **1** : the process of filtering **2** : the process of passing through or as if through a filter; *also* : DIFFUSION

fi·lum ter·mi·na·le \'fī-ləm-,tər-mə-'nā-(,)lē, 'fē-ləm-,ter-mə-'nä-,lā\ *n, pl* **fila ter·mi·na·lia** \'fī-lə-tər-mə-'nā-lē-ə, 'fē-lə-,ter-mə-'nä-lē-ə\ : the slender threadlike prolongation of the spinal cord below the origin of the lumbar nerves : the last portion of the pia mater

fim·bria \'fim-brē-ə\ *n, pl* **-bri·ae** \-brē-ˌē, -ˌī\ **1** : a bordering fringe esp. at the entrance of the fallopian tubes **2** : a band of nerve fibers bordering the hippocampus and joining the fornix — **fim·bri·al** \-brē-əl\ *adj*

fimbriata — see PLICA FIMBRIATA

fim·bri·at·ed \'fim-brē-ˌā-təd\ *also* **fim·bri·ate** \-ˌāt\ *adj* : having the edge or extremity fringed or bordered by slender processes

fi·nas·te·ride \fə-'nas-tə-ˌrīd\ *n* : a nitrogenous steroid derivative $C_{23}H_{36}$ N_2O_2 that is used esp. to treat symptoms of benign prostatic hyperplasia and to increase hair growth in male-pattern baldness — see PROPECIA, PROSCAR

fine needle *n* : a long thin hollow needle with a narrow bore used esp. to obtain samples by fine needle aspiration; *also* : a solid hairlike needle used in acupuncture

fine needle aspiration *n* : the process of obtaining a sample of cells and bits of tissue for examination by applying suction through a fine needle attached to a syringe — abbr. FNA

fin·ger \'fiŋ-gər\ *n* : any of the five terminating members of the hand : a digit of the forelimb; *esp* : one other than the thumb — **fin·gered** \'fiŋ-gərd\ *adj*

finger fracture *n* : valvulotomy of the mitral commissures performed by a finger thrust through the valve

fin·ger·nail \'fiŋ-gər-ˌnāl\ *n* : the nail of a finger

fin·ger·print \-ˌprint\ *n* **1** : an ink impression of the lines on the fingertip taken for purpose of identification **2** : the chromatogram or electrophoretogram obtained by cleaving a protein by enzymatic action and subjecting the resulting collection of peptides to two-dimensional chromatography or electrophoresis — compare DNA FINGERPRINTING — **fin·ger·print** *vb* — **fin·ger·print·ing** *n*

finger spelling *n* : the representation of individual letters and numbers using standardized finger positions

fin·ger·stall \-ˌstȯl\ *n* : ¹COT

finger–stick \-ˌstik\ *adj* : relating to or being a blood test for which blood is obtained by a finger stick

finger stick *n* : an instance of pricking the skin of a finger to obtain blood from a capillary

fin·ger·tip \-ˌtip\ *n* : the tip of a finger

fire \'fīr\ *vb* **fired; fir·ing** : to transmit or cause to transmit a nerve impulse

fire ant *n* : any ant of the genus *Solenopsis*; *esp* : IMPORTED FIRE ANT

fire·damp \-ˌdamp\ *n* : a combustible mine gas that consists chiefly of methane; *also* : the explosive mixture of this gas with air

first aid *n* : emergency care or treatment given to an ill or injured person before regular medical aid can be obtained

first cranial nerve *n* : OLFACTORY NERVE

first–degree burn *n* : a mild burn characterized by heat, pain, and reddening of the burned surface but not exhibiting blistering or charring of tissues

first intention *n* : the healing of an incised wound by the direct union of skin edges without granulations — compare SECOND INTENTION

first–line \'fərst-'līn\ *adj* : being the preferred, standard, or first choice ⟨~ treatment of advanced breast cancer⟩ — compare SECOND-LINE

first messenger *n* : an extracellular substance (as a hormone or neurotransmitter) that binds to a cell-surface receptor and initiates intracellular activity

first polar body *n* : POLAR BODY A

fish–liv·er oil \'fish-ˌli-vər-\ *n* : a fatty oil from the livers of various fishes (as cod, halibut, or sharks) used chiefly as a source of vitamin A

fish tapeworm *n* : a large tapeworm of the genus *Diphyllobothrium* (*D. latum*) that as an adult infests the human intestine and goes through its intermediate stages in freshwater fishes from which it is transmitted to humans when raw fish is eaten

fis·sion \'fi-shən, -zhən\ *n* **1** : a method of reproduction in which a living cell or body divides into two or more parts each of which grows into a whole new individual **2** : the splitting of an atomic nucleus resulting in the release of large amounts of energy — called also *nuclear fission* — **fis·sion·able** \'fi-shə-nə-bəl, -zhə-\ *adj*

fis·sure \'fi-shər\ *n* **1** : a natural cleft between body parts or in the substance of an organ: as **a** : any of several clefts separating the lobes of the liver **b** : any of various clefts between bones or parts of bones in the skull **c** : any of the deep clefts of the brain; *esp* : one of those located at points of elevation in the walls of the ventricles — compare SULCUS **d** : ANTERIOR MEDIAN FISSURE; *also* : POSTERIOR MEDIAN SEPTUM **2** : a break or slit in tissue usu. at the junction of skin and mucous membrane ⟨~ of the lip⟩ **3** : a linear developmental imperfection in the enamel of a tooth — **fis·sured** \'fi-shərd\ *adj*

fissure of Ro·lan·do \-rō-'lan-(ˌ)dō, -'län-\ *n* : CENTRAL SULCUS

Rolando, Luigi (1773–1831), Italian anatomist and physiologist.

fissure of syl·vi·us \-'sil-vē-əs\ *n* : SYLVIAN FISSURE

F. Dubois or **De Le Boë** — see SYLVIAN

fis·tu·la \'fis-chə-lə, -tyü-lə\ *n, pl* **-las** *or* **-lae** \-ˌlē, -ˌlī\ : an abnormal passage that leads from an abscess or hollow organ to the body surface or from one hollow organ or part to another and that may be surgically created to permit passage of fluids or secretions — **fis·tu·lat·ed** \-¸lā-tad\ *adj*

fis·tu·lec·to·my \¸fis-chə-'lek-tə-mē, -tyü-\ *n, pl* **-mies** : surgical excision of a fistula

fis·tu·li·za·tion \-lə-'zā-shən, -¸lī-\ *n* **1** : the condition of having a fistula **2** : surgical production of an artificial channel

fis·tu·lous \-ləs\ *adj* : of, relating to, or having the form or nature of a fistula

fistulous withers *n sing or pl* : a deep-seated chronic inflammation of the withers of the horse that discharges seropurulent or bloody fluid through one or more openings and is prob. associated with infection by bacteria of the genus *Brucella* (esp. *B. abortus*)

¹fit \'fit\ *n* **1** : a sudden violent attack of a disease (as epilepsy) esp. when marked by convulsions or unconsciousness : PAROXYSM **2** : a sudden but transient attack of a physical disturbance

²fit *adj* **fit·ter; fit·test** : sound physically and mentally : HEALTHY — **fit·ness** *n*

¹fix \'fiks\ *vb* **1 a** : to make firm, stable, or stationary **b** (1) : to change into a stable compound or available form ⟨bacteria that ~ nitrogen⟩ (2) : to kill, harden, and preserve for microscopic study **2** : SPAY, CASTRATE

²fix *n* : a shot of a narcotic

fix·at·ed \'fik-¸sā-təd\ *adj* : arrested in development or adjustment; *esp* : arrested at a pregenital level of psychosexual development

fix·a·tion \fik-'sā-shən\ *n* **1 a** : the act or an instance of focusing the eyes upon an object **b** (1) : a persistent concentration of libidinal energies upon objects characteristic of psychosexual stages of development preceding the genital stage (2) : an obsessive or unhealthy preoccupation or attachment **2** : the immobilization of the parts of a fractured bone esp. by the use of various metal attachments — **fix·ate** \'fik-¸sāt\ *vb*

fixation point *n* : the point in the visual field that is fixated by the two eyes in normal vision and for each eye is the point that directly stimulates the fovea of the retina

fix·a·tive \'fik-sə-tiv\ *n* : a substance used to fix living tissue

fix·a·tor \'fik-¸sā-tər\ *n* : a muscle that stabilizes or fixes a part of the body to which a muscle in the process of moving another part is attached

fixed idea *n* : IDÉE FIXE

fixed oil *n* : a nonvolatile oil; *esp* : FATTY OIL

fl *abbr* fluid

flac·cid \'fla-səd, 'flak-\ *adj* : not firm or stiff; *also* : lacking normal or youthful firmness ⟨~ muscles⟩ — **flac·cid·i·ty** \fla-'si-də-tē, flak-\ *n*

flaccid paralysis *n* : paralysis in which muscle tone is lacking in the affected muscles and in which tendon reflexes are decreased or absent

fla·gel·lant \'fla-jə-lənt, flə-'je-lənt\ *n* : a person who responds sexually to being beaten by or to beating another person — **flagellant** *adj* — **fla·gel·lant·ism** \-lən-¸ti-zəm\ *n*

fla·gel·lar \flə-'je-lər, 'fla-jə-\ *adj* : of or relating to a flagellum

¹fla·gel·late \'fla-jə-lət, -¸lāt; flə-'je-lət\ *adj* **1 a** *or* **flag·el·lat·ed** \'fla-jə-¸lā-təd\ : having flagella **b** : shaped like a flagellum **2** : of, relating to, or caused by flagellates ⟨~ diarrhea⟩

²flagellate *n* : a flagellate protozoan or alga

¹flag·el·la·tion \¸fla-jə-'lā-shən\ *n* : the practice of a flagellant

²flagellation *n* : the formation or arrangement of flagella

fla·gel·lum \flə-'je-ləm\ *n, pl* **-la** \-lə\ *also* **-lums** : a long tapering process that projects singly or in groups from a cell and is the primary organ of motion of many microorganisms

Flag·yl \'fla-gəl\ *trademark* — used for a preparation of metronidazole

flail \'flāl\ *adj* : exhibiting abnormal mobility and loss of response to normal controls — used of body parts (as joints) damaged by paralysis, accident, or surgery ⟨~ joint⟩

flammeus — see NEVUS FLAMMEUS

flank \'flaŋk\ *n* : the fleshy part of the side between the ribs and the hip; *broadly* : the side of a quadruped

flap \'flap\ *n* : a piece of tissue partly severed from its place of origin for use in surgical grafting

¹flare \'flar\ *vb* **flared; flar·ing** : to break out or intensify rapidly : become suddenly worse or more painful — often used with *up*

²flare *n* **1** : a sudden outburst or worsening of a disease — see FLARE-UP **2** : an area of skin flush resulting from and spreading out from a local center of vascular dilation and hyperemia ⟨urticaria ~⟩ **3** : the presence of floating particles in the fluid of the anterior chamber of the eye — called also *aqueous flare*

flare-up \-¸əp\ *n* : a sudden increase in the symptoms of a latent or subsiding disease ⟨a ~ of malaria⟩

flash \'flash\ *n* : RUSH **2** — see HOT FLASH

flat \'flat\ *adj* **flat·ter; flat·test** **1** : being or characterized by a horizontal line or tracing without peaks or depressions **2** : characterized by general impoverishment in the presence of emotion-evoking stimuli — **flat·ness** *n*

flat bone *n* : any of various bones (as of the skull, the jaw, the pelvis, or the rib cage) not rounded in cross section

flat·foot \-¸fut\ *n, pl* **flat·feet** \-¸fēt\ **1** : a condition in which the arch of the instep is flattened so that the entire sole rests upon the ground **2** : a foot affected with flatfoot — **flat–foot·ed** \-ˌfu̇-təd\ *adj*

flat plate *n* : a radiograph esp. of the abdomen taken with the subject lying flat

flat·u·lence \'fla-chə-ləns\ *n* : the quality or state of being flatulent

flat·u·lent \-lənt\ *adj* **1** : marked by or affected with gases generated in the intestine or stomach **2** : likely to cause digestive flatulence — **flat·u·lent·ly** *adv*

fla·tus \'flā-təs\ *n* : gas generated in the stomach or bowels

flat wart *n* : a small smooth slightly elevated wart found esp. on the face and back of the hands that occurs chiefly in children and adolescents — called also *plane wart, verruca plana*

flat·worm \'flat-ˌwərm\ *n* : any of a phylum (Platyhelminthes) of soft-bodied usu. much flattened worms (as the flukes and tapeworms) — called also *platyhelminth*

fla·vin \'flā-vən\ *n* : any of a class of yellow water-soluble nitrogenous pigments derived from isoalloxazine and occurring in the form of nucleotides as coenzymes of flavoproteins; *esp* : RIBOFLAVIN

flavin adenine di·nu·cle·o·tide \-ˌdī-'nü-klē-ō-ˌtīd, -'nyü-\ *n* : a coenzyme $C_{27}H_{33}N_9O_{15}P_2$ of some flavoproteins — called also *FAD*

flavin mononucleotide *n* : FMN

fla·vi·vi·rus \'flā-vi-ˌvī-rəs\ *n* **1** *cap* : a genus of single-stranded RNA viruses (family *Flaviviridae*) that are transmitted esp. by ticks and mosquitoes and that include the causative agents of dengue, Japanese B encephalitis, Saint Louis encephalitis, West Nile fever, and yellow fever **2** : any virus of the genus *Flavivirus*; *broadly* : any virus of the family (*Flaviviridae*) to which the genus *Flavivirus* belongs and which includes the causative agents of hepatitis C, bovine viral diarrhea, and cholera

fla·vo·bac·te·ri·um \ˌflā-vō-bak-'tir-ē-əm\ *n* : a genus of nonmotile aerobic gram-negative usu. rod-shaped bacteria including one (*F. meningosepticum*) that is found as a contaminant in hospitals and is associated with meningitis and septicemia esp. in newborn infants

fla·vo·noid \'flā-və-ˌnȯid, 'fla-\ *n* : any of a group of compounds that includes many common pigments — **flavonoid** *adj*

fla·vo·pro·tein \ˌflā-vō-'prō-ˌtēn, ˌfla-, -'prō-tē-ən\ *n* : a dehydrogenase that contains a flavin and often a metal and plays a major role in biological oxidations

flavum — see LIGAMENTUM FLAVUM

flax·seed \'flaks-ˌsēd\ *n* : the seed of flax (esp. *Linum usitatissimum*) used esp. as a demulcent and emollient and as a dietary supplement

flea \'flē\ *n* : any of an order (Siphonaptera) comprising small wingless bloodsucking insects that have a hard laterally compressed body and legs adapted to leaping and that feed on warm-blooded animals

flea-bite \-ˌbīt\ *n* : the bite of a flea; *also* : the red spot caused by such a bite — **flea–bit·ten** \-ˌbit-ᵊn\ *adj*

flea collar *n* : a collar for animals that contains insecticide for killing fleas

flea·wort \-ˌwȯrt, -ˌwört\ *n* : any of three Old World plantains of the genus *Plantago* (esp. *P. psyllium*) that are the source of psyllium seed — called also *psyllium*

fle·cai·nide \ˌfle-'kā-ˌnīd\ *n* : an antiarrhythmic drug used in the form of its acetate $C_{17}H_{20}F_6N_2O_3 \cdot C_2H_4O_2$ esp. to treat ventricular arrhythmias

flesh \'flesh\ *n* : the soft parts of the body; *esp* : the parts composed chiefly of skeletal muscle as distinguished from visceral structures, bone, and integuments — see PROUD FLESH — **fleshed** \'flesht\ *adj* — **fleshy** \'fle-shē\ *adj*

flesh fly *n* : any of a family (Sarcophagidae) of dipteran flies some of which cause myiasis

flesh wound *n* : an injury involving penetration of the body musculature without damage to bones or internal organs

Fletch·er·ism \'fle-chər-ˌi-zəm\ *n* : the practice of eating in small amounts and only when hungry and of chewing one's food thoroughly — **fletch·er·ize** \-ˌīz\ *vb*

Fletcher, Horace (1849–1919), American dietitian.

flex \'fleks\ *vb* **1** : to bend esp. repeatedly **2 a** : to move muscles so as to cause flexion of (a joint) **b** : to move or tense (a muscle) by contraction

flexibilitas — see CEREA FLEXIBILITAS

flex·i·ble \'flek-sə-bəl\ *adj* : capable of being flexed : capable of being turned, bowed, or twisted without breaking — **flex·i·bil·i·ty** \ˌflek-sə-'bi-lə-tē\ *n*

flex·ion *also* **flec·tion** \'flek-shən\ *n* **1** : a bending movement around a joint in a limb (as the knee or elbow) that decreases the angle between the bones of the limb at the joint — compare EXTENSION 2 **2** : a forward raising of the arm or leg by a movement at the shoulder or hip joint

flex·or \'flek-sər, -ˌsȯr\ *n* : a muscle serving to bend a body part (as a limb) — called also *flexor muscle*; compare EXTENSOR

flexor car·pi ra·di·al·is \-'kär-ˌpī-ˌrā-dē-'ā-ləs, -'kär-ˌpē-\ *n* : a superficial muscle of the palmar side of the forearm that flexes the hand and assists in abducting it

flexor carpi ul·nar·is \-ˌəl-'nar-əs\ *n* : a superficial muscle of the ulnar side of the forearm that flexes the hand and assists in adducting it

flexor dig·i·ti min·i·mi brev·is \-'di-jə-

ˌtī-ˈmi-nə-ˌmī-ˈbre-vəs, -ˈdi-jə-ˌtē-ˈmi-nə-ˌmē\ n 1 : a muscle of the ulnar side of the palm of the hand that flexes the little finger 2 : a muscle of the sole of the foot that flexes the first proximal phalanx of the little toe

flexor dig·i·to·rum brevis \-ˌdi-jə-ˈtōr-əm-\ n : a muscle of the middle part of the sole of the foot that flexes the second phalanx of each of the four small toes

flexor digitorum lon·gus \-ˈlȯŋ-gəs\ n : a muscle of the tibial side of the leg that flexes the terminal phalanx of each of the four small toes

flexor digitorum pro·fun·dus \-prō-ˈfən-dəs\ n : a deep muscle of the ulnar side of the forearm that flexes esp. the terminal phalanges of the four fingers

flexor digitorum su·per·fi·ci·al·is \-ˌsü-pər-ˌfi-shē-ˈā-ləs\ n : a superficial muscle of the palmar side of the forearm that flexes esp. the second phalanges of the four fingers

flexor hal·lu·cis brev·is \-ˈha-lü-səs-ˈbre-vəs, -lyü-, -ˈha-lə-kəs\ n : a short muscle of the sole of the foot that flexes the proximal phalanx of the big toe

flexor hallucis longus n : a long deep muscle of the fibular side of the leg that flexes esp. the second phalanx of the big toe

flexor muscle n : FLEXOR

flexor pol·li·cis brevis \-ˈpä-lə-səs-, -kəs-\ n : a short muscle of the palm that flexes and adducts the thumb

flexor pollicis longus n : a muscle of the radial side of the forearm that flexes esp. the second phalanx of the thumb

flexor ret·in·ac·u·lum \-ˌret-ᵊn-ˈa-kyə-ləm\ n 1 : a fibrous band of fascia on the medial side of the ankle that extends downward from the medial malleolus of the tibia to the calcaneus and that covers over the bony grooves containing the tendons of the flexor muscles, the posterior tibial artery and vein, and the tibial nerve as they pass into the sole of the foot 2 : a fibrous band of fascia on the palm side of the wrist and base of the hand that forms the roof of the carpal tunnel and covers the tendons of the flexor muscles and the median nerve as they pass into the hand — called also *transverse carpal ligament*

flex·ure \ˈflek-shər\ n 1 : the quality or state of being flexed : FLEXION 2 : an anatomical turn, bend, or fold; *esp* : one of three sharp bends of the anterior part of the primary axis of the vertebrate embryo that serve to establish the relationship of the parts of the developing brain — see CEPHALIC FLEXURE, HEPATIC FLEXURE, PONTINE FLEXURE, SPLENIC FLEXURE — **flex·ur·al** \-shər-əl\ adj

flick·er \ˈfli-kər\ n : the wavering or fluttering visual sensation produced by intermittent light when the interval between flashes is not small enough to produce complete fusion of the individual impressions

flicker fusion n : FUSION b(2)

flight of ideas n : a rapid shifting of ideas that is expressed as a disconnected rambling and occurs esp. in the manic phase of bipolar disorder

flight surgeon n : a medical officer (as in the U.S. Air Force) specializing in aerospace medicine

float·er \ˈflō-tər\ n : a bit of optical debris (as a dead cell or cell fragment) in the vitreous body or lens that may be perceived as a spot before the eye; *also* : a spot in the visual field due to such debris — usu. used in pl.; compare MUSCAE VOLITANTES

float·ing \ˈflōt-iŋ\ adj : located out of the normal position or abnormally movable ⟨a ~ kidney⟩

floating rib n : any rib in the last two pairs of ribs that have no attachment to the sternum — compare FALSE RIB

floc·cu·lar \ˈflä-kyə-lər\ adj : of or relating to a flocculus

floc·cu·late \ˈflä-kyə-ˌlāt\ vb **-lat·ed**; **-lat·ing** : to aggregate or cause to aggregate into a flocculent mass — **floc·cu·la·tion** \ˌflä-kyə-ˈlā-shən\ n

floc·cu·la·tion test \ˌflä-kyə-ˈlā-shən-\ n : any of various serological tests (as the Mazzini test for syphilis) in which a positive result depends on the combination of an antigen and antibody to produce a flocculent precipitate

floc·cu·lent \-kyə-lənt\ adj : made up of loosely aggregated particles ⟨a ~ precipitate⟩

floc·cu·lo·nod·u·lar lobe \ˌflä-kyə-(ˌ)lō-ˈnä-jə-lər-\ n : the posterior lobe of the cerebellum that consists of the nodulus and paired lateral flocculi and is concerned with equilibrium

floc·cu·lus \-ləs\ n, pl **-li** \-ˌlī, -ˌlē\ : a small irregular lobe on the undersurface of each hemisphere of the cerebellum that is linked with the corresponding side of the nodulus by a peduncle

Flo·max \ˈflō-ˌmaks\ trademark — used for a preparation of the hydrochloride of tamsulosin

Flo·nase \ˈflō-ˌnās\ trademark — used for a preparation of fluticasone propionate administered as a nasal spray

flood·ing \ˈflə-diŋ\ n : exposure therapy in which there is prolonged confrontation with an anxiety-provoking stimulus

floor \ˈflȯr\ n : the lower inside surface of a hollow anatomical structure ⟨the ~ of the pelvis⟩

flo·ra \ˈflȯr-ə\ n, pl **floras** also **flo·rae** \ˈflȯr-ˌē, -ˌī\ 1 : plant life; *esp* : the plant life characteristic of a region, period, or special environment — compare FAUNA 2 : the microorganisms (as bacteria) living in or on the body — **flo·ral** \ˈflȯr-əl\ adj

flor·id \ˈflȯr-əd, ˈflär-\ adj : fully developed : manifesting a complete and typical clinical syndrome ⟨~ hyperplasia⟩ — **flor·id·ly** adv

¹**floss** \'fläs, 'flòs\ n : DENTAL FLOSS

²**floss** vb : to use dental floss on (one's teeth)

Flo·vent \'flō-ˌvent\ trademark — used for a preparation of fluticasone propionate administered as an oral inhalant

¹**flow** \'flō\ vb **1** : to move with a continual change of place among the constituent particles : MENSTRUATE

²**flow** n **1** : the quantity that flows in a certain time **2** : MENSTRUATION

flow cytometry n : a technique for identifying and sorting cells and their components (as DNA) by staining with a fluorescent dye and detecting the fluorescence usu. by laser beam illumination — **flow cytometer** n

flowers of zinc n pl : zinc oxide esp. as obtained as a light white powder by burning zinc for use in pharmaceutical and cosmetic preparations

flow·me·ter \'flō-ˌmē-tər\ n : an instrument for measuring the velocity of flow of a fluid (as blood) in a tube or pipe

fl oz abbr fluid ounce

flu \'flü\ n **1** : INFLUENZA **2** : any of several virus or bacterial diseases marked esp. by respiratory or intestinal symptoms — see INTESTINAL FLU — **flu·like** \-ˌlīk\ adj

flu·con·a·zole \flü-'kä-nə-ˌzōl\ n : a triazole antifungal agent $C_{13}H_{12}F_2N_6O$ used to treat cryptococcal meningitis and local or systemic candida infections — see DIFLUCAN

fluc·tu·ant \'flək-chə-wənt\ adj : movable and compressible — used of abnormal body structures (as some abscesses or tumors)

fluc·tu·a·tion \ˌflək-chə-'wā-shən\ n : the wavelike motion of a fluid collected in a natural or artificial cavity of the body observed by palpation or percussion

flu·cy·to·sine \flü-'sī-tə-ˌsēn\ n : an antifungal agent $C_4H_4FN_3O$ used esp. against fungi of the genera Candida and Cryptococcus (esp. Cryptococcus neoformans)

flu·dar·a·bine \flü-'dar-ə-ˌbēn\ n : an antineoplastic agent administered intravenously in the form of its phosphate $C_{10}H_{13}FN_5O_7P$ esp. to treat chronic lymphocytic leukemia

flu·dro·cor·ti·sone \ˌflü-drō-'kòr-tə-ˌsōn, -ˌzōn\ n : a potent mineralocorticoid drug that possesses some glucocorticoid activity and is administered in the form of its acetate $C_{23}H_{31}FO_6$ to treat adrenocortical insufficiency

flu·id \'flü-əd\ n : a substance (as a liquid or gas) tending to flow or conform to the outline of its container; specif : one in the body of an animal or plant — see CEREBROSPINAL FLUID, SEMINAL FLUID — **fluid** adj

fluid dram or **flu·i·dram** \ˌflü-ə-'dram\

n : either of two units of liquid capacity: **a** : a U.S. unit equal to ⅛ U.S. fluid ounce **b** : a British unit equal to ⅛ British fluid ounce

flu·id·ex·tract \ˌflü-əd-'ek-ˌstrakt\ n : an alcohol preparation of a vegetable drug containing the active constituents of one gram of the dry drug in each milliliter

fluid ounce n **1** : a U.S. unit of liquid capacity equal to 1/16 pint **2** : a British unit of liquid capacity equal to 1/20 pint

fluke \'flük\ n : a flattened digenetic trematode worm; broadly : TREMATODE — see LIVER FLUKE

flu·nis·o·lide \flü-'ni-sə-ˌlīd\ n : a synthetic glucocorticoid $C_{24}H_{31}FO_6$·½H_2O administered as an oral inhalant to treat bronchial asthma and as a nasal spray to treat rhinitis

flu·ni·traz·e·pam \ˌflü-nə-'tra-zə-ˌpam\ n : a powerful benzodiazepine sedative and hypnotic drug $C_{16}H_{12}FN_3O_3$ that is not licensed for use in the U.S. but is used medically in other countries and that is a frequent illicit drug of abuse — see ROHYPNOL

flu·o·cin·o·lone ac·e·to·nide \ˌflü-ō-'sin-ᵊl-ˌōn-ˌa-sə-'tō-ˌnīd\ n : a glucocorticoid steroid $C_{24}H_{30}F_2O_6$ used esp. as an anti-inflammatory agent in the treatment of skin diseases

fluor- or **fluoro-** comb form **1** : fluorine ⟨fluorosis⟩ **2** also **fluori-** : fluorescence ⟨fluoroscope⟩

flu·o·res·ce·in \ˌflü-ər-'e-sē-ən, ˌflòr-\ n : a dye $C_{20}H_{12}O_5$ with a bright yellow-green fluorescence in alkaline solution that is used as the sodium salt as an aid in diagnosis

flu·o·res·cence \-'es-ᵊns\ n : luminescence that is caused by the absorption of radiation at one wavelength followed by the nearly immediate emission of radiation usu. at a different wavelength and that ceases almost at once when the source of radiation is removed; also : the radiation emitted — **flu·o·resce** \-'es\ vb — **flu·o·res·cent** \-'es-ᵊnt\ adj

fluorescence microscope n : ULTRAVIOLET MICROSCOPE

flu·o·ri·date \'flùr-ə-ˌdāt, 'flòr-\ vb **-dat·ed; -dat·ing** : to add a fluoride to (as drinking water) to reduce tooth decay — **flu·o·ri·da·tion** \ˌflùr-ə-'dā-shən, ˌflòr-\ n

flu·o·ride \'flü-ər-ˌīd\ n **1** : a compound of fluorine usu. with a more electrically positive element or radical **2** : the monovalent anion of fluorine — **fluoride** adj

flu·o·rine \'flü-ər-ˌēn, 'flòr-, -ən\ n : a nonmetallic monovalent halogen element that is normally a pale yellowish flammable irritating toxic gas — symbol F; see ELEMENT table

flu·o·rom·e·ter \ˌflü-ər-'ä-mə-tər\ or **flu·o·rim·e·ter** \-'i-mə-tər\ n : an instrument for measuring fluorescence and related phenomena (as intensity of radiation) — flu·o·ro·met·ric or flu·o·ri·met·ric \ˌflü-ər-ə-ˈme-trik, ˌflȯr-\ adj — flu·o·rom·e·try \-ˈä-mə-trē\ or flu·o·rim·e·try \-ˈi-mə-trē\ n

flu·o·ro·pho·tom·e·ter \ˌflü-ər-ō-fō-ˈtä-mə-tər, ˌflȯr-ō-\ n : FLUOROMETER — flu·o·ro·pho·to·met·ric \-ˌfō-tə-ˈme-trik\ adj — flu·o·ro·pho·tom·e·try \-ˌfō-ˈtä-mə-trē\ n

flu·o·ro·scope \ˈflu̇r-ə-ˌskōp, ˈflȯr-\ n : an instrument used in medical diagnosis for observing the internal structure of the body by means of X-rays — fluoroscope vb — flu·o·ro·scop·ic \ˌflu̇r-ə-ˈskä-pik, ˌflȯr-\ adj — flu·o·ro·scop·i·cal·ly \-pi-k(ə-)lē\ adv — flu·o·ros·co·pist \-ˈäs-kə-pist\ n — flu·o·ros·co·py \-pē\ n

flu·o·ro·sis \ˌflü-ər-ˈō-səs, ˌflȯr-\ n : an abnormal condition (as mottled enamel of human teeth) caused by fluorine or its compounds

flu·o·ro·ura·cil \ˌflü-ər-ō-ˈyu̇r-ə-ˌsil, -ˌsəl\ or 5-flu·o·ro·ura·cil \ˈfīv-\ n : a fluorine-containing pyrimidine base $C_4H_3FN_2O_2$ used to treat some kinds of cancer

flu·o·ro·quin·o·lone \-ˈkwi-nə-ˌlōn\ n : any of a group of fluorinated derivatives (as ciprofloxacin and levofloxacin) of quinolone that are used as antibacterial drugs

flu·ox·e·tine \ˌflü-ˈäk-sə-ˌtēn\ n : a drug that functions as an SSRI and is administered in the form of its hydrochloride $C_{17}H_{18}F_3NO·HCl$ esp. to treat depression, panic disorder, and obsessive-compulsive disorder — see PROZAC

flu·oxy·mes·te·rone \ˌflə-ˌwäk-sē-ˈme-stə-ˌrōn\ n : a synthetic androgen $C_{20}H_{29}FO_3$ used orally esp. in the treatment of testosterone deficiency in males and in the palliative treatment of breast cancer in females

flu·phen·azine \flü-ˈfe-nə-ˌzēn\ n : a phenothiazine tranquilizer used esp. in the form of its dihydrochloride $C_{22}H_{26}F_3N_3OS·2HCl$ — see PROLIXIN

flur·az·e·pam \ˌflu̇r-ˈa-zə-ˌpam\ n : a benzodiazepine closely related structurally to diazepam that is used as a hypnotic in the form of its hydrochloride $C_{21}H_{23}ClFN_3O·2HCl$ esp. to treat insomnia — see DALMANE

flur·bi·pro·fen \ˌflu̇r-ˈbi-prə-fən\ n : a nonsteroidal anti-inflammatory drug $C_{15}H_{13}FO_2$ used in the symptomatic treatment of rheumatoid arthritis and osteoarthritis — see ANSAID

flur·oth·yl \ˈflu̇r-ə-thil\ n : a liquid convulsant $C_4H_4F_6O$ that has been used in place of electroconvulsive therapy in the treatment of mental disorder

¹flush \ˈfləsh\ n : a transitory sensation of extreme heat (as in response to some physiological states)

²flush vb 1 : to blush or become suddenly suffused with color due to vasodilation 2 : to cleanse or wash out with or as if with a rush of liquid

flu·ta·mide \ˈflü-tə-ˌmīd\ n : a nonsteroidal antiandrogen $C_{11}H_{11}F_3N_2O_3$ used to treat prostate cancer

flu·ti·ca·sone propionate \flü-ˈti-kə-ˌsōn-\ n : a corticosteroid $C_{25}H_{31}F_3O_5S$ administered as a nasal spray to treat allergic rhinitis, as an oral inhalant to treat and prevent asthma, and topically as a cream or ointment to treat skin inflammation and itching — called also fluticasone; see ADVAIR DISKUS, FLONASE, FLOVENT

flut·ter \ˈflə-tər\ n : an abnormal rapid spasmodic and usu. rhythmic motion or contraction of a body part ⟨a serious ventricular ∼⟩ — flutter vb

flu·vox·a·mine \flü-ˈväk-sə-ˌmēn\ n : a drug that functions as an SSRI and is administered orally in the form of its maleate $C_{15}H_{21}O_2N_2F_3·C_4H_4O_4$ esp. to treat depression and obsessive-compulsive disorder — see LUVOX

flux \ˈfləks\ n 1 : a flowing or discharge of fluid from the body esp. when excessive or abnormal: as a : DIARRHEA b : DYSENTERY 2 : the matter discharged in a flux

fly \ˈflī\ n, pl flies 1 : any of a large order (Diptera) of usu. winged insects (as the housefly or a mosquito) that have the anterior wings functional, the posterior wings modified to function as sensory flight stabilizers, and segmented often headless, eyeless, and legless lavae 2 : a large stout-bodied fly (as a horsefly)

fly aga·ric \-ˈa-gə-rik, -ə-ˈgar-ik\ n : a poisonous mushroom of the genus Amanita (A. muscaria) that usu. has a bright red cap — called also fly amanita, fly mushroom

¹fly-blow \ˈflī-ˌblō\ vb -blew; -blown : to deposit eggs or young larvae of a flesh fly or blowfly in

²flyblow n : FLY-STRIKE

fly-blown \-ˌblōn\ adj 1 : infested with fly maggots 2 : covered with fly-specks

fly-strike \-ˌstrīk\ n : infestation with fly maggots — fly-struck \-ˌstrək\ adj

Fm symbol fermium

FM abbr fibromyalgia

FMN \ˌef-(ˌ)em-ˈen\ n : a yellow crystalline phosphoric ester $C_{17}H_{21}N_4O_9P$ of riboflavin that is a coenzyme of several flavoprotein enzymes — called also flavin mononucleotide, riboflavin phosphate

fMRI abbr functional magnetic resonance imaging

FMS abbr fibromyalgia syndrome

FNA abbr fine needle aspiration

foam \ˈfōm\ n : a light frothy mass of fine bubbles formed in or on the surface of a liquid — foam vb

foam cell n : a swollen vacuolated macrophage filled with lipid inclusions that often accumulates along arterial walls and is characteristic of some conditions of disturbed lipid metabolism

foamy virus \'fō-mē-\ *n* : any of a genus (*Spumavirus*) of nonpathogenic retroviruses that are sometimes transmitted to humans from nonhuman primates — called also *spumavirus*

FOBT *abbr* fecal occult blood test; fecal occult blood testing

fo·cal \'fō-kəl\ *adj* : of, relating to, being, or having a focus — **fo·cal·ly** \-kə-lē\ *adv*

focal epilepsy *n* : epilepsy characterized by partial seizures — called also *partial epilepsy*

focal infection *n* : a persistent bacterial infection of some organ or region; *esp* : one causing symptoms elsewhere in the body

focal length *n* : the distance of a focus from the surface of a lens or concave mirror — symbol *f*

focal point *n* : FOCUS 1

focal seizure *n* : PARTIAL SEIZURE

fo·cus \'fō-kəs\ *n, pl* **fo·ci** \'fō-ˌsī, -ˌkī\ *also* **fo·cus·es** **1** : a point at which rays (as of light) converge or from which they diverge or appear to diverge usu. giving rise to an image after reflection by a mirror or refraction by a lens or optical system **2** : a localized area of disease or the chief site of a generalized disease or infection — **focus** *vb*

foe·ti·cide *chiefly Brit var of* FETICIDE

foeto- *or* **foeti-** *chiefly Brit var of* FETO-

foe·tol·o·gy, foe·tus *chiefly Brit var of* FETOLOGY, FETUS

fog \'fäg, 'fòg\ *vb* **fogged; fog·ging** : to blur (a visual field) with lenses that prevent a sharp focus in order to relax accommodation before testing vision

foil \'fòil\ *n* : very thin sheet metal (as of gold) used esp. in filling teeth

fo·la·cin \'fō-lə-sən\ *n* : FOLIC ACID

fo·late \'fō-ˌlāt\ *n* : FOLIC ACID; *also* : a salt or ester of folic acid

fold \'fōld\ *n* : a margin formed by the doubling upon itself of a flat anatomical structure (as a membrane)

Fo·ley catheter \'fō-lē-\ *n* : a catheter with an inflatable balloon tip for retention in the bladder

Foley, Frederic Eugene Basil (1891–1966), American urologist.

fo·lic acid \'fō-lik-\ *n* : a crystalline vitamin $C_{19}H_{19}N_7O_6$ of the B complex that is used esp. in the treatment of nutritional anemias — called also *folacin, folate, pteroylglutamic acid, vitamin B_c, vitamin M*

folie à deux \fō-lē-(ˌ)ä-'dœ, -ˈdər\ *n, pl* **folies à deux** *same or* fō-'lēz-\ : the presence of the same or similar delusional ideas in two persons closely associated with one another

fo·lin·ic acid \fō-ˈli-nik-\ *n* : LEUCOVORIN

fo·li·um \'fō-lē-əm\ *n, pl* **fo·lia** \-lē-ə\ : one of the lamellae of the cerebellar cortex

folk medicine *n* : traditional medicine as practiced esp. by people isolated from modern medical services and usu. involving the use of plant-derived remedies on an empirical basis

fol·li·cle \'fä-li-kəl\ *n* **1** : a small anatomical cavity or deep narrow-mouthed depression; *esp* : a small simple or slightly branched gland : CRYPT **2** : a small lymph node **3** : a vesicle in the mammalian ovary that contains a developing egg surrounded by a covering of cells : OVARIAN FOLLICLE; *esp* : GRAAFIAN FOLLICLE — **fol·lic·u·lar** \fə-ˈli-kyə-lər, fä-\ *adj*

follicle mite *n* : any of several minute mites of the genus *Demodex* that are parasitic in the hair follicles

follicle–stimulating hormone *n* : a hormone from an anterior lobe of the pituitary gland that stimulates the growth of the ovum-containing follicles in the ovary and that activates sperm-forming cells

follicularis — see KERATOSIS FOLLICULARIS

folliculi — see LIQUOR FOLLICULI, THECA FOLLICULI

fol·lic·u·lin \fə-ˈli-kyə-lən, fä-\ *n* : ESTROGEN; *esp* : ESTRONE

fol·lic·u·li·tis \fə-ˌli-kyə-ˈlī-təs\ *n* : inflammation of one or more follicles esp. of the hair

fol·li·tro·pin \ˌfä-lə-ˈtrō-pən\ *n* : FOLLICLE-STIMULATING HORMONE

follow–up \'fä-lō-ˌəp\ *n* : maintenance of contact with or reexamination of a patient at usu. prescribed intervals following diagnosis or treatment; *also* : a patient with whom such contact is maintained — **follow–up** *adj* — **follow up** *vb*

fo·men·ta·tion \ˌfō-mən-ˈtā-shən, -ˌmen-\ *n* **1** : the application of hot moist substances to the body to ease pain **2** : the material applied in fomentation : POULTICE

fo·mite \'fō-ˌmīt\ *n, pl* **fo·mites** \-ˌmīts, 'fä-mə-ˌtēz\ : an inanimate object (as a dish or clothing) that may be contaminated with infectious organisms and serve in their transmission

F_1 generation *n* : the first filial generation produced by a cross and consisting of individuals heterozygous for characters in which the parents differ and are homozygous — compare F_2 GENERATION, P_1 GENERATION

fon·ta·nel *or* **fon·ta·nelle** \ˌfänt-ᵊn-ˈel\ *n* : any of the spaces closed by membranous structures between the uncompleted angles of the parietal bones and the neighboring bones of a fetal or young skull

food \'füd\ *n, often attrib* **1** : material consisting essentially of protein, carbohydrate, and fat used in the body of an organism to sustain growth, repair, and vital processes and to furnish energy; *also* : such food together with supplementary substances (as minerals, vitamins, and condiments) **2** : nutriment in solid form

food poisoning *n* **1** : either of two

acute gastrointestinal disorders caused by bacteria or their toxic products: **a** : a rapidly developing intoxication marked by nausea, vomiting, prostration, and often severe diarrhea and caused by the presence in food of toxic products produced by bacteria (as some staphylococci) **b** : a less rapidly developing infection esp. with salmonellae that has generally similar symptoms and results from multiplication of bacteria ingested with contaminated food **2** : a gastrointestinal disturbance occurring after consumption of food that is contaminated with chemical residues or food (as some fungi) that is inherently unsuitable for human consumption

food·stuff \'füd-ˌstəf\ *n* : a substance with food value; *esp* : a specific nutrient (as a fat or protein)

foot \'fut\ *n, pl* **feet** \'fēt\ **1** : the terminal part of the vertebrate leg upon which an individual stands **2** : a unit equal to ⅓ yard or 12 inches

foot–and–mouth disease *n* : an acute contagious febrile disease esp. of cloven-hoofed animals that is caused by serotypes of a picornavirus (species *Foot-and-mouth disease virus* of the genus *Aphthovirus*) and is marked by ulcerating vesicles in the mouth, about the hoofs, and on the udder and teats — called also *aftosa, aphthous fever, foot-and-mouth, hoof-and-mouth disease;* compare HAND, FOOT AND MOUTH DISEASE

foot·bath \'fut-ˌbath\ *n* : a bath for cleansing, warming, or disinfecting the feet

foot drop *n* : an extended position of the foot caused by paralysis of the flexor muscles of the leg

foot·ed \'fut-əd\ *adj* : having a foot or feet esp. of a specified kind or number — often used in combination ⟨a 4-*footed* animal⟩

foot·plate \'fut-ˌplāt\ *n* : the flat oval base of the stapes

foot–pound \-'paund\ *n, pl* **foot-pounds** : a unit of work equal to the work done by a force of one pound acting through a distance of one foot in the direction of the force

foot–pound–second \ˌfut-ˌpaund-'se-kənd\ *adj* : being or relating to a system of units based upon the foot as the unit of length, the pound as the unit of weight or mass, and the second as the unit of time — abbr. *fps*

foot rot *n* : a necrobacillosis of tissues of the foot esp. of sheep and cattle that is marked by sloughing, ulceration, suppuration, and sometimes loss of the hoof

fo·ra·men \fə-'rā-mən\ *n, pl* **fo·ram·i·na** \-'ra-mə-nə\ *or* **fo·ra·mens** \-'rā-mənz\ : a small opening, perforation, or orifice : FENESTRA 1 — **fo·ram·i·nal** \fə-'ra-mən-ᵊl\ *adj*

foramen ce·cum \-'sē-kəm\ *n* : a shallow depression in the posterior dorsal midline of the tongue that is the remnant of the more cranial part of the embryonic duct from which the thyroid gland developed

foramen lac·er·um \-'la-sər-əm\ *n* : an irregular aperture on the lower surface of the skull bounded by parts of the temporal, sphenoid, and occipital bones that gives passage to the internal carotid artery

foramen mag·num \-'mag-nəm\ *n* : the opening in the skull through which the spinal cord passes to become the medulla oblongata

foramen of Lusch·ka \-'lush-kə\ *n* : either of two openings each of which is situated on one side of the fourth ventricle of the brain and communicates with the subarachnoid space

Luschka, Hubert von (1820–1875), German anatomist.

foramen of Ma·gen·die \-mə-ˌzhän-'dē\ *n* : a passage through the midline of the roof of the fourth ventricle of the brain that gives passage to the cerebrospinal fluid from the ventricles to the subarachnoid space

Ma·gen·die, François \má-zhaⁿ-dē\ (1783–1855), French physiologist.

foramen of Mon·ro \-mən-'rō\ *n* : INTERVENTRICULAR FORAMEN

Monro, Alexander (Secundus) (1733–1817), British anatomist.

foramen of Wins·low \-'winz-ˌlō\ *n* : EPIPLOIC FORAMEN

Wins·low, Jacob (*or* Jacques–Bénigne) (1669–1760), Danish anatomist.

foramen ova·le \-ō-'va-(ˌ)lē, -'vä-, -'vä-\ *n* **1** : an opening in the septum between the two atria of the heart that is normally present only in the fetus **2** : an oval opening in the greater wing of the sphenoid for passage of the mandibular nerve

foramen ro·tun·dum \-rō-'tən-dəm\ *n* : a circular aperture in the anterior and medial part of the greater wing of the sphenoid that gives passage to the maxillary nerve

foramen spin·o·sum \-spi-'nō-səm\ *n* : an aperture in the greater wing of the sphenoid that gives passage to the middle meningeal artery

foramina *pl of* FORAMEN

for·ceps \'fȯr-səps, -ˌseps\ *n, pl* **forceps** : an instrument for grasping, holding firmly, or exerting traction upon objects esp. for delicate operations

For·dyce's disease \'fȯr-ˌdī-səz-\ *also* **For·dyce disease** \'fȯr-ˌdīs-\ *n* : a common anomaly of the oral mucosa in which misplaced sebaceous glands form yellowish white nodules on the lips or the lining of the mouth

Fordyce, John Addison (1858–1925), American dermatologist.

fore- *comb form* **1** : situated at the front : in front ⟨*fore*leg⟩ **2** : front part of (something specified) ⟨*fore*arm⟩

fore·arm \ˈfōr-ˌärm\ *n* : the part of the arm between the elbow and the wrist

fore·brain \-ˌbrān\ *n* : the anterior of the three primary divisions of the developing vertebrate brain or the corresponding part of the adult brain that includes esp. the cerebral hemispheres, the thalamus, and the hypothalamus and that esp. in higher vertebrates is the main control center for sensory and associative information processing, visceral functions, and voluntary motor functions — called also *prosencephalon*; see DIENCEPHALON, TELENCEPHALON

forebrain bundle — see MEDIAL FOREBRAIN BUNDLE

fore·fin·ger \ˈfōr-ˌfiŋ-gər\ *n* : INDEX FINGER

fore·foot \-ˌfůt\ *n* **1** : one of the anterior feet esp. of a quadruped **2** : the front part of the human foot

fore·gut \-ˌgət\ *n* : the anterior part of the digestive tract of a vertebrate embryo that develops into the pharynx, esophagus, stomach, and extreme anterior part of the intestine

fore·head \ˈfōr-əd, ˈfär-; ˈfōr-ˌhed\ *n* : the part of the face above the eyes — called also *brow*

for·eign \ˈfōr-ən, ˈfär-\ *adj* **1** : occurring in an abnormal situation in the living body and often introduced from outside **2** : not recognized by the immune system as part of the self

fore·leg \ˈfōr-ˌleg\ *n* : a front leg

fore·limb \-ˌlim\ *n* : a limb (as an arm, wing, fin, or leg) situated anteriorly

fo·ren·sic \fə-ˈren-sik, -zik\ *adj* : relating to or dealing with the application of scientific knowledge to legal problems ⟨a ~ pathologist⟩ ⟨~ experts⟩

forensic medicine *n* : a science that deals with the relation and application of medical facts to legal problems — called also *legal medicine*

forensic odontology *n* : a branch of forensic medicine dealing with teeth and marks left by teeth (as in identifying remains of a dead person)

forensic psychiatry *n* : the application of psychiatry in courts of law (as for the determination of criminal responsibility or liability to commitment for insanity) — **forensic psychiatrist** *n*

fore·play \ˈfōr-ˌplā\ *n* : erotic stimulation preceding sexual intercourse

fore·skin \-ˌskin\ *n* : a retractable fold of skin that covers the glans of the penis — called also *prepuce*

-form \ˌfōrm\ *adj comb form* : in the form or shape of : resembling ⟨choreiform⟩ ⟨epileptiform⟩

form·al·de·hyde \fōr-ˈmal-də-ˌhīd, fər-\ *n* : a colorless pungent irritating gas CH_2O used as a disinfectant and preservative

for·ma·lin \ˈfōr-mə-lən, -ˌlēn\ *n* : a clear aqueous solution of formaldehyde containing a small amount of methanol

formed element *n* : one of the red blood cells, white blood cells, or blood platelets as contrasted with the fluid portion of the blood

forme fruste \ˌfōrm-ˈfrēst, -ˈfrüst\ *n, pl* **formes frustes** *same or* -ˈfrüsts\ : an atypical and usu. incomplete manifestation of a disease

for·mic acid \ˈfōr-mik-\ *n* : a colorless pungent vesicant liquid acid CH_2O_2 found esp. in ants and in many plants

for·mi·ca·tion \ˌfōr-mə-ˈkā-shən\ *n* : an abnormal sensation resembling that made by insects creeping in or on the skin

for·mu·la \ˈfōr-myə-lə\ *n, pl* **-las** *or* **-lae** \-ˌlē, -ˌlī\ **1 a** : a recipe or prescription giving method and proportions of ingredients for the preparation of some material (as a medicine) **b** : a milk mixture or substitute (as one containing soybean protein) for feeding an infant; *also* : a batch of this made up at one time to meet an infant's future requirements (as during a 24-hour period) **2** : a symbolic expression showing the composition or constitution of a chemical substance and consisting of symbols for the elements present and subscripts to indicate the relative or total number of atoms present in a molecule ⟨the ~ for water is H_2O⟩ — see EMPIRICAL FORMULA, MOLECULAR FORMULA, STRUCTURAL FORMULA

for·mu·lary \ˈfōr-myə-ˌler-ē\ *n, pl* **-lar·ies** : a book containing a list of medicinal subtances and formulas

for·ni·ca·tion \ˌfōr-nə-ˈkā-shən\ *n* : consensual sexual intercourse between two persons not married to each other — **for·ni·cate** \ˈfōr-nə-ˌkāt\ *vb*

fornicis — see CRURA FORNICIS

for·nix \ˈfōr-niks\ *n, pl* **for·ni·ces** \-nə-ˌsēz\ : an anatomical arch or fold: as **a** : the vault of the cranium **b** : the part of the conjunctiva overlying the cornea **c** : a body of nerve fibers lying beneath the corpus callosum and serving to integrate the hippocampus with other parts of the brain **d** : the vaulted upper part of the vagina surrounding the uterine cervix **e** : the fundus of the stomach **f** : the vault of the pharynx

Fos·a·max \ˈfä-sə-ˌmaks\ *trademark* — used for a preparation of alendronate

fos·car·net \fäs-ˈkär-nət\ *n* : a hydrated sodium salt $Na_3CO_5P \cdot 6H_2O$ administered intravenously in individuals infected with HIV to treat retinitis caused by a cytomegalovirus — called also *foscarnet sodium*

fos·sa \ˈfä-sə\ *n, pl* **fos·sae** \-ˌsē, -ˌsī\ : an anatomical pit, groove, or depression ⟨the temporal ~ of the skull⟩

fossa na·vic·u·lar·is \-nə-ˌvi-kyə-ˈla-rəs\ *n* : a depression between the posterior margin of the vaginal opening and the fourchette

fossa oval·is \-ō-'va-ləs, -'vā-, -'vä-\ *n* **1** : a depression in the septum between the right and left atria that marks the position of the foramen ovale in the fetus **2** : SAPHENOUS OPENING

Fos·sar·ia \fä-'sar-ē-ə, fȯ-\ *n* : a genus of small freshwater snails (family Lymnaeidae) including intermediate hosts of liver flukes — compare GALBA, LYMNAEA

¹**foun·der** \'faun-dər\ *vb* **foun·dered**; **foun·der·ing 1** : to become disabled; *esp* : to go lame **2** : to disable (an animal) esp. by inducing laminitis through excessive feeding

²**founder** *n* : LAMINITIS

four·chette *or* **four·chet** \fur-'shet\ *n* : a small fold of membrane connecting the labia minora in the posterior part of the vulva

fourth cranial nerve *n* : TROCHLEAR NERVE

fourth ventricle *n* : a somewhat rhomboidal ventricle of the posterior part of the brain that connects at the front with the third ventricle through the aqueduct of Sylvius and at the back with the central canal of the spinal cord

fo·vea \'fō-vē-ə\ *n, pl* **fo·ve·ae** \-vē-ē, -ˌī\ **1** : a small fossa **2** : a small area of the retina without rods that affords acute vision — **fo·ve·al** \-əl\ *adj*

fovea cen·tra·lis \-sen-'tra-ləs, -'trä-, -'trā-\ *n* : FOVEA 2

fo·ve·o·la \fō-'vē-ə-lə\ *n, pl* **-lae** \-ˌlē, -ˌlī\ *or* **-las** : a small pit; *specif* : one of the pits in the embryonic gastric mucosa from which the gastric glands develop — **fo·ve·o·lar** \-lər\ *adj*

fowl cholera *n* : an acute contagious septicemic disease of birds that is marked by fever, weakness, diarrhea, and petechial hemorrhages in the mucous membranes and is caused by a bacterium of the genus *Pasteurella* (*P. multocida*)

fowl mite *n* : CHICKEN MITE — see NORTHERN FOWL MITE

fowl pest *n* : NEWCASTLE DISEASE

fowl plague *n* : BIRD FLU

fowl pox *n* : either of two forms of a disease esp. of chickens and turkeys that is caused by a poxvirus (species *Fowlpox virus* of the genus *Avipoxvirus*): **a** : a cutaneous form marked by pustules, warty growths, and scabs esp. on skin lacking feathers **b** : a more serious form occurring as cheesy lesions of the mucous membranes of the mouth, throat, and eyes

fowl tick *n* : any of several ticks of the genus *Argas* (as *A. persicus*) that attack fowl esp. in warm regions causing anemia and transmitting various diseases (as spirochetosis)

fowl typhoid *n* : an infectious disease of poultry characterized by diarrhea, anemia, and prostration and caused by a bacterium of the genus *Salmonella* (*S. gallinarum*)

fox·glove \'fäks-ˌgləv\ *n* : any plant of the genus *Digitalis*; *esp* : a common European biennial or perennial (*D. purpurea*) that is a source of digitalis

FP *abbr* **1** family physician; family practitioner **2** family practice

fps *abbr* foot-pound-second

Fr *symbol* francium

FR *abbr* flocculation reaction

frac·tion \'frak-shən\ *n* : one of several portions (as of a distillate) separable by fractionation

frac·tion·al \-shə-nəl\ *adj* : of, relating to, or involving a process for fractionating components of a mixture

frac·tion·ate \-shə-ˌnāt\ *vb* **-at·ed; -at·ing** : to separate (as a mixture) into different portions (as by precipitation) — **frac·tion·a·tion** \-ˈnā-shən\ *n*

frac·ture \'frak-chər, -shər\ *n* **1** : the act or process of breaking or the state of being broken; *specif* : the breaking of hard tissue (as bone) **2** : the rupture (as by tearing) of soft tissue ⟨kidney ∼⟩ — **fracture** *vb*

fragile X syndrome \-'eks-\ *n* : an inherited disorder that is associated with an abnormal X chromosome, that is characterized esp. by moderate to severe mental retardation, by large ears, chin, and forehead, and by enlarged testes in males, and that often has limited or no effect in heterozygous females — called also *fragile X*

fra·gil·i·tas os·si·um \frə-'ji-lə-təs-'ä-sē-əm\ *n* : OSTEOGENESIS IMPERFECTA

fram·be·sia \fram-'bē-zhə, -zhē-ə\ *n* : YAWS

frame \'frām\ *n* **1** : the physical makeup of an animal and esp. a human body : PHYSIQUE **2 a** : a part of a pair of glasses that holds one of the lenses **b** *pl* : that part of a pair of glasses other than the lenses

frame·shift \-ˌshift\ *adj* : relating to, being, or causing a mutation in which a number of nucleotides not divisible by three is inserted or deleted so that some triplet codons are read incorrectly during genetic translation — **frameshift** *n*

fran·ci·um \'fran-sē-əm\ *n* : a radioactive element discovered as a disintegration product of actinium and obtained artificially by the bombardment of thorium with protons — symbol *Fr*; see ELEMENT table

frank \'fraŋk\ *adj* : clinically evident ⟨∼ pus⟩ ⟨∼ gout⟩

Frank·fort horizontal plane \'fraŋk-fərt-\ *n* : a plane used in craniometry that is determined by the highest point on the upper margin of the opening of each external auditory canal and the low point on the lower margin of the left orbit — called also *Frankfort horizontal, Frankfort plane*

Frank–Star·ling law \'fraŋk-'stär-liŋ-\ *n* : STARLING'S LAW OF THE HEART

Frank, Otto (1865–1944), German physiologist.

Starling, Ernest Henry (1866–1927), British physiologist.

Frank–Starling law of the heart *n* : STARLING'S LAW OF THE HEART

fra·ter·nal \frə-'tərn-ᵊl\ *adj* : derived from two ova : DIZYGOTIC ⟨∼ twins⟩

FRCP *abbr* Fellow of the Royal College of Physicians

FRCS *abbr* Fellow of the Royal College of Surgeons

freck·le \'fre-kəl\ *n* : any of the small brownish spots in the skin that are due to augmented melanin production and that increase in number and intensity on exposure to sunlight — called also *ephelis;* compare LENTIGO — **freckle** *vb* — **freck·led** \-kəld\ *adj*

free \'frē\ *adj* **fre·er; fre·est 1 a** (1) : not united with, attached to, combined with, or mixed with something else ⟨a ∼ surface of a bodily part⟩ (2) : having the bare axon exposed in tissue ⟨a ∼ nerve ending⟩ **b** : not chemically combined ⟨∼ oxygen⟩ **2** : having all living connections severed before removal to another site ⟨a ∼ graft⟩

free association *n* **1 a** : the expression (as by speaking or writing) of the content of consciousness without censorship as an aid in gaining access to unconscious processes esp. in psychoanalysis **b** : the reporting of the first thought that comes to mind in response to a given stimulus (as a word) **2** : an idea or image elicited by free association **3** : a method using free association — **free–as·so·ci·ate** \'frē-ə-'sō-shē-ˌāt, -sē-\ *vb*

¹free·base \'frē-ˌbās\ *vb* **-based; -bas·ing** : to prepare or use (cocaine) as freebase — **free·bas·er** \-ˌbā-sər\ *n*

²freebase *n* : a purified solid form of cocaine (as crack) that is obtained by treating the powdered hydrochloride of cocaine with an alkaloid base (as sodium bicarbonate) and that can be smoked or heated to produce vapors for inhalation; *specif* : a form derived from treatment of the hydrochloride of cocaine with ammonia or similar alkaloid solution followed by extraction with a solvent (as ether)

free fall *n* : the condition of unrestrained motion in a gravitational field; *also* : such motion

free–float·ing \'frē-'flō-tiŋ\ *adj* : felt as an emotion without apparent cause ⟨∼ anxiety⟩

free–liv·ing \-'li-viŋ\ *adj* **1** : not fixed to the substrate but capable of motility ⟨a ∼ protozoan⟩ **2** : being metabolically independent : neither parasitic nor symbiotic

free–mar·tin \'frē-ˌmärt-ᵊn\ *n* : a sexually imperfect usu. sterile female calf born as a twin with a male

free radical *n* : an esp. reactive atom or group of atoms that has one or more unpaired electrons; *esp* : one that is produced in the body by natural biological processes or introduced from outside (as in tobacco smoke, toxins, or pollutants) and that can damage cells, proteins, and DNA by altering their chemical structure

free–stand·ing \'frē-'stan-diŋ\ *adj* : being independent; *esp* : not part of or affiliated with another organization ⟨a ∼ emergency clinic⟩

free–swimming *adj* : able to swim about : not attached ⟨∼ larvae⟩

freeze \'frēz\ *vb* **froze** \'frōz\; **fro·zen** \'frōz-ᵊn\; **freez·ing 1** : to harden or cause to harden into a solid (as ice) by loss of heat **2** : to chill or become chilled with cold **3** : to anesthetize (a part) by cold

freeze–dry \'frēz-'drī\ *vb* **freeze-dried; freeze–dry·ing** : to dry and preserve (as food, vaccines, or tissue) in a frozen state under high vacuum — **freeze–dried** *adj*

freeze–etch·ing \-'e-chiŋ\ *n* : FREEZE FRACTURE — **freeze–etch** \-'ech\ *adj* — **freeze–etched** \-ˌecht\ *adj*

freeze fracture *also* **freeze–fracturing** *n* : preparation of a specimen (as of tissue) for electron microscopic examination by freezing, fracturing along natural structural lines, and preparing a replica — **freeze–fracture** *vb*

freezing point *n* : the temperature at which a liquid solidifies

Frei test \'frī-\ *n* : a serological test for the identification of lymphogranuloma venereum — called also *Frei skin test*

Frei, Wilhelm Siegmund (1885–1943), German dermatologist.

frem·i·tus \'fre-mə-təs\ *n* : a sensation felt by a hand placed on a part of the body (as the chest) that vibrates during speech

French \'french\, *n, pl* **French** : a unit of measure equal to one-third millimeter used in measuring the outside diameter of a tubular instrument (as a catheter) inserted into a body cavity

fren·ec·to·my \frə-'nek-tə-mē\ *n, pl* **-mies** : excision of a frenulum

fren·u·lum \'fren-yə-ləm\ *n, pl* **-la** \-lə\ : a connecting fold of membrane serving to support or restrain a part (as the tongue)

fre·num \'frē-nəm\ *n, pl* **frenums** or **fre·na** \-nə\ : FRENULUM

freq *abbr* frequency

fre·quen·cy \'frē-kwən-sē\ *n, pl* **-cies 1** : the number of individuals in a single class when objects are classified according to variations in a set of one or more specified attributes **2** : the number of repetitions of a periodic process in a unit of time

Freud·ian \'froi-dē-ən\ *adj* : of, relating to, or according with the psychoanalytic theories or practices of Freud — **Freudian** *n* — **Freud·ian·ism** \-ə-ˌni-zəm\ *n*

Freud \'froid\, **Sigmund** (1856–1939), Austrian neurologist and psychiatrist.

Freudian slip *n* : a slip of the tongue that is motivated by and reveals some unconscious aspect of the mind

Freund's adjuvant \'froindz-\ *n* : any of several oil and water emulsions that contain antigens and are used to stimulate antibody production in experimental animals

    Freund \'froind\, **Jules Thomas** (1890–1960), American immunologist.

fri·a·ble \'frī-ə-bəl\ *adj* : easily crumbled or pulverized ⟨~ carcinomatous tissue⟩; *also* : marked by erosion and bleeding ⟨a ~ cervix⟩ — **fri·a·bil·i·ty** \ˌfrī-ə-'bi-lə-tē\ *n*

friar's balsam *n* : an alcoholic solution containing essentially benzoin, storax, balsam of Tolu, and aloes applied topically to the skin (as to relieve irritation) and after addition to hot water as an inhalant with expectorant activity — called also *compound benzoin tincture*

Fried·man test \'frēd-mən-\ *also* **Friedman's test** *n* : a modification of the Aschheim-Zondek test for pregnancy using rabbits as test animals

    Friedman, Maurice Harold (1903–1991), American physiologist.

Fried·reich's ataxia \'frēd-rīks-, 'frēt-rīks-\ *n* : a recessive hereditary degenerative disease affecting the spinal column, cerebellum, and medulla, marked by muscular incoordination and twitching, and usu. becoming manifest in the adult

    Friedreich \'frēt-rīk\, **Nikolaus** (1825–1882), German neurologist.

Friend virus \'frend\ *n* : a strain of murine leukemia virus that causes erythroleukemia in mice — called also *Friend leukemia virus*

    Friend, Charlotte (1921–1987), American microbiologist.

frig·id \'fri-jəd\ *adj* **1** : abnormally averse to sexual intercourse — used esp. of women **2** *of a female* : unable to achieve orgasm during sexual intercourse — **fri·gid·i·ty** \fri-'ji-də-tē\ *n*

fringed tapeworm *n* : a tapeworm of the genus *Thysanosoma* (*T. actinioides*) found in the intestine and bile ducts of ruminants esp. in the western U.S.

frog \'frog, 'fräg\ *n* **1** : the triangular elastic horny pad in the middle of the sole of the foot of a horse **2** : a condition in the throat that produces hoarseness ⟨had a ~ in his throat⟩

Fröh·lich's syndrome *or* **Froeh·lich's syndrome** \'frā-liks-, 'frœ-liks-\ *n* : ADIPOSOGENITAL DYSTROPHY

    Fröhlich \'frœ-lik\, **Alfred** (1871–1953), Austrian pharmacologist and neurologist.

frondosum — see CHORION FRONDOSUM

fron·tal \'frənt-əl\ *adj* **1** : of, relating to, or adjacent to the forehead or the frontal bone **2** : of, relating to, or situated at the front or anteriorly **3** : parallel to the main axis of the body and at right angles to the sagittal plane ⟨a ~ plane⟩ — **fron·tal·ly** *adv*

frontal bone *n* : a bone that forms the forehead and roofs over most of the orbits and nasal cavity and that at birth consists of two halves separated by a suture

frontal eminence *n* : the prominence of the human frontal bone above each superciliary ridge

frontal gyrus *n* : any of the convolutions of the outer surface of the frontal lobe of the brain — called also *frontal convolution*

fron·ta·lis \frən-'tā-ləs\ *n* : the muscle of the forehead that forms part of the occipitofrontalis — called also *frontalis muscle*

frontal lobe *n* : the anterior division of each cerebral hemisphere having its lower part in the anterior fossa of the skull and bordered behind by the central sulcus

frontal lobotomy *n* : PREFRONTAL LOBOTOMY

frontal nerve *n* : a branch of the ophthalmic nerve supplying the forehead, scalp, and adjoining parts

frontal process *n* **1** : a long plate that is part of the maxillary bone and contributes to the formation of the lateral part of the nose and of the nasal cavity — called also *nasal process* **2** : a process of the zygomatic bone articulating superiorly with the frontal bone, forming part of the orbit anteriorly, and articulating with the sphenoid bone posteriorly

frontal sinus *n* : either of two air spaces lined with mucous membrane each of which lies within the frontal bone above one of the orbits

fronto- *comb form* : frontal bone and ⟨*fronto*parietal⟩

fron·to·oc·cip·i·tal \ˌfrən-tō-äk-'sip-ət-əl, -ˌfrän-\ *adj* : of or relating to the forehead and occiput

fron·to·pa·ri·etal \-pə-'rī-ət-əl\ *adj* : of, relating to, or involving both frontal and parietal bones of the skull

frontoparietal suture *n* : CORONAL SUTURE

fron·to·tem·po·ral \-'tem-pə-rəl\ *adj* : of or relating to the frontal and the temporal bones

frost·bite \'frost-ˌbīt\ *n* : the superficial or deep freezing of the tissues of some part of the body (as the feet or hands); *also* : the damage to tissues caused by freezing — **frostbite** *vb*

frost·nip \'frost-ˌnip\ *n* : the reversible freezing of superficial skin layers that is usu. marked by numbness and whiteness of the skin

frot·tage \fro-'täzh\ *n* : FROTTEURISM

frot·teur \fro-'tər\ *n* : one who practices frotteurism

frot·teur·ism \-ˌi-zəm\ *n* : the paraphiliac practice of achieving sexual stimulation or orgasm by touching and rubbing against a person without the person's consent and usu. in a public place — called also *frottage*

froze *past of* FREEZE

frozen *past part of* FREEZE

frozen shoulder *n* : a shoulder affected by severe pain, stiffening, and restricted motion — called also *adhesive capsulitis*

fruc·to·kin·ase \ˌfrək-tō-ˈkī-ˌnās, -ˈki-, -ˌnāz, ˌfrùk-\ *n* : a kinase that catalyzes the transfer of phosphate groups to fructose

fruc·tose \ˈfrək-ˌtōs, ˈfrúk-, ˈfrúk-, -ˌtōz\ *n* **1** : a sugar $C_6H_{12}O_6$ sweeter and more soluble than glucose **2** : the very sweet soluble levorotatory D-form of fructose that occurs esp. in fruit juices and honey — called also *levulose*

fruc·tos·uria \ˌfrək-tə-ˈsùr-ē-ə\ *n* : the presence of fructose in the urine

fruit·ar·i·an \frü-ˈter-ē-ən\ *n* : one who lives chiefly on fruit

fruiting body *n* : a plant organ specialized for producing spores; *esp* : SPOROPHORE

fruit sugar *n* : FRUCTOSE 2

fru·se·mide \ˈfrü-sə-ˌmīd\ *n, chiefly Brit* : FUROSEMIDE

frus·trat·ed *adj* : filled with a sense of frustration : feeling deep insecurity, discouragement, or dissatisfaction

frus·tra·tion \(ˌ)frəs-ˈtrā-shən\ *n* **1** : a deep chronic sense or state of insecurity and dissatisfaction arising from unresolved problems or unfulfilled needs **2** : something that frustrates — **frus·trate** \ˈfrəs-ˌtrāt\ *vb*

FSH *abbr* follicle-stimulating hormone

ft *abbr* feet; foot

F_2 generation *n* : the generation produced by interbreeding individuals of an F_1 generation and consisting of individuals that exhibit the result of recombination and segregation of genes controlling traits for which stocks of the P_1 generation differ

fuch·sin *or* **fuch·sine** \ˈfyük-sən, -ˌsēn\ *n* : a dye that yields a brilliant bluish red and is used in carbolfuchsin paint, in Schiff's reagent, and as a biological stain

fu·cose \ˈfyü-ˌkōs, -ˌkōz\ *n* : an aldose sugar that occurs in bound form in the dextrorotatory D-form in various glycosides and in the levorotatory L-form in some brown algae and in mammalian polysaccharides typical of some blood groups

fu·co·si·dase \ˌfyü-ˈkō-sə-ˌdās, -ˌdāz\ *n* : an enzyme existing in stereoisomeric alpha and beta forms that catalyzes the metabolism of fucose

fu·co·si·do·sis \-ˌkō-sə-ˈdō-səs\ *n, pl* **-do·ses** \-ˌsēz\ : a disorder of metabolism inherited as a recessive trait and characterized by progressive neurological degeneration, deficiency of the alpha stereoisomer of fucosidase, and

accumulation of fucose-containing carbohydrates

fugax — see AMAUROSIS FUGAX, PROCTALGIA FUGAX

-fuge \ˌfyüj\ *n comb form* : one that drives away ⟨febri*fuge*⟩ ⟨vermi*fuge*⟩

fu·gi·tive \ˈfyü-jə-tiv\ *adj* : tending to be inconstant or transient

fu·gu \ˈfyü-(ˌ)gü, ˈfü-\ *n* : any of various very poisonous puffer fish that contain tetrodotoxin and that are used as food in Japan after the toxin-containing organs are removed

fugue \ˈfyüg\ *n* : a disturbed state of consciousness in which the one affected seems to perform acts in full awareness but upon recovery cannot recollect them

ful·gu·ra·tion \ˌfùl-gə-ˈrā-shən, fəl-, -gyə-, -jə-\ *n* : ELECTRODESICCATION — **ful·gu·rate** \ˈfùl-gə-ˌrāt, ˈfəl-, -gyə-, -jə-\ *vb*

full–blown *adj* : fully developed : being in its most extreme or serious form : possessing or exhibiting the characteristic symptoms ⟨a ∼ cold⟩

full–mouthed \ˈfùl-ˈmaúthd, -ˈmaútht\ *adj* : having a full complement of teeth — used esp. of sheep and cattle

ful·mi·nant \ˈfùl-mə-nənt, ˈfəl-\ *adj* : coming on suddenly with great severity ⟨∼ hepatitis⟩

ful·mi·nat·ing \-ˌnā-tiŋ\ *adj* : FULMINANT — **ful·mi·na·tion** \ˌfùl-mə-ˈnā-shən, ˌfəl-\ *n*

fu·ma·rate \ˈfyü-mə-ˌrāt\ *n* : a salt or ester of fumaric acid

fu·mar·ic acid \fyü-ˈmar-ik-\ *n* : a crystalline acid $C_4H_4O_4$ formed from succinic acid as an intermediate in the Krebs cycle

fu·mi·gant \ˈfyü-mi-gənt\ *n* : a substance used in fumigating

fu·mi·gate \ˈfyü-mə-ˌgāt\ *vb* **-gat·ed; -gat·ing** : to apply smoke, vapor, or gas to esp. for the purpose of disinfecting or of destroying pests — **fu·mi·ga·tion** \ˌfyü-mə-ˈgā-shən\ *n* — **fu·mi·ga·tor** \ˈfyü-mə-ˌgā-tər\ *n*

func·tion \ˈfəŋk-shən\ *n* : any of a group of related actions contributing to a larger action; *esp* : the normal and specific contribution of a bodily part to the economy of a living organism — **function** *vb* — **func·tion·less** \-ləs\ *adj*

func·tion·al \ˈfəŋk-shə-nəl\ *adj* **1 a** : of, connected with, or being a function — compare STRUCTURAL 1 **b** : affecting physiological or psychological functions but not organic structure ⟨∼ heart disease⟩ ⟨a ∼ psychosis⟩ — compare ORGANIC 1b **2** : performing or able to perform a regular function — **func·tion·al·ly** *adv*

functional food *n* : NUTRACEUTICAL

functional magnetic resonance imaging *n* : magnetic resonance imaging used to detect physical changes (as of blood flow) in the brain resulting from increased neuronal activity (as during performance of a specific cognitive task) — abbr. *fMRI;* called also *functional MRI*

fun·dal \'fənd-ᵊl\ *adj* : FUNDIC

fun·da·ment \'fən-də-mənt\ *n* **1** : BUTTOCKS **2** : ANUS

fun·dic \'fən-dik\ *adj* : of or relating to a fundus

fundic gland *n* : one of the tubular glands of the fundus of the stomach secreting pepsin and mucus — compare CHIEF CELL 1

fun·do·pli·ca·tion \ˌfən-dō-pli-'kā-shən\ *n* : a surgical procedure in which the upper portion of the stomach is wrapped around the lower end of the esophagus and sutured in place as a treatment for the reflux of stomach contents into the esophagus — see NISSEN FUNDOPLICATION

fun·dus \'fən-dəs\ *n, pl* **fun·di** \-ˌdī, -ˌdē\ : the bottom or part opposite the aperture of the internal surface of a hollow organ: as **a** : the greater curvature of the stomach **b** : the lower back part of the bladder **c** : the large upper end of the uterus **d** : the part of the eye opposite the pupil

fun·du·scop·ic *also* **fun·do·scop·ic** \ˌfən-də-'skä-pik\ *adj* : of, done by, or obtained by ophthalmoscopic examination of the fundus of the eye — **fun·dus·co·py** \ˌfən-'dəs-kə-pē\ *also* **fun·dos·co·py** \-'däs-\ *n*

fun·gae·mia Brit var of FUNGEMIA

fun·gal \'fən-gəl\ *adj* **1** : of, relating to, or having the characteristics of fungi **2** : caused by a fungus ⟨∼ infections⟩

fun·gate \'fən-ˌgāt\ *vb* **-gat·ed; -gat·ing** : to assume a fungal form or grow rapidly like a fungus — **fun·ga·tion** \ˌfən-'gā-shən\ *n*

fun·ge·mia \fən-'gē-mē-ə\ *n* : the presence of fungi in the blood

fungi *pl of* FUNGUS

fungi- *comb form* : fungus ⟨*fungi*cide⟩

fun·gi·cid·al \ˌfən-jə-'sīd-ᵊl, ˌfən-gə-\ *adj* : destroying fungi; *broadly* : inhibiting the growth of fungi — **fun·gi·cid·al·ly** *adv*

fun·gi·cide \'fən-jə-ˌsīd, 'fən-gə-\ *n* : an agent that destroys fungi or inhibits their growth

fun·gi·form \'fən-jə-ˌfȯrm, 'fən-gə-\ *adj* : shaped like a mushroom

fungiform papilla *n* : any of numerous papillae on the upper surface of the tongue that are flat-topped and are noticeably red from the richly vascular stroma and usu. contain taste buds

fun·gi·stat \'fən-jə-ˌstat, 'fən-gə-\ *n* : a fungistatic agent

fun·gi·stat·ic \ˌfən-jə-'sta-tik, ˌfən-gə-\ *adj* : capable of inhibiting the growth and reproduction of fungi without destroying them ⟨a ∼ agent⟩ — **fun·gi·stat·i·cal·ly** \-ti-k(ə-)lē\ *adv*

Fun·gi·zone \'fən-jə-ˌzōn\ *trademark* — used for a preparation of amphotericin B

fun·goid \'fən-ˌgȯid\ *adj* : resembling, characteristic of, caused by, or being a fungus ⟨a ∼ ulcer⟩ ⟨a ∼ growth⟩

fungoides — see MYCOSIS FUNGOIDES

fun·gous \'fən-gəs\ *adj* : FUNGAL

fun·gus \'fən-gəs\ *n, pl* **fun·gi** \'fən-ˌjī, 'fən-ˌgī\ *also* **fun·gus·es** \'fən-gə-səz\ *often attrib* **1** : any of a kingdom (Fungi) of saprophytic and parasitic spore-producing organisms formerly classified as plants that lack chlorophyll and include molds, rusts, mildews, smuts, mushrooms, and yeasts **2** : infection with a fungus

fu·nic·u·li·tis \fyü-ˌni-kyə-'lī-təs, fə-\ *n* : inflammation of the spermatic cord

fu·nic·u·lus \fyü-'ni-kyə-ləs, fə-\ *n, pl* **-li** \-ˌlī, -ˌlē\ : any of various bodily structures more or less like a cord in form: as **a** : one of the longitudinal subdivisions of white matter in each lateral half of the spinal cord — see ANTERIOR FUNICULUS, LATERAL FUNICULUS, POSTERIOR FUNICULUS; compare COLUMN a **b** : SPERMATIC CORD

funnel chest *n* : a depression of the anterior wall of the chest produced by a sinking in of the sternum — called also *funnel breast, pectus excavatum*

funny bone *n* : the place at the back of the elbow where the ulnar nerve rests against a prominence of the humerus — called also *crazy bone*

FUO *abbr* fever of undetermined origin

fur \'fər\ *n* : a coat of epithelial debris on the tongue

fu·ra·zol·i·done \ˌfyùr-ə-'zä-lə-ˌdōn\ *n* : an antimicrobial drug $C_8H_7N_3O_5$ used against bacteria and some protozoans esp. in infections of the gastrointestinal tract

furious rabies *n* : rabies characterized by spasm of the muscles of throat and diaphragm, choking, salivation, extreme excitement, and evidence of fear often manifested by indiscriminate snapping at objects — compare PARALYTIC RABIES

fu·ro·se·mide \fyü-'rō-sə-ˌmīd\ *n* : a powerful diuretic $C_{12}H_{11}ClN_2O_5S$ used esp. to treat edema — called also *frusemide, furosemide;* see LASIX

furred \'fərd\ *adj* : having a coating consisting chiefly of mucus and dead epithelial cells ⟨a ∼ tongue⟩

fur·row \'fər-(ˌ)ō\ *n* **1** : a marked narrow depression or groove **2** : a deep wrinkle

fur·se·mide \'fər-sə-ˌmīd\ *n* : FUROSEMIDE

fu·run·cle \'fyùr-ˌəŋ-kəl\ *n* : BOIL — **fu·run·cu·lar** \fyù-'rəŋ-kyə-lər\ *adj* — **fu·run·cu·lous** \-ləs\ *adj*

fu·run·cu·lo·sis \ˌfyü-ˌrəŋ-kyə-'lō-səs, *n, pl* **-lo·ses** \-ˌsēz\ **1** : the condition of having or tending to develop multiple furuncles **2** : a highly infectious disease of various salmon and trout (genera *Salmo* and *Oncorhynchus*) and their relatives that is caused by a bacterium (*Aeromonas salmonicida* of the family Vibrionaceae)

fuse \'fyüz\ *vb* **fused; fus·ing** : to undergo or cause to undergo fusion

fusi- *comb form* : spindle ⟨*fusi*form⟩

fu·si·form \'fyü-zə-ˌfȯrm\ *adj* : tapering toward each end ⟨a ~ aneurysm⟩

fu·sion \'fyü-zhən\ *n, often attrib* : a union by or as if by melting together: as **a** : a merging of diverse elements into a unified whole; *specif* : the blending of retinal images in binocular vision **b** (1) : a blend of sensations, perceptions, ideas, or attitudes such that the component elements can seldom be identified by introspective analysis (2) : the perception of light from a source that is intermittent

above a critical frequency as if the source were continuous — called also *flicker fusion;* compare FLICKER **c** : the surgical immobilization of a joint — see SPINAL FUSION

fu·so·bac·te·ri·um \ˌfyü-zō-bak-'tir-ē-əm\ *n* 1 *cap* : a genus of gram-negative anaerobic strictly parasitic rod-shaped bacteria that is placed in either of two families (Bacteroidaceae or Fusobacteriaceae) and includes some pathogens occurring esp. in purulent or gangrenous infections **2** *pl* **-ria** \-ē-ə\ : any bacterium of the genus *Fusobacterium*

fu·so·spi·ro·chet·al \-ˌspī-rə-'kēt-ᵊl\ *adj* : of, relating to, or caused by fusobacteria and spirochetes

g \'jē\ *n, pl* **g's** *or* **gs** \'jēz\ : a unit of force equal to the force exerted by gravity on a body at rest and used to indicate the force to which a body is subjected when accelerated

g *abbr* **1** gram **2** gravity

G *abbr* guanine

Ga *symbol* gallium

GABA *abbr* gamma-aminobutyric acid

gab·a·pen·tin \ˌga-bə-ˌpen-tin\ *n* : an anticonvulsant drug $C_9H_{17}NO_2$ that is administered orally in the treatment of partial seizures — see NEURONTIN

G–ac·tin \'jē-ˌak-tən\ *n* : a globular monomeric form of actin produced in solutions of low ionic concentration — compare F-ACTIN

GAD *abbr* generalized anxiety disorder

gad·fly \'gad-ˌflī\ *n, pl* **-flies** : any of various flies (as a horsefly or botfly) that bite or annoy livestock

gad·o·lin·i·um \ˌgad-ᵊl-'i-nē-əm\ *n* : a magnetic metallic element — symbol *Gd;* see ELEMENT table

gag reflex *n* : reflex contraction of the muscles of the throat caused esp. by stimulation (as by touch) of the pharynx

gal *abbr* gallon

galact- *or* **galacto-** *comb form* **1** : milk ⟨*galacto*rrhea⟩ **2** : galactose ⟨*galacto*kinase⟩

ga·lac·to·cele \gə-'lak-tə-ˌsēl\ *n* : a cystic tumor esp. of a mammary gland containing milk or a milky fluid

ga·lac·to·ki·nase \gə-ˌlak-tō-'kī-nās, -'ki-, -ˌnāz\ *n* : a kinase that catalyzes the transfer of phosphate groups to galactose

ga·lac·tor·rhea \gə-ˌlak-tə-'rē-ə\ *n* : a spontaneous flow of milk from the nipple

ga·lac·tor·rhoea *chiefly Brit var of* GALACTORRHEA

ga·lac·tos·ae·mia *chiefly Brit var of* GALACTOSEMIA

ga·lac·tos·amine \gə-ˌlak-'tō-sə-ˌmēn, -zə-\ *n* : an amino derivative $C_6H_{13}O_5N$ of galactose that occurs in cartilage

ga·lac·tose \gə-'lak-ˌtōs, -ˌtōz\ *n* : a sugar $C_6H_{12}O_6$ that is less soluble and less sweet than glucose and is known in dextrorotatory, levorotatory, and racemic forms

ga·lac·tos·emia \gə-ˌlak-tə-'sē-mē-ə\ *n* : a metabolic disorder inherited as an autosomal recessive trait in which galactose accumulates in the blood due to deficiency of an enzyme catalyzing its conversion to glucose — **ga·lac·tos·emic** \-mik\ *adj*

ga·lac·to·si·dase \gə-ˌlak-'tō-sə-ˌdās, -zə-ˌdāz\ *n* : an enzyme (as lactase) that hydrolyzes a galactoside

ga·lac·to·side \gə-'lak-tə-ˌsīd\ *n* : a glycoside that yields galactose on hydrolysis

ga·lac·tos·uria \gə-ˌlak-(ˌ)tō-'sùr-ē-ə, -'syùr-\ *n* : the presence of galactose in the urine

gal·a·nin \'ga-lə-nin\ *n* : a neurotransmitter that plays a role in regulating various physiological functions (as contraction of gastrointestinal muscle and inhibition of insulin)

Gal·ba \'gal-bə, 'gȯl-\ *n* : a genus of freshwater snails (family Lymnaeidae) that include hosts of a liver fluke of the genus *Fasciola* (*F. hepatica*) and that are sometimes considered indistinguishable from the genus *Lymnaea* — compare FOSSARIA

ga·lea \'gā-lē-ə, 'ga-\ *n* : GALEA APONEUROTICA

galea apo·neu·ro·ti·ca \-ˌa-pō-nù-'rä-ti-kə, -nyù-\ *n* : the aponeurosis underlying the scalp and linking the frontalis and occipitalis muscles — called also *epicranial aponeurosis*

ga·len·i·cal \gə-'le-ni-kəl\ *n* : a standard medicinal preparation (as an extract or tincture) containing usu. one or more active constituents of a plant — **ga·len·ic** \-nik\ *also* **galenical** *adj*

Ga·len \'gā-lən\ (*ca* 129–*ca* 199), Greek physician.

Ga·len·ist \'gā-lə-nist\ *n* : a follower or disciple of the ancient physician Galen — **Ga·len·ism** \-,ni-zəm\ *n*

Galen's vein *n* **1** : either of a pair of cerebral veins in the roof of the third ventricle that drain the interior of the brain **2** : GREAT CEREBRAL VEIN

¹gall \'gȯl\ *n* : BILE; *esp* : bile obtained from an animal and used in medicine

²gall *n* : a skin sore caused by chronic irritation

³gall *vb* : to rub and wear away by friction : CHAFE

gal·la·mine tri·eth·io·dide \'ga-lə-ˌmēn-ˌtrī-ˌe-'thī-ə-ˌdīd\ *n* : an iodide salt $C_{30}H_{60}I_3N_3O_3$ that is used to produce muscle relaxation esp. during anesthesia — called also *gallamine*

gal·late \'ga-ˌlāt, 'gȯ-\ *n* : a salt or ester of gallic acid — see PROPYL GALLATE

gall·blad·der \'gȯl-ˌbla-dər\ *n* : a membranous muscular sac in which bile from the liver is stored

galli — see CRISTA GALLI

gal·lic acid \'ga-lik-, 'gȯ-\ *n* : a white crystalline acid $C_7H_6O_5$ found widely in plants or combined in tannins

gal·li·um \'ga-lē-əm\ *n* : a rare bluish white metallic element that is used in the form of its hydrated nitrate salt $Ga(NO_3)_3 \cdot 9H_2O$ to treat hypercalcemia caused by certain cancers — symbol *Ga*; see ELEMENT table

gal·lon \'ga-lən\ *n* **1** : a U.S. unit of liquid capacity equal to four quarts or 231 cubic inches **2** : a British unit of liquid and dry capacity equal to four quarts or 277.42 cubic inches — called also *imperial gallon*

gal·lop \'ga-ləp\ *n* : GALLOP RHYTHM

galloping *adj, of a disease* : progressing rapidly toward a fatal conclusion

gallop rhythm *n* : an abnormal heart rhythm marked by the occurrence of three distinct sounds in each heartbeat like the sound of a galloping horse — called also *gallop*

gall sickness *n* : ANAPLASMOSIS

gall·stone \'gȯl-ˌstōn\ *n* : a calculus (as of cholesterol) formed in the gallbladder or biliary passages — called also *cholelith*

gal·van·ic \gal-'va-nik\ *adj* : of, relating to, involving, or producing a direct current of electricity 〈~ stimulation of flaccid muscles〉 — **gal·van·i·cal·ly** \-ni-k(ə-)lē\ *adv*

Gal·va·ni \gäl-'vä-nē\, **Luigi** (1737–1798), Italian physician and physicist.

galvanic skin response *n* : a change in the electrical resistance of the skin in response to emotional arousal which increases sympathetic nervous system activity — abbr. *GSR*

gal·va·nism \'gal-və-ˌni-zəm\ *n* : the therapeutic use of direct electric current (as to relieve pain)

gal·va·nom·e·ter \ˌgal-və-'nä-mə-tər\ *n* : an instrument for detecting or measuring a small electric current

gamet- *or* **gameto-** *comb form* : gamete 〈*gametic*〉 〈*gameto*genesis〉

gam·ete \'ga-ˌmēt, gə-'mēt\ *n* : a mature male or female germ cell usu. possessing a haploid chromosome set and capable of initiating formation of a new diploid individual by fusion with a gamete of the opposite sex — called also *sex cell* — **ga·met·ic** \gə-'me-tik\ *adj* — **ga·met·i·cal·ly** \-ti-k(ə-)lē\ *adv*

gamete in·tra·fal·lo·pi·an transfer \-ˌin-trə-fə-'lō-pē-ən-\ *n* : a method of assisting reproduction in cases of infertility in which eggs are obtained from an ovary, mixed with sperm, and inserted into a fallopian tube — abbr. *GIFT*; called also *gamete intrafallopian tube transfer*; compare ZYGOTE INTRAFALLOPIAN TRANSFER

ga·me·to·cide \gə-'mē-tə-ˌsīd\ *n* : an agent that destroys the gametocytes of a malaria parasite

ga·me·to·cyte \-ˌsīt\ *n* : a cell (as of a protozoan causing malaria) that divides to produce gametes

gam·e·to·gen·e·sis \ˌga-mə-tə-'je-nə-səs, gə-ˌmē-tə-\ *n, pl* **-e·ses** \-ˌsēz\ : the production of gametes — **gam·e·tog·e·nous** \ˌga-mə-'tä-jə-nəs\ *adj*

-gam·ic \'gam-ik\ *adj comb form* : -GAMOUS 〈mono*gamic*〉

¹gam·ma \'ga-mə\ *n* **1** : the third letter of the Greek alphabet — symbol Γ or γ **2** : GAMMA RAY

²gamma *or* **γ-** *adj* **1** : of or relating to one of three or more closely related chemical substances 〈the *gamma* chain of hemoglobin〉 — used somewhat arbitrarily to specify ordinal relationship or a particular physical form **2** *of streptococci* : producing no hemolysis on blood agar plates

gam·ma–ami·no·bu·tyr·ic acid *also* γ-ami·no·bu·tyr·ic acid \ˌga-mə-ə-ˌmē-(ˌ)nō-byü-'tir-ik-, ˌga-mə-ˌa-mə-()nō-\ *n* : an amino acid $C_4H_9NO_2$ that is a neurotransmitter that induces inhibition of postsynaptic neurons — abbr. *GABA*

gamma benzene hexa·chlo·ride \-ˌhek-sə-'klȯr-ˌīd\ *n* : the gamma isomer of benzene hexachloride that comprises the insecticide lindane and is used in medicine esp. as a scabicide and pediculicide in a one-percent cream, lotion, or shampoo — called also *gamma BHC*

gamma camera *n* : a camera that detects the gamma-ray photons emitted from a radioactive tracer injected into the body and is used esp. in medical diagnostic scanning

gamma globulin *n* **1 a** : a protein fraction of blood rich in antibodies **b** : a sterile solution of gamma globulin from pooled human blood administered esp. for passive immunity against measles, German measles, hepatitis A, or poliomyelitis **2** : any of numerous globulins of blood plasma or serum that have less electrophoretic mobility at alkaline pH than serum albumins, alpha globulins, or beta globulins and that include most antibodies

gamma hydroxybutyrate *n* : GHB

gamma interferon *n* : an interferon produced by T cells that regulates the immune response (as by the activation of macrophages and natural killer cells) and is used in a form obtained from recombinant DNA esp. in the control of infections associated with chronic granulomatous disease — called also *interferon gamma*

Gamma Knife *trademark* — used for a medical device that emits a highly focused beam of gamma radiation used in noninvasive surgery

gamma radiation *n* : radiation that is composed of gamma rays and is used in cancer radiotherapy

gamma ray *n* : a photon emitted spontaneously by a radioactive substance; *also* : a high-energy photon — usu. used in pl.

gam·mop·a·thy \ga-'mä-pǝ-thē\ *n*, *pl* **-thies** : a disorder characterized by a disturbance in the body's synthesis of antibodies

-g·a·mous \gǝ-mǝs\ *adj comb form* **1** : characterized by having or practicing (such) a marriage or (such or so many) marriages ⟨mono*gamous*⟩ **2** : having (such) gametes or reproductive organs or (such) a mode of fertilization ⟨hetero*gamous*⟩

-g·a·my \gǝ-mē\ *n comb form*, *pl* **g·a·mies 1** : marriage ⟨mono*gamy*⟩ **2** : possession of (such) gametes or reproductive organs or (such) a mode of fertilization ⟨hetero*gamy*⟩

gan·ci·clo·vir \gan-'sī-klǝ-ͺvir\ *n* : an antiviral drug $C_9H_{13}N_5O_4$ related to acyclovir and used esp. in the treatment of cytomegalovirus retinitis in immunocompromised patients — called also *DHPG*

gangli- *or* **ganglio-** *comb form* : ganglion ⟨*gangli*oma⟩ ⟨*ganglio*neuroma⟩

ganglia *pl of* GANGLION

gan·gli·al \'gaṇ-glē-ǝl\ *adj* : of, relating to, or resembling a ganglion

gan·gli·at·ed cord \ͺgaṇ-glē-ͺā-tǝd-\ *n* : either of the two main trunks of the sympathetic nervous system of which one lies on each side of the spinal column

gan·gli·o·ma \ͺgaṇ-glē-'ō-mǝ\ *n*, *pl* **-mas** *also* **-ma·ta** \-mǝ-tǝ\ : a tumor of a ganglion

gan·gli·on \'gaṇ-glē-ǝn\ *n*, *pl* **-glia** \-glē-ǝ\ *also* **-gli·ons 1** : a small cystic tumor (as on the back of the wrist) containing viscid fluid and connected either with a joint membrane or tendon sheath **2 a** : a mass of nerve tissue containing cell bodies of neurons that is located outside the central nervous system and forms an enlargement upon a nerve or upon two or more nerves at their point of junction or separation **b** : a mass of gray matter within the brain or spinal cord : NUCLEUS **2** — see BASAL GANGLION

gan·gli·on·at·ed \-ǝ-ͺnā-tǝd\ *adj* : furnished with ganglia

ganglion cell *n* : a nerve cell having its body outside the central nervous system

gan·gli·on·ec·to·my \ͺgaṇ-glē-ǝ-'nek-tǝ-mē\ *n*, *pl* **-mies** : surgical removal of a nerve ganglion

gan·glio·neu·ro·ma \-(ͺ)ō-nù-'rō-mǝ, -nyù-\ *n*, *pl* **-mas** *also* **-ma·ta** \-mǝ-tǝ\ : a neuroma derived from ganglion cells

gan·gli·on·ic \ͺgaṇ-glē-'ä-nik\ *adj* : of, relating to, or affecting ganglia or ganglion cells

ganglionic blocking agent *n* : a drug used to produce blockade at a ganglion

gan·gli·on·itis \ͺgaṇ-glē-ǝ-'nī-tǝs\ *n* : inflammation of a ganglion

gan·gli·o·side \'gaṇ-glē-ǝ-ͺsīd\ *n* : any of a group of glycolipids that are found esp. in the plasma membrane of cells of the gray matter and have sialic acid, hexoses, and hexosamines in the carbohydrate part and ceramide as the lipid

gan·gli·o·si·do·sis \ͺgaṇ-glē-ͺō-sī-'dō-sǝs\ *n*, *pl* **-do·ses** \-ͺsēz\ : any of several inherited metabolic diseases (as Tay-Sachs disease) characterized by an enzyme deficiency which causes accumulation of gangliosides in the tissues

gan·go·sa \gaṇ-'gō-sǝ\ *n* : a destructive ulcerative condition believed to be a manifestation of yaws that usu. originates about the soft palate and spreads into the hard palate, nasal structures, and outward to the face — compare GOUNDOU

gan·grene \'gaṇ-ͺgrēn, gaṇ-'\ *n* : local death of soft tissues due to loss of blood supply — **gangrene** *vb* — **gan·gre·nous** \'gaṇ-grǝ-nǝs\ *adj*

gangrenosum — see PYODERMA GANGRENOSUM

gangrenous stomatitis *n* : CANCRUM ORIS

gan·ja \'gän-jǝ, 'gan-\ *n* : a potent preparation of marijuana used esp. for smoking; *broadly* : MARIJUANA

Gan·ser syndrome \'gän-zǝr-\ *or* **Gan·ser's syndrome** *n* : a pattern of psychopathological behavior characterized by the giving of approximate answers (as 2 × 2 = about 5)

    Ganser, Sigbert Joseph Maria (1853–1931), German psychiatrist.

gapes \'gāps\ *n* : a disease of birds and esp. young birds in which gapeworms invade and irritate the trachea

gape·worm \'gāp-ͺwǝrm\ *n* : a nematode worm of the genus *Syngamus* (*S. trachea*) that causes gapes of birds

gap junction *n* : an area of contact between adjacent cells characterized by modification of the cell membranes for intercellular communication or transfer of low molecular-weight substances — **gap-junc·tion·al** \'gap-ˈjəŋk-shə-nəl\ adj

Gard·ner·el·la \ˌgärd-nə-ˈre-lə\ n : a genus of bacteria that includes one (*G. vaginalis* syn. *Haemophilus vaginalis*) often present in the flora of the healthy vagina and present in greatly increased numbers in bacterial vaginosis

Gard·ner \'gärd-nər\, **Herman L.** (fl 1955–80), American physician.

Gard·ner's syndrome \'gärd-nərz-\ n : a familial polyposis marked by numerous adenomatous polyps in the colon which typically become malignant if left untreated, by osteomas (as of the skull or mandible), and by skin tumors, that is inherited as an autosomal dominant trait, and that is sometimes considered a variant form of familial adenomatous polyposis

gar·get \'gär-gət\ n : mastitis of domestic animals; esp : chronic bovine mastitis

¹**gar·gle** \'gär-gəl\ vb **gar·gled; gar·gling** 1 : to hold (a liquid) in the mouth and agitate with air from the lungs 2 : to cleanse or disinfect (the oral cavity) by gargling

²**gargle** n : a liquid used in gargling

gar·goyl·ism \'gar-ˌgȯi-ˌli-zəm\ n : MUCOPOLYSACCHARIDOSIS; esp : HURLER'S SYNDROME

Gart·ner's duct \'gart-nərz-, 'gert-\ n : the remains in the female mammal of a part of the Wolffian duct of the embryo — called also *duct of Gartner*

Gart·ner \'gert-nər\, **Hermann Treschow** (1785–1827), Danish surgeon and anatomist.

gas \'gas\ n, pl **gas·es** also **gas·ses** 1 : a fluid (as air) that has neither independent shape nor volume but tends to expand indefinitely 2 : a gaseous product of digestion; also : discomfort from this 3 : a gas or gaseous mixture used to produce anesthesia 4 : a substance that can be used to produce a poisonous, asphyxiating, or irritant atmosphere

gas chromatograph n : an instrument used to separate a sample into components in gas chromatography

gas chromatography n : chromatography in which the sample mixture is vaporized and injected into a stream of carrier gas (as helium) moving through a column containing a stationary phase composed of a liquid or a particulate solid and is separated into its component compounds according to the affinity of the compounds for the stationary phase — **gas chromatographic** adj

gas·eous \'ga-sē-əs, 'ga-shəs\ adj : having the form of or being gas; also : of or relating to gases

gas gangrene n : progressive gangrene marked by impregnation of the dead and dying tissue with gas and caused by one or more toxin-producing bacteria of the genus *Clostridium*

gash \'gash\ n : a deep long cut esp. in flesh — **gash** vb

gas–liquid chromatography n : gas chromatography in which the stationary phase is a liquid — **gas–liquid chromatographic** adj

gas mask n : a mask connected to a chemical air filter and used to protect the face and lungs from toxic gases; broadly : RESPIRATOR 1

gas·se·ri·an ganglion \ga-ˈsir-ē-ən-\ n, often cap 1st G : TRIGEMINAL GANGLION

Gas·ser \'gä-sər\, **Johann Laurentius** (1723–1765), Austrian anatomist.

Gas·ter·oph·i·lus \ˌgas-tə-ˈrä-fə-ləs\ n : a genus of botflies including several (esp. *G. intestinalis* in the U.S.) that infest horses and rarely humans

gastr- or **gastro-** also **gastri-** comb form 1 : stomach ⟨*gastritis*⟩ 2 : gastric and ⟨*gastro*intestinal⟩

gas·tral \'gas-trəl\ adj : of or relating to the stomach or digestive tract

gas·tral·gia \ga-ˈstral-jə\ n : pain in the stomach or epigastrium esp. of a neuralgic type — **gas·tral·gic** \-jik\ adj

gas·trec·to·my \ga-ˈstrek-tə-mē\ n, pl **-mies** : surgical removal of all or part of the stomach

gas·tric \'gas-trik\ adj : of or relating to the stomach

gastrica — see ACHYLIA GASTRICA

gastric artery n 1 : a branch of the celiac artery that passes to the cardiac end of the stomach and along the lesser curvature — called also *left gastric artery*; see RIGHT GASTRIC ARTERY 2 : any of several branches of the splenic artery distributed to the greater curvature of the stomach

gastric bypass n : a surgical bypass operation performed to restrict food intake and reduce absorption of calories and nutrients in the treatment of severe obesity that typically involves reducing the size of the stomach and reconnecting the smaller stomach to bypass the first portion of the small intestine; esp : ROUX-EN-Y GASTRIC BYPASS

gastric gland n : any of various glands in the walls of the stomach that secrete gastric juice

gastric juice n : a thin watery acid digestive fluid secreted by the glands in the mucous membrane of the stomach and containing 0.2 to 0.4 percent free hydrochloric acid and several enzymes (as pepsin)

gastric pit n : any of the numerous depressions in the mucous membrane lining the stomach into which the gastric glands discharge their secretions

gastric ulcer n : a peptic ulcer situated in the stomach

gas·trin \'gas-trən\ n : any of various polypeptide hormones that are secreted by the gastric mucosa and induce secretion of gastric juice

gas·tri·no·ma \ˌgas-trə-ˈnō-mə\ *n, pl* **-mas** *also* **-ma·ta** \-mə-tə\ : a tumor that often involves blood vessels, usu. occurs in the pancreas or the wall of the duodenum, and produces excessive amounts of gastrin — see ZOLLINGER-ELLISON SYNDROME

gas·tri·tis \ga-ˈstrī-təs\ *n* : inflammation esp. of the mucous membrane of the stomach

gastro- — see GASTR-

gas·troc·ne·mi·us \ˌgas-(ˌ)träk-ˈnē-mē-əs, -trək-\ *n, pl* **-mii** \-mē-ˌī\ : the largest and most superficial muscle of the calf of the leg that arises by two heads from the condyles of the femur and has its tendon of insertion incorporated as part of the Achilles tendon — called also *gastrocnemius muscle*

gas·tro·co·lic \ˌgas-trō-ˈkä-lik, -ˈkō-\ *adj* : of, relating to, or uniting the stomach and colon ⟨a ∼ fistula⟩

gastrocolic reflex *n* : the occurrence of peristalsis following the entrance of food into the empty stomach

Gas·tro·dis·coi·des \ˌgas-trō-dis-ˈkòi-(ˌ)dēz\ *n* : a genus of amphistome trematode worms including an intestinal parasite (*G. hominis*) of humans and swine in southeastern Asia

gas·tro·du·o·de·nal \ˌgas-trō-ˌdü-ə-ˈdēn-ᵊl, -ˌdyü-; -dü-ˈäd-ᵊn-əl, -dyü-\ *adj* : of, relating to, or involving the stomach and the duodenum

gastroduodenal artery *n* : an artery that arises from the hepatic artery and divides to form the right gastroepiploic artery and a branch supplying the duodenum and pancreas

gas·tro·du·o·de·nos·to·my \ˌgas-trō-(ˌ)dü-ˈnäs-tə-mē, -ˌdyü-: -dü-ˌäd-ᵊn-ˈäs-tə-mē, -dyü-\ *n, pl* **-mies** : surgical formation of a passage between the stomach and the duodenum

gas·tro·en·ter·i·tis \-ˌen-tə-ˈrī-təs\ *n, pl* **-en·ter·it·i·des** \-ˈri-tə-ˌdēz\ : inflammation of the lining membrane of the stomach and the intestines

gas·tro·en·ter·ol·o·gist \-ˌen-tə-ˈrä-lə-jist\ *n* : a specialist in gastroenterology

gas·tro·en·ter·ol·o·gy \-ˌen-tə-ˈrä-lə-jē\ *n, pl* **-gies** : a branch of medicine concerned with the structure, functions, diseases, and pathology of the stomach and intestines — **gas·tro·en·ter·o·log·i·cal** \-rə-ˈlä-ji-kəl\ *or* **gas·tro·en·ter·o·log·ic** \-ˈlä-jik\ *adj*

gas·tro·en·ter·op·a·thy \-ˌen-tə-ˈrä-pə-thē\ *n, pl* **-thies** : a disease of the stomach and intestines

gas·tro·en·ter·os·to·my \-ˈräs-tə-mē\ *n, pl* **-mies** : the surgical formation of a passage between the stomach and small intestine

gas·tro·ep·i·plo·ic artery \-ˌe-pə-ˈplō-ik\ *n* : either of two arteries forming an anastomosis along the greater curvature of the stomach: **a** : one that is larger, arises as one of the two terminal branches of the gastroduodenal artery, and passes from right to left — called also *right gastroepiploic artery* **b** : one that is smaller, arises as a branch of the splenic artery, and passes from left to right — called also *left gastroepiploic artery*

gas·tro·esoph·a·ge·al \ˌgas-trō-i-ˌsä-fə-ˈjē-əl\ *adj* : of, relating to, or involving the stomach and esophagus

gastroesophageal reflux *n* : backward flow of the gastric contents into the esophagus due to improper functioning of a sphincter at the lower end of the esophagus and resulting esp. in heartburn

gastroesophageal reflux disease *n* : a highly variable chronic condition that is characterized by periodic episodes of gastroesophageal reflux usu. accompanied by heartburn and that may result in histopathologic changes in the esophagus — abbr. *GERD*

gas·tro·in·tes·ti·nal \-in-ˈtes-tən-ᵊl\ *adj* : of, relating to, or affecting both stomach and intestine

gastrointestinal tract *n* : the stomach and intestine as a functional unit

gas·tro·je·ju·nal \-ji-ˈjün-ᵊl\ *adj* : of, relating to, or involving both stomach and jejunum ⟨∼ lesions⟩

gas·tro·je·ju·nos·to·my \-ji-(ˌ)jü-ˈnäs-tə-mē\ *n, pl* **-mies** : the surgical formation of a passage between the stomach and jejunum : GASTROENTEROSTOMY

gas·tro·lith \ˈga-strə-ˌlith\ *n* : a gastric calculus

gas·tro·pa·re·sis \ˌgas-trō-pə-ˈrē-səs\ *n, pl* **-re·ses** \-ˌsēz\ : partial paralysis of the stomach

gas·trop·a·thy \ga-ˈsträ-pə-thē\ *n, pl* **-thies** : a disease of the stomach

gas·tro·pexy \ˈgas-trə-ˌpek-sē\ *n, pl* **-pex·ies** : a surgical operation in which the stomach is sutured to the abdominal wall

gas·tro·pod \ˈgas-trə-ˌpäd\ *n* : any of a large class (Gastropoda) of mollusks (as snails) with a one-piece shell or none and usu. a distinct head bearing sensory organs — **gastropod** *adj*

gas·tros·chi·sis \ga-ˈsträs-kə-səs\ *n, pl* **-chi·ses** \-ˌsēz\ : congenital fissure of the ventral abdominal wall

gas·tro·scope \ˈgas-trə-ˌskōp\ *n* : an endoscope for inspecting the interior of the stomach — **gas·tro·scop·ic** \ˌgas-trə-ˈskä-pik\ *adj* — **gas·tros·co·pist** \ga-ˈsträs-kə-pist\ *n* — **gas·tros·co·py** \-pē\ *n*

gas·tro·splen·ic ligament \ˌgas-trō-ˈsple-nik-\ *n* : a mesenteric fold passing from the greater curvature of the stomach to the spleen

gas·tros·to·my \ga-ˈsträs-tə-mē\ *n, pl* **-mies** **1** : the surgical formation of an opening through the abdominal wall into the stomach **2** : the opening made by gastrostomy

gas·trot·o·my \ga-'strä-tə-mē\ n, pl **-mies** : surgical incision into the stomach

gas·tru·la \'gas-trə-lə\ n, pl **-las** or **-lae** \-ˌlē, -ˌlī\ : an early embryo that develops from the blastula and in mammals is formed by the differentiation of the upper layer of the blastodisc into the ectoderm and the lower layer into the endoderm and by the inward migration of cells through the primitive streak to form the mesoderm — compare BLASTULA, MORULA — **gas·tru·lar** \-lər\ adj

gas·tru·la·tion \ˌgas-trə-'lā-shən\ n : the process of becoming or of forming a gastrula — **gas·tru·late** \'gas-trə-ˌlāt\ vb

gatch bed \'gach-\ n, often cap : a hospital bed with a frame in three movable sections equipped with mechanical spring parts that permit raising the head end, foot end, or middle as required; broadly : HOSPITAL BED

Gatch, Willis Dew (1878–1954), American surgeon.

gate·keep·er \'gāt-ˌkē-pər\ n : a health-care professional (as a primary care physician) who regulates access esp. to hospitals and specialists

gath·er \'ga-thər\ vb **gath·ered; gath·er·ing** : to swell and fill with pus

gathering n : a suppurating swelling : ABSCESS

Gau·cher's disease \gō-'shāz-\ n : a rare hereditary disorder of lipid metabolism that is caused by an enzyme deficiency of glucocerebrosidase, that is characterized by enormous enlargement of the spleen, pigmentation of the skin, and bone lesions, and that is marked by the presence of large amounts of glucocerebroside in the cells of the mononuclear phagocyte system

Gaucher, Philippe Charles Ernest (1854–1918), French physician.

gaul·the·ria \gȯl-'thir-ē-ə\ n **1** cap : a genus of evergreen shrubs of the heath family (Ericaceae) that includes the wintergreens **2** : a plant of the genus Gaultheria

Gaultier \gō-'tyā\, **Jean François** (1708–1756), Canadian physician and botanist.

gaultheria oil n : OIL OF WINTERGREEN

gauze \'gȯz\ n : a loosely woven cotton surgical dressing

ga·vage \gə-'väzh, gä-\ n : introduction of material into the stomach by a tube

gave past of GIVE

GB \ˌjē-'bē\ n : SARIN

GB abbr gallbladder

GC abbr **1** gas chromatograph; gas chromatography **2** gonococcus

G–CSF abbr granulocyte colony-stimulating factor

Gd symbol gadolinium

Ge symbol germanium

GE abbr gastroenterology

Gei·ger counter \'gī-gər-\ n : an instrument for detecting the presence and intensity of radiations (as particles from a radioactive substance) by means of the ionizing effect on an enclosed gas which results in a pulse that is amplified and fed to a device giving a visible or audible indication

Geiger, Hans (Johannes) Wilhelm (1882–1945), and **Müller** \'mue-ler\, **Walther** (fl 1928), German physicists.

Geiger–Mül·ler counter \-'myü-lər-\ n : GEIGER COUNTER

¹gel \'jel\ n : a colloid in a more solid form than a sol

²gel vb **gelled; gel·ling** : to change into or take on the form of a gel — **gel·able** \'je-lə-bəl\ adj

gel·ate \'je-ˌlāt\ vb **gel·at·ed; gel·at·ing** : GEL

gel·a·tin also **gel·a·tine** \'je-lə-tən\ n **1** : glutinous material obtained from animal tissues by boiling; esp : a colloidal protein used as a food and in medicine **2 a** : any of various substances (as agar) resembling gelatin **b** : an edible jelly made with gelatin — **ge·lat·i·nous** \jə-'lat-ᵊn-əs\ adj

gelatinosa — see SUBSTANTIA GELATINOSA

gel·ation \je-'lā-shən\ n : the formation of a gel from a sol

gel·cap \'jel-ˌkap\ n : a capsule-shaped tablet coated with gelatin for easy swallowing

geld \'geld\ vb : CASTRATE; also : SPAY

geld·ing \'gel-diŋ\ n : a castrated animal; specif : a castrated male horse

gel electrophoresis n : electrophoresis in which molecules (as proteins and nucleic acids) migrate through a gel and esp. a polyacrylamide gel and separate into bands according to size

gel filtration n : chromatography in which the material to be fractionated separates primarily according to molecular size as it moves into a column of a gel and is washed with a solvent so that the fractions appear successively at the end of the column — called also gel chromatography

ge·mel·lus \jə-'me-ləs\ n, pl **ge·mel·li** \-ˌlī\ also **ge·mel·lus·es** : either of two small muscles of the hip that insert into the tendon of the obturator internus: **a** : a superior one originating chiefly from the outer surface of the ischial spine — called also gemellus superior **b** : an inferior one originating chiefly from the ischial tuberosity — called also gemellus inferior

gem·fi·bro·zil \jem-'fī-brə-(ˌ)zil, -'fi-\ n : a drug $C_{15}H_{22}O_3$ that regulates blood serum lipids and is used esp. to lower the levels of triglycerides and increase the levels of HDLs in the treatment of hyperlipidemia — see LOPID

gem·i·na·tion \ˌje-mə-'nā-shən\ n : a doubling, duplication, or repetition;

esp : a formation of two teeth from a single tooth germ

gen- *or* **geno-** *comb form* : gene ⟨*genome*⟩

-gen \jən, ˌjen\ *also* **-gene** \ˌjēn\ *n comb form* **1** : producer ⟨carcino*gen*⟩ **2** : one that is (so) produced ⟨phos*gene*⟩

gen·der \'jen-dər\ *n* **1** : SEX 1 **2** : the behavioral, cultural, or psychological traits typically associated with one sex

gender identity *n* : the totality of physical and behavioral traits that are designated by a culture as masculine or feminine

gene \'jēn\ *n* : a specific sequence of nucleotides in DNA or RNA that is located usu. on a chromosome and that is the functional unit of inheritance controlling the transmission and expression of one or more traits by specifying the structure of a particular polypeptide and esp. a protein or controlling the function of other genetic material — called also *determinant, determiner, factor*

gene complex *n* : a group of genes of an individual or of a potentially interbreeding group that constitute an interacting functional unit

gene flow *n* : the passage and establishment of genes typical of one breeding population into the gene pool of another

gene frequency *n* : the ratio of the number of a specified allele in a population to the total of all alleles at its genetic locus

gene mutation *n* : mutation due to fundamental intramolecular reorganization of a gene — see POINT MUTATION

gene pool *n* : the collection of genes of all the individuals in an interbreeding population

genera *pl of* GENUS

gen·er·al \'je-nə-rəl, 'jen-rəl\ *adj* **1** : not confined by specialization or careful limitation ⟨a ∼ surgeon⟩ **2** : involving or affecting practically the entire organism : not local

general anesthesia *n* : anesthesia affecting the entire body and accompanied by loss of consciousness

general anesthetic *n* : an anesthetic used to produce general anesthesia

general hospital *n* : a hospital in which patients with many different types of ailments are given care

gen·er·al·ist \'jen-rə-list, 'je-nə-rə-\ *n* : one whose skills or interests extend to several different medical fields; *esp* : GENERAL PRACTITIONER

generalista — see OSTEITIS FIBROSA CYSTICA GENERALISTA

gen·er·al·iza·tion \ˌjen-rə-lə-'zā-shən, ˌje-nə-rə-\ *n* **1** : the action or process of generalizing **2** : the process whereby a response is made to a stimulus similar to but not identical with the conditioned stimulus

gen·er·al·ize \'jen-rə-ˌlīz, 'je-nə-rə-\ *vb* **-ized; -iz·ing** : to spread or extend throughout the body

generalized anxiety disorder *n* : an anxiety disorder marked by chronic excessive anxiety and worry that is difficult to control, causes distress or impairment in daily functioning, and is accompanied by three or more associated symptoms (as restlessness, irritability, poor concentration, and sleep disturbances) — abbr. *GAD*

generalized seizure *n* : a seizure (as an absence seizure or tonic-clonic seizure) that originates in both cerebral hemispheres — compare PARTIAL SEIZURE

general paresis *n* : insanity caused by syphilitic alteration of the brain that leads to dementia and paralysis — called also *dementia paralytica, general paralysis of the insane*

general practitioner *n* : a physician or veterinarian whose practice is not limited to a specialty

gen·er·a·tion \ˌje-nə-'rā-shən\ *n* **1** : a body of living beings constituting a single step in the line of descent from an ancestor **2** : the average span of time between the birth of parents and that of their offspring **3** : the action or process of producing offspring : PROCREATION

gen·er·a·tive \'je-nə-rə-tiv, -ˌrā-\ *adj* : having the power or function of propagating or reproducing

gen·er·a·tiv·i·ty \ˌje-nə-rə-'ti-və-tē\ *n, pl* **-ties** : a concern for persons besides self and family that usu. develops during middle age; *esp* : a need to nurture and guide younger people and contribute to the next generation — used in the psychology of Erik Erikson

¹ge·ner·ic \jə-'ner-ik\ *adj* **1** : not protected by trademark registration : NONPROPRIETARY **2** : relating to or having the rank of a biological genus — **ge·ner·i·cal·ly** \-i-k(ə-)lē\ *adv*

²generic *n* : a generic drug — usu. used in pl.

gene–splic·ing \'jēn-'splī-siŋ\ *n* : the process of preparing recombinant DNA

gene therapy *n* : the insertion of usu. genetically altered genes into cells esp. to replace defective genes in the treatment of genetic disorders or to provide a specialized disease-fighting function (as destruction of tumor cells)

ge·net·ic \jə-'ne-tik\ *also* **ge·net·i·cal** \-ti-kəl\ *adj* **1** : of, relating to, or involving genetics **2** : of, relating to, caused by, or controlled by genes ⟨a ∼ disease⟩ — compare ACQUIRED 1 — **ge·net·i·cal·ly** \-ti-k(ə-)lē\ *adv*

-ge·net·ic \jə-'ne-tik\ *adj comb form* : -GENIC ⟨osteo*genetic*⟩

genetic code *n* : the biochemical basis of heredity consisting of codons in DNA and RNA that determine the specific amino acid sequence in proteins and that appear to be uniform for all known forms of life — **genetic coding** n

genetic counseling n : guidance provided by a medical professional typically to individuals with an increased risk of having a child with a specific genetic disorder and that includes providing information concerning the probability of having a child with the disorder, prenatal diagnostic tests, and available treatment

genetic drift n : random changes in gene frequency esp. in small populations when leading to preservation or extinction of particular genes

genetic engineering n : the group of applied techniques of genetics and biotechnology used to cut up and join together genetic material and esp. DNA from one or more species of organism and to introduce the result into an organism in order to change one or more of its characteristics — **genetically engineered** adj — **genetic engineer** n

genetic fingerprint n : DNA FINGERPRINT

genetic fingerprinting n : DNA FINGERPRINTING

genetic imprinting n : GENOMIC IMPRINTING

genetic load n : the decrease in fitness of the average individual in a population due to the presence of deleterious genes or genotypes in the gene pool

genetic map n : MAP

genetic marker n : a readily recognizable genetic trait, gene, DNA segment, or gene product used for identification purposes esp. when closely linked to a trait or to genetic material that is difficult to identify

ge·net·ics \jə-'ne-tiks\ n **1 a** : a branch of biology that deals with the heredity and variation of organisms **b** : a treatise or textbook on genetics **2** : the genetic makeup and phenomena of an organism, type, group, or condition — **ge·net·i·cist** \-nə-tə-sist\ n

ge·ni·al \ji-'nī-əl\ adj : of or relating to the chin

genial tubercle n : MENTAL TUBERCLE

gen·ic \'jē-nik, 'je-\ adj : GENETIC 2 — **gen·i·cal·ly** \-nik(ə-)lē\ adv

-gen·ic \'je-nik, 'jē-\ adj comb form **1** : producing : forming ⟨carcinogenic⟩ **2** : produced by : formed from ⟨nephrogenic⟩

ge·nic·u·lar artery \jə-'ni-kyə-lər-\ n : any of several branches of the femoral and popliteal arteries that supply the region of the knee — called also genicular

ge·nic·u·late \-lət, -ˌlāt\ adj **1** : bent abruptly at an angle like a bent knee **2** : relating to, comprising, or belonging to a geniculate body or geniculate ganglion ⟨~ cells⟩ ⟨~ neurons⟩

geniculate body n : either of two prominences of the diencephalon that comprise the metathalamus: **a** : LATERAL GENICULATE BODY **b** : MEDIAL GENICULATE BODY

geniculate ganglion n : a small reddish ganglion consisting of sensory and sympathetic nerve cells located at the sharp backward bend of the facial nerve

ge·nic·u·lo·cal·ca·rine \jə-ˌni-kyə-(ˌ)kal-kə-ˌrīn\ adj : relating to or comprising the optic radiation from the lateral geniculate body and the pulvinar to the occipital lobe

genio- comb form : chin and ⟨genioglossus⟩

ge·nio·glos·sus \ˌjē-nē-ō-'glä-səs, -'glô-\ n, pl **-glos·si** \-ˌsī\ : a fanshaped muscle that arises from the superior mental spine, inserts on the hyoid bone and into the tongue, and serves to advance and retract and also to depress the tongue

ge·nio·hyo·glos·sus \-ˌhī-ō-'glä-səs, -'glô-\ n, pl **-glos·si** \-ˌsī\ : GENIOGLOSSUS

ge·nio·hy·oid \-'hī-ˌoid\ adj : of or relating to the chin and hyoid bone

ge·nio·hy·oid·e·us \-ˌhī-'oi-dē-əs\ n, pl **-oid·ei** \-dē-ˌī\ : GENIOHYOID MUSCLE

geniohyoid muscle n : a slender muscle that arises from the inferior mental spine, is inserted on the hyoid bone, and acts to raise the hyoid bone and draw it forward and to retract and depress the lower jaw — called also geniohyoid

ge·nis·tein \jə-'ni-stē-ən\ n : an isoflavone $C_{15}H_{10}O_5$ found esp. in soybeans and shown in laboratory experiments to have antitumor activity

gen·i·tal \'je-nə-t²l\ adj **1** : GENERATIVE **2** : of, relating to, or being a sexual organ **3** : of, relating to, or characterized by the stage of psychosexual development in psychoanalytic theory during which oral and anal impulses are subordinated to adaptive interpersonal mechanisms — compare ANAL 2a, ORAL 2a, PHALLIC 2 — **gen·i·tal·ly** adv

genital herpes n : herpes simplex of the type affecting the genitals — called also herpes genitalis, genital herpes simplex

gen·i·ta·lia \ˌje-nə-'tāl-yə\ n, pl : the organs of the reproductive system; esp : the external genital organs

genitalis — see HERPES GENITALIS

gen·i·tal·i·ty \-'ta-lə-tē\ n, pl **-ties** : possession of full genital sensitivity and capacity to develop orgasmic potency in relation to a sexual partner of the opposite sex

genital ridge n : a ridge of embryonic mesoblast developing from the mesonephros and giving rise to the gonad on either side of the body

gen·i·tals \'je-nə-t²lz\ n pl : GENITALIA

genital tubercle n : a conical protuberance on the belly wall of an embryo that develops into the penis in the male and the clitoris in the female

genital wart *n* : a wart on the skin or adjoining mucous membrane usu. near the anus and genital organs — called also *condyloma, condyloma acuminatum, venereal wart*

genito- *comb form* : genital and ⟨*genito*urinary⟩

gen·i·to·cru·ral nerve \jə-nə-(,)tō-ˈkrür-əl-\ *n* : GENITOFEMORAL NERVE

gen·i·to·fem·o·ral nerve \-ˈfe-mə-rəl-\ *n* : a nerve that arises from the first and second lumbar nerves and is distributed by way of branches to the skin of the scrotum or labia majora and to the upper anterior aspect of the thigh

gen·i·to·uri·nary \-ˈyu̇r-ə-,ner-ē\ *adj* : of, relating to, affecting, or being the organs of reproduction and urination : UROGENITAL

genitourinary system *n* : GENITOURINARY TRACT

genitourinary tract *n* : the system of organs comprising those concerned with the production and excretion of urine and those concerned with reproduction — called also *genitourinary system, urogenital system, urogenital tract*

geno- — see GEN-

ge·no·gram \ˈjē-nə-,gram, ˈje-\ *n* : a diagram outlining the behavioral or medical history of a family's members over several generations

ge·nome \ˈjē-,nōm\ *n* : one haploid set of chromosomes with the genes they contain

ge·nom·ic \ji-ˈnō-mik, -ˈnä-\ *adj* : of or relating to a genome or genomics

genomic imprinting *n* : genetic alteration of a gene or its expression that is inferred to take place from the observation that certain genes are expressed differently depending on whether they are inherited from the paternal or maternal parent — called also *genetic imprinting, imprinting*

ge·no·mics \jē-ˈnō-miks\ *n* : a branch of biotechnology concerned with the genetic mapping and DNA sequencing of sets of genes or the complete genomes of selected organisms using high-speed methods, with organizing the results in databases, and with applications of the data (as in medicine) — compare PROTEOMICS

ge·no·tox·ic \jē-nə-ˈtäk-sik\ *adj* : damaging to genetic material — **ge·no·tox·ic·i·ty** \-ˌtäk-ˈsi-sə-tē\ *n*

¹**ge·no·type** \ˈjē-nə-,tīp, ˈje-\ *n* : all or part of the genetic constitution of an individual or group — compare PHENOTYPE — **ge·no·typ·ic** \ˌjē-nə-ˈti-pik, ˌje-\ *also* **ge·no·typ·i·cal** \-pi-kəl\ *adj* — **ge·no·typ·i·cal·ly** \-pi-k(ə-)lē\ *adv*

²**genotype** *vb* **-typed; -typ·ing** : to determine the genotype of

-g·e·nous \jə-nəs\ *adj comb form* 1 : producing : yielding ⟨*erogenous*⟩ 2 : produced by : arising or originating in ⟨neuro*genous*⟩ ⟨endo*genous*⟩

gen·ta·mi·cin \ˌjen-tə-ˈmīs-ᵊn\ *n* : a broad-spectrum antibiotic mixture that is derived from an actinomycete of the genus *Micromonospora* (*M. purpurea* and *M. echinospora*) and is extensively used in the form of its sulfate in treating infections esp. of the urinary tract

gen·tian violet \ˈjen-chən-\ *n, often cap G&V* : a greenish mixture that contains not less than 96 percent of a pararosaniline derivative and is used esp. as a bactericide, fungicide, and anthelmintic

gen·tis·ic acid \jen-ˈti-sik-, -zik\ *n* : a crystalline acid $C_7H_6O_4$ used medicinally as an analgesic and diaphoretic

ge·nu \ˈjē-,nü, ˈjen-yü\ *n, pl* **gen·ua** \ˈjen-yə-wə\ : an abrupt flexure; *esp* : the bend in the anterior part of the corpus callosum — see GENU VALGUM, GENU VARUM

ge·nus \ˈjē-nəs, ˈje-\ *n, pl* **gen·era** \ˈje-nə-rə\ : a category of biological classification ranking between the family and the species, comprising structurally or phylogenetically related species or an isolated species exhibiting unusual differentiation, and being designated by a capitalized singular noun that is Latin or has a Latin form

genu val·gum \-ˈval-gəm\ *n* : KNOCK-KNEE

genu va·rum \-ˈvar-əm\ *n* : BOWLEG

-g·e·ny \jə-nē\ *n comb form, pl* **-g·e·nies** : generation : production ⟨embryo*geny*⟩ ⟨lyso*geny*⟩

geo·med·i·cine \ˌjē-ō-ˈme-də-sən\ *n* : a branch of medicine that deals with geographic factors in disease

ge·o·pha·gia \-ˈfā-jē-ə-, -jə\ *n* : GEOPHAGY

ge·oph·a·gy \jē-ˈä-fə-jē\ *n, pl* **-gies** : the practice of eating earthy substances (as clay) that in humans is performed esp. to augment a scanty or mineral-deficient diet or as part of a cultural tradition — compare PICA

ge·ot·ri·cho·sis \jē-ˌä-tra-ˈkō-səs\ *n* : infection of the bronchi or lungs and sometimes the mouth and intestines by a fungus of the genus *Geotrichum* (*G. candidum*)

Ge·ot·ri·chum \jē-ˈä-tri-kəm\ *n* : a genus of fungi (family Moniliaceae) including one (*G. candidum*) that causes human geotrichosis

GERD *abbr* gastroesophageal reflux disease

ger·i·at·ric \ˌjer-ē-ˈa-trik, ˌjir-\ *n* 1 **ger·i·at·rics** \-triks\ *pl* : a branch of medicine that deals with the problems and diseases of old age and aging people — compare GERONTOLOGY 2 : an aged person — **geriatric** *adj*

ger·i·a·tri·cian \ˌjer-ē-ə-ˈtri-shən, ˌjir-\ *n* : a specialist in geriatrics

ger·i·a·trist \ˌjer-ē-ˈa-trist, ˌjir-; jə-ˈrī-ə-\ *n* : GERIATRICIAN

germ \ˈjərm\ *n* 1 : a small mass of living substance capable of developing into an organism or one of its parts 2

: MICROORGANISM; *esp* : a microorganism causing disease

Ger·man cockroach \\'jər-mən-\\ *n* : a small active winged cockroach of the genus *Blattella* (*B. germanica*) that is prob. of African origin and is a common household pest in the U.S. — called also *Croton bug*

ger·ma·nin \\jər-'mā-nən\\ *n* : SURAMIN

ger·ma·ni·um \\(,)jər-'mā-nē-əm\\ *n* : a grayish white hard brittle element — symbol *Ge;* see ELEMENT table

German measles *n sing or pl* : an acute contagious virus disease that is milder than typical measles but is damaging to the fetus when occurring early in pregnancy and that is caused by a togavirus (species *Rubella virus* of the genus *Rubivirus*) — called also *rubella*

germ cell *n* : an egg or sperm cell or one of their antecedent cells

germ·free \\'jərm-,frē\\ *adj* : free of microorganisms : AXENIC

ger·mi·cid·al \\,jər-mə-'sīd-əl\\ *adj* : of or relating to a germicide; *also* : destroying germs

ger·mi·cide \\'jər-mə-,sīd\\ *n* : an agent that destroys germs

ger·mi·nal \\'jər-mə-nəl\\ *adj* : of, relating to, or having the characteristics of a germ cell or early embryo

germinal cell *n* : an embryonic cell of the early vertebrate nervous system that is the source of neuroblasts and glial cells

germinal center *n* : the lightly staining central proliferative area of a lymphoid follicle

germinal disk *n* **1** : BLASTODISC **2** : the part of the blastoderm that forms the embryo proper of an amniote vertebrate

germinal epithelium *n* : the epithelial covering of the genital ridges and of the gonads derived from them

germinal vesicle *n* : the enlarged nucleus of the egg before completion of meiosis

ger·mi·na·tive layer \\'jər-mə-,nā-tiv-, -nə-\\ *n* : the innermost layer of the epidermis from which new tissue is constantly formed

germinativum — see STRATUM GERMINATIVUM

ger·mi·no·ma \\,jər-mə-'nō-mə\\ *n, pl* **-mas** : a malignant tumor (as of the testis or pineal gland) originating from undifferentiated embryonic germ cells — see DYSGERMINOMA, SEMINOMA

germ layer *n* : any of the three primary layers of cells differentiated in most embryos during and immediately following gastrulation

germ line *n* : the cellular lineage from which eggs and sperm are derived and in which a cell undergoing mutation can be passed to the next generation

germ plasm *n* **1** : germ cells and their precursors serving as the bearers of heredity and being fundamentally independent of other cells **2** : the hereditary material of the germ cells : GENES

germ-proof \\'jərm-,prüf\\ *adj* : impervious to the penetration or action of germs

germ theory *n* : a theory in medicine: infections, contagious diseases, and various other conditions result from the action of microorganisms

geront- *or* **geronto-** *comb form* : aged one : old age ⟨*gerontology*⟩

ger·on·tol·o·gist \\,jer-ən-'tä-lə-jist\\ *n* : a specialist in gerontology

ger·on·tol·o·gy \\-jē\\ *n, pl* **-gies** : the comprehensive study of aging and the problems of the aged — compare GERIATRIC 1 — **ge·ron·to·log·i·cal** \\jə-,ränt-əl-'ä-ji-kəl\\ *also* **ge·ron·to·log·ic** \\-jik\\ *adj*

Gerst·mann's syndrome \\'gerst-mänz-, 'gərst-mənz-\\ *n* : cerebral dysfunction characterized esp. by finger agnosia, disorientation with respect to right and left, agraphia, and acalculia and caused by a lesion in the dominant cerebral hemisphere

Gerstmann, Josef (1887–1969), Austrian neurologist and psychiatrist.

Gerst·mann–Sträus·sler–Schein·ker syndrome \\'gerst-män-'shtrȯis-lər-'shīŋ-kər-\\ *n* : any of several rare fatal prion diseases that are inherited as autosomal dominant traits and are marked by progressive cognitive and motor impairment and by the accumulation of amyloid plaques in the brain — called also *Gerstmann=Sträussler-Scheinker disease*

Sträussler, Ernst (1872–1959), and **Scheinker, Ilya,** Austrian physicians.

ge·stalt \\gə-'stält, -'shtält, -'stȯlt, -'shtȯlt\\ *n, pl* **ge·stalt·en** \\-ən\\ *or* **gestalts** : a structure, arrangement, or pattern of physical, biological, or psychological phenomena so integrated as to constitute a functional unit with properties not derivable by summation of its parts

ge·stalt·ist \\gə-'stäl-tist, -'shtäl-, -'stȯl-, -'shtȯl-\\ *n, often cap* : a specialist in Gestalt psychology

Gestalt psychology *n* : the study of perception and behavior from the standpoint of an individual's response to gestalten with stress on the uniformity of psychological and physiological events and rejection of analysis into discrete events of stimulus, percept, and response — **Gestalt psychologist** *n*

Gestalt therapy *n* : psychotherapy that focuses on gaining self-awareness of emotions, perceptions, and behaviors in the immediate present

ges·ta·tion \\je-'stā-shən\\ *n* : the carrying of young in the uterus from conception to delivery : PREGNANCY **2** : GESTATION PERIOD — **ges·tate** \\'jes-,tāt\\ *vb* — **ges·ta·tion·al** \\-shə-nəl\\ *adj*

gestation period *n* : the length of time during which gestation takes place — called also *gestation*

ges·to·sis \je-ˈstō-səs\ *n, pl* **-to·ses** \-ˌsēz\ : any disorder of pregnancy; *esp* : TOXEMIA OF PREGNANCY

-geu·sia \ˈgü-zē-ə, ˈjü-, -sē-ə, -zhə\ *n comb form* : a ⟨specified⟩ condition of the sense of taste ⟨dys*geusia*⟩

GG *abbr* gamma globulin

GH *abbr* growth hormone

GHB \ˌjē-ˌāch-ˈbē\ *n* : a fatty acid $C_4H_8O_3$ that is a depressant of the central nervous system and is used illicitly to produce sedative and euphoric effects or to stimulate release of growth hormone to increase muscle mass — called also *gamma hydroxybutyrate*

ghost \ˈgōst\ *n* : a structure (as a cell or tissue) that does not stain normally because of degenerative changes; *specif* : a red blood cell that has lost its hemoglobin

ghrel·in \ˈgre-lən\ *n* : a peptide that is a growth hormone secretagogue released primarily by stomach cells and implicated in the stimulation of fat storage and food intake

GHRH *abbr* growth hormone-releasing hormone

GI *abbr* **1** gastrointestinal **2** glycemic index

giant cell *n* : a large multinucleate often phagocytic cell (as those characteristic of various sarcomas)

giant cell arteritis *n* : arterial inflammation that often involves the temporal arteries and may lead to blindness when the ophthalmic artery and its branches are affected, is characterized by the formation of giant cells, and may be accompanied by fever, malaise, fatigue, anorexia, weight loss, and arthralgia — called also *temporal arteritis*

giant–cell tumor *n* : an osteolytic tumor affecting the metaphyses and epiphyses of long bones that is usually benign but sometimes malignant — called also *osteoclastoma*

gi·ant·ism \ˈjī-ən-ˌti-zəm\ *n* : GIGANTISM

giant kidney worm *n* : a blood-red nematode worm of the genus *Dioctophyme* (*D. renale*) that sometimes exceeds a yard in length and invades mammalian kidneys esp. of the dog and occas. of humans

giant urticaria *n* : ANGIOEDEMA

giant water bug *n* : any of a family (Belostomatidae and esp. genus *Lethocerus*) of very large bugs capable of inflicting a painful bite

giar·dia \jē-ˈär-dē-ə, ˈjär-\ *n* **1** *cap* : a genus of flagellate protozoans inhabiting the intestines of various mammals and including one (*G. lamblia* syn. *G. intestinalis*) that is associated with diarrhea in humans **2** : any flagellate of the genus *Giardia*

Giard \zhē-ˈär\, **Alfred Mathieu** (1846–1908), French biologist.

giar·di·a·sis \ˌ(ˌ)jē-ˌär-ˈdī-ə-səs, jē-ər-, (ˌ)jär-\ *n, pl* **-a·ses** \-ˌsēz\ : infestation with or disease caused by a flagellate protozoan of the genus *Giardia* (esp. *G. lamblia*) that is often characterized by diarrhea — called also *lambliasis*

gid \ˈgid\ *n* : a disease esp. of sheep that is caused by the presence in the brain of the coenurus of a tapeworm of the genus *Multiceps* (*M. multiceps*) — called also *sturdy*

Gi·em·sa stain \gē-ˈem-zə-\ *also* **Giemsa's stain** *n* : a stain consisting of a mixture of eosin and a blue dye and used chiefly in differential staining of blood films — called also *Giemsa*

Giemsa, Gustav (1867–1948), German chemist and pharmacist.

GIFT *abbr* gamete intrafallopian transfer; gamete intrafallopian tube transfer

gi·gan·tism \jī-ˈgan-ˌti-zəm, jə-; ˈjī-gən-\ *n* : development to abnormally large size from excessive growth of the long bones accompanied by muscular weakness and sexual impotence and usu. caused by hyperpituitarism before normal ossification is complete — called also *macrosomia;* compare ACROMEGALY

Gi·la monster \ˈhē-lə-\ *n* : a large orange and black venomous lizard of the genus *Heloderma* (*H. suspectum*) of the southwestern U.S.

Gil·bert's syndrome \zhil-ˈberz-\ *n* : an inherited metabolic disorder that is characterized by elevated levels of serum bilirubin caused esp. by defective uptake of bilirubin by the liver — called also *Gilbert's disease*

Gilbert, Augustin–Nicholas (1858–1927), French physician.

Gil·christ's disease \ˈgil-ˌkrists-\ *n* : NORTH AMERICAN BLASTOMYCOSIS

Gilchrist, Thomas Caspar (1862–1927), American dermatologist.

¹**gill** \ˈjil\ *n* : either of two units of capacity: **a** : a British unit equal to ¼ imperial pint or 8.669 cubic inches **b** : a U.S. liquid unit equal to ¼ U.S. liquid pint or 7.218 cubic inches

²**gill** \ˈgil\ *n* **1** : an organ (as of a fish) for obtaining oxygen from water **2** : one of the radiating plates forming the undersurface of the cap of a mushroom — **gilled** \ˈgild\ *adj*

gill arch *n* : one of the bony or cartilaginous arches placed one behind the other on each side of the pharynx and supporting the gills of fishes and amphibians; *also* : BRANCHIAL ARCH

gill cleft *n* : GILL SLIT

Gilles de la Tou·rette syndrome \ˈzhēl-də-lä-tü-ˈret-\ *also* **Gilles de la Tourette's syndrome** *n* : TOURETTE'S SYNDROME

gill slit *n* : one of the openings or clefts between the gill arches in vertebrates that breathe by gills through which water taken in at the mouth passes to the exterior and bathes the gills; *also* : BRANCHIAL CLEFT

gin·ger \'jin-jər\ *n* : the aromatic rhizome of a tropical herb (*Zingiber officinale*) of the family Zingiberaceae, the ginger family) that is used as a spice and sometimes medicinally (as to relieve nausea); *also* : the plant

gingiv- *or* **gingivo-** *comb form* **1** : gum : gums ⟨*gingiv*itis⟩ **2** : gums and ⟨*gingivo*stomatitis⟩

gin·gi·va \'jin-jə-və, jin-'jī-\ *n, pl* **-vae** \-,vē, -,vī\ : GUM — **gin·gi·val** \'jin-jə-vəl\ *adj*

gingival crevice *n* : a narrow space between the free margin of the gingival epithelium and the adjacent enamel of a tooth — called also *gingival trough*

gingival papilla *n* : INTERDENTAL PAPILLA

gingival trough *n* : GINGIVAL CREVICE

gin·gi·vec·to·my \,jin-jə-'vek-tə-mē\ *n, pl* **-mies** : the excision of a portion of the gingiva

gin·gi·vi·tis \,jin-jə-'vī-təs\ *n* : inflammation of the gums that is often accompanied by tenderness or bleeding

gin·gi·vo·plas·ty \'jin-jə-və-,plas-tē\ *n, pl* **-ties** : a surgical procedure that involves reshaping the gums for aesthetic or functional purposes

gin·gi·vo·sto·ma·ti·tis \,jin-jə-vō-,stō-mə-'tī-təs\ *n, pl* **-ti·ides** \-'ti-tə-,dēz\ *or* **-ti·tis·es** : inflammation of the gums and of the mouth

gin·gly·mus \'jiŋ-glə-məs, 'giŋ-\ *n, pl* **gin·gly·mi** \-,mī, -,mē\ : a joint (as between the humerus and ulna) allowing motion in one plane only

gin·seng \'jin-,seŋ, -,siŋ\ *n* : the aromatic root of a Chinese perennial herb (*Panax schinseng* syn. *P. schinseng* of the family Araliaceae, the ginseng family) valued esp. locally as a medicine; *also* : the plant

gir·dle \'gərd-ᵊl\ *n* **1** : PECTORAL GIRDLE **2** : PELVIC GIRDLE

GI series \,jē-'ī-\ *n* : GASTROINTESTINAL SERIES

gi·tal·in \'ji-tə-lən; jə-'tā-lən, -'ta-\ *n* **1** : a crystalline glycoside $C_{35}H_{56}O_{12}$ obtained from digitalis **2** : a water-soluble mixture of glycosides of digitalis used similarly to digitalis

gi·tox·in \jə-'täk-sən\ *n* : a poisonous crystalline steroid glycoside $C_{41}H_{64}$-O_{14} that is obtained from digitalis and from lanatoside B by hydrolysis

give \'giv\ *vb* **gave** \'gāv\; **giv·en** \'giv-vən\; **giv·ing 1** : to administer as a medicine **2** : to cause a person to catch by contagion, infection, or exposure — **give birth** : to have a baby ⟨*gave birth* last Tuesday⟩ — **give birth to** : to produce as offspring ⟨*gave birth to* a daughter⟩

giz·zard \'gi-zərd\ *n* : the muscular usu. horny-lined enlargement of the digestive tract of a bird used for churning and grinding food

gla·bel·la \glə-'be-lə\ *n, pl* **-bel·lae** \-'be-(,)lē, -,lī\ : the smooth prominence between the eyebrows — **gla·bel·lar** \-'be-lər\ *adj*

gla·brous \'glā-brəs\ *adj* : having or being a smooth hairless surface ⟨~ skin⟩

glacial acetic acid *n* : acetic acid containing usu. less than 1 percent of water

glad·i·o·lus \,gla-dē-'ō-ləs\ *n, pl* **-li** \-(,)lē, -,lī\ : the large middle portion of the sternum lying between the upper manubrium and the lower xiphoid process — called also *mesosternum*

glairy \'glar-ē\ *adj* **glair·i·er; -est** : having a slimy viscid consistency suggestive of an egg white

gland \'gland\ *n* **1** : a cell, group of cells, or organ of endothelial origin that selectively removes materials from the blood, concentrates or alters them, and secretes them for further use in the body or for elimination from the body **2** : any of various animal structures (as a lymph node) suggestive of glands though not secretory in function — **gland·less** *adj*

glan·dered \'glan-dərd\ *adj* : affected with glanders

glan·ders \-dərz\ *n sing or pl* : a contagious and destructive disease esp. of horses caused by a bacterium of the genus *Burkholderia* (*B. mallei*) and characterized by caseating nodular lesions esp. of the respiratory mucosae, lungs, and skin

glandes *pl of* GLANS

gland of Bartholin *n* : BARTHOLIN'S GLAND

gland of Bow·man \-'bō-mən\ *n* : OLFACTORY GLAND

    W. Bowman — see BOWMAN'S CAPSULE

gland of Brunner *n* : BRUNNER'S GLAND

gland of external secretion *n* : EXOCRINE GLAND

gland of internal secretion *n* : ENDOCRINE GLAND

gland of Lit·tré \-lē-'trā\ *n* : any of the urethral glands of the male

    Littré, Alexis (1658–1726), French surgeon and anatomist.

gland of Moll \-'mōl, -'mȯl, -'mäl\ *n* : any of the small glands near the free margin of each eyelid regarded as modified sweat glands — called also *Moll's gland*

    Moll \'mȯl**, Jacob Antonius (1832–1914),** Dutch ophthalmologist.

gland of Ty·son \-'tīs-ᵊn\ *n* : PREPUTIAL GLAND

    Tyson, Edward (1650–1708), British anatomist.

glan·du·lar \'glan-jə-lər\ *adj* **1** : of, relating to, or involving glands, gland cells, or their products **2** : having the characteristics or function of a gland ⟨~ tissue⟩

glandular fever *n* : INFECTIOUS MONONUCLEOSIS

glan·du·lous \'glan-jə-ləs\ *adj* : GLANDULAR

glans \'glanz\ *n, pl* **glan·des** \'glan-ˌdēz\ **1** : a conical vascular body forming the extremity of the penis **2** : a conical vascular body that forms the extremity of the clitoris

glans cli·tor·i·dis \-klə-'tór-ə-(ˌ)dis\ *n* : GLANS 2

glans clitoris *n* : GLANS 2

glans penis *n* : GLANS 1

Gla·se·ri·an fissure \glə-'zir-ē-ən-\ *n* : PETROTYMPANIC FISSURE

Gla·ser \'glä-zər\, **Johann Heinrich** (1629–1675), Swiss anatomist and surgeon.

Glas·gow Coma Scale \'glas-(ˌ)kō-\ *n* : a scale that is used to assess the severity of a brain injury based on how a patient responds to certain standard stimuli (as by opening the eyes or giving a verbal response) and that for a low score (as 3 to 5) indicates a poor chance of recovery and for a high score (as 8 to 15) indicates a good chance of recovery

glass·es \'gla-səz\ *n pl* : a device used to correct defects of vision or to protect the eyes that consists typically of a pair of glass or plastic lenses and the frame by which they are held in place — called also *eyeglasses*

glass eye *n* **1** : an artificial eye made of glass **2** : an eye having a pale, whitish, or colorless iris — **glass-eyed** \-'īd\ *adj*

Glau·ber's salt \'glau̇-bərz-\ *also* **Glau·ber salt** \-bər-\ *n* : a colorless crystalline sodium sulfate Na₂SO₄·10H₂O used as a cathartic — sometimes used in pl.

Glauber, Johann Rudolf (1604–1670), German physician and chemist.

glau·co·ma \glau̇-'kō-mə, glȯ-\ *n* : a disease of the eye marked by increased pressure within the eyeball that can result in damage to the optic disk and gradual loss of vision — **glau·coma·tous** \-'kō-mə-təs, -'kä-\ *adj*

GLC *abbr* gas-liquid chromatography

Glea·son grade \'glē-sᵊn-\ *n* **1** : a grade given to each of the two most prevalent patterns of cancer cells in tissue obtained from biopsy of a prostate tumor that is based on a scale of 1 to 5 with 1 to 3 corresponding to well-differentiated cancer cells similar in appearance to normal cells in surrounding tissue and 4 to 5 corresponding to poorly differentiated cancer cells that look abnormal **2** : GLEASON SCORE

Gleason, Donald F. (*b* 1920), American pathologist.

Gleason score *n* : a score that is the sum of the two Gleason grades assigned to a prostate tumor and that is based on a scale of 2 to 10 with the lowest numbers indicating a slow-growing tumor unlikely to spread and the highest numbers indicating an aggressive tumor

gleet \'glēt\ *n* : a chronic inflammation (as gonorrhea) of a bodily orifice usu. accompanied by an abnormal discharge; *also* : the discharge itself

gle·no·hu·mer·al \ˌgle-(ˌ)nō-'hyü-mə-rəl, ˌglē-\ *adj* : of, relating to, or connecting the glenoid cavity and the humerus

glen·oid \'gle-ˌnȯid, 'glē-\ *adj* **1** : having the form of a smooth shallow depression — used chiefly of skeletal articulatory sockets **2** : of or relating to the glenoid cavity or glenoid fossa

glenoid cavity *n* : the shallow cavity of the upper part of the scapula by which the humerus articulates with the pectoral girdle

glenoid fossa *n* : the depression in each lateral wall of the skull with which the mandible articulates — called also *mandibular fossa*

glenoid labrum *or* **glen·oid·al labrum** \gli-'nȯid-ᵊl-\ *n* : a fibrocartilaginous ligament forming the margin of the glenoid cavity of the shoulder joint that serves to broaden and deepen the cavity and gives attachment to the long head of the biceps brachii — called also *labrum*

gli- *or* **glio-** *comb form* **1** : gliomatous ⟨*glio*blastoma⟩ **2** : neuroglial ⟨*gli*oma⟩

glia \'glē-ə, 'glī-ə\ *n* pl **glia** : supporting tissue that is intermingled with the essential elements of nervous tissue esp. in the brain, spinal cord, and ganglia and is composed of a network of fine fibrils and of flattened stellate cells with numerous radiating fibrillar processes — see MACROGLIA, MICROGLIA — **gli·al** \-əl\ *adj*

-g·lia \glē-ə\ *n comb form* : made up of a (specified) kind or size of element ⟨oligodendro*glia*⟩

gli·a·din \'glī-ə-dən\ *n* : PROLAMIN; *esp* : one obtained by alcoholic extraction of gluten from wheat and rye

gli·ben·cla·mide \glī-'ben-klə-ˌmīd\ *n* : GLYBURIDE

gliding joint *n* : a diarthrosis in which the articular surfaces glide upon each other without axial motion — called also *arthrodia, plane joint*

glio·blas·to·ma \ˌglī-(ˌ)ō-bla-'stō-mə\ *n, pl* **-mas** *also* **-ma·ta** \-mə-tə\ : a malignant rapidly growing astrocytoma of the central nervous system and usu. of a cerebral hemisphere — called also *spongioblastoma*

glioblastoma mul·ti·for·me \-ˌməl-tə-'fȯr-mē\ *n* : GLIOBLASTOMA

Glio·cla·di·um \ˌglī-ō-'klā-dē-əm\ *n* : a genus of molds resembling those of the genus *Penicillium*

gli·o·ma \glī-'ō-mə, glē-\ *n, pl* **-mas** *also* **-ma·ta** \-mə-tə\ : a tumor arising from glial cells — **gli·o·ma·tous** \-mə-təs\ *adj*

gli·o·ma·to·sis \glī-ˌō-mə-ˈtō-səs\ *n, pl* **-to·ses** \-ˌsēz\ : a glioma with diffuse proliferation of glial cells or with multiple foci

gli·o·sis \glī-ˈō-səs\ *n, pl* **gli·o·ses** \-ˌsēz\ : excessive development of glia — **gli·ot·ic** \-ˈä-tik\ *adj*

glio·tox·in \ˌglī-ō-ˈtäk-sən\ *n* : a toxic antibiotic $C_{13}H_{14}N_2O_4S_2$ that is produced by various fungi (as of the genera *Gliocladium* and *Aspergillus*)

glip·i·zide \ˈgli-pə-ˌzīd\ *n* : a sulfonylurea $C_{21}H_{27}N_5O_4S$ that lowers blood glucose levels and is used in the control of hyperglycemia associated with type 2 diabetes — see GLUCOTROL

Glis·son's capsule \ˈglis-ᵊnz-\ *n* : an investment of loose connective tissue entering the liver with the portal vessels and sheathing the larger vessels in their course through the organ

Glisson, Francis (1597–1677), British physician and anatomist.

Gln *abbr* glutamine

glob·al \ˈglō-bəl\ *adj* : being comprehensive, all-inclusive, or complete ⟨transient ∼ amnesia⟩

globe \ˈglōb\ *n* : EYEBALL

globe·fish \ˈglōb-ˌfish\ *n* : PUFFER FISH

glo·bin \ˈglō-bən\ *n* : a colorless protein obtained by removal of heme from a conjugated protein and esp. hemoglobin

glo·bo·side \ˈglō-bə-ˌsīd\ *n* : a complex glycolipid that occurs in the red blood cells, serum, liver, and spleen of humans and accumulates in traces in one of the variants of Tay-Sachs disease

glob·u·lar \ˈglä-byə-lər\ *adj* **1 a** : having the shape of a globe or globule **b** : having a compact folded molecular structure ⟨∼ proteins⟩ **2** : having or consisting of globules — **glob·u·lar·ly** \-lē\ *adv*

glob·ule \ˈglä-(ˌ)byül\ *n* : a small globular body or mass (as a drop of fat)

glob·u·lin \ˈglä-byə-lən\ *n* : any of a class of simple proteins (as myosin) that occur widely in plant and animal tissues — see ALPHA GLOBULIN, BETA GLOBULIN, GAMMA GLOBULIN

glo·bus hys·ter·i·cus \ˈglō-bəs-his-ˈter-i-kəs\ *n* : a choking sensation commonly experienced in hysteria

globus pal·li·dus \-ˈpa-lə-dəs\ *n* : the median portion of the lentiform nucleus — called also *pallidum*

glom·an·gi·o·ma \ˌglō-ˌman-jē-ˈō-ma\ *n, pl* **-mas** *also* **-ma·ta** \-mə-tə\ : GLOMUS TUMOR

glo·mec·to·my \ˌglō-ˈmek-tə-mē\ *n, pl* **-mies** : excision of a glomus (as the carotid body)

glomerul- *or* **glomerulo-** *comb form* : glomerulus of the kidney ⟨*glomeruli*tis⟩ ⟨*glomerulo*nephritis⟩

glo·mer·u·lar \glə-ˈmer-yə-lər, glō-, -ə-lər\ *adj* : of, relating to, or produced by a glomerulus ⟨∼ nephritis⟩

glomerular capsule *n* : BOWMAN'S CAPSULE

glo·mer·u·li·tis \glə-ˌmer-yə-ˈlī-təs, glō-, -ə-ˈlī-\ *n* : inflammation of the glomeruli of the kidney

glo·mer·u·lo·ne·phri·tis \-ˌmer-yə-lō-ni-ˈfrī-təs, -ə-lō-\ *n, pl* **-phri·ti·des** \-ˈfri-tə-ˌdēz\ : nephritis marked by inflammation of the capillaries of the renal glomeruli

glo·mer·u·lop·a·thy \-yə-ˈlä-pə-thē\ *n, pl* **-thies** : a disease (as glomerulonephritis) affecting the renal glomeruli

glo·mer·u·lo·sa \glə-ˌmer-yə-ˈlō-sə, -ə-ˈlō-, -zə\ *n, pl* **-sae** \-ˌsē, -ˌsī, -ˌzē, -ˌzī\ : ZONA GLOMERULOSA

glo·mer·u·lo·scle·ro·sis \-ˌlō-sklə-ˈrō-səs\ *n, pl* **-ro·ses** \-ˌsēz\ : nephrosclerosis involving the renal glomeruli

glo·mer·u·lus \glə-ˈmer-yə-ləs, glō-, -ə-ləs\ *n, pl* **-li** \-ˌlī, -ˌlē\ : a small convoluted or intertwined mass: as **a** : a tuft of capillaries at the point of origin of each nephron that passes a protein-free filtrate to the surrounding Bowman's capsule **b** : a dense entanglement of nerve fibers in the olfactory bulb that contains the primary synapses of the olfactory pathway

glo·mus \ˈglō-məs\ *n, pl* **glom·era** \ˈglä-mə-rə\ *also* **glo·mi** \ˈglō-ˌmī, -ˌmē\ : a small arteriovenous anastomosis together with its supporting structures: as **a** : a vascular tuft that suggests a renal glomerulus and that develops from the embryonic aorta in relation to the pronephros **b** : CAROTID BODY **c** : a tuft of the choroid plexus protruding into each lateral ventricle of the brain

glomus ca·rot·i·cum \-kə-ˈrä-ti-kəm\ *n* : CAROTID BODY

glomus coc·cy·ge·um \-käk-ˈsi-jē-əm\ *n* : a small mass of vascular tissue situated near the tip of the coccyx — called also *coccygeal body, coccygeal gland*

glomus jug·u·la·re \-jə-gyə-ˈlar-ē\ *n* : a mass of chemoreceptors in the adventitia of the dilation in the internal jugular vein where it arises from the transverse sinus in the jugular foramen

glomus tumor *n* : a painful benign tumor that develops by hypertrophy of a glomus — called also *glomangioma*

gloss- *or* **glosso-** *comb form* **1** : tongue ⟨*glossi*tis⟩ **2** : language ⟨*glosso*lalia⟩

glos·sal \ˈglä-səl, ˈglò-\ *adj* : of or relating to the tongue ⟨a ∼ cyst⟩

-glos·sia \ˈglä-sē-ə, ˈglò-\ *n comb form* : condition of having (such) a tongue ⟨micro*glossia*⟩

glos·si·na \glä-ˈsī-nə, glò-, -ˈsē-\ *n* **1** *cap* : an African genus of dipteran flies with a long slender sharp proboscis that includes the tsetse flies **2** : any dipteran fly of the genus *Glossina* : TSETSE FLY

glos·si·tis \glä-'sī-təs\ n : inflammation of the tongue

glosso- — see GLOSS-

gloss·odyn·ia \ˌglä-sō-'di-nē-ə, ˌglò-\ n : pain localized in the tongue

glos·so·la·lia \ˌglä-sə-'lä-lē-ə, ˌglò-\ n : profuse and often emotionally charged speech that mimics coherent speech but is usu. unintelligible to the listener and that is uttered in some states of religious ecstasy and in some schizophrenic states

glos·so·pal·a·tine arch \ˌglä-sō-'pa-lə-ˌtīn-, ˌglò-\ n : PALATOGLOSSAL ARCH

glossopalatine nerve n : NERVUS INTERMEDIUS

glos·so·pal·a·ti·nus \-ˌpa-lə-'tī-nəs\ n, pl -ni \-ˌnī, -ˌnē\ : PALATOGLOSSUS

glos·sop·a·thy \glä-'sä-pə-thē\ n, pl -thies : a disease of the tongue

glos·so·pha·ryn·geal \ˌglä-sō-fə-'rin-jē-əl, ˌglò-, -jəl; -ˌfar-ən-'jē-əl\ adj **1** : of or relating to both tongue and pharynx **2** : of, relating to, or affecting the glossopharyngeal nerve

glossopharyngeal nerve n : either of the ninth pair of cranial nerves that are mixed nerves and supply chiefly the pharynx, posterior tongue, and parotid gland with motor and sensory fibers — called also *glossopharyngeal, ninth cranial nerve*

glottidis — see RIMA GLOTTIDIS

glot·tis \'glä-təs\ n, pl **glot·tis·es** or **glot·ti·des** \-tə-ˌdēz\ : the space between one of the true vocal cords and the arytenoid cartilage on one side of the larynx and those on the other side; *also* : the structures that surround this space — compare EPIGLOTTIS

Glu abbr glutamic acid

gluc- or **gluco-** comb form : glucose ⟨*gluco*kinase⟩ ⟨*gluco*neogenesis⟩

glu·ca·gon \'glü-kə-ˌgän\ n : a protein hormone that is produced esp. by the pancreatic islets of Langerhans and that promotes an increase in the sugar content of the blood by increasing the rate of breakdown of glycogen in the liver — called also *hyperglycemic factor*

glu·can \'glü-ˌkan, -kən\ n : a polysaccharide (as glycogen) that is a polymer of glucose

glu·co·ce·re·bro·si·dase \ˌglü-kō-ˌser-ə-'brō-sə-ˌdās, -ˌdāz\ n : an enzyme that catalyzes the hydrolysis of the glucose part of a glucocerebroside and is deficient in patients affected with Gaucher's disease

glu·co·ce·re·bro·side \-'ser-ə-brə-ˌsīd, -sə-'rē-\ n : a lipid composed of a ceramide and glucose that accumulates in the tissues of patients affected with Gaucher's disease

glu·co·cor·ti·coid \-'kòr-ti-ˌkòid\ n : any of a group of corticosteroids (as cortisol or dexamethasone) that are involved esp. in carbohydrate, protein, and fat metabolism, that tend to increase liver glycogen and blood sugar by increasing gluconeogenesis, that are anti-inflammatory and immunosuppressive, and that are used widely in medicine (as to alleviate the symptoms of rheumatoid arthritis) — compare MINERALOCORTICOID

glu·co·ki·nase \-'kī-ˌnās, -ˌnāz\ n : a hexokinase found esp. in the liver that catalyzes the phosphorylation of glucose

glu·co·nate \'glü-kə-ˌnāt\ n : a salt or ester of a crystalline acid $C_6H_{12}O_7$ — see CALCIUM GLUCONATE, FERROUS GLUCONATE

glu·co·neo·gen·e·sis \ˌglü-kə-ˌnē-ə-'je-nə-səs\ n, pl **-e·ses** \-ˌsēz\ : formation of glucose esp. by the liver and kidney from precursors (as fats and proteins) other than carbohydrates — **glu·co·neo·gen·ic** \-'je-nik\ adj

Glu·co·phage \'glü-kō-ˌfāj\ trademark — used for a preparation of the hydrochloride of metformin

glu·cos·amine \glü-'kō-sə-ˌmēn, -zə-\ n : an amino derivative $C_6H_{13}NO_5$ of glucose that occurs esp. as a constituent of various polysaccharides that are components of structural substances (as cartilage and chitin)

glu·cose \'glü-ˌkōs, -ˌkōz\ n : a sugar $C_6H_{12}O_6$ known in dextrorotatory, levorotatory, and racemic forms; *esp* : the sweet soluble dextrorotatory form that occurs widely in nature and is the usual form in which carbohydrate is assimilated by animals

glucose–1–phosphate n : an ester $C_6H_{13}O_9P$ that reacts in the presence of a phosphorylase with aldoses and ketoses to yield disaccharides or with itself in liver and muscle to yield glycogen and phosphoric acid

glucose phosphate n : a phosphate ester of glucose: as **a** : GLUCOSE-1-PHOSPHATE **b** : GLUCOSE-6-PHOSPHATE

glucose–6–phosphate n : an ester $C_6H_{13}O_9P$ that is formed from glucose and ATP in the presence of a glucokinase and that is an essential early stage in glucose metabolism

glucose–6–phosphate dehydrogenase n : an enzyme found esp. in red blood cells that dehydrogenates glucose-6-phosphate in a glucose degradation pathway alternative to the Krebs cycle

glucose–6–phosphate dehydrogenase deficiency n : a hereditary metabolic disorder affecting red blood cells that is controlled by a variable gene on the X chromosome, that is characterized by a deficiency of glucose-6-phosphate dehydrogenase conferring marked susceptibility to hemolytic anemia which may be chronic, episodic, or induced by certain foods (as broad beans) or drugs (as primaquine), and that occurs esp. in individuals of Mediterranean or African descent

glucose tolerance test n : a test of the

body's ability to metabolize glucose that involves the administration of a measured dose of glucose to the fasting stomach and the determination of glucose levels in the blood and urine at measured intervals thereafter and that is used esp. to detect diabetes mellitus

glu·co·side \'glü-kə-ˌsīd\ *n* : GLYCO-SIDE; *esp* : a glycoside that yields glucose on hydrosis — **glu·co·sid·ic** \ˌglü-kə-'si-dik\ *adj*

glu·cos·uria \ˌglü-kō-'shùr-ē-ə, -'syùr-\ *n* : GLYCOSURIA

Glu·co·trol \'glü-kə-ˌtrōl\ *trademark* — used for a preparation of glipizide

Glu·co·vance \'glü-kō-ˌvans\ *trademark* — used for a preparation of glyburide and the hydrochloride of metformin

gluc·uron·ic acid \ˌglü-kyə-'rä-nik-\ *n* : a compound $C_6H_{10}O_7$ that occurs esp. as a constituent of glycosaminoglycans (as hyaluronic acid) and combined as a glucuronide

gluc·uron·i·dase \-'rä-nə-ˌdās, -ˌdāz\ *n* : an enzyme that hydrolyzes a glucuronide

gluc·uro·nide \glü-'kyùr-ə-ˌnīd\ *n* : any of various derivatives of glucuronic acid that are formed esp. as combinations with often toxic aromatic hydroxyl compounds (as phenols) and are excreted in the urine

glue–sniffing *n* : the deliberate inhalation of volatile organic solvents from plastic glues that may result in symptoms ranging from mild euphoria to disorientation and coma

glu·ta·mate \'glü-tə-ˌmāt\ *n* : a salt or ester of glutamic acid; *esp* : one that functions as an excitatory neurotransmitter — see MONOSODIUM GLUTAMATE

glutamate dehydrogenase *n* : an enzyme present esp. in liver mitochondria and cytosol that catalyzes the oxidation of glutamate to ammonia and α-ketoglutaric acid

glu·tam·ic acid \(ˌ)glü-'ta-mik-\ *n* : a crystalline amino acid $C_5H_9NO_4$ that is widely distributed in plant and animal proteins and acts esp. in the form of a salt or ester as a neurotransmitter which excites postsynaptic neurons — abbr. *Glu*

glutamic–ox·a·lo·ace·tic transami·nase \-ˌäk-sə-lō-ə-'sē-tik-\ *n* *also* **glu·tam·ic–ox·al·ace·tic transaminase** \-ˌäk-sə-lə-'sē-tik-\ *n* : ASPARTATE AMINOTRANSFERASE

glutamic pyruvic transaminase *n* : ALANINE AMINOTRANSFERASE

glu·ta·mine \'glü-tə-ˌmēn\ *n* : a crystalline amino acid $C_5H_{10}N_2O_3$ that is found both free and in proteins in plants and animals and that yields glutamic acid and ammonia on hydrolysis — abbr. *Gln*

glu·tar·al·de·hyde \ˌglü-tə-'ral-də-ˌhīd\ *n* : a compound $C_5H_8O_2$ used esp. as a

disinfectant and in fixing biological tissues

glu·tar·ic acid \glü-ˌtar-ik-\ *n* : a crystalline acid $C_5H_8O_4$ used esp. in organic synthesis

glu·ta·thi·one \ˌglü-tə-'thī-ˌōn\ *n* : a peptide $C_{10}H_{17}N_3O_6S$ that contains one amino-acid residue each of glutamic acid, cysteine, and glycine, that occurs widely in plant and animal tissues, and that plays an important role in biological oxidation-reduction processes and as a coenzyme

glute \'glüt\ *n* : GLUTEUS; *esp* : GLUTEUS MAXIMUS — usu. used in pl.

glu·te·al \'glü-tē-əl, glü-'tē-\ *adj* : of or relating to the buttocks or the gluteus muscles

gluteal artery *n* : either of two branches of the internal iliac artery that supply the gluteal region: **a** : the largest branch of the internal iliac artery that sends branches esp. to the gluteal muscles — called also *superior gluteal artery* **b** : a branch that is distributed esp. to the buttocks and the backs of the thighs — called also *inferior gluteal artery*

gluteal nerve *n* : either of two nerves arising from the sacral plexus and supplying the gluteal muscles and adjacent parts: **a** : one arising from the posterior part of the fourth and fifth lumbar nerves and from the first sacral nerve and distributed to the gluteus muscles and to the tensor fasciae latae — called also *superior gluteal nerve* **b** : one arising from the posterior part of the fifth lumbar nerve and from the first and second sacral nerves and distributed to the gluteus maximus — called also *inferior gluteal nerve*

gluteal tuberosity *n* : the lateral ridge of the linea aspera of the femur that gives attachment to the gluteus maximus

glu·ten \'glüt-ᵊn\ *n* : a gluey protein substance esp. of wheat flour that causes dough to be sticky

gluten–sensitive enteropathy *n* : CELIAC DISEASE

glutes *pl of* GLUTE

glu·teth·i·mide \glü-'te-thə-ˌmīd, -məd\ *n* : a sedative-hypnotic drug $C_{13}H_{15}NO_2$ that has pharmacological properties similar to the barbiturates

glu·te·us \'glü-tē-əs, glü-'tē-\ *n*, *pl* **glu·tei** \'glü-tē-ˌī, -tē-ˌē; glü-'tē-ˌī\ : any of three large muscles of the buttocks: **a** : GLUTEUS MAXIMUS **b** : GLUTEUS MEDIUS **c** : GLUTEUS MINIMUS

gluteus max·i·mus \-'mak-sə-məs\ *n*, *pl* **glutei max·i·mi** \-sə-ˌmī\ : the outermost of the three muscles in each buttock that acts to extend and laterally rotate the thigh

gluteus me·di·us \-'mē-dē-əs\ *n*, *pl* **glutei me·dii** \-dē-ˌī\ : the middle of the three muscles in each buttock that acts to abduct and medially rotate the thigh

glu·te·us min·i·mus \-'mi-nə-məs\ *n, pl* **glu·tei min·i·mi** \-,mī\ : the innermost of the three muscles in each buttock that acts similarly to the gluteus medius

Gly abbr glycine

gly·bur·ide \'gli-byə-,rīd\ *n* : a sulfonylurea $C_{23}H_{28}ClN_3O_5S$ used similarly to glipizide — called also *glibenclamide*; see DIAβETA, GLUCOVANCE, MICRONASE

glyc- *or* **glyco-** *comb form* : carbohydrate and esp. sugar ⟨*glyco*protein⟩

gly·cae·mia *chiefly Brit var of* GLYCEMIA

gly·can \'glī-,kan\ *n* : POLYSACCHARIDE

gly·cat·ed hemoglobin \'glī-,kā-təd\ *n* : HEMOGLOBIN A1C

gly·ce·mia \glī-'sē-mē-ə\ *n* : the presence of glucose in the blood — **gly·ce·mic** \-'sē-mik\ *adj*

glycemic index *n* : a measure of the rate at which an ingested food causes the level of glucose in the blood to rise; *also* : a ranking of foods according to their glycemic index — abbr. *GI*

glycer- *or* **glycero-** *comb form* **1** : glycerol ⟨*glyceryl*⟩ **2** : related to glycerol or glyceric acid ⟨*glycer*aldehyde⟩

glyc·er·al·de·hyde \,gli-sə-'ral-də-,hīd\ *n* : a sweet crystalline compound $C_3H_6O_3$ that is formed as an intermediate in carbohydrate metabolism

gly·cer·ic acid \gli-'ser-ik-\ *n* : a syrupy acid $C_3H_6O_4$ obtainable by oxidation of glycerol or glyceraldehyde

glyc·er·ide \'gli-sə-,rīd\ *n* : an ester of glycerol esp. with fatty acids

glyc·er·in *or* **glyc·er·ine** \'gli-sə-rən\ *n* : GLYCEROL

glycero- — see GLYCER-

glyc·er·ol \'gli-sə-,rȯl, -,rōl\ *n* : a sweet syrupy hygroscopic alcohol $C_3H_8O_3$ containing three hydroxy groups per molecule, usu. obtained by the saponification of fats, and used as a moistening agent, emollient, and lubricant, and as an emulsifying agent — called also *glycerin*

glyc·er·yl \'gli-sə-rəl\ *n* : a radical derived from glycerol by removal of hydroxide; *esp* : a trivalent radical CH_2CHCH_2

glyceryl guai·a·co·late \-'gwī-ə-,kò-,lāt, -'gī-, -kə-\ *n* : GUAIFENESIN

gly·cine \'glī-,sēn, 'glīs-ᵊn\ *n* : a sweet nonessential amino acid $C_2H_5NO_2$ that is a neurotransmitter which induces inhibition of postsynaptic neurons, is obtained by hydrolysis of proteins or is prepared synthetically, and is used in the form of its salt as an antacid — abbr. *Gly*

gly·cin·uria \,glīs-ᵊn-'ür-ē-ə, -'yūr-\ *n* : a kidney disorder characterized by the presence of excessive amounts of glycine in the urine

glyco- — see GLYC-

gly·co·bi·ar·sol \,glī-kō-(,)bī-'är-,sȯl, -,sȯl\ *n* : an antiprotozoal drug $C_8H_9AsBiNO_6$

gly·co·chol·ic acid \,glī-kō-'kä-lik-, -'kō-\ *n* : a crystalline acid $C_{26}H_{43}NO_6$ that occurs in bile

gly·co·con·ju·gate \,glī-kō-'kän-ji-gət, -,gāt\ *n* : any of a group of compounds (as the glycolipids and glycoproteins) consisting of sugars linked to proteins or lipids

gly·co·gen \'glī-kə-jən\ *n* : a white amorphous tasteless polysaccharide $(C_6H_{10}O_5)_x$ that constitutes the principal form in which carbohydrate is stored in animal tissues and esp. in muscle and liver tissue — called also *animal starch*

gly·co·ge·nase \glī-'kä-jə-,nās, -,nāz\ *n* : an enzyme that catalyzes the hydrolysis of glycogen

gly·co·gen·e·sis \,glī-kə-'je-nə-səs\ *n, pl* **-e·ses** \-,sēz\ : the formation and storage of glycogen — compare GLYCOGENOLYSIS

gly·co·gen·ic \-'je-nik\ *adj* : of, relating to, or involving glycogen or glycogenesis

gly·co·gen·ol·y·sis \,glī-kə-jə-'nä-lə-səs\ *n, pl* **-y·ses** \-,sēz\ : the breakdown of glycogen esp. to glucose in the body — compare GLYCOGENESIS — **gly·co·gen·o·lyt·ic** \-jən-ᵊl-'i-tik, -,jen-\ *adj*

gly·co·ge·no·sis \-jē-'nō-səs\ *n, pl* **-no·ses** \-,sēz\ : GLYCOGEN STORAGE DISEASE

glycogen storage disease *n* : any of several metabolic disorders (as McArdle's disease or Pompe's disease) that are characterized esp. by abnormal deposits of glycogen in tissue, are caused by enzyme deficiencies in glycogen metabolism, and are usu. inherited as an autosomal recessive trait

gly·co·he·mo·glo·bin \-'hē-mə-,glō-bən\ *n* : HEMOGLOBIN A1C

gly·col·ic acid *also* **gly·col·lic acid** \glī-'kä-lik-\ *n* : an alpha hydroxy acid $C_2H_4O_3$ that is used in chemical peels and that is the major toxic metabolite in ethylene glycol poisoning — called also *hydroxyacetic acid*

gly·co·lip·id \,glī-kō-'li-pəd\ *n* : a lipid (as a ganglioside or a cerebroside) that contains a carbohydrate radical

gly·col·y·sis \glī-'kä-lə-səs\ *n, pl* **-y·ses** \-,sēz\ : the enzymatic breakdown of a carbohydrate (as glucose) by way of phosphate derivatives with the production of pyruvic or lactic acid and energy stored in high-energy phosphate bonds of ATP — **gly·co·lyt·ic** \,glī-kə-'li-tik\ *adj* — **gly·co·lyt·i·cal·ly** *adv*

gly·co·pep·tide \,glī-kō-'pep-,tīd\ *n* : GLYCOPROTEIN

gly·co·pro·tein \-'prō-,tēn, -'prō-tē-ən\ *n* : a conjugated protein in which the nonprotein group is a carbohydrate — compare MUCOPROTEIN

gly·co·pyr·ro·late \-'pī-rə-,lāt\ *n* : a

synthetic anticholinergic drug $C_{19}H_{28}BrNO_3$ used in the treatment of gastrointestinal disorders (as peptic ulcer) esp. when associated with hyperacidity, hypermotility, or spasm — see ROBINUL

gly·cos·ami·no·gly·can \ˌglī-kō-sə-ˌmē-nō-ˈglī-ˌkan, -kō-ˌsa-mə-nō-\ *n* : any of various polysaccharides derived from an amino hexose that are constituents of mucoproteins, glycoproteins, and blood-group substances — called also *mucopolysaccharide*

gly·co·side \ˈglī-kə-ˌsīd\ *n* : any of numerous sugar derivatives that contain a nonsugar group attached through an oxygen or nitrogen bond and that on hydrolysis yield a sugar (as glucose) — **gly·co·sid·ic** \ˌglī-kə-ˈsi-dik\ *adj* — **gly·co·sid·i·cal·ly** *adv*

gly·co·sphin·go·lip·id \ˌglī-kō-ˌsfiŋ-gō-ˈli-pəd\ *n* : any of various lipids (as a cerebroside or a ganglioside) which are derivatives of ceramides and some of which accumulate in disorders of lipid metabolism (as Tay-Sachs disease)

gly·cos·uria \ˌglī-kō-ˈshùr-ē-ə, -ˈsyùr-\ *n* : the presence in the urine of abnormal amounts of sugar — called also *glucosuria* — **gly·cos·uric** \-ˈshùr-ik, -ˈsyùr-\ *adj*

gly·co·syl·at·ed hemoglobin \glī-ˈkō-sə-ˌlā-təd-\ *n* : HEMOGLOBIN A1C

glyc·yr·rhi·za \ˌgli-sə-ˈrī-zə\ *n* : the dried root of a licorice (*Glycyrrhiza glabra* of the legume family, Leguminosae) that is a source of extracts used to mask unpleasant flavors (as in drugs) or to give a pleasant taste (as to confections) — called also *licorice, licorice root*

gm *abbr* gram

GM and S *abbr* General Medicine and Surgery

GM–CSF *abbr* granulocyte-macrophage colony-stimulating factor

GN *abbr* graduate nurse

gnat \ˈnat\ *n* : any of various small usu. biting dipteran flies (as a midge or blackfly)

gna·thi·on \ˈnā-thē-ˌän, ˈna-\ *n* : the midpoint of the lower border of the human mandible

gna·thos·to·mi·a·sis \nə-ˌthäs-tə-ˈmī-ə-səs\ *n, pl* **-a·ses** \-ˌsēz\ : infestation with or disease caused by nematode worms (genus *Gnathostoma*) commonly acquired by eating raw fish

-g·na·thous \g-nə-thəs\ *adj comb form* : having (such) a jaw (prognathous)

-g·no·sia \g-ˈnō-zhə\ *n comb form* : -GNOSIS (agnosia) (prosopagnosia)

-g·no·sis \g-ˈnō-səs\ *n comb form, pl* **-g·no·ses** \-ˌsēz\ : knowledge : cognition : recognition (stereognosis)

-g·nos·tic \g-ˈnäs-tik\ *adj comb form* : characterized by or relating to (such) knowledge (pharmacognostic)

-g·no·sy \g-nə-sē\ *n comb form, pl* **-g·no·sies** : -GNOSIS (pharmacognosy)

GnRH *abbr* gonadotropin-releasing hormone

goal–directed *adj* : aimed toward a goal or toward completion of a task (~ behavior)

goblet cell *n* : a mucus-secreting epithelial cell (as of columnar epithelium) that is distended with secretion or its precursors at the free end

goi·ter \ˈgȯi-tər\ *n* : an enlargement of the thyroid gland that is commonly visible as a swelling of the anterior part of the neck, that often results from insufficient intake of iodine and then is usu. accompanied by hypothyroidism, and that in other cases is associated with hyperthyroidism usu. together with toxic symptoms and exophthalmos — called also *struma* — **goi·trous** \ˈgȯi-trəs\ *also* **goi·ter·ous** \ˈgȯi-tə-rəs\ *adj*

goi·tre *chiefly Brit var of* GOITER

goi·tro·gen \ˈgȯi-trə-jən\ *n* : a substance (as thiourea or thiouracil) that induces goiter formation

goi·tro·gen·ic \ˌgȯi-trə-ˈje-nik\ *also* **goi·ter·o·gen·ic** \ˌgȯi-tə-rō-ˈje-nik\ *adj* : producing or tending to produce goiter (a ~ agent) — **goi·tro·ge·nic·i·ty** \ˌgȯi-trə-jə-ˈni-sə-tē\ *n*

gold \ˈgōld\ *n, often attrib* : a malleable ductile yellow metallic element used in the form of its salts (as gold sodium thiomalate) esp. in the treatment of rheumatoid arthritis — symbol *Au*; see ELEMENT table

golden hour *n* : the hour immediately following traumatic injury in which medical treatment to prevent irreversible internal damage and optimize the chance of survival is most effective

gold sodium thio·ma·late \-ˌthī-ō-ˈma-lāt, -ˈmā-\ *n* : a mixture of two gold salts $C_4H_3AuNa_2O_4S$ and C_4H_4-$AuNaO_4S$ injected intramuscularly esp. in the treatment of rheumatoid arthritis — called also *gold thiomalate;* see MYOCHRYSINE

gold sodium thiosulfate *n* : a soluble gold compound $Na_3Au(S_2O_3)_2 \cdot 2H_2O$ administered by intravenous injection in the treatment of rheumatoid arthritis and lupus erythematosus

gold thio·glu·cose \-ˌthī-ō-ˈglü-ˌkōs\ *n* : an organic compound of gold $C_6H_{11}AuO_5S$ injected intramuscularly in the treatment of active rheumatoid arthritis and nondisseminated lupus erythematosus — called also *aurothioglucose*

Gol·gi \ˈgȯl-(ˌ)jē\ *adj* : of or relating to the Golgi apparatus, Golgi bodies, or the Golgi method of staining nerve tissue

Golgi, Camillo (1843 *or* 1844–1926), Italian histologist and pathologist.

Golgi apparatus *n* : a cytoplasmic organelle that consists of a stack of smooth membranous saccules and associated vesicles and that is active in the modification and transport of proteins — called also *Golgi complex*

Golgi body *n* : GOLGI APPARATUS; *also* : DICTYOSOME

Golgi cell *n* : a neuron with short dendrites and with either a long axon or an axon that breaks into processes soon after leaving the cell body

Golgi complex *n* : GOLGI APPARATUS

Golgi tendon organ *n* : a spindle-shaped sensory end organ within a tendon that provides information about muscle tension — called also *neurotendinous spindle*

go·mer \'gō-mər\ *n, med slang, usu disparaging* : a chronic problem patient who does not respond to treatment

gom·pho·sis \gäm-'fō-səs\ *n* : an immovable articulation in which a hard part is received into a bone cavity (as the teeth into the jaws)

go·nad \'gō-,nad\ *n* : a gamete-producing reproductive gland (as an ovary or testis) — **go·nad·al** \gō-'nad-ᵊl\ *adj*

go·nad·o·troph \gō-'nad-ə-,trōf\ *n* : a cell of the adenohypophysis that secretes a gonadotropic hormone (as luteinizing hormone)

go·nad·o·trop·ic \gō-,na-də-'trä-pik\ *also* **go·nad·o·tro·phic** \-'trō-fik, -'trä-\ *adj* : acting on or stimulating the gonads

go·nad·o·tro·pin \-'trō-pən\ *also* **go·nad·o·tro·phin** \-fən\ *n* : a gonadotropic hormone (as follicle-stimulating hormone) — see HUMAN CHORIONIC GONADOTROPIN

gonadotropin–releasing hormone *n* : a hormone produced by the hypothalamus that stimulates the adenohypophysis to release gonadotropins (as luteinizing hormone and follicle-stimulating hormone) — abbr. *GnRH*; called also *luteinizing hormone-releasing hormone*

G₁ phase \,jē-'wən-\ *n* : the period in the cell cycle from the end of cell division to the beginning of DNA replication — compare G₂ PHASE, M PHASE, S PHASE

goni- *or* **gonio-** *comb form* : corner : angle ⟨*gonio*meter⟩

gonial angle *n* : the angle formed by the junction of the posterior and lower borders of the human lower jaw — called also *angle of the jaw, angle of the mandible*

go·ni·om·e·ter \,gō-nē-'ä-mə-tər\ *n* : an instrument for measuring angles (as of a joint or the skull) — **go·nio·met·ric** \-nē-ə-'me-trik\ *adj* — **go·ni·om·e·try** \-nē-'ä-mə-trē\ *n*

go·nio·punc·ture \'gō-nē-ə-,pəŋk-chər\ *n* : a surgical operation for congenital glaucoma that involves making a puncture into the sclera with a knife at the site of discharge of aqueous fluid at the periphery of the anterior chamber of the eye

go·ni·o·scope \-,skōp\ *n* : an instrument consisting of a contact lens to be fitted over the cornea and an optical system with which the interior of the eye can be viewed — **go·ni·os·co·py** \,gō-nē-'äs-kə-pē\ *n*

go·ni·ot·o·my \,gō-nē-'ä-tə-mē\ *n, pl* **-mies** : surgical relief of glaucoma used in some congenital types and achieved by opening the canal of Schlemm

go·ni·tis \gō-'nī-təs\ *n* : inflammation of the knee

gono·coc·cae·mia *chiefly Brit var of* GONOCOCCEMIA

gono·coc·ce·mia \,gä-nə-,käk-'sē-mē-ə\ *n* : the presence of gonococci in the blood — **gono·coc·ce·mic** \-'sē-mik\ *adj*

gono·coc·cus \,gä-nə-'kä-kəs\ *n, pl* **-coc·ci** \-'käk-,sī, -,sē; -'kä-,kī, -,kē\ : a pus-producing bacterium of the genus *Neisseria* (*N. gonorrhoeae*) that causes gonorrhea — **gono·coc·cal** \-'kä-kəl\ *adj*

gon·or·rhea \,gä-nə-'rē-ə\ *n* : a contagious inflammation of the genital mucous membrane caused by the gonococcus — called also *clap* — **gon·or·rhe·al** \-'rē-əl\ *adj*

gon·or·rhoea *chiefly Brit var of* GONORRHEA

-g·o·ny \gə-nē\ *n comb form, pl* **-g·o·nies** : manner of generation or reproduction ⟨schizo*gony*⟩

go·ny·au·lax \,gō-nē-'ò-,laks\ *n* **1** *cap* : a large genus of phosphorescent marine dinoflagellates that when unusually abundant cause red tide **2** : any dinoflagellate of the genus *Gonyaulax*

good cholesterol *n* : HDL

Good·pas·ture's syndrome \'gùd-,pas-chərz-\ *also* **Good·pas·ture syndrome** \-chər-\ *n* : an autoimmune disorder of unknown cause that is characterized by the presence of circulating antibodies in the blood which attack the basement membrane of the kidney's glomeruli and the lung's alveoli and that is marked initially by coughing, fatigue, difficulty in breathing, and hemoptysis progressing to glomerulonephritis and pulmonary hemorrhages

Goodpasture, Ernest William (1886–1960), American pathologist.

goose bumps *n pl* : a roughness of the skin produced by erection of its papillae esp. from cold, fear, or a sudden feeling of excitement — called also *goose pimples*

goose-flesh \-,flesh\ *n* : GOOSE BUMPS

gork \'gòrk\ *n, med slang, usu disparaging* : a terminal patient whose brain is nonfunctional and the rest of whose body can be kept functioning only by the extensive use of mechanical devices and nutrient solutions — **gorked** \'gòrkt\ *adj, med slang*

goun·dou \'gün-(,)dü\ *n* : a tumorous swelling of the nose often considered a late lesion of yaws — compare GANGOSA

gout \'gaùt\ *n* : a metabolic disease

marked by a painful inflammation of the joints, deposits of urates in and around the joints, and usu. an excessive amount of uric acid in the blood — **gouty** \'gau̇-tē\ *adj*

gouty arthritis *n* : arthritis associated with gout and caused by the deposition of urate crystals in the articular cartilage of joints

GP *abbr* general practitioner

G₁ phase, G₂ phase — see entries alphabetized as G ONE PHASE, G TWO PHASE

gp120 \ˌjē-ˌpē-ˌwən-'twen-tē\ *n* : a glycoprotein that protrudes from the outer surface of the HIV virion and that must bind to a CD4 receptor on a T cell bearing such receptors before infection of the cell can occur

G protein \'jē-\ *n* : any of a class of cell membrane proteins that are coupled to cell surface receptors and upon stimulation of the receptor by a molecule (as a hormone) bind to GTP to form an active complex which mediates an intracellular event

gr *abbr* **1** grain **2** gram **3** gravity

graaf·ian follicle \'grä-fē-ən-, 'gra-\ *n, often cap G* : a mature follicle in a mammalian ovary that contains a liquid-filled cavity and that ruptures during ovulation to release an egg — called also *vesicular ovarian follicle*

de Graaf \də-'gräf\, **Reinier (1641–1673),** Dutch physician and anatomist.

grac·ile fasciculus \'gra-səl-, -ˌsīl-\ *n, pl* **gracile fasciculi** : FASCICULUS GRACILIS

grac·i·lis \'gra-sə-ləs\ *n* : the most superficial muscle of the inside of the thigh that acts to adduct the thigh and to flex the leg at the knee and assist in rotating it medially

grade \'grād\ *n* : a degree of severity of a disease or abnormal condition ⟨a ∼ III carcinoma⟩

gra·di·ent echo \'grä-dē-ənt-'e-kō\ *n* : a signal that is detected in a nuclear magnetic resonance spectrometer that is analogous to a spin echo but is produced by varying the magnetic field following application of a single radio-frequency pulse rather than by application of a series of radio-frequency pulses — usu. used attributively ⟨*gradient-echo* magnetic resonance imaging⟩; called also *gradient-recalled echo*

graduate nurse *n* : a person who has completed the regular course of study and practical hospital training in nursing school — abbr. *GN;* called also *trained nurse*

Graf·en·berg spot \'gra-fən-bərg-\ *n* : G-SPOT

Gräf·en·berg \'gre-fən-ˌberk\, **Ernst (1881–1957),** American (German-born) gynecologist.

¹**graft** \'graft\ *vb* : to implant (living tissue) surgically

²**graft** *n* **1** : the act of grafting **2** : something grafted; *specif* : living tissue used in grafting

graft–versus–host *adj* : of, relating to, or caused by graft-versus-host disease

graft–versus–host disease *n* : a bodily condition that results when T cells from a usu. allogeneic tissue or organ transplant and esp. a bone marrow transplant react immunologically against the recipient's antigens attacking cells and tissues (as of the skin and liver) and that may be fatal — abbr. *GVHD;* called also *graft-versus-host reaction*

grain \'grān\ *n* : a unit of avoirdupois, Troy, and apothecaries' weight equal to 0.0648 gram or 0.002286 avoirdupois ounce or 0.002083 Troy ounce — abbr. *gr*

grain alcohol *n* : ETHANOL

grain itch *n* : an itching rash caused by the bite of a mite of the genus *Pyemotes* (*P. ventricosus*) that occurs chiefly on grain, straw, or straw products — compare GROCER'S ITCH

gram \'gram\ *n* : a metric unit of mass equal to ¹/₁₀₀₀ kilogram and nearly equal to the mass of one cubic centimeter of water at its maximum density — abbr. *g*

-gram \ˌgram\ *n comb form* : drawing : writing : record ⟨cardio*gram*⟩

gram calorie *n* : CALORIE la

gram·i·ci·din \ˌgra-mə-'sīd-²n\ *n* : an antibacterial mixture produced by a soil bacterium of the genus *Bacillus* (*B. brevis*) and used topically against gram-positive bacteria in local infections esp. of the eye

gramme *chiefly Brit var of* GRAM

gram–negative *adj* : not holding the purple dye when stained by Gram's stain — used chiefly of bacteria

gram–positive *adj* : holding the purple dye when stained by Gram's stain — used chiefly of bacteria

Gram's solution \'gramz-\ *n* : a watery solution of iodine and the iodide of potassium used in staining bacteria by Gram's stain

Gram \'gräm\, **Hans Christian Joachim (1853–1938),** Danish physician.

Gram's stain *or* **Gram stain** \'gram-\ *n* **1** : a method for the differential staining of bacteria by treatment with Gram's solution after staining with a triphenylmethane dye — called also *Gram's method* **2** : the chemicals used in Gram's stain

gram–variable *adj* : staining irregularly or inconsistently by Gram's stain

gran·di·ose \'gran-dē-ˌōs, ˌgran-dē-'\ *adj* : characterized by affectation of grandeur or splendor or by absurd exaggeration ⟨∼ delusions⟩ — **gran·di·os·i·ty** \ˌgran-dē-'äs-ət-ē\ *n*

grand mal \'grän-ˌmäl, 'grän-, 'grand-, -'mal\ *n* : severe epilepsy characterized by tonic-clonic seizures; *also* : a tonic-clonic seizure

grand rounds *n pl* : rounds involving the formal presentation by an expert of a clinical issue sometimes in the presence of selected patients

granul- *or* **granuli-** *or* **granulo-** *comb form* \\'gran-yə-lər\\

gran·u·lar \\'gran-yə-lər\\ *adj* **1** : consisting of or appearing to consist of granules; *esp* : characterized by or being cytoplasm which contains granules ⟨∼ cells⟩ **2** : having or marked by granulations ⟨∼ tissue⟩ — **gran·u·lar·i·ty** \\,gran-yə-'lar-ə-tē\\ *n*

granular conjunctivitis *n* : TRACHOMA

gran·u·late \\'gran-yə-,lāt\\ *vb* **-lat·ed; -lat·ing** **1** : to form or crystallize (as sugar) into grains or granules **2** : to form granulations ⟨a *granulating* wound⟩

gran·u·la·tion \\,gran-yə-'lā-shən\\ *n* **1** : the act or process of granulating **2** : the condition of being granulated **2 a** (1) : a minute mass of tissue projecting from the surface of an organ (as on the eyelids in trachoma) (2) : one of the minute red granules made up of loops of newly formed capillaries that form on a raw surface (as of a wound) and that with fibroblasts are the active agents in the process of healing — see GRANULATION TISSUE **b** : the act or process of forming such elevations or granules

granulation tissue *n* : tissue made up of granulations that temporarily replaces lost tissue in a wound

gran·ule \\'gran-(,)yül\\ *n* : a little grain or small particle; *esp* : one of a number of particles forming a larger unit

granule cell *n* : one of the small neurons of the cortex of the cerebellum and cerebrum

granuli- — see GRANUL-

granulo- — see GRANUL-

gran·u·lo·cyte \\'gran-yə-lō-,sīt\\ *n* : a polymorphonuclear white blood cell (as an eosinophil or neutrophil) with granule-containing cytoplasm — compare AGRANULOCYTE — **gran·u·lo·cyt·ic** \\,gran-yə-lō-'si-tik\\ *adj*

granulocyte colony–stimulating factor *n* : a colony-stimulating factor that acts to promote the maturation of precursor cells into granulocytes — abbr. *G-CSF*

granulocyte–macrophage colony–stimulating factor *n* : a colony-stimulating factor that promotes the differentiation of bone marrow stem cells, stimulates the maturation of precursor cells into granulocytes and macrophages, and activates mature macrophages — abbr. *GM-CSF*

granulocytic leukemia *n* : MYELOGENOUS LEUKEMIA

gran·u·lo·cy·to·pe·nia \\,gran-yə-lō-,sī-tə-'pē-nē-ə\\ *n* : deficiency of blood granulocytes; *esp* : AGRANULOCYTO-

SIS — **gran·u·lo·cy·to·pe·nic** \\-'pē-nik\\ *adj*

gran·u·lo·cy·to·poi·e·sis \\-,sī-tə-pói-'ē-səs\\ *n, pl* **-e·ses** \\-,sēz\\ : GRANULOPOIESIS

gran·u·lo·cy·to·sis \\,gran-yə-lō-,sī-'tō-səs\\ *n, pl* **-to·ses** \\-,sēz\\ : an increase in the number of blood granulocytes — compare LYMPHOCYTOSIS, MONOCYTOSIS

gran·u·lo·ma \\,gran-yə-'lō-mə\\ *n, pl* **-mas** *also* **-ma·ta** \\-mə-tə\\ : a mass or nodule of chronically inflamed tissue with granulations that is usu. associated with an infective process

granuloma an·nu·la·re \\-,a-nyü-'lar-ē\\ *n* : a benign chronic rash of unknown cause characterized by one or more flat spreading ringlike spots with lighter centers esp. on the feet, legs, hands, or fingers

granuloma in·gui·na·le \\-,iŋ-gwə-'na-lē, -'nä-, -'nā-\\ *n* : a sexually transmitted disease characterized by ulceration and formation of granulations on the genitalia and in the groin area and caused by a bacterium of the genus *Calymmatobacterium* (*C. granulomatis* syn. *Donovania granulomatis*)

gran·u·lo·ma·to·sis \\,gran-yə-,lō-mə-'tō-səs\\ *n, pl* **-to·ses** \\-,sēz\\ : a chronic condition marked by the formation of numerous granulomas

gran·u·lo·ma·tous \\-'lō-mə-təs\\ *adj* : of, relating to, or characterized by granuloma — see CHRONIC GRANULOMATOUS DISEASE

gran·u·lo·poi·e·sis \\-(,)lō-,pói-'ē-səs\\ *n, pl* **-e·ses** \\-,sēz\\ : the formation of blood granulocytes typically in the bone marrow — **gran·u·lo·poi·et·ic** \\-,pói-'e-tik\\ *adj*

gran·u·lo·sa cell \\,gran-yə-'lō-sə-, -zə-\\ *n* : one of the estrogen-secreting cells of the epithelial lining of a graafian follicle or its follicular precursor

granulosum — see STRATUM GRANULOSUM

grapes \\'grāps\\ *n pl* **1** : a cluster of raw red nodules of granulation tissue in the hollow of the fetlock of horses that is characteristic of advanced or chronic grease heel **2** : tuberculous disease of the pleura in cattle — usu. used with a sing. verb; called also *grape disease*

grape sugar *n* : DEXTROSE

-graph \\,graf\\ *n comb form* **1** : something written ⟨monograph⟩ **2** : instrument for making or transmitting records ⟨electrocardiograph⟩

-gra·phia \\'gra-fē-ə\\ *n comb form* : writing characteristic of a (specified) usu. psychological abnormality ⟨dysgraphia⟩ ⟨dermographia⟩

grapho- *comb form* : writing ⟨graphology⟩

gra·phol·o·gy \\gra-'fä-lə-jē\\ *n, pl* **-gies** : the study of handwriting esp. for the purpose of character analysis — **graph·o·log·i·cal** \\,gra-fə-'lä-ji-kəl\\

adj — **gra·phol·o·gist** \gra-'fä-lə-jist\ *n*

grapho·ma·nia \ˌgra-fō-'mā-nē-ə, -nyə\ *n* : a compulsive urge to write — **grapho·ma·ni·ac** \-nē-ˌak\ *n*

grapho·spasm \'gra-fə-ˌspa-zəm\ *n* : WRITER'S CRAMP

gras — see TULLE GRAS

GRAS *abbr* generally recognized as safe

grass \'gras\ *n* : MARIJUANA

grass sickness *n* : a frequently fatal disease of grazing horses of unknown cause that affects gastrointestinal functioning by causing difficulty in swallowing, interruption of peristalsis, and fecal impaction — called also *grass disease*

grass staggers *n* : GRASS TETANY

grass tetany *n* : a disease of cattle and esp. milk cows marked by tetanic staggering, convulsions, coma, and frequently death and caused by reduction of blood calcium and magnesium when overeating on lush pasture — called also *hypomagnesia*

grav *abbr* gravida

grave \'grāv\ *adj* : very serious : dangerous to life — used of an illness or its prospects ⟨a ∼ prognosis⟩

grav·el \'gra-vəl\ *n* 1 : a deposit of small calculous concretions in the kidneys and urinary bladder 2 : the condition that results from the presence of deposits of gravel

Graves' disease \'grāvz-\ *n* : a common form of hyperthyroidism characterized by goiter and often a slight protrusion of the eyeballs — called also *Basedow's disease, exophthalmic goiter*

Graves, Robert James (1796–1853), British physician.

grav·id \'gra-vəd\ *adj* : PREGNANT

grav·i·da \'gra-və-də\ *n, pl* **-das** *also* **-dae** \-ˌdē\ : a pregnant woman — often used in combination with a number or figure to indicate the number of pregnancies a woman has had ⟨a ∼ four⟩; compare PARA — **grav·id·ic** \gra-'vi-dik\ *adj*

gravidarum — see HYPEREMESIS GRAVIDARUM

gra·vid·i·ty \gra-'vi-də-tē\ *n, pl* **-ties** 1 : PREGNANCY 2 : the number of times a female has been pregnant — compare PARITY 2

gravior — see ICHTHYOSIS HYSTRIX GRAVIOR

gravis — see ICTERUS GRAVIS, ICTERUS GRAVIS NEONATORUM, MYASTHENIA GRAVIS

grav·i·ta·tion \ˌgra-və-'tā-shən\ *n* : a natural force of attraction that tends to draw bodies together and that occurs because of the mass of the bodies — **grav·i·ta·tion·al** \-shə-nəl\ *adj* — **grav·i·ta·tion·al·ly** *adv*

gravitational field *n* : the space around an object having mass in which the object's gravitational influence can be detected

grav·i·ty \'gra-və-tē\ *n, pl* **-ties** : the gravitational attraction of the mass of a celestial object (as earth) for bodies close to it; *also* : GRAVITATION

gravity drip *n* : the administration of a fluid into the body using an apparatus in which gravity provides the force moving the fluid

gray \'grā\ *n* : the mks unit of absorbed dose of ionizing radiation equal to an energy of one joule per kilogram of irradiated material — abbr. *Gy*

Gray, Louis Harold (1905–1965), British radiobiologist.

gray column *n* : any of the longitudinal columns of gray matter in each lateral half of the spinal cord — called also *gray horn;* compare COLUMN a

gray commissure *n* : a transverse band of gray matter in the spinal cord appearing in sections as the transverse bar of the H-shaped mass of gray matter

gray matter *n* : neural tissue esp. of the brain and spinal cord that contains cell bodies as well as nerve fibers, has a brownish gray color, and forms most of the cortex and nuclei of the brain, the columns of the spinal cord, and the bodies of ganglia — called also *gray substance*

gray·out \'grā-ˌaůt\ *n* : a transient dimming or haziness of vision resulting from temporary impairment of cerebral circulation — compare BLACKOUT, REDOUT — **gray out** *vb*

gray ramus *n* : RAMUS COMMUNICANS b

gray substance *n* : GRAY MATTER

gray syndrome *n* : a potentially fatal toxic reaction to chloramphenicol esp. in premature infants that is characterized by abdominal distension, cyanosis, vasomotor collapse, and irregular respiration

GRE *abbr* gradient echo; gradient-recalled echo

grease heel *n* : a chronic inflammation of the skin of the fetlocks and pasterns of horses marked by an excess of oily secretion, ulcerations, and in severe cases general swelling of the legs, nodular excrescences, and a foul-smelling discharge — called also *greasy heel;* see GRAPES 1

great cerebral vein *n* : a broad unpaired vein formed by the junction of Galen's veins and uniting with the inferior sagittal sinus to form the straight sinus

greater cornu *n* : THYROHYAL

greater curvature *n* : the boundary of the stomach that forms a long usu. convex curve on the left from the opening for the esophagus to the opening into the duodenum — compare LESSER CURVATURE

greater multangular *n* : TRAPEZIUM — called also *greater multangular bone*

greater occipital nerve n : OCCIPITAL NERVE a

greater omentum n : a part of the peritoneum attached to the greater curvature of the stomach and to the colon and hanging down over the small intestine — called also *caul;* compare LESSER OMENTUM

greater palatine artery n : PALATINE ARTERY 1b

greater palatine foramen n : a foramen in each posterior side of the palate giving passage to the greater palatine artery and to a palatine nerve

greater petrosal nerve n : a mixed nerve that arises in the geniculate ganglion, joins with the deep petrosal nerve at the entrance of the pterygoid canal to form the Vidian nerve, and as part of this nerve sends sensory fibers to the soft palate with some to the eustachian tube and sends parasympathetic fibers forming the motor root of the pterygopalatine ganglion — called also *greater superficial petrosal nerve*

greater sciatic foramen n : SCIATIC FORAMEN a

greater sciatic notch n : SCIATIC NOTCH a

greater splanchnic nerve n : SPLANCHNIC NERVE a

greater superficial petrosal nerve n : GREATER PETROSAL NERVE

greater trochanter *also* **great trochanter** n : TROCHANTER a

greater tubercle n : a prominence on the upper lateral part of the end of the humerus that serves as the insertion for the supraspinatus, infraspinatus, and teres minor — compare LESSER TUBERCLE

greater vestibular gland n : BARTHOLIN'S GLAND

greater wing *also* **great wing** n : a broad curved winglike expanse on each side of the sphenoid bone — called also *alisphenoid;* compare LESSER WING

great ragweed n : RAGWEED b

great saphenous vein n : SAPHENOUS VEIN a

great toe n : BIG TOE

great white shark n : a large shark (*Carcharodon carcharias* of the family Lamnidae) that is bluish when young but becomes whitish with age and has been known to attack humans — called also *white shark*

green \'grēn\ *adj* **1** *of a wound:* being recently incurred and unhealed **2** *of hemolytic streptococci* : tending to produce green pigment when cultured on blood media

green monkey n : a long-tailed African monkey (*Cercopithecus aethiops*) having greenish-appearing hair and often used in medical research — called also *vervet*

green monkey disease n : MARBURG FEVER

green·sick·ness \'grēn‚sik-nəs\ n : CHLOROSIS — **green-sick** *adj*

green soap n : a soft soap made from vegetable oils and used esp. in the treatment of skin diseases

green·stick fracture \'grēn‚stik-\ n : a bone fracture in a young individual in which the bone is partly broken and partly bent

grew *past of* GROW

grey·out *chiefly Brit var of* GRAYOUT

¹gripe \'grīp\ *vb* **griped; grip·ing** : to cause or experience pinching and spasmodic pain in the bowels of

²gripe n : a pinching spasmodic intestinal pain — used in pl.

grippe \'grip\ n : an acute febrile contagious virus disease; *esp* : INFLUENZA 1a — **grippy** \'gri-pē\ *adj*

gris·eo·ful·vin \‚gri-zē-ō-'fůl-vən,-sē-, -'fəl-\ n : a fungistatic antibiotic $C_{17}H_{17}ClO_6$ used systemically in treating superficial infections by fungi esp. of the genera *Epidermophyton, Microsporum,* and *Trichophyton*

griseum — see INDUSIUM GRISEUM

grocer's itch n : an itching dermatitis that results from prolonged contact with some mites (esp. family Acaridae), their products, or materials infested with them — called also *baker's itch;* compare GRAIN ITCH

groin \'groin\ n : the fold or depression marking the juncture of the lower abdomen and the inner part of the thigh; *also* : the region of this line

groin pull n : a usu. sports-related injury characterized by intense pain in the region of the groin usu. due to abnormal straining or stretching of an adductor muscle of the thigh and esp. the adductor longus

groove \'grüv\ n : a long narrow depression occurring naturally on the surface of an anatomical part

gross \'grōs\ *adj* **1** : glaringly or flagrantly obvious **2** : visible without the aid of a microscope : MACROSCOPIC ⟨∼ lesions⟩ — compare OCCULT

gross anatomy n : a branch of anatomy that deals with the macroscopic structure of tissues and organs — compare HISTOLOGY — **gross anatomist** n

ground itch n : an itching inflammation of the skin marking the point of entrance into the body of larval hookworms

ground substance n : a more or less homogeneous matrix that forms the background in which the specific differentiated elements of a system are suspended: **a** : the intercellular substance of tissues **b** : CYTOSOL

Group A n : the Lancefield group of beta-hemolytic streptococci comprising all strains of a species of the genus *Streptococcus* (*S. pyogenes*) — usu. used attributively ⟨*Group A* streptococcal infection⟩

Group B n : the Lancefield group of

usu. beta-hemolytic streptococci comprising all strains of a species of the genus *Streptococcus* (*S. agalactiae*) — usu. used attributively ⟨*Group B* streptococcal sepsis of neonates⟩

group dynamics *n sing or pl* : the interacting forces within a small human group; *also* : the sociological study of these forces

group home *n* : a residence for persons (as developmentally disabled individuals) requiring care, assistance, or supervision

group practice *n* : medicine practiced by a group of associated physicians or dentists (as specialists in different fields) working as partners or as partners and employees

group psychotherapy *n* : GROUP THERAPY

group therapy *n* : therapy in the presence of a therapist in which several patients discuss and share their personal problems — **group therapist** *n*

grow \'grō\ *vb* **grew** \'grü\; **grown** \'grōn\; **grow·ing** **1 a** : to spring up and develop to maturity **b** : to be able to grow in some place or situation **c** : to assume some relation through or as if through a process of natural growth ⟨the cut edges of the wound *grew* together⟩ **2** : to increase in size by addition of material by assimilation into the living organism or by accretion in a nonbiological process (as crystallization)

growing pains *n pl* : pains occurring in the legs of growing children having no demonstrable relation to growth

growth \'grōth\ *n* **1 a** (1) : a stage in the process of growing (2) : full growth **b** : the process of growing **2 a** : something that grows or has grown **b** : an abnormal proliferation of tissue (as a tumor)

growth cone *n* : the specialized motile tip of an axon of a growing or regenerating neuron

growth factor *n* : a substance (as a vitamin B_{12} or an interleukin) that promotes growth and esp. cellular growth

growth hormone *n* : a polypeptide hormone that is secreted by the anterior lobe of the pituitary gland and regulates growth; *also* : a recombinant version of this hormone — called also *somatotropic hormone*, *somatotropin*; see BOVINE GROWTH HORMONE, HUMAN GROWTH HORMONE

growth hormone–releasing hormone *n* : a neuropeptide released by the hypothalamus that stimulates the release of growth hormone — abbr. *GHRH*; called also *growth hormone-releasing factor*

growth plate *n* : the region in a long bone between the epiphysis and diaphysis where growth in length occurs — called also *physis*

g's *or* **gs** *pl of* G

G6PD *abbr* glucose-6-phosphate dehydrogenase

G–spot \'jē-ˌspät\ *n* : a mass of tissue that is held to exist in the anterior vaginal wall and to be highly erogenous — called also *Grafenberg spot*

GSR *abbr* galvanic skin response

G suit *n* : a suit designed to counteract the physiological effects of acceleration on an aviator or astronaut

GSW *abbr* gunshot wound

GTH *abbr* gonadotropic hormone

GTP \ˌjē-(ˌ)tē-ˈpē\ *n* : an energy-rich nucleotide analogous to ATP that is composed of guanine linked to ribose and three phosphate groups and is necessary for peptide-bond formation during protein synthesis — called also *guanosine triphosphate*

G_2 phase \ˌjē-ˈtü-\ *n* : the period in the cell cycle from the completion of DNA replication to the beginning of cell division — compare G_1 PHASE, M PHASE, S PHASE

GU *abbr* genitourinary

guai·ac \'gwī-ˌak\ *n* : GUAIACUM

guai·a·col \'gwī-ə-ˌkȯl, -ˌkōl\ *n* : a liquid or solid compound $C_7H_8O_2$ with an aromatic odor used chiefly as an expectorant and as a local anesthetic

guaiac test *n* : a test for blood in urine or feces using a reagent containing guaiacum that yields a blue color when blood is present — see HEMOCCULT

guai·a·cum \'gwī-ə-kəm\ *n* : a resin with a faint balsamic odor obtained as tears or masses from the trunk of either of two trees (*Guaiacum officinale* and *G. sanctum* of the family Zygophyllaceae) and used in various tests (as the guaiac test)

guai·fen·e·sin \gwī-ˈfe-nə-sən\ *n* : the glyceryl ether of guaiacol $C_{10}H_{14}O_4$ that is used esp. as an expectorant — called also *glyceryl guaiacolate*

gua·neth·i·dine \gwä-ˈne-thə-ˌdēn\ *n* : a drug used esp. in the form of its sulfate $C_{10}H_{22}N_4 \cdot H_2SO_4$ in treating severe high blood pressure

gua·ni·dine \'gwä-nə-ˌdēn\ *n* : a base CH_5N_3 that is derived from guanine and is used in the form of its hydrochloride $CH_5N_3 \cdot HCl$ to enhance acetylcholine activity

gua·nine \'gwä-ˌnēn\ *n* : a purine base $C_5H_5N_5O$ that codes genetic information in the polynucleotide chain of DNA or RNA — compare ADENINE, CYTOSINE, THYMINE, URACIL

gua·no·sine \'gwä-nə-ˌsēn\ *n* : a nucleoside $C_{10}H_{13}N_5O_5$ composed of guanine and ribose

guanosine 3′, 5′–monophosphate *n* : CYCLIC GMP

guanosine triphosphate *n* : GTP

gua·nyl·ate cy·clase \'gwän-ᵊl-ˌāt-ˈsī-ˌklās, -ˌklāz\ *n* : an enzyme that catalyzes the formation of cyclic GMP from GTP

guard·ing \'gär-diŋ\ *n* : involuntary reaction to protect an area of pain (as by spasm of muscle on palpation of the abdomen over a painful lesion)

gu·ber·nac·u·lum \ˌgü-bər-ˈna-kyü-ləm\ *n, pl* **-la** \-lə\ : a fibrous cord that connects the fetal testis with the bottom of the scrotum and by failing to elongate in proportion to the rest of the fetus causes the descent of the testis

guide \ˈgīd\ *n* : a grooved director for a surgical probe or knife

guided imagery *n* : any of various techniques (as a series of verbal suggestions) used to guide another person or oneself in imagining sensations and esp. in visualizing an image in the mind to bring about a desired physical response (as a reduction in stress, anxiety, or pain)

Guil·lain–Bar·ré syndrome \ˌgē-ˈlan-ˌbä-ˈrā-, ˌgē-ˈyaⁿ-\ *n* : a polyneuritis of unknown cause characterized esp. by muscle weakness and paralysis — called also *Landry's paralysis*

   Guillain \gē-ˈyaⁿ\, **Georges Charles (1876–1961),** and **Barré** \bä-ˈrā\, **Jean Alexander (1880–1967),** French neurologists.

guil·lo·tine \ˈgi-lə-ˌtēn, ˈgē-ə-\ *n* : a surgical instrument that consists of a ring and handle with a knife blade which slides down the handle and across the ring and that is used for cutting out a protruding structure (as a tonsil) capable of being placed in the ring

   Guil·lo·tin \gē-yȯ-ˈtaⁿ\, **Joseph-Ignace (1738–1814),** French surgeon.

guillotine amputation *n* : an emergency surgical amputation (as of a leg) in which the skin is incised around the part being amputated and is allowed to retract, successive layers of muscle are then divided around the part, and finally the bone is divided

guilt \ˈgilt\ *n* : feelings of culpability esp. for imagined offenses or from a sense of inadequacy : morbid self-reproach often manifest in marked preoccupation with the moral correctness of one's behavior

guin·ea worm \ˈgi-nē-\ *n* : a slender tropical nematode worm of the genus *Dracunculus* (*D. medinensis*) that has an adult female that may attain a length of several feet and is characterized by a life cycle which includes larval development in small freshwater crustaceans (genus *Cyclops* of the order Copepoda), ingestion by humans in contaminated drinking water, passage from the intestine to the thorax and abdomen for maturation and mating, and migration of gravid females to subcutaneous tissues and then out through the skin — called also *Medina worm*

guinea worm disease *n* : DRACUNCULIASIS

Gulf War syndrome *n* : a syndrome of

uncertain cause including fatigue, joint pain, memory loss, skin rash, and headache that has been reported in veterans of the war fought in the Persian Gulf in 1991

gul·let \ˈgə-lət\ *n* : ESOPHAGUS; *broadly* : THROAT

gum \ˈgəm\ *n* : the tissue that surrounds the necks of teeth and covers the alveolar parts of the jaws; *broadly* : the alveolar portion of a jaw with its enveloping soft tissues

gum ar·a·bic \-ˈar-ə-bik\ *n* : a water-soluble gum obtained from several leguminous plants (genus *Acacia* and esp. *A. senegal* and *A. arabica*) and used esp. in pharmacy to suspend insoluble substances in water, to prepare emulsions, and to make pills and lozenges — called also *acacia, gum acacia*

gum·boil \ˈgəm-ˌbȯil\ *n* : an abscess in the gum

gum karaya *n* : KARAYA GUM

gum·line \ˈgəm-ˌlīn\ *n* : the line separating the gum from the exposed part of the tooth

gum·ma \ˈgə-mə\ *n, pl* **gummas** *also* **gum·ma·ta** \-mə-tə\ : a tumor of gummy or rubbery consistency that is characteristic of the tertiary stage of syphilis — **gum·ma·tous** \-mə-təs\ *adj*

gum tragacanth *n* : TRAGACANTH

gur·ney \ˈgər-nē\ *n, pl* **gurneys** : a wheeled cot or stretcher

gus·ta·tion \ˌgəs-ˈtā-shən\ *n* : the act or sensation of tasting

gus·ta·to·ry \ˈgəs-tə-ˌtȯr-ē\ *adj* : relating to, affecting, associated with, or being the sense of taste

gut \ˈgət\ *n* **1 a** : DIGESTIVE TRACT; *also* : part of the digestive tract and esp. the intestine or stomach **b** : ABDOMEN 1a, BELLY — usu. used in pl.; not often in formal use **2** : CATGUT

Guth·rie test \ˈgə-thrē-\ *n* : a test for phenylketonuria in which the plasma phenylalanine of an affected individual reverses the inhibition of a strain of bacteria of the genus *Bacillus* (*B. subtilis*) needing it for growth

   Guthrie, Robert (1916–1995), American microbiologist.

gut·ta-per·cha \ˌgə-tə-ˈpər-chə\ *n* : a tough plastic substance from the latex of several Malaysian trees (genera *Payena* and *Palaquium*) of the sapodilla family (Sapotaceae) that is used in dentistry esp. as a filling in root canals

gut·tate \ˈgə-ˌtāt\ *adj* : having small usu. colored spots or drops

gut·ter \ˈgə-tər\ *n* : a depressed furrow between body parts (as on the surface between a pair of adjacent ribs) — see PARACOLIC GUTTER

Gut·zeit test \ˈgüt-ˌsīt-\ *n* : a test for arsenic used esp. in toxicology

   Gutzeit, Ernst Wilhelm Heinrich (1845–1888), German chemist.

GVH *abbr* graft-versus-host

GVHD *abbr* graft-versus-host disease

Gy *abbr* gray

Gym·no·din·i·um \\,jim-nə-'di-nē-əm\ *n* : a large genus of marine and freshwater dinoflagellates (family Gymnodiniidae) that includes a few forms which cause red tide

gyn *abbr* gynecologic; gynecologist; gynecology

gynaec- *or* **gynaeco-** *chiefly Brit var of* GYNEC-

gy·nae·coid, gy·nae·col·o·gy *chiefly Brit var of* GYNECOID, GYNECOLOGY

gyn·an·dro·blas·to·ma \\,(,)gī-,nan-drə-bla-'stō-mə, (,)ji-, ,jī-\ *n, pl* **-mas** *also* **-ma·ta** \-mə-tə\ : a rare tumor of the ovary with both masculinizing and feminizing effects — compare ARRHENOBLASTOMA

gynec- *or* **gyneco-** *comb form* : woman ⟨*gynec*oid⟩ ⟨*gyneco*logy⟩

gy·ne·cog·ra·phy \\,gī-nə-'kä-grə-fē, ,ji-\ *n, pl* **-phies** : radiographic visualization of the female reproductive tract

gy·ne·coid \'gī-ni-,kóid, 'ji-\ *adj* **1** *of the pelvis* : having the rounded form typical of the human female — compare ANDROID, ANTHROPOID, PLATYPELLOID **2** : relating to or characterized by the distribution of body fat chiefly in the region of the hips and thighs ⟨∼ obesity⟩ — compare ANDROID

gy·ne·col·o·gist \\,gī-nə-'kä-lə-jist, ,ji-, ,jī-\ *n* : a specialist in gynecology

gy·ne·col·o·gy \\,gī-nə-'kä-lə-jē, ,ji-, ,jī-\ *n, pl* **-gies** : a branch of medicine that deals with the diseases and routine physical care of the reproductive system of women — **gy·ne·co·log·ic** \-ni-kə-'lä-jik\ *or* **gy·ne·co·log·i·cal** \-ji-kəl\ *adj*

gy·ne·co·mas·tia \'gī-nə-kō-'mas-tē-ə, 'ji-, 'jī-\ *n* : excessive development of the breast in the male

gy·noid \'gī-,nóid, 'ji-\ *adj* : GYNECOID 2

gyp·py tummy \'ji-pē-\ *n* : diarrhea contracted esp. by travelers

gy·rase \'jī-,rās, -,rāz\ *n* : a bacterial enzyme that catalyzes the breaking and rejoining of bonds linking adjacent nucleotides in circular DNA to generate supercoiled DNA helices

gy·rate \'jī-,rāt\ *adj* : winding or coiled around : CONVOLUTED

gyrate atrophy *n* : progressive degeneration of the choroid and pigment epithelium of the retina that is inherited as an autosomal recessive trait and is characterized esp. by myopia, constriction of the visual field, night blindness, and cataracts

gy·ra·tion \jī-'rā-shən\ *n* : the pattern of convolutions of the brain

Gy·ro·mi·tra \jī-rō-'mī-trə, jir-ə-\ *n* : a genus of ascomycetous fungi (family Helvellaceae) that typically contain toxins causing illness or death — see FALSE MOREL

gy·rus \'jī-rəs\ *n, pl* **gy·ri** \-,rī\ : a convoluted ridge between anatomical grooves; *esp* : CONVOLUTION

h *abbr* **1** height **2** [Latin *hora*] hour — used in writing prescriptions; see QH

H *abbr* heroin

H *symbol* hydrogen

ha·ben·u·la \hə-'ben-yə-lə\ *n, pl* **-lae** \-,lē, -,lī\ **1** : TRIGONUM HABENULAE **2** : either of two nuclei of which one lies on each side of the pineal gland under the corresponding trigonum habenulae, is composed of two groups of nerve cells, and forms a correlation center for olfactory stimuli — called also *habenular nucleus* — **ha·ben·u·lar** \-lər\ *adj*

habenular commissure *n* : a band of nerve fibers situated in front of the pineal gland that connects the habenular nucleus on one side with that on the other

hab·it \'ha-bət\ *n* **1** : a behavior pattern acquired by frequent repetition or physiological exposure that shows itself in regularity or increased facility of performance **2** : an acquired mode of behavior that has become nearly or completely involuntary **3** : ADDICTION

hab·i·tat \'ha-bə-,tat\ *n* : the place or environment where a plant or animal naturally occurs

habit-forming *adj* : inducing the formation of an addiction

ha·bit·u·al \hə-'bi-chə-wəl\ *adj* **1** : having the nature of a habit : being in accordance with habit **2** : doing, practicing, or acting in some manner by force of habit — **ha·bit·u·al·ly** *adv*

habitual abortion *n* : spontaneous abortion occurring in three or more successive pregnancies

ha·bit·u·a·tion \-,bi-chə-'wā-shən\ *n* **1** : the act or process of making habitual or accustomed **2 a** : tolerance to the effects of a drug acquired through continued use **b** : psychological dependence on a drug after a period of use — compare ADDICTION **3** : a form of nonassociative learning characterized by a decrease in responsiveness upon repeated exposure to a stimulus — compare SENSITIZATION 3 — **ha·bit·u·ate** \-'bi-chə-,wāt\ *vb*

hab·i·tus \'ha-bə-təs\ *n, pl* **habitus** \-təs, -,tüs\ : HABIT; *specif* : body-build and constitution esp. as related to predisposition to disease

Hab·ro·ne·ma \ˌha-brō-ˈnē-mə\ *n* : a genus of parasitic nematode worms (family Spiruridae) that live as adults in the stomach of the horse or the proventriculus of various birds — see HABRONEMIASIS, SUMMER SORES

hab·ro·ne·mi·a·sis \ˌha-brə-nē-ˈmī-ə-səs\ *n, pl* **-a·ses** \-ˌsēz\ : infestation with or disease caused by roundworms of the genus *Habronema*

hack \ˈhak\ *n* : a short dry cough — **hack** *vb*

haem- *or* **haemo-** *chiefly Brit var of* HEM-

haema- *chiefly Brit var of* HEMA-

hae·ma·cy·tom·e·ter, haemal, haem·an·gi·o·ma *chiefly Brit var of* HEMACYTOMETER, HEMAL, HEMANGIOMA

Hae·ma·phy·sa·lis \ˌhē-mə-ˈfī-sə-ləs, ˌhe-\ *n* : a cosmopolitan genus of small ixodid ticks including some that are disease carriers — see KYASANUR FOREST DISEASE

haemat- *or* **haemato-** *chiefly Brit var of* HEMAT-

hae·ma·tem·e·sis, hae·ma·tog·e·nous *chiefly Brit var of* HEMATEMESIS, HEMATOGENOUS

haematobium — see SCHISTOSOMIASIS HAEMATOBIUM

Hae·ma·to·pi·nus \-tə-ˈpī-nəs\ *n* : a genus of sucking lice including the hog louse (*H. suis*) and short-nosed cattle louse (*H. eurysternus*)

-hae·mia *chiefly Brit var of* -EMIA

hae·mo·bar·ton·el·la \ˌhē-mō-ˌbär-tə-ˈne-lə, ˌhe-\ *n* **1** *cap* : a genus of bacteria (family Anaplasmataceae) that are blood parasites in various mammals **2** *pl* **-lae** \-ˌlē, -ˌlī\ : a bacterium of the genus *Haemobartonella*

hae·mo·bar·ton·el·lo·sis *also* **he·mo·bar·ton·el·lo·sis** \-tə-nə-ˈlō-səs\ *n, pl* **-lo·ses** \-ˌsēz\ : an infection or disease caused by bacteria of the genus *Haemobartonella*

hae·mo·glo·bin *chiefly Brit var of* HEMOGLOBIN

Hae·mon·chus \hē-ˈmäŋ-kəs\ *n* : a genus of nematode worms (family Trichostrongylidae) including a parasite (*H. contortus*) of the abomasum of ruminants (as sheep)

hae·mo·phil·ia *chiefly Brit var of* HEMOPHILIA

hae·moph·i·lus \hē-ˈmä-fə-ləs\ *n* **1** *cap* : a genus of nonmotile gram-negative facultatively anaerobic rod bacteria (family Pasteurellaceae) that include several important pathogens (as *H. influenzae* associated with respiratory infections, conjunctivitis, and meningitis and *H. ducreyi* of chancroid) **2** *pl* **-li** \-ˌlī, -ˌlē\ : any bacterium of the genus *Haemophilus* — see HIB

Hae·mo·pro·te·us \ˌhē-mō-ˈprō-tē-əs, ˌhe-mə-\ *n* : a genus of protozoan parasites (family Haemoproteidae) occurring in the blood of some birds

haem·or·rhage, haem·or·rhoid *chiefly Brit var of* HEMORRHAGE, HEMORRHOID

haf·ni·um \ˈhaf-nē-əm\ *n* : a metallic element that readily absorbs neutrons — symbol *Hf*; see ELEMENT table

Hage·man factor \ˈha-gə-mən-, ˈhāg-mən-\ *n* : FACTOR XII

Hageman (*fl* 1963), hospital patient.

hair \ˈhar\ *n, often attrib* **1** : a slender threadlike outgrowth of the epidermis of an animal; *esp* : one of the usu. pigmented filaments that form the characteristic coat of a mammal **2** : the hairy covering of an animal or a body part; *esp* : the coating of hairs on a human head — **hairlike** *adj*

hair ball *n* : a compact mass of hair formed in the stomach esp. of a shedding animal (as a cat) that cleanses its coat by licking — called also *trichobezoar*

hair bulb *n* : the bulbous expansion at the base of a hair from which the hair shaft develops

hair cell *n* : a cell with hairlike processes; *esp* : one of the sensory cells in the auditory epithelium of the organ of Corti

haired \ˈhard\ *adj* : having hair esp. of a specified kind — usu. used in combination ⟨red-*haired*⟩

hair follicle *n* : the tubular epithelial sheath that surrounds the lower part of the hair shaft and encloses at the bottom a vascular papilla supplying the growing basal part of the hair with nourishment

hair·line \ˈhar-ˌlīn\ *n* : the outline of scalp hair esp. on the forehead

hairline fracture *n* : a fracture that appears as a narrow crack along the surface of a bone

hair puller *n* : an individual affected with trichotillomania

hair·pull·ing \ˈher-ˌpu̇-liŋ\ *n* : the often pathological habit of pulling out one's hair one or a few hairs at a time — see TRICHOTILLOMANIA

hair root *n* : ROOT 2

hair shaft *n* : the part of a hair projecting beyond the skin

hair·worm \ˈhar-ˌwərm\ *n* : any nematode worm of the genus *Capillaria*

hairy cell leukemia \ˈhar-ē-\ *n* : a chronic leukemia that is usu. of B cell origin and is characterized by malignant cells with a ciliated appearance that replace bone marrow and infiltrate the spleen causing splenomegaly

hairy leukoplakia *n* : a condition that affects the mouth and esp. the edges of the tongue, is characterized by poorly demarcated white raised lesions with a corrugated appearance, is caused by infection with the Epstein-Barr virus, and is associated with HIV infection and AIDS — called also *oral hairy leukoplakia*

hal·a·zone \ˈhal-ə-ˌzōn\ *n* : a white powdery acid $C_7H_5Cl_2NO_4S$ used as a disinfectant for drinking water

Hal·cion \'hal-sē-ˌän\ *trademark* — used for a preparation of triazolam

Hal·dol \'hal-ˌdȯl, -ˌdōl\ *trademark* — used for a preparation of haloperidol

half–life \'haf-ˌlīf\ *n* **1** : the time required for half of the atoms of a radioactive substance to become disintegrated **2** : the time required for half the amount of a substance (as a drug or radioactive tracer) in or introduced into a living system or ecosystem to be eliminated or disintegrated by natural processes

half–moon \-ˌmün\ *n* : LUNULA a

half–value layer *n* : the thickness of an absorbing substance necessary to reduce by one half the initial intensity of the radiation passing through it

halfway house *n* : a center for individuals after institutionalization (as for mental disorder or drug addiction) that is designed to facilitate their readjustment to private life

halibut–liver oil *n* : a yellowish to brownish fatty oil from the liver of the halibut used chiefly as a source of vitamin A

hal·i·to·sis \ˌha-lə-'tō-səs\ *n, pl* **-to·ses** \-ˌsēz\ : a condition of having fetid breath

hal·lu·ci·na·tion \hə-ˌlüs-ᵊn-'ā-shən\ *n* **1** : a perception of something (as a visual image or a sound) with no external cause usu. arising from a disorder of the nervous system (as in delirium tremens) or in response to drugs (as LSD) **2** : the object of an hallucinatory perception — **hal·lu·ci·nate** \-'lüs-ᵊn-ˌāt\ *vb* — **hal·lu·ci·na·tor** \-'lüs-ᵊn-ˌā-tər\ *n* — **hal·lu·ci·na·to·ry** \-'lüs-ᵊn-ə-ˌtōr-ē\ *adj*

hal·lu·ci·no·gen \hə-'lüs-ᵊn-ə-jən\ *n* : a substance and esp. a drug that induces hallucinations

¹hal·lu·ci·no·gen·ic \hə-ˌlüs-ᵊn-ə-'je-nik\ *adj* : causing hallucinations — **hal·lu·ci·no·gen·i·cal·ly** \-ni-k(ə-)lē\ *adv*

²hallucinogenic *n* : HALLUCINOGEN

hal·lu·ci·no·sis \hə-ˌlüs-ᵊn-'ō-səs\ *n, pl* **-no·ses** \-ˌsēz\ : a pathological mental state characterized by hallucinations

hallucis — see ABDUCTOR HALLUCIS, ADDUCTOR HALLUCIS, EXTENSOR HALLUCIS BREVIS, EXTENSOR HALLUCIS LONGUS, FLEXOR HALLUCIS BREVIS, FLEXOR HALLUCIS LONGUS

hal·lux \'ha-ləks\ *n, pl* **hal·lu·ces** \'ha-lə-ˌsēz, 'hal-yə-\ : the innermost digit of the foot : BIG TOE

hallux rig·id·us \-'ri-jə-dəs\ *n* : restricted mobility of the big toe due to stiffness of the metatarsophalangeal joint esp. when due to arthritic changes in the joint

hallux val·gus \-'val-gəs\ *n* : an abnormal deviation of the big toe away from the midline of the body or toward the other toes of the foot that is associated esp. with the wearing of ill=fitting shoes

ha·lo \'hā-(ˌ)lō\ *n, pl* **halos** *or* **haloes**
1 : a circle of light appearing to surround a luminous body; *esp* : one seen as the result of the presence of glaucoma **2** : a differentiated zone surrounding a central object : an orthopedic device used to immobilize the head and neck (as to treat fracture of neck vertebrae) that consists of a metal band placed around the head and fastened to the skull usu. with metal pins and that is attached by extensions to an inflexible vest — called also *halo brace*

halo effect *n* : generalization from the perception of one outstanding personality trait to an overly favorable evaluation of the whole personality

hal·o·fan·trine \ˌha-lə-'fan-ˌtrēn\ *n* : an antimalarial drug used in the form of its hydrochloride $C_{26}H_{30}Cl_2F_3NO·HCl$ esp. against chloroquine-resistant falciparum malaria

halo·gen \'ha-lə-jən\ *n* : any of the five elements fluorine, chlorine, bromine, iodine, and astatine that exist in the free state normally with two atoms per molecule

hal·o·ge·ton \ˌha-lə-'jē-ˌtän\ *n* : a coarse herb (*Halogeton glomeratus* of the family Chenopodiaceae) that in western U.S. ranges is dangerous to sheep and cattle because of its high oxalate content

halo·per·i·dol \ˌha-lō-'per-ə-ˌdȯl, -ˌdōl\ *n* : a butyrophenone antipsychotic drug $C_{21}H_{23}ClFNO_2$ used esp. to treat schizophrenia and to control the involuntary tics and vocalizations of Tourette's syndrome — see HALDOL

halo·thane \'ha-lə-ˌthān\ *n* : a nonexplosive inhalational anesthetic $C_2H·BrClF_3$

Hal·sted radical mastectomy \'hal-ˌsted-\ *n* : RADICAL MASTECTOMY — called also *Halsted radical*

  Halsted, William Stewart (1852–1922), American surgeon.

hal·zoun \ˌhal-'zün, 'hal-zün\ *n* : infestation of the larynx and pharynx esp. by tongue worms (genus *Linguatula* and esp. *L. serrata*) consumed in raw liver

ham \'ham\ *n* **1** : the part of the leg behind the knee : the hollow of the knee : POPLITEAL SPACE **2** : a buttock with its associated thigh or with the posterior part of a thigh — usu. used in pl.

hama·dry·ad \ˌha-mə-'drī-əd, -ˌad\ *n* : KING COBRA

ham·ar·to·ma \ˌha-ˌmär-'tō-mə\ *n, pl* **-mas** *also* **-ma·ta** \-mə-tə\ : a mass resembling a tumor that represents anomalous development of tissue natural to a part or organ rather than a true tumor

ha·mate \'hā-ˌmāt, 'ha-mət\ *n* : a bone on the little-finger side of the second row of the carpus — called also *unci·form, unciform bone*

ham·mer \'ha-mər\ *n* : MALLEUS

ham·mer·toe \'ha-mər-ˌtō\ *n* : a deformed claw-shaped toe and esp. the second that results from permanent angular flexion between one or both phalangeal joints — called also *claw toe*

¹ham·string \'ham-,striŋ\ *n* **1 a** : either of two groups of tendons bounding the upper part of the popliteal space at the back of the knee and forming the tendons of insertion of some muscles of the back of the thigh **b** : HAMSTRING MUSCLE **2** : a large tendon above and behind the hock of a quadruped

²hamstring *vb* **-strung** \-,strəŋ\; **-string·ing** \-,striŋ-iŋ\ : to cripple by cutting the leg tendons

hamstring muscle *n* : any of three muscles at the back of the thigh that function to flex and rotate the leg and extend the thigh: **a** : SEMIMEMBRANOSUS **b** : SEMITENDINOSUS **c** : BICEPS b

ham·u·lus \'ha-myə-ləs\ *n, pl* **-u·li** \-,lī, -,lē\ : a hook or hooked process

hand \'hand\ *n, often attrib* : the terminal part of the vertebrate forelimb when modified (as in humans) as a grasping organ

hand·ed \'han-dəd\ *adj* **1** : having a hand or hands esp. of a specified kind or number — usu. used in combination ⟨a large-*handed* man⟩ **2** : using a specified hand or number of hands — used in combination ⟨right-*handed*⟩

hand·ed·ness \-nəs\ *n* : a tendency to use one hand rather than the other

hand, foot and mouth disease *n* : a usu. mild contagious disease esp. of young children that is caused by an enterovirus (species *Human enterovirus A*, esp. serotype Human coxsackievirus A16) and is characterized by vesicular lesions in the mouth, on the hands and feet, and sometimes in the diaper-covered area — compare FOOT-AND-MOUTH DISEASE

hand·i·cap \'han-di-,kap, -dē-\ *n* **1** : a disadvantage that makes achievement unusually difficult **2** *sometimes offensive* : a physical disability

hand·i·capped \-,kapt\ *adj, sometimes offensive* : having a physical or mental disability; *also* : of or reserved for individuals with a physical disability

hand·piece \'hand-,pēs\ *n* : the handheld part of an electrically powered dental apparatus that holds the revolving instruments (as a bur)

Hand–Schül·ler–Chris·tian disease \'hand-'shü-lər-'kris-chən-\ *n* : an inflammatory histiocytosis associated with disturbances in cholesterol metabolism that occurs chiefly in young children and is marked by cystic defects of the skull and by exophthalmos and diabetes insipidus — called also *Schüller-Christian disease*

Hand, Alfred (1868–1949), American physician.

Schüller \'shue-ler\, Artur (1874–1958), Austrian neurologist.

Christian, Henry Asbury (1876–1951), American physician.

hang·nail \'haŋ-,nāl\ *n* : a bit of skin hanging loose at the side or root of a fingernail

hang·over \-,ō-vər\ *n* : disagreeable physical effects (as headache or nausea) following heavy consumption of alcohol or the use of drugs

hang–up \-,əp\ *n* : a source of mental or emotional difficulty

Han·sen's bacillus \'han-sənz-\ *n* : a bacterium of the genus *Mycobacterium* (*M. leprae*) that causes leprosy

Han·sen \'hän-sen\, Gerhard Henrik Armauer (1841–1912), Norwegian physician.

Hansen's disease *n* : LEPROSY

Han·ta·an virus \'han-tə-ən-\ *n* : a hantavirus (species *Hantaan virus*) that causes hemorrhagic fever with renal syndrome and esp. Korean hemorrhagic fever

han·ta·vi·rus \'han-tə-,vī-rəs\ *n* **1** *cap* : a genus of bunyaviruses that infect rodents as their natural hosts, are transmitted to humans esp. by exposure to the virus in airborne particles of rodent feces and urine, and include viruses causing hantavirus pulmonary syndrome and hemorrhagic fever with renal syndrome **2** : any virus of the genus *Hantavirus*

hantavirus pulmonary syndrome *n* : an acute respiratory disease caused by various hantaviruses and characterized initially esp. by fatigue, fever and muscle pain which rapidly progress to pulmonary edema and hypoxia often resulting in death from shock or cardiac complications

H antigen \'āch-\ *n* : any of various antigens associated with the flagella of motile bacteria and used in serological identification of various bacteria — compare O ANTIGEN

HA1c \,āch-,ā-,wən-'sē\ *n* : HEMOGLOBIN A1C

hap·a·lo·nych·ia \,ha-pə-lō-'ni-kē-ə\ *n* : abnormal softness of the fingernails or toenails

hap·loid \'ha-,plóid\ *adj* : having the gametic number of chromosomes or half the number characteristic of somatic cells : MONOPLOID — **haploid** *n* — **hap·loi·dy** \-,plói-dē\ *n*

hap·lo·scope \'ha-plə-,skōp\ *n* : a simple stereoscope that is used in the study of depth perception

hap·lo·type \-,tīp\ *n* : a group of alleles of different genes (as of the major histocompatibility complex) on a single chromosome that are closely enough linked to be inherited usu. as a unit

hapt- or **hapto-** *comb form* : contact : touch : combination ⟨*hapten*⟩

hap·ten \'hap-,ten\ *n* : a small separable part of an antigen that reacts specif. with an antibody but is incapable of stimulating antibody production except in combination with an associated protein molecule — **hap-ten-ic** \hap-'te-nik\ *adj*

hap-tic \'hap-tik\ *adj* **1** : relating to or based on the sense of touch **2** : characterized by a predilection for the sense of touch

hap-tics \-tiks\ *n* : a science concerned with the sense of touch

hap-to-glo-bin \'hap-tə-ˌglō-bən\ *n* : any of several forms of an alpha globulin found in blood serum that can combine with free hemoglobin in the plasma and thereby prevent the loss of iron into the urine

hard \'härd\ *adj* **1** : not easily penetrated : not easily yielding to pressure **2** : of or relating to radiation of relatively high penetrating power ⟨∼ X-rays⟩ **3** : being at once addictive and gravely detrimental to health ⟨such ∼ drugs as heroin⟩ **4** : resistant to biodegradation ⟨∼ pesticides like DDT⟩ — **hard·ness** *n*

hard·en·ing \'härd-ᵊn-iŋ\ *n* : SCLEROSIS 1 ⟨∼ of the arteries⟩

hard–of–hearing *adj* : of or relating to a defective but functional sense of hearing

hard pad *n* : a serious and frequently fatal virus disease of dogs now considered to be a form of distemper — called also *hard pad disease*

hard palate *n* : the bony anterior part of the palate forming the roof of the mouth

hardware disease *n* : traumatic damage to the viscera of cattle due to ingestion of a usu. sharp foreign body

Har·dy–Wein·berg law \'här-dē-'win-ˌbərg\ *n* : a fundamental principle of population genetics: population gene frequencies and population genotype frequencies remain constant from generation to generation if mating is random and if mutation, selection, immigration, and emigration do not occur — called also *Hardy-Weinberg principle*

    Hardy, Godfrey Harold (1877–1947), British mathematician.

    Wein·berg \'vīn-ˌberk\, **Wilhelm (1862–1937)**, German physician and geneticist.

hare·lip \'har-ˌlip\ *n, sometimes offensive* : CLEFT LIP — **hare·lipped** \-ˌlipt\ *adj*

har·ma·line \'här-mə-ˌlēn\ *n* : a hallucinogenic alkaloid $C_{13}H_{14}N_2O$ found in several plants (*Peganum harmala* of the family Zygophyllaceae and *Banisteriopsis* spp. of the family Malpighiaceae) that is a stimulant of the central nervous system

har·mine \'här-ˌmēn\ *n* : a hallucinogenic alkaloid $C_{13}H_{12}N_2O$ similar to harmaline

Hart·mann's solution \'härt-mənz-\ *n* : LACTATED RINGER'S SOLUTION

    Hartmann, Alexis Frank (1898–1964), American pediatrician.

Hart·nup disease \'härt-ˌnəp-\ *n* : an inherited metabolic disease that is caused by abnormalities of the renal tubules and is characterized by aminoaciduria, a dry red scaly rash, and episodic muscular incoordination

    Hartnup (*fl* 1950s), British family.

harts·horn \'härts-ˌhörn\ *n* : a preparation of ammonia used as smelling salts — see SPIRIT OF HARTSHORN

hash \'hash\ *n* : HASHISH

Ha·shi·mo·to's thyroiditis *also* **Hashimoto thyroiditis** \ˌhä-shē-'mō-(ˌ)tō(z)-\ *n* : a chronic autoimmune thyroiditis that is characterized by thyroid enlargement, thyroid fibrosis, lymphatic infiltration of thyroid tissue, and the production of antibodies which attack the thyroid — called also *Hashimoto's disease, Hashimoto's struma, struma lymphomatosa*

    Hashimoto, Hakaru (1881–1934), Japanese surgeon.

hash·ish \'ha-ˌshēsh, ha-'shēsh\ *n* : the concentrated resin from the flowering tops of the female hemp plant (*Cannabis sativa*) that is smoked, chewed, or drunk for its intoxicating effect — called also *charas*; compare BHANG, MARIJUANA

Has·sall's corpuscle \'ha-səlz-\ *n* : one of the small bodies of the medulla of the thymus having granular cells at the center surrounded by concentric layers of modified epithelial cells — called also *thymic corpuscle*

    Hassall, Arthur Hill (1817–1894), British physician and chemist.

has·si·um \'ha-sē-əm\ *n* : a short-lived radioactive element produced artificially — symbol *Hs*; see ELEMENT table

hatch·et \'ha-chət\ *n* : a dental excavator

hatha yoga \'hə-tə-\ *n* : a form of yoga emphasizing a system of physical postures for balancing, stretching, and strengthening the body

haus·tra·tion \hö-'strā-shən\ *n* **1** : the property or state of having haustra **2** : HAUSTRUM

haus·trum \'hö-strəm\ *n, pl* **haus·tra** \-strə\ : one of the pouches or sacculations into which the large intestine is divided — **haus·tral** \-strəl\ *adj*

ha·ver·sian canal \hə-'vər-zhən-\ *n, often cap H* : any of the small canals through which the blood vessels ramify in bone

    Ha·vers \'hā-vərz, 'ha-\, **Clopton (1655?–1702)**, British osteologist.

haversian system *n, often cap H* : a haversian canal with the laminae of bone that surround it — called also *osteon*

Hav·rix \'ha-riks\ *trademark* — used for a vaccine against hepatitis

haw \'hö\ *n* : NICTITATING MEMBRANE; *esp* : an inflamed nictitating membrane of a domesticated mammal

hawk \'hök\ *vb* : to make a harsh coughing sound in or as if in clearing the throat; *also* : to raise by hawking ⟨∼ up phlegm⟩ — **hawk** *n*

hay fever *n* : an acute allergic reaction to pollen that is usu. seasonal and is marked by sneezing, nasal discharge and congestion, and itching and watering of the eyes — called also *pollinosis*

haz·mat \'haz-ˌmat\ *n, often attrib* : a material (as one that is flammable) that would be a danger to life or to the environment if released without necessary precautions being taken

Hb *abbr* hemoglobin

H band \'āch-\ *n* : a relatively pale band in the middle of the A band of striated muscle

HbA1c \ˌāch-ˌbē-ˌā-ˌwən-'sē\ *n* : HEMOGLOBIN A1C

HBsAg *abbr* hepatitis B surface antigen

HBV *abbr* hepatitis B virus

HCG *abbr* human chorionic gonadotropin

HCM *abbr* hypertrophic cardiomyopathy

HCT *abbr* hematocrit

HCTZ *abbr* hydrochlorothiazide

HCV *abbr* hepatitis C virus

HDL \ˌāch-(ˌ)dē-'el\ *n* : a lipoprotein of blood plasma that is composed of a high proportion of protein with little triglyceride and cholesterol and that is associated with decreased probability of developing atherosclerosis — called also *alpha-lipoprotein, good cholesterol, high-density lipoprotein;* compare LDL, VLDL

He *symbol* helium

head \'hed\ *n* **1** : the division of the human body that contains the brain, the eyes, the ears, the nose, and the mouth; *also* : the corresponding anterior division of the body of all vertebrates, most arthropods, and many other animals **2** : HEADACHE **3** : a projection or extremity esp. of an anatomical part: as **a** : the rounded proximal end of a long bone (as the humerus) **b** : the end of a muscle nearest the origin **4** : the part of a boil, pimple, or abscess at which it is likely to break — **head** *adj*

head·ache \'he-ˌdāk\ *n* : pain in the head — called also *cephalalgia* — **head·achy** \-ˌdā-kē\ *adj*

head cold *n* : a common cold centered in the nasal passages and adjacent mucous tissues

head louse *n* : a sucking louse of the genus *Pediculus* (*P. humanus capitis*) that lives on the human scalp

head nurse *n* : CHARGE NURSE; *esp* : one with overall responsibility for the supervision of the administrative and clinical aspects of nursing care

head·shrink·er \'hed-ˌshriŋ-kər\ *n* : SHRINK

heal \'hēl\ *vb* **1** : to make or become sound or whole esp. in bodily condition **2** : to cure of disease or affliction — **heal·er** \'hē-lər\ *n*

¹heal·ing \'hē-liŋ\ *n* **1** : the act or process of curing or of restoring to health **2** : the process of getting well

²healing *adj* : tending to heal or cure : CURATIVE ⟨a ∼ art⟩

health \'helth\ *n, often attrib* **1** : the condition of an organism or one of its parts in which it performs its vital functions normally or properly : the state of being sound in body or mind; *esp* : freedom from physical disease and pain — compare DISEASE **2** : the condition of an organism with respect to the performance of its vital functions as evaluated subjectively ⟨how is your ∼ today⟩

health care *n* : the maintenance and restoration of health by the treatment and prevention of disease esp. by trained and licensed professionals — **health–care** *adj*

health department *n* : a division of a local or larger government responsible for the oversight and care of matters relating to public health

health·ful \'helth-fəl\ *adj* : beneficial to health of body or mind — **health·ful·ly** *adv* — **health·ful·ness** *n*

health insurance *n* : insurance against loss through illness of the insured; *esp* : insurance providing compensation for medical expenses

Health Insurance Portability and Accountability Act *n* : a federal law enacted in 1996 that protects continuity of health coverage (as when a person changes jobs), that limits health-plan exclusions for preexisting conditions, that requires patient medical information be kept private and secure, that standardizes electronic transactions involving health information, and that permits tax deduction of health insurance premiums by the self-employed — abbr. HIPAA

health maintenance organization *n* : HMO

health spa *n* : SPA 2; *esp* : one emphasizing health and fitness

health visitor *n, Brit* : a trained person who is usu. a qualified nurse and is employed by a local British authority to visit people in their homes and advise them on health matters

healthy \'hel-thē\ *adj* **health·i·er; -est 1** : enjoying health and vigor of body, mind, or spirit **2** : revealing a state of health **3** : conducive to health — **health·i·ly** \-thə-lē\ *adv* — **health·i·ness** \-thē-nəs\ *n*

hear \'hir\ *vb* **heard** \'hərd\; **hear·ing** : to perceive or have the capacity to perceive sound

hearing *n* : one of the senses that is concerned with the perception of sound, is mediated through the organ of Corti, is normally sensitive in humans to sound vibrations between 16 and 27,000 hertz but most receptive to those between 2000 and 5000 hertz, is conducted centrally by the cochlear branch of the auditory nerve, and is coordinated esp. in the medial geniculate body

hearing aid *n* : an electronic device usu. worn in or behind the ear of a hearing-impaired person for amplifying sound

hearing dog *n* : a dog trained to alert its deaf or hearing-impaired owner to sounds (as of a doorbell or telephone) — called also *hearing ear dog*

heart \'härt\ *n* : a hollow muscular organ of vertebrate animals that by its rhythmic contraction acts as a pump maintaining the circulation of the blood and that in the human adult is about five inches (13 centimeters) long and three and one half inches (9 centimeters) broad, is of conical form, is enclosed in a serous pericardium, and consists as in other mammals and in birds of four chambers divided into an upper pair of rather thin-walled atria which receive blood from the veins and a lower pair of thick-walled ventricles into which the blood is forced and which in turn pump it into the arteries

heart attack *n* : an acute episode of heart disease marked by the death or damage of heart muscle due to insufficient blood supply to the heart muscle itself usu. as a result of a coronary thrombosis or a coronary occlusion and that is characterized esp. by chest pain — called also *myocardial infarction;* compare ANGINA PECTORIS, CORONARY INSUFFICIENCY, HEART FAILURE 1

heart·beat \'härt-,bēt\ *n* : one complete pulsation of the heart

heart block *n* : incoordination of the heartbeat in which the atria and ventricles beat independently due to defective transmission through the bundle of His and which is marked by decreased cardiac output often with cerebral ischemia

heart·burn \-,bərn\ *n* : a burning discomfort behind the lower part of the sternum usu. related to spasm of the lower end of the esophagus or of the upper part of the stomach often in association with gastroesophageal reflux disease — called also *cardialgia, pyrosis;* compare WATER BRASH

heart disease *n* : an abnormal organic condition of the heart or of the heart and circulation

heart failure *n* **1** : a condition in which the heart is unable to pump blood at an adequate rate or in adequate volume — compare ANGINA PECTORIS, CONGESTIVE HEART FAILURE, CORONARY FAILURE, HEART ATTACK **2** : cessation of heartbeat : DEATH

heart–healthy \'härt-,hel-thē\ *adj* : conducive to a healthy heart and circulatory system ⟨a ∼ diet⟩

heart–lung machine *n* : a mechanical pump that maintains circulation during heart surgery by shunting blood away from the heart, oxygenating it, and returning it to the body

heart murmur *n* : MURMUR

heart rate *n* : a measure of cardiac activity usu. expressed as number of beats per minute

heart valve *n* : any of the valves (as the atrioventricular valves) that control blood flow to and from the heart — called also *cardiac valve*

heart·wa·ter \'härt-,wȯ-tər, -,wä-\ *n* : a serious febrile disease of sheep, goats, and cattle in southern Africa that is caused by a bacterium of the genus *Cowdria* (*C. ruminantium*) transmitted by a bont tick — called also *heartwater disease, heartwater fever*

heart·worm \-,wərm\ *n* : a filarial worm of the genus *Dirofilaria* (*D. immitis*) that is a parasite esp. in the right heart of dogs and is transmitted by mosquitoes; *also* : infestation with or disease caused by the heartworm

heat \'hēt\ *n* **1 a** : a feverish state of the body : pathological excessive bodily temperature (as from inflammation) **b** : a warm flushed condition of the body (as after exercise) **2** : sexual excitement esp. in a female mammal; *specif* : ESTRUS

heat cramps *n pl* : a condition that is marked by sudden development of cramps in skeletal muscles and that results from prolonged work in high temperatures accompanied by profuse perspiration with loss of sodium chloride from the body

heat exchanger *n* : a device (as in an apparatus for extracorporeal blood circulation) for transferring heat from one fluid to another without allowing them to mix

heat exhaustion *n* : a condition marked by weakness, nausea, dizziness, and profuse sweating that results from physical exertion in a hot environment — called also *heat prostration;* compare HEATSTROKE

heat prostration *n* : HEAT EXHAUSTION

heat rash *n* : PRICKLY HEAT

heat shock protein *n* : any of a group of proteins that are produced esp. in cells subjected to stressful conditions (as high temperature) and that serve to ensure proper protein folding

heat·stroke \'hēt-,strōk\ *n* : a condition marked esp. by cessation of sweating, extremely high body temperature, and collapse that results from prolonged exposure to high temperature — compare HEAT EXHAUSTION

heave \'hēv\ *vb* **heaved; heav·ing** : VOMIT, RETCH

heaves \'hēvz\ *n, sing or pl* **1** : chronic emphysema of the horse affecting the alveolae of the lungs — called also *broken wind* **2** : a spell of retching or vomiting

heavy chain *n* : either of the two larger of the four polypeptide chains comprising antibodies — compare LIGHT CHAIN

he·be·phre·nia \ˌhē-bə-ˈfrē-nē-ə, -ˈfre-\ n : a disorganized form of schizophrenia characterized esp. by incoherence, delusions lacking an underlying theme, and affect that is flat, inappropriate, or silly — **he·be·phre·nic** \-ˈfre-nik, -ˈfrē-\ adj or n

Heb·er·den's node \ˈhe-bər-dənz-\ n : any of the bony knots at joint margins (as at the terminal joints of the fingers) commonly associated with osteoarthritis — compare BOUCHARD'S NODE

Heberden, William (1710–1801), British physician.

hec·tic \ˈhek-tik\ adj 1 : of, relating to, or being a fluctuating but persistent fever (as in tuberculosis) 2 : having a hectic fever

heel \ˈhēl\ n 1 : the back of the human foot below the ankle and behind the arch 2 : the part of the palm of the hand nearest the wrist

heel bone n : CALCANEUS

heel fly n : CATTLE GRUB; esp : one in the adult stage

Heer·fordt's syndrome \ˈhär-ˌfôrts-\ n : UVEOPAROTID FEVER

Heerfordt, Christian Frederik (1871–1953), Danish ophthalmologist.

height \ˈhīt\ n : the distance from the bottom to the top of something standing upright; esp : the distance from the lowest to the highest point of an animal body esp. of a human being in a natural standing position or from the lowest point to an arbitrarily chosen upper point

Heim·lich maneuver \ˈhīm-lik-\ n : the manual application of sudden upward pressure on the upper abdomen of a choking victim to force a foreign object from the trachea

Heimlich, Henry Jay (b 1920), American surgeon.

Heinz body \ˈhīnts-, ˈhīnz-\ n : a cellular inclusion in a red blood cell that consists of damaged aggregated hemoglobin and is associated with some forms of hemolytic anemia

Heinz \ˈhīnts\, **Robert (1865–1924),** German physician.

hela cell \ˈhē-lə-\ n, often cap H & 1st L : a cell of a continuously cultured strain isolated from a human uterine cervical carcinoma in 1951 and used in biomedical research esp. to culture viruses

Lacks \ˈlaks\, **Henrietta (fl 1951),** American hospital patient.

heli- or **helio-** comb form : sun ⟨helio-therapy⟩

helic- or **helico-** comb form : helix : spiral ⟨helical⟩ ⟨helicotrema⟩

he·li·cal \ˈhe-li-kəl, ˈhē-\ adj : of, relating to, or having the form of a helix; broadly : SPIRAL 1a — **he·li·cal·ly** adv

he·li·case \ˈhe-lə-ˌkās, ˈhē-\ n : any of various enzymes that catalyze the unwinding and separation of double-stranded DNA or RNA during its replication

hel·i·cine artery \ˈhe-lə-ˌsēn-, ˈhe-lə-ˌsīn-\ n : any of various convoluted and dilated arterial vessels that empty directly into the cavernous spaces of erectile tissue and function in its erection

hel·i·co·bac·ter \ˈhe-li-kō-ˌbak-tər\ n 1 cap : a genus of bacteria formerly placed in the genus Campylobacter and including one (H. pylori) associated with gastritis and implicated as a causative agent of gastric and duodenal ulcers 2 : any bacterium of the genus Helicobacter

hel·i·co·trema \ˌhe-lə-kō-ˈtrē-mə\ n : the minute opening by which the scala tympani and scala vestibuli communicate at the top of the cochlea of the ear

he·lio·ther·a·py \ˌhē-lē-ō-ˈther-ə-pē\ n, pl -pies : the use of sunlight or of an artificial source of ultraviolet, visible, or infrared radiation for therapeutic purposes

he·li·um \ˈhē-lē-əm\ n : a light nonflammable gaseous element — symbol He; see ELEMENT table

he·lix \ˈhē-liks\ n, pl **he·li·ces** \ˈhe-lə-ˌsēz, ˈhē-\ also **he·lix·es** \ˈhē-lik-səz\ 1 : the inward curved rim of the external ear 2 : a curve traced on a cylinder by the rotation of a point crossing its right sections at a constant oblique angle; broadly : SPIRAL 2 — see ALPHA-HELIX, DOUBLE HELIX

hel·le·bore \ˈhe-lə-ˌbôr\ n 1 : any of a genus (Helleborus) of poisonous Eurasian herbs of the buttercup family (Ranunculaceae) that have showy flowers; also : the dried rhizome of a hellebore (as H. niger) formerly used in medicine 2 a : a poisonous herb of the genus Veratrum b : the dried rhizome of either of two hellebores (Veratrum viride of No. America and V. album of Eurasia) that is used as an insecticide and contains toxic alkaloids that are cardiac and respiratory depressants — called also veratrum

HELLP syndrome \ˈhelp-\ n [hemolysis elevated liver enzymes, and low platelet count] : a serious disorder of pregnancy that is of unknown etiology, that usu. occurs between the 23rd and 39th weeks, and that is characterized by a great reduction in the number of platelets per cubic millimeter, by hemolysis, and by abnormal liver function tests

hel·minth \ˈhel-ˌminth\ n : a parasitic worm (as a tapeworm, liver fluke, or ascarid); esp : an intestinal worm — **hel·min·thic** \hel-ˈmin-thik\ adj

helminth- or **helmintho-** comb form : helminth ⟨helminthiasis⟩

hel·min·thi·a·sis \ˌhel-mən-ˈthī-ə-səs\ n, pl **-a·ses** \-ˌsēz\ : infestation with or disease caused by parasitic worms

hel·min·thol·o·gy \-ˈthä-lə-jē\ n, pl **-gies** : a branch of zoology concerned with helminths; *esp* : the study of parasitic worms — **hel·min·thol·o·gist** \-'thä-lə-jist\ *n*

Helo·der·ma \ˌhē-lō-'dər-mə, ˌhe-\ *n* : a genus of lizards (family Helodermatidae) including the Gila monsters

helper/inducer T cell *n* : T4 CELL

helper T cell *n* : a T cell that participates in an immune response by recognizing a foreign antigen and secreting lymphokines to activate T cell and B cell proliferation, that usu. carries CD4 molecular markers on its cell surface, and that is reduced to 20 percent or less of normal numbers in AIDS — called also *helper cell, helper lymphocyte, helper T lymphocyte;* compare CYTOTOXIC T CELL, SUPPRESSOR T CELL

hem- *or* **hemo-** *comb form* : blood ⟨*hemal*⟩ ⟨*hemangioma*⟩ ⟨*hemophilia*⟩

hema- *comb form* : HEM- ⟨*hemacytometer*⟩

he·ma·cy·tom·e·ter \ˌhē-mə-sī-'tä-mə-tər\ *n* : an instrument for counting blood cells — called also *hemocytometer*

hem·ad·sorp·tion \ˌhē-(ˌ)mad-'sȯrp-shən, -'zȯrp-\ *n* : adherence of red blood cells to the surface of something (as a virus or cell) — **hem·ad·sorb·ing** \-'sȯrb-iŋ, -'zȯr-\ *adj*

hem·ag·glu·ti·na·tion \ˌhē-mə-ˌglüt-ᵊn-'ā-shən\ *n* : agglutination of red blood cells — **hem·ag·glu·ti·nate** \-'glüt-ᵊn-ˌāt\ *vb*

hem·ag·glu·ti·nin \ˌhē-mə-'glüt-ᵊn-ən\ *also* **he·mo·ag·glu·ti·nin** \ˌhē-mō-ə-\ *n* : an agglutinin (as an antibody or viral capsid protein) that causes hemagglutination — compare LEUKOAGGLUTININ

he·mal \'hē-məl\ *adj* **1** : of or relating to the blood or blood vessels **2** : relating to or situated on the side of the spinal cord where the heart and chief blood vessels are placed — compare NEURAL 2

hem·an·gio·blas·to·ma \ˌhē-ˌman-jē-ō-blas-'tō-mə\ *n, pl* **-mas** *also* **-ma·ta** \-mə-tə\ : a hemangioma esp. of the cerebellum that tends to be associated with von Hippel-Lindau disease

he·man·gio·en·do·the·li·o·ma \ˌhē-ˌman-jē-ō-ˌen-dō-ˌthē-lē-'ō-mə\ *n, pl* **-mas** *also* **-ma·ta** \-mə-tə\ : an often malignant tumor originating from proliferation of capillary endothelium

hem·an·gi·o·ma \ˌhē-ˌman-jē-'ō-mə\ *n, pl* **-mas** *also* **-ma·ta** \-mə-tə\ : a usu. benign tumor made up of blood vessels that typically occurs as a purplish or reddish slightly elevated area of skin

he·man·gi·o·ma·to·sis \-jē-ˌō-mə-'tō-səs\ *n, pl* **-to·ses** \-ˌsēz\ : a condition in which hemangiomas are present in several parts of the body

hem·an·gio·peri·cy·to·ma \-jē-ō-ˌper-ə-ˌsī-'tō-mə\ *n, pl* **-mas** *also* **-ma·ta** \-mə-tə\ : a vascular tumor composed of spindle cells that are held to be derived from pericytes

he·man·gio·sar·co·ma \-jē-ō-sär-'kō-mə\ *n, pl* **-mas** *also* **-ma·ta** \-mə-tə\ : a malignant hemangioma

he·mar·thro·sis \ˌhē-mär-'thrō-səs, ˌhe-\ *n, pl* **-thro·ses** \-ˌsēz\ : hemorrhage into a joint

hemat- *or* **hemato-** *comb form* : HEM- ⟨*hemat*emesis⟩ ⟨*hemato*genous⟩

he·ma·tem·e·sis \ˌhē-mə-'te-mə-səs, ˌhē-mə-tə-'mē-səs\ *n, pl* **-e·ses** \-ˌsēz\ : the vomiting of blood

he·ma·tin \'hē-mə-tən\ *n* **1** : a brownish black or bluish black derivative $C_4H_{33}N_4O_5Fe$ of oxidized heme; *also* : any of several similar compounds **2** : HEME

he·ma·tin·ic \ˌhē-mə-'ti-nik\ *n* : an agent tending to stimulate blood cell formation or to increase the hemoglobin in the blood — **hematinic** *adj*

he·ma·to·cele \'hē-mə-tə-ˌsēl, hi-'ma-tə-\ *n* : a blood-filled cavity of the body; *also* : the effusion of blood into a body cavity (as the scrotum)

he·ma·to·che·zia \ˌhē-mə-tə-'kē-zē-ə, ˌhe-; hi-ˌma-tə-\ *n* : the passage of blood in the feces — compare MELENA

he·ma·to·col·pos \ˌhē-mə-tō-'käl-pəs, ˌhe-, -ˌpäs; hi-ˌma-tə-\ *n* : an accumulation of blood within the vagina

he·mat·o·crit \hi-'ma-tə-krət, -ˌkrit\ *n* **1** : an instrument for determining usu. by centrifugation the relative amounts of plasma and corpuscles in blood **2** : the percent of the volume of whole blood that is composed of red blood cells as determined by separation of red blood cells from the plasma usu. by centrifugation — called also *packed cell volume*

he·ma·to·gen·ic \ˌhē-mə-tə-'je-nik\ *adj* : HEMATOGENOUS 2

he·ma·tog·e·nous \ˌhē-mə-'tä-jə-nəs\ *adj* **1** : producing blood **2** : involving, spread by, or arising in the blood — **he·ma·tog·e·nous·ly** *adv*

he·ma·to·log·ic \ˌhē-mət-ᵊl-'ä-jik\ *also* **he·ma·to·log·i·cal** \-ji-kəl\ *adj* : of or relating to blood or to hematology

he·ma·tol·o·gy \ˌhē-mə-'tä-lə-jē\ *n, pl* **-gies** : a medical science that deals with the blood and blood-forming organs — **he·ma·tol·o·gist** \-jist\ *n*

he·ma·to·ma \-'tō-mə\ *n, pl* **-mas** *also* **-ma·ta** \-mə-tə\ : a mass of usu. clotted blood that forms in a tissue, organ, or body space as a result of a broken blood vessel

he·ma·to·me·tra \ˌhē-mə-tə-'mē-trə, ˌhe-\ *n* : an accumulation of blood or menstrual fluid in the uterus

he·ma·to·my·e·lia \hi-ˌma-tə-ˌmī-'ē-lē-ə, ˌhē-mə-tō-\ *n* : a hemorrhage into the spinal cord

he·ma·to·pa·thol·o·gy \hi-ˌma-tə-pə-'thä-lə-jē, ˌhē-mə-tō-\ *n, pl* **-gies** : the medical science concerned with diseases of the blood and related tissues — **he·ma·to·pa·thol·o·gist** \-jist\ *n*

he·ma·toph·a·gous \ˌhē-mə-'tä-fə-gəs\ *adj* : feeding on blood ⟨~ insects⟩

he·ma·to·poi·e·sis \hi-ˌma-tə-ˌpoi-ˈē-səs, ˌhē-mə-tō-\ n, pl -e·ses \-ˌsēz\ : the formation of blood or of blood cells in the living body — called also *hemopoiesis* — **he·ma·to·poi·et·ic** \-ˈe-tik\ adj

hematopoietic growth factor n : any of a group of glycoproteins that promote the proliferation and maturation of blood cells; esp : COLONY-STIMULATING FACTOR

he·ma·to·por·phy·rin \ˌhē-mə-tə-ˈpòr-fə-rən, ˌhe-\ n : any of several isomeric porphyrins $C_{34}H_{38}O_6N_4$ that are hydrated derivatives of protoporphyrins

he·ma·to·sal·pinx \ˌhē-mə-tə-ˈsal-(ˌ)pinks, ˌhe-, hi-ˌma-tə-\ n, pl -sal·pin·ges \-sal-ˈpin-(ˌ)jēz\ : accumulation of blood in a fallopian tube

he·ma·tox·y·lin \ˌhē-mə-ˈtäk-sə-lən\ n : a crystalline phenolic compound $C_{16}H_{14}O_6$ used chiefly as a biological stain

he·ma·tu·ria \ˌhē-mə-ˈtùr-ē-ə, -ˈtyùr-\ n : the presence of blood or blood cells in the urine

heme \ˈhēm\ n : the deep red iron-containing prosthetic group $C_{34}H_{32}N_4O_4Fe$ of hemoglobin and myoglobin

hem·er·a·lo·pia \ˌhe-mə-rə-ˈlō-pē-ə\ n 1 : a defect of vision characterized by reduced visual capacity in bright lights 2 : NIGHT BLINDNESS — not considered correct medical usage

hemi- prefix : half ⟨*hemi*block⟩

-hemia — see -EMIA

hemi·an·es·the·sia \ˌhe-mē-ˌa-nəs-ˈthē-zhə\ n : loss of sensation in either lateral half of the body

hemi·an·o·pia \ˌə-ˈnō-pē-ə\ or hemi·an·op·sia \-ˈnäp-sē-ə\ n : blindness in one half of the visual field of one or both eyes — called also *hemiopia* — hemi·an·op·tic \-ə-ˈnäp-tik\ adj

hemi·at·ro·phy \-ˈa-trə-fē\ n, pl -phies : atrophy that affects one half of an organ or part or one side of the whole body — compare HEMIHYPERTROPHY

hemi·azy·gos vein \-(ˌ)ā-ˈzī-gəs-, -ˈa-zə-gəs-\ : a vein that receives blood from the lower half of the left thoracic wall and the left abdominal wall, ascends along the left side of the spinal column, and empties into the azygos vein near the middle of the thorax

hemi·bal·lis·mus \ˌhe-mi-ba-ˈliz-məs\ also hemi·bal·lism \-ˈba-li-zəm\ n : violent uncontrollable movements of one lateral half of the body usu. due to a lesion in the subthalamic nucleus of the contralateral side of the body

hemi·block \ˈhe-mi-ˌbläk\ n : inhibition or failure of conduction in either of the two divisions of the left branch of the bundle of His

he·mic \ˈhē-mik\ adj : of, relating to, or produced by the blood or the circulation of the blood ⟨a ~ murmur⟩

hemi·cho·lin·i·um \-kō-ˈli-nē-əm\ n : any of several blockers of the parasympathetic nervous system that interfere with the synthesis of acetylcholine

hemi·cho·rea \ˌhe-mi-kə-ˈrē-ə\ n : chorea affecting only one lateral half of the body

hemi·col·ec·to·my \-kə-ˈlek-tə-mē, -kō-\ n, pl -mies : surgical excision of part of the colon

hemi·cra·nia \-ˈkrā-nē-ə\ n : pain in one side of the head — hemi·cra·ni·al \-nē-əl\ adj

hemi·des·mo·some \-ˈdez-mə-ˌsōm\ n : a specialization of the plasma membrane of an epithelial cell that serves to connect the basal surface of the cell to the basement membrane

hemi·di·a·phragm \-ˈdī-ə-ˌfram\ n : one of the two lateral halves of the diaphragm separating the chest and abdominal cavities

hemi·fa·cial \-ˈfā-shəl\ adj : involving or affecting one lateral half of the face

hemi·field \ˈhe-mi-ˌfēld\ n : one of two halves of a sensory field (as of vision)

hemi·gas·trec·to·my \ˌhe-mi-ˌga-ˈstrek-tə-mē\ n, pl -mies : surgical removal of one half of the stomach

hemi·glos·sec·to·my \-ˌglä-ˈsek-tə-mē, -ˌglò-\ n, pl -mies : surgical excision of one lateral half of the tongue

hemi·hy·per·tro·phy \-hī-ˈpər-trə-fē\ n, pl -phies : hypertrophy of one half of an organ or part or of one side of the whole body ⟨facial ~⟩ — compare HEMIATROPHY

hemi·lam·i·nec·to·my \-ˌla-mə-ˈnek-tə-mē\ n, pl -mies : laminectomy involving the removal of vertebral laminae on only one side

hemi·me·lia \-ˈmē-lē-ə\ n : a congenital abnormality (as total or partial absence) affecting only the distal half of a limb

he·min \ˈhē-mən\ n : a crystalline salt $C_{34}H_{32}N_4O_4FeCl$ that inhibits the biosynthesis of porphyrin and is used to ameliorate the symptoms of some forms of porphyria

hemi·o·pia \ˌhe-mē-ˈō-pē-ə\ or hemi·op·sia \-ˈäp-sē-ə\ n : HEMIANOPIA

hemi·pa·re·sis \ˌhe-mi-pə-ˈrē-səs, -ˈpar-ə-\ n, pl -re·ses \-ˌsēz\ : muscular weakness or partial paralysis restricted to one side of the body — hemi·pa·ret·ic \-ˈre-tik\ adj

hemi·pel·vec·to·my \-pel-ˈvek-tə-mē\ n, pl -mies : amputation of one leg together with removal of the half of the pelvis on the same side of the body

hemi·ple·gia \ˌhe-mi-ˈplē-jə, -jē-ə\ n : total or partial paralysis of one side of the body that results from disease of or injury to the motor centers of the brain

¹hemi·ple·gic \-ˈplē-jik\ adj : relating to or marked by hemiplegia

²hemiplegic n : a hemiplegic individual

hemi·ret·i·na \,he-mi-'ret-ᵊn-ə\ *n, pl* **-i·nas** *or* **-i·nae** \-ᵊn-,ē, -,ī\ : one half of the retina of one eye

hemi·sect \'he-mi-,sekt\ *vb* : to divide along the mesial plane

hemi·sphere \-,sfir\ *n* : half of a spherical structure or organ: as **a** : CEREBRAL HEMISPHERE **b** : either of the two lobes of the cerebellum of which one projects laterally and posteriorly from each side of the vermis

hemi·spher·ec·to·my \-sfi-'rek-tə-mē\ *n, pl* **-mies** : surgical removal of a cerebral hemisphere

hemi·spher·ic \,he-mi-'sfir-ik, -'sfer-\ *adj* : of, relating to, or affecting a hemisphere (as a cerebral hemisphere) ⟨∼ lesions⟩

hemi·tho·rax \-'thōr-,aks\ *n, pl* **-rax·es** *or* **-tho·ra·ces** \-'thōr-ə-,sēz\ : a lateral half of the thorax

hemi·thy·roid·ec·to·my \-,thī-,ròi-'dek-tə-mē\ *n, pl* **-mies** : surgical removal of one lobe of the thyroid gland

hemi·zy·gote \-'zī-,gōt\ *n* : one that is hemizygous

hemi·zy·gous \-'zī-gəs\ *adj* : having or characterized by one or more genes (as in a genetic deficiency or in an X chromosome paired with a Y chromosome) that have no allelic counterparts — **hemi·zy·gos·i·ty** \-zī-'gä-sə-tē\ *n*

hem·lock \'hem-,läk\ *n* **1** : any of several poisonous herbs (as a poison hemlock or a water hemlock) of the carrot family (Umbelliferae) **2** : a drug or lethal drink prepared from the poison hemlock

hemo- — see HEM-

hemoagglutinin *var of* HEMAGGLUTININ

hemobartonellosis *var of* HAEMOBARTONELLOSIS

he·mo·bil·ia \,hē-mə-'bi-lē-ə\ *n* : bleeding into the bile ducts and gallbladder

he·mo·blas·to·sis \,hē-mə-,blas-'tō-səs\ *n, pl* **-to·ses** \-,sēz\ : abnormal proliferation of the blood-forming tissues

he·moc·cult \'hē-mə-,kəlt\ *adj* : relating to or being a modified guaiac test for occult blood

he·mo·cho·ri·al \,hē-mə-'kōr-ē-əl\ *adj, of a placenta* : having the fetal epithelium bathed in maternal blood

he·mo·chro·ma·to·sis \,hē-mə-,krō-mə-'tō-səs\ *n, pl* **-to·ses** \-,sēz\ : a hereditary disorder of metabolism that involves the deposition of iron-containing pigments in the tissues, is characterized esp. by joint or abdominal pain, weakness, and fatigue, and may lead to bronzing of the skin, arthritis, diabetes, cirrhosis, or heart disease if untreated — compare HEMOSIDEROSIS — **he·mo·chro·ma·tot·ic** \-'tä-tik\ *adj*

he·mo·co·ag·u·la·tion \,hē-mō-kō-,a-gyə-'lā-shən\ *n* : coagulation of blood

he·mo·con·cen·tra·tion \,hē-mō-,kän-sən-'trā-shən\ *n* : increased concentration of cells and solids in the blood usu. resulting from loss of fluid to the tissues — compare HEMODILUTION 1

he·mo·cul·ture \'hē-mə-,kəl-chər\ *n* : a culture made from blood to detect the presence of pathogenic microorganisms

he·mo·cy·to·blast \,hē-mə-'sī-tə-,blast\ *n* : a stem cell for blood-cellular elements; *esp* : one considered competent to produce all types of blood cell — **he·mo·cy·to·blas·tic** \-,sī-tə-'blas-tik\ *adj*

he·mo·cy·tom·e·ter \-sī-'tä-mə-tər\ *n* : HEMACYTOMETER

he·mo·di·al·y·sis \,hē-mō-dī-'a-lə-səs\ *n, pl* **-y·ses** \-,sēz\ : DIALYSIS 2a

he·mo·di·a·lyz·er \-'dī-ə-,lī-zər\ *n* : ARTIFICIAL KIDNEY

he·mo·di·lu·tion \-dī-'lü-shən, -də-\ *n* **1** : decreased concentration (as after hemorrhage) of cells and solids in the blood resulting from gain of fluid from the tissues — compare HEMOCONCENTRATION **2** : a medical procedure for producing hemodilution; *esp* : one performed esp. to reduce the number of red blood cells lost during surgery that involves the preoperative withdrawal of one or more units of whole blood, immediate replacement with an equal volume of intravenous fluid, and postoperative reinfusion of withdrawn blood — **he·mo·di·lute** \-'lüt\ *vb*

he·mo·dy·nam·ic \-dī-'na-mik, -də-\ *adj* **1** : of, relating to, or involving hemodynamics **2** : relating to or functioning in the mechanics of blood circulation — **he·mo·dy·nam·i·cal·ly** *adv*

he·mo·dy·nam·ics \-miks\ *n sing or pl* **1** : a branch of physiology that deals with the circulation of the blood **2 a** : the forces or mechanisms involved in circulation **b** : hemodynamic effect (as of a drug)

he·mo·fil·ter \'hē-mō-,fil-tər\ *n* : a filter used for hemofiltration

he·mo·fil·tra·tion \,hē-mō-fil-'trā-shən\ *n* : the process of removing blood from the living body, purifying it by passing it through a system of extracorporeal filters, and returning it to the body

he·mo·glo·bin \'hē-mə-,glō-bən\ *n* : an iron-containing respiratory pigment of red blood cells that functions primarily in the transport of oxygen from the lungs to the tissues of the body, that consists of a globin of four subunits each of which is linked to a heme molecule, that combines loosely and reversibly with oxygen in the lungs or gills to form oxyhemoglobin and with carbon dioxide in the tissues to form carbhemoglobin, and that in humans is present normally in blood to the extent of 14 to 16 grams in 100 milliliters — compare CARBOXYHEMOGLOBIN, METHEMOGLOBIN — **he·mo·glo·bin·ic** \,hē-mə-glō-'bi-nik\ *adj*

— **he·mo·glo·bi·nous** \-'glō-bə-nəs\ *adj*

hemoglobin A *n* : the hemoglobin in the red blood cells of the normal human adult that consists of two alpha chains and two beta chains

hemoglobin A1c \-ā-,wən-'sē\ *n* : a stable glycoprotein formed when glucose binds to hemoglobin A in the blood; *also* : a test that measures the level of hemoglobin A1c in the blood as a means of determining the average blood sugar concentrations for the preceding two to three months — called also *glycated hemoglobin, glycohemoglobin, glycosylated hemoglobin, HA1c, HbA1c*

hemoglobin C *n* : an abnormal hemoglobin that differs from hemoglobin A in having a lysine residue substituted for the glutamic-acid residue at position 6 in two of the four polypeptide chains making up the hemoglobin molecule

hemoglobin C disease *n* : an inherited hemolytic anemia that occurs esp. in individuals of African descent and is characterized esp. by splenomegaly and the presence of target cells and hemoglobin C in the blood

he·mo·glo·bin·emia \-,glō-bə-'nē-mē-ə\ *n* : the presence of free hemoglobin in the blood plasma resulting from the solution of hemoglobin out of the red blood cells or from their disintegration

hemoglobin F *n* : FETAL HEMOGLOBIN

he·mo·glo·bin·om·e·ter \-,glō-bə-'nä-mə-tər\ *n* : an instrument for the colorimetric determination of hemoglobin in blood — **he·mo·glo·bin·om·e·try** \-'nä-mə-trē\ *n*

he·mo·glo·bin·op·a·thy \hē-mə-,glō-bə-'nä-pə-thē\ *n, pl* **-thies** : a blood disorder (as sickle-cell anemia) caused by a genetically determined change in the molecular structure of hemoglobin

hemoglobin S *n* : an abnormal hemoglobin occurring in the red blood cells in sickle-cell anemia and sickle-cell trait and differing from hemoglobin A in having a valine residue substituted for the glutamic-acid residue in position 6 of two of the four polypeptide chains making up the hemoglobin molecule

he·mo·glo·bin·uria \,hē-mə-,glō-bə-'nùr-ē-ə, -'nyùr-\ *n* : the presence of free hemoglobin in the urine — **he·mo·glo·bin·uric** \-'nùr-ik, -'nyùr-\ *adj*

he·mo·gram \'hē-mə-,gram\ *n* : a systematic report of the findings from a blood examination

he·mol·y·sate *also* **he·mol·y·zate** \hi-'mäl-ə-,zāt, -,sāt\ *n* : a product of hemolysis

he·mo·ly·sin \,hē-mə-'līs-ᵊn, hi-'mäl-ə-sən\ *n* : a substance that causes the dissolution of red blood cells — called also *hemotoxin*

he·mo·ly·sis \hi-'mäl-ə-səs, ,hē-mə-'lī-

səs\ *n, pl* **-ly·ses** \-,sēz\ : lysis of red blood cells with liberation of hemoglobin — see BETA HEMOLYSIS — **he·mo·lyt·ic** \,hē-mə-'li-tik\ *adj*

hemolytic anemia *n* : anemia caused by excessive destruction (as in infection or sickle-cell anemia) of red blood cells

hemolytic disease of the newborn *n* : ERYTHROBLASTOSIS FETALIS

hemolytic jaundice *n* : a condition characterized by excessive destruction of red blood cells accompanied by jaundice

hemolytic uremic syndrome *n* : a rare disease that is marked by the formation of thrombi in the capillaries and arterioles esp. of the kidney, that is characterized clinically by hemolytic anemia, thrombocytopenia, and varying degrees of kidney failure, that is precipitated by a variety of etiologic factors (as infection with *Escherichia coli* or *Shigella dysenteriae*), and that primarily affects infants and young children — abbr. *HUS;* see THROMBOTIC THROMBOCYTOPENIC PURPURA

he·mo·lyze \'hē-mə-,līz\ *vb* **-lyzed; -lyz·ing** : to cause or undergo hemolysis of

he·mo·par·a·site \,hē-mō-'par-ə-,sīt\ *n* : an animal parasite (as a filarial worm) living in the blood of a vertebrate — **he·mo·par·a·sit·ic** \-,par-ə-'si-tik\ *adj*

he·mop·a·thy \hē-'mä-pə-thē\ *n, pl* **-thies** : a pathological state (as anemia or agranulocytosis) of the blood or blood-forming tissues

he·mo·per·fu·sion \,hē-mō-pər-'fyü-zhən\ *n* : blood cleansing by adsorption on an extracorporeal medium (as activated charcoal) of impurities (as of larger molecular size than are removed by dialysis

he·mo·peri·car·di·um \,hē-mō-,per-ə-'kär-dē-əm\ *n, pl* **-dia** \-dē-ə\ : blood in the pericardial cavity

he·mo·peri·to·ne·um \-,per-ət-ᵊn-'ē-əm\ *n* : blood in the peritoneal cavity

he·mo·pex·in \-'pek-sən\ *n* : a glycoprotein that binds heme preventing its excretion in urine and that is part of the beta-globulin fraction of human serum

¹**he·mo·phile** \'hē-mə-,fīl\ *adj* **1** : HEMOPHILIAC **2** : HEMOPHILIC **2**

²**hemophile** *n* **1** : HEMOPHILIAC **2** : a hemophilic organism (as a bacterium)

he·mo·phil·ia \,hē-mə-'fi-lē-ə\ *n* : a sex-linked hereditary blood defect that occurs almost exclusively in males and is characterized by delayed clotting of the blood and consequent difficulty in controlling hemorrhage even after minor injuries — compare CHRISTMAS DISEASE, HEMORRHAGIC DIATHESIS

hemophilia A *n* : hemophilia caused by the absence of factor VIII from the blood

hemophilia B n : CHRISTMAS DISEASE

¹**he·mo·phil·i·ac** \-'fi-lē-ˌak\ adj 1 : of, resembling, or affected with hemophilia

²**hemophiliac** n : one affected with hemophilia — called also *bleeder*

¹**he·mo·phil·ic** \-'fi-lik\ adj 1 : HEMOPHILIAC ⟨a ~ patient⟩ 2 : tending to thrive in blood ⟨~ bacteria⟩

²**hemophilic** n : HEMOPHILIAC

he·moph·i·lus \hē-'mä-fə-ləs\ n : HAEMOPHILUS 2

He·moph·i·lus \hē-'mä-fə-ləs\ n, syn of HAEMOPHILUS

he·mo·pneu·mo·tho·rax \ˌhē-mə-ˌnü-mə-'thōr-ˌaks, -ˌnyü-\ n, pl **-rax·es** or **-ra·ces** \-'thōr-ə-ˌsēz\ : the accumulation of blood and air in the pleural cavity

he·mo·poi·e·sis \ˌhē-mə-pói-'ē-səs\ n, pl **-e·ses** \-ˌsēz\ : HEMATOPOIESIS — **he·mo·poi·et·ic** \-'e-tik\ adj

he·mo·pro·tein \-'prō-ˌtēn\ n : a conjugated protein (as hemoglobin or cytochrome) whose prosthetic group is a porphyrin combined with iron

he·mop·ty·sis \hi-'mäp-tə-səs\ n, pl **-ty·ses** \-ˌsēz\ : expectoration of blood from some part of the respiratory tract

he·mor·rhe·ol·o·gy \ˌhē-mə-rē-'ä-lə-jē\ n, pl **-gies** : the science of the physical properties of blood flow in the circulatory system — **he·mo·rheo·log·i·cal** \-ˌrē-ə-'lä-ji-kəl\ also **he·mo·rheo·log·ic** \-'lä-jik\ adj

hem·or·rhage \'hem-rij, 'hem-ə-\ n : a copious discharge of blood from the blood vessels — **hemorrhage** vb — **hem·or·rhag·ic** \ˌhem-ə-'ra-jik\ adj

hemorrhagica — see PURPURA HEMORRHAGICA

hemorrhagic dengue n : DENGUE HEMORRHAGIC FEVER

hemorrhagic diathesis n : an abnormal tendency to spontaneous often severe bleeding — compare HEMOPHILIA, THROMBOCYTOPENIC PURPURA

hemorrhagic fever n : any of a diverse group of virus diseases (as Korean hemorrhagic fever, Lassa fever, and Ebola) usu. transmitted by arthropods or rodents and characterized by a sudden onset, fever, aching, bleeding in the internal organs, petechiae, and shock

hemorrhagic fever with renal syndrome n : any of several clinically similar diseases that are caused by hantaviruses (as the Hantaan virus) and are characterized by fever, renal insufficiency, thrombocytopenia, and hemorrhage but not usu. by pulmonary complications

hemorrhagic septicemia n : any of several pasteurelloses of domestic animals that are caused by a bacterium of the genus *Pasteurella* (P. multocida)

hemorrhagic shock n : shock resulting from reduction of the volume of blood in the body due to hemorrhage

hemorrhagic stroke n : stroke caused by the rupture of a blood vessel with bleeding into the tissue of the brain

hemorrhagicum — see CORPUS HEMORRHAGICUM

hem·or·rhoid \'hem-ˌrȯid, 'he-mə-\ n : a mass of dilated veins in swollen tissue at the margin of the anus or nearby within the rectum — usu. used in pl.; called also *piles*

¹**hem·or·rhoid·al** \ˌhem-'rȯid-³l, ˌhe-mə-\ adj 1 : of, relating to, or involving hemorrhoids 2 : RECTAL

²**hemorrhoidal** n : a hemorrhoidal part (as an artery or vein)

hemorrhoidal artery n : RECTAL ARTERY

hemorrhoidal vein n : RECTAL VEIN

hem·or·rhoid·ec·to·my \ˌhe-mə-ˌrȯi-dek-tə-mē\ n, pl **-mies** : surgical removal of a hemorrhoid

he·mo·sid·er·in \ˌhē-mō-'si-də-rən\ n : a yellowish brown granular pigment formed by breakdown of hemoglobin, found in phagocytes and in tissues esp. in disturbances of iron metabolism (as in hemochromatosis, hemosiderosis, or some anemias)

he·mo·sid·er·o·sis \-ˌsi-də-'rō-səs\ n, pl **-o·ses** \-ˌsēz\ : excessive deposition of hemosiderin in bodily tissues as a result of the breakdown of red blood cells — compare HEMOCHROMATOSIS

he·mo·sta·sis \ˌhē-mə-'stā-səs\ n, pl **-sta·ses** \-ˌsēz\ 1 : stoppage or sluggishness of blood flow 2 : the arrest of bleeding (as by a hemostatic agent)

he·mo·stat \'hē-mə-ˌstat\ n 1 : HEMOSTATIC 2 : an instrument and esp. forceps for compressing a bleeding vessel

¹**he·mo·stat·ic** \ˌhē-mə-'sta-tik\ n : an agent that checks bleeding; esp : one that shortens the clotting time of blood

²**hemostatic** adj 1 : of or caused by hemostasis 2 : serving to check bleeding

he·mo·ther·a·py \-'ther-ə-pē\ n, pl **-pies** : treatment involving the administration of fresh blood, a blood fraction, or a blood preparation

he·mo·tho·rax \ˌhē-mə-'thōr-ˌaks\ n, pl **-tho·rax·es** or **-tho·ra·ces** \-'thōr-ə-ˌsēz\ : blood in the pleural cavity

he·mo·tox·ic \-'täk-sik\ adj : destructive to red blood corpuscles

he·mo·tox·in \-'täk-sən\ n : HEMOLYSIN

he·mo·zo·in \ˌhē-mə-'zō-ən\ n : an iron-containing pigment which accumulates as cytoplasmic granules in malaria parasites and is a breakdown product of hemoglobin

hemp \'hemp\ n 1 : a tall widely grown Asian herb of the genus *Cannabis* (C. sativa) with a strong woody fiber used esp. for cordage 2 : the fiber of hemp 3 : a psychoactive drug (as marijuana or hashish) from hemp

hen·bane \'hen-ˌbān\ n : a poisonous fetid Old World herb of the genus

Hyoscyamus (*H. niger*) that contains the alkaloids hyoscyamine and scopolamine — called also *black henbane*

Hen·le's layer \\'hen-lēz-\ *n* : a single layer of cuboidal epithelium forming the outer boundary of the inner stratum of a hair follicle — compare HUXLEY'S LAYER

Hen·le \\'hen-lə\, **Friedrich Gustav Jacob (1809–1885),** German anatomist and histologist.

Henle's loop *n* : LOOP OF HENLE

He·noch–Schön·lein *adj* : SCHÖNLEIN≠ HENOCH ⟨~ purpura⟩

He·noch's purpura \\'he-nȯks-\ *n* : Schönlein-Henoch purpura that is characterized esp. by gastrointestinal bleeding and pain — compare SCHÖNLEIN'S DISEASE

E. H. Henoch — see SCHÖNLEIN≠ HENOCH

HEPA \\'he-pə\ *adj* [*h*igh *e*fficiency *p*articulate *air*] : being, using, or containing a filter usu. designed to remove 99.97% of airborne particles measuring 0.3 microns or greater in diameter passing through it

hep·a·ran sulfate \\'he-pə-₁ran-\ *n* : a sulfated glycosaminoglycan that accumulates in bodily tissues in abnormal amounts in some mucopolysaccharidoses — called also *heparitin sulfate*

hep·a·rin \\'he-pə-rən\ *n* : a glycosaminoglycan sulfuric acid ester that occurs esp. in the liver and lungs, that prolongs the clotting time of blood by preventing the formation of fibrin, and that is administered parenterally in the form of its sodium salt in vascular surgery and in the treatment of postoperative thrombosis and embolism — see LIQUAEMIN; compare ANTIPROTHROMBIN, ANTITHROMBIN

he·pa·rin·ase \\'he-pə-rə-₁nās, -₁nāz\ *n* : an enzyme that breaks down heparin

hep·a·rin·ize \\'he-pə-rə-₁nīz\ *vb* **-ized; -iz·ing** : to treat with heparin — **hep·a·rin·iza·tion** \-rə-nə-'zā-shən\ *n*

hep·a·rin·oid \-₁nȯid\ *n* : any of various sulfated polysaccharides that have anticoagulant activity resembling that of heparin — **heparinoid** *adj*

hep·a·ri·tin sulfate \\'he-pə-₁rī-tin-\ *n* : HEPARAN SULFATE

hepat- *or* **hepato-** *comb form* **1** : liver ⟨*hepat*itis⟩ ⟨*hepato*toxic⟩ **2** : hepatic and ⟨*hepato*biliary⟩

hep·a·tec·to·my \₁he-pə-'tek-tə-mē\ *n*, *pl* **-mies** : excision of the liver or of part of the liver — **hep·a·tec·to·mized** \-tə-₁mīzd\ *adj*

he·pat·ic \hi-'pa-tik\ *adj* : of, relating to, affecting, or associated with the liver ⟨~ injury⟩ ⟨~ insufficiency⟩

hepatic artery *n* : the branch of the celiac artery that supplies the liver with arterial blood

hepatic cell *n* : HEPATOCYTE

hepatic coma *n* : a coma that is induced by severe liver disease

hepatic duct *n* : a duct conveying the bile away from the liver and uniting with the cystic duct to form the common bile duct

hepatic flexure *n* : the right-angle bend in the colon on the right side of the body near the liver that marks the junction of the ascending colon and the transverse colon — called also *right colic flexure*

he·pat·i·cos·to·my \hi-₁pa-ti-'käs-tə-mē\ *n, pl* **-mies** : an operation to provide an artificial opening into the hepatic duct

he·pat·i·cot·o·my \-'kä-tə-mē\ *n, pl* **-mies** : surgical incision of the hepatic duct

hepatic portal system *n* : a group of veins that carry blood from the capillaries of the stomach, intestine, spleen, and pancreas to the sinusoids of the liver

hepatic portal vein *n* : a portal vein carrying blood from the digestive organs and spleen to the liver

hepaticus — see FETOR HEPATICUS

hepatic vein *n* : any of the veins that carry the blood received from the hepatic artery and from the hepatic portal vein away from the liver and that in humans are usu. three in number and open into the inferior vena cava

hepatis — see PORTA HEPATIS

hep·a·ti·tis \₁he-pə-'tī-təs\ *n, pl* **-tit·i·des** \-'ti-tə-₁dēz\ *also* **-ti·tis·es** \-'tī-tə-səz\ **1** : inflammation of the liver **2** : a disease or condition (as hepatitis A or hepatitis B) marked by inflammation of the liver — **hep·a·tit·ic** \-'ti-tik\ *adj*

hepatitis A *n* : an acute usu. benign hepatitis caused by a picornavirus (species *Hepatitis A virus* of the genus *Hepatovirus*) that does not persist in the blood serum and is transmitted esp. in food and water contaminated with infected fecal matter — called also *infectious hepatitis*

hepatitis B *n* : a sometimes fatal hepatitis caused by a double-stranded DNA virus (species *Hepatitis B virus* of the genus *Orthohepadnavirus*, family *Hepadnaviridae*) that tends to persist in the blood serum and is transmitted esp. by contact with infected blood (as by transfusion) or other infected bodily fluids (as semen) — called also *serum hepatitis*

hepatitis B surface antigen *n* : an antigen that is usu. a surface particle from the hepatitis B virus and that is found in the sera esp. of patients with hepatitis B — abbr. *HBsAg;* called also *Australia antigen*

hepatitis C *n* : hepatitis caused by a flavivirus (species *Hepatitis C virus* of the genus *Hepacivirus*) that tends to persist in the blood serum and is usu. transmitted by contact with infected blood (as by transfusion or by illicit intravenous drug use) and that is the cause of most cases of hepatitis diagnosed as non-A, non-B hepatitis

hepatitis D n : hepatitis that is similar to hepatitis B and is caused by coinfection with the hepatitis B virus and hepatitis D virus — called also *delta hepatitis, hepatitis delta*

hepatitis D virus n : a subviral particle lacking the protein coat and the surface antigens of the hepatitis B virus that is unable to invade cells except in the presence of the hepatitis B virus and together with this virus causes hepatitis D — called also *delta agent, delta virus, hepatitis delta virus*

hepatitis E n : a hepatitis that is rare in the U.S. but is common in some third-world countries, is usu. contracted from sewage-contaminated water, and is caused by a single-stranded RNA virus (species *Hepatitis E virus* of the genus *Hepevirus*) similar to the caliciviruses in its structural morphology and in the organization of its genome

hep·a·ti·za·tion \he-pə-tə-'zā-shən\ n : conversion of tissue (as of the lungs in pneumonia) into a substance which resembles liver tissue — **hep·a·tized** \'he-pə-ˌtīzd\ adj

hepato- — see HEPAT-

he·pa·to·bil·i·ary \he-pə-tō-'bi-lē-ˌer-ē, hi-ˌpa-tə-\ adj : of, relating to, situated in or near, produced in, or affecting the liver and bile, bile ducts, and gallbladder ⟨∼ disease⟩

he·pa·to·blas·to·ma \-blas-'tō-mə\ n, pl **-mas** also **-ma·ta** \-mə-tə\ : a malignant tumor of the liver esp. of infants and young children that is composed of cells resembling embryonic hepatocytes

he·pa·to·car·cin·o·gen \-kär-'si-nə-jən, -ˌkärs-ᵊn-ə-jen\ n : a substance or agent causing cancer of the liver — **he·pa·to·car·cin·o·gen·ic** \-ˌje-nik\ adj — **he·pa·to·car·cin·o·ge·nic·i·ty** \-jə-'ni-sə-tē\ n

he·pa·to·car·cin·o·gen·e·sis \-ˌkärs-ᵊn-ō-'je-nə-səs\ n, pl **-es·es** \-ˌsēz\ : the production of cancer of the liver

he·pa·to·car·ci·no·ma \-ˌkärs-ᵊn-'ō-mə\ n, pl **-mas** also **-ma·ta** \-mə-tə\ : carcinoma of the liver

he·pa·to·cel·lu·lar \ˌhep-ət-ō-'sel-yə-lər, hi-ˌpat-ō-'sel-\ adj : of or involving hepatocytes ⟨∼ carcinomas⟩

he·pa·to·cyte \hi-'pa-tə-ˌsīt, 'he-pə-tə-\ n : any of the polygonal epithelial parenchymatous cells of the liver that secrete bile — called also *hepatic cell, liver cell*

he·pa·to·gen·ic \ˌhe-pə-tō-'je-nik, hi-ˌpa-tə-\ or **hep·a·tog·e·nous** \ˌhe-pə-'tä-jə-nəs\ adj : produced or originating in the liver

he·pa·to·len·tic·u·lar degeneration \hi-ˌpa-tə-len-ˌti-kyə-lər-, ˌhe-pə-tō-\ n : WILSON'S DISEASE

hep·a·tol·o·gy \ˌhe-pə-'tä-lə-jē\ n, pl **-gies** : a branch of medicine concerned with the liver — **hep·a·tol·o·gist** \-jist\ n

hep·a·to·ma \ˌhe-pə-'tō-mə\ n, pl **-mas** also **-ma·ta** \-mə-tə\ : a usu. malignant tumor of the liver — **hep·a·to·ma·tous** \-mə-təs\ adj

he·pa·to·meg·a·ly \ˌhe-pə-tō-'me-gə-lē, hi-ˌpa-tə-'me-\ n, pl **-lies** : enlargement of the liver — **he·pa·to·meg·a·lic** \-'me-gə-lik\ adj

he·pa·to·pan·cre·at·ic \hi-ˌpa-tə-ˌpaŋ-krē-'a-tik, hi-ˌpə-tō-, -ˌpan-\ adj : of or relating to the liver and the pancreas

hep·a·top·a·thy \ˌhe-pə-'tä-pə-thē\ n, pl **-thies** : an abnormal or diseased state of the liver

he·pa·to·por·tal \ˌhe-pə-tō-'pórt-ᵊl, hi-ˌpa-tə-\ adj : of or relating to the hepatic portal system

he·pa·to·re·nal \-'rē-nəl\ adj : of, relating to, or affecting the liver and the kidneys ⟨fatal ∼ dysfunction⟩

hepatorenal syndrome n : functional kidney failure associated with cirrhosis of the liver and characterized typically by jaundice, ascites, hypoalbuminemia, hypoprothrombinemia, and encephalopathy

hep·a·tor·rha·phy \ˌhe-pə-'tór-ə-fē\ n, pl **-phies** : suture of a wound or injury to the liver

hep·a·to·sis \ˌhe-pə-'tō-səs\ n, pl **-to·ses** \-ˌsēz\ : any noninflammatory functional disorder of the liver

he·pa·to·splen·ic \ˌhe-pə-tō-'sple-nik, hi-ˌpa-tə-\ adj : of or affecting the liver and spleen ⟨∼ schistosomiasis⟩

he·pa·to·spleno·meg·a·ly \-ˌsple-nō-'me-gə-lē\ n, pl **-lies** : coincident enlargement of the liver and spleen

hep·a·tot·o·my \ˌhe-pə-'tä-tə-mē\ n, pl **-mies** : surgical incision of the liver

he·pa·to·tox·ic \ˌhe-pə-tō-'täk-sik, hi-ˌpa-tə-'täk-\ adj : relating to or causing injury to the liver — **he·pa·to·tox·ic·i·ty** \-täk-'si-sə-tē\ n

he·pa·to·tox·in \-'täk-sən\ n : a substance toxic to the liver

hep·ta·chlor \'hep-tə-ˌklór\ n : a persistent chlorinated hydrocarbon pesticide $C_{10}H_5Cl_7$ that causes liver disease in animals and is a suspected human carcinogen

herb \'ərb, 'hərb\ n, often attrib **1** : a seed plant that lacks woody tissue and dies to the ground at the end of a growing season **2** : a plant or plant part valued for medicinal, savory, or aromatic qualities

¹herb·al \'ər-bəl, 'hər-\ n **1** : a book about plants esp. with reference to their medical properties **2** : HERBAL REMEDY

²herbal adj : of, relating to, or made of herbs

herb·al·ism \'ər-bə-ˌli-zəm, 'hər-\ n : HERBAL MEDICINE 1

herb·al·ist \'ər-bə-list, 'hər-\ n **1** : one who collects or grows herbs **2** : one who practices herbal medicine

herbal medicine n **1** : the art or practice of using herbs and herbal remedies to maintain health and to prevent, alleviate, or cure disease — called also *herbalism* **2** : HERBAL REMEDY

herbal remedy *n* : a plant or plant part or an extract or mixture of these used to prevent, alleviate, or cure disease — called also *herbal, herbal medicine*

herb doctor *n* : HERBALIST 2

Her·cep·tin \härˈsep-tən\ *trademark* — used for a preparation of trastuzumab

herd immunity *n* : a reduction in the probability of infection that is held to apply to susceptible members of a population in which a significant proportion of the individuals are immune because the chance of coming in contact with an infected individual is less

he·red·i·tary \hə-ˈre-də-ˌter-ē\ *adj* **1** : genetically transmitted or transmittable from parent to offspring — compare ACQUIRED 2, CONGENITAL 2, FAMILIAL **2** : of or relating to inheritance or heredity — **he·red·i·tar·i·ly** \-ˌre-də-ˈter-ə-lē\ *adv*

hereditary hemorrhagic telangiectasia *n* : a hereditary abnormality that is characterized by multiple telangiectasias and by bleeding into the tissues and mucous membranes because of abnormal fragility of the capillaries — called also *Rendu-Osler-Weber disease*

hereditary spherocytosis *n* : a disorder of red blood cells that is inherited as a dominant trait and is characterized by anemia, small thick fragile spherocytes which are extremely susceptible to hemolysis, enlargement of the spleen, reticulocytosis, and mild jaundice

he·red·i·ty \hə-ˈre-də-tē\ *n, pl* **-ties 1** : the sum of the qualities and potentialities genetically derived from one's ancestors **2** : the transmission of traits from ancestor to descendant through the molecular mechanism lying primarily in the DNA or RNA of the genes — compare MEIOSIS

heredo- *comb form* : hereditary ⟨*heredo*familial⟩

her·e·do·fa·mil·ial \ˌher-ə-dō-fə-ˈmil-yəl\ *adj* : tending to occur in more than one member of a family and suspected of having a genetic basis

Her·ing–Breu·er reflex \ˈher-iŋ-ˈbrȯi-ər-\ *n* : any of several reflexes that control inflation and deflation of the lungs; *esp* : reflex inhibition of inspiration triggered by pulmonary muscle spindles upon expansion of the lungs and mediated by the vagus nerve

Hering, Karl Ewald Konstantin (1834–1918), German physiologist and psychologist.

Breuer, Josef (1842–1925), Austrian physician and physiologist.

her·i·ta·bil·i·ty \ˌher-ə-tə-ˈbil-ə-tē\ *n, pl* **-ties 1** : the quality or state of being heritable **2** : the proportion of observed variation in a particular trait (as intelligence) that can be attributed to inherited genetic factors in contrast to environmental ones

her·i·ta·ble \ˈher-ə-tə-bəl\ *adj* : HEREDITARY

her·maph·ro·dite \(ˌ)hər-ˈma-frə-ˌdīt\ *n* : an individual having both male and female reproductive organs — **hermaphrodite** *adj* — **her·maph·ro·dit·ic** \-ˌma-frə-ˈdi-tik\ *adj* — **her·maph·ro·dit·ism** \-ˈma-frə-ˌdī-ˌti-zəm\ *n*

her·met·ic \(ˌ)hər-ˈme-tik\ *adj* : being airtight or impervious to air — **her·met·i·cal·ly** \-ti-k(ə-)lē\ *adv*

her·nia \ˈhər-nē-ə\ *n, pl* **-ni·as** *or* **-ni·ae** \-nē-ˌē, -nē-ˌī\ : a protrusion of an organ or part through a wall of the cavity in which it is normally enclosed — called also *rupture*; see ABDOMINAL HERNIA, HIATAL HERNIA, STRANGULATED HERNIA — **her·ni·al** \-nē-əl\ *adj*

hernial sac *n* : a protruding pouch of peritoneum that contains a herniated organ or tissue

her·ni·ate \ˈhər-nē-ˌāt\ *vb* **-at·ed; -at·ing** : to protrude through an abnormal body opening : RUPTURE

her·ni·a·tion \ˌhər-nē-ˈā-shən\ *n* **1** : the act or process of herniating **2** : HERNIA

hernio- *comb form* : hernia ⟨*hernio*rrhaphy⟩ ⟨*hernio*tomy⟩

her·nio·plas·ty \ˈhər-nē-ə-ˌplas-tē\ *n, pl* **-ties** : HERNIORRHAPHY

her·ni·or·rha·phy \ˌhər-nē-ˈȯr-ə-fē\ *n, pl* **-phies** : an operation for hernia that involves opening the hernial sac, returning the contents to their normal place, obliterating the hernial sac, and closing the opening with strong sutures

her·ni·ot·o·my \-ˈä-tə-mē\ *n, pl* **-mies** : the operation of cutting through a band of tissue that constricts a strangulated hernia

he·ro·ic \hi-ˈrō-ik\ *adj* **1** : of a kind that is likely to be undertaken only to save life ⟨∼ surgery⟩ **2** : having a pronounced effect — used chiefly of medicaments or dosage ⟨∼ doses⟩

her·o·in \ˈher-ə-wən\ *n* : a strongly physiologically addictive narcotic $C_{21}H_{23}NO_5$ that is made by acetylation of but is more potent than morphine and that is prohibited for medical use in the U.S. but is used illicitly for its euphoric effects — called also *diacetylmorphine, diamorphine*

her·o·in·ism \-wə-ˌni-zəm\ *n* : addiction to heroin

her·pan·gi·na \ˌhər-ˌpan-ˈjī-nə, ˌhər-ˈpan-jə-nə\ *n* : a contagious disease of children characterized by fever, headache, and a vesicular eruption in the throat and caused by any of numerous coxsackieviruses and echoviruses

her·pes \'hər-(ˌ)pēz\ *n* : any of several inflammatory diseases of the skin caused by herpesviruses and characterized by clusters of vesicles; *esp* : HERPES SIMPLEX

her·pes gen·i·tal·is \ˌhər-(ˌ)pēz-ˌje-nə-'ta-ləs\ *n* : GENITAL HERPES

herpes keratitis *n* : keratitis caused by any of the herpesviruses that produce herpes simplex or shingles

herpes la·bi·al·is \-ˌlā-bē-'a-ləs\ *n* : herpes simplex affecting the lips and nose

herpes sim·plex \-'sim-ˌpleks\ *n* : either of two diseases caused by herpesviruses of the genus *Simplexvirus* that are marked esp. by watery blisters on the skin or mucous membranes of the lips, mouth, face, or genital region — see HSV-1, HSV-2

her·pes·vi·rus \-'vī-rəs\ *n* : any of a family (*Herpesviridae*) of double-stranded DNA viruses that include the cytomegalovirus and Epstein-Barr virus and the causative agents of chicken pox, equine coital exanthema, herpes simplex, infectious bovine rhinotracheitis, infectious laryngotracheitis, malignant catarrhal fever, Marek's disease, pseudorabies, rhinopneumonitis, roseola infantum, and shingles

herpes zos·ter \-'zäs-tər\ *n* : SHINGLES

herpet- *or* **herpeto-** *comb form* : herpes ⟨*herpeti*form⟩

her·pet·ic \(ˌ)hər-'pe-tik\ *adj* : of, relating to, or resembling herpes

her·pet·i·form \-'pe-tə-ˌfȯrm\ *adj* : resembling herpes

herpetiformis — see DERMATITIS HERPETIFORMIS

hertz \'hərts, 'herts\ *n* : a unit of frequency equal to one cycle per second — abbr. *Hz*

Herx·heim·er reaction \'hərks-ˌhī-mər-\ *n* : JARISCH-HERXHEIMER REACTION

Heschl's gyrus \'he-shəlz-\ *n* : a convolution of the temporal lobe that is the cortical center for hearing and runs obliquely outward and forward from the posterior part of the lateral sulcus

    Heschl, Richard Ladislaus (1824–1881), Austrian anatomist.

het·a·cil·lin \ˌhe-tə-'si-lən\ *n* : a semisynthetic oral penicillin $C_{19}H_{23}N_3O_4S$ that is converted to ampicillin in the body

heter- *or* **hetero-** *comb form* : other than usual : other : different ⟨*hetero*-graft⟩

Het·er·a·kis \-'ra-kəs\ *n* : a genus (family Heterakidae) of nematode worms including some (*H. gallinarum*) that infests esp. chickens and turkeys and serves as an intermediate host and transmitter of the protozoan causing blackhead

het·ero \'he-tə-ˌrō\ *n, pl* **-er·os** : HETEROSEXUAL

het·ero·an·ti·body \ˌhe-tə-rō-'an-ti-ˌbä-dē\ *n, pl* **-dies** : an antibody specific for a heterologous antigen

het·ero·an·ti·gen \-'an-ti-jən, -ˌjen\ *n* : an antibody that is produced by an individual of one species and is capable of stimulating an immune response in an individual of another species

het·ero·chro·ma·tin \-'krō-mə-tən\ *n* : densely staining chromatin that appears as nodules in or along chromosomes and contains relatively few genes — **het·ero·chro·mat·ic** \-krə-'ma-tik\ *adj*

het·ero·chro·mia \ˌhe-tə-rō-'krō-mē-ə\ *n* : a difference in coloration in two anatomical structures or two parts of the same structure which are normally alike in color ⟨~ of the iris⟩

heterochromia ir·i·dis \-'ir-i-dəs\ *n* : a difference in color between the irises of the two eyes or between parts of one iris

het·ero·cy·clic \ˌhe-tə-rō-'sī-klik, -'si-\ *adj* : relating to, characterized by, or being a ring composed of atoms of more than one kind

heterocyclic amine *n* : an amine containing one or more closed rings of carbon and nitrogen; *esp* : any of various carcinogenic amines formed when creatine or creatinine reacts with free amino acids and sugar in meat cooked at high temperature

het·ero·di·mer \-'dī-mər\ *n* : a protein composed of two polypeptide chains differing in composition in the order, number, or kind of their amino acid residues — **het·ero·di·mer·ic** \-dī-'mer-ik\ *adj*

het·ero·du·plex \ˌhe-tə-rō-'dü-ˌpleks, -'dyü-\ *n* : a nucleic-acid molecule composed of two chains with each derived from a different parent molecule — **heteroduplex** *adj*

het·ero·gam·ete \ˌhe-tə-rō-'ga-ˌmēt, -gə-'mēt\ *n* : either of a pair of gametes that differ in form, size, or behavior and occur typically as large nonmotile female gametes and small motile sperm

het·ero·ga·met·ic \-gə-'me-tik, -'mē-\ *adj* : forming two kinds of gametes of which one determines offspring of one sex and the other determines offspring of the opposite sex — **het·ero·gam·e·ty** \-'ga-mə-tē\ *n*

het·er·og·a·my \ˌhe-tə-'rä-gə-mē\ *n, pl* **-mies** 1 : sexual reproduction involving fusion of unlike gametes 2 : the condition of reproducing by heterogamy — **het·er·og·a·mous** \-məs\ *adj*

het·ero·ge·neous \ˌhe-tə-rə-'jē-nē-əs\ *adj* : not uniform in structure or composition — **het·ero·ge·ne·ity** \ˌhe-tə-rō-jə-'nē-ə-tē\ *n*

het·ero·gen·ic \ˌhe-tər-ə-'je-nik\ *adj* : derived from or involving individuals of a different species ⟨~ antigens⟩

het·er·og·e·nous \ˌhe-tə-'rä-jə-nəs\

adj **1** : originating in an outside source; *esp* : derived from another species ⟨∼ bone grafts⟩ **2** : HETEROGENEOUS

het·ero·graft \'he-tə-rō-ˌgráft\ *n* : XENOGRAFT

het·er·ol·o·gous \ˌhe-tə-'rä-lə-gəs\ *adj* **1** : derived from a different species ⟨∼ DNA⟩ — compare AUTOLOGOUS, HOMOLOGOUS 2 **2** : characterized by cross-reactivity ⟨a ∼ vaccine⟩ — **het·er·ol·o·gous·ly** *adv*

¹**het·ero·phile** \'he-tə-rə-ˌfīl\ *or* **het·er·o·phil** \-ˌfil\ *adj* : relating to or being any of a group of antigens in organisms of different species that induce the formation of antibodies which will cross-react with the other antigens of the group; *also* : being or relating to any of the antibodies produced and capable of cross-reacting in this way

²**heterophile** *or* **heterophil** *n* : NEUTROPHIL — used esp. in veterinary medicine

het·ero·pho·ria \ˌhe-tə-rō-'fōr-ē-ə\ *n* : latent strabismus in which one eye tends to deviate either medially or laterally — compare EXOPHORIA

het·ero·plas·tic \ˌhe-tə-rə-'plas-tik\ *adj* : HETEROLOGOUS — **het·er·o·plas·ti·cal·ly** *adv*

het·ero·plas·ty \'he-tə-rə-ˌplas-tē\ *n, pl* **-ties** : XENOGRAFT

¹**het·ero·sex·u·al** \ˌhe-tə-rō-'sek-shə-wəl\ *adj* **1 a** : of, relating to, or characterized by a tendency to direct sexual desire toward individuals of the opposite sex — compare HOMOSEXUAL 1 **b** : of, relating to, or involving sexual intercourse between individuals of the opposite sex — compare HOMOSEXUAL 2 **2** : of or relating to different sexes — **het·ero·sex·u·al·i·ty** \-ˌsek-shə-'wa-lə-tē\ *n* — **het·ero·sex·u·al·ly** *adv*

²**heterosexual** *n* : a heterosexual individual

het·ero·top·ic \ˌhe-tə-rə-'tä-pik\ *adj* **1** : occurring in an abnormal place ⟨∼ bone formation⟩ **2** : grafted or transplanted into an abnormal position ⟨∼ liver transplantation⟩ — **het·ero·to·pia** \-'tō-pē-ə\ *also* **het·er·ot·o·py** \ˌhe-tə-'rä-tə-pē\ *n* — **het·ero·top·i·cal·ly** *adv*

het·ero·trans·plant \ˌhe-tə-rō-'trans-ˌplant\ *n* : XENOGRAFT — **het·ero·trans·plan·ta·tion** \-ˌtrans-ˌplan-'tā-shən\ *n*

het·ero·tro·pia \-'trō-pē-ə\ *n* : STRABISMUS

het·ero·typ·ic \ˌhe-tə-rō-'ti-pik\ *adj* : different in kind, arrangement, or form ⟨∼ aggregations of cells⟩

het·ero·zy·go·sis \ˌhe-tə-rō-(ˌ)zī-'gō-səs\ *n, pl* **-go·ses** \-ˌsēz\ : HETEROZYGOSITY

het·ero·zy·gos·i·ty \-(ˌ)zī-'gä-sə-tē\ *n, pl* **-ties** : the state of being heterozygous

het·ero·zy·gote \-'zī-ˌgōt\ *n* : a heterozygous individual — **het·ero·zy·got·ic** \-(ˌ)zī-'gä-tik\ *adj*

het·ero·zy·gous \-'zī-gəs\ *adj* : having the two genes at corresponding loci on homologous chromosomes different for one or more loci — compare HOMOZYGOUS

HEW *abbr* Department of Health, Education, and Welfare

hex A \ˌheks-'ā\ *n* : HEXOSAMINIDASE A

hexachloride — see BENZENE HEXACHLORIDE, GAMMA BENZENE HEXACHLORIDE

hexa·chlo·ro·eth·ane \ˌhek-sə-ˌklōr-ō-'eth-ˌān\ *or* **hexa·chlor·eth·ane** \-ˌklōr-'eth-ˌān\ *n* : a toxic compound C_2Cl_6 used in the control of liver flukes in veterinary medicine

hexa·chlo·ro·phane \-'klōr-ə-ˌfān\ *n, Brit* : HEXACHLOROPHENE

hexa·chlo·ro·phene \-'klōr-ə-ˌfēn\ *n* : a powdered phenolic bacteria-inhibiting agent $C_{13}Cl_6H_6O_2$

hexa·dac·ty·ly \-'dak-tə-lē\ *n, pl* **-lies** : the condition of having six fingers or toes on a hand or foot

hexa·flu·o·re·ni·um \-ˌflü-ər-'ē-nē-əm\ *n* : a cholinesterase inhibitor used as the bromide $C_{36}H_{12}Br_2N_2$ in surgery to extend the skeletal-muscle relaxing activity of succinylcholine

hexa·me·tho·ni·um \ˌhek-sə-mə-'thō-nē-əm\ *n* : either of two compounds $C_{12}H_{30}Br_2N_2$ or $C_{12}H_{30}Cl_2N_2$ used as ganglionic blocking agents in the treatment of hypertension

hexa·meth·y·lene·tet·ra·mine \-ˌme-thə-ˌlēn-'te-trə-ˌmēn\ *n* : METHENAMINE

hex·amine \'hek-sə-ˌmēn\ *n* : METHENAMINE

hexanitrate — see MANNITOL HEXANITRATE

hex B \ˌheks-'bē\ *n* : HEXOSAMINIDASE B

hex·es·trol \'hek-sə-ˌströl, -ˌstrōl\ *n* : a synthetic derivative $C_{18}H_{22}O_2$ of diethylstilbestrol

hexo·bar·bi·tal \ˌhek-sə-'bär-bə-ˌtol\ *n* : a barbiturate $C_{12}H_{16}N_2O_3$ used as a sedative and hypnotic and in the form of its soluble sodium salt $C_{12}H_{15}N_2NaO_3$ as an intravenous anesthetic of short duration

hexo·bar·bi·tone \-'bär-bə-ˌtōn\ *n, chiefly Brit* : HEXOBARBITAL

hexo·cy·cli·um meth·yl·sul·fate \-'sī-klē-əm-ˌme-thəl-'səl-ˌfāt\ *n* : a white crystalline anticholinergic agent $C_{21}H_{36}N_2O_5S$ that tends to suppress gastric secretion and has been used in the treatment of peptic ulcers

hex·oes·trol \'hek-sē-ˌströl, -ˌstrōl\ *chiefly Brit var of* HEXESTROL

hexo·ki·nase \ˌhek-sə-'kī-ˌnās, -ˌnāz\ *n* : any of a group of enzymes that accelerate the phosphorylation of hexoses (as in the formation of glucose-6-phosphate from glucose and ATP) in carbohydrate metabolism

hex·os·a·mine \hek-ˈsä-sə-ˌmēn\ n : an amine (as glucosamine) derived from a hexose by replacement of hydroxyl by the amino group

hex·os·a·min·i·dase \ˌhek-ˌsä-sə-ˈmi-nə-ˌdās, -ˌdāz\ n : either of two hydrolytic enzymes that catalyze the splitting off of a hexose from a ganglioside and are deficient in some metabolic diseases: **a** : HEXOSAMINIDASE A **b** : HEXOSAMINIDASE B

hexosaminidase A n : the more thermolabile hexosaminidase that is deficient in Tay-Sachs disease and Sandhoff's disease — called also *hex A*

hexosaminidase B n : the more thermostable hexosaminidase that is deficient in Sandoff's disease but present in elevated quantities in Tay-Sachs disease — called also *hex B*

hex·ose \ˈhek-ˌsōs, -ˌsōz\ n : any monosaccharide (as glucose) containing six carbon atoms in the molecule

hex·yl·res·or·cin·ol \ˌhek-səl-rə-ˈzȯrs-ᵊn-ˌȯl, -ˌōl\ n : a crystalline phenol $C_{12}H_{18}O_2$ used as an anthelmintic and topical antiseptic

Hf symbol hafnium

Hg symbol [New Latin *hydrargyrum*] mercury — see MM HG

Hgb abbr hemoglobin

HGE abbr human granulocytic ehrlichiosis

HGH abbr human growth hormone

HHA abbr home health aide

HHS abbr Department of Health and Human Services

HHV–6 \ˌāch-ˌāch-vē-ˈsiks\ n : a human herpesvirus (species *Human herpesvirus 6* of the genus *Roseolovirus*) that causes roseola infantum

HI abbr hemagglutination inhibition

5–HIAA abbr 5-hydroxyindoleacetic acid

hi·a·tal \hī-ˈāt-ᵊl\ adj : of, relating to, or involving a hiatus

hiatal hernia n : a hernia in which an anatomical part (as the stomach) protrudes through the esophageal hiatus of the diaphragm — called also *hiatus hernia*

hi·a·tus \hī-ˈā-təs\ n : a gap or passage through an anatomical part or organ; *esp* : a gap through which another part or organ passes

hiatus semi·lu·nar·is \-ˌse-mi-lü-ˈnar-əs\ n : a curved fissure in the nasal passages into which the frontal and maxillary sinuses open

Hib n, often attrib : a serotype of a bacterium of the genus *Haemophilus* (*H. influenzae* type B) that causes bacterial meningitis and pneumonia esp. in children ⟨a ~ vaccine⟩ ⟨~ disease⟩ — see CONJUGATE VACCINE

hi·ber·no·ma \ˌhī-bər-ˈnō-mə\ n, pl **-mas** also **-ma·ta** \-mə-tə\ : a rare benign tumor that contains fat cells

hic·cup also **hic·cough** \ˈhi-(ˌ)kəp\ n 1 : a spasmodic inhalation with closure of the glottis accompanied by a peculiar sound 2 : an attack of hiccuping — usu. used in pl. but with a sing. or pl. verb — **hiccup** vb

hick·ey \ˈhi-kē\ n, pl **hickeys** : a temporary red mark on the skin produced esp. by biting and sucking (as during sexual activity)

Hick·man \ˈhik-mən\ trademark — used for an indwelling venous catheter

hide·bound \ˈhīd-ˌbau̇nd\ adj 1 : having a dry skin lacking in pliancy and adhering closely to the underlying flesh — used of domestic animals 2 : having scleroderma — used of human beings

hidr- or **hidro-** comb form : sweat glands ⟨*hidr*adenitis⟩

hi·drad·e·ni·tis \hi-ˌdrad-ᵊn-ˈī-təs, ˌhī-\ n : inflammation of a sweat gland

hidradenitis sup·pu·ra·ti·va \-ˌsə-pyür-ə-ˈtī-və\ n : a chronic suppurative inflammatory disease of the apocrine sweat glands

hi·drad·e·no·ma \hī-ˌdrad-ᵊn-ˈō-mə\ n, pl **-mas** also **-ma·ta** \-mə-tə\ : any benign tumor derived from epithelial cells of sweat glands

hidradenoma pa·pil·li·fer·um \-ˌpa-pi-lə-ˈfer-əm\ n : a benign solitary tumor of adult women that occurs in the anogenital region

hi·dro·sis \hi-ˈdrō-səs, hī-\ n, pl **-dro·ses** \-ˌsēz\ : excretion of sweat : PERSPIRATION

hi·drot·ic \hi-ˈdrät-ik, hī-\ adj : causing perspiration : DIAPHORETIC, SUDORIFIC

¹high \ˈhī\ adj 1 : having a complex organization : greatly differentiated or developed phylogenetically ⟨the ~er apes⟩ — compare LOW 2 **a** : exhibiting elation or euphoric excitement **b** : being intoxicated; also : excited or stupefied by or as if by a drug (as marijuana or heroin)

²high n : an excited, euphoric, or stupefied state; *esp* : one produced by or as if by a drug (as heroin)

high blood pressure n : HYPERTENSION

high colonic n : an enema injected deeply into the colon

high–density lipoprotein n : HDL

high forceps n : a rare procedure for delivery of an infant by the use of forceps before engagement has occurred — compare LOW FORCEPS, MIDFORCEPS

high–grade \ˈhī-ˈgrād\ adj : being near the upper, most serious, or most life-threatening extreme of a specified range — compare LOW-GRADE

high–performance liquid chromatography n : liquid chromatography in which the degree of separation is increased by forcing a solvent under pressure through a densely packed adsorbent — abbr. HPLC; called also *high-pressure liquid chromatography*

high–power adj : of, relating to, being, or made with a lens that magnifies an image a relatively large number of times and esp. about 40 times

high–strung \\'hī-'strəŋ\\ *adj* : having an extremely nervous or sensitive temperament

hi·lar \\'hī-lər\\ *adj* : of, relating to, affecting, or located near a hilum

hill·ock \\'hi-lək\\ *n* : any small anatomical prominence or elevation

hi·lum \\'hī-ləm\\ *n, pl* **hi·la** \\-lə\\ : a notch or opening from a bodily part esp. when it is where the blood vessels, nerves, or ducts leave and enter: as **a** : the indented part of a kidney **b** : the depression in the medial surface of a lung that forms the opening through which the bronchus, blood vessels, and nerves pass **c** : a shallow depression in one side of a lymph node through which blood vessels pass and efferent lymphatic vessels emerge

hi·lus \\-ləs\\ *n, pl* **hi·li** \\-₁lī\\ : HILUM

hind·brain \\'hīnd-₁brān\\ *n* : the posterior division of the three primary divisions of the developing vertebrate brain or the corresponding part of the adult brain that includes the cerebellum, pons, and medulla oblongata and that controls the autonomic functions and equilibrium — called also *rhombencephalon*; see METENCEPHALON, MYELENCEPHALON

hind·foot \\-₁fùt\\ *n* **1** *usu* **hind foot** : one of the posterior feet of a quadruped **2** : the posterior part of the human foot that contains the calcaneus, talus, navicular, and cuboid bones

hind·gut \\-₁gət\\ *n* : the posterior part of the embryonic digestive tract

hind leg *n* : the posterior leg of a quadruped

hind limb *n* : a posterior limb esp. of a quadruped

hinge joint \\'hinj-\\ *n* : a joint between bones (as at the elbow or knee) that permits motion in only one plane; *esp* : GINGLYMUS

hip \\'hip\\ *n* **1** : the laterally projecting region of each side of the lower or posterior part of the mammalian trunk formed by the lateral parts of the pelvis and upper part of the femur together with the fleshy parts covering them **2** : HIP JOINT

HIPAA *abbr* Health Insurance Portability and Accountability Act

hip bone \\-₁bōn\\ *n* : the large flaring bone that makes a lateral half of the pelvis in mammals and is composed of the ilium, ischium, and pubis which are consolidated into one bone in the adult — called also *innominate bone, os coxae, pelvic bone*

hip joint *n* : the ball-and-socket joint comprising the articulation between the femur and the hip bone

hipped \\'hipt\\ *adj* : having hips esp. of a specified kind — often used in combination ⟨broad-*hipped*⟩

hip·po·cam·pal \\₁hi-pə-'kam-pəl\\ *adj* : of or relating to the hippocampus

hippocampal commissure *n* : a triangular band of nerve fibers joining the two crura of the fornix of the rhinencephalon anteriorly before they fuse to form the body of the fornix — called also *psalterium*

hippocampal convolution *n* : PARAHIPPOCAMPAL GYRUS

hippocampal gyrus *n* : PARAHIPPOCAMPAL GYRUS

hippocampal sulcus *n* : a fissure of the mesial surface of each cerebral hemisphere extending from behind the posterior end of the corpus callosum forward and downward to the parahippocampal gyrus — called also *hippocampal fissure*

hip·po·cam·pus \\₁hi-pə-'kam-pəs\\ *n, pl* **-pi** \\-₁pī, -₁(₁)pē\\ : a curved elongated ridge that is an important part of the limbic system, extends over the floor of the descending horn of each lateral ventricle of the brain, consists of gray matter covered on the ventricular surface with white matter, and is involved in forming, storing, and processing memory

Hip·po·crat·ic \\₁hi-pə-'kra-tik\\ *adj* : of or relating to Hippocrates or to the school of medicine that took his name

Hip·poc·ra·tes \\hi-'pä-krə-₁tēz\\ (*ca* 460 BC–*ca* 370 BC), Greek physician.

Hippocratic facies *n* : the face as it appears near death and in some debilitating conditions marked by sunken eyes and temples, pinched nose, and tense hard skin

Hippocratic oath *n* : an oath that embodies a code of medical ethics and is usu. taken by those about to begin medical practice

hip pointer *n* : a deep bruise to the iliac crest or to the attachments of the muscles attached to it that occurs esp. in contact sports (as football)

hip·pu·ran \\'hi-pyù-₁ran\\ *n* : a white crystalline iodine-containing powder $C_9H_7INNaO_3·2H_2O$ used as a radiopaque agent in urography of the kidney — called also *iodohippurate sodium, sodium iodohippurate*

hip·pus \\'hi-pəs\\ *n* : a spasmodic variation in the size of the pupil of the eye caused by a tremor of the iris

Hirsch·sprung's disease \\'hirsh-₁prùŋz-\\ *n* : megacolon that is caused by congenital absence of ganglion cells in the muscular wall of the distal part of the colon with resulting loss of peristaltic function in this part and dilatation of the colon proximal to the aganglionic part — called also *congenital megacolon*

Hirschsprung, Harold (1830–1916), Danish pediatrician.

hir·sute \\'hər-₁süt, 'hir-, -₁hər-\\ *adj* : very hairy — **hir·sute·ness** *n*

hir·sut·ism \\'hər-sə-₁ti-zəm, 'hir-\\ *n* : excessive growth of hair of normal or abnormal distribution : HYPERTRICHOSIS

hi·ru·din \hir-ˈüd-ᵊn, ˈhir-yu̇-dən\ *n* : an anticoagulant extracted from the buccal glands of a leech

Hi·ru·do \hi-ˈrü-(ˌ)dō\ *n* : a genus of leeches (family Hirudinidae) that includes the common medicinal leech (*H. medicinalis*)

His bundle \ˈhis-\ *n* : BUNDLE OF HIS

hist- or **histo-** *comb form* : tissue ⟨*hist*amine⟩ ⟨*histo*compatibility⟩

his·ta·mine \ˈhis-tə-ˌmēn, -mən\ *n* : a compound $C_5H_9N_3$ esp. of mammalian tissues that causes dilatation of capillaries, contraction of smooth muscle, and stimulation of gastric acid secretion, that is released during allergic reactions, and that is formed by decarboxylation of histidine — **his·ta·min·ic** \ˌhis-tə-ˈmi-nik\ *adj*

histamine cephalalgia *n* : CLUSTER HEADACHE

his·ta·min·er·gic \ˌhis-tə-mə-ˈnər-jik\ *adj* : liberating or activated by histamine ⟨~ receptors⟩

his·ta·mi·no·lyt·ic \ˌhis-tə-ˌmi-nə-ˈli-tik, hi-ˌsta-mə-nə-\ *adj* : breaking down or tending to break down histamine

histi- or **histio-** *comb form* : tissue ⟨*histio*cyte⟩

his·ti·di·nae·mia *chiefly Brit var of* HISTIDINEMIA

his·ti·dine \ˈhis-tə-ˌdēn\ *n* : a crystalline essential amino acid $C_6H_9N_3O_2$ formed by the hydrolysis of most proteins

his·ti·di·ne·mia \ˌhis-tə-də-ˈnē-mē-ə\ *n* : a recessive autosomal metabolic defect that results in an excess amount of histidine in the blood and urine due to an enzyme deficiency

his·ti·din·uria \-ˈnu̇r-ē-ə, -ˈnyu̇r-\ *n* : the presence of an excessive amount of histidine in the urine

his·tio·cyte \ˈhis-tē-ə-ˌsīt\ *n* : MACROPHAGE; *esp* : a nonmotile macrophage of extravascular tissues and esp. connective tissue — **his·tio·cyt·ic** \ˌhis-tē-ə-ˈsi-tik\ *adj*

histiocytic lymphoma *n* : a non-Hodgkin's lymphoma marked by the presence of large cells that morphologically resemble histiocytes but are typically of B or T cell origin — called also *histiocytic sarcoma, reticulum cell sarcoma, reticulosarcoma*

his·tio·cy·to·ma \ˌhis-tē-ō-sī-ˈtō-mə\ *n, pl* **-mas** *also* **-ma·ta** \-mə-tə\ : a tumor that consists predominantly of macrophages

his·tio·cy·to·sis \-ˈtō-səs\ *n, pl* **-to·ses** \-ˌsēz\ : abnormal multiplication of macrophages; *broadly* : a condition characterized by such multiplication

histo- — *see* HIST-

his·to·chem·is·try \-ˈke-mə-strē\ *n, pl* **-tries** : a science that combines the techniques of biochemistry and histology in the study of the chemical constitution of cells and tissues —

his·to·chem·i·cal \-ˈke-mə-kəl\ *adj* — **his·to·chem·i·cal·ly** *adv*

his·to·com·pat·i·bil·i·ty \ˌhis-(ˌ)tō-kəm-ˌpa-tə-ˈbi-lə-tē\ *n, pl* **-ties** *often attrib* : a state of mutual tolerance between tissues that allows them to be grafted effectively — *see* MAJOR HISTOCOMPATIBILITY COMPLEX — **his·to·com·pat·i·ble** \-kəm-ˈpa-tə-bəl\ *adj*

histocompatibility antigen *n* : any of the polymorphic glycoprotein molecules on the surface membranes of cells that aid in the ability of the immune system to determine self from nonself, that bind to and display antigenic peptide fragments for T cell recognition, and that are determined by the major histocompatibility complex

his·to·flu·o·res·cence \-ˌflȯr-ˈes-ᵊns, -ˌflu̇r-\ *n* : fluorescence by a tissue upon radiation after introduction of a fluorescent substance into the body and its uptake by the tissue — **his·to·flu·o·res·cent** \-ˈes-ᵊnt\ *adj*

his·to·gen·e·sis \ˌhis-tə-ˈje-nə-səs\ *n, pl* **-e·ses** \-ˌsēz\ : the formation and differentiation of tissues — **his·to·ge·net·ic** \-jə-ˈne-tik\ *adj* — **his·to·ge·net·i·cal·ly** *adv*

his·toid \ˈhis-ˌtȯid\ *adj* **1** : resembling the normal tissues ⟨~ tumors⟩ **2** : developed from or consisting of but one tissue

his·to·in·com·pat·i·bil·i·ty \ˌhis-(ˌ)tō-ˌin-kəm-ˌpa-tə-ˈbi-lə-tē\ *n, pl* **-ties** : a state of mutual intolerance between tissues (as of a fetus and its mother or a graft and its host) that normally leads to reaction against or rejection of one by the other — **his·to·in·com·pat·i·ble** \-kəm-ˈpa-tə-bəl\ *adj*

his·tol·o·gy \hi-ˈstä-lə-jē\ *n, pl* **-gies 1** : a branch of anatomy that deals with the minute structure of animal and plant tissues as discernible with the microscope — compare GROSS ANATOMY **2** : a treatise on histology **3** : tissue structure or organization — **his·to·log·i·cal** \ˌhis-tə-ˈlä-ji-kəl\ *or* **his·to·log·ic** \-ˈlä-jik\ *adj* — **his·to·log·i·cal·ly** *adv* — **his·tol·o·gist** \hi-ˈstä-lə-jist\ *n*

His·to·mo·nas \ˌhis-tə-ˈmō-nəs\ *n* : a genus of flagellate protozoans (family Mastigamoebidae) that are parasites in the liver and intestinal mucosa esp. of poultry and are usu. considered to include a single species (*H. meleagridis*) that causes blackhead

his·to·mo·ni·a·sis \ˌhis-tə-mə-ˈnī-ə-səs\ *n, pl* **-a·ses** \-ˌsēz\ : infection with or disease caused by protozoans of the genus *Histomonas* : BLACKHEAD **2**

his·to·mor·phom·e·try \ˌhis-tō-mȯr-ˈfä-mə-trē\ *n, pl* **-tries** : the quantitative study of the microscopic organization and structure of a tissue (as bone) esp. by computer-assisted analysis of images formed by a microscope — **his·to·mor·pho·met·ric**

\-ˌmȯr-fə-'me-trik\ *also* **his·to·mor·pho·met·ri·cal** \-tri-kəl\ *adj*

his·tone \'his-ˌtōn\ *n* : any of various simple water-soluble proteins that are rich in the basic amino acids lysine and arginine and are complexed with DNA in nucleosomes

his·to·patho·gen·e·sis \ˌhis-tə-ˌpa-thə-'je-nə-səs\ *n, pl* **-e·ses** \-ˌsēz\ : the origin and development of diseased tissue

his·to·pa·thol·o·gist \ˌhis-tō-pə-'thä-lə-jist, -pa-\ *n* : a pathologist who specializes in the detection of the effects of disease on body tissues; *esp* : one who identifies tumors by their histological characteristics

his·to·pa·thol·o·gy \ˌhis-tō-pə-'thä-lə-jē, -pa-\ *n, pl* **-gies 1** : a branch of pathology concerned with the tissue changes characteristic of disease **2** : the tissue changes that affect a part or accompany a disease — **his·to·path·o·log·ic** \-ˌpa-thə-'lä-jik\ *or* **his·to·path·o·log·i·cal** \-ji-kəl\ *adj* — **his·to·path·o·log·i·cal·ly** *adv*

his·to·plas·ma \ˌhis-tə-'plaz-mə\ *n* **1** *cap* : a genus of imperfect fungi that includes one (*H. capsulatum*) causing histoplasmosis and another (*H. farciminosum*) causing epizootic lymphangitis **2** : any fungus of the genus *Histoplasma*

his·to·plas·min \-'plaz-mən\ *n* : a sterile filtrate of a culture of a fungus of the genus *Histoplasma* (*H. capsulatum*) used in a cutaneous test for histoplasmosis

his·to·plas·mo·sis \-ˌplaz-'mō-səs\ *n, pl* **-mo·ses** \-ˌsēz\ : a respiratory disease with symptoms like those of influenza that is endemic in the Mississippi and Ohio river valleys of the U.S., is caused by a fungus of the genus *Histoplasma* (*H. capsulatum*), and is marked by benign involvement of lymph nodes of the trachea and bronchi usu. without symptoms or by severe progressive generalized involvement of the lymph nodes and macrophage-rich tissue with fever, anemia, leukopenia and often with local lesions (as of the skin or mouth)

his·to·ry \'his-tə-rē\ *n, pl* **-ries** : an account of a patient's family and personal background and past and present health

his·to·tech·nol·o·gy \ˌhis-tə-tek-'nä-lə-jē\ *n, pl* **-gies** : technical histology concerned esp. with preparing and processing (as by sectioning, fixing, and staining) histological specimens — **his·to·tech·nol·o·gist** \-jəst\ *n*

his·to·tox·ic \ˌhis-tə-'täk-sik\ *adj* : toxic to tissues ⟨∼ agents⟩

histotoxic anoxia *n* : histotoxic hypoxia esp. of great severity

histotoxic hypoxia *n* : a deficiency of oxygen reaching the bodily tissues due to impairment of cellular respiration esp. by a toxic agent (as cyanide or alcohol)

HIV \ˌāch-(ˌ)ī-'vē\ *n* : either of two retroviruses that infect and destroy helper T cells of the immune system causing the marked reduction in their numbers that is diagnostic of AIDS — called also *AIDS virus, human immunodeficiency virus;* see HIV-1, HIV-2

hive \'hīv\ *n* : the raised edematous red patch of skin or mucous membrane characteristic of hives : an urticarial wheal

hives \'hīvz\ *n sing or pl* : an allergic disorder marked by raised edematous patches of skin or mucous membrane and usu. by intense itching and caused by contact with a specific precipitating factor (as a food, drug, or inhalant) either externally or internally — called also *urticaria*

HIV-1 \ˌāch-(ˌ)ī-(ˌ)vē-'wən\ *n* : a retrovirus of the genus *Lentivirus* (species *Human immunodeficiency virus 1*) that is the most prevalent HIV — called also *HTLV-III, LAV*

HIV-2 \-'tü\ *n* : a retrovirus of the genus *Lentivirus* (species *Human immunodeficiency virus 2*) that causes AIDS esp. in western Africa, is closely related in structure to SIV of monkeys, and is less virulent than HIV-1 and has a longer incubation period than HIV-1

HLA *also* **HL–A** \ˌāch-(ˌ)el-'ā\ *n* [*hu*man *l*eukocyte *a*ntigen] **1** : the major histocompatibility complex in humans **2** : a genetic locus, gene, or antigen of the major histocompatibility complex in humans — often used attributively ⟨*HLA* antigens⟩ ⟨*HLA* typing⟩; often used with one or more letters to designate a locus or with letters and a number to designate an allele at the locus or the antigen corresponding to the locus and allele ⟨*HLA*-B27 antigen⟩

HMD *abbr* hyaline membrane disease

HMO \ˌāch-(ˌ)em-'ō\ *n, pl* **HMOs** : an organization that provides comprehensive health care to voluntarily enrolled individuals and families in a particular geographic area by member physicians with limited referral to outside specialists and that is financed by fixed periodic payments determined in advance — called also *health maintenance organization*

HNPCC *abbr* hereditary nonpolyposis colon cancer; hereditary nonpolyposis colorectal cancer

Ho *symbol* holmium

hoarse \'hȯrs\ *adj* **hoars·er; hoars·est 1** : rough or harsh in sound ⟨a ∼ voice⟩ **2** : having a hoarse voice — **hoarse·ly** *adv* — **hoarse·ness** *n*

hob·nail liver \'häb-ˌnāl-\ *or* **hobnailed liver** \'häb-ˌnāld-\ *n* **1** : the liver as it appears in one form of cirrhosis in which it is shrunken and hard and covered with small projecting nodules **2** : the cirrhosis associated with hobnail liver : LAENNEC'S CIRRHOSIS

hock \'häk\ *n* : the joint or region of

the joint that unites the tarsal bones in the hind limb of a quadruped (as the horse) and that corresponds to the human ankle but is elevated and bends backward

hock disease *n* : PEROSIS

Hodg·kin's disease \'häj-kənz-\ *n* : a malignant lymphoma that is marked by the presence of Reed-Sternberg cells and is characterized by progressive enlargement of lymph nodes, spleen, and liver and by progressive anemia — called also *Hodgkin's, Hodgkin's anemia*

Hodgkin, Thomas (1798–1866), British physician.

Hodgkin's paragranuloma *n* : PARAGRANULOMA 2

hog cholera *n* : a highly infectious often fatal disease of swine caused by a flavivirus of the genus *Pestivirus* (species *Classical swine fever virus*) and characterized by fever, loss of appetite, weakness, erythematous lesions, and severe leukopenia — called also *swine fever;* see AFRICAN SWINE FEVER

hog louse *n* : a large sucking louse of the genus *Haematopinus (H. suis)* that is parasitic on the hog

hol- *or* **holo-** *comb form* **1** : complete : total ⟨*holo*enzyme⟩ **2** : completely : totally ⟨*holo*endemic⟩

hold·fast \'hōld-ˌfast\ *n* : an organ by which a parasitic animal (as a tapeworm) attaches itself to its host

ho·lism \'hō-ˌli-zəm\ *n* **1** : a theory that the universe and esp. living nature is correctly seen in terms of interacting wholes (as of living organisms) that are more than the mere sum of elementary particles **2** : a holistic study or method of treatment

ho·lis·tic \hō-'lis-tik\ *adj* **1** : of or relating to holism **2** : relating to or concerned with wholes or with complete systems rather than with the analysis of, treatment of, or dissection into parts ⟨~ medicine attempts to treat both the mind and the body⟩ — **ho·lis·ti·cal·ly** *adv*

Hol·land·er test \'hä-lən-dər-\ *n* : a test for function of the vagus nerve (as after vagotomy for peptic ulcer) in which insulin is administered to induce hypoglycemia and gastric acidity tends to increase if innervation by the vagus nerve remains and decrease if severance is complete

Hollander, Franklin (1899–1966), American physiologist.

hol·low \'hä-(ˌ)lō\ *n* : a depressed part of a surface or a concavity

hollow organ *n* : a visceral organ that is a hollow tube or pouch (as the stomach or intestine) or that includes a cavity (as of the heart or bladder) which serves a vital function

hol·mi·um \'hōl-mē-əm\ *n* : a metallic element that occurs with yttrium and forms highly magnetic compounds — symbol *Ho;* see ELEMENT table

ho·lo·blas·tic \ˌhō-lə-'blas-tik, ˌhä-\ *adj* : characterized by cleavage planes that divide the whole egg into distinct and separate though coherent blastomeres ⟨~ eggs⟩ — compare MEROBLASTIC

ho·lo·crine \'hō-lə-krən, 'hä-, -ˌkrīn, -ˌkrēn\ *adj* : producing or being a secretion resulting from lysis of secretory cells ⟨~ glands⟩ — compare APOCRINE, ECCRINE, MEROCRINE

ho·lo·en·dem·ic \ˌhō-lō-en-'de-mik\ *adj* : affecting all or characterized by the infection of essentially all the inhabitants of a particular area

ho·lo·en·zyme \ˌhō-lō-'en-ˌzīm\ *n* : a catalytically active enzyme consisting of an apoenzyme combined with its cofactor

ho·lo·sys·tol·ic \ˌhō-lō-sis-'tä-lik\ *adj* : relating to an entire systole ⟨a ~ murmur⟩

Hol·ter monitor \'hōl-tər-\ *n* : a portable device that makes a continuous record of electrical activity of the heart and that can be worn by an ambulatory patient during the course of daily activities in order to detect fleeting episodes of abnormal heart rhythms — **Holter monitoring** *n*

Holter, Norman Jefferis (1914–1983), American biophysicist.

hom- — see HOMO-

Ho·mans' sign \'hō-mənz-\ *n* : pain in the calf of the leg upon dorsiflexion of the foot with the leg extended that is diagnostic of thrombosis in the deep veins of the area

Homans, John (1877–1954), American surgeon.

hom·at·ro·pine \hō-'ma-trə-ˌpēn\ *n* : a poisonous drug used in the form of its hydrobromide $C_{16}H_{21}NO_3 \cdot HBr$ for dilating the pupil of the eye and in the form of its methyl bromide $C_{16}H_{21}NO_3 \cdot CH_3Br$ in combination with hydrocodone in cough suppressant preparations — see HYCODAN

home- *or* **homeo-** *also* **homoi-** *or* **homoio-** *comb form* : like : similar ⟨*homeo*stasis⟩ ⟨*homoio*thermy⟩

home care *n* : services (as nursing care) provided to individuals who are confined to the home

home health aide *n* : a trained and certified health-care worker who provides assistance to a patient in the home with personal care and light household duties and who monitors the patient's condition — abbr. HHA

ho·meo·box \'hō-mē-ō-ˌbäks\ *n* : a short usu. highly conserved DNA sequence in various genes and esp. homeotic genes that encodes a DNA=binding amino acid domain of some proteins

ho·meo·path \'hō-mē-ə-ˌpath\ *n* : a practitioner or adherent of homeopathy

ho·me·op·a·thy \ˌhō-mē-'ä-pə-thē, ˌhä-\ *n, pl* **-thies** : a system of medical practice that treats a disease esp. by the administration of minute doses of a remedy that would in healthy persons produce symptoms similar to those of the disease — compare ALLOPATHY 2 — **ho·meo·path·ic** \ˌhō-mē-ə-ˈpa-thik\ adj — **ho·meo·path·i·cal·ly** adv

ho·meo·sta·sis \ˌhō-mē-ō-ˈstā-səs\ n : the maintenance of relatively stable internal physiological conditions (as body temperature or the pH of blood) under fluctuating environmental conditions — **ho·meo·stat·ic** \-ˈsta-tik\ adj — **ho·meo·stat·i·cal·ly** adv

ho·meo·ther·my \ˈhō-mē-ə-ˌthər-mē\ also **ho·moio·ther·my** \hō-ˈmȯi-ə-\ n, pl **-mies** : the condition of being warm-blooded : WARM-BLOODEDNESS — **ho·meo·therm** \-ˌthərm\ also **ho·moio·therm** \hō-ˈmȯi-ə-\ n — **ho·meo·ther·mic** \ˌhō-mē-ō-ˈthər-mik\ also **ho·moio·ther·mic** \hō-ˌmȯi-ə-\ adj

ho·me·ot·ic also **ho·moe·ot·ic** \ˌhō-mē-ˈä-tik\ adj : relating to, caused by, or being a homeotic gene

homeotic gene n : a gene that produces a usu. major shift in the developmental fate of an organ or body part esp. to a homologous organ or part normally found elsewhere in the organism

home remedy n : a simply prepared medication or tonic often of unproven effectiveness administered without prescription or professional supervision

ho·mi·cid·al \ˌhä-mə-ˈsīd-ᵊl, ˌhō-\ adj : of, relating to, or tending toward homicide — **ho·mi·cid·al·ly** adv

ho·mi·cide \ˈhä-mə-ˌsīd, ˈhō-\ n : a killing of one human being by another

hom·i·nid \ˈhä-mə-nəd, -ˌnid\ n : any of a family (Hominidae) of bipedal primate mammals comprising recent humans together with extinct ancestral and related forms — **hominid** adj

ho·mo \ˈhō-(ˌ)mō\ n 1 cap : a genus of primate mammals (family Hominidae) that includes modern humans (H. sapiens) and several extinct related species (as H. erectus) 2 pl **mos** : any primate mammal of the genus Homo

homo- or **hom-** comb form 1 : one and the same : similar : alike ⟨homozygous⟩ 2 : derived from the same species ⟨homograft⟩ 3 : homosexual ⟨homophobia⟩

ho·mo·cys·te·ine \ˌhō-mō-ˈsis-tə-ˌēn, ˌhä-\ n : an amino acid $C_4H_9NO_2S$ that is produced in animal metabolism by removal of a methyl group from methionine and forms a complex with serine that breaks up to produce cysteine and homoserine and that appears to be associated with an increased risk of cardiovascular disease when occurring at high levels in the blood

ho·mo·cys·tine \-ˈsis-ˌtēn\ n : an amino acid $C_8H_{16}N_2O_4S_2$ formed by

oxidation of homocysteine and excreted in the urine in homocystinuria

ho·mo·cys·tin·uria \-ˌsis-ti-ˈnu̇r-ē-ə, -ˈnyu̇r-\ n : a metabolic disorder inherited as a recessive autosomal trait, caused by deficiency of an enzyme important in the metabolism of homocystine with resulting accumulation of homocystine in the body and its excretion in the urine, and characterized typically by mental retardation, dislocation of the crystalline lenses, skeletal abnormalities, and thromboembolic disease — **ho·mo·cys·tin·uric** \-ˈnu̇r-ik, -ˈnyu̇r-\ adj

ho·mo·cy·to·tro·pic \-ˌsī-tə-ˈtrō-pik\ adj : of, relating to, or being any antibody that attaches to cells of the species in which it originates but not to cells of other species

ho·mo·di·mer \-ˈdī-mər\ n : a protein composed of two polypeptide chains that are identical in the order, number, and kind of their amino acid residues — **ho·mo·di·mer·ic** \-ˈdī-ˈmer-ik\ adj

homoe- or **homoeo-** chiefly Brit var of HOME-

ho·moeo·path, ho·moe·op·a·thy, ho·moeo·sta·sis, ho·moec·ther·my chiefly Brit var of HOMEOPATH, HOMEOPATHY, HOMEOSTASIS, HOMEOTHERMY

homeotic var of HOMEOTIC

ho·mo·erot·ic \ˌhō-mō-i-ˈrä-tik\ adj : HOMOSEXUAL — **ho·mo·erot·i·cism** \-i-ˈrä-tə-ˌsi-zəm\ also **ho·mo·erot·ism** \-ˈer-ə-ˌti-zəm\ n

ho·mo·ga·met·ic \-gə-ˈme-tik, -ˈmē-\ adj : forming gametes which all have the same type of sex chromosome

ho·mog·e·nate \hō-ˈmä-jə-ˌnāt, hə-\ n : a product of homogenizing

ho·mo·ge·neous \ˌhō-mə-ˈjē-nē-əs, -nyəs\ adj : of uniform structure or composition throughout — **ho·mo·ge·ne·ity** \ˌhō-mə-jə-ˈnē-ə-tē, -ˌhä-, -ˈnā-\ adj — **ho·mo·ge·neous·ly** adv — **ho·mo·ge·neous·ness** n

ho·mog·e·nize \hō-ˈmä-jə-ˌnīz, hə-\ vb **-nized; -niz·ing** 1 : to reduce to small particles of uniform size and distribute evenly usu. in a liquid 2 : to reduce the particles of so that they are uniformly small and evenly distributed; specif : to break up the fat globules of (milk) into very fine particles — **ho·mog·e·ni·za·tion** \hō-ˌmä-jə-nə-ˈzā-shən, hə-\ n — **ho·mog·e·niz·er** \-ˈmä-jə-ˌnī-zər\ n

ho·mog·e·nous \-nəs\ adj 1 : HOMOPLASTIC 2 : HOMOGENEOUS

ho·mo·gen·tis·ic acid \ˌhō-mō-jen-ˈti-zik, ˌhä-\ n : a crystalline acid $C_8H_8O_4$ formed as an intermediate in the metabolism of phenylalanine and tyrosine and found esp. in the urine of those affected with alkaptonuria

ho·mo·graft \ˈhō-mə-ˌgraft, ˈhä-\ n : a graft of tissue from a donor of the same species as the recipient — called also *homotransplant;* compare XE-NOGRAFT — **homograft** *vb*

homoi- *or* **homoio-** — see HOME-

homoiothermy *var of* HOMEOTHERMY

ho·mo·lat·er·al \ˌhō-mō-ˈla-tər-əl, ˌhä-\ *adj* : IPSILATERAL

ho·mol·o·gous \hō-ˈmä-lə-gəs, hə-\ *adj* **1 a** : having the same relative position, value, or structure **b** : having the same or allelic genes with genetic loci usu. arranged in the same order ⟨∼ chromosomes⟩ **2** : derived from or involving organisms of the same species ⟨∼ tissue grafts⟩ — compare AUTOLOGOUS, HETEROLOGOUS 1 3 : relating to or being immunity or a serum produced by or containing a specific antibody corresponding to a specific antigen — **ho·mol·o·gous·ly** *adv*

ho·mo·logue *or* **ho·mo·log** \ˈhō-mə-ˌlȯg, ˈhä-, -ˌläg\ *n* : something (as a chromosome) that is homologous

ho·mol·o·gy \hō-ˈmä-lə-jē, hə-\ *n, pl* **-gies** **1** : likeness in structure between parts of different organisms due to evolutionary differentiation from the same or a corresponding part of a remote ancestor — compare ANALOGY **2** : correspondence in structure between different parts of the same individual **3** : similarity of nucleotide or amino acid sequence (as in nucleic acids or proteins)

hom·on·y·mous \hō-ˈmä-nə-məs\ *adj* **1** : affecting the same part of the visual field of each eye ⟨right ∼ hemianopia⟩ **2** : relating to or being diplopia in which the image that is seen by the right eye is to the right of the image that is seen by the left eye

¹ho·mo·phile \ˈhō-mə-ˌfīl\ *adj* : of, relating to, or concerned with homosexuals or homosexuality ⟨∼ lifestyles⟩; *also* : being homosexual

²homophile *n* : HOMOSEXUAL

ho·mo·pho·bia \ˌhō-mə-ˈfō-bē-ə\ *n* : irrational fear of, aversion to, or discrimination against homosexuality or homosexuals — **ho·mo·phobe** \ˈhō-mə-ˌfōb\ *n* — **ho·mo·pho·bic** \ˌhō-mə-ˈfō-bik\ *adj*

ho·mo·plas·tic \ˌhō-mə-ˈplas-tik, ˌhä-\ *adj* : of, relating to, or derived from another individual of the same species

ho·mo·sal·ate \ˌhō-mō-ˈsa-ˌlāt, ˌhä-\ *n* : a salicylate $C_{16}H_{22}O_3$ that is used in sunscreen lotions to absorb ultraviolet rays and promote tanning

ho·mo·ser·ine \ˌhō-mō-ˈser-ˌēn, ˌhä-, -ˈsir-\ *n* : an amino acid $C_4H_9NO_3$ that is formed in the conversion of methionine to cysteine — see HOMOCYSTEINE

¹ho·mo·sex·u·al \ˌhō-mə-ˈsek-shə-wəl\ *adj* **1** : of, relating to, or characterized by a tendency to direct sexual desire toward individuals of one's own sex — compare HETEROSEXUAL 1a **2** : of, relating to, or involving sexual intercourse between individuals of the same sex — compare HETEROSEXUAL 1b — **ho·mo·sex·u·al·ly** *adv*

²homosexual *n* : a homosexual individual and esp. a male

ho·mo·sex·u·al·i·ty \ˌhō-mə-ˌsek-shə-ˈwa-lə-tē\ *n, pl* **-ties** **1** : the quality or state of being homosexual **2** : erotic activity with another of the same sex

ho·mo·trans·plant \ˌhō-mō-ˈtrans-ˌplant, ˌhä-\ *n* : HOMOGRAFT — **ho·motransplant** *vb* — **ho·mo·trans·plan·ta·tion** \-ˌtrans-ˌplan-ˈtā-shən\ *n*

ho·mo·va·nil·lic acid \-və-ˈni-lik-\ *n* : a dopamine metabolite $C_9H_{10}O_4$ excreted in human urine

ho·mo·zy·go·sis \-ˌzī-ˈgō-səs\ *n, pl* **-go·ses** \-ˌsēz\ : HOMOZYGOSITY

ho·mo·zy·gos·i·ty \-ˈgä-sə-tē\ *n, pl* **-ties** : the state of being homozygous

ho·mo·zy·gote \-ˈzī-ˌgōt\ *n* : a homozygous individual

ho·mo·zy·gous \-ˈzī-gəs\ *adj* : having the two genes at corresponding loci on homologous chromosomes identical for one or more loci — compare HETEROZYGOUS

H_1 antagonist \ˈāch-ˈwən-\ *n* : any of various drugs (as cetirizine or loratadine) that bind competitively with histamine to H_1 receptors on cell membranes and are used variously as sedatives, antiemetics, and anticholinergics — called also *H_1 blocker, H_1 receptor antagonist*

H_1 receptor *n* : a receptor for histamine on cell membranes that modulates the dilation of blood vessels and the contraction of smooth muscle

hon·ey·bee \ˈhə-nē-ˌbē\ *n* : a honey=producing bee (genus *Apis*); *esp* : a European bee (*A. mellifera*) introduced worldwide and kept in hives for the honey it produces

hon·ey·comb \ˈhə-nē-ˌkōm\ *n* : RETICULUM 1

Hong Kong flu \ˈhäŋ-ˈkäŋ-\ *n* : influenza that is caused by a subtype (H3N2) of the orthomyxovirus causing influenza A and that was responsible for about 34,000 deaths in the U.S. in the influenza pandemic of 1968–1969 — called also *Hong Kong influenza;* compare ASIAN FLU, SPANISH FLU

hoof \ˈhu̇f, ˈhüf\ *n, pl* **hooves** \ˈhüvz, ˈhu̇vz\ *also* **hoofs** : a horny covering that protects the ends of the toes of ungulate mammals (as horses or cattle); *also* : a hoofed foot — **hoofed** \ˈhu̇ft, ˈhüft, ˈhu̇vd, ˈhüvd\ *or* **hooved** \ˈhu̇vd, ˈhüvd\ *adj*

hoof–and–mouth disease *n* : FOOT=AND-MOUTH DISEASE

hook \ˈhu̇k\ *n* **1** : an instrument used in surgery to take hold of tissue **2** : an anatomical part that resembles a hook

hook·worm \-ˌwərm\ *n* **1** : any of several parasitic nematode worms (family Ancylostomatidae) that have strong buccal hooks or plates for attaching to the host's intestinal lining and that include serious bloodsucking pests **2** : ANCYLOSTOMIASIS

hookworm disease *n* : ANCYLOSTOMIASIS

hoose \'hüz\ *n* : bronchitis of cattle, sheep, and goats caused by larval strongylid roundworms irritating the bronchial tubes — called also **husk**

hor·de·o·lum \hȯr-'dē-ə-ləm\ *n, pl* **-o·la** \-lə\ : STY

hore·hound \'hōr-ˌhaȯnd\ *n* **1** : an Old World bitter plant (*Marrubium vulgare*) of the mint family (Labiatae) that is used as a tonic and anthelmintic **2** : an extract or confection made from horehound and used as a remedy for coughs and colds

hor·i·zon·tal \ˌhȯr-ə-'zänt-ᵊl, ˌhär-\ *adj* **1** : relating to or being a transverse plane or section of the body **2** : relating to or being transmission (as of a disease) by physical contact or proximity — compare VERTICAL — **hor·i·zon·tal·ly** *adv*

horizontal cell *n* : any of the retinal neurons whose axons pass along a course in the plexiform layer following the contour of the retina and whose dendrites synapse with the rods and cones

horizontal fissure *n* : a fissure of the right lung that begins at the oblique fissure and runs horizontally dividing the lung into superior and middle lobes

horizontal plate *n* : a plate of the palatine bone that is situated horizontally, joins the bone of the opposite side, and forms the back part of the hard palate — compare PERPENDICULAR PLATE 2

hor·me·sis \hȯr-'mē-səs\ *n* : a theoretical phenomenon of dose-response relationships in which something (as a heavy metal or ionizing radiation) that produces harmful biological effects at moderate to high doses may produce beneficial effects at low doses — **hor·met·ic** \-'me-tik\ *adj*

hormonal therapy *n* : HORMONE THERAPY

hor·mone \'hȯr-ˌmōn\ *n* **1 a** : a product of living cells that circulates in body fluids and produces a specific often stimulatory effect on the activity of cells usu. remote from its point of origin **b** : a synthetic substance that acts like a hormone **2** : SEX HORMONE — **hor·mon·al** \hȯr-'mōn-ᵊl\ *adj* — **hor·mon·al·ly** *adv* — **hormone-like** *adj*

hormone replacement therapy *n* : the administration of estrogen along with a synthetic progestin esp. to ameliorate the symptoms of menopause and reduce the risk of postmenopausal osteoporosis — abbr. *HRT*

hormone therapy *n* : the therapeutic use of hormones: as **a** : the administration of hormones esp. to increase diminished levels in the body; *esp* : HORMONE REPLACEMENT THERAPY **b** : therapy involving the use of drugs or surgical procedures to suppress the production of or inhibit the effects of a hormone (as estrogen or testosterone) ⟨*hormone therapy* to treat breast or prostate cancer⟩

hor·mo·no·ther·a·py \hȯr-ˌmō-nə-'ther-ə-pē\ *n* : HORMONE THERAPY

horn \'hȯrn\ *n* **1** : one of the hard projections of bone or keratin on the head of many hoofed mammals; *also* : the material of which horns are composed or a similar material **2** : CORNU — **horned** \'hȯrnd\ *adj*

horn cell *n* : a nerve cell lying in one of the gray columns of the spinal cord

horned rattlesnake *n* : SIDEWINDER

Hor·ner's syndrome \'hȯr-nərz-\ *n* : a syndrome marked by sinking in of the eyeball, contraction of the pupil, drooping of the upper eyelid, and vasodilation and anhidrosis of the face, and caused by injury to the cervical sympathetic nerve fibers on the affected side

    Horner, Johann Friedrich (1831–1886), Swiss ophthalmologist.

horn fly *n* : a small black European dipteran fly (*Haematobia irritans* of the family Muscidae) that has been introduced into No. America where it is a bloodsucking pest of cattle

horny \'hȯr-nē\ *adj* **horn·i·er; -est 1** : composed of or resembling tough fibrous material consisting chiefly of keratin : KERATINOUS ⟨~ tissue⟩ **2** : being hard or callous

horny layer *n* : STRATUM CORNEUM

hor·rip·i·la·tion \hȯ-ˌri-pə-'lā-shən, hä-\ *n* : a bristling of the hair of the head or body : GOOSE BUMPS — **hor·rip·i·late** \-'ri-pə-ˌlāt\ *vb*

horror au·to·tox·i·cus \-ˌȯ-tō-'täk-sə-kəs\ *n* : SELF-TOLERANCE

horse \'hȯrs\ *n, pl* **hors·es** *also* **horse** : a large solid-hoofed herbivorous mammal (*Equus caballus* of the family Equidae) domesticated since prehistoric times

horse bot *n* : HORSE BOTFLY; *specif* : a larva of a horse botfly

horse botfly *n* : a cosmopolitan botfly of the genus *Gasterophilus* (*G. intestinalis*) whose larvae parasitize the stomach lining of the horse

horse·fly \'hȯrs-ˌflī\ *n, pl* **-flies** : any of a family (Tabanidae) of usu. large dipteran flies with bloodsucking females

horse·shoe kidney \-ˌshü\ *n* : a congenital partial fusion of the kidneys resulting in a horseshoe shape

Hor·ton's syndrome \'hȯr-tənz-\ *n* : CLUSTER HEADACHE

    Horton, Bayard Taylor (1895–1980), American physician.

hosp *abbr* hospital

hos·pice \'häs-pəs\ *n* : a facility or program designed to provide a caring environment for meeting the physical and emotional needs of the terminally ill

hos·pi·tal \'häs-ˌpit-ᵊl\ *n, often attrib* **1** : a charitable institution for the needy, aged, infirm, or young **2 a** : an institution where the sick or injured are given medical or surgical care — usu. used in British English without an article after a preposition **b** : a place for the care and treatment of sick and injured animals

hospital bed *n* : a bed used for patients (as in a hospital) that can be adjusted esp. to raise the head end, foot end, or middle as required — see GATCH BED

hos·pi·tal·ism \'häs-(ˌ)pit-ᵊl-ˌi-zəm\ *n* **1 a** : the factors and influences that adversely affect the health of hospitalized persons **b** : the effect of such factors on mental or physical health **2** : the deleterious physical and mental effects on infants and children resulting from their living in institutions without the benefit of a home environment and parents

hos·pi·tal·ist \'häs-(ˌ)pit-ᵊl-əst\ *n* : a physician who specializes in seeing and treating other physicians' hospitalized patients in order to minimize the number of hospital visits by the patients' regular physicians

hos·pi·tal·iza·tion \ˌhäs-(ˌ)pit-ᵊl-ə-'zā-shən\ *n* **1** : the act or process of being hospitalized **2** : the period of stay in a hospital

hospitalization insurance *n* : insurance that provides benefits to cover or partly cover hospital expenses

hos·pi·tal·ize \'häs-(ˌ)pit-ᵊl-ˌīz, häs-'pit-ᵊl-ˌīz\ *vb* **-ized; -iz·ing** : to place in a hospital as a patient

host \'hōst\ *n* **1** : a living animal or plant on or in which a parasite lives — see DEFINITIVE HOST, INTERMEDIATE HOST **2 a** : an individual into which a tissue or part is transplanted from another **b** : an individual in whom an abnormal growth (as a cancer) is proliferating

host cell *n* : a living cell invaded by or capable of being invaded by an infectious agent (as a virus)

hos·til·i·ty \hä-'sti-lə-tē\ *n, pl* **-ties** : conflict, opposition, or resistance in thought or principle — **hos·tile** \'häs-təl, -ˌtīl\ *adj*

hot \'hät\ *adj* **hot·ter; hot·test 1** : having heat in a degree exceeding normal body heat **2** : RADIOACTIVE; *esp* : exhibiting a relatively great amount of radioactivity when subjected to radionuclide scanning

hot flash *n* : a sudden brief flushing and sensation of heat caused by dilation of skin capillaries usu. associated with menopausal endocrine imbalance — called also *hot flush*

hot line *n* : a usu. toll-free telephone service available to the public for some specific purpose ⟨a poison control *hot line*⟩ ⟨an AIDS *hot line*⟩

hot pack *n* : absorbent material (as squares of gauze) wrung out in hot water, wrapped around the body or a portion of the body, and covered with dry material to hold in the moist heat — compare COLD PACK

hot spot *n* **1** : a patch of painful moist inflamed skin on a domestic animal and esp. a dog **2** : a site in genetic material having a high frequency of mutation or recombination

hot–water bottle *n* : a usu. rubber bag that has a stopper and is filled with hot water to provide warmth

hourglass stomach *n* : a stomach divided into two communicating cavities by a circular constriction usu. caused by the scar tissue around an ulcer

house·bro·ken \'haùs-ˌbrō-kən\ *adj* : trained to excretory habits acceptable in indoor living — used of a household pet — **house·break** \-ˌbrāk\ *vb*

house call *n* : a visit (as by a doctor) to a home to provide medical care

house doctor *n* : a physician in residence at an establishment (as a hotel) or on the premises temporarily in the event of a medical emergency

house–dust mite \'haùs-ˌdəst-\ *n* : either of two widely distributed mites (*Dermatophagoides farinae* and *D. pteronyssinus*) that commonly occur in house dust and often induce allergic responses esp. in children

house·fly \-ˌflī\ *n, pl* **-flies** : a cosmopolitan dipteran fly of the genus *Musca* (*M. domestica*) that is often found about human habitations and may act as a mechanical vector of diseases (as typhoid fever); *also* : any of various flies of similar appearance or habitat

house·maid's knee \'haùs-ˌmādz-\ *n* : a swelling over the knee due to an enlargement of the bursa in the front of the patella

house·man \'haùs-mən\ *n, pl* **-men** \-mən\ *chiefly Brit* : INTERN

house mouse *n* : a common mostly cosmopolitan mouse of the genus *Mus* (*M. musculus*) that usu. lives and breeds about buildings, is an important laboratory animal, and is an important pest as a consumer of human food and as a vector of diseases

house officer *n* : an intern or resident employed by a hospital

house physician *n* : a physician and esp. a resident employed by a hospital

house staff *n* : interns, residents, and fellows of a hospital

house surgeon *n* : a surgeon fully qualified in a specialty and resident in a hospital

Hous·ton's valve \'hü-stənz-\ *n* : any of the usu. three but sometimes four or two permanent transverse crescent-shaped folds of the rectum

Houston, John (1802–1845), British surgeon.

How·ard test \'haü-ərd-\ *n* : a test of renal function that involves the catheterization of each ureter so that the urinary output of each kidney can be determined and analyzed separately

    Howard, John Eager (1902–1985), American internist and endocrinologist.

How·ell–Jol·ly body \'haü-əl-zhȯ-'lē-, -'jä-lē-\ *n* : one of the basophilic granules that are prob. nuclear fragments, that sometimes occur in red blood cells, and that indicate by their appearance in circulating blood that red cells are leaving the marrow while incompletely mature (as in certain anemias)

    Howell, William Henry (1860–1945), American physiologist.

    Jolly \zhȯ-'lē\, **Justin–Marie–Jules (1870–1953),** French histologist.

How·ship's lacuna \'haü-,ships-\ *n* : a groove or cavity usu. containing osteoclasts that occurs in bone which is undergoing reabsorption

    Howship, John (1781–1841), British anatomist.

HPI *abbr* history of present illness

HPLC *abbr* high-performance liquid chromatography

hr *abbr* [Latin *hora*] hour — used in writing prescriptions; see QH

hs *abbr* [Latin *hora somni*] at bedtime — used esp. in writing prescriptions

HPV \,ăch-,pē-'vē\ *n* : HUMAN PAPILLOMAVIRUS

HRT *abbr* hormone replacement therapy

Hs *symbol* hassium

HS *abbr* house surgeon

HSA *abbr* human serum albumin

HSV \,ăch-,es-'vē\ *n* : either of two herpesviruses that cause herpes simplex — see HSV-1, HSV-2

HSV–1 \-,vē-'wən\ *n* : a herpesvirus of the genus *Simplexvirus* (species *Human herpesvirus 1*) that causes the type of herpes simplex typically involving the lips, mouth, and face

HSV–2 \-'tü\ *n* : a herpesvirus of the genus *Simplexvirus* (species *Human herpesvirus 2*) that causes the type of herpes simplex typically involving the genital region

ht *abbr* height

5–HT \'fiv-,ăch-'tē\ *n* : SEROTONIN

HTLV \,ăch-(,)tē-(,)el-'vē\ *n* : any of several retroviruses that formerly included the original strain of HIV — often used with a number or Roman numeral to indicate the type and order of discovery ⟨HTLV-III⟩; called also *human T-cell leukemia virus, human T-cell lymphotropic virus, human T-lymphotropic virus*

HTLV–1 \-,vē-'wən\ *n* : an HTLV (species *Primate T-lymphotropic virus 1* of the genus *Deltaretrovirus*) that is found in association with adult T-cell leukemia and a progressive paralyzing myelopathy

HTLV–III *n* : HIV-1

H₂ antagonist \-'tü-\ *n* : a drug (as famotidine or ranitidine) that reduces or inhibits the secretion of gastric acid by binding competitively with histamine to H₂ receptors on cell membranes — called also *H₂ blocker, H₂ receptor antagonist*

H₂ receptor *n* : a receptor for histamine on cell membranes that modulates the stimulation of heart rate and the secretion of gastric acid — called also *H₂ histamine receptor*

Hub·bard tank \'hə-bərd-\ *n* : a large tank in which a patient can easily be assisted in exercises while in the water

    Hubbard, Leroy Watkins (1857–1938), American orthopedic surgeon.

hue \'hyü\ *n* : the one of the three psychological dimensions of color perception that permits them to be classified as red, yellow, green, blue, or an intermediate between any contiguous pair of these colors and that is correlated with the wavelength or the combination of wavelengths comprising the stimulus — compare BRIGHTNESS, SATURATION 4

huff \'həf\ *vb* : to inhale (noxious fumes) through the mouth for the euphoric effect produced by the inhalant; *also* : to inhale the noxious fumes of (a substance) for their euphoric effect

Huh·ner test \'hyü-nər-\ *n* : a test used in sterility studies that involves postcoital examination of fluid aspirated from the vagina and cervix to determine the presence or survival of spermatozoa in these areas

    Huhner, Max (1873–1947), American surgeon.

¹hu·man \'hyü-mən, 'yü-\ *adj* **1 a** : of, relating to, or characteristic of humans **b** : primarily or usu. harbored by, affecting, or attacking humans ⟨~ parasites⟩ **2** : being or consisting of humans ⟨the ~ race⟩ **3** : consisting of hominids — **hu·man·ness** *n*

²human *n* : a bipedal primate mammal of the genus *Homo* (*H. sapiens*) : MAN; *broadly* : HOMINID — **hu·man·like** \-,līk\ *adj*

human being *n* : HUMAN

human botfly *n* : a large fly of the genus *Dermatobia* (*D. hominis*) that is widely distributed in tropical America and undergoes its larval development subcutaneously in some mammals including humans

human chorionic gonadotropin *n* : a glycoprotein hormone similar in structure to luteinizing hormone that is secreted by the placenta during early pregnancy to maintain corpus luteum function, is commonly tested for as an indicator of pregnancy, and is used medically to induce ovulation and to treat male hypogonadism and cryptorchidism — *abbr. HCG*

human ecology *n* : the ecology of human communities and populations esp. as concerned with preservation of environmental quality through proper application of conservation and civil engineering practices

human ehrlichiosis *n* : any of several ehrlichioses affecting humans; *esp* : HUMAN GRANULOCYTIC EHRLICHIOSIS

human engineering *n* : ERGONOMICS 1

human factors *n* : ERGONOMICS 1

human factors engineering *n* : ERGONOMICS 1

human granulocytic ehrlichiosis *n* : an ehrlichiosis of humans that is marked by fever, myalgia, headache, leukemia, and thrombocytopenia and that is caused by a rickettsial bacterium of the genus *Ehrlichia* which is transmitted by ixodid ticks — abbr. *HGE*

human growth hormone *n* : the naturally occurring growth hormone of humans or a recombinant version that is used to treat children with growth hormone deficiencies and has been used esp. by athletes to increase muscle mass — abbr. *HGH*; see SOMATROPIN

human immunodeficiency virus *n* : HIV

human leukocyte antigen *n* : any of various proteins that are encoded by genes of the major histocompatibility complex in humans and are found on the surface of many cell types (as white blood cells); *broadly* : HLA 2

human papillomavirus *n* : any of numerous papillomaviruses (as of the genera *Alphapapillomavirus*, *Betapapillomavirus*, and *Gammapapillomavirus*) that cause human papillomas (as plantar warts and genital warts) and include some associated with the production of cervical cancer — called also *HPV*

human relations *n* 1 : the social and interpersonal relations between humans 2 : a course, study, or program designed to develop better interpersonal and intergroup adjustments

human T–cell leukemia virus *n* : HTLV

human T–cell leukemia virus type III *n* : HIV-1

human T–cell lym·pho·tro·pic virus \-ˌlim-fə-ˈtrō-pik-\ *n* : HTLV

human T–cell lymphotropic virus type III *n* : HIV-1

human T–lymphotropic virus *n* : HTLV

human T–lymphotropic virus type III *n* : HIV-1

hu·mec·tant \hyü-ˈmek-tənt\ *n* : a substance (as sorbitol) that promotes retention of moisture — **humectant** *adj*

hu·mer·al \ˈhyü-mə-rəl\ *adj* : of, relating to, or situated in the region of the humerus or shoulder

humeral circumflex artery — see ANTERIOR HUMERAL CIRCUMFLEX ARTERY, POSTERIOR HUMERAL CIRCUMFLEX ARTERY

hu·mer·us \ˈhyü-mə-rəs\ *n*, *pl* **hu·meri** \-ˌrī, -ˌrē\ : the longest bone of the upper arm or forelimb extending from the shoulder to the elbow, articulating above by a rounded head with the glenoid fossa, having below a broad articular surface divided by a ridge into a medial pulley-shaped portion and a lateral rounded eminence that articulate with the ulna and radius respectively

hu·mid·i·fi·er \hyü-ˈmi-də-ˌfī-ər, yü-\ *n* : a device for supplying or maintaining humidity

hu·mid·i·fy \-ˌfī\ *vb* **-fied; -fy·ing** : to make humid — **hu·mid·i·fi·ca·tion** \-ˌmi-də-fə-ˈkā-shən\ *n*

hu·mid·i·ty \hyü-ˈmi-də-tē, yü-\ *n*, *pl* **-ties** : a moderate degree of wetness esp. of the atmosphere — see ABSOLUTE HUMIDITY, RELATIVE HUMIDITY

hu·mor \ˈhyü-mər, ˈyü-\ *n* 1 : a normal functioning bodily semifluid or fluid (as the blood or lymph) 2 : a secretion (as a hormone) that is an excitant of activity

hu·mor·al \ˈhyü-mə-rəl, ˈyü-\ *adj* 1 : of, relating to, proceeding from, or involving a bodily humor (as a hormone) 2 : relating to or being the part of immunity or the immune response that involves antibodies secreted by B cells and circulating in bodily fluids ⟨∼ immunity⟩ — compare CELL-MEDIATED

hu·mour *chiefly Brit var of* HUMOR

hump \ˈhəmp\ *n* : a rounded protuberance; *esp* : HUMPBACK

hump·back \-ˌbak, *for 1 also* -ˈbak\ *n* 1 : a humped or crooked back; *also* : KYPHOSIS 2 : HUNCHBACK 2 — **hump·backed** \-ˌbakt\ *adj*

Hu·mu·lin \ˈhyü-myü-lən\ *trademark* — used for a preparation of insulin produced by genetic engineering and structurally identical to insulin made by the human pancreas

hunch·back \ˈhənch-ˌbak\ *n* 1 : HUMPBACK 1 2 : a person with a humpback — **hunch·backed** \-ˌbakt\ *adj*

hun·ger \ˈhəŋ-gər\ *n* 1 : a craving, desire, or urgent need for food 2 : an uneasy sensation occasioned normally by the lack of food and resulting directly from stimulation of the sensory nerves of the stomach by the contraction and churning movement of the empty stomach 3 : a weakened disordered condition brought about by prolonged lack of food ⟨die of ∼⟩

hunger pangs *n pl* : pains in the abdominal region which occur in the early stages of hunger or fasting and are correlated with contractions of the empty stomach or intestines

Hun·ner's ulcer \ˈhə-nərz-\ *n* : a painful ulcer affecting all layers of the bladder wall and usu. associated with inflammation of the wall

Hunner, Guy Leroy (1868–1957), American gynecologist.

Hun·ter's canal \'hən-tərz-\ *n* : an aponeurotic canal in the middle third of the thigh through which the femoral artery passes

Hunter, John (1728–1793), British anatomist and surgeon.

Hunter's syndrome *or* **Hunter syndrome** \'hən-tər-\ *n* : a mucopolysaccharidosis that is similar to Hurler's syndrome but is inherited as a sex-linked recessive trait and has milder symptoms

Hunter, Charles (1873–1955), Canadian physician.

Hun·ting·ton's chorea \'hən-tiŋ-tənz-\ *n* : HUNTINGTON'S DISEASE

Huntington, George (1850–1916), American neurologist.

Huntington's disease *also* **Huntington disease** *n* : a progressive chorea that is inherited as an autosomal dominant trait, usu. begins in middle age, and is characterized by choreiform movements, emotional disturbances, and mental deterioration — called also *Huntington's*

Hur·ler's syndrome \'hər-lərz-, 'hur-\ *or* **Hur·ler syndrome** \-lər-\ *n* : a mucopolysaccharidosis that is inherited as an autosomal recessive trait and is characterized by deformities of the skeleton and features, hepatosplenomegaly, restricted joint flexibility, clouding of the cornea, mental deficiency, and deafness — called also *Hurler's disease*

Hur·ler \'hur-lər\, Gertrud (1889–1965), German pediatrician.

HUS *abbr* hemolytic uremic syndrome

husk \'həsk\ *n* : HOOSE

Hutch·in·son's teeth \'hə-chən-sənz-\ *n sing or pl* : peg-shaped teeth having a crescent-shaped notch in the cutting edge and occurring esp. in children with congenital syphilis

Hutchinson, Sir Jonathan (1828–1913), British surgeon and pathologist.

Hutchinson's triad *n* : a triad of symptoms that comprises Hutchinson's teeth, interstitial keratitis, and deafness and occurs in children with congenital syphilis

Hux·ley's layer \'həks-lēz-\ *n* : a layer of the inner stratum of a hair follicle composed of one or two layers of horny flattened epithelial cells with nuclei and situated between Henle's layer and the cuticle next to the hair

Huxley, Thomas Henry (1825–1895), British biologist.

hy- *or* **hyo-** *comb form* : of, relating to, or connecting with the hyoid bone ⟨*hyo*glossus⟩

hyal- *or* **hyalo-** *comb form* : glass : glassy : hyaline ⟨*hyal*uronic acid⟩

¹hy·a·line \'hī-ə-lən, -,līn\ *adj* : transparent or nearly transparent and usu. homogeneous

²hy·a·line \-ə-lən\ *n* : any of several translucent nitrogenous substances that collect around cells and are capable of being stained by eosin

hyaline cartilage *n* : translucent bluish white cartilage consisting of cells embedded in an apparently homogeneous matrix, present in joints and respiratory passages, and forming most of the fetal skeleton

hyaline cast *n* : a renal cast of mucoprotein characterized by homogeneity of structure

hyaline degeneration *n* : tissue degeneration chiefly of connective tissues in which structural elements of affected cells are replaced by homogeneous translucent material that stains intensely with acid stains

hyaline membrane disease *n* : RESPIRATORY DISTRESS SYNDROME

hy·a·lin·i·za·tion \,hī-ə-lə-nə-'zā-shən\ *n* : the process of becoming hyaline or of undergoing hyaline degeneration; *also* : the resulting state — **hy·a·lin·ized** \'hī-ə-lə-,nīzd\ *adj*

hy·a·li·no·sis \,hī-ə-lə-'nō-səs\ *n, pl* **-no·ses** \-,sēz\ **1** : HYALINE DEGENERATION **2** : a condition characterized by hyaline degeneration

hy·a·li·tis \,hī-ə-'lī-təs\ *n* **1** : inflammation of the vitreous body of the eye **2** : inflammation of the hyaloid membrane of the vitreous humor

hyalo- — see HYAL-

hy·a·loid \'hī-ə-,loid\ *adj* : being glassy or transparent ⟨a ~ appearance⟩

hyaloid membrane *n* : a very delicate membrane enclosing the vitreous body of the eye

hy·al·o·mere \'hī-ə-lə-,mir\ *n* : the pale portion of a blood platelet that is not refractile — compare CHROMOMERE

Hy·a·lom·ma \,hī-ə-'lä-mə\ *n* : a genus of Old World ticks that attack wild and domestic mammals and sometimes humans, produce severe lesions by their bites, and often serve as vectors of viral and protozoal diseases (as east coast fever)

hy·a·lo·plasm \hī-'a-lə-,pla-zəm, 'hī-ə-lō-\ *n* : CYTOSOL — **hy·a·lo·plas·mic** \,hī-,a-lə-'plaz-mik, ,hī-ə-lō-\ *adj*

hy·al·uron·ic acid \,hī(l)-yü-'rä-nik-, ,hī-əl-yü-\ *n* : a viscous glycosaminoglycan that occurs esp. in the vitreous body, the umbilical cord, and synovial fluid and as a cementing substance in the subcutaneous tissue

hy·al·uron·i·dase \-'rä-nə-,dās, -,dāz\ *n* : a mucolytic enzyme that facilitates the spread of fluids through tissues by lowering the viscosity of hyaluronic acid and is used esp. to aid in the dispersion of fluids (as local anesthetics) injected subcutaneously — called also *spreading factor*

H–Y antigen *n* : a male histocompatibility antigen determined by genes on the Y chromosome

hy·brid \'hī-brəd\ *n* **1** : an offspring of two animals or plants of different races, breeds, varieties, species, or genera **2** : something heterogeneous in origin or composition ⟨artificial ∼s of DNA and RNA⟩ — **hybrid** *adj* — **hy·brid·ism** \-brə-ˌdi-zəm\ *n*

hy·brid·ize \'hī-brə-ˌdīz\ *vb* **-ized; -iz·ing** : to cause to interbreed or combine so as to produce hybrids — **hy·brid·i·za·tion** \ˌhī-brə-də-'zā-shən\ *n*

hy·brid·oma \ˌhī-brə-'dō-mə\ *n* : a hybrid cell produced by the fusion of an antibody-producing lymphocyte with a tumor cell and used to culture continuously a specific monoclonal antibody

hy·can·thone \hī-'kan-ˌthōn\ *n* : a lucanthone analog $C_{20}H_{24}N_2O_2S$ used to treat schistosomiasis

Hy·co·dan \'hī-kə-ˌdan\ *trademark* — used for a preparation of the bitartrate of hydrocodone and the methyl bromide of homatropine

hy·dan·to·in \hī-'dan-tə-wən\ *n* **1** : a crystalline weakly acidic compound $C_3H_4N_2O_2$ with a sweetish taste that is found in beet juice **2** : a derivative of hydantoin (as phenytoin)

hy·dan·to·in·ate \-wə-ˌnāt\ *n* : a salt of hydantoin or of one of its derivatives

hy·da·tid \'hī-də-təd, -ˌtid\ *n* **1** : the larval cyst of a tapeworm of the genus *Echinococcus* that usu. occurs as a fluid-filled sac containing daughter cysts in which scolices develop but that occas. forms a proliferating spongy mass which actively metastasizes in the host's tissues — called also *hydatid cyst*; see ECHINOCOCCUS 1 **2 a** : an abnormal cyst or cystic structure; *esp* : HYDATIDIFORM MOLE **b** : HYDATID DISEASE

hydatid disease *n* : a form of echinococcosis caused by the development of hydatids of a tapeworm of the genus *Echinococcus* (*E. granulosus*) in the tissues esp. of the liver or lungs of humans and some domestic animals (as sheep and dogs)

hy·da·tid·i·form mole \ˌhī-də-'ti-də-ˌform-\ *n* : a mass in the uterus that consists of enlarged edematous degenerated chorionic villi growing in clusters resembling grapes, that typically develops following fertilization of an enucleate egg, and that may or may not contain fetal tissue

hy·da·tid·o·sis \ˌhī-də-ˌti-'dō-səs\ *n, pl* **-o·ses** \-ˌsēz\ : ECHINOCOCCOSIS; *specif* : HYDATID DISEASE

Hyd·er·gine \'hī-dər-ˌjēn\ *trademark* — used for a preparation of ergoloid mesylates

hydr- *or* **hydro-** *comb form* **1** : water ⟨*hydro*therapy⟩ **2** : an accumulation of fluid in a (specified) bodily part ⟨*hydro*cephalus⟩ ⟨*hydro*nephrosis⟩

hy·drae·mia *chiefly Brit var of* HYDREMIA

hy·dra·gogue \'hī-drə-ˌgäg\ *n* : a cathartic that causes copious watery discharges from the bowels

hy·dral·azine \hī-'dra-lə-ˌzēn\ *n* : an antihypertensive drug that is used in the form of its hydrochloride C_8H_8-N_4·HCl and produces peripheral arteriolar dilation by relaxing vascular smooth muscle

hy·dram·ni·os \hī-'dram-nē-ˌäs\ *n* : excessive accumulation of the amniotic fluid — called also *polyhydramnios* — **hy·dram·ni·ot·ic** \hī-ˌdram-nē-'ä-tik\ *adj*

hy·dran·en·ceph·a·ly \ˌhī-dra-nen-'se-fə-lē\ *n, pl* **-lies** : a congenital defect of the brain in which fluid-filled cavities take the place of the cerebral hemispheres

hy·drar·gy·rism \hī-'drär-jə-ˌri-zəm\ *n* : MERCURIALISM

hy·drar·thro·sis \ˌhī-(ˌ)drär-'thrō-səs\ *n, pl* **-thro·ses** : a watery effusion into a joint cavity

¹hy·drate \'hī-ˌdrāt\ *n* **1** : a compound or complex ion formed by the union of water with some other substance **2** : HYDROXIDE

²hydrate *vb* **hy·drat·ed; hy·drat·ing 1** : to cause to take up or combine with water or the elements of water **2** : to become a hydrate

hy·dra·tion \hī-'drā-shən\ *n* **1** : the act or process of combining or treating with water: as **a** : the introduction of additional fluid into the body **b** : a chemical reaction in which water takes part with the formation of only one product **2** : the quality or state of being hydrated; *esp* : the condition of having adequate fluid in body tissues

hy·dra·zide \'hī-drə-ˌzīd\ *n* : any of a class of compounds resulting from the replacement by an acid group of hydrogen in hydrazine or in one of its derivatives

hy·dra·zine \'hī-drə-ˌzēn\ *n* : a colorless fuming corrosive strongly reducing liquid base N_2H_4 used in the production of numerous materials (as pharmaceuticals and plastics); *also* : an organic base derived from this

hy·dra·zone \'hī-drə-ˌzōn\ *n* : any of a class of compounds containing the group >C=NNHR

hy·dre·mia \hī-'drē-mē-ə\ *n* : an abnormally watery state of the blood — **hy·dre·mic** \-mik\ *adj*

hy·dren·ceph·a·ly \ˌhī-dren-'se-fə-lē\ *n, pl* **-lies** : HYDROCEPHALUS

hydro- — see HYDR-

hy·droa \hī-'drō-ə\ *n* : an itching usu. vesicular eruption of the skin; *esp* : one induced by exposure to light

hy·dro·bro·mide \ˌhī-drō-'brō-ˌmīd\ *n* : a salt of hydrogen bromide with an organic base

hy·dro·car·bon \-'kär-bən\ *n* : an organic compound (as benzene) containing only carbon and hydrogen and often occurring esp. in petroleum, natural gas, and coal

hy·dro·cele \'hī-drə-ˌsēl\ *n* : an accumulation of serous fluid in a sacculated cavity (as the scrotum)

hy·dro·ce·lec·to·my \ˌhī-drə-sē-ˈlek-tə-mē\ *n, pl* **-mies** : surgical removal of a hydrocele

¹hy·dro·ce·phal·ic \ˌhī-drō-sə-ˈfa-lik\ *adj* : relating to, characterized by, or affected with hydrocephalus

²hydrocephalic *n* : an individual affected with hydrocephalus

hy·dro·ceph·a·lus \-ˈse-fə-ləs\ *n, pl* **-li** \-ˌlī\ : an abnormal increase in the amount of cerebrospinal fluid within the cranial cavity that is accompanied by expansion of the cerebral ventricles and enlargement of the skull

hy·dro·ceph·a·ly \ˌhī-drō-ˈse-fə-lē\ *n, pl* **-lies** : HYDROCEPHALUS

hy·dro·chlo·ric acid \ˌhī-drə-ˌklor-ik-\ *n* : an aqueous solution of hydrogen chloride HCl that is a strong corrosive irritating acid and is normally present in dilute form in gastric juice — called also *muriatic acid*

hy·dro·chlo·ride \-ˈklor-ˌīd\ *n* : a salt of hydrochloric acid with an organic base used esp. as a vehicle for the administration of a drug

hy·dro·chlo·ro·thi·a·zide \-ˌklor-ə-ˈthī-ə-ˌzīd\ *n* : a diuretic and antihypertensive drug $C_7H_8ClN_3O_4S_2$ — abbr. *HCTZ*; see DYAZIDE, HYDRODIURIL, HYZAAR, MAXZIDE, ORETIC

hy·dro·cho·le·re·sis \-ˌkō-lər-ˈē-səs, -ˌkä-\ *n, pl* **-re·ses** \-ˌsēz\ : increased production of watery liver bile without necessarily increased secretion of bile solids

¹hy·dro·cho·le·ret·ic \-ˈe-tik\ *adj* : of, relating to, or characterized by hydrocholeresis

²hydrocholeretic *n* : an agent that produces hydrocholeresis

hy·dro·co·done \ˌhī-drō-ˈkō-ˌdōn\ *n* : a habit-forming codeine derivative used in the form of its bitartrate $C_{18}H_{21}NO_3 \cdot C_4H_6O_6$ usu. in combination with other drugs (as acetaminophen) as an analgesic or cough sedative — called also *dihydrocodeinone*; see HYCODAN, VICODIN

hy·dro·cor·ti·sone \-ˈkor-tə-ˌsōn, -ˌzōn\ *n* : CORTISOL; *esp* : cortisol used pharmaceutically

hy·dro·cy·an·ic acid \ˌhī-drō-sī-ˈa-nik-\ *n* : an aqueous solution of hydrogen cyanide HCN that is an extremely poisonous weak acid used esp. in fumigating — called also *prussic acid*

Hy·dro·di·ur·il \-ˈdī-yə-ˌril\ *trademark* — used for a preparation of hydrochlorothiazide

hy·dro·dy·nam·ics \ˌhī-drō-dī-ˈna-miks\ *n* : a branch of physics that deals with the motion of fluids and the forces acting on solid bodies immersed in fluids and in motion relative to them — **hy·dro·dy·nam·ic** \-mik\ *adj*

hy·dro·flu·me·thi·a·zide \-ˌflü-mə-ˈthī-ə-ˌzīd\ *n* : a diuretic and antihypertensive drug $C_8H_8F_3N_3O_4S_2$

hy·dro·gel \ˈhī-drə-ˌjel\ *n* : a gel in which the liquid is water

hy·dro·gen \ˈhī-drə-jən\ *n* : a nonmetallic element that is the simplest and lightest of the elements and is normally a colorless odorless highly flammable gas having two atoms in a molecule — symbol *H*; see ELEMENT table — **hy·drog·e·nous** \hī-ˈdrä-jə-nəs\ *adj*

hy·dro·ge·nate \hī-ˈdrä-jə-ˌnāt, ˈhī-drə-jə-\ *vb* **-nat·ed; -nat·ing** : to add hydrogen to the molecule of (an unsaturated organic compound) — **hy·dro·ge·na·tion** \hī-ˌdrä-jə-ˈnā-shən, ˌhī-drə-jə-\ *n*

hydrogen bond *n* : an electrostatic attraction between a hydrogen atom in one polar molecule (as of water) and a small negatively charged atom (as of fluorine, oxygen, or nitrogen) in usu. another molecule of the same or a different polar substance

hydrogen bromide *n* : a colorless irritating gas HBr that fumes in moist air and yields a strong acid resembling hydrochloric acid when dissolved in water

hydrogen chloride *n* : a colorless pungent poisonous gas HCl that fumes in moist air and yields hydrochloric acid when dissolved in water

hydrogen cyanide *n* **1** : a poisonous usu. gaseous compound HCN that has the odor of bitter almonds **2** : HYDROCYANIC ACID

hydrogen peroxide *n* : an unstable compound H_2O_2 used esp. as an oxidizing and bleaching agent and as an antiseptic

hy·dro·lase \ˈhī-drə-ˌlās, -ˌlāz\ *n* : a hydrolytic enzyme (as an esterase)

hy·drol·o·gy \hī-ˈdrä-lə-jē\ *n, pl* **-gies** : the body of medical knowledge and practice concerned with the therapeutic use of bathing and water

hy·dro·ly·sate \hī-ˈdrä-lə-ˌsāt, ˌhī-drə-ˈlī-\ *or* **hy·dro·ly·zate** \-ˌzāt\ *n* : a product of hydrolysis

hy·drol·y·sis \hī-ˈdrä-lə-səs, ˌhī-drə-ˈlī-\ *n* : a chemical process of decomposition involving splitting of a bond and the addition of the hydrogen cation and the hydroxide anion of water — **hy·dro·lyt·ic** \ˌhī-drə-ˈli-tik\ *adj* — **hy·dro·lyze** \ˈhī-drə-ˌlīz\ *vb* — **hy·dro·lyz·able** \ˌhī-drə-ˈlī-zə-bəl\ *adj*

hy·dro·me·tro·col·pos \ˌhī-drō-ˌmē-trō-ˈkäl-ˌpäs\ *n* : an accumulation of watery fluid in the uterus and vagina

hy·dro·mor·phone \-ˈmor-ˌfōn\ *n* : a morphine derivative administered in the form of its hydrochloride $C_{17}H_{19}NO_3 \cdot HCl$ as an analgesic — called also *dihydromorphinone*

hy·dro·ne·phro·sis \ˌhī-drō-ni-ˈfrō-səs\ *n, pl* **-phro·ses** \-ˌsēz\ : cystic distension of the kidney caused by the accumulation of urine in the renal pelvis as a result of obstruction to outflow and accompanied by atrophy of the kidney structure and cyst formation — **hy·dro·ne·phrot·ic** \-ni-'frä-tik\ *adj*

hy·drop·a·thy \hī-'drä-pə-thē\ *n, pl* **-thies** : a method of treating disease by copious and frequent use of water both externally and internally — compare HYDROTHERAPY — **hy·dro·path·ic** \ˌhī-drə-'pa-thik\ *adj*

hy·dro·pe·nia \ˌhī-drə-'pē-nē-ə\ *n* : a condition in which the body is deficient in water — **hy·dro·pe·nic** \-'pē-nik\ *adj*

hy·dro·peri·car·di·um \ˌhī-drō-per-ə-'kär-dē-əm\ *n, pl* **-dia** \-dē-ə\ : an excess of watery fluid in the pericardial cavity

hy·dro·phil·ic \-'fi-lik\ *adj* : of, relating to, or having a strong affinity for water \~ colloids\ — compare LIPOPHILIC — **hy·dro·phi·lic·i·ty** \-fi-'li-sə-tē\ *n*

hy·dro·pho·bia \ˌhī-drə-'fō-bē-ə\ *n* 1 : a morbid dread of water 2 : RABIES

hy·dro·pho·bic \-'fō-bik\ *adj* 1 : of, relating to, or suffering from hydrophobia 2 : resistant to or avoiding wetting \a \~ lens\ 3 : of, relating to, or having a lack of affinity for water \~ colloids\ — **hy·dro·pho·bic·i·ty** \-ˌfō-'bi-sə-tē\ *n*

hy·droph·thal·mos \ˌhī-ˌdräf-'thal-mäs\ *n* : general enlargement of the eyeball due to a watery effusion within it

hy·drop·ic \hī-'drä-pik\ *adj* 1 : exhibiting hydrops; *esp* : EDEMATOUS 2 : characterized by swelling and taking up of fluid — used of a type of cellular degeneration

hy·dro·pneu·mo·tho·rax \ˌhī-drə-ˌnü-mə-'thȯr-ˌaks, -ˌnyü-\ *n, pl* **-tho·rax·es** *or* **-tho·ra·ces** \-'thȯr-ə-ˌsēz\ : the presence of gas and serous fluid in the pleural cavity

hy·drops \'hī-ˌdräps\ *n, pl* **hy·drop·ses** \-ˌdräp-ˌsēz\ 1 : EDEMA 2 : distension of a hollow organ with fluid 3 : HYDROPS FETALIS

hydrops fe·tal·is \-fē-'ta-ləs\ *n* : serious and extensive edema of the fetus (as in erythroblastosis fetalis)

hy·dro·qui·none \ˌhī-drō-kwi-'nōn, -'kwi-ˌnōn\ *n* : a bleaching agent $C_6H_6O_2$ used topically to remove pigmentation from hyperpigmented areas of skin (as a lentigo or freckle)

hy·dro·sal·pinx \-'sal-(ˌ)piŋks\ *n, pl* **-sal·pin·ges** \-sal-'pin-(ˌ)jēz\ : abnormal distension of one or both fallopian tubes with fluid usu. due to inflammation

hy·dro·ther·a·py \ˌhī-drō-'ther-ə-pē\ *n, pl* **-pies** : the therapeutic use of water (as in a whirlpool bath) — compare HYDROPATHY — **hy·dro·ther·a·peu·tic** \-ˌther-ə-'pyü-tik\ *adj*

hy·dro·tho·rax \-'thȯr-ˌaks\ *n, pl* **-tho·rax·es** *or* **-tho·ra·ces** \-'thȯr-ə-ˌsēz\ : an excess of serous fluid in the pleural cavity; *esp* : an effusion resulting from failing circulation (as in heart disease)

hy·dro·ure·ter \ˌhī-drō-'yur-ə-tər, -'yu-ˌrē-tər\ *n* : abnormal distension of the ureter with urine

hy·drox·ide \hī-'dräk-ˌsīd\ *n* 1 : the anion OH^- consisting of one atom of hydrogen and one of oxygen — called also *hydroxide ion* 2 : an ionic compound of hydroxide with an element or group

hy·droxo·co·bal·amin \hī-ˌdräk-(ˌ)sō-kō-'ba-lə-mən\ *n* : a member $C_{62}H_{89}CoN_{13}O_{15}P$ of the vitamin B_{12} group used in treating and preventing vitamin B_{12} deficiency

hy·droxy \hī-'dräk-sē\ *adj* : being or containing hydroxyl; *esp* : containing hydroxyl in place of hydrogen — often used in combination *hydroxy*butyric acid\

hy·droxy·am·phet·amine \hī-ˌdräk-sē-am-'fe-tə-ˌmēn, -mən\ *n* : a sympathomimetic drug administered in the form of its hydrobromide $C_9H_{13}NO$·HBr and used esp. as a mydriatic

hydroxyanisole — see BUTYLATED HYDROXYANISOLE

hy·droxy·ap·a·tite \hī-ˌdräk-sē-'a·pə-ˌtīt\ *also* **hy·drox·yl·ap·a·tite** \-sə-'la-\ *n* : a complex phosphate of calcium $Ca_5(PO_4)_3OH$ that is the chief structural element of bone

hy·droxy·ben·zo·ic acid \-ben-'zō-ik-\ *n* : SALICYLIC ACID

hy·droxy·bu·ty·rate \-'byü-tə-ˌrāt\ *n* : a salt or ester of hydroxybutyric acid — see GAMMA HYDROXYBUTYRATE

hy·droxy·bu·tyr·ic acid \-byü-'tir-ik-\ *or* **β–hy·droxy·bu·tyr·ic acid** \'bä-tə-\ *n* : a derivative $C_4H_8O_3$ of butyric acid that is excreted in urine in increased quantities in diabetes — called also *oxybutyric acid*

hy·droxy·chlor·o·quine \-'klȯr-ə-ˌkwēn, -kwin\ *n* : a drug derived from quinoline that is administered orally in the form of its sulfate $C_{18}H_{26}ClN_3O·H_2SO_4$ to treat malaria, rheumatoid arthritis, and lupus erythematosus — see PLAQUENIL

25–hy·droxy·cho·le·cal·cif·er·ol \'twen-tē-ˈfiv-hī-ˌdräk-sē-ˌkō-lə-(ˌ)kal-'si-fə-ˌrȯl, -ˌrōl\ *n* : a sterol $C_{27}H_{44}O_2$ that is a metabolite of cholecalciferol formed in the liver and that is the circulating form of vitamin D

17–hy·droxy·cor·ti·co·ste·roid \ˌse-vən-'tēn-hī-ˌdräk-sē-ˌkȯrt-i-kō-'stir-ˌȯid, -'ster-\ *n* : any of several adrenocorticosteroids (as cortisol) with an –OH group and an $HOCH_2CO$ group attached to carbon 17 of the fused ring structure of the steroid

hy·droxy·di·one sodium suc·ci·nate \hī-ˌdräk-sē-'dī-ˌōn . . . 'sək-sə-ˌnāt\ *n* : a steroid $C_{25}H_{35}NaO_6$ given intravenously as a general anesthetic

6–hy·droxy·do·pa·mine \'siks-hī-ˌdräk-sē-'dō-pə-ˌmēn\ *n* : an isomer of norepinephrine that is taken up by catecholaminergic nerve fibers and causes the degeneration of their terminals

5-hy·droxy·in·dole·ace·tic acid \'fiv-hī-ˌdräk-sē-ˌin-(ˌ)dō-lə-ˌsē-tik-\ n : a metabolite $C_{10}H_9NO_3$ of serotonin that is present in cerebrospinal fluid and in urine — abbr. *5-HIAA*

hy·drox·yl \hī-'dräk-səl\ n **1** : the chemical group or ion OH that consists of one atom of hydrogen and one of oxygen and is neutral or positively charged **2** : HYDROXIDE 1

hydroxylapatite *var of* HYDROXYAPATITE

hy·drox·y·lase \hī-'dräk-sə-ˌlās, -ˌlāz\ n : any of a group of enzymes that catalyze oxidation reactions in which one of the two atoms of molecular oxygen is incorporated into the substrate and the other is used to oxidize NADH or NADPH

hy·droxy·ly·sine \hī-ˌdräk-sē-'lī-ˌsēn\ n : an amino acid $C_6H_{14}N_2O_3$ that is found esp. in collagen

hy·droxy·pro·ges·ter·one \hī-ˌdräk-sē-prō-'jes-tə-ˌrōn\ *or* **17α-hydroxyprogesterone** \se-vən-ˌtēn-'al-fə-\ n : a synthetic derivative of progesterone used esp. in the form of the salt of caproic acid $C_{27}H_{40}O_4$ in progestational therapy (as for amenorrhea)

hy·droxy·pro·line \-'prō-ˌlēn\ n : an amino acid $C_5H_9NO_3$ that occurs naturally as a constituent of collagen

8-hy·droxy·quin·o·line \ˌāt-hī-ˌdräk-sē-'kwin-ᵊl-ˌēn\ n : a derivative of quinoline used esp. in the form of its sulfate $(C_9H_7NO)_2 \cdot H_2SO_4$ as a disinfectant, topical antiseptic, antiperspirant, and deodorant — called also *oxyquinoline*

hy·droxy·ste·roid \-'stir-ˌoid, -'ster-\ n : any of several ketosteroids (as androsterone) found esp. in urine

hydroxytoluene — see BUTYLATED HYDROXYTOLUENE

5-hy·droxy·tryp·ta·mine \'fiv-hī-ˌdräk-sē-'trip-tə-ˌmēn\ n : SEROTONIN

hy·droxy·urea \-yu̇-'rē-ə\ n : an antineoplastic drug $CH_4N_2O_2$ used esp. to treat myeloproliferative disorders (as chronic myelogenous leukemia, polycythemia vera, and thrombocythemia) and malignant tumors

hy·droxy·zine \hī-'dräk-sə-ˌzēn\ n : a compound that is administered usu. in the form of its dihydrochloride $C_{21}H_{27}ClN_2O_2 \cdot 2HCl$ or pamoate $C_{21}H_{27}ClN_2O_2 \cdot C_{23}H_{16}O_6$ and is used as an antihistamine and tranquilizer — see VISTARIL

hy·giene \'hī-ˌjēn\ n **1** : a science of the establishment and maintenance of health — see MENTAL HYGIENE **2** : conditions or practices (as of cleanliness) conducive to health — **hy·gien·ic** \ˌhī-jē-'e-nik, hī-'je-, hī-'jē-\ adj — **hy·gien·i·cal·ly** adv

hy·gien·ics \-iks\ n : HYGIENE 1

hy·gien·ist \hī-'jē-nist, -'je-; 'hī-ˌjē-\ n : a specialist in hygiene; *esp* : one

skilled in a specified branch of hygiene — see DENTAL HYGIENIST

hy·gro·ma \hī-'grō-mə\ n, pl **-mas** also **-ma·ta** \-mə-tə\ : a cystic tumor of lymphatic origin

hy·grom·e·ter \hī-'grä-mə-tər\ n : any of several instruments for measuring the humidity of the atmosphere — **hy·gro·met·ric** \ˌhī-grə-'me-trik\ adj

hy·gro·my·cin B \ˌhī-grə-'mīs-ᵊn-'bē\ n : an antibiotic $C_{20}H_{37}N_3O_{13}$ obtained from a bacterium of the genus *Streptomyces* (*S. hygroscopicus*) and used as an anthelmintic in swine and chickens

hy·gro·scop·ic \ˌhī-grə-'skä-pik\ adj : readily taking up and retaining moisture ⟨glycerol is ~⟩

Hy·gro·ton \'hī-grə-ˌtän\ n : a preparation of chlorthalidone — formerly a U.S. registered trademark

hy·men \'hī-mən\ n : a fold of mucous membrane partly or wholly closing the orifice of the vagina — **hy·men·al** \-mən-ᵊl\ adj

hymen- *or* **hymeno-** *comb form* : hymen : membrane ⟨*hymen*ectomy⟩

hy·men·ec·to·my \ˌhī-mə-'nek-tə-mē\ n, pl **-mies** : surgical removal of the hymen

Hy·me·nol·e·pis \ˌhī-mə-'nä-lə-pəs\ n : a genus of small taenioid tapeworms (family Hymenolepididae) that are parasites of mammals and birds and include one (*H. nana*) that is an intestinal parasite of humans

hy·me·nop·ter·an \ˌhī-mə-'näp-tə-rən\ n : any of an order (Hymenoptera) of highly specialized and often colonial insects (as bees, wasps, and ants) that have usu. four thin transparent wings and the abdomen on a slender stalk — **hymenopteran** adj — **hy·me·nop·ter·ous** \-tə-rəs\ adj

hy·me·nop·ter·ism \-'näp-tə-ˌri-zəm\ n : poisoning resulting from the bite or sting of a hymenopteran insect

hy·men·ot·o·my \ˌhī-mə-'nä-tə-mē\ n, pl **-mies** : surgical incision of the hymen

hyo- — see HY-

hyo·glos·sal \ˌhī-ō-'gläs-ᵊl, -'glòs-\ adj : of, relating to, or connecting the tongue and hyoid bone

hyo·glos·sus \-'glä-səs, -'glò-\ n, pl **-si** \-ˌsī, -ˌsē\ : a flat muscle on each side of the tongue

hy·oid \'hī-ˌoid\ adj : of or relating to the hyoid bone

hyoid bone n : a U-shaped bone or complex of bones that is situated between the base of the tongue and the larynx and that supports the tongue, the larynx, and their muscles — called also *hyoid*

hyo·man·dib·u·lar \ˌhī-ō-man-'di-byu̇-lər\ n : a bone or cartilage that forms the columella or stapes of the ear of higher vertebrates — **hyomandibular** adj

hyo·scine \'hī-ə-ˌsēn\ n : SCOPOLAMINE; *esp* : the levorotatory form of scopolamine

hyo·scy·a·mine \hī-ə-ˈsī-ə-ˌmēn\ n : a poisonous crystalline alkaloid $C_{17}H_{23}$-NO_3 of which atropine is a racemic mixture; *esp* : its levorotatory form found esp. in belladonna and henbane and used similarly to atropine

hyo·scy·a·mus \-məs\ n **1** *cap* : a genus of poisonous Eurasian herbs of the nightshade family (Solanaceae) that includes the henbane (*H. niger*) **2** : the dried leaves of the henbane containing the alkaloids hyoscyamine and scopolamine and used as an antispasmodic and sedative

Hyo·stron·gy·lus \ˌhī-ə-ˈsträn-jə-ləs\ n : a genus of nematode worms (family Trichostrongylidae) that includes the common small red stomach worm (*H. rubidus*) of swine

¹hyp·acu·sic \ˌhi-pə-ˈkü-sik, ˌhī-, -ˈkyü-\ adj : affected with hypoacusis

²hypacusic n : one affected with hypoacusis

hyp·acu·sis \-ˈkü-səs, -ˈkyü-\ n : HYPOACUSIS

hyp·aes·the·sia *Brit var of* HYPESTHESIA

hyp·al·ge·sia \ˌhip-ᵊl-ˈjē-zhə, ˌhī-pal-, -zē-ə, -zhē-ə\ n : diminished sensitivity to pain — **hyp·al·ge·sic** \-ˈjē-zik, -sik\ adj

Hy·paque \ˈhī-ˌpāk\ *trademark* — used for a diatrizoate preparation for use in radiographic diagnosis

hyper- *prefix* **1** : excessively ⟨*hyper*sensitive⟩ **2** : excessive ⟨*hyper*emia⟩

hy·per·acid·i·ty \ˌhī-pə-rə-ˈsi-də-tē\ n, pl **-ties** : the condition of containing more than the normal amount of acid — **hy·per·ac·id** \ˌhī-pə-ˈra-səd\ adj

¹hy·per·ac·tive \ˌhī-pə-ˈrak-tiv\ adj : affected with or exhibiting hyperactivity; *broadly* : more active than is usual or desirable

²hyperactive n : one who is hyperactive

hy·per·ac·tiv·i·ty \ˌhī-pə-ˌrak-ˈti-və-tē\ n, pl **-ties** : a state or condition of being excessively or pathologically active; *esp* : ATTENTION DEFICIT DISORDER

hy·per·acu·ity \ˌhī-pə-rə-ˈkyü-ə-tē\ n, pl **-ities** : greater than normal acuteness esp. of a sense; *specif* : visual acuity that is better than twenty-twenty

hy·per·acu·sis \ˌhī-pə-rə-ˈkü-səs, -ˈkyü-\ n : abnormally acute hearing

hy·per·acute \ˌhī-pə-rə-ˈkyüt\ adj : extremely or excessively acute ⟨∼ hearing⟩

hy·per·adren·a·lin·ae·mia *chiefly Brit var of* HYPERADRENALINEMIA

hy·per·adren·a·lin·emia \ˌhī-pə-rə-ˌdren-ᵊl-ə-ˈnē-mē-ə\ n : the presence of an excess of adrenal hormones (as epinephrine) in the blood

hy·per·ad·re·no·cor·ti·cism \ˌhī-pə-rə-ˌdrē-nō-ˈkór-tə-ˌsi-zəm\ n : the presence of an excess of adrenocortical products in the body

hy·per·ae·mia, hy·per·aes·the·sia *chiefly Brit var of* HYPEREMIA, HYPERESTHESIA

hy·per·ag·gres·sive \ˌhī-pə-rə-ˈgre-səv\ adj : extremely or excessively aggressive ⟨∼ patients⟩

hy·per·al·do·ste·ron·ae·mia *chiefly Brit var of* HYPERALDOSTERONEMIA

hy·per·al·do·ste·ron·emia \ˌhī-pə-ral-ˌdās-tə-ˌrō-ˈnē-mē-ə, -ˌral-dō-stə-ˌrō-\ n : the presence of an excess of aldosterone in the blood

hy·per·al·do·ste·ron·ism \ˌhī-pə-ˌral-ˈdās-tə-ˌrō-ˌni-zəm, -ˌral-dō-stə-ˈrō-\ n : ALDOSTERONISM

hy·per·al·ge·sia \ˌhī-pə-ral-ˈjē-zhə, -zē-ə, -zhē-ə\ n : increased sensitivity to pain or enhanced intensity of pain sensation — **hy·per·al·ge·sic** \-ˈjē-zik, -sik\ adj

hy·per·al·i·men·ta·tion \ˌhī-pə-ˌra-lə-mən-ˈtā-shən\ n : the administration of nutrients by intravenous feeding

hy·per·ami·no·ac·id·uria \ˌhī-pə-rə-ˌmē-nō-ˌa-sə-ˈdür-ē-ə, -ˈdyür-\ n : the presence of an excess of amino acids in the urine

hy·per·am·mo·nae·mia *also* **hy·per·am·mon·i·ae·mia** *chiefly Brit var of* HYPERAMMONEMIA

hy·per·am·mo·ne·mia \ˌhī-pə-ˌra-mə-ˈnē-mē-ə\ *also* **hy·per·am·mon·i·emia** \ˌhī-pə-rə-ˌmō-nē-ˈyē-mē-ə\ n : the presence of an excess of ammonia in the blood — **hy·per·am·mo·ne·mic** \ˌhī-pə-ˌra-mə-ˈnē-mik\ adj

hy·per·am·y·las·ae·mia *chiefly Brit var of* HYPERAMYLASEMIA

hy·per·am·y·las·emia \ˌhī-pə-ˌra-mə-ˌlā-ˈsē-mē-ə\ n : the presence of an excess of amylase in the blood

hy·per·arous·al \ˌhī-pə-rə-ˈrau-zəl\ n : excessive arousal

hy·per·bar·ic \ˌhī-pər-ˈbar-ik\ adj **1** : having a specific gravity greater than that of cerebrospinal fluid — used of solutions for spinal anesthesia; compare HYPOBARIC **2** : of, relating to, or utilizing greater than normal pressure esp. of oxygen ⟨a ∼ chamber⟩ ⟨∼ medicine⟩ — **hy·per·bar·i·cal·ly** adv

hy·per·be·ta·li·po·pro·tein·emia \-ˌbā-tə-ˌlī-pō-ˌprō-ˌtē-ˈnē-mē-ə, -ˌli-, -ˌprō-tē-ə-\ n : the presence of excess LDLs in the blood

hy·per·bil·i·ru·bin·emia \-ˌbi-lē-ˌrü-bi-ˈnē-mē-ə\ n : the presence of an excess of bilirubin in the blood — called also *bilirubinemia*

hy·per·cal·cae·mia *chiefly Brit var of* HYPERCALCEMIA

hy·per·cal·ce·mia \ˌhī-pər-ˌkal-ˈsē-mē-ə\ n : the presence of an excess of calcium in the blood — **hy·per·cal·ce·mic** \-ˈsē-mik\ adj

hy·per·cal·ci·uria \-ˌkal-sē-ˈyür-ē-ə\ *also* **hy·per·cal·cin·uria** \-ˌkal-sə-ˈnür-ē-ə\ n : the presence of an excess amount of calcium in the urine

hy·per·cap·nia \-ˈkap-nē-ə\ n : the presence of an excess of carbon dioxide in the blood — **hy·per·cap·nic** \-nik\ adj

hy·per·car·bia \-ˈkär-bē-ə\ n : HYPERCAPNIA

hy·per·cel·lu·lar·i·ty \-ˌsel-yə-ˈlar-ə-tē\ *n, pl* **-ties** : the presence of an abnormal excess of cells (as in bone marrow) — **hy·per·cel·lu·lar** \-ˈsel-yə-lər\ *adj*

hy·per·ce·men·to·sis \-ˌsē-men-ˈtō-səs\ *n, pl* **-to·ses** \-ˌsēz\ : excessive formation of cementum at the root of a tooth

hy·per·chlor·ae·mia *chiefly Brit var of* HYPERCHLOREMIA

hy·per·chlor·emia \-ˌklōr-ˈē-mē-ə\ *n* : the presence of excess chloride ions in the blood — **hy·per·chlor·emic** \-ˈē-mik\ *adj*

hy·per·chlor·hy·dria \-ˌklōr-ˈhī-drē-ə\ *n* : the presence of a greater than typical proportion of hydrochloric acid in gastric juice — compare ACHLORHYDRIA, HYPOCHLORHYDRIA

hy·per·cho·les·ter·ol·emia \ˌhī-pər-kə-ˌles-tə-rə-ˈlē-mē-ə\ *also* **hy·per·cho·les·ter·emia** \-tə-ˈrē-mē-ə\ *n* : the presence of excess cholesterol in the blood — see FAMILIAL HYPERCHOLESTEROLEMIA — **hy·per·cho·les·ter·ol·emic** \-tə-rə-ˈlē-mik\ *also* **hy·per·cho·les·ter·emic** \-tə-ˈrē-mik\ *adj*

hy·per·chro·ma·sia \-ˈkrō-ˈmā-zhə, -zē-ə, -zhē-ə\ *n* : HYPERCHROMATISM

hy·per·chro·ma·tism \-ˈkrō-mə-ˌti-zəm\ *n* : the development of excess chromatin or of excessive nuclear staining esp. as a part of a pathological process — **hy·per·chro·mat·ic** \-ˌkrō-ˈma-tik\ *adj*

hy·per·chro·mia \-ˈkrō-mē-ə\ *n* **1** : excessive pigmentation (as of the skin) **2** : a state of the red blood cells marked by increase in the hemoglobin content — **hy·per·chro·mic** \-ˈkrō-mik\ *adj*

hyperchromic anemia *n* : an anemia with increase of hemoglobin in individual red blood cells and reduction in the number of red blood cells — see PERNICIOUS ANEMIA; compare HYPOCHROMIC ANEMIA

hy·per·chy·lo·mi·cro·ne·mia \ˌhī-pər-ˌkī-lō-ˌmī-krō-ˈnē-mē-ə\ *n* : the presence of excess chylomicrons in the blood

hy·per·co·ag·u·la·bil·i·ty \-kō-ˌa-gyə-lə-ˈbi-lə-tē\ *n, pl* **-ties** : excessive coagulability — **hy·per·co·ag·u·la·ble** \-kō-ˈa-gyə-lə-bəl\ *adj*

hy·per·cor·ti·sol·ism \-ˈkȯr-ti-ˌsȯ-ˌli-zəm, -ˌsō-\ *n* : hyperadrenocorticism produced by excess cortisol in the body

hy·per·cu·prae·mia *chiefly Brit var of* HYPERCUPREMIA

hy·per·cu·pre·mia \-kü-ˈprē-mē-ə, -kyü-\ *n* : the presence of an excess of copper in the blood

hy·per·cy·thae·mia *chiefly Brit var of* HYPERCYTHEMIA

hy·per·cy·the·mia \-sī-ˈthē-mē-ə\ *n* : the presence of an excess of red blood cells in the blood : POLYCYTHEMIA — **hy·per·cy·the·mic** \-ˈthē-mik\ *adj*

hy·per·dip·loid \-ˈdi-ˌplȯid\ *adj* : having slightly more than the diploid number of chromosomes

hy·per·dy·nam·ic \-dī-ˈna-mik\ *adj* : marked by abnormally increased muscular activity esp. when of organic origin

hy·per·eme·sis \-ˈe-mə-səs, -i-ˈmē-\ *n, pl* **-eme·ses** \-ˌsēz\ : excessive vomiting

hyperemesis grav·i·dar·um \-ˌgra-və-ˈdar-əm\ *n* : excessive vomiting during pregnancy

hy·per·emia \ˌhī-pə-ˈrē-mē-ə\ *n* : excess of blood in a body part : CONGESTION — **hy·per·emic** \-mik\ *adj*

hy·per·en·dem·ic \-en-ˈde-mik, -in-\ *adj* **1** : exhibiting a high and continued incidence — used chiefly of human diseases **2** : marked by hyperendemic disease — used of geographic areas — **hy·per·en·de·mic·i·ty** \-ˌen-ˌde-ˈmi-sə-tē\ *n*

hy·per·er·gic \ˌhī-pər-ˈər-jik\ *adj* : characterized by or exhibiting a greater than normal sensitivity to an allergen — **hy·per·er·gy** \ˈhī-pər-ˌər-jē\ *n*

hy·per·es·the·sia \ˌhī-pər-es-ˈthē-zhə, -zhē-ə\ *n* : unusual or pathological sensitivity of the skin or of a particular sense to stimulation — **hy·per·es·thet·ic** \-ˈthe-tik\ *adj*

hy·per·es·trin·ism \-ˈes-trə-ˌni-zəm\ *n* : a condition marked by the presence of excess estrins in the body

hy·per·es·tro·gen·ism \-ˈes-trə-jə-ˌni-zəm\ *n* : a condition marked by the presence of excess estrogens in the body

hy·per·ex·cit·abil·i·ty \ˌhī-pər-ik-ˌsī-tə-ˈbi-lə-tē\ *n, pl* **-ties** : the state or condition of being unusually or excessively excitable — **hy·per·ex·cited** \-ik-ˈsī-təd\ *adj* — **hy·per·ex·cite·ment** *n*

hy·per·ex·tend \ˌhī-pər-ik-ˈstend\ *vb* : to extend so that the angle between bones of a joint is greater than normal 〈a ~ed elbow〉; *also* : to extend (as a body part) beyond the normal range of motion — **hy·per·ex·ten·sion** \-ˈsten-chən\ *n*

hy·per·ex·ten·si·ble \-ik-ˈsten-sə-bəl\ *adj* : having the capacity to be hyperextended or stretched to a greater than normal degree — **hy·per·ex·ten·si·bil·i·ty** \-sten-sə-ˈbi-lə-tē\ *n*

hy·per·fil·tra·tion \-fil-ˈtrā-shən\ *n* : a usu. abnormal increase in the filtration rate of the renal glomeruli

hy·per·flex \ˈhī-pər-ˌfleks\ *vb* : to flex so that the angle between the bones of a joint is smaller than normal — **hy·per·flex·ion** \-ˌflek-shən\ *n*

hy·per·func·tion \-ˌfəŋk-shən\ *n* : excessive or abnormal activity 〈cardiac ~〉 — **hy·per·func·tion·al** \-shə-nəl\ *adj* — **hy·per·func·tion·ing** *n*

hy·per·gam·ma·glob·u·lin·ae·mia
chiefly Brit var of HYPERGAMMAGLOB-
ULINEMIA

hy·per·gam·ma·glob·u·lin·emia \hī-
pər-ˌga-mə-ˌglä-byə-lə-ˈnē-mē-ə\ *n*
: the presence of an excess of gamma
globulins in the blood — **hy·per·gam·
ma·glob·u·lin·emic** \-ˈnē-mik\ *adj*

hy·per·gas·trin·ae·mia *chiefly Brit var
of* HYPERGASTRINEMIA

hy·per·gas·trin·emia \-ˌgas-trə-ˈnē-
mē-ə\ *n* : the presence of an excess of
gastrin in the blood — **hy·per·gas·
trin·emic** \-ˈnē-mik\ *adj*

hy·per·glob·u·lin·ae·mia *chiefly Brit
var of* HYPERGLOBULINEMIA

hy·per·glob·u·lin·emia \-ˌglä-byə-lə-
ˈnē-mē-ə\ *n* : the presence of excess
globulins in the blood — **hy·per·glob·
u·lin·emic** \-ˈnē-mik\ *adj*

hy·per·glu·ca·gon·ae·mia *chiefly Brit
var of* HYPERGLUCAGONEMIA

hy·per·glu·ca·gon·emia \-ˌglü-kə-gə-
ˈnē-mē-ə\ *n* : the presence of excess
glucagon in the blood

hy·per·gly·ce·mia \ˌhī-pər-glī-ˈsē-mē-
ə\ *n* : an excess of sugar in the blood
— **hy·per·gly·ce·mic** \-mik\ *adj*

hyperglycemic factor *n* : GLUCAGON

hy·per·gly·ci·nae·mia *chiefly Brit var
of* HYPERGLYCINEMIA

hy·per·gly·ci·ne·mia \ˌhī-pər-ˌglī-
ˈnē-mē-ə\ *n* : a hereditary disorder
characterized by the presence of excess glycine in the blood

hy·per·go·nad·ism \ˌhī-pər-ˈgō-ˌna-di-
zəm\ *n* : excessive hormonal secretion
by the gonads

hy·per·hi·dro·sis \-hi-ˈdrō-səs, -hī-\
also **hy·peri·dro·sis** \-i-ˈdrō-\ *n, pl*
-dro·ses \-ˌsēz\ : generalized or localized excessive sweating — compare
HYPOHIDROSIS

hy·per·hy·dra·tion \ˌhī-ˈdrā-shən\ *n*
: an excess of water in the body

hy·per·i·cism \hī-ˈper-ə-ˌsi-zəm\ *n* : a
severe dermatitis of domestic animals
due to photosensitivity resulting from
eating Saint-John's-wort

hy·per·im·mune \ˌhī-pər-i-ˈmyün\ *adj*
: exhibiting an unusual degree of immunization: **a** *of a serum*: containing
exceptional quantities of antibody **b**
of an antibody: having the characteristics of a blocking antibody

hy·per·im·mu·nize \-ˈi-myə-ˌnīz\ *vb*
-nized; -niz·ing : to induce a high
level of immunity or of circulating
antibodies in — **hy·per·im·mu·ni·za-
tion** \-ˌi-myə-nə-ˈzā-shən\ *n*

hy·per·in·fec·tion \-in-ˈfek-shən\ *n*
: repeated reinfection with larvae produced by parasitic worms already in
the body — compare AUTOINFEC-
TION

hy·per·in·fla·tion \-in-ˈflā-shən\ *n* : excessive inflation (as of the lungs)

hy·per·in·su·lin·ae·mia \ˌin-sə-lə-ˈnē-
mē-ə\ *n* : the presence of excess insulin in the blood — **hy·per·in·su·lin-
emic** \-mik\ *adj*

hy·per·in·su·lin·ism \-ˈin-sə-lə-ˌni-
zəm\ *n* : the presence of excess insulin
in the body resulting in hypoglycemia

hy·per·ir·ri·ta·bil·i·ty \ir-ə-tə-ˈbi-lə-tē\
n, pl **-ties** : abnormally great or unin-
hibited response to stimuli — **hy·per-
ir·ri·ta·ble** \-ˈir-ə-tə-bəl\ *adj*

hy·per·ka·lae·mia *chiefly Brit var of*
HYPERKALEMIA

hy·per·ka·le·mia \-kā-ˈlē-mē-ə\ *n* : the
presence of an abnormally high concentration of potassium in the blood
— called also *hyperpotassemia* — **hy·
per·ka·le·mic** \-ˈlē-mik\ *adj*

hy·per·ke·ra·ti·ni·za·tion \-ˌker-ə-tə-
nə-ˈzā-shən, -kə-ˌrat-ᵊn-ə-\ *n* : HYPER-
KERATOSIS

hy·per·ke·ra·to·sis \-ˌker-ə-ˈtō-səs, *n,
pl* **-to·ses** \-ˈtō-ˌsēz\ **1** : hypertrophy
of the stratum corneum of the skin **2**
: any of various conditions marked by
hyperkeratosis — **hy·per·ker·a·tot·ic**
\-ˈtät-ik\ *adj*

hy·per·ke·to·ne·mia \-ˌkē-tə-ˈnē-mē-ə\
n : KETONEMIA 1

hy·per·ki·ne·sia \-kə-ˈnē-zhə, -kī-,
-zhē-ə\ *n* : HYPERKINESIS

hy·per·ki·ne·sis \-ˈnē-səs\ *n* **1** : abnormally increased and sometimes uncontrollable activity or muscular
movements — compare HYPOKINE-
SIA **2** : a condition esp. of childhood
characterized by hyperactivity

hy·per·ki·net·ic \-kə-ˈne-tik, -kī-\ *adj*
: of, relating to, or affected with hyperkinesis or hyperactivity

hy·per·lex·ia \-ˈlek-sē-ə\ *n* : precocious
reading ability accompanied by difficulties in acquiring language and social skills — **hy·per·lex·ic** \-sik\ *adj*

hy·per·li·pe·mia \ˌhī-pər-li-ˈpē-mē-ə\ *n*
: HYPERLIPIDEMIA — **hy·per·li·pe·
mic** \-mik\ *adj*

hy·per·lip·id·ae·mia *chiefly Brit var of*
HYPERLIPIDEMIA

hy·per·lip·id·emia \-ˌli-pə-ˈdē-mē-ə\ *n*
: the presence of excess fat or lipids
in the blood — **hy·per·lip·id·emic**
\-mik\ *adj*

hy·per·li·po·pro·tein·ae·mia *chiefly
Brit var of* HYPERLIPOPROTEINEMIA

hy·per·li·po·pro·tein·emia \-ˌlī-pə-
ˌprō-tē-ˈnē-mē-ə, -ˌli-\ *n* : the presence
of excess lipoprotein in the blood

hy·per·lu·cent \-ˈlüs-ᵊnt\ *adj* : being
excessively radiolucent ⟨a ~ lung⟩
— **hy·per·lu·cen·cy** \-ˈlüs-ᵊn-sē\ *n*

hy·per·mag·ne·sae·mia *chiefly Brit var
of* HYPERMAGNESEMIA

hy·per·mag·ne·se·mia \-ˌmag-ni-ˈsē-
mē-ə\ *n* : the presence of excess magnesium in the blood serum

hy·per·men·or·rhea \-ˌme-nə-ˈrē-ə\ *n*
: abnormally profuse or prolonged
menstrual flow — compare MENOR-
RHAGIA

hy·per·me·tab·o·lism \-mə-ˈta-bə-ˌli-
zəm\ *n* : metabolism at an increased
or excessive rate — **hy·per·meta·bol-
ic** \-ˌme-tə-ˈbä-lik\ *adj*

hy·per·me·tria \-ˈmē-trē-ə\ *n* : a condition of cerebellar dysfunction in

which voluntary muscular movements tend to result in the movement of body parts (as the arm and hand) beyond the intended goal

hy·per·me·tro·pia \,hī-pər-mi-'trō-pē-ə\ *n* : HYPEROPIA — **hy·per·me·tro·pic** \-'trō-pik, -'trä-\ *adj*

hy·per·mne·sia \,hī-(,)pərm-'nē-zhə, -zhē-ə\ *n* : abnormally vivid or complete memory or recall of the past (as at times of extreme danger) — **hy·perm·ne·sic** \-'nē-zik, -sik\ *adj*

hy·per·mo·bil·i·ty \,hī-pər-mō-'bi-lə-tē\ *n, pl* **-ties** : an increase in the range of movement of which a bodily part and esp. a joint is capable — **hy·per·mo·bile** \-'mō-bəl, -,bīl, -,bēl\ *adj*

hy·per·mo·til·i·ty \,hī-pər-mō-'ti-lə-tē\ *n, pl* **-ties** : abnormal or excessive movement; *specif* : excessive motility of all or part of the gastrointestinal tract — compare HYPERPERISTALSIS, HYPOMOTILITY — **hy·per·mo·tile** \-'mōt-ᵊl, -'mō-,tīl\ *adj*

hy·per·na·trae·mia *chiefly Brit var of* HYPERNATREMIA

hy·per·na·tre·mia \-nā-'trē-mē-ə\ *n* : the presence of an abnormally high concentration of sodium in the blood — **hy·per·na·tre·mic** \-mik\ *adj*

hy·per·neph·roid \-'ne-,frȯid\ *adj* : resembling the adrenal cortex in histological structure (∼ tumors)

hy·per·ne·phro·ma \-ni-'frō-mə\ *n, pl* **-mas** *also* **-ma·ta** \-mə-tə\ : a tumor of the kidney resembling the adrenal cortex in its histological structure

hy·per·oes·trin·ism, hy·per·oes·tro·gen·ism *chiefly Brit var of* HYPERESTRINISM, HYPERESTROGENISM

hy·per·ope \'hī-pər-,ōp\ *n* : a person affected with hyperopia

hy·per·opia \,hī-pər-'ō-pē-ə\ *n* : a condition in which visual images come to a focus behind the retina of the eye and vision is better for distant than for near objects — called also *farsightedness, hypermetropia* — **hy·per·opic** \-'ō-pik, -'ä-\ *adj*

hy·per·os·mia \,hī-pər-'äz-mē-ə\ *n* : extreme acuteness of the sense of smell

hy·per·os·mo·lal·i·ty \-,äz-mō-'la-lə-tē\ *n, pl* **-ties** : the condition esp. of a bodily fluid of having abnormally high osmolality

hy·per·os·mo·lar·i·ty \-'lar-ə-tē\ *n, pl* **-ties** : the condition esp. of a bodily fluid of having abnormally high osmolarity — **hy·per·os·mo·lar** \-,äz-'mō-lər\ *adj*

hy·per·os·mot·ic \-,äz-'mä-tik\ *adj* : HYPERTONIC 2

hy·per·os·to·sis \-,äs-'tō-səs\ *n, pl* **-to·ses** \-,sēz\ : excessive growth or thickening of bone tissue — **hy·per·os·tot·ic** \-'tä-tik\ *adj*

hy·per·ox·al·uria \-,äk-sə-'luṙ-ē-ə\ *n* : the presence of excess oxalic acid or oxalates in the urine

hy·per·ox·ia \-'äk-sē-ə\ *n* : a bodily condition characterized by a greater

oxygen content of the tissues and organs than normally exists at sea level

hy·per·para·thy·roid·ism \,hī-pər-,par-ə-'thī-,rȯi-,di-zəm\ *n* : the presence of excess parathyroid hormone in the body resulting in disturbance of calcium metabolism

hy·per·path·ia \-'pa-thē-ə\ *n* **1** : disagreeable or painful sensation in response to a normally innocuous stimulus (as touch) **2** : a condition in which the sensations of hyperpathia occur — **hy·per·path·ic** \-thik\ *adj*

hy·per·peri·stal·sis \-,per-ə-'stȯl-səs, -'stäl-, -'stal-\ *n, pl* **-stal·ses** \-,sēz\ : excessive or excessively vigorous peristalsis — compare HYPERMOTILITY

hy·per·pha·gia \-'fā-jə, -jē-ə\ *n* : abnormally increased appetite for food frequently associated with injury to the hypothalamus — compare POLYPHAGIA — **hy·per·phag·ic** \-'fa-jik\ *adj*

hy·per·phe·nyl·al·a·nin·ae·mia *chiefly Brit var of* HYPERPHENYLALANINEMIA

hy·per·phe·nyl·al·a·nin·emia \-,fen-ᵊl-,a-lə-nə-'nē-mē-ə, -,fēn-\ *n* : the presence of excess phenylalanine in the blood (as in phenylketonuria) — **hy·per·phe·nyl·al·a·nin·emic** \-'nē-mik\ *adj*

hy·per·pho·ria \-'fōr-ē-ə\ *n* : latent strabismus in which one eye deviates upward in relation to the other

hy·per·phos·pha·tae·mia *chiefly Brit var of* HYPERPHOSPHATEMIA

hy·per·phos·pha·te·mia \-,fäs-fə-'tē-mē-ə\ *n* : the presence of excess phosphate in the blood

hy·per·phos·pha·tu·ria \-,fäs-fə-'tuṙ-ē-ə, -'tyuṙ-\ *n* : the presence of excess phosphate in the urine

hy·per·pi·e·sia \-,pī-'ē-zhə, -zhē-ə\ *n* : HYPERTENSION; *esp* : ESSENTIAL HYPERTENSION

hy·per·pig·men·ta·tion \-,pig-mən-'tā-shən, -,men-\ *n* : excess pigmentation in a bodily part or tissue (as the skin) — **hy·per·pig·ment·ed** \-'pig-mən-təd, -,men-\ *adj*

hy·per·pi·tu·ita·rism \-pə-'tü-ə-tə-,ri-zəm, -'tyü-, -,tri-zəm\ *n* : excessive production of growth hormones by the pituitary gland — **hy·per·pi·tu·itary** \-pə-'tü-ə-,ter-ē, -'tyü-\ *adj*

hy·per·pla·sia \,hī-pər-'plā-zhə, -zhē-ə\ *n* : an abnormal or unusual increase in the elements composing a part (as cells composing a tissue) — see BENIGN PROSTATIC HYPERPLASIA — **hy·per·plas·tic** \-'plas-tik\ *adj*

hy·per·ploid \'hī-pər-,plȯid\ *adj* : having a chromosome number slightly greater than an exact multiple of the haploid number — **hy·per·ploi·dy** \-,plȯid-ē\ *n*

hy·per·pnea \,hī-pərp-'nē-ə, -,pər-\ *n* : abnormally rapid or deep breathing — **hy·per·pne·ic** \-'nē-ik\ *adj*

hy·per·pnoea *chiefly Brit var of* HY-PERPNEA

hy·per·po·lar·ize \ˌhī-pər-ˈpō-lə-ˌrīz\ *vb* **-ized; -iz·ing 1 :** to produce an increase in potential difference across (a biological membrane) **2 :** to undergo or produce an increase in potential difference across something — **hy·per·po·lar·i·za·tion** \-ˌpō-lə-rə-ˈzā-shən\ *n*

hy·per·po·tas·sae·mia *chiefly Brit var of* HYPERPOTASSEMIA

hy·per·po·tas·se·mia \-ˌpə-ˌta-ˈsē-mē-ə\ *n* **:** HYPERKALEMIA — **hy·per·po·tas·se·mic** \-ˈsē-mik\ *adj*

hy·per·pro·duc·tion \-prə-ˈdək-shən, -prō-\ *n* **:** excessive production

hy·per·pro·lac·tin·ae·mia *chiefly Brit var of* HYPERPROLACTINAEMIA

hy·per·pro·lac·tin·emia \-prō-ˌlak-tə-ˈnē-mē-ə\ *n* **:** the presence of an abnormally high concentration of prolactin in the blood — **hy·per·pro·lac·tin·emic** \-ˈnē-mik\ *adj*

hy·per·pro·lin·ae·mia *chiefly Brit var of* HYPERPROLINEMIA

hy·per·pro·lin·emia \-ˌprō-lə-ˈnē-mē-ə\ *n* **:** a hereditary metabolic disorder characterized by an abnormally high concentration of proline in the blood and often associated with mental retardation

hy·per·py·rex·ia \-pī-ˈrek-sē-ə\ *n* **:** exceptionally high fever

hy·per·re·ac·tive \-rē-ˈak-tiv\ *adj* **:** having or showing abnormally high sensitivity to stimuli — **hy·per·re·ac·tiv·i·ty** \-(ˌ)rē-ˌak-ˈti-və-tē\ *n*

hy·per·re·flex·ia \-rē-ˈflek-sē-ə\ *n* **:** overactivity of physiological reflexes

hy·per·re·nin·ae·mia *chiefly Brit var of* HYPERRENINEMIA

hy·per·re·nin·emia \-ˌrē-nə-ˈnē-mē-ə, -ˌre-\ *n* **:** the presence of an abnormally high concentration of renin in the blood

hy·per·re·spon·sive \-ri-ˈspän-siv\ *adj* **:** characterized by an abnormal degree of responsiveness (as to a physical stimulus) — **hy·per·re·spon·siv·i·ty** \-ri-ˌspän-ˈsi-və-tē\ *n*

hy·per·sal·i·va·tion \-ˌsa-lə-ˈvā-shən\ *n* **:** excessive salivation

hy·per·se·cre·tion \-si-ˈkrē-shən\ *n* **:** excessive production of a bodily secretion — **hy·per·se·crete** \-si-ˈkrēt\ *vb* — **hy·per·se·cre·to·ry** \-ˈsē-krə-ˌtor-ē, -si-ˈkrē-tə-rē\ *adj*

hy·per·sen·si·tive \ˌhī-pər-ˈsen-sə-tiv\ *adj* **1 :** excessively or abnormally sensitive **2 :** abnormally susceptible physiologically to a specific agent (as a drug) — **hy·per·sen·si·tive·ness** *n* — **hy·per·sen·si·tiv·i·ty** \-ˌsen-sə-ˈti-və-tē\ *n* — **hy·per·sen·si·ti·za·tion** \-ˌsen-sə-tə-ˈzā-shən\ *n* — **hy·per·sen·si·tize** \-ˈsen-sə-ˌtīz\ *vb*

hy·per·sex·u·al \-ˈsek-shə-wəl\ *adj* **:** exhibiting unusual or excessive concern with or indulgence in sexual activity — **hy·per·sex·u·al·i·ty** \-ˌsek-shə-ˈwa-lə-tē\ *n*

hy·per·sid·er·ae·mia *chiefly Brit var of* HYPERSIDEREMIA

hy·per·sid·er·emia \-ˌsi-də-ˈrē-mē-ə\ *n* **:** the presence of an abnormally high concentration of iron in the blood — **hy·per·sid·er·e·mic** \-mik\ *adj*

hy·per·som·nia \-ˈsäm-nē-ə\ *n* **1 :** sleep of excessive depth or duration **2 :** the condition of sleeping for excessive periods at intervals with intervening periods of normal duration of sleeping and waking — *compare* NARCOLEPSY

hy·per·sple·nism \-ˈsplē-ˌni-zəm, -ˈsple-\ *n* **:** a condition marked by excessive destruction of one or more kinds of blood cells in the spleen

hy·per·sthen·ic \ˌhī-pərs-ˈthe-nik\ *adj* **:** of, relating to, or characterized by excessive muscle tone

hy·per·sus·cep·ti·ble \-sə-ˈsep-tə-bəl\ *adj* **:** HYPERSENSITIVE — **hy·per·sus·cep·ti·bil·i·ty** \-ˌsep-tə-ˈbi-lə-tē\ *n*

hy·per·tel·or·ism \-ˈte-lə-ˌri-zəm\ *n* **:** excessive width between two bodily parts or organs (as the eyes)

hy·per·tense \ˌhī-pər-ˈtens\ *adj* **:** excessively tense ⟨a ~ emotional state⟩

hy·per·ten·sin·ase \-ˈten-sə-ˌnās, -ˌnāz\ *n* **:** ANGIOTENSINASE

hy·per·ten·sin·o·gen \-ˈten-ˈsi-nə-jən, -ˌjen\ *n* **:** ANGIOTENSINOGEN

hy·per·ten·sion \ˌhī-pər-ˈten-chən\ *n* **1 :** abnormally high arterial blood pressure that is usu. indicated by an adult systolic blood pressure of 140 mm Hg or greater or a diastolic blood pressure of 90 mm Hg or greater, is chiefly of unknown cause but may be attributable to a preexisting condition (as renal or endocrine disorder), and that is a risk factor for various pathological conditions or events (as heart attack or stroke) — *see* ESSENTIAL HYPERTENSION, SECONDARY HYPERTENSION, WHITE COAT HYPERTENSION **2 :** a systemic condition resulting from hypertension that is either symptomless or is accompanied esp. by dizziness, palpitations, fainting, or headache

¹hy·per·ten·sive \-ˈten-siv\ *adj* **:** marked by or due to hypertension ⟨~ renal disease⟩; *also* **:** affected with hypertension ⟨a ~ patient⟩

²hypertensive *n* **:** a person affected with hypertension

hy·per·ther·mia \-ˈthər-mē-ə\ *n* **1 :** elevated temperature of the body (as that occurring in heatstroke) — *see* MALIGNANT HYPERTHERMIA **2 :** the artificial heating of all or part of the body (as in diathermy) for therapeutic purposes (as to treat cancer) — **hy·per·ther·mic** \-mik\ *adj*

hy·per·thy·roid \-ˈthī-ˌroid\ *adj* **:** of, relating to, or affected with hyperthyroidism ⟨a ~ state⟩

hy·per·thy·roid·ism \-ˌroi-di-zəm\ *n* **:** excessive functional activity of the thyroid gland; *also* **:** the resulting condition marked esp. by increased metabolic rate, enlargement of the thyroid gland, rapid heart rate, and high blood pressure — called also *thyrotoxicosis;* see GRAVES' DISEASE

hy·per·to·nia \ˌhī-pər-ˈtō-nē-ə\ *n* : HYPERTONICITY

hy·per·ton·ic \-ˈtä-nik\ *adj* 1 : exhibiting excessive tone or tension ⟨a ∼ bladder⟩ 2 : having a higher osmotic pressure than a surrounding medium or a fluid under comparison — compare HYPOTONIC 2, ISOTONIC 1

hy·per·to·nic·i·ty \-tə-ˈni-sə-tē\ *n, pl* **-ties** : the quality or state of being hypertonic

hy·per·to·nus \-ˈtō-nəs\ *n* : HYPERTONICITY

hy·per·tri·cho·sis \-tri-ˈkō-səs\ *n, pl* **-cho·ses** \-ˌsēz\ : excessive growth of hair

hy·per·tri·glyc·er·i·dae·mia *chiefly Brit var of* HYPERTRIGLYCERIDEMIA

hy·per·tri·glyc·er·i·de·mia \-ˌtrī-ˌgli-sə-ˌrī-ˈde-mē-ə\ *n* : the presence of an excess of triglycerides in the blood — **hy·per·tri·glyc·er·i·de·mic** \-ˈde-mik\ *adj*

hypertrophic arthritis *n* : OSTEOARTHRITIS

hypertrophic cardiomyopathy *n* : cardiomyopathy that is characterized by ventricular hypertrophy esp. of the left ventricle and is marked by chest pain, syncope, and palpitations — abbr. *HCM*

hy·per·tro·phy \hī-ˈpər-trə-fē\ *n, pl* **-phies** : excessive development of an organ or part; *specif* : increase in bulk (as by thickening of muscle fibers) without multiplication of parts — **hy·per·tro·phic** \ˌhī-pər-ˈtrō-fik\ *adj* — **hypertrophy** *vb*

hy·per·tro·pia \ˌhī-pər-ˈtrō-pē-ə\ *n* : elevation of the line of vision of one eye above that of the other : upward strabismus

hy·per·uri·ce·mia \ˌhī-pər-ˌyu̇r-ə-ˈsē-mē-ə\ *n* : excess uric acid in the blood (as in gout) — called also *uricemia* — **hy·per·uri·ce·mic** \-ˈsē-mik\ *adj*

hy·per·uri·cos·uria \-ˌyu̇r-i-kō-ˈshu̇r-ē-ə, -ˈsyu̇r-\ *n* : the excretion of excessive amounts of uric acid in the urine

hy·per·vari·able \-ˈvar-ē-ə-bəl\ *adj* : relating to or being any of the relatively short extremely variable polypeptide chain segments in the variable region of an antibody light chain or heavy chain; *also* : relating to, containing, or being a highly variable nucleotide sequence

hy·per·ven·ti·late \-ˈvent-ᵊl-ˌāt\ *vb* **-lat·ed; -lat·ing** : to breathe rapidly and deeply : undergo hyperventilation

hy·per·ven·ti·la·tion \-ˌvent-ᵊl-ˈā-shən\ *n* : excessive rate and depth of respiration leading to abnormal loss of carbon dioxide from the blood — called also *overventilation*

hy·per·vig·i·lance \-ˈvi-jə-ləns\ *n* : the condition of maintaining an abnor-

mal awareness of environmental stimuli — **hy·per·vig·i·lant** \-lənt\ *adj*

hy·per·vis·cos·i·ty \-vis-ˈkä-sə-tē\ *n, pl* **-ties** : excessive viscosity (of the blood)

hy·per·vi·ta·min·o·sis \-ˌvī-tə-mə-ˈnō-səs\ *n, pl* **-oses** \-ˌsēz\ : an abnormal state resulting from excessive intake of one or more vitamins

hy·per·vol·ae·mia *chiefly Brit var of* HYPERVOLEMIA

hy·per·vol·emia \-vä-ˈlē-mē-ə\ *n* : an excessive volume of blood in the body — **hy·per·vol·emic** \-ˈlē-mik\ *adj*

hyp·es·the·sia \ˌhī-pes-ˈthē-zhə, -hi-, -zhē-ə\ *or* **hy·po·es·the·sia** \ˌhī-pō-es-\ *n* : impaired or decreased tactile sensibility — **hyp·es·thet·ic** *or* **hy·po·es·thet·ic** \-ˈthe-tik\ *adj*

hy·phae·ma *chiefly Brit var of* HYPHEMA

hy·phe·ma \hī-ˈfē-mə\ *n* : a hemorrhage in the anterior chamber of the eye

hypn- *or* **hypno-** *comb form* 1 : sleep ⟨*hypn*agogic⟩ 2 : hypnotism ⟨*hyp*notherapy⟩

hyp·na·go·gic *also* **hyp·no·go·gic** \ˌhip-nə-ˈgä-jik, -ˈgō-\ *adj* : of, relating to, or occurring in the period of drowsiness immediately preceding sleep ⟨∼ hallucinations⟩ — compare HYPNOPOMPIC

hyp·no·anal·y·sis \ˌhip-nō-ə-ˈna-lə-səs\ *n, pl* **-y·ses** \-ˌsēz\ : the treatment of mental and emotional disorders by hypnosis and psychoanalytic methods

hyp·no·pom·pic \ˌhip-nə-ˈpäm-pik\ *adj* : associated with the semiconsciousness preceding waking ⟨∼ illusions⟩ — compare HYPNAGOGIC

hyp·no·sis \hip-ˈnō-səs\ *n, pl* **-no·ses** \-ˌsēz\ 1 : a trancelike state that resembles sleep but is induced by a person whose suggestions are readily accepted by the subject 2 : any of various conditions that resemble sleep 3 : HYPNOTISM 1

hyp·no·ther·a·pist \ˌhip-nō-ˈther-ə-pist\ *n* : a specialist in hypnotherapy

hyp·no·ther·a·py \-ˈther-ə-pē\ *n, pl* **-pies** 1 : treatment by hypnotism 2 : psychotherapy that facilitates suggestion, reeducation, or analysis by means of hypnosis

¹**hyp·not·ic** \hip-ˈnä-tik\ *adj* 1 : tending to produce sleep : SOPORIFIC 2 : of or relating to hypnosis or hypnotism — **hyp·not·i·cal·ly** *adv*

²**hypnotic** *n* 1 : a sleep-inducing agent : SOPORIFIC 2 : one that is or can be hypnotized

hyp·no·tism \ˈhip-nə-ˌti-zəm\ *n* 1 : the study or act of inducing hypnosis — compare MESMERISM 2 : HYPNOSIS 1

hyp·no·tist \-tist\ *n* : a person who induces hypnosis

hyp·no·tize \-ˌtīz\ *vb* **-tized; -tiz·ing** : to induce hypnosis in — **hyp·no·tiz·abil·i·ty** \ˌhip-nə-ˌtī-zə-ˈbi-lə-tē\ *n* — **hyp·no·tiz·able** \ˌhip-nə-ˈtī-zə-bəl\ *adj*

¹**hy·po** \ˈhī-(ˌ)pō\ *n, pl* **hypos** : HY-POCHONDRIA

²**hypo** *n, pl* **hypos** **1** : HYPODERMIC SYRINGE **2** : HYPODERMIC INJECTION

hypo- *or* **hyp-** *prefix* **1** : under : beneath : down ⟨*hypo*dermic⟩ **2** : less than normal or normally ⟨*hypo*tension⟩

hy·po·acid·i·ty \ˌhī-pō-a-ˈsi-də-tē\ *n, pl* **-ties** : abnormally low acidity

hy·po·ac·tive \-ˈak-tiv\ *adj* : less than normally active ⟨~ sexual desire⟩ — **hy·po·ac·tiv·i·ty** \-ak-ˈti-və-tē\ *n*

hy·po·acu·sis \-ə-ˈkü-səs, -ˈkyü-\ *n* : partial loss of hearing — called also *hypacusis*

hy·po·adren·al·ism \-ə-ˈdren-ᵊl-ˌi-zəm\ *n* : abnormally decreased activity of the adrenal glands; *specif* : HYPOADRENOCORTICISM

hy·po·ad·re·no·cor·ti·cism \-ə-ˌdrē-nō-ˈkór-tə-ˌsi-zəm\ *n* : abnormally decreased activity of the adrenal cortex (as in Addison's disease)

hy·po·aes·the·sia \ˌhī-pō-es-ˈthē-zhə, -hī-, -zhē-ə\ *Brit var of* HYPESTHESIA

hy·po·al·bu·min·ae·mia *chiefly Brit var of* HYPOALBUMINEMIA

hy·po·al·bu·min·emia \-al-ˌbyü-mə-ˈnē-mē-ə\ *n* : hypoproteinemia marked by reduction in serum albumins — **hy·po·al·bu·min·emic** \-ˈnē-mik\ *adj*

hy·po·al·ge·sia \-al-ˈjē-zhə, -zhē-ə, -zē-ə\ *n* : decreased sensitivity to pain

hy·po·al·ler·gen·ic \-ˌa-lər-ˈje-nik\ *adj* : having little likelihood of causing an allergic response ⟨~ food⟩

hy·po·ami·no·ac·id·emia \-ə-ˌmē-nō-ˌa-sə-ˈdē-mē-ə\ *n* : the presence of abnormally low concentrations of amino acids in the blood

hy·po·bar·ic \-ˈbar-ik\ *adj* : having a specific gravity less than that of cerebrospinal fluid — used of solutions for spinal anesthesia; compare HYPERBARIC 1

hy·po·bar·ism \-ˈbar-ˌi-zəm\ *n* : a condition which occurs when the ambient pressure is lower than the pressure of gases within the body and which may be marked by the distension of bodily cavities and the release of gas bubbles within bodily tissues

hy·po·blast \ˈhī-pə-ˌblast\ *n* : the endoderm of an embryo — **hy·po·blas·tic** \ˌhī-pə-ˈblas-tik\ *adj*

hy·po·cal·cae·mia *chiefly Brit var of* HYPOCALCEMIA

hy·po·cal·ce·mia \ˌhī-pō-ˌkal-ˈsē-mē-ə\ *n* : a deficiency of calcium in the blood — **hy·po·cal·ce·mic** \-mik\ *adj*

hy·po·cal·ci·fi·ca·tion \-ˌkal-sə-fə-ˈkā-shən\ *n* : decreased or deficient calcification (as of tooth enamel)

hy·po·ca·lor·ic \-kə-ˈlōr-ik, -ˈlär-; -kə-lə-rik\ *adj* : characterized by a low number of dietary calories

hy·po·cap·nia \-ˈkap-nē-ə\ *n* : a deficiency of carbon dioxide in the blood — **hy·po·cap·nic** \-nik\ *adj*

hy·po·chlor·ae·mia *chiefly Brit var of* HYPOCHLOREMIA

hy·po·chlor·emia \ˌhī-pō-klōr-ˈē-mē-ə\ *n* : abnormal decrease of chlorides in the blood — **hy·po·chlor·emic** \-klōr-ˈē-mik\ *adj*

hy·po·chlor·hy·dria \-klōr-ˈhī-drē-ə\ *n* : deficiency of hydrochloric acid in the gastric juice — compare ACHLORHYDRIA, HYPERCHLORHYDRIA — **hy·po·chlor·hy·dric** \-ˈhī-drik\ *adj*

hy·po·chlo·rite \ˌhī-pə-ˈklōr-ˌīt\ *n* : a salt or ester of hypochlorous acid

hy·po·chlo·rous acid \-ˈklōr-əs-\ *n* : an unstable strongly oxidizing but weak acid HClO obtained in solution along with hydrochloric acid by reaction of chlorine with water and used esp. in the form of salts as an oxidizing agent, bleaching agent, disinfectant, and chlorinating agent

hy·po·cho·les·ter·ol·emia \ˌhī-pō-kə-ˌles-tə-rə-ˈlē-mē-ə\ *also* **hy·po·cho·les·ter·emia** \-tə-ˈrē-mē-ə\ *n* : an abnormal deficiency of cholesterol in the blood — **hy·po·cho·les·ter·ol·emic** \-ˈlē-mik\ *also* **hy·po·cho·les·ter·emic** \-ˈrē-mik\ *adj*

hy·po·chon·dria \ˌhī-pə-ˈkän-drē-ə\ *n* : extreme depression of mind or spirits often centered on imaginary physical ailments; *specif* : HYPOCHONDRIASIS

¹**hy·po·chon·dri·ac** \-drē-ˌak\ *adj* **1** : HYPOCHONDRIACAL **2 a** : situated below the costal cartilages **b** : of, relating to, or being the two abdominal regions lying on either side of the epigastric region and above the lumbar regions

²**hypochondriac** *n* : a person affected by hypochondria or hypochondriasis

hy·po·chon·dri·a·cal \-kən-ˈdrī-ə-kəl, -ˌkän-\ *adj* : affected with or produced by hypochondria

hy·po·chon·dri·a·sis \-ˈdrī-ə-səs, -a·ses \-ˌsēz\ *n, pl* **-a·ses** : morbid concern about one's health esp. when accompanied by delusions of physical disease

hy·po·chon·dri·um \-ˈkän-drē-əm\ *n, pl* **-dria** \-drē-ə\ : either hypochondriac region of the body

hy·po·chro·mia \ˌhī-pə-ˈkrō-mē-ə\ *n* **1** : deficiency of color or pigmentation **2** : deficiency of hemoglobin in the red blood cells (as in nutritional anemia) — **hy·po·chro·mic** \-ˈkrō-mik\ *adj*

hypochromic anemia *n* : an anemia marked by deficient hemoglobin and usu. microcytic red blood cells — compare HYPERCHROMIC ANEMIA

hy·po·co·ag·u·la·bil·i·ty \ˌhī-pō-kō-ˌa-gyə-lə-ˈbi-lə-tē\ *n, pl* **-ties** : decreased or deficient coagulability of blood — **hy·po·co·ag·u·la·ble** \-kō-ˈa-gyə-lə-bəl\ *adj*

hy·po·com·ple·men·tae·mia *chiefly Brit var of* HYPOCOMPLEMENTEMIA

hy·po·com·ple·men·te·mia \-ˌkäm-plə-(ˌ)men-ˈtē-mē-ə\ *n* : an abnormal deficiency of complement in the blood — **hy·po·com·ple·men·te·mic** \-ˈtē-mik\ *adj*

hy·po·cu·prae·mia *chiefly Brit var of* HYPOCUPREMIA

hy·po·cu·pre·mia \-kü-ˈprē-mē-ə, -kyü-\ *n* : an abnormal deficiency of copper in the blood

hy·po·cu·pro·sis \-kü-ˈprō-səs, -kyü-\ *n, pl* **-pro·ses** \-ˌsēz\ : HYPOCUPREMIA

hy·po·der·ma \ˌhī-pə-ˈdər-mə\ *n* **1** *cap* : a genus (family Hypodermatidae) of dipteran flies that have parasitic larvae and include the common cattle grub (*H. lineatum*) **2** : any insect or maggot of the genus *Hypoderma*

hy·po·der·ma·to·sis \-ˌdər-mə-ˈtō-səs\ *n* : infestation with maggots of flies of the genus *Hypoderma*

hy·po·der·mi·a·sis \-dər-ˈmī-ə-səs\ *n, pl* **-a·ses** \-ˌsēz\ : HYPODERMATOSIS

¹hy·po·der·mic \ˌhī-pə-ˈdər-mik\ *adj* **1** : of or relating to the parts beneath the skin **2** : adapted for use in or administered by injection beneath the skin — **hy·po·der·mi·cal·ly** *adv*

²hypodermic *n* **1** : HYPODERMIC INJECTION **2** : HYPODERMIC SYRINGE

hypodermic injection *n* : an injection made into the subcutaneous tissues

hypodermic needle *n* : NEEDLE 2 2 : a hypodermic syringe complete with needle

hypodermic syringe *n* : a small syringe used with a hollow needle for injection of material into or beneath the skin

hy·po·der·mis \ˌhī-pə-ˈdər-məs\ *n* : SUPERFICIAL FASCIA

hy·po·der·moc·ly·sis \-dər-ˈmä-klə-səs\ *n, pl* **-ly·ses** \-ˌsēz\ : subcutaneous injection of fluids (as saline solution)

hy·po·dip·loid \ˌhī-pō-ˈdi-ˌplȯid\ *adj* : having slightly fewer than the diploid number of chromosomes — **hy·po·dip·loi·dy** \-ˌplȯi-dē\ *n*

hy·po·don·tia \-ˈdän-chə, -chē-ə\ *n* : an esp. congenital condition marked by a less than normal number of teeth : partial anodontia — **hy·po·don·tic** \-ˈdän-tik\ *adj*

hy·po·dy·nam·ic \-dī-ˈna-mik\ *adj* : marked by or exhibiting a decrease in strength or power ⟨the ∼ heart⟩

hypoesthesia *var of* HYPESTHESIA

hy·po·es·tro·ge·ne·mia \-ˌes-trə-jə-ˈnē-mē-ə\ *n* : a deficiency of one or more estrogens (as estrone or estradiol) in the blood

hy·po·es·tro·gen·ism \-ˈes-trə-jə-ˌni-zəm\ *n* : a deficiency of estrogen in the body — **hy·po·es·tro·gen·ic** \-ˌes-trə-ˈje-nik\ *adj*

hy·po·fer·rae·mia *chiefly Brit var of* HYPOFERREMIA

hy·po·fer·re·mia \ˌhī-pō-fə-ˈrē-mē-ə\ *n* : an abnormal deficiency of iron in the blood — **hy·po·fer·re·mic** \-ˈrē-mik\ *adj*

hy·po·fi·brin·o·gen·ae·mia *chiefly Brit var of* HYPOFIBRINOGENEMIA

hy·po·fi·brin·o·gen·emia \-ˌfī-ˌbri-nə-jə-ˈnē-mē-ə\ *n* : an abnormal deficiency of fibrinogen in the blood

hy·po·func·tion \ˈhī-pō-ˌfəŋk-shən\ *n* : decreased or insufficient function esp. of an endocrine gland

hy·po·gam·ma·glob·u·lin·emia \-ˌgam-ə-ˌglä-byə-lə-ˈnē-mē-ə\ *n* : a deficiency of gamma globulins in the blood — **hy·po·gam·ma·glob·u·lin·emic** \-ˈnē-mik\ *adj*

hy·po·gas·tric \ˌhī-pə-ˈgas-trik\ *adj* **1** : of or relating to the lower median abdominal region **2** : relating to or situated along or near the internal iliac arteries or the internal iliac veins

hypogastric artery *n* : ILIAC ARTERY 3

hypogastric nerve *n* : a nerve or several parallel nerve bundles situated dorsal and medial to the common and the internal iliac arteries

hypogastric plexus *n* : the sympathetic nerve plexus that supplies the pelvic viscera

hypogastric vein *n* : ILIAC VEIN c

hy·po·gas·tri·um \ˌhī-pə-ˈgas-trē-əm\ *n, pl* **-tria** \-trē-ə\ : the hypogastric region of the abdomen

hy·po·gen·i·tal·ism \-ˈje-nə-tə-ˌli-zəm\ *n* : subnormal development of genital organs : genital infantilism

hy·po·geu·sia \-ˈgü-sē-ə, -ˈjü-, -zē-ə\ *n* : decreased sensitivity to taste

hy·po·glos·sal \ˌhī-pə-ˈglä-səl\ *adj* : of or relating to the hypoglossal nerves

hypoglossal nerve *n* : either of the 12th and final pair of cranial nerves which are motor nerves arising from the medulla oblongata and supplying muscles of the tongue and hyoid apparatus — called also *hypoglossal, twelfth cranial nerve*

hypoglossal nucleus *n* : a nucleus in the floor of the fourth ventricle of the brain that is the origin of the hypoglossal nerve

hy·po·glos·sus \-ˈglä-səs\ *n, pl* **-glos·si** \-ˌsī, -ˌsē\ : HYPOGLOSSAL NERVE

hy·po·gly·ce·mia \ˌhī-pō-glī-ˈsē-mē-ə\ *n* : abnormal decrease of sugar in the blood

¹hy·po·gly·ce·mic \-ˈsē-mik\ *adj* **1** : of, relating to, caused by, or affected with hypoglycemia **2** : producing a decrease in the level of sugar in the blood ⟨∼ drugs⟩

²hypoglycemic *n* **1** : one affected with hypoglycemia **2** : an agent that lowers the level of sugar in the blood

hy·po·go·nad·al \-gō-ˈnad-ᵊl\ *adj* **1** : relating to or affected with hypogonadism **2** : marked by or exhibiting deficient development of secondary sex characteristics

hy·po·go·nad·ism \-ˈgō-ˌna-ˌdi-zəm\ *n* **1** : functional incompetence of the gonads esp. in the male **2** : a condition (as Klinefelter's syndrome) involving gonadal incompetence

hy·po·go·nad·o·trop·ic \-ˌgō-ˌna-də-

'trä-pik\ *or* **hy·po·go·nad·o·tro·phic** \-'trō-fik, -'trä-\ *adj* : characterized by a deficiency of gonadotropins

hy·po·hi·dro·sis \-hi-'drō-səs, -hī-\ *n, pl* **-dro·ses** \-₁sēz\ : abnormally diminished sweating — compare HYPERHIDROSIS

hy·po·his·ti·di·ne·mia \-₁his-tə-də-'nē-mē-ə\ *n* : a low concentration of histidine in the blood that is characteristic of rheumatoid arthritis — **hy·po·his·ti·di·ne·mic** \-'nē-mik\ *adj*

hy·po·in·su·lin·emia \-₁in-sə-lə-'nē-mē-ə\ *n* : an abnormally low concentration of insulin in the blood — **hy·po·in·su·lin·emic** \-'nē-mik\ *adj*

hy·po·ka·lae·mia *chiefly Brit var of* HYPOKALEMIA

hy·po·ka·le·mia \-kā-'lē-mē-ə\ *n* : a deficiency of potassium in the blood — called also *hypopotassemia* — **hy·po·ka·le·mic** \-'lē-mik\ *adj*

hy·po·ki·ne·sia \-kə-'nē-zhə, -kī-, -zhē-ə\ *n* : abnormally decreased muscular movement — compare HYPERKINESIS

hy·po·ki·ne·sis \-'nē-səs\ *n, pl* **-ne·ses** \-₁sēz\ : HYPOKINESIA

hy·po·ki·net·ic \-'ne-tik\ *adj* : characterized by, associated with, or caused by decreased motor activity

hy·po·lip·id·ae·mia *chiefly Brit var of* HYPOLIPIDEMIA

hy·po·lip·id·emia \-₁li-pə-'dē-mē-ə\ *n* : a deficiency of lipids in the blood — **hy·po·lip·id·emic** \-'dē-mik\ *adj*

hy·po·mag·ne·sae·mia *chiefly Brit var of* HYPOMAGNESEMIA

hy·po·mag·ne·se·mia \-₁hī-pə-₁mag-nə-'sē-mē-ə\ *n* : a deficiency of magnesium in the blood — **hy·po·mag·ne·se·mic** \-mik\ *adj*

hy·po·ma·nia \₁hī-pə-'mā-nē-ə, -nyə\ *n* : a mild mania esp. when part of bipolar disorder

¹**hy·po·man·ic** \-'ma-nik\ *adj* : of, relating to, or affected with hypomania

²**hypomanic** *n* : one affected with hypomania

hy·po·men·or·rhea \-₁me-nə-'rē-ə\ *n* : decreased menstrual flow

hy·po·me·tab·o·lism \₁hī-pō-mə-'ta-bə-₁li-zəm\ *n* : a condition (as in myxedema) marked by an abnormally low metabolic rate — **hy·po·meta·bol·ic** \-₁me-tə-'bä-lik\ *adj*

hy·po·me·tria \-'mē-trē-ə\ *n* : a condition of cerebellar dysfunction in which voluntary muscular movements tend to result in the movement of bodily parts (as the arm and hand) short of the intended goal

hy·po·min·er·al·ized \-'mi-nə-rə-₁līzd\ *adj* : relating to or characterized by a deficiency of minerals

hy·po·mo·til·i·ty \₁hī-pō-mō-'ti-lə-tē\ *n, pl* **-ties** : abnormal deficiency of movement; *specif* : decreased motility of all or part of the gastrointestinal tract — compare HYPERMOTILITY

hy·po·na·trae·mia *chiefly Brit var of* HYPONATREMIA

hy·po·na·tre·mia \-nā-'trē-mē-ə\ *n* : deficiency of sodium in the blood — **hy·po·na·tre·mic** \-mik\ *adj*

hy·po-oes·tro·ge·nae·mia, hypo-oes·tro·gen·ism *chiefly Brit var of* HYPO-ESTROGENEMIA, HYPOESTROGENISM

hypoosmolality *var of* HYPOSMOLALITY

hy·po·os·mot·ic \-₁äz-'mä-tik\ *or* **hy·pos·mot·ic** \₁hī-₁päz-\ *adj* : HYPOTONIC 2

hy·po·para·thy·roid·ism \-₁par-ə-'thī-₁roi-₁di-zəm\ *n* : deficiency of parathyroid hormone in the body; *also* : the resultant abnormal state marked by low serum calcium and a tendency to chronic tetany — **hy·po·para·thy·roid** \-'thī-₁roid\ *adj*

hy·po·per·fu·sion \₁hī-pō-pər-'fyü-zhən\ *n* : decreased blood flow through an organ ⟨cerebral ∼⟩

hy·po·phar·ynx \-'far-iŋks\ *n, pl* **-pha·ryn·ges** \-fə-'rin-(₁)jēz\ *also* **-phar·ynx·es** : the laryngeal part of the pharynx extending from the hyoid bone to the lower margin of the cricoid cartilage — **hy·po·pha·ryn·geal** \-₁far-ən-'jē-əl; -fə-'rin-jəl, -jē-əl\ *adj*

hy·po·phos·pha·tae·mia *chiefly Brit var of* HYPOPHOSPHATEMIA

hy·po·phos·pha·ta·sia \₁hī-pō-₁fäs-fə-'tā-zhə, -zhē-ə\ *n* : a congenital metabolic disorder characterized by a deficiency of alkaline phosphatase and usu. resulting in demineralization of bone

hy·po·phos·pha·te·mia \-₁fäs-fə-'tē-mē-ə\ *n* : deficiency of phosphates in the blood — **hy·po·phos·pha·te·mic** \-'tē-mik\ *adj*

hy·po·phys·e·al *also* **hy·po·phy·si·al** \(₁)hī-₁pä-fə-'sē-əl, ₁hī-pə-fə-; -'zē-; ₁hī-pə-'fi-zē-əl\ *adj* : of or relating to the hypophysis

hypophyseal fossa *n* : the depression in the sphenoid bone that contains the hypophysis

hy·poph·y·sec·to·mize \(₁)hī-₁pä-fə-'sek-tə-₁mīz\ *vb* **-mized; -miz·ing** : to remove the pituitary gland from

hy·poph·y·sec·to·my \-mē\ *n, pl* **-mies** : surgical removal of the pituitary gland

hy·po·phys·io·tro·pic \₁hī-pō-₁fi-zē-ō-'trō-pik, -'trä-\ *or* **hy·po·phys·io·tro·phic** \-'trō-fik\ *adj* : acting on or stimulating the hypophysis

hy·poph·y·sis \hī-'pä-fə-səs\ *n, pl* **-y·ses** \-₁sēz\ : PITUITARY GLAND

hypophysis ce·re·bri \-sə-'rē-₁brī, -'ser-ə-\ *n* : PITUITARY GLAND

hy·po·pig·men·ta·tion \₁hī-pō-₁pig-mən-'tā-shən, -₁men-\ *n* : diminished pigmentation in a bodily part or tissue (as the skin) — **hy·po·pig·ment·ed** \-'pig-mən-təd, -₁men-\ *adj*

hy·po·pi·tu·ita·rism \₁hī-pō-pə-'tü-ə-tə-₁ri-zəm, -'tyü-\ *n* : deficient production of growth hormones by the pituitary gland — **hy·po·pi·tu·itary** \-'tü-ə-ˌter-ē, -'tyü-\ *adj*

hy·po·pla·sia \-'plā-zhə, -zhē-ə\ *n* : a condition of arrested development in which an organ or part remains below the normal size or in an immature state — **hy·po·plas·tic** \-'plas-tik\ *adj*

hypoplastic anemia *n* : APLASTIC ANEMIA

hypoplastic left heart syndrome *n* : a congenital malformation of the heart in which the left side is underdeveloped resulting in insufficient blood flow

hy·po·pnea \ˌhī-pō-'nē-ə\ *n* : abnormally slow or esp. shallow respiration

hy·po·pnoea *chiefly Brit var of* HYPOPNEA

hy·po·po·tas·sae·mia *chiefly Brit var of* HYPOPOTASSEMIA

hy·po·po·tas·se·mia \-pə-ˌta-'sē-mē-ə\ *n* : HYPOKALEMIA — **hy·po·po·tas·se·mic** \-'sē-mik\ *adj*

hy·po·pro·lac·tin·ae·mia *chiefly Brit var of* HYPOPROLACTINEMIA

hy·po·pro·lac·tin·emia \-prō-ˌlak-tə-'nē-mē-ə\ *n* : a condition characterized by a deficiency of prolactin in the blood

hy·po·pro·tein·ae·mia *chiefly Brit var of* HYPOPROTEINEMIA

hy·po·pro·tein·emia \-ˌprō-tə-'nē-mē-ə, -ˌprō-ˌtē-, -ˌprō-tē-ə-\ *n* : abnormal deficiency of protein in the blood — **hy·po·pro·tein·emic** \-'nē-mik\ *adj*

hy·po·pro·throm·bin·ae·mia *chiefly Brit var of* HYPOPROTHROMBINEMIA

hy·po·pro·throm·bin·emia \-prō-ˌthräm-bə-'nē-mē-ə\ *n* : deficiency of prothrombin in the blood usu. due to vitamin K deficiency or liver disease and resulting in delayed clotting of blood or spontaneous bleeding (as from the nose) — **hy·po·pro·throm·bin·emic** \-'nē-mik\ *adj*

hy·po·py·on \hī-'pō-pē-ˌän\ *n* : an accumulation of white blood cells in the anterior chamber of the eye

hy·po·re·ac·tive \ˌhī-pō-rē-'ak-tiv\ *adj* : having or showing abnormally low sensitivity to stimuli — **hy·po·re·ac·tiv·i·ty** \-(ˌ)rē-ˌak-'ti-və-tē\ *n*

hy·po·re·flex·ia \-rē-'flek-sē-ə\ *n* : underactivity of bodily reflexes

hypos *pl of* HYPO

hy·po·sal·i·va·tion \-ˌsa-lə-'vā-shən\ *n* : diminished salivation

hy·po·se·cre·tion \ˌhī-pō-si-'krē-shən\ *n* : production of a bodily secretion at an abnormally slow rate or in abnormally small quantities

hy·po·sen·si·tive \-'sen-sə-tiv\ *adj* : exhibiting or marked by deficient response to stimulation — **hy·po·sen·si·tiv·i·ty** \-ˌsen-sə-'ti-və-tē\ *n*

hy·po·sen·si·ti·za·tion \-ˌsen-sə-tə-'zā-shən\ *n* : the state or process of being

reduced in sensitivity esp. to an allergen : DESENSITIZATION — **hy·po·sen·si·tize** \-'sen-sə-ˌtīz\ *vb*

hy·pos·mia \hī-'päz-mē-ə, hi-\ *n* : impairment of the sense of smell

hy·pos·mo·lal·i·ty \ˌhī-ˌpäz-mō-'la-lə-tē\ *or* **hy·po·os·mo·lal·i·ty** \ˌhī-pō-ˌäz-\ *n, pl* **-ties** : the condition esp. of a bodily fluid of having abnormally low osmolality

hy·pos·mo·lar·i·ty \ˌhī-ˌpäz-mō-'lar-ə-tē\ *n, pl* **-ties** : the condition esp. of a bodily fluid of having abnormally low osmolarity — **hy·pos·mo·lar** \ˌhī-ˌpäz-'mō-lər\ *adj*

hyposmotic *var of* HYPOOSMOTIC

hy·po·spa·di·as \ˌhī-pə-'spā-dē-əs\ *n* : an abnormality of the penis in which the urethra opens on the underside

hy·pos·ta·sis \hī-'päs-tə-səs\ *n, pl* **-ta·ses** \-ˌsēz\ : the settling of blood in relatively lower parts of an organ or the body due to impaired or absent circulation — **hy·po·stat·ic** \ˌhī-pə-'sta-tik\ *adj*

hypostatic pneumonia *n* : pneumonia that usu. results from the collection of fluid in the dorsal region of the lungs and occurs esp. in those (as the bedridden or elderly) confined to a supine position for extended periods

hy·po·sthe·nia \ˌhī-päs-'thē-nē-ə\ *n* : lack of strength : bodily weakness — **hy·po·sthen·ic** \ˌhī-pəs-'the-nik\ *adj*

hy·po·sthe·nu·ria \ˌhī-ˌpäs-thə-'nūr-ē-ə, -'nyur-\ *n* : the secretion of urine of low specific gravity due to inability of the kidney to concentrate the urine normally

hy·po·ten·sion \ˌhī-pō-'ten-chən\ *n* **1** : abnormally low pressure of the blood — called also *low blood pressure* **2** : abnormally low pressure of the intraocular fluid

¹**hy·po·ten·sive** \-'ten-siv\ *adj* **1** : characterized by or due to hypotension ⟨~ shock⟩ **2** : causing low blood pressure or a lowering of blood pressure ⟨~ drugs⟩

²**hypotensive** *n* : one with hypotension

hy·po·tha·lam·ic \ˌhī-pō-thə-'la-mik\ *adj* : of or relating to the hypothalamus — **hy·po·tha·lam·i·cal·ly** *adv*

hypothalamic releasing factor *n* : any hormone that is secreted by the hypothalamus and stimulates the pituitary gland directly to secrete a hormone — called also *hypothalamic releasing hormone, releasing factor*

hypothalamo- *comb form* : hypothalamus ⟨*hypothalamo*tomy⟩

hy·po·thal·a·mot·o·my \ˌhī-pō-ˌtha-lə-'mä-tə-mē\ *n, pl* **-mies** : psychosurgery in which lesions are made in the hypothalamus

hy·po·thal·a·mus \-'tha-lə-məs\ *n, pl* **-mi** \-ˌmī\ : a basal part of the diencephalon that lies beneath the thalamus on each side, forms the floor of the third ventricle, and includes vital autonomic regulatory centers

hy·po·the·nar eminence \ˌhī-pō-'thē-

‚när-, -nər-; hī-'pä-thə-‚när-, -nər-\ *n* : the prominent part of the palm of the hand above the base of the little finger

hypothenar muscle *n* : any of four muscles located in the area of the hypothenar eminence: **a** : ABDUCTOR DIGITI MINIMI **b** : FLEXOR DIGITI MINIMI BREVIS **c** : PALMARIS BREVIS **d** : OPPONENS DIGITI MINIMI

hy·po·ther·mia \-'thər-mē-ə\ *n* : subnormal temperature of the body — **hy·po·ther·mic** \-mik\ *adj*

hy·po·thy·re·o·sis \‚hī-pō-‚thī-rē-'ō-səs\ *n* : HYPOTHYROIDISM

hy·po·thy·roid·ism \‚hī-pō-'thī-‚rȯi-‚di-zəm\ *n* : deficient activity of the thyroid gland; *also* : a resultant bodily condition characterized by lowered metabolic rate and general loss of vigor — **hy·po·thy·roid** \-'rȯid\ *adj*

hy·po·thy·ro·sis \-‚thī-'rō-səs\ *n* : HYPOTHYROIDISM

hy·po·thy·rox·in·emia *chiefly Brit var of* HYPOTHYROXINEMIA

hy·po·thy·rox·in·emia \‚hī-pō-thī-‚räk-sə-'nē-mē-ə\ *n* : the presence of an abnormally low concentration of thyroxine in the blood — **hy·po·thy·rox·in·emic** \-'nē-mik\ *adj*

hy·po·to·nia \‚hī-pə-'tō-nē-ə, -pō-\ *n* **1** : abnormally low pressure of the intraocular fluid **2** : the state of having hypotonic muscle tone

hy·po·ton·ic \‚hī-pə-'tä-nik, -pō-\ *adj* **1** : having deficient tone or tension **2** : having a lower osmotic pressure than a surrounding medium or a fluid under comparison — compare HYPERTONIC 2

hy·po·to·nic·i·ty \-tə-'ni-sə-tē\ *n, pl* **-ties 1** : the state or condition of having hypotonic osmotic pressure **2** : HYPOTONIA

hy·pot·o·ny \hī-'pä-tə-nē\ *n, pl* **-onies** : HYPOTONIA

hy·po·tri·cho·sis \-tri-'kō-səs\ *n, pl* **-cho·ses** \-‚sēz\ : congenital deficiency of hair

hy·pot·ro·phy \hī-'pä-trə-fē\ *n, pl* **-phies** : subnormal growth

hy·po·tym·pa·num \‚hī-pō-'tim-pə-nəm\ *n, pl* **-na** \-nə\ *also* **-nums** : the lower part of the middle ear — compare EPITYMPANUM

hy·po·uri·ce·mia \-‚yu̇r-ə-'sē-mē-ə\ *n* : deficient uric acid in the blood — **hy·po·uri·ce·mic** \-'sē-mik\ *adj*

hy·po·ven·ti·la·tion \-‚vent-ᵊl-'ā-shən\ *n* : deficient ventilation of the lungs that results in reduction in the oxygen content or increase in the carbon dioxide content of the blood or both — **hy·po·ven·ti·lat·ed** \-'vent-ᵊl-‚ā-təd\ *adj*

hy·po·vi·ta·min·osis \-‚vī-tə-mə-'nō-səs\ *n* : AVITAMINOSIS — **hy·po·vi·ta·min·ot·ic** \-'nä-tik\ *adj*

hy·po·vo·lae·mia *chiefly Brit var of* HYPOVOLEMIA

hy·po·vo·le·mia \-vä-'lē-mē-ə\ *n* : decrease in the volume of the circulat-

ing blood — **hy·po·vo·le·mic** \-'lē-mik\ *adj*

hy·pox·ae·mia *chiefly Brit var of* HYPOXEMIA

hy·po·xan·thine \‚hī-pō-'zan-‚thēn\ *n* : a purine base $C_5H_4N_4O$ of plant and animal tissues that is an intermediate in uric acid synthesis

hypoxanthine–guanine phos·pho·ri·bo·syl·trans·fer·ase \-‚fäs-fō-‚rī-bō-sil-'trans-(‚)fər-‚ās, -‚āz\ *n* : an enzyme that conserves hypoxanthine in the body by limiting its conversion to uric acid and that is lacking in Lesch-Nyhan syndrome — called also *hypoxanthine phosphoribosyltransferase*

hyp·ox·emia \‚hī-‚päk-'sē-mē-ə, ‚hī-\ *n* : deficient oxygenation of the blood — **hyp·ox·emic** \-mik\ *adj*

hyp·ox·ia \hī-'päk-sē-ə, hī-\ *n* : a deficiency of oxygen reaching the tissues of the body — **hyp·ox·ic** \-sik\ *adj*

hyps- *or* **hypsi-** *or* **hypso-** *comb form* : high ⟨*hyps*arrhythmia⟩

hyps·ar·rhyth·mia *also* **hyps·arhyth·mia** \‚hips-ā-'rith-mē-ə\ *n* : an abnormal encephalogram that is characterized by slow waves of high voltage and a disorganized arrangement of spikes, occurs esp. in infants, and is indicative of a condition that leads to severe mental retardation if left untreated

hyster- *or* **hystero-** *comb form* **1** : womb ⟨*hystero*tomy⟩ **2** : hysteria ⟨*hyster*oid⟩

hys·ter·ec·to·my \‚his-tə-'rek-tə-mē\ *n, pl* **-mies** : surgical removal of the uterus — **hys·ter·ec·to·mized** \-tə-‚mīzd\ *adj*

hys·te·ria \hi-'ster-ē-ə, -'stir-\ *n* **1** : a psychoneurosis marked by emotional excitability and disturbances of the psychic, sensory, vasomotor, and visceral functions without an organic basis **2** : behavior exhibiting overwhelming or unmanageable fear or emotional excess

hys·ter·ic \hi-'ster-ik\ *n* : one subject to or affected with hysteria

hys·ter·i·cal \-i-kəl\ *also* **hys·ter·ic** \-'ster-ik\ *adj* : of, relating to, or marked by hysteria — **hys·ter·i·cal·ly** *adv*

hysterical personality *n* : a personality characterized by superficiality, egocentricity, vanity, dependence, and manipulativeness, by dramatic, reactive, and intensely expressed emotional behavior, and often by disturbed interpersonal relationships

hys·ter·ics \-iks\ *n sing or pl* : a fit of uncontrollable laughter or crying : HYSTERIA

hystericus — see GLOBUS HYSTERICUS

hys·ter·o·gram \'his-tə-rō-‚gram\ *n* : a radiograph of the uterus

hys·ter·og·ra·phy \‚his-tə-'rä-grə-fē\ *n, pl* **-phies** : examination of the uterus by radiography after the injection of an opaque medium

hys·ter·oid \'his-tə-ˌroid\ *adj* : resembling or tending toward hysteria

hys·ter·o·plas·ty \'his-tə-rō-ˌplas-tē\ *n, pl* **-ties** : plastic surgery of the uterus

hys·ter·or·rha·phy \ˌhis-tə-'ror-ə-fē\ *n, pl* **-phies** : a suturing of an incised or ruptured uterus

hys·ter·o·sal·pin·go·gram \ˌhis-tə-rō-ˌsal-'piŋ-gə-ˌgram\ *n* : a radiograph made by hysterosalpingography

hys·ter·o·sal·pin·gog·ra·phy \-ˌsal-ˌpiŋ-'gä-gre-fē\ *n, pl* **-phies** : examination of the uterus and fallopian tubes by radiography after injection of an opaque medium — called also *uterosalpingography*

hys·ter·o·sal·pin·gos·to·my \-'gäs-tə-mē\ *n, pl* **-mies** : surgical establishment of an anastomosis between the uterus and an occluded fallopian tube

hys·ter·o·scope \'his-tə-rō-ˌskōp\ *n* : an endoscope used for the visual examination of the cervix and the interior of the uterus — **hys·ter·o·scop·ic** \ˌhis-tə-rō-'skä-pik\ *adj* — **hys·ter·os·co·py** \ˌhis-tə-'räs-kə-pē\ *n*

hys·ter·o·sto·mat·o·my \ˌhis-tə-rō-ˌstō-'ma·tə-mē\ *n, pl* **-mies** : surgical incision of the uterine cervix

hys·ter·ot·o·my \ˌhis-tə-'rä-tə-mē\ *n, pl* **-mies** : surgical incision of the uterus; *esp* : CESAREAN SECTION

hystrix — see ICHTHYOSIS HYSTRIX GRAVIOR

Hy·trin \'hī-trin\ *trademark* — used for a preparation of the hydrated hydrochloride of terazosin

Hy·zaar \'hī-ˌzär\ *trademark* — used for a preparation of hydrochlorothiazide and the potassium salt of losartan

Hz *abbr* hertz

H zone \'āch-ˌzōn\ *n* : a narrow and less dense zone of myosin filaments bisecting the A band in striated muscle — compare M LINE

i *abbr* incisor

I *symbol* iodine

-i·a·sis \'ī-ə-səs\ *n suffix, pl* **-i·a·ses** \-ˌsēz\ : disease having characteristics of or produced by (something specified) ⟨amebiasis⟩ ⟨onchocerciasis⟩

-i·at·ric \ē-'a-trik\ *also* **-i·at·ri·cal** \-tri-kəl\ *adj comb form* : of or relating to (such) medical treatment or healing ⟨pediatric⟩

-i·at·rics \ē-'a-triks\ *n pl comb form* : medical treatment ⟨pediatrics⟩

-i·a·trist \'ī-ə-trəst\ *n comb form* : physician : healer ⟨podiatrist⟩

iatro- *comb form* : physician : medicine : healing ⟨iatrogenic⟩

iat·ro·gen·ic \(ˌ)ī-ˌa-trə-'je-nik\ *adj* : induced inadvertently by a physician or surgeon or by medical treatment or diagnostic procedures ⟨an ∼ rash⟩ — **iat·ro·gen·e·sis** \-'je-nə-səs\ *n* — **iat·ro·gen·i·cal·ly** *adv*

-i·a·try \'ī-ə-trē\ *n comb form, pl* **-ia·tries** : medical treatment : healing ⟨podiatry⟩ ⟨psychiatry⟩

I band \'ī-\ *n* : a pale band across a striated muscle fiber that consists of actin and is situated between two A bands — called also *isotropic band*

ibo·te·nic acid \ˌī-bō-'tē-nik-\ *n* : a neurotoxic compound $C_5H_6N_2O_4$ found esp. in fly agaric

IBS *abbr* irritable bowel syndrome

ibu·pro·fen \ˌī-byü-'prō-fən\ *n* : a nonsteroidal anti-inflammatory drug $C_{13}H_{18}O_2$ used in over-the-counter preparations to relieve pain and fever and in prescription strength esp. to relieve the symptoms of rheumatoid arthritis and degenerative arthritis — see ADVIL, MOTRIN

ICD *abbr* International Classification of Diseases — usu. used with an number indicating the revision ⟨ICD-9⟩

ice \'īs\ *n* : methamphetamine in the form of crystals of its hydrochloride salt $C_{10}H_{15}N\cdot HCl$ when used illicitly for smoking — called also *crystal, crystal meth*

ice bag *n* : a waterproof bag to hold ice for local application of cold to the body

ice pack *n* : crushed ice placed in a container (as in an ice bag) or folded in a towel and applied to the body

ich·tham·mol \'ik-thə-ˌmȯl, -ˌmōl\ *n* : a brownish black viscous tarry liquid prepared from a distillate of some hydrocarbon-containing rocks and used as an antiseptic and emollient — see ICHTHYOL

ichthy- *or* **ichthyo-** *comb form* : fish ⟨ichthyosarcotoxism⟩

Ich·thy·ol \'ik-thē-ˌȯl, -ˌōl\ *trademark* — used for a preparation of ichthammol

ich·thy·o·sar·co·tox·ism \ˌik-thē-ō-ˌsär-kə-'täk-ˌsi-zəm\ *n* : poisoning caused by the ingestion of fish whose flesh contains a toxic substance

ich·thy·o·si·form \ˌik-thē-'ō-sə-ˌfȯrm\ *adj* : resembling ichthyosis or that of ichthyosis ⟨∼ erythroderma⟩

ich·thy·o·sis \ˌik-thē-'ō-səs\ *n, pl* **-o·ses** \-ˌsēz\ : any of several diseases usu. of hereditary origin characterized by rough, thick, and scaly skin — **ich·thy·ot·ic** \-'ä-tik\ *adj*

ichthyosis hys·trix gra·vi·or \-'his-triks-'gra-vē-ȯr, -'grä-\ *n* : a rare hereditary disorder characterized by the formation of brown, verrucose, and often linear lesions of the skin

ichthyosis vul·gar·is \-,vəl-'gar-əs\ *n* : the common hereditary form of ichthyosis

ICN *abbr* International Council of Nurses

ICP *abbr* intracranial pressure

-ics \iks\ *n sing or pl suffix* **1** : study : knowledge : skill : practice ⟨*optics*⟩ ⟨*pediatrics*⟩ **2** : characteristic actions or activities ⟨*hysterics*⟩ **3** : characteristic qualities, operations, or phenomena ⟨*acoustics*⟩ ⟨*phonetics*⟩

ICSH *abbr* interstitial-cell stimulating hormone

ICSI *abbr* intracytoplasmic sperm injection

ICT *abbr* insulin coma therapy

ic·tal \'ik-tᵊl\ *adj* : of, relating to, or caused by ictus

icter- *or* **ictero-** *comb form* : jaundice ⟨*ictero*genic⟩

ic·ter·ic \ik-'ter-ik\ *adj* : of, relating to, or affected with jaundice

icteric index *n* : ICTERUS INDEX

ic·ter·o·gen·ic \,ik-tə-rō-'je-nik, ik-,ter-ə-\ *adj* : causing or tending to cause jaundice ⟨∼ drugs⟩

ic·ter·us \'ik-tə-rəs\ *n* : JAUNDICE

icterus gra·vis \-'gra-vəs, -'grä-\ *n* : ICTERUS GRAVIS NEONATORUM

icterus gravis neo·na·tor·um \-,nē-ō-nä-'tȯr-əm\ *n* : severe jaundice in a newborn child due esp. to erythroblastosis fetalis

icterus index *n* : a figure representing the amount of bilirubin in the blood as determined by comparing the color of a sample of test serum with a set of color standards ⟨an *icterus index* of 15 or above indicates active jaundice⟩ — called also *icteric index*

icterus neo·na·tor·um \-,nē-ō-nä-'tȯr-əm\ *n* : jaundice in a newborn

ic·tus \'ik-təs\ *n* **1** : a beat or pulsation esp. of the heart **2** : a sudden attack or seizure esp. of stroke

ICTV *abbr* International Committee on Taxonomy of Viruses

ICU *abbr* intensive care unit

¹id \'id\ *n* : the one of the three divisions of the psyche in psychoanalytic theory that is completely unconscious and is the source of psychic energy derived from instinctual needs and drives — compare EGO, SUPEREGO

²id *n* : a skin rash that is an allergic reaction to an agent causing an infection ⟨a syphilitic ∼⟩

ID *abbr* intradermal

¹-id \əd, ,()id\ *also* **-ide** \īd\ *n suffix* : skin rash caused by (something specified) ⟨syphil*id*⟩

²-id *n suffix* : structure, body, or particle of a (specified) kind ⟨chromat*id*⟩

IDA *abbr* iron-deficiency anemia

-i·da \ə-də\ *n pl suffix* : animals that are or have the form of — in names of

higher taxa (as orders and classes) ⟨Arach*nida*⟩ — **-i·dan** \ə-dən, əd-ᵊn\ *n or adj suffix*

-i·dae \ə-,dē\ *n pl suffix* : members of the family of — in names of zoological families ⟨Homin*idae*⟩ ⟨Ixod*idae*⟩

IDDM *abbr* insulin-dependent diabetes mellitus

idea \ī-'dē-ə\ *n* : something imagined or pictured in the mind

idea of reference *n* : a delusion that the remarks one overhears and people one encounters seem to be concerned with and usu. hostile to oneself — called also *delusion of reference*

ide·ation \,ī-dē-'ā-shən\ *n* : the capacity for or the act of forming or entertaining ideas ⟨suicidal ∼⟩ — **ide·ation·al** \-shə-nəl\ *adj*

idée fixe \(,)ē-,dā-'fēks\ *n, pl* **idées fixes** *same or* -'fēk-səz\ : a usu. delusional idea that dominates the whole mental life during a prolonged period (as in certain mental disorders) — called also *fixed idea*

iden·ti·cal \ī-'den-ti-kəl\ *adj* : MONOZYGOTIC ⟨∼ twins⟩

iden·ti·fi·ca·tion \ī-,den-tə-fə-'kā-shən\ *n* **1** : psychological orientation of the self in regard to something (as a person or group) with a resulting feeling of close emotional association **2** : a largely unconscious process whereby an individual models thoughts, feelings, and actions after those attributed to an object that has been incorporated as a mental image — **iden·ti·fy** \ī-'den-tə-,fī\ *vb*

iden·ti·ty \ī-'den-tə-tē\ *n, pl* **-ties** **1** : the distinguishing character or personality of an individual **2** : the relation established by psychological identification

identity crisis *n* : personal psychosocial conflict esp. in adolescence that involves confusion about one's social role and often a sense of loss of continuity to one's personality

ideo·mo·tor \,ī-dē-ə-'mō-tər, ,i-\ *adj* **1** : not reflex but motivated by an idea ⟨∼ action⟩ **2** : of, relating to, or concerned with ideomotor activity

ID₅₀ *symbol* — used for the dose of an infectious organism required to produce infection in 50 percent of the experimental subjects

idio- *comb form* **1** : one's own : personal : separate : distinct ⟨*idio*type⟩ ⟨*idio*syncrasy⟩ **2** : self-produced : arising within ⟨*idio*pathic⟩

id·i·o·cy \'i-dē-ə-sē\ *n, pl* **-cies** *usu offensive* : extreme mental retardation

id·io·path·ic \,i-dē-ə-'pa-thik\ *adj* : arising spontaneously or from an obscure or unknown cause : PRIMARY ⟨∼ epilepsy⟩ ⟨∼ thrombocytopenic purpura⟩ — **id·io·path·i·cal·ly** *adv*

idiopathic hypertension *n* : ESSENTIAL HYPERTENSION

id·io·syn·cra·sy \,i-dē-ə-'siŋ-krə-sē\ *n, pl* **-sies** **1** : a peculiarity of physical or mental constitution or temperament **2** : individual hypersensitiveness (as to a food) — **id·i·o·syn·crat·ic** \ˌi-dē-ō-sin-ˈkra-tik\ *adj*

id·i·ot \ˈi-dē-ət\ *n, usu offensive* : a person affected with extreme mental retardation — **idiot** *adj, usu offensive*

idiot sa·vant \ˈē-ˌdyō-sä-ˈvän⁰\ *n, pl* **idiots savants** *or* **idiot savants** *same or* -ˈvä⁰z\ : a person affected with a mental disability (as autism or mental retardation) who exhibits exceptional skill or brilliance in some limited field (as mathematics or music) — called also *savant*

id·io·type \ˈi-dē-ō-ˌtīp\ *n* : the molecular structure and conformation in the variable region of an antibody that confers its antigenic specificity — compare ALLOTYPE, ISOTYPE — **id·io·typ·ic** \ˌi-dē-ə-ˈti-pik\ *adj*

id·io·ven·tric·u·lar \ˌi-dē-ə-ven-ˈtri-kyə-lər, -vən-\ *adj* : of, relating to, associated with, or arising in the ventricles of the heart independently of the atria

idox·uri·dine \ˌī-ˌdäks-ˈyùr-ə-ˌdēn\ *n* : a drug $C_9H_{11}IN_2O_5$ used to treat keratitis caused by the herpesviruses producing herpes simplex — abbr. *IDU*; called also *iododeoxyuridine, IUDR*

-i·dro·sis \i-ˈdrō-səs\ *n comb form, pl* **-i·dro·ses** \-ˌsēz\ : a specified form of sweating ⟨brom*idrosis*⟩

IDU *abbr* idoxuridine

IF *abbr* interferon

IFN *abbr* interferon

ifos·fa·mide \ī-ˈfäs-fə-ˌmīd\ *n* : a synthetic cyclophosphamide analog $C_7H_{15}Cl_2N_2O_2P$ that is administered by injection for the treatment esp. of testicular cancer

Ig *abbr* immunoglobulin

IgA \ˌī-(ˌ)jē-ˈā\ *n* : a class of antibodies found in external bodily secretions (as saliva, tears, and sweat); *also* : an antibody of this class — called also *immunoglobulin A*

IgD \ˌī-(ˌ)jē-ˈdē\ *n* : a minor class of antibodies that are of undetermined function except as receptors for antigen; *also* : an antibody of this class — called also *immunoglobulin D*

IgE \ˌī-(ˌ)jē-ˈē\ *n* : a class of antibodies that function esp. in allergic reactions; *also* : an antibody of this class — called also *immunoglobulin E*

IGF *abbr* insulin-like growth factor

IGF–1 *abbr* insulin-like growth factor 1

IgG \ˌī-(ˌ)jē-ˈjē\ *n* : a class of antibodies that facilitate the phagocytic destruction of microorganisms foreign to the body, that bind to and activate complement, and that are the only antibodies to cross over the placenta from mother to fetus; *also* : an antibody of this class — called also *immunoglobulin G*

IgM \ˌī-(ˌ)jē-ˈem\ *n* : a class of antibodies of high molecular weight including those appearing early in the immune response to be replaced later by IgG and that are highly efficient in binding complement; *also* : an antibody of this class — called also *immunoglobulin M*

Il *symbol* illinium

IL *abbr* interleukin — often used with an identifying number ⟨*IL-2*⟩ ⟨*IL-6*⟩

il- — see IN-

Ile *abbr* isoleucine

ile- *also* **ileo-** *comb form* **1** : ileum ⟨*ileitis*⟩ **2** : ileal and ⟨*ileocecal*⟩

ilea *pl of* ILEUM

il·e·al \ˈi-lē-əl\ *also* **il·e·ac** \-ˌak\ *adj* : of, relating to, or affecting the ileum

il·e·itis \ˌi-lē-ˈī-təs\ *n, pl* **-it·i·des** \-ˈi-tə-dēz\ : inflammation of the ileum — see REGIONAL ILEITIS

il·eo·anal \ˌi-lē-ō-ˈā-n⁰l\ *adj* : of, relating to, or connecting the ileum and anus

il·eo·ce·cal \ˌi-lē-ō-ˈsē-kəl\ *adj* : of, relating to, or connecting the ileum and cecum

ileocecal valve *n* : the valve formed by two folds of mucous membrane at the opening of the ileum into the large intestine — called also *Bauhin's valve*

il·eo·col·ic \-ˈkō-lik, -ˈkä-\ *adj* : relating to, situated near, or involving the ileum and the colon

ileocolic artery *n* : a branch of the superior mesenteric artery that supplies the terminal part of the ileum and the beginning of the colon

il·eo·co·li·tis \ˌi-lē-ō-kō-ˈlī-təs\ *n* : inflammation of the mucous membrane of the ileum and colon

il·eo·co·los·to·my \-kə-ˈläs-tə-mē\ *n, pl* **-mies** : a surgical operation producing an artificial opening connecting the ileum and colon

il·eo·cyto·plas·ty \-ˈsī-tə-ˌplas-tē\ *n, pl* **-ties** : plastic surgery that involves anastomosing a segment of the ileum to the bladder esp. in order to increase bladder capacity and preserve the function of the kidneys and ureters

il·eo·il·e·al \-ˈi-lē-əl\ *adj* : relating to or involving two different parts of the ileum ⟨an ~ anastomosis⟩

il·eo·proc·tos·to·my \-ˌpräk-ˈtäs-tə-mē\ *n, pl* **-mies** : a surgical operation producing a permanent artificial opening connecting the ileum and rectum

il·e·os·to·my \ˌi-lē-ˈäs-tə-mē\ *n, pl* **-mies 1** : surgical formation of an artificial anus by connecting the ileum to an opening in the abdominal wall **2** : the artificial opening made by ileostomy

ileostomy bag *n* : a container designed to receive feces discharged through an ileostomy

Iletin \ˈī-lə-tən\ *trademark* — used for a preparation of insulin

il·e·um \ˈi-lē-əm\ *n, pl* **il·ea** \-lē-ə\ : the last portion of the small intestine extending between the jejunum and large intestine

il·e·us \'i-lē-əs\ *n* : obstruction of the bowel; *specif* : a condition that is commonly marked by a painful distended abdomen, vomiting of dark or fecal matter, toxemia, and dehydration and that results when the intestinal contents back up because peristalsis fails although the lumen is not occluded — compare VOLVULUS

ilia *pl of* ILIUM

il·i·ac \'i-lē-‚ak\ *also* **il·i·al** \-əl\ *adj* **1** : of, relating to, or located near the ilium ⟨the ~ bone⟩ **2** : of or relating to either of the lowest lateral abdominal regions

iliac artery *n* **1** : either of the large arteries supplying blood to the lower trunk and hind limbs and arising by bifurcation of the aorta to form one vessel for each side of the body — called also *common iliac artery* **2** : the outer branch of the common iliac artery on either side of the body that becomes the femoral artery — called also *external iliac artery* **3** : the inner branch of the common iliac artery on either side of the body that supplies blood chiefly to the pelvic and gluteal areas — called also *hypogastric artery, internal iliac artery*

iliac crest *n* : the thick curved upper border of the ilium

iliac fossa *n* : the inner concavity of the ilium

iliac node *n* : any of the lymph nodes grouped around the iliac arteries and the iliac veins — see EXTERNAL ILIAC NODE, INTERNAL ILIAC NODE

iliac spine *n* : any of four projections on the ilium: **a** : ANTERIOR INFERIOR ILIAC SPINE **b** : ANTERIOR SUPERIOR ILIAC SPINE **c** : POSTERIOR INFERIOR ILIAC SPINE **d** : POSTERIOR SUPERIOR ILIAC SPINE

ili·a·cus \i-'lī-ə-kəs\ *n, pl* **ili·a·ci** \-ə-‚sī\ : a muscle of the iliac region of the abdomen that flexes the thigh or bends the pelvis and lumbar region forward

iliac vein *n* : any of several veins on each side of the body corresponding to and accompanying the iliac arteries: **a** : either of two veins of which one is formed on each side of the body by the union of the external and internal iliac veins and which unite to form the inferior vena cava — called also *common iliac vein* **b** : a vein that drains the leg and lower part of the anterior abdominal wall, is an upward continuation of the femoral vein, and unites with the internal iliac vein — called also *external iliac vein* **c** : a vein that drains the pelvis and gluteal and perineal regions and that unites with the external iliac vein to form the common iliac vein — called also *hypogastric vein, internal iliac vein*

ilio- *comb form* : iliac and ⟨*ilio*inguinal⟩

il·io·coc·cy·geus \‚i-lē-ō-käk-'si-jəs, -jē-əs\ *n* : a muscle of the pelvis that is

a subdivision of the levator ani and helps support the pelvic viscera — compare PUBOCOCCYGEUS

il·io·cos·ta·lis \-käs-'tā-ləs\ *n* : the lateral division of the sacrospinalis muscle that helps to keep the trunk erect and consists of three parts: **a** : ILIOCOSTALIS CERVICIS **b** : ILIOCOSTALIS LUMBORUM **c** : ILIOCOSTALIS THORACIS

iliocostalis cer·vi·cis \-'sər-və-səs\ *n* : a muscle that extends from the ribs to the cervical transverse processes and acts to draw the neck to the same side and to elevate the ribs

iliocostalis dor·si \-'dòr-‚sī\ *n* : ILIOCOSTALIS THORACIS

iliocostalis lum·bor·um \-‚ləm-'bòr-əm\ *n* : a muscle that extends from the ilium to the lower ribs and acts to draw the trunk to the same side or to depress the ribs

iliocostalis tho·ra·cis \-thə-'rā-səs\ *n* : a muscle that extends from the lower to the upper ribs and acts to draw the trunk to the same side and to approximate the ribs

il·io·fem·o·ral \‚i-lē-ō-'fe-mə-rəl\ *adj* **1** : of or relating to the ilium and the femur **2** : relating to or involving an iliac vein and a femoral vein

iliofemoral ligament *n* : a ligament that extends from the anterior inferior iliac spine to the intertrochanteric line of the femur and divides below into two branches — called also *Y ligament*

il·io·hy·po·gas·tric nerve \‚i-lē-ō-‚hī-pə-'gas-trik-\ *n* : a branch of the first lumbar nerve distributed to the skin of the lateral part of the buttocks, the skin of the pubic region, and the muscles of the anterolateral abdominal wall

il·io·in·gui·nal \-'iŋ-gwən-ᵊl\ *adj* : of, relating to, or affecting the iliac and inguinal abdominal regions

ilioinguinal nerve *n* : a branch of the first lumbar nerve distributed to the muscles of the anterolateral wall of the abdomen, the skin of the proximal and medial part of the thigh, the base of the penis and the scrotum in the male, and the mons veneris and labia majora in the female

il·io·lum·bar artery \‚i-lē-ō-'ləm-bər-, -‚bär-\ *n* : a branch of the internal iliac artery that supplies muscles in the lumbar region and the iliac fossa

iliolumbar ligament *n* : a ligament connecting the transverse process of the last lumbar vertebra with the iliac crest

il·io·pec·tin·e·al eminence \‚i-lē-ō-pek-'ti-nē-əl-\ *n* : a ridge on the hip bone marking the junction of the ilium and the pubis

iliopectineal line *n* : a line or ridge on the inner surface of the hip bone marking the border between the true and false pelvis

il·io·pso·as \ˌi-lē-ō-ˈsō-əs, -lē-ˈäp-sō-əs\ n : a muscle consisting of the iliacus and psoas major muscles

iliopsoas tendon n : the tendon that is common to the iliacus and psoas major

il·io·tib·i·al \ˌi-lē-ō-ˈti-bē-əl\ adj : of or relating to the ilium and the tibia

iliotibial band n : a fibrous thickening of the fascia lata that extends from the iliac crest down the lateral part of the thigh to the lateral condyle of the tibia and that provides stability to the knee and assists with flexion and extension of the knee — called also *iliotibial tract, IT band*

iliotibial band friction syndrome n : a sports injury that is marked by pain in the lateral part of the knee and results from inflammation of the iliotibial band due to overuse (as in long-distance running) as it slides across the lateral condyle of the femur as the knee is flexed and extended repeatedly — called also *iliotibial band syndrome*

il·i·um \ˈi-lē-əm\ n, pl **il·ia** \-lē-ə\ : the dorsal, upper, and largest one of the three bones composing either lateral half of the pelvis that is broad and expanded above and narrower below where it joins with the ischium and pubis to form part of the acetabulum

¹ill \ˈil\ adj worse \ˈwərs\ also **ill·er; worst** \ˈwərst\ **1** : affected with some ailment : not in good health ⟨incurably ∼⟩ **2** : affected with nausea often to the point of vomiting

²ill n : AILMENT, SICKNESS

ill·ness \ˈil-nəs\ n : an unhealthy condition of body or mind : SICKNESS

il·lu·sion \i-ˈlü-zhən\ n **1** : perception of something objectively existing in such a way as to cause misinterpretation of its actual nature; *esp* : OPTICAL ILLUSION **2** : HALLUCINATION 1 **3** : a pattern capable of reversible perspective

Il·o·sone \ˈi-lə-ˌsōn\ *trademark* — used for a preparation of a salt of erythromycin

Il·o·ty·cin \ˌi-lə-ˈtī-sən\ n : a preparation of erythromycin — formerly a U.S. registered trademark

IM *abbr* **1** internal medicine **2** intramuscular; intramuscularly

im- — see IN-

¹im·age \ˈi-mij\ n : a mental picture or impression of something: as **a** : an idealized conception of a person and esp. a parent that is formed by an infant or child, that is retained in the unconscious, and influences behavior in later life — called also *imago* **b** : the memory of a perception in psychology that is modified by subsequent experience; *also* : the representation of the source of a stimulus on a receptor mechanism

²image vb **im·aged; im·ag·ing 1** : to call up a mental picture of **2** : to create a representation of; *also* : to form an image of

image intensifier n : a device used esp. for diagnosis in radiology that provides a more intense image for a given amount of radiation than can be obtained by the usual fluorometric methods — **image intensification** n

im·ag·ery \ˈi-mij-rē, -mi-jə-\ n, pl **-er·ies** : mental images; *esp* : the products of imagination ⟨psychotic ∼⟩

im·ag·ing n : the action or process of producing an image esp. of a part of the body by radiographic techniques ⟨diagnostic ∼⟩ ⟨cardiac ∼⟩ — see MAGNETIC RESONANCE IMAGING

ima·go \i-ˈmā-(ˌ)gō, -ˈmä-\ n, pl **ima·goes** or **ima·gi·nes** \-ˈmä-gə-ˌnēz, -ˈmä-\ : IMAGE a

im·bal·ance \(ˌ)im-ˈba-ləns\ n : lack of balance : the state of being out of equilibrium or out of proportion: as **a** : loss of parallel relation between the optical axes of the eyes caused by faulty action of the extrinsic muscles and often resulting in diplopia **b** : absence of biological equilibrium ⟨a vitamin ∼⟩ — **im·bal·anced** \-lənst\ adj

im·be·cile \ˈim-bə-səl, -ˌsil\ n, usu offensive : a person affected with moderate mental retardation — **imbecile** or **im·be·cil·ic** \ˌim-bə-ˈsi-lik\ adj, usu offensive — **im·be·cil·i·ty** \ˌim-bə-ˈsi-lə-tē\ n, usu offensive

imbed var of EMBED

im·bri·ca·tion \ˌim-brə-ˈkā-shən\ n : an overlapping esp. of successive layers of tissue in the surgical closure of a wound — **im·bri·cate** \ˈim-brə-ˌkāt\ vb

im·id·az·ole \ˌi-mə-ˈda-ˌzōl\ n **1** : a white crystalline heterocyclic base $C_3H_4N_2$ that is an antimetabolite related to histidine **2** : any of a large class of derivatives of imidazole including histidine and histamine

im·id·az·o·line \ˌi-mə-ˈda-zə-ˌlēn\ n : any of three derivatives $C_3H_6N_2$ of imidazole with adrenergic blocking activity

im·i·no·gly·cin·uria \ˌi-mə-ˌnō-ˌglī-sə-ˈnu̇r-ē-ə, -ˈnyu̇r-\ n : an abnormal inherited condition of the kidney associated esp. with hyperprolinemia and characterized by the presence of proline, hydroxyproline, and glycine in the urine

im·i·pen·em \ˌi-mə-ˈpe-nəm\ n : a semisynthetic beta-lactam $C_{12}H_{17}N_3$-$O_4S \cdot H_2O$ that is derived from an antibiotic produced by a bacterium of the genus *Streptomyces* (*S. cattleya*) and is effective against gram-negative and gram-positive bacteria

imip·ra·mine \i-ˈmi-prə-ˌmēn\ n : a tricyclic antidepressant drug used esp. in the form of its hydrochloride $C_{19}H_{24}N_2 \cdot HCl$ or pamoate $(C_{19}H_{24}N_2)_2$-$C_{23}H_{16}O_6$ — see TOFRANIL

Im·i·trex \ˈi-mə-ˌtreks\ *trademark* — used for a preparation of the succinate of sumatriptan

im·ma·ture \ˌi-mə-ˈtu̇r, -ˈtyu̇r, -ˈchu̇r\ *adj* : lacking complete growth, differentiation, or development — **im·ma·ture·ly** *adv* — **im·ma·tu·ri·ty** \-ˈtu̇r-ə-tē, -ˈtyu̇r-, -ˈchu̇r-\ *n*

im·me·di·ate \i-ˈmē-dē-ət\ *adj* **1** : acting or being without the intervention of another object, cause, or agency : being direct ⟨the ∼ cause of death⟩ **2** : present to the mind independently of other states or factors ⟨∼ awareness⟩

immediate auscultation *n* : auscultation performed without a stethoscope by laying the ear directly against the patient's body

immediate hypersensitivity *n, pl* **-ties** : hypersensitivity in which exposure to an antigen produces an immediate or almost immediate reaction

immersion foot *n* : a painful condition of the feet marked by inflammation and stabbing pain and followed by discoloration, swelling, ulcers, and numbness due to prolonged exposure to moist cold usu. without actual freezing

im·mo·bile \ˌi-ˈmō-bəl, -ˌbēl, -ˌbīl\ *adj* **1** : incapable of being moved **2** : not moving ⟨keep the patient ∼⟩ — **im·mo·bil·i·ty** \ˌi-mō-ˈbi-lə-tē\ *n*

im·mo·bi·lize \i-ˈmō-bə-ˌlīz\ *vb* **-ized; -iz·ing** : to make immobile; *esp* : to fix (as a body part) so as to reduce or eliminate motion usu. by means of a cast or splint, by strapping, or by strict bed rest — **im·mo·bi·li·za·tion** \-ˌmō-bə-lə-ˈzā-shən\ *n*

im·mune \i-ˈmyün\ *adj* **1** : not susceptible or responsive; *esp* : having a high degree of resistance to a disease **2 a** : having or producing antibodies or lymphocytes capable of reacting with a specific antigen ⟨an ∼ serum⟩ **b** : produced by, involved in, or concerned with immunity or an immune response ⟨∼ agglutinins⟩

immune complex *n* : any of various molecular complexes formed in the blood by combination of an antigen and an antibody that tend to accumulate in bodily tissue and are associated with various pathological conditions (as glomerulonephritis and systemic lupus erythematosus)

immune globulin *n* : globulin from the blood of a person or animal immune to a particular disease — called also *immune serum globulin*

immune response *n* : a bodily response to an antigen that occurs when lymphocytes identify the antigenic molecule as foreign and induce the formation of antibodies and lymphocytes capable of reacting with it and rendering it harmless — called also *immune reaction*

immune serum *n* : ANTISERUM

immune system *n* : the bodily system that protects the body from foreign substances, cells, and tissues by producing the immune response and that includes esp. the thymus, spleen, lymph nodes, special deposits of lymphoid tissue (as in the gastrointestinal tract and bone marrow), lymphocytes including the B cells and T cells, and antibodies

immune therapy *n* : IMMUNOTHERAPY

im·mu·ni·ty \i-ˈmyü-nə-tē\ *n, pl* **-ties** : the quality or state of being immune; *esp* : a condition of being able to resist a particular disease esp. through preventing development of a pathogenic microorganism or by counteracting the effects of its products — see ACQUIRED IMMUNITY, ACTIVE IMMUNITY, NATURAL IMMUNITY, PASSIVE IMMUNITY

im·mu·ni·za·tion \ˌi-myə-nə-ˈzā-shən\ *n* : the creation of immunity usu. against a particular disease; *esp* : treatment (as by vaccination) of an organism for the purpose of making it immune to a particular pathogen — **im·mu·nize** \ˈi-myə-ˌnīz\ *vb*

immuno- *comb form* **1** : physiological immunity ⟨*immuno*logy⟩ **2** : immunologic ⟨*immuno*chemistry⟩ : immunologically ⟨*immuno*compromised⟩ : immunology and ⟨*immuno*genetics⟩

im·mu·no·ad·sor·bent \ˌi-myə-nō-ad-ˈsȯr-bənt, i-ˌmyü-nō-, -ˈzȯr-\ *n* : IMMUNOSORBENT — **immunoadsorbent** *adj*

im·mu·no·as·say \ˈi-myə-nō-ˈas-ˌā, -a-ˈsā\ *n* : a technique or test (as the enzyme-linked immunosorbent assay) used to detect the presence or quantity of a substance (as a protein) based on its capacity to act as an antigen or antibody — **immunoassay** *vb* — **im·mu·no·as·say·able** \-a-ˈsā-ə-bəl\ *adj*

im·mu·no·bi·ol·o·gy \-bī-ˈä-lə-jē\ *n, pl* **-gies** : a branch of biology concerned with the physiological reactions characteristic of the immune state — **im·mu·no·bi·o·log·i·cal** \-bī-ə-ˈlä-ji-kəl\ *or* **im·mu·no·bi·o·log·ic** \-ˈlä-jik\ *adj* — **im·mu·no·bi·ol·o·gist** \-bī-ˈä-lə-jist\ *n*

im·mu·no·blast \i-ˈmyü-nō-ˌblast, ˈi-myə-nō-\ *n* : a lymphocyte that has enlarged following antigenic stimulation : LYMPHOBLAST

im·mu·no·blas·tic \ˌi-myə-nō-ˈblas-tik, i-ˌmyü-nō-\ *adj* : marked by the proliferation of immunoblasts

immunoblastic lymphadenopathy *n* : ANGIOIMMUNOBLASTIC LYMPHADENOPATHY

im·mu·no·blot \-ˌblät\ *n* : a blot (as a Western blot) in which a radioactively labeled antibody is used as the molecular probe — **im·mu·no·blot·ting** *n*

im·mu·no·chem·is·try \-ˈke-mə-strē\ *n, pl* **-tries** : a branch of chemistry that deals with the chemical aspects of immunology — **im·mu·no·chem·i·cal** \-ˈke-mə-kəl\ *adj* — **im·mu·no·chem·i·cal·ly** *adv* — **im·mu·no·chem·ist** \-ˈke-mist\ *n*

im·mu·no·che·mo·ther·a·py \-ˌkē-mō-

'ther-ə-pē\ *n, pl* **-pies** : the combined use of immunotherapy and chemotherapy in the treatment or control of disease

im·mu·no·com·pe·tence \-'käm-pə-təns\ *n* : the capacity for a normal immune response — **im·mu·no·com·pe·tent** \-tənt\ *adj*

im·mu·no·com·pro·mised \-'käm-prə-ˌmīzd\ *adj* : having the immune system impaired or weakened (as by drugs or illness) ⟨∼ patients⟩

im·mu·no·con·ju·gate \-'kän-ji-gət, -'kän-jə-ˌgät\ *n* : a complex of an antibody and a toxic agent (as a drug) used to kill or destroy a targeted antigen (as a cancer cell)

im·mu·no·cyte \i-'myü-nō-ˌsīt, 'i-myə-nō-\ *n* : a cell (as a lymphocyte) that has an immunologic function

im·mu·no·cy·to·chem·is·try \ˌi-myə-nō-ˌsī-tō-'ke-mə-strē, i-ˌmyü-nō-\ *n, pl* **-tries** : the application of biochemistry to cellular immunology — **im·mu·no·cy·to·chem·i·cal** \-'ke-mi-kəl\ *adj*

im·mu·no·de·fi·cien·cy \-di-'fi-shən-sē\ *n, pl* **-cies** : inability to produce a normal complement of antibodies or immunologically sensitized T cells esp. in response to specific antigens — **im·mu·no·de·fi·cient** \-shənt\ *adj*

im·mu·no·de·pres·sion \-di-'pre-shən\ *n* : IMMUNOSUPPRESSION — **im·mu·no·de·pres·sant** \-di-'pres-ᵊnt\ *n*

im·mu·no·di·ag·no·sis \ˌi-ˌdī-ig-'nō-səs\ *n, pl* **-no·ses** \-ˌsēz\ : diagnosis (as of cancer) by immunological methods — **im·mu·no·di·ag·nos·tic** \-'näs-tik\ *adj*

im·mu·no·dif·fu·sion \-di-'fyü-zhən\ *n* : any of several techniques for obtaining a precipitate between an antibody and its specific antigen by suspending one in a gel and letting the other migrate through it from a well or by letting both antibody and antigen migrate through the gel from separate wells to form an area of precipitation

im·mu·no·elec·tro·pho·re·sis \-ə-ˌlek-trə-fə-'rē-səs\ *n, pl* **-re·ses** \-ˌsēz\ : electrophoretic separation of proteins followed by identification by the formation of precipitates through specific immunologic reactions — **im·mu·no·elec·tro·pho·ret·ic** \-'re-tik\ *adj* — **im·mu·no·elec·tro·pho·ret·i·cal·ly** *adv*

im·mu·no·flu·o·res·cence \-flȯ-'res-ᵊns, -flü-\ *n* : the labeling of antibodies or antigens with fluorescent dyes esp. for the purpose of demonstrating the presence of a particular antigen or antibody in a tissue preparation or smear — **im·mu·no·flu·o·res·cent** \-ᵊnt\ *adj*

im·mu·no·gen \i-'myü-nə-jən, 'i-myə-nə-, -ˌjen\ *n* : an antigen that provokes an immune response

im·mu·no·ge·net·ics \-jə-'ne-tiks\ *n* : a branch of immunology concerned with the interrelations of heredity, disease, and the immune system and its components (as antibodies) — **im·mu·no·ge·net·ic** \-tik\ *adj* — **im·mu·no·ge·net·i·cal·ly** *adv* — **im·mu·no·ge·net·i·cist** \-jə-'ne-tə-sist\ *n*

im·mu·no·gen·ic \ˌi-myə-nō-'jen-ik, i-ˌmyü-nō-\ *adj* : relating to or producing an immune response ⟨∼ substances⟩ — **im·mu·no·gen·i·cal·ly** *adv* — **im·mu·no·ge·nic·i·ty** \-jə-'ni-sə-tē\ *n*

im·mu·no·glob·u·lin \-'glä-byə-lən\ *n* : ANTIBODY — abbr. *Ig*

immunoglobulin A *n* : IGA
immunoglobulin D *n* : IGD
immunoglobulin E *n* : IGE
immunoglobulin G *n* : IGG
immunoglobulin M *n* : IGM

im·mu·no·he·ma·tol·o·gy \-ˌhē-mə-'tä-lə-jē\ *n, pl* **-gies** : a branch of immunology that deals with the immunologic properties of blood — **im·mu·no·he·ma·to·log·ic** \-ˌhē-mə-tə-'lä-jik\ *or* **im·mu·no·he·ma·to·log·i·cal** \-ji-kəl\ *adj* — **im·mu·no·he·ma·tol·o·gist** \-ˌhē-mə-'tä-lə-jist\ *n*

im·mu·no·his·to·chem·i·cal \-ˌhis-tō-'ke-mi-kəl\ *adj* : of or relating to the application of histochemical and immunologic methods to chemical analysis of tissues and cells — **im·mu·no·his·to·chem·i·cal·ly** *adv* — **im·mu·no·his·to·chem·is·try** \-'ke-mə-strē\ *n*

im·mu·no·his·to·log·i·cal \-ˌhis-tə-'lä-ji-kəl\ *also* **im·mu·no·his·to·log·ic** \-'lä-jik\ *adj* : of or relating to the application of immunologic methods to histology — **im·mu·no·his·tol·o·gy** \-hi-'stä-lə-jē\ *n*

immunological surveillance *n* : IMMUNOSURVEILLANCE

im·mu·nol·o·gist \ˌi-myə-'nä-lə-jist\ *n* : a specialist in immunology

im·mu·nol·o·gy \ˌi-myə-'nä-lə-jē\ *n, pl* **-gies** : a science that deals with the immune system and the cell-mediated and humoral aspects of immunity and immune responses — **im·mu·no·log·ic** \-nə-'lä-jik\ *or* **im·mu·no·log·i·cal** \-ji-kəl\ *adj* — **im·mu·no·log·i·cal·ly** *adv*

im·mu·no·mod·u·lat·ing \ˌi-myə-nō-'mä-jə-ˌlā-tiŋ, i-ˌmyü-nō-\ *adj* : of, relating to, being, or involving an immunomodulator ⟨∼ agents⟩

im·mu·no·mod·u·la·tion \-ˌmä-jə-'lā-shən\ *n* : modification of the immune response or the functioning of the immune system by the action of an immunomodulator

im·mu·no·mod·u·la·tor \ˌi-myə-nō-'mä-jə-ˌlā-tər, i-ˌmyü-nō-\ *n* : a chemical agent (as methotrexate) that modifies the immune response or the functioning of the immune system — **im·mu·no·mod·u·la·to·ry** \-'mä-jə-lə-ˌtōr-ē\ *adj*

im·mu·no·patho·gen·e·sis \-ˌpa-thə-'je-nə-səs\ *n, pl* **-e·ses** \-ˌsēz\ : the development of disease as affected by the immune system — **im·mu·no·path·o·gen·ic** \-'je-nik\ *adj*

im·mu·no·pa·thol·o·gist \-pə-'thä-lə-jist, -pa-\ *n* : a specialist in immunopathology

im·mu·no·pa·thol·o·gy \-pə-'thä-lə-jē, -pa-\ *n, pl* **-gies** 1 : a branch of medicine that deals with immune responses associated with disease 2 : the pathology of an organism, organ system, or disease with respect to the immune system, immunity, and immune responses — **im·mu·no·path·o·log·ic** \-,pa-thə-'lä-jik\ *or* **im·mu·no·path·o·log·i·cal** \-ji-kəl\ *adj*

im·mu·no·phe·no·type \-'fē-nə-,tīp\ *n* : the immunochemical and immunohistological characteristics of a cell or group of cells — **im·mu·no·phe·no·typ·ic** \-,fē-nə-'ti-pik\ *also* **im·mu·no·phe·no·typ·i·cal** \-pi-kəl\ *adj* — **im·mu·no·phe·no·typ·i·cal·ly** \-pi-k(ə-)lē\ *adv*

im·mu·no·phe·no·typ·ing \-'fē-nə-,tī-piŋ\ *n* : the process of determining the immunophenotype of a cell or group of cells

im·mu·no·phil·in \-'fi-lən\ *n* : any of a group of proteins that exhibit high specificity in binding to immunosuppressive agents (as cyclosporine)

im·mu·no·pre·cip·i·ta·tion \-pri-,si-pə-'tā-shən\ *n* : precipitation of a complex of an antibody and its specific antigen — **im·mu·no·pre·cip·i·tate** \-'si-pə-tət, -,tāt\ *n* — **im·mu·no·pre·cip·i·tate** \-,tāt\ *vb*

im·mu·no·pro·lif·er·a·tive \-prə-'li-fə-,rā-tiv\ *adj* : of, relating to, or characterized by the proliferation of lymphocytes and esp. plasma cells ⟨~ disorders⟩

immunoproliferative small intestinal disease *n* : a lymphoma that arises in the small intestine, is marked esp. by abdominal pain, diarrhea, and malabsorption, is associated with the secretion by proliferating plasma cells of truncated IgA heavy chains without the accompanying light chains, and that chiefly affects individuals in Mediterranean regions — abbr. *IPSID*; called also *alpha chain disease, Mediterranean lymphoma*

im·mu·no·pro·phy·lax·is \-,prō-fə-'lak-səs, -,prä-\ *n, pl* **-lax·es** \-,sēz\ : the prevention of disease by the production of active or passive immunity

im·mu·no·ra·dio·met·ric assay \-,rā-dē-ō-'me-trik-\ *n* : immunoassay of a substance by combining it with a radioactively labeled antibody

im·mu·no·re·ac·tive \-rē-'ak-tiv\ *adj* : reacting to particular antigens or haptens ⟨serum ~ insulin⟩ ⟨~ lymphocytes⟩ — **im·mu·no·re·ac·tion** \-'ak-shən\ *n* — **im·mu·no·re·ac·tiv·i·ty** \-(,)rē-,ak-'ti-və-tē\ *n*

im·mu·no·reg·u·la·to·ry \-'re-gyə-lə-,tōr-ē\ *adj* : of or relating to the regulation of the immune system ⟨~ T

cells⟩ — **im·mu·no·reg·u·la·tion** \-,re-gyə-'lā-shən\ *n*

im·mu·no·sor·bent \-'sòr-bənt, -'zòr-\ *adj* : relating to or using a substrate consisting of a specific antibody or antigen chemically combined with an insoluble substance (as cellulose) to selectively remove the corresponding specific antigen or antibody from solution — **immunosorbent** *n*

im·mu·no·stim·u·la·tion \-,sti-myə-'lā-shən\ *n* : stimulation of an immune response — **im·mu·no·stim·u·lant** \-'sti-myə-lənt\ *n or adj* — **im·mu·no·stim·u·la·to·ry** \-'sti-myə-lə-,tōr-ē\ *adj*

im·mu·no·sup·pres·sion \-sə-'pre-shən\ *n* : suppression (as by drugs) of natural immune responses — **im·mu·no·sup·press** \-sə-'pres\ *vb* — **im·mu·no·sup·pres·sant** \-'pres-ə nt\ *n or adj* — **im·mu·no·sup·pres·sive** \-'pre-səv\ *adj*

im·mu·no·sur·veil·lance \-sər-'vā-ləns\ *n* : a monitoring process of the immune system which detects and destroys neoplastic cells and which tends to break down in immunosuppressed individuals — called also *immunological surveillance*

im·mu·no·ther·a·py \-'ther-ə-pē\ *n, pl* **-pies** : treatment of or prophylaxis against disease by attempting to produce active or passive immunity — called also *immune therapy* — **im·mu·no·ther·a·peu·tic** \-,ther-ə-'pyü-tik\ *adj*

im·mu·no·tox·ic·i·ty \-täk-'si-sə-sə-tē\ *n, pl* **-ties** : toxicity to the immune system — **im·mu·no·tox·ic** \-'täk-sik\ *adj*

im·mu·no·tox·i·col·o·gy \-,täk-si-'kä-lə-jē\ *n, pl* **-gies** : the study of the effects of toxic substances on the immune system

im·mu·no·tox·in \-'mye-nō-,täk-sən, i-'myü-nō-\ *n* : a toxin that is linked to a monoclonal antibody and is delivered to only those cells (as cancer cells) targeted by the monoclonal antibody to which it is linked

Imo·di·um \i-'mō-dē-əm\ *trademark* — used for a preparation of the hydrochloride of loperamide

IMP \,ī-(,)em-'pē\ *n* : INOSINIC ACID

im·pact·ed \im-'pak-təd\ *adj* 1 a : blocked by material (as feces) that is firmly packed or wedged in position ⟨an ~ colon⟩ b : wedged or lodged in a bodily passage ⟨an ~ mass of feces⟩ 2 : characterized by broken ends of bone driven together ⟨an ~ fracture⟩ 3 *of a tooth* : wedged between the jawbone and another tooth ⟨an ~ wisdom tooth⟩ — **im·pac·tion** \im-'pak-shən\ *n*

impaction fracture *n* : a fracture that is impacted

im·paired \im-'pard\ *adj* : being in a less than perfect or whole condition: as **a** : disabled or functionally defective — often used in combination ⟨hearing-*impaired*⟩ **b** : intoxicated by alcohol or narcotics ⟨driving while ∼⟩ — **im·pair·ment** \-'par-mənt\ n

im·pal·pa·ble \(ˌ)im-'pal-pə-bəl\ adj : incapable of being felt by touch

im·ped·ance \im-'pēd-ᵊns\ n : opposition to blood flow in the circulatory system

im·ped·i·ment \im-'pe-də-mənt\ n : something that impedes ⟨a hearing ∼⟩; esp : an impairment (as a stutter or a lisp) that interferes with the proper articulation of speech

imperfecta — see AMELOGENESIS IMPERFECTA, OSTEOGENESIS IMPERFECTA, OSTEOGENESIS IMPERFECTA CONGENITA, OSTEOGENESIS IMPERFECTA TARDA

im·per·fect fungus \(ˌ)im-'pər-fikt-\ n : any of various fungi of which only the asexual spore-producing stage is known

im·per·fo·rate \(ˌ)im-'pər-fə-rət, -ˌrāt\ adj : having no opening or aperture; specif : lacking the usual or normal opening ⟨an ∼ hymen⟩ ⟨an ∼ anus⟩

im·pe·ri·al gallon \im-'pir-ē-əl-\ n : GALLON 2

im·per·me·able \(ˌ)im-'pər-mē-ə-bəl\ adj : not permitting passage (as of a fluid) through its substance — **im·per·me·abil·i·ty** \-ˌmē-ə-'bi-lə-tē\ n

im·pe·tig·i·nized \ˌim-pə-'ti-jə-ˌnīzd\ adj : affected with impetigo on top of an underlying dermatologic condition

im·pe·tig·i·nous \ˌim-pə-'ti-jə-nəs\ adj : of, relating to, or resembling impetigo ⟨∼ skin lesions⟩

im·pe·ti·go \ˌim-pə-'tē-(ˌ)gō, -'tī-\ n : an acute contagious staphylococcal or streptococcal skin disease characterized by vesicles, pustules, and yellowish crusts

impetigo con·ta·gi·o·sa \-kən-ˌtā-jē-'ō-sə\ n : IMPETIGO

im·plant \'im-ˌplant\ n : something (as a graft, a small container of radioactive material for treatment of cancer, or a pellet containing hormones to be gradually absorbed) that is implanted esp. in tissue — **im·plant** \im-'plant\ vb — **im·plant·able** \-'plan-tə-bəl\ adj

im·plan·ta·tion \ˌim-ˌplan-'tā-shən\ n : the act or process of implanting or the state of being implanted: as **a** : the placement of a natural or artificial tooth in an artificially prepared socket in the jawbone **b** in placental mammals : the process of attachment of the embryo to the maternal uterine wall — called also nidation **c** : medical treatment by the insertion of an implant

im·plant·ee \ˌim-ˌplan-'tē\ n : the recipient of an implant

im·plan·tol·o·gist \ˌim-ˌplan-'tä-lə-jist\ n : a dentist who specializes in implantology

im·plan·tol·o·gy \-'tä-lə-jē\ n, pl -gies : a branch of dentistry dealing with dental implantation

im·plo·sion therapy \im-'plō-zhən-\ n : IMPLOSIVE THERAPY

im·plo·sive therapy \im-'plō-siv-\ n : exposure therapy in which visualization is utilized by the patient

imported fire ant n : either of two mound-building So. American fire ants of the genus Solenopsis (S. invicta and S. richteri) that have been introduced into the southeastern U.S. and can inflict stings requiring medical attention

im·po·tence \'im-pə-təns\ n **1** : the quality or state of not being potent ⟨the growing ∼ of antibiotics⟩ **2** : an abnormal physical or psychological state of a male characterized by inability to engage in sexual intercourse because of failure to have or maintain an erection — called also erectile dysfunction

im·po·ten·cy \-tən-sē\ n, pl -cies : IMPOTENCE

im·po·tent \'im-pə-tənt\ adj **1** : not potent **2** : unable to engage in sexual intercourse because of inability to have and maintain an erection; broadly : STERILE

im·preg·nate \im-'preg-ˌnāt, 'im-ˌ\ vb -nat·ed; -nat·ing **1 a** : to make pregnant **b** : to introduce sperm cells into : FERTILIZE **2** : to cause to be filled, imbued, permeated, or saturated — **im·preg·na·tion** \(ˌ)im-ˌpreg-'nā-shən\ n

im·pres·sion \im-'pre-shən\ n : an imprint in plastic material of the surfaces of the teeth and adjacent portions of the jaw from which a likeness may be produced in dentistry

im·print·ing \'im-ˌprint-iŋ, im-'\ n **1** : a rapid learning process that takes place early in the life of a social animal and establishes a behavior pattern (as recognition of and attraction to its own kind or a substitute) **2** : GENOMIC IMPRINTING — **imprint** vb

im·pulse \'im-ˌpəls\ n **1** : a wave of excitation transmitted through tissues and esp. nerve fibers and muscles that results in physiological activity or inhibition **2** : a sudden spontaneous inclination or incitement to some usu. unpremeditated action — **im·pul·sive** \im-'pəl-siv\ adj

Im·u·ran \'i-myə-ˌran\ trademark — used for a preparation of azathioprine

in abbr inch

In symbol indium

¹in- or **il-** or **im-** or **ir-** prefix : not — usu. il- before l ⟨illegitimate⟩ and im- before b, m, or p ⟨imbalance⟩ ⟨immobile⟩ ⟨impalpable⟩ and ir- before r ⟨irreducible⟩ and in- before other sounds ⟨inoperable⟩

²in- or **il-** or **im-** or **ir-** prefix : in : within : into : toward : on ⟨irradiation⟩ — usu. il- before l, im- before b, m, or p, ir- before r, and in- before other sounds

-in \ən,ᵊn, ˌin\ n suffix **1 a** : neutral chemical compound ⟨insulin⟩ **b** : enzyme ⟨pancreatin⟩ **c** : antibiotic

⟨penicill*in*⟩ **2** : pharmaceutical product ⟨niac*in*⟩

in·ac·ti·vate \(ˌ)i-'nak-tə-ˌvāt\ *vb* **-vat·ed; -vat·ing** : to make inactive: as **a** : to destroy certain biological activities of (~ the complement of normal serum by heat) **b** : to cause (as an infective agent) to lose disease-producing capacity (~ bacteria) — **in·ac·ti·va·tion** \i-ˌnak-tə-'vā-shən\ *n*

in·ac·tive \i-'nak-tiv\ *adj* : not active: as **a** : marked by deliberate or enforced absence of activity or effort ⟨forced by illness to lead an ~ life⟩ **b** *of a disease* : not progressing or fulminant : QUIESCENT **c** : chemically inert (~ charcoal) **d** : biologically inert esp. because of the loss of some quality (as infectivity or antigenicity) — **in·ac·tiv·i·ty** \i-ˌnak-'ti-və-tē\ *n*

in·ad·e·quate \i-'na-də-kwət\ *adj* : not adequate; *specif* : lacking the capacity for psychological maturity or adequate social adjustment

in·a·ni·tion \i-nə-'ni-shən\ *n* : the exhausted condition that results from lack of food and water

in·ap·pe·tence \i-'na-pə-təns\ *n* : loss or lack of appetite

in·ap·pro·pri·ate \i-ə-'prō-prē-ət\ *adj* : ABNORMAL 1

in·born \'in-'bȯrn\ *adj* : HEREDITARY, INHERITED (~ errors of metabolism)

in·breed·ing \'in-ˌbrē-diŋ\ *n* : the interbreeding of closely related individuals — compare OUTBREEDING — **in·bred** \-ˌbred\ *adj* — **in·breed** \-ˌbrēd\ *vb*

in·ca·pac·i·tant \ˌin-kə-'pa-sə-tənt\ *n* : a chemical or biological agent (as tear gas) used to temporarily incapacitate people or animals (as in a riot)

in·car·cer·at·ed \in-'kär-sə-ˌrā-təd\ *adj, of a hernia* : constricted but not strangulated

in·car·cer·a·tion \in-ˌkär-sə-'rā-shən\ *n* **1** : a confining or state of being confined **2** : abnormal retention or confinement of a body part; *specif* : a constriction of the neck of a hernial sac so that the hernial contents become irreducible

in·cest \'in-ˌsest\ *n* : sexual intercourse between persons so closely related that they are forbidden by law to marry; *also* : the statutory crime of engaging in such sexual intercourse — **in·ces·tu·ous** \in-'ses-chə-wəs\ *adj*

inch \'inch\ *n* : a unit of length equal to 1/36 yard or 2.54 centimeters

in·ci·dence \'in-sə-dəns, -ˌdens\ *n* : rate of occurrence or influence; *esp* : the rate of occurrence of new cases of a particular disease in a population being studied — compare PREVALENCE

in·cip·i·ent \in-'si-pē-ənt\ *adj* : beginning to come into being or to become apparent ⟨the ~ stage of a fever⟩

in·ci·sal \in-'sī-zəl\ *adj* : relating to, being, or involving the cutting edge or surface of a tooth (as an incisor)

in·cise \in-'sīz, -'sīs\ *vb* **in·cised; in·cis·ing** : to cut into : make an incision in ⟨*incised* the swollen tissue⟩

incised *adj, of a cut or wound* : made with or as if with a sharp knife or scalpel : clean and well-defined

in·ci·sion \in-'si-zhən\ *n* **1** : a cut or wound of body tissue made esp. in surgery **2** : an act of incising something — **in·ci·sion·al** \-zhə-nəl\ *adj*

in·ci·sive \in-'sī-siv\ *adj* : INCISAL; *also* : of, relating to, or situated near the incisors

incisive canal *n* : a narrow branched passage that extends from the floor of the nasal cavity to the incisive fossa and transmits the nasopalatine nerve and a branch of the greater palatine artery

incisive fossa *n* : a depression on the front of the maxillary bone above the incisor teeth

in·ci·sor \in-'sī-zər\ *n* : a front tooth adapted for cutting; *esp* : any of the eight cutting human teeth that are located between the canines with four in the lower and four in the upper jaw

in·ci·su·ra \ˌin-ˌsī-'zhu̇r-ə, -sə-\ *n, pl* **in·ci·su·rae** \-ˌē, -ˌī\ **1** : a notch, cleft, or fissure of a body part or organ **2** : a downward notch in the curve recording aortic blood pressure that occurs between systole and diastole and is caused by backward flow of blood for a short time before the aortic valve closes

incisura an·gu·lar·is \-ˌaŋ-gyə-'lar-əs\ *n* : a notch or bend in the lesser curvature of the stomach near its pyloric end

in·cli·na·tion \ˌin-klə-'nā-shən\ *n* : a deviation from the true vertical or horizontal; *esp* : the deviation of the long axis of a tooth or of the slope of a cusp from the vertical

in·clu·sion \in-'klü-zhən\ *n* : something that is included; *esp* : a passive usu. temporary product of cell activity (as a starch grain) within the cytoplasm or nucleus

inclusion blennorrhea *n* : INCLUSION CONJUNCTIVITIS

inclusion body *n* : an inclusion, abnormal structure, or foreign cell within a cell; *specif* : an intracellular body that is characteristic of some virus diseases and that is the site of virus multiplication

inclusion body myositis *n* : an inflammatory muscle disease of unknown cause that is marked physically by slowly progressive muscle weakness and atrophy esp. of the limbs and histologically by abnormal inclusions (as vacuoles, amyloid deposits, or T cell infiltrates) in muscle fibers

inclusion conjunctivitis *n* : an infectious disease esp. of newborn infants characterized by acute conjunctivitis and the presence of large inclusion bodies and caused by a chlamydia (*C. trachomatis*)

in·clu·sion disease *n* : CYTOMEGALIC INCLUSION DISEASE

in·co·her·ent \ˌin-kō-ˈhir-ənt, -ˈher-\ *adj* : lacking clarity or intelligibility usu. by reason of some emotional stress ⟨∼ speech⟩ — **in·co·her·ence** \-əns\ *n* — **in·co·her·ent·ly** *adv*

in·com·pat·i·ble \ˌin-kəm-ˈpa-tə-bəl\ *adj* **1** : unsuitable for use together because of chemical interaction or antagonistic physiological effects ⟨∼ drugs⟩ **2** *of blood or serum* : unsuitable for use in a particular transfusion because of the presence of agglutinins that act against the recipient's red blood cells — **in·com·pat·i·bil·i·ty** \-ˌpa-tə-ˈbi-lə-tē\ *n*

in·com·pe·tence \in-ˈkäm-pə-təns\ *n* **1** : lack of legal qualification **2** : inability of an organ or part to perform its function adequately ⟨venous ∼⟩ — **in·com·pe·tent** \-tənt\ *adj*

in·com·pe·ten·cy \-tən-sē\ *n, pl* **-cies** : INCOMPETENCE

in·com·plete \ˌin-kəm-ˈplēt\ *adj* **1** *of insect metamorphosis* : having no pupal stage between the immature stages and the adult with the young insect usu. resembling the adult — compare COMPLETE 1 **2** *of a bone fracture* : not broken entirely across — compare COMPLETE 2

incomplete dominance *n* : the property of being expressed or inherited as a semidominant gene or trait

in·con·stant \in-ˈkän-stənt\ *adj* : not always present ⟨an ∼ muscle⟩

in·con·ti·nence \in-ˈkänt-ᵊn-əns\ *n* **1** : inability or failure to restrain sexual appetite **2** : inability of the body to control the evacuative functions — see STRESS INCONTINENCE, URGE INCONTINENCE — **in·con·ti·nent** \-ənt\ *adj*

in·co·or·di·na·tion \ˌin-kō-ˌȯrd-ᵊn-ˈā-shən\ *n* : lack of coordination esp. of muscular movements resulting from loss of voluntary control

in·cre·men·tal lines \ˌin-krə-ˈment-ᵊl-, ˌin-\ *n pl* : lines seen in a tooth in section showing the periodic depositions of dentin, enamel, and cementum occurring during growth

incremental lines of Ret·zi·us \-ˈret-sē-əs\ *n pl* : incremental lines in the enamel of a tooth

    Retzius, Magnus Gustaf (1842–1919), Swedish anatomist and anthropologist.

in·crus·ta·tion \ˌin-ˌkrəs-ˈtā-shən\ *or* **en·crus·ta·tion** \ˌen-\ *n* **1** : the act of encrusting : the state of being encrusted **2** : a crust or hard coating

in·cu·bate \ˈin-kyə-ˌbāt, ˈin-\ *vb* **-bat·ed; -bat·ing 1** : to maintain (as embryos or bacteria) under conditions favorable for hatching or development **2** : to undergo incubation

in·cu·ba·tion \ˌin-kyə-ˈbā-shən, ˌin-\ *n* **1** : the act or process of incubating **2** : INCUBATION PERIOD

incubation period *n* : the period between the infection of an individual by a pathogen and the manifestation of the disease it causes

in·cu·ba·tor \ˈin-kyə-ˌbā-tər, ˈin-\ *n* : one that incubates; *esp* : an apparatus with a chamber used to provide controlled environmental conditions esp. for the cultivation of microorganisms or the care and protection of premature or sick babies

in·cur·able \in-ˈkyu̇r-ə-bəl\ *adj* : impossible to cure ⟨∼ diseases⟩ — **in·cur·ably** \-blē\ *adv*

in·cus \ˈiŋ-kəs\ *n, pl* **in·cu·des** \iŋ-ˈkyü-(ˌ)dēz, ˈiŋ-kyə-ˌdēz\ : the middle bone of a chain of three small bones in the middle ear — called also *anvil*

IND \ˌī-(ˌ)en-ˈdē\ *abbr* investigational new drug

in·dane·di·one \ˌin-dān-ˈdī-ˌōn\ *or* **in·dan·di·one** \ˌin-dan-\ *n* : any of a group of synthetic anticoagulants

indecent assault *n* : an offensive sexual act or series of acts exclusive of rape committed against another person without consent

indecent exposure *n* : intentional exposure of part of one's body (as the genitalia) in a place where such exposure is likely to be an offense against the generally accepted standards of decency in a community

independent assortment *n* : formation of random combinations of chromosomes in meiosis and of genes on different pairs of homologous chromosomes by the passage at random of one of each diploid pair of homologous chromosomes into each gamete independently of each other pair

independent practice association *n* : an organization providing health care by doctors who maintain their own offices and continue to see their own patients but agree to treat enrolled members of the organization for a negotiated lump sum payment or a fixed payment per member or per service provided — abbr. *IPA*

In·der·al \ˈin-də-ˌral\ *trademark* — used for a preparation of the hydrochloride of propranolol

in·de·ter·mi·nate \ˌin-di-ˈtər-mə-nət\ *adj* : relating to, being, or undergoing indeterminate cleavage ⟨an ∼ egg⟩

indeterminate cleavage *n* : cleavage in which all the early divisions produce blastomeres with the potencies of the entire zygote — compare DETERMINATE CLEAVAGE

in·dex \ˈin-ˌdeks\ *n, pl* **in·dex·es** *or* **in·di·ces** \-də-ˌsēz\ **1** : a number (as a ratio) derived from a series of observations and used as an indicator or measure (as of a condition, property, or phenomenon) **2** : the ratio of one dimension of a thing (as an anatomical structure) to another dimension — see CEPHALIC INDEX, CRANIAL INDEX

index case *n* **1** : an instance of a disease or a genetically determined condition that is discovered first and leads to the discovery of others in a family or group **2** : INDEX PATIENT

index finger *n* : the finger next to the thumb — called also *forefinger*

index of refraction *n* : the ratio of the speed of radiation (as light) in one medium to that in another medium — called also *refractive index*

index patient *n* : a patient whose disease or condition provides an index case — called also *index case-patient*

Indian hemp *n* : HEMP 1

indica — see CANNABIS INDICA

in·di·can \'in-də-ˌkan\ *n* : an indigo-forming substance $C_8H_7NO_4S$ found as a salt in urine and other animal fluids; *also* : its potassium salt C_8H_6-KNO_4S

in·di·cate \'in-də-ˌkāt\ *vb* **-cat·ed; -cat·ing 1** : to be a fairly certain symptom of : show the presence or existence of **2** : to call for esp. as treatment for a particular condition ⟨radical surgery is *indicated*⟩

in·di·ca·tion \ˌin-də-'kā-shən\ *n* **1** : a symptom or particular circumstance that indicates the advisability or necessity of a specific medical treatment or procedure **2** : something that is indicated as advisable or necessary

in·di·ca·tor \'in-də-ˌkā-tər\ *n* : a substance (as a dye) used to show visually (as by change of color) the condition of a solution with respect to the presence of a particular material (as a free acid or alkali)

indices *pl of* INDEX

indicis — see EXTENSOR INDICIS, EXTENSOR INDICIS PROPRIUS

in·dig·e·nous \in-'di-jə-nəs\ *adj* : having originated in and being produced, growing, or living naturally in a particular region or environment ⟨a disease ~ to the tropics⟩

in·di·gest·ible \ˌin-(ˌ)dī-'jes-tə-bəl, -də-\ *adj* : not digestible : not easily digested ⟨~ fiber⟩ — **in·di·gest·ibil·ity** \-ˌjes-tə-'bi-lə-tē\ *n*

in·di·ges·tion \-'jes-chən\ *n* **1** : inability to digest or difficulty in digesting food : incomplete or imperfect digestion of food **2** : a case or attack of indigestion marked esp. by pain, discomfort, or a burning sensation in the upper abdomen often accompanied by abdominal bloating, nausea, belching, flatulence, or uncomfortable fullness

in·di·go car·mine \'in-di-ˌgō-'kär-mən, -ˌmīn\ *n* : a soluble blue dye $C_{16}H_8$-$N_2Na_2O_8S_2$ that is used chiefly as a biological stain and food color and since it is rapidly excreted by the kidneys is used as a dye to mark ureteral structures (as in cystoscopy and catheterization)

in·din·a·vir \in-'di-nə-ˌvir\ *n* : a protease inhibitor used in the form of its sulfate $C_{36}H_{47}N_5O_4·H_2SO_4$ in combination therapy with antiretroviral

drugs (as lamivudine) to treat HIV infection — see CRIXIVAN

in·dis·posed \ˌin-di-'spōzd\ *adj* : being usu. temporarily in poor physical health : slightly ill — **in·dis·po·si·tion** \(ˌ)in-ˌdis-pə-'zi-shən\ *n*

in·di·um \'in-dē-əm\ *n* : a malleable fusible silvery metallic element — symbol *In*; see ELEMENT table

individual psychology *n* : a modification of psychoanalysis developed by the Austrian psychologist Alfred Adler emphasizing feelings of inferiority and a desire for power as the primary motivating forces in human behavior

in·di·vid·u·a·tion \ˌin-də-ˌvi-jə-'wā-shən\ *n* : the process in the analytic psychology of C. G. Jung by which the self is formed by integrating elements of the conscious and unconscious mind — **in·di·vid·u·ate** \-'vi-jə-ˌwāt\ *vb*

In·do·cin \'in-də-sən\ *trademark* — used for a preparation of indomethacin

in·do·cy·a·nine green \ˌin-dō-'sī-ə-ˌnēn-, -nən-\ *n* : a green dye $C_{43}H_{47}$-$N_2NaO_6S_2$ used esp. in testing liver blood flow and cardiac output

in·dole \'in-ˌdōl\ *n* : a crystalline compound C_8H_7N that is found in the intestines and feces as a decomposition product of proteins containing tryptophan; *also* : a derivative of indole

in·dole·ace·tic acid \ˌin-ˌdō-lə-ˌsē-tik-\ *n* : a compound $C_{10}H_9NO_2$ formed from tryptophan in plants and animals that is present in small amounts in normal urine and acts as a growth hormone in plants

in·do·lent \'in-də-lənt\ *adj* **1** : causing little or no pain ⟨an ~ tumor⟩ **2 a** : growing or progressing slowly ⟨an ~ disease⟩ **b** : slow to heal ⟨an ~ ulcer⟩ — **in·do·lence** \-ləns\ *n*

in·do·meth·a·cin \ˌin-dō-'me-thə-sən\ *n* : an NSAID $C_{19}H_{16}ClNO_4$ with analgesic and antipyretic properties used esp. to treat painful inflammatory conditions (as rheumatoid arthritis and osteoarthritis) — see INDOCIN

in·duce \in-'düs, -'dyüs\ *vb* **in·duced; in·duc·ing 1** : to cause or bring about: as **a** : to cause to form through embryonic induction **b** : to cause or initiate by artificial means ⟨*induced* labor⟩ **2** : to produce anesthesia in

in·duc·er \-'dü-sər, -'dyü-\ *n* : one that induces; *specif* : a substance capable of activating the transcription of a gene by combining with and inactivating a genetic repressor

in·duc·ible \in-'dü-sə-bəl, -'dyü-\ *adj* : capable of being formed, activated, or expressed in response to a stimulus esp. of a molecular kind ⟨~ enzymes⟩ — **in·duc·ibil·i·ty** \in-ˌdü-sə-'bi-lə-tē, -ˌdyü-\ *n*

in·duc·tion \in-'dək-shən\ *n* **1** : the act of causing or bringing on or about ⟨~ of labor⟩; *specif* : the establishment of the initial state of anesthesia often with an agent other than that used subsequently to maintain the anesthetic state **2 a** : arousal of a part or area (as of the retina) by stimulation of an adjacent part or area **b** : the sum of the processes by which the fate of embryonic cells is determined and differentiation brought about — **in·duct** \in-'dəkt\ *vb* — **in·duc·tive** \in-'dək-tiv\ *adj* — **in·duc·tive·ly** *adv*

induction chemotherapy *n* : chemotherapy usu. with high doses of anticancer drugs in the initial treatment esp. of advanced cancers in order to make subsequent treatment (as surgery or radiotherapy) more effective

in·duc·tor \in-'dək-tər\ *n* : one that inducts; *esp* : ORGANIZER

in·du·rat·ed \'in-dü-₁rā-təd, -dyü-\ *adj* : having become firm or hard esp. by increase of fibrous elements ⟨∼ tissue⟩ ⟨an ulcer with an ∼ border⟩

in·du·ra·tion \₁in-dü-'rā-shən, -dyü-\ *n* **1** : an increase in the fibrous elements in tissue commonly associated with inflammation and marked by loss of elasticity and pliability : SCLEROSIS **2** : a hardened mass or formation — **in·du·ra·tive** \'in-dü-₁rā-tiv, -dyü-; in-'dür-ə-tiv, -'dyür-\ *adj*

in·du·si·um gris·e·um \in-'dü-zē-əm-'gri-zē-əm, -'dyü-, -zhē-\ *n* : a thin layer of gray matter over the dorsal surface of the corpus callosum

industrial disease *n* : OCCUPATIONAL DISEASE

industrial hygiene *n* : a science concerned with the protection and improvement of the health and well-being of workers in their vocational environment — **industrial hygienist** *n*

industrial psychologist *n* : a psychologist who specializes in workplace problems and issues (as employee satisfaction and motivation)

in·dwell·ing \'in-₁dwe-liŋ\ *adj* : left within a bodily organ or passage to maintain drainage, prevent obstruction, or provide a route for administration of food or drugs — used of an implanted tube (as a catheter)

in·elas·tic \₁i-nə-'las-tik\ *adj* : not elastic

in·ert \i-'nərt\ *adj* **1** : lacking the power to move **2** : deficient in active properties; *esp* : lacking a usual or anticipated chemical or biological action ⟨an ∼ drug⟩ — **in·ert·ness** *n*

inert gas *n* : NOBLE GAS

in·er·tia \i-'nər-shə\ *n* : lack of activity or movement — used esp. of the uterus in labor when its contractions are weak or irregular

in ex·tre·mis \₁in-ik-'strē-məs, -'strā-\ *adv* : at the point of death

in·fan·cy \'in-fən-sē\ *n*, *pl* **-cies 1** : early childhood **2** : the legal status of an infant

in·fant \'in-fənt\ *n* **1 a** : a child in the first year of life : BABY **b** : a child several years of age **2** : a person who is not of full age : MINOR — **infant** *adj*

in·fan·ti·cide \in-'fan-tə-₁sīd\ *n* : the killing of an infant — **in·fan·ti·ci·dal** \-₁fan-tə-'sīd-⁰l\ *adj*

in·fan·tile \'in-fən-₁tīl, -₁tēl, -(₁)til\ *adj* **1** : of, relating to, or occurring in infants or infancy ⟨∼ eczema⟩ **2** : suitable to or characteristic of an infant; *esp* : very immature

infantile amaurotic idiocy *n* **1** : TAY-SACHS DISEASE **2** : SANDHOFF'S DISEASE

infantile autism *n* : a severe autism that first occurs before 30 months of age — called also *Kanner's syndrome*

infantile paralysis *n* : POLIOMYELITIS

infantile scurvy *n* : acute scurvy during infancy caused by malnutrition — called also *Barlow's disease*

in·fan·til·ism \'in-fən-₁tī-₁li-zəm, -tə-; in-'fant-⁰l-₁i-\ *n* : retention of childish physical, mental, or emotional qualities in adult life; *esp* : failure to attain sexual maturity

infantum — see ROSEOLA INFANTUM

in·farct \'in-₁färkt, in-'\ *n* : an area of necrosis in a tissue or organ resulting from obstruction of the local circulation by a thrombus or embolus — **in·farct·ed** \in-'färk-təd\ *adj*

in·farc·tion \in-'färk-shən\ *n* **1** : the process of forming an infarct **2** : INFARCT

in·fect \in-'fekt\ *vb* **1** : to contaminate with a disease-producing substance or agent (as bacteria) **2 a** : to communicate a pathogen or a disease to **b** *of a pathogenic organism* : to invade (an individual or organ) usu. by penetration — compare INFEST

in·fec·tant \in-'fek-tənt\ *n* : an agent of infection (as a bacterium or virus)

in·fec·tion \in-'fek-shən\ *n* **1** : an infective agent or material contaminated with an infective agent **2 a** : the state produced by the establishment of an infective agent in or on a suitable host **b** : a disease resulting from infection : INFECTIOUS DISEASE **3** : an act or process of infecting; *also* : the establishment of a pathogen in its host after invasion

infection stone *n* : a kidney stone composed of struvite

infectiosum — see ERYTHEMA INFECTIOSUM

in·fec·tious \in-'fek-shəs\ *adj* **1** : capable of causing infection **2** : communicable by invasion of the body of a susceptible organism — compare CONTAGIOUS 1 — **in·fec·tious·ly** *adv* — **in·fec·tious·ness** *n*

infectious abortion *n* : CONTAGIOUS ABORTION

infectious anemia *n* **1** : EQUINE INFECTIOUS ANEMIA **2** : FELINE INFECTIOUS ANEMIA

infectious bovine rhinotracheitis *n* : a highly contagious disease of cattle caused by a herpesvirus of the genus

Varicellovirus (species *Bovine herpesvirus 1*) and characterized esp. by fever and by inflammation and ulceration of the nasal cavities and trachea

infectious coryza *n* : an acute infectious respiratory disease of chickens that is caused by a bacterium of the genus *Haemophilus* (*H. paragallinarum* syn. *H. gallinarum*)

infectious disease *n* : a disease caused by the entrance into the body of organisms (as bacteria) which grow and multiply there — see COMMUNICABLE DISEASE, CONTAGIOUS DISEASE

infectious enterohepatitis *n* : BLACKHEAD 2

infectious hepatitis *n* : HEPATITIS A

infectious jaundice *n* **1** : HEPATITIS A **2** : WEIL'S DISEASE

infectious laryngotracheitis *n* : a severe highly contagious and often fatal respiratory disease of chickens and pheasants that is caused by a herpesvirus (species *Gallid herpesvirus 1* of the genus *Iltovirus*)

infectious mononucleosis *n* : an acute infectious disease associated with Epstein-Barr virus and characterized by fever, swelling of lymph nodes, and lymphocytosis — called also *glandular fever, kissing disease, mono*

in·fec·tive \in-ˈfek-tiv\ *adj* : producing or capable of producing infection : INFECTIOUS

in·fec·tiv·i·ty \ˌin-ˌfek-ˈti-və-tē\ *n, pl* **-ties** : the quality of being infective : the ability to produce infection; *specif* : a tendency to spread rapidly from host to host — compare VIRULENCE b

in·fec·tor \in-ˈfek-tər\ *n* : one that infects

in·fe·ri·or \in-ˈfir-ē-ər\ *adj* **1** : situated below and closer to the feet than another and esp. another similar part of an upright body esp. of a human being — compare SUPERIOR 1 **2** : situated in a more posterior or ventral position in the body of a quadruped — compare SUPERIOR 2

inferior alveolar artery *n* : a branch of the maxillary artery that is distributed to the mucous membrane of the mouth and to the teeth of the lower jaw — called also *mandibular artery, inferior dental artery*

inferior alveolar nerve *n* : a branch of the mandibular nerve that is distributed to the teeth of the lower jaw and to the skin of the chin and the skin and mucous membrane of the lower lip — called also *inferior alveolar, inferior dental nerve*

inferior alveolar vein *n* : a vein that accompanies the inferior alveolar artery and drains the lower jaw and lower teeth

inferior articular process *n* : ARTICULAR PROCESS b

inferior cerebellar peduncle *n* : CEREBELLAR PEDUNCLE c

inferior colliculus *n* : either member of the posterior and lower pair of corpora quadrigemina that are situated next to the pons and together constitute one of the lower centers for hearing — compare SUPERIOR COLLICULUS

inferior concha *n* : NASAL CONCHA a

inferior constrictor *n* : a muscle of the pharynx that acts to constrict part of the pharynx in swallowing — called also *constrictor pharyngis inferior, inferior pharyngeal constrictor muscle;* compare MIDDLE CONSTRICTOR, SUPERIOR CONSTRICTOR

inferior dental artery *n* : INFERIOR ALVEOLAR ARTERY

inferior dental nerve *n* : INFERIOR ALVEOLAR NERVE

inferior extensor retinaculum *n* : EXTENSOR RETINACULUM 1a

inferior ganglion *n* **1** : the lower and larger of the two sensory ganglia of the glossopharyngeal nerve — called also *petrosal ganglion;* compare SUPERIOR GANGLION 1 **2** : the lower of the two ganglia of the vagus nerve that forms a swelling just beyond the exit of the nerve from the jugular foramen — called also *inferior vagal ganglion, nodose ganglion;* compare SUPERIOR GANGLION 2

inferior gluteal artery *n* : GLUTEAL ARTERY b

inferior gluteal nerve *n* : GLUTEAL NERVE b

inferior hemorrhoidal artery *n* : RECTAL ARTERY a

inferior hemorrhoidal vein *n* : RECTAL VEIN a

inferior horn *n* : the cornu in the lateral ventricle of each cerebral hemisphere that curves downward into the temporal lobe — compare ANTERIOR HORN 2, POSTERIOR HORN 2

in·fe·ri·or·i·ty \(ˌ)in-ˌfir-ē-ˈôr-ə-tē, -ˈär-\ *n, pl* **-ties** : a condition or state of being inferior or having a sense of being inferior or inadequate esp. with respect to one's apparent equals or to the world at large

inferiority complex *n* : an acute sense of personal inferiority resulting either in timidity or through overcompensation in exaggerated aggressiveness

inferior laryngeal artery *n* : LARYNGEAL ARTERY a

inferior laryngeal nerve *n* **1** : LARYNGEAL NERVE b — called also *inferior laryngeal* **2** : any of the terminal branches of the inferior laryngeal nerve

inferior longitudinal fasciculus *n* : a band of association fibers in each cerebral hemisphere that connects the occipital and temporal lobes

in·fe·ri·or·ly *adv* : in a lower position

inferior maxillary bone *n* : JAW 1b

inferior maxillary nerve *n* : MANDIBULAR NERVE

inferior meatus *n* : a space extending along the lateral wall of the nasal cavity between the inferior nasal concha and the floor of the nasal cavity — compare MIDDLE MEATUS, SUPERIOR MEATUS

inferior mesenteric artery *n* : MESENTERIC ARTERY a

inferior mesenteric ganglion *n* : MESENTERIC GANGLION a

inferior mesenteric plexus *n* : MESENTERIC PLEXUS a

inferior mesenteric vein *n* : MESENTERIC VEIN a

inferior nasal concha *n* : NASAL CONCHA a

inferior nuchal line *n* : NUCHAL LINE c

inferior oblique *n* : OBLIQUE b(2)

inferior olive *n* : a large gray nucleus that forms the interior of the olive on each side of the medulla oblongata — called also *inferior olivary nucleus;* see ACCESSORY OLIVARY NUCLEUS; compare SUPERIOR OLIVE

inferior ophthalmic vein *n* : OPHTHALMIC VEIN b

inferior orbital fissure *n* : ORBITAL FISSURE b

inferior pancreaticoduodenal artery *n* : PANCREATICODUODENAL ARTERY a

inferior pectoral nerve *n* : PECTORAL NERVE b

inferior peroneal retinaculum *n* : PERONEAL RETINACULUM b

inferior petrosal sinus *n* : PETROSAL SINUS b

inferior pharyngeal constrictor muscle *n* : INFERIOR PHARYNGEAL CONSTRICTOR

inferior phrenic artery *n* : PHRENIC ARTERY b

inferior phrenic vein *n* : PHRENIC VEIN b

inferior radioulnar joint *n* : DISTAL RADIOULNAR JOINT

inferior ramus *n* : RAMUS b(2), c

inferior rectal artery *n* : RECTAL ARTERY a

inferior rectal vein *n* : RECTAL VEIN a

inferior rectus *n* : RECTUS 2d

inferior sagittal sinus *n* : SAGITTAL SINUS b

inferior temporal gyrus *n* : TEMPORAL GYRUS c

inferior thyroarytenoid ligament *n* : VOCAL LIGAMENT

inferior thyroid artery *n* : THYROID ARTERY b

inferior turbinate *n* : NASAL CONCHA a

inferior turbinate bone *also* **inferior tur·bi·nat·ed bone** \-'tər-bə-ˌnā-təd-\ *n* : NASAL CONCHA a

inferior ulnar collateral artery *n* : a small artery that arises from the brachial artery just above the elbow and branches to anastomose with other arteries in the region of the elbow — compare SUPERIOR ULNAR COLLATERAL ARTERY

inferior vagal ganglion *n* : INFERIOR GANGLION 2

inferior vena cava *n* : a vein that is the largest vein in the human body, is formed by the union of the two common iliac veins at the level of the fifth lumbar vertebra, and returns blood to the right atrium of the heart from bodily parts below the diaphragm

inferior vermis *n* : VERMIS 1b

inferior vesical *n* : VESICAL ARTERY b

inferior vesical artery *n* : VESICAL ARTERY b

inferior vestibular nucleus *n* : the one of the four vestibular nuclei on each side of the medulla oblongata that sends fibers down both sides of the spinal cord to synapse with motor neurons of the ventral roots

inferior vocal cords *n pl* : TRUE VOCAL CORDS

infero- *comb form* : below and 〈*infero*medial〉

in·fe·ro·me·di·al \ˌin-fə-rō-'mē-dē-əl\ *adj* : situated below and in the middle

in·fe·ro·tem·po·ral \-'tem-p(ə-)rəl\ *adj* 1 : being the inferior part of the temporal lobe of the cerebral cortex; *also* : situated or occurring in, on, or under this part 2 : of, relating to, or being the lower lateral quadrant of the eye or visual field

in·fer·tile \in-'fərt-ᵊl\ *adj* : not fertile : incapable of or unsuccessful in achieving pregnancy over a considerable period of time (as a year) in spite of determined attempts by heterosexual intercourse without contraception — **in·fer·til·i·ty** \ˌin-(ˌ)fər-'til-ə-tē\ *n*

in·fest \in-'fest\ *vb* : to live in or on as a parasite — compare INFECT — **in·fes·tant** \in-'fes-tənt\ *n* — **in·fes·ta·tion** \ˌin-ˌfes-'tā-shən\ *n*

in·fib·u·la·tion \(ˌ)in-ˌfi-byə-'lā-shən\ *n* : an act or practice of fastening by ring, clasp, or stitches the labia majora in girls and the foreskin in boys in order to prevent sexual intercourse

in·fil·trate \in-'fil-ˌtrāt, 'in-(ˌ)fil-\ *n* : something that passes or is caused to pass into or through something by permeating or filtering; *esp* : a substance that passes into the bodily tissues and forms an abnormal accumulation 〈a lung ∼〉 — **infiltrate** *vb* — **in·fil·tra·tion** \ˌin-(ˌ)fil-'trā-shən\ *n* — **in·fil·tra·tive** \'in-fil-ˌtrā-tiv, in-'fil-trə-\ *adj*

infiltration anesthesia *n* : anesthesia of an operative site accomplished by local injection of anesthetics

in·firm \in-'fərm\ *adj* : of poor or deteriorated vitality; *esp* : feeble from age

in·fir·ma·ry \in-'fər-mə-rē\ *n, pl* **-ries** : a place esp. in a school or college for the care and treatment of the sick

in·fir·mi·ty \in-'fər-mə-tē\ *n, pl* **-ties** : the quality or state of being infirm; *esp* : an unsound, unhealthy, or debilitated state

in·flame \in-'flām\ *vb* **in·flamed; in·flam·ing** 1 : to cause inflammation in (bodily tissue) **2** : to become affected with inflammation

in·flam·ma·tion \ˌin-flə-'mā-shən\ *n* : a local response to cellular injury that is marked by capillary dilatation, leukocytic infiltration, redness, heat, pain, swelling, and often loss of function and that serves as a mechanism initiating the elimination of noxious agents and of damaged tissue — **in·flam·ma·to·ry** \in-'fla-mə-ˌtōr-ē\ *adj*

inflammatory bowel disease *n* : either of two inflammatory diseases of the bowel: **a** : CROHN'S DISEASE **b** : ULCERATIVE COLITIS

in·flu·en·za \ˌin-(ˌ)flü-'en-zə\ *n* **1 a** : an acute highly contagious respiratory disease caused by an orthomyxovirus: (1) : INFLUENZA A (2) : INFLUENZA B (3) : INFLUENZA C **b** : any human respiratory infection of undetermined cause — not used technically **2** : any of various febrile virus diseases of domestic animals marked esp. by respiratory symptoms — **in·flu·en·zal** \-zəl\ *adj*

influenza A *n* : moderate to severe influenza that affects humans and some other vertebrates (as birds) sometimes in pandemics following mutation in the causative virus, that in humans is characterized by sudden onset, fever, prostration, severe aches and pains, and progressive inflammation of the respiratory mucous membranes, and that has numerous variants caused by subtypes (as H1N1, H2N2, or H3N2) of an orthomyxovirus (species *Influenza A virus* of the genus *Influenzavirus A*) — see ASIAN FLU, BIRD FLU, HONG KONG FLU, SPANISH FLU, SWINE INFLUENZA

influenza B *n* : influenza that is usu. milder than influenza A, that may occur in epidemics but not pandemics, and that is caused by an orthomyxovirus (species *Influenza B virus* of the genus *Influenzavirus B*) infecting only humans and esp. children

influenza C *n* : influenza that is restricted to humans, that usu. occurs as a subclinical infection, that occurs in neither epidemics or pandemics, and that is caused by an orthomyxovirus (species *Influenza C virus* of the genus *Influenzavirus C*)

influenza vaccine *n* : a vaccine against influenza; *specif* : a mixture of strains of inactivated influenza virus from chick embryo culture

influenza virus *n* : any of the orthomyxoviruses that belong to three genera (*Influenzavirus A, Influenzavirus B,* and *Influenzavirus C*) and that cause influenza A, influenza B, and influenza C in vertebrates

informed consent *n* : consent to surgery by a patient or to participation in a medical experiment by a subject after achieving an understanding of what is involved

infra- *prefix* **1** : below ⟨*infra*hyoid⟩ **2** : below in a scale or series ⟨*infra*red⟩

in·fra·car·di·ac \ˌin-frə-'kär-dē-ˌak\ *adj* : situated below the heart

in·fra·cla·vic·u·lar \ˌin-frə-kla-'vi-kyə-lər\ *adj* : situated or occurring below the clavicle

in·fra·dia·phrag·mat·ic \ˌin-frə-ˌdī-ə-frə-'ma-tik, -ˌfrag-\ *adj* : situated, occurring, or performed below the diaphragm ⟨an ~ abscess⟩

in·fra·gle·noid tubercle \ˌin-frə-'glē-ˌnōid-, -'gle-\ *n* : a tubercle on the scapula for the attachment of the long head of the triceps muscle

in·fra·hy·oid \ˌin-frə-'hī-ˌóid\ *adj* : situated below the hyoid bone

infrahyoid muscle *n* : any of four muscles on each side that are situated next to the larynx and comprise the sternohyoid, sternothyroid, thyrohyoid, and omohyoid muscles

in·fra·mam·ma·ry \ˌin-frə-'ma-mə-rē\ *adj* : situated or occurring below the mammary gland ⟨~ pain⟩

in·fra·or·bit·al \ˌin-frə-'ór-bət-ᵊl\ *adj* : situated beneath the orbit

infraorbital artery *n* : a branch or continuation of the maxillary artery that runs along the infraorbital groove with the infraorbital nerve and passes through the infraorbital foramen to give off branches which supply the face just below the eye

infraorbital fissure *n* : ORBITAL FISSURE B

infraorbital foramen *n* : an opening in the maxillary bone just below the lower rim of the orbit that gives passage to the infraorbital artery, nerve, and vein

infraorbital groove *n* : a groove in the middle of the posterior part of the bony floor of the orbit that gives passage to the infraorbital artery, vein, and nerve

infraorbital nerve *n* : a branch of the maxillary nerve that divides into branches distributed to the skin of the upper part of the cheek, the upper lip, and the lower eyelid

infraorbital vein *n* : a vein that drains the inferior structures of the orbit and the adjacent area of the face and that empties into the pterygoid plexus

in·fra·pa·tel·lar \ˌin-frə-pə-'te-lər\ *adj* : situated below the patella or its ligament

in·fra·red \ˌin-frə-'red\ *adj* **1** : lying outside the visible spectrum at its red end — used of radiation having a wavelength between about 700 nanometers and 1 millimeter **2** : relating to, producing, or employing infrared radiation ⟨~ therapy⟩ — **infrared** *n*

in·fra·re·nal \ˌin-frə-'rēn-ᵊl\ *adj* : situated or occurring below the kidneys

in·fra·spi·na·tus \ˌin-frə-spī-'nā-təs\ *n, pl* **-na·ti** \-'nā-ˌtī\ : a muscle that occupies the chief part of the infraspinous fossa of the scapula and rotates the arm laterally

in·fra·spi·nous \ˌin-frə-'spī-nəs\ *adj* : lying below a spine; *esp* : lying below the spine of the scapula

infraspinous fossa *n* : the part of the dorsal surface of the scapula below the spine of the scapula

in·fra·tem·po·ral \ˌin-frə-'tem-pə-rəl\ *adj* : situated below the temporal fossa

infratemporal crest *n* : a transverse ridge on the outer surface of the greater wing of the sphenoid bone that divides it into a superior portion that contributes to the formation of the temporal fossa and an inferior portion that contributes to the formation of the infratemporal fossa

infratemporal fossa *n* : a fossa that is bounded above by the plane of the zygomatic arch, laterally by the ramus of the mandible, and medially by the pterygoid plate, and that contains the masseter and pterygoid muscles and the mandibular nerve

in·fra·ten·to·ri·al \ˌin-frə-ten-'tōr-ē-əl\ *adj* : occurring or made below the tentorium cerebelli 〈~ burr holes〉

in·fun·dib·u·lar \ˌin-(ˌ)fən-'di-byə-lər\ *adj* : of, relating to, affecting, situated near, or having an infundibulum

infundibular process *n* : NEURAL LOBE

infundibular recess *n* : a funnel-shaped downward prolongation of the floor of the third ventricle of the brain

in·fun·dib·u·lo·pel·vic ligament \ˌin-fən-ˌdi-byə-lō-'pel-vik-\ *n* : SUSPENSORY LIGAMENT OF THE OVARY

in·fun·dib·u·lum \ˌin-(ˌ)fən-'di-byə-ləm\ *n, pl* **-la** \-lə\ : any of various conical or dilated organs or parts: **a** : the hollow conical process of gray matter that constitutes the stalk of the neurohypophysis by which the pituitary gland is continuous with the brain **b** : any of the small spaces having walls with alveoli in which the bronchial tubes terminate in the lungs **c** : CONUS ARTERIOSUS **d** : the abdominal opening of a fallopian tube

in·fu·sion \in-'fyü-zhən\ *n* 1 : the introducing of a solution (as of glucose) esp. into a vein; *also* : the solution so used 2 **a** : the steeping or soaking usu. in water of a substance (as a plant drug) in order to extract its soluble constituents or principles — compare DECOCTION 1 **b** : the liquid extract obtained by this process — **in·fuse** \in-'fyüz\ *vb*

infusion pump *n* : a device that releases a measured amount of a substance in a specific period of time

in·ges·ta \in-'jes-tə\ *n pl* : material taken into the body by way of the digestive tract

in·gest·ible \in-'jes-tə-bəl\ *adj* : capable of being ingested 〈~ capsules〉

in·ges·tion \in-'jes-chən\ *n* : the taking of material (as food) into the digestive system — **in·gest** \-'jest\ *vb* — **in·gest·ive** \in-'jes-tiv\ *adj*

in·grow·ing \'in-ˌgrō-iŋ\ *adj* : INGROWN

in·grown \'in-ˌgrōn\ *adj* : grown in; *specif* : having the normally free tip or edge embedded in the flesh 〈an ~ toenail〉

in·growth \'in-ˌgrōth\ *n* 1 : a growing inward (as to fill a void) 〈~ of cells〉 2 : something that grows in or into a space 〈lymphoid ~s〉

in·gui·nal \'iŋ-gwən-ᵊl\ *adj* 1 : of, relating to, or situated in the region of the groin 2 : ILIAC 2

inguinal canal *n* 1 : a passage in the male through which the testis descends into the scrotum and in which the spermatic cord lies 2 : a passage in the female accommodating the round ligament

inguinale — see GRANULOMA INGUINALE, LYMPHOGRANULOMA INGUINALE

inguinal hernia *n* : a hernia in which part of the intestine protrudes into the inguinal canal

inguinal ligament *n* : the thickened lower border of the aponeurosis of the external oblique muscle of the abdomen — called also *Poupart's ligament*

inguinal node *n* : any of the superficial lymph nodes of the groin

inguinal ring *n* : either of two openings in the fasciae of the abdominal muscles on each side of the body that are the inlet and outlet of the inguinal canal, give passage to the spermatic cord in the male and the round ligament in the female, and are a frequent site of hernia formation: **a** : DEEP INGUINAL RING **b** : SUPERFICIAL INGUINAL RING

INH *abbr* isoniazid

¹**in·hal·ant** *also* **in·hal·ent** \in-'hā-lənt\ *n* 1 : something (as an allergen) that is inhaled 2 : any of various often toxic volatile substances (as spray paint or glue) whose fumes are sometimes inhaled for their euphoric effect

²**inhalant** *also* **inhalent** *adj* : used for inhaling or constituting an inhalant 〈~ anesthetics〉

in·ha·la·tion \ˌin-hə-'lā-shən, ˌin-ᵊl-'ā-\ *n* 1 : the act or an instance of inhaling; *specif* : the action of drawing air into the lungs by means of a complex of essentially reflex actions 2 : material (as medication) to be taken in by inhaling — **in·ha·la·tion·al** \-shə-nəl\ *adj*

inhalation therapist *n* : a specialist in inhalation therapy

inhalation therapy *n* : the therapeutic use of inhaled gases and esp. oxygen (as in the treatment of respiratory disease)

in·ha·la·tor \'in-hə-ˌlā-tər, 'in-ᵊl-ˌā-\ *n* : a device providing a mixture of oxygen and carbon dioxide for breathing that is used esp. in conjunction with artificial respiration

in·hale \in-'hāl\ *vb* **in·haled; in·hal·ing** : to breathe in

in·hal·er \in-'hā-lər\ *n* : a device by means of which usu. medicinal material is inhaled

in·her·it \in-'her-ət\ *vb* : to receive from a parent or ancestor by genetic transmission — **in·her·it·able** \in-'her-ə-tə-bəl\ *adj* — **in·her·it·abil·i·ty** \-,her-ə-tə-'bi-lə-tē\ *n*

in·her·i·tance \in-'her-ə-təns\ *n* **1** : the reception of genetic qualities by transmission from parent to offspring **2** : all the genetic characters or qualities transmitted from parent to offspring

in·hib·in \in-'hi-bən\ *n* : a hormone that is secreted by the pituitary gland and in the male by the Sertoli cells and in the female by the granulosa cells and that inhibits the secretion of follicle-stimulating hormone

in·hib·it \in-'hi-bət\ *vb* **1 a** : to restrain from free or spontaneous activity esp. through the operation of inner psychological or external social constraints **b** : to check or restrain the force or vitality of ⟨∼ aggressive tendencies⟩ **2 a** : to reduce or suppress the activity of ⟨∼ a nerve⟩ **b** : to retard or prevent the formation of **c** : to retard, interfere with, or prevent (a process or reaction) ⟨∼ ovulation⟩ — **in·hib·i·tor** \in-'hi-bə-tər\ *n* — **in·hib·i·to·ry** \in-'hi-bə-,tōr-ē\ *adj*

in·hib·it·able \-bə-tə-bəl\ *adj* : capable of being inhibited

in·hi·bi·tion \,in-hə-'bi-shən, ,i-nə-\ *n* : the act or an instance of inhibiting or the state of being inhibited: as **a** (1) : a restraining of the function of a bodily organ or an agent (as an enzyme) ⟨∼ of the heartbeat⟩ (2) : interference with or retardation or prevention of a process or activity ⟨∼ of bacterial growth⟩ **b** (1) : a desirable restraint or check upon the free or spontaneous instincts or impulses of an individual guided or directed by social and cultural forces (2) : a neurotic restraint upon a normal or beneficial impulse or activity caused by psychological inner conflicts or by sociocultural forces

inhibitory postsynaptic potential *n* : increased negativity of the membrane potential of a neuron on the postsynaptic side of a nerve synapse that is caused by a neurotransmitter and that tends to inhibit the neuron — abbr. *IPSP*

in·i·en·ceph·a·lus \,i-nē-in-'se-fə-ləs\ *n* : a teratological fetus with a fissure in the occiput through which the brain protrudes — **in·i·en·ceph·a·ly** \-lē\ *n*

in·i·on \'i-nē-,än, -ən\ *n* : OCCIPITAL PROTUBERANCE a

initiation codon *n* : a codon that stimulates the binding of a transfer RNA which starts protein synthesis — called also *initiator codon*

ini·ti·a·tor \i-'ni-shē-,ā-tər\ *n* **1** : a substance that initiates a chemical reaction **2** : a substance that produces an irreversible change in bodily tissue causing it to respond to other substances which promote the growth of tumors

in·ject \in-'jekt\ *vb* : to introduce a fluid into (a living body); *also* : to treat (an individual) with injections

¹**in·ject·able** \-'jek-tə-bəl\ *adj* : capable of being injected ⟨∼ medications⟩

²**injectable** *n* : an injectable substance

in·jec·tion \in-'jek-shən\ *n* **1 a** : the act or an instance of injecting a drug or other substance into the body **b** : a solution (as of a drug) intended for injection (as by catheter or hypodermic syringe) either under or through the skin or into the tissues, a vein, or a body cavity **2** : CONGESTION — see CIRCUMCORNEAL INJECTION

in·jure \'in-jər\ *vb* **in·jured; in·jur·ing** **1** : to inflict bodily hurt on **2** : to impair the soundness of — **in·ju·ri·ous** \in-'jùr-ē-əs\ *adj* — **in·ju·ri·ous·ly** *adv*

in·ju·ry \'in-jə-rē\ *n, pl* **-ries** : hurt, damage, or loss sustained

injury potential *n* : the difference in electrical potential between the injured and uninjured parts of a nerve or muscle

inkblot test *n* : any of several psychological tests (as a Rorschach test) based on the interpretation of irregular figures (as blots of ink)

in·lay \'in-,lā\ *n* **1** : a tooth filling shaped to fit a cavity and then cemented into place **2** : a piece of tissue (as bone) laid into the site of missing tissue to cover a defect

in·let \'in-,let, -lət\ *n* : the upper opening of a bodily cavity; *esp* : that of the cavity of the true pelvis bounded by the pelvic brim

in·mate \'in-,māt\ *n* : a person confined (as in a psychiatric hospital) esp. for a long time

in·nards \'i-nərdz\ *n pl* : the internal organs of a human being or animal; *esp* : VISCERA

in·nate \i-'nāt, 'i-,\ *adj* : existing in, belonging to, or determined by factors present in an individual from birth : INBORN ⟨∼ behavior⟩ — **in·nate·ly** *adv* — **in·nate·ness** *n*

innate immunity *n* : NATURAL IMMUNITY

inner cell mass *n* : the portion of the blastocyst of an embryo that is destined to become the embryo proper

inner–directed *adj* : directed in thought and action by one's own scale of values as opposed to external norms — compare OTHER-DIRECTED — **inner-direction** *n*

inner ear *n* : the essential part of the organ of hearing and equilibrium that is typically located in the temporal bone, is innervated by the auditory nerve, and includes the vestibule, the semicircular canals, and the cochlea — called also *internal ear*

in·ner·vate \'i-nər-ˌvāt, 'i-(ˌ)nər-\ *vb* **-vat·ed; -vat·ing 1 :** to supply with nerves **2 :** to arouse or stimulate (a nerve or an organ) to activity — **in·ner·va·tion** \ˌi-(ˌ)nər-'vā-shən, ˌi,nər-\ *n*

in·no·cent \'i-nə-sənt\ *adj* **:** lacking capacity to injure : BENIGN ⟨an ∼ tumor⟩ ⟨∼ heart murmurs⟩

innominata — see SUBSTANTIA INNOMINATA

in·nom·i·nate artery \i-'nä-mə-nət-\ *n* **:** BRACHIOCEPHALIC ARTERY

innominate bone *n* **:** HIP BONE

innominate vein *n* **:** BRACHIOCEPHALIC VEIN

ino- *comb form* **:** fiber : fibrous ⟨*ino*tropic⟩

in·oc·u·lant \i-'nä-kyə-lənt\ *n* **:** INOCULUM

in·oc·u·late \-ˌlāt\ *vb* **-lat·ed; -lat·ing 1 :** to introduce a microorganism or virus into ⟨∼ mice with anthrax⟩ **2 :** to introduce (as a microorganism) into a suitable situation for growth **3 :** to introduce immunologically active material (as an antibody or antigen) into esp. in order to treat or prevent a disease ⟨∼ children against diphtheria⟩

in·oc·u·la·tion \i-ˌnä-kyə-'lā-shən\ *n* **1 :** the act or process or an instance of inoculating: as **a :** the introduction of a pathogen or antigen into a living organism to stimulate the production of antibodies **b :** the introduction of a vaccine or serum into a living organism to confer immunity **2 :** INOCULUM

in·oc·u·lum \i-'nä-kyə-ləm\ *n, pl* **-la** \-lə\ **:** material used for inoculation

in·op·er·a·ble \i-'nä-pə-rə-bəl\ *adj* **:** not treatable or remediable by surgery ⟨∼ cancer⟩ — **in·op·er·a·bil·i·ty** \i-ˌnä-pə-rə-'bi-lə-tē\ *n*

in·or·gan·ic \ˌin-ˌȯr-'ga-nik\ *adj* **1 :** being or composed of matter other than plant or animal ⟨an ∼ heart⟩ **2 :** of, relating to, or dealt with by a branch of chemistry concerned with substances not usu. classed as organic — **in·or·gan·i·cal·ly** *adv*

in·or·gas·mic \ˌin-ˌȯr-'gaz-mik\ *adj* **:** not experiencing or having experienced orgasm

ino·sin·ate \i-'nō-si-ˌnāt\ *n* **:** a salt or ester of inosinic acid

ino·sine \'i-nə-ˌsēn, 'ī-, -sən\ *n* **:** a crystalline nucleoside $C_{10}H_{12}N_4O_5$

ino·sin·ic acid \ˌi-nə-'si-nik-, ˌī-\ *n* **:** a nucleotide $C_{10}H_{13}N_4O_8P$ that is found in muscle and is formed by deamination of AMP — called also *IMP*

ino·si·tol \i-'nō-sə-ˌtȯl, ī-, -ˌtōl\ *n* **:** any of several stereoisomeric cyclic alcohols $C_6H_{12}O_6$; *esp* **:** MYOINOSITOL

ino·tro·pic \ˌē-nə-'trō-pik, ˌi-, -'trä-\ *adj* **:** relating to or influencing the force of muscular contractions

in·pa·tient \'in-ˌpā-shənt\ *n* **:** a hospital patient who receives lodging and food as well as treatment — compare OUTPATIENT

in·quest \'in-ˌkwest\ *n* **:** a judicial or official inquiry esp. before a jury to determine the cause of a violent or unexpected death ⟨a coroner's ∼⟩

in·sane \(ˌ)in-'sān\ *adj* **1 :** mentally disordered : exhibiting insanity **2 :** used by, typical of, or intended for insane persons — **in·sane·ly** *adv*

in·san·i·tary \(ˌ)in-'sa-nə-ˌter-ē\ *adj* **:** unclean enough to endanger health

in·san·i·ty \in-'sa-nə-tē\ *n, pl* **-ties 1 :** a severely disordered state of the mind usu. occurring as a specific disorder (as paranoid schizophrenia) **2 :** unsoundness of mind or lack of the ability to understand that prevents one from having the mental capacity required by law to enter into a particular relationship, status, or transaction or that removes one from criminal or civil responsibility

in·scrip·tion \in-'skrip-shən\ *n* **:** the part of a medical prescription that contains the names and quantities of the drugs to be compounded

in·sect \'in-ˌsekt\ *n* **:** any of a class (Insecta) of arthropods with well-defined head, thorax, and abdomen, three pairs of legs, and typically one or two pairs of wings — **insect** *adj*

in·sec·ti·cide \in-'sek-tə-ˌsīd\ *n* **:** an agent that destroys insects — **in·sec·ti·cid·al** \(ˌ)in-ˌsek-tə-'sīd-ᵊl\ *adj*

in·se·cu·ri·ty \ˌin-si-'kyúr-ə-tē\ *n, pl* **-ties :** a feeling of apprehensiveness and uncertainty : lack of assurance or stability — **in·se·cure** \-'kyúr\ *adj*

in·sem·i·nate \in-'se-mə-ˌnāt\ *vb* **-nat·ed; -nat·ing :** to introduce semen into the genital tract of (a female) — **in·sem·i·na·tion** \-ˌse-mə-'nā-shən\ *n*

in·sem·i·na·tor \-ˌnā-tər\ *n* **:** one that inseminates cattle artificially

in·sen·si·ble \(ˌ)in-'sen-sə-bəl\ *adj* **:** incapable or bereft of feeling or sensation: as **a :** UNCONSCIOUS **b :** lacking sensory perception or ability to react **c :** lacking emotional response : APATHETIC **2 :** not perceived by the senses ⟨∼ perspiration⟩ — **in·sen·si·bil·i·ty** \(ˌ)in-ˌsen-sə-'bi-lə-tē\ *n*

in·sert \in-'sərt\ *vb, of a muscle* **:** to be in attachment to the part to be moved

inserted *adj* **:** attached by natural growth (as a muscle or tendon)

in·ser·tion \in-'sər-shən\ *n* **1 :** the part of a muscle by which it is attached to the part to be moved — compare ORIGIN 2 **2 :** the mode or place of attachment of an organ or part **3 a :** a section of genetic material inserted into an existing gene sequence **b :** the mutational process producing a genetic insertion — **in·ser·tion·al** \-shə-nᵊl\ *adj*

in·sid·i·ous \in-'si-dē-əs\ *adj* **:** developing so gradually as to be well established before becoming apparent ⟨an ∼ disease⟩ — **in·sid·i·ous·ly** *adv*

in·sight \'in-ˌsīt\ *n* **1** : understanding or awareness of one's mental or emotional condition **2** : immediate and clear understanding (as seeing the solution to a problem or the means to reaching a goal) that takes place without recourse to overt trial-and-error behavior — **in·sight·ful** \'in-ˌsīt-fəl, in-'\ *adj* — **in·sight·ful·ly** *adv*

insipidus — see CENTRAL DIABETES INSIPIDUS, DIABETES INSIPIDUS, NEPHROGENIC DIABETES INSIPIDUS

in si·tu \in-'sī-(ˌ)tü, -'si-, -'sē-, -(ˌ)tyü, -(ˌ)chü\ *adv or adj* : in the natural or original position or place — see CARCINOMA IN SITU

in·sol·u·ble \(ˌ)in-'säl-yə-bəl\ *adj* : incapable of being dissolved in a liquid; *also* : soluble only with difficulty or to a slight degree

in·som·nia \in-'säm-nē-ə\ *n* : prolonged and usu. abnormal inability to obtain adequate sleep

¹in·som·ni·ac \-nē-ˌak\ *n* : one affected with insomnia

²insomniac *adj* : affected with insomnia ⟨an ∼ patient⟩

in·spec·tion \in-'spek-shən\ *n* : visual observation of the body during a medical examination — compare PALPATION 2 — **in·spect** \in-'spekt\ *vb*

in·spi·ra·tion \ˌin-spə-'rā-shən\ *n* : the drawing of air into the lungs — **in·spi·ra·to·ry** \in-'spī-rə-ˌtōr-ē, 'in-spə-rə-\ *adj*

inspiratory capacity *n* : the total amount of air that can be drawn into the lungs after normal expiration

inspiratory reserve volume *n* : the maximal amount of additional air that can be drawn into the lungs by determined effort after normal inspiration — compare EXPIRATORY RESERVE VOLUME

in·spire \in-'spīr\ *vb* **in·spired; in·spir·ing** : to draw in by breathing : breathe in : INHALE

in·spis·sat·ed \in-'spi-ˌsā-təd, 'in-spə-ˌsā-\ *adj* : thick or thickened in consistency

in·sta·bil·i·ty \ˌin-stə-'bi-lə-tē\ *n, pl* **-ties** : lack of emotional or mental stability

in·step \'in-ˌstep\ *n* : the arched middle portion of the human foot in front of the ankle joint; *esp* : its upper surface

in·still \in-'stil\ *vb* **in·stilled; in·still·ing** : to cause to enter esp. drop by drop ⟨∼ medication into the eye⟩ — **in·stil·la·tion** \ˌin-stə-'lā-shən\ *n*

in·stinct \'in-ˌstiŋkt\ *n* **1** : a largely inheritable and unalterable tendency of an organism to make a complex and specific response to environmental stimuli without involving reason **2** : behavior that is mediated by reactions below the conscious level — **in·stinc·tive** \in-'stiŋk-tiv\ *adj* — **in·stinc·tive·ly** *adv* — **in·stinc·tu·al** \in-'stiŋk-chə-wəl\ *adj*

in·sti·tu·tion·al·ize \ˌin-stə-'tü-shə-nə-

ˌlīz, -'tyü-\ *vb* **1** : to place in or commit to an institution (as a nursing home or hospital) offering specialized care **2** : to accustom (a person) so firmly to the care and supervised routine of an institution as to make incapable of managing a life outside — **in·sti·tu·tion·al·iza·tion** \-ˌtü-shə-nə-lə-'zā-shən, -ˌtyü-\ *n*

in·stru·men·tal \ˌin-strə-'men-təl\ *adj* : OPERANT ⟨∼ conditioning⟩

in·stru·men·ta·tion \ˌin-strə-mən-'tā-shən, -ˌmen-\ *n* : a use of or operation with instruments

in·suf·fi·cien·cy \ˌin-sə-'fi-shən-sē\ *n, pl* **-cies** : the quality or state of not being sufficient: as **a** : lack of adequate supply of something **b** : lack of physical power or capacity; *esp* : inability of an organ or bodily part to function normally — **in·suf·fi·cient** \-shənt\ *adj*

in·suf·fla·tion \ˌin-sə-'flā-shən\ *n* : the act of blowing something (as a drug in powdered form) into a body cavity; *specif* : the introduction of a flow of gas into a body cavity ⟨oxygen for tracheal gas ∼⟩ ⟨abdominal ∼ with carbon dioxide⟩ — **in·suf·flate** \'in-sə-ˌflāt, in-'sə-ˌflāt\ *vb* — **in·suf·fla·tor** \'in-sə-ˌflā-tər, in-'sə-ˌflā-tər\ *n*

in·su·la \'in-sü-lə, -syü-, -shü-\ *n, pl* **su·lae** \-ˌlē, -ˌlī\ : the lobe in the center of the cerebral hemisphere that is situated deeply between the lips of the sylvian fissure — called also *central lobe, island of Reil*

in·su·lar \-lər\ *adj* : of or relating to an island of cells or tissue (as the islets of Langerhans or the insula)

in·su·lin \'in-sə-lən\ *n* : a protein hormone that is synthesized in the pancreas from proinsulin and secreted by the beta cells of the islets of Langerhans, that is essential for the metabolism of carbohydrates, lipids, and proteins, that regulates blood sugar levels by facilitating the uptake of glucose into tissues, by promoting its conversion into glycogen, fatty acids, and triglycerides, and by reducing the release of glucose from the liver, and that when produced in insufficient quantities results in diabetes mellitus — see ILETIN

in·su·lin·ae·mia *chiefly Brit var of* INSULINEMIA

in·su·lin·ase \-lə-ˌnās, -ˌnāz\ *n* : an enzyme found esp. in liver that inactivates insulin

insulin coma therapy *n* : INSULIN SHOCK THERAPY

insulin–dependent diabetes *n* : TYPE 1 DIABETES

insulin–dependent diabetes mellitus *n* : TYPE 1 DIABETES — *abbr. IDDM*

in·su·lin·emia \ˌin-sə-lə-'nē-mē-ə\ *n* : the presence of an abnormally high concentration of insulin in the blood

insulin glar·gine \-'glär-ˌjēn\ *n* : a long-acting recombinant form of insulin

insulin isophane *n* : ISOPHANE INSULIN

insulin–like growth factor *n* : either of two polypeptides structurally similar to insulin that are secreted either during fetal development or during childhood and that mediate growth hormone activity; *esp* : INSULINLIKE GROWTH FACTOR 1

insulin–like growth factor 1 *n* : the juvenile form of insulin-like growth factor that is produced chiefly by the liver with production declining after puberty — abbr. *IGF-1*

in·su·lin·o·ma \ˌin-sə-lə-ˈnō-mə\ *n, pl* **-mas** *also* **-ma·ta** \-mə-tə\ : a usu. benign insulin-secreting tumor of the islets of Langerhans

in·su·li·no·tro·pic \ˌin-sə-ˌli-nə-ˈtrō-pik, -ˈträ-\ *adj* : stimulating or affecting the production and activity of insulin ⟨an ∼ hormone⟩

insulin resistance *n* : reduced sensitivity to insulin by the body's insulindependent processes (as glucose uptake, lipolysis, and inhibition of glucose production by the liver) that is typical of type 2 diabetes but often occurs in the absence of diabetes

insulin resistance syndrome *n* : METABOLIC SYNDROME

insulin shock *n* : severe hypoglycemia that is associated with the presence of excessive insulin in the system and that if left untreated may result in convulsions and progressive development of coma

insulin shock therapy *n* : the treatment of mental disorder (as schizophrenia) by insulin in doses sufficient to produce deep coma — called also *insulin coma therapy*

insulin zinc suspension *n* : a suspension of insulin in a solution containing zinc in the form of a salt that is used for injection and has a slow onset and long duration of action — called also *Lente insulin*

in·su·li·tis \ˌin-sə-ˈlī-təs\ *n* : invasion of the pancreatic islets of Langerhans by lymphocytes that results in destruction of the beta cells of the pancreas

in·su·lo·ma \ˌin-sə-ˈlō-mə\ *n, pl* **-mas** *also* **-ma·ta** \-mə-tə\ : INSULINOMA

in·sult \ˈin-ˌsəlt\ *n* **1** : injury to the body or one of its parts **2** : something that causes or has a potential for causing insult to the body — **insult** *vb*

in·tact \in-ˈtakt\ *adj* **1** : physically and functionally complete **2** : mentally unimpaired — **in·tact·ness** *n*

In·tal *trademark* — used for a preparation of cromolyn sodium

in·te·gra·tion \ˌin-tə-ˈgrā-shən\ *n* **1** : coordination of mental processes into a normal effective personality or with the individual's environment **2** : the process by which the different parts of an organism are made a functional and structural whole esp. through the activity of the nervous system and of hormones — **in·tegrate** \ˈin-tə-ˌgrāt\ *vb* — **in·te·gra·tive** \ˈin-tə-ˌgrā-tiv\ *adj*

integrative medicine *n* : medicine that integrates the therapies of alternative medicine with those practiced by mainstream medical practitioners

in·te·grin \ˈin-tə-grən\ *n* : any of various glycoproteins found on cell surfaces (as of white blood cells or platelets) that promote adhesion of cells (as T cells) to other cells (as endothelial cells) or to extracellular material (as fibronectin) and that mediate various biological processes (as phagocytosis and wound healing)

in·teg·ri·ty \in-ˈte-grə-tē\ *n, pl* **-ties** : an unimpaired condition ⟨vascular ∼⟩

in·teg·u·ment \in-ˈte-gyə-mənt\ *n* : an enveloping layer (as a skin or membrane) of an organism or one of its parts — **in·teg·u·men·ta·ry** \-ˈmen-tə-rē\ *adj*

in·tel·lec·tu·al·ize \ˌint-ᵊl-ˈek-chə-wə-ˌlīz\ *vb* **-ized; -iz·ing** : to avoid conscious recognition of the emotional basis of (an act or feeling) by substituting a superficially plausible explanation — **in·tel·lec·tu·al·iza·tion** \-ˌek-chə-wə-lə-ˈzā-shən\ *n*

in·tel·li·gence \in-ˈte-lə-jəns\ *n* **1 a** : the ability to learn or understand or to deal with new or trying situations **b** : the ability to apply knowledge to manipulate one's environment or to think abstractly as measured by objective criteria (as tests) **2** : mental acuteness — **in·tel·li·gent** \-jənt\ *adj* — **in·tel·li·gent·ly** *adv*

intelligence quotient *n* : IQ

intelligence test *n* : a test designed to determine the relative mental capacity of a person

intensifying screen *n* : a fluorescent screen placed next to an X-ray photographic film in order to intensify the image initially produced on the film by the action of X-rays

in·ten·si·ty \in-ˈten-sə-tē\ *n, pl* **-ties** : SATURATION 4

in·ten·sive \in-ˈten-siv\ *adj* : of, relating to, or marked by an extreme degree esp. of dosage, duration, or frequency ⟨high-dose ∼ chemotherapy⟩ ⟨∼ counseling for eating disorders⟩ — **in·ten·sive·ly** *adv*

intensive care *adj* : having special medical facilities, services, and monitoring devices to meet the needs of gravely ill patients ⟨an *intensive care* unit⟩ — **intensive care** *n*

in·ten·siv·ist \in-ˈten-sə-vəst\ *n* : a physician specializing in the care and treatment of patients in intensive care

in·ten·tion \in-ˈten-chən\ *n* : a process or manner of healing of incised wounds — see FIRST INTENTION, SECOND INTENTION

intention tremor *n* : a slow tremor of the extremities that increases on attempted voluntary movement and is observed in certain diseases (as multiple sclerosis) of the nervous system

inter- *comb form* : between : among ⟨*inter*cellular⟩ ⟨*inter*costal⟩

in·ter·al·ve·o·lar \ˌin-tə-ral-'vē-ə-lər\ *adj* : situated between alveoli esp. of the lungs

in·ter·atri·al \ˌin-tər-'ā-trē-əl\ *adj* : situated between the atria of the heart

interatrial septum *n* : the wall separating the right and left atria of the heart — called also *atrial septum*

in·ter·au·ral \-'ȯr-əl\ *adj* **1** : situated between or connecting the ears **2** : of or relating to sound reception and perception by each ear considered separately

in·ter·body \'in-tər-ˌbä-dē\ *adj* : performed between the bodies of two contiguous vertebrae ⟨an ∼ fusion⟩

in·ter·breed \ˌin-tər-'brēd\ *vb* **-bred** \-'bred\; **-breed·ing** : to breed together: as **a** : CROSSBREED **b** : to breed within a closed population

in·ter·ca·lat·ed disk \in-'tər-kə-ˌlā-təd-\ *n* : any of the regions of the sarcolemma and underlying cytoplasm that comprise the junctions between adjacent cells and that function to connect them mechanically and electrically across cardiac muscle that are actually membranes separating adjacent cells

intercalated duct *n* : a duct from a tubule or acinus of the pancreas that drains into an intralobular duct

in·ter·cap·il·lary \ˌin-tər-'ka-pə-ˌler-ē\ *adj* : situated between capillaries

in·ter·car·pal \-'kär-pəl\ *adj* : situated between, occurring between, or connecting carpal bones ⟨an ∼ joint⟩

in·ter·cav·ern·ous \-'ka-vər-nəs\ *adj* : situated between and connecting the cavernous sinuses behind and in front of the pituitary gland ⟨an ∼ sinus⟩

in·ter·cel·lu·lar \-'sel-yə-lər\ *adj* : occurring between cells ⟨∼ spaces⟩ — **in·ter·cel·lu·lar·ly** *adv*

in·ter·con·dy·lar \-'kän-də-lər\ *adj* : situated between two condyles

in·ter·con·dy·loid \-'kän-də-ˌlȯid\ *adj* : INTERCONDYLAR

¹in·ter·cos·tal \ˌin-tər-'käs-tᵊl\ *adj* : situated or extending between the ribs

²intercostal *n* : an intercostal part or structure (as a muscle or nerve)

intercostal artery *n* : any of the arteries supplying or lying in the intercostal spaces: **a** : any of the arteries branching in front directly from the internal thoracic artery — called also *anterior intercostal artery* **b** : any of the arteries that branch from the costocervical trunk of the subclavian artery — called also *posterior intercostal artery*

intercostal muscle *n* : any of the short muscles that extend between the ribs and serve to move the ribs in respiration: **a** : any of 11 muscles on each side between the vertebrae and the junction of the ribs and their cartilages — called also *external intercostal muscle* **b** : any of 11 muscles on

each side between the sternum and the line on a rib marking an insertion of the iliocostalis — called also *internal intercostal muscle*

intercostal nerve *n* : any of 11 nerves on each side of which each is an anterior division of a thoracic nerve lying between a pair of adjacent ribs

intercostal vein *n* : any of the veins of the intercostal spaces — see SUPERIOR INTERCOSTAL VEIN

in·ter·cos·to·bra·chi·al nerve \ˌin-tər-ˌkäs-tō-'brā-kē-əl-\ *n* : a branch of the second intercostal nerve that supplies the skin of the inner and back part of the upper half of the arm

in·ter·course \'int-ər-ˌkȯrs\ *n* : physical sexual contact between individuals that involves the genitalia of at least one person ⟨anal ∼⟩; *esp* : SEXUAL INTERCOURSE 1 ⟨heterosexual ∼⟩

in·ter·cris·tal \ˌin-tər-'kris-tᵊl\ *adj* : measured between two crests (as of bone)

in·ter·crit·i·cal \-'kri-ti-kəl\ *adj* : being in the period between attacks ⟨∼ gout⟩

in·ter·cur·rent \-'kər-ənt\ *adj* : occurring during and modifying the course of another disease ⟨an ∼ infection⟩

in·ter·den·tal \-'dent-ᵊl\ *adj* : situated or intended for use between the teeth — **in·ter·den·tal·ly** \-ᵊl-ē\ *adv*

interdental papilla *n* : the triangular wedge of gingiva between two adjacent teeth — called also *gingival papilla*

in·ter·dig·i·tal \-'di-jə-tᵊl\ *adj* : occurring between digits ⟨an ∼ space⟩

in·ter·dig·i·tate \-'di-jə-ˌtāt\ *vb* **-tat·ed**; **-tat·ing** : to become interlocked like the fingers of folded hands — **in·ter·dig·i·ta·tion** \-ˌdij-ə-'tā-shən\ *n*

in·ter·fere \ˌin-tər-'fir\ *vb* **-fered**; **-fer·ing** : to be inconsistent with and disturb the performance of previously learned behavior

in·ter·fer·ence \-'fir-əns\ *n* **1** : partial or complete inhibition or sometimes facilitation of other genetic crossovers in the vicinity of a chromosomal locus where a preceding crossover has occurred **2** : the disturbing effect of new learning on the performance of previously learned behavior with which it is inconsistent — compare NEGATIVE TRANSFER **3** : prevention of typical growth and development of a virus in a suitable host by the presence of another virus in the same host individual

in·ter·fer·on \ˌin-tər-'fir-ˌän\ *n* : any of a group of heat-stable soluble basic antiviral glycoproteins of low molecular weight that are produced usu. by cells exposed to the action of a virus, sometimes to the action of another intracellular parasite (as a bacterium), or experimentally to the action of some chemicals, and that include some used medically as antiviral or antineoplastic agents — see ALPHA INTERFERON, BETA INTERFERON, GAMMA INTERFERON

in·ter·fer·on al·fa \-\\'al-fə\\ *n* : alpha interferon produced by recombinant DNA technology

interferon alpha *n* : ALPHA INTERFERON

interferon gamma *n* : GAMMA INTERFERON

in·ter·fi·bril·lar \\in-tər-\\'fi-brə-lər, -\\'fī-\\ *or* **in·ter·fi·bril·lary** \\-\\'fī-brə-\\ler-ē, -\\'fī\\ *adj* : situated between fibrils

in·ter·gen·ic \\-\\'jē-nik\\ *adj* : occurring between genes : involving more than one gene

in·ter·glob·u·lar \\-\\'glä-byə-lər\\ *adj* : resulting from or situated in an area of faulty dentin formation ⟨~ dentin⟩

in·ter·hemi·spher·ic \\-\\he-mə-\\'sfir-ik, -\\'sfer-\\ *also* **in·ter·hemi·spher·al** \\-əl\\ *adj* : extending or occurring between hemispheres (as of the cerebrum)

in·ter·ic·tal \\-\\'ik-təl\\ *adj* : occurring between seizures (as of epilepsy)

in·ter·ki·ne·sis \\-kə-\\'nē-səs, -kī-\\ *n, pl* **-ne·ses** \\-\\sēz\\ : the period between the first and second meiotic divisions

in·ter·leu·kin \\in-tər-\\'lü-kən\\ *n* : any of several compounds of low molecular weight that are produced by lymphocytes, macrophages, and monocytes and that function esp. in regulation of the immune system and esp. cell-mediated immunity — often used with an identifying number ⟨*interleukin*-6 induces maturation of B cells and proliferation of T cells⟩

in·ter·lo·bar \\int-ər-\\'lō-bər, -\\bär\\ *adj* : situated between the lobes of an organ or structure

interlobar artery *n* : any of various secondary branches of the renal arteries that branch to form the arcuate arteries

interlobar vein *n* : any of the veins of the kidney that are formed by convergence of arcuate veins and empty into the renal veins or their branches

in·ter·lob·u·lar \\-\\'lä-byə-lər\\ *adj* : lying between, connecting, or transporting the secretions of lobules

interlobular artery *n* : any of the branches of an arcuate artery that pass radially in the cortex of the kidney toward the surface

interlobular vein *n* : any of the veins in the cortex of the kidney that empty into the arcuate veins

in·ter·max·il·lary \\-\\'mak-sə-\\ler-ē\\ *adj* **1** : lying between maxillae; *esp* : joining the two maxillary bones ⟨~ sutures⟩ **2** : of or relating to the premaxillae

intermedia — see MASSA INTERMEDIA, PARS INTERMEDIA

intermediary metabolism *n* : the intracellular process by which nutritive material is converted into cellular components

intermediate cuneiform bone *n* : CUNEIFORM BONE 1b — called also *intermediate cuneiform*

intermediate filament *n* : any of a class of usu. insoluble cellular protein fibers (as a neurofilament or cytokeratin) that serve esp. to provide structural stability and strength to the cytoskeleton and are intermediate in diameter between microfilaments and microtubules

intermediate host *n* **1** : a host which is normally used by a parasite in the course of its life cycle and in which it may multiply asexually but not sexually — compare DEFINITIVE HOST **2 a** : RESERVOIR 2 b : VECTOR 1

intermediate metabolism *n* : INTERMEDIARY METABOLISM

intermediate temporal artery *n* : TEMPORAL ARTERY 3b

in·ter·me·din \\in-tər-\\'mēd-ən\\ *n* : MELANOCYTE-STIMULATING HORMONE

in·ter·me·dio·lat·er·al \\in-tər-\\mē-dē-ō-\\'la-tə-rəl\\ *adj* : of, relating to, or being the lateral column of gray matter in the spinal cord

intermedium — see STRATUM INTERMEDIUM

intermedius — see NERVUS INTERMEDIUS, VASTUS INTERMEDIUS

in·ter·men·stru·al \\-\\'men-strə-wəl\\ *adj* : occurring between menstrual periods ⟨~ pain⟩

in·ter·mis·sion \\in-tər-\\'mi-shən\\ *n* : the space of time between two paroxysms of a disease

in·ter·mit·tent \\-\\'mit-ənt\\ *adj* : coming and going at intervals : not continuous ⟨~ fever⟩ — **in·ter·mit·tence** \\-əns\\ *n*

intermittent claudication *n* : cramping pain and weakness in the legs and esp. the calves on walking that disappears after rest and is usu. associated with inadequate blood supply to the muscles

intermittent explosive disorder *n* : a personality disorder characterized by repeated episodes of violent aggressive behavior that is out of proportion to the events provoking it

intermittent positive pressure breathing *n* : enforced periodic inflation of the lungs by the intermittent application of an increase of pressure to a reservoir of air (as in a bag) supplying the lungs — abbr. *IPPB*

in·ter·mus·cu·lar \\-\\'məs-kyə-lər\\ *adj* : lying between and separating muscles ⟨~ fat⟩

in·tern *also* **in·terne** \\'in-ˌtərn\\ *n* : a physician gaining supervised practical experience in a hospital after graduating from medical school — **intern** *vb*

interna — see THECA INTERNA

in·ter·nal \\in-\\'tərn-əl\\ *adj* **1 a** : situated near the inside of the body **b** : situated on the side toward the midsagittal plane of the body ⟨the ~ surface of the lung⟩ **2** : present or arising within an organism or one of its parts ⟨~ stimulus⟩ **3** : applied or intended for application through the stomach by being swallowed ⟨an ~ remedy⟩ — **in·ter·nal·ly** *adv*

internal acoustic meatus *n* : INTERNAL AUDITORY CANAL

internal anal sphincter *n* : ANAL SPHINCTER b

internal auditory artery *n* : a long slender artery that arises from the basilar artery or one of its branches and is distributed to the inner ear — called also *internal auditory*, *labyrinthine artery*

internal auditory canal *n* : a short auditory canal in the petrous portion of the temporal bone through which pass the facial and auditory nerves and the nervus intermedius — called also *internal acoustic meatus, internal auditory meatus*

internal capsule *n* : CAPSULE 1b(1)

internal carotid artery *n* : the inner branch of the carotid artery that supplies the brain, eyes, and other internal structures of the head — called also *internal carotid*

internal ear *n* : INNER EAR

internal iliac artery *n* : ILIAC ARTERY 3

internal iliac node *n* : any of the lymph nodes grouped around the internal iliac artery and the internal iliac vein — compare EXTERNAL ILIAC NODE

internal iliac vein *n* : ILIAC VEIN c

internal inguinal ring *n* : DEEP INGUINAL RING

internal intercostal muscle *n* : INTERCOSTAL MUSCLE b — called also *internal intercostal*

in·ter·nal·ize \in-'tərn-ᵊl-ˌīz\ *vb* **-ized; -iz·ing** : to incorporate (as values) within the self as conscious or subconscious guiding principles through learning or socialization — **in·ter·nal·iza·tion** \-ˌtərn-ᵊl-ə-'zā-shən\ *n*

internal jugular vein *n* : JUGULAR VEIN a — called also *internal jugular*

internal malleolus *n* : MALLEOLUS b

internal mammary artery *n* : INTERNAL THORACIC ARTERY

internal maxillary artery *n* : MAXILLARY ARTERY

internal medicine *n* : a branch of medicine that deals with the diagnosis and treatment of nonsurgical diseases — abbr. *IM*

internal oblique *n* : OBLIQUE a(2)

internal occipital crest *n* : OCCIPITAL CREST b

internal occipital protuberance *n* : OCCIPITAL PROTUBERANCE b

internal os *n* : the opening of the cervix into the body of the uterus

internal pterygoid muscle *n* : PTERYGOID MUSCLE b

internal pudendal artery *n* : a branch of the internal iliac artery that is distributed esp. to the external genitalia and the perineum — compare EXTERNAL PUDENDAL ARTERY

internal pudendal vein *n* : any of several veins that receive blood from the external genitalia and the perineum and unite to form a single vein that empties into the internal iliac vein

internal respiration *n* : the exchange of gases (as oxygen and carbon dioxide) between the cells of the body and the blood — compare EXTERNAL RESPIRATION

internal spermatic artery *n* : TESTICULAR ARTERY

internal thoracic artery *n* : a branch of the subclavian artery of each side that runs down along the anterior wall of the thorax — called also *internal mammary artery*

internal thoracic vein *n* : a vein of the trunk on each side of the body that accompanies the corresponding internal thoracic artery and empties into the brachiocephalic vein

In·ter·na·tion·al System of Units \ˌin-tər-'nash-nəl-, -ən-ᵊl-\ *n* : a system of units based on the metric system and developed and refined by international convention esp. for scientific work

international unit *n* : a quantity of a biologic (as a vitamin) that produces a particular biological effect agreed upon as an international standard

interne, interneship *var of* INTERN, INTERNSHIP

in·ter·neu·ron \ˌin-tər-'nü-ˌrän, -'nyü-\ *n* : a neuron that conveys impulses from one neuron to another — called also *associative neuron, internuncial, internuncial neuron;* compare MOTOR NEURON, SENSORY NEURON — **in·ter·neu·ro·nal** \-'nùr-ən-ᵊl, -'nyùr-ən-, -nyù-'rōn-\ *adj*

in·ter·nist \'in-ˌtər-nist\ *n* : a specialist in internal medicine esp. as distinguished from a surgeon

in·tern·ship *also* **in·terne·ship** *n* **1** : the state or position of being an intern **2 a** : a period of service as an intern **b** : the phase of medical training covered during such service

¹**in·ter·nun·ci·al** \ˌin-tər-'nən-sē-əl, -'nùn-\ *adj* : of, relating to, or being interneurons ⟨~ fibers⟩

²**internuncial** *n* : INTERNEURON

internuncial neuron *n* : INTERNEURON

internus — see MEATUS ACUSTICUS INTERNUS, OBLIQUUS INTERNUS ABDOMINIS, OBTURATOR INTERNUS, SPHINCTER ANI INTERNUS, VASTUS INTERNUS

in·ter·oc·clu·sal \-ə-'klü-səl, -zəl\ *adj* : situated or occurring between the occlusal surfaces of opposing teeth

in·tero·cep·tive \ˌin-tə-rō-'sep-tiv\ *adj* : of, relating to, or being stimuli arising within the body and esp. in the viscera

in·tero·cep·tor \-tər\ *n* : a sensory receptor excited by interoceptive stimuli — compare EXTEROCEPTOR

in·ter·os·se·ous \ˌin-tər-ˈä-sē-əs\ *adj* : situated between bones

interosseous artery — see COMMON INTEROSSEOUS ARTERY

interosseous membrane *n* : either of two thin strong sheets of fibrous tissue: **a** : one extending between and connecting the shafts of the radius and ulna **b** : one extending between and connecting the shafts of the tibia and fibula

interosseous muscle *n* : INTEROSSEUS

in·ter·os·se·us \ˌin-tər-ˈä-sē-əs\ *n, pl* **-sei** \-sē-ˌī\ : any of various small muscles arising from the metacarpals and metatarsals and inserted into the bases of the first phalanges: **a** : DORSAL INTEROSSEUS **b** : PALMAR INTEROSSEUS **c** : PLANTAR INTEROSSEUS

interosseus dorsalis *n, pl* **interossei dorsales** : DORSAL INTEROSSEUS

interosseus palmaris *n, pl* **interossei palmares** : PALMAR INTEROSSEUS

interosseus plantaris *n, pl* **interossei plantares** : PLANTAR INTEROSSEUS

in·ter·par·ox·ys·mal \-ˌpar-ək-ˈsiz-məl, -pə-ˌräk-\ *adj* : occurring between paroxysms

in·ter·pe·dun·cu·lar nucleus \ˌin-tər-pi-ˈdəŋ-kyə-lər-\ *n* : a mass of nerve cells lying between the cerebral peduncles in the midsagittal plane just dorsal to the pons — called also *interpeduncular ganglion*

in·ter·per·son·al \-ˈpərs-ᵊn-əl\ *adj* : being, relating to, or involving relations between persons — **in·ter·per·son·al·ly** *adv*

interpersonal therapy *n* : psychotherapy that focuses on a patient's interpersonal relationships and is used esp. to treat depression — abbr. *IPT*; called also *interpersonal psychotherapy*

in·ter·pha·lan·ge·al \ˌin-tər-ˌfā-lən-ˈjē-əl, -ˌfa-; -fə-ˈlan-jē-əl, -fā-\ *adj* : situated or occurring between phalanges; *also* : of or relating to an interphalangeal joint

in·ter·phase \ˈin-tər-ˌfāz\ *n* : the interval between the end of one mitotic or meiotic division and the beginning of another — called also *resting stage*

in·ter·po·lat·ed \in-ˈtər-pə-ˌlā-təd\ *adj* : occurring between normal heartbeats without disturbing the succeeding beat or the basic rhythm of the heart ⟨an ~ ventricular extrasystole⟩

in·ter·pris·mat·ic \ˌin-tər-priz-ˈma-tik\ *adj* : situated or occurring between prisms esp. of enamel

in·ter·prox·i·mal \-ˈpräk-sə-məl\ *adj* : situated, occurring, or used in the areas between adjoining teeth

in·ter·pu·pil·lary \-ˈpyü-pə-ˌler-ē\ *adj* : extending between the pupils of the eyes; *also* : extending between the centers of a pair of spectacle lenses ⟨~ distance⟩

in·ter·ra·dic·u·lar \-rə-ˈdi-kyə-lər\ *adj* : situated between the roots of a tooth

interruptus — see COITUS INTERRUPTUS

in·ter·scap·u·lar \ˌin-tər-ˈska-pyə-lər\ *adj* : of, relating to, situated in, or occurring in the region between the scapulae ⟨~ pain⟩

in·ter·sen·so·ry \-ˈsens-ə-rē\ *adj* : involving two or more sensory systems

in·ter·sep·tal \-ˈsept-ᵊl\ *adj* : situated between septa

in·ter·sex \ˈin-tər-ˌseks\ *n* : an intersexual individual

in·ter·sex·u·al \ˌin-tər-ˈsek-shə-wəl\ *adj* **1** : existing between sexes ⟨~ hostility⟩ **2** : intermediate in sexual characters between a typical male and a typical female — **in·ter·sex·u·al·i·ty** \-ˌsek-shə-ˈwa-lə-tē\ *n*

in·ter·space \ˈin-tər-ˌspās\ *n* : the space between two related body parts whether void or filled by another kind of structure

in·ter·spi·na·lis \ˌint-ər-ˌspī-ˈna-ləs, -ˈnä-\ *n, pl* **-na·les** \-ˌlēz\ : any of various short muscles that have their origin on the superior surface of the spinous process of one vertebra and their insertion on the inferior surface of the contiguous vertebra above

in·ter·spi·nal ligament \ˌin-tər-ˈspīn-ᵊl-\ *n* : any of the thin membranous ligaments that connect the spinous processes of contiguous vertebrae — called also *interspinous ligament*

in·ter·stim·u·lus \-ˈstim-yə-ləs\ *adj* : of, relating to, or being the interval between the presentation of two discrete stimuli

in·ter·sti·tial \-ˈsti-shəl\ *adj* **1** : situated within but not restricted to or characteristic of a particular organ or tissue — used esp. of fibrous tissue **2** : affecting the interstitial tissues of an organ or part ⟨~ hepatitis⟩ **3** : occurring in the part of a fallopian tube in the wall of the uterus ⟨~ pregnancy⟩ — **in·ter·sti·tial·ly** *adv*

interstitial cell *n* : a cell situated between the germ cells of the gonads; *esp* : LEYDIG CELL

interstitial cell of Leydig *n* : LEYDIG CELL

interstitial–cell stimulating hormone *n* : LUTEINIZING HORMONE

interstitial cystitis *n* : a chronic idiopathic cystitis characterized by painful inflammation of the subepithelial connective tissue and often accompanied by Hunner's ulcer

interstitial keratitis *n* : a chronic progressive keratitis of the corneal stroma often resulting in blindness and frequently associated with congenital syphilis

interstitial pneumonia *n* : any of several chronic lung diseases of unknown etiology that affect interstitial tissues of the lung

in·ter·sti·tium \ˌin-tər-ˈsti-shē-əm\ *n, pl* **-tia** \-ē-ə\ : interstitial tissue

in·ter·sub·ject \'in-tər-ˌsəb-jekt\ *adj* : occurring between subjects in an experiment ⟨∼ variability⟩

in·ter·tar·sal \ˌin-tər-'tär-səl\ *adj* : situated, occurring, or performed between tarsal bones ⟨∼ joint⟩

in·ter·trans·ver·sar·ii \-ˌtrans-vər-'ser-ē-ˌī\ *n pl* : a series of small muscles connecting the transverse processes of contiguous vertebrae

in·ter·tri·go \-'trī-ˌgō\ *n* : inflammation produced by chafing of adjacent areas of skin — **in·ter·trig·i·nous** \-'tri-jə-nəs\ *adj*

in·ter·tro·chan·ter·ic \-ˌtrō-kən-'ter-ik, -ˌkan-\ *adj* : situated, performed, or occurring between trochanters ⟨∼ fractures⟩

intertrochanteric line *n* : a line on the anterior surface of the femur that runs obliquely from the greater trochanter to the lesser trochanter

in·ter·tu·ber·cu·lar groove \ˌin-tər-tü-'bər-kyə-lər-, -tyü-\ *n* : BICIPITAL GROOVE

intertubercular line *n* : an imaginary line passing through the iliac crests of the hip bones that separates the umbilical and lumbar regions of the abdomen from the hypogastric and iliac regions

in·ter·ven·tion \ˌin-tər-'ven-chən\ *n* : the act or fact or a method of interfering with the outcome or course esp. of a condition or process (as to prevent harm or improve functioning) — **in·ter·ven·tion·al** \-'ven-chə-nəl\ *adj*

in·ter·ven·tric·u·lar \-ven-'tri-kyə-lər\ *adj* : situated between ventricles

interventricular foramen *n* : the opening from each lateral ventricle into the third ventricle of the brain — called also *foramen of Monro*

interventricular groove *n* : INTERVENTRICULAR SULCUS

interventricular septum *n* : the curved slanting wall that separates the right and left ventricles of the heart

interventricular sulcus *n* : either of the anterior and posterior grooves on the surface of the heart that lie over the interventricular septum and join at the apex

in·ter·ver·te·bral \ˌin-tər-'vər-tə-brəl, -(ˌ)vər-'tē-\ *adj* : situated between vertebrae — **in·ter·ver·te·bral·ly** *adv*

intervertebral disk *n* : any of the tough elastic disks that are interposed between the centra of adjoining vertebrae

intervertebral foramen *n* : any of the openings that give passage to the spinal nerves from the vertebral canal

in·tes·ti·nal \in-'tes-tən-ᵊl\ *adj* **1 a** : affecting or occurring in the intestine **b** : living in the intestine ⟨the ∼ flora⟩ **2** : of, relating to, or being the intestine ⟨the ∼ canal⟩ — **in·tes·ti·nal·ly** *adv*

intestinal artery *n* : any of 12 to 15 arteries that arise from the superior mesenteric artery and supply the jejunum and ileum

intestinal flu *n* : an acute usu. transitory attack of gastroenteritis that is marked by nausea, vomiting, diarrhea, and abdominal cramping and is typically caused by a virus (as the Norwalk virus) or a bacterium (as E. coli) — not usu. used technically

intestinal gland *n* : CRYPT OF LIEBERKÜHN

intestinal juice *n* : a fluid that is secreted in small quantity by the small intestine and contains various enzymes (as lipase and amylase) — called also *succus entericus*

intestinal lipodystrophy *n* : WHIPPLE'S DISEASE

in·tes·tine \in-'tes-tən\ *n* : the tubular portion of the digestive tract that lies posterior to the stomach from which it is separated by the pyloric sphincter and consists of a slender but long anterior part made up of the duodenum, jejunum, and ileum and a broader shorter posterior part made up of cecum, colon, and rectum — often used in pl.; see LARGE INTESTINE, SMALL INTESTINE

in·ti·ma \'in-tə-mə\ *n, pl* **-mae** \-ˌmē, -ˌmī\ *or* **-mas** : the innermost coat of an organ (as a blood vessel) consisting usu. of an endothelial layer backed by connective tissue and elastic tissue — called also *tunica intima* — **in·ti·mal** \-məl\ *adj*

in·tol·er·ance \(ˌ)in-'tä-lə-rəns\ *n* **1** : lack of an ability to endure ⟨an ∼ to light⟩ **2** : exceptional sensitivity (as to a drug); *specif* : inability to properly metabolize or absorb a substance ⟨glucose ∼⟩ — **in·tol·er·ant** \-rənt\ *adj*

in·tox·i·cant \in-'täk-si-kənt\ *n* : something that intoxicates; *esp* : an alcoholic drink — **intoxicant** *adj*

in·tox·i·cate \-sə-ˌkāt\ *vb* **-cat·ed; -cat·ing** **1** : POISON **2** : to excite or stupefy by alcohol or a drug esp. to the point where physical and mental control is markedly diminished

in·tox·i·cat·ed \-ˌkā-təd\ *adj* : affected by an intoxicant and esp. by alcohol

in·tox·i·ca·tion \in-ˌtäk-sə-'kā-shən\ *n* **1** : an abnormal state that is essentially a poisoning ⟨intestinal ∼⟩ **2** : the condition of being drunk

in·tra- \ˌin-trə, -(ˌ)trä\ *prefix* **1 a** : within ⟨*intra*cerebellar⟩ **b** : during ⟨*intra*operative⟩ **c** : between layers of ⟨*intra*dermal⟩ **2** : INTRO- ⟨an *intra*muscular injection⟩

in·tra-ab·dom·i·nal \ˌin-trə-ab-'dä-mən-ᵊl\ *adj* : situated within, occurring within, or administered by entering the abdomen ⟨∼ pressure⟩

in·tra-al·ve·o·lar \ˌin-trə-al-'vē-ə-lər\ *adj* : situated or occurring within an alveolus ⟨∼ hemorrhage⟩

in·tra-am·ni·ot·ic \-ˌam-nē-'ä-tik\ *adj* : situated within, occurring within, or administered by entering the amnion — **in·tra-am·ni·ot·i·cal·ly** *adv*

in·tra-aor·tic \-ā-'ȯr-tik\ *adj* **1** : situated or occurring within the aorta **2** : of, relating to, or used in intra-aortic balloon counterpulsation

intra-aortic balloon counterpulsation *n* : counterpulsation in which cardiocirculatory assistance is provided by a balloon inserted in the thoracic aorta which is inflated during diastole and deflated just before systole

in·tra-ar·te·ri·al \-är-'tir-ē-əl\ *adj* : situated or occurring within, administered into, or involving entry by way of an artery ⟨an ∼ catheter⟩ — **in·tra-ar·te·ri·al·ly** *adv*

in·tra-ar·tic·u·lar \-är-'ti-kyə-lər\ *adj* : situated within, occurring within, or administered by entering a joint — **in·tra-ar·tic·u·lar·ly** *adv*

in·tra-atri·al \-'ā-trē-əl\ *adj* : situated or occurring within an atrium esp. of the heart ⟨an ∼ block⟩

in·tra-bron·chi·al \-'brän-kē-əl\ *adj* : situated or occurring within the bronchial tubes ⟨∼ foreign bodies⟩

in·tra-can·a·lic·u·lar \-ˌkan-ᵊl-'i-kyə-lər\ *adj* : situated or occurring within a canaliculus ⟨∼ biliary stasis⟩

in·tra-cap·su·lar \-'kap-sə-lər\ *adj* **1** : situated or occurring within a capsule **2** *of a cataract operation* : involving removal of the entire lens and its capsule — compare EXTRACAPSULAR 2

in·tra-car·di·ac \-'kär-dē-ˌak\ *also* **in·tra-car·di·al** \-dē-əl\ *adj* : situated within, occurring within, introduced into, or involving entry into the heart

in·tra-ca·rot·id \-kə-'rä-təd\ *adj* : situated within, occurring within, or administered by entering a carotid artery

in·tra-cav·i·tary \-'ka-və-ˌter-ē\ *adj* : situated or occurring within a body cavity; *esp* : of, relating to, or being treatment (as of cancer) characterized by the insertion of esp. radioactive substances in a cavity

in·tra-cel·lu·lar \-'sel-yə-lər\ *adj* : existing, occurring, or functioning within a cell — **in·tra-cel·lu·lar·ly** *adv*

in·tra-cer·e·bel·lar \-ˌser-ə-'be-lər\ *adj* : situated or occurring within the cerebellum ⟨∼ hemorrhage⟩

in·tra-ce·re·bral \-sə-'rē-brəl, -'ser-ə-\ *adj* : situated within, occurring within, or administered by entering the cerebrum ⟨∼ injections⟩ ⟨∼ bleeding⟩ — **in·tra-ce·re·bral·ly** *adv*

in·tra-cis·ter·nal \-sis-'tər-nəl\ *adj* : situated within, occurring within, or administered by entering a cisterna — **in·tra-cis·ter·nal·ly** *adv*

in·tra-cor·ne·al \-'kȯr-nē-əl\ *adj* : occurring within, situated within, or implanted in the cornea ⟨an ∼ lens⟩

in·tra-co·ro·nal \-'kȯr-ən-ᵊl, -'kär-; -kə-'rōn-\ *adj* : situated or made within the crown of a tooth

in·tra-cor·o·nary \-'kȯr-ə-ˌner-ē, -'kär-\

adj : situated within, occurring within, or administered by entering the heart ⟨∼ pressure⟩

in·tra-cor·ti·cal \-'kȯr-ti-kəl\ *adj* : situated or occurring within a cortex and esp. the cerebral cortex ⟨∼ injection⟩

in·tra-cra·ni·al \-'krā-nē-əl\ *adj* : situated or occurring within the cranium ⟨∼ pressure⟩; *also* : affecting or involving intracranial structures — **in·tra-cra·ni·al·ly** *adv*

in·trac·ta·ble \(ˌ)in-'trak-tə-bəl\ *adj* **1** : not easily managed or controlled (as by antibiotics or psychotherapy) **2** : not easily relieved or cured ⟨∼ pain⟩ — **in·trac·ta·bil·i·ty** \(ˌ)in-ˌtrak-tə-'bi-lə-tē\ *n*

in·tra-cu·ta·ne·ous \ˌin-trə-kyù-'tā-nē-əs, -(ˌ)trā-\ *adj* : INTRADERMAL ⟨∼ lesions⟩ — **in·tra-cu·ta·ne·ous·ly** *adv*

intracutaneous test *n* : INTRADERMAL TEST

in·tra·cy·to·plas·mic \-ˌsī-tə-'plaz-mik\ *adj* : lying or occurring in the cytoplasm ⟨∼ inclusions⟩

intracytoplasmic sperm injection *n* : injection of a single sperm into an egg that has been obtained from an ovary followed by transfer of the egg to an incubator where fertilization takes place and then by introduction of the fertilized egg into a female's uterus — abbr. *ICSI*

in·tra·der·mal \-'dər-məl\ *adj* : situated, occurring, or done within or between the layers of the skin; *also* : administered by entering the skin ⟨∼ injections⟩ — **in·tra·der·mal·ly** *adv*

intradermal test *n* : a test for immunity or hypersensitivity made by injecting a minute amount of diluted antigen into the skin — called also *intracutaneous test*; compare PATCH TEST, PRICK TEST, SCRATCH TEST

in·tra·di·a·lyt·ic \ˌin-ə-'li-tik\ *adj* : occurring or carried out during hemodialysis ⟨∼ hypotension⟩

in·tra·duc·tal \ˌin-trə-'dək-tᵊl\ *adj* : situated within, occurring within, or introduced into a duct ⟨∼ carcinoma⟩

in·tra·du·o·de·nal \-ˌdü-ə-'dēn-ᵊl, -ˌdyü-; -'äd-ᵊn-əl\ *adj* : situated in or introduced into the duodenum

in·tra·du·ral \-'dùr-əl, -'dyùr-\ *adj* : situated, occurring, or performed within or between the membranes of the dura mater ⟨an ∼ tumor⟩

in·tra·epi·der·mal \-ˌe-pə-'dər-məl\ *adj* : located or occurring within the epidermis ⟨∼ nerve fibers⟩

in·tra·epi·the·li·al \-ˌe-pə-'thē-lē-əl\ *adj* : occurring in or situated among the cells of the epithelium — see PROSTATIC INTRAEPITHELIAL NEOPLASIA

in·tra·eryth·ro·cyt·ic \-i-ˌri-thrə-'si-tik\ *adj* : situated or occurring within the red blood cells

in·tra·esoph·a·ge·al \-i-ˌsä-fə-'jē-əl\ *adj* : occurring within the esophagus

intra·fal·lo·pi·an — see GAMETE INTRAFALLOPIAN TRANSFER, ZYGOTE INTRAFALLOPIAN TRANSFER

in·tra·fa·mil·ial \-fə-'mil-yəl\ *adj* : occurring within a family ⟨∼ conflict⟩

in·tra·fol·lic·u·lar \-fə-'li-kyə-lər, -fä-\ *adj* : situated within a follicle

in·tra·fu·sal \-'fyü-zəl\ *adj* : situated within a muscle spindle ⟨∼ muscle fibers⟩ — compare EXTRAFUSAL

in·tra·gas·tric \-'gas-trik\ *adj* : situated or occurring within the stomach

in·tra·gen·ic \-'je-nik\ *adj* : being or occurring within a gene

in·tra·he·pat·ic \-hi-'pa-tik\ *adj* : situated or occurring within or originating in the liver ⟨∼ cholestasis⟩

in·tra·le·sion·al \-'lē-zhən-ᵊl\ *adj* : introduced into or performed within a lesion — **in·tra·le·sion·al·ly** *adv*

in·tra·lo·bar \-'lō-bər, -,bär\ *adj* : situated within a lobe

in·tra·lob·u·lar \-'lä-byə-lər\ *adj* : situated or occurring within a lobule (as of the liver or pancreas)

intralobular vein *n* : CENTRAL VEIN

in·tra·lu·mi·nal \-'lü-mən-ᵊl\ *adj* : situated within, occurring within, or introduced into the lumen

in·tra·mam·ma·ry \-'ma-mə-rē\ *adj* : situated or introduced within the mammary tissue ⟨an ∼ infusion⟩

in·tra·med·ul·lary \-'med-ᵊl-,er-ē, -'mej-ᵊl-; -mə-'də-lə-rē\ *adj* : situated or occurring within a medulla; *esp* : involving use of the marrow space of a bone for support ⟨∼ pinning of a fracture⟩

in·tra·mem·brane \-'mem-,brān\ *adj* : INTRAMEMBRANOUS 2

in·tra·mem·bra·nous \-'mem-brə-nəs\ *adj* **1** : relating to, formed by, or being ossification of a membrane ⟨∼ bone development⟩ **2** : situated within a membrane

in·tra·mi·to·chon·dri·al \-,mī-tə-'kän-drē-əl\ *adj* : situated or occurring within mitochondria ⟨∼ inclusions⟩

in·tra·mu·co·sal \-myü-'kō-zəl\ *adj* : situated within, occurring within, or administered by entering a mucous membrane ⟨∼ gastric carcinoma⟩

in·tra·mu·ral \-'myür-əl\ *adj* : situated or occurring within the substance of the walls of an organ ⟨∼ infarction⟩

in·tra·mus·cu·lar \-'məs-kyə-lər\ *adj* : situated within, occurring within, or administered by entering a muscle — **in·tra·mus·cu·lar·ly** *adv*

in·tra·myo·car·di·al \-,mī-ə-'kär-dē-əl\ *adj* : situated within, occurring within, or administered by entering the myocardium ⟨an ∼ injection⟩

in·tra·na·sal \-'nā-zəl\ *adj* : lying within or administered by way of the nasal structures ⟨∼ corticosteroids⟩ — **in·tra·na·sal·ly** *adv*

in·tra·neu·ral \-'nùr-əl, -'nyùr-\ *adj* : situated within, occurring within, or administered by entering a nerve or nervous tissue — **in·tra·neu·ral·ly** *adv*

in·tra·neu·ro·nal \-'nùr-ən-ᵊl, -'nyùr-; -nù-'rōn-ᵊl, -nyù-\ *adj* : situated or occurring within a neuron

in·tra·nu·cle·ar \-'nü-klē-ər, -'nyü-\ *adj* : situated or occurring within a nucleus ⟨cells with ∼ inclusions⟩

in·tra·oc·u·lar \,in-trə-'ä-kyə-lər\ *adj* : implanted in, occurring within, or administered by entering the eyeball — **in·tra·oc·u·lar·ly** *adv*

intraocular pressure *n* : the pressure within the eyeball that gives it a round firm shape and is caused by the aqueous humor and vitreous body — called also *intraocular tension*

in·tra·op·er·a·tive \,in-trə-'ä-pə-rə-tiv\ *adj* : occurring, carried out, or encountered in the course of surgery ⟨∼ irradiation⟩ ⟨∼ infarction⟩ — **in·tra·op·er·a·tive·ly** *adv*

in·tra·oral \-'ōr-əl, -'är-\ *adj* : situated, occurring, or performed within the mouth ⟨∼ ulcerations⟩

in·tra·os·se·ous \-'ä-sē-əs\ *adj* : situated within, occurring within, or administered by entering a bone

in·tra·ovar·i·an \-ō-'var-ē-ən\ *adj* : situated or occurring within the ovary

in·tra·ovu·lar \-'ä-vyə-lər, -'ō-\ *adj* : situated or occurring within the ovum

in·tra·pan·cre·at·ic \-,pan-krē-'a-tik, -,pan-\ *adj* : situated or occurring within the pancreas

in·tra·pa·ren·chy·mal \-pə-'ren-kə-məl, -,par-ən-'kī-\ *adj* : situated or occurring within the parenchyma of an organ

in·tra·par·tum \-'pär-təm\ *adj* : occurring or provided during the act of birth ⟨∼ fetal monitoring⟩ ⟨∼ care⟩

in·tra·pel·vic \-'pel-vik\ *adj* : situated or performed within the pelvis

in·tra·peri·car·di·al \-,per-ə-'kär-dē-əl\ *adj* : situated within or administered by entering the pericardium

in·tra·per·i·to·ne·al \,in-trə-,per-ət-ᵊn-'ē-əl\ *adj* : situated within or administered by entering the peritoneum — **in·tra·per·i·to·ne·al·ly** *adv*

in·tra·pleu·ral \-'plùr-əl\ *adj* : situated within, occurring within, or administered by entering the pleura or pleural cavity — **in·tra·pleu·ral·ly** *adv*

intrapleural pneumonolysis *n* : PNEUMONOLYSIS b

in·tra·psy·chic \,in-trə-'sī-kik\ *adj* : being or occurring within the psyche, mind, or personality

in·tra·pul·mo·nary \-'pùl-mə-,ner-ē, -'pəl-\ *also* **in·tra·pul·mon·ic** \-,pùl-'mä-nik, -,pəl-\ *adj* : situated within, occurring within, or administered by entering the lungs — **in·tra·pul·mo·nar·i·ly** \-,pùl-mə-'ner-ə-,lē\ *adv*

in·tra·rec·tal \-'rekt-ᵊl\ *adj* : situated within, occurring within, or administered by entering the rectum

in·tra·re·nal \-'rēn-ᵊl\ *adj* : situated within, occurring within, or administered by entering the kidney — **in·tra·re·nal·ly** *adv*

in·tra·ret·i·nal \-'ret-ᵊn-əl\ *adj* : situated or occurring within the retina

in·tra·scro·tal \-'skrōt-ᵊl\ *adj* : situated or occurring within the scrotum

in·tra·spi·nal \-'spīn-ᵊl\ *adj* : situated within, occurring within, or introduced into the spine and esp. the vertebral canal ⟨∼ nerve terminals⟩

in·tra·splen·ic \-'sple-nik\ *adj* : situated within or introduced into the spleen — **in·tra·splen·i·cal·ly** *adv*

in·tra·tes·tic·u·lar \-tes-'ti-kyə-lər\ *adj* : situated within, performed within, or administered into a testis — **in·tra·tes·tic·u·lar·ly** *adv*

in·tra·the·cal \-'thē-kəl\ *adj* : introduced into or occurring in the space under the arachnoid membrane of the brain or spinal cord — **in·tra·the·cal·ly** *adv*

in·tra·tho·rac·ic \-thə-'ra-sik\ *adj* : situated, occurring, or performed within the thorax ⟨∼ pressure⟩

in·tra·thy·roi·dal \-thī-'roid-ᵊl\ *adj* : situated within or occurring within the thyroid

in·tra·tra·che·al \-'trā-kē-əl\ *adj* : occurring within or introduced into the trachea — **in·tra·tra·che·al·ly** *adv*

in·tra·ure·thral \-yü-'rē-thrəl\ *adj* : situated within, introduced into, or done in the urethra

in·tra·uter·ine \-'yü-tə-rən, -₁rīn\ *adj* : of, situated in, used in, or occurring within the uterus; *also* : involving or occurring during the part of development that takes place in the uterus

intrauterine contraceptive device *n* : INTRAUTERINE DEVICE

intrauterine device *n* : a device (as of metal or plastic) inserted and left in the uterus to prevent effective conception — called also *IUCD, IUD*

in·tra·vag·i·nal \-'va-jən-ᵊl\ *adj* : situated within, occurring within, or introduced into the vagina — **in·tra·vag·i·nal·ly** *adv*

in·trav·a·sa·tion \in-₁tra-və-'sā-shən\ *n* : the entrance of foreign matter into a vessel of the body and esp. a blood vessel

in·tra·vas·cu·lar \₁in-trə-'vas-kyə-lər\ *adj* : situated in, occurring in, or administered by entry into a blood vessel — **in·tra·vas·cu·lar·ly** *adv*

in·tra·ve·nous \₁in-trə-'vē-nəs\ *adj* **1** : situated within, performed within, occurring within, or entering by way of the interior of a vein ⟨an ∼ feeding⟩ **2** : used in intravenous procedures ⟨an ∼ needle⟩ — **in·tra·ve·nous·ly** *adv*

intravenous pyelogram *n* : a pyelogram in which radiographic visualization is obtained after intravenous administration of a radiopaque medium which collects in the kidneys

in·tra·ven·tric·u·lar \₁in-trə-ven-'tri-kyə-lər\ *adj* : situated within, occurring within, or administered into a ventricle — **in·tra·ven·tric·u·lar·ly** *adv*

in·tra·ver·te·bral \-(₁)vər-'tē-brəl, -'vər-tə-\ *adj* : situated or occurring within a vertebra

in·tra·ves·i·cal \-'ve-si-kəl\ *adj* : situated or occurring within the bladder

in·tra·vi·tal \-'vīt-ᵊl\ *adj* **1** : performed upon or found in a living subject **2** : having or utilizing the property of staining cells without killing them — compare SUPRAVITAL — **in·tra·vi·tal·ly** *adv*

in·tra·vi·tam \-'vī-₁tam, -'wē-₁täm\ *adj* : INTRAVITAL

in·tra·vit·re·al \-'vi-trē-əl\ *adj* : INTRAVITREOUS ⟨∼ injection⟩

in·tra·vit·re·ous \-'vi-trē-əs\ *adj* : situated within, occurring within, or introduced into the vitreous body ⟨∼ hemorrhage⟩

in·trin·sic \in-'trin-zik, -sik\ *adj* **1** : originating or due to causes or factors within a body, organ, or part ⟨∼ asthma⟩ **2** : originating and included wholly within an organ or part ⟨∼ muscles⟩ — compare EXTRINSIC

intrinsic factor *n* : a substance produced by the normal gastrointestinal mucosa that facilitates absorption of vitamin B_{12}

intro- *prefix* **1** : in : into ⟨*intro*jection⟩ **2** : inward : within ⟨*intro*vert⟩ — compare EXTRO-

in·troi·tus \in-'trō-ə-təs\ *n, pl* **introitus** : the vaginal opening — **in·troi·tal** \in-'trō-ət-ᵊl\ *adj*

in·tro·ject \₁in-trə-'jekt\ *vb* **1** : to incorporate (attitudes or ideas) into one's personality unconsciously **2** : to turn toward oneself (the love felt for another) or against oneself (the hostility felt toward another) — **in·tro·jec·tion** \-'jek-shən\ *n*

in·tro·mis·sion \₁in-trə-'mi-shən\ *n* : the insertion or period of insertion of the penis in the vagina in copulation

in·tron \'in-₁trän\ *n* : a polynucleotide sequence in a nucleic acid that does not code information for protein synthesis and is removed before translation of messenger RNA — compare EXON — **in·tron·ic** \in-'trä-nik\ *adj*

In·tro·pin \'in-trə-₁pin\ *trademark* — used for a preparation of the hydrochloride of dopamine

in·tro·spec·tion \₁in-trə-'spek-shən\ *n* : an examination of one's own thoughts and feelings — **in·tro·spec·tive** \-tiv\ *adj*

in·tro·ver·sion \₁in-trə-'vər-zhən, -shən\ *n* **1** : the act of directing one's attention toward or getting gratification from one's own interests, thoughts, and feelings **2** : the state or tendency toward being wholly or predominantly concerned with and interested in one's own mental life — compare EXTROVERSION

in·tro·vert \'in-trə-₁vərt\ *n* : one whose personality is characterized by introversion; *broadly* : a reserved or shy person — compare EXTROVERT — **in·tro·vert·ed** \'in-trə-₁vər-təd\ *also* **in·tro·vert** \'in-trə-₁vərt\ *adj*

in·tu·ba·tion \₁in-tü-'bā-shən, -tyü-\ *n*

: the introduction of a tube into a hollow organ (as the trachea or intestine) to keep it open or restore its patency if obstructed — compare EXTUBATION — **in·tu·bate** \'in-tü-ˌbāt, -tyü-\ vb

in·tu·mes·cence \ˌin-tü-'mes-³ns, -tyü-\ n 1 a : the action or process of becoming enlarged or swollen b : the state of being swollen 2 : something (as a tumor) that is swollen or enlarged

in·tus·sus·cep·tion \ˌin-tə-sə-'sep-shən\ n : INVAGINATION; esp : the slipping of a length of intestine into an adjacent portion usu. producing obstruction — **in·tus·sus·cept** \ˌin-tə-sə-'sept\ vb

in·u·lin \'in-yə-lən\ n : a white mildly sweet plant polysaccharide that is used as a source of levulose, as a diagnostic agent in a test for kidney function, and as an additive in low-fat and low-sugar processed foods

in·unc·tion \i-'nəŋk-shən\ n 1 : the rubbing of an ointment into the skin for therapeutic purposes 2 : OINTMENT, UNGUENT

in utero \in-'yü-tə-ˌrō\ adv or adj : in the uterus : before birth

in·vade \in-'vād\ vb **in·vad·ed; in·vad·ing** 1 : to enter and spread within either normally (as in development) or abnormally (as in infection) often with harmful effects 2 : to affect injuriously and progressively

in·vag·i·na·tion \ˌin-ˌva-jə-'nā-shən\ n 1 : an act or process of folding in so that an outer surface becomes an inner surface: as a : the formation of a gastrula by an infolding of part of the wall of the blastula b : intestinal intussusception 2 : an invaginated part — **in·vag·i·nate** \in-'va-jə-ˌnāt\ vb

¹**in·val·id** \'in-və-ləd\ adj 1 : suffering from disease or disability : SICKLY 2 : of, relating to, or suited to one that is sick ⟨an ~ chair⟩

²**invalid** n : one that is sickly or disabled

³**in·val·id** \'in-və-ləd, -ˌlid\ vb 1 : to remove from active duty by reason of sickness or disability 2 : to make sickly or disabled

in·va·lid·ism \'in-və-lə-ˌdi-zəm\ n : a chronic condition of being an invalid

in·va·sion \in-'vā-zhən\ n : the act of invading: as a : the penetration of the body of a host by a microorganism b : the spread and multiplication of a pathogenic microorganism or of malignant cells in the body of a host

in·va·sive \-siv, -ziv\ adj 1 : tending to spread; esp : tending to invade healthy tissue ⟨~ cancer cells⟩ 2 : involving entry into the living body (as by incision or by insertion of an instrument) ⟨~ diagnostic techniques⟩ — **in·va·sive·ness** n

in·ven·to·ry \'in-vən-ˌtōr-ē\ n, pl -ries 1 : a questionnaire designed to provide an index of individual interests or personality traits 2 : a list of traits, preferences, attitudes, interests, or abilities that is used in evaluating personal characteristics or skills

in·ver·sion \in-'vər-zhən, -shən\ n 1 : a reversal of position, order, form, or relationship: as a : a dislocation of a bodily structure in which it is turned partially or wholly inside out ⟨~ of the uterus⟩ b : the condition (as of the foot) of being turned or rotated inward — compare EVERSION 2 c : a breaking off of a chromosome section and its subsequent reattachment in inverted position; also : a chromosomal section that has undergone this process 2 : HOMOSEXUALITY — **in·vert** \in-'vərt\ vb

inversus — see SITUS INVERSUS

in·ver·tase \in-'vər-ˌtās, 'in-vər-, -ˌtāz\ n : an enzyme found in many microorganisms and plants and in animal intestines that catalyzes the hydrolysis of sucrose — called also saccharase, sucrase

¹**in·ver·te·brate** \(ˌ)in-'vər-tə-brət, -ˌbrāt\ n : an animal having no backbone or internal skeleton

²**invertebrate** adj : lacking a spinal column; also : of or relating to invertebrate animals

in·vest \in-'vest\ vb : to envelop or cover completely ⟨the pleura ~s the lung⟩

in·ves·ti·ga·tion·al new drug \in-ˌves-ti-'gā-shə-nəl-\ n : a drug that has not been approved for general use by the Food and Drug Administration but is under investigation in clinical trials regarding its safety and efficacy first by clinical investigators and then by practicing physicians using subjects who have given informed consent to participate — abbr. IND; called also investigational drug

in·vest·ment \-mənt\ n : an external covering of a cell, part, or organism

in·vi·a·ble \(ˌ)in-'vī-ə-bəl\ adj : incapable of surviving esp. because of a deleterious genetic constitution — **in·vi·a·bil·i·ty** \-ˌvī-ə-'bi-lə-tē\ n

in vi·tro \in-'vē-(ˌ)trō, -'vi-\ adv or adj : outside the living body and in an artificial environment

in vitro fertilization n : mixture usu. in a laboratory dish of sperm with eggs which have been obtained from an ovary that is followed by transfer of one or more of the resulting fertilized eggs into the uterus — abbr. IVF

in vi·vo \in-'vē-(ˌ)vō\ adv or adj 1 : in the living body of a plant or animal 2 : in a real-life situation

in·vo·lu·crum \ˌin-və-'lü-krəm\ n, pl **-cra** \-krə\ : a formation of new bone about a sequestrum (as in osteomyelitis)

in·vol·un·tary \(ˌ)in-'vä-lən-ˌter-ē\ adj : not subject to control of the will : REFLEX ⟨~ contractions⟩

involuntary muscle n : muscle governing reflex functions and not under direct voluntary control; *esp* : SMOOTH MUSCLE

in·vo·lute \ˌin-və-ˈlüt\ *vb* **-lut·ed; -lut·ing 1** : to return to a former condition **2** : to become cleared up

in·vo·lu·tion \ˌin-və-ˈlü-shən\ *n* **1 a** : an inward curvature or penetration **b** : the formation of a gastrula by ingrowth of cells formed at the dorsal lip **2** : a shrinking or return to a former size ⟨∼ of the uterus after pregnancy⟩ **3** : the regressive alterations of a body or its parts characteristic of the aging process; *specif* : decline marked by a decrease of bodily vigor and in women by menopause

in·vo·lu·tion·al \ˌin-və-ˈlü-shə-nəl\ *adj* **1** : of or relating to involutional melancholia **2** : of or relating to the climacterium and its associated bodily and mental changes

involutional melancholia *n* : agitated depression occurring at about the time of menopause or andropause — called also *involutional psychosis*

in·volve \in-ˈvälv, -ˈvolv\ *vb* **in·volved; in·volv·ing** : to affect with a disease or condition : include in an area of damage, trauma, or insult ⟨herpes *involved* the trigeminal nerve⟩ — **in·volve·ment** \-mənt\ *n*

Iod·amoe·ba \(ˌ)ī-ˌō-də-ˈmē-bə\ *n* : a genus of amoebas including one (*I. butschlii*) commensal in the intestine of mammals including humans

io·dide \ˈī-ə-ˌdīd\ *n* : a compound of iodine usu. with a more electrically positive element or radical

io·dine \ˈī-ə-ˌdīn, -dən, -ˌdēn\ *n* **1** : a nonmetallic halogen element used in medicine (as in antisepsis and in the treatment of goiter) — symbol *I;* see ELEMENT table **2** : a tincture of iodine used esp. as a topical antiseptic

iodine–131 *n* : a heavy radioactive isotope of iodine that has the mass number 131 and a half-life of eight days, gives off beta and gamma rays, and is used esp. in the form of its sodium salt in the diagnosis of thyroid disease and the treatment of goiter

iodine–125 *n* : a light radioactive isotope of iodine that has the mass number of 125 and a half-life of 60 days, gives off soft gamma rays, and is used as a tracer in thyroid studies and as therapy in hyperthyroidism

io·dip·amide \ˌī-ə-ˈdi-pə-ˌmīd\ *n* : a radiopaque substance $C_{20}H_{14}I_6N_2O_6$ used as the sodium or meglumine salts esp. in cholecystography

io·dism \ˈī-ə-ˌdi-zəm\ *n* : an abnormal local and systemic condition resulting from overdosage with, prolonged use of, or sensitivity to iodine or iodine compounds and marked by ptyalism, coryza, frontal headache, emaciation, and skin eruptions

io·dize \ˈī-ə-ˌdīz\ *vb* **io·dized; io·diz·ing** : to treat with iodine or an iodide ⟨*iodized* salt⟩

io·do·chlor·hy·droxy·quin \ī-ˌō-də-

ˌklor-hi-ˈdräk-sē-ˌkwin, ī-ˌä-də-\ *n* : an antimicrobial and mildly irritant drug C_9H_5ClINO formerly used esp. as an antidiarrheal but now used mainly as an antiseptic

io·do·de·oxy·uri·dine \ī-ˌō-də-dē-ˌäk-sē-ˈyur-ə-ˌdēn\ *or* **5–io·do·de·oxy·uri·dine** \ˈfīv-\ *n* : IDOXURIDINE

io·do·form \ī-ˈō-də-ˌform, -ˈä-\ *n* : a yellow crystalline volatile compound CHI_3 used as an antiseptic dressing

io·do·hip·pur·ate sodium \ī-ˌō-də-ˈhi-pyə-ˌrāt-, ī-ˌä-, -hi-ˈpyur-ˌāt-\ *n* : HIPPURAN

io·do·phor \ī-ˈō-də-ˌfor, ī-ˈä-\ *n* : a complex of iodine and a surface-active agent that releases iodine gradually and serves as a disinfectant

io·dop·sin \ˌī-ə-ˈdäp-sən\ *n* : a photosensitive violet pigment in the retinal cones that is similar to rhodopsin but more labile, is formed from vitamin A, and is important in photopic vision

io·do·pyr·a·cet \ˌī-ˌō-də-ˈpir-ə-ˌset, ī-ˌä-\ *n* : a salt $C_8H_{19}I_2N_2O_3$ used as a radiopaque medium esp. in urography

io·do·quin·ol \ˌī-ˌō-də-ˈkwi-ˌnol, -ˌä-, -ˌnol\ *n* : a drug $C_9H_5I_2NO$ used esp. in the treatment of amebic dysentery — called also *diiodohydroxyquin, diiodohydroxyquinoline*

IOM *abbr* Institute of Medicine

ion \ˈī-ˌän, ˈī-ən\ *n* : an electrically charged particle, atom, or group of atoms — **ion·ic** \ī-ˈä-nik\ *adj* — **ion·i·cal·ly** *adv*

ion channel *n* : a cell membrane channel that is selectively permeable to certain ions (as of calcium or sodium)

ion·ize \ˈī-ə-ˌnīz\ *vb* **ion·ized; ion·iz·ing 1** : to convert wholly or partly into ions **2** : to become ionized — **ion·iz·able** \ˌī-ə-ˈnī-zə-bəl\ *adj* — **ion·iza·tion** \ˌī-ə-nə-ˈzā-shən\ *n*

ion·o·phore \ī-ˈä-nə-ˌfor\ *n* : a compound that facilitates transmission of an ion (as of calcium) across a lipid barrier (as in a cell membrane) by combining with the ion or by increasing the permeability of the barrier to it — **ion·oph·o·rous** \ˌī-ə-ˈnä-fə-rəs\ *adj*

ion·to·pho·re·sis \(ˌ)ī-ˌän-tə-fə-ˈrē-səs\ *n, pl* **-re·ses** \-ˌsēz\ : the introduction of an ionized substance (as a drug) through intact skin by the application of a direct electric current — **ion·to·pho·ret·ic** \-ˈre-tik\ *adj* — **ion·to·pho·ret·i·cal·ly** *adv*

io·pa·no·ic acid \ˌī-ə-pə-ˈnō-ik-\ *n* : a crystalline powder $C_{11}H_{12}I_3NO_2$ used as a radiopaque medium in cholecystography

io·phen·dyl·ate \ˌī-ə-ˈfen-də-ˌlāt\ *n* : a radiopaque liquid $C_{19}H_{29}IO_2$ used esp. in myelography

io·thal·a·mate \ˌī-ə-ˈtha-lə-ˌmāt\ *n* : any of several salts of iothalamic acid that are administered by injection as radiopaque media

io·tha·lam·ic acid \ī-ə-thə-ˈla-mik-\ *n* : a white odorless powder $C_{11}H_9I_3N_2O_4$ used as a radiopaque medium

IP *abbr* intraperitoneal; intraperitoneally

IPA *abbr* independent practice association

ip·e·cac \'i-pi-ˌkak\ *also* **ipe·ca·cu·anha** \ˌi-pi-ˌka-kü-'a-nə\ *n* **1** : the dried rhizome and roots of either of two tropical American plants (*Cephaelis acuminata* and *C. ipecacuanha*) of the madder family (Rubiaceae) used esp. as a source of emetine **2** : an emetic and expectorant preparation of ipecac; *esp* : IPECAC SYRUP

ipecac syrup *n* : an emetic and expectorant liquid preparation that is used to induce vomiting in accidental poisoning and is prepared by extracting the ether-soluble alkaloids from powdered ipecac and mixing them with glycerol and a syrup — called also *syrup of ipecac*

ipo·date \'i-pə-ˌdāt\ *n* : a compound $C_{12}H_{13}I_3N_2O_2$ that is administered as the sodium or calcium salt for use as a radiopaque medium in cholecystography and cholangiography

IPPB *abbr* intermittent positive pressure breathing

ip·ra·tro·pi·um bromide \ˌi-prə-ˌtrō-pē-əm-\ *n* : an anticholinergic bronchodilator used $C_{20}H_{30}BrNO_3 \cdot H_2O$ used esp. in the treatment of chronic obstructive pulmonary disease — see COMBIVENT

ipri·fla·vone \ˌī-pri-'flā-ˌvōn\ *n* : a semisynthetic isoflavone $C_{18}H_{16}O_3$ used to prevent postmenopausal bone loss

ipro·ni·a·zid \ˌī-prə-'nī-ə-zəd\ *n* : a derivative $C_9H_{13}N_3O$ of isoniazid that is a monoamine oxidase inhibitor used as an antidepressant and formerly used in treating tuberculosis

IPSID *abbr* immunoproliferative small intestinal disease

ip·si·lat·er·al \ˌip-si-'la-tə-rəl\ *adj* : situated or appearing on or affecting the same side of the body — compare CONTRALATERAL — **ip·si·lat·er·al·ly** *adv*

IPSP *abbr* inhibitory postsynaptic potential

IPT *abbr* interpersonal psychotherapy; interpersonal therapy

IQ \ˌī-'kyü\ *n* [*intelligence quotient*] : a number used to express the apparent relative intelligence of a person: as **a** : the ratio of the mental age (as reported on a standardized test) to the chronological age multiplied by 100 **b** : a score determined by one's performance on a standardized intelligence test relative to the average performance of others of the same age

Ir *symbol* iridium

IR *abbr* infrared

ir- — see IN-

irid- *or* **irido-** *comb form* **1** : iris of the eye ⟨*iridectomy*⟩ **2** : iris and ⟨*iridocyclitis*⟩

iri·dec·to·my \ˌir-ə-'dek-tə-mē, ˌīr-\ *n, pl* **-mies** : the surgical removal of part of the iris of the eye

iri·den·clei·sis \ˌir-ə-den-'klī-səs, ˌīr-\ *n, pl* **-clei·ses** \-ˌsēz\ : a surgical procedure esp. for relief of glaucoma in which a small portion of the iris is implanted in a corneal incision to facilitate drainage of aqueous humor

irides *pl of* IRIS

irid·ic \i-'ri-dik, ī-\ *adj* : of or relating to the iris of the eye

iridis — see HETEROCHROMIA IRIDIS, RUBEOSIS IRIDIS

irid·i·um \ir-'i-dē-əm\ *n* : a silver-white brittle metallic element of the platinum group — symbol *Ir;* see ELEMENT table

iri·do·cy·cli·tis \ˌir-ə-dō-sī-'klī-təs, ˌīr-, -si-\ *n* : inflammation of the iris and the ciliary body

iri·do·di·al·y·sis \ˌir-ə-dō-dī-'a-lə-səs, ˌīr-\ *n, pl* **-y·ses** \-ˌsēz\ : separation of the iris from its attachments to the ciliary body

iri·dol·o·gy \ˌī-rə-'dä-lə-jē\ *n, pl* **-gies** : the study of the iris of the eye for indications of bodily health and disease — **iri·dol·o·gist** \-jist\ *n*

iri·do·ple·gia \ˌir-ə-dō-'plē-jə, ˌīr-, -jē-ə\ *n* : paralysis of the sphincter of the iris

iri·dot·o·my \ˌir-ə-'dä-tə-mē, ˌīr-\ *n, pl* **-mies** : incision of the iris

iris \'ī-rəs\ *n, pl* **iris·es** *or* **iri·des** \'ī-rə-ˌdēz, 'ir-ə-\ : the opaque muscular contractile diaphragm that is suspended in the aqueous humor in front of the lens of the eye, is perforated by the pupil and is continuous peripherally with the ciliary body, has a deeply pigmented posterior surface which excludes the entrance of light except through the pupil and a colored anterior surface which determines the color of the eyes

iris bom·bé \-ˌbäm-'bā\ *n* : a condition in which the iris is bowed forward by an accumulation of fluid between the iris and the lens

Irish moss *n* **1** : the dried and bleached plants of a red alga (esp. *Chondrus crispus*) used as an agent for thickening or emulsifying or as a demulcent **2** : a red alga (esp. *Chondrus crispus*) that is a source of Irish moss

iri·tis \ī-'rī-təs\ *n* : inflammation of the iris of the eye

iron \'ī(-)rn, 'ī-ərn\ *n* **1** : a heavy malleable ductile magnetic silver-white metallic element vital to biological processes (as in transport of oxygen in the body) — symbol *Fe;* see ELEMENT table **2** : iron chemically combined ⟨~ in the blood⟩ — **iron** *adj*

iron–deficiency anemia *n* : anemia that is caused by a deficiency of iron and characterized by hypochromic microcytic red blood cells

iron lung *n* : a device for artificial respiration in which rhythmic alternations in the air pressure in a chamber surrounding a patient's chest force air into and out of the lungs esp. when the nerves governing the chest muscles fail to function because of poliomyelitis — called also *Drinker respirator*

ir·ra·di·ate \i-'rā-dē-,āt\ *vb* **-at·ed; -at·ing** : to affect or treat by radiant energy (as heat); *specif* : to treat by exposure to radiation (as ultraviolet light or gamma rays) — **ir·ra·di·a·tor** \-ā-tər\ *n*

ir·ra·di·a·tion \ir-,ā-dē-'ā-shən\ *n* **1** : the radiation of a physiologically active agent from a point of origin within the body; *esp* : the spread of a nervous impulse beyond the usual conduction path **2 a** : exposure to radiation (as ultraviolet light, X-rays, or alpha particles) **b** : application of radiation (as X-rays or gamma rays) esp. for therapeutic purposes

ir·re·duc·ible \,ir-i-'düs-sə-bəl, -'dyü-\ *adj* : impossible to bring into a desired or normal position or state (an ~ hernia)

ir·reg·u·lar \i-'re-gyə-lər\ *adj* **1** : lacking perfect symmetry of form : not straight, smooth, even, or regular (~ teeth) **2 a** : lacking continuity or regularity of occurrence, activity, or function (~ breathing) **b** *of a physiological function* : failing to occur at regular or normal intervals **c** *of an individual* : failing to defecate at regular or normal intervals — **ir·reg·u·lar·i·ty** \i-,re-gyə-'lar-ə-tē\ *n* — **ir·reg·u·lar·ly** *adv*

ir·re·me·di·a·ble \,ir-i-'mē-dē-ə-bəl\ *adj* : impossible to remedy or cure

ir·re·vers·ible \,ir-i-'vər-sə-bəl\ *adj, of a pathological process* : of such severity that recovery is impossible (~ brain damage) — **ir·re·vers·ibil·i·ty** \-,vər-sə-'bi-lə-tē\ *n* — **ir·re·vers·ibly** \-'vər-sə-blē\ *adv*

ir·ri·gate \'ir-ə-,gāt\ *vb* **-gat·ed; -gat·ing** : to flush (a body part) with a stream of liquid (as in removing a foreign body or medicating) — **ir·ri·ga·tion** \,ir-ə-'gā-shən\ *n* — **ir·ri·ga·tor** \'ir-ə-,gā-tər\ *n*

ir·ri·ta·bil·i·ty \,ir-ə-tə-'bi-lə-tē\ *n, pl* **-ties 1** : the property of protoplasm and of living organisms that permits them to react to stimuli **2 a** : quick excitability to annoyance, impatience, or anger **b** : abnormal or excessive excitability of an organ or part of the body (as the stomach or bladder) — **ir·ri·ta·ble** \'ir-ə-tə-bəl\ *adj*

irritable bowel syndrome *n* : a chronic functional disorder of the colon that is of unknown etiology but is often associated with abnormal intestinal motility and increased sensitivity to visceral pain and that is characterized by diarrhea or constipation or diarrhea alternating with constipation, abdominal pain or discomfort, abdominal bloating, and passage of mucus in the stool — called also *irritable colon, irritable colon syndrome, mucous colitis, spastic colon*

ir·ri·tant \'ir-ə-tənt\ *adj* : causing irritation; *specif* : tending to produce inflammation — **irritant** *n*

ir·ri·tate \'ir-ə-,tāt\ *vb* **-tat·ed; -tat·ing 1** : to provoke impatience, anger, or displeasure in **2** : to cause (an organ or tissue) to be irritable : produce irritation in **3** : to produce excitation in (as a nerve) : cause (as a muscle) to contract — **ir·ri·ta·tion** \,ir-ə-'tā-shən\ *n*

ir·ri·ta·tive \'ir-ə-,tā-tiv\ *adj* **1** : serving to excite : IRRITATING (an ~ agent) **2** : accompanied with or produced by irritation (~ coughing)

is- *or* **iso-** *comb form* **1** : equal : homogeneous : uniform (*iso*smotic) **2** : for or from different individuals of the same species (*iso*agglutinin)

isch·ae·mia *chiefly Brit var of* ISCHEMIA

isch·emia \is-'kē-mē-ə\ *n* : deficient supply of blood to a body part (as the heart or brain) that is due to obstruction of the inflow of arterial blood (as by the narrowing of arteries by spasm or disease) — **isch·emic** \-mik\ *adj* — **isch·emi·cal·ly** *adv*

ischemic stroke *n* : stroke caused by thrombosis or embolism

ischi- *or* **ischio-** *comb form* **1** : ischium (*ischi*ectomy) **2** : ischial and (*ischio*rectal)

ischia *pl of* ISCHIUM

is·chi·al \'is-kē-əl\ *adj* : of, relating to, or situated near the ischium

ischial spine *n* : a thin pointed triangular eminence that projects from the dorsal border of the ischium and gives attachment to the gemellus superior on its external surface and to the coccygeus, levator ani, and pelvic fascia on its internal surface

ischial tuberosity *n* : a bony swelling on the posterior part of the superior ramus of the ischium that gives attachment to various muscles and bears the weight of the body in sitting

is·chi·ec·to·my \,is-kē-'ek-tə-mē\ *n, pl* **-mies** : surgical removal of a segment of the hip bone including the ischium

is·chio·cav·er·no·sus \,is-kē-ō-,ka-vər-'nō-səs\ *n, pl* **-no·si** \-,sī\ : a muscle on each side that arises from the ischium near the crus of the penis or clitoris and is inserted on the crus near the pubic symphysis

is·chio·coc·cy·geus \-käk-'si-jē-əs\ *n, pl* **-cy·gei** \-jē-,ī, -,ē\ : COCCYGEUS

is·chio·fem·o·ral \-'fe-mə-rəl\ *adj* : of, relating to, or being an accessory ligament of the hip joint passing from the ischium below the acetabulum to the hip joint capsule

is·chio·pu·bic ramus \,is-kē-ō-'pyü-bik-\ *n* : the flattened inferior projection of the hip bone below the obturator foramen consisting of the united inferior rami of the pubis and ischium

is·chio·rec·tal \ˌis-kē-ō-ˈrekt-ᵊl\ *adj* : of, relating to, or adjacent to both ischium and rectum ⟨an ∼ abscess⟩

is·chi·um \ˈis-kē-əm\ *n, pl* **is·chia** \-ə\ : the dorsal and posterior of the three principal bones composing either half of the pelvis consisting in humans of a thick portion, a large rough eminence on which the body rests when sitting, and a forwardly directed ramus which joins that of the pubis

Ishi·ha·ra \ˌi-shē-ˈhär-ə\ *adj* : of, relating to, or used in an Ishihara test

Ishihara, Shinobu (1879–1963), Japanese ophthalmologist.

Ishihara test *n* : a widely used test for color blindness that consists of a set of plates covered with colored dots which the test subject views in order to find a number composed of dots of one color which a person with various defects of color vision will confuse with surrounding dots of color

is·land \ˈī-lənd\ *n* : an isolated anatomical structure, tissue, or group of cells

island of Lang·er·hans \-ˈläŋ-ər-ˌhänz, -ˌhäns\ *n* : ISLET OF LANGERHANS

island of Reil \-ˈrīl\ *n* : INSULA

Reil, Johann Christian (1759–1813), German anatomist.

is·let \ˈī-lət\ *n* : ISLET OF LANGERHANS

islet cell *n* : one of the endocrine cells making up an islet of Langerhans

islet of Lang·er·hans \-ˈläŋ-ər-ˌhänz, -ˌhäns\ *n* : any of the groups of small slightly granular endocrine cells that form anastomosing trabeculae among the tubules and alveoli of the pancreas and secrete insulin and glucagon — called also *islet*

Langerhans, Paul (1847–1888), German pathologist.

-ism \ˌi-zəm\ *n suffix* **1** : act, practice, or process ⟨hypnot*ism*⟩ **2 a** : state, condition, or property ⟨polymorph*ism*⟩ **b** : abnormal state or condition resulting from excess of a (specified) thing or marked by resemblance to a (specified) person or thing ⟨alcohol*ism*⟩ ⟨morphin*ism*⟩

iso- — see IS-

iso·ag·glu·ti·na·tion \ˌī-(ˌ)sō-ə-ˌglüt-ᵊn-ˈā-shən\ *n* : agglutination of an agglutinogen of one individual by the serum of another of the same species

iso·ag·glu·ti·nin \-ə-ˈglüt-ᵊn-ən\ *n* : an antibody produced by one individual that causes agglutination of cells (as red blood cells) of other individuals of the same species

iso·ag·glu·tin·o·gen \-ˌa-glü-ˈti-nə-jən\ *n* : an antigenic substance capable of provoking formation of or reacting with an isoagglutinin

iso·al·lox·a·zine \-ə-ˈläk-sə-ˌzēn\ *n* : a yellow solid $C_{10}H_6N_4O_2$ that is the precursor of various flavins (as riboflavin)

iso·am·yl nitrite \ˌī-sō-ˈa-məl-\ *n* : AMYL NITRITE

iso·an·ti·body \ˌī-(ˌ)sō-ˈan-ti-ˌbä-dē\ *n, pl* **-bod·ies** : ALLOANTIBODY

iso·an·ti·gen \-ˈan-ti-jən\ *n* : ALLOANTIGEN

iso·bor·nyl thio·cy·ano·ace·tate \ˌī-sō-ˈbȯr-nil-ˌthī-ō-ˌsī-ə-nō-ˈa-sə-ˌtāt, -sī-ə-nō-\ *n* : a yellow oily liquid $C_{13}H_{19}N_2OS$ used as a pediculicide

iso·bu·tyl nitrite \ˌī-sō-ˈbyüt-ᵊl-\ *n* : BUTYL NITRITE

iso·car·box·az·id \-ˌkär-ˈbäk-sə-zəd\ *n* : a hydrazide monoamine oxidase inhibitor $C_{12}H_{13}N_3O_2$ used as an antidepressant — see MARPLAN

iso·chro·mo·some \-ˈkrō-mə-ˌsōm, -ˌzōm\ *n* : a chromosome produced by transverse splitting of the centromere so that both arms are from the same side of the centromere, are of equal length, and possess identical genes

iso·ci·trate \ˌī-sō-ˈsi-ˌtrāt\ *n* : any salt or ester of isocitric acid; *also* : ISOCITRIC ACID

iso·cit·rate de·hy·dro·ge·nase \-ˌdē-(ˌ)hī-ˈdrä-je-ˌnās, -ˈhī-drə-jə-, -ˌnāz\ *n* : either of two enzymes which catalyze the oxidation of isocitric acid (as in the Krebs cycle) — called also *isocitric dehydrogenase*

iso·cit·ric acid \ˌī-sə-ˈsi-trik-\ *n* : a crystalline isomer of citric acid that occurs esp. as an intermediate stage in the Krebs cycle

isocitric dehydrogenase *n* : ISOCITRATE DEHYDROGENASE

iso·dose \ˈī-sə-ˌdōs\ *adj* : of or relating to points or zones in a medium that receive equal doses of radiation

iso·elec·tric \ˌī-sō-i-ˈlek-trik\ *adj* : being the pH at which the electrolyte will not migrate in an electrical field ⟨the ∼ point of a protein⟩

isoelectric focusing *n* : an electrophoretic technique for separating proteins by causing them to migrate under the influence of an electric field through a medium (as a gel) having a pH gradient to locations with pH values corresponding to their isoelectric points

iso·en·zyme \ˌī-sō-ˈen-ˌzīm\ *n* : any of two or more chemically distinct but functionally similar enzymes — called also *isozyme* — **iso·en·zy·mat·ic** \ˌī-sō-ˌen-zə-ˈma-tik, -zī-\ *adj* — **iso·en·zy·mic** \-en-ˈzī-mik\ *adj*

iso·eth·a·rine \-ˈe-thə-ˌrēn\ *n* : a beta₂-adrenergic bronchodilator administered by oral inhalation esp. in the form of its hydrochloride $C_{13}H_{21}NO_3$·HCl to treat asthma and bronchospasm

iso·fla·vone \-ˈflā-ˌvōn\ *n* : a bioactive ketone $C_{15}H_{10}O_2$ having numerous derivatives that are found in plants (as the soybean) and have antioxidant and estrogenic activity; *also* : any of these derivatives (as genistein)

iso·fluro·phate \-ˈflur-ə-ˌfāt\ *n* : a volatile irritating liquid ester C_6H_{14}-

FO_3P that acts as a nerve gas by inhibiting cholinesterases and as a miotic and that is used chiefly in treating glaucoma — called also *DFP, diisopropyl fluorophosphate*

iso·form \'ī-sə-ˌfȯrm\ *n* : any of two or more functionally similar proteins that have a similar but not identical amino acid sequence

iso·ge·ne·ic \ˌī-sō-jə-'nē-ik, -'nā-\ *adj* : SYNGENEIC ⟨an ∼ graft⟩

iso·gen·ic \-'je-nik\ *adj* : characterized by essentially identical genes

iso·graft \'ī-sə-ˌgraft\ *n* : a homograft between genetically identical or nearly identical individuals — **isograft** *vb*

iso·hem·ag·glu·ti·nin \ˌī-sō-ˌhē-mə-'glüt-ᵊn-ən\ *n* : a hemagglutinin causing isoagglutination

iso·hy·dric shift \ˌī-sō-'hī-drik-\ *n* : the set of chemical reactions in a red blood cell by which oxygen is released to the tissues and carbon dioxide is taken up while the blood remains at constant pH

iso·im·mu·ni·za·tion \ˌī-sō-ˌi-myə-nə-'zā-shən\ *n* : production by an individual of antibodies against constituents of the tissues of another individual of the same species (as when transfused with blood from one belonging to a different blood group)

¹iso·late \'ī-sə-ˌlāt\ *vb* **-lat·ed; -lat·ing** : to set apart from others: as **a** : to separate (one with a contagious disease) from others not similarly infected **b** : to separate (as a chemical compound) from all other substances : obtain pure or in a free state

²iso·late \'ī-sə-lət, -ˌlāt\ *n* **1** : an individual (as a single organism), a viable part of an organism (as a cell), or a strain that has been isolated (as from diseased tissue); *also* : a pure culture produced from such an isolate **2** : a socially maladjusted individual

iso·la·tion \ˌī-sə-'lā-shən\ *n* **1** : the action of isolating or condition of being isolated **2** : a psychological defense mechanism consisting of the separating of ideas or memories from the emotions connected with them

Iso·lette \ˌī-sə-'let\ *trademark* — used for an incubator for premature infants that provides controlled temperature and humidity and an oxygen supply

iso·leu·cine \ˌī-sō-'lü-ˌsēn\ *n* : a crystalline essential amino acid $C_6H_{13}NO_2$ isomeric with leucine — abbr. *Ile*

isol·o·gous \ī-'sä-lə-gəs\ *adj* : SYNGENEIC

iso·mer \'ī-sə-mər\ *n* : any of two or more compounds, radicals, or ions that contain the same number of atoms of the same elements but differ in structural arrangement and properties — **iso·mer·ic** \ˌī-sə-'mer-ik\ *adj* — **isom·er·ism** \ī-'sä-mə-ˌri-zəm\ *n*

iso·me·thep·tene \ˌī-sō-me-'thep-ˌtēn\ *n* : a vasoconstrictive and antispas-

modic drug administered esp. in the form of its mucate $C_{24}H_{48}N_2O_8$

iso·met·ric \ˌī-sə-'me-trik\ *adj* : of, relating to, involving, or being muscular contraction (as in isometrics) against resistance, without significant change of length of muscle fibers, and with marked increase in muscle tone — compare ISOTONIC 2 — **iso·met·ri·cal·ly** *adv*

iso·met·rics \ˌī-sə-'me-triks\ *n sing or pl* : isometric exercise or an isometric system of exercises

iso·ni·a·zid \ˌī-sə-'nī-ə-zəd\ *n* : a crystalline compound $C_6H_7N_3O$ used in treating tuberculosis

isonicotinic acid hydrazide *n* : ISONIAZID

iso·nip·e·caine \ˌī-sō-'ni-pə-ˌkān\ *n* : MEPERIDINE

iso·os·mot·ic \ˌī-sō-äz-'mä-tik\ *adj* : ISOTONIC 1

Iso·paque \ˌī-sō-'pāk\ *trademark* — used for a preparation of metrizoate sodium

iso·peri·stal·tic \ˌī-sō-ˌper-ə-'stȯl-tik, -'stäl-, -'stal-\ *adj* : performed or arranged so that the grafted or anastomosed parts exhibit peristalsis in the same direction ⟨∼ gastroenterostomy⟩ — **iso·peri·stal·ti·cal·ly** *adv*

iso·phane insulin \'ī-sō-ˌfān-\ *n* : a crystalline suspension of insulin, protamine, and zinc in a buffered aqueous solution that is used for injection and has a slow onset and long duration of action — called also *insulin isophane, isophane, NPH insulin*

iso·preg·nen·one \-'preg-ne-ˌnōn\ *n* : DYDROGESTERONE

iso·pren·a·line \ˌī-sə-'pren-ᵊl-ən\ *n* : ISOPROTERENOL

iso·pro·pa·mide iodide \ˌī-sō-'prō-pə-ˌmēd-\ *n* : an anticholinergic $C_{23}H_{33}IN_2O$ used esp. for its antispasmodic and antisecretory effect on the gastrointestinal tract — called also *isopropamide*

iso·pro·pa·nol \-'prō-pə-ˌnȯl, -ˌnōl\ *n* : ISOPROPYL ALCOHOL

iso·pro·pyl alcohol \ˌī-sə-'prō-pəl-\ *n* : a volatile flammable alcohol C_3H_8O used as a rubbing alcohol

iso·pro·pyl·ar·te·re·nol \ˌī-sə-ˌprō-pə-ˌlär-tə-'rē-ˌnȯl, -ˌnōl\ *n* : ISOPROTERENOL

isopropyl my·ris·tate \-mə-'ris-ˌtāt\ *n* : an ester $C_{17}H_{34}O_2$ of isopropyl alcohol that is used as an emollient to promote absorption through the skin

iso·pro·ter·e·nol \ˌī-sō-prō-'ter-ə-ˌnȯl, -nəl\ *n* : a sympathomimetic agent that is used in the form of its hydrochloride $C_{11}H_{17}NO_3 \cdot HCl$ or sulfate $(C_{11}H_{17}NO_3)_2 \cdot H_2SO_4$ esp. as a bronchodilator in the treatment of asthma, bronchitis, and emphysema — called also *isoprenaline, isopropylarterenol*; see ISUPREL

isop·ter \ī-'säp-tər\ *n* : a contour line in a representation of the visual field around the points representing the macula lutea that passes through the points of equal visual acuity

Isor·dil \ˈī-sȯr-ˌdil\ *trademark* — used for a preparation of isosorbide dinitrate

is·os·mot·ic \ˌī-ˌsäz-ˈmä-tik, -ˌsäs-\ *adj* : ISOTONIC 1 — **is·os·mot·i·cal·ly** *adv*

iso·sor·bide \ˌī-sō-ˈsȯr-ˌbīd\ *n* 1 : a diuretic $C_6H_{10}O_4$ 2 : ISOSORBIDE DINITRATE

isosorbide di·ni·trate \-dī-ˈnī-ˌtrāt\ *n* : a coronary vasodilator $C_6H_8N_2O_8$ used esp. in the treatment of angina pectoris — see ISORDIL

Isos·po·ra \ī-ˈsäs-pə-rə\ *n* : a genus of coccidian protozoans closely related to the genus *Eimeria* and including the only coccidian (*I. hominis*) known to be parasitic in humans

isothiocyanate — see ALLYL ISOTHIOCYANATE

iso·thi·pen·dyl \ˌī-sō-ˌthī-ˈpen-ˌdil\ *n* : an antihistaminic drug $C_{16}H_{19}N_3S$

iso·ton·ic \ˌī-sə-ˈtä-nik\ *adj* 1 : of, relating to, or exhibiting equal osmotic pressure (~ solutions) — compare HYPERTONIC 2, HYPOTONIC 2 2 : of, relating to, or being muscular contraction in the absence of significant resistance, with marked shortening of muscle fibers, and without great increase in muscle tone — compare ISOMETRIC — **iso·ton·i·cal·ly** *adv* — **iso·to·nic·i·ty** \-tō-ˈni-sə-tē\ *n*

iso·tope \ˈī-sə-ˌtōp\ *n* 1 : any of two or more species of atoms of a chemical element with the same atomic number that differ in the number of neutrons in an atom and have different physical properties 2 : NUCLIDE — **iso·to·pic** \ˌī-sə-ˈtä-pik, -ˈtō-\ *adj* — **iso·to·pi·cal·ly** *adv*

iso·trans·plant \ˌī-sō-ˈtrans-ˌplant\ *n* : a graft between syngeneic individuals

iso·tret·i·no·in \ˌī-sō-ˈtre-tə-ˌnȯin\ *n* : an isomer of retinoic acid that is a synthetic derivative of vitamin A, that inhibits sebaceous gland function and keratinization, and that is used in the treatment of severe inflammatory acne but is contraindicated in pregnancy because of its implication as a cause of birth defects — called also *13-cis-retinoic acid, retinoic acid*; see ACCUTANE

isotropic band *n* : I BAND

iso·type \ˈī-sə-ˌtīp\ *n* : any of the categories of antibodies determined by their physicochemical properties (as molecular weight) and antigenic characteristics that occur in all individuals of a species — compare ALLOTYPE, IDIOTYPE — **iso·typ·ic** \ˌī-sə-ˈti-pik\ *adj*

iso·va·ler·ic acid \ˌī-sō-və-ˈlir-ik-, -ˈler-\ *n* : a liquid acid $C_5H_{10}O_2$ that has a disagreeable odor

isovaleric ac·i·de·mia \-ˌa-sə-ˈdē-mē-ə\ *n* : a metabolic disorder characterized by the presence of an abnormally high concentration of isovaleric acid in the blood causing acidosis, coma, and an unpleasant body odor

iso·vol·ume \ˈī-sə-ˌväl-yəm, -ˌ(ˌ)yüm\ *adj* : ISOVOLUMETRIC

iso·vol·u·met·ric \ˌī-sə-ˌväl-yü-ˈme-trik\ *adj* : of, relating to, or characterized by unchanging volume; *esp* : relating to or being an early phase of ventricular systole in which the cardiac muscle exerts increasing pressure on the contents of the ventricle without significant change in the muscle fiber length and the ventricular volume remains constant

iso·vo·lu·mic \-və-ˈlü-mik\ *adj* : ISOVOLUMETRIC

is·ox·az·o·lyl \(ˌ)ī-ˌsäk-ˈsa-zə-ˌlil\ *adj* : relating to or being any of a group of semisynthetic penicillins (as oxacillin and cloxacillin) that are resistant to beta-lactamase, stable in acids, and active against gram-positive bacteria

is·ox·su·prine \ī-ˈsäk-sə-ˌprēn\ *n* : a sympathomimetic drug $C_{18}H_{23}NO_3$ used chiefly as a vasodilator

iso·zyme \ˈī-sə-ˌzīm\ *n* : ISOENZYME — **iso·zy·mic** \ˌī-sə-ˈzī-mik\ *adj*

is·sue \ˈi-(ˌ)shü\ *n* : a discharge (as of blood) from the body that is caused by disease or other physical disorder or that is produced artificially; *also* : an incision made to produce such a discharge

isth·mus \ˈis-məs\ *n* : a contracted anatomical part or passage connecting two larger structures or cavities: as **a** : an embryonic constriction separating the midbrain from the hindbrain **b** : the lower portion of the uterine corpus — **isth·mic** \ˈis-mik\ *adj*

isthmus of the fauces *n* : FAUCES

Isu·prel \ˈī-sü-ˌprel\ *trademark* — used for a preparation of the hydrochloride of isoproterenol

itai–itai \ī-ˈtī-i-ˌtī\ *n* : an extremely painful condition caused by poisoning following the ingestion of cadmium and characterized by bone decalcification — called also *itai-itai disease*

IT band \ˌī-ˈtē-\ *n* : ILIOTIBIAL BAND

itch \ˈich\ *n* 1 : an uneasy irritating sensation in the upper surface of the skin usu. held to result from mild stimulation of pain receptors 2 : a skin disorder accompanied by an itch; *esp* : a contagious eruption caused by an itch mite of the genus *Sarcoptes* (*S. scabiei*) that burrows in the skin and causes intense itching — **itch** *vb* — **itch·i·ness** \ˈi-chē-nəs\ *n* — **itchy** \ˈi-chē\ *adj*

¹**itch·ing** *adj* : having, producing, or marked by an uneasy sensation in the skin (an ~ skin eruption)

²**itching** *n* : ITCH 1

itch mite *n* : any of several minute parasitic mites that burrow into the skin and cause itch; *esp* : a mite of any of several varieties of a species of the genus *Sarcoptes* (*S. scabiei*) that causes the itch

-ite \ˌīt\ *n suffix* **1** : substance produced through some (specified) process ⟨catabol*ite*⟩ **2** : segment or constituent part of a body or of a bodily part ⟨som*ite*⟩ ⟨dendr*ite*⟩

-it·ic \ˈi-tik\ *adj suffix* : of, resembling, or marked by — in adjectives formed from nouns usu. ending in *-ite* ⟨den-dr*itic*⟩ and *-itis* ⟨bronch*itic*⟩

-i·tis \ˈī-təs\ *n suffix, pl* **-it·is·es** *also* **-it·i·des** \ˈi-tə-ˌdēz\ *or* **-i·tes** \ˈī-(ˌ)tēz\ : disease usu. inflammatory of a (specified) part or organ : inflammation of ⟨laryng*itis*⟩ ⟨appendic*itis*⟩

ITP *abbr* idiopathic thrombocytopenic purpura

it·ra·con·a·zole \i-trə-ˈkä-nə-ˌzōl\ *n* : a triazole antifungal agent $C_{35}H_{38}Cl_2N_8O_4$ used orally esp. to treat blastomycosis and histoplasmosis — see SPORANOX

IU *abbr* international unit

IUCD \ˌī-(ˌ)yü-(ˌ)sē-ˈdē\ *n* : INTRAUTERINE DEVICE

IUD \ˌī-(ˌ)yü-ˈdē\ *n* : INTRAUTERINE DEVICE

IUDR \ˌī-(ˌ)yü-(ˌ)dē-ˈär\ *n* : IDOXURIDINE

IV \ˈī-ˈvē\ *n, pl* **IVs** : an apparatus used to administer a fluid (as of medication, blood, or nutrients) intravenously; *also* : a fluid administered by IV

IV *abbr* **1** intravenous; intravenously **2** intraventricular

iver·mec·tin \ˌī-vər-ˈmek-tən\ *n* : a drug mixture of two structurally similar semisynthetic lactones that is used in veterinary medicine as an anthelmintic, acaricide, and insecticide and in human medicine to treat onchocerciasis

IVF *abbr* in vitro fertilization

IVP *abbr* intravenous pyelogram

Ix·o·des \ik-ˈsō-(ˌ)dēz\ *n* : a widespread genus of ixodid ticks (as the deer tick) many of which are bloodsucking parasites of humans and animals, and sometimes cause paralysis or other severe reactions

ix·od·i·cide \ik-ˈsä-di-ˌsīd, -ˈsō-\ *n* : an agent that destroys ticks

ixo·did \ik-ˈsä-did, -ˈsō-\ *adj* : of or relating to a family (Ixodidae) of ticks (as the deer tick and American dog tick) having a hard outer shell and feeding on two or three hosts during the life cycle — **ixodid** *n*

J

jaag·siek·te *also* **jag·siek·te** *or* **jaag-ziek·te** *or* **jag·ziek·te** \ˈyäg-ˌsēk-tə, -ˌzēk-\ *n* : a chronic contagious pneumonitis of sheep and sometimes goats that is caused by a retrovirus (species *Ovine pulmonary adenocarcinoma virus* of the genus *Betaretrovirus*) — called also *pulmonary adenomatosis*

jack·et \ˈja-kət\ *n* **1** : a rigid covering that envelops the upper body and provides support, correction, or restraint **2** : JACKET CROWN

jacket crown *n* : an artificial crown that is placed over the remains of a natural tooth

jack·so·ni·an \jak-ˈsō-nē-ən\ *adj, often cap* : of, relating to, associated with, or resembling Jacksonian epilepsy

Jack·son \ˈjak-sən\, **John Hughlings (1835–1911),** British neurologist.

Jacksonian epilepsy *n* : epilepsy that is characterized by progressive spreading of the abnormal movements or sensations from a focus affecting a muscle group on one side of the body to adjacent muscles or by becoming generalized and that corresponds to the spread of epileptic activity in the motor cortex

Ja·cob·son's nerve \ˈjä-kəb-sənz-\ *n* : TYMPANIC NERVE

Jacobson \ˈyä-kȯp-sən\, **Ludwig Levin (1783–1843),** Danish anatomist.

Jacobson's organ *n* : VOMERONASAL ORGAN

jac·ti·ta·tion \ˌjak-tə-ˈtā-shən\ *n* : a tossing to and fro or jerking and twitching of the body or its parts : excessive restlessness esp. in certain psychiatric disorders — **jac·ti·tate** \ˈjak-tə-ˌtāt\ *vb*

Jaf·fé reaction \yä-ˈfā-, zhä-\ *also* **Jaf·fé's reaction** \-ˈfāz-\ *n* : a reaction between creatinine and picric acid in alkaline solution that results in the formation of a red compound and is used to measure the amount of creatinine (as in creatinuria)

Jaffé \yä-ˈfā\, **Max (1841–1911),** German biochemist.

jail fever \ˈjāl-\ *n* : TYPHUS a

jake leg \ˈjāk-\ *n* : a paralysis caused by drinking improperly distilled or contaminated liquor

Ja·kob–Creutz·feldt disease \ˈyä-(ˌ)kȯb-ˈkrȯits-ˌfelt-\ *n* : CREUTZFELDT-JAKOB DISEASE

jal·ap \ˈja-ləp, ˈjä-\ *n* **1** : the dried tuberous root of a Mexican plant (*Ipomoea purga*) of the morning-glory family (Convolvulaceae); *also* : a powdered purgative drug prepared from it that contains resinous glycosides **2** : a plant yielding jalap

JAMA *abbr* Journal of the American Medical Association

ja·mais vu \ˌzhä-ˌme-ˈvᵫ, jä-ˌmä-ˈvᵫ\

n : a disorder of memory characterized by the illusion that the familiar is being encountered for the first time — compare PARAMNESIA b

James·town weed \'jāmz-taún-\ n : JIMSONWEED

jani·ceps \'ja-nə-,seps, 'jā-\ n : a malformed double fetus joined at the thorax and skull and having two equal faces looking in opposite directions

Japanese B encephalitis n : an encephalitis that occurs epidemically in Japan and other Asian countries in the summer, is caused by a virus of the genus *Flavivirus* (species *Japanese encephalitis virus*) transmitted by mosquitoes (esp. *Culex tritaeniorhynchus*) and usu. produces a subclinical infection but may cause acute meningoencephalomyelitis — called also *Japanese encephalitis*

japonica — see SCHISTOSOMIASIS JAPONICA

jar·gon \'jär-gən\ n : unintelligible, meaningless, or incoherent speech (as that associated with Wernicke's aphasia or some forms of schizophrenia)

Ja·risch–Herx·hei·mer reaction \'yä-rish-'herks-,hī-mər-\ n : an increase in the symptoms of a spirochetal disease (as syphilis or Lyme disease) occurring in some persons when treatment with spirocheticidal drugs is started — called also *Herxheimer reaction*
Jarisch, Adolf (1850–1902), Austrian dermatologist.
Herxheimer, Karl (1861–1944), German dermatologist.

Jar·vik-7 \jär-vik-'se-vən\ n : an air-driven artificial heart that remains tethered to an external console after implantation and that was formerly implanted in human patients in a clinical study — called also *Jarvik heart*
Jarvik, Robert Koffler (b 1946), American physician and inventor.

jaun·dice \'jȯn-dəs, 'jän-\ n 1 : a yellowish pigmentation of the skin, tissues, and certain body fluids caused by the deposition of bile pigments that follows interference with normal production and discharge of bile (as in certain liver diseases) or excessive breakdown of red blood cells (as after internal hemorrhage or in various hemolytic states) 2 : any disease or abnormal condition (as hepatitis A or leptospirosis) that is characterized by jaundice — **jaun·diced** \-dəst\ adj

jaw \'jȯ\ n 1 : either of two complex cartilaginous or bony structures in most vertebrates that border the mouth, support the soft parts enclosing it, and usu. bear teeth on their oral margin: **a** : an upper structure more or less firmly fused with the skull — called also *upper jaw, maxilla* **b** : a lower structure that consists of a single bone or of completely fused bones and that is hinged, movable, and articulated by a pair of condyles with the temporal bone of either side

— called also *inferior maxillary bone, lower jaw, mandible* 2 : the parts constituting the walls of the mouth and serving to open and close it — usu. used in pl.

jaw·bone \'jȯ-,bōn\ n : JAW 1; esp : MANDIBLE

jawed \'jȯd\ adj : having jaws — usu. used in combination ⟨square-*jawed*⟩

Jaws of Life trademark — used for a hydraulic tool that is used esp. to free victims trapped inside wrecked motor vehicles

JCAH abbr Joint Commission on Accreditation of Hospitals

JCAHO abbr Joint Commission on Accreditation of Healthcare Organizations

J chain \'jā-\ n : a relatively short polypeptide chain with a high number of cysteine residues that is found in antibodies of the IgM and IgA classes

jejun- or **jejuno-** comb form 1 : jejunum ⟨*jeju*nitis⟩ 2 : jejunum and ⟨*jejuno*ileitis⟩

je·ju·nal \ji-'jün-ᵊl\ adj : of or relating to the jejunum

je·ju·ni·tis \je-jü-'nī-təs\ n : inflammation of the jejunum

je·ju·no·il·e·al bypass \ji-jü-nō-'i-lē-əl-\ n : a surgical bypass operation performed esp. to reduce absorption in the small intestine that involves joining the first part of the jejunum with the more distal segment of the ileum

je·ju·no·il·e·itis \ji-jü-nō-,i-lē-'ī-təs, je-jü-nō-\ n : inflammation of the jejunum and the ileum

je·ju·no·il·e·os·to·my \ji-jü-nō-,i-lē-'äs-tə-mē, je-jü-nō-\ n, pl -mies : the formation of an anastomosis between the jejunum and the ileum

je·ju·nos·to·my \ji-jü-'näs-tə-mē, je-jü-\ n, pl -mies 1 : the surgical formation of an opening through the abdominal wall into the jejunum 2 : the opening made by jejunostomy

je·ju·num \ji-'jü-nəm\ n, pl **je·ju·na** \-na\ : the section of the small intestine that comprises the first two fifths beyond the duodenum and that is larger, thicker-walled, and more vascular and has more circular folds and fewer Peyer's patches than the ileum

jel·ly \'je-lē\ n, pl **jellies** : a semisolid gelatinous substance: as **a** : a medicated preparation usu. intended for local application ⟨ephedrine ~⟩ **b** : a jellylike preparation used in electrocardiography to obtain better conduction of electricity ⟨electrode ~⟩

jel·ly·fish \-,fish\ n : a free-swimming marine sexually reproducing coelenterate of either of two classes (Hydrozoa and Scyphozoa) that has a nearly transparent saucer-shaped body and tentacles studded with stinging cells

je·quir·i·ty bean \jə-'kwir-ə-tē-\ n 1 : the poisonous scarlet and black seed of the rosary pea 2 : ROSARY PEA 1

jerk \'jərk\ n : an involuntary spasmodic muscular movement due to reflex action; *esp* : one induced by an external stimulus — see KNEE JERK

jet fatigue \'jet-fə-ˌtēg\ *n* : JET LAG

jet in·jec·tor \-in-'jek-tər\ *n* : a device used to inject subcutaneously a fine stream of fluid under high pressure without puncturing the skin — **jet injec·tion** \-'jek-shən\ *n*

jet lag \'jet-ˌlag\ *n* : a condition that is characterized by various psychological and physiological effects (as fatigue and irritability), occurs following long flight through several time zones, and prob. results from disruption of circadian rhythms in the human body — called also *jet fatigue* — **jet–lagged** *adj*

jig·ger \'ji-gər\ *n* : CHIGGER

jim·son·weed \'jim-sən-ˌwēd\ *n* : a poisonous tall annual weed of the genus *Datura* (*D. stramonium*) with rank-smelling foliage and globe-shaped prickly fruits — called also *Jamestown weed*; see STRAMONIUM 1

jit·ters \'ji-tərz\ *n pl* : a state of extreme nervousness or nervous shaking — **jit·ter** \-tər\ *vb* — **jit·teri·ness** \-tə-rē-nəs\ *n* — **jit·tery** *adj*

JND *abbr* just noticeable difference

job \'jäb\ *n* : plastic surgery for cosmetic purposes ⟨an eye ∼⟩

jock itch \'jäk-\ *n* : ringworm of the crotch : TINEA CRURIS — called also *jockey itch*

jock·strap \'jäk-ˌstrap\ *n* : ATHLETIC SUPPORTER

jogger's nipple *n* : pain and often dermatitis due to chafing of the nipples by clothing worn while jogging — called also *jogger's nipples*

Johne's bacillus \'yō-nēz-\ *n* : a bacillus of the genus *Mycobacterium* (*M. paratuberculosis*) that causes Johne's disease

Johne \'yō-nə\, **Heinrich Albert** (1839–1910), German bacteriologist.

Johne's disease \'yō-nəz-\ *n* : a chronic often fatal enteritis esp. of cattle that is caused by Johne's bacillus — called also *paratuberculosis*

john·ny *also* **john·nie** \'jä-nē\ *n, pl* **johnnies** : a short-sleeved collarless gown that is open in the back and is worn by persons (as hospital patients) undergoing medical examination or treatment

joint \'jȯint\ *n* : the point of contact between skeletal elements whether movable or rigidly fixed together with the surrounding and supporting parts (as membranes, tendons, and ligaments) — **out of joint** *of a bone* : having the head slipped from its socket

joint capsule *n* : a ligamentous sac that surrounds the articular cavity of a freely movable joint, is attached to the bones, completely encloses the joint, and is composed of an outer fibrous membrane and an inner synovial membrane — called also *articular capsule*

joint·ed \'jȯin-təd\ *adj* : having joints

joint fluid *n* : SYNOVIAL FLUID

joint ill *n* : NAVEL ILL

joint mouse \-'maůs\ *n* : a loose fragment (as of cartilage) within a synovial space

joule \'jül\ *n* : a unit of work or energy equal to the work done by a force of one newton acting through a distance of one meter

Joule, James Prescott (1818–1889), British physicist.

¹**ju·gal** \'jü-gəl\ *adj* : MALAR

²**jugal** *n* : ZYGOMATIC BONE — called also *jugal bone*

¹**jug·u·lar** \'jə-gyə-lər, 'jü-\ *adj* **1** : of or relating to the throat or neck **2** : of or relating to the jugular vein

²**jugular** *n* : JUGULAR VEIN

jugulare — see GLOMUS JUGULARE

jugular foramen *n* : a large irregular opening from the posterior cranial fossa that is bounded anteriorly by the petrous part of the temporal bone and posteriorly by the jugular notch of the occipital bone and that transmits the inferior petrosal sinus, the glossopharyngeal, vagus, and accessory nerves, and the internal jugular vein

jugular fossa *n* : a depression on the basilar surface of the petrous portion of the temporal bone that contains a dilation of the internal jugular vein

jugular ganglion *n* : SUPERIOR GANGLION

jugular notch \-'näch\ *n* **1** : SUPRASTERNAL NOTCH **2 a** : a notch in the inferior border of the occipital bone behind the jugular process that forms the posterior part of the jugular foramen **b** : a notch in the petrous portion of the temporal bone that corresponds to the jugular notch of the occipital bone and with it makes up the jugular foramen

jugular process *n* : a quadrilateral or triangular process of the occipital bone on each side that articulates with the temporal bone and is situated lateral to the condyle of the occipital bone on each side articulating with the atlas

jugular trunk *n* : either of two major lymph vessels of which one lies on each side of the body and drains the head and neck

jugular vein *n* : any of several veins of each side of the neck: as **a** : a vein that collects the blood from the interior of the cranium, the superficial part of the face, and the neck, runs down the neck on the outside of the internal and common carotid arteries, and unites with the subclavian vein to form the brachiocephalic vein — called also *internal jugular vein* **b** : a smaller and more superficial vein that collects most of the blood from the exterior of the cranium and deep parts of the face and opens into the subclavian vein — called also *external* *jugular vein* **c** : a vein that commences near the hyoid bone and joins the terminal part of the external jugular vein or the subclavian vein — called also *anterior jugular vein*

juice \ˈjüs\ *n* : a natural bodily fluid — see GASTRIC JUICE, INTESTINAL JUICE, PANCREATIC JUICE

jumping gene *n* : TRANSPOSABLE ELEMENT; *also* : TRANSPOSON

junc·tion \ˈjəŋk-shən\ *n* : a place or point of meeting — see NEUROMUSCULAR JUNCTION — **junc·tion·al** \-shə-nəl\ *adj*

junctional epidermolysis bullosa *n* : any of several forms of epidermolysis bullosa that are marked esp. by usu. severe blister formation between the epidermis and basement membrane often accompanied by involvement of the mucous membranes (as of the mouth) and that are inherited as an autosomal recessive trait

junctional nevus *n* : a nevus that develops at the junction of the dermis and epidermis and is potentially cancerous — called also *junction nevus*

junctional rhythm *n* : a cardiac rhythm resulting from impulses coming from a locus of tissue in the area of the atrioventricular node

junctional tachycardia *n* : tachycardia associated with the generation of impulses in a locus in the region of the atrioventricular node

Jung·ian \ˈyu̇n-ē-ən\ *adj* : of, relating to, or characteristic of C. G. Jung or his psychological doctrines — **Jungian** *n*

   Jung \ˈyu̇n\, **Carl Gustav (1875–1961),** Swiss psychologist and psychiatrist.

jungle fever *n* : a severe form of malaria or yellow fever — compare JUNGLE YELLOW FEVER

jungle rot *n* : any of various esp. pyogenic skin infections contracted in tropical environments

jungle yellow fever *n* : yellow fever endemic in or near forest or jungle areas in Africa and So. America and transmitted by mosquitoes (esp. genus *Haemagogus*) other than members of the genus *Aedes*

Ju·nin virus \hü-ˈnēn-\ *n* : a virus of the genus *Arenavirus* (species *Junin virus*) that is the causative agent of a hemorrhagic fever endemic in Argentina and that is transmitted to humans chiefly by rodents

ju·ni·per \ˈjü-nə-pər\ *n* : an evergreen shrub or tree (genus *Juniperus*) of the cypress family (Cupressaceae)

juniper tar *n* : a dark tarry liquid used topically in treating skin diseases and obtained by distillation from the wood of a Eurasian juniper (*Juniperus oxycedrus*) — called also *cade oil, juniper tar oil*

junk DNA *n* : a region of DNA that usu. consists of a repeating DNA sequence, does not code for a protein, and has no known function

just noticeable difference *n* : the minimum amount of change in a physical stimulus required for a subject to detect reliably a difference in the level of stimulation

jus·to ma·jor \ˈjəs-tō-ˈmā-jər\ *adj, of pelvic dimensions* : greater than normal

justo mi·nor \-ˈmī-nər\ *adj, of pelvic dimensions* : smaller than normal

ju·ve·nile \ˈjü-və-ˌnīl, -nəl\ *adj* **1** : physiologically immature or undeveloped **2** : of, relating to, characteristic of, or affecting children or young people ⟨~ arthritis⟩ **3** : reflecting psychological or intellectual immaturity — **juvenile** *n*

juvenile amaurotic idiocy *n* : BATTEN DISEASE

juvenile delinquency *n* **1** : conduct by a juvenile characterized by antisocial behavior that is subject to legal action **2** : a violation of the law committed by a juvenile that would have been a crime if committed by an adult — **juvenile delinquent** *n*

juvenile diabetes *n* : TYPE 1 DIABETES

juvenile myoclonic epilepsy *n* : epilepsy that typically begins during adolescence or late childhood and is marked by myoclonic seizures which occur shortly after awakening and are often followed by tonic-clonic seizures or sometimes by absence seizures

juvenile–onset diabetes *n* : TYPE 1 DIABETES

juxta- *comb form* : situated near ⟨*juxta*glomerular⟩

jux·ta·ar·tic·u·lar \ˌjək-stə-är-ˈti-kyə-lər\ *adj* : situated near a joint

jux·ta·glo·mer·u·lar \-glə-ˈmer-yə-lər, -glō-, -ə-lər\ *adj* : situated near a kidney glomerulus

juxtaglomerular apparatus *n* : a functional unit near a kidney glomerulus that controls renin release and is composed of juxtaglomerular cells and a macula densa

juxtaglomerular cell *n* : any of a group of cells that are situated in the wall of each afferent arteriole of a kidney glomerulus near its point of entry adjacent to a macula densa and that produce and secrete renin

jux·ta·med·ul·lary \ˌjək-stə-ˈmed-ᵊl-ˌer-ē, -ˈmej-ᵊl-; -mə-ˈdə-lə-rē\ *adj* : situated or occurring near the edge of the medulla of the kidney

K *symbol* [New Latin *kalium*] potassium

Kahn test \'kän-\ *n* : a serum-precipitation reaction for the diagnosis of syphilis — called also *Kahn, Kahn reaction*

Kahn, Reuben Leon (1887–1979), American immunologist.

kai·nate \'kī-ˌnāt, 'kā-\ *n* : KAINIC ACID

kai·nic acid \'kī-nik-, 'kā-\ *n* : an excitatory neurotoxin $C_{10}H_{15}NO_4$ that is a glutamate analog orig. isolated from a dried red alga (*Digenia simplex*) and is used as an anthelmintic and experimentally to induce seizures and neurodegeneration in laboratory animals

kala–azar \'kä-lə-ə-ˈzär, ˌka-\ *n* : a severe parasitic disease chiefly of Asia marked by fever, progressive anemia, leukopenia, and enlargement of the spleen and liver and caused by a flagellate of the genus *Leishmania* (*L. donovani*) that is transmitted by the bite of sand flies — called also *dumdum fever*; see LEISHMAN-DONOVAN BODY

ka·li·ure·sis \ˌka-lē-yù-ˈrē-səs, ˌka-\ *also* **kal·ure·sis** \ˌkāl-(y)ù-ˈre-, ˌkal-\ *n, pl* **-ure·ses** \-ˌsēz\ : excretion of potassium in the urine esp. in excessive amounts — **ka·li·uret·ic** \-ˈre-tik\ *adj*

kal·li·din \'ka-lə-din\ *n* : either of two vasodilator kinins formed from blood plasma globulin by the action of kallikrein

kal·li·kre·in \ˌka-lə-ˈkrē-ən, kə-ˈli-krē-ən\ *n* : a hypotensive protease that liberates kinins from blood plasma proteins and is used therapeutically for vasodilation

Kall·mann syndrome \'kȯl-mən-\ *or* **Kall·mann's syndrome** \-mənz-\ *n* : a hereditary condition marked by hypogonadism caused by a deficiency of gonadotropins and anosmia caused by failure of the olfactory lobes to develop

Kallmann, Franz Josef (1897–1965), American geneticist and psychiatrist.

kana·my·cin \ˌka-nə-ˈmīs-ᵊn\ *n* : a broad-spectrum antibiotic from a Japanese soil bacterium of the genus *Streptomyces* (*S. kanamyceticus*)

Kan·ner's syndrome \'ka-nərz-\ *n* : INFANTILE AUTISM

Kanner, Leo (1894–1981), American psychiatrist.

Kan·trex \'kan-ˌtreks\ *trademark* — used for a preparation of kanamycin

ka·olin \'kā-ə-lin\ *n* : a fine usu. white clay that is used in medicine esp. as an adsorbent in the treatment of diarrhea (as from food poisoning)

Kao·pec·tate \ˌkā-ō-ˈpek-ˌtāt\ *trademark* — used for a preparation of kaolin used as an antidiarrheal

Ka·po·si's sarcoma \'ka-pə-zēz-, kə-'pō-, -sēz-\ *n* : a neoplastic disease that occurs esp. in individuals coinfected with HIV and a specific herpesvirus (species *Human herpesvirus 8* of the genus *Rhadinovirus*), that affects esp. the skin and mucous membranes, and is marked usu. by pink to reddish-brown or bluish plaques, macules, papules, or nodules esp. on the lower extremities — abbr. *KS*

Kaposi, Moritz (1837–1902), Hungarian dermatologist.

LAMBDA CHAIN

kap·pa chain *or* **κ chain** \'ka-pə-\ *n* : a polypeptide chain of one of the two types of light chain that are found in antibodies and can be distinguished antigenically and by the sequence of amino acids in the chain — compare LAMBDA CHAIN

ka·ra·ya gum \kə-ˈrī-ə-\ *n* : any of several laxative vegetable gums obtained from tropical Asian trees (genera *Sterculia* of the family Sterculiaceae and *Cochlospermum* of the family Bixaceae) — called also *gum karaya, karaya, sterculia gum*

ka·rez·za \kä-ˈret-sə\ *n* : COITUS RESERVATUS

Kar·ta·ge·ner's syndrome \kär-ˈtä-gə-nərz-, ˌkär-tə-ˈgā-nərz-\ *n* : an abnormal condition inherited as an autosomal recessive trait and characterized by situs inversus, abnormalities in the protein structure of cilia, and chronic bronchiectasis and sinusitis

Kartagener, Manes (1897–1975), Swiss physician.

kary- *or* **karyo-** *also* **cary-** *or* **caryo-** *comb form* : nucleus of a cell ⟨*karyo*kinesis⟩ ⟨*karyo*type⟩

kary·og·a·my \ˌkar-ē-ˈä-gə-mē\ *n, pl* **-mies** : the fusion of cell nuclei (as in fertilization)

karyo·gram \'kar-ē-ō-ˌgram\ *n* : KARYOTYPE; *esp* : a diagrammatic representation of the chromosome complement of an organism

karyo·ki·ne·sis \ˌkar-ē-ō-kə-ˈnē-səs, -kī-\ *n, pl* **-ne·ses** \-ˌsēz\ **1** : the nuclear phenomena characteristic of mitosis **2** : the whole process of mitosis — compare CYTOKINESIS — **karyo·ki·net·ic** \-ˈne-tik\ *adj*

kary·ol·o·gy \ˌkar-ē-ˈä-lə-jē\ *n, pl* **-gies** **1** : the minute cytological characteristics of the cell nucleus esp. with regard to the chromosomes of a single cell or of the cells of an organism or group of organisms **2** : a branch of cytology concerned with the karyology of cell nuclei — **karyo·log·i·cal** \-ē-ə-ˈlä-ji-kəl\ *also* **karyo·log·ic** \-jik\ *adj* — **karyo·log·i·cal·ly** *adv*

karyo·lymph \'kar-ē-ō-ˌlimf\ *n* : NUCLEOPLASM

kary·ol·y·sis \ˌkar-ē-ˈä-lə-səs\ *n, pl* **-y-**

ses \-ˌsēz\ : dissolution of the cell nucleus with loss of its affinity for basic stains sometimes occurring normally but usu. in necrosis — compare KARYORRHEXIS

karyo·plasm \'kar-ē-ō-ˌpla-zəm\ *n* : NUCLEOPLASM

karyo·pyk·no·sis \ˌkar-ē-(ˌ)ō-pik-'nō-səs\ *n* : shrinkage of the cell nuclei of epithelial cells (as of the vagina) with breakup of the chromatin into unstructured granules — **karyo·pyk·not·ic** \-'nä-tik\ *adj*

karyopyknotic index *n* : an index that is calculated as the percentage of epithelial cells with karyopyknotic nuclei exfoliated from the vagina and is used in the hormonal evaluation of a patient

kary·or·rhex·is \ˌkar-ē-ō-'rek-səs\ *n, pl* **-rhex·es** \-ˌsēz\ : a degenerative cellular process involving fragmentation of the nucleus and the breakup of the chromatin into unstructured granules — compare KARYOLYSIS

karyo·some \'kar-ē-ə-ˌsōm\ *n* : a mass of chromatin in a cell nucleus that resembles a nucleolus

¹karyo·type \'kar-ē-ə-ˌtīp\ *n* : the chromosomal characteristics of a cell; *also* : the chromosomes themselves or a representation of them — **karyo·typ·ic** \ˌkar-ē-ə-'ti-pik\ *adj* — **karyo·typ·i·cal·ly** *adv*

²karyotype *vb* **-typed; -typ·ing** : to determine the karyotype of

karyo·typ·ing \-ˌtīp-iŋ\ *n* : the action or process of studying karyotypes or of making representations of them

Ka·ta·ya·ma syndrome \ˌkä-tə-'yä-mə-\ *n ; specif* : an acute form usu. occurring several weeks after initial infection with the causative schistosome (*Schistosoma japonicum*) — called also *Katayama disease, Katayama fever*

ka·va \'kä-və\ *n* **1** : an Australasian pepper (*Piper methysticum*) from whose crushed root an intoxicating beverage is made; *also* : the beverage **2** : a preparation consisting of the ground dried rhizome and roots of the kava plant that is used esp. as a dietary supplement chiefly to relieve stress, anxiety, and sleeplessness and that has been linked to cases of severe liver injury

kava kava \'kä-və-'kä-və\ *n* : KAVA

Ka·wa·sa·ki disease \ˌkä-wə-'sä-kē-\ *also* **Ka·wa·sa·ki's disease** \-kēz-\ *n* : an acute febrile disease of unknown cause affecting esp. infants and children that is characterized by a reddish macular rash esp. on the trunk, conjunctivitis, inflammation of mucous membranes (as of the tongue), erythema of the palms and soles followed by desquamation, edema of the hands and feet, and swollen lymph nodes in the neck — called also *Kawasaki syndrome, mucocutaneous lymph node disease, mucocutaneous lymph node syndrome*

Kawasaki, Tomisaku (*fl* 1961), Japanese pediatrician.

Kay·ser–Flei·scher ring \'kī-zər-'flī-shər-\ *n* : a brown or greenish brown ring of copper deposits around the cornea that is characteristic of Wilson's disease

Kayser, Bernhard (1869–1954), and **Fleischer, Bruno Otto (1874–1965),** German ophthalmologists.

kb *abbr* kilobase

K–Dur \'kä-ˌdůr\ *trademark* — used for a sustained-release preparation of potassium chloride for oral administration

ked \'ked\ *n* : SHEEP KED

Ke·gel exercises \'kā-gəl-, 'kē-\ *n pl* : repetitive contractions by a woman of the muscles that are used to stop the urinary flow in urination in order to increase the tone of the pubococcygeal muscle esp. to control incontinence or to enhance sexual responsiveness during intercourse

Kegel, Arnold Henry (1894–1976), American physician.

Kell \'kel\ *adj* : of, relating to, or being a group of allelic red-blood-cell antigens of which some are important causes of transfusion reactions and some forms of erythroblastosis fetalis

Kell, medical patient.

Kel·ler \'ke-lər\ *adj* : relating to or being an operation to correct hallux valgus by excision of the proximal part of the proximal phalanx of the big toe with resulting shortening of the toe

Keller, William Lorden (1874–1959), American surgeon.

ke·loid \'kē-ˌlȯid\ *n* : a thick scar resulting from excessive growth of fibrous tissue and occurring esp. after burns or radiation injury — **keloid** *adj* — **ke·loi·dal** \kē-'lȯid-ᵊl\ *adj*

kelp \'kelp\ *n* : any of various large brown seaweeds (order Laminariales) and esp. laminarias

kel·vin \'kel-vin\ *n* : the base unit of temperature in the International System of Units that is equal to $1/273.16$ of the Kelvin scale temperature of the triple point of water

Thom·son \'täm-sən\, **Sir William (1st Baron Kelvin of Largs) (1824–1907),** British physicist.

Kelvin *adj* : relating to, conforming to, or being a temperature scale according to which absolute zero is 0 K, the equivalent of $-273.15°C$

Ken·a·cort \'ke-nə-ˌkȯrt\ *n* : a preparation of triamcinolone — formerly a U.S. registered trademark

Ken·ne·dy's disease \'ke-nə-dēz-\ *also* **Ken·ne·dy disease** \-dē-\ *n* : a progressive muscular and neurological disorder that is characterized esp. by muscular weakness and atrophy and by neural degeneration, that is inherited as an X-linked recessive trait, and that chiefly affects adult males —

called also *spinal and bulbar muscular atrophy*

Kennedy, William Robert (*b* 1927), American neurologist.

kennel cough *n* : tracheobronchitis of dogs or cats

Ken·ny method \'ke-nē-\ *n* : a method of treating poliomyelitis consisting basically of application of hot fomentations and rehabilitation of muscular activity by passive movement and then guided active coordination — called also *Kenny treatment*

Kenny, Elizabeth (1880–1952), Australian nurse.

ker·a·sin \'ker-ə-sən\ *n* : a cerebroside $C_{48}H_{93}NO_8$ that occurs esp. in Gaucher's disease

ker·a·tan sulfate \'ker-ə-,tan-\ *n* : any of several sulfated glycosaminoglycans that have been found esp. in the cornea, cartilage, and bone

ker·a·tec·to·my \,ker-ə-'tek-tə-mē\ *n, pl* **-mies** : surgical excision of part of the cornea

ke·rat·ic precipitates \kə-'ra-tik-\ *n pl* : accumulations on the posterior surface of the cornea esp. of macrophages and epithelial cells that occur in chronic inflammatory conditions — called also *keratitis punctata*

ker·a·tin \'ker-ət-ᵊn\ *n* : any of various sulfur-containing fibrous proteins that form the chemical basis of horny epidermal tissues (as hair and nails)

ke·ra·ti·ni·za·tion \,ker-ə-tə-nə-'zā-shən, kə-,rat-ᵊn-ə-\ *n* : conversion into keratin or keratinous tissue — **ker·a·ti·nize** \'ker-ə-tə-,nīz, kə-'rat-ᵊn-,īz\ *vb*

ke·ra·ti·no·cyte \kə-'rat-ᵊn-ə-,sīt, ,ker-ə-'ti-nə-\ *n* : an epidermal cell that produces keratin

ke·ra·ti·nous \kə-'rat-ᵊn-əs, ,ker-ə-'tī-nəs\ *adj* : composed of or containing keratin : HORNY

ker·a·ti·tis \,ker-ə-'tī-təs\ *n, pl* **-tit·i·des** \-'ti-tə-,dēz\ : inflammation of the cornea of the eye characterized by burning or smarting, blurring of vision, and sensitiveness to light and caused by infectious or noninfectious agents

keratitis punc·ta·ta \-pəŋk-'tä-tə, -'tä-\ *n* : KERATIC PRECIPITATES

ker·a·to·ac·an·tho·ma \,ker-ə-tō-,a-,kan-'thō-mə\ *n, pl* **-mas** *also* **-ma·ta** \-mə-tə\ : a rapidly growing skin tumor that occurs esp. in elderly individuals, resembles a carcinoma of squamous epithelial cells but does not spread, and tends to heal spontaneously with some scarring if left untreated

ker·a·to·con·junc·ti·vi·tis \'ker-ə-(,)tō-kən-,jəŋk-tə-'vī-təs\ *n* : combined inflammation of the cornea and conjunctiva; *esp* : EPIDEMIC KERATOCONJUNCTIVITIS

keratoconjunctivitis sic·ca \-'si-kə\ *n* : DRY EYE

ker·a·to·co·nus \,ker-ə-tō-'kō-nəs\ *n* : cone-shaped protrusion of the cornea

ker·a·to·der·ma \-'dər-mə\ *n* : a horny condition of the skin

keratoderma blen·nor·rhag·i·cum \-,ble-nó-'ra-ji-kəm\ *n* : KERATOSIS BLENNORRHAGICA

ker·a·to·der·mia \,ker-ə-tō-'dər-mē-ə\ *n* : KERATODERMA

ker·a·to·hy·a·lin \-'hī-ə-lən\ *also* **ker·a·to·hy·a·line** \-lən, -,lēn\ *n* : a colorless translucent protein that occurs esp. in granules of the stratum granulosum of the epidermis

ker·a·tol·y·sis \,ker-ə-'tä-lə-səs\ *n, pl* **-y·ses** \-,sēz\ **1** : the process of breaking down or dissolving keratin **2** : a skin disease marked by peeling of the horny layer of the epidermis

¹ker·a·to·lyt·ic \,ker-ə-tō-'li-tik\ *adj* : relating to or causing keratolysis

²keratolytic *n* : a keratolytic agent

ker·a·to·ma·la·cia \,ker-ə-tō-mə-'lā-sh(ē-)ə, -sē-ə\ *n* : a softening and ulceration of the cornea of the eye resulting from severe systemic deficiency of vitamin A — compare XEROPHTHALMIA

ker·a·tome \'ker-ə-,tōm\ *n* : a surgical instrument used for making an incision in the cornea in cataract operations

ker·a·tom·e·ter \,ker-ə-'tä-mə-tər\ *n* : an instrument for measuring the curvature of the cornea

ker·a·tom·e·try \,ker-ə-'tä-mə-trē\ *n, pl* **-tries** : measurement of the form and curvature of the cornea — **ker·a·to·met·ric** \-tō-'me-trik\ *adj*

ker·at·o·mil·eu·sis \,ker-ət-ō-mi-'lü-səs, -'lyü-\ *n* : keratoplasty in which a piece of the cornea is removed, frozen, shaped to correct refractive error, and reinserted

ker·a·top·a·thy \,ker-ə-'tä-pə-thē\ *n, pl* **-thies** : any noninflammatory disease of the eye — see BAND KERATOPATHY

ker·a·to·pha·kia \,ker-ə-tō-'fā-kē-ə\ *n* : keratoplasty in which corneal tissue from a donor is frozen, shaped, and inserted into the cornea of a recipient

ker·a·to·plas·ty \'ker-ə-tō-,plas-tē\ *n, pl* **-ties** : plastic surgery on the cornea; *esp* : corneal grafting

ker·a·to·pros·the·sis \,ker-ə-tō-präs-'thē-səs, -'präs-thə-\ *n, pl* **-the·ses** \-,sēz\ : a plastic replacement for an opacified inner part of a cornea

ker·a·to·scope \'ker-ə-tō-,skōp\ *n* : an instrument for examining the cornea esp. to detect irregularities of its anterior surface

ker·a·to·sis \,ker-ə-'tō-səs\ *n, pl* **-to·ses** \-,sēz\ **1** : a disease of the skin marked by overgrowth of horny tissue **2** : an area of the skin affected with keratosis — **ker·a·tot·ic** \-'tä-tik\ *adj*

keratosis blen·nor·rhag·i·ca \-,ble-nó-'ra-ji-kə\ *n* : a disease that is characterized by a scaly rash esp. on the palms and soles and is associated esp. with Reiter's syndrome — called also *keratoderma blennorrhagicum*

ker·a·to·sis fol·li·cu·lar·is \-ˌfä-lə-kyə-'ler-əs\ *n* : DARIER'S DISEASE

keratosis pi·lar·is \-pi-'ler-əs\ *n* : a condition marked by the formation of hard conical elevations in the openings of the sebaceous glands esp. of the thighs and arms that resemble permanent goose bumps

ker·a·tot·o·mist \ˌker-ə-'tä-tə-mist\ *n* : a surgeon who performs keratotomies

ker·a·tot·o·my \-mē\ *n, pl* **-mies** : incision of the cornea

ke·ri·on \'kir-ē-ˌän\ *n* : inflammatory ringworm of the hair follicles of the beard and scalp usu. accompanied by secondary bacterial infection

ker·nic·ter·us \kər-'nik-tə-rəs\ *n* : a condition marked by the deposit of bile pigments in the nuclei of the brain and spinal cord and by degeneration of nerve cells that occurs usu. in infants as a part of the syndrome of erythroblastosis fetalis — **ker·nic·ter·ic** \-rik\ *adj*

Ker·nig sign \'ker-nig-\ *or* **Kernig's sign** \'ker-nigz-\ *n* : an indication usu. present in meningitis that consists of pain and resistance on attempting to extend the leg at the knee with the thigh flexed at the hip

Kernig, Vladimir Mikhailovich (1840–1917), Russian physician.

ke·ta·mine \'kē-tə-ˌmēn\ *n* : a general anesthetic that is administered intravenously and intramuscularly in the form of its hydrochloride $C_{13}H_{16}$-ClNO·HCl — see SPECIAL K

ke·thox·al \kē-'thäk-səl\ *n* : an antiviral agent $C_6H_{12}O_4$

ke·to \'kē-(ˌ)tō\ *adj* : of or relating to a ketone; *also* : containing a ketone group

keto acid *n* : a compound that is both a ketone and an acid

ke·to·ac·i·do·sis \ˌkē-tō-ˌa-sə-'dō-səs\ *n, pl* **-do·ses** \-ˌsēz\ : acidosis accompanied by ketosis ⟨diabetic ∼⟩ — **ke·to·ac·i·dot·ic** \-'dä-tik\ *adj*

ke·to·con·a·zole \ˌkē-tō-'kō-nə-ˌzōl\ *n* : a synthetic broad-spectrum antifungal agent $C_{26}H_{28}Cl_2N_4O_4$ used to treat chronic internal and cutaneous disorders — see NIZORAL

ke·to·gen·e·sis \ˌkē-tō-'je-nə-səs\ *n, pl* **-e·ses** \-ˌsēz\ : the production of ketone bodies (as in diabetes mellitus) — **ke·to·gen·ic** \-'je-nik\ *adj*

ketogenic diet *n* : a diet supplying a large amount of fat and minimal amounts of carbohydrate and protein

ke·to·glu·tar·ic acid \ˌkē-tō-glü-'tar-ik-\ *n* : either of two crystalline keto derivatives $C_5H_6O_5$ of glutaric acid; *esp* : ALPHA-KETOGLUTARIC ACID

α–ketoglutaric acid *var of* ALPHA-KETOGLUTARIC ACID

ke·to·nae·mia *chiefly Brit var of* KETONEMIA

ke·tone \'kē-ˌtōn\ *n* : an organic compound (as acetone) with a CO group attached to two carbon atoms

ketone body *n* : any of the three compounds acetoacetic acid, acetone, and the beta derivative of hydroxybutyric acid which are normal intermediates in lipid metabolism and accumulate in the blood and urine in abnormal amounts in conditions of impaired metabolism (as in diabetes mellitus) — called also *acetone body*

ke·to·ne·mia \ˌkē-tə-'nē-mē-ə\ *n* **1** : a condition marked by an abnormal increase of ketone bodies in the circulating blood — called also *hyperketonemia* **2** : KETOSIS 2 — **ke·to·ne·mic** \-'nē-mik\ *adj*

ke·ton·uria \ˌkē-tə-'núr-ē-ə, -'nyúr-\ *n* : the presence of excess ketone bodies in the urine in conditions (as diabetes mellitus and starvation acidosis) involving reduced or disturbed carbohydrate metabolism — called also *acetonuria*

ke·to·pro·fen \ˌkē-tə-'prō-fən\ *n* : an analgesic nonsteroidal anti-inflammatory drug $C_{16}H_{14}O_3$ used to treat dysmenorrhea and the symptoms of rheumatoid arthritis and osteoarthritis

ke·tose \'kē-ˌtōs, -ˌtōz\ *n* : a sugar (as fructose) containing one ketone group per molecule

ke·to·sis \kē-'tō-səs\ *n, pl* **-to·ses** \-ˌsēz\ **1** : an abnormal increase of ketone bodies in the body in conditions of reduced or disturbed carbohydrate metabolism (as in diabetes mellitus) — compare ACIDOSIS, ALKALOSIS **2** : a nutritional disease esp. of cattle that is marked by reduction of blood sugar and the presence of ketone bodies in the blood, tissues, milk, and urine — **ke·tot·ic** \-'tä-tik\ *adj*

ke·to·ste·roid \ˌkē-tō-'stir-ˌóid, -'ster-\ *n* : a steroid (as cortisone or estrone) containing a ketone group; *esp* : 17=KETOSTEROID

17–ketosteroid *n* : any of the ketosteroids (as androsterone, dehydroepiandrosterone, and estrone) that have the keto group attached to carbon atom 17 of the steroid ring structure, are present in normal human urine, and may be an indication of a tumor of the adrenal cortex or ovary when present in excess

Ke·ty method \'kē-tē-\ *n* : a method of determining coronary blood flow by measurement of nitrous oxide levels in the blood of a patient breathing nitrous oxide

Kety, Seymour Solomon (1915–2000), American physiologist.

kg *abbr* kilogram

khel·lin \'ke-lən\ *n* : a crystalline compound $C_{14}H_{12}O_5$ obtained from the fruit of a Middle Eastern plant (*Ammi visnaga*) of the carrot family (Umbelliferae) and used esp. as a coronary vasodilator

kid·ney \'kid-nē\ *n, pl* **kidneys** : one of a pair of vertebrate organs situated in the body cavity near the spinal column that excrete waste products of metabolism, in humans are bean-shaped organs about 4½ inches (11½ centimeters) long lying behind the peritoneum in a mass of fatty tissue, and consist chiefly of nephrons by which urine is secreted, collected, and discharged into the pelvis of the kidney where it is conveyed by the ureter to the bladder — compare MESO-NEPHROS, METANEPHROS, PRO-NEPHROS

kidney stone *n* : a calculus in the kidney — called also *renal calculus*

kidney worm *n* : any of several nematode worms parasitic in the kidneys: as **a** : GIANT KIDNEY WORM **b** : a common worm of the genus *Stephanurus* (*S. dentatus*) that is related to the gapeworm and is parasitic in the kidneys, lungs, and other viscera of the hog in warm regions

Kien·böck's disease \'kēn-ˌbeks-\ *n* : osteochondrosis affecting the lunate bone
  Kien·böck \'kēn-ˌbœk\, **Robert** (1871–1953), Austrian radiologist.

killed \'kild\ *adj* : being or containing a virus that has been inactivated (as by chemicals) so that it is no longer effective ⟨~ vaccines⟩

killer bee *n* : AFRICANIZED BEE

killer cell *n* : a lymphocyte (as a cytotoxic T cell or a natural killer cell) with cytotoxic activity

killer T cell *n* : CYTOTOXIC T CELL

killer T lymphocyte *n* : CYTOTOXIC T CELL

ki·lo·base \'ki-lə-ˌbās\ *n* : a unit of measure of the length of a nucleic-acid chain (as of DNA or RNA) that equals one thousand base pairs

ki·lo·cal·o·rie \-ˌka-lə-rē\ *n* : CALORIE 1b

ki·lo·gram \'ki-lə-ˌgram, 'kē-\ *n* **1** : the base unit of mass in the International System of Units that is nearly equal to the mass of 1000 cubic centimeters of water at the temperature of its maximum density **2** : a unit of force or weight equal to the weight of a kilogram mass under a gravitational attraction equal to that of the earth

kilogram calorie *n* : CALORIE 1b

ki·lo·joule \'ki-lə-ˌjül\ *n* : 1000 joules

ki·lo·me·ter \'ki-lə-ˌmē-tər, kə-'lä-mə-tər\ *n* : 1000 meters

ki·lo·rad \'ki-lə-ˌrad\ *n* : 1000 rads

ki·lo·volt \-ˌvōlt\ *n* : a unit of potential difference equal to 1000 volts

kin- or **kine-** or **kino-** or **cin-** or **cino-** *comb form* : motion : action ⟨*kines*thesia⟩

kin·aes·the·sia *chiefly Brit var of* KINESTHESIA

ki·nase \'kī-ˌnās, -ˌnāz\ *n* : an enzyme that catalyzes the transfer of phosphate groups from a high-energy phosphate-containing molecule (as ATP or ADP) to a substrate — called also *phosphokinase*

kind·ling \'kin-dliŋ\ *n* : the electro-physiological changes that occur in the brain as a result of repeated intermittent exposure to a subthreshold electrical or chemical stimulus (as one causing seizures) so that there develops a usu. permanent decrease in the threshold of excitability

ki·ne·mat·ics \ˌki-nə-'ma-tiks, ˌkī-\ *n* **1** : a science that deals with aspects of motion apart from considerations of mass and force **2** : the properties and phenomena of an object or system in motion of interest to kinematics ⟨the ~ of a joint⟩ — **ki·ne·mat·ic** \-tik\ *or* **ki·ne·mat·i·cal** \-ti-kəl\ *adj*

kineplasty *var of* CINEPLASTY

kinesi- *or* **kinesio-** *comb form* : movement ⟨*kinesio*logy⟩

-ki·ne·sia \kə-'nē-zhə, kī-, -zhē-ə\ *comb form* : movement : motion ⟨hyper*kinesia*⟩

ki·ne·sin \ki-'nē-sən\ *n* : an ATPase similar to dynein that functions as a motor protein in the intracellular transport esp. of cell organelles and molecules along microtubules

ki·ne·si·ol·o·gy \kə-ˌnē-sē-'ä-lə-jē, kī-, -zē-\ *n, pl* **-gies** : the study of the principles of mechanics and anatomy in relation to human movement — **ki·ne·si·o·log·ic** \-ō-'lä-jik\ *or* **ki·ne·si·o·log·i·cal** \-ji-kəl\ *adj* — **ki·ne·si·ol·o·gist** \kə-ˌnē-sē-'ä-lə-jist, kī-, -zē-\ *n*

ki·ne·sis \kə-'nē-səs, kī-\ *n, pl* **ki·ne·ses** \-ˌsēz\ : a movement that lacks directional orientation and depends upon the intensity of stimulation

-ki·ne·sis \kə-'nē-sis, kī-\ *n, pl* **-ki·ne·ses** \-ˌsēz\ **1** : division ⟨karyo*kinesis*⟩ **2** : production of motion ⟨psycho*kinesis*⟩ ⟨tele*kinesis*⟩

kin·es·the·sia \ˌki-nəs-'thē-zhə, -zhē-ə\ *or* **kin·es·the·sis** \-'thē-səs\, *n, pl* **-the·sias** *or* **-the·ses** \-ˌsēz\ : a sense mediated by end organs located in muscles, tendons, and joints and stimulated by bodily movements and tensions; *also* : sensory experience derived from this sense — see MUSCLE SENSE — **kin·es·thet·ic** \-'thē-tik\ *adj* — **kin·es·thet·i·cal·ly** *adv*

kinet- *or* **kineto-** *comb form* : movement : motion ⟨*kineto*chore⟩

ki·net·ic \kə-'ne-tik, kī-\ *adj* : of or relating to the motion of material bodies and the forces and energy associated therewith — **ki·net·i·cal·ly** *adv*

ki·net·ics \kə-'ne-tiks, kī-\ *n sing or pl* **1 a** : a science that deals with the effects of forces upon the motions of material bodies or with changes in a physical or chemical system **b** : the rate of change in such a system **2** : the mechanism by which a physical or chemical change is effected

ki·net·o·chore \kə-'ne-tə-ˌkōr, kī-\ *n* **1** : CENTROMERE **2** : a specialized structure on the centromere to which the microtubular spindle fibers attach during mitosis and meiosis

king co·bra \-'kō-brə\ *n* : a large cobra

(*Ophiophagus hannah* syn. *Naja hannah*) of southeastern Asia and the Philippines — called also *hamadryad*

king·dom \'kiŋ-dəm\ *n* : any of the three primary divisions of lifeless material, plants, and animals into which natural objects are grouped; *also* : a biological category (as Animalia) that ranks above the phylum and below the domain

king's evil *n, often cap K&E* : SCROFULA

ki·nin \'kī-nən\ *n* : any of various polypeptide hormones that are formed locally in the tissues and cause dilation of blood vessels and contraction of smooth muscle

ki·ni·nase \'kī-nə-ˌnās, -ˌnāz\ *n* : an enzyme in blood that destroys a kinin

ki·nin·o·gen \kī-'ni-nə-jən\ *n* : an inactive precursor of a kinin — **ki·nin·o·gen·ic** \(ˌ)kī-ˌni-nə-'je-nik\ *adj*

kino- — see KIN-

ki·no·cil·i·um \ˌkī-nō-'si-lē-əm\ *n, pl* **-cil·ia** \-lē-ə\ : a motile cilium that occurs alone at the end of a sensory hair cell of the inner ear among numerous nonmotile stereocilia

Kirsch·ner wire \'kərsh-nər-\ *n* : metal wire inserted through bone and used to achieve internal traction or immobilization of bone fractures

    Kirschner, Martin (1879–1942), German surgeon.

kissing bug *n* : CONENOSE

kissing disease *n* : INFECTIOUS MONONUCLEOSIS

kiss of life *n, chiefly Brit* : artificial respiration by the mouth-to-mouth method

kleb·si·el·la \ˌkleb-zē-'e-lə\ *n* 1 *cap* : a genus of nonmotile gram-negative rod-shaped bacteria (family Enterobacteriaceae) that include causative agents of respiratory and urinary infections — see PNEUMOBACILLUS 2 : any bacterium of the genus *Klebsiella*

    Klebs \'kleps\, **(Theodor Albrecht) Edwin** (1834–1913), German bacteriologist.

Klebs–Löff·ler bacillus \'kleps-'lef-lər-, 'klebz-\ *n* : a bacterium of the genus *Corynebacterium* (*C. diphtheriae*) that causes human diphtheria

    Löff·ler \'lüf-lər\, **Friedrich August Johannes** (1852–1915), German bacteriologist.

klee·blatt·schä·del \'klā-ˌblät-ˌshäd-ᵊl\ *n* : CLOVERLEAF SKULL

Klein·ian \'klī-nē-ən\ *adj* : of, relating to, or according with the psychoanalytic theories or practices of Melanie Klein — **Kleinian** *n*

    Klein \'klīn\, **Melanie** (1882–1960), Austrian psychoanalyst.

klept- *or* **klepto-** *comb form* : stealing : theft ⟨*klepto*mania⟩

klep·to·lag·nia \ˌklep-tə-'lag-nē-ə\ *n* : sexual arousal and gratification produced by committing an act of theft

klep·to·ma·nia \ˌklep-tə-'mā-nē-ə, -nyə\ *n* : a persistent neurotic impulse to steal esp. without economic motive

klep·to·ma·ni·ac \-nē-ˌak\ *n* : an individual exhibiting kleptomania

Kline·fel·ter's syndrome \'klīn-ˌfel-tərz-\ *also* **Kline·fel·ter syndrome** \-tər-\ *n* : an abnormal condition in a male characterized by two X chromosomes and one Y chromosome, infertility, smallness of the testes, sparse facial and body hair, and gynecomastia

    Klinefelter, Harry Fitch (1912–1990), American physician.

Kline reaction \'klīn-\ *n* : KLINE TEST

Kline test *n* : a rapid precipitation test for the diagnosis of syphilis

    Kline, Benjamin Schoenbrun (*b* 1886), American pathologist.

Klip·pel–Feil syndrome \kli-'pel-'fīl-\ *n* : congenital fusion of the cervical vertebrae resulting in a short and relatively immobile neck

    Klip·pel \klē-'pel\, **Maurice** (1858–1942), and **Feil** \'fāl\, **André** (*b* 1884), French neurologists.

Klor–Con \'klȯr-ˌkän\ *trademark* — used for a preparation of potassium chloride or potassium bicarbonate

Klump·ke's paralysis \'klümp-kēz-\ *n* : atrophic paralysis of the forearm and the hand due to injury to the eighth cervical and first thoracic nerves

    Dé·jé·rine–Klump·ke \dā-zhā-ˌrēn-klüm-'kē\, **Augusta** (1859–1927), French neurologist.

Klü·ver–Bu·cy syndrome \'klü-vər-'b(y)ü-sē-\ *n* : a group of symptoms (as excessive reactivity to visual stimuli, hypersexuality, and diminished emotional responses) that are caused by bilateral removal of the temporal lobes induced experimentally in monkeys and that sometimes occur in humans with severe injuries to the temporal lobes

    Klüver, Heinrich (1897–1979), American neurologist and psychologist.

    Bucy, Paul Clancy (1904–1992), American neurologist.

km *abbr* kilometer

knee \'nē\ *n* 1 : a joint in the middle part of the leg that is the articulation between the femur, tibia, and patella — called also *knee joint* 2 : the part of the leg that includes this joint — **kneed** \'nēd\ *adj*

knee-cap \'nē-ˌkap\ *n* : PATELLA

knee jerk *n* : an involuntary forward jerk or kick produced by a light blow or sudden strain upon the patellar ligament of the knee that causes a reflex contraction of the quadriceps muscle — called also *patellar reflex*

knee joint *n* : KNEE 1

Kne·mi·do·kop·tes \ˌnē-mə-dō-'käp-(ˌ)tēz\ *n* : a genus of itch mites (family Sarcoptidae) that attack birds

knife \'nīf\ *n, pl* **knives** \'nīvz\ 1 : any of various instruments used in surgery primarily to sever tissues: as **a** : a cutting instrument consisting of a sharp blade attached to a handle **b** : an instrument that cuts by means of an electrical current **2** : SURGERY 3 — usu. used in the phrase *under the knife* ⟨went under the ~ this morning⟩

knit \'nit\ *vb* **knit** *or* **knit·ted; knit·ting** : to grow or cause to grow together ⟨a fracture that *knitted* slowly⟩

knock–knee \'näk-,nē\ *n* : a condition in which the legs curve inward at the knees — called also *genu valgum* — **knock–kneed** \-,nēd\ *adj*

knock·out \'näk-,aùt\ *adj* : having all or part of a gene eliminated or inactivated by genetic engineering ⟨~ mice⟩

knot \'nät\ *n* **1** : an interlacing of the parts of one or more flexible bodies (as threads or sutures) in a lump to prevent their spontaneous separation — see SURGEON'S KNOT **2** : a usu. firm or hard lump, swelling, or protuberance in or on a part of the body or a bone or process — compare SURFER'S KNOT — **knot** *vb*

knuck·le \'nə-kəl\ *n* **1 a** : the rounded prominence formed by the ends of the two adjacent bones at a joint — used esp. of those at the joints of the fingers **b** : the joint of a knuckle **2** : a sharply flexed loop of intestines incarcerated in a hernia

Koch·er's forceps \'kō-kərz-\ *n* : a strong forceps for controlling bleeding in surgery having serrated blades with interlocking teeth at the tips

Kocher \'kō-kər\, **Emil Theodor** (1841–1917), Swiss surgeon.

Koch's bacillus \'kōks-, 'kōch-\ *or* **Koch bacillus** \'kōk-, 'kōch-\ *n* : a bacillus of the genus *Mycobacterium* (*M. tuberculosis*) that causes human tuberculosis

Koch \'kōk\, (Heinrich Hermann) **Robert** (1843–1910), German bacteriologist.

Koch's postulates *n pl* : a statement of the steps required to establish a microorganism as the cause of a disease: (1) it must be found in all cases of the disease; (2) it must be isolated from the host and grown in pure culture; (3) it must reproduce the original disease when introduced into a susceptible host; (4) it must be found present in the experimental host so infected — called also *Koch's laws*

Koch–Weeks bacillus \-'wēks-\ *n* : a bacterium of the genus *Haemophilus* (*H. aegyptius*) associated with an infectious form of human conjunctivitis

Weeks, John Elmer (1853–1949), American ophthalmologist.

Koch–Weeks conjunctivitis *n* : conjunctivitis caused by the Koch-Weeks bacillus

koi·lo·cyte \'kói-lə-,sīt\ *n* : a vacuolated pyknotic epithelial cell associated with certain human papillomavirus infections (as of the genitals)

koi·lo·cy·to·sis \,kói-lə-sī-'tō-səs\ *n* : the presence of koilocytes usu. in the anogenital region or the uterine cervix

koil·onych·ia \,kói-lō-'ni-kē-ə\ *n* : abnormal thinness and concavity of fingernails occurring esp. in hypochromic anemias — called also *spoon nails*

Kop·lik's spots \'kä-pliks-\ *or* **Kop·lik spots** \-plik-\ *n pl* : small bluish white dots surrounded by a reddish zone that appear on the mucous membrane of the cheeks and lips before the appearance of the skin eruption in a case of measles

Koplik, Henry (1858–1927), American pediatrician.

Korean hemorrhagic fever *n* : a hemorrhagic fever that is endemic in Korea, Manchuria, and Siberia, is caused by the Hantaan virus, and is characterized by acute renal failure in addition to the usual symptoms of the hemorrhagic fevers — called also *epidemic hemorrhagic fever*

Ko·rot·koff sounds *also* **Ko·rot·kow sounds** *or* **Ko·rot·kov sounds** \kō-'rót-kòf-\ *n pl* : arterial sounds heard through a stethoscope applied to the brachial artery distal to the cuff of a sphygmomanometer that change with varying cuff pressure and that are used to determine systolic and diastolic blood pressure

Korotkoff, Nikolai Sergeievich (1874–1920), Russian physician.

Kor·sa·koff's psychosis \'kòr-sə-,kòfs-\ *n* : an abnormal mental condition that is usu. a sequel of chronic alcoholism, is often associated with polyneuritis, and is characterized by an impaired ability to acquire new information and by an irregular memory loss for which the patient often attempts to compensate through confabulation

Korsakoff *or* **Korsakov, Sergei Sergeievich** (1853–1900), Russian psychiatrist.

Korsakoff's syndrome *or* **Korsakoff syndrome** *n* : KORSAKOFF'S PSYCHOSIS

Kr *symbol* krypton

Krab·be's disease \'kra-bēz-\ *n* : a rapidly progressive demyelinating familial leukoencephalopathy with onset in infancy characterized by irritability followed by tonic convulsions, quadriplegia, blindness, deafness, dementia, and death

Krabbe \'krä-bə\, **Knud H.** (1885–1961), Danish neurologist.

krad \'kä-,rad\ *n, pl* **krad** *also* **krads** : KILORAD

krait \'krīt\ *n* : any of a genus (*Bungarus*) of brightly banded extremely venomous nocturnal elapid snakes of southern Asia and adjacent islands

krau·ro·sis \krò-'rō-səs\ *n, pl* **-ro·ses** \-,sēz\ : atrophy and shriveling of the skin or mucous membrane esp. of the vulva where it is often a precancerous lesion — **krau·rot·ic** \-'rä-tik\ *adj*

krau·ro·sis vul·vae \-'vəl-vē\ *n* : kraurosis of the vulva

Krau·se's corpuscle \'kraủ-zəz-\ *n* : any of various rounded sensory end organs occurring in mucous membranes (as of the conjunctiva or genitals) — called also *corpuscle of Krause*

Krause, Wilhelm Johann Friedrich (1833–1910), German anatomist.

Krause's end–bulb *n* : KRAUSE'S CORPUSCLE

kre·bi·o·zen \krə-'bī-ə-zən\ *n* : a drug formerly used in the treatment of cancer that was of unproved effectiveness and was of undisclosed formulation but was reported to contain creatine

Krebs cycle \'krebz-\ *n* : a sequence of reactions in the living organism in which oxidation of acetic acid or acetyl equivalent provides energy for storage in phosphate bonds (as in ATP) — called also *citric acid cycle, tricarboxylic acid cycle*

Krebs, Sir Hans Adolf (1900–1981), German-British biochemist.

Kru·ken·berg tumor \'krü-kən-,bərg-\ *n* : a metastatic ovarian tumor of mucin-producing epithelial cells usu. derived from a primary gastrointestinal tumor

Kru·ken·berg \-,berk\, **Friedrich Ernst (1871–1946),** German pathologist.

kryp·ton \'krip-,tän\ *n* : a colorless relatively inert gaseous element — symbol *Kr;* see ELEMENT table

KS *abbr* Kaposi's sarcoma

KUB *abbr* kidney, ureter, and bladder

Ku·gel·berg–Wel·an·der disease \'kü-gəl-,bərg-'ve-lən-dər-\ *n* : muscular weakness and atrophy that is caused by degeneration of motor neurons in the ventral horn of the spinal cord, is usu. inherited as an autosomal recessive trait, and that becomes symptomatic during childhood or adolescence typically progressing slowly during adulthood — compare WERDNIG-HOFFMANN DISEASE

Kugelberg, Eric Klas Henrik (1913–1983), and **Welander, Lisa (1909–2001),** Swedish neurologists.

Kupf·fer cell \'kủp-fər-\ *also* **Kupffer's cell** \-fərz-\ *n* : a fixed macrophage of the walls of the liver sinusoids that is stellate with a large oval nucleus and the cytoplasm commonly packed with fragments resulting from phagocytic action

Kupffer, Karl Wilhelm von (1829–1902), German anatomist.

ku·ru \'kü-,rü, 'kúr-ü\ *n* : a rare progressive fatal prion disease that resembles Creutzfeldt-Jakob disease and has occurred among tribespeople in eastern New Guinea who engaged in a form of ritual cannibalism — called also *laughing death, laughing sickness*

Kuss·maul breathing \'kủs-,maủl-\ *or* **Kuss·maul's breathing** \-,maủlz-\ *n* : abnormally slow deep respiration characteristic of air hunger and occurring esp. in acidotic states — called also *Kussmaul respiration*

Kussmaul, Adolf (1822–1902), German physician.

Kveim test \'kvām-\ *n* : a test for sarcoidosis used esp. formerly in which a suspension of sarcoid-containing tissue (as of the lymph nodes or spleen) is injected intradermally and which is positive when the formation of sarcoid granulomas are detected at the site of injection

Kveim, Morten Ansgar (1892–1966), Norwegian physician.

kwa·shi·or·kor \,kwä-shē-'ôr-kòr, -ôr-'kòr\ *n* : severe malnutrition chiefly affecting young children esp. of impoverished regions that is characterized by failure to grow and develop, changes in the pigmentation of the skin and hair, edema, fatty degeneration of the liver, anemia, and apathy and is caused by a diet excessively high in carbohydrate and extremely low in protein — compare PELLAGRA

Kwell \'kwel\ *trademark* — used for a preparation of lindane

Kya·sa·nur For·est disease \,kya-sə-'nủr-'fòr-əst-\ *n* : a disease caused by a virus of the genus *Flavivirus* (*Kyasanur Forest disease virus*) that is characterized by fever, headache, diarrhea, and intestinal bleeding and is transmitted by immature ticks of the genus *Haemaphysalis*

ky·mo·gram \'kī-mə-,gram\ *n* : a record made by a kymograph

ky·mo·graph \-,graf\ *n* : a device which graphically records motion or pressure (as of blood) — **ky·mo·graph·ic** \,kī-mə-'gra-fik\ *adj* — **ky·mog·ra·phy** \kī-'mä-grə-fē\ *n*

ky·pho·plas·ty \'kī-fō-,plas-tē\ *n, pl* **-ties** : a medical procedure that is similar to vertebroplasty in the use of acrylic cement to stabilize and reduce pain associated with a vertebral compression fracture but that additionally restores vertebral height and lessens spinal deformity by injecting the cement into a cavity created in the fractured bone by the insertion and inflation of a special balloon

ky·pho·sco·li·o·sis \,kī-fō-,skō-lē-'ō-səs\ *n, pl* **-o·ses** \-,sēz\ : backward and lateral curvature of the spine

ky·pho·sis \kī-'fō-səs\ *n, pl* **-pho·ses** \-,sēz\ : exaggerated backward curvature of the thoracic region of the spinal column — compare LORDOSIS, SCOLIOSIS — **ky·phot·ic** \-'fä-tik\ *adj*

L

L *abbr* lumbar — used esp. with a number from 1 to 5 to indicate a vertebra or segment of the spinal cord in the lumbar region

L *symbol* lithium

l- *prefix* **1** \ˈlē-(ˌ)vō, ˌel, ˈel\ : levorotatory — usu. printed in italic ⟨*l*-tartaric acid⟩ **2** \ˌel, ˈel\ : having a similar configuration at a selected carbon atom to the configuration of levorotatory glyceraldehyde — usu. printed as a small capital ⟨L-fructose⟩

La *symbol* lanthanum

lab \ˈlab\ *n* : LABORATORY

¹la·bel \ˈlā-bəl\ *n* : a usu. radioactive isotope used in labeling

²label *vb* **la·beled** *or* **la·belled**; **la·bel·ing** *or* **la·bel·ling** **1** : to distinguish (an element or atom) by using an isotope distinctive in some manner (as in mass or radioactivity) **2** : to distinguish (as a compound or cell) by introducing a traceable constituent (as a dye or labeled atom)

la·bet·a·lol \lə-ˈbe-tə-ˌlȯl, -ˌlōl\ *n* : a beta-adrenergic blocking agent used in the form of its hydrochloride $C_{19}H_{24}O_3 \cdot HCl$ to treat hypertension

labia *pl of* LABIUM

la·bi·al \ˈlā-bē-əl\ *adj* : of, relating to, or situated near the lips or labia — **la·bi·al·ly** *adv*

labial artery *n* : either of two branches of the facial artery of which one is distributed to the upper and one to the lower lip

labial gland *n* : one of the small tubular mucous and serous glands lying beneath the mucous membrane of the lips

labialis — see HERPES LABIALIS

la·bia ma·jo·ra \ˈlā-bē-ə-mə-ˈjȯr-ə\ *n pl* : the outer fatty folds of the vulva bounding the vestibule

labia mi·no·ra \-mə-ˈnȯr-ə\ *n pl* : the inner highly vascular largely connective-tissue folds of the vulva bounding the vestibule — called also *nymphae*

labii — see LEVATOR LABII SUPERIORIS, LEVATOR LABII SUPERIORIS ALAEQUE NASI, QUADRATUS LABII SUPERIORIS

la·bile \ˈlā-ˌbīl, -bəl\ *adj* : readily or frequently changing: as **a** : readily or continually undergoing chemical, physical, or biological change or breakdown ⟨a ~ antigen⟩ **b** : characterized by wide fluctuations (as in blood pressure or glucose tolerance) ⟨~ hypertension⟩ **c** : emotionally unstable — **la·bil·i·ty** \lā-ˈbi-lə-tē\ *n*

labile factor *n* : FACTOR V

labio- *comb form* : labial and ⟨*labio*lingual⟩

la·bio-buc·cal \ˌlā-bē-ō-ˈbə-kəl\ *adj* : of, relating to, or lying against the inner surface of the lips and cheeks; also : administered to labio-buccal tissue ⟨a ~ injection⟩

la·bio·glos·so·pha·ryn·geal \ˌlā-bē-ō-ˌgläs-ō-ˌfar-ən-ˈjē-əl, -ˌglös-, -fə-ˈrin-jəl, -jē-əl\ *adj* : of, relating to, or affecting the lips, tongue, and pharynx

la·bio·lin·gual \-ˈliŋ-gwəl, -gyə-wəl\ *adj* **1** : of or relating to the lips and the tongue **2** : of or relating to the labial and lingual aspects of a tooth — **la·bio·lin·gual·ly** *adv*

la·bio·scro·tal \-ˈskrōt-ᵊl\ *adj* : relating to or being a swelling or ridge on each side of the embryonic rudiment of the penis or clitoris which develops into one of the scrotal sacs in the male and one of the labia majora in the female

la·bi·um \ˈlā-bē-əm\ *n, pl* **la·bia** \-ə\ : any of the folds at the margin of the vulva — compare LABIA MAJORA, LABIA MINORA

la·bor \ˈlā-bər\ *n* : the physical activities involved in parturition consisting essentially of a prolonged series of involuntary contractions of the uterine musculature together with both reflex and voluntary contractions of the abdominal wall; also : the period of time during which such labor takes place — **labor** *vb*

lab·o·ra·to·ry \ˈla-brə-ˌtōr-ē\ *n, pl* **-ries** *often attrib* : a place equipped for experimental study in a science or for testing and analysis

la·bored \ˈlā-bərd\ *adj* : produced or performed with difficulty or strain ⟨~ breathing⟩

labor room *n* : a hospital room where a woman in labor stays before being taken to the delivery room

la·brum \ˈlā-brəm\ *n* : a fibrous ring of cartilage attached to the rim of a joint; *esp* : GLENOID LABRUM

lab·y·rinth \ˈla-bə-ˌrinth\ *n* : a tortuous anatomical structure; *esp* : the internal ear or its bony or membranous part — see BONY LABYRINTH, MEMBRANOUS LABYRINTH

lab·y·rin·thec·to·my \ˌlab-ə-rin-ˈthek-tə-mē\ *n, pl* **-mies** : surgical removal of the labyrinth of the ear

lab·y·rin·thine \-ˈrin-thən, -ˌthīn, -ˌthēn\ *adj* : of, relating to, affecting, or originating in the internal ear

labyrinthine artery *n* : INTERNAL AUDITORY ARTERY

labyrinthine sense *n* : VESTIBULAR SENSE

lab·y·rin·thi·tis \ˌla-bə-rin-ˈthī-təs\ *n* : inflammation of the labyrinth of the internal ear

lab·y·rin·thot·o·my \ˌla-bə-rin-ˈthä-tə-mē\ *n, pl* **-mies** : surgical incision into the labyrinth of the internal ear

lac·er·a·tion \ˌla-sə-ˈrā-shən\ *n* **1** : the act of making a rough or jagged wound or tear **2** : a torn and ragged wound — **lac·er·ate** \ˈla-sə-ˌrāt\ *vb*

lacerum — see FORAMEN LACERUM

lachrymal, lachrymation, lachrymator, lachrymatory var of LACRIMAL, LACRIMATION, LACRIMATOR, LACRIMATORY

lac operon \'lak-\ n : the operon which controls lactose metabolism and has been isolated from E. coli

¹**lac·ri·mal** also **lach·ry·mal** \'la-krə-məl\ adj 1 : of, relating to, associated with, located near, or constituting the glands that produce tears 2 : of or relating to tears (∼ effusions)

²**lacrimal** also **lachrymal** n : a lacrimal anatomical part (as a lacrimal bone)

lacrimal apparatus n : the bodily parts which function in the production of tears including the lacrimal glands, lacrimal ducts, lacrimal sacs, nasolacrimal ducts, and lacrimal puncta

lacrimal artery n : a large branch of the ophthalmic artery that arises near the optic foramen and supplies the lacrimal gland

lacrimal bone n : a small thin bone making up part of the front inner wall of each orbit and providing a groove for the passage of the lacrimal ducts

lacrimal canal n : LACRIMAL DUCT 1

lacrimal canaliculus n : LACRIMAL DUCT 1

lacrimal caruncle n : a small reddish follicular elevation at the medial angle of the eye

lacrimal duct n 1 : a short canal leading from a minute orifice on a small elevation at the medial angle of each eyelid to the lacrimal sac — called also lacrimal canal, lacrimal canaliculus 2 : any of several small ducts that carry tears from the lacrimal gland to the fornix of the conjunctiva

lacrimal gland n : an acinous gland that is about the size and shape of an almond, secretes tears, and is situated laterally and superiorly to the bulb of the eye in a shallow depression on the inner surface of the frontal bone — called also tear gland

lacrimal nerve n : a small branch of the ophthalmic nerve that enters the lacrimal gland with the lacrimal artery and supplies the lacrimal gland and the adjacent conjunctiva and the skin of the upper eyelid

lacrimal punc·tum \-'pəŋk-təm\ n : the opening of either the upper or the lower lacrimal duct at the inner canthus of the eye

lacrimal sac n : the dilated oval upper end of the nasolacrimal duct that is situated in a groove formed by the lacrimal bone and the frontal process of the maxilla, is closed at its upper end, and receives the lacrimal ducts

lac·ri·ma·tion also **lach·ry·ma·tion** \,la-krə-'mā-shən\ n : the secretion of tears; specif : abnormal or excessive secretion of tears due to local or systemic disease

lac·ri·ma·tor also **lach·ry·ma·tor** \'la-krə-,mā-tər\ n : a tear-producing substance (as tear gas)

lac·ri·ma·to·ry also **lach·ry·ma·to·ry** \'la-kri-mə-,tōr-ē\ adj : of, relating to, or prompting tears

La Crosse encephalitis \lə-'krȯs-\ n : an encephalitis typically affecting children that is caused by the La Crosse virus transmitted esp. by a mosquito of the genus Aedes (A. triseriatus)

La Crosse virus n : a virus that causes La Crosse encephalitis and that belongs to a strain of a virus of the genus Orthobunyavirus (species California encephalitis virus)

lact- or **lacti-** or **lacto-** comb form 1 : milk (lactogenesis) 2 a : lactic acid (lactate) b : lactose (lactase)

lact·ac·i·de·mia \,lak-,ta-sə-'dē-mē-ə\ n : the presence of excess lactic acid in the blood

lact·al·bu·min \,lak-,tal-'byü-mən\ n : an albumin that is found in milk and is similar to serum albumin; esp : a protein fraction from whey

lac·tam \'lak-,tam\ n : any of a class of amides of amino carboxylic acids that are characterized by the group –CONH– in a ring and that include many antibiotics

β–lactam var of BETA-LACTAM

β–lactamase var of BETA-LACTAMASE

lac·tase \'lak-,tās, -,tāz\ n : an enzyme that hydrolyzes lactose to glucose and galactose and occurs esp. in the intestines of young mammals and in yeasts

¹**lac·tate** \'lak-,tāt\ n : a salt or ester of lactic acid

²**lactate** vb **lac·tat·ed; lac·tat·ing** : to secrete milk

lactate dehydrogenase n : any of a group of isoenzymes that catalyze reversibly the conversion of pyruvic acid to lactic acid, are found esp. in the liver, kidneys, striated muscle, and the myocardium, and tend to accumulate in the body when these organs or tissues are diseased or injured — called also lactic dehydrogenase

lactated Ringer's solution n : a sterile aqueous solution that is similar to Ringer's solution but contains sodium lactate in addition to calcium chloride, sodium chloride, and potassium chloride — called also Hartmann's solution, lactated Ringer's, Ringer's lactate, Ringer's lactate solution

S. Ringer — see RINGER'S FLUID

lac·ta·tion \lak-'tā-shən\ n 1 : the secretion and yielding of milk by the mammary gland 2 : one complete period of lactation extending from about the time of parturition to weaning

lactation tetany n : MILK FEVER 1

¹**lac·te·al** \'lak-tē-əl\ adj 1 : relating to, consisting of, producing, or resembling milk (∼ fluid) 2 a : conveying or containing a milky fluid (as chyle)

⟨a ∼ channel⟩ **b** : of or relating to the lacteals ⟨impaired ∼ function⟩

²**lacteal** *n* : any of the lymphatic vessels arising from the villi of the small intestine and conveying chyle to the thoracic duct

lacti- — see LACT-

lac·tic ac·id \'lak-tik-\ *n* : an organic acid $C_3H_6O_3$ that is known in three optically isomeric forms: **a** *or* D—**lactic acid** \'dē-\ : the dextrorotatory form present normally in blood and muscle tissue as a product of the metabolism of glucose and glycogen **b** *or* L—**lactic acid** \'el-\ : the levorotatory form obtained by biological fermentation of sucrose **c** *or* DL—**lactic acid** \'dē-'el-\ : the racemic form present in food products and made usu. by bacterial fermentation

lactic acidosis *n* : a condition characterized by the accumulation of lactic acid in bodily tissues

lactic dehydrogenase *n* : LACTATE DEHYDROGENASE

lac·tif·er·ous duct \lak-'ti-fə-rəs-\ *n* : any of the milk-carrying ducts of the mammary gland that open on the nipple

lactiferous sinus *n* : an expansion in a lactiferous duct at the base of the nipple in which milk accumulates

lacto- — see LACT-

lac·to·ba·cil·lus \,lak-tō-bə-'si-ləs\ *n* **1** *cap* : a genus of gram-positive nonmotile lactic-acid-forming bacteria (family Lactobacillaceae) **2** *pl* **-li** \-,lī *also* -,ē\ : any bacterium of the genus Lactobacillus

lac·to·fer·rin \,lak-tō-'fer-ən\ *n* : a red iron-binding protein synthesized by neutrophils and glandular epithelial cells, found in many human secretions (as tears and milk), and retarding bacterial and fungal growth

lac·to·fla·vin \,lak-tō-'flā-vən\ *n* : RIBOFLAVIN

lac·to·gen \'lak-tə-jən, -,jen\ *n* : any hormone (as prolactin) that stimulates the production of milk — see PLACENTAL LACTOGEN

lac·to·gen·e·sis \,lak-tō-'je-nə-səs\ *n*, *pl* **-e·ses** \-,sēz\ : initiation of lactation

lac·to·gen·ic \,lak-tō-'je-nik\ *adj* : stimulating lactation

lactogenic hormone *n* : LACTOGEN; *esp* : PROLACTIN

lac·tone \'lak-,tōn\ *n* : any of various cyclic esters formed from acids containing one or more OH groups

lac·to—ovo—veg·e·tar·i·an \,lak-tō-,ō-vō-,ve-jə-'ter-ē-ən\ *n* : a vegetarian whose diet includes milk, eggs, vegetables, fruits, grains, and nuts — compare LACTO-VEGETARIAN — **lacto–ovo–vegetarian** *adj*

lac·to·per·ox·i·dase \,lak-tō-pə-'räk-sə-,dās, -,dāz\ *n* : a peroxidase found in milk and saliva that catalyzes the oxidation of the anions thiocyanate or iodide by hydrogen peroxide resulting in the production of antimicrobial compounds

lac·tose \'lak-,tōs, -,tōz\ *n* : a disaccharide sugar $C_{12}H_{22}O_{11}$ that is present in milk, yields glucose and galactose upon hydrolysis, yields esp. lactic acid upon fermentation, and is used chiefly in foods, medicines, and culture media (as for the production of penicillin) — called also *milk sugar*

lac·tos·uria \,lak-tō-'shùr-ē-ə, -'syùr-\ *n* : the presence of lactose in the urine

lac·to—veg·e·tar·i·an \,lak-tō-,ve-jə-'ter-ē-ən\ *n* : a vegetarian whose diet includes milk, vegetables, fruits, grains, and nuts — compare LACTO-OVO-VEGETARIAN — **lacto–vegetarian** *adj*

lac·tu·lose \'lak-tyù-,lōs, -tù-, -,lōz\ *n* : a cathartic disaccharide $C_{12}H_{22}O_{11}$ used to treat chronic constipation and disturbances of function in the central nervous system accompanying severe liver disease

la·cu·na \lə-'kü-nə, -'kyü-\ *n*, *pl* **la·cu·nae** \-,nē, -,nī\ : a small cavity, pit, or discontinuity in an anatomical structure: as **a** : one of the follicles in the mucous membrane of the urethra **b** : one of the minute cavities in bone or cartilage occupied by the osteocytes — **la·cu·nar** \-nər\ *adj*

Laen·nec's cirrhosis *or* **Laën·nec's cirrhosis** \'lā-neks-\ *n* : hepatic cirrhosis in which increased connective tissue spreads out from the portal spaces compressing and distorting the lobules, causing impairment of liver function, and ultimately producing the typical hobnail liver — called also *portal cirrhosis*

   Laennec, René–Théophile–Hyacinthe (1781–1826), French physician.

la·e·trile \'lā-ə-(,)tril\ *n*, *often cap* : a drug that is derived esp. from pits of the apricot (*Prunus armeniaca* of the rose family, Rosaceae), that contains amygdalin, and that has been used in the treatment of cancer although of unproved effectiveness

laev- *or* **laevo-** *Brit var of* LEV-

lae·vo·car·dia, lae·vo·do·pa *Brit var of* LEVOCARDIA, LEVODOPA

La·fo·ra body \lä-'fōr-ə-\ *n* : any of the cytoplasmic inclusion bodies found in neurons of parts of the central nervous system in Lafora disease and consisting of a complex of glycoprotein and glycosaminoglycan

   Lafora, Gonzalo Rodríguez (1886–1971), Spanish neurologist.

Lafora disease *or* **Lafora's disease** *n* : an inherited form of myoclonic epilepsy that typically begins during adolescence or late childhood and is characterized by progressive neurological deterioration and the presence of Lafora bodies in parts of the central nervous system

-lag·nia \'lag-nē-ə\ *comb form* : sexual excitement ⟨uro*lagnia*⟩

lag·oph·thal·mos or **lag·oph·thal·mus** \la-ˌgäf-'thal-məs\ n : pathological incomplete closure of the eyelids : inability to close the eyelids fully

la grippe \lä-'grip\ n : INFLUENZA

LAK \'lak; ˌel-(ˌ)ā-'kā\ n : LYM-PHOKINE-ACTIVATED KILLER CELL

LAK cell n : LYMPHOKINE-ACTIVATED KILLER CELL

lake \'lāk\ vb **laked; lak·ing** : to undergo or cause (blood) to undergo a physiological change in which the hemoglobin becomes dissolved in the plasma

-la·lia \'lā-lē-ə\ n comb form : speech disorder (of a specified type) 〈echolalia〉

lal·la·tion \la-'lā-shən\ n **1** : infantile speech whether in infants or in older speakers (as from mental retardation) **2** : a defective articulation of the letter l, the substitution of \l\ for another sound, or the substitution of another sound for \l\

La·maze \lə-'mäz\ adj : relating to or being a method of childbirth that involves psychological and physical preparation by the mother in order to suppress pain and facilitate delivery without drugs

Lamaze, Fernand (1890–1957), French obstetrician.

lamb·da \'lam-də\ n **1** : the point of junction of the sagittal and lambdoid sutures of the skull **2** : PHAGE LAMB-DA

lambda chain or **λ chain** n : a polypeptide chain of one of the two types of light chain that are found in antibodies and can be distinguished antigenically and by the sequence of amino acids in the chain — compare KAPPA CHAIN

lamb·da·cism \'lam-də-ˌsi-zəm\ n : a defective articulation of \l\, the substitution of other sounds for it, or the substitution of \l\ for another sound

lambda phage n : PHAGE LAMBDA

lamb·doid \'lam-ˌdȯid\ or **lamb·doi·dal** \ˌlam-'dȯid-ᵊl\ adj : of, relating to, or being the suture shaped like the Greek letter lambda (λ) that connects the occipital and parietal bones

Lam·bert–Ea·ton syndrome \'lam-bərt-'ē-tᵊn-\ n : an autoimmune disorder that is caused by impaired presynaptic release of acetylcholine at nerve synapses, that is characterized by progressive weakness esp. of the limbs, and that is often associated with a malignant condition (as small-cell lung cancer) — called also *Eaton-Lambert syndrome, Lambert-Eaton myasthenic syndrome*

Lambert, Edward Howard (b 1915), and Eaton, Lealdes McKendree (1905–1958), American physicians.

lam·bli·a·sis \lam-'blī-ə-səs\ n, pl **-a·ses** \-ˌsēz\ : GIARDIASIS

Lambl, \'läm-bᵊl\, Wilhelm Dusan (1824–1895), Austrian physician.

lame \'lām\ adj **lam·er; lam·est** : having a body part and esp. a limb so disabled as to impair freedom of movement : physically disabled — **lame·ly** adv — **lame·ness** n

la·mel·la \lə-'me-lə\ n, pl **la·mel·lae** \-ˌlē, -ˌlī\ also **lamellas 1** : an organ, process, or part resembling a plate: as **a** : one of the bony concentric layers surrounding the haversian canals in bone **b** (1) : one of the incremental layers of cementum laid down in a tooth (2) : a thin sheetlike organic structure in the enamel of a tooth extending inward from a surface crack **2** : a small medicated disk prepared from gelatin and glycerin for use esp. in the eyes — **la·mel·lar** \lə-'me-lər\ adj — **lam·el·lat·ed** \'la-mə-ˌlā-təd\ adj

lamellar ichthyosis n : a rare inherited form of ichthyosis characterized by large coarse scales

lamin- or **lamini-** or **lamino-** comb form : lamina 〈lamin*itis*〉

lam·i·na \'la-mə-nə\ n, pl **-nae** \-ˌnē, -ˌnī\ or **-nas** : a thin plate or layer esp. of an anatomical part

lamina cri·bro·sa \-kri-'brō-sə\ n, pl **laminae cri·bro·sae** \-ˌsē, -ˌsī\ : any of several anatomical structures having the form of a perforated plate: as **a** : CRIBRIFORM PLATE 1 **b** : the part of the sclera of the eye penetrated by the fibers of the optic nerve **c** : a perforated plate that closes the internal auditory canal

lamina du·ra \-'dur-ə, -'dyur-\ n : the thin hard layer of bone that lines the socket of a tooth and that appears as a dark line in radiography

laminagram, laminagraph var of LAMINOGRAM, LAMINOGRAPH

lamina pro·pria \-'prō-prē-ə\ n, pl **laminae pro·pri·ae** \-prē-ˌē, -ˌī\ : a highly vascular layer of connective tissue under the basement membrane lining a layer of epithelium

lam·i·nar \'la-mə-nər\ adj : arranged in, consisting of, or resembling laminae

lam·i·nar·ia \ˌla-mə-'nar-ē-ə\ n : any of a genus (*Laminaria*) of kelps of which some have been used to dilate the cervix in performing an abortion

lamina spi·ral·is \-spə-'ra-ləs, -'rā-\ n : SPIRAL LAMINA

lam·i·nat·ed \'la-mə-ˌnā-təd\ adj : composed or arranged in layers or laminae 〈~ membranes〉

lamina ter·mi·nal·is \-ˌtər-mi-'na-ləs, -'nā-\ n : a thin layer of gray matter in the telencephalon that extends backward from the corpus callosum above the optic chiasma and forms the median portion of the rostral wall of the third ventricle of the cerebrum

lam·i·na·tion \ˌla-mə-'nā-shən\ n : a laminated structure or arrangement

lam·i·nec·to·my \ˌla-mə-'nek-tə-mē\ n, pl **-mies** : surgical removal of the posterior arch of a vertebra

lamini- or **lamino-** — see LAMIN-

lam·i·nin \'la-mə-nən\ *n* : a glycoprotein that is a component of connective tissue basement membrane and that promotes cell adhesion

lam·i·ni·tis \ₗla-mə-'nī-təs\ *n* : inflammation of a lamina esp. in the hoof of a horse, cow, or goat that is typically caused by excessive ingestion of a dietary substance (as carbohydrate) — called also *founder*

lam·i·no·gram *or* **lam·i·na·gram** \'la-mə-nə-ₗgram\ *n* : a radiograph of a layer of the body made by means of a laminograph; *broadly* : TOMOGRAM

lam·i·no·graph *or* **lam·i·na·graph** \-ₗgraf\ *n* : an X-ray machine that makes radiography of body tissue possible at any desired depth; *broadly* : TOMOGRAPH — **lam·i·no·graph·ic** \ₗla-mə-nə-'gra-fik\ *adj* — **lam·i·nog·ra·phy** \ₗla-mə-'nä-grə-fē\ *n*

lam·i·not·o·my \ₗla-mə-'nä-tə-mē\ *n, pl* **-mies** : surgical division of a vertebral lamina

Lam·i·sil \'la-mə-ₗsil\ *trademark* — used for a preparation of the hydrochloride of terbinafine

la·miv·u·dine \lə-'mi-vyü-ₗdēn\ *n* : an antiviral drug $C_8H_{11}N_3O_3S$ that acts against HIV by inhibiting reverse transcriptase — see EPIVIR, 3TC

lamp \'lamp\ *n* : any of various devices for producing light or heat — see SLIT LAMP

lam·pas \'lam-pəs\ *n* : a congestion of the mucous membrane of the hard palate just posterior to the incisor teeth of the horse due to irritation and bruising from harsh coarse feeds

la·nat·o·side \lə-'na-tə-ₗsīd\ *n* : any of three poisonous crystalline cardiac steroid glycosides occurring in the leaves of a foxglove (*Digitalis lanata*): **a** : the glycoside $C_{49}H_{76}O_{19}$ yielding digitoxin, glucose, and acetic acid on hydrolysis — called also *digilanid A, lanatoside A* **b** : the glycoside $C_{49}H_{76}O_{20}$ yielding gitoxin, glucose, and acetic acid on hydrolysis — called also *digilanid B, lanatoside B* **c** : the bitter glycoside $C_{49}H_{76}O_{20}$ yielding digoxin, glucose, and acetic acid on hydrolysis — and used similarly to digitalis — called also *digilanid C, lanatoside C*

¹lance \'lans\ *n* : LANCET

²lance *vb* **lanced; lanc·ing** : to open with a lancet : make an incision in or into ⟨∼ a boil⟩ ⟨∼ a vein⟩

Lance·field group \'lans-ₗfēld-\ *also* **Lance·field's group** \-ₗfēldz-\ *n* : any of the serologically distinguishable groups into which streptococci can be divided — see GROUP A, GROUP B
Lancefield, Rebecca Craighill (1895–1981), American bacteriologist.

lan·cet \'lan-sət\ *n* : a sharp-pointed and commonly two-edged surgical instrument used to make small incisions

lancet fluke *n* : a small liver fluke of the genus *Dicrocoelium* (*D. den-*

driticum) widely distributed in sheep and cattle and rarely infecting humans

lan·ci·nat·ing \'lan-sə-ₗnā-tiŋ\ *adj* : characterized by piercing or stabbing sensations ⟨∼ pain⟩

land·mark \'land-ₗmärk\ *n* : an anatomical structure used as a point of orientation in locating other structures (as in surgical procedures)

Lan·dolt ring \'län-dōlt-\ *n* : one of a series of incomplete rings or circles used in some eye charts to determine visual discrimination or acuity
Landolt, Edmond (1846–1926), French ophthalmologist.

Lan·dry's paralysis \län-drēz-\ *n* : GUILLAIN-BARRÉ SYNDROME
Landry, Jean-Baptiste-Octave (1826–1865), French physician.

Lang·er·hans cell \'läŋ-ər-ₗhäns-\ *n* : a dendritic cell of the interstitial spaces of the epidermis that functions as an antigen-presenting cell
P. Langerhans, — see ISLET OF LANGERHANS

Lang·hans cell \'läŋ-häns-\ *n* : any of the cells of cuboidal epithelium that make up the cytotrophoblast
Langhans, Theodor (1839–1915), German pathologist and anatomist.

Langhans giant cell *n* : any of the large cells found in the lesions of some granulomatous conditions (as leprosy) and containing a number of peripheral nuclei arranged in a circle or in the shape of a horseshoe

lan·o·lin \'lan-ᵊl-ən\ *n* : wool grease esp. when refined for use in ointments and cosmetics

Lan·ox·in \lə-'näk-sən\ *trademark* — used for a preparation of digoxin

lan·so·praz·ole \lan-'sō-prə-ₗzōl\ *n* : a benzimidazole derivative $C_{16}H_{14}F_3$-N_3O_2S that inhibits gastric acid secretion and is used similarly to omeprazole — see PREVACID

lan·tha·num \'lan-thə-nəm\ *n* : a white soft malleable metallic element — symbol *La*; see ELEMENT table

la·nu·go \lə-'nü-(ₗ)gō, -'nyü-\ *n* : a dense cottony or downy growth; *specif* : the soft downy hair that covers the fetus

lap *abbr* laparotomy

lap·a·ro·scope \'la-pə-rə-ₗskōp\ *n* : a usu. rigid endoscope that is inserted through an incision in the abdominal wall and is used to examine visually the interior of the peritoneal cavity — called also *peritoneoscope*

lap·a·ros·co·pist \ₗla-pə-'räs-kə-pist\ *n* : a physician or surgeon who performs laparoscopies

lap·a·ros·co·py \-pē\ *n, pl* **-pies 1** : visual examination of the abdomen by means of a laparoscope **2** : an operation (as tubal ligation or gallbladder removal) involving laparoscopy — **lap·a·ro·scop·ic** \-rə-'skä-pik\ *adj* — **lap·a·ro·scop·i·cal·ly** *adv*

lap·a·rot·o·my \ˌla-pə-ˈrä-tə-mē\ *n, pl* **-mies** : surgical section of the abdominal wall

La·place's law \lä-ˈpläs-səz-\ *n* : LAW OF LAPLACE

Lar·gac·til \lär-ˈgak-til\ *n* : a preparation of the hydrochloride of chlorpromazine — formerly a U.S. registered trademark

large bowel *n* : LARGE INTESTINE

large calorie *n* : CALORIE 1b

large–cell carcinoma *n* : a non-small cell lung cancer usu. arising in the bronchi and composed of large undifferentiated cells — called also *large=cell lung carcinoma*

large intestine *n* : the more terminal division of the intestine that is wider and shorter than the small intestine, typically divided into cecum, colon, and rectum, and concerned esp. with the resorption of water and the formation of feces

lark·spur \ˈlärk-ˌspər\ *n* : DELPHINIUM 2

Lar·sen's syndrome \ˈlär-sənz-\ *n* : a syndrome characterized by cleft palate, flattened facies, multiple congenital joint dislocations and deformities of the foot

  Larsen, Loren Joseph (b 1914), American orthopedic surgeon.

lar·va \ˈlär-və\ *n, pl* **lar·vae** \-(ˌ)vē, -ˌvī\ *also* **larvas** : the immature, wingless, and often wormlike feeding form that hatches from the egg of many insects — **lar·val** \-vəl\ *adj*

larval mi·grans \-ˈmī-ˌgranz\ *n* : CREEPING ERUPTION

larva migrans *n, pl* **larvae mi·gran·tes** \-ˌmī-ˈgran-ˌtēz\ : CREEPING ERUPTION

lar·vi·cide *also* **lar·va·cide** \ˈlär-və-ˌsīd\ *n* : an agent for killing larvae — **lar·vi·cid·al** \ˌlär-və-ˈsīd-ᵊl\ *adj* — **lar·vi·cid·al·ly** *adv*

laryng- *or* **laryngo-** *comb form* 1 : larynx ⟨*laryng*itis⟩ **2 a** : laryngeal ⟨*laryngo*spasm⟩ **b** : laryngeal and ⟨*laryngo*pharyngeal⟩

¹la·ryn·ge·al \lə-ˈrin-jəl, -jē-əl; ˌlar-ən-ˈjē-əl\ *adj* : of, relating to, affecting, or used on the larynx — **la·ryn·ge·al·ly** *adv*

²laryngeal *n* : an anatomical part (as a nerve or artery) that supplies or is associated with the larynx

laryngeal artery *n* : either of two arteries supplying blood to the larynx: **a** : a branch of the inferior thyroid artery that supplies the muscles and mucous membranes of the dorsal part of the larynx — called also *inferior laryngeal artery* **b** : a branch of the superior thyroid artery or sometimes of the external carotid artery that supplies the muscles, mucous membranes, and glands of the larynx — called also *superior laryngeal artery*

laryngeal nerve *n* : either of two branches of the vagus nerve supplying the larynx: **a** : one that arises from

the ganglion of the vagus situated below the jugular foramen and supplies the cricothyroid muscle — called also *superior laryngeal nerve* **b** : one that arises below the larynx and supplies all the muscles of the thyroid except the cricothyroid — called also *inferior laryngeal nerve, recurrent laryngeal nerve;* — see INFERIOR LARYNGEAL NERVE 2

lar·yn·gec·to·mee \ˌlar-ən-jek-tə-ˈmē\ *n* : a person who has undergone laryngectomy

lar·yn·gec·to·my \-ˈjek-tə-mē\ *n, pl* **-mies** : surgical removal of all or part of the larynx — **lar·yn·gec·to·mized** \-tə-ˌmīzd\ *adj*

larynges *pl of* LARYNX

lar·yn·gis·mus stri·du·lus \ˌlar-ən-ˈjiz-məs-ˈstri-jə-ləs\ *n, pl* **lar·yn·gis·mi strid·u·li** \-ˌmī-ˈstri-jə-ˌlī\ : a sudden spasm of the larynx that occurs in children esp. in rickets and is marked by difficult breathing with prolonged noisy inspiration — compare LARYNGOSPASM

lar·yn·gi·tis \ˌlar-ən-ˈjī-təs\ *n, pl* **-git·i·des** \-ˈji-tə-ˌdēz\ : inflammation of the larynx

laryngo- — see LARYNG-

la·ryn·go·cele \lə-ˈriŋ-gə-ˌsēl\ *n* : an air-containing evagination of laryngeal mucous membrane having its opening communicating with the ventricle of the larynx

la·ryn·go·fis·sure \lə-ˌriŋ-gō-ˈfi-shər\ *n* : surgical opening of the larynx by an incision through the thyroid cartilage esp. for the removal of a tumor

lar·yn·gog·ra·phy \ˌlar-ən-ˈgä-grə-fē\ *n, pl* **-phies** : X-ray depiction of the larynx after use of a radiopaque material

laryngol *abbr* laryngological

la·ryn·go·log·i·cal \lə-ˌriŋ-gə-ˈlä-ji-kəl\ *also* **la·ryn·go·log·ic** \-ˈlä-jik\ *adj* : of or relating to laryngology or the larynx

lar·yn·gol·o·gist \ˌlar-ən-ˈgä-lə-jist\ *n* : a physician specializing in laryngology

lar·yn·gol·o·gy \ˌlar-ən-ˈgä-lə-jē\ *n, pl* **-gies** : a branch of medicine dealing with diseases of the larynx and nasopharynx

la·ryn·go·pha·ryn·ge·al \lə-ˌriŋ-gō-ˌfar-ən-ˈjē-əl, -fə-ˈrin-jəl, -jē-əl\ *adj* : of or common to both the larynx and the pharynx ⟨∼ cancer⟩

la·ryn·go·phar·yn·gi·tis \-ˌfar-ən-ˈjī-təs\ *n, pl* **-git·i·des** \-ˈji-tə-ˌdēz\ : inflammation of both the larynx and the pharynx

la·ryn·go·phar·ynx \-ˈfar-iŋks\ *n* : the lower part of the pharynx lying behind or adjacent to the larynx — compare NASOPHARYNX

la·ryn·go·plas·ty \lə-ˈriŋ-gə-ˌplas-tē\ *n, pl* **-ties** : plastic surgery to repair laryngeal defects

la·ryn·go·scope \lə-ˈriŋ-gə-ˌskōp, -ˈrin-jə-\ *n* : an endoscope for visually examining the interior of the larynx — **la·ryn·go·scop·ic** \-ˌriŋ-gə-ˈskä-pik, -ˌrin-jə-\ *or* **la·ryn·go·scop·i·cal** \-pi-kəl\ *adj*

lar·yn·gos·co·py \ˌlar-ən-ˈgäs-kə-pē\ *n, pl* **-pies** : examination of the interior of the larynx (as with a laryngoscope)

la·ryn·go·spasm \lə-ˈriŋ-gə-ˌspa-zəm\ *n* : spasmodic closure of the larynx — compare LARYNGISMUS STRIDULUS

lar·yn·got·o·my \ˌlar-ən-ˈgä-tə-mē\ *n, pl* **-mies** : surgical incision of the larynx

la·ryn·go·tra·che·al \lə-ˌriŋ-gō-ˈtrā-kē-əl\ *adj* : of or common to the larynx and trachea ⟨∼ stenosis⟩

la·ryn·go·tra·che·itis \-ˌtrā-kē-ˈī-təs\ *n* : inflammation of both larynx and trachea — see INFECTIOUS LARYNGOTRACHEITIS

la·ryn·go·tra·cheo·bron·chi·tis \-ˌtrā-kē-ō-brän-ˈkī-təs, -brän-\ *n, pl* **-chit·i·des** \-tə-ˌdēz\ : inflammation of the larynx, trachea, and bronchi

lar·ynx \ˈlar-iŋks\ *n, pl* **la·ryn·ges** \lə-ˈrin-(ˌ)jēz\ *or* **lar·ynx·es** : the modified upper part of the respiratory passage that is bounded above by the glottis, is continuous below with the trachea, has a complex cartilaginous or bony skeleton capable of limited motion through the action of associated muscles, and has a set of elastic vocal cords that play a major role in sound production and speech — called also *voice box*

¹la·ser \ˈlā-zər\ *n* : a device that utilizes the natural oscillations of atoms or molecules between energy levels for generating coherent electromagnetic radiation usu. in the ultraviolet, visible, or infrared regions of the spectrum

²laser *vb* : to subject to the action of a laser : treat with a laser

laser–assisted in–situ keratomileusis *n* : LASIK

lash \ˈlash\ *n* : EYELASH

LA·SIK \ˈlā-sik\ *n* : a surgical operation to reshape the cornea for correction of nearsightedness, farsightedness, or astigmatism that involves use of an excimer laser to remove varying degrees of tissue from the inner part of the cornea — called also *laser-assisted in-situ keratomileusis*

La·six \ˈlā-ziks, -siks\ *trademark* — used for a preparation of furosemide

L–as·par·a·gi·nase \ˈel-as-ˈpar-ə-jə-ˌnās, -ˌnāz\ *n* : an enzyme that breaks down the physiological commoner form of asparagine, is obtained esp. from bacteria, and is used esp. to treat leukemia

Las·sa fever \ˈla-sə-\ *n* : a disease esp. of Africa that is caused by the Lassa virus and is characterized by a high fever, headaches, mouth ulcers, muscle aches, small hemorrhages under the skin, heart and kidney failure, and a high mortality rate

Lassa virus *n* : a virus of the genus *Arenavirus* (species *Lassa virus*) that causes Lassa fever

las·si·tude \ˈla-sə-ˌtüd, -ˌtyüd\ *n* : a condition of weariness, debility, or fatigue

lat \ˈlat\ *n* : LATISSIMUS DORSI — usu. used in pl.

lata — see FASCIA LATA

latae — see FASCIA LATA, TENSOR FASCIAE LATAE

la·tah \ˈlä-tə\ *n* : a neurotic condition marked by automatic obedience, echolalia, and echopraxia observed esp. among the Malayan people

la·tan·o·prost \lə-ˈta-nə-ˌpräst\ *n* : a prostaglandin analog $C_{26}H_{40}O_5$ used topically to reduce elevated intraocular pressure — see XALATAN

la·ten·cy \ˈlāt-ᵊn-sē\ *n, pl* **-cies** 1 : the quality or state of being latent; *esp* : the state or period of living or developing in a host without producing symptoms — used of an infective agent or disease 2 : LATENCY PERIOD 1 3 : the interval between stimulation and response — called also *latent period*

latency period *n* 1 : a stage of psychosexual development following the phallic stage that extends from about the age of five to the beginning of puberty and during which sexual urges often appear to lie dormant — called also *latency* 2 : LATENT PERIOD

la·tent \ˈlāt-ᵊnt\ *adj* : existing in hidden or dormant form: as **a** : present or capable of living or developing in a host without producing visible symptoms of disease ⟨a ∼ virus⟩ **b** : not consciously expressed **c** : relating to or being the latent content of a dream or thought — **la·tent·ly** *adv*

latent content *n* : the underlying meaning of a dream or thought that is exposed in psychoanalysis by interpretation of its symbols or by free association — compare MANIFEST CONTENT

latent learning *n* : learning that is not demonstrated by behavior at the time it is held to take place but that is inferred to exist based on a greater than expected number of favorable or desired responses at a later time when reinforcement is given

latent period *n* 1 : the period between exposure to a disease-causing agent or process and the appearance of symptoms 2 : LATENCY 3

late–onset diabetes *n* : TYPE 2 DIABETES

lat·er·al \ˈla-tə-rəl, -trəl\ *adj* : of or relating to the side; *esp, of a body part* : lying at or extending toward the right or left side : lying away from the median axis of the body

lateral arcuate ligament *n* : a fascial band that extends from the tip of the transverse process of the first lumbar vertebra to the twelfth rib and provides attachment for part of the diaphragm — compare MEDIAL ARCUATE LIGAMENT, MEDIAN ARCUATE LIGAMENT

lateral brachial cutaneous nerve *n* : a continuation of the posterior branch of the axillary nerve that supplies the skin of the lateral aspect of the upper arm over the distal part of the deltoid muscle and the adjacent head of the triceps brachii

lateral collateral ligament *n* : a ligament that connects the lateral epicondyle of the femur with the lateral side of the head of the fibula and helps to stabilize the knee by preventing lateral dislocation — called also *fibular collateral ligament, LCL*; compare MEDIAL COLLATERAL LIGAMENT

lateral column *n* **1** : a lateral extension of the gray matter in each lateral half of the spinal cord present in the thoracic and upper lumbar regions — called also *lateral horn;* compare DORSAL HORN, VENTRAL HORN **2** : LATERAL FUNICULUS

lateral condyle *n* : a condyle on the outer side of the lower extremity of the femur; *also* : a corresponding eminence on the upper part of the tibia that articulates with the lateral condyle of the femur — compare MEDIAL CONDYLE

lateral cord *n* : a cord of nerve tissue that is formed by union of the superior and middle trunks of the brachial plexus and that forms one of the two roots of the median nerve — compare MEDIAL CORD, POSTERIOR CORD

lateral corticospinal tract *n* : a band of nerve fibers that descends in the posterolateral part of each side of the spinal cord and consists mostly of fibers arising in the motor cortex of the contralateral side of the brain

lateral cricoarytenoid *n* : CRICOARYTENOID 1

lateral cuneiform bone *n* : CUNEIFORM BONE 1c — called also *lateral cuneiform*

lateral decubitus *n* : a position in which a patient lies on his or her side and which is used esp. in radiography and in making a lumbar puncture

lateral epicondyle *n* : EPICONDYLE a

lateral epicondylitis *n* : TENNIS ELBOW

lateral femoral circumflex artery *n* : an artery that branches from the deep femoral artery or from the femoral artery itself and that supplies the muscles of the lateral part of the thigh and hip joint — compare MEDIAL FEMORAL CIRCUMFLEX ARTERY

lateral femoral circumflex vein *n* : a vein accompanying the lateral femoral circumflex artery and emptying into the femoral vein — compare MEDIAL FEMORAL CIRCUMFLEX VEIN

lateral femoral cutaneous nerve *n* : a nerve that arises from the lumbar plexus and that supplies the anterior and lateral aspects of the thigh down to the knee — compare POSTERIOR FEMORAL CUTANEOUS NERVE

lateral fissure *n* : SYLVIAN FISSURE

lateral funiculus *n* : a longitudinal division on each side of the spinal cord comprising white matter between the dorsal and ventral roots — compare ANTERIOR FUNICULUS, POSTERIOR FUNICULUS

lateral gastrocnemius bursa *n* : a bursa of the knee joint that is situated between the lateral head of the gastrocnemius muscle and the joint capsule

lateral geniculate body *n* : a part of the metathalamus that is the terminus of most fibers of the optic tract and receives nerve impulses from the retinas which are relayed to the visual cortex by way of the geniculocalcarine tracts — compare MEDIAL GENICULATE BODY

lateral geniculate nucleus *n* : a nucleus of the lateral geniculate body

lateral horn *n* : LATERAL COLUMN 1

lateral humeral epicondylitis *n* : TENNIS ELBOW

lateral inhibition *n* : a visual process in which the firing of a retinal cell inhibits the firing of surrounding retinal cells and which is held to enhance the perception of areas of contrast

lateralis — see RECTUS LATERALIS, VASTUS LATERALIS

lat·er·al·i·ty \ˌla-tə-ˈra-lə-tē\ *n, pl* **-ties** : preference in use of homologous parts on one lateral half of the body over those on the other : dominance in function of one of a pair of lateral homologous parts

lat·er·al·i·za·tion \ˌla-tə-rə-lə-ˈzā-shən, ˌla-trə-lə-\ *n* : localization of function or activity (as of verbal processes in the brain) on one side of the body in preference to the other — **lat·er·al·ize** \ˈla-tə-rə-ˌlīz, -trə-\ *vb*

lateral lemniscus *n* : a band of nerve fibers that arises in the cochlear nuclei and terminates in the inferior colliculus and the lateral geniculate body of the opposite side of the brain

lateral ligament *n* : any of various ligaments (as the lateral collateral ligament of the knee) that are in a lateral position or that prevent lateral dislocation of a joint

lateral malleolus *n* : MALLEOLUS a

lateral meniscus *n* : MENISCUS a(1)

lateral nucleus *n* : any of a group of nuclei of the thalamus situated in the dorsolateral region extending from its anterior to posterior ends

lateral pectoral nerve *n* : PECTORAL NERVE a

lateral plantar artery *n* : PLANTAR ARTERY a

lateral plantar nerve *n* : PLANTAR NERVE a

lateral plantar vein *n* : PLANTAR VEIN a

lateral popliteal nerve *n* : COMMON PERONEAL NERVE

lateral pterygoid muscle *n* : PTERYGOID MUSCLE a

lateral pterygoid nerve *n* : PTERYGOID NERVE a

lateral pterygoid plate *n* : PTERYGOID PLATE a

lateral rectus *n* : RECTUS 2b

lateral reticular nucleus *n* : a nucleus of the reticular formation that receives fibers esp. from the dorsal horn of the spinal cord and sends axons to the cerebellum on the same side of the body

lateral sacral artery *n* : either of two arteries on each side which arise from the posterior division of the internal iliac artery and supply muscles and skin in the area

lateral sacral crest *n* : SACRAL CREST b

lateral sacral vein *n* : any of several veins that accompany the corresponding lateral sacral arteries and empty into the internal iliac veins

lateral semilunar cartilage *n* : MENISCUS a(1)

lateral spinothalamic tract *n* : SPINOTHALAMIC TRACT b

lateral sulcus *n* : SYLVIAN FISSURE

lateral thoracic artery *n* : THORACIC ARTERY 1b

lateral umbilical ligament *n* : MEDIAL UMBILICAL LIGAMENT

lateral ventricle *n* : an internal cavity in each cerebral hemisphere that consists of a central body and three cornua — see ANTERIOR HORN 2, INFERIOR HORN, POSTERIOR HORN 2

lateral vestibular nucleus *n* : the one of the four vestibular nuclei on each side of the medulla oblongata that sends fibers down the same side of the spinal cord through the vestibulospinal tract — called also *Deiters' nucleus*

latex agglutination test *n* : a test for a specific antibody and esp. rheumatoid factor in which the corresponding antigen is adsorbed on spherical polystyrene latex particles which undergo agglutination upon addition of the specific antibody — called also *latex fixation test, latex test*

lath·y·rism \'la-thə-ˌri-zəm\ *n* : a diseased condition of humans and domestic animals that results from poisoning by an amino acid found in some legumes (genus *Lathyrus* and esp. *L. sativus*) and is characterized esp. by spastic paralysis of the hind or lower limbs — **lath·y·rit·ic** \ˌla-thə-'ri-tik\ *adj*

lath·y·ro·gen \'la-thə-rə-jən, -ˌjen\ *n* : any of a group of compounds that tend to cause lathyrism and inhibit the formation of links between chains of collagen

la·tis·si·mus dor·si \lə-'ti-sə-məs-'dòr-ˌsī\ *n, pl* **la·tis·si·mi dorsi** \-ˌmī-\ : a broad flat superficial muscle of the lower part of the back that extends, adducts, and rotates the arm medially and draws the shoulder downward and backward

Lat·ro·dec·tus \ˌla-trō-'dek-təs\ *n* : a genus of venomous spiders (family Theridiidae) including the black widow (*L. mactans*)

lats \'lats\ *pl of* LAT

LATS *abbr* long-acting thyroid stimulator

latum — see CONDYLOMA LATUM

laud·able pus \'lò-də-bəl-\ *n* : pus discharged freely (as from a wound) and formerly supposed to facilitate the elimination of unhealthy humors from the injured body

lau·da·num \'lòd-nəm, -ˀn-əm\ *n* **1** : any of various formerly used preparations of opium **2** : a tincture of opium

laughing death *n* : KURU

laughing gas *n* : NITROUS OXIDE

laughing sickness *n* : KURU

Lau·rence–Moon–Biedl syndrome \'lòr-əns-'mün-'bēd-ᵊl-, 'lär-\ *n* : an inherited disorder affecting esp. males and characterized by obesity, mental retardation, the presence of extra fingers or toes, subnormal development of the genital organs, and sometimes by retinitis pigmentosa

Laurence, John Zachariah (1830–1874), British physician.

Moon, Robert Charles (1844–1914), American ophthalmologist.

Biedl, Artur (1869–1933), German physician.

lau·ryl \'lòr-əl, 'lär-\ *n* : the monovalent chemical group $C_{12}H_{25}$ — see SODIUM LAURYL SULFATE

LAV \ˌel-(ˌ)ā-'vē\ *n* : HIV-1

la·vage \lə-'väzh, 'la-vij\ *n* : the act or action of washing; *esp* : the therapeutic washing out of an organ or part ⟨gastric ∼⟩ — **lavage** *vb*

law of dominance *n* : MENDEL'S LAW 3

law of independent assortment *n* : MENDEL'S LAW 2

law of La·place \-lä-'pläs\ *n* : a law in physics that in medicine is applied in the physiology of blood flow: under equilibrium conditions the pressure tangent to the circumference of a vessel storing or transmitting fluid equals the product of the pressure across the wall and the radius of the vessel for a sphere and half this for a tube — called also *Laplace's law*

Laplace, Pierre–Simon (1749–1827), French astronomer and mathematician.

law of segregation *n* : MENDEL'S LAW 1

law·ren·ci·um \lò-'ren-sē-əm\ *n* : a short-lived radioactive element that is produced artificially from californium — symbol *Lr;* see ELEMENT table

Lawrence, Ernest Orlando \'lòr-əns, 'lär-\ (1901–1958), American physicist.

lax \'laks\ *adj* **1** of the bowels : LOOSE 3 **2** : having loose bowels
lax·a·tion \lak-'sā-shən\ *n* : a bowel movement
¹lax·a·tive \'lak-sə-tiv\ *adj* **1** : having a tendency to loosen or relax; *specif* : relieving constipation **2** : LAX 2 — **lax·a·tive·ly** *adv*
²laxative *n* : a usu. mild laxative drug
lax·i·ty \'lak-sə-tē\ *n, pl* **-ties** : the quality or state of being loose ⟨a certain ~ of the bowels⟩ ⟨ligamentous ~⟩
la·zar \'la-zər, 'lā-\ *n* : LEPER
laz·a·ret·to \₁la-zə-'re-(₁)tō\ *or* **laz·a·ret** \-'re, -'rē\ *n, pl* **-rettos** *or* **-rets** **1** *usu* **lazaretto** : an institution (as a hospital) for those with contagious diseases **2** : a building or a ship used for detention in quarantine
lazy eye *n* : AMBLYOPIA; *also* : an eye affected with amblyopia
lazy–eye blindness *n* : AMBLYOPIA
lb *abbr* pound
LC *abbr* liquid chromatography
L chain *n* : LIGHT CHAIN
LCL \₁el-₁sē-'el\ *n* : LATERAL COLLATERAL LIGAMENT
LCMV *abbr* lymphocytic choriomeningitis virus
LD *abbr* **1** learning disability; learning disabled **2** lethal dose
LD50 *or* **LD₅₀** \₁el-₁dē-'fif-tē\ *n* : the amount of a toxic agent (as a poison, virus, or radiation) that is sufficient to kill 50 percent of a population of animals usu. within a certain time — called also *median lethal dose*
LDH *abbr* lactate dehydrogenase; lactic dehydrogenase
LDL \₁el-(₁)dē-'el\ *n* : a lipoprotein of blood plasma that is composed of a moderate proportion of protein with little triglyceride and a high proportion of cholesterol and that is associated with increased probability of developing atherosclerosis — called also *bad cholesterol, beta-lipoprotein, low-density lipoprotein*; compare HDL, VLDL
L–do·pa \'el-'dō-pə\ *n* : the levorotatory form of dopa that is obtained esp. from broad beans or prepared synthetically, is converted to dopamine in the brain, and is used in treating Parkinson's disease — called also *levodopa*; see SINEMET
LE *abbr* lupus erythematosus
¹lead \'lēd\ *n* : a flexible or solid insulated conductor connected to or leading out from an electrical device (as an electroencephalograph)
²lead \'led\ *n, often attrib* : a heavy soft malleable bluish white metallic element found mostly in combination and used esp. in pipes, cable sheaths, batteries, solder, type metal, and shields against radioactivity — symbol *Pb*; see ELEMENT table
lead acetate \'led-\ *n* : a poisonous soluble lead salt $PbC_4H_6O_4 \cdot 3H_2O$ used in medicine esp. formerly as an astringent

lead arsenate *n* : an arsenate of lead; *esp* : either of the two salts $PbHAsO_4$ and $Pb_3(AsO_4)_2$ formerly used as insecticides
lead carbonate *n* : a carbonate of lead; *esp* : a poisonous basic salt $Pb_3(OH)_2(CO_3)_2$ that was formerly used as a white pigment in paints
lead palsy *n* : localized paralysis caused by lead poisoning esp. of the extensor muscles of the forearm
lead poisoning *n* : chronic intoxication that is produced by the absorption of lead into the system and is characterized esp. by fatigue, abdominal pain, nausea, diarrhea, loss of appetite, anemia, a dark line along the gums, and muscular paralysis or weakness of limbs — called also *plumbism, saturnism*
leaf·let \'lē-flət\ *n* : a leaflike organ, structure, or part; *esp* : any of the flaps of the biscuspid valve or the tricuspid valve
learn·ing \'lər-niŋ\ *n* : the process of acquiring a modification in a behavioral tendency by experience (as exposure to conditioning); *also* : the modified behavioral tendency thus induced — **learn** \'lərn\ *vb*
learning disability *n* : any of various disorders (as dyslexia or dysgraphia) that interfere with an individual's ability to learn resulting in impaired functioning in verbal language, reasoning, or academic skills (as reading and mathematics) and are thought to be caused by difficulties in processing and integrating information — **learning disabled** *adj*
least splanchnic nerve \'lēst-\ *n* : SPLANCHNIC NERVE C
Le·boy·er \lə-bói-'ā\ *adj* : of or relating to a method of childbirth designed to reduce trauma for the newborn esp. by avoiding use of forceps and bright lights in the delivery room and by giving the newborn a warm bath
Leboyer, **Frédéric** (*b* **1918**), French obstetrician.
LE cell \₁el-'ē-₁sel\ *n* : a polymorphonuclear leukocyte that is found esp. in patients with lupus erythematosus — called also *lupus erythematosus cell*
lecith- *or* **lecitho-** *comb form* : yolk of an egg ⟨*lecith*al⟩ ⟨ovo*lecith*in⟩
lec·i·thal \'le-sə-thəl\ *adj* : having a yolk — often used in combination
lec·i·thin \'le-sə-thən\ *n* : any of several waxy hygroscopic phospholipids that are widely distributed in animals and plants, form colloidal solutions in water, and have emulsifying, wetting, and antioxidant properties; *also* : a mixture of or a substance rich in lecithins — called also *phosphatidylcholine*
lec·i·thin·ase \-thə-₁nās, -₁nāz\ *n* : PHOSPHOLIPASE
lec·tin \'lek-tin\ *n* : any of a group of proteins esp. of plants that are not an-

tibodies and do not originate in an immune system but bind specifically to carbohydrate-containing receptors on cell surfaces (as of red blood cells)

leech \'lēch\ *n* : any of numerous carnivorous or bloodsucking worms. freshwater annelid worms (class Hirudinea) that typically have a flattened segmented lance-shaped body with a sucker at each end — see MEDICINAL LEECH

LE factor \ˌel-'ē-\ *n* : an antibody found in the serum esp. of patients with systemic lupus erythematosus

Le-Fort \lə-'fôrt\ *n* **1** : a fracture of the maxilla and associated bones of the middle face region — used with the Roman numeral I to III to indicate type and severity; often used attributively ⟨*Lefort* III fractures involve complete separation of the maxilla and one or more facial bones from the skull⟩ **2** : an operation that involves reconstructing the middle face region by moving the maxilla and associated bones forward — used with the Roman numeral I to III to indicate type; often used attributively ⟨*LeFort* II osteotomy in which the maxilla and adjacent nasal bones are repositioned⟩

Le Fort, René (1869–1951), French surgeon.

left atrioventricular valve *n* : MITRAL VALVE

left colic flexure *n* : SPLENIC FLEXURE

left gastric artery *n* : GASTRIC ARTERY 1

left gastroepiploic artery *n* : GASTROEPIPLOIC ARTERY b

left–hand·ed \'left-'han-dəd\ *adj* **1** : using the left hand habitually or more easily than the right **2** : relating to, designed for, or done with the left hand **3** : having a direction contrary to that of movement of the hands of a watch viewed from in front **4** : LEVOROTATORY — **left–handed** *adv* — **left–hand·ed·ness** *n*

left heart *n* : the left atrium and ventricle : the half of the heart that receives oxygenated blood from the pulmonary circulation and passes it to the aorta

left lymphatic duct *n* : THORACIC DUCT

left pulmonary artery *n* : PULMONARY ARTERY c

left subcostal vein *n* : SUBCOSTAL VEIN b

leg \'leg\ *n* : a limb of an animal used esp. for supporting the body and for walking: as **a** : either of the two lower human limbs that extend from the top of the thigh to the foot and esp. the part between the knee and the ankle **b** : any of the rather generalized appendages of an arthropod used in walking and crawling — **leg·ged** \'legəd, 'legd\ *adj*

legal age *n* : the age at which a person enters into full adult legal rights and responsibilities

legal blindness *n* : blindness as recognized by law which in most states of the U.S. means that the better eye using the best possible methods of correction has visual acuity of 20/200 or worse or that the visual field is restricted to 20 degrees or less — **le·gal·ly blind** *adj*

legal medicine *n* : FORENSIC MEDICINE

Legg–Cal·vé–Per·thes disease \'legˌkal-'vā-'pər-ˌtēz-\ *n* : osteochondritis affecting the bony knob at the upper end of the femur — called also *Legg-Perthes disease, Perthes disease*

Legg, Arthur Thornton (1874–1939), American orthopedic surgeon.

Calvé, Jacques (1875–1954), French surgeon.

Perthes, Georg Clemens (1869–1927), German surgeon.

Legg–Perthes disease *n* : LEGG-CALVÉ-PERTHES DISEASE

le·gion·el·la \ˌlē-jə-'ne-lə\ *n* **1** *cap* : a genus of gram-negative rod-shaped bacteria (family Legionellaceae) that includes the causative agent (*L. pneumophila*) of Legionnaires' disease **2** *pl* **-lae** *also* **-las** : a bacterium of the genus *Legionella*

le·gion·el·lo·sis \ˌlē-jə-ˌne-'lō-səs\ *n* : LEGIONNAIRES' DISEASE

Le·gion·naires' bacillus \ˌlē-jə-'narz-\ *n* : a bacterium of the genus *Legionella* (*L. pneumophila*) that causes Legionnaires' disease

Legionnaires' disease *also* **Legionnaire's disease** *n* : pneumonia that is caused by a bacterium of the genus *Legionella* (*L. pneumophila*), that is characterized initially by symptoms resembling influenza (as malaise and muscular aches) followed by high fever, cough, diarrhea, lobar pneumonia, and mental confusion, and that may be fatal esp. in elderly and immunocompromised individuals — see PONTIAC FEVER

le·gume \'le-ˌgyüm, li-'gyüm\ *n* : any of a large family (Leguminosae) of plants having fruits that are dry pods and split when ripe and including important food and forage plants (as beans and clover); *also* : the fruit or seed of a legume used as food — **le·gu·mi·nous** \li-'gyü-mə-nəs, le-\ *adj*

leio- or **lio-** *comb form* : smooth ⟨*leio*myoma⟩

leio·myo·blas·to·ma \ˌlī-ō-ˌmī-ō-blas-'tō-mə\ *n, pl* **-mas** *also* **-ma·ta** \-mə-tə\ : LEIOMYOMA; *esp* : one resembling epithelium

leio·my·o·ma \ˌlī-ō-mī-'ō-mə\ *n, pl* **-mas** *also* **-ma·ta** \-mə-tə\ : a benign tumor (as a fibroid) consisting of smooth muscle fibers — **leio·my·o·ma·tous** \-mə-təs\ *adj*

leio·myo·sar·co·ma \ˌlī-ō-ˌmī-ō-sär-'kō-mə\ *n, pl* **-mas** *also* **-ma·ta** \-mə-tə\ : a sarcoma composed in part of smooth muscle cells

Leish·man–Don·o·van body \'lēsh-mən-'dä-nə-vən-\ *n* : a protozoan of the genus *Leishmania* (esp. *L. donovani*) in its nonmotile stage that is found esp. in cells of the skin, spleen, and liver of individuals affected with leishmaniasis and esp. kala-azar — compare DONOVAN BODY

Leishman, Sir William Boog (1865–1926), British bacteriologist.

Donovan, Charles (1863–1951), British surgeon.

leish·man·ia \lēsh-'ma-nē-ə, -'mä-\ *n* **1** *cap* : a genus of flagellate protozoans (family Trypanosomatidae) that are parasitic in the tissues of vertebrates, are transmitted by sand flies (genera *Phlebotomus* and *Lutzomyia*), and include one (*L. donovani*) causing kala-azar and another (*L. tropica*) causing oriental sore **2** : any protozoan of the genus *Leishmania*; *broadly* : a protozoan resembling the leishmanias that is included in the family (Trypanosomatidae) to which they belong — **leish·man·ial** \-nē-əl\ *adj*

leish·man·i·a·sis \lēsh-mə-'nī-ə-səs\ *n, pl* **-a·ses** \-ˌsēz\ : infection with or disease (as kala-azar or oriental sore) caused by leishmanias

lem·nis·cus \lem-'nis-kəs\ *n, pl* **-nis·ci** \-'nis-ˌkī, -ˌkē; -'ni-ˌsī\ : a band of fibers and esp. nerve fibers — called also *fillet*; see LATERAL LEMNISCUS, MEDIAL LEMNISCUS — **lem·nis·cal** \-'nis-kəl\ *adj*

len·i·tive \'le-nə-tiv\ *adj* : alleviating pain or harshness — **lenitive** *n*

Len·nox–Gas·taut syndrome \'le-nəks-gas-'tō-\ *n* : an epileptic syndrome esp. of young children that is marked by tonic, atonic, and myoclonic seizures and by atypical absence seizures and that is associated with impaired intellectual functioning and developmental delays

Lennox, William Gordon (1884–1960), American neurologist.

Gas·taut \gás-tō\, **Henri Jean-Pascal (1915–1995)**, French neurologist.

lens *also* **lense** \'lenz\ *n* **1** : a curved piece of glass or plastic used singly or combined in eyeglasses or an optical instrument (as a microscope) for forming an image; *also* : a device for focusing radiation other than light **2** : a highly transparent biconvex lens-shaped or nearly spherical body in the eye that focuses light rays entering the eye typically onto the retina and that lies immediately behind the pupil — **lensed** *adj* — **lens·less** *adj*

lens·om·e·ter \len-'zä-mə-tər\ *n* : an instrument used to determine the optical properties (as the focal length and axis) of ophthalmic lenses

Len·te insulin \'len-tā-\ *n* : INSULIN ZINC SUSPENSION

len·ti·co·nus \ˌlen-tə-'kō-nəs\ *n* : a rare abnormal and usu. congenital condition of the lens of the eye in which the surface is conical esp. on the posterior side

len·tic·u·lar \len-'ti-kyə-lər\ *adj* **1** : having the shape of a double-convex lens **2** : of or relating to a lens esp. of the eye **3** : relating to or being the lentiform nucleus of the brain

lenticular nucleus *n* : LENTIFORM NUCLEUS

lenticular process *n* : the tip of the long process of the incus which articulates with the stapes

lentiform nucleus *n* : the one of the four basal ganglia in each cerebral hemisphere that comprises the larger and external nucleus of the corpus striatum — called also *lenticular nucleus*

len·ti·go \len-'tī-(ˌ)gō, -'tē-\ *n, pl* **len·tig·i·nes** \len-'ti-jə-ˌnēz\ **1** : a small melanotic spot in the skin in which the formation of pigment is unrelated to exposure to sunlight and which is potentially malignant; *esp* : NEVUS — compare FRECKLE **2** : FRECKLE

lentigo ma·lig·na \-mə-'lig-nə\ *n* : a precancerous lesion on the skin esp. in areas exposed to the sun (as the face) that is flat, mottled, and brownish with an irregular outline and grows slowly over a period of years

lentigo se·nil·is \-sə-'ni-ləs\ *n* : AGE SPOTS

len·ti·vi·rus \'len-tə-ˌvī-rəs\ *n* **1** *cap* : a genus of retroviruses that include SIV and HIV **2** : any retrovirus of the genus *Lentivirus* — **len·ti·vi·ral** \-rəl\ *adj*

le·on·ti·a·sis os·sea \ˌlē-ən-'tī-ə-səs-'ä-sē-ə\ *n* : an overgrowth of the bones of the head producing enlargement and distortion of the face

lep·er \'le-pər\ *n* : an individual affected with leprosy

LE phenomenon \ˌel-'ē-\ *n* : the process which a white blood cell undergoes in becoming a lupus erythematosus cell

lep·ra \'le-prə\ *n* : LEPROSY

lep·re·chaun·ism \'le-prə-ˌkä-ˌni-zəm, -ˌkô-\ *n* : a rare inherited disorder characterized by mental and physical retardation, by endocrine disorders, by hirsutism, and esp. by a facies marked by large wide-set eyes and large low-set ears

lep·rol·o·gist \le-'prä-lə-jist\ *n* : a specialist in the study of leprosy and its treatment — **lep·rol·o·gy** \-jē\ *n*

lep·ro·ma \le-'prō-mə\ *n, pl* **-mas** *also* **-ma·ta** \-mə-tə\ : a nodular lesion of leprosy

le·pro·ma·tous \lə-'prä-mə-təs, -'prō-\ *adj* : of, relating to, characterized by, or affected with lepromas or lepromatous leprosy ⟨~ patients⟩

lepromatous leprosy *n* : the one of the two major forms of leprosy that is characterized by the formation of lepromas, the presence of numerous Hansen's bacilli in the lesions, and a negative skin reaction to lepromin and that remains infectious to others until treated — compare TUBERCULOID LEPROSY

lep·ro·min \le-'prō-mən\ *n* : an extract of human leprous tissue used in a skin test for leprosy infection

lep·ro·sar·i·um \ˌle-prə-'ser-ē-əm\ *n, pl* **-i·ums** *or* **-ia** \-ē-ə\ : a hospital for leprosy patients

lep·ro·stat·ic \ˌle-prə-'sta-tik\ *n* : an agent that inhibits the growth of Hansen's bacillus

lep·ro·sy \'le-prə-sē\ *n, pl* **-sies** : a chronic disease caused by infection with an acid-fast bacillus of the genus *Mycobacterium* (*M. leprae*) and characterized by the formation of nodules on the surface of the body and esp. on the face or by the appearance of tuberculoid macules on the skin that enlarge and spread and are accompanied by loss of sensation followed sooner or later in both types if not treated by involvement of nerves with eventual paralysis, wasting of muscle, and production of deformities and mutilations — called also *Hansen's disease, lepra*; see LEPROMATOUS LEPROSY, TUBERCULOID LEPROSY

lep·rot·ic \le-'prä-tik\ *adj* : of, caused by, or infected with leprosy

lep·rous \'le-prəs\ *adj* **1** : infected with leprosy **2** : of, relating to, or associated with leprosy or a leper

-lep·sy \ˌlep-sē\ *n comb form, pl* **-lep·sies** : taking : seizure ⟨narco*lepsy*⟩

lept- *or* **lepto-** *comb form* : small : weak : thin : fine ⟨*lepto*meninges⟩

lep·ta·zol \'lep-tə-ˌzōl, -ˌzōl\ *n, chiefly Brit* : PENTYLENETETRAZOL

lep·tin \'lep-tən\ *n* : a peptide hormone that is produced by fat cells and plays a role in body weight regulation by acting on the hypothalamus to suppress appetite and burn fat stored in adipose tissue

lep·to \'lep-ˌtō\ *n* : LEPTOSPIROSIS

lep·to·me·nin·ges \ˌlep-tō-mə-'nin-(ˌ)jēz\ *n pl* : the pia mater and the arachnoid considered together as investing the brain and spinal cord — called also *pia-arachnoid* — **lep·to·men·in·ge·al** \-ˌme-nən-'jē-əl\ *adj*

lep·to·men·in·gi·tis \-ˌme-nən-'jī-təs\ *n, pl* **-git·i·des** \-'ji-tə-ˌdēz\ : inflammation of the pia mater and the arachnoid membrane

lep·to·ne·ma \ˌlep-tə-'nē-mə\ *n* : a chromatin thread or chromosome at the leptotene stage of meiotic prophase

lep·to·phos \'lep-tō-ˌfäs\ *n* : an organophosphorus pesticide $C_{13}H_{10}BrCl_2O_2PS$ that has been associated with the occurrence of neurological damage in individuals exposed to it esp. in the early and mid 1970s

lep·to·spi·ra \ˌlep-tō-'spī-rə\ *n* **1** *cap* : a genus of extremely slender aerobic spirochetes (family Leptospiraceae) that are free-living or parasitic in

mammals and include a number of important pathogens (as *L. icterohaemorrhagiae* of Weil's disease or *L. canicola* of canicola fever) **2** *pl* **-ra** *or* **-ras** *or* **-rae** \-ˌrē\ : LEPTOSPIRE

lep·to·spire \'lep-tə-ˌspīr\ *n* : any spirochete of the genus *Leptospira* — called also *leptospira* — **lep·to·spi·ral** \ˌlep-tə-'spī-rəl\ *adj*

lep·to·spi·ro·sis \ˌlep-tə-spī-'rō-səs\ *n, pl* **-ro·ses** \-ˌsēz\ : any of several diseases of humans and domestic animals that are caused by infection with spirochetes of the genus *Leptospira* — called also *lepto*; see WEIL'S DISEASE

lep·to·tene \'lep-tə-ˌtēn\ *n* : a stage of meiotic prophase immediately preceding synapsis in which the chromosomes appear as fine discrete threads — **leptotene** *adj*

Le·riche's syndrome \lə-'rē-shəz-\ *n* : occlusion of the descending continuation of the aorta in the abdomen typically resulting in impotence, the absence of a pulse in the femoral arteries, and weakness and numbness in the lower back, buttocks, hips, thighs, and calves

Leriche, René (1879–1955), French surgeon.

¹les·bi·an \'lez-bē-ən\ *adj* : of or relating to homosexuality between females

²lesbian *n* : a female homosexual

les·bi·an·ism \'lez-bē-ə-ˌni-zəm\ *n* : female homosexuality

Lesch–Ny·han syndrome \'lesh-'nī-ən-\ *n* : a rare and usu. fatal genetic disorder of male children that is inherited as an X-linked recessive trait and is characterized by hyperuricemia, mental retardation, spasticity, compulsive biting of the lips and fingers, and a deficiency of hypoxanthine-guanine phosphoribosyltransferase — called also *Lesch-Nyhan disease*

Lesch, Michael (b 1939), and Nyhan, William Leo (b 1926), American pediatricians.

¹le·sion \'lē-zhən\ *n* : an abnormal change in structure of an organ or part due to injury or disease; *esp* : one that is circumscribed and well defined — **le·sioned** \-zhənd\ *adj*

²lesion *vb* : to produce lesions in

lesser cornu *n* : CERATOHYAL

lesser curvature *n* : the boundary of the stomach that in humans forms a relatively short concave curve on the right from the opening for the esophagus to the opening into the duodenum — compare GREATER CURVATURE

lesser multangular *n* : TRAPEZOID — called also *lesser multangular bone*

lesser occipital nerve *n* : OCCIPITAL NERVE b

lesser omentum *n* : a part of the peritoneum attached to the liver and to the lesser curvature of the stomach and supporting the hepatic vessels — compare GREATER OMENTUM

lesser petrosal nerve *n* : the continuation of the tympanic nerve beyond the inferior ganglion of the glossopharyngeal nerve that terminates in the otic ganglion which it supplies with preganglionic parasympathetic fibers

lesser sciatic foramen *n* : SCIATIC FORAMEN b

lesser sciatic notch *n* : SCIATIC NOTCH b

lesser splanchnic nerve *n* : SPLANCHNIC NERVE b

lesser trochanter *n* : TROCHANTER b

lesser tubercle *n* : a prominence on the upper anterior part of the end of the humerus that serves as the insertion for the subscapularis — compare GREATER TUBERCLE

lesser wing *n* : an anterior triangular process on each side of the sphenoid bone in front of and much smaller than the corresponding greater wing

let-down \'let-ˌdau̇n\ *n* : a physiological response of a lactating mammal to suckling and allied stimuli whereby increased intramammary pressure forces previously secreted milk from the acini and finer tubules into larger ducts from where it can be drawn through the nipple

let down *vb* : to release (formed milk) within the mammary gland or udder

¹**le·thal** \'lē-thəl\ *adj* : of, relating to, or causing death ⟨a ~ injury⟩; *also* : capable of causing death ⟨~ chemicals⟩ ⟨a ~ dose⟩ — **le·thal·i·ty** \lē-'tha-lə-tē\ *n* — **le·thal·ly** *adv*

²**lethal** *n* 1 : an abnormality of genetic origin causing the death of the organism possessing it usu. before maturity **2** : LETHAL GENE

lethal gene *n* : a gene that in some (as homozygous) conditions may prevent development or cause the death of an organism or its germ cells — called also *lethal factor, lethal mutant, lethal mutation*

lethargica — see ENCEPHALITIS LETHARGICA

leth·ar·gy \'le-thər-jē\ *n, pl* **-gies 1** : abnormal drowsiness **2** : the quality or state of being lazy, sluggish, or indifferent — **lethargic** *adj*

let·ro·zole \'le-trə-ˌzōl\ *n* : a nonsteroidal aromatase inhibitor $C_{17}H_{11}N_5$ that is administered orally to treat breast cancer in postmenopausal women — see FEMARA

Let·ter·er–Si·we disease \'le-tər-ər-'sē-və-\ *n* : an acute often fatal disease of young children that is marked by proliferation of Langerhans cells and is characterized esp. by fever, anemia, hepatosplenomegaly, and a eczematous skin rash

Letterer, Erich (1895–1982), German physician.

Siwe, Sture August (1897–1966), Swedish pediatrician.

Leu *abbr* leucine

leuc- or **leuco-** *chiefly Brit var of* LEUK-

leu·cine \'lü-ˌsēn\ *n* : a white crystalline essential amino acid $C_6H_{13}NO_2$ obtained by the hydrolysis of most dietary proteins — abbr. *Leu*

leucine aminopeptidase *n* : an aminopeptidase that is found in all bodily tissues and is increased in the serum in some conditions or diseases (as pancreatic carcinoma)

leucine–en·keph·a·lin \-en-'kef-ə-lən\ *n* : a pentapeptide having a terminal leucine residue that is one of the two enkephalins occurring naturally in the brain — called also *Leu= enkephalin*

leu·ci·no·sis \ˌlü-sə-'nō-səs\ *n, pl* **-no·ses** \-ˌsēz\ *or* **-no·sis·es** : a condition characterized by an abnormally high concentration of leucine in bodily tissues and the presence of leucine in the urine

leucocyt- or **leucocyto-** *chiefly Brit var of* LEUKOCYT-

leu·co·cy·to·zo·on \ˌlü-kō-ˌsī-tə-'zō-ˌän, -ən\ *n* **1** *cap* : a genus of sporozoans parasitic in birds **2** *pl* **-zoa** \-'zō-ə\ : any sporozoan of the genus *Leucocytozoon*

leu·co·cy·to·zoo·no·sis \-ˌzō-ə-'nō-səs\ *n, pl* **-no·ses** \-ˌsēz\ : a disease of birds caused by infection with sporozoans of the genus *Leucocytozoon*

leu·cov·o·rin \lü-'kä-və-rin\ *n* : a metabolically active form of folic acid that has been used in cancer therapy to protect normal cells against methotrexate — called also *citrovorum factor, folinic acid*

Leu–en·keph·a·lin \ˌlü-en-'ke-fə-lin\ *n* : LEUCINE-ENKEPHALIN

leuk- or **leuko-** *comb form* **1** : white : colorless : weakly colored ⟨*leuko*cyte⟩ ⟨*leuko*rrhea⟩ **2** : leukocyte ⟨*leuk*emia⟩ **3** : white matter of the brain ⟨*leuko*encephalopathy⟩

leu·kae·mia, leu·kae·mic *chiefly Brit var of* LEUKEMIA, LEUKEMIC

leu·ka·phe·re·sis \ˌlü-kə-fə-'rē-səs\ *n, pl* **-phe·re·ses** \-ˌsēz\ : apheresis used to remove white blood cells (as in the treatment of chronic lymphocytic leukemia) — called also *leukopheresis*

leu·ke·mia \lü-'kē-mē-ə\ *n* : an acute or chronic disease characterized by an abnormal increase in the number of white blood cells in bodily tissues with or without a corresponding increase of those in the circulating blood — see ACUTE LYMPHOBLASTIC LEUKEMIA, ACUTE MYELOGENOUS LEUKEMIA, CHRONIC LYMPHOCYTIC LEUKEMIA, CHRONIC MYELOGENOUS LEUKEMIA, FELINE LEUKEMIA, LYMPHOBLASTIC LEUKEMIA, LYMPHOCYTIC LEUKEMIA, MONOCYTIC LEUKEMIA, MYELOGENOUS LEUKEMIA, PROMYELOCYTIC LEUKEMIA

¹**leu·ke·mic** \lü-'kē-mik\ *adj* **1** : of, relating to, or affected by leukemia **2**

: characterized by an increase in white blood cells ⟨∼ blood⟩

²**leukemic** *n* : a person affected with leukemia

leu·ke·mo·gen·e·sis \ˌlü-ˌkē-mə-ˈje-nə-səs\, *n, pl* **-e·ses** \-ˌsēz\ : induction or production of leukemia — **leu·ke·mo·gen·ic** \-ˈjen-ik\ *adj*

leu·ke·moid \lü-ˈkē-ˌmȯid\ *adj* : resembling leukemia

leuko- — see LEUK-

leu·ko·ag·glu·ti·nin \ˌlü-kə-ə-ˈglüt-ᵊn-ən\ *n* : an antibody that agglutinates leukocytes — compare HEMAGGLUTININ

leukocyt- *or* **leukocyto-** *comb form* : leukocyte ⟨*leukocyto*sis⟩

leu·ko·cyte \ˈlü-kə-ˌsīt\ *n* **1** : WHITE BLOOD CELL **2** : a cell (as a macrophage) of the tissues comparable to or derived from a leukocyte

leu·ko·cyt·ic \ˌlü-kə-ˈsi-tik\ *adj* **1** : of, relating to, or involving leukocytes **2** : characterized by an excess of leukocytes

leu·ko·cy·to·sis \ˌlü-kə-sī-ˈtō-səs, -kə-sə-\ *n, pl* **-to·ses** \-ˌsēz\ : an increase in the number of white blood cells in the circulating blood that occurs normally (as after meals) or abnormally (as in some infections) — **leu·ko·cy·tot·ic** \-ˈtä-tik\ *adj*

leu·ko·der·ma \ˌlü-kə-ˈdər-mə\ *n* : partial or total loss or absence of pigmentation that is marked esp. by white patches of skin — see VITILIGO

leu·ko·dys·tro·phy \ˌlü-kō-ˈdis-trə-fē\ *n, pl* **-phies** : any of several inherited diseases characterized by progressive degeneration of myelin in the brain, spinal cord, and peripheral nerves

leu·ko·en·ceph·a·lop·a·thy \ˌin-ˌse-fə-ˈlä-pə-thē\ *n, pl* **-thies** : any of various diseases affecting the brain's white matter; *esp* : PROGRESSIVE MULTIFOCAL LEUKOENCEPHALOPATHY

leuk·onych·ia \ˌlü-kō-ˈni-kē-ə\ *n* : a white spotting, streaking, or discoloration of the fingernails caused by injury or ill health

leu·ko·pe·nia \ˌlü-kō-ˈpē-nē-ə\ *n* : a condition in which the number of white blood cells circulating in the blood is abnormally low and which is most commonly due to a decreased production of new cells in conjunction with various infectious diseases, as a reaction to various drugs or other chemicals, or in response to irradiation — **leu·ko·pe·nic** \-ˈpē-nik\ *adj*

leu·ko·phe·re·sis \-fə-ˈrē-səs\ *n, pl* **-re·ses** \-ˌsēz\ : LEUKAPHERESIS

leu·ko·pla·kia \ˌlü-kō-ˈplā-kē-ə\ *n* : a condition commonly considered precancerous in which thickened white patches of epithelium occur on the mucous membranes esp. of the mouth, vulva, and renal pelvis; *also* : a lesion or lesioned area of leukoplakia — **leu·ko·pla·kic** \-ˈplā-kik\ *adj*

leu·ko·poi·e·sis \-ˌpȯi-ˈē-səs\ *n, pl* **-e·ses** \-ˌsēz\ : the formation of white blood cells — **leu·ko·poi·et·ic** \-ˈe-tik\ *adj*

leu·kor·rhea \ˌlü-kə-ˈrē-ə\ *n* : a white, yellowish, or greenish white viscid discharge from the vagina resulting from inflammation or congestion of the uterine or vaginal mucous membrane — **leu·kor·rhe·al** \-ˈrē-əl\ *adj*

leu·ko·sar·co·ma \ˌlü-kō-sär-ˈkō-mə\ *n, pl* **-mas** *also* **-ma·ta** \-mə-tə\ : lymphosarcoma accompanied by leukemia — **leu·ko·sar·co·ma·to·sis** \-ˌsär-ˌkō-mə-ˈtō-səs\ *n*

leu·ko·sis \lü-ˈkō-səs\ *n, pl* **-ko·ses** \-ˌsēz\ : LEUKEMIA; *esp* : any of various leukemic diseases of poultry — **leu·kot·ic** \-ˈkä-tik\ *adj*

leu·ko·tac·tic \ˌlü-kō-ˈtak-tik\ *adj* : tending to attract leukocytes

leu·ko·tome \ˈlü-kə-ˌtōm\ *n* : a cannula through which a wire is inserted and used to cut the white matter in the brain in lobotomy

leu·kot·o·my \lü-ˈkä-tə-mē\ *n, pl* **-mies** : LOBOTOMY

leu·ko·tox·in \ˌlü-kə-ˈtäk-sən\ *n* : a substance specif. destructive to leukocytes

leu·ko·tri·ene \ˌlü-kə-ˈtrī-ˌēn\ *n* : any of a group of eicosanoids that are generated in basophils, mast cells, macrophages, and human lung tissue by lipoxygenase-catalyzed oxygenation esp. of arachidonic acid and that participate in allergic responses (as bronchoconstriction in asthma) — see SLOW-REACTING SUBSTANCE OF ANAPHYLAXIS

leu·pro·lide \lü-ˈprō-ˌlīd\ *n* : a synthetic analog of gonadotropin-releasing hormone used in the form of its acetate $C_{59}H_{84}N_{16}O_{12} \cdot C_2H_4O_2$ to treat cancer of the prostate gland — see LUPRON

leu·ro·cris·tine \ˌlùr-ō-ˈkris-ˌtēn\ *n* : VINCRISTINE

lev- *or* **levo-** *comb form* : left : on the left side : to the left ⟨*levo*cardia⟩

lev·al·lor·phan \ˌle-və-ˈlȯr-ˌfan, -fən\ *n* : a drug $C_{19}H_{25}NO$ related to morphine that is used to counteract morphine poisoning

le·vam·i·sole \lə-ˈva-mə-ˌsōl\ *n* : an anthelmintic drug administered in the form of its hydrochloride $C_{11}H_{12}$-$N_2S \cdot HCl$ that also possesses immunostimulant properties and is used esp. in the treatment of colon cancer

Le·vant storax \lə-ˈvant-\ *n* : STORAX 1

Le·va·quin \ˈle-və-kwən\ *trademark* — used for a preparation of levofloxacin

lev·ar·ter·e·nol \ˌle-vär-ˈtir-ə-ˌnȯl, -ˌter-, -ˌnȯl\ *n* : levorotatory norepinephrine

le·va·tor \li-ˈvā-tər\ *n, pl* **lev·a·to·res** \ˌle-və-ˈtōr-(ˌ)ēz\ *or* **le·va·tors** \li-ˈvā-tərz\ : a muscle that serves to raise a body part — compare DEPRESSOR a

levator an·gu·li oris \-ˈaŋ-gyə-ˌlī-ˈȯr-əs\ *n* : a facial muscle that arises from the maxilla, inclines downward to be inserted into the corner of the mouth, and draws the lips up and back — called also *caninus*

le·va·tor ani \-ˈā-ˌnī\ *n* : a broad thin muscle that is attached in a sheet to each side of the inner surface of the pelvis and descends to form the floor of the pelvic cavity where it supports the viscera and surrounds structures which pass through it and inserts into the sides of the apex of the coccyx, the margins of the anus, the side of the rectum, and the central tendinous point of the perineum — see ILIO-COCCYGEUS, PUBOCOCCYGEUS

le·va·to·res cos·tar·um \-ˌkäs-ˈtär-əm, -ˈtär-\ *n pl* : a series of 12 muscles on each side that arise from the transverse processes of the seventh cervical and upper 11 thoracic vertebrae, that insert into the ribs, and that raise the ribs increasing the volume of the thoracic cavity and extend, bend, and rotate the spinal column

le·va·tor la·bii su·pe·ri·or·is \-ˈlā-bē-ˌī-sù-ˌpir-ē-ˈór-əs\ *n* : a facial muscle arising from the lower margin of the orbit and inserting into the muscular substance of the upper lip which it elevates — called also *quadratus labii superioris*

levator labii superioris alae·que na·si \-ā-ˈlē-kwē-ˈnā-ˌzī\ *n* : a muscle that arises from the nasal process of the maxilla, that passes downward and laterally, that divides into a part inserting into the alar cartilage and one inserting into the upper lip, and that dilates the nostril and raises the upper lip

levator pal·pe·brae su·pe·ri·or·is \-ˌpal-ˈpē-ˌbrē-sù-ˌpir-ē-ˈór-əs\ *n* : a thin flat extrinsic muscle of the eye arising from the lesser wing of the sphenoid bone and inserting into the tarsal plate of the skin of the upper eyelid which it raises

levator pros·ta·tae \-ˈpräs-tə-ˌtē\ *n* : a part of the pubococcygeus comprising the more medial and ventral fasciculi that insert into the tissue in front of the anus and serve to support and elevate the prostate gland

levator scap·u·lae \-ˈska-pyə-ˌlē\ *n* : a back muscle that arises in the transverse processes of the first four cervical vertebrae and descends to insert into the vertebral border of the scapula which it elevates

levator ve·li pal·a·ti·ni \-ˈvē-ˌlī-ˌpa-lə-ˈtī-ˌnī\ *n* : a muscle arising from the temporal bone and the cartilage of the eustachian tube and descending to insert into the midline of the soft palate which it elevates esp. to close the nasopharynx while swallowing is taking place

Le·Veen shunt \lə-ˈvēn-ˈshənt\ *n* : a plastic tube that passes from the jugular vein to the peritoneal cavity where a valve permits absorption of ascitic fluid which is carried back to venous circulation by way of the superior vena cava

LeVeen, Harry Henry (1914–1996), American surgeon.

Le·vin tube \lə-ˈvēn-, lə-ˈvin-\ *n* : a tube designed to be passed into the stomach or duodenum through the nose

Levin, Abraham Louis (1880–1940), American physician.

Le·vi·tra \lə-ˈvē-trə\ *trademark* — used for a preparation of the hydrated hydrochloride of vardenafil

le·vo \ˈlē-(ˌ)vō\ *adj* : LEVOROTATORY

levo- — see LEV-

le·vo·car·dia \ˌlē-və-ˈkär-dē-ə\ *n* : normal position of the heart when associated with situs inversus of other abdominal viscera and usu. with structural defects of the heart itself

le·vo·di·hy·droxy·phe·nyl·al·a·nine \ˌlē-vō-ˌdī-hī-ˌdräk-sē-ˌfen-ᵊl-ˈa-lə-ˌnēn, -ˌfēn-\ *n* : L-DOPA

le·vo·do·pa \ˌlē-və-ˈdō-pə, ˌlē-və-ˈdō-pə\ *n* : L-DOPA

Le·vo–Dro·mo·ran \ˌlē-vō-ˈdrō-mə-ˌran\ *trademark* — used for a preparation of levorphanol

le·vo·flox·a·cin \ˌlē-və-ˈfläk-sə-sən\ *n* : a broad-spectrum antibacterial agent that is the levorotatory isomer of ofloxacin — see LEVAQUIN

le·vo·nor·ges·trel \ˌlē-və-nór-ˈjes-trəl\ *n* : the levorotatory form of norgestrel used in birth control pills and contraceptive implants — see NORPLANT

Levo·phed \ˈle-və-ˌfed\ *trademark* — used for a preparation of norepinephrine

Le·vo·prome \ˈlē-və-ˌprōm\ *trademark* — used for a preparation of methotrimeprazine

le·vo·pro·poxy·phene \ˌlē-və-prō-ˈpäk-si-ˌfēn\ *n* : a drug used esp. in the form of the napsylate $C_{22}H_{29}NO_2 \cdot C_{10}H_8SO_3$ as an antitussive

le·vo·ro·ta·to·ry \ˌlē-rō-tə-ˌtōr-ē\ *or* **le·vo·ro·ta·ry** \-ˈrō-tə-rē\ *adj* : turning toward the left or counterclockwise; *esp* : rotating the plane of polarization of light to the left — compare DEXTROROTATORY

lev·or·pha·nol \ˌle-ˈvór-fə-ˌnól\ *n* : an addictive drug used esp. in the form of its hydrated tartrate $C_{17}H_{23}NO \cdot C_4H_6O_6 \cdot 2H_2O$ as a potent analgesic with properties similar to morphine — see LEVO-DROMORAN

Le·vo·throid \ˈlē-və-ˌthrȯid\ *trademark* — used for a preparation of the sodium salt of levothyroxine

le·vo·thy·rox·ine \ˌlē-vō-thī-ˈräk-ˌsēn, -sən\ *n* : the levorotatory isomer of thyroxine that is administered in the form of its sodium salt $C_{15}H_{10}I_4N\text{-}NaO_4$ in the treatment of hypothyroidism — see LEVOTHROID, LEVOXYL, SYNTHROID

Le·vox·yl \lə-ˈväk-səl\ *trademark* — used for a preparation of the sodium salt of levothyroxine

lev·u·lose \'le-vyə-ˌlōs, -ˌlōz\ *n* : FRUCTOSE 2

lev·u·los·uria \ˌle-vyə-lō-'syúr-ē-ə, -'shúr-\ *n* : the presence of fructose in the urine

Lew·is blood group \'lü-əs-\ *n* : any of a system of blood groups controlled by a pair of dominant-recessive alleles and characterized by antigens which are adsorbed onto the surface of red blood cells and tend to interreact with the antigens produced by secretors although they are genetically independent of them

Lewis, H. D. G., British hospital patient.

lew·is·ite \'lü-ə-ˌsīt\ *n* : a colorless or brown vesicant liquid $C_2H_2AsCl_3$ developed as a poison gas for war use

Lewis, Winford Lee (1878–1943), American chemist.

Lewy body \'lü-ē-, 'lā-vē-\ *n* : an eosinophilic inclusion body found in the cytoplasm of neurons of the cortex and brain stem in Parkinson's disease and some forms of dementia

Lew·ey \'lü-ē\ **Frederic Henry** (*orig.* **Friedrich Heinrich Lewy**) (1885–1950), American neurologist.

Lex·a·pro \'lek-sə-ˌprō\ *trademark* — used for a preparation of the oxalate of escitalopram

-lex·ia \'lek-sē-ə\ *n comb form* : reading of (such) a kind or with (such) an impairment ⟨dys*lexia*⟩

Ley·dig cell \'lī-dig-\ *also* **Ley·dig's cell** \-digz-\ *n* : a cell of interstitial tissue of the testis that is usu. considered the chief source of testicular androgens and esp. testosterone — called also *cell of Leydig, interstitial cell of Leydig*

Leydig, Franz von (1821–1908), German anatomist.

L-form \'el-ˌfórm\ *n* : a variant form of some bacteria that usu. lacks a cell wall — called also *L-phase*

LGL syndrome \ˌel-ˌjē-'el-\ *n* : LOWN-GANONG-LEVINE SYNDROME

LH *abbr* luteinizing hormone

LHRH *abbr* luteinizing hormone-releasing hormone

Li *symbol* lithium

lib — see AD LIB

li·bi·do \lə-'bē-(ˌ)dō, -'bī-, 'li-bə-ˌdō\ *n, pl* **-dos** 1 : instinctual psychic energy that in psychoanalytic theory is derived from primitive biological urges (as for sexual pleasure or self-preservation) and is expressed in conscious activity 2 : sexual drive — **li·bid·i·nal** \lə-'bid-ᵊn-əl\ *adj*

libitum — see AD LIBITUM

Lib·man–Sacks endocarditis \'lib-mən-'saks-\ *n* : a noninfectious form of verrucous endocarditis associated with systemic lupus erythematosus — called also *Libman-Sacks disease, Libman-Sacks syndrome*

Libman, Emanuel (1872–1946), and **Sacks, Benjamin** (1896–1939), American physicians.

li·brary \'lī-ˌbrer-ē\ *n, pl* **-brar·ies** : a collection of cloned DNA fragments that are maintained in a suitable cellular environment and that represent the genetic material of a particular organism or tissue

Lib·ri·um \'li-brē-əm\ *trademark* — used for a preparation of the hydrochloride of chlordiazepoxide

lice *pl of* LOUSE

licensed practical nurse *n* : a person who has undergone training and obtained a license (as from a state) to provide routine care for the sick — called also *LPN*

licensed vocational nurse *n* : a licensed practical nurse authorized by license to practice in the states of California or Texas — called also *LVN*

li·cen·sure \'lī-sᵊn-shər\ *n* : the state or condition of having a license granted by official or legal authority to perform medical acts and procedures not permitted by persons without such a license ⟨RN ∼⟩; *also* : the granting of such licenses

li·chen \'lī-kən\ *n* 1 : any of several skin diseases characterized by the eruption of flat papules; *esp* : LICHEN PLANUS 2 : any of numerous complex plantlike organisms made up of an alga and a fungus growing in symbiotic association

li·chen·i·fi·ca·tion \lī-ˌke-nə-fə-'kā-shən, ˌlī-kə-\ *n* : the process by which skin becomes hardened and leathery or lichenoid usu. as a result of chronic irritation; *also* : a patch of skin so modified — **li·chen·i·fied** \lī-'ke-nə-ˌfīd, 'lī-kə-\ *adj*

li·chen·oid \'lī-kə-ˌnóid\ *adj* : resembling lichen ⟨a ∼ eruption⟩

lichenoides — see PITYRIASIS LICHENOIDES ET VARIOLIFORMIS ACUTA

lichen pla·nus \-'plā-nəs\ *n* : a skin disease characterized by an eruption of wide flat papules covered by a horny glazed film, marked by intense itching, and often accompanied by lesions on the oral mucosa

lichen scle·ro·sus et atro·phi·cus \-ˌsklə-'rō-səs-et-ˌā-'trō-fi-kəs\ *n* : a chronic skin disease that is characterized by the eruption of flat white hardened papules with central hair follicles often having black keratotic plugs

lichen sim·plex chron·i·cus \-'sim-ˌpleks-'krä-ni-kəs\ *n* : NEURODERMATITIS; *specif* : neurodermatitis marked by raised scaly patches of thickened leathery skin

lic·o·rice \'li-kə-rish, -ris\ *n* : GLYCYRRHIZA

licorice root *n* : GLYCYRRHIZA

lid \'lid\ *n* : EYELID

li·do·caine \'lī-də-ˌkān\ *n* : a crystalline compound $C_{14}H_{22}N_2O$ used as a local anesthetic often in the form of its hydrochloride $C_{14}H_{22}N_2O \cdot HCl$ — called also *lignocaine*; see XYLOCAINE

Lie·ber·mann–Bur·chard test \ˈlē-bər-mən-ˈbu̇r-ˌkärt-\ *n* : a test for unsaturated steroids (as cholesterol) and for terpenes having the formula $C_{30}H_{48}$ — called also *Liebermann-Burchard reaction*

Liebermann, Carl Theodore (1842–1914), German chemist. H. Burchard may have been one of his many student-research assistants.

lie detector \ˈlī-di-ˌtek-tər\ *n* : a polygraph for detecting physiological evidence (as changes in heart rate) of the tension that accompanies lying

li·en \ˈlī-ən, ˈlī-ˌen\ *n* : SPLEEN — **li·en·al** \-ᵊl\ *adj*

lienal vein *n* : SPLENIC VEIN

life \ˈlīf\ *n, pl* **lives** \ˈlīvz\ **1 a** : the quality that distinguishes a vital and functional plant or animal from a dead body **b** : a state of living characterized by capacity for metabolism, growth, reaction to stimuli, and reproduction **2 a** : the sequence of physical and mental experiences that make up the existence of an individual **b** : a specific part or aspect of the process of living ⟨sex ∼⟩ ⟨adult ∼⟩ — **life·less** \ˈlīf-ləs\ *adj*

life cycle *n* : the series of stages in form and functional activity through which an organism passes between successive recurrences of a specified primary stage

life expectancy *n* : an expected number of years of life based on statistical probability

¹life-sav·ing \ˈlīf-ˌsā-viŋ\ *adj* : designed for or used in saving lives ⟨∼ drugs⟩

²lifesaving *n* : the skill or practice of saving or protecting the lives esp. of drowning persons

life science *n* : a branch of science (as biology or medicine) that deals with living organisms and life processes — usu. used in pl. — **life scientist** *n*

life space *n* : the physical and psychological environment of an individual or group

life span \ˈlīf-ˌspan\ *n* **1** : the duration of existence of an individual **2** : the average length of life of a kind of organism or of a material object

life–sup·port \ˈlīf-sə-ˌpȯrt\ *adj* : providing support necessary to sustain life; *esp* : of, relating to, or being a life-support system ⟨∼ equipment⟩

life support *n* : equipment, material, and treatment needed to keep a seriously ill or injured patient alive ⟨the patient was placed on *life support*⟩

life–support system *n* : a system that provides all or some of the items (as oxygen, food, water, and disposition of carbon dioxide and body wastes) necessary for maintaining life or health

Li–Frau·me·ni syndrome \ˈlē-frau̇-ˈmē-nē-\ *n* : a rare familial syndrome that is characterized esp. by a high risk of developing early breast cancer and sarcomas of soft tissue

Li, Frederick P. (*b* 1940), and **Fraumeni, Joseph F., Jr.** (*b* 1933), American epidemiologists.

lift \ˈlift\ *n* **1** : FACE-LIFT **2** : BREAST LIFT — **lift** *vb*

lig·a·ment \ˈli-gə-mənt\ *n* **1** : a tough band of tissue that serves to connect the articular extremities of bones or to support or retain an organ in place and is usu. composed of coarse bundles of dense white fibrous tissue parallel or closely interlaced, pliant, and flexible, but not extensible **2** : any of various folds or bands of pleura, peritoneum, or mesentery connecting parts or organs

ligament of the ovary *n* : a rounded cord of fibrous and muscular tissue extending from each superior angle of the uterus to the inner extremity of the ovary of the same side — called also *ovarian ligament*; see SUSPENSORY LIGAMENT OF THE OVARY

ligament of Treitz \-ˈtrīts\ *n* : a band of smooth muscle extending from the junction of the duodenum and jejunum to the left crus of the diaphragm and functioning as a suspensory ligament

Treitz, Wenzel (1819–1872), Austrian physician.

ligament of Zinn \-ˈzin, -ˈtsin\ *n* : the common tendon of the inferior rectus and the internal rectus muscles of the eye — called also *tendon of Zinn*

Zinn, Johann Gottfried (1727–1759), German anatomist and botanist.

lig·a·men·tous \ˌli-gə-ˈmen-təs\ *adj* **1** : of or relating to a ligament **2** : forming or formed of a ligament

lig·a·men·tum \ˌli-gə-ˈmen-təm\ *n, pl* **-ta** \-tə\ : LIGAMENT

ligamentum ar·te·rio·sum \-är-ˌtir-ē-ˈō-səm\ *n* : a cord of tissue that connects the pulmonary trunk and the aorta and that is the vestige of the ductus arteriosus

ligamentum fla·vum \-ˈflā-vəm\ *n, pl* **ligamenta fla·va** \-və\ : any of a series of ligaments of yellow elastic tissue connecting the laminae of adjacent vertebrae from the axis to the sacrum

ligamentum nu·chae \-ˈnü-ˌkē, -ˈnyü-, -ˌkī\ *n, pl* **ligamenta nuchae** : a medium ligament of the back of the neck that is rudimentary in humans but highly developed and composed of yellow elastic tissue in many quadrupeds where it assists in supporting the head

ligamentum te·res \-ˈtē-ˌrēz\ *n* : ROUND LIGAMENT; *esp* : ROUND LIGAMENT 1

ligamentum ve·no·sum \-vē-ˈnō-səm\ *n* : a cord of tissue connected to the liver that is the vestige of the ductus venosus

li·gase \ˈlī-ˌgās, -ˌgāz\ *n* : SYNTHETASE

li·ga·tion \lī-ˈgā-shən\ *n* **1 a** : the surgical process of tying up an anatomical channel (as a blood vessel) **b** : the process of joining together chemical chains (as of DNA or protein) **2** : something that binds : LIGATURE —

lig·a·ture \'lig-ə-ˌchu̇r, -chər, -ˌtyu̇r\ *n* **1** : something that is used to bind; *specif* : a filament (as a thread) used in surgery (as for tying blood vessels) **2** : the action or result of binding or tying — **ligature** *vb*

¹**light** \'līt\ *n* **1 a** : the sensation aroused by stimulation of the visual receptors **b** : an electromagnetic radiation in the wavelength range including infrared, visible, ultraviolet, and X-rays and traveling in a vacuum with a speed of about 186,281 miles (300,000 kilometers) per second; *specif* : the part of this range that is visible to the human eye **2** : a source of light

²**light** *or* **lite** *adj* : made with a lower calorie content or with less of some ingredient (as salt, fat, or alcohol) than usual ⟨∼ salad dressing⟩

light adaptation *n* : the adjustments including narrowing of the pupillary opening and decrease in rhodopsin by which the retina of the eye is made efficient as a visual receptor under conditions of strong illumination — compare DARK ADAPTATION — **light–adapt·ed** \'līt-ə-ˌdap-təd\ *adj*

light chain *n* : either of the two smaller of the four polypeptide chains that are subunits of antibodies — called also *L chain;* compare HEAVY CHAIN

light·en·ing \'līt-ᵊn-iŋ\ *n* : a sense of decreased weight and abdominal tension felt by a pregnant woman on descent of the fetus into the pelvic cavity prior to labor

light–head·ed·ness \'līt-'he-dəd-nəs\ *n* : the condition of being dizzy or on the verge of fainting — **light–head·ed** *adj*

light microscope *n* : an ordinary microscope that uses light as distinguished from an electron microscope — **light microscopy** *n*

light·ning pains \'līt-niŋ-\ *n pl* : intense shooting or lancinating pains occurring in tabes dorsalis

light therapy *n* : PHOTOTHERAPY; *esp* : the use of strong light for the treatment of depression (as in seasonal affective disorder) — called also *light treatment*

lig·nan \'lig-ˌnan\ *n* : any of a class of dimeric compounds including many found in plants and noted for having antioxidant and estrogenic activity

lig·no·caine \'lig-nə-ˌkān\ *n, Brit* : LIDOCAINE

limb \'lim\ *n* **1** : one of the projecting paired appendages of an animal body concerned esp. with movement and grasping; *esp* : a human leg or arm **2** : a branch or arm of something (as an anatomical part)

lim·bal \'lim-bəl\ *adj* : of or relating to the limbus ⟨a ∼ incision⟩

limb bud *n* : a proliferation of embryonic tissue shaped like a mound from which a limb develops

lim·ber·neck \'lim-bər-ˌnek\ *n* : a botulism of birds (esp. poultry) characterized by paralysis of the neck muscles and pharynx

lim·bic \'lim-bik\ *adj* : of, relating to, or being the limbic system of the brain

limbic lobe *n* : the marginal medial portion of the cortex of a cerebral hemisphere

limbic system *n* : a group of subcortical structures (as the hypothalamus, the hippocampus, and the amygdala) of the brain that are concerned esp. with emotion and motivation

lim·bus \'lim-bəs\ *n* : a border distinguished by color or structure; *esp* : the marginal region of the cornea of the eye by which it is continuous with the sclera

lime \'līm\ *n* : a caustic powdery white solid that consists of the oxide of calcium often together with magnesia

li·men \'lī-mən\ *n* : THRESHOLD

lim·i·nal \'li-mə-nəl\ *adj* **1** : of or relating to a sensory threshold **2** : barely perceptible

limp \'limp\ *vb* **1** : to walk lamely; : to walk favoring one leg **2** : to go unsteadily — **limp** *n*

Lin·co·cin \liŋ-'kō-sən\ *trademark* — used for a preparation of the hydrated hydrochloride of lincomycin

lin·co·my·cin \ˌliŋ-kə-'mīs-ᵊn\ *n* : an antibiotic effective esp. against gram-positive bacteria that is obtained from an actinomycete of the genus *Streptomyces* (*S. lincolnensis*) and is used in the form of its hydrated hydrochloride $C_{18}H_{34}N_2O_6S \cdot HCl \cdot H_2O$

linc·tus \'liŋk-təs\ *n, pl* **linc·tus·es** : a syrupy or sticky medicated preparation exerting a local action on the mucous membrane of the throat

lin·dane \'lin-ˌdān\ *n* : an insecticide consisting of not less than 99 percent gamma benzene hexachloride that is biodegraded very slowly

Lin·dau's disease \'lin-ˌdau̇z-\ *n* : VON HIPPEL-LINDAU DISEASE

line \'līn\ *n* **1** : a strain produced and maintained esp. by selective breeding or biological culture **2** : a narrow short synthetic tube (as of plastic) that is inserted approximately one inch into a vein (as of the arm) to provide temporary intravenous access for the administration of fluid, medication, or nutrients

lin·ea al·ba \'li-nē-ə-'al-bə\ *n, pl* **lin·e·ae al·bae** \'li-nē-ˌē-'al-ˌbē\ : a median vertical tendinous line on the abdomen formed of fibers from the aponeuroses of the two rectus abdominis muscles and extending from the xiphoid process to the pubic symphysis

linea as·pe·ra \-'as-pə-rə\ *n, pl* **lineae as·pe·rae** \-ˌrē\ : a longitudinal ridge on the posterior surface of the middle third of the femur

lineae al·bi·can·tes \-,al-bə-ˈkan-,tēz\ *n pl* : whitish marks in the skin esp. of the abdomen and breasts that often follow pregnancy

linea semi·lu·nar·is \-,se-mi-lü-ˈnar-əs\ *n, pl* **lineae semi·lu·nar·es** \-ˈnar-,ēz\ : a curved line on the ventral abdominal wall parallel to the midline and halfway between it and the side of the body that marks the lateral border of the rectus abdominis muscle — called also *semilunar line*

line of sight *n* : a line from an observer's eye to a distant point

line of vision *n* : a straight line joining the fovea of the eye with the fixation point

linguae — see LONGITUDINALIS LINGUAE

lin·gual \ˈliŋ-gwəl, -gyə-wəl\ *adj* **1** : of, relating to, or resembling the tongue **2** : lying near or next to the tongue; *esp* : relating to or being the surface of a tooth next to the tongue

lingual artery *n* : an artery arising from the external carotid artery between the superior thyroid and facial arteries and supplying the tongue

lingual gland *n* : any of the mucous, serous, or mixed glands that empty their secretions onto the surface of the tongue

lin·gual·ly \ˈliŋ-gwə-lē\ *adv* : toward the tongue ⟨a tooth displaced ∼⟩

lingual nerve *n* : a branch of the mandibular division of the trigeminal nerve supplying the anterior two thirds of the tongue and responding to stimuli of pressure, touch, and temperature

lingual tonsil *n* : a variable mass or group of small nodules of lymphoid tissue lying at the base of the tongue just anterior to the epiglottis

lin·gu·la \ˈliŋ-gyə-lə\ *n, pl* **lin·gu·lae** \-,lē\ : a tongue-shaped process or part: as **a** : a ridge of bone in the angle between the body and the greater wing of the sphenoid **b** : an elongated prominence of the superior vermis of the cerebellum **c** : a dependent projection of the upper lobe of the left lung — **lin·gu·lar** \-lər\ *adj*

lin·i·ment \ˈli-nə-mənt\ *n* : a liquid or semifluid preparation that is applied to the skin as an anodyne or a counterirritant — called also *embrocation*

li·ni·tis plas·ti·ca \lə-ˈnī-təs-ˈplas-ti-kə\ *n* : carcinoma of the stomach marked by thickening and diffuse infiltration of the wall rather than localization of the tumor in a discrete lump

link·age \ˈliŋ-kij\ *n* : the relationship between genes on the same chromosome that causes them to be inherited together — compare MENDEL'S LAW 2

linkage group *n* : a set of linked genes at different loci on the same chromosome

linked \ˈliŋkt\ *adj* : marked by linkage ⟨∼ genes⟩

Li·nog·na·thus \li-ˈnäg-nə-thəs\ *n* : a genus of sucking lice including parasites of several domestic mammals

lio- — see LEIO-

li·o·thy·ro·nine \ˌlī-ō-ˈthī-rə-,nēn\ *n* : TRIIODOTHYRONINE

lip \ˈlip\ *n* **1** : either of the two fleshy folds which surround the mouth and in humans are organs of speech essential to certain articulations; *also* : the pink or reddish margin of the human lip composed of nonglandular mucous membrane **2** : an edge of a wound **3** : either of a pair of fleshy folds surrounding an orifice **4** : an anatomical part or structure (as a labium) resembling a lip — **lip·like** \ˈlip-,līk\ *adj*

lip- or **lipo-** *comb form* : fat : fatty tissue : fatty ⟨*lipoid*⟩ ⟨*lipoprotein*⟩

li·pae·mia *chiefly Brit var of* LIPEMIA

li·pase \ˈli-,pās, ˈlī-, -,pāz\ *n* : an enzyme (as one secreted by the pancreas) that catalyzes the breakdown of fats and lipoproteins usu. into fatty acids and glycerol

li·pec·to·my \li-ˈpek-tə-mē, lī-\ *n, pl* **-mies** : the excision of subcutaneous fatty tissue esp. as a cosmetic surgical procedure

li·pe·mia \li-ˈpē-mē-ə\ *n* : the presence of an excess of fats or lipids in the blood; *specif* : HYPERCHOLESTEROLEMIA — **li·pe·mic** \-mik\ *adj*

lip·id \ˈli-pəd\ *also* **lip·ide** \-,pīd\ *n* : any of various substances that are soluble in nonpolar organic solvents, that with proteins and carbohydrates constitute the principal structural components of living cells, and that include fats, waxes, phospholipids, cerebrosides, and related and derived compounds — **li·pid·ic** \li-ˈpi-dik\ *adj*

lip·i·do·sis \,li-pə-ˈdō-səs\ *n, pl* **-do·ses** \-,sēz\ : a disorder of fat metabolism esp. involving the deposition of fat in an organ (as the liver or spleen) — called also *lipoidosis*

Lip·i·tor \ˈli-pə-,tór\ *trademark* — used for a preparation of the calcium salt of atorvastatin

li·po·at·ro·phy \,li-pō-ˈa-trə-fē\ *n, pl* **-phies** : an allergic reaction to insulin medication that is manifested as a loss of subcutaneous fat — **li·po·atro·phic** \-(,)ā-ˈtrō-fik\ *adj*

li·po·chon·dro·dys·tro·phy \-,kän-drə-ˈdis-trə-fē\ *n, pl* **-phies** : MUCOPOLYSACCHARIDOSIS; *esp* : HURLER'S SYNDROME

li·po·chrome \ˈli-pə-,krōm, ˈlī-\ *n* : any of the naturally occurring pigments soluble in fats or in solvents for fats; *esp* : CAROTENOID

li·po·dys·tro·phy \,li-pō-ˈdis-trə-fē, ,lī-\ *n, pl* **-phies** : a disorder of fat metabolism esp. involving loss of fat from or deposition of fat in tissue

lipodystrophy syndrome *n* : a group of side effects of antiretroviral therapy for HIV infection that include high triglyceride levels in the blood, diabetes, and redistribution of fat in the body

li·po·fi·bro·ma \ˌli-pō-fī-'brō-mə, ˌlī-\ *n, pl* **-mas** *also* **-ma·ta** \-mə-tə\ : a lipoma containing fibrous tissue

li·po·fus·cin \ˌli-pə-'fəs-ᵊn, ˌlī-, -'fyü-sᵊn\ *n* : a dark brown lipochrome found esp. in the tissue (as of the heart) of the aged

li·po·fus·cin·o·sis \-ˌfə-sə-'nō-səs, -ˌfyü-\ *n* : a storage disease (as Batten disease) marked by abnormal accumulation of lipofuscins

li·po·gen·e·sis \-'je-nə-səs\ *n, pl* **-e·ses** \-ˌsēz\ **1** : formation of fat in the living body esp. when excessive or abnormal **2** : the formation of fatty acids from acetyl coenzyme A in the living body

li·po·ic acid \li-'pō-ik-, lī-\ *n* : any of several microbial growth factors; *esp* : a crystalline compound $C_8H_{14}O_2S_2$ that is essential for the oxidation of alpha-keto acids (as pyruvic acid) in metabolism

¹li·poid \'lī-ˌpȯid, 'lī-\ *or* **li·poi·dal** \li-'pȯid-ᵊl\ *adj* : resembling fat

²lipoid *n* : LIPID

lipoidica — *see* NECROBIOSIS LIPOIDICA, NECROBIOSIS LIPOIDICA DIABETICORUM

li·poid·o·sis \ˌli-ˌpȯi-'dō-səs, ˌlī-\ *n, pl* **-o·ses** \-ˌsēz\ : LIPIDOSIS

li·pol·y·sis \li-'pä-lə-səs, lī-\ *n, pl* **-y·ses** \-ˌsēz\ : the hydrolysis of fat — **li·po·lyt·ic** \ˌli-pə-'li-tik, ˌlī-\ *adj*

li·po·ma \li-'pō-mə, lī-\ *n, pl* **-mas** *also* **-ma·ta** \-mə-tə\ : a tumor of fatty tissue — **li·po·ma·tous** \-mə-təs\ *adj*

li·po·ma·to·sis \ˌli-ˌpō-mə-'tō-səs, lī-\ *n, pl* **-to·ses** \-ˌsēz\ : any of several abnormal conditions marked by local or generalized deposits of fat or replacement of other tissue by fat; *specif* : the presence of multiple lipomas

li·po·phil·ic \ˌli-pə-'fi-lik, ˌlī-\ *adj* : having an affinity for lipids (as fats) ⟨a ∼ metabolite⟩ — *compare* HYDROPHILIC — **li·po·phi·lic·i·ty** \-fi-'li-sə-tē\ *n*

li·po·poly·sac·cha·ride \ˌli-pō-ˌpä-li-'sa-kə-ˌrīd, ˌlī-\ *n* : a large molecule consisting of lipids and sugars joined by chemical bonds

li·po·pro·tein \-'prō-ˌtēn\ *n* : any of a large class of conjugated proteins composed of a complex of protein and lipid — *see* HDL, LDL, VLDL

li·po·sar·co·ma \-sär-'kō-mə\ *n, pl* **-mas** *also* **-ma·ta** \-mə-tə\ : a sarcoma arising from immature fat cells of the bone marrow

li·po·some \'li-pə-ˌsōm, 'lī-\ *n* **1** : one of the fatty droplets in the cytoplasm of a cell **2** : an artificial vesicle that is composed of one or more concentric phospholipid bilayers and is used esp. to deliver microscopic substances (as DNA or drugs) to body cells — **li·po·so·mal** \ˌli-pə-'sō-məl, ˌlī-\ *adj*

li·po·suc·tion \-ˌsək-shən\ *n* : surgical removal of local fat deposits (as in the thighs) esp. for cosmetic purposes by applying suction through a small tube inserted into the body — **liposuction** *vb*

li·po·tro·pin \ˌli-pə-'trō-pən, ˌlī-\ *n* : either of two protein hormones of the anterior part of the pituitary gland that function in the mobilization of fat reserves; *esp* : BETA-LIPOTROPIN

li·pox·y·gen·ase \li-'päk-sə-jə-ˌnās, lī-, -ˌnāz\ *n* : a crystallizable enzyme that catalyzes the oxidation primarily of unsaturated fatty acids or unsaturated fats by oxygen

Lippes loop \'li-pēz-\ *n* : an S-shaped plastic intrauterine device

Lippes, Jack (*b* 1924), American obstetrician and gynecologist.

lip–read \'lip-ˌrēd\ *vb* **-read** \-ˌred\; **-read·ing** \-ˌrē-diŋ\ : to understand by lipreading; *also* : to use lipreading — **lip–read·er** \-ˌrē-dər\ *n*

lip·read·ing \-ˌrē-diŋ\ *n* : the interpreting of spoken words by watching the speaker's lip and facial movements without hearing the voice

Li·quae·min \'li-kwə-ˌmin\ *n* : a preparation of heparin — formerly a U.S. registered trademark

liq·ue·fac·tion \ˌli-kwə-'fak-shən\ *n* **1** : the process of making or becoming liquid **2** : the state of being liquid

¹liq·uid \'lik-wəd\ *adj* **1** : flowing freely like water **2** : having the properties of a liquid

²liquid *n* : a fluid (as water) that has no independent shape but has a definite volume, does not expand indefinitely, and is only slightly compressible

liq·uid·am·bar \ˌli-kwə-'dam-bər\ *n* **1** *cap* : a genus of trees of the witch hazel family (Hamamelidaceae) **2** : STORAX 2

liquid chromatography *n* : chromatography in which the mobile phase is a liquid

liquid protein diet *n* : a reducing diet consisting of high-protein liquids

Li·qui·prin \'li-kwə-ˌprin\ *n* : a preparation of acetaminophen — formerly a U.S. registered trademark

li·quor \'li-kər\ *n* : a liquid substance (as a medicinal solution usu. in water) — *compare* TINCTURE

li·quor am·nii \'lī-ˌkwȯr-'am-nē-ˌi, 'li-\ *n* : AMNIOTIC FLUID

liquor fol·li·cu·li \-fä-'li-kyə-ˌlī\ *n* : the fluid surrounding the ovum in the ovarian follicle

li·quo·rice *chiefly Brit var of* LICORICE

li·sin·o·pril \li-'si-nə-ˌpril, lī-\ *n* : an antihypertensive drug $C_{21}H_{31}N_3O_5 \cdot 2H_2O$ that is an ACE inhibitor — *see* PRINIVIL, ZESTRIL

lisp \'lisp\ *vb* **1** : to pronounce the sibilants \s\ and \z\ imperfectly esp. by giving them the sounds \th\ and \t͟h\ **2** : to speak with a lisp — **lisp** *n* — **lisp·er** \'lis-pər\ *n*

liss- *or* **lisso-** *comb form* : smooth ⟨*liss*encephaly⟩

lis·sen·ceph·a·ly \ˌli-sen-ˈse-fə-lē\ *n, pl* **-lies** : the condition of having a smooth cerebrum without convolutions — **lis·sen·ce·phal·ic** \-sə-ˈfa-lik\ *adj*

lis·te·ria \li-ˈstir-ē-ə\ *n* **1** *cap* : a genus of small gram-positive flagellated rod-shaped bacteria including one (*L. monocytogenes*) causing listeriosis **2** : any bacterium of the genus *Listeria* — **lis·te·ri·al** \li-ˈstir-ē-əl\ *adj* — **lis·te·ric** \-ik\ *adj*

Lis·ter \ˈlis-tər\, **Joseph (1827–1912)**, British surgeon and medical scientist.

lis·te·ri·o·sis \(ˌ)li-ˌstir-ē-ˈō-səs\ *n, pl* **-ri·o·ses** \-ˌsēz\ : a serious disease that is caused by a bacterium of the genus *Listeria* (*L. monocytogenes*), that in animals causes severe encephalitis and is often fatal, that is contracted by humans esp. from contaminated food (as processed meats or unpasteurized milk), that in otherwise healthy people typically takes the form of a mild flulike illness or has no noticeable symptoms, that in neonates, the elderly, and the immunocompromised often causes serious sometimes fatal illness with symptoms including meningitis and sepsis, and that in pregnant women usu. causes only mild illness in the mother but often results in miscarriage, stillbirth, or premature birth

li·ter \ˈlē-tər\ *n* : a metric unit of capacity equal to the volume of one kilogram of water at 4°C (39°F) and at standard atmospheric pressure of 760 millimeters of mercury

lith- *or* **litho-** *comb form* : calculus ⟨*lith*iasis⟩ ⟨*litho*tripsy⟩

-lith \ˌlith\ *n comb form* : calculus ⟨uro*lith*⟩

li·thi·a·sis \li-ˈthī-ə-səs\ *n, pl* **-a·ses** \-ˌsēz\ : the formation of stony concretions in the body (as in the urinary tract or gallbladder) — often used in combination ⟨chole*lithiasis*⟩

lith·i·um \ˈli-thē-əm\ *n* **1** : a soft silver-white element that is the lightest metal known — symbol *Li*; see ELEMENT table **2** : a lithium salt and esp. lithium carbonate used in psychiatric medicine

lithium carbonate *n* : a crystalline salt Li_2CO_3 used in medicine in the treatment of mania and hypomania in bipolar disorder

lith·o·gen·ic \ˌli-thə-ˈje-nik\ *adj* : of, promoting, or undergoing the formation of calculi ⟨a ~ diet⟩ — **lith·o·gen·e·sis** \-ˈje-nə-səs\ *n*

lith·o·la·paxy \ˈli-thə-lə-ˌpak-sē, ˈli-thə-lə-\ *n, pl* **-pax·ies** : LITHOTRIPSY

lith·o·pe·di·on \ˌli-thə-ˈpē-dē-ˌän\ *n* : a fetus calcified in the body of the mother

li·thot·o·my \li-ˈthä-tə-mē\ *n, pl* **-mies** : surgical incision of the urinary bladder for removal of a calculus

lith·o·trip·sy \ˈli-thə-ˌtrip-sē\ *n, pl* **-sies** : the breaking of a calculus (as by shock waves or crushing with a surgical instrument) in the urinary system into pieces small enough to be voided or washed out — called also *litholapaxy*

lith·o·trip·ter *also* **lith·o·trip·tor** \ˈli-thə-ˌtrip-tər\ *n* : a device for performing lithotripsy; *esp* : a noninvasive device that pulverizes calculi by focusing shock waves on a patient immersed in a water bath

lit·mus \ˈlit-məs\ *n* : a coloring matter from lichens that turns red in acid solutions and blue in alkaline solutions and is used as an acid-base indicator

litmus paper *n* : paper colored with litmus and used as an acid-base indicator

li·tre \ˈlē-tər\ *chiefly Brit var of* LITER

¹lit·ter \ˈli-tər\ *n* **1** : a device (as a stretcher) for carrying a sick or injured person **2** : the offspring at one birth of a multiparous animal

²litter *vb* : to give birth to young

little finger *n* : the fourth and smallest finger of the hand counting the index finger as the first

Little League elbow *n* : inflammation of the medial epicondyle and adjacent tissues of the elbow esp. in preteen and teenage baseball players who make too strenuous use of the muscles of the forearm — called also *Little Leaguer's elbow*

Lit·tle's disease \ˈli-tᵊlz-\ *n* : a form of spastic cerebral palsy marked by spastic diplegia in which the legs are typically more severely affected than the arms; *broadly* : CEREBRAL PALSY

Little, William John (1810–1894), British physician.

little stroke *n* : TRANSIENT ISCHEMIC ATTACK

little toe *n* : the outermost and smallest digit of the foot

live birth \ˈlīv-\ *n* : birth in such a state that processes of life are manifested after the emergence of the whole body : birth of a live fetus — compare STILLBIRTH

live-born \ˈlīv-ˈbȯrn\ *adj* : born alive — compare STILLBORN

li·ve·do re·tic·u·lar·is \li-ˈvē-dō-ri-ˌti-kyə-ˈlar-əs\ *n* : a condition of the peripheral blood vessels characterized by reddish blue mottling of the skin esp. of the extremities usu. upon exposure to cold

liv·er \ˈli-vər\ *n* : a large very vascular glandular organ of vertebrates that secretes bile and causes important changes in many of the substances contained in the blood which passes through it (as by converting sugars into glycogen which it stores up until required and by forming urea) that in humans is the largest gland in the body, weighs from 40 to 60 ounces (1100 to 1700 grams), is a dark red color, and occupies the upper right portion of the abdominal cavity immediately below the diaphragm

liver cell *n* : HEPATOCYTE

liver fluke *n* : any of various trematode worms that invade the mammalian liver; *esp* : one of the genus *Fasciola* (*F. hepatica*) that is a major parasite of the liver, bile ducts, and gallbladder of cattle and sheep, causes fascioliasis in humans, and uses snails of the genus *Lymnaea* as an intermediate host — see CHINESE LIVER FLUKE

liver rot *n* : a disease caused by liver flukes esp. in sheep and cattle and marked by great local damage to the liver — see DISTOMATOSIS

liver spots *n pl* : AGE SPOTS

lives *pl of* LIFE

liv·id \'li-vəd\ *adj* : discolored by bruising : BLACK-AND-BLUE — **li·vid·i·ty** \li-'vi-də-tē\ *n*

living will *n* : a document in which the signer requests to be allowed to die rather than be kept alive by artificial means in the event of becoming disabled beyond a reasonable expectation of recovery

li·vor mor·tis \'li-ˌvȯr-'mȯr-təs\ *n* : hypostasis of the blood following death that causes a purplish red discoloration of the skin — called also *dependent lividity, postmortem lividity*

LLQ *abbr* left lower quadrant (abdomen)

LMP *abbr* last menstrual period

Loa \'lō-ə\ *n* : a genus of African filarial worms (family Dipetalonematidae) that infect the subcutaneous tissues and blood, include the eye worm (*L. loa*) causing Calabar swellings, and are transmitted by the bite of flies of the genus *Chrysops*

load \'lōd\ *n* 1 : the amount of a deleterious microorganism, parasite, growth, or substance present in a human or animal body ⟨measure viral ∼ in the blood⟩ — called also *burden* 2 : GENETIC LOAD

load·ing \'lō-diŋ\ *n* 1 : administration of a factor or substance to the body or a bodily system in sufficient quantity to test capacity to deal with it 2 : the relative contribution of each component factor in a psychological test or in an experimental, clinical, or social situation

lo·a·i·a·sis \ˌlō-ə-'ī-ə-səs\ *or* **lo·i·a·sis** \lō-'ī-\ *n, pl* **-a·ses** \-ˌsēz\ : infestation with or disease caused by an eye worm of the genus *Loa* (*L. loa*) that migrates through the subcutaneous tissue and across the cornea of the eye — compare CALABAR SWELLING

loa loa \'lō-ə-'lō-ə\ *n* : LOAIASIS

lob- *or* **lobi-** *or* **lobo-** *comb form* : lobe ⟨*lobectomy*⟩ ⟨*lobotomy*⟩

lo·bar \'lō-bər, -ˌbär\ *adj* : of or relating to a lobe

lobar pneumonia *n* : acute pneumonia involving one or more lobes of the lung characterized by sudden onset,

chill, fever, difficulty in breathing, cough, and blood-stained sputum, marked by consolidation, and normally followed by resolution and return to normal of the lung tissue

lobe \'lōb\ *n* : a curved or rounded projection or division: as **a** : a more or less rounded projection of a body organ or part ⟨∼ of the ear⟩ **b** : a division of a body organ (as the brain or lungs) marked off by a fissure on the surface — **lobed** \'lōbd\ *adj*

lo·bec·to·my \lō-'bek-tə-mē\ *n, pl* **-mies** : surgical removal of a lobe of an organ (as a lung) or gland (as the thyroid); *specif* : excision of a lobe of the lung

lo·be·line \'lō-bə-ˌlēn\ *n* : an alkaloid $C_{22}H_{27}NO_2$ that is obtained from an American herb (*Lobelia inflata* of the family Lobeliaceae) and is used esp. as a smoking deterrent

lobi-, lobo- — see LOB-

lo·bot·o·my \lō-'bä-tə-mē\ *n, pl* **-mies** : surgical severance of nerve fibers connecting the frontal lobes to the thalamus for the relief of some mental disorders — called also *leukotomy* — **lo·bot·o·mize** \-ˌmīz\ *vb*

lobster claw \'läb-stər-ˌklȯ\ *n* : an incompletely dominant genetic anomaly marked by variable reduction of the skeleton of the extremities and cleaving of the hands and feet into two segments

lob·u·lar \'lä-byə-lər\ *adj* : of, relating to, affecting, or resembling a lobule

lob·u·lat·ed \'lä-byə-ˌlā-təd\ *adj* : made up of, provided with, or divided into lobules ⟨a ∼ tumor⟩ — **lob·u·la·tion** \ˌlä-byə-'lā-shən\ *n*

lob·ule \'lä-ˌbyül\ *n* 1 : a small lobe ⟨the ∼ of the ear⟩ 2 : a subdivision of a lobe; *specif* : one of the small masses of tissue of which various organs (as the liver) are made up

lob·u·lus \'lä-byə-ləs\ *n, pl* **lob·u·li** \-ˌlī\ 1 : LOBE 2 : LOBULE

¹lo·cal \'lō-kəl\ *adj* : involving or affecting only a restricted part of the organism ⟨∼ inflammation⟩ — compare SYSTEMIC a — **lo·cal·ly** *adv*

²local *n* : LOCAL ANESTHETIC; *also* : LOCAL ANESTHESIA

local anesthesia *n* : loss of sensation in a limited and usu. superficial area esp. from the effect of a local anesthetic

local anesthetic *n* : an anesthetic for use on a limited and usu. superficial area of the body

lo·cal·ize \'lō-kə-ˌlīz\ *vb* **-ized; -iz·ing** 1 : to make local; *esp* : to fix in or confine to a definite place or part 2 : to accumulate in or be restricted to a specific or limited area — **lo·cal·i·za·tion** \ˌlō-kə-lə-'zā-shən\ *n*

lo·chia \'lō-kē-ə, 'lä-\ *n, pl* **lochia** : a discharge from the uterus and vagina following delivery — **lo·chi·al** \-əl\ *adj*

loci *pl of* LOCUS

loci cerulei, loci coerulei *pl of* LOCUS CERULEUS, LOCUS COERULEUS

locked \ˈläkt\ *adj, of the knee joint* : having a restricted mobility and incapable of complete extension

locked–in syndrome *n* : the condition of a conscious patient who because of motor paralysis throughout the body is unable to communicate except possibly by coded eye movements

lock·jaw \ˈläk-ˌjȯ\ *n* : an early symptom of tetanus marked by spasm of the jaw muscles and inability to open the jaws; *also* : TETANUS 1a

lo·co·ism \ˈlō-kō-ˌi-zəm\ *n* 1 : a disease of horses, cattle, and sheep caused by chronic poisoning with locoweeds and characterized by motor and sensory nerve damage 2 : any of several intoxications of domestic animals (as selenosis) that are sometimes mistaken for locoweed poisoning

lo·co·mo·tion \ˌlō-kə-ˈmō-shən\ *n* : an act or the power of moving from place to place : progressive movement (as of an animal body) — **lo·co·mo·tor** \ˌlō-kə-ˈmō-tər\ *adj* — **lo·co·mo·to·ry** \ˌlō-kə-ˈmō-tə-rē\ *adj*

locomotor ataxia *n* : TABES DORSALIS

lo·co·re·gion·al \ˌ-ˈrēj-ən-ᵊl\ *adj* : restricted to a localized region of the body (∼ anesthesia)

lo·co·weed \ˈlō-(ˌ)kō-ˌwēd\ *n* : any of several leguminous plants (genera *Astragalus* and *Oxytropis*) of western No. America that cause locoism

loc·u·lus \ˈlä-kyə-ləs\ *n, pl* **-li** \-ˌlī, -ˌlē\ : a small chamber or cavity esp. in a plant or animal body — **loc·u·lat·ed** \ˈlä-kyə-ˌlā-təd\ *adj* — **loc·u·la·tion** \ˌlä-kyə-ˈlā-shən\ *n*

lo·cum te·nens \ˌlō-kəm-ˈtē-nenz, -nənz\ *n, pl* **locum te·nen·tes** \-ti-ˈnen-ˌtēz\ : a medical practitioner who temporarily takes the place of another

lo·cus \ˈlō-kəs\ *n, pl* **lo·ci** \ˈlō-ˌsī, -ˌkī, -ˌkē\ 1 : a place or site of an event, activity, or thing 2 : the position in a chromosome of a particular gene or allele

lo·cus ce·ru·le·us *also* **lo·cus ce·ru·le·us** \ˌlō-kəs-si-ˈrü-lē-əs\ *n, pl* **loci coe·ru·lei** *also* **loci ce·ru·lei** \-lē-ˌī\ : a blue area of the brain stem with many norepinephrine-containing neurons

Loef·fler's syndrome \ˈle-flərz-\ *n* : a mild pneumonitis marked by transitory pulmonary infiltration and eosinophilia and usu. considered to be basically an allergic reaction — called also *Loeffler's pneumonia*

   Löf·fler \ˈlœ-flər\, **Wilhelm** (1887–1972), Swiss physician.

log- *or* **logo-** *comb form* : word : thought : speech : discourse (*logorrhea*)

log·o·pe·dics \ˌlȯ-gə-ˈpē-diks, ˌlä-\ *n sing or pl* : the scientific study and treatment of speech defects

log·or·rhea \ˌlȯ-gə-ˈrē-ə, ˌlä-\ *n* : pathologically excessive and often incoherent talkativeness or wordiness

log·or·rhoea *chiefly Brit var of* LOGORRHEA

log·o·ther·a·py \ˌlȯ-gə-ˈther-ə-pē, ˌlä-\ *n, pl* **-pies** : a highly directive existential psychotherapy that emphasizes the importance of meaning in the patient's life esp. as gained through spiritual values

-l·o·gy \l-ə-jē\ *n comb form, pl* **-logies** : doctrine : theory : science (*physiology*)

loi·a·sis *var of* LOAIASIS

loin \ˈlȯin\ *n* 1 : the part of the body on each side of the spinal column between the hip bone and the false ribs 2 *pl* **a** : the upper and lower abdominal regions and the region about the hips **b** (1) : the pubic region (2) : the generative organs — not usu. used technically in senses 2a, b

loin disease *n* : aphosphorosis of cattle often complicated by botulism

Lo·mo·til \ˈlō-mə-ˌtil, lō-ˈmōt-ᵊl\ *trademark* — used for a preparation of the hydrochloride of diphenoxylate and the sulfate of atropine

lo·mus·tine \lō-ˈməs-ˌtēn\ *n* : an antineoplastic drug $C_9H_{16}ClN_3O_2$ used esp. in the treatment of brain tumors and Hodgkin's disease

lone star tick *n* : an ixodid tick of the genus *Amblyomma* (*A. americanum*) of the southern, central, and eastern U.S. that is a vector of several diseases (as Rocky Mountain spotted fever and ehrlichiosis) and in which the adult female has a single white spot on the back

long–acting thyroid stimulator *n* : a protein that often occurs in the plasma of patients with Graves' disease and may be an IgG immunoglobulin — abbr. *LATS*

long bone *n* : any of the elongated bones supporting a limb and consisting of an essentially cylindrical shaft that contains marrow and ends in enlarged heads for articulation with other bones

long ciliary nerve *n* : any of two or three nerves that are given off by the nasociliary nerve and are distributed to the iris and cornea — compare SHORT CILIARY NERVE

long head *n* : the longest of the three heads of the triceps muscle that arises from the infraglenoid tubercle of the scapula

longi *pl of* LONGUS

lon·gis·si·mus \län-ˈji-si-məs\ *n, pl* **lon·gis·si·mi** \-ˌmī\ : the intermediate division of the sacrospinalis muscle that consists of the longissimus capitis, longissimus cervicis, and longissimus thoracis; *also* : any of these three muscles

longissimus cap·i·tis \-ˈka-pi-təs\ *n* : a muscle that arises by tendons from the upper thoracic and lower cervical vertebrae, is inserted into the posterior margin of the mastoid process, and extends the head and bends and rotates it to one side — called also *trachelomastoid muscle*

longissimus cer·vi·cis \-'sər-vi-səs\ *n* : a muscle medial to the longissimus thoracis that arises by long thin tendons from the transverse processes of the upper four or five thoracic vertebrae, is inserted by similar tendons into the transverse processes of the second to sixth cervical vertebrae, and extends the spinal column and bends it to one side

longissimus dor·si \-'dȯr-sī\ *n* : LONGISSIMUS THORACIS

longissimus thor·a·cis \-'thȯr-ə-səs, -thō-'rā-səs\ *n* : a muscle that arises as the middle and largest division of the sacrospinalis muscle, that is attached by some of its fibers to the lumbar vertebrae, that is inserted into all the thoracic vertebrae and the lower 9 or 10 ribs, and that depresses the ribs and with the longissimus cervicis extends the spinal column and bends it to one side

lon·gi·tu·di·nal \,län-jə-'tüd-ᵊn-əl, -'tyüd-\ *adj* **1** : of, relating to, or occurring in the lengthwise dimension ⟨a ∼ fracture⟩ **2** : extending along or relating to the anteroposterior axis of a body or part **3** : involving the repeated observation or examination of a set of subjects over time with respect to one or more study variables — **lon·gi·tu·di·nal·ly** *adv*

longitudinal fissure *n* : the deep groove that divides the cerebrum into right and left hemispheres

lon·gi·tu·di·na·lis linguae \,län-jə-,tü-də-'nā-ləs-, -,tyü-\ *n* : either of two bands of muscle comprising the intrinsic musculature of the tongue — called also *longitudinalis*

long–nosed cattle louse *n* : a sucking louse of the genus *Linognathus* (*L. vituli*) that feeds on cattle

long posterior ciliary artery *n* : either of usu. two arteries of which one arises from the ophthalmic artery on each side of the optic nerve, passes forward along the optic nerve, enters the sclera, and at the junction of the ciliary process and the iris divides into upper and lower branches which form a ring of arteries around the iris — compare SHORT POSTERIOR CILIARY ARTERY

long QT syndrome *n* : any of several inherited cardiac arrhythmias that are characterized by abnormal duration and shape of the QT interval and that place the subject at risk for torsades de pointes — abbr. *LQTS*

long saphenous vein *n* : SAPHENOUS VEIN a

long·sight·ed \'lȯŋ-'sī-təd\ *adj* : FARSIGHTED — **long·sight·ed·ness** *n*

long terminal repeat *n* : an identical sequence of several hundred base pairs at each end of the DNA synthesized by the reverse transcriptase of a retrovirus that controls integration of

the viral DNA into the host DNA and expression of the genes of the virus — called also *LTR*

long–term memory *n* : memory that involves the storage and recall of information over a long period of time (as days, weeks, or years)

long–term nonprogressor *n* : an HIV-infected individual who remains symptom-free over the long term and does not progress to develop AIDS — called also *nonprogressor*

long–term potentiation *n* : a long-lasting strengthening of the response of a postsynaptic neuron to stimulation across the synapse that occurs with repeated stimulation and is thought to be related to learning and long-term memory — abbr. *LTP*

lon·gus \'lȯŋ-gəs\ *n, pl* **lon·gi** \,gī\ : a long structure (as a muscle) in the body — see ABDUCTOR POLLICIS LONGUS, ADDUCTOR LONGUS, EXTENSOR CARPI RADIALIS LONGUS, EXTENSOR DIGITORUM LONGUS, EXTENSOR HALLUCIS LONGUS, FLEXOR DIGITORUM LONGUS, FLEXOR HALLUCIS LONGUS, FLEXOR POLLICIS LONGUS, PALMARIS LONGUS, PERONEUS LONGUS

longus cap·i·tis \-'ka·pi-təs\ *n* : a muscle of either side of the front and upper portion of the neck that arises from the third to sixth cervical vertebrae, is inserted into the basilar portion of the occipital bone, and bends the neck forward

Lon·i·ten \'lä-ni-tən\ *trademark* — used for a preparation of minoxidil

loop — see LIPPES LOOP

loop diuretic *n* : a diuretic that inhibits reabsorption in the ascending limb of the loop of Henle causing greatly increased excretion of sodium chloride in the urine

loop of Hen·le \-'hen-lē\ *n* : the U-shaped part of a nephron that lies between and is continuous with the proximal and distal convoluted tubules, that leaves the cortex of the kidney descending into the medullary tissue and then bending back and reentering the cortex, and that functions in water resorption — called also *Henle's loop*

F. G. J. Henle — see HENLE'S LAYER

loose \'lüs\ *adj* **loos·er; loos·est** **1 a** (1) : having worked partly free from attachments ⟨a ∼ tooth⟩ (2) : having relative freedom of movement **b** : produced freely and accompanied by raising of mucus ⟨a ∼ cough⟩ **2 a** : not dense, close, or compact in structure or arrangement ⟨∼ connective tissue⟩ **b** : not solid : WATERY ⟨∼ stools⟩ **3** : OVERACTIVE; *specif* : marked by frequent voiding esp. of watery stools ⟨∼ bowels⟩ **4** : not tightly drawn or stretched ⟨∼ skin⟩ — **loose·ly** *adv* — **loose·ness** *n*

lo·per·a·mide \lō-'per-ə-,mīd\ *n* : a

synthetic antidiarrheal agent that slows intestinal peristalsis and is used in the form of its hydrochloride $C_{29}H_{33}ClN_2O_2 \cdot HCl$ — see IMODIUM

Lo·pid \'lō-pid\ *trademark* — used for a preparation of gemfibrozil

Lo·pres·sor \lō-'pre-sər, -,sór\ *trademark* — used for a preparation of the tartrate of metoprolol

lo·rat·a·dine \lə-'ra-tə-,dēn\ n : a long-acting H_1 antagonist $C_{22}H_{23}ClN_2O_2$ used esp. to relieve the symptoms of seasonal allergic rhinitis — see CLARITIN

lor·az·e·pam \lór-'a-zə-,pam\ n : an anxiolytic benzodiazepine $C_{15}H_{10}Cl_2$-N_2O_2 — see ATIVAN

lor·do·sis \lór-'dō-səs\ n : exaggerated forward curvature of the lumbar and cervical regions of the spinal column — compare KYPHOSIS, SCOLIOSIS — **lor·dot·ic** \-'dä-tik\ adj

lo·sar·tan \lō-'sär-,tan\ n : an antihypertensive drug that is administered in the form of its potassium salt $C_{22}H_{22}ClKN_6O$ and blocks the effects of angiotensin II — see COZAAR, HYZAAR

Lo·ten·sin \lō-'ten-sən\ *trademark* — used for a preparation of the hydrochloride of benazepril

lo·tion \'lō-shən\ n **1** : a liquid usu. aqueous medicinal preparation containing one or more insoluble substances and applied externally for skin disorders **2** : a liquid cosmetic preparation usu. containing a cleansing, softening, or astringent agent and applied to the skin

Lo·trel \'lō-,trel\ *trademark* — used for a preparation of amlodipine and benazepril

Lo·tri·min \'lō-trə-min\ *trademark* — used for a preparation of clotrimazole

Lou Geh·rig's disease \'lü-'ger-igz-\ n : AMYOTROPHIC LATERAL SCLEROSIS
   Gehrig, Lou (1903–1941), American baseball player.

loupe \'lüp\ n : a magnifying lens worn esp. by surgeons performing microsurgery; *also* : two such lenses mounted on a single frame

loup·ing ill \'laù-piŋ-, 'lō-\ n : a variable tick-borne virus disease that occurs esp. in sheep and other domestic animals and sporadically in humans, that affects primarily the central nervous system, and that is caused by a virus of the genus *Flavivirus* (species *Louping ill*)

louse \'laùs\ n, pl **lice** \'līs\ : any of the small wingless usu. flattened insects that are parasitic on warm-blooded animals and constitute two orders (Anoplura and Mallophaga)

louse–borne typhus n : TYPHUS a

lousy \'laù-zē\ adj **lous·i·er**; **-est** : infested with lice — **lous·i·ness** \'laù-zē-nəs\ n

lov·a·stat·in \'lō-və-,sta-tən, 'lə-\ n : a statin $C_{24}H_{36}O_5$ that decreases the level of cholesterol in the blood stream by inhibiting the liver enzyme that controls cholesterol synthesis and is used in the treatment of hypercholesterolemia — see MEVACOR

love handles n pl : fatty bulges along the sides at the waist

love object n : a person on whom affection is centered or on whom one is dependent for affection or needed help

low \'lō\ adj **low·er** \'lō-ər\; **low·est** \'lō-əst\ : having a relatively less complex organization : not greatly differentiated or developed phylogenetically ⟨the ∼*er* vertebrates⟩ — compare HIGH 1

low–back \'lō-'bak\ adj : of, relating to, suffering, or being pain in the lowest portion of the back ⟨∼ pain⟩

low blood pressure n : HYPOTENSION 1

low–density lipoprotein n : LDL

low·er \'lō-ər\ n : the lower member of a pair; *esp* : a lower denture

lower jaw n : JAW 1b

lower respiratory adj : of, relating to, or affecting the lower respiratory tract ⟨*lower respiratory* infections⟩

lower respiratory tract n : the part of the respiratory system including the larynx, trachea, bronchi, and lungs — compare UPPER RESPIRATORY TRACT

lowest splanchnic nerve n : SPLANCHNIC NERVE c

Lowe syndrome *also* **Lowe's syndrome** \'lō(z)-\ n : OCULOCEREBRORENAL SYNDROME
   Lowe, Charles Upton (b 1921), American pediatrician.

low forceps n : a procedure for delivery of an infant by the use of forceps when the head is visible at the outlet of the birth canal — called also *outlet forceps*; compare HIGH FORCEPS, MIDFORCEPS

low–grade \'lō-'grād\ adj : being near that extreme of a specified range which is lowest, least intense, or least competent ⟨a ∼ fever⟩ ⟨a ∼ infection⟩ — compare HIGH-GRADE

Lown–Gan·ong–Le·vine syndrome \'laùn-'gan-,óŋ-lə-'vīn-, -'vēn-\ n : a preexcitation syndrome characterized by atrial tachycardia together with a short P-R interval and a QRS complex of normal duration — called also *LGL syndrome*
   Lown \'laùn\, Bernard (b 1921), American cardiologist.
   Gan·ong \'gan-,óŋ\, William Francis (b 1924), American physiologist.
   Le·vine \lə-'vīn, -'vēn\, Samuel Albert (1891–1966), American cardiologist.

low–power adj : of, relating to, or being a lens that magnifies an image a relatively small number of times and esp. 10 times — compare HIGH=POWER

low–salt diet n : LOW-SODIUM DIET

low–sodium diet n : a diet restricted to foods naturally low in sodium content and prepared without added salt that is used esp. in the management of hypertension, heart failure, and kidney or liver dysfunction

low vision *n* : impaired vision in which there is a significant reduction in visual function that cannot be corrected by conventional glasses but which may be improved with special aids or devices

Lox·os·ce·les \läk-'sä-sə-ˌlēz\ *n* : a genus of spiders (family Loxoscelidae) that includes the brown recluse spider (*L. reclusa*)

lox·os·ce·lism \läk-'sä-sə-ˌli-zəm\ *n* : a painful condition resulting from the bite of a spider of the genus *Loxosceles* and esp. the brown recluse spider (*L. reclusa*) that is characterized esp. by local necrosis of tissue

loz·enge \'läz-ᵊnj\ *n* : a small usu. sweetened solid piece of medicated material that is designed to be held in the mouth for slow dissolution and often contains a demulcent — called also **pastille, troche**

L–PAM \'el-ˌpam\ *n* : MELPHALAN

L–phase \'el-ˌfāz\ *n* : L-FORM

LPN \ˌel-(ˌ)pē-'en\ *n* : LICENSED PRACTICAL NURSE

LQTS *abbr* long QT syndrome

Lr *symbol* lawrencium

LSD \ˌel-(ˌ)es-'dē\ *n* : a semisynthetic illicit organic compound $C_{20}H_{25}N_3O$ derived from ergot that induces extreme sensory distortions, altered perceptions of reality, and intense emotional states, that may also produce delusions or paranoia, and that may sometimes cause panic reactions in response to the effects experienced — called also *acid, lysergic acid diethylamide, lysergide*

LSD–25 *n* : LSD

LTH *abbr* luteotropic hormone

LTP *abbr* long-term potentiation

LTR \ˌel-ˌtē-'är\ *n* : LONG TERMINAL REPEAT

L–tryp·to·phan \'el-'trip-tə-ˌfan\ *n* : the levorotatory form of tryptophan that is a precursor of serotonin and was formerly used in some health food preparations in the belief that it promoted sleep and relieved depression — see EOSINOPHILIA-MYALGIA SYNDROME

Lu *symbol* lutetium

lubb–dupp *also* **lub–dup** *or* **lub–dub** \ˌləb-'dəp, -'dəb\ *n* : the characteristic sounds of a normal heartbeat as heard in auscultation

lu·can·thone \lü-'kan-ˌthōn\ *n* : an antischistosomal drug administered in the form of its hydrochloride $C_{20}H_{24}$-$N_2OS·HCl$ — called also *miracil D*

lu·cid \'lü-səd\ *adj* : having, showing, or characterized by an ability to think clearly and rationally — **lu·cid·i·ty** \lü-'si-də-tē\ *n*

lucid interval *n* : a temporary period of rationality or neurological normality (as between periods of dementia or immediately following a fatal head injury)

lucidum — see STRATUM LUCIDUM

Lu·cil·ia \lü-'si-lē-ə\ *n* : a genus of blowflies whose larvae are sometimes the cause of intestinal myiasis and infest open wounds

lüc·ken·schä·del \'lue-kən-ˌshād-ᵊl\ *n* : a condition characterized by incomplete ossification of the bones of the skull

Lud·wig's angina \'lüd-(ˌ)vigz-\ *n* : an acute streptococcal or sometimes staphylococcal infection of the deep tissues of the floor of the mouth and adjoining parts of the neck and lower jaw that is marked by severe rapid swelling which may close the respiratory passage and that is accompanied by chills and fever

Ludwig, Wilhelm Friedrich von (1790–1865), German surgeon.

Lu·er syringe \'lü-ər-\ *n* : a glass syringe with a glass piston that has the apposing surfaces ground and that is used esp. for hypodermic injection

Luer (d 1883), German instrument maker.

lu·es \'lü-(ˌ)ēz\ *n, pl* **lues** : SYPHILIS

lu·et·ic \lü-'e-tik\ *adj* : SYPHILITIC

Lu·gol's solution \lü-ˈgōlz-\ *n* : any of several deep brown solutions of iodine and potassium iodide in water or alcohol — called also *Lugol's iodine, Lugol's iodine solution*

Lugol, Jean Guillaume Auguste (1786–1851), French physician.

lumb- *or* **lumbo-** *comb form* : lumbar and ⟨*lumbo*sacral⟩

lum·ba·go \ˌləm-'bā-(ˌ)gō\ *n* : acute or chronic pain (as that caused by muscle strain) in the lower back

lum·bar \'ləm-bər, -ˌbär\ *adj* **1** : of, relating to, or constituting the loins or the vertebrae between the thoracic vertebrae and sacrum **2** : of, relating to, or being the abdominal region lying on either side of the umbilical region and above the corresponding iliac region

lumbar artery *n* : any artery of the usu. four pairs that arise from the back of the aorta opposite the lumbar vertebrae and supply the muscles of the loins, the skin of the sides of the abdomen, and the spinal cord

lumbar nerve *n* : any nerve of the five pairs of spinal nerves of the lumbar region of which one on each side passes out below each lumbar vertebra and the upper four unite by connecting branches into a lumbar plexus

lumbar plexus *n* : a plexus embedded in the psoas major and formed by the anterior or ventral divisions of the four upper lumbar nerves of which the first is usu. supplemented by a communication from the twelfth thoracic nerve

lumbar puncture *n* : puncture of the subarachnoid space in the lumbar region of the spinal cord to withdraw cerebrospinal fluid or inject anesthetic drugs — called also *spinal tap*

lumbar vein *n* : any vein of the four pairs collecting blood from the muscles and integument of the loins, the walls of the abdomen, and adjacent parts and emptying into the dorsal part of the inferior vena cava — see ASCENDING LUMBAR VEIN

lumbar vertebra *n* : any of the five vertebrae situated between the thoracic vertebrae above and the sacrum below

lumbo- — see LUMB-

lum·bo·dor·sal fascia \ˌləm-bō-ˈdȯr-səl-\ *n* : a large fascial band on each side of the back extending from the iliac crest and the sacrum to the ribs and the intermuscular septa of the muscles of the neck

lumborum — see ILIOCOSTALIS LUMBORUM, QUADRATUS LUMBORUM

lum·bo·sa·cral \ˌləm-bō-ˈsa-krəl, -ˈsā-\ *adj* : of, relating to, or being the lumbar and sacral regions or parts

lumbosacral joint *n* : the joint between the fifth lumbar vertebra and the sacrum

lumbosacral plexus *n* : a network of nerves comprising the lumbar plexus and the sacral plexus

lumbosacral trunk *n* : a nerve trunk formed by the fifth lumbar nerve and a smaller branch of the fourth lumbar nerve and connecting the lumbar plexus to the sacral plexus

lum·bri·ca·lis \ˌləm-brə-ˈkā-ləs\ *n, pl* **-les** \-ˌlēz\ **1** : any of the four small muscles of the palm of the hand that arise from tendons of the flexor digitorum profundus, are inserted at the base of the digit to which the tendon passes, and flex the proximal phalanx and extend the two distal phalanges of each finger **2** : any of four small muscles of the foot homologous to the lumbricales of the hand that arise from tendons of the flexor digitorum longus and are inserted into the first phalanges of the four small toes of which they flex the proximal phalanges and extend the two distal phalanges — **lum·bri·cal** \ˈləm-bri-kəl\ *adj*

lu·men \ˈlü-mən\ *n, pl* **lu·mi·na** \-mə-nə\ *or* **lumens** **1** : the cavity of a tubular organ or part ⟨the ∼ of a blood vessel⟩ **2** : the bore of a tube (as of a catheter) — **lu·mi·nal** *also* **lu·me·nal** \ˈlü-mən-ᵊl\ *adj*

Lu·mi·nal \ˈlü-mə-ˌnal, -ˌnȯl\ *trademark* — used for a preparation of the sodium salt of phenobarbital

lump \ˈləmp\ *n* **1** : a piece or mass of indefinite size and shape **2** : an abnormal mass or swelling

lump·ec·to·my \ˌləm-ˈpek-tə-mē\ *n, pl* **-mies** : excision of a breast tumor with a limited amount of associated tissue — called also *tylectomy*

lumpy jaw \ˈləm-pē-\ *also* **lump jaw** *n*

: ACTINOMYCOSIS; *esp* : actinomycosis of the head in cattle

lu·na·cy \ˈlü-nə-sē\ *n, pl* **-cies** : INSANITY; *also* : intermittent insanity once believed to be related to phases of the moon

lu·nar caustic \ˈlü-nər-, -ˌnär-\ *n* : silver nitrate esp. when fused and molded into sticks or small cones for use as a caustic

lu·nate bone \ˈlü-ˌnāt-\ *n* : a crescent-shaped bone that is the middle bone in the proximal row of the carpus between the scaphoid bone and the triquetral bone and that has a deep concavity on the distal surface articulating with the capitate — called also *lunate, semilunar bone*

lunate sulcus *n* : a sulcus of the cerebrum on the lateral part of the occipital lobe that marks the front boundary of the visual cortex

¹lu·na·tic \ˈlü-nə-ˌtik\ *adj* : INSANE

²lunatic *n* : an insane individual

Lu·nes·ta \lü-ˈnes-tə\ *trademark* — used for a preparation of eszopiclone

lung \ˈləŋ\ *n* **1** : one of the usu. two compound saccular organs that constitute the basic respiratory organ of air-breathing vertebrates, that normally occupy the entire lateral parts of the thorax and consist essentially of an inverted tree of intricately branched bronchioles communicating with thin-walled terminal alveoli swathed in a network of delicate capillaries where the actual gaseous exchange of respiration takes place, and that in humans are somewhat flattened with a broad base resting against the diaphragm and have the right lung divided into three lobes and the left into two lobes **2** : a mechanical device for regularly introducing fresh air into and withdrawing stale air from the lungs : RESPIRATOR — see IRON LUNG — **lunged** *adj*

lung·er \ˈləŋ-ər\ *n* : one affected with a chronic disease of the lungs; *esp* : one who is tubercular

lung fluke *n* : a fluke invading the lungs; *esp* : either of two forms of the genus *Paragonimus* (*P. westermani* and *P. kellicotti*) that produce lesions in humans which are comparable to those of tuberculosis and that are acquired by eating inadequately cooked freshwater crustaceans which act as intermediate hosts

lung·worm \ˈləŋ-ˌwərm\ *n* : any of various nematodes (esp. genera *Dictyocaulus* and *Metastrongylus* of the family Metastrongylidae) that infest the lungs and air passages of mammals

lu·nu·la \ˈlü-nyə-lə\ *n, pl* **-lae** \-ˌ(ˌ)lē\ *also* **-ˌlī** : a crescent-shaped body part: as **a** : the whitish mark at the base of a fingernail — called also *half-moon* **b** : the crescentic unattached border of a semilunar valve

lu·nule \ˈlü-ˌ(ˌ)nyül\ *n* : LUNULA

lupin • Lymnaea

418

lu·pine *also* **lu·pin** \ˈlü-pən\ *n* : any of a genus (*Lupinus*) of leguminous herbs some of which cause lupinosis

lu·pi·no·sis \ˌlü-pə-ˈnō-səs\ *n, pl* **-no·ses** \-ˌsēz\ : acute liver atrophy of domestic animals (as sheep) due to poisoning by ingestion of various lupines

lu·poid hepatitis \ˈlü-ˌpöid-\ *n* : chronic active hepatitis associated with lupus erythematosus

Lu·pron \ˈlü-ˌprän\ *trademark* — used for a preparation of the acetate of leuprolide

lu·pus \ˈlü-pəs\ *n* : any of several diseases (as lupus vulgaris or systemic lupus erythematosus) characterized by skin lesions

lupus band test *n* : a test to determine the presence of antibodies and complement deposits at the junction of the dermal and epidermal skin layers of patients with systemic lupus erythematosus

lupus er·y·the·ma·to·sus \ˌer-ə-ˌthē-mə-ˈtō-səs\ *n* : a disorder characterized by skin inflammation; *esp* : SYSTEMIC LUPUS ERYTHEMATOSUS

lupus erythematosus cell *n* : LE CELL

lupus ne·phri·tis \-ni-ˈfrī-təs\ *n* : glomerulonephritis associated with systemic lupus erythematosus that is typically characterized by proteinuria and hematuria and that often leads to renal failure

lupus vul·gar·is \-ˌvəl-ˈgar-əs\ *n* : a tuberculous disease of the skin marked by formation of soft brownish nodules with ulceration and scarring

LUQ *abbr* left upper quadrant (abdomen)

Lur·ide \ˈlür-ˌīd\ *trademark* — used for a preparation of sodium fluoride

lute- *or* **luteo-** *comb form* : corpus luteum ⟨*luteal*⟩ ⟨*luteo*lysis⟩

lutea — see MACULA LUTEA

lu·te·al \ˈlü-tē-əl\ *adj* : of, relating to, characterized by, or involving the corpus luteum ⟨~ activity⟩

lutecium *var of* LUTETIUM

lu·tein \ˈlü-tē-ən, ˈlü-ˌtēn\ *n* : an orange xanthophyll C₄₀H₅₆O₂ occurring in plants usu. with carotenes and chlorophylls and in animal fat, egg yolk, and the corpus luteum

lu·tein·i·za·tion \ˌlü-tē-ə-nə-ˈzā-shən, ˌlü-ˌtē-\ *n* : the process of forming corpora lutea — **lu·tein·ize** \ˈlü-tē-ə-ˌnīz, ˈlü-ˌtē-ˌnīz\ *vb*

luteinizing hormone *n* : a hormone that is secreted by the adenohypophysis of the pituitary gland and that in the female stimulates ovulation and the development of the corpora lutea and together with follicle-stimulating hormone the secretion of estrogen from developing ovarian follicles and in the male the development of interstitial tissue in the testis and the secretion of testosterone — abbr. *LH*; called also *interstitial-cell stimulating hormone, lutropin*

luteinizing hormone–releasing factor *n* : GONADOTROPIN-RELEASING HORMONE

luteinizing hormone–releasing hormone *n* : GONADOTROPIN-RELEASING HORMONE

lu·te·ol·y·sis \ˌlü-tē-ˈä-lə-səs\ *n, pl* **-y·ses** \-ˌsēz\ : regression of the corpus luteum — **lu·teo·lyt·ic** \ˌlü-tē-ə-ˈli-tik\ *adj*

lu·te·o·ma \ˌlü-tē-ˈō-mə\ *n, pl* **-mas** *also* **-ma·ta** \-mə-tə\ : an ovarian tumor derived from a corpus luteum — **lu·te·o·ma·tous** \-mə-təs\ *adj*

lu·teo·tro·pic \ˌlü-tē-ə-ˈtrō-pik, -ˈträ-\ *or* **lu·teo·tro·phic** \-ˈtrō-fik, -ˈträ-\ *adj* : acting on the corpora lutea

luteotropic hormone *n* : PROLACTIN

lu·teo·tro·pin \ˌlü-tē-ə-ˈtrō-pən\ *or* **lu·teo·tro·phin** \-fən\ *n* : PROLACTIN

lu·te·tium *also* **lu·te·cium** \lü-ˈtē-shē-əm, -shəm\ *n* : a metallic element — symbol *Lu*; see ELEMENT table

luteum — see CORPUS LUTEUM

lu·tro·pin \lü-ˈtrō-pən\ *n* : LUTEINIZING HORMONE

Lu·vox \ˈlü-ˌväks\ *trademark* — used for a preparation of the maleate of fluvoxamine

lux·a·tion \ˌlək-ˈsā-shən\ *n* : dislocation of an anatomical part — **lux·ate** \ˈlək-ˌsāt\ *vb*

LV *abbr* left ventricle

LVN \ˌel-(ˌ)vē-ˈen\ *n* : LICENSED VOCATIONAL NURSE

ly·can·thro·py \lī-ˈkan-thrə-pē\ *n, pl* **-pies** : a delusion that one has become or has assumed the characteristics of a wolf

Ly·ell's syndrome \ˈlī-əlz-\ *n* : TOXIC EPIDERMAL NECROLYSIS

Lyell, Alan (fl 1950–1972), British dermatologist.

ly·co·pene \ˈlī-kə-ˌpēn\ *n* : a red pigment C₄₀H₅₆ isomeric with carotene

ly·ing–in \ˌlī-iŋ-ˈin\ *n, pl* **lyings–in** *or* **lying–ins** : the state attending and consequent to childbirth : CONFINEMENT

Lyme arthritis \ˈlīm-\ *n* : arthritis as a symptom of or caused by Lyme disease; *also* : LYME DISEASE

Lyme disease *n* : an acute inflammatory disease that is usu. characterized initially by the skin lesion erythema migrans and by fatigue, fever, and chills and if left untreated may later manifest itself in cardiac and neurological disorders, joint pain, and arthritis and that is caused by a spirochete of the genus *Borrelia* (*B. burgdorferi*) transmitted by the bite of a tick esp. of the genus *Ixodes* (*I. scapularis* syn. *I. dammini* in the eastern and midwestern U.S., *I. pacificus* esp. in some parts of the Pacific coastal states of the U.S., and *I. ricinus* in Europe) — called also *Lyme, Lyme borreliosis*

Lym·naea \lim-ˈnē-ə, ˈlim-nē-ə\ *n* : a genus of snails (family Lymnaeidae) including some medically important intermediate hosts of flukes — compare FOSSARIA, GALBA

lymph \ˈlimf\ *n* : a usu. clear coagulable fluid that passes from intercellular spaces of body tissue into lymphatic vessels, is discharged into the blood by way of the thoracic duct, and resembles blood plasma in containing white blood cells but normally few red blood cells and no platelets — see CHYLE

lymph- *or* **lympho-** *comb form* : lymph : lymphatic tissue ⟨*lymph*edema⟩

lymph·ad·e·nec·to·my \ˌlim-ˌfad-ᵊn-ˈek-tə-mē\ *n, pl* **-mies** : surgical removal of a lymph node

lymph·ad·e·ni·tis \ˌlim-ˌfad-ᵊn-ˈī-təs\ *n* : inflammation of lymph nodes — **lymph·ad·e·nit·ic** \-ˈi-tik\ *adj*

lymph·ad·e·nop·a·thy \ˌlim-ˌfad-ᵊn-ˈä-pə-thē\ *n, pl* **-thies** : abnormal enlargement of the lymph nodes — **lymph·ad·e·no·path·ic** \ˌlim-ˌfad-ᵊn-ō-ˈpa-thik\ *adj*

lymphadenopathy–associated virus *n* : HIV-1

lymph·ad·e·no·sis \ˌlim-ˌfad-ᵊn-ˈō-səs\ *n, pl* **-no·ses** \-ˌsēz\ : any of certain abnormalities or diseases affecting the lymphatic system: as **a** : leukosis involving lymphatic tissues **b** : LYMPHOCYTIC LEUKEMIA

lymphangi- *or* **lymphangio-** *comb form* : lymphatic vessels ⟨*lymphangi*oma⟩

lymph·an·gi·ec·ta·sia \ˌlim-ˌfan-jē-ek-ˈtā-zhə, -zhē-ə\ *or* **lymph·an·gi·ec·ta·sis** \-ˈek-tə-səs\ *n, pl* **-ta·sias** *or* **-ta·ses** \-ˌsēz\ : dilatation of the lymphatic vessels

lymph·an·gio·gram \(ˌ)lim-ˈfan-jē-ə-ˌgram\ *n* : an X-ray picture made by lymphangiography

lymph·an·gi·og·ra·phy \ˌlim-ˌfan-jē-ˈä-grə-fē\ *n, pl* **-phies** : X-ray depiction of lymphatic vessels and lymph nodes after use of a radiopaque material — called also *lymphography* — **lymph·an·gio·graph·ic** \ˌlim-ˌfan-jē-ə-ˈgra-fik\ *adj*

lymph·an·gi·o·ma \ˌlim-ˌfan-jē-ˈō-mə\ *n, pl* **-mas** *also* **-ma·ta** \-mə-tə\ : a tumor formed of dilated lymphatic vessels

lymph·an·gio·sar·co·ma \ˌlim-ˌfan-jē-ō-(ˌ)sär-ˈkō-mə\ *n, pl* **-mas** *also* **-ma·ta** \-mə-tə\ : a sarcoma arising from the endothelial cells of lymphatic vessels

lymph·an·gi·ot·o·my \ˌlim-ˌfan-jē-ˈä-tə-mē\ *n, pl* **-mies** : incision of a lymphatic vessel

lymph·an·gi·tis \ˌlim-fan-ˈjī-təs\ *n, pl* **-git·i·des** \-ˈji-tə-ˌdēz\ : inflammation of the lymphatic vessels

¹lym·phat·ic \lim-ˈfa-tik\ *adj* **1** : of, relating to, or produced by lymph, lymphoid tissue, or lymphocytes **2** : conveying lymph — **lym·phat·i·cal·ly** *adv*

²lymphatic *n* : a vessel that contains or conveys lymph, that originates as an interfibrillar or intercellular cleft or space in a tissue or organ, and that if small has no distinct walls or walls composed only of endothelial cells and if large resembles a vein in structure — called also *lymphatic vessel, lymph vessel;* see THORACIC DUCT

lymphatic capillary *n* : any of the smallest lymphatic vessels that are blind at one end and collect lymph in organs and tissues — called also *lymph capillary*

lymphatic duct *n* : any of the lymphatic vessels that are part of the system collecting lymph from the lymphatic capillaries and draining it into the subclavian veins by way of the right lymphatic duct and the thoracic duct — called also *lymph duct*

lymphatic leukemia *n* : LYMPHOCYTIC LEUKEMIA

lym·phat·i·co·ve·nous \lim-ˌfa-ti-kō-ˈvē-nəs\ *adj* : of, relating to, or connecting the veins and lymphatic vessels ⟨~ anastomoses⟩

lymphatic system *n* : the part of the circulatory system that is concerned esp. with scavenging fluids and proteins that have escaped from cells and tissues and returning them to the blood, with the phagocytic removal of cellular debris and foreign material, and with immune responses, and that consists esp. of the thymus, spleen, tonsils, lymph, lymph nodes, lymphatic vessels, lymphocytes, and bone marrow — called also *lymphoid system, lymph system*

lymphatic vessel *n* : LYMPHATIC

lymph capillary *n* : LYMPHATIC CAPILLARY

lymph duct *n* : LYMPHATIC DUCT

lymph·ede·ma \ˌlim-fi-ˈdē-mə\ *n* : edema due to faulty lymphatic drainage — **lymph·edem·a·tous** \ˌlim-fi-ˈde-mə-təs\ *adj*

lymph follicle *n* : LYMPH NODE; *esp* : LYMPH NODULE

lymph gland *n* : LYMPH NODE

lymph node *n* : any of the rounded masses of lymphoid tissue that are surrounded by a capsule of connective tissue, are distributed along the lymphatic vessels, and contain numerous lymphocytes which filter the flow of lymph passing through the node — called also *lymph gland*

lymph nodule *n* : a small simple lymph node

lympho- — see LYMPH-

lym·pho·blast \ˈlim-fə-ˌblast\ *n* : a lymphocyte that has enlarged following stimulation by an antigen, has the capacity to recognize the stimulating antigen, and is undergoing proliferation and differentiation either to an effector state in which it functions to eliminate the antigen or to a memory state in which it functions to recognize the future reappearance of the antigen — called also *immunoblast* — **lym·pho·blas·tic** \ˌlim-fə-ˈblas-tik\ *adj*

lymphoblastic leukemia *n* : lymphocytic leukemia characterized by an abnormal increase in the number of lymphoblasts; *specif* : ACUTE LYMPHOBLASTIC LEUKEMIA

lym·pho·blas·toid \lim-fə-'blas-,tóid\ *adj* : resembling a lymphoblast

lym·pho·blas·to·ma \lim-fə-,blas-'tō-mə\ *n, pl* **-mas** *also* **-ma·ta** \-mə-tə\ : any of several diseases of lymph nodes marked by the formation of tumorous masses composed of mature or immature lymphocytes

lym·pho·blas·to·sis \-,blas-'tō-səs\ *n, pl* **-to·ses** \-,sēz\ : the presence of lymphoblasts in the peripheral blood

lym·pho·cele \'lim-fə-,sēl\ *n* : a cyst containing lymph

lym·pho·cyte \'lim-fə-,sīt\ *n* : any of the colorless weakly motile cells originating from stem cells and differentiating in lymphoid tissue (as of the thymus or bone marrow) that are the typical cellular elements of lymph, include the cellular mediators of immunity, and constitute 20 to 30 percent of the white blood cells of normal human blood — see B CELL, T CELL — **lym·pho·cyt·ic** \,lim-fə-'si-tik\ *adj*

lymphocyte transformation *n* : a transformation caused in lymphocytes by a mitosis-inducing agent (as phytohemagglutinin) or by a second exposure to an antigen and characterized by an increase in size and in the amount of cytoplasm, by visibility of nucleoli in the nucleus, and after about 72 hours by a marked resemblance to blast cells

lymphocytic cho·rio·men·in·gi·tis \-,kòr-ē-ō-,me-nən-'jī-təs\ *n* : an acute disease caused by a virus of the genus *Arenavirus* (species *Lymphocytic choriomeningitis virus*), characterized by fever, nausea and vomiting, headache, stiff neck, and slow pulse, and transmitted esp. by rodents

lymphocytic leukemia *n* : leukemia of either of two types marked by an abnormal increase in the number of white blood cells (as lymphocytes) which accumulate in bone marrow, lymphoid tissue (as of the lymph nodes and spleen), and circulating blood — called also *lymphatic leukemia, lymphoid leukemia;* see ACUTE LYMPHOBLASTIC LEUKEMIA, CHRONIC LYMPHOCYTIC LEUKEMIA

lym·pho·cy·to·pe·nia \,lim-fō-,sī-tə-'pē-nē-ə\ *n* : a decrease in the normal number of lymphocytes in the circulating blood

lym·pho·cy·to·poi·e·sis \-,pói-'ē-səs\ *n, pl* **-e·ses** \-,sēz\ : formation of lymphocytes usu. in the lymph nodes

lym·pho·cy·to·sis \,lim-fə-,sī-'tō-səs, -fə-sə-\ *n, pl* **-to·ses** \-,sēz\ : an increase in the number of lymphocytes in the blood usu. associated with chronic infections or inflammations — compare GRANULOCYTOSIS, MONOCYTOSIS

lym·pho·cy·to·tox·ic \,lim-fə-,sī-tə-'täk-sik\ *adj* 1 : being or relating to toxic effects on lymphocytes 2 : being toxic to lymphocytes — **lym·phocy·to·tox·ic·i·ty** \-täk-'si-sə-tē\ *n*

lym·phog·e·nous \lim-'fä-jə-nəs\ *also* **lym·pho·gen·ic** \,lim-fə-'je-nik\ *adj* 1 : producing lymph or lymphocytes 2 : arising, resulting from, or spread by way of lymphocytes or lymphatic vessels ⟨~ metastases⟩

lym·pho·gran·u·lo·ma \,lim-fō-,gran-yə-'lō-mə\ *n, pl* **-mas** *also* **-ma·ta** \-mə-tə\ 1 : a nodular swelling of a lymph node 2 : LYMPHOGRANULOMA VENEREUM — **lym·pho·gran·u·lo·mat·ous** \-'lō-mə-təs\ *adj*

lymphogranuloma in·gui·na·le \-,iŋ-gwə-'nä-lē, -'na-, -'nä-\ *n* : LYMPHOGRANULOMA VENEREUM

lym·pho·gran·u·lo·ma·to·sis \-,lō-mə-'tō-səs\ *n, pl* **-to·ses** \-,sēz\ : the development of benign or malignant lymphogranulomas in various parts of the body; *also* : a condition characterized by lymphogranulomas

lymphogranuloma ve·ne·re·um \-və-'nir-ē-əm\ *n* : a contagious venereal disease that is caused by various strains of a bacterium of the genus *Chlamydia* (*C. trachomatis*) and is marked by painful swelling and inflammation of the lymph nodes esp. in the region of the groin — called also *lymphogranuloma inguinale, lymphopathia venereum*

lym·phog·ra·phy \lim-'fä-grə-fē\ *n, pl* **-phies** : LYMPHANGIOGRAPHY — **lym·pho·graph·ic** \,lim-fə-'gra-fik\ *adj*

lym·phoid \'lim-,fóid\ *adj* 1 : of, relating to, or being tissue (as the lymph nodes or thymus) containing lymphocytes 2 : of, relating to, or resembling lymph

lymphoid cell *n* : any of the cells responsible for the production of immunity mediated by cells or antibodies and including lymphocytes, lymphoblasts, and plasma cells

lymphoid leukemia *n* : LYMPHOCYTIC LEUKEMIA

lymphoid system *n* : LYMPHATIC SYSTEM

lym·pho·kine \'lim-fə-,kīn\ *n* : any of various substances (an interleukin) of low molecular weight that are not antibodies, are secreted by T cells in response to stimulation by antigens, and have a role (as the activation of macrophages or the enhancement or inhibition of antibody production) in cell-mediated immunity

lym·pho·kine–activated killer cell *n* : a lymphocyte that has been turned into a tumor-killing cell by being cultured with interleukin-2 — called also LAK

lym·pho·ma \lim-'fō-mə\ *n, pl* **-mas** *also* **-ma·ta** \-mə-tə\ : a usu. malignant tumor of lymphoid tissue — see HODGKIN'S DISEASE, NON-

HODGKIN'S LYMPHOMA — **lym·pho·ma·tous** \-mə-təs\ *adj*

lym·pho·ma·toid \lim-'fō-mə-ˌtóid\ *adj* : characterized by or resembling lymphomas ⟨a ~ tumor⟩

lymphomatosa — see STRUMA LYMPHOMATOSA

lym·pho·ma·to·sis \(ˌ)lim-ˌfō-mə-'tō-səs\ *n, pl* **-to·ses** \-ˌsēz\ : the presence of multiple lymphomas in the body

lym·pho·path·ia ve·ne·re·um \lim-fə-ˌpa-thē-ə-və-'nir-ē-əm\ *n* : LYMPHOGRANULOMA VENEREUM

lym·pho·pe·nia \lim-fə-'pē-nē-ə\ *n* : reduction in the number of lymphocytes circulating in the blood — **lym·pho·pe·nic** \-'pē-nik\ *adj*

lym·pho·plas·ma·cyt·ic *also* **lym·pho·plas·mo·cyt·ic** \-ˌplaz-mə-'si-tik\ *adj* : of, relating to, or consisting of lymphocytes and plasma cells

lymphoplasmacytic lymphoma *n* : a slowly progressive non-Hodgkin's lymphoma marked by proliferation of small lymphocytes, plasmacytoid lymphocytes, and plasma cells — see WALDENSTRÖM'S MACROGLOBULINEMIA

lym·pho·poi·e·sis \ˌlim-fə-pói-'ē-səs\ *n, pl* **-e·ses** \-ˌsēz\ : the formation of lymphocytes or lymphatic tissue — **lym·pho·poi·et·ic** \-'pói-'e-tik\ *adj*

lym·pho·pro·lif·er·a·tive \lim-fō-prə-'li-fə-ˌrā-tiv, -rə-tiv\ *adj* : of or relating to the proliferation of lymphoid tissue ⟨a ~ disorder⟩ — **lym·pho·pro·lif·er·a·tion** \prə-ˌli-fə-'rā-shən\ *n*

lym·pho·re·tic·u·lar \lim-fō-ri-'ti-kyə-lər\ *adj* : RETICULOENDOTHELIAL

lymphoreticular system *n* : RETICULOENDOTHELIAL SYSTEM

lym·pho·sar·co·ma \ˌlim-fō-sär-'kō-mə\ *n, pl* **-mas** *also* **-ma·ta** \-mə-tə\ : a malignant lymphoma that tends to metastasize freely

lym·pho·tox·in \lim-fō-'täk-sən\ *n* : a lymphokine that lyses various cells and esp. tumor cells — **lym·pho·tox·ic** \-'täk-sik\ *adj*

lym·pho·tro·pic \-'trō-pik, -'trä-pik\ *adj* : having an affinity for lymphocytes — see HUMAN T-CELL LYMPHOTROPIC VIRUS, HUMAN T-LYMPHOTROPIC VIRUS

lymph system *n* : LYMPHATIC SYSTEM

lymph vessel *n* : LYMPHATIC

lyn·es·tre·nol \lin-'es-trə-ˌnól\ *n* : a progestational steroid $C_{20}H_{28}O$ used esp. in birth control pills

ly·oph·i·lize \lī-'ä-fə-ˌlīz\ *vb* **-lized; -liz·ing** : FREEZE–DRY — **ly·oph·i·li·za·tion** *n*

ly·pres·sin \ˌlī-'pres-ᵊn\ *n* : a lysine-containing vasopressin $C_{46}H_{65}N_{13}$-$O_{12}S_2$ used esp. as a nasal spray in the control of diabetes insipidus

Lys *abbr* lysine

lys- *or* **lysi-** *or* **lyso-** *comb form* : lysis ⟨*lysin*⟩ ⟨*lyso*lecithin⟩

lyse \'līs, 'līz\ *vb* **lysed; lys·ing** : to cause to undergo lysis : produce lysis in ⟨cells were *lysed*⟩

ly·ser·gic acid \lə-'sər-jik-, (ˌ)lī-\ *n* : a crystalline acid $C_{16}H_{16}N_2O_2$ that is an ergot alkaloid; *also* : LSD

lysergic acid di·eth·yl·am·ide \-ˌdī-ˌe-thə-'la-ˌmīd\ *n* : LSD

ly·ser·gide \lə-'sər-ˌjīd, lī-\ *n* : LSD

lysi- — see LYS-

ly·sin \'līs-ᵊn\ *n* : a substance (as an antibody) capable of causing lysis

ly·sine \'lī-ˌsēn\ *n* : a crystalline essential amino acid $C_6H_{14}N_2O_2$ obtained from the hydrolysis of various proteins — abbr. Lys

lysine vasopressin *n* : LYPRESSIN

ly·sis \'lī-səs\ *n, pl* **ly·ses** \-ˌsēz\ 1 : the gradual decline of a disease process (as fever) — compare CRISIS 1 2 : a process of disintegration or dissolution (as of cells)

-ly·sis \l-ə-səs, 'lī-səs\ *n comb form, pl* **-ly·ses** \-ə-ˌsēz\ 1 : decomposition ⟨hydro*lysis*⟩ 2 : disintegration : breaking down ⟨auto*lysis*⟩ 3 **a** : relief or reduction ⟨neuro*lysis*⟩ **b** : detachment ⟨epidermo*lysis*⟩

lyso- — see LYS-

ly·so·gen \'lī-sə-jən\ *n* : a lysogenic bacterium or bacterial strain

ly·so·gen·ic \ˌlī-sə-'je-nik\ *adj* 1 : harboring a prophage as hereditary material ⟨~ bacteria⟩ 2 : TEMPERATE ⟨~ bacteria⟩ — **ly·sog·e·ny** \lī-'sä-jə-nē\ *n*

Ly·sol \'lī-ˌsól, -ˌsōl\ *trademark* — used for a disinfectant consisting of a brown solution containing cresols

ly·so·lec·i·thin \ˌlī-sə-'le-sə-thən\ *n* : LYSOPHOSPHATIDYLCHOLINE

ly·so·phos·pha·ti·dyl·cho·line \ˌlī-sō-ˌfäs-fə-ˌtīd-ᵊl-'kō-ˌlēn, -(ˌ)fäs-ˌfa-təd-ᵊl-\ *n* : a hemolytic substance produced by the removal of a fatty acid group from a lecithin

ly·so·some \'lī-sə-ˌsōm\ *n* : a saclike cellular organelle that contains various hydrolytic enzymes — **ly·so·som·al** \ˌlī-sə-'sō-məl\ *adj* — **ly·so·mal·ly** *adv*

ly·so·zyme \'lī-sə-ˌzīm\ *n* : a basic bacteriolytic protein that hydrolyzes peptidoglycan and is present in egg white and in saliva and tears — called also *muramidase*

-lyte \ˌlīt\ *n comb form* : substance capable of undergoing (such) decomposition ⟨electro*lyte*⟩

lyt·ic \'li-tik\ *adj* : of or relating to lysis or a lysin; *also* : productive of or effecting lysis (as of cells) ⟨~ viruses⟩ — **ly·ti·cal·ly** *adv*

-lyt·ic \'li-tik\ *adj suffix* : of, relating to, or effecting (such) decomposition ⟨hydro*lytic*⟩

m *abbr* **1** meter **2** molar **3** molarity **4** mole **5** muscle

M *abbr* [Latin *misce*] mix — used in writing prescriptions

MA *abbr* mental age

McArdle's disease, McBurney's point — see entries alphabetized as MC-

Mace \'mās\ *trademark* — used for a temporarily disabling liquid that when sprayed in the face of a person causes tears, dizziness, immobilization, and sometimes nausea

¹**mac·er·ate** \'ma-sə-,rāt\ *vb* **-at·ed; -at·ing** : to soften (as tissue) by steeping or soaking so as to separate into constituent elements — **mac·er·at·ed** \-,rā-təd\ *adj* — **mac·er·a·tion** \,ma-sə-'rā-shən\ *n*

²**mac·er·ate** \-rət\ *n* : a product of macerating : something prepared by maceration

Ma·cha·do-Jo·seph disease \mə-,shä-dō-'jō-səf-\ *n* : ataxia of any of several phenotypically variant forms that are inherited as autosomal dominant traits, have an onset usu. early in adult life, tend to occur in families of Portuguese and esp. Azorean ancestry, and are characterized by progressive degeneration of the central nervous system

  Machado, and **Joseph,** (*fl* 1970s), Azorean-Portuguese families.

Ma·chu·po virus \mä-'chü-pō-\ *n* : a virus of the genus *Arenavirus* (species *Machupo virus*) that causes a hemorrhagic fever endemic in Bolivia where its natural reservoir is a murid rodent (*Calomys callosus*)

mackerel shark *n* : any of a family (Lamnidae) of large aggressive sharks including the great white shark

Mac·leod's syndrome \mə-'klaùdz-\ *n* : abnormally increased translucence of one lung usu. accompanied by reduction in ventilation and in perfusion with blood

  Macleod, William Mathieson (1911–1977), British physician.

macr- *or* **macro-** *comb form* : large ⟨*macro*molecule⟩ ⟨*macro*cyte⟩

Mac·ra·can·tho·rhyn·chus \,ma-krə-,kan-thə-'riŋ-kəs\ *n* : a genus of intestinal worms (phylum Acanthocephala) including the common acanthocephalan (*M. hirudinaceus*) of swine

mac·ro·ad·e·no·ma \,ma-krō-,a-d⁰n-'ō-mə\ *n, pl* **-mas** *also* **-ma·ta** \-mə-tə\ : an adenoma of the pituitary gland that is greater than ten millimeters in diameter

mac·ro·al·bu·min·uria \,ma-krō-al-,byü-mə-'nùr-ē-ə, -'nyùr-\ *n* : albuminuria characterized by a relatively high rate of urinary excretion of albumin typically greater than 300 milligrams per 24-hour period — compare MICROALBUMINURIA

mac·ro·an·gi·op·a·thy \,ma-krō-,an-jē-'ä-pə-thē\ *n, pl* **-thies** : an angiopathy affecting blood vessels of large and medium size

Mac·rob·del·la \,ma-,kräb-'de-lə\ *n* : a genus of large bloodsucking leeches including one (*M. decora*) that has been used medicinally

mac·ro·bi·ot·ic \,ma-krō-bī-'ä-tik, -bē-\ *adj* : of, relating to, or being a diet that consists of whole cereals and grains supplemented esp. with beans and vegetables

mac·ro·bi·ot·ics \-tiks\ *n* : a macrobiotic dietary system

mac·ro·ceph·a·lous \,ma-krō-'se-fə-ləs\ *or* **mac·ro·ceph·al·ic** \-sə-'fa-lik\ *adj* : having or being an exceptionally large head or cranium — **mac·ro·ceph·a·ly** \-'se-fə-lē\ *n*

mac·ro·cy·clic \,ma-krō-'si-klik, -'sī-\ *adj* : containing or being a chemical ring that consists usu. of 15 or more atoms ⟨∼ esters⟩ — **macrocyclic** *n*

mac·ro·cyte \'ma-krə-,sīt\ *n* : an exceptionally large red blood cell occurring chiefly in anemias (as pernicious anemia) — called also *megalocyte*

mac·ro·cyt·ic \,ma-krə-'si-tik\ *adj* : of or relating to macrocytes; *specif, of an anemia* : characterized by macrocytes in the blood

mac·ro·cy·to·sis \,ma-krə-sī-'tō-səs\ *n, pl* **-to·ses** \-,sēz\ : the occurrence of macrocytes in the blood

mac·ro·ga·mete \,ma-krō-gə-'mēt, -'ga-,mēt\ *n* : the larger and usu. female gamete of a heterogamous organism — compare MICROGAMETE

mac·ro·ga·me·to·cyte \-gə-'mē-tə-,sīt\ *n* : a gametocyte producing macrogametes

mac·ro·gen·i·to·so·mia \,ma-krō-,je-ni-tə-'sō-mē-ə\ *n* : premature excessive development of the external genitalia

mac·ro·glia \ma-'krä-glē-ə, ,ma-krō-'glī-ə\ *n* : glia of ectodermal origin made up of astrocytes and oligodendrocytes — **mac·ro·gli·al** \-əl\ *adj*

mac·ro·glob·u·lin \,ma-krō-'glä-byə-lən\ *n* : a highly polymerized globulin (as IgM) of high molecular weight

mac·ro·glob·u·lin·ae·mia *chiefly Brit var of* MACROGLOBULINEMIA

mac·ro·glob·u·lin·emia \-,glä-byə-lə-'nē-mē-ə\ *n* : a disorder characterized by increased blood serum viscosity and the presence of macroglobulins in the serum — **mac·ro·glob·u·lin·emic** \-mik\ *adj*

mac·ro·glos·sia \,ma-krō-'glä-sē-ə, -'glò-\ *n* : pathological and commonly congenital enlargement of the tongue

mac·ro·lide \'ma-krə-,līd\ *n* : any of several antibiotics (as erythromycin) that are produced by actinomycetes of the genus *Streptomyces*

mac·ro·mol·e·cule \ˌma-krō-ˈmä-li-ˌkyül\ *n* : a very large molecule (as of a protein) built up from smaller chemical structures — compare MICROMOLECULE — **mac·ro·mo·lec·u·lar** \-mə-ˈle-kyə-lər\ *adj*

mac·ro·nu·tri·ent \-ˈnü-trē-ənt, ˈnyü-\ *n* : a chemical element or substance (as protein, carbohydrate, or fat) required in relatively large quantities in nutrition

mac·ro·or·chid·ism \-ˈȯr-kə-ˌdi-zəm\ *n* : the condition (as in fragile X syndrome) of having large testicles

mac·ro·phage \ˈma-krə-ˌfäj, -ˌfäzh\ *n* : a phagocytic tissue cell of the immune system that may be fixed or freely motile, is derived from a monocyte, functions in the destruction of foreign antigens (as bacteria and viruses), and serves as an antigen-presenting cell — see HISTIOCYTE, MONONUCLEAR PHAGOCYTE SYSTEM — **mac·ro·phag·ic** \ˌma-krə-ˈfa-jik\ *adj*

macrophage colony–stimulating factor *n* : a colony-stimulating factor produced by macrophages, endothelial cells, and fibroblasts that stimulates production and maturation of macrophages — abbr. *M-CSF*

mac·ro·scop·ic \ˌma-krə-ˈskä-pik\ *adj* : large enough to be observed by the naked eye — compare MICROSCOPIC 2 — **mac·ro·scop·i·cal·ly** *adv*

mac·ro·so·mia \ˌma-krə-ˈsō-mē-ə\ *n* : GIGANTISM — **mac·ro·so·mic** \-ˈsō-mik\ *adj*

mac·ro·struc·ture \ˈma-krō-ˌstrək-chər\ *n* : the structure (as of a body part) revealed by visual examination with little or no magnification — **mac·ro·struc·tur·al** \ˌma-krō-ˈstrək-chə-rəl, -shə-rəl\ *adj*

macul- *or* **maculo-** *comb form* : macule : macular and ⟨*maculo*papular⟩

mac·u·la \ˈma-kyə-lə\ *n, pl* **-lae** \-ˌlē, -ˌlī\ *also* **-las** 1 : a spot or blotch; *esp* : MACULE 2 2 : an anatomical structure having the form of a spot differentiated from surrounding tissues: as **a** : MACULA ACUSTICA **b** : MACULA LUTEA

macula acu·sti·ca \-ə-ˈküs-ti-kə\ *n, pl* **maculae acu·sti·cae** \-ti-ˌsē\ : either of two small areas of sensory hair cells in the ear that are covered with gelatinous material on which are located crystals or concretions of calcium carbonate and that are associated with the perception of equilibrium: **a** : one located in the saccule — called also *macula sacculi* **b** : one located in the utricle — called also *macula utriculi*

macula den·sa \-ˈden-sə\ *n* : a group of modified epithelial cells in the distal convoluted tubule of the kidney that control renin release by relaying information about the sodium concentration in the fluid passing through the convoluted tubule to the renin-producing juxtaglomerular cells of the afferent arteriole

macula lu·tea \-ˈlü-tē-ə-\ *n, pl* **maculae lu·te·ae** \-tē-ˌē, -tē-ˌī\ : a small yellowish area lying slightly lateral to the center of the retina that constitutes the region of maximum visual acuity and is made up almost wholly of retinal cones

mac·u·lar \ˈma-kyə-lər\ *adj* 1 : of, relating to, or characterized by a spot or spots ⟨a ∼ skin rash⟩ 2 : of, relating to, affecting, or mediated by the macula lutea ⟨∼ vision⟩

macular degeneration *n* : progressive deterioration of the macula lutea resulting in the gradual loss of the central part of the visual field; *esp* : AGE-RELATED MACULAR DEGENERATION

macula sac·cu·li \-ˈsa-kyə-ˌlī\ *n* : MACULA ACUSTICA a

macula utriculi \-yü-ˈtri-kyə-ˌlī\ *n* : MACULA ACUSTICA b

mac·ule \ˈma-(ˌ)kyül\ *n* 1 : MACULA 2 2 : a patch of skin that is altered in color but usu. not elevated

maculo- — see MACUL-

mac·u·lo·pap·u·lar \ˌma-kyə-(ˌ)lō-ˈpa-pyə-lər\ *adj* : combining the characteristics of macules and papules ⟨a ∼ rash⟩ ⟨a ∼ lesion⟩

mac·u·lo·pap·ule \-ˈpa-(ˌ)pyül\ *n* : a maculopapular elevation of the skin

mac·u·lop·a·thy \ˌma-kyə-ˈlä-pə-thē\ *n, pl* **-thies** : any pathological condition of the macula lutea of the eye

¹mad \ˈmad\ *adj* **mad·der; mad·dest** 1 : arising from, indicative of, or marked by mental disorder 2 : affected with rabies : RABID

Mad·a·gas·car periwinkle \ˌma-də-ˈgas-kər-\ *n* : ROSY PERIWINKLE

mad cow disease *n* : BOVINE SPONGIFORM ENCEPHALOPATHY

mad itch *n* : PSEUDORABIES

²mad·ness \ˈmad-nəs\ *n* 1 : INSANITY 2 : any of several ailments of animals marked by frenzied behavior; *specif* : RABIES

Ma·du·ra foot \ˈma-dyur-ə-, -dur-; mə-ˈ\ *n* : maduromycosis of the foot

mad·u·ro·my·co·sis \ˌma-dyu-rō-mī-ˈkō-səs, -du-\ *n, pl* **-co·ses** \-ˌsēz\ : a destructive chronic disease usu. restricted to the feet, marked by swelling and deformity resulting from the formation of granulomatous nodules and caused by various actinomycetes (as of the genus *Nocardia*) and fungi (as of the genus *Madurella*) — called also *mycetoma* — **mad·u·ro·my·cot·ic** \-ˈkä-tik\ *adj*

mae·di \ˈmī-thē\ *n* : ovine progressive pneumonia esp. as manifested by respiratory symptoms

maf·e·nide \ˈma-fə-ˌnīd\ *n* : a sulfonamide applied topically in the form of its acetate $C_7H_{10}N_2O_2S·C_2H_4O_2$ as an antibacterial ointment esp. in the

treatment of burns — see SULFAMY-
LON

ma·ga·i·nin \mə-'gā-(ə-)nən\ n : any of
a group of peptide antibiotics isolated
from the skin of frogs (esp. *Xenopus
laevis*)

mag·got \'ma-gət\ n : a soft-bodied
legless grub that is the larva of a
dipteran fly (as the housefly) and develops usu. in decaying organic matter or as a parasite in plants or
animals

magic bullet n : a substance or therapy capable of destroying pathogens
(as cancer cells) or providing an effective remedy for a disease or condition
without deleterious side effects

magic mushroom n : any fungus containing hallucinogenic alkaloids (as
psilocybin)

mag·ma \'mag-mə\ n : a suspension of
a large amount of precipitated material (as in milk of magnesia) in a small
volume of a watery vehicle

magna — see CISTERNA MAGNA

mag·ne·sia \mag-'nē-shə, -'nē-zhə\ n
: MAGNESIUM OXIDE

magnesia magma n : MILK OF MAG-
NESIA

mag·ne·sium \mag-'nē-zē-əm, -zhəm\
n : a silver-white light malleable ductile metallic element that occurs
abundantly in nature (as in bones) —
symbol *Mg*; see ELEMENT table

magnesium carbonate n : a carbonate of magnesium; *esp* : the very white
crystalline salt $MgCO_3$ used as an
antacid and laxative

magnesium chloride n : a bitter crystalline salt $MgCl_2$ used esp. to replenish body electrolytes

magnesium citrate n : a crystalline
salt $C_{12}H_{10}Mg_3O_{14}$ used in the form of
a lemony effervescent solution as a
saline laxative

magnesium hydroxide n : a slightly
alkaline crystalline compound
$Mg(OH)_2$ used as an antacid and laxative — see MILK OF MAGNESIA

magnesium oxide n : a white compound MgO used as an antacid and
mild laxative

magnesium sil·i·cate \-'si-lə-,kāt,
-kət\ n : a silicate that is approximately $Mg_2Si_3O_8 \cdot nH_2O$ and that is
used chiefly in medicine as a gastric
antacid adsorbent and coating (as in
the treatment of ulcers)

magnesium sulfate n : a white anhy-
drous salt $MgSO_4$ that occurs naturally in hydrated form as Epsom salts
and that in the hydrated form
$MgSO_4 \cdot 7H_2O$ is used esp. to relieve
constipation, to treat magnesium deficiency, and to control convulsions
(as those associated with eclampsia)

magnetic field n : the portion of space
near a magnetic body or a current-
carrying body in which the magnetic
forces due to the body or current can
be detected

magnetic resonance n : the excitation of particles (as atomic nuclei or
electrons) in a magnetic field by exposure to electromagnetic radiation
of a specific frequency — abbr. *MR;*
see NUCLEAR MAGNETIC RESONANCE

magnetic resonance angiography n
: magnetic resonance imaging used to
visualize noninvasively the heart,
blood vessels, or blood flow in the circulatory system — abbr. *MRA;* called
also *MR angiography*

magnetic resonance imaging n : a
noninvasive diagnostic technique that
produces computerized images of internal body tissues and is based on
nuclear magnetic resonance of atoms
within the body induced by the application of radio waves — abbr. *MRI*

magnetic resonance spectroscopy n
: a noninvasive technique that is similar to magnetic resonance imaging
but uses a stronger field and is used to
monitor body chemistry (as in metabolism or blood flow) — abbr. *MRS*

mag·ne·to·en·ceph·a·log·ra·phy
\mag-,nē-tō-in-,se-fə-'lä-grə-fē\ n, pl
-phies : a noninvasive technique that
detects and records the magnetic field
associated with electrical activity in
the brain

mag·ni·fi·ca·tion \,mag-nə-fə-'kā-
shən\ n : the apparent enlargement of
an object by an optical instrument
that is the ratio of the dimensions of
an image formed by the instrument to
the corresponding dimensions of the
object — called also *power* — **mag·
ni·fy** \'mag-nə-,fī\ vb

mag·no·cel·lu·lar \,mag-nō-'sel-yə-lər\
adj : being or containing neurons with
large cell bodies — compare PARVO-
CELLULAR

magnum — see FORAMEN MAGNUM

magnus — see ADDUCTOR MAGNUS

ma huang \'mä-'hwäŋ\ n **1** : any of
several eastern Asian plants of the
genus *Ephedra* (esp. *E. sinica*) having
stems and roots yielding ephedrine **2**
: EPHEDRA 2

maid·en·head \'mād-ᵊn-,hed\ n : HY-
MEN

maim \'mām\ vb **1** : to commit the
felony of mayhem upon **2** : to wound
seriously : MUTILATE, DISABLE

main-line \'mān-,līn\ vb **-lined; -lin-
ing** *slang* : to inject a narcotic drug
(as heroin) into a vein

main·stream \-,strēm\ adj : relating to
or being tobacco smoke that is drawn
(as from a cigarette) directly into the
mouth of the smoker and is usu. inhaled into the lungs — compare SIDE-
STREAM

main·te·nance \'mānt-ᵊn-əns\ adj : designed or adequate to maintain a patient in a stable condition : serving to
maintain a gradual process of healing
or to prevent a relapse ⟨a ∼ dose⟩

ma·jor \'mā-jər\ adj : involving grave
risk : SERIOUS ⟨a ∼ illness⟩ — compare MINOR

majora — see LABIA MAJORA

major basic protein *n* : a toxic cationic protein that is the principal protein found in the granules of eosinophils and that is capable of damaging tissue (as of the eye) if released into extracellular spaces

major depression *n* **1** : MAJOR DEPRESSIVE DISORDER **2** : an episode of depression characteristic of major depressive disorder

¹**major depressive** *adj* : of, relating to, or affected with major depressive disorder

²**major depressive** *n* : an individual affected by or subject to episodes of major depressive disorder

major depressive disorder *n* : a mood disorder having a clinical course involving one or more episodes of serious psychological depression that last two or more weeks each and do not have intervening episodes of mania or hypomania

major histocompatibility complex *n* : a group of genes that function esp. in determining the histocompatibility antigens found on cell surfaces and that in humans comprise the alleles occurring at four loci on the short arm of chromosome 6 — abbr. *MHC*

major labia *n pl* : LABIA MAJORA

major–medical *adj* : of, relating to, or being a form of insurance designed to pay all or part of the medical bills of major illnesses usu. after deduction of a fixed initial sum

major surgery *n* : surgery involving a risk to the life of the patient; *specif* : an operation upon an organ within the cranium, chest, abdomen, or pelvic cavity — compare MINOR SURGERY

mal \'mäl, 'mȧl\ *n* : DISEASE, SICKNESS

mal- *comb form* **1** : bad ⟨*mal*practice⟩ **2 a** : abnormal ⟨*mal*formation⟩ **b** : abnormally ⟨*mal*formed⟩ **3 a** : inadequate ⟨*mal*adjustment⟩ **b** : inadequately ⟨*mal*nourished⟩

mal·ab·sorp·tion \ˌma-lȧb-'sȯrp-shən, -'zȯrp-\ *n* : faulty absorption of nutrient materials from the digestive tract — **mal·ab·sorp·tive** \-tiv\ *adj*

malabsorption syndrome *n* : a syndrome resulting from malabsorption that is typically characterized by weakness, diarrhea, muscle cramps, edema, and loss of weight

malac- *or* **malaco-** *comb form* : soft ⟨*malaco*plakia⟩

ma·la·cia \mə-'lā-shə, -shē-ə\ *n* : abnormal softening of a tissue — often used in combination ⟨osteo*malacia*⟩ — **ma·lac·ic** \-sik\ *adj*

mal·a·co·pla·kia *also* **mal·a·ko·pla·kia** \ˌma-lə-kō-'plā-kē-ə\ *n* : inflammation of the mucous membrane of a hollow organ (as the urinary bladder) characterized by the formation of soft granulomatous lesions

mal·ad·ap·ta·tion \ˌmal-ˌa-ˌdap-'tā-shən\ *n* : poor or inadequate adaptation ⟨psychological ∼⟩ — **mal·adap-**

tive \ˌma-lə-'dap-tiv\ *adj* — **mal·adap·tive·ly** *adv*

mal·a·die de Ro·ger \ˌma-lə-'dē-də-rō-'zhā\ *n* : a small usu. asymptomatic ventricular septal defect

    Roger, Henri–Louis (1809–1891), French physician.

mal·ad·just·ment \ˌma-lə-'jəst-mənt\ *n* : poor, faulty, or inadequate adjustment — **mal·ad·just·ed** \-'jəs-təd\ *adj*

mal·ad·min·is·tra·tion \ˌma-ləd-ˌmi-nə-'strā-shən\ *n* : incorrect administration (as of a drug)

mal·a·dy \'ma-lə-dē\ *n, pl* **-dies** : DISEASE, SICKNESS ⟨a fatal ∼⟩

mal·aise \mə-'lāz, ma-, -'lez\ *n* : an indefinite feeling of debility or lack of health often indicative of or accompanying the onset of an illness

mal·align·ment \ˌma-lə-'līn-mənt\ *n* : incorrect or imperfect alignment (as of teeth) — **mal·aligned** \-'līnd\ *adj*

ma·lar \'mā-lər, -ˌlär\ *adj* : of or relating to the cheek, the side of the head, or the zygomatic bone

malar bone *n* : ZYGOMATIC BONE — called also *malar*

malari- *or* **malario-** *comb form* : malaria ⟨*malario*logy⟩

ma·lar·ia \mə-'ler-ē-ə\ *n* **1** : an acute or chronic disease caused by the presence of sporozoan parasites of the genus *Plasmodium* in the red blood cells, transmitted from an infected to an uninfected individual by the bite of anopheline mosquitoes, and characterized by periodic attacks of chills and fever that coincide with mass destruction of blood cells and the release of toxic substances by the parasite at the end of each reproductive cycle — see FALCIPARUM MALARIA, VIVAX MALARIA **2** : any of various diseases of birds and mammals that are more or less similar to malaria of humans and are caused by blood protozoans — **ma·lar·i·al** \-əl\ *adj*

ma·lar·i·ae malaria \mə-'ler-ē-ˌē-\ *n* : malaria caused by a malaria parasite (*Plasmodium malariae*) and marked by recurrence of paroxysms at 72-hour intervals — called also *quartan malaria*

malarial mosquito *or* **malaria mosquito** *n* : a mosquito of the genus *Anopheles* (esp. *A. quadrimaculatus*) that transmits the malaria parasite

malaria parasite *n* : a protozoan of the sporozoan genus *Plasmodium* that is transmitted to humans or to certain other mammals or birds by the bite of a mosquito in which its sexual reproduction takes place, that multiplies asexually in the vertebrate host by schizogony in the red blood cells or in certain tissue cells, and that causes destruction of red blood cells and the febrile disease malaria — see MEROZOITE, PHANEROZOITE, SCHIZONT, SPOROZOITE

ma·lar·i·ol·o·gy \mə-ˌler-ē-'ä-lə-jē\ n, pl **-gies** : the scientific study of malaria — **ma·lar·i·ol·o·gist** \-jist\ n

ma·lar·i·ous \mə-'ler-ē-əs\ adj : characterized by the presence of or infected with malaria ⟨∼ regions⟩

Mal·as·se·zia \ˌma-lə-'sä-zē-ə\ n : a genus of lipophilic typically nonpathogenic yeastlike imperfect fungi including one (M. furfur syn. Pityrosporum oribiculare) that causes tinea versicolor and another (M. ovalis syn. Pityrosporum ovale) that is associated with seborrheic dermatitis

ma·late \'ma-ˌlāt, 'mā-\ n : a salt or ester of malic acid

mal·a·thi·on \ˌma-lə-'thī-ən, -ˌän\ n : an insecticide $C_{10}H_{19}O_6PS_2$ that is less toxic to mammals than parathion

mal del pin·to \ˌmal-del-'pin-tō\ n : PINTA

mal de mer \ˌmal-də-'mer\ n : SEA-SICKNESS

mal·des·cent \ˌmal-di-'sent\ n : an improper or incomplete descent of a testis into the scrotum — **mal·des·cend·ed** \-'sen-dəd\ adj

mal·de·vel·op·ment \ˌmal-di-'ve-ləp-mənt\ n : abnormal growth or development : DYSPLASIA

¹**male** \'māl\ n : an individual that produces small usu. motile gametes (as sperm or spermatozoa) which fertilize the eggs of a female

²**male** adj : of, relating to, or being the sex that produces gametes which fertilize the eggs of a female

ma·le·ate \'mā-lē-ˌāt, -lē-ət\ n : a salt or ester of maleic acid

male bonding n : bonding between males through shared activities excluding females

male climacteric n : ANDROPAUSE

ma·le·ic acid \mə-'lē-ik-, -'lā-\ n : an isomer of fumaric acid

male menopause n : ANDROPAUSE

male–pattern baldness n : androgenetic alopecia in the male characterized by loss of hair on the crown and temples

mal·for·ma·tion \ˌmal-fòr-'mā-shən\ n : irregular, anomalous, abnormal, or faulty formation or structure — **mal·formed** \(ˌ)mal-'fòrmd\ adj

mal·func·tion \(ˌ)mal-'fəŋk-shən\ vb : to function imperfectly or badly : fail to operate in the normal or usual manner — **malfunction** n

ma·lic acid \'ma-lik, 'mā-\ n : any of three optical isomers of an acid $C_4H_6O_5$; esp : the one formed as an intermediate in the Krebs cycle

maligna — see LENTIGO MALIGNA

ma·lig·nan·cy \mə-'lig-nən-sē\ n, pl **-cies** 1 : the quality or state of being malignant **2 a** : exhibition (as by a tumor) of malignant qualities : VIRULENCE **b** : a malignant tumor

ma·lig·nant \-nənt\ adj 1 : tending to produce death or deterioration; esp : tending to infiltrate, metastasize, and terminate fatally ⟨∼ tumors⟩ —

compare BENIGN 1 **2** : of unfavorable prognosis : not responding favorably to treatment ⟨a ∼ trend⟩

malignant catarrhal fever n : an acute infectious often fatal disease esp. of cattle and deer that is caused by several herpesviruses (genus Rhadinovirus) and is characterized esp. by fever, depression, enlarged lymph nodes, and discharge from the eyes and nose — called also catarrhal fever, malignant catarrh

malignant edema n : an acute often fatal toxemia of wild and domestic animals that follows wound infection by an anaerobic toxin-producing bacterium of the genus Clostridium (C. septicum)

malignant hypertension n : essential hypertension characterized by acute onset, severe symptoms, rapidly progressive course, and poor prognosis

malignant hyperthermia n : a rare inherited condition characterized by a rapid, extreme, and often fatal rise in body temperature following the administration of general anesthesia

malignant malaria n : FALCIPARUM MALARIA

malignant malnutrition n : KWASHIORKOR

malignant melanoma n : MELANOMA 2

malignant pustule n : localized anthrax of the skin taking the form of a pimple surrounded by a zone of edema and hyperemia and tending to become necrotic and ulcerated

malignant tertian malaria n : FALCIPARUM MALARIA

malignant transformation n : the transformation that a cell undergoes to become a rapidly dividing tumor-producing cell; also : the transformation of a mass of cells or a tissue into a rapidly growing tumor

ma·lig·ni·za·tion \mə-ˌlig-nə-'zā-shən\ n : a process or instance of becoming malignant ⟨∼ of a tumor⟩

ma·lin·ger \mə-'liŋ-gər\ vb **-gered**; **-ger·ing** : to pretend or exaggerate incapacity or illness (as to avoid duty or work) — **ma·lin·ger·er** \-ər\ n

mal·le·o·lar \mə-'lē-ə-lər\ adj : of or relating to a malleolus ⟨∼ fracture⟩

mal·le·o·lus \mə-'lē-ə-ləs\ n, pl **-li** \-ˌlī\ : an expanded projection or process at the distal extremity of each bone of the leg: **a** : the expanded lower extremity of the fibula situated on the lateral side of the leg at the ankle — called also external malleolus, lateral malleolus **b** : a strong pyramid-shaped process of the tibia that projects distally on the medial side of its lower extremity at the ankle — called also internal malleolus, medial malleolus

mal·let finger \'ma-lət-\ n : involuntary flexion of the distal phalanx of a finger caused by avulsion of the extensor tendon

mal·le·us \\'ma-lē-əs\\ *n, pl* **mal·lei** \\-lē-ˌī, -lē-ˌē\\ : the outermost of the chain of three ossicles in the middle ear consisting of a head, neck, short process, long process, and handle with the short process and handle being fastened to the tympanic membrane and the head articulating with the head of the incus — called also *hammer*

mal·nour·ished \\(ˌ)mal-'nər-isht\\ *adj* : UNDERNOURISHED

mal·nour·ish·ment \\-'nər-ish-mənt\\ *n* : MALNUTRITION

mal·nu·tri·tion \\ˌmal-nü-'tri-shən, -nyü-\\ *n* : faulty nutrition due to inadequate or unbalanced intake of nutrients or their impaired assimilation or utilization — **mal·nu·tri·tion·al** \\-'əl\\ *adj*

mal·oc·clu·sion \\ˌma-lə-'klü-zhən\\ *n* : improper occlusion; *esp* : abnormality in the coming together of teeth — **mal·oc·clud·ed** \\-'klü-dəd\\ *adj*

Mal·pi·ghi·an body \\mal-'pi-gē-ən-, -'pē-\\ *n* : RENAL CORPUSCLE; *also* : MALPIGHIAN CORPUSCLE 2

Malpighi \\mäl-'pē-gē\\, **Marcello (1628–1694),** Italian anatomist.

Malpighian corpuscle *n* 1 : RENAL CORPUSCLE 2 : any of the small masses of adenoid tissue formed around the branches of the splenic artery in the spleen

Malpighian layer *n* : the deepest part of the epidermis that consists of the stratum basale and stratum spinosum and is the site of mitotic activity

Malpighian pyramid *n* : RENAL PYRAMID

mal·posed \\ˌmal-'pōzd\\ *adj* : characterized by malposition \\~ teeth\\

mal·po·si·tion \\ˌmal-pə-'zi-shən\\ *n* : wrong or faulty position — **mal·po·si·tion·ing** \\-shə-niŋ\\ *n*

mal·prac·tice \\(ˌ)mal-'prak-təs\\ *n* : a dereliction of professional duty or a failure to exercise an accepted degree of professional skill or learning by a physician rendering professional services which results in injury, loss, or damage — **malpractice** *vb*

mal·pre·sen·ta·tion \\ˌmal-ˌprē-zen-'tā-shən, -ˌpre-\\ *n* : abnormal presentation of the fetus at birth

mal·ro·ta·tion \\ˌmal-rō-'tā-shən\\ *n* : improper rotation of a bodily part and esp. of the intestines — **mal·ro·tat·ed** \\-'rō-ˌtāt-əd\\ *adj*

MALT *abbr* mucosa-associated lymphoid tissue

Mal·ta fever \\'mȯl-tə-\\ *n* : BRUCELLOSIS a

malt·ase \\'mȯl-ˌtās, -ˌtāz\\ *n* : an enzyme that catalyzes the hydrolysis of maltose to glucose

malt·ose \\'mȯl-ˌtōs, -ˌtōz\\ *n* : a crystalline dextrorotatory sugar $C_{12}H_{22}O_{11}$ formed esp. from starch by amylase (as in saliva)

mal·union \\ˌmal-'yün-yən\\ *n* : incomplete or faulty union (as of the fragments of a fractured bone)

mam·ba \\'mäm-bə, 'mam-\\ *n* : any of several venomous elapid snakes (genus *Dendroaspis*) of sub-Saharan Africa

mamillary, mamillated, mamillothalamic tract *var of* MAMMILLARY, MAMMILLATED, MAMMILLOTHALAMIC TRACT

mamm- *or* **mamma-** *or* **mammi-** *or* **mammo-** *comb form* : breast *mammogram*\\

mam·ma \\'ma-mə\\, *n, pl* **mam·mae** \\'ma-ˌmē, -ˌmī\\ : a mammary gland and its accessory parts

mam·mal \\'ma-məl\\ *n* : any of a class (Mammalia) of warm-blooded higher vertebrates (as dogs, cats, and humans) that nourish their young with milk secreted by mammary glands and have the skin more or less covered by hair — **mam·ma·li·an** \\mə-'mā-lē-ən, ma-\\ *adj or n*

mam·ma·plas·ty *or* **mam·mo·plas·ty** \\'ma-mə-ˌplas-tē\\ *n, pl* **-ties** : plastic surgery of the breast

[1]**mam·ma·ry** \\'ma-mə-rē\\ *adj* : of, relating to, lying near, or affecting the mammae

[2]**mammary** *n, pl* **-aries** : MAMMARY GLAND

mammary artery — see INTERNAL THORACIC ARTERY

mammary gland *n* : any of the large compound sebaceous glands that in female mammals are modified to secrete milk, are situated ventrally in pairs, and usu. terminate in a nipple

mam·mil·la·ry *or* **mam·il·la·ry** \\'ma-mə-ˌler-ē, ma-'mi-lə-rē\\ *adj* 1 : of, relating to, or resembling the breasts 2 : studded with breast-shaped protuberances

mammillary body *n* : either of two small rounded eminences on the underside of the brain behind the tuber cinereum

mam·mil·lat·ed *or* **mam·il·lat·ed** \\'ma-mə-ˌlā-təd\\ *adj* 1 : having nipples or small protuberances 2 : having the form of a bluntly rounded protuberance

mam·mil·lo·tha·lam·ic tract *or* **ma·mil·lo·tha·lam·ic tract** \\mə-ˌmi-lō-thə-'la-mik-\\ *n* : a bundle of nerve fibers that runs from the mammillary body to the anterior nucleus of the thalamus — called also *mammillothalamic fasciculus*

mammo- — see MAMM-

mam·mo·gram \\'ma-mə-ˌgram\\ *n* 1 : a photograph of the breasts made by X-rays 2 : the procedure for producing a mammogram

mam·mo·graph \\-ˌgraf\\ *n* : MAMMOGRAM 1

mam·mog·ra·pher \\ma-'mä-grə-fər\\ *n* : a physician or radiological technologist who prepares and interprets mammograms

mam·mog·ra·phy \ma-'mä-grə-fē\ *n, pl* **-phies** : X-ray examination of the breasts (as for early detection of cancer) — **mam·mo·graph·ic** \₁ma-mə-'gra-fik\ *adj*

mammoplasty *var of* MAMMAPLASTY

mam·mo·tro·pin \₁ma-mə-'trōp-ᵊn\ *n* : PROLACTIN

man \'man\ *n, pl* **men** \'men\ : a bipedal primate mammal of the genus *Homo* (*H. sapiens*) that is anatomically related to the great apes (family Pongidae) but is distinguished esp. by notable development of the brain with a resultant capacity for articulate speech and abstract reasoning, is usu. considered to form a variable number of freely interbreeding races, and is the sole living representative of the hominid family; *broadly* : any living or extinct hominid

managed care *n* : a system of providing health care (as by an HMO or a PPO) that is designed to control costs through managed programs in which the physician accepts constraints on the amount charged for medical care and the patient is limited in the choice of a physician

managed care organization *n* : a company (as an HMO or PPO) offering health-care plans with cost controls using managed care — called also *MCO*

man·age·ment \'ma-nij-mənt\ *n* : the whole system of care and treatment of a disease or a sick individual — **man·age** \'ma-nij\ *vb*

Man·del·amine \man-'de-lə-mēn\ *trademark* — used for a preparation of the mandelate of methenamine

man·del·ate \'man-də-₁lāt\ *n* : a salt or ester of mandelic acid

man·del·ic acid \man-'de-lik-\ *n* : an acid $C_8H_8O_3$ that is used chiefly in the form of its salts as a urinary antiseptic

man·di·ble \'man-də-bəl\ *n* 1 : JAW 1; *esp* : JAW 1b 2 : the lower jaw with its investing soft parts — **man·dib·u·lar** \man-'di-byə-lər\ *adj*

mandibular *or* **mandibuli-** *or* **mandibulo-** *comb form* : mandibular and ⟨*mandibulo*facial dysostosis⟩

mandibular arch *n* : the first branchial arch of the vertebrate embryo from which in humans are developed the lower lip, the mandible, the masticatory muscles, and the anterior part of the tongue

mandibular artery *n* : INFERIOR ALVEOLAR ARTERY

mandibular canal *n* : a bony canal within the mandible that gives passage to blood vessels and nerves supplying the lower teeth

mandibular foramen *n* : the opening on the medial surface of the ramus of the mandible that leads into the mandibular canal and transmits blood vessels and nerves supplying the lower teeth

mandibular fossa *n* : GLENOID FOSSA

mandibular nerve *n* : the one of the three major branches or divisions of the trigeminal nerve that supplies sensory fibers to the lower jaw, the floor of the mouth, the anterior two-thirds of the tongue, and the lower teeth and motor fibers to the muscles of mastication — called also *inferior maxillary nerve;* compare MAXILLARY NERVE, OPHTHALMIC NERVE

mandibular notch *n* : a curved depression on the upper border of the lower jaw between the coronoid process and the condyloid process — called also *sigmoid notch*

mandibuli-, mandibulo- — see MANDIBUL-

man·di·bu·lo·fa·cial dysostosis \man-₁di-byə-lō-'fā-shəl-\ *n* : a dysostosis of the face and lower jaw inherited as an autosomal dominant trait and characterized by bilateral malformations, deformities of the outer and middle ear, and a usu. smaller lower jaw — called also *Treacher Collins syndrome*

man–eat·er \'man-₁ē-tər\ *n* : one (as a great white shark) that has or is thought to have an appetite for human flesh — **man–eat·ing** *adj*

man–eating shark *n* : MACKEREL SHARK; *esp* : GREAT WHITE SHARK

ma·neu·ver \mə-'nü-vər, -'nyü-\ *n* 1 : a movement, procedure, or method performed to achieve a desired result and esp. to restore a normal physiological state or to promote normal function — see HEIMLICH MANEUVER, VALSALVA MANEUVER 2 : a manipulation to accomplish a change of position; *specif* : rotational or other movement applied to a fetus within the uterus to alter its position and facilitate delivery — see SCANZONI MANEUVER

man·ga·nese \'maŋ-gə-₁nēz, -₁nēs\ *n* : a grayish white usu. hard and brittle metallic element — symbol *Mn;* see ELEMENT table

mange \'mānj\ *n* : any of various persistent contagious skin diseases that are marked esp. by eczematous inflammation and loss of hair, that affect domestic animals or sometimes humans, and that are caused by a minute parasitic mite of *Sarcoptes, Psoroptes, Chorioptes,* or related genera which burrows in or lives on the skin or by one of the genus *Demodex* which lives in the hair follicles or sebaceous glands — see CHORIOPTIC MANGE, DEMODECTIC MANGE, SARCOPTIC MANGE, SCABIES

mange mite *n* : any of the small parasitic mites that infest the skin of animals and cause mange

man·go fly \'maŋ-gō-\ *n* : any of various horseflies of the genus *Chrysops* that are vectors of filarial worms

man·gy \'mān-jē\ *adj* **man·gi·er; -est** 1 : infected with mange ⟨a ∼ dog⟩ 2

: relating to, characteristic of, or resulting from mange ⟨a ∼ itch⟩

ma·nia \'mā-nē-ə, -nyə\ n : excitement of psychotic proportions manifested by mental and physical hyperactivity, disorganization of behavior, and elevation of mood; *specif* : the manic phase of bipolar disorder

ma·ni·ac \'mā-nē-ˌak\ n : an individual affected with or exhibiting insanity — **ma·ni·a·cal** \mə-'nī-ə-kəl\ *also* **ma·ni·ac** \'mā-nē-ak\ *adj*

¹**man·ic** \'ma-nik\ *adj* : affected with, relating to, or resembling mania — **man·i·cal·ly** *adv*

²**manic** n : an individual affected with mania

manic–depression n : BIPOLAR DISORDER

¹**manic–depressive** *adj* : characterized by or affected with either mania or depression or alternating mania and depression (as in bipolar disorder)

²**manic–depressive** n : a manic-depressive person

manic–depressive illness n : BIPOLAR DISORDER

manic–depressive psychosis n : BIPOLAR DISORDER

man·i·fes·ta·tion \ˌma-nə-fə-'stā-shən, -ˌfe-\ n : a perceptible, outward, or visible expression (as of a disease or abnormal condition)

manifest content n : the content of a dream as it is recalled by the dreamer in psychoanalysis — compare LATENT CONTENT

ma·nip·u·late \mə-'ni-pyə-ˌlāt\ vb **-lated; -lat·ing 1** : to treat or operate with the hands or by mechanical means esp. in a skillful manner **2** : to control or play upon by artful, unfair, or insidious means esp. to one's own advantage — **ma·nip·u·la·tive** \mə-'ni-pyə-ˌlā-tiv, -lə-\ *adj* — **ma·nip·u·la·tive·ness** n

ma·nip·u·la·tion \mə-ˌni-pyə-'lā-shən\ n **1** : the act, process, or an instance of manipulating esp. a body part by manual examination and treatment; *esp* : adjustment of faulty structural relationships by manual means (as in the reduction of fractures or dislocations) **2** : the condition of being manipulated

man·ner·ism \'ma-nə-ˌri-zəm\ n : a characteristic and often unconscious mode or peculiarity of action, bearing, or treatment; *esp* : any pointless and compulsive activity performed repeatedly

man·ni·tol \'ma-nə-ˌtòl, -ˌtōl\ n : a slightly sweet crystalline alcohol $C_6H_{14}O_6$ found in many plants and used esp. as a diuretic and in testing kidney function

mannitol hexa·ni·trate \-ˌhek-sə-'nī-ˌträt\ n : an explosive crystalline ester $C_6H_8(NO_3)_6$ made from mannitol and used mixed with a carbohydrate (as lactose) in the treatment of angina pectoris and vascular hypertension

man·nose \'ma-ˌnōs, -ˌnōz\ n : an aldose $C_6H_{12}O_6$ found esp. in plants

man·nos·i·do·sis \mə-ˌnō-sə-'dō-səs\ n, pl **-do·ses** \-ˌsēz\ : a rare inherited metabolic disease characterized by deficiency of an enzyme catalyzing the metabolism of mannose with resulting accumulation of mannose in the body and marked esp. by facial and skeletal deformities and by mental retardation

ma·noeu·vre *chiefly Brit var of* MANEUVER

ma·nom·e·ter \mə-'nä-mə-tər\ n **1** : an instrument for measuring the pressure of gases and vapors **2** : SPHYGMOMANOMETER — **mano·met·ric** \ˌma-nə-'me-trik\ *adj* — **mano·met·ri·cal·ly** *adv* — **ma·nom·e·try** \mə-'nä-mə-trē\ n

Man·son·el·la \ˌman-sə-'ne-lə\ n : a genus of filarial worms (superfamily Filarioidea) including one (*M. ozzardi*) that is common and typically nonpathogenic in human visceral fat and mesenteries in So. and Central America

Man·son \'man-sən\, **Sir Patrick** (1844–1922), British parasitologist.

mansoni — see SCHISTOSOMIASIS MANSONI

Man·son's disease \'man-sənz-\ n : SCHISTOSOMIASIS MANSONI

man·tle \'mant-ᵊl\ n **1** : something that covers, enfolds, or envelops **2** : CEREBRAL CORTEX

Man·toux test \ˌman-'tü-, ˌmän-\ n : an intradermal test for hypersensitivity to tuberculin that indicates past or present infection with tubercle bacilli — see TUBERCULIN TEST

Mantoux, Charles (1877–1947), French physician.

ma·nu·bri·um \mə-'nü-brē-əm, -'nyü-\ n, pl **-bria** \-brē-ə\ *also* **-bri·ums** : an anatomical process or part shaped like a handle: as **a** : the uppermost segment of the sternum that is a somewhat triangular flattened bone with anterolateral borders which articulate with the clavicles **b** : the process of the malleus of the ear

ma·nus \'mā-nəs, 'ma-\ n, pl **ma·nus** \-nəs, -ˌnüs\ : the part of the vertebrate forelimb from the carpus to the distal end

many·plies \'me-nē-ˌplīz\ n : OMASUM

MAO *abbr* monoamine oxidase

MAOI *abbr* monoamine oxidase inhibitor

MAO inhibitor \ˌem-ˌā-'ō-\ n : MONOAMINE OXIDASE INHIBITOR

¹**map** \'map\ n : the arrangement of genes on a chromosome — called also *genetic map*

²**map** vb **mapped; map·ping 1** : to locate (a gene) on a chromosome **2** of a gene : to be located ⟨a repressor ∼s near the corresponding structural gene⟩

maple syrup urine disease n : a hereditary aminoaciduria caused by a deficiency of decarboxylase leading to high concentrations of valine, leucine, isoleucine, and alloisoleucine in the blood, urine, and cerebrospinal fluid and characterized by an odor of maple syrup to the urine, vomiting, hypertonicity, severe mental retardation, seizures, and eventually death unless the condition is treated with dietary measures

ma·pro·ti·line \mə-'prō-tə-ˌlēn\ *n* : an antidepressant drug used in the form of its hydrochloride $C_{20}H_{23}N \cdot HCl$ to relieve major depression (as in bipolar disorder) and anxiety associated with depression

ma·ras·mus \mə-'raz-məs\ *n* : severe malnutrition affecting infants and children esp. of impoverished regions that is characterized by poor growth, loss of subcutaneous fat, muscle atrophy, apathy, and pronounced weight loss and is usu. caused by a diet deficient in calories and proteins but sometimes by disease (as dysentery or giardiasis) — **ma·ras·mic** \-mik\ *adj*

marble bone disease *n* : OSTEOPETROSIS

Mar·burg fever \'mär-bərg-\ *n* : an often fatal hemorrhagic fever that is caused by the Marburg virus, is an acute febrile illness often progressing to severe hemorrhaging, is spread esp. by contact with the body fluids (as blood or saliva) of infected individuals, and was orig. reported in humans infected with green monkeys — called also *green monkey disease, Marburg disease, Marburg hemorrhagic fever*

Marburg virus *n* : a filovirus (species *Lake Victoria marburgvirus* of the genus *Marburgvirus*) that causes Marburg fever

march \'märch\ *n* : the progression of epileptic activity through the motor centers of the cerebral cortex that is manifested in localized convulsions in first one and then an adjacent part of the body

Mar·ek's disease \'mar-iks-\ *n* : a highly contagious virus disease of poultry that is characterized esp. by proliferation of lymphoid cells and is caused by either of two herpesviruses (species *Gallid herpesvirus 2* and *Gallid herpesvirus 3* of the genus *Mardivirus*)

Marek, Jozsef (1867–1952), Hungarian veterinarian.

Ma·rey's law \mə-'rāz-\ *n* : a statement in physiology: heart rate is related inversely to arterial blood pressure

Marey, Etienne–Jules (1830–1904), French physiologist.

Mar·e·zine \'mar-ə-ˌzēn\ *n* : a preparation of the hydrochloride of cyclizine — formerly a U.S. registered trademark

mar·fa·noid \'mär-fə-ˌnȯid\ *adj* : exhibiting the typical characteristics of Marfan syndrome ⟨~ habitus⟩

Mar·fan syndrome \'mär-ˌfan-\ *or*

Mar·fan's syndrome \-ˌfanz-\ *n* : a disorder of connective tissue that is inherited as a simple dominant trait, is caused by a defect in the gene controlling the production of fibrillin, and is characterized by abnormal elongation of the long bones and often by ocular and circulatory defects

Marfan \mär-'fäⁿ\, Antonin Bernard Jean (1858–1942), French pediatrician.

mar·gin \'mär-jən\ *n* **1** : the outside limit or edge of something (as a bodily part or a wound) **2** : the part of consciousness at a particular moment that is felt only vaguely and dimly — **mar·gin·al** \'mär-jə-nəl\ *adj*

mar·gin·ation \ˌmär-jə-'nā-shən\ *n* **1** : the act or process of forming a margin; *specif* : the adhesion of white blood cells to the walls of damaged blood vessels **2** : the action of finishing a dental restoration or a filling for a cavity

Ma·rie–Strüm·pell disease *also* **Ma·rie–Strüm·pell's disease** \mä-ˌrē-'strüm-pəl(z)-\ *n* : ANKYLOSING SPONDYLITIS

Marie, Pierre (1853–1940), French neurologist.

Strümpell \'shtruem-pəl\, Ernst Adolf Gustav Gottfried von (1853–1925), German neurologist.

mar·i·jua·na *also* **mar·i·hua·na** \ˌmar-ə-'wä-nə, -'hwä-\ *n* **1** : HEMP **1 2** : the dried leaves and flowering tops of the hemp plant that yield THC and are sometimes smoked in cigarettes for their intoxicating effect — compare BHANG, CANNABIS, HASHISH

Mar·i·nol \'mar-ə-ˌnȯl\ *trademark* — used for a preparation of dronabinol

mark \'märk\ *n* : an impression or trace made or occurring on something — see BIRTHMARK, STRAWBERRY MARK

mark·er \'mär-kər\ *n* : something that serves to identify, predict, or characterize: as **a** : BIOMARKER **b** : GENETIC MARKER — called also *marker gene*

Mar·o·teaux–La·my syndrome \ˌmär-ō-'tō-lä-'mē-\ *n* : a mucopolysaccharidosis that is inherited as an autosomal recessive trait and that is similar to Hurler's syndrome except that intellectual development is not retarded

Maroteaux, Pierre (*b* 1926), French physician.

Lamy, Maurice Emile Joseph (1895–1975), French physician.

Mar·plan \'mär-ˌplan\ *trademark* — used for a preparation of isocarboxazid

mar·row \'mar-(ˌ)ō\ *n* **1** : BONE MARROW **2** : the substance of the spinal cord

Mar·seilles fever \mär-'sā-\ *n* : BOUTONNEUSE FEVER

mar·su·pi·al·ize \mär-'sü-pē-ə-ˌlīz\ *vb* **-ized; -iz·ing** : to open (as the bladder or a cyst) and sew by the edges to the abdominal wound to permit further treatment (as of an enclosed tumor) or to discharge pathological matter (as from a hydatid cyst) — **mar·su·pi·al·i·za·tion** \-ˌsü-pē-ə-li-ˈzā-shən\ n

mas·cu·line \ˈmas-kyə-lən\ adj 1 : MALE 2 : having the qualities distinctive of or appropriate to a male 3 : having a mannish bearing or quality — **mas·cu·lin·i·ty** \ˌmas-kyə-ˈli-nə-tē\ n

mas·cu·lin·ize \ˈmas-kyə-lə-ˌnīz\ vb **-ized; -iz·ing** : to give a preponderantly masculine character to; esp : to cause (a female) to take on male characteristics — **mas·cu·lin·i·za·tion** \ˌmas-kyə-lə-nə-ˈzā-shən\ n

MASH abbr mobile army surgical hospital

¹**mask** \ˈmask\ n 1 : a protective covering for the face 2 a : any of various devices that cover the mouth and nose and are used to prevent inhalation of dangerous substances, to facilitate delivery of a gas, or to prevent the dispersal of exhaled infective material — see GAS MASK, OXYGEN MASK b : a cosmetic preparation for the skin of the face that produces a tightening effect as it dries

²**mask** vb 1 : to modify or reduce the effect or activity of (as a process or a reaction) 2 : to raise the audibility threshold of (a sound) by the simultaneous presentation of another sound

masked adj : failing to present or produce the usual symptoms : not obvious : LATENT ⟨a ∼ fever⟩

mas·och·ism \ˈma-sə-ˌki-zəm, ˈma-zə-, ˈmä-sə-\ n : a sexual perversion characterized by pleasure in being subjected to pain or humiliation esp. by a love object — compare ALGOLAGNIA, SADISM — **mas·och·is·tic** \ˌma-sə-ˈkis-tik, ˌma-zə-, ˌmä-sə-\ adj — **mas·och·is·ti·cal·ly** adv

Sa·cher–Ma·soch \ˈzä-kər-ˈmä-zȯk\, **Leopold von (1836–1895),** Austrian novelist.

mas·och·ist \-kist\ n : an individual who is given to masochism

mass \ˈmas\ n 1 : the property of a body that is a measure of its inertia, that is commonly taken as a measure of the amount of material it contains and causes it to have weight in a gravitational field 2 : a homogeneous pasty mixture compounded for making pills, lozenges, and plasters

mas·sage \mə-ˈsäzh, -ˈsäj\ n : manipulation of tissues (as by rubbing, stroking, kneading, or tapping) with the hand or an instrument for therapeutic purposes — **massage** vb

mas·sa in·ter·me·dia \ˈma-sə-ˌin-tər-ˈmē-dē-ə\ n : an apparently functionless mass of gray matter in the midline of the third ventricle that is found in many but not all human brains and is formed when the surfaces of the thalami protruding inward from opposite sides of the third ventricle make contact and fuse

mas·sa·sau·ga \ˌma-sə-ˈsȯ-gə\ n : a

medium-sized No. American rattlesnake of the genus *Sistrurus* (*S. catenatus*)

mas·se·ter \mə-ˈsē-tər, ma-\ n : a large muscle that raises the lower jaw and assists in mastication, arises from the zygomatic arch and the zygomatic process of the temporal bone, and is inserted into the mandibular ramus and gonial angle — **mas·se·ter·ic** \ˌma-sə-ˈter-ik\ adj

mas·seur \ma-ˈsər, mə-\ n : a man who practices massage

mas·seuse \-ˈsərz, -ˈsüz\ n : a woman who practices massage

mas·sive \ˈma-siv\ adj 1 : large in comparison to what is typical — used esp. of medical dosage or of an infective agent ⟨a ∼ dose of penicillin⟩ 2 : being extensive and severe — used of a pathologic condition ⟨a ∼ hemorrhage⟩

mass number n : an integer that approximates the mass of an isotope and designates the total number of protons and neutrons in the nucleus ⟨the symbol for carbon of *mass number* 14 is ^{14}C or C^{14}⟩

mas·so·ther·a·py \ˌma-sō-ˈther-ə-pē\ n, pl **-pies** : the practice of therapeutic massage

mass spectrometry n : an instrumental method for identifying the chemical constitution of a substance by means of the separation of gaseous ions according to their differing mass and charge — **mass spectrometer** n — **mass spectrometric** adj

mass spectroscopy n : MASS SPECTROMETRY — **mass spectroscope** n — **mass spectroscopic** adj

mast- or **masto-** comb form : breast : nipple : mammary gland ⟨*mast*itis⟩

Mas·tad·e·no·vi·rus \ˌma-ˈsta-də-nō-ˌvī-rəs\ n : a genus of adenoviruses that infect only mammals and include the causative agents of epidemic keratoconjunctivitis and pharyngoconjunctival fever

mas·tal·gia \mas-ˈtal-jə\ n : MASTODYNIA

mast cell \ˈmast-\ n : a large cell that occurs esp. in connective tissue and has basophilic granules containing substances (as histamine and heparin) which mediate allergic reactions

mas·tec·to·mee \ma-ˌstek-tə-ˈmē\ n : a person who has had a mastectomy

mas·tec·to·my \ma-ˈstek-tə-mē\ n, pl **-mies** : surgical removal of all or part of the breast and sometimes associated lymph nodes and muscles

master gland n : PITUITARY GLAND

-mas·tia \ˈmas-tē-ə\ n comb form : condition of having (such or so many) breasts or mammary glands ⟨gyneco*mastia*⟩

mas·ti·cate \ˈmas-tə-ˌkāt\ vb **-cat·ed; -cat·ing** 1 : to grind, crush, and chew (food) with or as if with the teeth in preparation for swallowing 2 : to soften or reduce to pulp by crushing or kneading — **mas·ti·ca·tion** \ˌmas-tə-'kā-shən\ n — **mas·ti·ca·to·ry** \'mas-ti-kə-ˌtōr-ē\ adj

mas·ti·tis \ma-'stī-təs\ n, pl **-tit·i·des** \-'ti-tə-ˌdēz\ : inflammation of the mammary gland or udder usu. caused by infection — **mas·tit·ic** \ma-'sti-tik\ adj

masto- — see MAST-

mas·to·cy·to·ma \ˌmas-tə-ˌsī-'tō-mə\ n, pl **-mas** also **-ma·ta** \-mə-tə\ : a tumorous mass produced by proliferation of mast cells

mas·to·cy·to·sis \-'tō-səs\ n, pl **-to·ses** \-ˌsēz\ : excessive proliferation of mast cells in the tissues

mas·to·dyn·ia \ˌmas-tə-'dī-nē-ə\ n : pain in the breast — called also *mastalgia*

¹**mas·toid** \'mas-ˌtȯid\ adj : of, relating to, or being the mastoid process; *also* : occurring in the region of the mastoid process

²**mastoid** n : a mastoid bone or process

mastoid air cell n : MASTOID CELL

mastoid antrum n : TYMPANIC ANTRUM

mastoid cell n : one of the small cavities in the mastoid process that develop after birth and are filled with air — called also *mastoid air cell*

mas·toid·ec·to·my \ˌmas-ˌtȯi-'dek-tə-mē\ n, pl **-mies** : surgical removal of the mastoid cells or of the mastoid process of the temporal bone

mas·toid·itis \ˌmas-ˌtȯi-'dī-təs\ n, pl **-it·i·des** \-'di-tə-ˌdēz\ : inflammation of the mastoid and esp. of the mastoid cells

mas·toid·ot·o·my \ˌmas-ˌtȯi-'dä-tə-mē\ n, pl **-mies** : incision of the mastoid

mastoid process n : the process of the temporal bone behind the ear that is well developed and of somewhat conical form in adults but inconspicuous in children

mas·top·a·thy \ma-'stä-pə-thē\ n, pl **-thies** : a disorder of the breast; *esp* : a painful disorder of the breast

mas·to·pexy \'mas-tō-ˌpek-sē\ n, pl **-pex·ies** : BREAST LIFT

mas·tot·o·my \ma-'stä-tə-mē\ n, pl **-mies** : incision of the breast

mas·tur·ba·tion \ˌmas-tər-'bā-shən\ n : erotic stimulation esp. of one's own genital organs commonly resulting in orgasm and achieved by manual or other bodily contact exclusive of sexual intercourse, by instrumental manipulation, occasionally by sexual fantasies, or by various combinations of these agencies — **mas·tur·bate** \'mas-tər-ˌbāt\ vb — **mas·tur·ba·tor** \-ˌbā-tər\ n

mas·tur·ba·to·ry \'mas-tər-bə-ˌtōr-ē\ adj : of, relating to, or associated with masturbation ⟨∼ fantasies⟩

mate vb **mat·ed; mat·ing** 1 : to pair or join for breeding 2 : COPULATE

ma·te·ria al·ba \mə-'tir-ē-ə-'al-bə\ n pl : a soft whitish deposit of epithelial cells, white blood cells, and microorganisms esp. at the gumline

materia med·i·ca \-'me-di-kə\ n 1 : substances used in the composition of medical remedies : DRUGS, MEDICINE 2 a : a branch of medical science that deals with the sources, nature, properties, and preparation of drugs b : a treatise on materia medica

ma·ter·nal \mə-'tərn-əl\ adj 1 : of, relating, belonging to, or characteristic of a mother ⟨∼ instinct⟩ 2 a : related through a mother b : inherited or derived from the female parent ⟨∼ genes⟩ — **ma·ter·nal·ly** adv

maternal inheritance n : inheritance of characters transmitted through extranuclear elements (as mitochondrial DNA) in the cytoplasm of the egg

maternal rubella n : German measles in a pregnant woman that may cause developmental anomalies in the fetus when occurring during the first trimester

¹**ma·ter·ni·ty** \mə-'tər-nə-tē\ n, pl **-ties** : a hospital facility designed for the care of women before and during childbirth and for the care of newborn babies

²**maternity** adj 1 : being or providing care during and immediately before and after childbirth ⟨a ∼ unit⟩ 2 : designed for wear during pregnancy 3 : effective for the period close to and including childbirth ⟨∼ leave⟩

ma·ter·no·fe·tal \me-ˌtər-nō-'fēt-əl\ adj : involving a fetus and its mother ⟨the human ∼ interface⟩; *also* : passing or transferred from the mother to the fetus ⟨∼ transmission of HIV⟩

ma·tri·cide \'ma-trə-ˌsīd, 'mā-\ n : murder of a mother by her son or daughter

ma·trix \'mā-triks\ n, pl **ma·tri·ces** \'mā-trə-ˌsēz, 'ma-\ or **matrixes** 1 a : the extracellular substance in which tissue cells (as of connective tissue) are embedded b : the thickened epithelium at the base of a fingernail or toenail from which new nail substance develops — called also *nail bed, nail matrix* 2 : a mass by which something is enclosed or in which something is embedded 3 a : a strip or band placed so as to serve as a retaining outer wall of a tooth in filling a cavity b : a metal or porcelain pattern in which an inlay is cast or fused

mat·ter \'ma-tər\ n 1 : material (as feces or urine) discharged or for discharge from the living body 2 : material discharged by suppuration : PUS

mattress suture n : a surgical stitch in which the suture is passed back and forth through both edges of a wound so that the needle is reinserted each time on the side of exit and passes through to the side of insertion

mat·u·rate \'ma-chə-ˌrāt\ vb **-rat·ed; -rat·ing** : MATURE

mat·u·ra·tion \ˌma-chə-'rā-shən\ n 1 a

: the process of becoming mature **b** : the emergence of personal and behavioral characteristics through growth processes **c** : the final stages of differentiation of cells, tissues, or organs **d** : the achievement of intellectual or emotional maturity **2 a** : the entire process by which diploid gamete-producing cells are transformed into haploid gametes that includes both meiosis and physiological and structural changes fitting the gamete for its future role **b** : SPERMIOGENESIS 2 — **mat·u·ra·tion·al** \ˌma-chə-ˈrā-shə-nəl\ *adj*

maturation promoting factor *n* : a protein complex that in its active form causes eukaryotic cells to undergo mitosis

ma·ture \mə-ˈtu̇r, -ˈtyu̇r, -ˈchu̇r\ *adj* **ma·tur·er; -est 1** : having completed natural growth and development ⟨a ∼ ovary⟩ **2** : having undergone maturation ⟨∼ germ cells⟩ — **mature** *vb*

ma·tu·ri·ty \mə-ˈtu̇r-ə-tē, -ˈtyu̇r-, -ˈchu̇r-\ *n, pl* **-ties** : the quality or state of being mature; *esp* : full development

maturity–onset diabetes *n* : TYPE 2 DIABETES

maturity–onset diabetes of the young *n* : type 2 diabetes of a relatively mild form that is inherited as an autosomal dominant trait and occurs in late adolescence or early adulthood — *abbr. MODY*

max *abbr* maximum

Max·ib·o·lin \mak-ˈsi-bə-lin, ˌmak-si-ˈbō-lin\ *n* : a preparation of ethylestrenol — formerly a U.S. registered trademark

maxill- *or* **maxilli-** *or* **maxillo-** *comb form* **1** : maxilla ⟨*maxill*ectomy⟩ **2** : maxillary and ⟨*maxillo*facial⟩

max·il·la \mak-ˈsi-lə\ *n, pl* **max·il·lae** \-ˈsi-(ˌ)lē, -ˌlī\ *or* **maxillas 1** : JAW 1a **2 a** : an upper jaw esp. of humans or other mammals in which the bony elements are closely fused **b** : either of two membrane bone elements of the upper jaw that lie lateral to the premaxillae and bear most of the teeth

¹**max·il·lary** \ˈmak-sə-ˌler-ē\ *adj* : of, relating to, being, or associated with a maxilla ⟨∼ blood vessels⟩

²**maxillary** *n, pl* **-lar·ies 1** : MAXILLA 2b **2** : a maxillary part (as a nerve or blood vessel)

maxillary air sinus *n* : MAXILLARY SINUS

maxillary artery *n* : an artery supplying the deep structures of the face (as the nasal cavities, palate, tonsils, and pharynx) and sending a branch to the meninges of the brain — called also *internal maxillary artery;* compare FACIAL ARTERY

maxillary bone *n* : MAXILLA 2b

maxillary nerve *n* : the one of the three major branches or divisions of the trigeminal nerve that supplies sensory fibers to the skin areas of the middle part of the face, the upper jaw and its teeth, and the mucous membranes of the palate, nasal cavities, and nasopharynx — called also *maxillary division;* compare MANDIBULAR NERVE, OPHTHALMIC NERVE

maxillary process *n* : a triangular embryonic process that grows out from the dorsal end of the mandibular arch on each side and forms the lateral part of the upper lip, the cheek, and the upper jaw except the premaxilla

maxillary sinus *n* : an air cavity in the body of the maxilla that communicates with the middle meatus of the nose — called also *antrum of Highmore*

maxillary vein *n* : a short venous trunk of the face that is formed by the union of veins from the pterygoid plexus and that joins with the superficial temporal vein to form a vein which contributes to the formation of the external jugular vein

max·il·lec·to·my \ˌmak-sə-ˈlek-tə-mē\ *n, pl* **-mies** : surgical removal of the maxilla

maxilli-, maxillo- — see MAXILL-

max·il·lo·fa·cial \mak-ˌsi-(ˌ)lō-ˈfā-shəl, ˌmak-sə-(ˌ)lō-\ *adj* : of, relating to, treating, or affecting the maxilla and the face ⟨∼ lesions⟩

max·i·mal \ˈmak-sə-məl\ *adj* **1** : most complete or effective ⟨∼ vasodilation⟩ **2** : being an upper limit — **max·i·mal·ly** *adv*

maximal oxygen consumption *or* **maximum oxygen consumption** *n* : VO₂ MAX

maximal oxygen uptake *or* **maximum oxygen uptake** *n* : VO₂ MAX

max·i·mum \ˈmak-sə-məm\ *n, pl* **max·i·ma** \-sə-mə\ *or* **maximums 1 a** : the greatest quantity or value attainable or attained **b** : the period of highest, greatest, or utmost development **2** : an upper limit allowed (as by a legal authority) or allowable (as by the circumstances of a particular case) — **maximum** *adj*

maximum heart rate *n* : the age-related number of beats per minute of the heart when working at its maximum that is usu. estimated as 220 minus one's age

maximum permissible concentration *n* : the maximum concentration of radioactive material in body tissue that is regarded as acceptable and not producing significant deleterious effects on the human organism — *abbr. MPC*

maximum permissible dose *n* : the amount of ionizing radiation a person may be exposed to supposedly without being harmed

max VO₂ *n* : VO₂ MAX

Max·zide \ˈmaks-ˌzīd\ *trademark* — used for a preparation of triamterene and hydrochlorothiazide

may·ap·ple \ˈmā-ˌap-ᵊl\ *n, often cap* : a No. American herb of the genus

Podophyllum (*P. peltatum*) having a poisonous rootstock and rootlets that are a source of the drug podophyllum

Ma·ya·ro virus \mä-'yä-rō-\ n : a So. American togavirus of the genus *Alphavirus* (species *Mayaro virus*) that causes a febrile disease

May·er–Ro·ki·tan·sky–Kü·ster–Hau·ser syndrome \'mī-ər-,rō-kə-'tän-skē-'kes-tər-'haú-zər-\ n : a congenital disorder that is marked esp. by absence of the vagina, primary amenorrhea, and absent or rudimentary uterus and that results from arrested development of the Müllerian ducts during early embryogenesis — called also *Mayer-Rokitansky syndrome*, *MRKH syndrome*, *müllerian agenesis*

   Mayer, August Franz Josef Karl (1787–1865), German anatomist and physiologist.

   Rokitansky, Karl Freiherr von (1804–1878), Austrian pathologist.

   Küster, Hermann (*b* 1897), German gynecologist.

   Hauser, G. A. (*fl* 1961), Swiss gynecologist.

may·hem \'mā-,hem, 'mā-əm\ n : willful and permanent crippling, mutilation, or disfiguring of any part of another's body; *also* : the crime of engaging in mayhem

may·tan·sine \'mā-,tan-,sēn\ n : an antineoplastic agent $C_{34}H_{46}ClN_3O_{10}$ isolated from any of several tropical shrubs and trees (genus *Maytenus* of the family Celastraceae)

maz- *or* **mazo-** *comb form* : breast ⟨*mazo*plasia⟩

ma·zin·dol \'mā-zin-,dōl\ n : an adrenergic drug $C_{16}H_{13}ClN_2O$ used as an appetite suppressant

ma·zo·pla·sia \,mā-zə-'plā-zhə, -zhē-ə\ n : a degenerative condition of breast tissue

Maz·zi·ni test \mə-'zē-nē-\ n : a flocculation test for the diagnosis of syphilis

   Mazzini, Louis Yolando (1894–1973), American serologist.

MB *abbr* [New Latin *medicinae baccalaureus*] bachelor of medicine

M band \'em-,band\ n : M LINE

MBD *abbr* minimal brain dysfunction

mc *abbr* millicurie

MC *abbr* 1 medical corps 2 [New Latin *magister chirurgiae*] master of surgery

Mc·Ar·dle's disease \mə-'kärd-ᵊlz-\ n : a glycogen storage disease that is inherited as an autosomal recessive trait, is marked esp. by muscle weakness and myoglobinuria, and is caused by a deficiency of muscle phosphorylase — called also *McArdle's syndrome*

   McArdle, Brian (1911–2002), British physician.

MCAT *abbr* Medical College Admissions Test

Mc·Bur·ney's point \mək-'bər-nēz-\ n : a point on the abdominal wall that lies between the navel and the right

anterior superior iliac spine and that is the point where most pain is elicited by pressure in acute appendicitis

   McBurney, Charles (1845–1913), American surgeon.

mcg *abbr* microgram

MCh *abbr* [New Latin *magister chirurgiae*] master of surgery

MCH *abbr* 1 maternal and child health 2 mean corpuscular hemoglobin (concentration)

MCHC *abbr* mean corpuscular hemoglobin concentration

mCi *abbr* millicurie

MCL \,em-,sē-'el\ n : MEDIAL COLLATERAL LIGAMENT

MCO \,em-,sē-'ō\ n : MANAGED CARE ORGANIZATION

M–CSF *abbr* macrophage colony-stimulating factor

MCV *abbr* mean corpuscular volume

Md *symbol* mendelevium

MD \,em-'dē\ n 1 [Latin *medicinae doctor*] : an earned academic degree conferring the rank and title of doctor of medicine 2 : a person who has a doctor of medicine

MD *abbr* muscular dystrophy

MDA \,em-,dē-'ā\ n : a synthetic amphetamine derivative $C_{10}H_{13}NO_2$ used illicitly for its mood-enhancing and hallucinogenic properties — called also *methylenedioxyamphetamine*

MDI *abbr* metered-dose inhaler

MDMA \,em-(,)dē-(,)em-'ā\ n : ECSTASY 2

MDR *abbr* minimum daily requirement

MDS *abbr* master of dental surgery

ME *abbr* medical examiner

meadow mushroom n : a common edible brown-spored mushroom (*Agaricus campestris*) that occurs naturally in moist open organically rich soil

mean corpuscular hemoglobin concentration n : the number of grams of hemoglobin per unit volume and usu. 100 milliliters of packed red blood cells that is found by multiplying the number of grams of hemoglobin per unit volume of the original blood sample of whole blood by 100 and dividing by the hematocrit — abbr. *MCHC*

mean corpuscular volume n : the volume of the average red blood cell in a given blood sample that is found by multiplying the hematocrit by 10 and dividing by the estimated number of red blood cells — abbr. *MCV*

mea·sle \'mē-zəl\ n : CYSTICERCUS; *specif* : one found in the muscles of a domesticated mammal

mea·sles \'mē-zəlz\ n sing or pl 1 a : an acute contagious disease that is caused by a paramyxovirus of the genus *Morbillivirus* (species *Measles virus*), that commences with catarrhal symptoms, conjunctivitis, cough, and Koplik's spots on the oral mucous membrane, and that is marked by the appearance on the third or fourth day of an eruption of distinct red circular spots which coalesce in a crescentic form, are slightly raised, and after the fourth day of the eruption gradually decline — called also *rubeola* **b** : any of various eruptive diseases (as German measles) **2** : infestation with or disease caused by larval tapeworms in the muscles and tissues; *specif* : infestation of cattle and swine with cysticerci of tapeworms that as adults parasitize humans

mea·sly \'mē-zə-lē, 'mēz-lē\ *adj* **measli·er; -est 1** : infected with measles **2 a** : containing larval tapeworms **b** : infected with trichinae

meat- *or* **meato-** *comb form* : meatus ⟨*meato*plasty⟩

me·a·tal \mē-'āt-ᵊl\ *adj* : of, relating to, or forming a meatus

me·a·to·plas·ty \mē-'a-tə-ˌplast-ē\ *n, pl* **-ties** : plastic surgery of a meatus

me·a·tot·o·my \ˌmē-ə-'tä-tə-mē\ *n, pl* **-mies** : incision of the urethral meatus esp. to enlarge it

me·a·tus \mē-'ā-təs\ *n, pl* **me·atus·es** \-tə-səz\ *or* **me·atus** \-'ā-təs, -ˌtüs\ : a natural body passage : CANAL, DUCT

me·ban·a·zine \me-'ba-nə-ˌzēn\ *n* : a monoamine oxidase inhibitor C₈H₁₂N₂ used as an antidepressant

Meb·a·ral \'me-bə-ˌral\ *trademark* — used for a preparation of mephobarbital

me·ben·da·zole \me-'ben-də-ˌzōl\ *n* : a broad-spectrum anthelmintic agent C₁₆H₁₃N₃O₃

me·bu·ta·mate \me-'byü-tə-ˌmāt\ *n* : a central nervous system depressant C₁₀H₂₀N₂O₄ used to treat mild hypertension

mec·a·myl·a·mine \ˌme-kə-'mi-lə-ˌmēn\ *n* : a drug administered orally in the form of its hydrochloride C₁₁H₂₁N·HCl as a ganglionic blocking agent to effect a rapid lowering of severely elevated blood pressure

me·chan·i·cal \mi-'ka-ni-kəl\ *adj* : caused by, resulting from, or relating to physical as opposed to biological or chemical processes or change ⟨∼ injury⟩ ⟨∼ asphyxiation⟩ — **me·chan·i·cal·ly** *adv*

mechanical heart *n* : a mechanism designed to maintain the flow of blood to the tissues of the body esp. during a surgical operation on the heart; *also* : an artificial heart

mechanical ventilation *n* : artificial ventilation of the lungs (as by positive end-expiratory pressure) using means external to the body

mech·a·nism \'me-kə-ˌni-zəm\ *n* **1** : a piece of machinery **2 a** : a bodily process or function ⟨the ∼ of healing⟩ **b** : the combination of mental processes by which a result is obtained ⟨psychological ∼s⟩ **3** : the fundamental physical or chemical processes involved in or responsible for an action, reaction, or other natural phenomenon — **mech·a·nis·tic** \ˌme-kə-'nis-tik\ *adj*

mech·a·no·chem·is·try \ˌme-kə-nō-'ke-mə-strē\ *n, pl* **-tries** : chemistry that deals with the conversion of chemical energy into mechanical work (as in the contraction of a muscle) — **mech·a·no·chem·i·cal** \-'ke-mi-kəl\ *adj*

mech·a·no·re·cep·tor \-ri-'sep-tər\ *n* : a neural end organ (as a tactile receptor) that responds to a mechanical stimulus (as a change in pressure) — **mech·a·no·re·cep·tion** \-'sep-shən\ *n* — **mech·a·no·re·cep·tive** \-'sep-tiv\ *adj*

mech·a·no·sen·so·ry \-'sen-sə-rē\ *adj* : of, relating to, or functioning in the sensing of mechanical stimuli ⟨∼ neurons⟩ ⟨∼ cells⟩

mech·lor·eth·amine \ˌme-ˌklȯr-'e-thə-ˌmēn\ *n* : a nitrogen mustard administered by injection in the form of its hydrochloride C₅H₁₁Cl₂N·HCl in the palliative treatment of neoplastic diseases (as Hodgkin's disease)

mech·o·lyl \'me-kə-ˌlil\ *n* : a preparation of the chloride of methacholine

Me·cis·to·cir·rus \mə-ˌsis-tō-'sir-əs\ *n* : a genus of nematode worms (family Trichostrongylidae) including a common parasite (*M. digitatus*) of the abomasum of domesticated ruminants and the stomach of swine

Meck·el–Gru·ber syndrome \'me-kəl-'grü-bər-\ *n* : a syndrome inherited as an autosomal recessive trait and typically characterized by occipital encephalocele, microcephaly, cleft palate, polydactyly, and polycystic kidneys — called also *Meckel's syndrome*
  Meckel, Johann Friedrich, the Younger (1781–1833), German anatomist.
  Gruber, Georg Benno Otto (1884–1977), German pathologist.

Meck·el's cartilage \'me-kəlz-\ *n* : the cartilaginous bar of the embryonic mandibular arch of which the distal end ossifies to form the malleus
  J. F. Meckel the Younger — see MECKEL–GRUBER SYNDROME

Meckel's diverticulum *n* : the proximal part of the omphalomesenteric duct when persistent as a blind fibrous tube connected with the lower ileum
  J. F. Meckel the Younger — see MECKEL–GRUBER SYNDROME

Meckel's ganglion *n* : PTERYGOPALATINE GANGLION
  Meckel, Johann Friedrich, the Elder (1724–1774), German anatomist.

mec·li·zine \'me-klə-ˌzēn\ *n* : a drug used usu. in the form of its hydrated hydrochloride C₂₅H₂₇ClN₂·2HCl·H₂O to treat nausea and vertigo — see ANTIVERT

mec·lo·fen·a·mate sodium \ˌme-klō-'fe-nə-ˌmāt-\ *n* : a mild analgesic and anti-inflammatory drug C₁₄H₁₀Cl₂N-

$NaO_2 \cdot H_2O$ used orally to treat rheumatoid arthritis and osteoarthritis — called also *meclofenamate*

mec·lo·zine \'me-klō-ˌzēn\ *Brit var of* MECLIZINE

me·co·ni·um \mi-'kō-nē-əm\ *n* : a dark greenish mass of desquamated cells, mucus, and bile that accumulates in the bowel of a fetus and is typically discharged shortly after birth

meconium ileus *n* : congenital intestinal obstruction by thickened viscous meconium that is often associated with cystic fibrosis of newborn infants

¹**med** \'med\ *adj* : MEDICAL ⟨~ school⟩

²**med** *n* : MEDICATION 2 — usu. used in pl. ⟨took pain ~s⟩

me·daz·e·pam \me-'da-zə-ˌpam\ *n* : a drug used in the form of its hydrochloride $C_{16}H_{15}ClN_2 \cdot HCl$ esp. formerly as a tranquilizer

med·e·vac *also* **med·i·vac** \'me-də-ˌvak\ *n* **1** : emergency evacuation of the sick or wounded (as from a combat area) **2** : a helicopter used for medevac — **medevac** *vb*

medi- *or* **medio-** *comb form* : middle ⟨*medio*lateral⟩

¹**media** *pl of* MEDIUM

²**me·dia** \'mē-dē-ə\ *n, pl* **me·di·ae** \-dē-ˌē\ : the middle coat of the wall of a blood or lymph vessel consisting chiefly of circular muscle fibers — called also *tunica media*

media — see AERO-OTITIS MEDIA, OTITIS MEDIA, SCALA MEDIA, SEROUS OTITIS MEDIA

me·di·ad \'mē-dē-ˌad\ *adv* : toward the median line or plane of a body or part

me·di·al \'mē-dē-əl\ *adj* **1** : lying or extending in the middle; *esp, of a body part* : lying or extending toward the median axis of the body ⟨the ~ surface of the tibia⟩ **2** : of or relating to the media of a blood vessel — **me·di·al·ly** *adv*

medial arcuate ligament *n* : an arched band of fascia that covers the upper part of the psoas major muscle, extends from the body of the first or second lumbar vertebra to the transverse process of the first and sometimes also the second lumbar vertebra, and provides attachment for part of the lumbar portion of the diaphragm — compare LATERAL ARCUATE LIGAMENT

medial collateral ligament *n* **1** : a ligament that connects the medial epicondyle of the femur with the medial condyle and medial surface of the tibia and that helps to stabilize the knee by preventing lateral dislocation — called also *MCL, tibial collateral ligament*; compare LATERAL COLLATERAL LIGAMENT **2** : ULNAR COLLATERAL LIGAMENT

medial condyle *n* : a condyle on the inner side of the lower extremity of the femur; *also* : a corresponding eminence on the upper part of the tibia that articulates with the medial condyle of the femur — compare LATERAL CONDYLE

medial cord *n* : a cord of nerve tissue that is continuous with the anterior division of the inferior trunk of the brachial plexus and that is one of the two roots forming the median nerve — compare LATERAL CORD, POSTERIOR CORD

medial cuneiform bone *n* : CUNEIFORM BONE 1a — called also *medial cuneiform*

medial epicondyle *n* : EPICONDYLE b

medial femoral circumflex artery *n* : an artery that branches from the deep femoral artery or from the femoral artery itself and that supplies the muscles of the medial part of the thigh and hip joint — compare LATERAL FEMORAL CIRCUMFLEX ARTERY

medial femoral circumflex vein *n* : a vein accompanying the medial femoral circumflex artery and emptying into the femoral vein or sometimes into one of its tributaries corresponding to the deep femoral artery — compare LATERAL FEMORAL CIRCUMFLEX VEIN

medial forebrain bundle *n* : a prominent tract of nerve fibers that connects the subcallosal area of the cerebral cortex with the lateral areas of the hypothalamus and that has fibers passing to the tuber cinereum, the brain stem, and the mammillary bodies

medial geniculate body *n* : a part of the metathalamus consisting of a small oval tubercle situated between the pulvinar, colliculi, and cerebral peduncle that receives nerve impulses from the inferior colliculus and relays them to the auditory cortex — compare LATERAL GENICULATE BODY

medialis — see RECTUS MEDIALIS, VASTUS MEDIALIS

medial lemniscus *n* : a band of nerve fibers that transmits proprioceptive impulses from the spinal cord to the thalamus

medial longitudinal fasciculus *n* : any of four longitudinal bundles of white matter of which there are two on each side that extend from the midbrain to the upper parts of the spinal cord where they are located close to the midline ventral to the gray commissure and that are composed of fibers esp. from the vestibular nuclei

medial malleolus *n* : MALLEOLUS b

medial meniscus *n* : MENISCUS a(2)

medial pectoral nerve *n* : PECTORAL NERVE b

medial plantar artery *n* : PLANTAR ARTERY b

medial plantar nerve *n* : PLANTAR NERVE b

medial plantar vein *n* : PLANTAR VEIN b

medial popliteal nerve *n* : TIBIAL NERVE

medial pterygoid muscle *n* : PTERYGOID MUSCLE b

medial pterygoid nerve *n* : PTERYGOID NERVE b

medial pterygoid plate *n* : PTERYGOID PLATE b

medial rectus *n* : RECTUS 2c

medial semilunar cartilage *n* : MENISCUS a(2)

medial umbilical ligament *n* : a fibrous cord sheathed in peritoneum and extending from the pelvis to the navel that is a remnant of part of the umbilical artery in the fetus — called also *lateral umbilical ligament*

medial vestibular nucleus : the one of the four vestibular nuclei on each side of the medulla oblongata that sends ascending fibers to the oculomotor and trochlear nuclei on the opposite side of the brain and sends descending fibers down both sides of the spinal cord to synapse with motor neurons of the ventral roots

¹**me·di·an** \'mē-dē-ən\ *n* : a medial part (as a vein or nerve)

²**median** *adj* : situated in the middle; *specif* : lying in a plane dividing a bilateral animal into right and left halves

median an·te·bra·chi·al vein \-ˌan-ti-'brā-kē-əl-\ *n* : a vein usu. present in the forearm that drains the perforating veins in the palm of the hand and that runs up the little finger side of the forearm

median arcuate ligament *n* : a tendinous arch that lies in front of the aorta and that connects the attachments of the lumbar portion of the diaphragm to the lumbar vertebrae on each side — compare LATERAL ARCUATE LIGAMENT

median cubital vein *n* : a continuation of the cephalic vein of the forearm that passes obliquely toward the inner side of the arm in the bend of the elbow to join with the ulnar veins in forming the basilic vein and is often selected for venipuncture

median eminence *n* : a raised area in the floor of the third ventricle of the brain produced by the infundibulum of the hypothalamus

median lethal dose *n* : LD50

median nerve *n* : a nerve that arises by two roots from the brachial plexus and passes down the middle of the front of the arm

median nuchal line *n* : OCCIPITAL CREST a

median plane *n* : MIDSAGITTAL PLANE

median sacral crest *n* : SACRAL CREST a

median sacral vein *n* : an unpaired vein that accompanies the middle sacral artery and usu. empties into the left common iliac vein

median umbilical ligament : a fibrous cord extending from the urinary bladder to the umbilicus that is the remnant of the fetal urachus

me·di·as·ti·nal \ˌmē-dē-ə-'stī-nəl\ *adj* : of, relating to, or affecting the mediastinum (~ fibrosis)

me·di·as·ti·ni·tis \ˌmē-dē-ˌas-tə-'nī-təs\ *n, pl* **-nit·i·des** \-'ni-tə-ˌdēz\ : inflammation of the tissues of the mediastinum

me·di·as·tin·o·scope \ˌmē-dē-ə-'sti-nə-ˌskōp\ *n* : an endoscope used in mediastinoscopy

me·di·as·ti·nos·co·py \ˌmē-dē-ˌas-tə-'näs-kə-pē\ *n, pl* **-pies** : examination of the mediastinum through an incision above the sternum

me·di·as·ti·not·o·my \-'nä-tə-mē\ *n, pl* **-mies** : surgical incision into the mediastinum

me·di·as·ti·num \ˌmē-dē-ə-'stī-nəm\ *n, pl* **-na** \-nə\ **1** : the space in the chest between the pleural sacs of the lungs that contains all the viscera of the chest except the lungs and pleurae; *also* : this space with its contents **2** : MEDIASTINUM TESTIS

mediastinum testis *n* : a mass of connective tissue at the back of the testis that is continuous externally with the tunica albuginea and internally with the interlobular septa and encloses the rete testis

¹**me·di·ate** \'mē-dē-ət\ *adj* **1** : occupying a middle position **2** : acting through an intervening agency : exhibiting indirect causation, connection, or relation

²**me·di·ate** \'mē-dē-ˌāt\ *vb* **-at·ed; -at·ing** : to transmit or carry (as a physical process or effect) as an intermediate mechanism or agency — **me·di·a·tion** \ˌmē-dē-'ā-shən\ *n*

me·di·a·tor \'mē-dē-ˌā-tər\ *n* : one that mediates; *esp* : a mediating agent (as an enzyme or hormone) in a chemical or biological process

med·ic \'me-dik\ *n* : one engaged in medical work; *esp* : CORPSMAN

medica — see MATERIA MEDICA

med·i·ca·ble \'me-di-kə-bəl\ *adj* : CURABLE, REMEDIABLE

Med·ic·aid \'me-di-ˌkād\ *n* : a program of medical aid designed for those unable to afford regular medical service and financed jointly by the state and federal governments

¹**med·i·cal** \'me-di-kəl\ *adj* **1** : of, relating to, or concerned with physicians or the practice of medicine often as distinguished from surgery **2** : requiring or devoted to medical treatment — **med·i·cal·ly** *adv*

²**medical** *n* : a medical examination

med·i·cal·ese \ˌme-di-kə-'lēz\ *n* : the specialized terminology of the medical profession

medical examiner *n* **1** : a usu. appointed public officer with duties similar to those of a coroner but who is required to have specific medical training (as in pathology) and is qualified to conduct medical examinations and autopsies **2** : a physician employed to make medical examinations (as of applicants for military service or of claimants of workers' compensation) **3** : a physician appointed to examine and license candidates for the practice of medicine in a political jurisdiction (as a state)

med·i·cal·ise *Brit var of* MEDICALIZE

med·i·cal·ize \'me-də-kə-ˌlīz\ *vb* **-ized;** **-iz·ing** : to view or treat as a medical concern, problem, or disorder — **med·i·cal·za·tion** \ˌme-də-kə-lə-'zā-shən\ *n*

medical jurisprudence *n* : FORENSIC MEDICINE

medical mall *n* : a facility offering comprehensive ambulatory medical services (as primary and secondary care, diagnostic procedures, outpatient surgery, and rehabilitation)

medical psychology *n* : theories of personality and behavior not necessarily derived from academic psychology that provide a basis for psychotherapy in psychiatry and in general medicine

medical record *n* : a record of a patient's medical information (as past diagnoses and treatments received)

medical tran·scrip·tion·ist \-tran-'skrip-shə-nist\ *n* : a typist who transcribes dictated medical reports

me·di·ca·ment \mi-'di-kə-mənt, 'me-di-kə-\ *n* : a substance used in therapy — **med·i·ca·men·tous** \mi-ˌdi-kə-'men-təs, ˌme-di-kə-\ *adj*

med·i·cant \'me-di-kənt\ *n* : a medicinal substance

Medi·care \'me-di-ˌkär\ *n* : a government program of medical care esp. for the elderly

med·i·cate \'me-də-ˌkāt\ *vb* **-cat·ed;** **-cat·ing 1** : to treat medicinally **2** : to impregnate with a medicinal substance ⟨*medicated* soap⟩

med·i·ca·tion \ˌme-də-'kā-shən\ *n* **1** : the act or process of medicating **2** : a medicinal substance : MEDICAMENT

¹**me·dic·i·nal** \mə-'dis-ᵊn-əl\ *adj* : of, relating to, or being medicine : tending or used to cure disease or relieve pain — **me·dic·i·nal·ly** *adv*

²**medicinal** *n* : a medicinal substance : MEDICINE

medicinal leech *n* : a large European freshwater leech of the genus *Hirudo* (*H. medicinalis*) that is a source of hirudin, is now sometimes used to drain blood (as from a hematoma), and was formerly used to bleed patients thought to have excess blood

med·i·cine \'me-də-sən\ *n* **1** : a substance or preparation used in treating disease **2 a** : the science and art dealing with the maintenance of health and the prevention, alleviation, or cure of disease **b** : the branch of medicine concerned with the nonsurgical treatment of disease

medicine chest *n* : a cupboard used esp. for storing medicines or first-aid supplies — called also *medicine cabinet*

medicine dropper *n* : DROPPER

med·i·co \'me-di-ˌkō\ *n, pl* **-cos** : a medical practitioner : PHYSICIAN; *also* : a medical student

medico- *comb form* : medical : medical and ⟨*medico*legal⟩

med·i·co·le·gal \ˌme-di-kō-'lē-gəl\ *adj* : of or relating to both medicine and law

med·i·gap \'me-də-ˌgap\ *n, often attrib* : supplemental health insurance that covers costs (as of a hospital stay) not covered by Medicare ⟨∼ plans⟩

Me·di·na worm \mə-'dē-nə-\ *n* : GUINEA WORM

medio- — see MEDI-

me·dio·car·pal \ˌmē-dē-ō-'kär-pəl\ *adj* : located between the two rows of the bones of the carpus ⟨the ∼ joint⟩

me·dio·lat·er·al \-'la-tə-rəl\ *adj* : relating to, extending along, or being a direction or axis from side to side or from median to lateral — **me·dio·lat·er·al·ly** *adv*

Med·i·ter·ra·nean anemia \ˌme-də-tə-'rā-nē-ən-\ *n* : THALASSEMIA

Mediterranean fever *n* : any of several febrile conditions often endemic in parts of the Mediterranean region; *specif* : BRUCELLOSIS a

Mediterranean lymphoma *n* : IMMUNOPROLIFERATIVE SMALL INTESTINAL DISEASE

me·di·um \'mē-dē-əm\ *n, pl* **mediums** *or* **me·dia** \-dē-ə\ **1** : a means of effecting or conveying something **2** *pl* **media** : a nutrient system for the artificial cultivation of cells or organisms and esp. bacteria

medius — see CONSTRICTOR PHARYNGIS MEDIUS, GLUTEUS MEDIUS, PEDUNCULUS CEREBELLARIS MEDIUS, SCALENUS MEDIUS

medivac *var of* MEDEVAC

MED·LARS \'med-ˌlärz\ *service mark* — used for a computer system for the search and retrieval of biomedical abstracts and bibliographical information from various databases

MED·LINE \'med-ˌlīn\ *service mark* — used for an online computer database of abstracts and references from biomedical journals that is searched by the MEDLARS system

med·ro·ges·tone \ˌme-drō-'jes-ˌtōn\ *n* : a synthetic progestin $C_{23}H_{32}O_2$ that has been used in the treatment of fibroid uterine tumors

Med·rol \'me-ˌdrōl\ *trademark* — used for a preparation of methylprednisolone

me·droxy·pro·ges·ter·one acetate \me-ˌdräk-sē-prō-'jes-tə-ˌrōn-\ *n* : a synthetic steroid progestational hormone $C_{24}H_{34}O_4$ that is used esp. in the treatment of amenorrhea and abnormal uterine bleeding, in conjunction with conjugated estrogens to relieve the symptoms of menopause and to prevent osteoporosis, and as an injectable contraceptive — called also *medroxyprogesterone;* see DEPO-PROVERA

me·dul·la \mə-'dəl-ə, -'du̇l-\ *n, pl* **-las** *or* **-lae** \-(ˌ)lē, -ˌlī\ **1** *pl* **medullae a** : BONE MARROW **b** : MEDULLA OBLONGATA **2 a** : the inner or deep part of an organ or structure **b** : MYELIN SHEATH

medulla ob·lon·ga·ta \-ˌä-ˌblȯŋ-'gä-tə\ *n, pl* **medulla oblongatas** *or* **medullae ob·lon·ga·tae** \-'gä-tē, -ˌtī\ : the somewhat pyramidal last part of the vertebrate brain developed from the posterior portion of the hindbrain and continuous posteriorly with the spinal cord, enclosing the fourth ventricle, and containing nuclei associated with most of the cranial nerves, major fiber tracts and decussations that link spinal with higher centers, and various centers mediating the control of involuntary vital functions (as respiration)

medullaris — see CONUS MEDULLARIS

med·ul·lary \'med-ᵊl-ˌer-ē, 'me-jə-ˌler-ē; mə-'də-lə-rē\ *adj* **1 a** : of or relating to the medulla of any body part or organ **b** : containing, consisting of, or resembling bone marrow **c** : of or relating to the medulla oblongata or the spinal cord **d** : of, relating to, or formed of the dorsally located embryonic ectoderm destined to sink below the surface and become neural tissue **2** : resembling bone marrow in consistency — used of cancers

medullary canal *n* : the marrow cavity of a bone

medullary cavity *n* : MEDULLARY CANAL

medullary cystic disease *n* : a progressive familial kidney disease that is characterized by renal medullary cysts and that manifests itself in anemia and uremia

medullary fold *n* : NEURAL FOLD

medullary groove *n* : NEURAL GROOVE

medullary plate *n* : the longitudinal dorsal zone of epiblast in the early vertebrate embryo that constitutes the primordium of the neural tissue

medulla spi·na·lis \-ˌspī-'nä-ləs\ *n* : SPINAL CORD

med·ul·lat·ed \'med-ᵊl-ˌā-təd, 'me-jə-ˌlā-\ *adj* **1** : MYELINATED **2** : having a medulla — used of fibers other than nerve fibers

med·ul·lec·to·my \ˌmed-ᵊl-'ek-tə-mē, ˌme-jə-'lek-\ *n, pl* **-mies** : surgical excision of a medulla (as of the adrenal glands)

me·dul·lin \me-'də-lən, 'med-ᵊl-in, 'me-jə-lin\ *n* : a renal prostaglandin effective in reducing blood pressure

me·dul·lo·blas·to·ma \mə-ˌdə-lō-ˌblas-'tō-mə\ *n, pl* **-tomas** *also* **-to·ma·ta** \-'tō-mə-tə\ : a malignant tumor of

the central nervous system arising in the cerebellum esp. in children

mef·e·nam·ic acid \ˌme-fə-'na-mik-\ *n* : a drug $C_{15}H_{15}NO_2$ used as an anti-inflammatory

mef·lo·quine \'me-flə-ˌkwīn\ *n* : an antimalarial drug similar to quinine that is administered in the form of its hydrochloride $C_{17}H_{16}F_6N_2O \cdot HCl$ esp. for the prevention and treatment of falciparum malaria

mega- *or* **meg-** *comb form* **1** : great : large ⟨*mega*colon⟩ ⟨*mega*dose⟩ **2** : million : multiplied by one million ⟨*mega*curie⟩

mega·co·lon \'me-gə-ˌkō-lən\ *n* : extreme dilation of the colon that may be congenital or acquired — see HIRSCHSPRUNG'S DISEASE

mega·cu·rie \'me-gə-ˌkyu̇r-ē, -kyu̇-ˌrē\ *n* : one million curies

mega·dose \-ˌdōs\ *n* : a large dose (as of a vitamin) — **mega·dos·ing** \-ˌdō-siŋ\ *n*

mega·esoph·a·gus \ˌme-gə-i-'sä-fə-gəs\ *n, pl* **-gi** \-ˌgī, -ˌjī\ : enlargement and hypertrophy of the lower portion of the esophagus

mega·kary·o·blast \ˌme-gə-'kar-ē-ō-ˌblast\ *n* : a large cell with large reticulate nucleus that gives rise to megakaryocytes

mega·kary·o·cyte \ˌme-gə-'kar-ē-ō-ˌsīt\ *n* : a large cell that has a lobulated nucleus, is found esp. in the bone marrow, and is the source of blood platelets — **mega·kary·o·cyt·ic** \-ˌkar-ē-ō-'si-tik\ *adj*

megal- *or* **megalo-** *comb form* **1** : large ⟨*megalo*cyte⟩ : abnormally large ⟨*megalo*cephaly⟩ **2** : grandiose ⟨*megalo*mania⟩

meg·a·lo·blast \'me-gə-lō-ˌblast\ *n* : a large erythroblast that appears in the blood esp. in pernicious anemia — **meg·a·lo·blas·tic** \ˌme-gə-lō-'blas-tik\ *adj*

megaloblastic anemia *n* : an anemia (as pernicious anemia) characterized by the presence of megaloblasts in the circulating blood

meg·a·lo·ceph·a·ly \ˌme-gə-lō-'se-fə-lē\ *n, pl* **-lies** : largeness and esp. abnormal largeness of the head

meg·a·lo·cyte \'me-gə-lə-ˌsīt\ *n* : MACROCYTE — **meg·a·lo·cyt·ic** \ˌme-gə-lə-'si-tik\ *adj*

meg·a·lo·ma·nia \ˌme-gə-lō-'mā-nē-ə, -nyə\ *n* : a delusional mental disorder that is marked by infantile feelings of personal omnipotence and grandeur — **meg·a·lo·ma·ni·a·cal** \-mə-'nī-ə-kəl\ *or* **megalomaniac** *also* **meg·a·lo·man·ic** \-'ma-nik\ *adj* — **meg·a·lo·ma·ni·a·cal·ly** *adv*

meg·a·lo·ma·ni·ac \-'mā-nē-ˌak\ *n* : an individual affected with or exhibiting megalomania

-meg·a·ly \'me-gə-lē\ *n comb form, pl* **-meg·a·lies** : abnormal enlargement (of a specified part) ⟨hepato*megaly*⟩

mega·rad \'me-gə-ˌrad\ *n* : one million rads — abbr. *Mrad*

mega·vi·ta·min \ˌme-gə-'vī-tə-mən\ *adj* : relating to or consisting of very large doses of vitamins and esp. doses many times greater than the recommended daily allowances

mega·vi·ta·mins \-mənz\ *n pl* : a large quantity of vitamins

me·ges·trol acetate \me-'jes-ˌtról-\ *n* : a synthetic progestational hormone $C_{24}H_{32}O_4$ used in palliative treatment of advanced carcinoma of the breast and in endometriosis

meg·lu·mine \'me-glü-ˌmēn, me-'glü-\ *n* : a crystalline base $C_7H_{17}NO_5$ used to prepare salts used in radiopaque and therapeutic substances — see IODIPAMIDE

me·grim \'mē-grəm\ *n* **1 a** : MIGRAINE **b** : VERTIGO **2** : any of numerous diseases of animals marked by disturbance of equilibrium and abnormal gait and behavior — usu. used in pl.

mei·bo·mian gland \mī-'bō-mē-ən-\ *n, often cap M* : one of the long sebaceous glands of the eyelids that discharge a fatty secretion which lubricates the eyelids — called also *tarsal gland;* see CHALAZION
> **Mei·bom** \'mī-ˌbóm\, **Heinrich (1638–1700),** German physician.

mei·o·sis \mī-'ō-səs\ *n, pl* **mei·o·ses** \-ˌsēz\ : the cellular process that results in the number of chromosomes in gamete-producing cells being reduced to one half and that involves a reduction division in which one of each pair of homologous chromosomes passes to each daughter cell and a mitotic division — compare MITOSIS 1 — **mei·ot·ic** \mī-'ä-tik\ *adj* — **mei·ot·i·cal·ly** *adv*

Meiss·ner's corpuscle \'mīs-nərz-\ *n* : any of the small elliptical tactile end organs in hairless skin containing numerous transversely placed tactile cells and fine flattened nerve endings
> **Meissner, Georg (1829–1905),** German anatomist and physiologist.

Meissner's plexus *n* : a plexus of ganglionated nerve fibers lying between the muscular and mucous coats of the intestine — compare MYENTERIC PLEXUS

meit·ner·i·um \mīt-'nir-ē-əm\ *n* : a short-lived radioactive element produced artificially — symbol *Mt;* see ELEMENT table
> **Meitner, Lise (1878–1968),** German physicist.

mel \'mel\ *n* : a subjective unit of tone pitch equal to $1/1000$ of the pitch of a tone having a frequency of 1000 hertz — used esp. in audiology

me·lae·na *chiefly Brit var of* MELENA

melan- *or* **melano-** *comb form* **1** : black : dark ⟨*melanin*⟩ ⟨*melano*ma⟩ **2** : melanin ⟨*melano*genesis⟩

mel·an·cho·lia \ˌme-lən-'kō-lē-ə\ *n* : a mental condition and esp. a manic-depressive condition characterized by extreme depression, bodily complaints, and often hallucinations and delusions

mel·an·cho·li·ac \-lē-ˌak\ *n* : an individual affected with melancholia

¹mel·an·chol·ic \ˌme-lən-'kä-lik\ *adj* **1** : of, relating to, or subject to melancholy : DEPRESSED **2** : of or relating to melancholia

²melancholic *n* **1** : a melancholy person **2** : MELANCHOLIAC

mel·an·choly \'me-lən-ˌkä-lē\ *n, pl* **-chol·ies 1** : MELANCHOLIA **2** : depression or dejection of spirits — **melancholy** *adj*

mel·a·nin \'me-lə-nən\ *n* : any of various black, dark brown, reddish brown, or yellow pigments of animal or plant structures (as skin or hair); *esp* : any of numerous animal pigments that are essentially polymeric derivatives of indole formed by enzymatic modification of tyrosine

mel·a·nism \'me-lə-ˌni-zəm\ *n* **1** : an increased amount of black or nearly black pigmentation (as of skin, feathers, or hair) of an individual or kind of organism **2** : intense human pigmentation in skin, eyes, and hair — **mel·a·nis·tic** \ˌme-lə-'nis-tik\ *adj*

mel·a·nize \'me-lə-ˌnīz\ *vb* **-nized; -niz·ing** : to convert into or infiltrate with melanin ⟨*melanized* cell granules⟩ — **mel·a·ni·za·tion** \ˌme-lə-nə-'zā-shən\ *n*

melano- — see MELAN-

me·la·no·blast \mə-'la-nə-ˌblast, 'me-lə-nō-\ *n* : a cell that is a precursor of a melanocyte

me·la·no·blas·to·ma \mə-ˌla-nə-blas-'tō-mə, ˌme-lə-nō-\ *n, pl* **-mas** *also* **-ma·ta** \-mə-tə\ : a malignant tumor derived from melanoblasts

mel·a·no·car·ci·no·ma \-ˌkärs-ᵊn-'ō-mə\ *n, pl* **-mas** *also* **-ma·ta** \-mə-tə\ : MELANOMA 2

me·la·no·cyte \mə-'la-nə-ˌsīt, 'me-lə-nō-\ *n* : an epidermal cell that produces melanin

melanocyte–stimulating hormone *n* : either of two vertebrate hormones of the pituitary gland that darken the skin by stimulating melanin dispersion in pigment-containing cells — abbr. *MSH;* called also *intermedin, melanophore-stimulating hormone, melanotropin*

me·la·no·cyt·ic \mə-ˌla-nə-'si-tik, ˌme-lə-nō-\ *adj* : similar to or characterized by the presence of melanocytes

me·la·no·cy·to·ma \-ˌsī-'tō-mə\ *n, pl* **-mas** *also* **-ma·ta** \-mə-tə\ : a benign tumor composed of melanocytes

me·la·no·der·ma \ˌme-lə-nō-'dər-mə, mə-ˌla-\ *n* : abnormally intense pigmentation of the skin

me·la·no·gen·e·sis \mə-ˌla-nə-'je-nə-səs, ˌme-lə-nō-\ *n, pl* **-e·ses** \-ˌsēz\ : the formation of melanin

me·la·no·gen·ic \-'je-nik\ *adj* **1** : of, relating to, or characteristic of melanogenesis **2** : producing melanin

mel·a·no·ma \,me-lə-'nō-mə\ *n, pl* **-mas** *also* **-ma·ta** \-mə-tə\ **1** : a benign or malignant skin tumor containing dark pigment **2** : a tumor of high malignancy that starts in melanocytes of normal skin or moles and metastasizes rapidly and widely — called also *malignant melanoma, melanocarcinoma, melanosarcoma*

me·la·no·phage \mə-'la-nə-,fāj, 'me-lə-nə-\ *n* : a melanin-containing cell which obtains the pigment by phagocytosis

me·la·no·phore–stimulating hormone \mə-'la-nə-,fōr-, 'me-lə-nə-\, *n* : MELANOCYTE-STIMULATING HORMONE

me·la·no·sar·co·ma \-sär-'kō-mə\ *n, pl* **-mas** *also* **-ma·ta** \-mə-tə\ : MELANOMA 2

mel·a·no·sis \,me-lə-'nō-səs\ *n, pl* **-no·ses** \-'nō-,sēz\ : a condition characterized by abnormal deposition of melanins or sometimes other pigments in the tissues of the body

melanosis co·li \-'kō-,lī\ *n* : dark brownish black pigmentation of the mucous membrane of the colon due to the deposition of pigment in macrophages

me·la·no·some \mə-'la-nə-,sōm, 'me-lə-nō-\ *n* : a melanin-producing granule in a melanocyte — **me·la·no·som·al** \mə-,la-nə-'sō-məl, ,me-lə-nō-\ *adj*

mel·a·not·ic \,me-lə-'nä-tik\ *adj* : having or characterized by black pigmentation ⟨a ~ sarcoma⟩

me·la·no·tro·pin \mə-,la-nə-'trō-pən, ,me-lə-nō-\ *n* : MELANOCYTE-STIMULATING HORMONE

me·lar·so·prol \me-'lar-sə-,prol\ *n* : a drug $C_{12}H_{15}AsN_6OS_2$ used in the treatment of trypanosomiasis esp. in advanced stages

me·las·ma \mə-'laz-mə\ *n* : a dark pigmentation of the skin (as in Addison's disease) — **me·las·mic** \-mik\ *adj*

mel·a·to·nin \,me-lə-'tō-nən\ *n* : a vertebrate hormone $C_{13}H_{16}N_2O_2$ that is derived from serotonin, is secreted by the pineal gland esp. in response to darkness, and has been linked to the regulation of circadian rhythms

me·le·na \mə-'lē-nə\ *n* : the passage of dark tarry stools containing decomposing blood that is usu. an indication of bleeding in the upper part of the digestive tract and esp. the esophagus, stomach, and duodenum — compare HEMATOCHEZIA — **me·le·nic** \-nik\ *adj*

mel·en·ges·trol acetate \,me-lən-'jes-,trōl-, -,trōl-\ *n* : a progestational and antineoplastic agent $C_{25}H_{32}O_4$ that has been used as a growth-stimulating feed additive for beef cattle

-me·lia \'mē-lē-ə\ *n comb form* : condition of the limbs ⟨micro*melia*⟩

mel·i·oi·do·sis \,me-lē-,òi-'dō-səs\, *n, pl* **-do·ses** \-,sēz\ : an infectious disease chiefly of southeastern Asia that is closely related to glanders, that is caused by a bacterium of the genus *Burkholderia* (*B. pseudomallei* syn. *Peudomonas pseudomallei*) which is readily transmitted to mammals including humans esp. by direct contact with infected areas (as soil or water), and that may occur as an acute pulmonary infection, as a localized infection (as of the skin), or as a sometimes fatal septicemia

me·lit·tin \mə-'lit-ᵊn\ *n* : a toxic protein in bee venom that causes localized pain and inflammation

Mel·la·ril \'me-lə-,ril\ *trademark* — used for a preparation of thioridazine

mellitus — see DIABETES MELLITUS, INSULIN-DEPENDENT DIABETES MELLITUS, NON-INSULIN-DEPENDENT DIABETES MELLITUS

Me·loph·a·gus \mə-'lä-fə-gəs\ *n* : a genus of wingless flies (family Hippoboscidae) that includes the sheep ked (*M. ovinus*)

melo·rhe·os·to·sis \,me-lə-,rē-ä-'stō-səs\, *n, pl* **-to·ses** \-,sēz\ *or* **-tosises** : an extremely rare form of osteosclerosis characterized by asymmetrical or local enlargement and sclerotic changes in the long bones of one extremity

mel·pha·lan \'mel-fə-,lan\ *n* : an antineoplastic drug $C_{13}H_{18}Cl_2N_2O_2$ that is a derivative of nitrogen mustard and is used esp. in the treatment of multiple myeloma — called also *L-PAM, phenylalanine mustard, sarcolysin*

melting point *n* : the temperature at which a solid melts

-me·lus \mə-ləs\ *n comb form, pl* **-me·li** \-,lī\ : one having a (specified) abnormality of the limbs ⟨phoco*melus*⟩

mem·ber \'mem-bər\ *n* : a body part or organ: as **a** : LIMB **b** : PENIS

membran- *or* **membrani-** *or* **membrano-** *comb form* : membrane ⟨*membrano*proliferative glomerulonephritis⟩

mem·bra·na \mem-'brā-nə, -'brä-\ *n, pl* **mem·bra·nae** \-,nē, -,nī\ : MEMBRANE

membrana nic·ti·tans \-'nik-tə-,tanz\ *n* : NICTITATING MEMBRANE

mem·brane \'mem-,brān\ *n* **1** : a thin soft pliable sheet or layer esp. of animal or plant origin **2** : a limiting protoplasmic surface or interface — see NUCLEAR MEMBRANE, PLASMA MEMBRANE — **mem·braned** \'mem-,brānd\ *adj*

membrane bone *n* : a bone that ossifies directly in connective tissue without previous existence as cartilage

membrane of Descemet *n* : DESCEMET'S MEMBRANE

membrane potential *n* : the difference in electrical potential between the interior of a cell and the interstitial fluid beyond the membrane

mem·bra·no·pro·lif·er·a·tive glomerulonephritis \,mem-,brā-nō-prə-'li-fə-rə-tiv-\ *n* : a slowly progressive chronic glomerulonephritis characterized by proliferation of mesangial cells and irregular thickening of glomerular capillary walls and narrowing of the capillary lumina

mem·bra·nous \'mem-brə-nəs\ *adj* **1** : of, relating to, or resembling membranes **2** : characterized or accompanied by the formation of a usu. abnormal membrane or membranous layer — **mem·bra·nous·ly** *adv*

membranous glomerulonephritis *n* : a form of glomerulonephritis characterized by thickening of glomerular capillary basement membranes and nephrotic syndrome

membranous labyrinth *n* : the system of membrane-lined interconnected sacs and passages that is suspended within the bony labyrinth of the inner ear, is filled with endolymph and is surrounded by perilymph, and includes the cochlear duct, utricle, saccule, and semicircular ducts

membranous urethra *n* : the part of the male urethra that is situated between the layers of the urogenital diaphragm and that connects the parts of the urethra passing through the prostate gland and the penis

mem·o·ry \'mem-rē, 'me-mə-\ *n, pl* **-ries** **1** : the power or process of reproducing or recalling what has been learned and retained esp. through associative mechanisms **2** : the store of things learned and retained from an organism's activity or experience as indicated by modification of structure or behavior or by recall and recognition

memory cell *n* : a long-lived lymphocyte that carries the antibody or receptor for a specific antigen after a first exposure to the antigen and that remains in a less than mature state until stimulated by a second exposure to the antigen at which time it mounts a more effective immune response than a cell which has not been exposed previously

memory trace *n* : ENGRAM

men *pl of* MAN

men- *or* **meno-** *comb form* : menstruation ⟨*meno*pause⟩ ⟨*meno*rrhagia⟩

men·a·di·one \ˌme-nə-'dī-ˌōn, -dī-'\ *n* : a yellow crystalline compound $C_{11}H_8O_2$ with the biological activity of natural vitamin K — called also *vitamin K₃*

me·naph·thone \mə-'naf-ˌthōn\ *n, Brit* : MENADIONE

men·a·quin·one \ˌme-nə-'kwi-ˌnōn\ *n* : VITAMIN K 1b; *also* : a synthetic derivative of vitamin K₂

men·ar·che \'me-ˌnär-kē\ *n* : the beginning of the menstrual function; *esp* : the first menstrual period of an individual — **men·ar·che·al** \ˌme-'när-kē-əl\ *or* **men·ar·chal** \-kəl\ *adj*

¹mend \'mend\ *vb* **1** : to restore to health : CURE **2** : to improve in health; *also* : HEAL

²mend *n* : an act of mending or repair — **on the mend** : getting better or improving esp. in health

men·de·le·vi·um \ˌmen-də-'lē-vē-əm, -'lā-\ *n* : a radioactive element that is artificially produced — symbol *Md*; see ELEMENT table

Men·de·lian \men-'dē-lē-ən, -'dēl-yən\ *adj* : of, relating to, or according with Mendel's laws or Mendelism — **Mendelian** *n*
Men·del \'mend-ᵊl\, **Gregor Johann (1822–1884),** Austrian botanist and geneticist.

Mendelian factor *n* : GENE

Mendelian inheritance *n* : inheritance of characters specif. transmitted by genes in accord with Mendel's law — called also *particulate inheritance*

Men·del·ism \'mend-ᵊl-ˌi-zəm\ *n* : the principles or the operations of Mendel's laws; *also* : MENDELIAN INHERITANCE

Men·del's law \'men-dᵊlz-\ *n* **1** : a principle in genetics: hereditary units occur in pairs that separate during gamete formation so that every gamete receives but one member of a pair — called also *law of segregation* **2** : a principle in genetics limited and modified by the subsequent discovery of the phenomenon of linkage: the different pairs of hereditary units are distributed to the gametes independently of each other, the gametes combine at random, and the various combinations of hereditary pairs occur in the zygotes according to the laws of chance — called also *law of independent assortment* **3** : a principle in genetics proved subsequently to be subject to many limitations: because one of each pair of hereditary units dominates the other in expression, characters are inherited as alternatives on an all or nothing basis — called also *law of dominance*

men·go·vi·rus \'meŋ-gō-ˌvī-rəs\ *n* : a picornavirus (species *Encephalomyocarditis virus* of the genus *Cardiovirus*) that causes encephalomyocarditis

Mé·nière's disease \mən-'yerz-, 'men-yərz-\ *n* : a disorder of the membranous labyrinth of the inner ear that is marked by recurrent attacks of dizziness, tinnitus, and deafness — called also *Ménière's syndrome*
Ménière, Prosper (1799–1862), French physician.

mening- *or* **meningo-** *also* **meningi-** *comb form* **1** : meninges ⟨*meningo*coccus⟩ ⟨*meningi*tis⟩ **2** : meninges and ⟨*meningo*encephalitis⟩

men·in·ge·al \ˌme-nən-'jē-əl\ *adj* : of, relating to, or affecting the meninges

meningeal artery *n* : any of several arteries supplying the meninges of the brain and neighboring structures; *esp* : MIDDLE MENINGEAL ARTERY

meningeal vein *n* : any of several veins draining the meninges of the brain and neighboring structures

meninges *pl of* MENINX

me·nin·gi·o·ma \mə-ˌnin-jē-ˈō-mə\ *n*, *pl* **-mas** *also* **-ma·ta** \-tə\ : a slow-growing encapsulated tumor arising from the meninges and often causing damage by pressing upon the brain and adjacent parts

men·in·gism \ˈme-nən-ˌji-zəm, mə-ˈnin-\ *n* : MENINGISMUS

men·in·gis·mus \ˌme-nən-ˈjiz-məs\, *pl* **-gis·mi** \-ˌmī\ : a state of meningeal irritation with symptoms suggesting meningitis that often occurs at the onset of acute febrile diseases esp. in children

men·in·gi·tis \ˌme-nən-ˈjī-təs\ *n*, *pl* **-git·i·des** \-ˈji-tə-ˌdēz\ **1** : inflammation of the meninges and esp. of the pia mater and the arachnoid **2** : a disease that may be either a mild illness caused by any of numerous viruses (as various coxsackieviruses) or a more severe one. life-threatening illness caused by a bacterium (esp. the meningococcus or the serotype designated B of *Haemophilus influenzae*), that may be associated with fever, headache, vomiting, malaise, and stiff neck — **men·in·git·ic** \-ˈji-tik\ *adj*

me·nin·go·cele *also* **me·nin·go·coele** \mə-ˈniŋ-gə-ˌsēl, mə-ˈnin-jə-\ *n* : a protrusion of meninges through a defect in the skull or spinal column forming a cyst filled with cerebrospinal fluid

me·nin·go·coc·cae·mia *chiefly Brit var of* MENINGOCOCCEMIA

me·nin·go·coc·ce·mia \mə-ˌniŋ-gō-ˌkäk-ˈsē-mē-ə, -ˌnin-jə-\ *n* : an abnormal condition characterized by the presence of meningococci in the blood

me·nin·go·coc·cus \mə-ˌniŋ-gə-ˈkä-kəs, -ˌnin-jə-\ *n*, *pl* **-coc·ci** \-ˈkä-ˌkī, -ˌkē; -ˈkäk-ˌsī, -ˌsē\ : a bacterium of the genus *Neisseria* (*N. meningitidis*) that causes cerebrospinal meningitis — **me·nin·go·coc·cal** \-ˈkä-kəl\ *also* **me·nin·go·coc·cic** \-ˈkä-kik, -ˈkäk-sik\ *adj*

me·nin·go·en·ceph·a·li·tis \-in-ˌse-fə-ˈlī-təs\ *n*, *pl* **-lit·i·des** \-ˈli-tə-ˌdēz\ : inflammation of the brain and meninges — **me·nin·go·en·ceph·a·lit·ic** \mə-ˌnin-gō-ən-ˌse-fə-ˈli-tik, -ˌnin-(ˌ)jō-\ *adj*

me·nin·go·en·ceph·a·lo·cele \-in-ˈse-fə-lō-ˌsēl\ *n* : a protrusion of meninges and brain through a defect in the skull

me·nin·go·en·ceph·a·lo·my·eli·tis \-in-ˌse-fə-lō-ˌmī-ə-ˈlī-təs\ *n*, *pl* **-elit·i·des** \-ə-ˈli-tə-ˌdēz\ : inflammation of the meninges, brain, and spinal cord

me·nin·go·my·elo·cele \-ˈmī-ə-lō-ˌsēl\ *n* : a protrusion of meninges and spinal cord through a defect in the spinal column

me·nin·go·vas·cu·lar \-ˈvas-kyə-lər\ *adj* : of, relating to, or affecting the meninges and the cerebral blood vessels

me·ninx \ˈmē-niŋks, ˈme-\ *n*, *pl* **me·nin·ges** \mə-ˈnin-(ˌ)jēz\ : any of the three membranes that envelop the brain and spinal cord and include the arachnoid, dura mater, and pia mater

me·nis·cal \mə-ˈnis-kəl\ *adj* : of or relating to a meniscus ⟨a ∼ tear⟩

men·is·cec·to·my \ˌme-ni-ˈsek-tə-mē\ *n*, *pl* **-mies** : surgical excision of a meniscus of the knee or temporomandibular joint

me·nis·cus \mə-ˈnis-kəs\ *n*, *pl* **me·nis·ci** \-ˈnis-ˌkī, -ˌkē; -ˈni-ˌsī\ *also* **me·nis·cus·es** : a fibrous cartilage within a joint: **a** : either of two crescent-shaped lamellae of fibrocartilage that border and partly cover the articulating surfaces of the tibia and femur at the knee : SEMILUNAR CARTILAGE: (1) : one mostly between the lateral condyles of the tibia and femur — called also *lateral meniscus, lateral semilunar cartilage* (2) : one mostly between the medial condyles of the tibia and femur — called also *medial meniscus, medial semilunar cartilage* **b** : a thin oval ligament of the temporomandibular joint that is situated between the condyle of the mandible and the mandibular fossa and separates the joint into two cavities

Men·kes' disease \ˈmeŋ-kəz-\ *n* : a disorder of copper metabolism that is inherited as a recessive X-linked trait and is characterized by a deficiency of copper in the liver and of copper-containing proteins (as ceruloplasmin) which results in mental retardation, brittle kinky hair, and a fatal outcome early in life — called also *Menkes' syndrome*

Menkes, John Hans (*b* 1928), American (Austrian-born) pediatric neurologist.

meno·met·ror·rha·gia \ˌme-nō-ˌmē-trə-ˈrā-jə, -ˈrä-, -jē-ə, -zhə\ *n* : a combination of menorrhagia and metrorrhagia

meno·pause \ˈme-nə-ˌpoz, ˈmē-\ *n* **1 a** (1) : the of natural cessation of menstruation occurring usu. between the ages of 45 and 55 with a mean in Western cultures of approximately 51 (2) : the physiological period in the life of a woman in which such cessation occurs — called also *climacteric, climax;* compare PERIMENOPAUSE **b** : cessation of menstruation from other than natural causes (as from surgical removal of the ovaries) **2** : ANDROPAUSE — **meno·paus·al** \ˌme-nə-ˈpo-zəl, ˌmē-\ *adj*

Men·o·pon \ˈme-nə-ˌpän\ *n* : a genus of biting lice that includes the shaft louse (*M. gallinae*) of poultry

men·or·rha·gia \ˌme-nə-ˈrä-jə, -ˈrä-, -jē-ə, -zhə\ *n* : abnormally profuse menstrual flow — compare HYPERMENORRHEA, METRORRHAGIA — **men·or·rhag·ic** \-ˈra-jik\ *adj*

men·or·rhea \ˌme-nə-ˈrē-ə\ *n* : normal menstrual flow

men·or·rhoea *chiefly Brit var of* MENORRHEA

men·ses \'men-ˌsēz\ *n sing or pl* : the menstrual flow

men·stru·al \'men-strə-wəl\ *adj* : of or relating to menstruation — **men·stru·al·ly** *adv*

menstrual cycle *n* : the whole cycle of physiologic changes from the beginning of one menstrual period to the beginning of the next

menstrual extraction *n* : a procedure for early termination of pregnancy by withdrawing the uterine lining and a fertilized egg if present by means of suction

men·stru·a·tion \ˌmen-strə-'wā-shən\ *n* : a discharging of blood, secretions, and tissue debris from the uterus that recurs in nonpregnant human and other primate females of breeding age at approximately monthly intervals and that is considered to represent a readjustment of the uterus to the nonpregnant state following proliferative changes accompanying the preceding ovulation; *also* : PERIOD 1b — **men·stru·ate** \'men-strə-ˌwāt\ *vb* — **men·stru·ous** \'men-strə-wəs\ *adj*

men·stru·um \'men-strə-wəm\ *n, pl* **-stru·ums** *or* **-strua** \-strə-wə\ : a substance that dissolves a solid or holds it in suspension : SOLVENT

menta *pl of* MENTUM

¹**men·tal** \'ment-ᵊl\ *adj* **1 a** : of or relating to the mind; *specif* : of or relating to the total emotional and intellectual response of an individual to external reality **b** : of or relating to intellectual as contrasted with emotional activity **2 a** : of, relating to, or affected by a psychiatric disorder **b** : intended for the care or treatment of persons affected by psychiatric disorders ⟨∼ hospitals⟩ — **men·tal·ly** *adv*

²**mental** *adj* : of or relating to the chin : GENIAL

mental age *n* : a measure used in psychological testing that expresses an individual's mental attainment in terms of the number of years it takes an average child to reach the same level

mental alienation *n* : mental disorder or derangement : INSANITY

mental artery *n* : a branch of the inferior alveolar artery on each side that emerges from the mental foramen and supplies blood to the chin — called also *mental branch*

mental capacity *n* **1** : sufficient understanding and memory to comprehend in a general way the situation in which one finds oneself and the nature, purpose, and consequence of any act or transaction into which one proposes to enter **2** : the degree of understanding and memory the law requires to uphold the validity of or to charge one with responsibility for a particular act or transaction

mental competence *n* : MENTAL CAPACITY

mental deficiency *n* : MENTAL RETARDATION

mental disorder *n* : a mental or bodily condition marked primarily by sufficient disorganization of personality, mind, and emotions to seriously impair the normal psychological functioning of the individual — called also *mental illness*

mental foramen *n* : a foramen for the passage of blood vessels and a nerve on the outside of the lower jaw on each side near the chin

mental health *n* : the condition of being sound mentally and emotionally that is characterized by the absence of mental disorder (as neurosis or psychosis) and by adequate adjustment esp. as reflected in feeling comfortable about oneself, positive feelings about others, and ability to meet the demands of life; *also* : the field of mental health : MENTAL HYGIENE

mental hygiene *n* : the science of maintaining mental health and preventing the development of mental disorder

mental illness *n* : MENTAL DISORDER

mental incapacity *n* **1** : an absence of mental capacity **2** : an inability through mental disorder or mental retardation to carry on the everyday affairs of life or to care for one's person or property with reasonable discretion — called also *mental incompetence*

men·ta·lis \men-'tā-lis\ *n, pl* **men·ta·les** \-ˌlēz\ : a muscle that originates in the incisive fossa of the mandible, inserts in the skin of the chin, and raises the chin and pushes up the lower lip

men·tal·i·ty \men-'ta-lə-tē\ *n, pl* **-ties** **1** : mental power or capacity **2** : mode or way of thought

mental nerve *n* : a branch of the inferior alveolar nerve that emerges from the bone of the mandible near the mental protuberance and divides into branches which are distributed to the skin of the chin and to the skin and mucous membranes of the lower lip

mental protuberance *n* : the bony protuberance at the front of the lower jaw forming the chin

mental retardation *n* : subaverage intellectual ability equivalent to or less than an IQ of 70 that is accompanied by significant deficits in abilities (as in communication or self-care) necessary for independent daily living, is present from birth or infancy, and is manifested esp. by delayed or abnormal development, by learning difficulties, and by problems in social adjustment — **mentally retarded** *adj*

mental spine *n* : either of two small elevations on the inner surface of each side of the symphysis of the lower jaw of which the superior one on each side provides attachment for the ge-

nioglossus and the inferior for the geniohyoid muscle

mental test *n* : any of various standardized procedures applied to an individual in order to ascertain ability
or evaluate behavior

mental tubercle *n* : a prominence on
each side of the mental protuberance
of the mandible — called also *genial
tubercle*

men·ta·tion \men-'tā-shən\ *n* : mental
activity ⟨unconscious ∼⟩

men·thol \'men-ˌthȯl, -ˌthōl\ *n* : a crystalline alcohol $C_{10}H_{20}O$ that occurs
esp. in mint oils, has the odor and
cooling properties of peppermint, and
is used in flavoring and in medicine
(as locally to relieve pain, itching, and
nasal congestion)

men·tho·lat·ed \'men-thə-ˌlā-təd\ *adj*
: containing or impregnated with
menthol ⟨a ∼ salve⟩

mentis — see COMPOS MENTIS, NON
COMPOS MENTIS

men·tum \'men-təm\ *n, pl* **men·ta** \-tə\
: CHIN

mep·a·crine \'me-pə-ˌkrēn, -krən\ *n,
chiefly Brit* : QUINACRINE

mep·a·zine \'me-pə-ˌzēn\ *n* : a phenothiazine $C_{19}H_{22}N_2S$ formerly used
as a tranquilizer

me·pen·zo·late bromide \mə-'pen-zə-
ˌlāt-\ *n* : an anticholinergic drug
$C_{21}H_{26}BrNO_3$

me·per·i·dine \mə-'per-ə-ˌdēn\ *n* : a
synthetic narcotic drug used in the
form of its hydrochloride $C_{15}H_{21}$-
$NO_2·HCl$ as an analgesic, sedative,
and antispasmodic — called also
isonipecaine, pethidine

me·phen·e·sin \mə-'fe-nə-sin\ *n* : a
compound $C_{10}H_{14}O_3$ used chiefly in
the treatment of neuromuscular conditions — called also *myanesin*

meph·en·ox·a·lone \ˌme-fə-'näk-sə-
ˌlōn\ *n* : a tranquilizing drug $C_{11}H_{13}$-
NO_4

me·phen·ter·mine \mə-'fen-tər-ˌmēn\
n : an adrenergic drug administered
often in the form of the sulfate
$C_{11}H_{17}N·H_2SO_4$ as a vasopressor and
nasal decongestant

me·phen·y·to·in \mə-'fe-ni-ˌtō-in\ *n*
: an anticonvulsant drug $C_{12}H_{14}N_2O_2$
— see MESANTOIN

mepho·bar·bi·tal \ˌme-fō-'bär-bə-ˌtäl\
n : a crystalline barbiturate
$C_{13}H_{14}N_2O_3$ used as a sedative and in
the treatment of epilepsy

Meph·y·ton \'me-fə-ˌtän\ *trademark* —
used for a preparation of vitamin K_1

me·piv·a·caine \me-'pi-və-ˌkān\ *n* : a
drug used esp. in the form of the hydrochloride $C_{15}H_{22}N_2O·HCl$ as a local
anesthetic

mep·ro·bam·ate \ˌme-prō-'ba-ˌmāt,
mə-'prō-bə-ˌmāt\ *n* : a bitter carbamate $C_9H_{18}N_2O_4$ used as a tranquilizer — see EQUANIL, MILTOWN

mer \'mər, 'mer\ *n* : the repeating
structural unit of a polymer — often
prefixed with a number indicating the

number of units in the polymer ⟨syn-
thesized two 20-*mers*⟩

¹**mer-** *or* **mero-** *comb form* : thigh ⟨*meralgia*⟩

²**mer-** *or* **mero-** *comb form* : part : partial ⟨*meroblastic*⟩

me·ral·gia \mə-'ral-jə, -jē-ə\ *n* : pain
esp. of a neuralgic kind in the thigh

meralgia par·aes·thet·i·ca *Brit var of*
MERALGIA PARESTHETICA

meralgia par·es·thet·i·ca \-ˌpar-əs-
'the-ti-kə\ *n* : an abnormal condition
characterized by pain and paresthesia
in the outer surface of the thigh

mer·al·lu·ride \mə-'ral-yə-ˌrīd, -ˌrid\ *n*
: a chemical combination of a mercurial compound $C_9H_{16}HgN_2O_6$ and
theophylline formerly used as a diuretic

mer·bro·min \ˌmər-'brō-mən\ *n* : a
green crystalline mercurial compound $C_{20}H_8Br_2HgNa_2O_6$ used as a
topical antiseptic and germicide in
the form of its red solution — see
MERCUROCHROME

mer·cap·tom·er·in \mər-ˌkap-'tä-
mə-rən\ *n* : a mercurial compound
$C_{16}H_{25}HgNNa_2O_6S$ formerly used as a
diuretic

mer·cap·to·pu·rine \ˌmər-ˌkap-tə-
'pyu̇r-ˌēn\ *n* : an antimetabolite
$C_5H_4N_4S$ that interferes esp. with the
metabolism of purine bases and the
biosynthesis of nucleic acids and that
is sometimes useful in the treatment
of acute leukemia

mer·cu·mat·i·lin \ˌmər-kyù-'mat-əl-ən,
mər-ˌkyü-mə-'ti-lən\ *n* : a chemical
combination of a mercury-containing
acid $C_{14}H_{14}HgO_6$ and theophylline
formerly used as a diuretic

¹**mer·cu·ri·al** \ˌmər-'kyu̇r-ē-əl\ *adj*
: of, relating to, containing, or caused
by mercury ⟨∼ salves⟩

²**mercurial** *n* : a pharmaceutical or
chemical containing mercury

mer·cu·ri·al·ism \ˌmər-'kyu̇r-ē-ə-ˌli-
zəm\ *n* : chronic poisoning with mercury — called also *hydrargyrism*

mer·cu·ric chloride \ˌmər-'kyu̇r-ik-\
n : a heavy crystalline poisonous compound $HgCl_2$ used as a disinfectant
and fungicide — called also *bichloride
of mercury, corrosive sublimate, mercury bichloride*

mercuric cyanide *n* : the mercury
cyanide $Hg(CN)_2$ which has been used
as an antiseptic

mercuric iodide *n* : a red crystalline
poisonous salt HgI_2 which has been
used as a topical antiseptic

mercuric oxide *n* : either of two forms
of a slightly water-soluble crystalline
poisonous compound HgO which
have been used in antiseptic ointments

Mer·cu·ro·chrome \ˌmər-'kyu̇r-ə-
ˌkrōm\ *trademark* — used for a
preparation of merbromin

mer·cu·ro·phyl·line \ˌmər-kyə-rō-'fi-
ˌlēn, -lən\ *n* : a chemical combination
of a mercurial compound $C_{14}H_{24}$-

HgNNaO₅ and theophylline formerly used as a diuretic

mer·cu·rous chloride \mər-ˈkyùr-əs-, ˈmər-kyə-rəs-\ *n* : CALOMEL

mer·cu·ry \ˈmər-kyə-rē\ *n, pl* **-ries 1** : a heavy silver-white poisonous metallic element that is liquid at ordinary temperatures — symbol *Hg*; called also *quicksilver*; see ELEMENT table **2** : a pharmaceutical preparation containing mercury or a compound of it

mercury bi·chlo·ride \-ˌbī-ˈklȯr-ˌīd\ *n* : MERCURIC CHLORIDE

mercury chloride *n* : a chloride of mercury: as **a** : CALOMEL **b** : MERCURIC CHLORIDE

mercury–vapor lamp *n* : an electric lamp in which the discharge takes place through mercury vapor and which has been used therapeutically as a source of ultraviolet radiation

mercy killing *n* : EUTHANASIA

-mere \ˌmir\ *n comb form* : part : segment ⟨blastomere⟩ ⟨centromere⟩

me·rid·i·an \mə-ˈri-dē-ən\ *n* **1** : an imaginary circle or closed curve on the surface of a sphere or globe-shaped body (as the eyeball) that lies in a plane passing through the poles **2** : any of the pathways along which the body's vital energy flows according to the theory of acupuncture — **meridian** *adj* — **me·rid·i·o·nal** \mə-ˈri-dē-ən-ᵊl\ *adj*

Mer·kel cell *also* **Merkel's cell** \ˈmər-kəl(z)-\ *n* : a cell that occurs in the basal part of the epidermis, is characterized by dense granules in its cytoplasm, is closely associated with the unmyelinated tip of a nerve fiber, and prob. functions in tactile sensory perception

Merkel, Friedrich Siegmund (1845–1919), German anatomist.

Merkel's disk *n* : the disklike expansion of the end of a nerve fiber together with a closely associated Merkel cell that has a presumed tactile function — called also *Merkel's corpuscle*

mero- — see MER-

mero·blas·tic \ˌmer-ə-ˈblas-tik\ *adj* : characterized by or being incomplete cleavage as a result of the presence of an impeding mass of yolk material (as in the eggs of birds) — compare HOLOBLASTIC — **mero·blas·ti·cal·ly** *adv*

mero·crine \ˈmer-ə-krən, -ˌkrīn, -ˌkrēn\ *adj* : producing a secretion that is discharged without major damage to the secreting cells ⟨~ glands⟩; *also* : of or produced by a merocrine gland ⟨a ~ secretion⟩ — compare APOCRINE, ECCRINE, HOLOCRINE

mero·my·o·sin \ˌmer-ə-ˈmī-ə-sən\ *n* : either of two structural subunits of myosin that are obtained esp. by tryptic digestion

mero·zo·ite \ˌmer-ə-ˈzō-ˌīt\ *n* : a small amoeboid sporozoan trophozoite (as

of a malaria parasite) produced by schizogony that is capable of initiating a new sexual or asexual cycle of development

mer·sal·yl \ˌmər-ˈsa-lil\ *n* : an organic mercurial C₁₃H₁₆HgNNaO₆ administered by injection in combination with theophylline as a diuretic

Mer·thi·o·late \ˌmər-ˈthī-ə-ˌlāt, -lət\ *n* : a preparaton of thimerosal — formerly a U.S. registered trademark

mes- *or* **meso-** *comb form* **1 a** : mid : in the middle ⟨mesoderm⟩ **b** : mesentery or membrane supporting a (specified) part ⟨mesoappendix⟩ ⟨mesocolon⟩ **2** : intermediate (as in size or type) ⟨mesomorph⟩

mes·an·gi·um \ˌme-ˈsan-jē-əm, ˌmē-\ *n, pl* **-gia** \-jē-ə\ : a thin membrane that gives support to the capillaries surrounding the tubule of a nephron — **mes·an·gi·al** \-jē-əl\ *adj*

Mes·an·to·in \me-ˈsan-tō-in\ *trademark* — used for a preparation of mephenytoin

mes·aor·ti·tis \ˌme-ˌsā-ȯr-ˈtī-təs, ˌmē-\ *n, pl* **-tit·i·des** \-ˈti-tə-ˌdēz\ : inflammation of the middle layer of the aorta

mes·ar·ter·i·tis \-ˌsär-tə-ˈrī-təs\ *n, pl* **-it·i·des** \-ˈri-tə-ˌdēz\ : inflammation of the middle layer of an artery

mes·cal \me-ˈskal, mə-\ *n* **1** : PEYOTE **2 2** : a usu. colorless Mexican liquor distilled esp. from the central leaves of any of various fleshy-leaved agaves (genus *Agave* of the family Agavaceae); *also* : a plant from which mescal is produced

mescal button *n* : PEYOTE BUTTON

mes·ca·line \ˈmes-kə-lən, -ˌlēn\ *n* : a hallucinogenic crystalline alkaloid C₁₁H₁₇NO₃ that is the chief active principle in peyote buttons

mes·en·ceph·a·lon \ˌme-zən-ˈse-fə-ˌlän, ˌmē-, -sən-, -lən\ *n* : MIDBRAIN — **mes·en·ce·phal·ic** \-zen-sə-ˈfa-lik, -sen-\ *adj*

mes·en·chyme \ˈme-zən-ˌkīm, ˈmē-, -sən-\ *n* : loosely organized undifferentiated mesodermal cells that give rise to such structures as connective tissues, blood, lymphatics, bone, and cartilage — **mes·en·chy·mal** \ˌme-zən-ˈkī-məl, ˌmē-, -sən-\ *adj* — **mes·en·chy·ma·tous** \-mə-təs\ *adj*

mes·en·chy·mo·ma \ˌme-zən-ˌkī-ˈmō-mə, ˌmē-, -sən-\ *n, pl* **-mas** *also* **-ma·ta** \-mə-tə\ : a benign or malignant tumor consisting of a mixture of at least two types of embryonic connective tissue

¹mes·en·ter·ic \ˌme-zən-ˈter-ik, -sən-\ *adj* : of, relating to, or located in or near a mesentery

²mesenteric *n* : a mesenteric part; *esp* : MESENTERIC ARTERY

mesenteric artery *n* : either of two arteries arising from the aorta and passing between the two layers of the mesentery to the intestine: **a** : one that arises just above the bifurcation of the abdominal aorta into the common iliac arteries and supplies the left half of the transverse colon, the descending colon, the sigmoid colon, and most of the rectum — called also *inferior mesenteric artery* **b** : one that arises from the aorta just below the celiac artery at the level of the first lumbar vertebra and supplies the greater part of the small intestine, the cecum, the ascending colon, and the right half of the transverse colon — called also *superior mesenteric artery*

mesenteric ganglion *n* : either of two ganglionic masses of the sympathetic nervous system associated with the corresponding mesenteric plexus: **a** : a variable amount of massed ganglionic tissue of the inferior mesenteric plexus near the origin of the inferior mesenteric artery — called also *inferior mesenteric ganglion* **b** : a usu. discrete ganglionic mass of the superior mesenteric plexus near the origin of the superior mesenteric artery — called also *superior mesenteric ganglion*

mesenteric node *n* : any of the lymphatic glands of the mesentery — called also *mesenteric gland, mesenteric lymph node*

mesenteric plexus *n* : either of two plexuses of the sympathetic nervous system lying mostly in the mesentery in close proximity to and distributed to the same structures as the corresponding mesenteric arteries: **a** : one associated with the inferior mesenteric artery — called also *inferior mesenteric plexus* **b** : a subdivision of the celiac plexus associated with the superior mesenteric artery — called also *superior mesenteric plexus*

mesenteric vein *n* : either of two veins draining the intestine, passing between the two layers of the mesentery, and associated with the corresponding mesenteric arteries: **a** : one that is a continuation of the superior rectal vein, that returns blood from the rectum, the sigmoid colon, and the descending colon, that accompanies the inferior mesenteric artery, and that usu. empties into the splenic vein — called also *inferior mesenteric vein* **b** : one that drains blood from the small intestine, the cecum, the ascending colon, and the transverse colon, that accompanies the superior mesenteric artery, and that joins with the splenic vein to form the portal vein — called also *superior mesenteric vein*

mes·en·tery \'mes-zən-ˌter-ē, -sən-\ *n, pl* **-ter·ies 1** : one or more vertebrate membranes that consist of a double fold of the peritoneum and invest the intestines and their appendages and connect them with the dorsal wall of the abdominal cavity; *specif* : such membranes connected with the jejunum and ileum in humans **2** : a fold of membrane comparable to a mesen-tery and supporting a viscus (as the heart) that is not a part of the digestive tract

mesh \'mesh\ *n* : a flexible netting of fine wire used in surgery esp. in the repair of large hernias and other body defects

me·si·al \'mē-zē-əl, -sē-\ *adj* **1** : being or located in the middle or a median part 〈the ∼ aspect of the metacarpal head〉 **2** : situated in or near or directed toward the median plane of the body 〈the heart is ∼ to the lungs〉 — compare DISTAL 1b **3** : of, relating to, or being the surface of a tooth that is next to the tooth in front of it or that is closest to the middle of the front of the jaw — compare DISTAL 1c, PROXIMAL 1b — **me·si·al·ly** *adv*

mesio- *comb form* : mesial and 〈*mesio*distal〉 〈*mesio*buccal〉

me·sio·buc·cal \ˌmē-zē-ō-'bək-ᵊl, -sē-\ *adj* : of or relating to the mesial and buccal surfaces of a tooth — **me·sio·buc·cal·ly** *adv*

me·sio·clu·sion *also* **me·si·oc·clu·sion** \ˌmē-zē-ə-'klü-zhən, -sē-\ *n* : malocclusion characterized by mesial displacement of one or more of the lower teeth

me·sio·dis·tal \ˌmē-zē-ō-'dist-ᵊl\ *adj* : of or relating to the mesial and distal surfaces of a tooth; *esp* : relating to, lying along, containing, or being a diameter joining the mesial and distal surfaces — **me·sio·dis·tal·ly** *adv*

me·sio·lin·gual \-'liŋ-gwəl\ *adj* : of or relating to the mesial and lingual surfaces of a tooth — **me·sio·lin·gual·ly** *adv*

mes·mer·ism \'mez-mə-ˌri-zəm, 'mes-\ *n* : hypnotic induction by the practices of F. A. Mesmer; *broadly* : HYPNOTISM — **mes·mer·ist** \-rist\ *n* — **mes·mer·ize** \-ˌrīz\ *vb*

Mes·mer \'mes-mər\, **Franz** *or* **Friedrich Anton (1734–1815),** German physician.

meso- — see MES-

me·so·ap·pen·dix \ˌme-zō-ə-'pen-diks, ˌmē-, -sō-\ *n, pl* **-dix·es** *or* **-di·ces** \-də-ˌsēz\ : the mesentery of the vermiform appendix — **me·so·ap·pen·di·ce·al** \-ˌpen-də-'sē-əl\ *adj*

me·so·blast \'me-zə-ˌblast, 'mē-, -sə-\ *n* : the embryonic cells that give rise to mesoderm; *broadly* : MESODERM — **me·so·blas·tic** \ˌme-zō-'blas-tik, ˌmē-, -sō-\ *adj*

me·so·car·di·um \ˌme-zō-'kär-dē-əm, ˌmē-, -sō-\ *n* **1** : the transitory mesentery of the embryonic heart **2** : either of two tubular prolongations of the epicardium that enclose the aorta and pulmonary trunk and the venae cavae and pulmonary veins

Me·so·ces·toi·des \-ˌses-'toi-(ˌ)dēz\ *n* : a genus (family Mesocestoididae) of tapeworms having the adults parasitic in mammals and birds and a slender threadlike contractile larva free in

me·so·co·lon \,me-zə-'kō-lən, ,mē-, -sə-\ n : a mesentery joining the colon to the dorsal abdominal wall

me·so·derm \'me-zə-,dərm, 'mē-, -sə-\ n : the middle of the three primary germ layers of an embryo that is the source esp. of bone, muscle, connective tissue, and dermis; *broadly* : tissue derived from this germ layer — **me·so·der·mal** \,me-zə-'dər-məl, ,mē-, -sə-\ adj — **me·so·der·mal·ly** adv

me·so·duo·de·num \,me-zə-,dü-ə-'dē-nəm, ,mē-, -sə-, -,dyü-; -dü-'äd-ᵊn-əm, -dyü-\ n, pl -**de·na** \-ə-'dē-nə, -'äd-ᵊn-ə\ or -**de·nums** : the mesentery of the duodenum usu. not persisting in adult life in humans and other mammals in which the developing intestine undergoes a counterclockwise rotation

me·so·gas·tri·um \,-'gas-trē-əm\ n, pl -**tria** \-trē-ə\ **1** : a ventral mesentery of the embryonic stomach that persists as the falciform ligament and the lesser omentum — called also *ventral mesogastrium* **2** : a dorsal mesentery of the embryonic stomach that gives rise to ligaments between the stomach and spleen and the spleen and kidney — called also *dorsal mesogastrium*

me·so·ino·si·tol \,me-zō-i-'nō-sə-,tól, ,mē-, -ī-'nō-, -,tōl\ n : MYOINOSITOL

me·so·lim·bic \-'lim-bik\ adj : of, relating to, or being the more central portion of the limbic system of the brain that arises mainly in the ventral tegmental area, consists esp. of dopaminergic neurons, and innervates the amygdala, nucleus accumbens, and olfactory tubercle

me·so·morph \'me-zə-,mórf, 'mē-, -sə-\ n : a mesomorphic body or person

me·so·mor·phic \,me-zə-'mór-fik, ,mē-, -sə-\ adj : having a husky muscular body build — compare ECTOMORPHIC, ENDOMORPHIC — **me·so·mor·phy** \'me-zə-,mór-fē, 'mē-, -sə-\ n

me·so·neph·ric \,me-zə-'ne-frik, ,mē-, -sə-\ adj : of or relating to the mesonephros

mesonephric duct n : WOLFFIAN DUCT

me·so·ne·phro·ma \-ni-'frō-mə\ n, pl -**mas** also -**ma·ta** \-mə-tə\ : a benign or malignant tumor esp. of the female genital tract held to be derived from the mesonephros

me·so·neph·ros \,me-zə-'ne-frəs, ,mē-, -sə-, -,fräs\ n, pl -**neph·roi** \-'ne-,frói\ : either member of the second and midmost of the three paired vertebrate renal organs that functions in adult fishes and amphibians but functions only in the embryo of reptiles, birds, and mammals in which it is replaced by a metanephros in the adult — called also *Wolffian body*; compare PRONEPHROS

me·sor·chi·um \mə-'zór-kē-əm\ n, pl -**chia** \-kē-ə\ : the fold of peritoneum that attaches the testis to the dorsal wall in the fetus

me·so·rec·tum \,me-zə-'rek-təm, ,mē-, -sə-\ n, pl -**tums** or -**ta** \-tə\ : the mesentery that supports the rectum

mes·orid·a·zine \,me-zó-'ri-də-,zēn, ,mē-, -só-\ n : a phenothiazine tranquilizer $C_{21}H_{26}N_2OS_2$ used in the treatment of schizophrenia, organic brain disorders, alcoholism, and psychoneuroses

me·so·sal·pinx \,me-zō-'sal-(,)piŋks, ,mē-, -sō-\ n, pl -**sal·pin·ges** \-sal-'pin-(,)jēz\ : a fold of the broad ligament investing and supporting the fallopian tube

me·so·sig·moid \-'sig-,móid\ n : the mesentery of the sigmoid part of the descending colon

me·so·ster·num \,me-zə-'stər-nəm, ,mē-, -sə-\ n, pl -**ster·na** \-nə\ : GLADIOLUS

me·so·ten·don \-'ten-dən\ n : a fold of synovial membrane connecting a tendon to its synovial sheath

me·so·the·li·o·ma \,me-zə-,thē-lē-'ō-mə, ,mē-, -sə-\ n, pl -**mas** also -**ma·ta** \-mə-tə\ : a tumor derived from mesothelial tissue (as that lining the peritoneum or pleura)

me·so·the·li·um \-'thē-lē-əm\ n, pl -**lia** \-lē-ə\ : epithelium derived from mesoderm that lines the body cavity of a vertebrate embryo and gives rise to epithelia (as of the peritoneum, pericardium, and pleurae), striated muscle, heart muscle, and several minor structures — **me·so·the·li·al** \-lē-əl\ adj

mes·ovar·i·um \-'var-ē-əm\ n, pl -**ovar·ia** \-ē-ə\ : the mesentery uniting the ovary with the body wall

mes·ox·a·lyl·urea \,-,äk-sə-li-'lúr-ē-ə, -,lil-'yúr-\ n : ALLOXAN

mes·sen·ger \'mes-ᵊn-jər\ n **1** : a substance (as a hormone) that mediates a biological effect — see FIRST MESSENGER, SECOND MESSENGER **2** : MESSENGER RNA

messenger RNA n : an RNA produced by transcription that carries the code for a particular protein from the nuclear DNA to a ribosome in the cytoplasm and acts as a template for the formation of that protein — called also *mRNA*; compare TRANSFER RNA

mes·ter·o·lone \me-'ster-ə-,lōn\ n : an androgen $C_{20}H_{32}O_2$ used in the treatment of male infertility

Mes·ti·non \'mes-tə-,nän\ trademark — used for a preparation of the bromide of pyridostigmine

mes·tra·nol \'mes-trə-,nól, -,nōl\ n : a synthetic estrogen $C_{21}H_{26}O_2$ used in birth control pills — see ENOVID, ORTHO-NOVUM

mes·y·late \'me-si-,lāt\ n : any of the esters of an acid CH_4SO_3 including some in which it is combined with a drug — see ERGOLOID MESYLATES

met \'met, ˌem-(ˌ)ē-'tē\ *n, often all cap* : a unit of measure of the rate at which the body expends energy that is based on the energy expenditure while sitting at rest and is equal to 3.5 milliliters of oxygen per kilogram of body weight per minute — called also *metabolic equivalent*

Met *abbr* methionine

meta- *or* **met-** *prefix* **1** : situated behind or beyond ⟨*met*encephalon⟩ **2** : change in : transformation of ⟨*meta*plasia⟩

meta–anal·y·sis \ˌme-tə-ə-'na-lə-səs\ *n* : a quantitative statistical analysis of several separate but similar experiments or studies in order to test the pooled data for statistical significance

met·a·bol·ic \ˌme-tə-'bä-lik\ *adj* **1** : of, relating to, or based on metabolism **2** : VEGETATIVE 1a(2) — used esp. of a cell nucleus that is not dividing — **met·a·bol·i·cal·ly** *adv*

metabolic acidosis *n* : acidosis resulting from excess acid due to abnormal metabolism, excessive acid intake, or renal retention or from excessive loss of bicarbonate (as in diarrhea)

metabolic alkalosis *n* : alkalosis resulting from excessive alkali intake or excessive acid loss (as from vomiting)

metabolic equivalent *n* : MET

metabolic pathway *n* : PATHWAY 2

metabolic rate *n* : metabolism per unit time esp. as estimated by food consumption, energy released as heat, or oxygen used in metabolic processes — see BASAL METABOLIC RATE

metabolic syndrome *n* : a syndrome marked by the presence of usu. three or more of a group of factors (as high blood pressure, abdominal obesity, high triglyceride levels, low HDL levels, and high fasting levels of blood sugar) that are linked to an increased risk of cardiovascular disease and type 2 diabetes — called also *insulin resistance syndrome, syndrome X*

me·tab·o·lism \mə-'ta-bə-ˌli-zəm\ *n* **1** : the sum of the processes in the buildup and destruction of protoplasm; *specif* : the chemical changes in living cells by which energy is provided for vital processes and activities and new material is assimilated — see ANABOLISM, CATABOLISM **2** : the sum of the processes by which a particular substance is handled (as by assimilation and incorporation or by detoxification and excretion) in the living body

me·tab·o·lite \-ˌlīt\ *n* **1** : a product of metabolism: **a** : a metabolic waste usu. more or less toxic to the organism producing it : EXCRETION **b** : a product of one metabolic process that is essential to another such process in the same organism **c** : a metabolic waste of one organism that is markedly toxic to another : ANTIBIOTIC **2** : a substance essential to the metabolism of a particular organism or to a particular metabolic process

me·tab·o·lize \-ˌlīz\ *vb* **-lized; -liz·ing** : to subject to metabolism — **me·tab·o·liz·able** \mə-ˌta-bə-'lī-zə-bəl\ *adj*

me·tab·o·tro·pic \mə-ˌta-bə-'trō-pik, -'trä\ *adj* : relating to or being receptor for glutamate that when complexed with G protein triggers increased production of certian intracellular messengers

¹**meta·car·pal** \ˌme-tə-'kär-pəl\ *adj* : of, relating to, or being the metacarpus or a metacarpal

²**metacarpal** *n* : any bone of the metacarpus of the human hand or the front foot in quadrupeds

meta·car·po·pha·lan·ge·al \ˌme-tə-ˌkär-pō-ˌfā-lən-'jē-əl, -ˌfa-, -fə-'lan-jē-\ *adj* : of, relating to, or involving both the metacarpus and the phalanges

meta·car·pus \-'kär-pəs\ *n* : the part of the human hand or the front foot in quadrupeds between the carpus and the phalanges that contains five more or less elongated bones when all the digits are present (as in humans) but is modified in many animals by the loss or reduction of some bones or the fusing of adjacent bones

meta·cen·tric \ˌme-tə-'sen-trik\ *adj* : having the centromere medially situated so that the two chromosomal arms are of roughly equal length — compare ACROCENTRIC, TELOCENTRIC — **metacentric** *n*

meta·cer·car·ia \ˌme-tə-(ˌ)sər-'kar-ē-ə\ *n, pl* **-i·ae** \-ē-ˌē\ : a tailless encysted late larva of a digenetic trematode that is usu. the form which is infective for the definitive host — **meta·cer·car·i·al** \-ē-əl\ *adj*

meta·ces·tode \-'ses-ˌtōd\ *n* : a stage of a tapeworm occurring in an intermediate host : a larval tapeworm

metachromatic leukodystrophy *n* : a genetic neurodegenerative disorder that is inherited as an autosomal recessive trait and is marked by the accumulation of sulfatides resulting in the loss of myelin in the central nervous system and leading to progressive deterioration of cognitive and motor functioning

me·tach·ro·nous \mə-'ta-krə-nəs\ *adj* : occurring or starting at different times ⟨∼ cancers⟩

meta·cre·sol \ˌme-tə-'krē-ˌsol, -ˌsōl\ *n* : an isomer of cresol that has antiseptic properties

meta·cryp·to·zo·ite \-ˌkrip-tō-'zō-ˌīt\ *n* : a member of a second or subsequent generation of tissue-dwelling forms of a malaria parasite derived from the sporozoite without intervening generations of blood parasites — compare CRYPTOZOITE

Meta·gon·i·mus \-'gä-nə-məs\ *n* : a genus of small intestinal flukes (family Heterophyidae) that includes one (*M. yokogawai*) common in humans, dogs, and cats in parts of eastern Asia as a result of the eating of raw fish containing the larva

Meta·hy·drin \'me-'hī-drin\ *trademark* — used for a preparation of trichlormethiazide

metall- *or* **metallo-** *comb form* : containing a metal atom or ion in the molecule ⟨*metallo*porphyrin⟩

me·tal·lo·en·zyme \mə-ˌta-lō-'en-ˌzīm\ *n* : an enzyme consisting of a protein linked with a specific metal

met·al·loid \'met-ᵊl-ˌȯid\ *n* : an element (as boron, silicon, or arsenic) intermediate in properties between the typical metals and nonmetals

me·tal·lo·por·phy·rin \-'pȯr-fə-rən\ *n* : a compound (as heme) formed from a porphyrin and a metal ion

me·tal·lo·pro·tein \-'prō-ˌtēn, -'prōt-ē-ən\ *n* : a conjugated protein in which the prosthetic group is a metal

me·tal·lo·thio·ne·in \-ˌthī-ə-'nē-ən\ *n* : any of various metal-binding proteins involved in the metabolism of copper and zinc in body tissue (as of the liver) and in the binding of toxic metals (as cadmium)

meta·mere \'me-tə-ˌmir\ *n* : any of a linear series of primitively similar segments into which the body of a higher invertebrate or vertebrate is divisible : SOMITE — **meta·mer·ic** \ˌme-tə-'mer-ik\ *adj*

meta·mor·phic \ˌme-tə-'mȯr-fik\ *adj* : of or relating to metamorphosis

meta·mor·pho·sis \ˌme-tə-'mȯr-fə-səs\ *n, pl* **-pho·ses** \-ˌsēz\ **1** : change of physical form, structure, or substance **2** : a marked and more or less abrupt developmental change in the form or structure of an animal (as a butterfly or a frog) occurring subsequent to birth or hatching — **meta·mor·phose** \-ˌfōz, -ˌfōs\ *vb*

Met·a·mu·cil \ˌme-tə-'myüs-ᵊl\ *trademark* — used for a laxative preparation of a hydrophilic mucilloid from the husk of psyllium seed

meta·my·elo·cyte \ˌme-tə-'mī-ə-lə-ˌsīt\ *n* : any of the most immature granulocytes present in normal blood that are distinguished by typical cytoplasmic granulation in combination with a simple kidney-shaped nucleus

meta·neph·ric \ˌme-tə-'ne-frik\ *adj* : of or relating to the metanephros

meta·neph·rine \-'ne-ˌfrēn\ *n* : a catabolite of epinephrine that is found in the urine and some tissues

meta·neph·ro·gen·ic \-ˌne-frə-'je-nik\ *adj* : giving rise to the metanephroi

meta·neph·ros \-'ne-frəs, -ˌfräs\ *n, pl* **-neph·roi** \-'ne-ˌfrȯi\ : either member of the final and most caudal pair of the three successive pairs of vertebrate renal organs that functions as a permanent adult kidney in reptiles, birds, and mammals but is not present at all in lower forms — compare MESONEPHROS, PRONEPHROS

meta·phase \'me-tə-ˌfāz\ *n* : the stage of mitosis and meiosis in which the chromosomes become arranged in the equatorial plane of the spindle

metaphase plate *n* : a section in the equatorial plane of the metaphase spindle having the chromosomes oriented upon it

me·taph·y·se·al *also* **me·taph·y·si·al** \mə-ˌta-fə-'sē-əl, -'zē-, ˌme-tə-'fi-zē-əl\ *adj* : of or relating to a metaphysis

me·taph·y·sis \mə-'ta-fə-səs\ *n, pl* **-y·ses** \-ˌsēz\ : the transitional zone at which the diaphysis and epiphysis of a bone come together

meta·pla·sia \ˌme-tə-'plā-zhə, -zhē-ə\ *n* **1** : transformation of one tissue into another ⟨~ of cartilage into bone⟩ **2** : abnormal replacement of cells of one type by cells of another — **meta·plas·tic** \-'plas-tik\ *adj*

meta·pro·ter·e·nol \ˌme-tə-prō-'ter-ə-ˌnȯl, -ˌnōl\ *n* : a beta-adrenergic bronchodilator that is administered in the form of its sulfate $(C_{11}H_{17}NO_3)_2 \cdot H_2SO_4$ in the treatment of bronchial asthma and reversible bronchospasm associated with bronchitis and emphysema — see ALUPENT

meta·ram·i·nol \ˌme-tə-'ra-mə-ˌnȯl, -ˌnōl\ *n* : a sympathomimetic drug used in the form of its bitartrate $C_9H_{13}NO_2 \cdot C_4H_6O_6$ esp. as a vasoconstrictor to raise or maintain blood pressure

met·ar·te·ri·ole \ˌmet-ˌär-'tir-ē-ˌōl\ *n* : any of the delicate blood vessels that branch from the smallest arterioles and connect with the capillary bed — called also *precapillary*

me·tas·ta·sis \mə-'tas-tə-səs\ *n, pl* **-ta·ses** \-ˌsēz\ **1 a** : change of position, state, or form **b** : the spread of a disease-producing agency (as cancer cells or bacteria) from the initial or primary site of disease to another part of the body; *also* : the process by which such spreading occurs **2** : a secondary malignant tumor resulting from metastasis — **me·tas·ta·size** \mə-'tas-tə-ˌsīz\ *vb* — **met·a·sta·tic** \ˌme-tə-'sta-tik\ *adj*

Meta·stron·gy·lus \ˌme-tə-'strän-jə-ləs\ *n* : a genus of nematode worms (family Metastrongylidae) parasitizing as adults the lungs and sometimes other organs of mammals

¹meta·tar·sal \ˌme-tə-'tär-səl\ *adj* : of, relating to, or being the part of the human foot or of the hind foot in quadrupeds between the tarsus and the phalanges that in humans comprises five elongated bones which form the front of the instep and ball of the foot

²metatarsal *n* : a metatarsal bone

meta·tar·sal·gia \-ˌtär-'sal-jə, -jē-ə\ *n* : a cramping burning pain below and between the metatarsal bones where they join the toe bones — see MORTON'S TOE

meta·tar·sec·to·my \-ˌtär-'sek-tə-mē\ *n, pl* **-mies** : surgical removal of the metatarsus or a metatarsal bone

meta·tar·so·pha·lan·ge·al joint \-ˌtär-sō-ˌfā-lən-ˈjē-əl-, -ˌfa-, -fə-ˈlan-jē-\ *n* : any of the joints between the metatarsals and the phalanges

meta·tar·sus \ˌme-tə-ˈtär-səs\ *n* : the part of the human foot or of the hind foot in quadrupeds that is between the tarsus and phalanges, contains when all the digits are present (as in humans) five more or less elongated bones but is modified in many animals with loss or reduction of some bones or fusing of others, and in humans forms the instep

meta·thal·a·mus \-ˈtha-lə-məs\ *n, pl* **-mi** \-ˌmī\ : the part of the diencephalon on each side that comprises the lateral and medial geniculate bodies

met·ax·a·lone \mə-ˈtak-sə-ˌlōn\ *n* : a drug $C_{12}H_{15}NO_3$ used as a skeletal muscle relaxant

meta·zo·an \ˌme-tə-ˈzō-ən\ *n* : any of a group (*Metazoa*) that comprises all animals having the body composed of cells differentiated into tissues and organs and usu. a digestive cavity lined with specialized cells — **metazoan** *adj*

met·en·ceph·a·lon \ˌmet-ˌen-ˈse-fə-ˌlän, -lən\ *n* : the anterior segment of the developing vertebrate hindbrain or the corresponding part of the adult brain composed of the cerebellum and pons — **met·en·ce·phal·ic** \-ˌen-sə-ˈfa-lik\ *adj*

Met–en·keph·a·lin \ˌme-ten-ˈke-fə-lin\ *n* : METHIONINE-ENKEPHALIN

me·te·or·ism \ˈmē-tē-ə-ˌri-zəm\ *n* : gaseous distension of the stomach or intestine : TYMPANITES

me·ter \ˈmē-tər\ *n* : the base unit of length in the International System of Units that is equal to the distance traveled by light in a vacuum in $^{1}/_{299,792,458}$ second or to about 39.37 inches

-meter *n comb form* : instrument or means for measuring ⟨calori*meter*⟩

metered–dose inhaler *n* : a pocket-sized handheld inhaler that delivers a standardized dose of medication for bronchodilation — abbr. *MDI*

meter–kilogram–second *adj* : MKS

met·for·min \met-ˈfȯr-mən\ *n* : an antidiabetic drug used in the form of its hydrochloride $C_4H_{11}N_5 \cdot HCl$ esp. to treat type 2 diabetes in patients unresponsive to or intolerant of approved sulfonylurea drugs — see GLUCOPHAGE, GLUCOVANCE

meth \ˈmeth\ *n* : METHAMPHETAMINE

meth- *or* **metho-** *comb form* : methyl ⟨*meth*amphetamine⟩

metha·cho·line \ˌme-thə-ˈkō-ˌlēn\ *n* : a parasympathomimetic drug administered in the form of its crystalline chloride $C_8H_{18}ClNO_2$ esp. to diagnose hypersensitivity of the bronchial air passages (as in asthma) — see MECHOLYL, PROVOCHOLINE

metha·cy·cline \ˌme-thə-ˈsī-ˌklēn\ *n* : a semisynthetic tetracycline $C_{22}H_{22}$-N_2O_8 with longer duration of action than most other tetracyclines and used in the treatment of gonorrhea esp. in penicillin-sensitive subjects

meth·a·done \ˈme-thə-ˌdōn\ *also* **meth·a·don** \-ˌdän\ *n* : a synthetic addictive narcotic drug used esp. in the form of its hydrochloride $C_{21}H_{27}$-$NO \cdot HCl$ for the relief of pain and as a substitute narcotic in the treatment of heroin addiction — called also *amidone*

met·haem·al·bu·min, met·hae·mo·glo·bin, met·hae·mo·glo·bi·nae·mia *chiefly Brit var of* METHEMALBUMIN, METHEMOGLOBIN, METHEMOGLOBINEMIA

meth·am·phet·amine \ˌme-tham-ˈfe-tə-ˌmēn, -thəm-, -mən\ *n* : an amine $C_{10}H_{15}N$ that is used medically in the form of its hydrochloride $C_{10}H_{15}N \cdot$ HCl esp. to treat attention deficit disorder and obesity and that is often abused illicitly as a stimulant — called also *meth, methedrine, methylamphetamine, speed*

meth·an·dro·sten·o·lone \ˌme-ˌthan-drō-ˈste-nə-ˌlōn\ *n* : an anabolic steroid $C_{20}H_{28}O_2$

meth·ane \ˈme-ˌthān\ *n* : a colorless odorless flammable gaseous hydrocarbon CH_4 that is lighter than air, forms explosive mixtures with air or oxygen, and occurs naturally as a by-product of the decomposition of organic matter by anaerobic bacteria

meth·a·nol \ˈme-thə-ˌnȯl, -ˌnōl\ *n* : a light volatile pungent flammable poisonous liquid alcohol CH_3OH used esp. as a solvent, antifreeze, or denaturant for ethyl alcohol and in the synthesis of other chemicals — called also *methyl alcohol, wood alcohol*

meth·an·the·line \me-ˈthan-thə-ˌlēn, -lən\ *n* : an anticholinergic drug usu. administered in the form of its crystalline bromide $C_{21}H_{26}BrNO_3$ in the treatment of peptic ulcers

meth·a·phen·i·lene \ˌme-thə-ˈfen-ᵊl-ˌēn\ *n* : a chemical preparation $C_{15}H_{20}N_2S$ formerly used as an antihistamine

meth·a·pyr·i·lene \-ˈpir-ə-ˌlēn\ *n* : an antihistamine drug $C_{14}H_{19}N_3S$ formerly used as a mild sedative in proprietary sleep-inducing drugs

meth·aqua·lone \me-ˈtha-kwə-ˌlōn\ *n* : a sedative and hypnotic nonbarbiturate drug $C_{16}H_{14}N_2O$ that is habit-forming — see QUAALUDE

meth·ar·bi·tal \me-ˈthär-bə-ˌtȯl, -ˌtäl\ *n* : an anticonvulsant barbiturate $C_9H_{14}N_2O_3$

meth·a·zol·amide \ˌme-thə-ˈzȯl-ə-ˌmīd\ *n* : a sulfonamide $C_5H_8N_4O_3S_2$ that inhibits the production of carbonic anhydrase, reduces intraocular pressure, and is used in the treatment of glaucoma — see NEPTAZANE

meth·di·la·zine \meth-ˈdi-lə-ˌzēn, -ˈdī-lə-ˌzīn\ n : a phenothiazine antihistamine used in the form of its hydrochloride $C_{18}H_{20}N_2S\cdot HCl$ as an antipruritic

meth·e·drine \ˈme-thə-drən, -ˌdrēn\ n : METHAMPHETAMINE

met·hem·al·bu·min \ˌmet-ˌhē-mal-ˈbyü-mən\ n : an albumin complex with hematin found in plasma during diseases (as blackwater fever) associated with extensive hemolysis

met·he·mo·glo·bin \(ˌ)met-ˈhē-mə-ˌglō-bin\ n : a soluble brown crystalline basic blood pigment that is found in normal blood in much smaller amounts than hemoglobin, that is formed from blood, hemoglobin, or oxyhemoglobin by oxidation, and that differs from hemoglobin in containing ferric iron and in being unable to combine reversibly with molecular oxygen — called also *ferrihemoglobin*

met·he·mo·glo·bi·ne·mia \ˌmet-ˌhē-mə-ˌglō-bə-ˈnē-mē-ə\ n : the presence of methemoglobin in the blood due to conversion of part of the hemoglobin to this inactive form

me·the·na·mine \mə-ˈthē-nə-ˌmēn, -mən\ n : a crystalline compound used esp. in the form of its mandelate $C_6H_{12}N_4\cdot C_8H_8O_3$ as a urinary antiseptic esp. to treat bacteriuria associated with cystitis and pyelitis — called also *hexamethylenetetramine, hexamine*; see MANDELAMINE

me·the·no·lone \mə-ˈthē-nə-lōn, me-ˈthe-\ n : a hormone $C_{20}H_{30}O_2$ that is an anabolic steroid

Meth·er·gine \ˈme-thər-jən\ *trademark* — used for a preparation of the maleate of methylergonovine

meth·i·cil·lin \ˌme-thə-ˈsi-lən\ n : a semisynthetic penicillin $C_{17}H_{19}N_2O_6$-NaS that is esp. effective against betalactamase producing staphylococci

me·thi·ma·zole \me-ˈthī-mə-ˌzōl, mə-\ n : a drug $C_4H_6N_2S$ used to inhibit activity of the thyroid gland

meth·io·dal sodium \mə-ˈthī-ə-ˌdal-\ n : a crystalline salt CH_2ISO_3Na used as a radiopaque contrast medium in intravenous urography

me·thi·o·nine \mə-ˈthī-ə-ˌnēn\ n : a crystalline sulfur-containing essential amino acid $C_5H_{11}NO_2S$ that occurs in the L-form as a constituent of many proteins (as casein and egg albumin) and that is used as a dietary supplement and in the treatment of fatty infiltration of the liver

methionine–en·keph·a·lin \-en-ˈkə-fə-lin\ n : a pentapeptide having a terminal methionine residue that is one of the two enkephalins occurring naturally in the brain — called also *Metenkephalin*

meth·is·a·zone \me-ˈthi-sə-ˌzōn\ n : an antiviral drug $C_{10}H_{10}N_4OS$ formerly used in the preventive treatment of smallpox

me·thix·ene \me-ˈthik-ˌsēn\ n : an anticholinergic drug $C_{20}H_{23}NS$ used as an antispasmodic in the treatment of functional bowel hypermotility and spasm

metho- — see METH-

meth·o·car·ba·mol \ˌme-thə-ˈkär-bə-ˌmȯl\ n : a skeletal muscle relaxant drug $C_{11}H_{15}NO_5$

meth·o·hex·i·tal \ˌme-thə-ˈhek-sə-ˌtȯl, -ˌtal\ n : a barbiturate with a short period of action usu. used in the form of its sodium salt $C_{14}H_{17}N_2NaO_3$ as an intravenous general anesthetic

meth·o·hex·i·tone \-ˌtōn\ n, *Brit* : METHOHEXITAL

meth·o·trex·ate \ˌme-thə-ˈtrek-ˌsāt\ n : a toxic drug $C_{20}H_{22}N_8O_5$ that is an analog of folic acid and is used to treat certain cancers, severe psoriasis, and rheumatoid arthritis — called also *amethopterin*

meth·o·tri·mep·ra·zine \-ˌtrī-ˈme-prə-ˌzēn\ n : a nonnarcotic analgesic and tranquilizer $C_{19}H_{24}N_2OS$ — see LEVOPROME

me·thox·amine \me-ˈthäk-sə-ˌmēn, -mən\ n : a sympathomimetic amine used in the form of its hydrochloride $C_{11}H_{17}NO_3\cdot HCl$ esp. to raise or maintain blood pressure (as during surgery) by its vasoconstrictor effects

me·thox·sa·len \me-ˈthäk-sə-lən\ n : a drug $C_{12}H_8O_4$ used to increase the production of melanin in the skin upon exposure to ultraviolet light and in the treatment of vitiligo — called also *8-methoxsalen, xanthotoxin*

me·thoxy·flu·rane \me-ˌthäk-sē-ˈflùr-ˌān\ n : a potent inhalational general anesthetic $C_3H_4Cl_2F_2O$ withdrawn from the U.S. market because of its link to liver and kidney damage

8–meth·oxy·psor·a·len \ˈāt-ˌme-ˌthäk-sē-ˈsȯr-ə-lən\ n : METHOXSALEN

meth·sco·pol·amine \ˌmeth-skō-ˈpä-lə-ˌmēn, -mən\ n : an anticholinergic derivative of scopolamine that is usu. used in the form of its bromide $C_{18}H_{24}BrNO_4$ for its inhibitory effect on gastric secretion and gastrointestinal motility esp. in the treatment of peptic ulcer and gastric disorders — see PAMINE

meth·sux·i·mide \-ˈsək-si-ˌmīd\ n : an anticonvulsant drug $C_{12}H_{13}NO_2$ used esp. in the control of absence seizures

meth·y·clo·thi·azide \ˌme-thi-klō-ˈthī-ə-ˌzīd\ n : a thiazide drug C_9H_{11}-$Cl_2N_3O_4S_2$ used as a diuretic and antihypertensive agent

meth·yl \ˈme-thəl, *Brit also* ˈmē-ˌthīl\ n : an alkyl group CH_3 that is derived from methane by removal of one hydrogen atom

meth·yl·al \ˈme-thə-ˌlal\ n : a volatile flammable liquid $C_3H_8O_2$ used as a hypnotic and anesthetic

methyl alcohol : METHANOL

me·thyl·am·phet·amine \ˌme-thəl-ˌam-ˈfe-tə-ˌmēn\ n : METHAMPHETAMINE

methylated spirit *n* : ethyl alcohol denatured with methanol — often used in pl. with a sing. verb

meth·yl·ation \ˌme-thə-ˈlā-shən\ *n* : introduction of the methyl group into a chemical compound; *esp* : DNA METHYLATION — **meth·yl·ate** \ˈme-thə-ˌlāt\ *vb*

meth·yl·ben·ze·tho·ni·um chloride \ˌme-thəl-ˌben-zə-ˌthō-nē-əm-\ *n* : a quaternary ammonium salt $C_{28}H_{54}ClNO_2$ used as a bactericide and antiseptic esp. in the treatment of diaper rash — called also *methylbenzethonium*

methyl bromide *n* : a poisonous gaseous compound CH_3Br

meth·yl·cel·lu·lose \ˌme-thəl-ˈsel-yə-ˌlōs, -ˌlōz\ *n* : any of various gummy products of cellulose methylation that swell in water and are used as bulk laxatives

meth·yl·cho·lan·threne \-kə-ˈlan-ˌthrēn\ *n* : a potent carcinogenic hydrocarbon $C_{21}H_{16}$ obtained from certain bile acids and cholesterol as well as synthetically

N–meth·yl–D–as·par·tate \ˈen-ˌme-thəl-ˌdē-ə-ˈspär-ˌtāt\ *n* : NMDA

meth·yl·do·pa \-ˈdō-pə\ *n* : an antihypertensive drug $C_{10}H_{13}NO_4$

meth·y·lene blue \ˈme-thə-ˌlēn-, -lən-\ *n* : a basic thiazine dye $C_{16}H_{18}ClN_3S·3H_2O$ used in the treatment of methemoglobinemia and as an antidote in cyanide poisoning

meth·y·lene·di·oxy·am·phet·amine \ˌme-thə-ˌlēn-dī-ˌäk-sē-am-ˈfe-tə-ˌmēn\ *also* **3,4–methylenedioxyamphetamine** \ˈthrē-ˌfōr-\ *n* : MDA

meth·y·lene·di·oxy·meth·am·phet·amine \-ˌme-tham-ˈfe-tə-ˌmēn\ *also* **3,4–methylenedioxymethamphetamine** *n* : ECSTASY 2

meth·yl·er·go·no·vine \ˌme-thəl-ˌər-gə-ˈnō-ˌvēn\ *n* : an oxytocic drug that is usu. administered in the form of its maleate $C_{20}H_{25}N_3O_2·C_4H_4O_4$ and is used similarly to ergonovine — see METHERGINE

meth·yl·glu·ca·mine \-ˈglü-kə-ˌmēn\ *n* : MEGLUMINE

meth·yl·hex·ane·amine \ˌme-thəl-ˌhek-sā-ˈna-mēn\ *n* : an amine base $C_7H_{17}N$ used as a local vasoconstrictor of nasal mucosa in the treatment of nasal congestion

meth·yl iso·cy·a·nate \-ˌī-sō-ˈsī-ə-ˌnāt\ *n* : an extremely toxic chemical CH_3NCO that is used esp. in the manufacture of pesticides and was the cause of numerous deaths and injuries in a leak at a chemical plant in Bhopal, India, in 1984 — abbr. *MIC*

meth·yl·ma·lon·ic acid \ˌme-thəl-mə-ˈlä-nik-\ *n* : a structural isomer of succinic acid present in minute amounts in healthy human urine but excreted in large quantities in the urine of individuals with a vitamin B_{12} deficiency

methylmalonic aciduria *n* : a metabolic defect which is controlled by an

autosomal recessive gene and in which methylmalonic acid is not converted to succinic acid with chronic metabolic acidosis resulting

meth·yl mer·cap·tan \ˌme-thəl-mər-ˈkap-ˌtan\ *n* : a pungent gas CH_4S produced in the intestine by the decomposition of certain proteins and responsible for the characteristic odor of fetor hepaticus

meth·yl·mer·cury \ˌme-thəl-ˈmər-kya-rē\ *n, pl* **-cu·ries** : any of various toxic compounds of mercury containing the complex $CH_3Hg–$ that often occur as pollutants formed as industrial by-products or pesticide residues, tend to accumulate in living organisms (as fish) esp. in higher levels of a food chain, are rapidly and easily absorbed through the human intestinal wall, and cause neurological dysfunction in humans — see MINAMATA DISEASE

meth·yl·mor·phine \ˌme-thəl-ˈmȯr-ˌfēn\ *n* : CODEINE

meth·yl·para·ben \ˌme-thəl-ˈpar-ə-ˌben\ *n* : a crystalline compound $C_8H_8O_3$ used as an antifungal preservative (as in pharmaceutical ointments and cosmetic creams)

methyl parathion *n* : a potent synthetic organophosphate insecticide $C_8H_{10}NO_5PS$ that is more toxic than parathion

meth·yl·phe·ni·date \ˌme-thəl-ˈfe-nə-ˌdāt, -ˈfē-\ *n* : a mild stimulant of the central nervous system that is administered orally in the form of its hydrochloride $C_{14}H_{19}NO_2·HCl$ to treat narcolepsy and attention deficit disorder — see CONCERTA, RITALIN

meth·yl·pred·nis·o·lone \-pred-ˈni-sə-ˌlōn\ *n* : a glucocorticoid $C_{22}H_{30}O_5$ that is a derivative of prednisolone and is used as an anti-inflammatory agent; *also* : any of several of its salts used similarly — see MEDROL

methyl salicylate *n* : a liquid ester $C_8H_8O_3$ that is obtained from the leaves of a wintergreen (*Gaultheria procumbens*) or the bark of a birch (*Betula lenta*), but is usu. made synthetically, and that is used as a flavoring and a counterirritant — see OIL OF WINTERGREEN

methylsulfate — see PENTAPIPERIUM METHYLSULFATE

meth·yl·tes·tos·ter·one \-te-ˈstäs-tə-ˌrōn\ *n* : a synthetic androgen $C_{20}H_{30}O_2$ administered orally esp. in the treatment of male testosterone deficiency

meth·yl·thio·ura·cil \-ˌthī-ō-ˈyu̇r-ə-ˌsil\ *n* : a crystalline compound $C_5H_6N_2OS$ used in the suppression of hyperactivity of the thyroid

α–meth·yl·ty·ro·sine \ˌal-fə-ˌme-thəl-ˈtī-rə-ˌsēn\ *n* : a compound $C_{10}H_{13}NO_3$ that inhibits the synthesis of catecholamines but not of serotonin

meth·yl·xan·thine \ˌme-thəl-ˈzan-ˌthēn\ *n* : a methylated xanthine derivative (as caffeine, theobromine, or theophylline)

meth·y·pry·lon \\,me-thə-'prī-,län\ *n* : a sedative and hypnotic drug $C_{10}H_{17}$NO$_2$

meth·y·ser·gide \\,me-thə-'sər-,jīd\ *n* : a serotonin antagonist used in the form of its maleate $C_{21}H_{27}N_3O_2 \cdot C_4H_4O_4$ esp. in the treatment and prevention of migraine headaches

met·o·clo·pra·mide \\,me-tə-'klō-prə-,mīd\ *n* : an antiemetic drug used in the form of its hydrated hydrochloride $C_{14}H_{22}ClN_3O_2 \cdot HCl \cdot H_2O$

met·o·cur·ine iodide \\,me-tə-'kyùr-,ēn-\ *n* : a crystalline iodine-containing powder $C_{40}H_{48}I_2N_2O_6$ that is derived from the dextrorotatory form of tubocurarine and is a potent skeletal muscle relaxant — called also *metocurine*

me·to·la·zone \me-'tō-lə-,zōn\ *n* : a diuretic and antihypertensive drug $C_{16}H_{16}ClN_3O_3S$

me·top·ic \me-'tä-pik\ *adj* : of or relating to the forehead : FRONTAL; *esp* : of, relating to, or being a suture uniting the frontal bones in the fetus and sometimes persistent after birth

met·o·pim·a·zine \\,me-tə-'pi-mə-,zēn\ *n* : an antiemetic drug $C_{22}H_{27}N_3O_3S_2$

Met·o·pi·rone \\,me-tə-'pir-,ōn\ *trademark* — used for a preparation of metyrapone

met·o·pon \'me-tə-,pän\ *n* : a narcotic drug that is derived from morphine and is used in the form of the hydrochloride $C_{18}H_{21}NO_3 \cdot HCl$ to relieve pain

met·o·pro·lol \me-'tō-prə-,lòl, -,lōl\ *n* : a beta-blocker $C_{15}H_{25}NO_3$ used in the form of its tartrate $(C_{15}H_{25}NO_3)_2 \cdot C_4H_6O_6$ or succinate $(C_{15}H_{25}NO_3)_2 \cdot C_4H_6O_4$ to treat hypertension, angina pectoris, and congestive heart failure — see LOPRESSOR, TOPROL

metr- or **metro-** *comb form* : uterus ⟨*metritis*⟩

-me·tra \'mē-trə\ *n comb form* : a (specified) condition of the uterus ⟨hemato*metra*⟩

Met·ra·zol \'me-trə-,zòl, -,zōl\ *n* : a preparation of pentylenetetrazol — formerly a U.S. registered trademark

me·tre *chiefly Brit var of* METER

met·ric \'me-trik\ *adj* : of, relating to, or using the metric system — **met·ri·cal·ly** *adv*

-met·ric \'me-trik\ *or* **-met·ri·cal** \'me-tri-kəl\ *adj comb form* 1 : of, employing, or obtained by (such) a meter ⟨calori*metric*⟩ 2 : of or relating to (such) an art, process, or science of measuring ⟨psycho*metric*⟩

metric system *n* : a decimal system of weights and measures based on the meter and on the kilogram — compare CGS, MKS

me·tri·tis \mə-'trī-təs\ *n* : inflammation of the uterus

-me·tri·um \'mē-trē-əm\ *n comb form, pl* **-me·tria** : part or layer of the uterus ⟨endo*metrium*⟩

me·triz·a·mide \me-'tri-za-,mīd\ *n* : a radiopaque medium $C_{18}H_{22}I_3N_3O_8$

me·ri·zo·ate sodium \me-tri-'zō-āt-\ *n* : a radiopaque medium $C_{12}H_{10}I_3$-N_2NaO_4 — see ISOPAQUE

met·ro·ni·da·zole \\,me-trə-'nī-də-,zōl\ *n* : an antiprotozoal and antibacterial drug $C_6H_9N_3O_3$ used esp. to treat vaginal trichomoniasis, amebiasis, and infections by anaerobic bacteria

met·ro·nom·ic \\,me-trə-'nä-mik\ *adj* : of, relating to, or being a drug or regimen of drugs administered in low doses at regular intervals over a prolonged period of time ⟨~ chemotherapy⟩

me·tror·rha·gia \\,mē-trə-'rä-jə, -jē-ə, -zhə; -'rä-\ *n* : irregular uterine bleeding esp. between menstrual periods — compare MENORRHAGIA — **me·tror·rhag·ic** \-'ra-jik\ *adj*

-me·try \mə-trē\ *n comb form, pl* **-me·tries** : art, process, or science of measuring (something specified) ⟨audio*metry*⟩

me·tu·re·de·pa \mə-,tùr-ə-'de-pə, ,me-tyə-rə-\ *n* : an antineoplastic drug $C_{11}H_{22}N_3O_3P$

me·tyr·a·pone \mə-'tir-ə-,pōn, -'tir-\ *n* : a metabolic hormone $C_{14}H_{14}N_2O$ that inhibits biosynthesis of cortisol and corticosterone and is used to test for normal functioning of the pituitary gland — see METOPIRONE

Met·zen·baum scissors \'met-sən-,bòm-\ *n* : surgical scissors having curved blades with blunt ends

Metzenbaum, Myron Firth (1876–1944), American surgeon.

Mev·a·cor \'me-və-,kòr\ *trademark* — used for a preparation of lovastatin

me·ze·re·um \mə-'zir-ē-əm\ *n* : the dried bark of various European shrubs (genus *Daphne* and esp. *D. mezereum* of the family Thymelaeaceae) used externally as a vesicant and irritant

mg *abbr* milligram

Mg *symbol* magnesium

MHC *abbr* major histocompatibility complex

MHPG \\,em-,āch-,pē-'jē\ *n* : a metabolite of norepinephrine that is reported for some patients to fall to lower levels during periods of depression

MI *abbr* 1 mitral incompetence; mitral insufficiency 2 myocardial infarction

mi·an·ser·in \mī-'an-sər-in\ *n* : a drug administered in the form of its hydrochloride $C_{18}H_{20}N_2 \cdot HCl$ esp. as an antidepressant

MIC *abbr* 1 methyl isocyanate 2 minimal inhibitory concentration; minimum inhibitory concentration

Mi·ca·tin \'mī-kə-,tin\ *trademark* — used for a preparation of the nitrate of miconazole

mice *pl of* MOUSE

mi·con·a·zole \mī-'kä-nə-,zōl\ *n* : an antifungal agent administered esp. in the form of its nitrate $C_{18}H_{14}Cl_4$-$N_2O \cdot HNO_3$ — see MICATIN

micr- *or* **micro-** *comb form* **1 a** : small : minute ⟨*micro*aneurysm⟩ **b** : used for or involving minute quantities or variations ⟨*micro*analysis⟩ **2 a** : using microscopy ⟨*micro*dissection⟩ : used in microscopy ⟨*micro*needle⟩ **b** : revealed by or having its structure discernible only by microscopical examination ⟨*micro*organism⟩ **3** : abnormally small ⟨*micro*cyte⟩

micra *pl of* MICRON

mi·cren·ceph·a·ly \ˌmī-ˌkren-'se-fə-lē\ *n, pl* **-lies** : the condition of having an abnormally small brain

mi·cro·ab·scess \'mī-krō-ˌab-ses\ *n* : a very small abscess

mi·cro·ad·e·no·ma \ˌmī-krō-ˌad-ᵊn-'ō-mə\ *n, pl* **-mas** *also* **-ma·ta** \-mə-tə\ : a very small adenoma

mi·cro·ag·gre·gate \-'a-gri-gət\ *n* : an aggregate of microscopic particles (as of fibrin) formed esp. in stored blood

mi·cro·al·bu·min·uria \-al-ˌbyü-mə-'nür-ē-ə, -'nyür-\ *n* : albuminuria characterized by a relatively low rate of urinary excretion of albumin typically between 30 and 300 milligrams per 24-hour period — compare MACROALBUMINURIA

mi·cro·anal·y·sis \ˌmī-krō-ə-'na-lə-səs\ *n, pl* **-y·ses** \-ˌsēz\ : chemical analysis on a small or minute scale that usu. requires special, very sensitive, or small-scale apparatus — **mi·cro·an·a·lyt·i·cal** \-ˌa-nᵊl-'i-ti-kəl\ *also* **mi·cro·an·a·lyt·ic** \-'i-tik\ *adj*

mi·cro·anat·o·my \-ə-'na-tə-mē\ *n, pl* **-mies** : HISTOLOGY — **mi·cro·ana·tom·i·cal** \-ˌa-nə-'tä-mi-kəl\ *adj*

mi·cro·an·eu·rysm *also* **mi·cro·an·eu·rism** \-'a-nyə-ˌri-zəm\ *n* : a saccular enlargement of the venous end of a retinal capillary associated esp. with diabetic retinopathy — **mi·cro·an·eu·rys·mal** \-ˌa-nyə-'riz-məl\ *adj*

mi·cro·an·gi·og·ra·phy \-ˌan-jē-'ä-grə-fē\ *n, pl* **-phies** : minutely detailed angiography — **mi·cro·an·gio·graph·ic** \-ˌan-jē-ə-'gra-fik\ *adj*

mi·cro·an·gi·op·a·thy \-'ä-pə-thē\ *n, pl* **-thies** : a disease of very fine blood vessels ⟨thrombotic ∼⟩ — **mi·cro·an·gio·path·ic** \-ˌan-jē-ə-'pa-thik\ *adj*

mi·cro·ar·ray \-ə-'rā\ *n* : a supporting material (as a glass or plastic slide) onto which numerous molecules or molecular fragments usu. of DNA or protein are attached in a regular pattern for use in biochemical or genetic analysis

mi·cro·ar·te·ri·og·ra·phy \-är-ˌtir-ē-'ä-grə-fē\ *n, pl* **-phies** : minutely detailed arteriography

mi·crobe \'mī-ˌkrōb\ *n* : MICROORGANISM, GERM; *used esp. of* pathogenic bacteria

mi·cro·bi·al \mī-'krō-bē-əl\ *adj* : of, relating to, caused by, or being microbes ⟨∼ infection⟩ ⟨∼ agents⟩ — **mi·cro·bi·al·ly** \-ē\ *adv*

mi·cro·bic \mī-'krō-bik\ *adj* : MICROBIAL

mi·cro·bi·cide \mī-'krō-bə-ˌsīd\ *n* : an agent that destroys microbes — **mi·cro·bi·ci·dal** \ˌmī-ˌkrō-bə-'sīd-ᵊl\ *adj*

mi·cro·bi·ol·o·gy \ˌmī-krō-bī-'ä-lə-jē\ *n, pl* **-gies** : a branch of biology dealing esp. with microorganisms (as bacteria and protozoa) — **mi·cro·bi·o·log·i·cal** \-ˌkrō-ˌbī-ə-'lä-ji-kəl\ *also* **mi·cro·bi·o·log·ic** \-'lä-jik\ *adj* — **mi·cro·bi·o·log·i·cal·ly** *adv* — **mi·cro·bi·ol·o·gist** \-'jist\ *n*

mi·cro·body \'mī-krō-ˌbä-dē\ *n, pl* **-bod·ies** : PEROXISOME

mi·cro·cal·ci·fi·ca·tion \-ˌkal-sə-fə-'kā-shən\ *n* : a tiny abnormal deposit of calcium salts esp. in the breast that in females is often an indicator of breast cancer

mi·cro·cap·sule \'mī-krō-ˌkap-səl, -(ˌ)sül\ *n* : a tiny capsule containing material (as a medicine) that is released when the capsule is broken, melted, or dissolved

¹**mi·cro·ce·phal·ic** \ˌmī-krō-sə-'fa-lik\ *adj* : having a small head; *specif* : having an abnormally small head

²**microcephalic** *n* : an individual with an abnormally small head

mi·cro·ceph·a·lus \-'se-fə-ləs\ *n, pl* **-li** \-ˌlī\ : MICROCEPHALY

mi·cro·ceph·a·ly \-'se-fə-lē\ *n, pl* **-lies** : a condition of abnormal smallness of the head usu. associated with mental retardation

mi·cro·cir·cu·la·tion \-ˌsər-kyə-'lā-shən\ *n* : blood circulation in the microvascular system; *also* : the microvascular system itself — **mi·cro·cir·cu·la·to·ry** \-'sər-kyə-lə-ˌtōr-ē\ *adj*

mi·cro·coc·cus \ˌmī-krō-'kä-kəs\ *n* **1** *cap* : a genus of nonmotile gram-positive spherical bacteria (family Micrococcaceae) that occur in tetrads or irregular clusters and include nonpathogenic forms found on human and animal skin **2** *pl* **-coc·ci** \-'kä-ˌkī, -'käk-ˌsī\ : a small spherical bacterium; *esp* : any bacterium of the genus *Micrococcus* — **mi·cro·coc·cal** \ˌmī-krō-'kä-kəl\ *adj*

mi·cro·cul·ture \'mī-krō-ˌkəl-chər\ *n* : a microscopic culture of cells or organisms — **mi·cro·cul·tur·al** \ˌmī-krō-'kəlch-(ə-)rəl\ *adj*

mi·cro·cu·rie \'mī-krō-ˌkyùr-ē, ˌmī-krō-kyù-'rē\ *n* : a unit of quantity or of radioactivity equal to one millionth of a curie

mi·cro·cyte \'mī-krə-ˌsīt\ *n* : an abnormally small red blood cell present esp. in some anemias

mi·cro·cyt·ic \ˌmī-krə-'si-tik\ *adj* : of, relating to, being, or characterized by the presence of microcytes

microcytic anemia *n* : an anemia characterized by the presence of microcytes in the blood

mi·cro·cy·to·sis \-sī-'tō-səs\ *n, pl* **-to·ses** \-ˌsēz\ : decrease in the size of red blood cells

mi·cro·cy·to·tox·ic·i·ty test \-ˌsī-tō-ˌtäk-ˈsi-sə-tē\ n : a procedure using microscopic quantities of materials (as complement and lymphocytes in cell-mediated immunity) to determine cytotoxicity (as to cancer cells or cells of transplanted tissue) — called also *microcytotoxicity assay*

mi·cro·dis·sec·tion \ˌmī-krō-di-ˈsek-shən, -dī-\ n : dissection under the microscope; *specif* : dissection of cells and tissues by means of fine needles that are precisely manipulated by levers — **mi·cro·dis·sect·ed** \-ˈsek-təd\ adj

mi·cro·dose \ˈmī-krō-ˌdōs\ n : an extremely small dose

mi·cro·do·sim·e·try \ˌmī-krō-dō-ˈsi-mə-trē\ n, pl -tries : dosimetry involving microdoses of radiation or minute amounts of radioactive materials

mi·cro·drop \ˈmī-krō-ˌdräp\ n : a very small drop or minute droplet (as 0.1 to 0.01 of a drop)

mi·cro·drop·let \-ˌdrä-plət\ n : MICRODROP

mi·cro·elec·trode \ˌmī-krō-i-ˈlek-ˌtrōd\ n : a minute electrode; *esp* : one that is inserted in a living biological cell or tissue in studying its electrical characteristics

mi·cro·elec·tro·pho·re·sis \-ˌlek-trə-fə-ˈrē-səs\ n, pl -re·ses \-ˌsēz\ : electrophoresis in which the movement of single particles is observed in a microscope — **mi·cro·elec·tro·pho·ret·ic** \-ˈre-tik\ adj — **mi·cro·elec·tro·pho·ret·i·cal·ly** adv

mi·cro·el·e·ment \ˌmī-krō-ˈe-lə-mənt\ n : TRACE ELEMENT

mi·cro·em·bo·lism \-ˈem-bə-ˌli-zəm\ n : a small embolism (as one consisting of an aggregation of platelets) that blocks an arteriole or the terminal part of an artery

mi·cro·em·bo·lus \-ˈem-bə-ləs\ n, pl -li \-ˌlī\ : an extremely small embolus

mi·cro·en·cap·su·late \-in-ˈkap-sə-ˌlāt\ vb -lat·ed; -lat·ing : to enclose in a microcapsule — **mi·cro·en·cap·su·la·tion** \-in-ˌkap-sə-ˈlā-shən\ n

mi·cro·en·vi·ron·ment \-in-ˈvī-rən-mənt, -ˈvī-ərn-\ n : a small usu. distinctly specialized and effectively isolated habitat or environment (as of a nerve cell) — **mi·cro·en·vi·ron·men·tal** \-ˌvī-rən-ˈment-ᵊl\ adj

mi·cro·fi·bril \-ˈfī-brəl, -ˈfi-\ n : an extremely fine fibril — **mi·cro·fi·bril·lar** \-brə-lər\ adj

mi·cro·fil·a·ment \ˌmī-krō-ˈfi-lə-mənt\ n : any of the minute actin-containing protein filaments that are widely distributed in the cytoplasm of eukaryotic cells, help maintain their structural framework, and play a role in the movement of cell components — **mi·cro·fil·a·men·tous** \-ˌfi-ˈmen-təs\ adj

mi·cro·fil·a·rae·mia chiefly Brit var of MICROFILAREMIA

mi·cro·fil·a·re·mia \-ˌfi-lə-ˈrē-mē-ə\ n : the presence of microfilariae in the blood of one affected with some forms of filariasis

mi·cro·fi·lar·ia \ˌmī-krō-fə-ˈlar-ē-ə\ n, pl -i·ae \-ē-ē\ : a minute larval filaria — **mi·cro·fi·lar·i·al** \-ē-əl\ adj

mi·cro·flo·ra \ˌmī-krə-ˈflōr-ə\ n : a small or strictly localized flora ⟨intestinal ∼⟩ — **mi·cro·flo·ral** \-əl\ adj

mi·cro·flu·o·rom·e·try \-ˌflü-ˈrä-mə-trē\ n, pl -tries : the detection and measurement of the fluorescence produced by minute quantities of materials (as in cells) — **mi·cro·flu·o·rom·e·ter** \-ər\ n — **mi·cro·flu·o·ro·met·ric** \-rə-ˈme-trik\ adj

mi·cro·ga·mete \ˌga-ˌmēt, -gə-ˈmēt\ n : the smaller and usu. male gamete of an organism producing two types of gametes — compare MACROGAMETE

mi·cro·ga·me·to·cyte \-gə-ˈmē-tə-ˌsīt\ n : a gametocyte producing microgametes

mi·crog·lia \mī-ˈkrä-glē-ə\ n : glia consisting of small cells with few processes that are scattered throughout the central nervous system, that are of mesodermal origin and are thought to be derived from fetal monocytes, and that have a phagocytic function as part of mononuclear phagocyte system — **mi·crog·li·al** \-glē-əl\ adj

β₂-mi·cro·glob·u·lin \ˌbā-tə-ˌtü-ˌmī-krō-ˈglä-byə-lən\ n : a beta globulin of low molecular weight that is present at a low level in plasma, is normally excreted in the urine, comprises the light chain in certain histocompatibility antigens, and occurs at elevated levels in blood serum or urine in some pathological conditions (as tubulointerstitial disease)

mi·cro·glos·sia \ˌmī-krō-ˈglä-sē-ə, -ˈglò-\ n : abnormal smallness of the tongue

mi·cro·gna·thia \ˌmī-krō-ˈnā-thē-ə, -ˈna-, ˌmī-ˌkräg-\ n : abnormal smallness of one or both jaws

mi·cro·gram \ˈmī-krə-ˌgram\ n : one millionth of a gram

mi·cro·graph \-ˌgraf\ n : a graphic reproduction (as a photograph) of the image of an object formed by a microscope — **micrograph** vb

mi·cro·hab·i·tat \ˌmī-krō-ˈha-bə-ˌtat\ n : the microenvironment in which an organism lives

mi·cro·he·mat·o·crit \-hi-ˈma-tə-ˌkrit\ n 1 : a procedure for determining the ratio of the volume of packed red blood cells to the volume of whole blood by centrifuging a minute quantity of blood in a capillary tube coated with heparin 2 : a hematocrit value obtained by microhematocrit

mi·cro·in·farct \-in-ˈfärkt\ n : a very small infarct

mi·cro·in·jec·tion \ˌmī-krō-in-ˈjek-shən\ n : injection under the microscope; *specif* : injection esp. by a micropipette into a tissue or single cell — **mi·cro·in·ject** \-in-'jekt\ *vb*

mi·cro·in·va·sive \-in-'vā-siv\ *adj* : of, relating to, or characterized by very slight invasion into adjacent tissues by malignant cells of a carcinoma in situ — **mi·cro·in·va·sion** \-'vā-zhən\ *n*

mi·cro·ion·to·pho·re·sis \-(,)ī-,än-tə-fə-'rē-səs\ *n, pl* **-re·ses** \-,sēz\ : a process for observing or recording the effect of an ionized substance on nerve cells that involves inserting a double micropipette into the brain close to a nerve cell, injecting an ionized fluid through one barrel of the pipette, and using a concentrated saline solution in the other tube as an electrical conductor to pick up and transmit back to an oscilloscope any change in neural activity — **mi·cro·ion·to·pho·ret·ic** \-'re-tik\ *adj* — **mi·cro·ion·to·pho·ret·i·cal·ly** *adv*

mi·cro·li·ter \'mī-krō-'lē-tər\ *n* : a unit of capacity equal to one millionth of a liter

mi·cro·lith \'mī-krō-,lith\ *n* : a microscopic calculus or concretion — compare GRAVEL 1

mi·cro·li·thi·a·sis \,mī-krō-li-'thī-ə-səs\ *n, pl* **-a·ses** \-,sēz\ : the formation or presence of microliths or gravel

mi·cro·ma·nip·u·la·tion \,mī-krō-mə-,ni-pyə-'lā-shən\ *n* : the technique or practice of manipulating cells or tissues (as by microdissection or microinjection) — **mi·cro·ma·nip·u·late** \-'ni-pyə-,lāt\ *vb* — **mi·cro·ma·nip·u·la·tor** \-'ni-pyə-,lā-tər\ *n*

mi·cro·mas·tia \-'mas-tē-ə\ *n* : postpubertal immaturity and abnormal smallness of the breasts

mi·cro·me·lia \-'mē-lē-ə\ *n* : a condition characterized by abnormally small and imperfectly developed extremities — **mi·cro·me·lic** \-'mē-lik\ *adj*

mi·cro·me·tas·ta·sis \,mī-krō-mə-'tas-tə-səs\ *n, pl* **-ta·ses** \-,sēz\ : the spread of cancer cells from a primary site and the formation of microscopic tumors at secondary sites; *also* : one of the microscopic tumors resulting from micrometastasis — **mi·cro·met·a·stat·ic** \-,me-tə-'sta-tik\ *adj*

mi·cro·me·ter \'mī-krō-,mē-tər\ *n* : MICRON

mi·cro·meth·od \'mī-krō-,me-thəd\ *n* : a method (as of microanalysis) that requires only very small quantities of material or that involves the use of the microscope

mi·cro·mi·cro·cu·rie \,mī-krō-'mī-krō-,kyür-ē\ *n* : one millionth of a microcurie

mi·cro·mol·e·cule \-'mä-lə-,kyül\ *n* : a molecule (as of an amino acid or a fatty acid) of relatively low molecular weight — compare MACROMOLECULE — **mi·cro·mo·lec·u·lar** \-mə-'lekyə-lər\ *adj*

mi·cro·mono·spo·ra \-,mä-nə-'spór-ə\ *n* **1** *cap* : a genus of actinomycetes that includes several antibiotic-producing forms (as *M. purpurea*, the source of gentamicin) **2** *pl* **-rae** \-rē\ : any bacterium of the genus *Micromonospora*

mi·cron \'mī-,krän\ *n* : a unit of length equal to one millionth of a meter — called also *micrometer, mu*

Mi·cro·nase \'mī-krō-,nās\ *trademark* — used for a preparation of glyburide

mi·cro·nee·dle \'mī-krō-,nēd-ᵊl\ *n* : a needle for micromanipulation

mi·cro·nod·u·lar \,mī-krō-'nä-jə-lər\ *adj* : characterized by the presence of extremely small nodules

mi·cro·nu·tri·ent \-'nü-trē-ənt, -'nyü-\ *n* **1** : TRACE ELEMENT **2** : an organic compound (as a vitamin) essential in minute amounts to the growth and health of an animal

mi·cro·or·gan·ism \-'ór-gə-,ni-zəm\ *n* : an organism of microscopic or submicroscopic size — **mi·cro·or·gan·is·mal** \-,ór-gə-'niz-məl\ *adj*

mi·cro·par·a·site \-'par-ə-,sīt\ *n* : a parasitic microorganism — **mi·cro·par·a·sit·ic** \-,par-ə-'si-tik\ *adj*

mi·cro·pe·nis \-'pē-nəs\ *n, pl* **-pe·nes** \-(,)nēz\ *or* **-pe·nis·es** : MICROPHALLUS

mi·cro·per·fu·sion \-pər-'fyü-zhən\ *n* : an act or instance of forcing a fluid through a small organ or tissue by way of a tubule or blood vessel — **mi·cro·per·fused** \-'fyüzd\ *adj*

mi·cro·phage \'mī-krə-,fāj\ *n* : a small phagocyte

mi·cro·pha·kia \,mī-krō-'fā-kē-ə\ *n* : abnormal smallness of the lens of the eye

mi·cro·phal·lus \-'fa-ləs\ *n* : smallness of the penis esp. to an abnormal degree — called also *micropenis*

mi·cro·phon·ic \,mī-krō-'fä-nik\ *n* : COCHLEAR MICROPHONIC — **microphonic** *adj*

mi·cro·pho·to·graph \-'fō-tə-,graf\ *n* : PHOTOMICROGRAPH — **mi·cro·pho·tog·ra·phy** \-fə-'tä-grə-fē\ *n*

mi·croph·thal·mia \,mī-,kräf-'thal-mē-ə\ *n* : abnormal smallness of the eye usu. occurring as a congenital anomaly

mi·croph·thal·mic \-'thal-mik\ *adj* : exhibiting microphthalmia : having small eyes

mi·croph·thal·mos \-məs, -,mäs\ *or* **mi·croph·thal·mus** \-'thal-məs\ *n, pl* **-moi** \-,mói\ *or* **-mi** \-,mī, -,mē\ : MICROPHTHALMIA

mi·cro·pi·pette *also* **mi·cro·pi·pet** \,mī-krō-pī-'pet\ *n* **1** : a pipette for the measurement of minute volumes **2** : a small and extremely fine-pointed pipette used in making microinjections — **micropipette** *vb*

mi·cro·po·rous \'mī-krō-,pōr-əs\ *adj* : characterized by very small pores or channels with diameters in the micron or nanometer range ⟨~ membranes⟩

mi·cro·probe \'mī-krō-ˌprōb\ n : a device for microanalysis that operates by exciting radiation in a minute area or volume of material so that the composition may be determined from the emission spectrum

mi·crop·sia \mī-'kräp-sē-ə\ also **mi·crop·sy** \'mī-ˌkräp-sē\ n, pl -**sias** also -**sies** : a pathological condition in which objects appear to be smaller than they are in reality

mi·cro·punc·ture \ˌmī-krō-'pəŋk-chər\ n : an extremely small puncture (as of a nephron); also : an act of making such a puncture

mi·cro·pyle \'mī-krə-ˌpīl\ n : a differentiated area of surface in an egg through which a sperm enters — **mi·cro·py·lar** \ˌmī-krə-'pī-lər\ adj

mi·cro·ra·dio·gram \ˌmī-krō-'rā-dē-ə-ˌgram\ n : MICRORADIOGRAPH

mi·cro·ra·dio·graph \-ˌgraf\ n : an X-ray photograph prepared by microradiography

mi·cro·ra·di·og·ra·phy \-ˌrā-dē-'ä-grə-fē\ n, pl -**phies** : radiography in which an X-ray photograph is prepared showing minute internal structure — **mi·cro·ra·dio·graph·ic** \-ˌrā-dē-ə-'gra-fik\ adj

mi·cro·sat·el·lite \-'sa-tᵊl-ˌit\ n : any of numerous short segments of DNA that are distributed throughout the genome, that consist of repeated sequences of usu. two to five nucleotides, and that are often useful markers in studies of genetic linkage because they tend to vary from one individual to another — compare MINISATELLITE

mi·cro·scis·sors \'mī-krō-ˌsi-zərz\ n sing or pl : extremely small scissors for use in microsurgery

mi·cro·scope \'mī-krə-ˌskōp\ n 1 : an optical instrument consisting of a lens or combination of lenses for making enlarged images of minute objects; esp : COMPOUND MICROSCOPE — see LIGHT MICROSCOPE, PHASE-CONTRAST MICROSCOPE, POLARIZING MICROSCOPE 2 : a non-optical instrument (as one using radiations other than light) for making enlarged images of minute objects — see ELECTRON MICROSCOPE, SCANNING ELECTRON MICROSCOPE

mi·cro·scop·ic \ˌmī-krə-'skä-pik\ also **mi·cro·scop·i·cal** \-pi-kəl\ adj 1 : of, relating to, or conducted with the microscope or microscopy 2 : so small or fine as to be invisible or indistinguishable without the use of a microscope — compare MACROSCOPIC, SUBMICROSCOPIC — **mi·cro·scop·i·cal·ly** adv

microscopic anatomy n : HISTOLOGY

mi·cros·co·py \mī-'kräs-kə-pē\ n, pl -**pies** : the use of or investigation with the microscope — **mi·cros·co·pist** \-pist\ n

mi·cro·sec·ond \'mī-krō-ˌse-kənd, -kənt\ n : one millionth of a second

mi·cro·sec·tion \-ˌsek-shən\ n : a thin section (as of tissue) prepared for microscopic examination — **microsection** vb

mi·cro·slide \'mī-krō-ˌslīd\ n : a slip of glass on which a preparation is mounted for microscopic examination

mi·cro·some \'mī-krə-ˌsōm\ n 1 : any of various minute cellular structures (as a ribosome) 2 : a particle in a particulate fraction that is obtained by heavy centrifugation of broken cells and consists of various amounts of ribosomes, fragmented endoplasmic reticulum, and mitochondrial cristae — **mi·cro·som·al** \ˌmī-krə-'sō-məl\ adj

mi·cro·so·mia \ˌmī-krə-'sō-mē-ə\ n : abnormal smallness of the body

mi·cro·sphe·ro·cy·to·sis \-ˌsfir-ō-sī-'tō-səs, -ˌsfer-\ n, pl -**to·ses** \-ˌtō-ˌsēz\ : spherocytosis esp. when marked by very small spherocytes

mi·cro·spo·rid·i·an \ˌmī-krō-spə-'ri-dē-ən\ n : any of an order (Microsporidia) of spore-forming parasitic protozoans that typically invade and destroy host cells and include some (as of the genera Enterocytozoon and Nosema) that cause infections in immunocompromised humans — **microsporidian** adj

mi·cro·spo·rid·i·o·sis \-spə-ˌri-dē-'ō-səs\ n, pl -**o·ses** \-ˌsēz\ : infestation with or disease caused by microsporidian protozoans

mi·cros·po·rum \mī-'kräs-pə-rəm\ n 1 cap : a genus of fungi (family Moniliaceae) producing both small, nearly oval single-celled spores and large spindle-shaped multicellular spores with a usu. rough outer wall and including several that cause ringworm, tinea capitis, and tinea corporis 2 pl -**ra** : any fungus of the genus Microsporum

mi·cro·struc·ture \'mī-krō-ˌstrək-chər\ n : microscopic structure (as of a cell) — **mi·cro·struc·tur·al** \ˌmī-krō-'strək-chə-rəl, -'strək-shrəl\ adj

mi·cro·sur·gery \ˌmī-krō-'sər-jə-rē\ n, pl -**ger·ies** : minute dissection or manipulation (as by a micromanipulator or laser beam) of living structures or tissue — **mi·cro·sur·geon** \'mī-krō-ˌsər-jən\ n — **mi·cro·sur·gi·cal** \ˌmī-krō-'sər-ji-kəl\ adj — **mi·cro·sur·gi·cal·ly** adv

mi·cro·sy·ringe \-sə-'rinj\ n : a hypodermic syringe equipped for the precise measurement and injection of minute quantities of fluid

mi·cro·tech·nique \ˌmī-krō-tek-'nēk\ also **mi·cro·tech·nic** \'mī-krō-ˌtek-nik, ˌmī-krō-tek-'nēk\ n : any of various methods of handling and preparing material for microscopic observation and study

mi·cro·throm·bus \-'thräm-bəs\ n, pl -**bi** \-ˌbī\ : a very small thrombus

mi·cro·tia \mī-ˈkrō-shə, -shē-ə\ n : abnormal smallness of the external ear

mi·cro·tome \ˈmī-krə-ˌtōm\ n : an instrument for cutting sections (as of organic tissues) for microscopic examination — **microtome** vb

mi·cro·trau·ma \ˈmī-krō-ˌtrau̇-mə, -ˌtrȯ-\ n : a very slight injury or lesion

mi·cro·tu·bule \ˌmī-krō-ˈtü-ˌbyül, -ˈtyü-\ n : any of the minute tubules in eukaryotic cytoplasm that are composed of the protein tubulin and form an important component of the cytoskeleton, mitotic spindle, cilia, and flagella — **mi·cro·tu·bu·lar** \-byə-lər\ adj

mi·cro·unit \ˈmī-krō-ˌyü-nət\ n : one millionth of a standard unit and esp. an international unit ⟨∼s of insulin⟩

mi·cro·vas·cu·lar \-ˈvas-kyə-lər\ adj : of, relating to, or constituting the part of the circulatory system made up of minute vessels (as venules or capillaries) that average less than 0.3 millimeters in diameter — **mi·cro·vas·cu·la·ture** \-lə-ˌchu̇r, -ˌtyu̇r\ n

mi·cro·ves·i·cle \-ˈve-si-kəl\ n : a very small vesicle

mi·cro·ves·sel \-ˈve-səl\ n : a blood vessel (as a capillary, arteriole, or venule) of the microcirculatory system

mi·cro·vil·lus \-ˈvi-ləs\ n, pl **-vil·li** \-ˌlī\ : a microscopic projection of a tissue, cell, or cell organelle; esp : any of the fingerlike outward projections of some cell surfaces — **mi·cro·vil·lar** \-ˈvi-lər\ adj — **mi·cro·vil·lous** \-ˈvi-ləs\ adj

mi·cro·wave \ˈmī-krō-ˌwāv\ n, often attrib : a comparatively short electromagnetic wave; esp : one between about 1 millimeter and 1 meter in wavelength

microwave sickness n : a condition of impaired health reported esp. in the Russian medical literature that is held to be caused by prolonged exposure to low-intensity microwave radiation

Mi·cru·rus \mī-ˈkru̇r-əs\ n : a genus of small venomous elapid snakes comprising the American coral snakes

mic·tu·ri·tion \ˌmik-chə-ˈri-shən, ˌmik-tyü-\ n : URINATION — **mic·tu·rate** \ˈmik-chə-ˌrāt, -tyü-\ vb

MID abbr minimal infective dose

mid·ax·il·lary line \ˌmid-ˈak-sə-ˌler-ē-\ n : an imaginary line through the axilla parallel to the long axis of the body and midway between its ventral and dorsal surfaces

mid·azo·lam \mi-ˈdā-zō-ˌlam\ n : a benzodiazepine tranquilizer administered in the form of its hydrochloride $C_{18}H_{13}ClFN_3 \cdot HCl$ esp. to produce sedation before an operation

mid·brain \ˈmid-ˌbrān\ n : the middle of the three primary divisions of the developing vertebrate brain or the corresponding part of the adult brain that includes a ventral part containing the cerebral peduncles and a dorsal tectum containing the corpora quadrigemina and that surrounds the aqueduct of Sylvius connecting the third and fourth ventricles — called also *mesencephalon*

mid·cla·vic·u·lar line \-kla-ˈvi-kyə-lər-, -klə-\ n : an imaginary line parallel to the long axis of the body and passing through the midpoint of the clavicle on the ventral surface of the body

middle age n : the period of life from about 45 to about 64 years of age — **mid·dle–aged** \ˌmid-ᵊl-ˈājd\ adj — **mid·dle–ag·er** \-ˈā-jər\ n

middle cerebellar peduncle n : CEREBELLAR PEDUNCLE b

middle cerebral artery n : CEREBRAL ARTERY b

middle concha n : NASAL CONCHA b

middle constrictor n : a fan-shaped muscle of the pharynx that arises from the ceratohyal and thyrohyal of the hyoid bone and from the stylohyoid ligament, inserts into the median line at the back of the pharynx, and acts to constrict part of the pharynx in swallowing — called also *constrictor pharyngis medius, middle pharyngeal constrictor muscle;* compare INFERIOR CONSTRICTOR, SUPERIOR CONSTRICTOR

middle ear n : the intermediate portion of the ear of higher vertebrates consisting typically of a small air-filled membrane-lined chamber in the temporal bone continuous with the nasopharynx through the eustachian tube, separated from the external ear by the tympanic membrane and from the inner ear by fenestrae, and containing a chain of three ossicles that extends from the tympanic membrane to the oval window and transmits vibrations to the inner ear — called also *tympanic cavity;* compare INCUS, MALLEUS, STAPES

middle finger n : the midmost of the five digits of the hand

middle hemorrhoidal artery n : RECTAL ARTERY b

middle hemorrhoidal vein n : RECTAL VEIN b

middle meatus n : a curved anteroposterior passage in each nasal cavity that is situated below the middle nasal concha and extends along the entire superior border of the inferior nasal concha — compare INFERIOR MEATUS, SUPERIOR MEATUS

middle meningeal artery n : a branch of the first portion of the maxillary artery that is the largest artery supplying the dura mater, enters the cranium through the foramen spinosum, and divides into anterior and posterior branches in a groove in the greater wing of the sphenoid bone

middle nasal concha n : NASAL CONCHA b

middle peduncle n : CEREBELLAR PEDUNCLE b

middle pharyngeal constrictor muscle *n* : MIDDLE CONSTRICTOR

middle rectal artery *n* : RECTAL ARTERY b

middle rectal vein *n* : RECTAL VEIN b

middle sacral artery *n* : a small artery that arises from the back of the abdominal part of the aorta just before it forks into the two common iliac arteries and that descends near the midline in front of the fourth and fifth lumbar vertebrae, the sacrum, and the coccyx to the glomus coccygeum

middle temporal artery *n* : TEMPORAL ARTERY 2b

middle temporal gyrus *n* : TEMPORAL GYRUS b

middle temporal vein *n* : TEMPORAL VEIN a (2)

middle turbinate *n* : NASAL CONCHA b

middle turbinate bone *also* **middle turbinated bone** *n* : NASAL CONCHA b

mid·dor·sal \(ˌ)mid-ˈdȯr-səl\ *adj* : of, relating to, or situated in the middle part or median line of the back

mid·epi·gas·tric \-ˌe-pi-ˈgas-trik\ *adj* : of, relating to, or located in the middle of the epigastric region of the abdomen ⟨∼ tenderness⟩

mid·face \ˈmid-ˌfās\ *n* : the middle of the face including the nose and its associated bony structures — **mid·fa·cial** \ˌmid-ˈfā-shəl\ *adj*

mid·for·ceps \-ˈfȯr-səps, -ˌseps\ *n* : a procedure for delivery of an infant by the use of forceps after engagement has occurred but before the head has reached the lower part of the birth canal — compare HIGH FORCEPS, LOW FORCEPS

midge \ˈmij\ *n* : any of numerous tiny dipteran flies (esp. families Ceratopogonidae, Cecidomyiidae, and Chironomidae) many of which are capable of giving painful bites and some of which are vectors or intermediate hosts of parasites of humans and various other vertebrates — see BITING MIDGE

midg·et \ˈmi-jət\ *n, sometimes offensive* : a very small person; *specif* : a person of unusually small size who is physically well-proportioned

midg·et·ism \ˈmi-jə-ˌti-zəm\ *n* : the state of being a midget

mid·gut \ˈmid-ˌgət\ *n* : the middle part of the digestive tract of a vertebrate embryo that in humans gives rise to the more distal part of the duodenum and to the jejunum, ileum, cecum and appendix, ascending colon, and much of the transverse colon

mid·life \ˈmid-ˈlīf\ *n* : MIDDLE AGE

midlife crisis *n* : a period of emotional turmoil in middle age caused by the realization that one is no longer young and characterized esp. by a strong desire for change

mid·line \ˈmid-ˌlīn, ˌmid-ˈlīn\ *n* : a median line; *esp* : the median line or median plane of the body or some part of the body

mid·preg·nan·cy \(ˌ)mid-ˈpreg-nən-sē\ *n, pl* **-cies** : the middle period of a term of pregnancy

mid·riff \ˈmi-ˌdrif\ *n* **1** : DIAPHRAGM 1 **2** : the mid-region of the human torso

mid·sag·it·tal \(ˌ)mid-ˈsa-jət-ᵊl\ *adj* : median and sagittal

midsagittal plane *n* : the median vertical longitudinal plane that divides a bilaterally symmetrical animal into right and left halves — called also *median plane*

mid·sec·tion \ˈmid-ˌsek-shən\ *n* : a section midway between the extremes; *esp* : MIDRIFF 2

mid·stream \ˌmid-ˈstrēm\ *adj* : of, relating to, or being urine passed during the middle of an act of urination and not at the beginning or end ⟨a ∼ specimen⟩

mid·tar·sal \-ˈtär-səl\ *adj* : of, relating to, or being the articulation between the two rows of tarsal bones

midtarsal amputation *n* : amputation of the forepart of the foot through the midtarsal joint

mid·tri·mes·ter \-(ˌ)trī-ˈmes-tər\ *adj* : of, performed during, or occurring during the fourth through sixth months of human pregnancy

mid·ven·tral \-ˈven-trəl\ *adj* : of, relating to, or being the middle of the ventral surface — **mid·ven·tral·ly** *adv*

mid·wife \ˈmid-ˌwīf\ *n* : one who assists women in childbirth — see NURSE-MIDWIFE

mid·wife·ry \ˌmid-ˈwi-fə-rē, -ˈwī-; ˈmid-ˌwī-\ *n, pl* **-ries** : the art or act of assisting at childbirth; *also* : OBSTETRICS — see NURSE-MIDWIFERY

mi·fep·ris·tone \ˌmi-ˈfe-pri-ˌstōn\ *n* : RU-486

mi·graine \ˈmī-ˌgrān\ *n* **1** : a condition that is marked by recurrent usu. unilateral severe headache often accompanied by nausea and vomiting and followed by sleep, that tends to occur in more than one member of a family, and that is of uncertain origin though attacks appear to be precipitated by dilatation of intracranial blood vessels **2** : an episode or attack of migraine ⟨suffers from ∼s⟩ — called also *sick headache* — **mi·grain·ous** \-ˌgrā-nəs\ *adj*

mi·grain·eur \ˌmē-gre-ˈnər\ *n* : a person who experiences migraines

mi·grain·oid \ˈmī-ˌgrā-ˌnȯid, mī-ˈgrā-\ *adj* : resembling migraine

migrans — see ERYTHEMA CHRONICUM MIGRANS, LARVAL MIGRANS, LARVA MIGRANS

migrantes — see LARVA MIGRANS

mi·grate \ˈmī-ˌgrāt, mī-ˈ\ *vb* **mi·grat·ed; mi·grat·ing** : to move from one place to another: as **a** : to move from one site to another in a host organism esp. as part of a life cycle **b** *of an atom or group* : to shift position within a molecule — **mi·gra·tion** \mī-ˈgrā-shən\ *n* — **mi·gra·to·ry** \'mī-grə-ˌtōr-ē\ *adj*

migration inhibitory factor *n* : a lymphokine which inhibits the migration of macrophages away from the site of interaction between lymphocytes and antigens

mi·ka·my·cin \ˌmī-kə-'mī-sən\ *n* : an antibiotic complex isolated from a bacterium of the genus *Streptomyces* (*S. mitakaensis*)

Mi·ku·licz resection \'me-kù-ˌlich-\ *n* : an operation for removal of part of the intestine and esp. the colon that involves bringing the diseased portion out of the body, closing the wound around the two parts of the loop which have been sutured together, and cutting off the diseased part leaving a double opening which is later joined by crushing the common wall and closed from the exterior

Mikulicz–Ra·dec·ki \-ra-'det-skē\, **Johann von** (1850–1905), Polish surgeon.

Mi·ku·licz's disease \-ˌli-chəz-\ *n* : abnormal enlargement of the lacrimal and salivary glands

Mikulicz's syndrome *n* : Mikulicz's disease esp. when occurring as a complication of another disease (as leukemia or sarcoidosis)

mild \'mīld\ *adj* **1** : moderate in action or effect ⟨a ~ drug⟩ **2** : not severe

mil·dew \'mil-ˌdü, -ˌdyü\ *n* **1** : a superficial usu. whitish growth produced esp. on organic matter or living plants by fungi (as of the families Erysiphaceae and Peronosporaceae) **2** : a fungus producing mildew

mild silver protein *n* : SILVER PROTEIN a

mil·i·ar·ia \ˌmi-lē-'ar-ē-ə\ *n* : an inflammatory disorder of the skin characterized by redness, eruption, burning or itching, and the release of sweat in abnormal ways (as by the eruption of vesicles) due to blockage of the ducts of the sweat glands; *esp* : PRICKLY HEAT — **mil·i·ar·i·al** \-əl\ *adj*

miliaria crys·tal·li·na \-ˌkris-tə-'lē-nə\ *n* : SUDAMINA

mil·i·ary \'mi-lē-ˌer-ē\ *adj* **1** : resembling or suggesting a small seed or many small seeds ⟨a ~ aneurysm⟩ ⟨~ tubercles⟩ **2** : characterized by the formation of numerous small lesions ⟨~ pneumonia⟩

miliary tuberculosis *n* : acute tuberculosis in which minute tubercles are formed in one or more organs of the body by tubercle bacilli usu. spread by way of the blood

mi·lieu \mēl-'yə(r), -'yü; 'mēl-ˌyü, mē-'lyœ̄\ *n*, *pl* **milieus** or **mi·lieux** *same or* -'yə(r)z, -'yüz; -ˌyüz, -'lyœ̄z\ : ENVIRONMENT

milieu therapy *n* : psychiatric treatment involving manipulation of the environment of a patient for therapeutic purposes

mil·i·um \'mi-lē-əm\ *n*, *pl* **mil·ia** \-lē-ə\

: a small pearly firm noninflammatory elevation of the skin (as of the face) due to retention of keratin in an oil gland duct blocked by a thin layer of epithelium — called also *whitehead;* compare BLACKHEAD 1

¹milk \'milk\ *n* : a fluid secreted by the mammary glands of females for the nourishment of their young; *esp* : cow's milk used as a food by humans

²milk *vb* : to draw off the milk of

milk·er's nodules \'mil-kərz-\ *n* : a mild virus infection characterized by reddish blue nodules on the hands, arms, face, or neck acquired by direct contact with the udders of cows infected with a poxvirus (species *Pseudocowpox virus* of the genus *Parapoxvirus*) — called also *paravaccinia, pseudocowpox*

milk fever *n* **1** : a febrile disorder following parturition **2** : a disease of newly lactating cows, sheep, or goats that is caused by excessive drain on the body mineral reserves during the establishment of the milk flow — called also *parturient paresis*

milk leg *n* : postpartum thrombophlebitis of a femoral vein — called also *phlegmasia alba dolens*

Milk·man's syndrome \'milk-mənz-\ *n* : an abnormal condition marked by porosity of bone and tendency to spontaneous often symmetrical fractures

Milkman, Louis Arthur (1895–1951), American radiologist.

milk of bismuth *n* : a thick white suspension in water of the hydroxide of bismuth and bismuth subcarbonate that is used esp. in the treatment of diarrhea

milk of magnesia *n* : a milk-white suspension of magnesium hydroxide in water used as an antacid and laxative — called also *magnesia magma*

milk sickness *n* : an acute disease characterized by weakness, vomiting, and constipation and caused by eating dairy products or meat from cattle affected with trembles

milk sugar *n* : LACTOSE

milk thistle *n* : a tall purple-flowered thistle (*Silybum marianum*) that is the source of silymarin; *also* : SILYMARIN

milk tooth *n* : a temporary tooth of a young mammal; *esp* : one of the human dentition including four incisors, two canines, and four molars in each jaw which fall out during childhood and are replaced by the permanent teeth — called also *baby tooth, deciduous tooth, primary tooth*

Mil·ler–Ab·bott tube \'mi-lər-'a-bət-\ *n* : a double-lumen balloon-tipped rubber tube used for the purpose of decompression in treating intestinal obstruction

Miller, Thomas Grier (1886–1981), **and Abbott, William Osler** (1902–1943), American physicians.

milli- *comb form* : thousandth — used esp. in terms belonging to the metric system ⟨*milli*rad⟩

mil·li·bar \\'mi-lə-ˌbär\ *n* : a unit of atmospheric pressure equal to ¹⁄₁₀₀₀ bar or 1000 dynes per square centimeter

mil·li·cu·rie \ˌmi-lə-ˈkyu̇r-(ˌ)ē, -kyu̇-ˈrē\ *n* : one thousandth of a curie — abbr. *mCi*

mil·li·gram \\'mi-lə-ˌgram\ *n* : one thousandth of a gram — abbr. *mg*

mil·li·li·ter \-ˌlē-tər\ *n* : one thousandth of a liter — abbr. *ml*

mil·li·me·ter \-ˌmē-tər\ *n* : one thousandth of a meter — abbr. *mm*

mil·li·mi·cron \ˌmi-lə-ˈmī-ˌkrän\ *n* : NANOMETER

mil·li·os·mol *or* **mil·li·os·mole** \ˌmi-lē-ˈäz-ˌmōl, -ˈäs-\ *n* : one thousandth of an osmol

mil·li·pede \\'mi-lə-ˌpēd\ *n* : any of a class (Diplopoda) of arthropods having usu. a cylindrical segmented body, two pairs of legs on most segments, and including some forms that secrete toxic substances causing skin irritation but that unlike centipedes possess no poison fangs

mil·li·rad \-ˌrad\ *n* : one thousandth of a rad — abbr. *mrad*

mil·li·rem \-ˌrem\ *n* : one thousandth of a rem — abbr. *mrem*

mil·li·roent·gen \ˌmi-lə-ˈrent-gən, -ˈrənt-, -jən; -ˈren-chən, -ˈrən-\ *n* : one thousandth of a roentgen — abbr. *mR*

mil·li·unit \\'mi-lə-ˌyü-nət\ *n* : one thousandth of a standard unit and esp. of an international unit

mil·ri·none \\'mil-rə-ˌnōn\ *n* : an inotropic vasodilator used in the form of its lactate $C_{12}H_9N_3O \cdot C_3H_6O_3$ esp. in short-term intravenous therapy for congestive heart failure

Mil·roy's disease \\'mil-ˌroiz-\ *n* : a hereditary lymphedema esp. of the legs
    Mil·roy, William Forsyth (1855–1942), American physician.

Mil·town \\'mil-ˌtau̇n\ *trademark* — used for a preparation of meprobamate

Mil·wau·kee brace \mil-ˈwȯ-kē-, -ˈwä-\ *n* : an orthopedic brace that extends from the pelvis to the neck and is used esp. in the treatment of scoliosis

mi·met·ic \mə-ˈme-tik, mī-\ *adj* : simulating the action or effect of — usu. used in combination ⟨sympatho*mimetic* drugs⟩

mim·ic \\'mi-mik\ *vb* **mim·icked** \-ˌmikt\; **mim·ick·ing** : to imitate or resemble closely: as **a** : to imitate the symptoms of **b** : to produce an effect and esp. a physiological effect similar to — **mimic** *n* — **mim·ic·ry** \\'mi-mi-krē\ *n*

min *abbr* minim

Min·a·ma·ta disease \ˌmi-nə-ˈmä-tə-\ *n* : a toxic neuropathy caused by the ingestion of methylmercury compounds (as in contaminated seafood) and characterized by impairment of cerebral functions, constriction of the visual field, and progressive weakening of muscles

mind \\'mīnd\ *n* **1** : the element or complex of elements in an individual that feels, perceives, thinks, wills, and esp. reasons **2** : the conscious mental events and capabilities in an organism **3** : the organized conscious and unconscious adaptive mental activity of an organism

mind–altering *adj* : PSYCHOACTIVE

mind–set \\'mīnd-ˌset\ *n* : a mental inclination, tendency, or habit

¹min·er·al \\'mi-nə-rəl\ *n* **1** : a solid homogeneous crystalline chemical element or compound that results from the inorganic processes of nature

²mineral *adj* **1** : of or relating to minerals; *also* : INORGANIC **2** : impregnated with mineral substances

min·er·al·ize \\'mi-nə-rə-ˌlīz\ *vb* **-ized; -iz·ing** : to impregnate or supply with minerals or an inorganic compound — **min·er·al·i·za·tion** \ˌmi-nə-rəl-ə-ˈzā-shən\ *n*

min·er·al·o·cor·ti·coid \ˌmi-nə-rə-lō-ˈkȯr-tə-ˌkȯid\ *n* : a corticosteroid (as aldosterone) that affects chiefly the electrolyte and fluid balance in the body — compare GLUCOCORTICOID

mineral oil *n* : a transparent oily liquid obtained usu. by distilling petroleum and used in medicine esp. for treating constipation

min·er's asthma \\'mī-nərz-\ *n* : PNEUMOCONIOSIS

miner's elbow *n* : bursitis of the elbow that tends to occur in miners who work in small tunnels and rest their weight on their elbows

miner's phthisis *n* : an occupational respiratory disease (as pneumoconiosis or anthracosilicosis) of miners

mini·lap·a·rot·o·my \ˌmi-nē-ˌla-pə-ˈrä-tə-mē\ *n, pl* **-mies** : a ligation of the Fallopian tubes performed through a small incision in the abdominal wall

min·im \\'mi-nəm\ *n* : either of two units of capacity equal to ¹⁄₆₀ fluid dram: **a** : a U.S. unit of liquid capacity equivalent to 0.003760 cubic inch or 0.061610 milliliter **b** : a British unit of liquid capacity and dry measure equivalent to 0.003612 cubic inch or 0.059194 milliliter

minimae — see VENAE CORDIS MINIMAE

min·i·mal \\'mi-nə-məl\ *adj* : relating to or being a minimum : constituting the least possible with respect to size, number, degree, or certain stated conditions

minimal brain damage *n* : ATTENTION DEFICIT DISORDER

minimal brain dysfunction *n* : ATTENTION DEFICIT DISORDER — abbr. *MBD*

minimal infective dose *n* : the smallest quantity of infective material that regularly produces infection — abbr. *MID*

minimal inhibitory concentration n : the smallest concentration of an antibiotic that regularly inhibits growth of a bacterium in vitro — abbr. *MIC*

minimi — see ABDUCTOR DIGITI MINIMI, EXTENSOR DIGITI MINIMI, FLEXOR DIGITI MINIMI BREVIS, GLUTEUS MINIMUS, OPPONENS DIGITI MINIMI

min·i·mum \'mi-nə-məm\ n, pl **-i·ma** \-mə\ or **-i·mums** 1 : the least quantity assignable, admissible, or possible 2 : the lowest degree or amount of variation (as of temperature) reached or recorded — **minimum** adj

minimum dose n : the smallest dose of a medicine or drug that will produce an effect

minimum inhibitory concentration n : MINIMAL INHIBITORY CONCENTRATION

minimum lethal dose n : the smallest dose experimentally found to kill any one animal of a test group

minimus — see GLUTEUS MINIMUS

mini-pill \'mi-nē-ˌpill\ n : a birth control pill that is intended to minimize side effects, contains a very low dose of a progestogen and esp. norethindrone but no estrogen, and is taken daily

Mini·press \-ˌpres\ trademark — used for a preparation of the hydrochloride of prazosin

mini·sat·el·lite \-'sa-t°l-ˌīt\ n : any of numerous DNA segments located mainly near the ends of chromosomes that consist of repeating sequences of at least five but usu. not more than 100 nucleotides and that are useful in DNA fingerprinting — compare MICROSATELLITE

mini–stroke n : TRANSIENT ISCHEMIC ATTACK

Min·ne·so·ta Mul·ti·pha·sic Personality Inventory \ˌmi-nə-ˌsō-tə-ˌməl-ti-'fā-zik-, -ˌməl-ˌtī-\ n : a test of personal and social adjustment based on a complex scaling of the answers to an elaborate true or false test

Mi·no·cin \mi-'nō-sin\ trademark — used for a preparation of the hydrochloride of minocycline

min·o·cy·cline \ˌmi-nō-'sī-ˌklēn\ n : a broad-spectrum tetracycline antibiotic administered in the form of its hydrochloride $C_{23}H_{27}N_3O_7 \cdot HCl$

¹**mi·nor** \'mī-nər\ adj : not serious or involving risk to life ⟨~ illness⟩ ⟨a ~ operation⟩ — compare MAJOR

²**minor** n : a person of either sex under the age of legal qualification for adult rights and responsibilities

minora — see LABIA MINORA

minor surgery n : surgery involving little risk to the life of the patient; specif : an operation on the superficial structures of the body or a manipulative procedure that does not involve a serious risk — compare MAJOR SURGERY

min·ox·i·dil \mi-'näk-sə-ˌdil\ n : a peripheral vasodilator $C_9H_{15}N_5O$ used orally to treat hypertension and topically in a propylene glycol solution to promote hair regrowth in male-pattern baldness — see LONITEN, ROGAINE

minute volume n : CARDIAC OUTPUT

mi·o·sis also **my·o·sis** \mī-'ō-səs, mē-\ n, pl **mi·o·ses** also **my·o·ses** \-ˌsēz\ : excessive smallness or contraction of the pupil of the eye

¹**mi·ot·ic** also **my·ot·ic** \-'ä-tik\ n : an agent that causes miosis

²**miotic** also **my·ot·ic** adj : relating to or characterized by miosis

mi·ra·cid·i·um \ˌmir-ə-'si-dē-əm, ˌmī-rə-\ n, pl **-cid·ia** \-dē-ə\ : the free-swimming ciliated first larva of a digenetic trematode that develops into a sporocyst after penetrating a suitable intermediate host — **mi·ra·cid·i·al** \-dē-əl\ adj

mir·a·cil D \'mir-ə-ˌsil-'dē\ n : LUCANTHONE

mir·a·cle drug \'mir-ə-kəl-\ n : a drug usu. newly discovered that elicits a dramatic response in a patient's condition — called also **wonder drug**

mi·rage \mə-'räzh\ n : an optical effect that is sometimes seen at sea, in the desert, or over a hot pavement, that may have the appearance of a pool of water or a mirror in which distant objects are seen inverted, and that is caused by the bending or reflection of rays of light by a layer of heated air of varying density

mi·rex \'mī-ˌreks\ n : an organochlorine insecticide $C_{10}Cl_{12}$ formerly used esp. against ants that is a suspected carcinogen

mirror writing n : backward writing resembling in slant and order of letters the reflection of ordinary writing in a mirror

mis- prefix : badly : wrongly ⟨misdiagnose⟩

mis·car·riage \mis-'kar-ij\ n : spontaneous expulsion of a human fetus before it is viable and esp. between the 12th and 28th weeks of gestation — compare ABORTION 1a — **mis·car·ry** \(ˌ)mis-'kar-ē\ vb

mis·di·ag·nose \(ˌ)mis-'dī-ig-ˌnōs, -ˌnōz\ vb **-nosed; -nos·ing** : to diagnose incorrectly — **mis·di·ag·no·sis** \(ˌ)mis-ˌdī-ig-'nō-səs\ n

mi·sog·y·nist \mə-'sä-jə-nist\ n : one who hates women — **misogynist** adj — **mi·sog·y·ny** \mə-'sä-jə-nē\ n

mi·so·pros·tol \ˌmī-sō-'präs-ˌtōl, -ˌtȯl\ n : a prostaglandin analog $C_{22}H_{38}O_5$ used to prevent stomach ulcers associated with NSAID use and to induce abortion in conjunction with RU-486

missed abortion \'mist-\ n : an intrauterine death of a fetus that is not followed by its immediate expulsion

missed labor n : a retention of a fetus in the uterus beyond the normal period of pregnancy

¹**mis·sense** \'mis-ˌsens\ adj : relating to

or being a genetic mutation involving alteration of one or more codons so that different amino acids are determined — compare ANTISENSE, NONSENSE

²**missense** *n* : missense genetic mutation

missionary position *n* : a coital position in which the female lies on her back with the male on top and with his face opposite hers

mit- *or* **mito-** *comb form* **1** : thread ⟨*mito*chondrion⟩ **2** : mitosis ⟨*mito*genesis⟩

mite \ˈmīt\ *n* : any of numerous small to very minute acarid arachnids that include parasites of insects and vertebrates some of which are important disease vectors, parasites of plants, pests of various stored products, and free-living aquatic and terrestrial forms — see ITCH MITE

mith·ra·my·cin \ˌmi-thrə-ˈmīs-ᵊn\ *n* : PLICAMYCIN

mith·ri·da·tism \ˌmi-thrə-ˈdā-ˌti-zəm\ *n* : tolerance to a poison acquired by taking gradually increased doses of it

Mith·ra·da·tes VI Eu·pa·tor \ˌmi-thrə-ˈdā-tēz-ˈsiks-ˈyü-pə-ˌtȯr\, **(d 63 BC),** king of Pontus.

mi·ti·cide \ˈmī-tə-ˌsīd\ *n* : an agent used to kill mites — **mi·ti·ci·dal** \ˌmī-tə-ˈsīd-ᵊl\ *adj*

mi·to·chon·dri·on \ˌmī-tə-ˈkän-drē-ən\ *n, pl* **-dria** \-drē-ə\ : any of various round or long cellular organelles of most eukaryotes that are found outside the nucleus, produce energy for the cell through cellular respiration, and are rich in fats, proteins, and enzymes — **mi·to·chon·dri·al** \-drē-əl\ *adj* — **mi·to·chon·dri·al·ly** *adv*

mitochondrial DNA *n* : an extranuclear double-stranded DNA found exclusively in mitochondria that in most eukaryotes is a circular molecule and is maternally inherited — called also *mtDNA*

mi·to·gen \ˈmī-tə-jən\ *n* : a substance that induces mitosis

mi·to·gen·e·sis \ˌmī-tə-ˈje-nə-səs\ *n, pl* **-e·ses** \-ˌsēz\ : the production of cell mitosis

mi·to·gen·ic \-ˈje-nik\ *adj* : of, producing, or stimulating mitosis

mi·to·my·cin \ˌmī-tə-ˈmīs-ᵊn\ *n* **1** : a complex of antibiotic substances which is produced by a Japanese bacterium of the genus *Streptomyces* (*S. caespitosus*) **2** : a component C_{15}-$H_{18}N_4O_5$ of mitomycin that inhibits DNA synthesis and is used as an antineoplastic in the palliative treatment of some carcinomas — called also *mitomycin C*

mi·to·sis \mī-ˈtō-səs\ *n, pl* **-to·ses** \-ˌsēz\ **1** : a process that takes place in the nucleus of a dividing cell, involves typically a series of steps consisting of prophase, metaphase, anaphase, and telophase, and results in the formation of two new nuclei each having the same number of chromosomes as the parent nucleus — compare MEIOSIS **2** : cell division in which mitosis occurs — **mi·tot·ic** \-ˈtä-tik\ *adj* — **mi·tot·i·cal·ly** *adv*

mitotic index *n* : the number of cells per thousand cells actively dividing at a particular time

mi·to·xan·trone \ˌmī-tō-ˈzan-ˌtrōn\ *n* : an antineoplastic drug that is used in the form of its dihydrochloride C_{22}-$H_{28}N_4O_6$·2HCl either alone or in combination in the treatment of some leukemias and carcinomas

mi·tral \ˈmī-trəl\ *adj* : of, relating to, being, or adjoining a mitral valve or orifice

mitral cell *n* : any of the pyramidal cells of the olfactory bulb about which terminate numerous fibers from the olfactory cells of the nasal mucosa

mitral insufficiency *n* : inability of the mitral valve to close perfectly permitting blood to flow back into the atrium and leading to varying degrees of heart failure — called also *mitral incompetence*

mitral orifice *n* : the left atrioventricular orifice

mitral regurgitation *n* : backward flow of blood into the atrium due to mitral insufficiency

mitral stenosis *n* : a condition usu. the result of disease in which the mitral valve is abnormally narrow

mitral valve *n* : a valve in the heart consisting of two triangular flaps which allow only unidirectional blood flow from the left atrium to the left ventricle — called also *bicuspid valve, left antrioventricular valve*

mitral valve prolapse *n* : a valvular heart disorder in which one or both mitral valve flaps close incompletely during systole usu. producing either a click or murmur and sometimes minor mitral regurgitation and which is often a benign symptomless condition but may be marked by varied symptoms (as chest pain, fatigue, or palpitations) — abbr. *MVP*; called also *Barlow's syndrome*

mit·tel·schmerz \ˈmit-ᵊl-ˌshmertz\ *n* : abdominal pain occurring between the menstrual periods and usu. considered to be associated with ovulation

mixed \ˈmikst\ *adj* **1** : combining features or exhibiting symptoms of more than one condition or disease ⟨a ∼ tumor⟩ **2** : producing more than one kind of secretion ⟨∼ salivary glands⟩

mixed connective tissue disease *n* : a syndrome characterized by symptoms of various rheumatic diseases (as systemic lupus erythematosus, scleroderma, and polymyositis) and by high concentrations of antibodies to extractable nuclear antigens

mixed dementia *n* : dementia involving both Alzheimer's disease and vascular dementia

mixed glioma *n* : a glioma consisting of more than one cell type

mixed nerve *n* : a nerve containing both sensory and motor fibers

mix·ture \'miks-chər\ *n* : a product of mixing: as **a** : a portion of matter consisting of two or more components in varying proportions that retain their own properties **b** : an aqueous liquid medicine; *specif* : a preparation in which insoluble substances are suspended in watery fluids by the addition of a viscid material (as gum, sugar, or glycerol)

mks \,em-,kā-'es\ *adj, often cap M&K&S* : of, relating to, or being a system of units based on the meter, the kilogram, and the second ⟨∼ system⟩ ⟨∼ units⟩

ml *abbr* milliliter

MLD *abbr* **1** median lethal dose **2** minimum lethal dose

M line \'em-,līn\ *n* : a thin dark line across the center of the H zone of a striated muscle fiber — called also *M band*

MLT *abbr* medical laboratory technician

mm *abbr* millimeter

mm Hg \,mi-lə-,mē-tər-əv-'mər-kyə-rē\ *n* : a unit of pressure equal to the pressure exerted by a column of mercury 1 millimeter high at 0°C and under the acceleration of gravity and nearly equivalent to 1 torr

M–mode \'em-,mōd\ *adj* : of, relating to, or being an ultrasonographic technique that is used for studying the movement of internal body structures

MMPI *abbr* Minnesota Multiphasic Personality Inventory

MMR *abbr* measles-mumps-rubella (vaccine)

Mn *symbol* manganese

MN *abbr* master of nursing

-m·ne·sia \m-'nē-zhə\ *n comb form* : a (specified) type or condition of memory ⟨para*mnesia*⟩

Mo *symbol* molybdenum

MO *abbr* medical officer

mo·bile \'mō-bəl, -,bīl\ *adj* **1** : capable of moving or being moved about readily **2** : characterized by an extreme degree of fluidity — **mo·bil·i·ty** \mō-'bi-lə-tē\ *n*

mo·bi·lize \'mō-bə-,līz\ *vb* **-lized; -liz·ing 1** : to put into movement or circulation : make mobile; *specif* : to release (something stored in the body) for body use **2** : to assemble (as resources) and make ready for use **3** : to separate (an organ or part) from associated structures so as to make more accessible for operative procedures **4** : to develop to a state of acute activity — **mo·bi·li·za·tion** \,mō-bə-lə-'zā-shən\ *n*

Mö·bius syndrome *or* **Moe·bius syndrome** \'mü-bē-əs-, 'mœ-\ *n* : congenital bilateral paralysis of the facial muscles associated with other neurological disorders

Möbius, Paul Julius (1853–1907), German neurologist.

moc·ca·sin \'mä-kə-sən\ *n* **1** : WATER MOCCASIN **2** : a snake (as of the genus *Natrix*) resembling a water moccasin

mo·dal·i·ty \mō-'da-lə-tē\ *n, pl* **-ties 1** : one of the main avenues of sensation (as vision) **2 a** : a usu. physical therapeutic agency **b** : an apparatus for applying a modality

¹mod·el \'mäd-°l\ *n* **1 a** : a pattern of something to be made **b** : a cast of a tooth or oral cavity **2** : something (as a similar object or a construct) used to help visualize or explore something else (as the living human body) that cannot be directly observed or experimented on — see ANIMAL MODEL

²model *vb* **mod·eled** *or* **mod·elled; mod·el·ing** *or* **mod·el·ling** : to produce (as by computer) a representation or simulation of

mod·er·ate \'mä-də-rət\ *adj* **1** : avoiding extremes of behavior : observing reasonable limits ⟨a ∼ drinker⟩ **2** : not severe in effect ⟨∼ pain⟩

modified radical mastectomy *n* : a mastectomy that is similar to a radical mastectomy but does not include removal of the pectoral muscles

mod·i·fi·er \'mä-də-,fī-ər\ *n* **1** : one that modifies **2** : a gene that modifies the effect of another

mod·i·fy \'mä-də-,fī\ *vb* **-fied; -fy·ing** : to make a change in ⟨∼ behavior by the use of drugs⟩ — **mod·i·fi·ca·tion** \,mä-də-fə-'kā-shən\ *n*

mo·di·o·lar \mə-'dī-ə-lər\ *adj* : of or relating to the modiolus of the ear

mo·di·o·lus \mə-'dī-ə-ləs\ *n, pl* **-li** \-,lī\ : a central bony column in the cochlea of the ear

MODS *abbr* multiple organ dysfunction syndrome

mod·u·late \'mä-jə-,lāt\ *vb* **-lat·ed; -lat·ing** : to adjust to or keep in proper measure or proportion ⟨∼ an immune response⟩ ⟨∼ cell activity⟩ — **mod·u·la·tion** \,mä-jə-'lā-shən\ *n* — **mod·u·la·tor** \'mä-jə-,lā-tər\ *n* — **mod·u·la·to·ry** \-lə-,tōr-ē\ *adj*

MODY *abbr* maturity-onset diabetes of the young

Moebius syndrome *var of* MÖBIUS SYNDROME

Mohs' technique \'mōz-\ *n* : a chemosurgical technique for the removal of skin malignancies in which excision is made to a depth at which the tissue is microscopically free of cancer — called also *Mohs' chemosurgery*

Mohs, Frederic Edward (1910–2002), American surgeon.

moist \'moist\ *adj* **1** : slightly or moderately wet **2 a** : marked by a discharge or exudation of liquid ⟨∼ eczema⟩ **b** : suggestive of the pres-

ence of liquid — used of sounds
heard in auscultation ⟨∼ rales⟩

moist gangrene n : gangrene that develops in the presence of combined
arterial and venous obstruction, is
usu. accompanied by an infection,
and is characterized by a watery discharge usu. of foul odor

mo·lal \'mō-ləl\ adj : of, relating to, or
containing a mole of solute per 1000
grams of solvent ⟨a ∼ solution⟩ —
mo·lal·i·ty \mō-'la-lə-tē\ n

¹**mo·lar** \'mō-lər\ n : a tooth with a
rounded or flattened surface adapted
for grinding; specif : one of the mammalian teeth behind the incisors and
canines sometimes including the premolars but more exactly restricted to
the three posterior pairs in each human jaw on each side which are not
preceded by milk teeth

²**molar** adj **1 a** : pulverizing by friction
⟨∼ teeth⟩ **b** : of, relating to, or located near the molar teeth ⟨∼ gland⟩
2 : of, relating to, possessing the qualities of, or characterized by a hydatidiform mole ⟨∼ pregnancy⟩

³**molar** adj **1** : of or relating to a mole
of a substance ⟨the ∼ volume of a
gas⟩ **2** : containing one mole of solute
in one liter of solution — **mo·lar·i·ty**
\mō-'lar-ə-tē\ n

¹**mold** \'mōld\ n : a cavity in which a
fluid or malleable substance is shaped

²**mold** vb : to give shape to esp. in a
mold

³**mold** vb : to become moldy

⁴**mold** n **1** : a superficial often woolly
growth produced esp. on damp or decaying organic matter or on living organisms by a fungus (as of the order
Mucorales) **2** : a fungus that produces mold

mold·ing \'mōl-diŋ\ n : the shaping of
the fetal head to allow it to pass
through the birth canal during birth

moldy \'mōl-dē\ adj **mold·i·er; -est**
: covered with a mold-producing fungus ⟨∼ bread⟩

¹**mole** \'mōl\ n : a pigmented spot,
mark, or small permanent protuberance on the human body; esp : NEVUS

²**mole** n : an abnormal mass in the
uterus: **a** : a blood clot containing a
degenerated fetus and its membranes
b : HYDATIDIFORM MOLE

³**mole** also **mol** \'mōl\ n : the base unit
in the International System of Units
for the amount of pure substance that
contains the same number of elementary entities as there are atoms in exactly 12 grams of the isotope carbon
12

mo·lec·u·lar \mə-'le-kyə-lər\ adj : of,
relating to, consisting of, or produced
by molecules — **mo·lec·u·lar·ly** adv

molecular biology n : a branch of biology dealing with the ultimate
physicochemical organization of living matter and esp. with the molecular basis of inheritance and protein
synthesis — **molecular biologist** n

molecular formula n : a chemical formula that gives the total number of
atoms of each element in a molecule
⟨the *molecular formula* of water is
H_2O⟩ — see STRUCTURAL FORMULA

molecular genetics n pl : a branch of
genetics dealing with the structure
and activity of genetic material at the
molecular level — **molecular geneticist** n

molecular weight n : the mass of a
molecule that may be calculated as
the sum of the atomic weights of its
constituent atoms

mol·e·cule \'mä-li-ˌkyül\ n : the smallest particle of a substance that retains
all the properties of the substance and
is composed of one or more atoms

mol·in·done \mō-'lin-ˌdōn\ n : an antipsychotic drug used in the form of
its hydrochloride $C_{16}H_{24}N_2O_2 \cdot HCl$
esp. in the treatment of schizophrenia

Moll's gland \'mälz\ n : GLAND OF
MOLL

mol·lus·ci·cide \mə-'ləs-kə-ˌsīd, -'lə-si-
ˌsīd\ n : an agent for destroying mollusks (as snails) — **mol·lus·ci·cid·al**
\-ˌləs-kə-'sīd-ᵊl, -ˌlə-si-'sīd-\ adj

mol·lus·cum \mə-'ləs-kəm\ n, pl **-ca**
\-kə\ : any of several skin diseases
marked by soft pulpy nodules; esp
: MOLLUSCUM CONTAGIOSUM

molluscum body n : any of the
rounded cytoplasmic bodies found in
the central opening of the nodules
characteristic of molluscum contagiosum

molluscum con·ta·gi·o·sum \-kən-ˌtā-
jē-'ō-səm\ n, pl **mollusca con·ta·gi·o·-
sa** \-sə\ : a mild chronic disease of the
skin caused by a poxvirus (species
Molluscum contagiosum virus of the
genus *Molluscipoxvirus*) and characterized by the formation of small nodules with a central opening and
contents resembling curd

mol·lusk or **mol·lusc** \'mä-ləsk\ n
: any of a large phylum (Mollusca) of
invertebrate animals (as snails) with a
soft unsegmented body usu. enclosed
in a calcareous shell — **mol·lus·can**
also **mol·lus·kan** \mə-'les-kən, mä-\
adj

molt \'mōlt\ vb : to shed hair, feathers,
shell, horns, or an outer layer periodically — **molt** n

mo·lyb·de·num \mə-'lib-də-nəm\ n : a
metallic element that is a trace element in plant and animal metabolism
— symbol *Mo;* see ELEMENT table

mo·met·a·sone fu·ro·ate \mō-'me-tə-
ˌsōn-'fyür-ə-ˌwāt\ n : a synthetic corticosteroid $C_{27}H_{30}Cl_2O_6$ used topically
in a cream or ointment base to treat
inflammatory and pruritic der-
matoses or intranasally in aqueous
suspension to relieve the nasal symptoms of allergic rhinitis — see NA-
SONEX

mom·ism \'mä-ˌmi-zəm\ n : an excessive popular adoration and sentimen-

talizing of mothers that is held to be oedipal in nature

mon- *or* **mono-** *comb form* **1** : one : single ⟨*mono*filament⟩ **2** : affecting a single part ⟨*mono*plegia⟩

monarticular *var of* MONOARTICULAR

mon·au·ral \(ˌ)mä-ˈnȯr-əl\ *adj* : of, relating to, affecting, or designed for use with one ear ⟨~ hearing aid systems⟩ — **mon·au·ral·ly** *adv*

Möncke·berg's sclerosis \ˈmün-kə-ˌbȯrgz-, ˈmeŋ-\ *n* : arteriosclerosis characterized by the formation of calcium deposits in the mediae of esp. the peripheral arteries

   Möncke·berg \ˈmœŋ-kə-ˌberk\, **Johann Georg** (1877–1925), German pathologist.

Monday morning disease *n* : azoturia of horses caused by heavy feeding during a period of inactivity — called also *Monday disease*

mo·nen·sin \mȯ-ˈnen-sən\ *n* : an antibiotic $C_{36}H_{62}O_{11}$ obtained from a bacterium of the genus *Streptomyces* (*S. cinnamonensis*) and used as an antiprotozoal, antibacterial, and antifungal agent and as an additive to cattle feed

mo·ne·ran \mə-ˈnir-ən\ *n* : PROKARYOTE — **moneran** *adj*

mon·es·trous \(ˌ)mä-ˈnes-trəs\ *adj* : experiencing estrus once each year or breeding season

mon·gol \ˈmäŋ-gəl, ˈmän-ˌgōl, ˈmäŋ-\ *n, often cap, usu offensive* : one affected with Down syndrome

mon·go·lian \mäŋ-ˈgōl-yən, mäŋ-, -ˈgō-lē-ən\ *adj, often cap, usu offensive* : MONGOLOID

Mongolian spot *n* : a bluish pigmented area near the base of the spine that is present at birth esp. in Asian, southern European, American Indian, and black infants and that usu. disappears during childhood

mon·gol·ism \ˈmäŋ-gə-ˌli-zəm\ *n, usu offensive* : DOWN SYNDROME

mon·gol·oid \ˈmäŋ-gə-ˌlȯid\ *adj, often cap, usu offensive* : of, relating to, or affected with Down syndrome — **mongoloid** *n, often cap, usu offensive*

mo·nie·zia \ˌmä-nē-ˈe-zē-ə\ *n* **1** *cap* : a genus of tapeworms (family Anoplocephalidae) parasitizing the intestine of various ruminants **2** : any tapeworm of the genus *Moniezia*

   Moniez \mȯn-ˈyä\, **Romain–Louis** (1852–1936), French parasitologist.

mo·nil·e·thrix \mə-ˈni-lə-ˌthriks\ *n, pl* **mon·i·let·ri·ches** \ˌmä-nə-ˈle-trə-ˌkēz\ : an inherited disease of the hair in which each hair appears as if strung with small beads or nodes

mo·nil·ia \mə-ˈni-lē-ə\ *n, pl* **monilias** *or* **monilia** *also* **mo·nil·i·ae** \-lē-ˌē\ **1** : any fungus of the genus *Candida* **2** *pl* **monilias** : CANDIDIASIS

Mo·nil·ia \mə-ˈni-lē-ə\ *n, syn of* CANDIDA

mo·nil·i·al \mə-ˈni-lē-əl\ *adj* : of, relating to, or caused by a fungus of the genus *Candida* ⟨~ vaginitis⟩

mo·nil·i·a·sis \ˌmō-nə-ˈlī-ə-səs, ˌmä-\ *n, pl* **-a·ses** \-ˌsēz\ : CANDIDIASIS

mo·nil·iid \mə-ˈni-lē-əd\ *n* : a secondary commonly generalized dermatitis resulting from hypersensitivity developed in response to a primary focus of infection with a fungus of the genus *Candida*

¹mon·i·tor \ˈmä-nə-tər\ *n* : one that monitors; *esp* : a device for observing or measuring a biologically important condition or function ⟨a heart ~⟩

²monitor *vb* **1** : to watch, observe, or check closely or continuously ⟨~ a patient's vital signs⟩ **2** : to test for intensity of radiations esp. if due to radioactivity

mon·key \ˈməŋ-kē\ *n* : a nonhuman primate mammal with the exception of the smaller more primitive species (as the lemurs, family Lemuridae)

mon·key·pox \ˈməŋ-kē-ˌpäks\ *n* : a rare virus disease esp. of central and western Africa that is caused by a poxvirus of the genus *Orthopoxvirus* (species *Monkeypox virus*), occurs chiefly in wild rodents and primates, and when transmitted to humans resembles smallpox but is milder

mono \ˈmä-(ˌ)nō\ *n* : INFECTIOUS MONONUCLEOSIS

mono- — see MON-

monoacetate — see RESORCINOL MONOACETATE

mono·am·ine \ˌmä-nō-ə-ˈmēn, -ˈa-ˌmēn\ *n* : an amine RNH_2 that has one organic substituent attached to the nitrogen atom; *esp* : one (as serotonin) that is functionally important in neural transmission

monoamine oxidase *n* : an enzyme that deaminates monoamines oxidatively and that functions in the nervous system by breaking down monoamine neurotransmitters oxidatively

monoamine oxidase inhibitor *n* : any of various antidepressant drugs which increase the concentration of monoamines in the brain by inhibiting the action of monoamine oxidase

mono·am·in·er·gic \ˌmä-nō-ˌa-mə-ˈnər-jik\ *adj* : liberating or involving monoamines (as serotonin or norepinephrine) in neural transmission ⟨~ neurons⟩ ⟨~ mechanisms⟩

mono·ar·tic·u·lar \ˌmä-nō-är-ˈti-kyə-lər\ *also* **mon·ar·tic·u·lar** \ˌmä-när-\ *adj* : affecting only one joint of the body ⟨~ arthritis⟩ — compare OLIGOARTICULAR, POLYARTICULAR

mono·bac·tam \ˌmä-nō-ˈbak-tam\ *n* : any of the class of beta-lactam antibiotics (as aztreonam) containing one ring in their molecular structure

mono·ben·zone \ˌmä-nō-ˈben-ˌzōn\ *n* : a drug $C_{13}H_{12}O_2$ applied topically as a melanin inhibitor in the treatment of hyperpigmentation

mono·blast \'mä-nō-ˌblast\ n : a motile cell of the spleen and bone marrow that gives rise to the monocyte of the circulating blood

mono·cho·ri·on·ic \ˌmä-nō-ˌkōr-ē-'ä-nik\ *also* **mono·cho·ri·al** \-'kō-rē-əl\ *adj, of twins* : sharing or developed with a common chorion

mono·chro·ma·cy \-'krō-mə-sē\ n, pl **-cies** : MONOCHROMATISM

mono·chro·mat \'mä-nō-krō-ˌmat, ˌmä-'\ n : a person who is completely color-blind

mono·chro·mat·ic \ˌmä-nō-krō-'ma-tik\ *adj* **1** : having or consisting of one color or hue **2** : consisting of radiation of a single wavelength or of a very small range of wavelengths **3** : of, relating to, or exhibiting monochromatism

mono·chro·ma·tism \-'krō-mə-ˌti-zəm\ n : complete color blindness in which all colors appear as shades of gray — called also *monochromacy*

mon·o·cle \'mä-ni-kəl\ n : an eyeglass for one eye

¹mono·clo·nal \ˌmä-nō-'klōn-ᵊl\ *adj* : produced by, being, or composed of cells derived from a single cell ⟨a ~ tumor⟩; *esp* : relating to or being an antibody derived from a single cell in large quantities for use against a specific antigen (as a cancer cell)

²monoclonal n : a monoclonal antibody

monoclonal gammopathy n : any of various disorders marked by proliferation of a single clone of antibody-producing lymphoid cells resulting in an abnormal increase of a monoclonal antibody in the blood serum and urine and that include both benign or asymptomatic conditions and neoplastic conditions (as multiple myeloma) — called also *plasma-cell dyscrasia*; see M PROTEIN 2

mono·crot·ic \-'krä-tik\ *adj, of the pulse* : having a simple beat and forming a smooth single-crested curve on a sphygmogram — compare DICROTIC 1

mon·oc·u·lar \mä-'nä-kyə-lər, mə-\ *adj* **1** : of, involving, or affecting a single eye ⟨a ~ cataract⟩ **2** : suitable for use with only one eye ⟨a ~ microscope⟩ — **mon·oc·u·lar·ly** *adv*

mono·cyte \'mä-nə-ˌsīt\ n : a large white blood cell with finely granulated chromatin dispersed throughout the nucleus that is formed in the bone marrow, enters the blood, and migrates into the connective tissue where it differentiates into a macrophage — **mono·cyt·ic** \ˌmä-nə-'si-tik\ *adj*

monocytic leukemia n : leukemia characterized by the presence of large numbers of monocytes in the circulating blood

mono·cy·to·sis \ˌmä-nō-sī-'tō-səs\ n, pl **-to·ses** \-ˌsēz\ : an abnormal increase in the number of monocytes in

the circulating blood — compare GRANULOCYTOSIS, LYMPHOCYTOSIS

mono·fac·to·ri·al \-fak-'tōr-ē-əl\ *adj* : MONOGENIC

mono·fil·a·ment \-'fi-lə-mənt\ n : a single untwisted filament (as of nylon) used to make surgical sutures

mo·nog·a·mist \mə-'nä-gə-mist\ n : one who practices or upholds monogamy

mo·nog·a·my \-mē\ n, pl **-mies** : the state or custom of being married to one person at a time or of having only one mate at a time — **mo·nog·a·mous** \mə-'nä-gə-məs\ *also* **mono·gam·ic** \ˌmä-nə-'ga-mik\ *adj*

mono·gas·tric \ˌmä-nō-'gas-trik\ *adj* : having a stomach with only a single compartment (as in humans)

mono·gen·ic \-'je-nik, -'jē-\ *adj* : of, relating to, or controlled by a single gene and esp. by either of an allelic pair — **mono·gen·i·cal·ly** *adv*

mono·graph \'mä-nə-ˌgraf\ n **1** : a learned detailed treatise covering a small area of a field of learning **2** : a description (as in the *U.S. Pharmacopeia*) of the name, chemical formula, and uniform method for determining the strength and purity of a drug — **monograph** *vb*

mono·iodo·ty·ro·sine \ˌmä-nō-ī-ˌō-də-'tī-rə-ˌsēn, -ī-ˌä-\ n : an iodine-containing tyrosine $C_9H_{10}INO_3$ that is produced in the thyroid gland and that combines with diiodotyrosine to form triiodothyronine

mono·lay·er \'mä-nō-ˌlā-ər\ n : a single continuous layer or film that is one cell or molecule in thickness

mono·ma·nia \ˌmä-nō-'mā-nē-ə, -nyə\ n : mental disorder esp. when limited in expression to one idea or area of thought — **mono·ma·ni·a·cal** \-mə-'nī-ə-kəl\ *adj*

mono·ma·ni·ac \-nē-ˌak\ n : an individual affected by monomania

mono·me·lic \-'mē-lik\ *adj* : relating to or affecting only one limb

mono·mer \'mä-nə-mər\ n : a chemical compound that can undergo polymerization — **mono·mer·ic** \ˌmä-nə-'mer-ik, -mō-\ *adj*

mono·neu·ri·tis \ˌmä-nō-nu̇-'rī-təs, -nyu̇-\ n, pl **-rit·i·des** \-'ri-tə-ˌdēz\ *or* **-ri·tis·es** : neuritis of a single nerve

mononeuritis mul·ti·plex \-'məl-ti-ˌpleks\ n : neuritis that affects several separate nerves — called also *mononeuropathy multiplex*

mono·neu·rop·a·thy \-nu̇-'rä-pə-thē, -nyu̇-\ n, pl **-thies** : a nerve disease affecting only a single nerve

¹mono·nu·cle·ar \ˌmä-nō-'nü-klē-ər, -'nyü-\ *adj* : having only one nucleus

²mononuclear n : a mononuclear cell; *esp* : MONOCYTE

mononuclear phagocyte system n : a system of cells comprising all free and fixed phagocytes and esp. macrophages together with their ancestral cells including monocytes and their precursors in the bone marrow — compare RETICULOENDOTHELIAL SYSTEM

mono·nu·cle·at·ed \-'nü-klē-₁ā-təd, -'nyü-\ *also* **mono·nu·cle·ate** \-klē-ət, -₁āt\ *adj* : MONONUCLEAR

mono·nu·cle·o·sis \-₁nü-klē-'ō-səs, -₁nyü-\ *n* : an abnormal increase of mononuclear white blood cells in the blood; *specif* : INFECTIOUS MONONUCLEOSIS

mono·nu·cle·o·tide \-'nü-klē-ə-₁tīd, -'nyü-\ *n* : a nucleotide that is derived from one molecule each of a nitrogenous base, a sugar, and a phosphoric acid

mono·pha·sic \-'fā-zik\ *adj* : having a single phase; *specif* : relating to or being a record of a nerve impulse that is negative or positive but not both ⟨a ∼ action potential⟩ — compare DIPHASIC b, POLYPHASIC 1 **2** : having a single period of activity followed by a period of rest in each 24-hour period

mono·phos·phate \-'fäs-₁fāt\ *n* : a phosphate containing a single phosphate group

mono·ple·gia \-'plē-jə, -jē-ə\ *n* : paralysis affecting a single limb, body part, or group of muscles — **mono·ple·gic** \-jik\ *adj*

mono·ploid \'mä-nō-₁plȯid\ *adj* : HAPLOID

mono·po·lar \₁mä-nō-'pō-lər\ *adj* : UNIPOLAR

mon·or·chid \mä-'nȯr-kəd\ *n* : an individual who has only one testis or only one descended into the scrotum — compare CRYPTORCHID — **monorchid** *adj*

mon·or·chid·ism \-kə-₁di-zəm\ *also* **mon·or·chism** \mä-'nȯr-₁ki-zəm\ *n* : the quality or state of being monorchid — compare CRYPTORCHIDISM

mono·sac·cha·ride \₁mä-nō-'sa-kə-₁rīd\ *n* : a sugar not decomposable to simpler sugars by hydrolysis — called also *simple sugar*

mono·so·di·um glu·ta·mate \₁mä-nō-'sō-dē-əm-'glü-tə-₁māt\ *n* : a crystalline salt $C_5H_8NO_4Na$ used to enhance the flavor of food and medicinally to reduce ammonia levels in blood and tissues in ammoniacal azotemia (as in hepatic insufficiency) — abbr. *MSG*; called also *sodium glutamate*; see CHINESE RESTAURANT SYNDROME

monosodium urate *n* : a salt of uric acid that precipitates out in cartilage as tophi in gout

mono·some \'mä-nō-₁sōm\ *n* **1** : a chromosome lacking a synaptic mate; *esp* : an unpaired X chromosome **2** : a single ribosome

mono·so·mic \₁mä-nə-'sō-mik\ *adj* : having one less than the diploid number of chromosomes — **mono·so·my** \'mä-nə-₁sō-mē\ *n*

mono·spe·cif·ic \₁mä-nō-spə-'si-fik\ *adj* : specific for a single antigen or receptor site on an antigen — **mono·spec·i·fic·i·ty** \₁spe-sə-'fi-sə-tē\ *n*

mono·sper·mic \-'spər-mik\ *adj* : involving or resulting from a single sperm cell ⟨∼ fertilization⟩

mono·sper·my \'mä-nə-₁spər-mē\ *n, pl* **-mies** : the entry of a single fertilizing sperm into an egg — compare POLYSPERMY

mon·os·tot·ic \₁mä-₁näs-'tä-tik\ *adj* : relating to or affecting a single bone

mono·symp·tom·at·ic \₁mä-nō-₁simp-tə-'ma-tik\ *adj* : exhibiting or manifested by a single principal symptom

mono·syn·ap·tic \-sə-'nap-tik\ *adj* : having or involving a single neural synapse — **mono·syn·ap·ti·cal·ly** *adv*

mono·ther·a·py \₁mä-nə-'ther-ə-pē\ *n, pl* **-pies** : the use of a single drug to treat a particular disorder or disease

mono·un·sat·u·rate \-₁ən-'sa-chə-rət\ *n* : a monounsaturated oil or fatty acid

mono·un·sat·u·rat·ed \-₁ən-'sa-chə-₁rā-təd\ *adj, of an oil, fat, or fatty acid* : containing one double or triple bond per molecule — compare POLYUNSATURATED

mono·va·lent \₁mä-nə-'vā-lənt\ *adj* **1** : having a chemical valence of one **2** : containing antibodies specific for or antigens of a single strain of a microorganism ⟨a ∼ vaccine⟩

mon·ovu·lar \(₁)mä-'nä-vyə-lər, -'nō-\ *adj* : MONOZYGOTIC ⟨∼ twins⟩

mon·ox·ide \mə-'näk-₁sīd\ *n* : an oxide containing one atom of oxygen per molecule — see CARBON MONOXIDE

mono·zy·got·ic \₁mä-nō-zī-'gä-tik\ *adj* : derived from a single egg ⟨∼ twins⟩ — **mono·zy·gos·i·ty** \-'gä-sə-tē\ *n* — **mono·zy·gote** \-'zī-₁gōt\ *n*

mono·zy·gous \₁mä-nō-'zī-gəs, (₁)mä-'nä-zə-gəs\ *adj* : MONOZYGOTIC

mons \'mänz\ *n, pl* **mon·tes** \'män-₁tēz\ : a body part or area raised above or demarcated from surrounding structures (as the papilla of mucosa through which the ureter enters the bladder)

mons pubis *n, pl* **montes pubis** : a rounded eminence of fatty tissue upon the pubic symphysis esp. of the human female — see MONS VENERIS

mon·ster \'män-stər\ *n* : an animal or plant of abnormal form or structure; *esp* : a fetus or offspring with a major developmental abnormality

mon·stros·i·ty \män-'strä-sə-tē\ *n, pl* **-ties 1 a** : a malformation of a plant or animal **b** : MONSTER **2** : the quality or state of deviating greatly from the natural form or character — **mon·strous** \'män-strəs\ *adj*

mons ve·ne·ris \-'ve-nə-rəs\ *n, pl* **montes veneris** : the mons pubis of a female

Mon·teg·gia fracture \män-'te-jə-\ or **Mon·teg·gia's fracture** \-'te-jəz-\ *n* : a fracture in the proximal part of the ulna with dislocation of the head of the radius

Monteggia, Giovanni Battista (1762–1815), Italian surgeon.

mon·te·lu·kast \ˌmän-tə-ˈlü-ˌkast\ n : a leukotriene antagonist used orally in the form of its sodium salt C₃₅H₃₅ClNNaO₃S to treat asthma or to relieve the symptoms of seasonal allergic rhinitis — see SINGULAIR

Mon·te·zu·ma's revenge \ˌmän-tə-ˈzü-məz-\ n : traveler's diarrhea esp. when contracted in Mexico

Montezuma II (1466–1520), Aztec emperor of Mexico.

Mont·gom·ery's gland \(ˌ)mənt-ˈgəm-rēz-, mänt-ˈgäm-\ n : an apocrine gland in the areola of the mammary gland

Montgomery, William Fetherston (1797–1859), British obstetrician.

month·lies \ˈmənth-lēz\ n pl : a menstrual period

mon·tic·u·lus \män-ˈtik-yə-ləs\ n : the median dorsal ridge of the cerebellum formed by the vermis

mood \ˈmüd\ n : a conscious state of mind or predominant emotion : affective state : FEELING 3

mood disorder n : any of several psychological disorders characterized by abnormalities of emotional state and including esp. major depressive disorder, dysthymia, and bipolar disorder — called also *affective disorder*

moon \ˈmün\ n : LUNULA

moon blindness n : a recurrent inflammation of the eye of the horse — called also *periodic ophthalmia*

moon facies n : the full rounded facies characteristic of hyperadrenocorticism — called also *moon face*

Moon's molar or **Moon molar** n : a first molar tooth which has become dome-shaped due to malformation by congenital syphilis; *also* : MULBERRY MOLAR

Moon, Henry (1845–1892), British surgeon.

MOPP \ˌem-(ˌ)ō-(ˌ)pē-ˈpē\ n : a drug regimen that includes mechlorethamine, vincristine, procarbazine, and prednisone and is used in the treatment of some forms of cancer (as Hodgkin's disease)

Mor·ax–Ax·en·feld bacillus \ˈmòr-äks-ˈäk-sən-ˌfeld-\ n : a rod-shaped bacterium of the genus *Moraxella* (M. lacunata) that causes Morax-Axenfeld conjunctivitis

Morax, Victor (1866–1935), French ophthalmologist.

Axenfeld, Karl Theodor Paul Polykarpos (1867–1930), German ophthalmologist.

Morax–Axenfeld conjunctivitis n : a chronic conjunctivitis caused by a rod-shaped bacterium of the genus *Moraxella* (M. lacunata) and now occurring rarely but formerly more prevalent in persons living under poor hygienic conditions

Mor·ax·el·la \ˌmòr-ak-ˈse-lə\ n : a genus of short rod-shaped gram-negative bacteria that is placed in either of two families (Moraxellaceae or Neisseriaceae) and includes the causative agent (M. lacunata) of Morax-Axenfeld conjunctivitis

mor·bid \ˈmòr-bəd\ adj 1 a : of, relating to, or characteristic of disease b : affected with or induced by disease ⟨a ∼ condition⟩ c : productive of disease ⟨∼ substances⟩ 2 : abnormally susceptible to or characterized by gloomy or unwholesome feelings

mor·bid·i·ty \mòr-ˈbi-də-tē\ n, pl -ties 1 : a diseased state or symptom 2 : the incidence of disease : the rate of sickness (as in a specified community or group) — compare MORTALITY 2

mor·bil·li \mòr-ˈbi-ˌlī\ n pl : MEASLES 1

mor·bil·li·form \mòr-ˈbi-lə-ˌfòrm\ adj : resembling the eruption of measles ⟨a ∼ pruritic rash⟩

mor·bil·li·vi·rus \-ˌvī-rəs\ n 1 cap : a genus of paramyxoviruses that includes the causative agents of canine distemper, measles, and rinderpest 2 : any virus of the genus *Morbillivirus*

mor·bus \ˈmòr-bəs\ n, pl mor·bi \-ˌbī\ : DISEASE — see CHOLERA MORBUS

mor·cel·la·tion \ˌmòr-sə-ˈlā-shən\ n : division and removal in small pieces (as of a tumor)

mor·gan \ˈmòr-gən\ n : a unit of inferred distance between genes on a chromosome that is used in constructing genetic maps and is equal to the distance for which the frequency of crossing-over between specific pairs of genes is 100 percent

Morgan, Thomas Hunt (1866–1945), American geneticist.

morgue \ˈmòrg\ n : a place where the bodies of persons found dead are kept until identified and claimed by relatives or are released for burial

mor·i·bund \ˈmòr-ə-(ˌ)bənd, ˈmär-\ adj : being in the state of dying : approaching death

mo·ric·i·zine \mə-ˈri-sə-ˌzēn\ n : an antiarrhythmic drug used in the form of its hydrochloride C₂₂H₂₅N₃O₄S·HCl esp. in the treatment of life-threatening ventricular arrhythmias

morning–after pill n : an oral drug typically containing high doses of estrogen taken up to usu. three days after unprotected sexual intercourse that interferes with pregnancy by inhibiting ovulation or by blocking implantation of a fertilized egg in the human uterus

morning breath n : halitosis upon awakening from sleep that is caused by the buildup of bacteria in the mouth due to decreased saliva production

morning sickness n : nausea and vomiting that occurs typically in the morning esp. during the earlier months of pregnancy

mo·ron \ˈmòr-ˌän\ n, usu offensive : a person affected with mild mental retardation

Moro reflex \\'mȯr-ō-\ *n* : a reflex reaction of infants upon being startled (as by a loud noise or a bright light) that is characterized by extension of the arms and legs away from the body and to the side and then by drawing them together as if in an embrace

Moro, Ernst (1874–1951), German pediatrician.

Moro test *n* : a diagnostic skin test formerly used to detect infection or past infection by the tubercle bacillus and involving the rubbing of an ointment containing tuberculin directly on the skin with the appearance of reddish papules after one or two days indicating a positive result

morph- *or* **morpho-** *comb form* : form : shape : structure : type ⟨*morphology*⟩

-morph \\,mȯrf\ *n comb form* : one having (such) a form ⟨ecto*morph*⟩

mor·phea \mȯr-'fē-ə\ *n, pl* **mor·phe·ae** \-'fē-ē\ : localized scleroderma

mor·phia \\'mȯr-fē-ə\ *n* : MORPHINE

-mor·phic \\'mȯr-fik\ *adj comb form* : having (such) a form ⟨endo*morphic*⟩

mor·phine \\'mȯr-,fēn\ *n* : a bitter crystalline addictive narcotic base $C_{17}H_{19}NO_3$ that is the principal alkaloid of opium and is used in the form of its hydrated sulfate $(C_{17}H_{19}NO_3)_2$·H_2SO_4·$5H_2O$ or hydrated hydrochloride $C_{17}H_{19}NO_3$·HCl·$3H_2O$ as an analgesic and sedative

mor·phin·ism \\'mȯr-,fē-,ni-zəm, -fə-\ *n* : a disordered condition of health produced by habitual use of morphine

mor·phi·no·mi·met·ic \\,mȯr-fē-nə-mə-'me-tik, -fə-, -mī-\ *adj* : resembling opiates in their affinity for opiate receptors in the brain

-mor·phism \\'mȯr-,fi-zəm\ *n comb form* : quality or state of having (such) a form ⟨poly*morphism*⟩

mor·pho·dif·fer·en·ti·a·tion \\,mȯr-fō-,di-fə-,ren-chē-'ā-shən\ *n* : structure or organ differentiation (as in tooth development)

mor·phoea *Brit var of* MORPHEA

mor·pho·gen \\'mȯr-fə-jən, -,jen\ *n* : a diffusible chemical substance that exerts control over morphogenesis esp. by forming a gradient in concentration

mor·pho·gen·e·sis \\,mȯr-fə-'je-nə-səs\ *n, pl* **-e·ses** \-,sēz\ : the formation and differentiation of tissues and organs — compare ORGANOGENESIS

mor·pho·ge·net·ic \-jə-'ne-tik\ *adj* : relating to or concerned with the development of normal organic form — **mor·pho·ge·net·i·cal·ly** *adv*

mor·pho·gen·ic \-'je-nik\ *adj* : MORPHOGENETIC

mor·pho·log·i·cal \\,mȯr-fə-'lä-ji-kəl\ *also* **mor·pho·log·ic** \-'lä-jik\ *adj* : of, relating to, or concerned with form or structure — **mor·pho·log·i·cal·ly** *adv*

mor·phol·o·gy \mȯr-'fä-lə-jē\ *n, pl* **-gies 1** : a branch of biology that deals with the form and structure of animals and plants esp. with respect to the forms, relations, metamorphoses, and phylogenetic development of organs apart from their functions — see ANATOMY 1; compare PHYSIOLOGY 1 **2** : the form and structure of an organism or any of its parts — **mor·phol·o·gist** \-jist\ *n*

-mor·phous \\'mȯr-fəs\ *adj comb form* : having (such) a form ⟨poly*morphous*⟩

-mor·phy \\,mȯr-fē\ *n comb form, pl* **-mor·phies** : quality or state of having (such) a form ⟨meso*morphy*⟩

Mor·quio's disease \\'mȯr-kē-,ōz-\ *n* : a mucopolysaccharidosis that is inherited as an autosomal recessive trait and is characterized by excretion of keratan sulfate in the urine, dwarfism, a short neck, protruding sternum, kyphosis, scoliosis, a flat nose, prominent upper jaw, and a waddling gait

Morquio, Luis (1867–1935), Uruguayan physician.

mor·rhu·ate sodium \\'mȯr-ə-,wāt-\ *n* : a granular mixture of the salts of fatty acids obtained from cod-liver oil that is administered in solution intravenously as a sclerosing agent esp. in the treatment of varicose veins

mor·tal \\'mȯrt-ᵊl\ *adj* **1** : having caused or being about to cause death : FATAL ⟨a ~ injury⟩ **2** : of, relating to, or connected with death

mor·tal·i·ty \mȯr-'ta-lə-tē\ *n, pl* **-ties 1** : the quality or state of being mortal **2 a** : the number of deaths in a given time or place **b** : the proportion of deaths to population : DEATH RATE — called also *mortality rate*; compare FERTILITY 2, MORBIDITY 2

mor·tar \\'mȯr-tər\ *n* : a strong vessel in which material is pounded or rubbed with a pestle

mor·ti·cian \mȯr-'ti-shən\ *n* : UNDERTAKER

mor·ti·fi·ca·tion \\,mȯr-tə-fə-'kā-shən\ *n* : local death of tissue in the animal body : NECROSIS, GANGRENE

mortis — see ALGOR MORTIS, RIGOR MORTIS

Mor·ton's neuroma \\,mȯr-tᵊnz-\ *n* : a neuroma formed in conjunction with Morton's toe

Morton, Thomas George (1835–1903), American surgeon.

Morton's toe *n* : metatarsalgia that is caused by compression of a branch of the plantar nerve between the heads of the metatarsal bones — called also *Morton's disease, Morton's foot*

mor·tu·ary \\'mȯr-chə-,wer-ē\ *n, pl* **-ar·ies** : a place in which dead bodies are kept and prepared for burial or cremation

mor·u·la \\'mȯr-yü-lə, 'mär-\ *n, pl* **-lae** \-,lē, -,lī\ : a globular solid mass of blastomeres formed by cleavage of a zygote that typically precedes the blastula — compare GASTRULA —

mor·u·la·tion \ˌmȯr-yu̇-'lā-shən, ˌmär-\ n

¹mo·sa·ic \mō-'zā-ik\ n : an organism or one of its parts composed of cells of more than one genotype : CHIMERA

²mosaic adj **1** : exhibiting mosaicism **2** : DETERMINATE — **mo·sa·i·cal·ly** adv

mo·sa·icism \mō-'zā-ə-ˌsi-zəm\ n : the condition of possessing cells of two or more different genetic constitutions

mos·qui·to \mə-'skē-tō\ n, pl **-toes** also **-tos** : any of a family (Culicidae) of dipteran flies with females that have a set of needlelike organs in the proboscis adapted to puncture the skin of animals and to suck their blood and that are in some cases vectors of serious diseases — see AEDES, ANOPHELES, CULEX

mosquito forceps n : a very small surgical forceps — called also *mosquito clamp*

mossy fiber n : any of the complexly branched axons that innervate the granule cells of the cerebellar cortex

mother cell n : a cell that gives rise to other cells usu. of a different sort

mo·tile \'mōt-ᵊl, 'mō-ˌtīl\ adj : exhibiting or capable of movement

mo·til·in \mō-'ti-lən\ n : a polypeptide hormone secreted by the small intestine that increases gastrointestinal motility and stimulates the production of pepsin

mo·til·i·ty \mō-'ti-lə-tē\ n, pl **-ties** : the quality or state of being motile : CONTRACTILITY ⟨gastrointestinal ∼⟩

mo·tion \'mō-shən\ n **1** : an act, process, or instance of changing place : MOVEMENT **2 a** : an evacuation of the bowels **b** : the matter evacuated — often used in pl. ⟨blood in the ∼s⟩

motion sickness n : sickness induced by motion (as in travel by air, car, or ship) and characterized by nausea

mo·ti·vate \'mō-tə-ˌvāt\ vb **-vat·ed; -vat·ing** : to provide with a motive or serve as a motive for — **mo·ti·va·tion** \ˌmō-tə-'vā-shən\ n — **mo·ti·va·tion·al** \-shnəl, -shən-ᵊl\ adj — **mo·ti·va·tion·al·ly** adv

mo·tive \'mō-tiv\ n : something (as a need or desire) that causes a person to act

moto- comb form : motion : motor ⟨*moto*neuron⟩

mo·to·neu·ron \ˌmō-tō-'nü-ˌrän, -'nyü-\ n : MOTOR NEURON — **mo·to·neu·ro·nal** \-'nür-ən-ᵊl, -'nyür-; -ˌnü-'rōn-, -nyü-\ adj

mo·tor \'mō-tər\ adj **1** : causing or imparting motion **2** : of, relating to, or being a motor neuron or a nerve containing motor neurons ⟨∼ fibers⟩ **3** : of, relating to, concerned with, or involving muscular movement

motor aphasia n : the inability to speak or to organize the muscular movements of speech — called also *Broca's aphasia*

motor area n : any of various areas of cerebral cortex believed to be associated with the initiation, coordination, and transmission of motor impulses to lower centers; *specif* : a region immediately anterior to the central sulcus having an unusually thick zone of cortical gray matter and communicating with lower centers chiefly through the corticospinal tracts — see PRECENTRAL GYRUS

motor center n : a nervous center that controls or modifies (as by inhibiting or reinforcing) a motor impulse

motor cortex n : the cortex of a motor area; *also* : the motor areas as a functional whole

motor end plate n : the terminal arborization of a motor axon on a muscle fiber

mo·tor·ic \mō-'tȯr-ik, -'tär-\ adj : MOTOR 3 — **mo·tor·i·cal·ly** adv

motor neuron n : a neuron that passes from the central nervous system or a ganglion toward or to a muscle and conducts an impulse that causes movement — called also *motoneuron*; compare INTERNEURON, SENSORY NEURON

motor paralysis n : paralysis of the voluntary muscles

motor protein n : a protein (as dynein, kinesin, or myosin) that moves itself along a filament or polymeric molecule using energy generated by the hydrolysis of ATP

motor root n : a nerve root containing only motor fibers; *specif* : VENTRAL ROOT — compare SENSORY ROOT

motor unit n : a motor neuron together with the muscle fibers on which it acts

Mo·trin \'mō-trən\ trademark — used for a preparation of ibuprofen

mottled enamel n : spotted tooth enamel typically caused by drinking water containing excessive fluorides during the time teeth are calcifying

mou·lage \mü-'läzh\ n : a mold of a lesion or defect used as a guide in applying medical treatment (as in radiotherapy) or in performing reconstructive surgery esp. on the face

mould, mould·ing, mouldy chiefly Brit var of MOLD, MOLDING, MOLDY

moult chiefly Brit var of MOLT

mount \'maunt\ n **1** : a glass slide with its accessories on which objects are placed for examination with a microscope **2** : a specimen mounted on a slide for microscopic examination — **mount** vb

mountain fever n : any of various febrile diseases occurring in mountainous regions

mountain sickness n : altitude sickness experienced esp. above 10,000 feet (about 3000 meters) and caused by insufficient oxygen in the air

mouse \'maus\ n, pl **mice** \'mīs\ **1** : any of numerous small rodents (as of the genus *Mus*) with pointed snout, rather small ears, elongated body, and slender hairless or sparsely haired tail **2** : a dark-colored swelling caused by a blow; *specif* : BLACK EYE

mouse·pox \'maůs-ˌpäks\ *n* : a highly contagious disease of mice that is caused by a poxvirus of the genus *Orthopoxvirus* (species *Ectromelia virus*) — called also *ectromelia*

mouth \'maůth\ *n, pl* **mouths** \'maůthz\ : the natural opening through which food passes into the animal body and which in vertebrates is typically bounded externally by the lips and internally by the pharynx and encloses the tongue, gums, and teeth

mouth breather *n* : a person who habitually inhales and exhales through the mouth rather than through the nose

mouth–to–mouth *adj* : of, relating to, or being a method of artificial respiration in which the rescuer's mouth is placed tightly over the victim's mouth in order to force air into the victim's lungs by blowing forcefully enough every few seconds to inflate them ⟨~ resuscitation⟩

mouth·wash \'maůth-ˌwȯsh, -ˌwäsh\ *n* : a liquid preparation (as an antiseptic solution) for cleansing the mouth and teeth — called also *collutorium*

move \'müv\ *vb* **moved; mov·ing** **1** : to go or pass from one place to another **2** *of the bowels* : to eject fecal matter : EVACUATE

move·ment \'müv-mənt\ *n* **1** : the act or process of moving **2 a** : an act of voiding the bowels **b** : matter expelled from the bowels at one passage : STOOL

moxa \'mäk-sə\ *n* : a soft woolly mass prepared from the ground young leaves of an aromatic Eurasian plant (genus *Artemesia*, esp. *A. vulgaris*) that is used in traditional Chinese and Japanese medicine typically in the form of sticks or cones which are ignited and placed on or close to the skin or used to heat acupuncture needles

mox·i·bus·tion \ˌmäk-si-'bəs-chən\ *n* : the therapeutic use of moxa

moxa·lac·tam \ˌmäk-sə-'lak-ˌtam\ *n* : a cephalosporin antibiotic administered parenterally in the form of its disodium salt $C_{20}H_{18}N_6Na_2O_9S$

MPC *abbr* maximum permissible concentration

MPD *abbr* multiple personality disorder

MPH *abbr* master of public health

M phase \'em-ˌfāz\ *n* : the period in the cell cycle during which cell division takes place — compare G_1 PHASE, G_2 PHASE, S PHASE

M protein *n* **1** : an antigenic protein of Group A streptococci that is found on the cell wall extending into the surrounding capsule and confers streptococcal virulence by protecting the cell from phagocytotic action — called

also *M substance* **2** : a monoclonal antibody that is produced by plasma cells abnormally proliferating from a single clone and that is characteristic of monoclonal gammopathy

MPTP \ˌem-ˌpē-ˌtē-'pē\ *n* [1-methyl-4-phenyl-1,2,3,6-*t*etrahydropyridine] : a neurotoxin $C_{12}H_{15}N$ that destroys dopamine-producing neurons of the substantia nigra and causes symptoms (as tremors and rigidity) similar to those of Parkinson's disease

mR *abbr* milliroentgen

MR *abbr* magnetic resonance

MRA *abbr* magnetic resonance angiography

mrad *abbr* milliradian

Mrad *abbr* megarad

MR angiography \ˌem-ˌär-\ *n* : MAGNETIC RESONANCE ANGIOGRAPHY

mrem *abbr* millirem

MRI \ˌem-ˌär-'ī\ *n* : MAGNETIC RESONANCE IMAGING; *also* : the procedure in which magnetic resonance imaging is used

MRKH syndrome \ˌem-ˌär-ˌkā-'āch-\ *n* : MAYER-ROKITANSKY-KÜSTER-HAUSER SYNDROME

mRNA \ˌem-(ˌ)är-(ˌ)en-'ā\ *n* : MESSENGER RNA

MRS *abbr* magnetic resonance spectroscopy

MRSA \ˌem-ˌär-ˌes-'ā\ *n* [*m*ethicillin-*r*esistant *S*taphylococcus *a*ureus] : any of several bacterial strains of the genus *Staphylococcus* (*S. aureus*) that are resistant to beta-lactam antibiotics and that are typically benign colonizers of the skin and mucous membranes but may cause severe infections esp. in immunocompromised individuals

MS *abbr* multiple sclerosis

MSA *abbr* multiple system atrophy

MSG *abbr* monosodium glutamate

MSH *abbr* melanocyte-stimulating hormone

MSN *abbr* master of science in nursing

M substance \'em-ˌ\ *n* : M PROTEIN 1

MSW *abbr* master of social work

Mt *symbol* meitnerium

MT *abbr* medical technologist

mtDNA \ˌem-ˌtē-ˌdē-ˌen-'ā\ *n* : MITOCHONDRIAL DNA

mu \'myü, 'mü\ *n, pl* mu : MICRON

muc- *or* **muci-** *or* **muco-** *comb form* **1** : mucus ⟨*muc*in⟩ ⟨*muco*protein⟩ **2** : mucous and ⟨*muco*purulent⟩

mu·cate \'myü-ˌkāt\ *n* : a salt of a crystalline acid $C_6H_{10}O_8$ esp. when formed by combination with a drug that is an organic base and used as a vehicle for administration of the drug

mu·ci·lage \'myü-sə-lij\ *n* **1** : a gelatinous substance of various plants (as legumes or seaweeds) that contains protein and polysaccharides and is similar to plant gums **2** : an aqueous usu. viscid solution (as of a gum) used in pharmacy as an excipient and in medicine as a demulcent — **mu·ci·lag·i·nous** \ˌmyü-sə-'la-jə-nəs\ *adj*

mu·cil·loid \'myü-sə-ˌlóid\ *n* : a mucilaginous substance

mu·cin \'myüs-ᵊn\ *n* : any of a group of mucoproteins that are found in various human and animal secretions and tissues (as in saliva, the lining of the stomach, and the skin) and that are white or yellowish powders when dry and viscid when moist

mu·cin·o·gen \myü-'si-nə-jən, -ˌjen\ *n* : any of various substances which undergo conversion into mucins

mu·ci·nous \'myüs-ᵊn-əs\ *adj* : of, relating to, resembling, or containing mucin 〈~ fluid〉 〈~ carcinoma〉

muco- — see MUC-

mu·co·buc·cal fold \ˌmyü-kō-'bə-kəl-\ *n* : the fold formed by the oral mucosa where it passes from the mandible or maxilla to the cheek

mu·co·cele \'myü-kə-ˌsēl\ *n* : a swelling like a sac that is due to distension of a hollow organ or cavity with mucus 〈a ~ of the appendix〉; *specif* : a dilated lacrimal sac

mu·co·cil·i·ary \ˌmyü-kō-'si-lē-ˌer-ē\ *adj* : of, relating to, or involving cilia of the mucous membranes of the respiratory system

mu·co·cu·ta·ne·ous \ˌmyü-kō-kyù-'tā-nē-əs\ *adj* : made up of or involving both typical skin and mucous membrane 〈~ candidiasis〉

mucocutaneous lymph node disease *n* : KAWASAKI DISEASE

mucocutaneous lymph node syndrome *n* : KAWASAKI DISEASE

mu·co·epi·der·moid \ˌmyü-kō-ˌe-pə-'dər-ˌmoid\ *adj* : of, relating to, or consisting of both mucous and squamous epithelial cells; *esp* : being a tumor of the salivary glands made up of mucous and epithelial elements 〈~ carcinoma〉

mu·co·gin·gi·val \-ˈjin-jə-vəl\ *adj* : of, relating to, or being the junction between the oral mucosa and the gingiva 〈the ~ line〉

¹**mu·coid** \'myü-ˌkóid\ *adj* : resembling mucus

²**mucoid** *n* : MUCOPROTEIN

mu·co·lip·i·do·sis \ˌmyü-kō-ˌli-pə-'dō-səs\ *n, pl* **-do·ses** \-ˌsēz\ : any of several metabolic disorders that are marked by the accumulation of glycosaminoglycans and lipids in tissues and by lysosomal enzymes which are produced in deficient amounts or which fail to be incorporated into lysosomes, that are inherited as autosomal recessive traits, and that have characteristics (as mental retardation) resembling Hurler's syndrome

mu·co·lyt·ic \ˌmyü-kə-'li-tik\ *adj* : hydrolyzing glycosaminoglycans : tending to break down or lower the viscosity of mucin-containing body secretions or components

Mu·co·myst \'myü-kə-ˌmist\ *trademark* — used for a preparation of acetylcysteine

mu·co·pep·tide \ˌmyü-kō-'pep-ˌtīd\ *n* : PEPTIDOGLYCAN

mu·co·peri·os·te·um \-ˌper-ē-'äs-tē-əm\ *n* : a periosteum backed with mucous membrane (as that of the palatine surface of the mouth) — **mu·co·peri·os·te·al** \-'äs-tē-əl\ *adj*

mu·co·poly·sac·cha·ride \ˌmyü-kō-ˌpä-li-'sa-kə-ˌrīd\ *n* : GLYCOSAMINOGLYCAN

mu·co·poly·sac·cha·ri·do·sis \-ˌsa-kə-rī-'dō-səs\ *n, pl* **-do·ses** \-ˌsēz\ : any of a group of inherited disorders (as Hunter's syndrome and Hurler's syndrome) of glycosaminoglycan metabolism that are characterized by the accumulation of glycosaminoglycans in the tissues and their excretion in the urine — called also *gargoylism, lipochondrodystrophy*

mu·co·pro·tein \ˌmyü-kə-'prō-ˌtēn\ *n* : any of a group of various complex conjugated proteins (as mucins) that contain glycosaminoglycans (as chondroitin sulfate) combined with amino acid units or polypeptides and that occur in body fluids and tissues — called also *mucoid;* compare GLYCOPROTEIN

mu·co·pu·ru·lent \-'pyùr-yə-lənt\ *adj* : containing both mucus and pus 〈a ~ discharge〉

mu·co·pus \'myü-kō-ˌpəs\ *n* : mucus mixed with pus

mu·cor \'myü-ˌkór\ *n* **1** *cap* : a genus (family Mucoraceae) of molds including several (as *M. corymbifer*) causing infections in humans and animals **2** : any mold of the genus *Mucor*

mu·cor·my·co·sis \ˌmyü-kər-mī-'kō-səs\ *n, pl* **-co·ses** \-ˌsēz\ : mycosis caused by fungi of the genus *Mucor* usu. primarily involving the lungs and invading other tissues by means of metastatic lesions — **mu·cor·my·cot·ic** \-'kä-tik\ *adj*

mu·co·sa \myü-'kō-zə\ *n, pl* **-sae** \-(ˌ)zē, -ˌzī\ *or* **-sas** : MUCOUS MEMBRANE — **mu·co·sal** \-zəl\ *adj*

mucosae — see MUSCULARIS MUCOSAE

mucosal disease *n* : a usu. fatal form of bovine viral diarrhea marked esp. by high fever, diarrhea, and ulcers of the digestive tract mucosa; *broadly* : BOVINE VIRAL DIARRHEA

mu·co·si·tis \ˌmyü-kə-'sī-təs\ *n* : inflammation of a mucous membrane

mu·co·stat·ic \ˌmyü-kə-'sta-tik\ *adj* **1** : of, relating to, or representing the mucosal tissues of the jaws as they are in a state of rest **2** : stopping the secretion of mucus

mu·cous \'myü-kəs\ *adj* **1** : covered with or as if with mucus 〈a ~ surface〉 **2** : of, relating to, or resembling mucus 〈a ~ secretion〉 **3** : secreting or containing mucus 〈~ glands〉

mucous cell *n* : a cell that secretes mucus

mucous colitis *n* : IRRITABLE BOWEL SYNDROME; *esp* : irritable bowel syndrome characterized by the passage of unusually large amounts of mucus

mucous membrane *n* : a membrane rich in mucous glands; *specif* : one that lines body passages and cavities which communicate directly or indirectly with the exterior (as the digestive, respiratory, and genitourinary tracts), that functions in protection, support, nutrient absorption, and secretion of mucus, enzymes, and salts, and that consists of a deep vascular connective-tissue stroma and a superficial epithelium — compare SEROUS MEMBRANE

mu·co·vis·ci·do·sis \ˌmyü-kō-ˌvi-sə-ˈdō-səs\ *n, pl* **-do·ses** \-ˌsēz\ : CYSTIC FIBROSIS

mu·cus \ˈmyü-kəs\ *n* : a viscid slippery secretion that is usu. rich in mucins and is produced by mucous membranes which it moistens and protects

mud bath *n* : an immersion of the body or a part of it in mud (as for the alleviation of rheumatism or gout)

mud fever *n* **1** : a chapped inflamed condition of the skin of the legs and belly of a horse due to irritation from mud or drying resulting from washing off mud spatters and closely related or identical in nature to grease heel **2** : a mild leptospirosis that occurs chiefly in European agricultural and other workers in wet soil, is caused by infection with a spirochete of the genus *Leptospira* (*L. interrogans*) present in native field mice, and is marked by fever and headache without accompanying jaundice

Muel·le·ri·us \myü-ˈlir-ē-əs\ *n* : a genus of lungworms (family Metastrongylidae) including one (*M. capillaris*) that infects the lungs of sheep and goats and has larval stages in various snails and slugs

Mül·ler \ˈmue-ler\, **Fritz (Johann Friedrich Theodor) (1822–1897),** German zoologist.

MUFA \ˈməfə, ˈm(y)ü-\ *n* : a monounsaturated fatty acid

mulberry molar *n* : a first molar tooth whose occlusal surface is pitted due to congenital syphilis with nodules replacing the cusps — see MOON'S MOLAR

mules·ing \ˈmyül-ziŋ\ *n* : the use of Mules operation to reduce the occurrence of blowfly strike

Mules operation \ˈmyülz-\ *n* : removal of excess loose skin from either side of the crutch of a sheep to reduce the incidence of blowfly strike

Mules, J. H. W., Australian sheep rancher.

Mül·ler cell \ˈmyü-lər-, ˈmi-, ˈmə-\ *also* **Mül·ler's cell** \-lərz-\ *n* : FIBER OF MÜLLER

Mül·ler \ˈmue-lər, ˈmyü-\, **Heinrich (1820–1864),** German anatomist.

mül·le·ri·an agenesis \myü-ˈlir-ē-ən-, mi-, mə-\ *n* : MAYER-ROKITANSKY-KÜSTER-HAUSER SYNDROME

Müllerian duct *also* **Muel·le·ri·an duct** *n* : either of a pair of ducts parallel to the Wolffian ducts and giving rise in the female to the fallopian tubes, uterus, cervix, and upper portion of the vagina — called also *paramesonephric duct*

Mül·ler \ˈmue-lər, ˈmyü-\, **Johannes Peter (1801–1858),** German physiologist and anatomist.

Müllerian inhibiting substance *n* : a glycoprotein hormone produced by the Sertoli cells of the male during fetal development that causes regression and atrophy of the Müllerian ducts

Müllerian tubercle *n* : an elevation on the wall of the embryonic urogenital sinus where the Müllerian ducts enter

¹mult·an·gu·lar \ˌməl-ˈtaŋ-gyə-lər\ *adj* : having many angles ⟨a ~ bone⟩

²multangular *n* : a multangular bone — see TRAPEZIUM, TRAPEZOID

multi- *comb form* **1 a** : many : multiple : much ⟨*multi*neuronal⟩ **b** : consisting of, containing, or having more than two ⟨*multi*nucleate⟩ **c** : more than one ⟨*multi*parous⟩ **2** : affecting many parts ⟨*multi*glandular⟩

mul·ti·an·gu·lar \ˌməl-tē-ˈaŋ-gyə-lər, ˌməl-ˌtī-\ *adj* : MULTANGULAR

mul·ti·cel·lu·lar \-ˈsel-yə-lər\ *adj* : having or consisting of many cells — **mul·ti·cel·lu·lar·i·ty** \-ˌsel-yə-ˈlar-ə-tē\ *n*

mul·ti·cen·ter \-ˈsen-tər\ *adj* : involving more than one medical or research institution ⟨a ~ study⟩

mul·ti·cen·tric \-ˈsen-trik\ *adj* : having multiple centers of origin ⟨a ~ tumor⟩

mul·ti·ceps \ˈməl-tə-ˌseps\ *n* **1** *cap* : a genus of taeniid tapeworms that have a coenurus larva parasitic in ruminants, rodents, and rarely humans and that include the parasite of gid (*M. multiceps*) and other worms typically parasitic on carnivores **2** : COENURUS

mul·ti·clo·nal \ˌməl-tē-ˈklō-nəl, -ˌtī-\ *adj* : POLYCLONAL

mul·ti·cus·pid \-ˈkəs-pəd\ *adj* : having several cusps ⟨a ~ tooth⟩

mul·ti·cys·tic \-ˈsis-tik\ *adj* : POLYCYSTIC

mul·ti·dose \ˈməl-tē-ˌdōs, -ˌtī-\ *adj* : utilizing or containing more than one dose

mul·ti·drug \-ˌdrəg\ *adj* : utilizing or relating to more than one drug ⟨~ therapy⟩

mul·ti·en·zyme \ˌməl-tē-ˈen-ˌzīm, -ˌtī-\ *adj* : composed of or involving two or more enzymes that function in a biosynthetic pathway ⟨a ~ complex⟩

mul·ti·fac·to·ri·al \-fak-ˈtōr-ē-əl\ *adj* **1** : having characters or a mode of inheritance dependent on a number of genes at different loci **2** *or* **mul·ti·fac·tor** \-ˈfak-tər\ : having, involving, or produced by a variety of elements or causes ⟨a ∼ study⟩ ⟨a ∼ etiology⟩ — **mul·ti·fac·to·ri·al·ly** adv

mul·tif·i·dus \ˌməl-ˈti-fə-dəs\ n, pl **-di** \-ˌdī\ : a muscle of the fifth and deepest layer of the back filling up the groove on each side of the spinous processes of the vertebrae from the sacrum to the skull and consisting of many fasciculi that pass upward and inward to the spinous processes and help to erect and rotate the spine

mul·ti·fo·cal \ˌməl-tē-ˈfō-kəl\ adj **1** : having more than one focal length ⟨∼ lenses⟩ **2** : arising from or occurring in more than one focus or location ⟨∼ seizures⟩

multifocal leukoencephalopathy — see PROGRESSIVE MULTIFOCAL LEUKOENCEPHALOPATHY

mul·ti·form \ˈməl-ti-ˌfȯrm\ adj : having or occurring in many forms

multiforme — see ERYTHEMA MULTIFORME, GLIOBLASTOMA MULTIFORME

mul·ti·gene \ˌməl-tē-ˈjēn, -ˌtī-\ adj : relating to or determined by a group of genes which were originally copies of the same gene but evolved by mutation to become different from each other

mul·ti·gen·ic \-ˈje-nik, -ˈjē-\ adj : MULTIFACTORIAL 1

mul·ti·glan·du·lar \-ˈglan-jə-lər\ adj : POLYGLANDULAR

mul·ti·grav·i·da \-ˈgra-vi-də\ n, pl **-dae** \-ˌdē\ also **-das** : a woman who has been pregnant more than once — compare MULTIPARA

mul·ti·han·di·capped \ˌməl-tē-ˈhan-di-ˌkapt, -ˌtī-\ adj, sometimes offensive : affected by more than one mental or physical disability

mul·ti·hos·pi·tal \-ˈhäs-ˌpit-ᵊl\ adj : involving or affiliated with more than one hospital

multi–infarct dementia n : irreversible vascular dementia of gradual progression that results from a series of small strokes in which cerebral infarction occurs

mul·ti·lobed \-ˈlōbd\ adj : having two or more lobes

mul·ti·loc·u·lar \-ˈlä-kyə-lər\ adj : having or divided into many small chambers or vesicles ⟨a ∼ cyst⟩

mul·ti·mam·mate rat \-ˈma-ˌmāt-\ n : any of several African rodents (genus *Mastomys*) that are vectors of disease (as Lassa fever) and are used in medical research — called also *multimammate mouse*

mul·ti·mo·dal \-ˈmōd-ᵊl\ adj : relating to, having, or utilizing more than one mode or modality (as of stimulation or treatment)

mul·ti·neu·ro·nal \-ˈnu̇r-ən-ᵊl, -ˈnyu̇r-; -nu̇-ˈrōn-, -nyu̇-\ adj : made up of or involving more than one neuron

mul·ti·nod·u·lar \-ˈnä-jə-lər\ adj : having many nodules ⟨∼ goiter⟩

mul·ti·nu·cle·ate \-ˈnü-klē-ət, -ˈnyü-\ or **mul·ti·nu·cle·at·ed** \-klē-ˌā-təd\ adj : having more than two nuclei

mul·ti·or·gan \-ˈȯr-gən\ adj : of, involving, or affecting more than one organ ⟨∼ failure⟩

mul·ti·or·gas·mic \-ȯr-ˈgaz-mik\ adj : experiencing one orgasm after another with little or no recovery period between them

mul·tip·a·ra \ˌməl-ˈti-pə-rə\ n : a woman who has borne more than one child — compare MULTIGRAVIDA

mul·ti·par·i·ty \ˌməl-ti-ˈpar-ə-tē\ n, pl **-ties 1** : the production of two or more young at a birth **2** : the condition of having borne a number of children

mul·tip·a·rous \ˌməl-ˈti-pər-əs\ adj **1** : producing many or more than one at a birth **2** : having experienced one or more previous parturitions — compare PRIMIPAROUS

Multiphasic — see MINNESOTA MULTIPHASIC PERSONALITY INVENTORY

mul·ti·ple \ˈməl-tə-pəl\ adj **1** : consisting of, including, or involving more than one ⟨∼ births⟩ **2** : affecting many parts of the body at once

multiple allele n : an allele of a genetic locus having more than two allelic forms within a population

multiple factor n : POLYGENE

multiple myeloma n : a disease of bone marrow that is characterized by the presence of numerous myelomas in various bones of the body — called also *myelomatosis*

multiple organ dysfunction syndrome n : progressive dysfunction of two or more major organ systems in a critically ill patient that makes it impossible to maintain homeostasis without medical intervention and that is typically a complication of sepsis and is a major factor in predicting mortality — abbr. *MODS*

multiple personality disorder n : a dissociative disorder that is characterized by the presence of two or more distinct and complex identities or personality states each of which becomes dominant and controls behavior from time to time to the exclusion of the others — called also *alternating personality, dissociative identity disorder, multiple personality*

multiple sclerosis n : a demyelinating disease marked by patches of hardened tissue in the brain or the spinal cord and associated esp. with partial or complete paralysis and jerking muscle tremor

multiple system atrophy n : any of several progressive neurodegenerative diseases that are of unknown cause, have an onset usu. during middle age and are characterized by a combination of symptoms (as orthostatic hypotension, urinary incontinence, rigidity, and loss of balance) indicative of autonomic dysfunction, parkinsonism, and cerebellar ataxia — abbr. **MSA**; see SHY-DRAGER SYNDROME

multiplex — see ARTHROGRYPOSIS MULTIPLEX CONGENITA, MONONEURITIS MULTIPLEX, PARAMYOCLONUS MULTIPLEX

mul·ti·po·lar \ˌməl-tē-ˈpō-lər, -ˌtī-\ *adj* **1** : having several poles ⟨∼ mitoses⟩ **2** : having several dendrites ⟨∼ neurons⟩ — **mul·ti·po·lar·i·ty** \-ˌpō-ˈlar-ə-tē\ *n*

mul·tip·o·tent \ˌməl-ˈti-pə-tənt\ *adj* : having the potential of becoming any of several mature cell types ⟨∼ stem cells⟩

mul·ti·po·ten·tial \ˌməl-tē-pə-ˈten-chəl, -ˌtī-\ *adj* : MULTIPOTENT

mul·ti·re·sis·tant \-ri-ˈzis-tənt\ *adj* : biologically resistant to several toxic agents ⟨∼ strains of bacteria⟩

mul·ti·spe·cial·ty \-ˈspe-shəl-tē\ *adj* : providing service in or staffed by members of several medical specialties ⟨∼ health centers⟩

mul·ti·syn·ap·tic \-sə-ˈnap-tik\ *adj* : relating to or consisting of more than one synapse ⟨∼ pathways⟩

mul·ti·sys·tem \-ˈsis-təm\ *also* **mul·ti·sys·te·mic** \-sis-ˈtē-mik\ *adj* : relating to, consisting of, or involving more than one bodily system

¹**mul·ti·va·lent** \-ˈvā-lənt\ *adj* **1** : represented more than twice in the somatic chromosome number ⟨∼ chromosomes⟩ **2** : POLYVALENT

²**multivalent** *n* : a multivalent group of chromosomes

mul·ti·ve·sic·u·lar \-və-ˈsi-kyə-lər, -ve-\ *adj* : having, containing, or composed of many vesicles ⟨a ∼ cyst⟩

multivesicular body *n* : a lysosome that is a membranous sac containing numerous small endocytic vesicles

mul·ti·ves·sel \-ˈve-səl\ *adj* : affecting more than one blood vessel ⟨∼ coronary artery disease⟩

¹**mul·ti·vi·ta·min** \-ˈvī-tə-mən, -ˈvi-\ *adj* : containing several vitamins and esp. all known to be essential to health

²**multivitamin** *n* : a multivitamin preparation

mum·mi·fy \ˈmə-mi-ˌfī\ *vb* **-fied; -fy·ing** : to dry up and shrivel like a mummy ⟨a *mummified* fetus⟩ — **mum·mi·fi·ca·tion** \ˌmə-mi-fə-ˈkā-shən\ *n*

mumps \ˈməmps\ *n sing or pl* : an acute contagious virus disease caused by a paramyxovirus of the genus *Rubulavirus* (species *Mumps virus*) and marked by fever and by swelling esp. of the parotid gland — called also *epidemic parotitis*

Mun·chau·sen syndrome \ˈmən-ˌchaů-zən-\ *or* **Mun·chau·sen's syndrome** \-zənz-\ *n* : a psychological disorder characterized by the feigning of the symptoms of a disease or injury in order to undergo diagnostic tests, hospitalization, or medical or surgical treatment

Münch·hau·sen \ˈmᵫnk-ˌhaů-zən,

Karl Friedrich Hieronymous, Freiherr von (1720–1797), German soldier.

Munchausen syndrome by proxy *also* **Munchausen's syndrome by proxy** *n* : a psychological disorder in which a parent and typically a mother harms her child (as by poisoning), falsifies the child's medical history, or tampers with the child's medical specimens in order to create a situation that requires or seems to require medical attention

mu·pir·o·cin \myü-ˈpir-ō-sən\ *n* : an antibacterial drug $C_{26}H_{44}O_9$ or its hydrated calcium salt $(C_{26}H_{43}O_9)_2Ca\cdot 2H_2O$ that is derived from a bacterium of the genus *Pseudomonas* (*P. fluorescens*) and is used esp. in the topical treatment of impetigo caused by bacteria of the genus *Streptococcus* (*S. pyogenes*) and *Staphylococcus* (*S. aureus*) — see BACTROBAN

mu·ral \ˈmyůr-əl\ *adj* : attached to or limited to a wall or a cavity ⟨a ∼ thrombus⟩ ⟨∼ abscesses⟩

mu·ram·i·dase \myü-ˈra-mə-ˌdās, -ˌdāz\ *n* : LYSOZYME

mu·rein \ˈmyůr-ē-ən, ˈmyůr-ˌēn\ *n* : PEPTIDOGLYCAN

mu·ri·at·ic acid \ˌmyůr-ē-ˈa-tik-\ *n* : HYDROCHLORIC ACID

mu·rid \ˈmyůr-id\ *n* : any of a large family (Muridae) of relatively small rodents including various Old World forms (as the house mouse and the common rats) — **murid** *adj*

¹**mu·rine** \ˈmyůr-ˌīn\ *adj* **1 a** : of or relating to the genus *Mus* or its subfamily (Murinae) that includes the common household rats and mice **b** : of, relating to, or produced by the house mouse ⟨a ∼ odor⟩ **2** : affecting or transmitted by rats or mice ⟨∼ rickettsial diseases⟩

²**murine** *n* : a murine animal

murine leukemia virus *n* : a retrovirus (species *Murine leukemia virus* of the genus *Gammaretrovirus*) that includes several strains producing leukemia in mice — see FRIEND VIRUS

murine typhus *n* : a mild febrile disease that is marked by headache and rash, is caused by a bacterium of the genus *Rickettsia* (*R. typhi*), is widespread in nature in rodents, and is transmitted to humans by a flea — called also *endemic typhus*

mur·mur \ˈmər-mər\ *n* : an atypical sound of the heart indicating a functional or structural abnormality — called also *heart murmur*

Mur·ray Val·ley encephalitis \ˈmər-ē-ˈva-lē-\ *n* : an encephalitis endemic in northern Australia and Papua New Guinea that is caused by a virus of the genus *Flavivirus* (species *Murray Valley encephalitis virus*) transmitted by mosquitoes (esp. *Culex annulirostris*) and that is often asymptomatic but may cause serious potentially fatal disease

Mus \\'məs\\ *n* : a genus of rodents (family Muridae) that includes the house mouse (*M. musculus*)

Mus·ca \\'məs-kə\\ *n* : a genus of flies (family Muscidae) that is now restricted to the common housefly (*M. domestica*) and closely related flies

mus·cae vo·li·tan·tes \\'məs-ˌkē-vä-lə-'tan-ˌtēz, 'məs-ˌsē-\\ *n pl* : spots before the eyes due to cells and cell fragments in the vitreous humor and lens — compare FLOATER

mus·ca·rine \\'məs-kə-ˌrēn\\ *n* : a toxic ammonium base [$C_9H_{20}NO_2$]⁺ that is biochemically related to acetylcholine, was orig. extracted from fly agaric but also occurs in other mushrooms (as of the genus *Inocybe*), and when ingested produces symptoms of peripheral nervous system stimulation (as excessive salivation, lacrimation, bronchial secretion, diarrhea, miosis, and bradycardia)

mus·ca·rin·ic \\ˌməs-kə-'ri-nik\\ *adj* : relating to, resembling, producing, or mediating the parasympathetic effects (as a slowed heart rate and increased activity of smooth muscle) produced by muscarine (∼ receptors) — compare NICOTINIC

mus·cle \\'mə-səl\\ *n, often attrib* 1 : a body tissue consisting of long cells that contract when stimulated and produce motion — see CARDIAC MUSCLE, SMOOTH MUSCLE, STRIATED MUSCLE 2 : an organ that is essentially a mass of muscle tissue attached at either end to a fixed point and that by contracting moves or checks the movement of a body part — see AGONIST 1, ANTAGONIST a, SYNERGIST 2

mus·cle-bound \\'mə-səl-ˌba͝und\\ *adj* : having some of the muscles tense and enlarged and of impaired elasticity sometimes as a result of excessive exercise

muscle fiber *n* : any of the elongated cells characteristic of muscle

muscle sense *n* : the part of kinesthesia mediated by end organs located in muscles

muscle spasm *n* : persistent involuntary hypertonicity of one or more muscles usu. of central origin and commonly associated with pain and excessive irritability

muscle spindle *n* : a sensory end organ in a muscle that is sensitive to stretch in the muscle, consists of small striated muscle fibers richly supplied with nerve fibers, and is enclosed in a connective tissue sheath — called also *stretch receptor*

muscle tone *n* : TONUS 2

muscul- *or* **musculo-** *comb form* 1 : muscle ⟨*muscular*⟩ 2 : muscular and ⟨*musculoskeletal*⟩

mus·cu·lar \\'məs-kyə-lər\\ *adj* 1 a : of, relating to, or constituting muscle b : of, relating to, or performed by the muscles 2 : having well-developed musculature — **mus·cu·lar·ly** *adv*

muscular coat *n* : an outer layer of smooth muscle surrounding a hollow or tubular organ (as the bladder, esophagus, large intestine, small intestine, stomach, ureter, uterus, and vagina) that often consists of an inner layer of circular fibers serving to narrow the lumen of the organ and an outer layer of longitudinal fibers serving to shorten its length — called also *muscularis externa, tunica muscularis*

muscular dystrophy *n* : any of a group of hereditary diseases characterized by progressive wasting of muscles — see BECKER MUSCULAR DYSTROPHY, DUCHENNE MUSCULAR DYSTROPHY

mus·cu·la·ris \\ˌməs-kyə-'lar-is\\ *n* 1 : the smooth muscular layer of the wall of various more or less contractile organs (as the bladder) 2 : the thin layer of smooth muscle that forms part of a mucous membrane

muscularis ex·ter·na \\-eks-'tər-nə\\ *n* : MUSCULAR COAT

muscularis mu·co·sae \\-myü-'kō-sē\\ *also* **muscularis mu·co·sa** \\-sə\\ *n* : MUSCULARIS 2

mus·cu·lar·i·ty \\ˌməs-kyə-'lar-ə-tē\\ *n, pl* **-ties** : the quality or state of being muscular

mus·cu·la·ture \\'məs-kyə-lə-ˌchu̇r, -chər, -ˌtyu̇r\\ *n* : the muscles of all or a part of the body

mus·cu·li pec·ti·na·ti \\'məs-kyə-ˌlī-ˌpek-ti-'nā-ˌtī\\ *n pl* : small muscular ridges on the inner wall of the auricular appendage of the left and the right atria of the heart

musculo- — see MUSCUL-

mus·cu·lo·cu·ta·ne·ous \\ˌməs-kyə-lō-kyü-'tā-nē-əs\\ *adj* : of, relating to, supplying, or consisting of both muscle and skin (∼ flaps)

musculocutaneous nerve *n* 1 : a large branch of the brachial plexus supplying various parts of the upper arm (as flexor muscles) and forearm (as the skin) 2 : SUPERFICIAL PERONEAL NERVE

mus·cu·lo·fas·cial \\-'fa-shəl, -shē-əl\\ *adj* : relating to or consisting of both muscular and fascial tissue

mus·cu·lo·fi·brous \\-'fī-brəs\\ *adj* : relating to or consisting of both muscular and fibrous connective tissue

mus·cu·lo·mem·bra·nous \\-'mem-brə-nəs\\ *adj* : relating to or consisting of both muscle and membrane

mus·cu·lo·phren·ic artery \\-'fre-nik\\ *n* : a branch of the internal thoracic artery that gives off branches to the seventh, eighth, and ninth intercostal spaces as anterior intercostal arteries, to the pericardium, to the diaphragm, and to the abdominal muscles — called also *musculophrenic, musculophrenic branch*

musculorum — see DYSTONIA MUSCULORUM DEFORMANS

mus·cu·lo·skel·e·tal \\ˌməs-kyə-lō-'ske-lət-əl\\ *adj* : of, relating to, or involving both musculature and skeleton

mus·cu·lo·ten·di·nous \-'ten-də-nəs\ *adj* : of, relating to, or affecting muscular and tendinous tissue

musculotendinous cuff *n* : ROTATOR CUFF

mus·cu·lus \'məs-kyə-ləs\ *n, pl* **-li** \-ˌlī\ : MUSCLE

mush·room \'məsh-ˌrüm, -ˌrùm\ *n* **1** : an enlarged complex fleshy fruiting body of a fungus (as a basidiomycete) that arises from an underground mycelium and consists typically of a stem bearing a spore-bearing structure; *esp* : one that is edible — compare TOADSTOOL **2** : FUNGUS 1

mu·si·co·gen·ic \ˌmyü-zi-kō-'je-nik\ *adj* : of, relating to, or being epileptic seizures precipitated by music

music therapy *n* : the treatment of disease (as mental disorder) by means of music — **music therapist** *n*

mussel poisoning *n* : a toxic reaction and esp. paralytic shellfish poisoning following the consumption of mussels

mus·tard \'məs-tərd\ *n* **1** : a pungent yellow powder of the seeds of any of several herbs (*Brassica nigra, B. hirta,* or *B. juncea* of the family Cruciferae syn. Brassicaceae, the mustard family) used as a condiment or in medicine as a stimulant and diuretic, an emetic, and a counterirritant **2 a** : MUSTARD GAS **b** : NITROGEN MUSTARD

mustard gas *n* : an irritant oily liquid $C_4H_8Cl_2S$ used esp. as a chemical weapon that causes blistering, attacks the eyes and lungs, and is a systemic poison — called also *sulfur mustard*

mustard oil *n* **1** : a colorless to pale yellow pungent irritating essential oil that is obtained by distillation from mustard seeds, that consists largely of allyl isothiocyanate, and that is used esp. in liniments and medicinal plasters **2** : ALLYL ISOTHIOCYANATE

mustard plaster *n* : a counterirritant and rubefacient plaster containing powdered mustard — called also *mustard paper*

mu·ta·gen \'myü-tə-jən\ *n* : a substance (as a chemical or various radiations) that tends to increase the frequency or extent of mutation

mu·ta·gen·e·sis \ˌmyü-tə-'je-nə-səs\ *n, pl* **-e·ses** \-ˌsēz\ : the occurrence or induction of mutation — **mu·ta·gen·ic** \-'je-nik\ *adj* — **mu·ta·ge·nic·i·ty** \-jə-'ni-sə-tē\ *n*

mu·ta·gen·ize \'myü-tə-jə-ˌnīz\ *vb* **-ized; -iz·ing** : MUTATE

¹mu·tant \'myü-ᵊnt\ *adj* : of, relating to, or produced by mutation

²mutant *n* : a mutant individual

mu·ta·tion \myü-'tā-shən\ *n* **1** : a relatively permanent change in hereditary material involving either a physical change in chromosome relations or a biochemical change in the codons that make up genes; *also* : the process

of producing a mutation **2** : an individual, strain, or trait resulting from mutation — **mu·tate** \'myü-ˌtāt, myü-'\ *vb* — **mu·ta·tion·al** \-'shə-nəl\ *adj* — **mu·ta·tion·al·ly** *adv*

¹mute \'myüt\ *adj* **mut·er; mut·est** : unable to speak : lacking the power of speech — **mute·ness** *n*

²mute *n* : a person who cannot or does not speak

mu·ti·late \'myüt-ᵊl-ˌāt\ *vb* **-lat·ed; -lat·ing** : to cut off or permanently destroy a limb or essential part of; *also* : CASTRATE — **mu·ti·la·tion** \ˌmyüt-ᵊl-'ā-shən\ *n*

mut·ism \'myü-ˌti-zəm\ *n* : the condition of being mute whether from physical, functional, or psychological cause

¹muz·zle \'mə-zəl\ *n* **1** : the projecting jaws and nose of an animal **2** : a fastening or covering for the mouth of an animal used to prevent eating or biting

²muzzle *vb* **muz·zled; muz·zling** : to fit with a muzzle

Mv *symbol* mendelevium

MVP *abbr* mitral valve prolapse

my- *or* **myo-** *comb form* **1 a** : muscle ⟨*my*asthenia⟩ ⟨*myo*globin⟩ **b** : muscular and ⟨*myo*neural⟩ **2** : myoma and ⟨*myo*edema⟩

my·al·gia \mī-'al-jē, -jē-ə\ *n* : pain in one or more muscles — **my·al·gic** \-jik\ *adj*

myalgic encephalomyelitis *n, chiefly Brit* : CHRONIC FATIGUE SYNDROME

My·am·bu·tol \mī-'am-byù-ˌtòl, -ˌtōl\ *trademark* — used for a preparation of the dihydrochloride of ethambutol

my·an·e·sin \mī-'a-nə-sən\ *n* : ME-PHENESIN

my·as·the·nia \ˌmī-əs-'thē-nē-ə\ *n* : muscular debility; *also* : MYASTHENIA GRAVIS — **my·as·then·ic** \-'thē-nik\ *adj*

myasthenia gra·vis \-'gra-vis, -'grä-\ *n* : a disease characterized by progressive weakness of voluntary muscles without atrophy or sensory disturbance and caused by an autoimmune attack on acetylcholine receptors at neuromuscular junctions

my·a·to·nia \ˌmī-ə-'tō-nē-ə\ *n* : lack of muscle tone : muscular flabbiness

myc- *or* **myco-** *comb form* : fungus ⟨*myc*elium⟩ ⟨*myco*logy⟩ ⟨*myco*sis⟩

my·ce·li·um \mī-'sē-lē-əm\ *n, pl* **-lia** \-lē-ə\ : the mass of interwoven filaments that forms esp. the vegetative body of a fungus and is often submerged in another body (as of soil or organic matter or the tissues of a host); *also* : a similar mass of filaments formed by some bacteria (as of the genus *Streptomyces*) — **my·ce·li·al** \-lē-əl\ *adj*

-my·ces \'mī-ˌsēz\ *n comb form* : fungus — used esp. in taxonomic names of fungi and certain bacteria resembling fungi and in their corresponding vernacular names ⟨Strepto*myces*⟩

mycet- *or* **myceto-** *comb form* : fungus ⟨*mycetoma*⟩

-my·cete \'mī-ˌsēt, ˌmī-'sēt\ *n comb form* : fungus ⟨actino*mycete*⟩

my·ce·tis·mus \ˌmī-sə-'tiz-məs\ *n, pl* **-mi** \-ˌmī\ : mushroom poisoning

my·ce·to·ma \ˌmī-sə-'tō-mə\ *n, pl* **-mas** *also* **-ma·ta** \-mə-tə\ **1** : a condition marked by invasion of the deep subcutaneous tissues with fungi and actinomycetes: **a** : MADUROMYCOSIS **b** : NOCARDIOSIS **2** : a tumorous mass occurring in mycetoma — **my·ce·to·ma·tous** \-mə-təs\ *adj*

-my·cin \'mīs-ᵊn\ *n comb form* : substance obtained from a fungus ⟨erythro*mycin*⟩

my·co·bac·te·ri·o·sis \ˌmī-kō-bak-ˌtir-ē-'ō-səs\ *n, pl* **-o·ses** \-ˌsēz\ : a disease caused by bacteria of the genus *Mycobacterium*

my·co·bac·te·ri·um \-bak-'tir-ē-əm\ *n* **1** *cap* : a genus of nonmotile acid-fast aerobic bacteria (family Mycobacteriaceae) that include the causative agents of tuberculosis (*M. tuberculosis*) and leprosy (*M. leprae*) as well as numerous purely saprophytic forms **2** *pl* **-ria** : any bacterium of the genus *Mycobacterium* or a closely related genus — **my·co·bac·te·ri·al** \-ē-əl\ *adj*

Mycobacterium avi·um complex \-'ā-vē-əm-\ *n* : two bacteria of the genus *Mycobacterium* (*M. avium* and *M. intracellulare*) that account for most mycobacterial infections in humans other than tuberculosis, that usu. affect the lungs, and that may cause disseminated disease in immunosuppressed conditions (as AIDS)

Mycobacterium avium–in·tra·cel·lu·la·re complex \-ˌin-trə-ˌsel-yə-'lär-ē-\ *n* : MYCOBACTERIUM AVIUM COMPLEX

my·col·o·gy \mī-'kä-lə-jē\ *n, pl* **-gies** **1** : a branch of biology dealing with fungi **2** : fungal life — **my·co·log·i·cal** \ˌmī-kə-'läj-i-kəl\ *adj* — **my·col·o·gist** \mī-'kä-lə-jist\ *n*

my·co·my·cin \ˌmī-kə-'mīs-ᵊn\ *n* : an antibiotic acid C₁₃H₁₀O₂ obtained from an actinomycete of the genus *Nocardia* (*N. acidophilus*)

my·co·phe·no·lic acid \ˌmī-kō-fi-'nō-lik, -'nä-\ *n* : a crystalline antibiotic C₁₇H₂₀O₆ obtained from fungi of the genus *Penicillium*

my·co·plas·ma \ˌmī-kō-'plaz-mə\ *n* **1** *cap* : a genus of minute pleomorphic gram-negative chiefly nonmotile bacteria (family Mycoplasmataceae) that are mostly parasitic usu. in mammals — see PLEUROPNEUMONIA **2** *pl* **-mas** *also* **-ma·ta** \-mə-tə\ : any bacterium of the genus *Mycoplasma* or of the family (Mycoplasmataceae) to which it belongs — called also *pleuropneumonia-like organism, PPLO* — **my·co·plas·mal** \-məl\ *adj*

my·co·sis \mī-'kō-səs\ *n, pl* **my·co·ses** \-ˌsēz\ : infection with or disease caused by a fungus

mycosis fun·goi·des \-fən-'gȯi-ˌdēz\ *n* : cutaneous T-cell lymphoma characterized by a chronic patchy red scaly irregular and often eczematous dermatitis that progresses over a period of years to form elevated plaques and then tumors

my·co·stat \'mī-kə-stat\ *n* : an agent that inhibits the growth of molds — **my·co·stat·ic** \ˌmī-kə-'sta-tik\ *adj*

My·co·stat·in \-'sta-tən\ *trademark* — used for a preparation of nystatin

my·cot·ic \mī-'kä-tik\ *adj* : of, relating to, or characterized by mycosis

my·co·tox·ic \ˌmī-kō-'täk-sik\ *adj* : of, relating to, or caused by a mycotoxin — **my·co·tox·ic·i·ty** \-ˌtäk-'si-sə-tē\ *n*

my·co·tox·i·co·sis \ˌmī-kō-ˌtäk-sə-'kō-səs\ *n, pl* **-co·ses** \-ˌkō-ˌsēz\ : poisoning caused by a mycotoxin

my·co·tox·in \-'täk-sən\ *n* : a poisonous substance produced by a fungus and esp. a mold — see AFLATOXIN

My·dri·a·cyl \mə-'drī-ə-ˌsil\ *trademark* — used for a preparation of tropicamide

my·dri·a·sis \mə-'drī-ə-səs\ *n, pl* **-a·ses** \-ˌsēz\ : excessive or prolonged dilation of the pupil of the eye

¹myd·ri·at·ic \ˌmi-drē-'a-tik\ *adj* : causing or involving dilation of the pupil of the eye

²mydriatic *n* : a drug that produces dilation of the pupil of the eye

my·ec·to·my \mī-'ek-tə-mē\ *n, pl* **-mies** : surgical excision of part of a muscle

myel- *or* **myelo-** *comb form* : marrow: as **a** : bone marrow ⟨*myelo*cyte⟩ **b** : spinal cord ⟨*myelo*dysplasia⟩

my·el·en·ceph·a·lon \ˌmī-ə-len-'se-fə-ˌlän, -lən\ *n* : the posterior part of the developing vertebrate hindbrain or the corresponding part of the adult brain composed of the medulla oblongata — **my·el·en·ce·phal·ic** \-ˌlen-sə-'fa-lik\ *adj*

-my·e·lia \ˌmī-'ē-lē-ə\ *n comb form* : a (specified) condition of the spinal cord ⟨hemato*myelia*⟩ ⟨syringo*myelia*⟩

my·elin \'mī-ə-lən\ *n* : a soft white material of lipid and protein that is secreted by oligodendrocytes and Schwann cells and forms a thick sheath about axons — see MYELIN SHEATH — **my·elin·ic** \ˌmī-ə-'li-nik\ *adj*

my·elin·at·ed \'mī-ə-lə-ˌnā-təd\ *adj* : having a myelin sheath

my·e·li·na·tion \ˌmī-ə-lə-'nā-shən\ *n* **1** : the process of acquiring a myelin sheath **2** : the condition of being myelinated

myelin basic protein *n* : a protein that is a constituent of myelin and is often found in higher than normal amounts in the cerebrospinal fluid of people affected with some demyelinating disease (as multiple sclerosis)

my·e·lin·i·za·tion \ˌmī-ə-ˌli-nə-'zā-shən\ *n* : MYELINATION

my·e·li·nol·y·sis \-'nä-lə-səs\ *n* : DE-MYELINATION — see CENTRAL PONTINE MYELINOLYSIS

myelin sheath *n* : the insulating covering that surrounds an axon with multiple spiral layers of myelin, that is discontinuous at the nodes of Ranvier, and that increases the speed at which a nerve impulse can travel along an axon

my·e·li·tis \ˌmī-ə-'lī-təs\ *n, pl* **my·elit·i·des** \-'li-tə-ˌdēz\ : inflammation of the spinal cord or of the bone marrow — **my·elit·ic** \-'li-tik\ *adj*

my·e·lo·blast \'mī-ə-lə-ˌblast\ *n* : a large mononuclear nongranular bone marrow cell; *esp* : one that is a precursor of a myelocyte — **my·e·lo·blas·tic** \ˌmī-ə-lə-'blas-tik\ *adj*

myeloblastic leukemia *n* : MYELOGE-NOUS LEUKEMIA

my·e·lo·blas·to·sis \ˌmī-ə-lō-blas-'tō-səs\ *n, pl* **-to·ses** \-ˌsēz\ : the presence of an abnormally large number of myeloblasts in the tissues, organs, or circulating blood

my·e·lo·cele \'mī-ə-lə-ˌsēl\ *n* : spina bifida in which the neural tissue of the spinal cord is exposed

my·e·lo·cyte \'mī-ə-lə-ˌsīt\ *n* : a bone marrow cell; *esp* : a motile cell with cytoplasmic granules that gives rise to the blood granulocytes and occurs abnormally in the circulating blood (as in myelogenous leukemia) — **my·e·lo·cyt·ic** \ˌmī-ə-lə-'si-tik\ *adj*

myelocytic leukemia *n* : MYELOGE-NOUS LEUKEMIA

my·e·lo·cy·to·ma \-sī-'tō-mə\ *n, pl* **-mas** *also* **-ma·ta** \-mə-tə\ : a tumor esp. of fowl in which the typical cellular element is a myelocyte or a cell of similar differentiation

my·e·lo·cy·to·sis \-sī-'tō-səs\ *n, pl* **-to·ses** \-ˌsēz\ : the presence of excess numbers of myelocytes esp. in the blood or bone marrow

my·e·lo·dys·pla·sia \-dis-'plā-zhə, -zhē-ə\ *n* 1 : a developmental anomaly of the spinal cord 2 : MYELODYSPLAS-TIC SYNDROME — **my·e·lo·dys·plas·tic** \-'plas-tik\ *adj*

myelodysplastic syndrome *n* : any of a group of bone marrow disorders that are marked esp. by an abnormal reduction in one or more types of circulating blood cells due to defective growth and maturation of blood-forming cells in the bone marrow and that sometimes progress to acute myelogenous leukemia — called also *myelodysplasia, preleukemia*

my·e·lo·fi·bro·sis \ˌmī-ə-lō-fī-'brō-səs\ *n, pl* **-bro·ses** \-ˌsēz\ : an anemic condition in which bone marrow becomes fibrotic and the liver and spleen usu. exhibit a development of blood cell precursors — **my·e·lo·fi·brot·ic** \-'brä-tik\ *adj*

my·e·log·e·nous \ˌmī-ə-'lä-jə-nəs\ *also* **my·e·lo·gen·ic** \ˌmī-ə-lə-'je-nik\ *adj*

: of, relating to, originating in, or produced by the bone marrow

myelogenous leukemia *n* : leukemia characterized by proliferation of myeloid tissue (as of the bone marrow and spleen) and an abnormal increase in the number of granulocytes, myelocytes, and myeloblasts in the circulating blood — called also *granulocytic leukemia, myeloblastic leukemia, myelocytic leukemia, myeloid leukemia*; see ACUTE MYELOGENOUS LEUKEMIA, ACUTE NONLYMPHO-CYTIC LEUKEMIA, CHRONIC MYEL-OGENOUS LEUKEMIA

my·e·lo·gram \'mī-ə-lə-ˌgram\ *n* 1 : a differential study of the cellular elements present in bone marrow usu. made on material obtained by sternal biopsy 2 : a radiograph of the spinal cord made by myelography

my·e·lo·graph·ic \ˌmī-ə-lə-'gra-fik\ *adj* : of, relating to, or made by means of a myelogram or myelography — **my·e·lo·graph·i·cal·ly** *adv*

my·e·log·ra·phy \ˌmī-ə-'lä-grə-fē\ *n, pl* **-phies** : radiographic visualization of the spinal cord after injection of a contrast medium into the spinal subarachnoid space

my·e·loid \'mī-ə-ˌlȯid\ *adj* 1 : of or relating to the spinal cord 2 : of, relating to, or resembling bone marrow

myeloid leukemia *n* : MYELOGENOUS LEUKEMIA

my·e·lo·li·po·ma \ˌmī-ə-lō-lī-'pō-mə, -lī-\ *n, pl* **-mas** *also* **-ma·ta** \-mə-tə\ : a benign tumor esp. of the adrenal glands that consists of fat and hematopoietic tissue

my·e·lo·ma \ˌmī-ə-'lō-mə\ *n, pl* **-mas** *also* **-ma·ta** \-mə-tə\ : a primary tumor of the bone marrow formed of any one of the bone marrow cells (as myelocytes or plasma cells) and usu. involving several different bones at the same time — see MULTIPLE MYELOMA

my·e·lo·ma·to·sis \ˌmī-ə-lō-mə-'tō-səs\ *n, pl* **-to·ses** \-ˌsēz\ : MULTIPLE MYELOMA

my·e·lo·me·nin·go·cele \ˌmī-ə-lō-mə-'nin-gə-ˌsēl, -mə-'nin-jə-\ *n* : spina bifida in which neural tissue and the investing meninges protrude from the spinal column forming a sac under the skin

my·e·lo·mono·cyt·ic \-ˌmä-nə-'si-tik\ *adj* : relating to or being a blood cell that has the characteristics of both monocytes and granulocytes

myelomonocytic leukemia *n* : a kind of monocytic leukemia in which the cells resemble granulocytes

my·e·lop·a·thy \ˌmī-ə-'lä-pə-thē\ *n, pl* **-thies** : any disease or disorder of the spinal cord or bone marrow — **my·e·lo·path·ic** \ˌmī-ə-lō-'pa-thik\ *adj*

myelophthisic anemia \ˌmī-ə-lō-'ti-zik-, -'ti-sik-\ *n* : anemia in which the blood-forming elements of the bone marrow are unable to reproduce normal blood cells and which is commonly caused by specific toxins or by overgrowth of tumor cells

my·elo·poi·e·sis \ˌmī-ə-lō-(ˌ)pȯi-ˈē-səs\ *n, pl* **-poi·e·ses** \-ˈē-ˌsēz\ **1** : production of marrow or marrow cells **2** : production of blood cells in bone marrow; *esp* : formation of blood granulocytes — **my·elo·poi·et·ic** \-(ˌ)pȯi-ˈe-tik\ *adj*

my·elo·pro·lif·er·a·tive \ˈmī-ə-lō-prə-ˈli-fə-ˌrā-tiv, -rə-\ *adj* : of, relating to, or being a disorder (as leukemia) marked by excessive proliferation of bone marrow elements and esp. blood cell precursors

my·elo·sis \ˌmī-ə-ˈlō-səs\ *n, pl* **-elo·ses** \-ˌsēz\ **1** : the proliferation of marrow tissue to produce the changes in cell distribution typical of myelogenous leukemia **2** : MYELOGENOUS LEUKEMIA

my·elo·sup·pres·sion \ˌmī-ə-lō-sə-ˈpre-shən\ *n* : suppression of the bone marrow's production of blood cells and platelets — **my·elo·sup·pres·sive** \-sə-ˈpre-siv\ *adj*

my·elot·o·my \ˌmī-ə-ˈlä-tə-mē\ *n, pl* **-mies** : surgical incision of the spinal cord; *esp* : section of crossing nerve fibers at the midline of the spinal cord and esp. of sensory fibers for the relief of intractable pain

my·elo·tox·ic \ˌmī-ə-lō-ˈtäk-sik\ *adj* : destructive to bone marrow or any of its elements ⟨a ~ agent⟩ — **my·elo·tox·ic·i·ty** \-täk-ˈsi-sə-tē\ *n*

my·en·ter·ic \ˌmī-ən-ˈter-ik\ *adj* : of or relating to the muscular coat of the intestinal wall

myenteric plexus *n* : a network of nerve fibers and ganglia between the longitudinal and circular muscle layers of the intestine — called also *Auerbach's plexus;* compare MEISSNER'S PLEXUS

myenteric plexus of Auerbach *n* : MYENTERIC PLEXUS

myenteric reflex *n* : a reflex that is responsible for the wave of peristalsis moving along the intestine and that involves contraction of the digestive tube above and relaxation below the place where it is stimulated by an accumulated mass of food

my·ia·sis \mī-ˈī-ə-səs, mē-\ *n, pl* **my·ia·ses** \-ˌsēz\ : infestation with fly maggots

myl- *or* **mylo-** *comb form* : molar ⟨*my*lohyoid⟩

My·lan·ta \mī-ˈlan-tə\ *trademark* — used for an antacid and antiflatulent preparation of aluminum hydroxide, magnesium hydroxide, and simethicone

Myl·e·ran \ˈmil-ə-ˌran\ *trademark* — used for a preparation of busulfan

My·li·con \ˈmil-ə-ˌkän\ *trademark* — used for a preparation of simethicone

my·lo·hy·oid \ˌmī-lō-ˈhī-ˌȯid\ *adj* : of, indicating, or adjoining the mylohyoid muscle

my·lo·hy·oi·de·us \-hī-ˈȯi-dē-əs\ *n, pl* **-dei** \-dē-ˌī\ : MYLOHYOID MUSCLE

mylohyoid line *n* : a ridge on the inner side of the bone of the lower jaw giving attachment to the mylohyoid muscle and to the superior constrictor of the pharynx — called also *mylohyoid ridge*

mylohyoid muscle *n* : a flat triangular muscle on each side of the mouth that is located above the anterior belly of the digastric muscle, extends from the inner surface of the mandible to the hyoid bone, and with its mate on the opposite side forms the floor of the mouth — called also *mylohyoid, mylohyoideus*

myo- — see MY-

myo·blast \ˈmī-ə-ˌblast\ *n* : an undifferentiated cell capable of giving rise to muscle cells

myo·blas·to·ma \ˌmī-ə-(ˌ)blas-ˈtō-mə\ *n, pl* **-mas** *also* **-ma·ta** \-mə-tə\ : a tumor that is composed of cells resembling primitive myoblasts and is associated with striated muscle

myo·car·di·al \ˌmī-ə-ˈkär-dē-əl\ *adj* : of, relating to, or involving the myocardium — **myo·car·di·al·ly** *adv*

myocardial infarction *n* : HEART ATTACK

myocardial insufficiency *n* : inability of the myocardium to perform its function : HEART FAILURE

myo·car·di·op·a·thy \-ˌkär-dē-ˈä-pə-thē\ *n, pl* **-thies** : disease of the myocardium

myo·car·di·tis \ˌmī-ə-(ˌ)kär-ˈdī-təs\ *n* : inflammation of the myocardium

myo·car·di·um \ˌmī-ə-ˈkär-dē-əm\ *n, pl* **-dia** \-dē-ə\ : the middle muscular layer of the heart wall

Myo·chrys·ine \ˌmī-ō-ˈkrī-ˌsēn, -sən\ *trademark* — used for a preparation of gold sodium thiomalate

myo·clo·nia \ˌmī-ə-ˈklō-nē-ə\ *n* : MYOCLONUS

myo·clon·ic \-ˈklä-nik\ *adj* : of, relating to, characterized by, or being myoclonus ⟨~ seizures⟩

myoclonic epilepsy *n* : epilepsy marked by myoclonic seizures: as **a** : JUVENILE MYOCLONIC EPILEPSY **b** : LAFORA DISEASE

my·oc·lo·nus \mī-ˈä-klə-nəs\ *n* : irregular involuntary contraction of a muscle usu. resulting from functional disorder of controlling motor neurons; *also* : a condition characterized by myoclonus

myoclonus epilepsy *n* : MYOCLONIC EPILEPSY

myo·cyte \ˈmī-ə-ˌsīt\ *n* : a contractile cell; *specif* : a muscle cell

myo·ede·ma \ˌmī-ō-i-ˈdē-mə\ *n, pl* **-mas** *also* **-ma·ta** \-mə-tə\ : the formation of a lump in a muscle when struck a slight blow that occurs in states of exhaustion or in certain diseases

myo·elec·tric \ˌmī-ō-i-ˈlek-trik\ *also* **myo·elec·tri·cal** \-tri-kəl\ *adj* : of, relating to, or utilizing electricity generated by muscle

myo·epi·the·li·al \-,e-pə-'thē-lē-əl\ *adj* : of, relating to, or being large contractile cells of epithelial origin which are located at the base of the secretory cells of various glands (as the salivary and mammary glands)

myo·epi·the·li·o·ma \-,e-pə-,thē-lē-'ō-mə\ *n, pl* **-mas** *also* **-ma·ta** \-mə-tə\ : a tumor arising from myoepithelial cells esp. of the sweat glands

myo·epi·the·li·um \-'thē-lē-əm\ *n, pl* **-lia** : tissue made up of myoepithelial cells

myo·fas·cial \-'fa-shəl, -shē-əl\ *adj* : of or relating to the fasciae of muscles

myo·fi·ber \'mī-ō-,fī-bər\ *n* : MUSCLE FIBER

myo·fi·bre *chiefly Brit var of* MYOFIBER

myo·fi·bril \,mī-ō-'fī-brəl, -'fi-\ *n* : one of the longitudinal parallel contractile elements of a muscle cell that are composed of myosin and actin — **myo·fi·bril·lar** \-brə-lər\ *adj*

myo·fi·bro·blast \-'fī-brə-,blast, -'fi-\ *n* : a fibroblast that has developed some of the functional and structural characteristics (as the presence of myofilaments) of smooth muscle cells

myo·fil·a·ment \-'fi-lə-mənt\ *n* : one of the individual filaments of actin or myosin that make up a myofibril

myo·func·tion·al \-'fəŋk-shə-nəl\ *adj* : of, relating to, or concerned with muscle function esp. in the treatment of orthodontic problems

myo·gen·e·sis \,mī-ə-'je-nə-səs\ *n, pl* **-e·ses** \-,sēz\ : the development of muscle tissue

myo·gen·ic \,mī-ə-'je-nik\ *also* **my·og·e·nous** \mī-'ä-jə-nəs\ *adj* **1** : originating in muscle ⟨a ~ pain⟩ **2** : taking place or functioning in ordered rhythmic fashion because of the inherent properties of cardiac muscle rather than specific neural stimuli ⟨a ~ heartbeat⟩ — compare NEUROGENIC 2b — **myo·ge·nic·i·ty** \-jə-'ni-sə-tē\ *n*

myo·glo·bin \,mī-ə-'glō-bən, 'mī-ə-,\ *n* : a red iron-containing protein pigment in muscles that is similar to hemoglobin

myo·glo·bin·uria \-,glō-bi-'nùr-ē-ə, -'nyùr-\ *n* : the presence of myoglobin in the urine

myo·gram \'mī-ə-,gram\ *n* : a graphic representation of the phenomena (as intensity) of muscular contractions

myo·graph \-,graf\ *n* : an apparatus for producing myograms

my·oid \'mī-,ȯid\ *adj* : resembling muscle

myo·ino·si·tol \,mī-ō-i-'nō-sə-,tȯl, -,tōl\ *n* : a biologically active inositol that is a component of many phospholipids — called also *mesoinositol*

myo·in·ti·mal \-'in-tə-məl\ *adj* : of, relating to, or being the smooth muscle cells of the intima of a blood vessel

myom- *or* **myomo-** *comb form* : myoma ⟨*myom*ectomy⟩

my·o·ma \mī-'ō-mə\ *n, pl* **-mas** *also* **-ma·ta** \-mə-tə\ : a tumor consisting of muscle tissue

myo·mec·to·my \,mī-ə-'mek-tə-mē, *pl* **-mies** : surgical excision of a myoma or fibroid

myo·me·tri·tis \-mə-'trī-təs\ *n* : inflammation of the uterine myometrium

myo·me·tri·um \,mī-ə-'mē-trē-əm\ *n* : the muscular layer of the wall of the uterus — **myo·me·tri·al** \-'mē-trē-əl\ *adj*

myo·ne·cro·sis \-nə-'krō-səs, -ne-\ *n, pl* **-cro·ses** \-,sēz\ : necrosis of muscle

myo·neu·ral \,mī-ə-'nùr-əl, -'nyùr-\ *adj* : of, relating to, or connecting muscles and nerves ⟨~ effects⟩

myoneural junction *n* : NEUROMUSCULAR JUNCTION

myo·path·ic \,mī-ə-'pa-thik\ *adj* **1** : involving abnormality of the muscles ⟨~ syndrome⟩ **2** : of or relating to myopathy ⟨~ dystrophy⟩

my·op·a·thy \mī-'ä-pə-thē\ *n, pl* **-thies** : a disorder of muscle tissue or muscles

my·ope \'mī-,ōp\ *n* : a myopic person — called also *myopic*

myo·peri·car·di·tis \,mī-ō-,per-ə-,kär-'dī-təs\ *n, pl* **-dit·i·des** \-'di-tə-,dēz\ : inflammation of both the myocardium and pericardium

my·o·pia \mī-'ō-pē-ə\ *n* : a condition in which the visual images come to a focus in front of the retina of the eye because of defects in the refractive media of the eye or of abnormal length of the eyeball resulting esp. in defective vision of distant objects — called also *nearsightedness*; compare ASTIGMATISM 2, EMMETROPIA

¹my·o·pic \-'ō-pik, -'ä-\ *adj* : affected by myopia : of, relating to, or exhibiting myopia — **my·o·pi·cal·ly** *adv*

²myopic *n* : MYOPE

myo·plasm \'mī-ə-,pla-zəm\ *n* : the contractile portion of muscle tissue — compare SARCOPLASM — **myo·plas·mic** \,mī-ə-'plaz-mik\ *adj*

¹myo·re·lax·ant \,mī-ō-ri-'lak-sənt\ *n* : a drug that causes relaxation of muscle

²myorelaxant *adj* : relating to or causing relaxation of muscle ⟨~ effects⟩ — **myo·re·lax·ation** \,-rē-,lak-'sā-shən, -ri-,lak-\ *n*

myo·sar·co·ma \-sär-'kō-mə\ *n, pl* **-mas** *also* **-ma·ta** \-mə-tə\ : a sarcomatous myoma

my·o·sin \'mī-ə-sən\ *n* : a fibrous globulin of muscle that can split ATP and that reacts with actin to form actomyosin

myosis *var of* MIOSIS

myo·si·tis \,mī-ə-'sī-təs\ *n* : muscular discomfort or pain

myositis os·sif·i·cans \-ä-'si-fə-,kanz\ *n* : myositis accompanied by ossification of muscle tissue or bony deposits in the muscles

myo·tat·ic reflex \,mī-ə-'ta-tik-\ *n* : STRETCH REFLEX

myotic *var of* MIOTIC

myo·tome \'mī-ə-ˌtōm\ *n* **1** : the portion of an embryonic somite from which skeletal musculature is produced **2** : an instrument for myotomy — **myo·to·mal** \ˌmī-ə-'tō-məl\ *adj*

my·ot·o·my \mī-'ä-tə-mē\ *n, pl* **-mies** : incision or division of a muscle

myo·to·nia \ˌmī-ə-'tō-nē-ə\ *n* : tonic spasm of one or more muscles; *also* : a condition characterized by such spasms — **myo·ton·ic** \-'tä-nik\ *adj*

myotonia con·gen·i·ta \-kän-'je-nə-tə\ *n* : an inherited condition that is characterized by delay in the ability to relax muscles after forceful contractions but not by wasting of muscle — called also *Thomsen's disease*

myotonia dys·tro·phi·ca \-dis-'trä-fi-kə, -'trō-\ *n* : MYOTONIC DYSTROPHY

myotonic dystrophy *n* : an inherited condition characterized by delay in the ability to relax muscles after forceful contraction, wasting of muscles, the formation of cataracts, premature baldness, atrophy of the gonads, endocrine and cardiac abnormalities, and often mental retardation — abbr. *DM;* called also *myotonic muscular dystrophy*

my·ot·o·nus \mī-'ä-tə-nəs\ *n* : sustained spasm of a muscle or muscle group

myo·tox·ic \ˌmī-ō-'täk-sik\ *adj* : having or being a toxic effect on muscle — **myo·tox·ic·i·ty** \-täk-'si-sə-tē\ *n*

myo·trop·ic \ˌmī-ə-'trä-pik, -'trō-\ *adj* : affecting or tending to invade muscles ⟨a ∼ infection⟩

myo·tube \'mī-ə-ˌtüb, -ˌtyüb\ *n* : a developmental stage of a muscle fiber

myring- or **myringo-** *comb form* : tympanic membrane ⟨*myringo*tomy⟩

my·rin·go·plas·ty \mə-'riŋ-gə-ˌplas-tē\ *n, pl* **-ties** : a surgical operation for the repair of perforations in the tympanic membrane

myr·in·got·o·my \ˌmir-ən-'gä-tə-mē\ *n, pl* **-mies** : incision of the tympanic membrane — called also *tympanotomy*

my·ris·tate \mi-'ris-ˌtāt\ — see ISO-PROPYL MYRISTATE

myx- or **myxo-** *comb form* **1** : mucus ⟨*myxo*ma⟩ **2** : myxoma ⟨*myxo*sarcoma⟩

myx·ede·ma \ˌmik-sə-'dē-mə\ *n* : severe hypothyroidism characterized by firm inelastic edema, dry skin and hair, and loss of mental and physical vigor — **myx·ede·ma·tous** \-'de-mə-təs, -'dē-\ *adj*

myx·oid \'mik-ˌsȯid\ *adj* : resembling mucus

myx·o·ma \mik-'sō-mə\ *n, pl* **-mas** *also* **-ma·ta** \-mə-tə\ : a soft tumor made up of gelatinous connective tissue resembling that found in the umbilical cord — **myx·o·ma·tous** \-mə-təs\ *adj*

myx·o·ma·to·sis \ˌmik-ˌsō-mə-'tō-səs\ *n, pl* **-to·ses** \-ˌsēz\ : a condition characterized by the presence of myxomas in the body; *specif* : a severe disease of rabbits that is caused by a poxvirus (species *Myxoma virus* of the genus *Leporipoxvirus*), is transmitted by mosquitoes, biting flies, and direct contact, and has been used in the biological control of wild rabbit populations

myxo·sar·co·ma \-sär-'kō-mə\ *n, pl* **-mas** *also* **-ma·ta** \-mə-tə\ : a sarcoma with myxomatous elements

myxo·vi·rus \'mik-sə-ˌvī-rəs\ *n* : any of the viruses classified as orthomyxoviruses and paramyxoviruses that were formerly included in a single now rejected family (Myxoviridae) — **myxo·vi·ral** \ˌmik-sə-'vī-rəl\ *adj*

n \'en\ *n, pl* **n's** or **ns** \'enz\ : the haploid or gametic number of chromosomes — compare X

N *symbol* nitrogen — usu. italicized when used as a prefix ⟨*N*-allylnormorphine⟩

Na *symbol* sodium

NA *abbr* **1** Nomina Anatomica **2** nurse's aide

na·bo·thi·an cyst \nə-'bō-thē-ən-\ *n* : a mucous gland of the uterine cervix esp. when occluded and dilated — called also *nabothian follicle*

Na·both \'nä-ˌbȯt\, **Martin (1675–1721)**, German anatomist and physician.

NAD \ˌen-(ˌ)ā-'dē\ *n* : a coenzyme $C_{21}H_{27}N_7O_{14}P_2$ of numerous dehydrogenases that occurs in most cells and plays an important role in all phases of intermediary metabolism as an oxidizing agent or when in the reduced form as a reducing agent for various metabolites — called also *nicotinamide adenine dinucleotide, diphosphopyridine nucleotide*

NADH \ˌen-(ˌ)ā-(ˌ)dē-'āch\ *n* : the reduced form of NAD

na·do·lol \nā-'dō-ˌlȯl, -ˌlōl\ *n* : a beta-blocker $C_{17}H_{27}NO_4$ used in the treatment of hypertension and angina pectoris

NADP \ˌen-(ˌ)ā-(ˌ)dē-'pē\ *n* : a coenzyme $C_{21}H_{28}N_7O_{17}P_3$ of numerous dehydrogenases (as that acting on glucose-6-phosphate) that occurs esp. in red blood cells and plays a role in intermediary metabolism similar to

NAD but acting often on different metabolites — called also *nicotinamide adenine dinucleotide phosphate*, *TPN*, *triphosphopyridine nucleotide*

NADPH \\,en-(,)ā-(,)dē-(,)pē-'āch\ *n* : the reduced form of NADP

Nae·gle·ria \nā-'glir-ē-ə\ *n* : a genus of protozoans occurring esp. in stagnant water and including one (*N. fowleri*) causing meningoencephalitis

nae·void, nae·vus *chiefly Brit var of* NEVOID, NEVUS

naf·cil·lin \naf-'si-lən\ *n* : a semisynthetic penicillin that is resistant to beta-lactamase and is used esp. in the form of its hydrated sodium salt $C_{21}H_{21}N_2NaO_5S \cdot H_2O$ as an antibiotic

naf·ox·i·dine \na-'fäk-sə-,dēn\ *n* : an antiestrogen administered in the form of its hydrochloride $C_{29}H_{31}NO_2 \cdot HCl$

na·ga·na *also* **na·ga·na** \nə-'gä-nə\ *n* : a highly fatal disease of domestic animals in tropical Africa caused by a flagellated protozoan of the genus *Trypanosoma* and transmitted by tsetse and other biting flies; *broadly* : trypanosomiasis of domestic animals

nail \'nāl\ *n* **1** : a horny sheath of thickened and condensed epithelial stratum lucidum that grows out from a vascular matrix of dermis and protects the upper surface of the end of each finger and toe — called also *nail plate* **2** : a rod (as of metal) used to fix the parts of a broken bone in normal relation ⟨a medullary ~⟩

nail bed *n* : the vascular epidermis upon which most of the fingernail or toenail rests that has a longitudinally ridged surface often visible through the nail; *also* : MATRIX 1b

nail–biting *n* : habitual biting at the fingernails usu. being symptomatic of emotional tensions and frustrations

nail fold *n* : the fold of the dermis at the margin of a fingernail or toenail

nail·ing \'nā-liŋ\ *n* : the act or process of fixing the parts of a broken bone by means of a nail

nail matrix *n* : MATRIX 1b

nail plate *n* : NAIL 1

na·ive *or* **na·ïve** \nä-'ēv\ *adj* **na·iv·er; -est** **1** : not previously subjected to experimentation or a particular experimental situation ⟨~ laboratory rats⟩ **2** : not having previously used a particular drug (as marijuana) **3** : not having been exposed previously to an antigen ⟨~ T cells⟩

Na·ja \'nä-jə\ *n* : a genus of elapid snakes comprising the true cobras

na·ked \'nä-kəd\ *adj* : lacking some natural external covering (as of hair or myelin) — used of the animal body or one of its parts ⟨~ nerve endings⟩

na·li·dix·ic acid \,nä-lə-'dik-sik-\ *n* : an antibacterial agent $C_{12}H_{12}N_2O_3$ that is used esp. in the treatment of genitourinary infections — see NEGGRAM

Nal·line \'na-,lēn\ *trademark* — used for a preparation of the hydrochloride of nalorphine

na·lor·phine \na-'lòr-,fēn\ *n* : a white crystalline compound that is derived from morphine and is used in the form of its hydrochloride $C_{19}H_{21}NO_3 \cdot HCl$ as a respiratory stimulant to counteract poisoning by morphine and similar narcotic drugs — called also *N-allylnormorphine*; see NALLINE

nal·ox·one \na-'läk-,sōn, 'na-lək-,sōn\ *n* : a potent antagonist of narcotic drugs and esp. morphine that is used esp. in the form of its hydrochloride $C_{19}H_{21}NO_4 \cdot HCl$ — see NARCAN

nal·trex·one \nal-'trek-,sōn\ *n* : a synthetic opiate antagonist used in the form of its hydrochloride $C_{20}H_{23}NO_4 \cdot HCl$ esp. to maintain detoxified opiate addicts in a drug-free state

nan- *or* **nano-** *comb form* : dwarf ⟨*nano*cephalic⟩

nan·dro·lone \'nan-drə-,lōn\ *n* : a semisynthetic anabolic steroid $C_{18}H_{26}O_2$ derived from testosterone

na·nism \'na-,ni-zəm, 'nā-\ *n* : the condition of being abnormally or exceptionally small in stature : DWARFISM

nano- *comb form* : one billionth (10^{-9}) part of ⟨*nano*second⟩

nano·ce·phal·ic \,na-nō-si-'fa-lik\ *adj* : having an abnormally small head

nano·cu·rie \'na-nō-,kyùr-ē, -,kyù-,rē\ *n* : one billionth of a curie

nano·gram \-,gram\ *n* : one billionth of a gram — abbr. *ng*

nano·me·ter \-,mē-tər\ *n* : one billionth of a meter — abbr. *nm*

nano·sec·ond \-,se-kənd, -kənt\ *n* : one billionth of a second — abbr. *ns*, *nsec*

nape \'nāp, 'nap\ *n* : the back of the neck

na·phaz·o·line \nə-'fa-zə-,lēn\ *n* : a base used topically in the form of its hydrochloride $C_{14}H_{14}N_2 \cdot HCl$ esp. to relieve nasal congestion and itching and redness of the eyes

naphthoate — see PAMAQUINE NAPHTHOATE

naph·tho·qui·none *also* **naph·tha·qui·none** \,naf-thə-kwi-'nōn, -'kwi-,nōn\ *n* : any of three isomeric yellow to red crystalline compounds $C_{10}H_6O_2$; *esp* : one that occurs naturally in the form of derivatives (as vitamin K)

naph·thyl·amine \naf-'thi-lə-,mēn\ *n* : either of two isomeric crystalline bases $C_{10}H_9N$ that are used esp. in synthesizing dyes; *esp* : one (*β-naphthylamine*) with the amino group in the beta position that has been demonstrated to cause bladder cancer in individuals exposed to it while working in the dye industry

nap·kin \'nap-kən\ *n* : SANITARY NAPKIN

nap·ra·path \'nap-rə-,path\ *n* : a practitioner of naprapathy

na·prap·a·thy \nə-'pra-pə-thē\ *n*, *pl* **-thies** : a system of treatment by manipulation of connective tissue and adjoining structures (as ligaments, joints, and muscles) and by dietary measures that is held to facilitate the recuperative and regenerative processes of the body

Na·pro·syn \nə-ˈpräs-ᵊn\ *trademark* — used for a preparation of naproxen

na·prox·en \nə-ˈpräk-sᵊn\ *n* : an antiinflammatory analgesic antipyretic drug $C_{14}H_{14}O_3$ used esp. to treat arthritis often in the form of its sodium salt $C_{14}H_{13}NaO_3$ — see ALEVE, NAPROSYN

nap·syl·ate \ˈnap-sə-ˌlāt\ *n* : a salt of either of two crystalline acids $C_{10}H_7$-SO_3H

Naqua \ˈna-kwə\ *trademark* — used for a preparation of trichlormethiazide

narc- *or* **narco-** *comb form* **1** : numbness : stupor ⟨*narcosis*⟩ **2** : deep sleep ⟨*narcolepsy*⟩

Nar·can \ˈnär-ˌkan\ *trademark* — used for a preparation of naloxone

nar·cis·sism \ˈnär-sə-ˌsi-zəm\ *n* **1** : love of or sexual desire for one's own body **2** : the state or stage of development in psychoanalytic theory in which there is considerable erotic interest in one's own body and ego and which in abnormal forms persists through fixation or reappears through regression — **nar·cis·sist** \-sist\ *n* — **nar·cis·sis·tic** \ˌnär-sə-ˈsis-tik\ *adj*

narcissistic personality disorder *n* : a personality disorder characterized esp. by an exaggerated sense of self-importance, persistent need for admiration, lack of empathy for others, excessive pride in achievements, and snobbish, disdainful, or patronizing attitudes

nar·co·anal·y·sis \ˌnär-kō-ə-ˈna-lə-səs\ *n, pl* **-y·ses** \-ˌsēz\ : psychotherapy that is performed under sedation for the recovery of repressed memories together with the emotion accompanying the experience

nar·co·lep·sy \ˈnär-kə-ˌlep-sē\ *n, pl* **-sies** : a condition characterized by brief attacks of deep sleep often occurring with cataplexy and hypnagogic hallucinations — compare HYPERSOMNIA 2

¹nar·co·lep·tic \ˌnär-kə-ˈlep-tik\ *adj* : of, relating to, or affected with narcolepsy

²narcoleptic *n* : an individual who is subject to attacks of narcolepsy

nar·co·sis \när-ˈkō-səs\ *n, pl* **-co·ses** \-ˌsēz\ : a state of stupor, unconsciousness, or arrested activity produced by the influence of narcotics or other chemicals or physical agents — see NITROGEN NARCOSIS

nar·co·syn·the·sis \ˌnär-kō-ˈsin-thə-səs\ *n, pl* **-the·ses** \-ˌsēz\ : NARCOANALYSIS

¹nar·cot·ic \när-ˈkä-tik\ *n* **1** : a drug (as codeine, methadone, or morphine) that in moderate doses dulls the senses, relieves pain, and induces profound sleep but in excessive doses causes stupor, coma, or convulsions **2** : a drug (as marijuana or LSD) subject to restriction similar to that of addictive narcotics whether physiologically addictive and narcotic or not

²narcotic *adj* **1** : having the properties of or yielding a narcotic **2** : of, induced by, or concerned with narcotics **3** : of, involving, or intended for narcotic addicts

nar·co·ti·za·tion \ˌnär-kə-tə-ˈzā-shən\ *n* : the act or process of inducing narcosis

nar·co·tize \ˈnär-kə-ˌtīz\ *vb* **-tized; -tiz·ing** **1** : to treat with or subject to a narcotic **2** : to put into a state of narcosis

Nar·dil \ˈnär-ˌdil\ *trademark* — used for a preparation of phenelzine

na·ris \ˈnar-əs\ *n pl* : either of the pair of openings of the nose

narrow–angle glaucoma *n* : ANGLE-CLOSURE GLAUCOMA

narrow–spectrum *adj* : effective against only a limited range of organisms — compare BROAD-SPECTRUM

nas- *or* **naso-** *comb form* **1** : nose : nasal ⟨*naso*pharyngoscope⟩ **2** : nasal and ⟨*naso*tracheal⟩

Na·sa·cort \ˈnā-zə-ˌkórt\ *trademark* — used for a preparation of triamcinolone

¹na·sal \ˈnā-zəl\ *n* : a nasal part (as a bone)

²nasal *adj* : of or relating to the nose — **na·sal·ly** *adv*

nasal bone *n* : either of two bones of the skull of vertebrates above the fishes that lie in front of the frontal bones and in humans are oblong in shape forming by their junction the bridge of the nose and partly covering the nasal cavity

nasal cavity *n* : the vaulted chamber that lies between the floor of the cranium and the roof of the mouth extending from the external nares to the pharynx, being enclosed by bone or cartilage and usu. incompletely divided into lateral halves by the septum of the nose, and having its walls lined with mucous membrane that is rich in venous plexuses and ciliated in the lower part which forms the beginning of the respiratory passage and warms and filters the inhaled air and that is modified as sensory epithelium in the upper olfactory part

nasal concha *n* : any of three thin bony plates on the lateral wall of the nasal fossa on each side with or without their covering of mucous membrane: **a** : a separate curved bony plate that is the largest of the three and separates the inferior and middle meatuses of the nose — called also *inferior concha, inferior nasal concha, inferior turbinate, inferior turbinate* *bone* **b** : the lower of two thin bony processes of the ethmoid bone on the lateral wall of each nasal fossa that separates the superior and middle meatuses of the nose — called also *middle concha, middle nasal concha, middle turbinate, middle turbinate bone* **c** : the upper of two thin bony processes of the ethmoid bone on the lateral wall of each nasal fossa that forms the upper boundary of the superior meatus of the nose — called also *superior concha, superior nasal concha, superior turbinate, superior turbinate bone*

nasal fossa *n* : either lateral half of the nasal cavity

na·sa·lis \nā-ˈzā-ləs, -ˈsā-\ *n* : a small muscle on each side of the nose that constricts the nasal aperture

nasal nerve *n* : NASOCILIARY NERVE

nasal notch *n* : the rough surface on the anterior lower border of the frontal bone between the orbits which articulates with the nasal bones and the maxillae

nasal process *n* : FRONTAL PROCESS 1

nasal septum *n* : the bony and cartilaginous partition between the nasal passages

nasal spine *n* : any of several median bony processes adjacent to the nasal passages: as **a** : ANTERIOR NASAL SPINE **b** : POSTERIOR NASAL SPINE

nasi — see ALA NASI, LEVATOR LABII SUPERIORIS ALAEQUE NASI

nasi- — see NAS-

na·si·on \ˈnā-zē-ˌän\ *n* : the middle point of the nasofrontal suture

naso- — see NAS-

na·so·al·ve·o·lar \ˌnā-zō-al-ˈvē-ə-lər\ *adj* : of, relating to, or affecting the nose and one or more maxillary alveoli ⟨a ~ cyst⟩

na·so·cil·i·ary \ˌnā-zō-ˈsil-lē-ˌer-ē\ *adj* : nasal and ciliary

nasociliary nerve *n* : a branch of the ophthalmic nerve distributed in part to the ciliary ganglion and in part to the mucous membrane and skin of the nose — called also *nasal nerve*

na·so·fron·tal \-ˈfrənt-ᵊl\ *adj* : of or relating to the nasal and frontal bones

nasofrontal suture *n* : the cranial suture between the nasal and frontal bones

na·so·gas·tric \-ˈgas-trik\ *adj* : of, relating to, being, or performed by intubation of the stomach by way of the nasal passages ⟨insert a ~ tube⟩

na·so·la·bi·al \-ˈlā-bē-əl\ *adj* : of, relating to, located between, or affecting the nose and the upper lip

na·so·lac·ri·mal *also* **na·so·lach·ry·mal** \-ˈla-krə-məl\ *adj* : of or relating to the lacrimal apparatus and nose

nasolacrimal duct *n* : a duct that transmits tears from the lacrimal sac to the inferior meatus of the nose

na·so·max·il·lary \-ˈmak-sə-ˌler-ē\ *adj* : of, relating to, or located between the nasal bone and the maxilla

Na·so·nex \ˈnā-zə-ˌneks\ *trademark* — used for a preparation of mometasone furoate used intranasally

na·so·pal·a·tine \-ˈpa-lə-ˌtīn\ *adj* : of, relating to, or connecting the nose and the palate

nasopalatine nerve *n* : a parasympathetic and sensory nerve that arises in the pterygopalatine ganglion, passes through the sphenopalatine foramen, across the roof of the nasal cavity to the nasal septum, and obliquely downward to and through the incisive canal, and innervates esp. the glands and mucosa of the nasal septum and the anterior part of the hard palate

na·so·pha·ryn·geal \ˌnā-zō-fə-ˈrin-jəl, -jē-əl; -ˌfar-ən-ˈjē-əl\ *adj* : of, relating to, or affecting the nose and pharynx or the nasopharynx ⟨~ cancer⟩

nasopharyngeal tonsil *n* : PHARYNGEAL TONSIL

na·so·pha·ryn·go·scope \-fə-ˈriŋ-gə-ˌskōp\ *n* : an endoscope for visually examining the nasal passages and pharynx — **na·so·pha·ryn·go·scop·ic** \-fə-ˌriŋ-gə-ˈskä-pik\ *adj* — **na·so·phar·yn·gos·co·py** \-ˌfar-ən-ˈgäs-kə-pē\

na·so·phar·ynx \-ˈfar-iŋks\ *n, pl* **-pha·ryn·ges** \-fə-ˈrin-(ˌ)jēz\ *also* **-phar·ynx·es** : the upper part of the pharynx continuous with the nasal passages — compare LARYNGOPHARYNX

na·so·tra·che·al \-ˈtrā-kē-əl\ *adj* : of, relating to, being, or performed by means of intubation of the trachea by way of the nasal passage

na·tal \ˈnāt-ᵊl\ *adj* : of or relating to birth ⟨the ~ death rate⟩

na·tal·i·ty \nā-ˈta-lə-tē, nə-\ *n, pl* **-ties** : BIRTHRATE

na·tes \ˈnā-ˌtēz\ *n pl* : BUTTOCKS

National Formulary *n* : a periodically revised book of officially established and recognized drug names and standards — abbr. *NF*

na·tri·ure·sis \ˌnā-trē-yù-ˈrē-səs\ *n* : excessive loss of cations and esp. sodium in the urine — **na·tri·uret·ic** \-ˈre-tik\ *adj or n*

natural childbirth *n* : a system of managing childbirth in which the mother receives preparatory education in order to remain conscious during and assist in delivery with minimal or no use of drugs or anesthetics

natural family planning *n* : a method of birth control that involves abstention from sexual intercourse during the period of ovulation which is determined through observation and measurement of bodily signs (as cervical mucus and body temperature)

natural food *n* : food that has undergone minimal processing and contains no preservatives or artificial additives (as synthetic flavorings)

natural history *n* : the natural development of something (as an organism or disease) over a period of time

natural immunity *n* : immunity possessed by a group (as a species or race) that is present in an individual at birth prior to exposure to a pathogen or antigen and that includes components (as intact skin, salivary enzymes, neutrophils, natural killer cells, and complement) which provide an initial response against infection — called also *innate immunity;* compare ACQUIRED IMMUNITY, ACTIVE IMMUNITY, PASSIVE IMMUNITY

natural killer cell *n* : a large granular lymphocyte esp. of destroying tumor cells or virally infected cells without prior exposure to the target cell and without having it presented with or marked by a histocompatibility antigen — called also *NK cell*

na·tu·ro·path \ˈnā-chə-rə-ˌpath, nə-ˈtyur-ə-\ *n* : a practitioner of naturopathy

na·tu·rop·a·thy \ˌnā-chə-ˈrä-pə-thē\ *n, pl* **-thies** : a system of treatment of disease that avoids drugs and surgery and emphasizes the use of natural agents (as air, water, and herbs) and physical means (as tissue manipulation and electrotherapy) — **na·tu·ro·path·ic** \ˌnā-chə-rə-ˈpa-thik, nə-ˌtyur-ə-\ *adj*

nau·sea \ˈnȯ-zē-ə, -sē-ə; ˈnȯ-zhə, -shə\ *n* : a stomach distress with distaste for food and an urge to vomit

nau·se·ant \ˈnȯ-zhənt, -zhē-ənt, -shənt, -shē-ənt\ *adj* : inducing nausea : NAUSEATING

nau·se·ate \ˈnȯ-zē-ˌāt, -zhē-, -sē-, -shē-\ *vb* **-at·ed; -at·ing** : to affect or become affected with nausea

nau·seous \ˈnȯ-shəs, ˈnȯ-zē-əs\ *adj* **1** : causing nausea **2** : affected with nausea

Nav·ane \ˈna-ˌvān\ *trademark* — used for a preparation of thiothixene

na·vel \ˈnā-vəl\ *n* : a depression in the middle of the abdomen that marks the point of former attachment of the umbilical cord to the embryo — called also *umbilicus*

navel ill *n* : a serious septicemia of newborn animals caused by pus-producing bacteria entering the body through the umbilical cord or opening — called also *joint ill*

¹na·vic·u·lar \nə-ˈvi-kyə-lər\ *n* : a navicular bone: **a** : the one of the seven tarsal bones of the human foot that is situated on the big-toe side between the talus and the cuneiform bones — called also *scaphoid* **b** : SCAPHOID 2

²navicular *adj* **1** : resembling or having the shape of a boat ⟨a ∼ bone⟩ **2** : of, relating to, or involving a navicular bone ⟨∼ fractures⟩

navicular disease *n* : inflammation of the navicular bone and forefoot of the horse

navicular fossa *n* : the dilated terminal portion of the urethra in the glans penis

navicularis — see FOSSA NAVICULARIS

Nb *symbol* niobium

NBRT *abbr* National Board for Respiratory Therapy

NCI *abbr* National Cancer Institute

Nd *symbol* neodymium

ND *abbr* doctor of naturopathy

NDT *abbr* neurodevelopmental treatment

Ne *symbol* neon

ne- *or* **neo-** *comb form* **1 a** : new : recent ⟨*neonatal*⟩ **b** : chemically new — used for compounds isomeric with or otherwise related to an indicated compound ⟨*neostigmine*⟩ **2** : new and abnormal ⟨*neoplasm*⟩

near point *n* : the point nearest the eye at which an object is accurately focused on the retina when the maximum degree of accommodation is employed — compare FAR POINT

near·sight·ed \ˈnir-ˈsī-təd\ *adj* : able to see near things more clearly than distant ones : MYOPIC — **near·sight·ed·ly** *adv*

near·sight·ed·ness *n* : MYOPIA

neb·u·li·za·tion \ˌne-byə-lə-ˈzā-shən\ *n* **1** : reduction of a medicinal solution to a fine spray **2** : treatment (as of asthma) by means of a fine spray — **neb·u·lize** \ˈne-byə-ˌlīz\ *vb*

neb·u·liz·er \-ˌlī-zər\ *n* : ATOMIZER; *specif* : an atomizer equipped to produce an extremely fine spray for deep penetration of the lungs

Ne·ca·tor \nə-ˈkā-tər\ *n* : a genus of common hookworms that include internal parasites of humans and various other mammals — compare ANCYLOSTOMA

neck \ˈnek\ *n* **1 a** : the usu. narrowed part of an animal that connects the head with the body; *specif* : the cervical region of a vertebrate **b** : the part of a tapeworm immediately behind the scolex from which new proglottids are produced **2** : a relatively narrow part suggestive of a neck: as **a** : a narrow part of a bone ⟨the ∼ of the femur⟩ **b** : CERVIX 2 **c** : the part of a tooth between the crown and the root

necr- *or* **necro-** *comb form* **1 a** : those that are dead : the dead : corpses ⟨*necrophilia*⟩ **b** : one that is dead : corpse ⟨*necropsy*⟩ **2** : death : conversion to dead tissue : atrophy ⟨*necrosis*⟩

necro \ˈne-(ˌ)krō\ *n* : NECROTIC ENTERITIS a

nec·ro·bac·il·lo·sis \ˌne-krō-ˌba-sə-ˈlō-səs\ *n, pl* **-lo·ses** \-ˌsēz\ : any of several diseases or infections (as bullnose, calf diphtheria, or foot rot) that are characterized by inflammation and ulcerative or necrotic lesions and are caused by or associated with a bacterium of the genus *Fusobacterium* (*F. necrophorum*)

nec·ro·bi·o·sis \-bī-ˈō-səs\ *n, pl* **-o·ses** \-ˌsēz\ : death of a cell or group of cells within a tissue whether normal (as in various epithelial tissues) or part of a pathologic process — compare NECROSIS

nec·ro·bi·o·sis li·poid·i·ca \-li-ˈpȯi-di-kə\ *n* : a disease of the skin that is characterized by the formation of multiple necrobiotic lesions esp. on the legs and that is often associated with diabetes mellitus

necrobiosis lipoidica dia·bet·i·co·rum \-ˌdī-ə-ˌbe-ti-ˈkȯr-əm\ *n* : NECROBIOSIS LIPOIDICA

nec·ro·bi·ot·ic \ˌne-krə-bī-ˈä-tik\ *adj* : of, relating to, or being in a state of necrobiosis

nec·ro·phile \ˈne-krə-ˌfīl\ *n* : one that is affected with necrophilia

nec·ro·phil·ia \ˌne-krə-ˈfi-lē-ə\ *n* : obsession with and usu. erotic interest in or stimulation by corpses

¹nec·ro·phil·i·ac \-ˈfi-lē-ˌak\ *adj* : of, relating to, or affected with necrophilia

²necrophiliac *n* : NECROPHILE

nec·ro·phil·ic \-ˈfi-lik\ *adj* : NECROPHILIAC

¹nec·rop·sy \ˈne-ˌkräp-sē\ *n, pl* **-sies** : AUTOPSY; *esp* : an autopsy performed on an animal

²necropsy *vb* **-sied; -sy·ing** : AUTOPSY

nec·rose \ˈne-ˌkrōs, -ˌkrōz, ne-ˈkrōz\ *vb* **nec·rosed; nec·ros·ing** : to undergo or cause to undergo necrosis

ne·cro·sis \nə-ˈkrō-sis, ne-\ *n, pl* **ne·cro·ses** \-ˌsēz\ : death of living tissue; *specif* : death of a portion of tissue differentially affected by local injury (as loss of blood supply, corrosion, burning, or the local lesion of a disease) — compare NECROBIOSIS

nec·ro·sper·mia \ˌne-krə-ˈspər-mē-ə\ *n* : a condition in which the spermatozoa in seminal fluid are dead or motionless

ne·crot·ic \nə-ˈkrä-tik, ne-\ *adj* : affected with, characterized by, or producing necrosis ⟨a ∼ gall bladder⟩

necrotic enteritis *n* : either of two often fatal infectious diseases marked esp. by intestinal inflammation and necrosis and by diarrhea: **a** : one affecting young swine and caused by a bacterium of the genus *Salmonella* (*S. choleraesuis*) — called also *necro* **b** : one affecting poultry and caused by a bacterium of the genus *Clostridium* (*C. perfringens*)

necrotic rhinitis *n* : BULLNOSE

nec·ro·tiz·ing \ˈne-krə-ˌtī-zin\ *adj* : causing, associated with, or undergoing necrosis ⟨∼ infections⟩

necrotizing angiitis *n* : NECROTIZING VASCULITIS

necrotizing fasciitis *n* : a severe soft tissue infection typically by Group A streptococci or by a mixture of aerobic and anaerobic bacteria that is marked by edema and necrosis of subcutaneous tissue with involvement of the fascia and widespread undermining of adjacent tissue, by painful

red swollen skin over affected areas, and by polymorphonuclear leukocytosis

necrotizing papillitis *n* : necrosis of the papillae of the kidney — called also *necrotizing renal papillitis*

necrotizing ulcerative gingivitis *n* : ACUTE NECROTIZING ULCERATIVE GINGIVITIS

necrotizing vasculitis *n* : an inflammatory condition of the blood vessels characterized by necrosis of vascular tissue — called also *necrotizing angiitis, systemic necrotizing vasculitis*

ne·do·cro·mil sodium \nə-ˈdä-krə-mil-\ *n* : a disodium salt $C_{19}H_{15}N$-Na_2O_7 that is similar in action to cromolyn sodium and is administered either as an aerosol by oral inhalation for the treatment of mild to moderate asthma or as eyedrops for the treatment of itching associated with allergic conjunctivitis — called also *nedocromil*

¹nee·dle \ˈnēd-ᵊl\ *n* **1** : a small slender usu. steel instrument designed to carry sutures when sewing tissues in surgery **2** : a slender hollow instrument for introducing material into or removing material from the body parenterally

²needle *vb* **nee·dled; nee·dling** : to puncture, operate on, or inject with a needle

needle biopsy *n* : any of several methods (as fine needle aspiration or core biopsy) for obtaining a sample of cells or tissue by inserting a hollow needle through the skin and withdrawing the sample from the tissue or organ to be examined

nee·dle·stick \ˈnēd-ᵊl-ˌstik\ *n* : an accidental puncture of the skin with an unsterile instrument (as a syringe) — called also *needlestick injury*

neg·a·tive \ˈne-gə-tiv\ *adj* **1** : marked by denial, prohibition, or refusal **2** : marked by features (as hostility or pessimism) that hinder or oppose constructive treatment or development **3** : being, relating to, or charged with electricity of which the electron is the elementary unit **4** : not affirming the presence of a condition, substance, or organism suspected to be present; *also* : having a test result indicating the absence esp. of a condition, substance, or organism ⟨she is HIV ∼⟩ — **negative** *n* — **neg·a·tive·ly** *adv* — **neg·a·tiv·i·ty** \ˌne-gə-ˈti-və-tē\ *n*

negative feedback *n* : feedback that tends to stabilize a process by reducing its rate or output when its effects are too great

negative pressure *n* : pressure that is less than existing atmospheric pressure

negative reinforcement *n* : psychological reinforcement by removal of an unpleasant stimulus when a desired response occurs

negative transfer *n* : the impeding of learning or performance in a situation by the carry-over of learned responses from another situation — compare INTERFERENCE 2

neg·a·tiv·ism \'ne-gə-ti-,vi-zəm\ *n* **1** : an attitude of mind marked by skepticism about nearly everything affirmed by others **2** : a tendency to refuse to do, to do the opposite of, or to do something at variance with what is asked — **neg·a·tiv·ist·ic** \,ne-gə-ti-'vis-tik\ *adj*

Neg·Gram \'neg-,gram\ *trademark* — used for a preparation of nalidixic acid

Ne·gri body \'nā-grē-\ *n* : an inclusion body found in the nerve cells in rabies

Negri, Adelchi (1876–1912), Italian physician and pathologist.

Neis·se·ria \nī-'sir-ē-ə\ *n* : a genus (family Neisseriaceae) of parasitic bacteria that grow in pairs and occas. tetrads and include the gonococcus (*N. gonorrhoeae*) and meningococcus (*N. meningitidis*)

Neis·ser \'nī-sər\, **Albert Ludwig Sigesmund (1855–1916),** German dermatologist.

neis·se·ri·an \nī-'sir-ē-ən\ *or* **neis·se·ri·al** \-ē-əl\ *adj* : of, relating to, or caused by bacteria of the genus *Neisseria* (~ infections)

nel·fin·a·vir \nel-'fi-nə-,vir\ *n* : a protease inhibitor that is administered in the form of its mesylate $C_{32}H_{45}N_3O_4S \cdot CH_4O_3S$ in the treatment of HIV infection — see VIRACEPT

nemat- *or* **nemato-** *comb form* **1** : thread 〈*nemato*cyst〉 **2** : nematode 〈*nemato*logy〉

ne·ma·ti·cide *or* **ne·ma·to·cide** \'ne-mə-tə-,sīd, ni-'ma-tə-\ *n* : a substance or preparation used to destroy nematodes — **ne·ma·to·cid·al** *also* **ne·ma·ti·cid·al** \,ne-mə-tə-'sīd-əl, ni-,ma-tə-\ *adj*

ne·ma·to·cyst \'ne-mə-tə-,sist, ni-'ma-tə-\ *n* : one of the minute stinging organelles of various coelenterates

nem·a·tode \'ne-mə-,tōd\ *n* : any of a phylum (Nematoda) of elongated cylindrical worms parasitic in animals or plants or free-living in soil or water

Nem·a·to·di·rus \,ne-mə-tə-'dī-rəs\ *n* : a genus of reddish strongylid nematode worms parasitic in the small intestine of ruminants and sometimes other mammals

nem·a·tol·o·gy \,ne-mə-'tä-lə-jē\ *n, pl* **-gies** : a branch of zoology that deals with nematodes — **nem·a·tol·o·gist** \-jist\ *n*

Nem·bu·tal \'nem-byə-,tòl\ *trademark* — used for the sodium salt of pentobarbital

neo- — see NE-

neo·ars·phen·a·mine \,nē-ō-ärs-'fe-nə-,mēn\ *n* : a yellow powder $C_{13}H_{13}As_2N_2NaO_4S$ similar to arsphenamine in structure and use — called also *neosalvarsan*

neo·cer·e·bel·lum \,nē-ō-,ser-ə-'be-ləm\ *n, pl* **-bellums** *or* **-bel·la** : the part of the cerebellum associated with the cerebral cortex in the integration of voluntary limb movements and comprising most of the cerebellar hemispheres and the superior vermis — compare PALEOCEREBELLUM — **neo·cer·e·bel·lar** \,nē-ō-,ser-ə-'bel-ər\ *adj*

neo·cin·cho·phen \,nē-ō-'siŋ-kə-,fen\ *n* : a white crystalline compound $C_{19}H_{17}NO_2$ used as an analgesic and in the treatment of gout

neo·cor·tex \,nē-ō-'kȯr-,teks\ *n, pl* **-cor·ti·ces** \-'kȯr-tə-,sēz\ *or* **-cor·texes** : the dorsal region of the cerebral cortex that is unique to mammals — **neo·cor·ti·cal** \-'kȯr-ti-kəl\ *adj*

neo·dym·i·um \,nē-ō-'di-mē-əm\ *n* : a yellow metallic element — symbol *Nd*; see ELEMENT table

¹**neo–Freud·ian** \-'frȯi-dē-ən\ *adj, often cap N* : of or relating to a school of psychoanalysis that differs from Freudian orthodoxy in emphasizing the importance of social and cultural factors in the development of an individual's personality

S. Freud, — see FREUDIAN

²**neo–Freudian** *n, often cap N* : a member of or advocate of a neo-Freudian school of psychoanalysis

neo·in·ti·ma \-'in-tə-mə\ *n* : a new or thickened layer of arterial intima formed esp. on a prosthesis or in atherosclerosis by migration and proliferation of cells from the media — **neo·in·ti·mal** \-məl\ *adj*

ne·ol·o·gism \nē-'ä-lə-,ji-zəm\ *n* **1** : a new word, usage, or expression **2** : a word coined by a psychotic individual that is meaningless except to the coiner

neo·my·cin \,nē-ə-'mīs-²n\ *n* : a broad-spectrum highly toxic mixture of antibiotics produced by a bacterium of the genus *Streptomyces* (*S. fradiae*) and used esp. to treat topical infections

ne·on \'nē-,än\ *n* : a colorless odorless primarily inert gaseous element — symbol *Ne*; see ELEMENT table

neo·na·tal \,nē-ō-'nāt-²l\ *adj* : of, relating to, or affecting the newborn and esp. the human infant during the first month after birth — compare PRENATAL, POSTNATAL — **neo·na·tal·ly** *adv*

ne·o·nate \'nē-ə-,nāt\ *n* : a newborn infant; *esp* : an infant less than a month old

neo·na·tol·o·gist \,nē-ō-nā-'tä-lə-jist\ *n* : a specialist in neonatology

neo·na·tol·o·gy \-jē\ *n, pl* **-gies** : a branch of medicine concerned with the care, development, and diseases of newborn infants

neonatorum — see ICTERUS GRAVIS NEONATORUM, ICTERUS NEONATORUM, OPHTHALMIA NEONATORUM, SCLEREMA NEONATORUM

neo·pal·li·um \nē-ō-'pa-lē-əm\ *n, pl* **-lia** \-lē-ə\ : the part of the cerebral cortex that develops from the area between the piriform lobe and the hippocampus, comprises the nonolfactory region of the cortex, and attains its maximum development in humans where it makes up the greater part of the cerebral hemisphere on each side — compare ARCHIPALLIUM

neo·pho·bia \nē-ə-'fō-bē-ə\ *n* : dread of or aversion to novelty

neo·pla·sia \nē-ə-'plā-zhə, -zhē-ə\ *n* 1 : the process of tumor formation 2 : a tumorous condition of the body — see PROSTATIC INTRAEPITHELIAL NEOPLASIA

neo·plasm \'nē-ə-ˌpla-zəm\ *n* : a new growth of tissue serving no physiological function : TUMOR

neo·plas·tic \ˌnē-ə-'plas-tik\ *adj* : of, relating to, or constituting a neoplasm or neoplasia — **neo·plas·ti·cal·ly** *adv*

neo·sal·var·san \ˌnē-ō-'sal-vər-ˌsan\ *n* : NEOARSPHENAMINE

neo·stig·mine \ˌnē-ə-'stig-ˌmēn\ *n* : an anticholinesterase that is used in the form of its bromide $C_{12}H_{19}BrN_2O_2$ or a sulfate derivative $C_{13}H_{22}N_2O_6S$ esp. in the diagnosis and treatment of myasthenia gravis and in the treatment of urinary bladder or bowel atony — see PROSTIGMIN

neo·stri·a·tum \ˌnē-ō-(ˌ)strī-'ā-təm\ *n, pl* **-tums** *or* **-ta** \-tə\ : the evolutionarily newer part of the corpus striatum consisting of the caudate nucleus and putamen — **neo·stri·a·tal** \-'āt-ᵊl\ *adj*

Neo-Sy·neph·rine \ˌnē-ō-si-'ne-frən, -ˌfrēn\ *trademark* — used for a preparation of the hydrochloride of phenylephrine

neo·vas·cu·lar·iza·tion \-ˌvas-kyə-lə-rə-'zā-shən\ *n* : vascularization esp. in abnormal quantity (as in some conditions of the retina) or in abnormal tissue (as a tumor) — **neo·vas·cu·lar** \ˌnē-ō-'vas-kyə-lər\ *adj* — **neo·vas·cu·lar·i·ty** \-ˌvas-kyə-'lar-ə-tē\ *n*

neph·e·lom·e·ter \ˌne-fə-'lä-mə-tər\ *n* : an instrument for measuring turbidity (as to determine the number of bacteria suspended in a fluid) — **neph·e·lo·met·ric** \ˌne-fə-lō-'me-trik\ *adj* — **neph·e·lom·e·try** \-'läm-ə-trē\ *n*

nephr- *or* **nephro-** *comb form* : kidney 〈*nephr*ectomy〉 〈*nephro*logy〉

ne·phrec·to·my \ni-'frek-tə-mē\ *n, pl* **-mies** : the surgical removal of a kidney — **ne·phrec·to·mize** \-ˌmīz\ *vb*

neph·ric \'ne-frik\ *adj* : RENAL

ne·phrit·ic \ni-'fri-tik\ *adj* 1 : RENAL 2 : of, relating to, or affected with nephritis

ne·phri·tis \ni-'frī-təs\ *n, pl* **ne·phrit·i·des** \-'fri-tə-ˌdēz\ : acute or chronic inflammation of the kidney affecting the structure (as of the glomerulus or parenchyma) and caused by infection, a degenerative process, or vascu-

lar disease — compare NEPHROSCLE-ROSIS, NEPHROSIS

neph·ri·to·gen·ic \ˌne-frə-tə-'je-nik, -ˌfri-tə-\ *adj* : causing nephritis

neph·ro·blas·to·ma \ˌne-frō-blas-'tō-mə\ *n, pl* **-mas** *also* **-ma·ta** \-mə-tə\ : WILMS' TUMOR

neph·ro·cal·ci·no·sis \ˌne-frō-ˌkal-si-'nō-səs\ *n, pl* **-no·ses** \-ˌsēz\ : a condition marked by calcification of the tubules of the kidney

neph·ro·gen·ic \ˌne-frə-'je-nik\ *adj* 1 : originating in the kidney : caused by factors originating in the kidney 〈~ hypertension〉 2 : developing into or producing kidney tissue

nephrogenic diabetes insipidus *n* : diabetes insipidus that is caused by partial or complete failure of the kidneys to respond to vasopressin

neph·ro·gram \'ne-frə-ˌgram\ *n* : an X-ray of the kidney

ne·phrog·ra·phy \ni-'frä-grə-fē\ *n, pl* **-phies** : radiography of the kidney

-nephroi *pl of* -NEPHROS

neph·ro·li·thi·a·sis \ˌne-frō-li-'thī-ə-səs\ *n, pl* **-a·ses** \-ˌsēz\ : a condition marked by the presence of renal calculi

neph·ro·li·thot·o·my \-li-'thä-tə-mē\ *n, pl* **-mies** : the surgical operation of removing a calculus from the kidney

ne·phrol·o·gist \ni-'frä-lə-jist\ *n* : a specialist in nephrology

ne·phrol·o·gy \ni-'frä-lə-jē\ *n, pl* **-gies** : a medical specialty concerned with the kidneys and esp. with their structure, functions, or diseases

ne·phro·ma \ni-'frō-mə\ *n, pl* **-mas** *also* **-ma·ta** \-mə-tə\ : a malignant tumor of the renal cortex

neph·ron \'ne-ˌfrän\ *n* : a single excretory unit of the vertebrate kidney typically consisting of a Malpighian corpuscle, proximal convoluted tubule, loop of Henle, distal convoluted tubule, collecting tubule, and vascular and supporting tissues and discharging by way of a renal papilla into the renal pelvis

ne·phrop·a·thy \ni-'frä-pə-thē\ *n, pl* **-thies** : an abnormal state of the kidney; *esp* : one associated with or secondary to some other pathological process — **neph·ro·path·ic** \ˌne-frə-'pa-thik\ *adj*

neph·ro·pexy \'ne-frə-ˌpek-sē\ *n, pl* **-pex·ies** : surgical fixation of a floating kidney

neph·rop·to·sis \ˌne-ˌfräp-'tō-səs\ *n, pl* **-to·ses** \-ˌsēz\ : abnormal mobility of the kidney : floating kidney

ne·phror·rha·phy \ne-'frȯr-ə-fē\ *n, pl* **-phies** 1 : the fixation of a floating kidney by suturing it to the posterior abdominal wall 2 : the suturing of a kidney wound

-nephros \'ne-frəs, -ˌfräs\ *n comb form, pl* **-neph·roi** \'ne-ˌfrȯi\ : kidney 〈pronephros〉

neph·ro·scle·ro·sis \ˌne-frō-sklə-'rō-səs\ *n, pl* **-ro·ses** \-ˌsēz\ : hardening of the kidney; *specif* : a condition that is characterized by sclerosis of the renal arterioles with reduced blood flow and contraction of the kidney, that is associated usu. with hypertension, and that terminates in renal failure and uremia — compare NEPHRITIS — **neph·ro·scle·rot·ic** \-'rä-tik\ *adj*

neph·ro·scope \'ne-frə-ˌskōp\ *n* : an endoscope used for inspecting and passing instruments into the interior of the kidney — **neph·ros·co·py** \ni-'frä-skə-pē\ *n*

ne·phro·sis \ni-'frō-səs\ *n, pl* **ne·phro·ses** \-ˌsēz\ : a noninflammatory disease of the kidneys chiefly affecting function of the nephrons; *esp* : NEPHROTIC SYNDROME — compare NEPHRITIS

ne·phros·to·gram \ni-'fräs-tə-ˌgram\ *n* : a radiograph of the renal pelvis after injection of a radiopaque substance through an opening formed by nephrostomy

ne·phros·to·my \ni-'fräs-tə-mē\ *n, pl* **-mies** : the surgical formation of an opening between a renal pelvis and the outside of the body

ne·phrot·ic \ni-'frä-tik\ *adj* : of, relating to, affected by, or associated with nephrosis ⟨∼ edema⟩ ⟨a ∼ patient⟩

nephrotic syndrome *n* : an abnormal condition that is marked by deficiency of albumin in the blood and by excess excretion of proteins in the urine due to altered permeability of the glomerular basement membranes

neph·ro·to·mo·gram \ˌne-frō-'tō-mə-ˌgram\ *n* : a radiograph made by nephrotomography

neph·ro·to·mog·ra·phy \-tō-'mä-grə-fē\ *n, pl* **-phies** : tomographic visualization of the kidney usu. combined with intravenous nephrography — **neph·ro·to·mo·graph·ic** \-ˌtō-mə-'gra-fik\ *adj*

ne·phrot·o·my \ni-'frä-tə-mē\ *n, pl* **-mies** : surgical incision of a kidney (as for the extraction of a calculus)

neph·ro·tox·ic \ˌne-frə-'täk-sik\ *adj* : poisonous to the kidney ⟨∼ drugs⟩; *also* : resulting from or marked by poisoning of the kidney ⟨∼ effects⟩ — **neph·ro·tox·ic·i·ty** \-täk-'si-sə-tē\ *n*

neph·ro·tox·in \-'täk-sən\ *n* : a cytotoxin that is destructive to kidney cells

Nep·ta·zane \'nep-tə-ˌzān\ *trademark* — used for a preparation of methazolamide

nep·tu·ni·um \nep-'tü-nē-əm, -'tyü-\ *n* : a radioactive metallic element — symbol *Np*; see ELEMENT table

nerve \'nərv\ *n* **1** : any of the filamentous bands of nervous tissue that connect parts of the nervous system with the other organs, conduct nervous impulses, and are made up of axons and dendrites together with protective and supportive structures and that for the larger nerves have the fibers gathered into funiculi surrounded by a perineurium and the funiculi enclosed in a common epineurium **2 nerves** *pl* : a state or condition of nervous agitation or irritability **3** : the sensitive pulp of a tooth

nerve block *n* **1** : an interruption of the passage of impulses through a nerve (as with pressure or narcotization) — called also *nerve blocking* **2** : BLOCK ANESTHESIA

nerve cell *n* : NEURON; *also* : CELL BODY

nerve center *n* : CENTER

nerve cord *n* : the dorsal tubular cord of nervous tissue above the notochord that in vertebrates includes or develops an anterior enlargement comprising the brain and a more posterior part comprising the spinal cord with the two together making up the central nervous system

nerve deafness *n* : hearing loss or impairment resulting from injury to or loss of function of the organ of Corti or the auditory nerve — called also *perceptive deafness;* compare CENTRAL DEAFNESS, CONDUCTION DEAFNESS

nerve ending *n* : the structure in which the distal end of the axon of a nerve fiber terminates

nerve fiber *n* : any of the processes (as an axon or a dendrite) of a neuron

nerve gas *n* : an organophosphate chemical weapon that interferes with normal nerve transmission and induces intense bronchial spasm with resulting inhibition of respiration

nerve growth factor *n* : a protein that promotes development of the sensory and sympathetic nervous systems and is required for maintenance of sympathetic neurons — abbr. *NGF*

nerve impulse *n* : the progressive physicochemical change in the membrane of a nerve fiber that follows stimulation and serves to transmit a record of sensation from a receptor or an instruction to act to an effector — called also *nervous impulse*

nerve of Her·ing \-'her-iŋ\ *n* : a nerve that arises from the main trunk of the glossopharyngeal nerve and runs along the internal carotid artery to supply afferent fibers esp. to the baroreceptors of the carotid sinus

    Hering, Heinrich Ewald (1866–1948), German physiologist.

nerve sheath *n* : NEURILEMMA

nerve trunk *n* : a bundle of nerve fibers enclosed in a connective tissue sheath

nervi *pl of* NERVUS

nerv·ing \'nər-viŋ\ *n* : the removal of part of a nerve trunk in chronic inflammation in order to cure lameness (as of a horse) by destroying sensation in the parts supplied

nervosa — see ANOREXIA NERVOSA, PARS NERVOSA

ner·vous \'nər-vəs\ *adj* **1** : of, relating to, or composed of neurons ⟨the ∼ layer of the eye⟩ **2 a** : of or relating to the nerves; *also* : originating in or affected by the nerves ⟨∼ energy⟩ **b** : easily excited or irritated — **ner·vous·ly** *adv* — **ner·vous·ness** *n*

nervous breakdown *n* : an attack of mental or emotional disorder esp. when of sufficient severity to require hospitalization

nervous impulse *n* : NERVE IMPULSE

nervous system *n* : the bodily system that in vertebrates is made up of the brain and spinal cord, nerves, ganglia, and parts of the receptor organs and that receives and interprets stimuli and transmits impulses to the effector organs — see AUTONOMIC NERVOUS SYSTEM, CENTRAL NERVOUS SYSTEM, PERIPHERAL NERVOUS SYSTEM

ner·vus \'nər-vəs, 'ner-\ *n, pl* **ner·vi** \'nər-,vī, 'ner-,vē\ : NERVE 1

nervus er·i·gens \-'er-i-jenz\ *n, pl* **nervi er·i·gen·tes** \-,er-i-'jen-(,)tēz\ : PELVIC SPLANCHNIC NERVE

nervus in·ter·me·di·us \-,in-tər-'mē-dē-əs\ *n* : the branch of the facial nerve that contains sensory and parasympathetic fibers and that supplies the anterior tongue and parts of the palate and fauces — called also *glossopalatine nerve*

nervus ra·di·a·lis \-,rā-dē-'ā-ləs\ *n, pl* **nervi ra·di·a·les** \-(,)lēz\ : RADIAL NERVE

nervus ter·mi·na·lis \-,tər-mə-'nā-ləs\ *n, pl* **nervi ter·mi·na·les** \-(,)lēz\ : a group of ganglionated nerve fibers that arise in the cerebral hemisphere near where the nerve tract leading from the olfactory bulb joins the temporal lobe and that pass anteriorly along this tract and the olfactory bulb through the cribriform plate to the nasal mucosa — called also *terminal nerve*

Nes·a·caine \'ne-sə-,kān\ *trademark* — used for a preparation of chloroprocaine

net·tle \'net-ᵊl\ *n* **1** : any plant of the genus *Urtica* **2** : any of various prickly or stinging plants other than one of the genus *Urtica*

nettle rash *n* : an eruption on the skin caused by or resembling the condition produced by stinging with nettles : HIVES

Neu·po·gen \'nü-pə-jən, 'nyü-\ *trademark* — used for a preparation of filgrastim

neur- *or* **neuro-** *comb form* **1** : nerve ⟨*neural*⟩ ⟨*neurology*⟩ **2** : neural : neural and ⟨*neuromuscular*⟩

neu·ral \'nùr-əl, -'nyùr-\ *adj* **1** : of, relating to, or affecting a nerve or the nervous system **2** : situated in the region of or on the same side of the body as the brain and spinal cord : DORSAL — compare HEMAL 2 — **neu·ral·ly** *adv*

neural arch *n* : the cartilaginous or bony arch enclosing the spinal cord on the dorsal side of a vertebra — called also *vertebral arch*

neural canal *n* **1** : VERTEBRAL CANAL **2** : the cavity or system of cavities in a vertebrate embryo that form the central canal of the spinal cord and the ventricles of the brain

neural crest *n* : the ridge of one of the folds forming the neural tube that gives rise to the spinal ganglia and various structures of the autonomic nervous system — called also *neural ridge;* compare NEURAL PLATE

neural fold *n* : the lateral longitudinal fold on each side of the neural plate that by folding over and fusing with the opposite fold gives rise to the neural tube

neu·ral·gia \nù-'ral-jə, nyù-\ *n* : acute paroxysmal pain radiating along the course of one or more nerves usu. without demonstrable changes in the nerve structure — compare NEURITIS — **neu·ral·gic** \-jik\ *adj*

neural groove *n* : the median dorsal longitudinal groove formed in the vertebrate embryo by the neural plate after the appearance of the neural folds — called also *medullary groove*

neural lobe *n* : the expanded distal portion of the neurohypophysis — called also *infundibular process, pars nervosa*

neural plate *n* : a thickened plate of ectoderm along the dorsal midline of the early embryo that gives rise to the neural tube and crests

neural ridge *n* : NEURAL CREST

neural tube *n* : the hollow longitudinal dorsal tube that is formed by infolding and subsequent fusion of the opposite ectodermal folds in the vertebrate embryo and gives rise to the brain and spinal cord

neural tube defect *n* : any of various congenital defects (as anencephaly and spina bifida) caused by incomplete closure of the neural tube during the early stages of embryonic development

neur·amin·ic acid \,nùr-ə-'mi-nik-, ,nyùr-\ *n* : an amino acid $C_9H_{17}NO_8$ that is essentially a carbohydrate and occurs in the form of acyl derivatives

neur·amin·i·dase \,nùr-ə-'mi-nə-,dās, ,nyùr-, -,dāz\ *n* : a hydrolytic enzyme that occurs on the surface of the pneumococcus, the orthomyxoviruses, and some paramyxoviruses and that cleaves terminal acetylated neuraminic acids from sugar residues (as in glycoproteins and mucoproteins)

neuraminidase inhibitor *n* : any of a class of antiviral drugs (as oseltamivir or zanamir) used for prophylaxis against or treatment of influenza A or B that inhibit the action of viral neuraminidase so that the release of newly formed viruses from infected cells is impeded

neur·aprax·ia \ˌn(y)ùr-ə-'prak-sē-ə, ˌnyùr-, -ˌ(ˌ)ā-\ *n* : an injury to a nerve that interrupts conduction causing temporary paralysis but not degeneration and that is followed by a complete and rapid recovery

neur·as·the·nic \-'the-nik\ *adj* : of, relating to, or having neurasthenia

¹**neur·as·the·nia** \ˌnùr-əs-'thē-nē-ə, ˌnyùr-\ *n* : a condition that is characterized esp. by physical and mental exhaustion usu. with accompanying symptoms (as headaches, insomnia, and irritability), is believed to result from psychological factors (as emotional stress), and is sometimes considered similar to or identical with chronic fatigue syndrome

²**neurasthenic** *n* : a person affected with neurasthenia

neur·ax·is \nùr-'ak-səs, nyùr-\ *n, pl* **neur·ax·es** \-ˌsēz\ : CENTRAL NERVOUS SYSTEM

neu·rec·to·my \nù-'rek-tə-mē, nyù-\ *n, pl* **-mies** : the surgical excision of part of a nerve

neu·ri·lem·ma \ˌnùr-ə-'le-mə, ˌnyùr-\ *n* : the outer layer surrounding a Schwann cell of a myelinated axon — called also *nerve sheath, Schwann's sheath, sheath of Schwann* — **neu·ri·lem·mal** \-'le-məl\ *adj*

neu·ri·lem·mo·ma or **neu·ri·le·mo·ma** or **neu·ro·lem·mo·ma** \-lə-'mō-mə\ *n, pl* **-mas** *also* **-ma·ta** \-mə-tə\ : a tumor of the myelinated sheaths of nerve fibers that consist of Schwann cells in a matrix — called also *neurinoma, schwannoma*

neu·ri·no·ma \ˌnùr-ə-'nō-mə, ˌnyùr-\ *n, pl* **-mas** *also* **-ma·ta** \-mə-tə\ : NEURILEMMOMA

neu·rite \'n(y)ù-ˌrīt\ *n* : AXON; *also* : DENDRITE

neu·ri·tis \nù-'rī-təs, nyù-\ *n, pl* **-rit·i·des** \-'ri-tə-ˌdēz\ *or* **-ri·tis·es** : an inflammatory or degenerative lesion of a nerve marked esp. by pain, sensory disturbances, and impaired or lost reflexes — compare NEURALGIA — **neu·rit·ic** \-'ri-tik\ *adj*

neu·ro \'nù-ˌrō, 'nyù-\ *adj* : NEUROLOGICAL

neuro- see NEUR-

neu·ro·ac·tive \ˌnùr-ō-'ak-tiv, ˌnyùr-\ *adj* : stimulating neural tissue

neu·ro·anat·o·my \-ə-'na-tə-mē\ *n, pl* **-mies** : the anatomy of nervous tissue and the nervous system — **neu·ro·ana·tom·i·cal** \-ˌa-nə-'tä-mi-kəl\ *also* **neu·ro·ana·tom·ic** \-mik\ *adj* — **neu·ro·ana·tom·i·cal·ly** \-mi-k(ə-)lē\ *adv* — **neu·ro·anat·o·mist** \-'na-tə-mist\ *n*

neu·ro·ar·throp·a·thy \-är-'thrä-pə-thē\ *n, pl* **-thies** : a joint disease (as Charcot's joint) that is associated with a disorder of the nervous system

neu·ro·be·hav·ior·al \-bi-'hā-vyə-rəl\ *adj* : of or relating to the relationship between the action of the nervous system and behavior

neu·ro·bi·ol·o·gy \-bī-'ä-lə-jē\ *n, pl* **-gies** : a branch of biology that deals with the anatomy, physiology, and pathology of the nervous system — **neu·ro·bi·o·log·i·cal** \-ˌbī-ə-'lä-ji-kəl\ *also* **neu·ro·bi·o·log·ic** \-jik\ *adj* — **neu·ro·bi·o·log·i·cal·ly** \-ji-k(ə-)lē\ *adv* — **neu·ro·bi·ol·o·gist** \-bī-'ä-lə-jist\ *n*

neu·ro·blast \'nùr-ə-ˌblast, 'nyùr-\ *n* : a cellular precursor of a nerve cell; *esp* : an undifferentiated embryonic nerve cell — **neu·ro·blas·tic** \ˌnùr-ə-'blas-tik, ˌnyùr-\ *adj*

neu·ro·blas·to·ma \ˌnùr-ō-blas-'tō-mə, ˌnyùr-\ *n, pl* **-mas** *also* **-ma·ta** \-mə-tə\ : a malignant tumor formed of embryonic ganglion cells

neu·ro·bor·rel·i·o·sis \-bə-ˌre-lē-'ō-səs\ *n, pl* **-o·ses** \-ˌsēz\ : disease of the central nervous system caused by infection with a spirochete of the genus *Borrelia*; *esp* : a late stage of Lyme disease typically involving the skin, joints, and central nervous system

neu·ro·car·dio·gen·ic syncope \-ˌkär-dē-(ˌ)ō-'je-nik-\ : VASOVAGAL SYNCOPE

neu·ro·cen·trum \-'sen-trəm\ *n, pl* **-trums** *or* **-tra** \-tra\ : either of the two dorsal elements of a vertebra that unite to form a neural arch from which the vertebral spine is developed — **neu·ro·cen·tral** \-'sen-trəl\ *adj*

neu·ro·chem·is·try \-'ke-mə-strē\ *n, pl* **-tries 1** : the study of the chemical makeup and activities of nervous tissue **2** : chemical processes and phenomena related to the nervous system — **neu·ro·chem·i·cal** \-'ke-mi-kəl\ *adj or n* — **neu·ro·chem·i·cal·ly** \-mi-k(ə-)lē\ *adv* — **neu·ro·chem·ist** \-'ke-mist\ *n*

neu·ro·cir·cu·la·to·ry \-'sər-kyə-lə-ˌtōr-ē\ *adj* : of or relating to the nervous and circulatory systems

neurocirculatory asthenia *n* : a condition marked by shortness of breath, fatigue, rapid pulse, and heart palpitation sometimes with extra beats that occurs chiefly with exertion and is not due to physical disease of the heart — called also *cardiac neurosis, effort syndrome, soldier's heart*

neu·ro·cog·ni·tive \-'käg-nə-tiv\ *n* : of, relating to, or involving the central nervous system and cognitive abilities ⟨∼ deficits⟩

neu·ro·cra·ni·um \-'krā-nē-əm\ *n, pl* **-ni·ums** *or* **-nia** \-nē-ə\ : the portion of the skull that encloses and protects the brain — **neu·ro·cra·ni·al** \-nē-əl\ *adj*

neu·ro·cu·ta·ne·ous \-kyù-'tā-nē-əs\ *adj* : of, relating to, or affecting the skin and nerves ⟨a ∼ syndrome⟩

neu·ro·cys·ti·cer·co·sis \-ˌsi-stə-(ˌ)sər-'kō-səs\ *n, pl* **-co·ses** \-ˌsēz\ : infection of the central nervous system with cysticerci of the pork tapeworm

neu·ro·cy·to·ma \-sī-'tō-mə\ *n, pl* **-mas** *also* **-ma·ta** \-mə-tə\ : any of various tumors of nerve tissue arising in the central or sympathetic nervous system

neu·ro·de·gen·er·a·tive \-di-'je-nə-rə-tiv, -,rā-\ *adj* : relating to or characterized by degeneration of nervous tissue — **neu·ro·de·gen·er·a·tion** \-je-nə-'rā-shən\ *n*

neu·ro·der·ma·ti·tis \-,dər-mə-'tī-təs\ *n, pl* **-ti·tis·es** *or* **-tit·i·des** \-'ti-tə-,dēz\ : chronic eczematous dermatitis arising from repeated rubbing or scratching of a real or imagined irritation of the skin — see LICHEN SIMPLEX CHRONICUS

neu·ro·de·vel·op·ment \-di-'ve-ləp-mənt\ *n* : the development of the nervous system — **neu·ro·de·vel·op·ment·al** \-,ve-ləp-'ment-°l\ *adj*

neu·ro·di·ag·nos·tic \-,dī-ig-'näs-tik\ *adj* : of or relating to the diagnosis of diseases of the nervous system

neu·ro·dy·nam·ic \-dī-'na-mik\ *adj* : of, relating to, or involving communication between different parts of the nervous system — **neu·ro·dy·nam·ics** \-miks\ *n*

neu·ro·ec·to·derm \-'ek-tə-,dərm\ *n* : embryonic ectoderm that gives rise to nervous tissue — **neu·ro·ec·to·der·mal** \-,ek-tə-'dər-məl\ *adj*

neu·ro·ef·fec·tor \-i-'fek-tər, -,tòr\ *adj* : of, relating to, or involving both neural and effector components

neu·ro·elec·tric \-i-'lek-trik\ *also* **neu·ro·elec·tri·cal** \-tri-kəl\ *adj* : of or relating to the electrical phenomena (as potentials or signals) generated by the nervous system

neu·ro·en·do·crine \-'en-də-krən, -,krīn, -,krēn\ *adj* **1** : of, relating to, or being a hormonal substance that influences the activity of nerves **2** : of, relating to, or functioning in neurosecretion

neu·ro·en·do·cri·nol·o·gy \-,en-də-kri-'nä-lə-jē, -(,)krī-\ *n, pl* **-gies** : a branch of biology dealing with neurosecretion and the physiological interaction between the central nervous system and the endocrine system — **neu·ro·en·do·cri·no·log·i·cal** \-,kri-nəl-'äj-i-kəl, -,krī-, -,krē-\ *also* **neu·ro·en·do·cri·no·log·ic** \-nə-'lä-jik\ *adj* — **neu·ro·en·do·cri·nol·o·gist** \-'nä-lə-jist\ *n*

neu·ro·ep·i·the·li·al \,nùr-ō-,e-pə-'thē-lē-əl, ,nyùr-\ *adj* **1** : of or relating to neuroepithelium **2** : having qualities of both neural and epithelial cells

neu·ro·ep·i·the·li·o·ma \-,thē-lē-'ō-mə\ *n, pl* **-mas** *also* **-ma·ta** \-mə-tə\ : a neurocytoma or glioma esp. of the retina

neu·ro·ep·i·the·li·um \-'thē-lē-əm\ *n, pl* **-lia** \-lē-ə\ **1** : the part of the embryonic ectoderm that gives rise to the nervous system **2** : the modified epithelium of an organ of special sense

neu·ro·fi·bril \,nùr-ō-'fī-brəl, ,nyùr-, -'fi-\ *n* : a fine proteinaceous fibril found in cytoplasm (as of a neuron) and capable of conducting excitation — **neu·ro·fi·bril·lary** \-brə-,ler-ē\ *also* **neu·ro·fi·bril·lar** \-brə-lər\ *adj*

neurofibrillary tangle *n* : a pathological accumulation of paired helical filaments composed of abnormally formed tau protein that is found chiefly in the cytoplasm of nerve cells of the brain and esp. the cerebral cortex and hippocampus and that occurs typically in Alzheimer's disease

neu·ro·fi·bro·ma \-fī-'brō-mə\ *n, pl* **-mas** *also* **-ma·ta** \-mə-tə\ : a fibroma composed of nervous and connective tissue and produced by proliferation of Schwann cells

neu·ro·fi·bro·ma·to·sis \-fī-,brō-mə-'tō-səs\ *n, pl* **-to·ses** \-,sēz\ : a disorder inherited as an autosomal dominant and characterized by brown spots on the skin, neurofibromas of peripheral nerves, and deformities of subcutaneous tissues and bone — abbr. *NF;* called also *Recklinghausen's disease, von Recklinghausen's disease*

neu·ro·fi·bro·sar·co·ma \-fī-,brō-sär-'kō-mə\ *n, pl* **-mas** *also* **-ma·ta** \-mə-tə\ : a malignant neurofibroma

neu·ro·fil·a·ment \-'fi-lə-mənt\ *n* : a microscopic filament of protein that is found in the cytoplasm of neurons and that with neurotubules makes up the structure of neurofibrils — **neu·ro·fil·a·men·tous** \-,fi-lə-'men-təs\ *adj*

neu·ro·gen·e·sis \,nùr-ə-'je-nə-səs, ,nyùr-\ *n, pl* **-e·ses** \-,sēz\ : development of nerves, nervous tissue, or the nervous system

neu·ro·ge·net·ics \-jə-'ne-tiks\ *n* : a branch of genetics dealing with the nervous system and esp. with its development

neu·ro·gen·ic \,nùr-ō-'je-nik, ,nyùr-\ *also* **neu·ro·ge·nous** \nù-'rä-jə-nəs, nyù-\ *adj* **1 a** : originating in nervous tissue ⟨a ∼ tumor⟩ **b** : induced, controlled, or modified by nervous factors; *esp* : disordered because of abnormally altered neural relations ⟨the ∼ kidney⟩ **2 a** : constituting the neural component of a bodily process ⟨∼ factors in disease⟩ **b** : taking place in or viewed as taking place in ordered rhythmic fashion under the control of a network of nerve cells scattered in the cardiac muscle ⟨a ∼ heartbeat⟩ — compare MYOGENIC 2 — **neu·ro·gen·i·cal·ly** *adv*

neu·ro·glia \nù-'rō-glē-ə, nyù-, -'rä-; ,nùr-ə-'glē-ə, ,nyùr-, -'glī-\ *n* : GLIA — **neu·ro·gli·al** \-əl\ *adj*

neu·ro·his·tol·o·gy \,nùr-ō-hi-'stä-lə-jē, nyùr-\ *n, pl* **-gies** : a branch of histology concerned with the nervous system — **neu·ro·his·to·log·i·cal** \-,his-tə-'lä-ji-kəl\ *also* **neu·ro·his·to·log·ic** \-'lä-jik\ *adj* — **neu·ro·his·tol·o·gist** \-hi-'stä-lə-jist\ *n*

neu·ro·hor·mon·al \-hòr-'mōn-°l\ *adj* **1** : involving both neural and hormonal mechanisms **2** : of, relating to, or being a neurohormone

neu·ro·hor·mone \-'hȯr-ˌmōn\ *n* : a hormone (as norepinephrine) produced by or acting on nervous tissue

neu·ro·hu·mor \-'hyü-mər, -'yü-\ *n* : NEUROHORMONE; *esp* : NEUROTRANSMITTER — **neu·ro·hu·mor·al** \-mə-rəl\ *adj*

neu·ro·hy·po·phy·se·al *or* **neu·ro·hy·po·phy·si·al** \-(ˌ)hī-pä-fə-'sē-əl, -ˌhī-pə-fə-, -ˌzē-; -ˌhī-pə-'fi-zē-əl\ *adj* : of, relating to, or secreted by the neurohypophysis ⟨~ hormones⟩

neu·ro·hy·poph·y·sis \-hī-'pä-fə-səs\ *n* : the portion of the pituitary gland that is derived from the embryonic brain, is composed of the infundibulum and neural lobe, and is concerned with the secretion of various hormones — called also *posterior pituitary gland*; compare ADENOHYPOPHYSIS

neu·ro·im·ag·ing \-'i-mə-jiŋ\ *n* : a clinical specialty concerned with producing images of the brain by noninvasive techniques (as computed tomography, magnetic resonance imaging, and positron-emission tomography); *also* : imaging of the brain by these techniques

neu·ro·im·mu·nol·o·gy \-ˌi-myə-'nä-lə-jē\ *n, pl* **-gies** : a branch of immunology that deals esp. with the interrelationships of the nervous system and immune responses and autoimmune disorders — **neu·ro·im·mu·no·log·i·cal** \-nə-'lä-ji-kəl\ *adj*

neurolemmoma *var of* NEURILEMMOMA

neu·ro·lept·an·al·ge·sia \-ˌlep-tan-əl-'jē-zhə, -zhē-ə, -zē-ə\ *also* **neu·ro·lep·to·an·al·ge·sia** \-ˌlep-tō-ˌan-əl-\ *n* : joint administration of a tranquilizing drug and an analgesic esp. for relief of surgical pain — **neu·ro·lept·an·al·ge·sic** \-'jē-zik, -sik\ *adj*

neu·ro·lep·tic \-'lep-tik\ *n* : ANTIPSYCHOTIC

neu·ro·lin·guis·tics \-liŋ-'gwis-tiks\ *n* : the study of the relationships between the human nervous system and language esp. with respect to the correspondence between disorders of language and the nervous system — **neu·ro·lin·guis·tic** \-tik\ *adj*

neu·rol·o·gist \nu̇-'rä-lə-jist, nyu̇-\ *n* : a person specializing in neurology; *esp* : a physician skilled in the diagnosis and treatment of disease of the nervous system

neu·rol·o·gy \-jē\ *n, pl* **-gies** : a branch of medicine concerned esp. with the structure, function, and diseases of the nervous system — **neu·ro·log·i·cal** \ˌnu̇r-ə-'lä-ji-kəl, ˌnyu̇r-\ *or* **neu·ro·log·ic** \-jik\ *adj* — **neu·ro·log·i·cal·ly** *adv*

neu·rol·y·sis \nu̇-'rä-lə-səs, nyu̇-\ *n, pl* **-y·ses** \-ˌsēz\ **1 a** : the breaking down of nervous tissue (as from disease or injury) **b** : destruction of nervous tissue (as by the use of chemicals or radio frequencies) to temporarily or permanently block nerve pathways esp. to relieve pain or spasticity **2** : the surgical operation of freeing a nerve from perineural adhesions — **neu·ro·lyt·ic** \ˌnu̇r-ə-'li-tik, ˌnyu̇r-\ *adj*

neu·ro·ma \nu̇-'rō-mə, nyu̇-\ *n, pl* **-mas** *also* **-ma·ta** \-mə-tə\ **1** : a tumor or mass growing from a nerve and usu. consisting of nerve fibers **2** : a mass of nerve tissue in an amputation stump resulting from abnormal regrowth of the stumps of severed nerves — called also *amputation neuroma*

neu·ro·mod·u·la·tor \ˌnu̇r-ō-'mä-jə-ˌlā-tər, ˌnyu̇r-\ *n* : something (as a polypeptide) that potentiates or inhibits the transmission of a nerve impulse but is not the actual means of transmission itself — **neu·ro·mod·u·la·to·ry** \-lə-ˌtȯr-ē\ *adj*

neu·ro·mo·tor \-'mō-tər\ *adj* : relating to efferent nervous impulses

neu·ro·mus·cu·lar \-'məs-kyə-lər\ *adj* : of or relating to nerves and muscles; *esp* : jointly involving nervous and muscular elements ⟨~ disease⟩

neuromuscular junction *n* : the junction of an efferent nerve fiber and the muscle fiber plasma membrane — called also *myoneural junction*

neuromuscular spindle *n* : MUSCLE SPINDLE

neu·ro·my·eli·tis \ˌnu̇r-ō-ˌmī-ə-'lī-təs, ˌnyu̇r-\ *n* **1** : inflammation of the medullary substance of the nerves **2** : inflammation of both spinal cord and nerves

neu·ro·my·op·a·thy \-ˌmī-'ä-pə-thē\ *n, pl* **-thies** : a disease of nerves and associated muscle tissue

neu·ron \'nu̇-ˌrän, 'nyü-ˌrän, 'nyü-\ *also* **neu·rone** \-ˌrōn\ *n* : one of the cells that constitute nervous tissue, that have the property of transmitting and receiving nervous impulses, and that possess cytoplasmic processes which are highly differentiated frequently as multiple dendrites or usu. as solitary axons and which conduct impulses toward and away from the cell body — called also *nerve cell* — **neu·ro·nal** \'nu̇-rən-əl, 'nyu̇-; nu̇-'rōn-əl, nyu̇-\ *also* **neu·ron·ic** \nu̇-'rä-nik, nyu̇-\ *adj*

neu·ro·neu·ro·nal \ˌnu̇r-ō-'nu̇-rən-əl, ˌnyu̇r-ō-'nyu̇-; ˌnu̇r-ō-nu̇-'rōn-əl, ˌnyu̇r-ō-nyu̇-\ *adj* : between neurons or nerve fibers

neu·ron·itis \ˌnu̇r-ō-'nī-təs, ˌnyu̇r-\ *n* : inflammation of neurons; *esp* : neuritis involving nerve roots and neurons within the spinal cord

neu·ro·no·tro·pic \-'trō-pik, -'trä-\ *adj* : having an affinity for neurons : NEUROTROPIC

Neu·ron·tin \'nu̇r-än-tin\ *trademark* — used for a preparation of gabapentin

neu·ro·oph·thal·mol·o·gy \-ˌäf-thəl-'mä-lə-jē, -ˌäp-\ *n, pl* **-gies** : the neurological study of the eye — **neu·ro-**

oph·thal·mo·log·ic \-mə-'lä-jik\ or **neu·ro—oph·thal·mo·log·i·cal** \-'lä-ji-kəl\ adj

neu·ro—otology var of NEUROTOLOGY

neu·ro·par·a·lyt·ic \-,par-ə-'li-tik\ adj : of, relating to, causing, or characterized by paralysis or loss of sensation due to a lesion in a nerve

neu·ro·path·ic \,nŭr-ə-'pa-thik, ,nyŭr-\ adj : of, relating to, characterized by, or being a neuropathy ⟨~ pain⟩ ⟨~ disorders⟩ — **neu·ro·path·i·cal·ly** adv

neu·ro·patho·gen·e·sis \-,pa-thə-'je-nə-səs\ n, pl **-e·ses** \-,sēz\ : the pathogenesis of a nervous disease

neu·ro·patho·gen·ic \-'je-nik\ adj : causing or capable of causing disease of nervous tissue ⟨~ viruses⟩

neu·ro·pa·thol·o·gist \,nŭr-ō-pə-'thä-lə-jist, ,nyŭr-\ n : a specialist in neuropathology

neu·ro·pa·thol·o·gy \-pə-'thä-lə-jē, -pa-\ n, pl **-gies** : pathology of the nervous system — **neu·ro·patho·log·ic** \-,pa-thə-'lä-jik\ or **neu·ro·patho·log·i·cal** \-ji-kəl\ adj — **neu·ro·patho·log·i·cal·ly** \-k(ə-)lē\ adv

neu·rop·a·thy \nŭ-'rä-pə-thē, nyŭ-\ n, pl **-thies** : an abnormal and usu. degenerative state of the nervous system or nerves; also : a systemic condition that stems from a neuropathy

neu·ro·pep·tide \,nŭr-ō-'pep-,tīd, ,nyŭr-\ n : an endogenous peptide (as an endorphin) that influences neural activity or functioning

neuropeptide Y n : a neurotransmitter that has a vasoconstrictive effect on blood vessels and is held to play a role in regulating eating behavior

neu·ro·phar·ma·ceu·ti·cal \-,fär-mə-'sü-ti-kəl\ n : a drug used to treat neuropsychiatric, neuropsychological, or nervous-system disorders (as depression or schizophrenia)

neu·ro·phar·ma·col·o·gist \-,fär-mə-'kä-lə-jist\ n : a specialist in neuropharmacology

neu·ro·phar·ma·col·o·gy \-,fär-mə-'kä-lə-jē\ n, pl **-gies** **1** : a branch of medical science dealing with the action of drugs on and in the nervous system **2** : the properties and reactions of a drug on and in the nervous system — **neu·ro·phar·ma·co·log·i·cal** \-kə-'lä-ji-kəl\ also **neu·ro·phar·ma·co·log·ic** \-jik\ adj

neu·ro·phy·sin \-'fī-sᵊn\ n : any of several brain hormones that bind with and carry either oxytocin or vasopressin

neu·ro·phys·i·ol·o·gist \-,fi-zē-'ä-lə-jist\ n : a specialist in neurophysiology

neu·ro·phys·i·ol·o·gy \-,fi-zē-'ä-lə-jē\ n, pl **-gies** : physiology of the nervous system — **neu·ro·phys·i·o·log·i·cal** \-zē-ə-'lä-ji-kəl\ also **neu·ro·phys·i·o·log·ic** \-jik\ adj — **neu·ro·phys·i·o·log·i·cal·ly** adv

neu·ro·pil \'nŭr-ō-,pil, 'nyŭr-\ also **neu·ro·pile** \-,pīl\ n : a fibrous network of delicate unmyelinated nerve fibers found in concentrations of nervous tissue that is highly developed — **neu·ro·pi·lar** \,nŭr-ō-'pī-lər, ,nyŭr-\ adj

neu·ro·pro·tec·tant \,nŭr-ō-prə-'tek-tənt, ,nyŭr-\ n : a neuroprotective drug that protects against or helps repair the damaging effects of a stroke

neu·ro·pro·tec·tive \,nŭr-ō-prə-'tek-tiv\ adj : serving to protect neurons from injury or degeneration — **neu·ro·pro·tec·tion** \-shən\ n

neu·ro·psy·chi·a·trist \,nŭr-ō-sə-'kī-ə-trist, ,nyŭr-, -sī-\ n : a specialist in neuropsychiatry

neu·ro·psy·chi·a·try \-sə-'kī-ə-trē, -sī-\ n, pl **-tries** : a branch of medicine concerned with both neurology and psychiatry — **neu·ro·psy·chi·at·ric** \-,sī-kē-'a-trik\ adj — **neu·ro·psy·chi·at·ri·cal·ly** adv

neu·ro·psy·chol·o·gist \-sī-'kä-lə-jist\ n : a specialist in neuropsychology

neu·ro·psy·chol·o·gy \-jē\ n, pl **-gies** : a science concerned with the integration of psychological observations on behavior and the mind with neurological observations on the brain and nervous system — **neu·ro·psy·cho·log·i·cal** \-,sī-kə-'lä-ji-kəl\ adj — **neu·ro·psy·cho·log·i·cal·ly** adv

neu·ro·psy·cho·phar·ma·col·o·gy \-,sī-kō-,fär-mə-'kä-lə-jē\ n, pl **-gies** : a branch of medical science combining neuropharmacology and psychopharmacology

neu·ro·ra·di·ol·o·gist \-,rā-dē-'ä-lə-jist\ n : a specialist in neuroradiology

neu·ro·ra·di·ol·o·gy \-,rā-dē-'ä-lə-jē\ n, pl **-gies** : radiology of the nervous system — **neu·ro·ra·dio·log·i·cal** \-dē-ə-'lä-ji-kəl\ also **neu·ro·ra·dio·log·ic** \-jik\ adj

neu·ro·ret·i·ni·tis \-,ret-ᵊn-'ī-təs\ n, pl **-nit·i·des** \-'ni-tə-,dēz\ : inflammation of the optic nerve and the retina

neu·ror·rha·phy \nŭ-'rȯr-ə-fē, nyŭ-\ n, pl **-phies** : the surgical suturing of a divided nerve

neu·ro·sci·ence \,nŭr-ō-'sī-əns, ,nyŭr-\ n : a branch (as neurophysiology) of biology that deals with the anatomy, physiology, biochemistry, or molecular biology of nerves and nervous tissue and esp. their relation to behavior and learning — **neu·ro·sci·en·tif·ic** \-,sī-ən-'ti-fik\ adj — **neu·ro·sci·en·tist** \-'sī-ən-tist\ n

neu·ro·se·cre·tion \-si-'krē-shən\ n **1** : the process of producing a secretion by neurons **2** : a secretion produced by neurosecretion — **neu·ro·se·cre·to·ry** \-'sē-krə-,tȯr-ē\ adj

neu·ro·sen·so·ry \-'sen-sə-rē\ adj : of or relating to afferent nerves

neu·ro·sis \nŭ-'rō-səs, nyŭ-\ n, pl **-ro·ses** \-,sēz\ : a mental and emotional disorder that affects only part of the personality, is accompanied by a less distorted perception of reality than in a psychosis, does not result in disturbance of the use of language, and is accompanied by various physical, physiological, and mental disturbances (as visceral symptoms, anxieties, or phobias)

neu·ro·stim·u·la·tor \ˌnŭr-ō-ˈsti-myə-ˌlā-tər, ˌnyŭr-\ *n* : a device that provides electrical stimulation to nerves

neu·ro·sur·geon \-ˈsər-jən\ *n* : a surgeon specializing in neurosurgery

neu·ro·sur·gery \ˌnŭr-ō-ˈsər-jə-rē\ *n, pl* **-ger·ies** : surgery of nervous structures (as nerves, the brain, or the spinal cord) — **neu·ro·sur·gi·cal** \-ˈsər-ji-kəl\ *adj* — **neu·ro·sur·gi·cal·ly** *adv*

neu·ro·syph·i·lis \-ˈsi-fə-ləs\ *n* : syphilis of the central nervous system — **neu·ro·syph·i·lit·ic** \-ˌsi-fə-ˈli-tik\ *adj*

neu·ro·ten·di·nous spindle \-ˈten-di-nəs-\ *n* : GOLGI TENDON ORGAN

neu·ro·ten·sin \-ˈten-sən\ *n* : a protein composed of 13 amino acid residues that causes hypertension and vasodilation and is present in the brain

¹**neu·rot·ic** \nŭ-ˈrä-tik, nyŭ-\ *adj* **1 a** : of, relating to, or involving the nerves ⟨a ∼ disorder⟩ **b** : being a neurosis : NERVOUS **2** : affected with, relating to, or characterized by neurosis ⟨a ∼ person⟩ — **neu·rot·i·cal·ly** *adv*

²**neurotic** *n* **1** : one affected with a neurosis **2** : an emotionally unstable individual

neu·rot·i·cism \-ˈrä-tə-ˌsi-zəm\ *n* : a neurotic character, condition, or trait

neu·rot·ol·o·gy \ˌnŭr-ō-ˈtä-lə-jē, ˌnyŭr-\ *or* **neu·ro·otol·o·gy** \-ō-ˈtä-lə-jē\ *n, pl* **-gies** : the neurological study of the ear — **neu·ro·to·log·ic** \-tə-ˈlä-jik\ *or* **neu·ro·oto·log·i·cal** \-ˌō-tə-ˈlä-ji-kəl\ *also* **neu·ro·oto·log·ic** \-ˌō-tə-ˈlä-jik\ *or* **neu·ro·oto·log·i·cal** \-tə-ˈlä-ji-kəl\ *adj*

neu·rot·o·my \-ˈrä-tə-mē\ *n, pl* **-mies** **1** : the dissection or cutting of nerves **2** : the division of a nerve (as to relieve neuralgia)

neu·ro·tox·ic \ˌnŭr-ō-ˈtäk-sik, ˌnyŭr-\ *adj* : toxic to the nerves or nervous tissue — **neu·ro·tox·ic·i·ty** \-ˌtäk-ˈsi-sə-tē\ *n*

neu·ro·tox·i·col·o·gist \-ˌtäk-sə-ˈkä-lə-jist\ *n* : a specialist in the study of neurotoxins and their effects

neu·ro·tox·i·col·o·gy \-jē\ *n, pl* **-gies** : the study of neurotoxins and their effects — **neu·ro·tox·i·co·log·i·cal** \-kə-ˈlä-jə-kəl\ *adj*

neu·ro·tox·in \-ˈtäk-sən\ *n* : a poisonous protein complex that acts on the nervous system

neu·ro·trans·mis·sion \-trans-ˈmi-shən, -tranz-\ *n* : the transmission of nerve impulses across a synapse

neu·ro·trans·mit·ter \-trans-ˈmi-tər, -tranz-; -ˈtrans-ˌmi-, -ˈtranz-\ *n* : a substance (as norepinephrine or acetyl-choline) that transmits nerve impulses across a synapse — see FALSE NEUROTRANSMITTER

neu·ro·trau·ma \-ˈtrō-mə, -ˈtraů-\ *n* : injury to a nerve or to the nervous system

neu·ro·troph·ic \-ˈträ-fik, -ˈtrō-\ *adj* **1** : relating to or dependent on the influence of nerves on the nutrition of tissue **2** : NEUROTROPIC

neurotrophic factor *n* : any of a group of neuropeptides (as nerve growth factor) that regulate the growth, differentiation, and survival of certain neurons in the peripheral and central nervous systems

neu·ro·tro·phin \-ˈtrō-fən\ *n* : NEUROTROPHIC FACTOR

neu·ro·trop·ic \-ˈträ-pik\ *adj* : having an affinity for or localizing selectively in nerve tissue ⟨∼ viruses⟩ — compare PANTROPIC — **neu·ro·tro·pism** \nŭ-ˈrä-trə-ˌpi-zəm, nyŭ-\ *n*

neu·ro·tu·bule \ˌnŭr-ō-ˈtü-ˌbyül, ˌnyŭr-ō-ˈtyü-\ *n* : a microtubule occurring in a neuron — see NEUROFILAMENT

neu·ro·vas·cu·lar \-ˈvas-kyə-lər\ *adj* : of, relating to, or involving both nerves and blood vessels

neu·ro·vi·rol·o·gy \-vī-ˈrä-lə-jē\ *n, pl* **-gies** : virology concerned with viral infections of the nervous system

neu·ro·vir·u·lence \-ˈvir-yə-ləns, -ˈvir-ə-\ *n* : the tendency or capacity of a microorganism to cause disease of the nervous system — **neu·ro·vir·u·lent** \-lənt\ *adj*

neu·ru·la \ˈnŭr-yü-lə, ˈnyŭr-, -ů-lə\ *n, pl* **-lae** \-ˌlē\ *or* **-las** : an early vertebrate embryo which follows the gastrula and in which nervous tissue begins to differentiate — **neu·ru·la·tion** \ˌnŭr-yü-ˈlā-shən, ˌnyŭr-, -ů-\ *n*

¹**neu·ter** \ˈnü-tər, ˈnyü-\ *n* : a spayed or castrated animal (as a cat)

²**neuter** *vb* : CASTRATE 1, ALTER

neu·tral \ˈnü-trəl, ˈnyü-\ *adj* **1** : not decided or pronounced as to characteristics **2** : neither acid nor basic : neither acid nor alkaline; *specif* : having a pH value of 7.0 **3** : not electrically charged

neutral fat *n* : TRIGLYCERIDE

neu·tral·ize \ˈnü-trə-ˌlīz, ˈnyü-\ *vb* **-ized; -iz·ing 1** : to make chemically neutral **2** : to counteract the activity or effect of : make ineffective **3** : to make electrically inert by combining equal positive and negative quantities — **neu·tral·i·za·tion** \ˌnü-trə-lə-ˈzā-shən, ˌnyü-\ *n*

neutro- *comb form* **1** : neutral ⟨*neu*trophil⟩ **2** : neutrophil ⟨*neutro*penia⟩

neu·tron \ˈnü-ˌträn, ˈnyü-\ *n* : an uncharged atomic particle that is nearly equal in mass to the proton

neu·tro·pe·nia \ˌnü-trə-ˈpē-nē-ə, ˌnyü-\ *n* : leukopenia in which the decrease in white blood cells is chiefly in neutrophils — **neu·tro·pe·nic** \-'pē-nik\ *adj*

¹neu·tro·phil \'nü-trə-,fil, 'nyü-\ *or* **neu·tro·phil·ic** \,nü-trə-'fi-lik, ,nyü-\ *adj* : staining to the same degree with acid or basic dyes ⟨∼ granulocytes⟩

²neutrophil *n* : a granulocyte that is the chief phagocytic white blood cell

neu·tro·phil·ia \,nü-trə-'fi-lē-ə, ,nyü-\ *n* : leukocytosis in which the increase in white blood cells is chiefly in neutrophils

ne·vi·ra·pine \nə-'vir-ə-,pēn, -'vī-rə-\ *n* : a reverse transcriptase inhibitor $C_{15}H_{14}N_4O$ that is administered orally in combination with at least one other antiretroviral agent in the treatment of infection by HIV-1

ne·void \'nē-,vȯid\ *adj* : resembling a nevus ⟨a ∼ tumor⟩; *also* : accompanied by nevi or similar superficial lesions

ne·vus \'nē-vəs\ *n, pl* **ne·vi** \-,vī\ : a congenital or acquired usu. highly pigmented area on the skin that is either flat or raised : MOLE — see BLUE NEVUS, SPIDER NEVUS

nevus flam·me·us \-'fla-mē-əs\ *n* : PORT-WINE STAIN

¹new·born \'nü-'bȯrn, 'nyü-\ *adj* **1** : recently born ⟨a ∼ infant⟩ **2** : affecting or relating to the newborn

²new·born \-,bȯrn\ *n, pl* **newborn** *or* **newborns** : a newborn individual : NEONATE

New·cas·tle disease \'nü-,ka-səl-, 'nyü-; 'nü-'ka-səl-, ,nyü-\ *n* : a contagious mild to fatal virus disease of birds and esp. the domestic chicken that is caused by a paramyxovirus (species *Newcastle disease virus* of the genus *Avulavirus*) and is marked by highly variable symptoms (as coughing, diarrhea, and tremors)

new drug *n* : a drug that has not been declared safe and effective by qualified experts under the conditions prescribed, recommended, or suggested in the label and that may be a new chemical formula or an established drug prescribed for use in a new way

New Latin *n* : Latin as used since the end of the medieval period esp. in scientific description and classification

new·ton \'nü-tən, 'nyü-\ *n* : the unit of force in the metric system equal to the force required to impart an acceleration of one meter per second per second to a mass of one kilogram

Newton, Sir Issac (1642–1727), British physicist and mathematician.

new variant Creutzfeldt–Jakob disease *n* : VARIANT CREUTZFELDT–JAKOB DISEASE — abbr. *nvCJD*

Nex·i·um \'nek-sē-əm\ *trademark* — used for a preparation of the magnesium salt of esomeprazole

NF *abbr* **1** National Formulary **2** neurofibromatosis

NFP *abbr* natural family planning

ng *abbr* nanogram

NG *abbr* nasogastric

n'gana *var of* NAGANA

NGF *abbr* nerve growth factor

NGU *abbr* nongonococcal urethritis

NHS *abbr* National Health Service

Ni *symbol* nickel

ni·a·cin \'nī-ə-sən\ *n* : a crystalline acid $C_6H_5NO_2$ of the vitamin B complex that occurs usu. in the form of a complex of niacinamide in various animal and plant parts (as blood, liver, yeast, bran, and legumes) and is effective in preventing and treating human pellagra and blacktongue of dogs — called also *nicotinic acid*

ni·a·cin·amide \,nī-ə-'si-nə-,mīd\ *n* : a crystalline amide $C_6H_6N_2O$ of the vitamin B complex that is formed from and converted to niacin in the living organism, occurs naturally usu. as a constituent of coenzymes, and is used similarly to niacin — called also *nicotinamide*

ni·al·amide \nī-'a-lə-,mīd\ *n* : a synthetic antidepressant drug $C_{16}H_{18}$-N_4O_2 that is an inhibitor of monoamine oxidase

ni·car·di·pine \nī-'kär-də-,pēn\ *n* : a calcium channel blocker administered orally in the form of its hydrochloride $C_{26}H_{29}N_3O_6\cdot HCl$ to treat angina pectoris and hypertension

nick \'nik\ *n* : a break in one strand of two-stranded DNA caused by a missing phosphodiester bond — **nick** *vb*

nick·el \'ni-kəl\ *n* : a silver-white hard malleable ductile metallic element — symbol *Ni*; see ELEMENT table

nick·ing \'ni-kiŋ\ *n* : localized constriction of a retinal vein by the pressure from an artery crossing it seen esp. in arterial hypertension

nicotin- *or* **nicoti-** *comb form* **1** : nicotine ⟨*nicotinic*⟩ **2** : nicotinic acid ⟨*nicotinamide*⟩

nic·o·tin·amide \,ni-kə-'tē-nə-,mīd, -'ti-\ *n* : NIACINAMIDE

nicotinamide adenine dinucleotide *n* : NAD

nicotinamide adenine dinucleotide phosphate *n* : NADP

nic·o·tine \'ni-kə-,tēn\ *n* : a poisonous alkaloid $C_{10}H_{14}N_2$ that is the chief active principle of tobacco

Ni·cot \nē-'kō\, Jean (1530?–1600), French diplomat.

nic·o·tin·ic \,ni-kə-'tē-nik, -'ti-\ *adj* : relating to, resembling, producing, or mediating the effects that are produced by acetylcholine liberated by nerve fibers at autonomic ganglia and at the neuromuscular junctions of voluntary muscle and that are mimicked by nicotine which increases activity in small doses and inhibits it in larger doses ⟨∼ receptors⟩ — compare MUSCARINIC

nicotinic acid *n* : NIACIN

nictitans — see MEMBRANA NICTITANS

nic·ti·tat·ing membrane \'nik-tə-,tā-tiŋ-\ *n* : a thin membrane found in many vertebrate animals at the inner angle or beneath the lower lid of the eye and capable of extending across the eyeball — called also *membrana nictitans, third eyelid*

NICU *abbr* neonatal intensive care unit

ni-da-tion \nī-'dā-shən\ *n* **1** : the development of the epithelial membrane lining the inner surface of the uterus following menstruation **2** : IMPLANTATION b

NIDDK *abbr* National Institute of Diabetes and Digestive and Kidney Diseases

NIDDM *abbr* non-insulin-dependent diabetes mellitus

ni-dus \'nī-dəs\ *n, pl* **ni-di** \-ˌdī\ *or* **ni-dus-es** : a place where something originates or is fostered or develops; *specif* : the point of origin or focus of an infection or disease process

Nie-mann–Pick disease \'nē-ˌmän-'pik-\ *n* : an error in lipid metabolism that is inherited as an autosomal recessive trait, is characterized by accumulation of phospholipid in macrophages of the liver, spleen, lymph glands, and bone marrow, and leads to gastrointestinal disturbances, malnutrition, enlargement of the spleen, liver, and lymph nodes, and abnormalities of the blood-forming organs

Niemann, Albert (1880–1921), and Pick, Ludwig (1868–1944), German physicians.

ni-fed-i-pine \nī-'fe-də-ˌpēn\ *n* : a calcium channel blocker $C_{17}H_{18}N_2O_6$ that is a coronary vasodilator used esp. in the treatment of angina pectoris — see ADALAT, PROCARDIA

night blindness *n* : reduced visual capacity in faint light (as at night) — called also *nyctalopia* — **night–blind** \'nīt-ˌblīnd\ *adj*

night-mare \'nīt-ˌmar\ *n* : a frightening or distressing dream that usu. awakens the sleeper

night-shade \'nīt-ˌshād\ *n* **1** : any plant of the genus *Solanum* (family Solanaceae, the nightshade family) including some poisonous weeds and important crop plants (as the potato and eggplant) **2** : BELLADONNA 1

night sweat *n* : profuse sweating during sleep (as that associated with menopause or tuberculosis)

night terror *n* : a sudden awakening in dazed terror that occurs in children during slow-wave sleep, is often preceded by a sudden shrill cry uttered in sleep, and is not remembered when the child awakes — usu. used in pl.; called also *pavor nocturnus*

night vision *n* : ability to see in dim light (as provided by moon and stars)

ni-gra \'nī-grə\ *n* : SUBSTANTIA NIGRA — **ni-gral** \-grəl\ *adj*

nigricans — see ACANTHOSIS NIGRICANS

ni-gro-stri-a-tal \ˌnī-grō-strī-'āt-ᵊl\ *adj* : of, relating to, or joining the corpus striatum and the substantia nigra

NIH *abbr* National Institutes of Health

ni-hi-lism \'nī-ə-ˌli-zəm, 'nē-, -hə-\ *n* : NIHILISTIC DELUSION **2** : skepticism as to the value of a drug or method of treatment ⟨therapeutic ∼⟩ — **ni-hi-lis-tic** \ˌnī-ə-'lis-tik, ˌnē-, -hə-\ *adj*

nihilistic delusion *n* : the belief that oneself, a part of one's body, or the real world does not exist or has been destroyed

nik-eth-amide \ni-'ke-thə-ˌmīd\ *n* : a bitter viscous liquid or crystalline compound $C_{10}H_{14}N_2O$ used esp. formerly as a respiratory stimulant

NIMH *abbr* National Institute of Mental Health

ni-mo-di-pine \ni-'mō-də-ˌpēn\ *n* : a calcium channel blocker $C_{21}H_{26}N_2O_7$

ninth cranial nerve *n* : GLOSSOPHARYNGEAL NERVE

ni-o-bi-um \nī-'ō-bē-əm\ *n* : a lustrous ductile metallic element — symbol *Nb*; see ELEMENT table

NIOSH *abbr* National Institute of Occupational Safety and Health

Ni-pah virus \'nē-pə-\ *n* : a paramyxovirus (species *Nipah virus* of the genus *Henipavirus*) that has caused epidemics of respiratory disease in pigs and an often fatal encephalitis in humans in Malaysia, Singapore, and Bangladesh

nip-per \'ni-pər\ *n* : an incisor of a horse; *esp* : one of the middle four incisors — compare CORNER TOOTH, DIVIDER

nip-ple \'ni-pəl\ *n* **1** : the protuberance of a mammary gland upon which in the female the lactiferous ducts open and from which milk is drawn **2** : an artificial teat through which a bottle-fed infant nurses

Ni-pride \'nī-ˌprīd\ *n* : a preparation of sodium nitroprusside — formerly a U.S. registered trademark

ni-sin \'nī-sən\ *n* : a polypeptide antibiotic that is produced by a bacterium (*Lactococcus lactis* syn. *Streptococcus lactis*) and is used as a food preservative

Nis-sen fundoplication \'ni-sᵊn-\ *n* : fundoplication in which the fundus of the stomach is wrapped completely around the lower end of the esophagus

Nissen, Rudolph (1896–1981), Swiss (German-born) surgeon.

Nissl bodies \'ni-səl-\ *n pl* : discrete granular bodies of variable size that occur in the cell body and dendrites but not the axon of neurons and are composed of RNA and polyribosomes — called also *Nissl granules, tigroid substance*

Nissl, Franz (1860–1919), German neurologist.

Nissl substance *n* : the nucleoprotein material of Nissl bodies — called also *chromidial substance*

nit \'nit\ *n* : the egg of a louse or other parasitic insect; *also* : the insect itself when young

ni·trate \'nī-ˌtrāt, -trət\ *n* : a salt or ester of nitric acid

ni·tric acid \'nī-trik-\ *n* : a corrosive liquid inorganic acid HNO_3

nitric oxide *n* : a poisonous colorless gas NO that occurs as a common air pollutant formed by the oxidation of atmospheric nitrogen and that is also formed by the oxidation of arginine in the body where it regulates numerous biological processes (as vasodilation and neurotransmission)

nitric oxide syn·thase \-ˈsin-ˌthās, -ˌthāz\ *n* : any of various enzymes that catalyze the oxidation of arginine to form nitric oxide and citrulline

ni·trite \'nī-ˌtrīt\ *n* : a salt or ester of nitrous acid

ni·tri·toid reaction \'nī-trə-ˌtȯid-\ *n* : an acute reaction sometimes occurring to certain drugs (as gold sodium thiomalate) and resembling poisoning by nitrite esp. in the presence of flushing, tachycardia, and faintness — called also *nitritoid crisis*

ni·tro \'nī-(ˌ)trō\ *n, pl* **nitros** : any of various nitrated products; *specif* : NITROGLYCERIN

Ni·tro–Dur \'nī-trō-ˌdər\ *trademark* — used for a preparation of nitroglycerin

ni·tro·fu·ran \ˌnī-trō-ˈfyur-ˌan, -ˌfyur-ˈran\ *n* : any of several compounds containing a nitro group that are used as bacteria-inhibiting agents

ni·tro·fu·ran·to·in \-fyu-ˈran-tō-in\ *n* : a nitrofuran derivative $C_8H_6N_4O_5$ that is a broad-spectrum antimicrobial agent used esp. in treating urinary tract infections

ni·tro·fu·ra·zone \-ˈfyur-ə-ˌzōn\ *n* : a pale yellow crystalline compound $C_6H_6N_4O_4$ used topically as a bacteriostatic or bactericidal dressing (as for wounds and infections)

ni·tro·gen \'nī-trə-jən\ *n* : a nonmetallic element that in the free form is normally a colorless odorless tasteless inert gas containing two atoms per molecule and comprising 78 percent of the atmosphere and that in the combined form is a constituent of biologically important compounds (as proteins and nucleic acids) — symbol *N;* see ELEMENT table

nitrogen balance *n* : the difference between nitrogen intake and nitrogen excretion in the animal body such that a greater intake results in a positive balance and an increased excretion causes a negative balance

nitrogen base *or* **nitrogenous base** *n* : a nitrogen-containing molecule with basic properties; *esp* : one that is a purine or pyrimidine

nitrogen dioxide *n* : a poisonous strongly oxidizing reddish brown gas NO_2

nitrogen mustard *n* : any of various toxic blistering compounds analogous to mustard gas but containing nitrogen instead of sulfur; *esp* : MECHLORETHAMINE

nitrogen narcosis *n* : a state of euphoria and confusion similar to alcohol intoxication which occurs when nitrogen in normal air enters the bloodstream at increased partial pressure (as in deepwater diving) — called also *rapture of the deep*

ni·trog·e·nous \nī-ˈträ-jə-nəs\ *adj* : of, relating to, or containing nitrogen in combined form (as in proteins)

ni·tro·glyc·er·in *or* **ni·tro·glyc·er·ine** \ˌnī-trə-ˈgli-sə-rən\ *n* : a heavy oily explosive poisonous liquid $C_3H_5N_3O_9$ used in medicine as a vasodilator (as in angina pectoris) — see NITRO-DUR, NITROSTAT

ni·tro·mer·sol \ˌnī-trō-ˈmər-ˌsȯl, -ˌsōl\ *n* : a brownish yellow to yellow solid organic mercurial $C_7H_5HgNO_3$ used esp. formerly as an antiseptic and disinfectant

nitroprusside — see SODIUM NITROPRUSSIDE

ni·tro·sa·mine \nī-ˈtrō-sə-ˌmēn\ *n* : any of various neutral compounds which are characterized by the group NNO and of which some are powerful carcinogens

ni·tro·so·di·meth·yl·amine \nī-ˌtrō-sō-ˌdī-ˌme-thə-ˈla-ˌmēn, -ə-ˌmēn\ *n* : DIMETHYLNITROSAMINE

ni·tro·so·urea \-yü-ˈrē-ə\ *n* : any of a group of lipid-soluble antineoplastic drugs that function as alkylating agents with the ability to cross the blood-brain barrier — see CARMUSTINE

Ni·tro·stat \'nī-trə-ˌstat\ *trademark* — used for a preparation of nitroglycerin

ni·trous oxide \'nī-trəs-\ *n* : a colorless gas N_2O that when inhaled produces loss of sensibility to pain preceded by exhilaration and sometimes laughter and is used esp. as an anesthetic in dentistry — called also *laughing gas*

ni·zat·i·dine \nī-ˈza-tə-ˌdīn, -ˌdēn\ *n* : an H_2 antagonist $C_{12}H_{21}N_5O_2S_2$ that inhibits gastric acid secretion and is used in the treatment of duodenal ulcers — see AXID

Ni·zo·ral \'nī-zə-ˌral\ *trademark* — used for a preparation of ketoconazole

NK cell \ˌen-ˈkā-\ *n* : NATURAL KILLER CELL

nm *abbr* nanometer

NMDA \ˌen-ˌem-ˌdē-ˈā\ *n* : a synthetic amino acid $C_5H_9NO_4$ that binds selectively to glutamate receptors on neurons resulting in the opening of calcium channels — called also *N-methyl-D-aspartate*

NMR *abbr* nuclear magnetic resonance

NNK \ˌen-ˌen-ˈkā\ *n* : a nitrosamine $C_{10}H_{13}N_3O_2$ in tobacco smoke that is derived from nicotine and is a powerful carcinogen

No *symbol* nobelium

no·bel·i·um \nō-'be-lē-əm\ n : a radioactive element produced artificially — symbol *No;* see ELEMENT table

No·bel \nō-'bel\, **Alfred Bernhard** (1833–1896), Swedish inventor and philanthropist.

no·ble gas \'nō-bəl-\ n : any of a group of rare gases that include helium, neon, argon, krypton, xenon, and sometimes radon that exhibit great stability and extremely low reaction rates — called also *inert gas*

no·car·dia \nō-'kär-dē-ə\ n **1** *cap* : a genus of aerobic actinomycetes (family Actinomycetaceae) that include various pathogens as well as some soil-dwelling saprophytes **2** : any actinomycete of the genus *Nocardia* — **no·car·di·al** \-əl\ *adj*

No·card \nō-'kär\, **Edmond–Isidore–Étienne** (1850–1903), French veterinarian and biologist.

no·car·di·o·sis \nō-ˌkär-dē-'ō-səs\ n, pl **-o·ses** \-ˌsēz\ : actinomycosis caused by a bacteria of the genus *Nocardia* and characterized by production of spreading granulomatous lesions

no·ce·bo \nō-'sē-(ˌ)bō\ n : a harmless substance that when taken by a patient is associated with harmful effects due to negative expectations or the psychological condition of the patient

noci- *comb form* : pain ⟨*noci*ceptor⟩

no·ci·cep·tive \ˌnō-si-'sep-tiv\ *adj* **1** of *a stimulus* : causing pain or injury **2** : of, induced by, or responding to a nociceptive stimulus — used esp. of receptors or protective reflexes

no·ci·cep·tor \-'sep-tər\ n : a receptor for injurious or painful stimuli : a pain sense organ

no code n : an order not to revive or sustain a patient who experiences a life-threating event (as heart stoppage); *also* : a patient assigned a no code

noc·tu·ria \näk-'tùr-ē-ə, -'tyùr-\ n : urination at night esp. when excessive

noc·tur·nal \näk-'tərn-əl\ *adj* **1** : of, relating to, or occurring at night ⟨~ myoclonus⟩ **2** : characterized by nocturnal activity

nocturnal emission n : an involuntary discharge of semen during sleep often accompanied by an erotic dream

nocturnus — see PAVOR NOCTURNUS

noc·u·ous \'nä-kyə-wəs\ *adj* : likely to cause injury ⟨a ~ stimulus⟩

nod·al \'nōd-əl\ *adj* : being, relating to, or located at or near a node — **nod·al·ly** *adv*

node \'nōd\ n **1** : a pathological swelling or enlargement (as of a rheumatic joint) **2** : a body part resembling a knot; *esp* : a discrete mass of one kind of tissue enclosed in tissue of a different kind — see ATRIOVENTRICULAR NODE, LYMPH NODE

cancer that has not spread to nearby lymph nodes ⟨~ breast cancer⟩

node of Ran·vier \-'rän-vē-ˌā\ n : a small gap in the myelin sheath of a myelinated axon

Ran·vier \räⁿ-vyā\, **Louis–Antoine** (1835–1922), French histologist.

nodosa — see PERIARTERITIS NODOSA, POLYARTERITIS NODOSA

no·dose ganglion \'nō-ˌdōs-\ n : INFERIOR GANGLION 2

nodosum — see ERYTHEMA NODOSUM

nod·u·lar \'nä-jə-lər\ *adj* : of, relating to, characterized by, or occurring in the form of nodules ⟨~ lesions⟩ — **nod·u·lar·i·ty** \ˌnä-jə-'lar-ə-tē\ n

nodular disease n : infestation with or disease caused by nodular worms of the genus *Oesophagostomum* — called also *nodule worm disease*

nodular worm n : any of several nematode worms of the genus *Oesophagostomum* that are parasitic in the large intestine of ruminants and swine — called also *nodule worm*

nod·ule \'nä-(ˌ)jül\ n : a small mass of rounded or irregular shape: as **a** : a small abnormal knobby bodily protuberance (as a tumorous growth or a calcification near an arthritic joint) **b** : the nodulus of the cerebellum

nod·u·lo·cys·tic \ˌnä-jə-lō-'sis-stik\ *adj* : characterized by the formation of nodules and cystic lesions ⟨~ acne⟩

nod·u·lus \'nä-jə-ləs\ n, pl **nod·u·li** \-ˌlī\ : NODULE; *esp* : a prominence on the inferior surface of the cerebellum forming the anterior end of the vermis

noire — see TACHE NOIRE

noise pollution n : environmental pollution consisting of annoying or harmful noise (as of cars or airplanes) — called also *sound pollution*

Nol·va·dex \'näl-və-ˌdeks\ *trademark* — used for a preparation of the citrate of tamoxifen

no·ma \'nō-mə\ n : a spreading invasive gangrene chiefly of the lining of the cheek and lips that is usu. fatal and occurs most often in persons severely debilitated by disease or profound nutritional deficiency — see CANCRUM ORIS

no·men·cla·ture \'nō-mən-ˌklā-chər\ n : a system of terms used in a particular science; *esp* : an international system of standardized New Latin names used in biology for kinds and groups of kinds of animals and plants — see BINOMIAL NOMENCLATURE — **no·men·cla·tur·al** \ˌnō-mən-'klā-chə-rəl\ *adj*

No·mi·na An·a·tom·i·ca \'nä-mi-nə-ˌa-nə-'tä-mi-kə, 'nō-\ n : the Latin anatomical nomenclature that was prepared by revising the Basle Nomina Anatomica, adopted in 1955 at the Sixth International Congress of Anatomists, and modified at subsequent Congresses — abbr. *NA*

no·mo·top·ic \nä-mə-'tō-pik, ˌnō-, -'tä-\ *adj* : occurring in the normal place

-n·o·my \n-ə-mē\ *n comb form, pl* **-n·o·mies** : system of laws or sum of knowledge regarding a (specified) field ⟨taxo*nomy*⟩

non- *prefix* : not : reverse of : absence of ⟨*non*allergic⟩

non·ab·sorb·able \ˌnän-əb-'sȯr-bə-bəl, -'zȯr-\ *adj* : not capable of being absorbed ⟨~ silk sutures⟩

non·ac·id \-'a-səd\ *adj* : not acid : being without acid properties

non·adap·tive \ˌnän-ə-'dap-tiv\ *adj* : not serving to adapt the individual to the environment ⟨~ traits⟩

non·ad·dict \-'a-dikt\ *n* : a person who is not addicted to a drug

non·ad·dict·ing \-ə-'dik-tiŋ\ *adj* : NON-ADDICTIVE

non·ad·dic·tive \-ə-'dik-tiv\ *adj* : not causing addiction ⟨~ painkillers⟩

non·al·le·lic \ˌnän-ə-'lē-lik, -'le-\ *adj* : not behaving as alleles toward one another ⟨~ genes⟩

non·al·ler·gen·ic \ˌ,a-lər-'je-nik\ *adj* : not causing an allergic reaction

non·al·ler·gic \-ə-'lər-jik\ *adj* : not allergic; *also* : not caused by an allergic reaction ⟨~ rhinitis⟩

non·am·bu·la·tory \-'am-byə-lə-ˌtȯr-ē\ *adj* : not able to walk about ⟨~ patients⟩

non–A, non–B hepatitis \ˌnän-'ā-ˌnän-'bē-\ *n* : hepatitis clinically and immunologically similar to hepatitis A and hepatitis B but caused by different viruses; *esp* : HEPATITIS C

non·an·ti·bi·ot·ic \ˌnän-ˌan-tē-bī-'ä-tik, -ˌan-ˌtī-\ *adj* : not antibiotic

non·an·ti·gen·ic \ˌan-ti-'je-nik\ *adj* : not antigenic ⟨~ materials⟩

non·ar·tic·u·lar \ˌnän-är-'ti-kyə-lər\ *adj* : affecting or involving soft tissues (as muscles and connective tissues) rather than joints ⟨~ rheumatism⟩

non·as·so·cia·tive \-ə-'sō-shē-ˌā-tiv, -sē-ˌā-tiv, -shə-tiv\ *adj* : relating to or being learning (as habituation and sensitization) that is not associative learning

non·ato·pic \-(ˌ)ā-'tä-pik, -'tō-\ *adj* : not affecting with atopy ⟨~ patients⟩

non·bac·te·ri·al \-bak-'tir-ē-əl\ *adj* : not of, relating to, caused by, or being bacteria ⟨~ pneumonia⟩

non·bar·bi·tu·rate \-bär-'bi-chə-rət, -ˌrāt\ *adj* : not derived from barbituric acid ⟨~ sedatives⟩

non·bi·o·log·i·cal \-ˌbī-ə-'lä-ji-kəl\ *adj* : not biological ⟨~ factors⟩

non·cal·ci·fied \-'kal-sə-ˌfīd\ *adj* : not calcified ⟨a ~ lesion⟩

non·ca·lo·ric \-kə-'lȯr-ik, -'lär-; -ˌka-lə-rik\ *adj* : not providing calories when consumed as part of a diet ⟨~ beverages⟩

non·can·cer·ous \-'kan-sə-rəs\ *adj* : not affected with or being cancer

non·car·ci·no·gen·ic \-ˌkär-ˌsi-nə-'je-nik, -ˌkärs-ᵊn-ə-\ *adj* : not causing cancer — **non·car·cin·o·gen** \-kär-'si-nə-jən, -'kärs-ᵊn-ə-jən\ *n*

non·car·di·ac \-'kär-dē-ˌak\ *adj* : not cardiac: as **a** : not affected with heart disease **b** : not relating to the heart or heart disease ⟨~ disorders⟩

non·ca·se·at·ing \-'kā-sē-ˌā-tiŋ\ *adj* : not exhibiting caseation ⟨~ granulomas⟩

non·cel·lu·lar \-'sel-yə-lər\ *adj* : not made up of or divided into cells

non·chro·mo·som·al \-ˌkrō-mə-'sō-məl\ *adj* **1** : not situated on a chromosome ⟨~ DNA⟩ **2** : not involving chromosomes ⟨~ mutations⟩

non·cod·ing \-'kō-diŋ\ *adj* : not specifying the genetic code ⟨~ introns⟩

non·co·ital \-'kō-ət-ᵊl, -kō-'ēt-\ *adj* : not involving heterosexual copulation

non·com·e·do·gen·ic \-ˌkä-mə-dō-'je-nik\ *adj* : not tending to clog pores (as by the formation of blackheads)

non·com·mu·ni·ca·ble \-kə-'myü-ni-kə-bəl\ *adj* : not capable of being communicated; *specif* : not transmissible by direct contact ⟨a ~ disease⟩

non·com·pli·ance \-kəm-'plī-əns\ *n* : failure or refusal to comply (as in the taking of prescribed medication) — **non·com·pli·ant** \-ənt\ *adj*

non com·pos men·tis \ˌnän-ˌkäm-pəs-'men-təs, ˌnōn-\ *adj* : not of sound mind

non·con·scious \-'kän-chəs\ *adj* : not conscious

non·con·ta·gious \ˌnän-kən-'tā-jəs\ *adj* : not contagious ⟨a ~ disease⟩

non·con·trac·tile \-kən-'trakt-ᵊl, -ˌīl\ *adj* : not contractile ⟨~ fibers⟩

non·con·vul·sive \-kən-'vəl-siv\ *adj* : not convulsive ⟨~ seizures⟩

non·cor·o·nary \-'kȯr-ə-ˌner-ē, -'kär-\ *adj* : not affecting, affected with disease of, or involving the coronary vessels of the heart ⟨~ patients⟩

non·cy·to·tox·ic \-ˌsī-tə-'täk-sik\ *adj* : not toxic to cells ⟨~ drug doses⟩

non·de·form·ing \-di-'fȯr-miŋ\ *adj* : not causing deformation ⟨~ arthritis⟩

non·de·pressed \-di-'prest\ *adj* : not depressed ⟨~ adults⟩

¹non·di·a·bet·ic \-ˌdī-ə-'be-tik\ *adj* : not affected with diabetes ⟨~ persons⟩

²nondiabetic *n* : an individual not affected with diabetes

non·di·ag·nos·tic \-ˌdī-ig-'näs-tik, -əg-\ *adj* : not diagnostic ⟨a ~ lung scan⟩

non·di·a·lyz·able \-ˌdī-ə-'lī-zə-bəl\ *adj* : not dialyzable

non·di·rec·tive \ˌnän-də-'rek-tiv, -(ˌ)dī-\ *adj* : of, relating to, or being psychotherapy, counseling, or interviewing in which the counselor refrains from interpretation or explanation but encourages the patient (as by repeating phrases) to talk freely

non·dis·junc·tion \-dis-'jəŋk-shən\ *n* : failure of homologous chromosomes or sister chromatids to separate subsequent to metaphase in meiosis or mitosis so that one daughter cell has both and the other neither of the chromosomes

non·dis·sem·i·nat·ed \-di-ˈse-mə-ˌnā-təd\ *adj* : not disseminated ⟨∼ lupus erythematosus⟩

non·di·vid·ing \-də-ˈvī-diŋ\ *adj* : not undergoing cell division ⟨∼ cells⟩

non·drowsy \-ˈdrau̇-zē\ *adj* : not causing or accompanied by drowsiness

non·drug \(ˌ)nän-ˈdrəg\ *adj* : not relating to, being, or employing drugs

non·elas·tic \-i-ˈlas-tik\ *adj* : not elastic ⟨∼ fibrous tissue⟩

non·emer·gency \-i-ˈmər-jən-sē\ *adj* : not requiring emergency care ⟨∼ surgery⟩ ⟨∼ patients⟩

non·en·zy·mat·ic \-ˌen-zə-ˈma-tik\ *or* **non·en·zy·mic** \-en-ˈzī-mik\ *also* **non·en·zyme** \-ˈen-ˌzīm\ *adj* : not involving the action of enzymes

non·ero·sive \-i-ˈrō-siv, -ziv\ *adj* : not characterized by erosion of tissue

non·es·sen·tial \-i-ˈsen-chəl\ *adj* : being a substance synthesized by the body in sufficient quantity for normal health and growth ⟨a ∼ fatty acid⟩ — compare ESSENTIAL

nonessential amino acid *n* : any of various amino acids that are required for normal health and growth, that can be synthesized within the body or derived in the body from essential amino acids, and that include alanine, asparagine, aspartic acid, cystine, glutamic acid, glutamine, glycine, proline, serine, and tyrosine

non·fa·mil·ial \-fə-ˈmil-yəl\ *adj* : not familial ⟨∼ colon cancer⟩

non·fat \ˌnän-ˈfat\ *adj* : lacking fat solids : having fat solids removed ⟨∼ milk⟩

non·fa·tal \-ˈfāt-əl\ *adj* : not fatal

non·fe·brile \-ˈfe-ˌbrīl, -ˈfē-\ *adj* : not marked or affected by a fever ⟨∼ illnesses⟩ ⟨∼ patients⟩; *also* : not occurring with a fever ⟨∼ seizures⟩

non·flag·el·lat·ed \-ˈfla-jə-ˌlā-təd\ *adj* : not having flagella

non·func·tion·al \-ˈfəŋk-shə-nəl\ *adj* : not performing or able to perform a regular function ⟨a ∼ muscle⟩

non·ge·net·ic \-jə-ˈne-tik\ *adj* : not genetic ⟨∼ diseases⟩

non·glan·du·lar \-ˈglan-jə-lər\ *adj* : not glandular ⟨the ∼ mucosa⟩

non·gono·coc·cal \-ˌgä-nə-ˈkä-kəl\ *adj* : not caused by a gonococcus

nongonococcal urethritis *n* : urethritis caused by a microorganism other than a gonococcus; *esp* : urethritis that is sexually transmitted and is caused esp. by a bacterium of the genus *Chlamydia* (*C. trachomatis*) or of the genus *Ureaplasma* (*U. urealyticum*) — called also *nonspecific urethritis*

non·gran·u·lar \-ˈgra-nyə-lər\ *adj* : not granular; *esp* : characterized by or being cytoplasm which does not contain granules ⟨∼ white blood cells⟩

non·grav·id \-ˈgra-vid\ *adj* : not pregnant

non·heal·ing \-ˈhē-liŋ\ *adj* : not healing ⟨∼ ulcers⟩

non·heme \-ˈhēm\ *adj* : not containing or being iron that is bound in a porphyrin ring like that of heme

non·he·mo·lyt·ic \-ˌhē-mə-ˈli-tik\ *adj* : not causing or characterized by hemolysis ⟨a ∼ streptococcus⟩

non·hem·or·rhag·ic \-ˌhe-mə-ˈra-jik\ *adj* : not causing or associated with hemorrhage ⟨∼ shock⟩

non·he·red·i·tary \-hə-ˈre-də-ˌter-ē\ *adj* : not hereditary

non·her·i·ta·ble \-ˈher-ə-tə-bəl\ *adj* : not heritable ⟨∼ diseases⟩

non·his·tone \-ˈhis-ˌtōn\ *adj* : relating to or being any of the eukaryotic proteins (as DNA polymerase) that form complexes with DNA but are not considered histones

non–Hodg·kin's lymphoma \-ˈhäj-kinz-\ *n* : any of various malignant lymphomas (as Burkitt's lymphoma) that are not classified as Hodgkin's disease, have malignant cells derived from B cells, T cells, or natural killer cells, and are characterized esp. by enlarged lymph nodes, fever, night sweats, fatigue, and weight loss — compare HODGKIN'S DISEASE

non·ho·mol·o·gous \-hō-ˈmä-lə-gəs, -hə-\ *adj* : being of unlike genetic constitution — used of chromosomes of one set containing nonallelic genes

non·hor·mo·nal \-hȯr-ˈmōn-əl\ *adj* : not hormonal ⟨∼ therapies⟩

non·hos·pi·tal \-ˈhäs-ˌpit-əl\ *adj* : not relating to, associated with, or occurring within a hospital ⟨∼ clinics⟩

non·hos·pi·tal·ized \-ˈhäs-ˌpit-əl-ˌīzd\ *adj* : not hospitalized ⟨∼ patients⟩

non·iden·ti·cal \-(ˌ)ī-ˈden-ti-kəl\ *adj* : not identical; *esp* : FRATERNAL

non·im·mune \-i-ˈmyün\ *adj* **1** : not immune : lacking immunity ⟨∼ people⟩ **2** : not caused or mediated by the immune system ⟨drug-induced ∼ thrombocytopenia⟩

non·in·fect·ed \-in-ˈfek-təd\ *adj* : not having been subjected to infection

non·in·fec·tious \-in-ˈfek-shəs\ *adj* : not infectious ⟨∼ diseases⟩

non·in·fec·tive \-tiv\ *adj* : not infective ⟨∼ enteritis⟩

non·in·flam·ma·to·ry \-in-ˈfla-mə-ˌtȯr-ē\ *adj* : not inflammatory

non·in·sti·tu·tion·al·ized \-ˌin-stə-ˈtü-shə-nə-ˌlīzd, -ˈtyü-\ *adj* : not institutionalized

non–insulin–dependent diabetes *n* : TYPE 2 DIABETES

non–insulin–dependent diabetes mellitus *n* : TYPE 2 DIABETES — abbr. *NIDDM*

non·in·va·sive \-in-ˈvā-siv, -ziv\ *adj* **1** : not tending to spread; *specif* : not tending to infiltrate and destroy healthy tissue ⟨∼ cancer of the bladder⟩ **2** : not being or involving an invasive medical procedure ⟨∼ imaging techniques that do not require the injection of dyes⟩ — **non·in·va·sive·ly** adv — **non·in·va·sive·ness** n

non·ir·ra·di·at·ed \-i-'rā-dē-ˌā-tad\ adj : not having been exposed to radiation

non·isch·emic \-is-'kē-mik\ adj : not marked by or resulting from ischemia ⟨∼ tissue⟩

non·ke·ra·ti·nized \-'ker-ə-tə-ˌnīzd, -kə-'ra-tᵊn-ˌīzd\ adj : not keratinous ⟨∼ epithelium⟩

non·ke·tot·ic \-kē-'tä-tik\ adj : not associated with ketosis ⟨∼ coma⟩

non·liv·ing \-'li-viŋ\ adj : not having or characterized by life

non·lym·pho·cyt·ic \-ˌlim-fə-'si-tik\ adj : not lymphocytic — see ACUTE NONLYMPHOCYTIC LEUKEMIA

non·lym·phoid \-'lim-ˌfȯid\ adj : not derived from or being lymphoid tissue ⟨∼ cells⟩; also : not composed of lymphoid cells ⟨a ∼ tumor⟩

non·ma·lig·nant \-mə-'lig-nənt\ adj : not malignant ⟨a ∼ tumor⟩

non·med·ul·lat·ed \-'med-ᵊl-ˌā-təd, -'me-jə-ˌlā-\ adj : UNMYELINATED

non·mel·a·no·ma \-ˌme-lə-'nō-mə\ n, often attrib : a tumor that is not a melanoma ⟨∼ skin cancer⟩

non·met·al \-'met-ᵊl\ n : a chemical element (as carbon) that lacks the characteristics of a metal — **non·me·tal·lic** \-mə-'ta-lik\ adj

non·met·a·stat·ic \-ˌme-tə-'sta-tik\ adj : not metastatic ⟨∼ tumors⟩

non·mi·cro·bi·al \-mī-'krō-bē-əl\ adj : not microbial ⟨∼ diseases⟩

non·mo·tile \-'mōt-ᵊl, -'mō-ˌtīl\ adj : not motile ⟨∼ gametes⟩

non·my·elin·at·ed \-'mī-ə-lə-ˌnā-təd\ adj : UNMYELINATED

non·my·eloid \-'mī-ə-ˌlȯid\ adj : not being, involving, or affecting bone marrow ⟨∼ malignancies⟩

non·nar·cot·ic \-när-'kä-tik\ adj : not narcotic ⟨∼ analgesics⟩

non·neo·plas·tic \-ˌnē-ə-'plas-tik\ adj : not being or not caused by neoplasms ⟨∼ diseases⟩

non·ner·vous \-ˌnȯr-vəs\ adj : not nervous ⟨∼ tissue⟩

non·neu·ro·nal \-'nu̇r-ə-nᵊl, -'nyu̇-, -nü-'rōn-ᵊl, -nyü-\ adj : of, relating to, or being cells other than neurons

non·nu·cle·at·ed \-'nü-klē-ˌā-təd, -'nyü-\ adj : not nucleated ⟨∼ cells⟩

non·nu·tri·tive \-'nü-trə-tiv, -'nyü-\ adj : not relating to or providing nutrition

non·obese \-ō-'bēs\ adj : not obese

non·ob·struc·tive \-əb-'strək-tiv\ adj : not causing or characterized by obstruction (as of a bodily passage)

non·oc·clu·sive \-ə-'klü-siv\ adj : not causing or characterized by occlusion

non·of·fi·cial \-ə-'fi-shəl\ adj : not described in the current U.S. Pharmacopeia and National Formulary and never having been described therein — compare OFFICIAL

non·ol·fac·to·ry \-äl-'fak-tə-rē, -ōl-\ adj : not olfactory

non·op·er·a·tive \-'ä-pə-rə-tiv, -ˌrā-\ adj : not involving an operation ⟨∼ treatment⟩

non·or·gas·mic \-ȯr-'gaz-mik\ adj : not capable of experiencing orgasm

non·oxy·nol-9 \nä-'näk-sə-ˌnȯl-'nīn, -ˌnȯl-\ n : a spermicide used in contraceptive products that consists of a mixture of compounds having the general formula $C_{15}H_{23}(OCH_2CH_2)_n$-OH with an average of nine ethylene oxide groups per molecule

non·par·a·sit·ic \-ˌpar-ə-'si-tik\ adj : not parasitic; esp : not caused by parasites ⟨∼ diseases⟩

non·patho·gen·ic \-ˌpa-thə-'je-nik\ adj : not capable of inducing disease

non·per·sis·tent \-pər-'sis-tənt\ adj : not persistent; esp : decomposed rapidly by environmental action ⟨∼ insecticides⟩

non·phy·si·cian \-fə-'zi-shən\ n : a person who is not a legally qualified physician

non·pig·ment·ed \-'pig-mən-təd\ adj : not pigmented ⟨∼ skin lesions⟩

non·poi·son·ous \-'pȯi-zə-nəs\ adj : not poisonous ⟨∼ snakes⟩

non·po·lar \-'pō-lər\ adj : not polar; esp : consisting of molecules not having a dipole

non·pol·yp·o·sis \-ˌpä-li-'pō-səs\ adj : characterized by the absence of polyps ⟨hereditary ∼ colorectal cancer⟩

non·preg·nant \-'preg-nənt\ adj : not pregnant

non·pre·scrip·tion \-pri-'skrip-shən\ adj : available for purchase without a doctor's prescription ⟨∼ drugs⟩

non·pro·duc·tive \-prə-'dək-tiv\ adj, of a cough : not effective in raising mucus or exudate from the respiratory tract : DRY 2

non·pro·gres·sor \-prə-'gre-sər\ n : LONG-TERM NONPROGRESSOR

non·pro·pri·etary \-prə-'prī-ə-ˌter-ē\ adj : not proprietary ⟨a drug's ∼ name⟩

non·pro·tein \-'prō-ˌtēn\ adj : not being or derived from protein

non·psy·chi·at·ric \-ˌsī-kē-'a-trik\ adj : not psychiatric ⟨∼ patients⟩

non·psy·chi·a·trist \-sə-'kī-ə-trist, -sī-\ adj : not specializing in psychiatry ⟨∼ physicians⟩ — **nonpsychiatrist** n

non·psy·chot·ic \-sī-'kä-tik\ adj : not psychotic ⟨∼ emotional disorders⟩

non·ra·dio·ac·tive \-ˌrä-dē-ō-'ak-tiv\ adj : not radioactive ⟨∼ probes⟩

non·re·ac·tive \-rē-'ak-tiv\ adj : not reactive; esp : not exhibiting a positive reaction in a particular laboratory test ⟨all of the serums were ∼⟩

non–REM sleep \-ˌrem-\ n : SLOW-WAVE SLEEP

non·re·nal \-'rēn-ᵊl\ adj : not renal; esp : not resulting from dysfunction of the kidneys ⟨∼ alkalosis⟩

non·re·spond·er \-ri-'spän-dər\ *n* : one (as a patient) that does not respond (as to medical treatment)

non·rheu·ma·toid \-'rü-mə-ˌtȯid\ *adj* : not relating to, affected with, or being rheumatoid arthritis

non·rhyth·mic \-'rith-mik\ *adj* : not rhythmic ⟨∼ contractions⟩

¹**non·schizo·phren·ic** \-ˌskit-sə-'fre-nik\ *adj* : not relating to, affected with, or being schizophrenia

²**nonschizophrenic** *n* : a nonschizophrenic individual

non·se·cre·tor \-si-'krē-tər\ *n* : an individual of blood group A, B, or AB who does not secrete the antigens characteristic of these blood groups in bodily fluids (as saliva)

non·se·cre·to·ry \-'sē-krə-ˌtȯr-ē\ *adj* : not secretory ⟨∼ cells⟩

non·se·dat·ing \-si-'dā-tiŋ\ *adj* : not producing sedation ⟨∼ antihistamines⟩

¹**non·sed·a·tive** \-'se-də-tiv\ *adj* : NONSEDATING

²**nonsedative** *n* : a nonsedating drug

non·se·lec·tive \-sə-'lek-tiv\ *adj* : not selective; *esp* : not limited (as to a single body part or organism) in action or effect ⟨∼ anti-infective agents⟩

non·self \ˌnän-'self\ *n* : material that is foreign to the body of an organism — **nonself** *adj*

¹**non·sense** \'nän-ˌsens, -səns\ *n* : genetic information consisting of one or more codons that do not code for any amino acid and usu. cause termination of the molecular chain in protein synthesis — compare ANTISENSE, MISSENSE

²**nonsense** *adj* : consisting of one or more codons that are genetic nonsense ⟨∼ mutations⟩

non·sen·si·tive \-'sen-sə-tiv\ *adj* : not sensitive ⟨∼ skin⟩

non·sex·u·al \-'sek-shə-wəl\ *adj* : not sexual ⟨∼ reproduction⟩

non–small cell lung cancer *n* : any carcinoma (as an adenocarcinoma or squamous cell carcinoma) of the lungs that is not a small-cell lung cancer — called also *non-small cell cancer, non-small cell carcinoma, non-small cell lung carcinoma;* see LARGE-CELL CARCINOMA

non·smok·er \-'smō-kər\ *n* : a person who does not smoke tobacco

non·spe·cif·ic \-spi-'si-fik\ *adj* : not specific: as **a** : not caused by a specific agent ⟨∼ enteritis⟩ **b** : having a general purpose or effect — **non·spe·cif·i·cal·ly** *adv*

nonspecific urethritis *n* : NONGONO-COCCAL URETHRITIS

nonspecific vaginitis *n* : BACTERIAL VAGINOSIS

non·ste·roi·dal \-stə-'rȯid-ᵊl\ *also* **non·ste·roid** \-'stir-ˌȯid, -'ster-\ *adj* : of, relating to, or being a compound and esp. a drug that is not a steroid — see NSAID — **nonsteroid** *n*

non·stress test \'nän-'stres\ *n* : a test of fetal well-being that is performed by ultrasound monitoring of the increase in fetal heartbeat following fetal movement

nonstriated muscle *n* : SMOOTH MUSCLE

non·sug·ar \-'shů-gər\ *n* : a substance that is not a sugar; *esp* : AGLYCONE

non·sup·pu·ra·tive \-'sə-pyə-ˌrā-tiv\ *adj* : not characterized by or accompanied by suppuration

non·sur·gi·cal \-'sər-ji-kəl\ *adj* : not surgical ⟨∼ hospital care⟩ — **non·sur·gi·cal·ly** *adv*

non·sys·tem·ic \-sis-'te-mik\ *adj* : not systemic ⟨∼ infections⟩

non·tast·er \-'tā-stər\ *n* : a person unable to taste the chemical phenylthiocarbamide

non·ther·a·peu·tic \-ˌther-ə-'pyü-tik\ *adj* : not relating to or being therapy

non·throm·bo·cy·to·pe·nic \-ˌthräm-bə-ˌsī-tə-'pē-nik\ *adj* : not relating to, affected with, or associated with thrombocytopenia ⟨∼ purpura⟩

non·tox·ic \-'täk-sik\ *adj* **1** : not toxic ⟨∼ chemicals⟩ **2** *of goiter* : not associated with hyperthyroidism

non·trau·mat·ic \-trə-'ma-tik, -trȯ-, -trau\ *adj* : not causing, caused by, or associated with trauma and esp. traumatic injury ⟨∼ hemorrhage⟩

non·trop·i·cal sprue \-'trä-pi-kəl-\ *n* : CELIAC DISEASE

non·tu·ber·cu·lous \-tů-'bər-kyə-ləs, -tyů-\ *adj* : not causing, caused by, or affected with tuberculosis ⟨∼ mycobacteria⟩

non·union \-'yün-yən\ *n* : failure of the fragments of a broken bone to knit together

non·vas·cu·lar \-'vas-kyə-lər\ *adj* : lacking blood vessels or a vascular system ⟨a ∼ layer of the skin⟩

non·ven·om·ous \-'ve-nə-məs\ *adj* : not venomous

non·vi·a·ble \-'vī-ə-bəl\ *adj* : not capable of living, growing, or developing and functioning successfully

no·o·tro·pic \ˌnō-ə-'trō-pik, -'trä-\ *n* : a drug that promotes the enhancement of cognition and memory and the facilitation of learning — called also *smart drug* — **nootropic** *adj*

NOPHN *abbr* National Organization for Public Health Nursing

nor·adren·a·line *also* **nor·adren·a·lin** \ˌnȯr-ə-'dren-ᵊl-ən\ *n* : NOREPINEPHRINE

nor·ad·ren·er·gic \ˌnȯr-ˌa-drə-'nər-jik\ *adj* : liberating, activated by, or involving norepinephrine in the transmission of nerve impulses — compare ADRENERGIC 1, CHOLINERGIC 1

nor·el·ges·tro·min \ˌnȯr-el-'jes-trə-mən\ *n* : a synthetic progestogen $C_{21}H_{29}NO_2$ that is used in combination with ethinyl estradiol in a contraceptive transdermal patch — see ORTHO EVRA

nor·epi·neph·rine \ˌnȯr-ˌe-pə-'ne-frən, -ˌfrēn\ *n* : a catecholamine $C_8H_{11}NO_3$

that is the chemical means of transmission across synapses in postganglionic neurons of the sympathetic nervous system and in some parts of the central nervous system, is a vasopressor hormone of the adrenal medulla, and is a precursor of epinephrine in its major biosynthetic pathway — called also *noradrenaline*; see LEVOPHED

nor·eth·in·drone \nȯ-'re-thən-ˌdrōn\ *n* : a synthetic progestational hormone $C_{20}H_{26}O_2$ used in birth control pills often in the form of its acetate $C_{22}H_{28}O_3$ — see ORTHO-NOVUM

nor·ethis·ter·one \ˌnȯr-ə-'this-tə-ˌrōn\ *n, chiefly Brit* : NORETHINDRONE

nor·ethyn·o·drel \ˌnȯr-ə-'thi-nə-ˌdrəl\ *n* : a progesterone derivative $C_{20}H_{26}O_2$ used in birth control pills and in the treatment of endometriosis and hypermenorrhea — see ENOVID

nor·flox·a·cin \nȯr-'fläk-sə-ˌsin\ *n* : a fluoroquinolone $C_{16}H_{18}FN_3O_3$ used topically to treat conjunctivitis and orally to treat various bacterial infections (as of the urinary tract)

nor·ges·ti·mate \nȯr-'jes-tə-ˌmāt\ *n* : a synthetic progestogen $C_{23}H_{31}NO_3$ that is used in combination with an estrogen (as ethinyl estradiol) in birth control pills — see ORTHO TRI-CYCLEN

nor·ges·trel \nȯr-'jes-trel\ *n* : a synthetic progestogen $C_{21}H_{28}O_2$ having two optically active forms of which the biologically active levorotatory form is used in birth control pills — see LEVONORGESTREL

norm \'nȯrm\ *n* : an established standard or average: as **a** : a set standard of development or achievement usu. derived from the average or median achievement of a large group **b** : a pattern or trait taken to be typical in the behavior of a social group

norm- *or* **normo-** *comb form* : normal ⟨*normo*blast⟩ ⟨*normo*tensive⟩

¹**nor·mal** \'nȯr-məl\ *adj* **1 a** : according with, constituting, or not deviating from a norm, rule, or principle **b** : conforming to a type, standard, or regular pattern **2** : occurring naturally and not because of disease, inoculation, or any experimental treatment ⟨∼ immunity⟩ **3 a** : of, relating to, or characterized by average intelligence or development **b** : free from mental disorder : SANE **c** : characterized by balanced well-integrated functioning of the organism as a whole — **nor·mal·ize** \'nȯr-mə-ˌlīz\ *vb* — **nor·mal·ly** \'nȯr-mə-lē\ *adv*

²**normal** *n* : a subject who is normal

nor·meta·neph·rine \ˌnȯr-ˌme-tə-'ne-fran, -ˌfren\ *n* : a metabolite of norepinephrine $C_9H_{13}NO_3$ found esp. in the urine

nor·mo·ac·tive \ˌnȯr-mō-'ak-tiv\ *adj* : normally active ⟨∼ children⟩; *also* : indicating normal activity ⟨∼ bowel sounds⟩

nor·mo·blast \'nȯr-mə-ˌblast\ *n* : an

immature red blood cell containing hemoglobin and a pyknotic nucleus and normally present in bone marrow but appearing in the blood in many anemias — compare ERYTHROBLAST — **nor·mo·blas·tic** \ˌnȯr-mə-'blas-tik\ *adj*

nor·mo·cal·cae·mia *chiefly Brit var of* NORMOCALCEMIA

nor·mo·cal·ce·mia \ˌnȯr-mō-kal-'sē-mē-ə\ *n* : the presence of a normal concentration of calcium in the blood — **nor·mo·cal·ce·mic** \-mik\ *adj*

nor·mo·chro·mia \ˌnȯr-mə-'krō-mē-ə\ *n* : the color of red blood cells that contain a normal amount of hemoglobin — **nor·mo·chro·mic** \-'krō-mik\ *adj*

normochromic anemia *n* : an anemia marked by reduced numbers of normochromic red blood cells in the circulating blood

nor·mo·cyte \'nȯr-mə-ˌsīt\ *n* : a red blood cell that is normal in size and in hemoglobin content

nor·mo·cyt·ic \ˌnȯr-mə-'si-tik\ *adj* : characterized by red blood cells that are normal in size and usu. in hemoglobin content ⟨∼ blood⟩

normocytic anemia *n* : an anemia marked by reduced numbers of normal red blood cells in the circulating blood

nor·mo·gly·ce·mia \ˌnȯr-mō-glī-'sē-mē-ə\ *n* : the presence of a normal concentration of glucose in the blood — **nor·mo·gly·ce·mic** \-mik\ *adj*

nor·mo·ka·le·mic \ˌnȯr-mō-kā-'lē-mik\ *adj* : having or characterized by a normal concentration of potassium in the blood ⟨∼ patients⟩

nor·mo·ten·sive \ˌnȯr-mō-'ten-siv\ *adj* : having normal blood pressure

nor·mo·ther·mia \-'thər-mē-ə\ *n* : normal body temperature — **nor·mo·ther·mic** \-mik\ *adj*

nor·mo·vo·lae·mia *chiefly Brit var of* NORMOVOLEMIA

nor·mo·vol·emia \ˌnȯr-mō-ˌvä-'lē-mē-ə\ *n* : a normal volume of blood in the body — **nor·mo·vol·emic** \-mik\ *adj*

Nor·plant \'nȯr-ˌplant\ *trademark* — used for contraceptive implants of encapsulated levonorgestrel

Nor·pra·min \'nȯr-prə-mən\ *trademark* — used for a preparation of the hydrochloride of desipramine

Nor·rie disease *also* **Nor·rie's disease** \'nȯr-ē(z)-\ *n* : a rare congenital X-linked disease that affects males and is characterized esp. by retinal malformation and opacification of the vitreous body leading to blindness, by progressive mental deterioration, and by deafness

Norrie, Gordon (1855–1941), Danish ophthalmologist.

19–nor·tes·tos·ter·one \(ˌ)nīn-'ten-ˌnȯr-te-'stäs-tə-ˌrōn\ *n* : NANDROLONE

North American blastomycosis *n* : blastomycosis that involves esp. the skin, lymph nodes, and lungs and is caused by infection with a fungus of the genus *Blastomyces* (*B. dermatitidis*) — called also *Gilchrist's disease*

Northern blot *n* : a blot consisting of a sheet of a cellulose derivative that contains spots of RNA for identification by a suitable molecular probe — compare SOUTHERN BLOT, WESTERN BLOT — **Northern blotting** *n*

northern cattle grub *n* : an immature form or adult of a warble fly of the genus *Hypoderma* (*H. bovis*) — called also *cattle grub*

northern fowl mite *n* : a parasitic mite (*Ornithonyssus sylviarum*) that is a pest of birds and esp. poultry

northern rat flea *n* : a common and widely distributed flea of the genus *Nosopsyllus* (*N. fasciatus*) that is parasitic on rats and transmits murine typhus and possibly plague

nor·trip·ty·line \nȯr-ˈtrip-tə-ˌlēn\ *n* : a tricyclic antidepressant administered in the form of its hydrochloride $C_{19}H_{21}N \cdot HCl$ — see AVENTYL

Nor·vasc \ˈnȯr-ˌvask\ *trademark* — used for a preparation of the salt of amlodipine

Nor·vir \ˈnȯr-ˌvir\ *trademark* — used for a preparation of ritonavir

Nor·walk virus \ˈnȯr-ˌwȯk-\ *n* : a calicivirus (species *Norwalk virus* of the genus *Norovirus*) that causes an infectious human gastroenteritis — called also *Norwalk agent*

Nor·way rat \ˈnȯr-wā-\ *n* : BROWN RAT

Nor·wood procedure \ˈnȯr-ˌwud-\ *n* : a complex surgical procedure esp. for the palliative treatment of hypoplastic left heart syndrome — called also *Norwood operation*

  Norwood, William I. (*b* 1941), American surgeon.

nos- or **noso-** *comb form* : disease ⟨*nosology*⟩

nose \ˈnōz\ *n* **1 a** : the part of the face that bears the nostrils and covers the anterior part of the nasal cavity; *broadly* : this part together with the nasal cavity **b** : the anterior part of the head above or projecting beyond the muzzle **2** : the sense of smell : OLFACTION **3** : OLFACTORY ORGAN

nose·bleed \-ˌblēd\ *n* : an attack of bleeding from the nose — called also *epistaxis*

nose botfly *n* : a botfly of the genus *Gasterophilus* (*G. haemorrhoidalis*) that is parasitic in the larval stage esp. on horses and mules — called also *nose fly*

nose job *n* : RHINOPLASTY

nose·piece \ˈnōz-ˌpēs\ *n* : the bridge of a pair of eyeglasses

nos·o·co·mi·al \ˌnä-sə-ˈkō-mē-əl\ *adj* : acquired or occurring in a hospital ⟨∼ infection⟩ — **nos·o·co·mi·al·ly** \-ē\ *adv*

no·sol·o·gy \nō-ˈsä-lə-jē, -ˈzä-\ *n, pl* **-gies 1** : a classification or list of diseases **2** : a branch of medical science that deals with classification of diseases — **no·so·log·i·cal** \ˌnō-sə-ˈlä-ji-kəl\ or **no·so·log·ic** \-jik\ *adj* — **no·so·log·i·cal·ly** *adv* — **no·sol·o·gist** \ˌnō-ˈsä-lə-jist\ *n*

Nos·o·psyl·lus \ˌnä-sə-ˈsi-ləs\ *n* : a genus of fleas that includes the northern rat flea (*N. fasciatus*)

nos·tril \ˈnäs-trəl\ *n* **1** : either of the external nares; *broadly* : either of the nares with the adjoining passage on the same side of the nasal septum **2** : either fleshy lateral wall of the nose

nos·trum \ˈnäs-trəm\ *n* : a medicine of secret composition recommended by its preparer but usu. without scientific proof of its effectiveness

not- or **noto-** *comb form* : back : back part ⟨*notochord*⟩

notch \ˈnäch\ *n* : a V-shaped indentation (as on a bone) — **notched** \ˈnächt\ *adj*

no·ti·fi·able \ˌnō-tə-ˈfī-ə-bəl\ *adj* : required by law to be reported to official health authorities ⟨a ∼ disease⟩

no·ti·fi·ca·tion \ˌnō-tə-fə-ˈkā-shən\ *n* : the act of reporting the occurrence of a communicable disease or of an individual affected with such a disease — **no·ti·fy** \ˈnō-tə-ˌfī\ *vb*

no·to·chord \ˈnō-tə-ˌkȯrd\ *n* : a longitudinal flexible rod of cells that in all vertebrates and some more primitive forms provides the supporting axis of the body, that is almost obliterated in the adult of higher vertebrates as the body develops from the dorsal lip of the blastopore extending forward between epiblast and hypoblast in the middorsal line — **no·to·chord·al** \ˌnō-tə-ˈkȯrd-ᵊl\ *adj*

No·to·ed·res \ˌnō-tō-ˈe-ˌdrēz\ *n* : a genus of mites (family Sarcoptidae) containing mange mites that attack various mammals and esp. cats and occas. infest humans usu. through contact with cats

nour·ish \ˈnər-ish\ *vb* : to furnish or sustain with nutriment

nour·ish·ing *adj* : giving nourishment : NUTRITIOUS

nour·ish·ment \ˈnər-ish-mənt\ *n* **1** : FOOD 1, NUTRIMENT **2** : the act of nourishing or the state of being nourished

no·vo·bi·o·cin \ˌnō-və-ˈbī-ə-sən\ *n* : a highly toxic antibiotic $C_{31}H_{36}N_2O_{11}$ used in some serious cases of staphylococcal and urinary tract infection

No·vo·cain \ˈnō-və-ˌkān\ *trademark* — used for a preparation of the hydrochloride of procaine

no·vo·caine \-ˌkān\ *n* : procaine in the form of its hydrochloride; *broadly* : a local anesthetic

noxa \ˈnäk-sə\ *n, pl* **nox·ae** \-ˌsē, -ˌsī\ : something that exerts a harmful effect on the body

nox·ious \ˈnäk-shəs\ *adj* : physically harmful or destructive to living beings

Np *symbol* neptunium

NP *abbr* **1** neuropsychiatric; neuropsychiatry **2** nurse practitioner

NPH insulin \,en-,pē-'āch-\ *n* [*neutral protamine of *H*agedorn*] : ISOPHANE INSULIN

NPN *abbr* nonprotein nitrogen

NPO *abbr* [Latin *nil per os*] nothing by mouth

NR *abbr* no refill

NREM sleep \'en-,rem\ *n* : SLOW-WAVE SLEEP

ns *abbr* nanosecond

NSAID \'en-,sed, -,sād\ *n* : a non-steroidal anti-inflammatory drug (as ibuprofen)

nsec *abbr* nanosecond

NSU *abbr* nonspecific urethritis

NTD *abbr* neural tube defect

nu·chae \'nü-kē, 'nyü-\ — see LIGA-MENTUM NUCHAE

nu·chal \'nü-kəl, 'nyü-\ *adj* : of, relating to, or lying in the region of the nape

nuchal line *n* : any of several ridges on the outside of the skull: as **a** : one on each side that extends laterally in a curve from the external occipital protuberance to the mastoid process of the temporal bone — called also *superior nuchal line* **b** : OCCIPITAL CREST a **c** : one on each side that extends laterally from the middle of the external occipital crest below and roughly parallel to the superior nuchal line — called also *inferior nuchal line*

nucle- *or* **nucleo-** *comb form* **1** : nucleus ⟨*nucleon*⟩ ⟨*nucleo*plasm⟩ **2** : nucleic acid ⟨*nucleo*protein⟩

nu·cle·ar \'nü-klē-ər, 'nyü-\ *adj* **1** : of, relating to, or constituting a nucleus **2** : of, relating to, or utilizing the atomic nucleus, atomic energy, the atomic bomb, or atomic power

nuclear family *n* : a family group that consists only of father, mother, and children — see EXTENDED FAMILY

nuclear fission *n* : FISSION 2

nuclear magnetic resonance *n* **1** : the magnetic resonance of an atomic nucleus **2** : chemical analysis that uses nuclear magnetic resonance esp. to study molecular structure — abbr. *NMR;* see MAGNETIC RESONANCE IMAGING

nuclear medicine *n* : a branch of medicine dealing with the use of radioactive materials in the diagnosis and treatment of disease

nuclear membrane *n* : a double membrane enclosing a cell nucleus and having its outer part continuous with the endoplasmic reticulum

nuclear sap *n* : NUCLEOPLASM

nu·cle·ase \'nü-klē-,ās, 'nyü-, -,āz\ *n* : any of various enzymes that promote hydrolysis of nucleic acids

nu·cle·at·ed \-,ā-təd\ *or* **nu·cle·ate** \-klē-ət\ *adj* : having a nucleus or nuclei

nuclei *pl of* NUCLEUS

nu·cle·ic acid \nü-'klē-ik-, nyü-, -'klā-\

n : any of various acids (as an RNA or a DNA) composed of nucleotide chains

nu·cle·in \'nü-klē-in, 'nyü-\ *n* **1** : NU-CLEOPROTEIN **2** : NUCLEIC ACID

nucleo- — see NUCLE-

nu·cleo·cap·sid \,nü-klē-ō-'kap-səd, ,nyü-\ *n* : the nucleic acid and surrounding protein coat of a virus

nu·cleo·cy·to·plas·mic \-,sī-tə-'plaz-mik\ *adj* : of or relating to the nucleus and cytoplasm

nu·cleo·his·tone \-'his-,tōn\ *n* : a nucleoprotein in which the protein is a histone

nu·cle·oid \'nü-klē-,óid, 'nyü-\ *n* : the DNA-containing area of a prokaryotic cell (as a bacterium)

nucleol- *or* **nucleolo-** *comb form* : nucleolus ⟨*nucleolar*⟩

nu·cle·o·lar \nü-'klē-ə-lər, nyü-, ,nü-klē-'ō-lər, ,nyü-\ *adj* : of, relating to, or constituting a nucleolus

nucleolar organizer *n* : NUCLEOLUS ORGANIZER

nu·cle·o·lus \nü-'klē-ə-ləs, nyü-\ *n, pl* **-li** \-,lī\ : a spherical body of the nucleus of most eukaryotes that becomes enlarged during protein synthesis, is associated with a nucleolus organizer, and contains the DNA templates for ribosomal RNA

nucleolus organizer *n* : the specific part of a chromosome with which a nucleolus is associated esp. during its reorganization after nuclear division — called also *nucleolar organizer*

nu·cleo·plasm \'nü-klē-ə-,pla-zəm, 'nyü-\ *n* : the fluid or semifluid portion of a cell nucleus

nu·cleo·pro·tein \,nü-klē-ō-'prō-,tēn, ,nyü-\ *n* : a compound that consists of a protein (as a histone) conjugated with a nucleic acid (as a DNA) and that is the principal constituent of the hereditary material in chromosomes

nu·cle·o·side \'nü-klē-ə-,sīd, 'nyü-\ *n* : a compound (as guanosine or adenosine) that consists of a purine or pyrimidine base combined with deoxyribose or ribose and is found esp. in DNA or RNA

nu·cleo·some \-,sōm\ *n* : any of the repeating globular subunits of chromatin that consist of a complex of DNA and histone — **nu·cleo·so·mal** \,nü-klē-ə-'sō-məl, ,nyü-\ *adj*

nu·cle·o·tide \'nü-klē-ə-,tīd, 'nyü-\ *n* : any of several compounds that consist of a ribose or deoxyribose sugar joined to a purine or pyrimidine base and to a phosphate group and that are the basic structural units of RNA and DNA

nu·cle·us \'nü-klē-əs, 'nyü-\ *n, pl* **nu·clei** \-klē-,ī\ *also* **nu·cle·us·es** **1** : a cellular organelle of eukaryotes that is essential to cell functions (as reproduction and protein synthesis), is composed of a fluid or semifluid portion and a nucleoprotein-rich network from which chromosomes and nucleoli arise, and is enclosed in a definite membrane **2** : a mass of gray matter or group of nerve cells in the central nervous system **3** : the positively charged central portion of an atom that comprises nearly all of the atomic mass and that consists of protons and usu. neutrons

nucleus ac·cum·bens \-ə-'kəm-bənz\ *n* : a nucleus forming the floor of the caudal part of the anterior prolongation of the lateral ventricle of the brain

nucleus am·big·u·us \-am-'bi-gyə-wəs\ *n* : an elongated nucleus in the medulla oblongata that is a continuation of a group of cells in the ventral horn of the spinal cord and gives rise to the motor fibers of the glossopharyngeal, vagus, and accessory nerves supplying striated muscle of the larynx and pharynx

nucleus ba·sa·lis \-bə-'sä-ləs\ *n* : the gray matter of the substantia innominata of the forebrain that consists mostly of cholinergic neurons

nucleus basalis of Mey·nert \-'mī-nert\ *n* : NUCLEUS BASALIS
  Meynert, Theodor Hermann (1833–1892), Austrian psychiatrist and neurologist.

nucleus cu·ne·a·tus \-,kyü-nē-'ä-təs\ *n* : the nucleus in the medulla oblongata in which the fibers of the fasciculus cuneatus terminate and synapse with a component of the medial lemniscus — called also *cuneate nucleus*

nucleus grac·i·lis \-'gra-sə-ləs\ *n* : a nucleus in the posterior part of the medulla oblongata in which the fibers of the fasciculus gracilis terminate

nucleus pul·po·sus \-,pəl-'pō-səs\ *n, pl* **nuclei pul·po·si** \-,sī\ : an elastic pulpy mass lying in the center of each intervertebral fibrocartilage

nu·clide \'nü-,klīd, 'nyü-\ *n* : a species of atom characterized by the constitution of its nucleus and hence by the number of protons, the number of neutrons, and the energy content

null cell \'nəl-\ *n* : a lymphocyte in the blood that does not have on its surface the receptors typical of either mature B cells or T cells

nul·li·grav·i·da \,nə-lə-'gra-və-də\ *n, pl* **-dae** \-,dī, -,dē\ *also* **-das** : a woman who has never been pregnant

nul·lip·a·ra \nə-'li-pə-rə\ *n, pl* **-ras** *or* **-rae** \-,rē\ : a woman who has never borne a child

nul·lip·a·rous \,nə-'li-pə-rəs\ *adj* : of, relating to, or being a female that has not borne offspring — **nul·li·par·i·ty** \,nə-lə-'par-ə-tē\ *n*

numb \'nəm\ *adj* : devoid of sensation (as from the administration of anesthesia or exposure to cold) — **numb** *vb* — **numb·ness** *n*

num·mu·lar \'nə-myə-lər\ *adj* **1** : circular or oval in shape ⟨∼ lesions⟩ **2** : characterized by circular or oval lesions or drops ⟨∼ dermatitis⟩

¹**nurse** \'nərs\ *n* **1** : a woman who suckles an infant not her own : WET NURSE **2** : a licensed health-care professional who practices independently or is supervised by a physician, surgeon, or dentist and who is skilled in promoting and maintaining health — see LICENSED PRACTICAL NURSE, LICENSED VOCATIONAL NURSE, REGISTERED NURSE

²**nurse** *vb* **nursed; nurs·ing 1 a** : to nourish at the breast : SUCKLE **b** : to take nourishment from the breast : SUCK **2 a** : to care for and wait on (as an injured or infirm person) **b** : to attempt a cure of (as an ailment) by care and treatment

nurse–anes·the·tist \-ə-'nes-thə-tist\ *n* : a registered nurse who has completed two years of additional training in anesthesia and is qualified to serve as an anesthetist under the supervision of a physician

nurse clinician *n* : NURSE-PRACTITIONER

nurse–midwife *n, pl* **nurse–midwives** : a registered nurse with additional training as a midwife who is certified to deliver infants and provide prenatal and postpartum care, newborn care, and some routine care (as gynecological exams) of women — **nurse–midwifery** *n*

nurse practitioner *n* : a registered nurse who through advanced training is qualified to assume some of the duties and responsibilities formerly assumed only by a physician — abbr. *NP;* called also *nurse clinician*

nurs·ery \'nər-sə-rē\ *n, pl* **-er·ies** : the department of a hospital where newborn infants are cared for

nurse's aide *n* : a worker who assists trained nurses in a hospital by performing general services (as giving baths or taking vital signs)

nurs·ing \'nər-sin\ *n* **1** : the profession of a nurse **2** : the duties of a nurse

nursing bottle *n* : a bottle with a nipple (as of rubber) used in supplying food to infants

nursing home *n* : a privately operated establishment where maintenance and personal or nursing care are provided for persons (as the aged or the chronically ill) who are unable to care for themselves properly

nur·tur·ance \'nər-chə-rəns\ *n* : affectionate care and attention — **nur·tur·ant** \-rənt\ *adj*

nu·tra·ceu·ti·cal *also* **nu·tri·ceu·ti·cal** \,nü-trə-'sü-ti-kəl, ,nyü-\ *n* : a foodstuff (as a fortified food or a dietary supplement) that is held to provide health or medical benefits in addition to its basic nutritional value — called also *functional food*

Nu·tra·Sweet \'nü-trə-,swēt, 'nyü-\ *trademark* — used for a preparation of aspartame

¹**nu·tri·ent** \'nü-trē-ənt, 'nyü-\ *adj* : furnishing nourishment

²**nutrient** *n* : a nutritive substance or ingredient

nu·tri·ment \'nü-trə-mənt, 'nyü-\ *n* : something that nourishes or promotes growth, provides energy, repairs body tissues, and maintains life

nu·tri·tion \nü-'tri-shən, nyü-\ *n* **1** : the act or process of nourishing or being nourished; *specif* : the sum of the processes by which an animal or plant takes in and utilizes food substances **2** : FOOD 1, NOURISHMENT — **nu·tri·tion·al** \-'tri-shə-nəl\ *adj* — **nu·tri·tion·al·ly** *adv*

nutritional anemia *n* : anemia (as hypochromic anemia) that results from inadequate intake or assimilation of materials essential for the production of red blood cells and hemoglobin — called also *deficiency anemia*

nu·tri·tion·ist \-'tri-shə-nist\ *n* : a specialist in the study of nutrition

nu·tri·tious \nü-'tri-shəs, nyü-\ *adj* : providing nourishment

nu·tri·tive \'nü-trə-tiv, 'nyü-\ *adj* **1** : of or relating to nutrition **2** : NOURISHING

nu·tri·ture \'nü-trə-ˌchùr, 'nyü-, -ˌchər\ *n* : bodily condition with respect to nutrition and esp. with respect to a given nutrient (as zinc)

nux vom·i·ca \'nəks-'vä-mi-kə\ *n, pl* **nux vomica 1** : the poisonous seed of an Asian tree of the genus *Strychnos* (*S. nux-vomica*) that contains the alkaloids strychnine and brucine **2** : a drug containing nux vomica

nvCJD *abbr* new variant Creutzfeldt-Jakob disease

nyc·ta·lo·pia \ˌnik-tə-'lō-pē-ə\ *n* : NIGHT BLINDNESS

ny·li·drin \'nī-li-drən\ *n* : a synthetic adrenergic drug that acts as a peripheral vasodilator and is usu. administered in the form of its hydrochloride $C_{19}H_{25}NO_2\cdot HCl$

nymph \'nimf\ *n* **1** : any of various immature insects; *esp* : a larva of an insect (as a true bug) with incomplete metamorphosis that differs from the adult esp. in size and in its incompletely developed wings and genitalia **2** : a mite or tick in the first eight-legged form that immediately follows the last larval molt — **nymph·al** \'nim-fəl\ *adj*

nymph- *or* **nympho-** *also* **nymphi-** *comb form* : nymph : nymphae ⟨*nympho*mania⟩

nym·phae \'nim-(ˌ)fē\ *n pl* : LABIA MINORA

nym·pho \'nim-(ˌ)fō\ *n, pl* **nymphos** : NYMPHOMANIAC

nym·pho·ma·nia \ˌnim-fə-'mā-nē-ə, -nyə\ *n* : excessive sexual desire by a female — compare SATYRIASIS

¹**nym·pho·ma·ni·ac** \-nē-ˌak\ *n* : one affected with nymphomania

²**nymphomaniac** *or* **nym·pho·ma·ni·a·cal** \-mə-'nī-ə-kəl\ *adj* : of, affected with, or characterized by nymphomania

nys·tag·mus \ni-'stag-məs\ *n* : involuntary usu. rapid movement of the eyeballs occurring normally with dizziness during and after bodily rotation or abnormally following head injury or as a symptom of disease

nys·ta·tin \'nis-tət-ən\ *n* : an antibiotic that is derived from a soil actinomycete of the genus *Streptomyces* (*S. noursei*) and is used esp. in the treatment of candidiasis

O \'ō\ *n* : the one of the four ABO blood groups characterized by the absence of antigens designated by the letters A and B and by the presence of antibodies against these antigens

O *abbr* [Latin *octarius*] pint — used in writing prescriptions

O *symbol* oxygen

o- *or* **oo-** *comb form* : egg : ovum ⟨*oocyte*⟩

OA *abbr* osteoarthritis

O antigen \'ō-\ *n* : an antigen that occurs in the body of a gram-negative bacterial cell — compare H ANTIGEN

oat cell \'ōt-\ *n* : any of the small round or oval cells with a high ratio of nuclear protoplasm to cytoplasm that resemble oat grains and are characteristic of small-cell lung cancer

oat–cell cancer *n* : SMALL-CELL LUNG CANCER

oat–cell carcinoma *n* : SMALL-CELL LUNG CANCER

oath — see HIPPOCRATIC OATH

OB *abbr* **1** obstetric **2** obstetrician **3** obstetrics

obese \ō-'bēs\ *adj* : having excessive body fat : affected by obesity

obe·si·ty \ō-'bē-sə-tē\ *n, pl* **-ties** : a condition that is characterized by excessive accumulation and storage of fat in the body and that in an adult is typically indicated by a body mass index of 30 or greater

obex \'ō-ˌbeks\ *n* : a thin triangular lamina of gray matter in the roof of the fourth ventricle of the brain

ob–gyn \ˌō-(ˌ)bē-'jin, -(ˌ)jē-(ˌ)wī-'en\ *n, pl* **ob–gyns** : a physician who specializes in obstetrics and gynecology

OB-GYN *abbr* obstetrics-gynecology

ob·jec·tive \əb-'jek-tiv, äb-\ *adj* **1** : of, relating to, or being an object, phenomenon, or condition in the realm of sensible experience independent of individual thought and perceptible by all observers ⟨∼ reality⟩ **2** : perceptible to persons other than the affected individual ⟨an ∼ symptom of disease⟩ — compare SUBJECTIVE 2b — **ob·jec·tive·ly** adv

ob·li·gate \'ä-bli-gət, -ˌgāt\ adj **1** : restricted to one particularly characteristic mode of life or way of functioning **2** : biologically essential for survival — **ob·li·gate·ly** adv

oblig·a·to·ry \ə-'bli-gə-ˌtōr-ē, ä-\ adj : OBLIGATE 1

¹oblique \ō-'blēk, ə-, -'blīk\ adj **1** : neither perpendicular nor parallel : being on an incline **2** : situated obliquely and having one end not inserted on bone ⟨∼ muscles⟩ — **oblique·ly** adv

²oblique n : any of several oblique muscles: as **a** : either of two flat muscles on each side that form the middle and outer layers of the lateral walls of the abdomen and that act to compress the abdominal contents and to assist in expelling the contents of various visceral organs (as in urination and expiration): (1) : one that forms the outer layer of the lateral abdominal wall — called also external oblique, obliquus externus abdominis (2) : one situated under the external oblique in the lateral and ventral part of the abdominal wall — called also internal oblique, obliquus internus abdominis **b** (1) : a long thin muscle that arises just above the margin of the optic foramen, is inserted on the upper part of the eyeball, and moves the eye downward and laterally — called also superior oblique, obliquus superior oculi (2) : a short muscle that arises from the orbital surface of the maxilla, is inserted slightly in front of and below the superior oblique, and moves the eye upward and laterally — called also inferior oblique, obliquus inferior oculi **c** (1) : a muscle that arises from the superior surface of the transverse process of the atlas, passes medially upward to insert into the occipital bone, and functions to extend the head and bend it to the side — called also obliquus capitis superior, obliquus superior (2) : a muscle that arises from the apex of the spinous process of the axis, inserts into the transverse process of the atlas, and rotates the atlas turning the face in the same direction — called also obliquus capitis inferior, obliquus inferior

oblique fissure n : either of two fissures of the lungs of which the one on the left side of the body separates the superior lobe of the left lung from the inferior lobe and the one on the right separates the superior and middle lobes of the right lung from the inferior lobe

oblique popliteal ligament n : a strong broad flat fibrous ligament that passes obliquely across and strengthens the posterior part of the knee — compare ARCUATE POPLITEAL LIGAMENT

oblique vein of Mar·shall \-'mär-shəl\ n : OBLIQUE VEIN OF THE LEFT ATRIUM

Marshall, John (1818–1891), British anatomist and surgeon.

oblique vein of the left atrium n : a small vein that passes obliquely down the posterior surface of the left atrium and empties into the coronary sinus — called also oblique vein, oblique vein of left atrium

ob·li·quus \ō-'blī-kwəs\ n, pl **ob·li·qui** \-ˌkwī\ : OBLIQUE

obliquus cap·i·tis inferior \-'ka-pə-təs-\ n : OBLIQUE c(2)

obliquus capitis superior n : OBLIQUE c(1)

obliquus externus ab·dom·i·nis \-ab-'dä-mə-nəs\ n : OBLIQUE a(1)

obliquus inferior n : OBLIQUE c(2)

obliquus inferior oc·u·li \-'ä-kyu̇-ˌlī, -ˌlē\ n : OBLIQUE b(2)

obliquus internus ab·dom·i·nis \-ab-'dä-mə-nəs\ n : OBLIQUE a(2)

obliquus superior n : OBLIQUE c(1)

obliquus superior oc·u·li \-'ä-kyu̇-ˌlī, -ˌlē\ n : OBLIQUE b(1)

obliterans — see ARTERIOSCLEROSIS OBLITERANS, ENDARTERITIS OBLITERANS, THROMBOANGIITIS OBLITERANS

oblit·er·ate \ə-'bli-tə-ˌrāt, ō-\ vb **-at·ed; -at·ing** : to cause to disappear (as a bodily part or a scar) or collapse (as a duct conveying body fluid) — **oblit·er·a·tion** \-ˌbli-tə-'rā-shən\ n — **oblit·er·a·tive** \ə-'bli-tə-ˌrā-tiv, ō-, -rə-\ adj

obliterating endarteritis n : ENDARTERITIS OBLITERANS

ob·lon·ga·ta \ˌä-ˌblȯŋ-'gä-tə\ n, pl **-tas** or **-tae** \-ˌtē\ : MEDULLA OBLONGATA

OBS abbr **1** obstetrician **2** obstetrics

ob·ser·va·tion \ˌäb-sər-'vā-shən, -zər-\ n **1** : the noting of a fact or occurrence (as in nature) often involving the measurement of some magnitude with suitable instruments; also : a record so obtained **2** : close watch or examination (as to monitor or diagnose a condition) ⟨postoperative ∼⟩

ob·sess \əb-'ses, äb-\ vb **1** : to preoccupy intensely or abnormally **2** : to engage in obsessive thinking : become obsessed with an idea

ob·ses·sion \äb-'se-shən, əb-\ n : a persistent disturbing preoccupation with an often unreasonable idea or feeling; also : something that causes such preoccupation — compare COMPULSION, PHOBIA — **ob·ses·sion·al** \-'se-shə-nəl\ adj

obsessional neurosis n : an obsessive-compulsive disorder in which obsessive thinking predominates with little need to perform compulsive acts

¹ob·ses·sive \äb-'se-siv, əb-\ adj : of, relating to, causing, or characterized by obsession : deriving from obsession ⟨∼ behavior⟩ — **ob·ses·sive·ly** *adv* — **ob·ses·sive·ness** *n*

²**obsessive** *n* : an obsessive individual

¹**obsessive–compulsive** *adj* : relating to or characterized by recurring obsessions and compulsions esp. as symptoms of an obsessive-compulsive disorder

²**obsessive–compulsive** *n* : an individual affected with an obsessive-compulsive disorder

obsessive–compulsive disorder *n* : a psychoneurotic disorder in which the patient is beset with obsessions or compulsions or both and suffers extreme anxiety or depression through failure to think the obsessive thoughts or perform the compelling acts — abbr. *OCD*; called also *obsessive-compulsive neurosis, obsessive-compulsive reaction*

ob·stet·ric \əb-'ste-trik, äb-\ *or* **ob·stet·ri·cal** \-tri-kəl\ *adj* : of, relating to, or associated with childbirth or obstetrics — **ob·stet·ri·cal·ly** *adv*

obstetric forceps *n* : a forceps for grasping the fetal head or other part to facilitate delivery in difficult labor

ob·ste·tri·cian \ˌäb-stə-'tri-shən\ *n* : a physician specializing in obstetrics

ob·stet·rics \əb-'ste-triks, äb-\ *n sing or pl* : a branch of medical science that deals with birth and with its antecedents and sequelae

ob·sti·pa·tion \ˌäb-stə-'pā-shən\ *n* : severe and intractable constipation

ob·struct \əb-'strəkt, äb-\ *vb* : to block or close up by an obstacle

ob·struc·tion \əb-'strək-shən, äb-\ *n* **1 a** : an act of obstructing **b** : a condition of being clogged or blocked ⟨intestinal ∼⟩ **2** : something that obstructs ⟨an airway ∼⟩ — **ob·struc·tive** \-tiv\ *adj*

obstructive jaundice *n* : jaundice due to obstruction of the biliary passages

obstructive sleep apnea *n* : sleep apnea that is caused by recurring interruption of breathing during sleep due to obstruction usu. of the upper airway esp. by weak, redundant, or malformed pharyngeal tissues, that occurs chiefly in overweight middle-aged and elderly individuals, and that results in hypoxemia and frequent arousals during the night and in excessive sleepiness during the day — abbr. *OSA;* called also *obstructive sleep apnea syndrome*

ob·tund \äb-'tənd\ *vb* : to reduce the intensity or sensitivity of : make dull ⟨agents that ∼ pain⟩ — **ob·tun·da·tion** \ˌäb-ˌ(ˌ)tən-'dā-shən\ *n*

ob·tu·ra·tor \'äb-tyə-ˌrā-tər, -tə-\ *n* **1 a** : either of two muscles arising from the obturator membrane and adjacent bony surfaces: (1) : OBTURATOR EXTERNUS (2) : OBTURATOR INTERNUS **b** : OBTURATOR NERVE **2 a** : a prosthetic device that closes or blocks up an opening (as a fissure in the palate) **b** : a device that blocks the opening of an instrument (as a sigmoidoscope) that is being introduced into the body

obturator artery *n* : an artery that arises from the internal iliac artery or one of its branches, passes out through the obturator canal, and divides into two branches which are distributed to the muscles and fasciae of the hip and thigh

obturator canal *n* : the small opening of the obturator foramen through which nerves and vessels pass

obturator ex·ter·nus \-ek-'stər-nəs\ *n* : a flat triangular muscle that arises esp. from the medial side of the obturator foramen and from the medial part of the obturator membrane, that inserts by a tendon into the trochanteric fossa of the femur, and that acts to rotate the thigh laterally

obturator foramen *n* : an opening that is situated between the ischium and pubis of the hip bone

obturator in·ter·nus \-in-'tər-nəs\ *n* : a muscle that arises from the margin of the obturator foramen and from the obturator membrane, that inserts into the greater trochanter of the femur, and that acts to rotate the thigh laterally when it is extended and to abduct it in the flexed position

obturator membrane *n* : a firm fibrous membrane covering most of the obturator foramen except for the obturator canal

obturator nerve *n* : a branch of the lumbar plexus that arises from the second, third, and fourth lumbar nerves and that supplies the hip and knee joints, the adductor muscles of the thigh, and the skin

obturator vein *n* : a tributary of the internal iliac vein that accompanies the obturator artery

occipit- *or* **occipito-** *comb form* : occipital and ⟨*occipito*temporal⟩

occipita *pl of* OCCIPUT

¹**oc·cip·i·tal** \äk-'si-pət-ᵊl\ *adj* : of, relating to, or located within or near the occiput or the occipital bone

²**occipital** *n* : OCCIPITAL BONE

occipital artery *n* : an artery that arises from the external carotid artery, ascends within the superficial fascia of the scalp, and supplies or gives off branches supplying structures and esp. muscles of the back of the neck and head

occipital bone *n* : a compound bone that forms the posterior part of the skull and surrounds the foramen magnum, bears the condyles for articulation with the atlas, is composed of four united elements, is much curved and roughly trapezoidal in outline, and ends in front of the foramen magnum in the basilar process

occipital condyle *n* : an articular surface on the occipital bone by which the skull articulates with the atlas

occipital crest *n* : either of the two ridges on the occipital bone: **a** : a median ridge on the outer surface of the occipital bone that with the external occipital protuberance gives attachment to the ligamentum nuchae — called also *external occipital crest, median nuchal line* **b** : a median ridge similarly situated on the inner surface of the occipital bone that bifurcates near the foramen magnum to give attachment to the falx cerebelli — called also *internal occipital crest*

occipital fontanel *n* : a triangular fontanel at the meeting of the sutures between the parietal and occipital bones

oc·cip·i·ta·lis \ăk-ˌsi-pə-ˈtā-ləs\ *n* : the posterior belly of the occipitofrontalis that arises from the lateral two-thirds of the superior nuchal lines and from the mastoid part of the temporal bone, inserts into the galea aponeurotica, and acts to move the scalp

occipital lobe *n* : the posterior lobe of each cerebral hemisphere that bears the visual areas and has the form of a 3-sided pyramid

occipital nerve *n* : either of two nerves that arise mostly from the second cervical nerve: **a** : one that innervates the scalp at the top of the head — called also *greater occipital nerve* **b** : one that innervates the scalp esp. in the lateral area of the head behind the ear — called also *lesser occipital nerve*

occipital protuberance *n* : either of two prominences on the occipital bone: **a** : a prominence on the outer surface of the occipital bone midway between the upper border and the foramen magnum — called also *external occipital protuberance, inion* **b** : a prominence similarly situated on the inner surface of the occipital bone — called also *internal occipital protuberance*

occipital sinus *n* : a single or paired venous sinus that arises near the margin of the foramen magnum by the union of several small veins and empties into the confluence of sinuses or sometimes into one of the transverse sinuses

occipito- — see OCCIPIT-

oc·cip·i·to·fron·ta·lis \ăk-ˌsi-pə-tō-frən-ˈtā-ləs\ *n* : a fibrous and muscular sheet on each side of the vertex of the skull that extends from the eyebrow to the occiput, that is composed of the frontalis muscle in front and the occipitalis muscle in back with the galea aponeurotica in between, and that acts to draw back the scalp to raise the eyebrow and wrinkle the forehead — called also *epicranius*

oc·cip·i·to·pa·ri·etal \-pə-ˈrī-ət-ᵊl\ *adj* : of or relating to the occipital and parietal bones of the skull

oc·cip·i·to·tem·po·ral \-ˈtem-pə-rəl\ *adj* : of, relating to, or distributed to

the occipital and temporal lobes of a cerebral hemisphere ⟨the ∼ cortex⟩

oc·ci·put \ˈäk-sə-(ˌ)pət\ *n, pl* **occiputs** *or* **oc·cip·i·ta** \äk-ˈsi-pə-tə\ : the back part of the head or skull

oc·clude \ə-ˈklüd, ä-\ *vb* **oc·clud·ed; oc·clud·ing 1** : to close up or block off : OBSTRUCT **2** : to bring (upper and lower teeth) into occlusion **3** : SORB

occlus- *or* **occluso-** *comb form* : occlusion ⟨*occlusal*⟩

oc·clu·sal \ə-ˈklü-səl, ä-, -zəl\ *adj* : of, relating to, or being the grinding or biting surface of a tooth; *also* : of or relating to occlusion of the teeth ⟨∼ abnormalities⟩ — **oc·clu·sal·ly** *adv*

occlusal disharmony *n* : a condition in which incorrect positioning of one or more teeth causes an abnormal increase in or change of direction of the force applied to one or more teeth when the upper and lower teeth are occluded

occlusal plane *n* : an imaginary plane formed by the occlusal surfaces of the teeth when the jaw is closed

oc·clu·sion \ə-ˈklü-zhən\ *n* **1** : the act of occluding or the state of being occluded : a shutting off or obstruction of something ⟨a coronary ∼⟩; *esp* : a blocking of the central passage of one reflex by the passage of another **2 a** : the bringing of the opposing surfaces of the teeth of the two jaws into contact; *also* : the relation between the surfaces when in contact **b** : the transient approximation of the edges of a natural opening ⟨∼ of the eyelids⟩ — **oc·clu·sive** \-siv\ *adj*

occlusive dressing *n* : a dressing that seals a wound to protect against infection

oc·cult \ə-ˈkəlt, ˈä-ˌkəlt\ *adj* : not manifest or detectable by clinical methods alone ⟨∼ carcinoma⟩; *also* : not present in macroscopic amounts ⟨∼ blood in a stool specimen⟩ ⟨fecal ∼ blood testing⟩ — compare GROSS 2

occulta — see SPINA BIFIDA OCCULTA

oc·cu·pa·tion·al \ˌä-kyə-ˈpā-shə-nəl\ *adj* : relating to or being an occupational disease ⟨∼ asthma⟩ — **oc·cu·pa·tion·al·ly** *adv*

occupational disease *n* : an illness caused by factors arising from one's occupation — called also *industrial disease*

occupational medicine *n* : a branch of medicine concerned with the prevention and treatment of occupational diseases

occupational therapist *n* : a person trained and licensed in the practice of occupational therapy

occupational therapy *n* : therapy based on engagement in meaningful activities of daily life (as self-care skills, education, work, or social interaction) esp. to enable or encourage participation in such activities despite impairments or limitations in physical or mental functioning

OCD *abbr* obsessive-compulsive disorder

och·ra·tox·in \ˌō-krə-'täk-sən\ *n* : a mycotoxin produced by a fungus of the genus *Aspergillus* (*A. ochraceus*)

ochro·no·sis \ˌō-krə-'nō-səs\ *n, pl* **-no·ses** \-ˌsēz\ : a condition often associated with alkaptonuria and marked by pigment deposits in cartilages, ligaments, and tendons — **ochro·not·ic** \-'nä-tik\ *adj*

oc·tre·o·tide \äk-'trē-ə-ˌtīd\ *n* : a long-acting synthetic analog of somatostatin that is administered esp. by subcutaneous injection in the form of its acetate $C_{49}H_{66}N_{10}O_{10}S_2$ and is used to treat acromegaly and to treat severe diarrhea associated with metastatic carcinoid tumors and vipomas

ocul- *or* **oculo-** *comb form* 1 : eye ⟨*oculo*motor⟩ 2 : ocular and ⟨*oculo*cutaneous⟩

oc·u·lar \'ä-kyə-lər\ *adj* : of or relating to the eye ⟨~ muscles⟩ ⟨~ diseases⟩

oc·u·lar·ist \'ä-kyə-lə-rist\ *n* : a person who makes and fits artificial eyes

oculi — *see* OBLIQUUS INFERIOR OCULI, OBLIQUUS SUPERIOR OCULI, ORBICULARIS OCULI, RECTUS OCULI

oc·u·list \'ä-kyə-list\ *n* 1 : OPHTHALMOLOGIST 2 : OPTOMETRIST

oc·u·lo·ce·re·bro·re·nal syndrome \ˌä-kyə-lō-sə-ˌrē-brō-'rē-nᵊl-\ *n* : a rare disorder that is inherited as an X-linked recessive trait and is marked esp. by congenital cataracts, mental retardation, generalized hypotonia, and dysfunction of the renal tubules — called also *Lowe syndrome*

oc·u·lo·cu·ta·ne·ous \ˌä-kyə-(ˌ)lō-kyü-'tā-nē-əs\ *adj* : relating to or affecting both the eyes and the skin

oc·u·lo·glan·du·lar \-'glan-jə-lər\ *adj* : affecting or producing symptoms in the eye and lymph nodes — see PARINAUD'S OCULOGLANDULAR SYNDROME

oc·u·lo·gy·ric crisis \ˌä-kyə-lō-'jī-rik-\ *n* : a spasmodic attack that occurs in some nervous diseases and is marked by fixation of the eyeballs in one position usu. upward — called also *oculogyric spasm*

oc·u·lo·mo·tor \ˌä-kyə-lə-'mō-tər\ *adj* 1 : moving or tending to move the eyeball 2 : of or relating to the oculomotor nerve

oculomotor nerve *n* : either nerve of the third pair of cranial nerves with some associated autonomic fibers, arise from the midbrain, supply most muscles of the eye with motor fibers, and supply the ciliary body and iris with autonomic fibers by way of the ciliary ganglion — called also *third cranial nerve*

oculomotor nucleus *n* : a nucleus that is situated under the aqueduct of Sylvius rostral to the trochlear nucleus and is the source of the motor fibers of the oculomotor nerve

oc·u·lo·plas·tic \ˌä-kyə-lō-'plas-tik\ *adj* : of, relating to, or being plastic surgery of the eye and associated structures

od *abbr* [Latin *omnes dies*] every day — used in writing prescriptions

¹OD \(ˌ)ō-'dē\ *n* 1 : an overdose of a narcotic 2 : one who has taken an OD

²OD *vb* **OD'd** *or* **ODed; OD'ing; OD's** : to become ill or die of an OD

OD *abbr* 1 : doctor of optometry 2 [Latin *oculus dexter*] right eye — used in writing prescriptions

ODD *abbr* oppositional defiant disorder

Od·di's sphincter \'ä-dēz-\ *n* : SPHINCTER OF ODDI

odont- *or* **odonto-** *comb form* : tooth ⟨*odont*itis⟩ ⟨*odonto*blast⟩

odon·tal·gia \(ˌ)ō-ˌdän-'tal-jə, -jē-ə\ *n* : TOOTHACHE — **odon·tal·gic** \-jik\ *adj*

-odon·tia \ə-'dän-chə, -chē-ə\ *n comb form* : form, condition, or mode of treatment of the teeth ⟨ortho*dontia*⟩

odon·ti·tis \-'tī-təs\ *n, pl* **odon·tit·i·des** \-'tī-tə-ˌdēz\ : inflammation of a tooth

odon·to·blast \ō-'dän-tə-ˌblast\ *n* : one of the elongated radially arranged outer cells of the dental pulp that secrete dentin — **odon·to·blas·tic** \-ˌdän-tə-'blas-tik\ *adj*

odon·to·gen·e·sis \ō-ˌdän-tə-'je-nə-səs\ *n, pl* **-e·ses** \-ˌsēz\ : the formation and development of teeth

odon·to·gen·ic \ō-ˌdän-tə-'je-nik\ *adj* 1 : forming or capable of forming teeth ⟨~ tissues⟩ 2 : containing or arising from odontogenic tissues ⟨~ tumors⟩

odon·toid process \ō-'dän-ˌtoid-\ *n* : DENS

odon·tol·o·gist \(ˌ)ō-ˌdän-'tä-lə-jist\ *n* : a specialist in odontology

odon·tol·o·gy \ō-ˌdän-'tä-lə-jē\ *n, pl* **-gies** 1 : a science dealing with the teeth, their structure and development, and their diseases 2 : FORENSIC ODONTOLOGY — **odon·to·log·i·cal** \-ˌdänt-ᵊl-'ä-ji-kəl\ *adj*

odon·to·ma \ˌō-(ˌ)dän-'tō-mə\ *n, pl* **-mas** *also* **-ma·ta** \-mə-tə\ : a tumor originating from a tooth and containing dental tissue (as enamel)

odon·tome \ō-'dän-ˌtōm\ *n* : ODONTOMA

odor \'ō-dər\ *n* 1 : a quality of something that stimulates the olfactory organ : SMELL 2 : a sensation resulting from adequate chemical stimulation of the olfactory organ ⟨a disagreeable ~⟩ — **odored** *adj* — **odor·less** *adj*

odour *chiefly Brit var of* ODOR

-o·dyn·ia \ə-'di-nē-ə\ *n comb form* : pain ⟨pleuro*dynia*⟩

odyno·pha·gia \ō-ˌdi-nō-'fā-jə, -jē-ə\ *n* : pain produced by swallowing

oe·de·ma *chiefly Brit var of* EDEMA

oe·di·pal \'e-də-pəl, 'ē-\ *adj, often cap* : of, relating to, or resulting from the

Oedipus complex — **oe·di·pal·ly** *adv*, *often cap*

¹**Oe·di·pus** \-pəs\ *adj* : OEDIPAL

²**Oedipus** *n* : OEDIPUS COMPLEX

Oedipus complex *n* : the positive libidinal feelings of a child toward the parent of the opposite sex and hostile or jealous feelings toward the parent of the same sex that may be a source of adult personality disorder when unresolved — used esp. of the male child; see ELECTRA COMPLEX

oesophag- or **oesophago-** *chiefly Brit var of* ESOPHAG-

oe·soph·a·ge·al, **oe·soph·a·gec·to·my,** **oe·soph·a·go·gas·trec·to·my,** **oe·soph·a·go·plas·ty,** **oe·soph·a·gus** *chiefly Brit var of* ESOPHAGEAL, ESOPHAGECTOMY, ESOPHAGOGAS-TRECTOMY, ESOPHAGOPLASTY, ESOPHAGUS

oe·soph·a·go·sto·mi·a·sis *also* **esoph·a·go·sto·mi·a·sis** \i-ˌsä-fə-ˌ(ˌ)gō-stə-ˈmī-ə-səs\ *n, pl* **-a·ses** \-ˌsēz\ : infestation with or disease caused by nematode worms of the genus *Oesophagostomum* : NODULAR DISEASE

Oe·soph·a·gos·to·mum \i-ˌsä-fə-ˈgäs-tə-məm\ *n* : a genus of strongylid nematode worms comprising the nodular worms of ruminants and swine and other worms affecting primates including humans esp. in Africa

oestr- or **oestro-** *chiefly Brit var of* ESTR-

oes·tra·di·ol \ˌēs-trə-ˈdī-ˌȯl, -ˌōl\, **oes·tro·gen** \ˈē-strə-jən\, **oes·trus** \ˈē-strəs\ *chiefly Brit var of* ESTRADIOL, ESTROGEN, ESTRUS

Oes·trus \ˈes-trəs, ˈēs-\ *n* : a genus (family *Oestridae*) of dipteran flies including the sheep botfly (*O. ovis*)

of·fi·cial \ə-ˈfi-shəl\ *adj* : prescribed or recognized as authorized; *specif* : described by the *U.S. Pharmacopeia* or the *National Formulary* — compare NONOFFICIAL, UNOFFICIAL — **of·fi·cial·ly** *adv*

¹**of·fic·i·nal** \ə-ˈfis-ᵊn-əl, ȯ-, ä-; ˌȯ-fə-ˈsīn-ᵊl, ˌä-\ *adj* **1 a** : available without special preparation or compounding ⟨~ medicine⟩ **b** : OFFICIAL 2 **c** *of a plant* : MEDICINAL ⟨~ herbs⟩

²**officinal** *n* : an official drug, medicine, or plant

off-la·bel \ˌȯf-ˈlā-bəl\ *adj* : of, relating to, or being an approved drug legally prescribed by a physician or a medical device legally used by a physician for a purpose (as the treatment of children or of a certain disease or condition) for which it has not specifically been approved

off·spring \ˈȯf-ˌspriŋ\ *n, pl* **offspring** *also* **offsprings** : the progeny of an animal or plant

oflox·a·cin \ō-ˈfläk-sə-sən\ *n* : a fluoroquinolone $C_{18}H_{20}FN_3O_4$ that is a broad-spectrum antibacterial agent that is used in topical solution for otic or ophthalmic use or is administered orally or intravenously for other uses — see LEVOFLOXACIN

Ogil·vie's syndrome \ˈō-gəl-vēz-\ *n* : distension of the colon that is similar to that occurring as a consequence of bowel obstruction but in which no physical obstruction exists and that occurs esp. in seriously ill individuals and as a complication of abdominal surgery

Ogilvie, Sir William Heneage (1887–1971), British surgeon.

ohm \ˈōm\ *n* : a unit of electrical resistance equal to the resistance of a circuit in which a potential difference of one volt produces a current of one ampere

Ohm, Georg Simon (1789–1854), German physicist.

OI *abbr* opportunistic infection

oid·i·um \ō-ˈi-dē-əm\ *n* **1** *cap* : a genus of imperfect fungi (family Moniliaceae) including many which are now considered to be asexual spore-producing stages of various powdery mildews **2** *pl* **oid·ia** \-dē-ə\ : any fungus of the genus *Oidium*

oil \ˈȯil\ *n* **1** : any of numerous fatty combustible substances that are liquid or can be liquefied easily on warming, are soluble in ether but not in water, and leave a greasy stain on paper or cloth — see ESSENTIAL OIL, FATTY OIL, VOLATILE OIL **2** : a substance (as a cosmetic preparation) of oily consistency — **oil** *adj*

oil gland *n* : a gland (as of the skin) that produces an oily secretion; *specif* : SEBACEOUS GLAND

oil of wintergreen *n* : a preparation of methyl salicylate obtained by distilling the leaves of wintergreen (*Gaultheria procumbens*) — called also wintergreen oil

oily \ˈȯi-lē\ *adj* **oil·i·er; -est 1** : of, relating to, or consisting of oil **2** : excessively high in naturally secreted oils ⟨~ hair⟩ ⟨~ skin⟩

oint·ment \ˈȯint-mənt\ *n* : a salve or unguent for application to the skin; *specif* : a semisolid medicinal preparation usu. having a base of fatty or greasy material

-ol \ˌȯl, ˌōl\ *n suffix* : chemical compound (as an alcohol or phenol) containing hydroxyl ⟨glycerol⟩

OL *abbr* [Latin *oculus laevus*] left eye — used in writing prescriptions

olan·za·pine \ō-ˈlan-zə-ˌpēn\ *n* : an antipsychotic drug $C_{17}H_{20}N_4S$ used esp. in the short-term treatment of schizophrenia and acute manic episodes of bipolar disorder — see ZYPREXA

ole- or **oleo-** *also* **olei-** *comb form* : oil ⟨olein⟩

olea *pl of* OLEUM

ole·an·der \ˈō-lē-ˌan-dər, ˌō-lē-ˈ\ *n* : a poisonous evergreen shrub (*Nerium oleander*) of the dogbane family (Apocynaceae) that contains the cardiac glycoside oleandrin

ole·an·do·my·cin \ˌō-lē-ˌan-də-ˈmīs-ᵊn\ *n* : an antibiotic $C_{35}H_{61}NO_{12}$ produced by a bacterium of the genus *Streptomyces* (*S. antibioticus*)

ole·an·drin \ˌō-lē-ˈan-drən\ *n* : a poisonous crystalline glycoside $C_{32}H_{48}O_9$ found in oleander leaves and resembling digitalis in its action

ole·ate \ˈō-lē-ˌāt\ *n* **1** : a salt or ester of oleic acid **2** : a liquid or semisolid preparation of a medicinal dissolved in an excess of oleic acid

olec·ra·non \ō-ˈle-krə-ˌnän\ *n* : the large process of the ulna that projects behind the elbow, forms the bony prominence of the elbow, and receives the insertion of the triceps muscle

olecranon fossa *n* : the fossa at the distal end of the humerus into which the olecranon fits when the arm is in full extension — compare CORONOID FOSSA

ole·ic acid \ō-ˈlē-ik-, -ˈlā-\ *n* : a monounsaturated fatty acid $C_{18}H_{34}O_2$ found in natural fats and oils

ole·in \ˈō-lē-ən\ *n* : an ester of glycerol and oleic acid

oleo- *see* OLE-

oleo·res·in \ˌō-lē-ō-ˈrez-ᵊn\ *n* **1** : a natural plant product containing chiefly essential oil and resin **2** : a preparation consisting essentially of oil holding resin in solution — **oleo·res·in·ous** \-ˈrez-ᵊn-əs\ *adj*

oleo·tho·rax \-ˈthōr-ˌaks\ *n, pl* **-tho·rax·es** *or* **-tho·ra·ces** \-ˈthōr-ə-ˌsēz\ : a state in which oil is present in the pleural cavity usu. as a result of injection — compare PNEUMOTHORAX

oles·tra \ō-ˈles-trə\ *n* : a noncaloric fat substitute that consists of sucrose esters resistant to absorption by the digestive system due to their large size

ole·um \ˈō-lē-əm\ *n, pl* **olea** \-lē-ə\ : OIL 1

ol·fac·tion \äl-ˈfak-shən, ōl-\ *n* **1** : the sense of smell **2** : the act or process of smelling

ol·fac·to·ry \äl-ˈfak-tə-rē, ōl-\ *adj* : of, relating to, or connected with the sense of smell

olfactory area *n* **1** : the sensory area for olfaction lying in the parahippocampal gyrus **2** : the area of nasal mucosa in which the olfactory organ is situated

olfactory bulb *n* : a bulbous anterior projection of the olfactory lobe that is the place of termination of the olfactory nerves

olfactory cell *n* : a sensory cell specialized for the reception of sensory stimuli caused by odors; *specif* : any of the spindle-shaped neurons in the nasal mucous membrane of vertebrates — see OLFACTORY ORGAN

olfactory cortex *n* : a group of cortical areas of the cerebrum that receive sensory input from the olfactory bulb via the olfactory tract and includes the piriform cortex and parts of the

olfactory tubercle, amygdala, and entorhinal cortex

olfactory epithelium *n* : the nasal mucosa containing olfactory cells

olfactory gland *n* : any of the tubular and often branched glands occurring beneath the olfactory epithelium of the nose — called also *Bowman's gland, gland of Bowman*

olfactory gyrus *n* : either a lateral or a medial gyrus on each side of the brain by which the olfactory tract on the corresponding side communicates with the olfactory area

olfactory lobe *n* : a lobe of the brain that rests on the lower surface of a temporal lobe and projects forward from the anterior lower part of each cerebral hemisphere and that consists of an olfactory bulb, an olfactory tract, and an olfactory trigone

olfactory nerve *n* : either of the pair of nerves that are the first cranial nerves, that serve to conduct sensory stimuli from the olfactory organ to the brain, and that arise from the olfactory cells and terminate in the olfactory bulb — called also *first cranial nerve*

olfactory organ *n* : an organ of chemical sense that receives stimuli interpreted as odors, that lies in the walls of the upper part of the nasal cavity, and that forms a mucous membrane continuous with the rest of the lining of the nasal cavity

olfactory pit *n* : a depression on the head of an embryo that becomes converted into a nasal passage

olfactory tract *n* : a tract of nerve fibers in the olfactory lobe on the inferior surface of the frontal lobe of the brain that passes from the olfactory bulb to the olfactory trigone

olfactory trigone *n* : a triangular area of gray matter on each side of the brain forming the junction of an olfactory tract with a cerebral hemisphere near the optic chiasma

olfactory tubercle *n* : a small area of gray matter behind the olfactory trigone that is innervated by dopaminergic neurons from the ventral tegmental area

olig- *or* **oligo-** *comb form* **1** : few ⟨*oligo*peptide⟩ **2** : deficiency : insufficiency ⟨*olig*uria⟩

ol·i·gae·mia *chiefly Brit var of* OLIGEMIA

ol·i·ge·mia \ˌä-lə-ˈgē-mē-ə, -ˈjē-\ *n* : a condition in which the total volume of the blood is reduced — **ol·i·ge·mic** \-mik\ *adj*

oli·go·ar·tic·u·lar \ˌä-li-gō-är-ˈti-kyə-lər, ə-ˌli-gə-\ *adj* : affecting a few joints ⟨∼ arthritis⟩ — compare MONOARTICULAR, POLYARTICULAR

oli·go·dac·tyl·ism \ˌä-li-gō-ˈdak-tə-ˌli-zəm, ə-ˌli-gō-\ *also* **oli·go·dac·tyly** \-lē\ *n, pl* **-tyl·isms** *also* **-tylies** : the presence of fewer than five digits on a hand or foot

oli·go·den·dro·cyte \-'den-drə-ˌsīt\ *n* : a glial cell resembling an astrocyte but smaller with few and slender processes having few branches and forming the myelin sheath around axons in the central nervous system

oli·go·den·drog·lia \ˌä-li-gō-den-'drä-glē-ə, ˌō-li-, -'drō-\ *n* : glia made up of oligodendrocytes — **oli·go·den·drog·li·al** \-lē-əl\ *adj*

oli·go·den·dro·gli·o·ma \-ˌden-drō-glī-'ō-mə\ *n, pl* **-mas** *also* **-ma·ta** \-mə-tə\ : a tumor of the nervous system composed of oligodendroglia

oli·go·fruc·tose \-'frŭk-ˌtōs, -'frŭk-, -'frŭk, -ˌtōz\ *n* : a short-chain polysaccharide produced by partial enzymatic hydrolysis of inulin and used similarly to inulin in processed foods

oli·go·hy·dram·ni·os \-ˌhī-'dram-nē-ˌäs\ *n* : deficiency of amniotic fluid sometimes resulting in an embryonic defect through adherence between embryo and amnion

oli·go·men·or·rhea \-ˌme-nə-'rē-ə\ *n* : abnormally infrequent or scanty menstrual flow

oli·go·men·or·rhoea *chiefly Brit var of* OLIGOMENORRHEA

oli·go·nu·cle·o·tide \-'nü-klē-ə-ˌtīd, -'nyü-\ *n* : a nucleic-acid chain usu. consisting of up to 20 nucleotides

oli·go·pep·tide \ˌä-li-gō-'pep-ˌtīd, ˌō-li-\ *n* : a protein fragment or molecule that usu. consists of less than 25 amino acid residues linked in a polypeptide chain

oli·go·phre·nia \-'frē-nē-ə\ *n* : MENTAL RETARDATION

oli·go·sper·mia \-'spər-mē-ə\ *n* : deficiency of sperm in the semen — **oli·go·sper·mic** \-mik\ *adj*

ol·i·gu·ria \ˌä-lə-'gŭr-ē-ə, -'gyŭr-\ *n* : reduced excretion of urine — **ol·i·gur·ic** \-ik\ *adj*

ol·i·vary \'ä-lə-ˌver-ē\ *adj* **1** : shaped like an olive **2** : of, relating to, situated near, or comprising one or more of the olives, inferior olives, or superior olives ⟨the ∼ complex⟩

olivary body *n* : OLIVE

olivary nucleus *n* **1** : INFERIOR OLIVE **2** : SUPERIOR OLIVE

ol·ive \'ä-liv\ *n* : an oval eminence on each ventrolateral aspect of the medulla oblongata that contains the inferior olive of the same side — called also *olivary body*

olive oil *n* : a pale yellow to yellowish green edible oil obtained from the pulp of olives that is high in monounsaturated fatty acids and is used chiefly in cooking, in soaps, and as an emollient

ol·i·vo·cer·e·bel·lar tract \ˌä-li-vō-ˌser-ə-'be-lər-\ *n* : a tract of fibers that arises in the olive on one side, crosses to the olive on the other, and enters the cerebellum by way of the inferior cerebellar peduncle

ol·i·vo·pon·to·cer·e·bel·lar atrophy \-ˌpän-tō-ˌser-ə-'be-lər-\ *n* : an inherited disease esp. of mid to late life that is characterized by ataxia, hypotonia, dysarthria, and degeneration of the cerebellar cortex, middle cerebellar peduncles, and inferior olives — called also *olivopontocerebellar degeneration*

ol·i·vo·spi·nal tract \-'spīn-ᵊl-\ *n* : a tract of fibers on the peripheral aspect of the ventral side of the cervical part of the spinal cord that communicates with the inferior olive

ol·sal·a·zine \ōl-'sal-ə-ˌzēn\ *n* : a disodium salicylate salt $C_{14}H_8N_2Na_2O_6$ administered orally as an anti-inflammatory agent to treat ulcerative colitis — called also *olsalazine sodium*

-o·ma \'ō-mə\ *n suffix, pl* **-o·mas** \-məz\ *also* **-o·ma·ta** \-mə-tə\ : tumor ⟨aden*oma*⟩ ⟨fibr*oma*⟩

oma·sum \ō-'mä-səm\ *n, pl* **oma·sa** \-sə\ : the third chamber of the ruminant stomach that is situated between the reticulum and the abomasum — called also *manyplies, psalterium*

oma·sal \-səl\ *adj*

ome·ga-6 \ō-'me-gə-'siks, -'mä-\ *adj* : being or composed of polyunsaturated fatty acids in which the first double bond in the hydrocarbon chain occurs between the sixth and seventh carbon atoms from the end of the molecule most distant from the carboxylic acid group and which are found esp. in vegetable oils, nuts, beans, seeds, and grains — **omega-6** *n*

ome·ga-3 \-'thrē\ *adj* : being or composed of polyunsaturated fatty acids in which the first double bond in the hydrocarbon chain occurs between the third and fourth carbon atoms from the end of the molecule most distant from the carboxylic acid group and which are found esp. in fish (as tuna and salmon), fish oils, green leafy vegetables, and some vegetable oils — **omega-3** *n*

oment- *or* **omento-** *comb form* : omentum ⟨*oment*ectomy⟩ ⟨*omento*pexy⟩

omen·tec·to·my \ˌō-men-'tek-tə-mē\ *n, pl* **-mies** : excision or resection of all or part of an omentum — called also *epiploectomy*

omen·to·pexy \ō-'men-tə-ˌpek-sē\ *n, pl* **-pex·ies** : the operation of suturing the omentum esp. to another organ

omen·to·plas·ty \-ˌplas-tē\ *n, pl* **-ties** : the use of a piece or flap of tissue from an omentum as a graft

omen·tor·rha·phy \ˌō-men-'tȯr-ə-fē\ *n, pl* **-phies** : surgical repair of an omentum by suturing

omen·tum \ō-'men-təm\ *n, pl* **-ta** \-tə\ *or* **-tums** : a fold of peritoneum connecting or supporting abdominal structures (as the stomach or liver) — see GREATER OMENTUM, LESSER OMENTUM — **omen·tal** \-'ment-ᵊl\ *adj*

omep·ra·zole \ō-'me-prə-ˌzōl\ *n* : a benzimidazole derivative $C_{17}H_{19}N_3$-

O₃S that is used to inhibit gastric acid secretion (as in the treatment of duodenal and gastric ulcers and gastroesophageal reflux) — see PRILOSEC

omo·hy·oi·de·us \ˌhī-ˈōi-dē-əs\ *n, pl* **-dei** \-dē-ˌī\ : OMOHYOID MUSCLE

omo·hy·oid muscle \ˌō-mō-ˈhī-ˌōid-\ *n* : a muscle that arises from the upper border of the scapula, is inserted in the body of the hyoid bone, and acts to draw the hyoid bone in a caudal direction — called also *omohyoid*

omphal- *or* **omphalo-** *comb form* **1** : umbilicus ⟨*omphal*itis⟩ **2** : umbilical and ⟨*omphal*omesenteric duct⟩

om·pha·lec·to·my \ˌäm-fə-ˈlek-tə-mē\ *n, pl* **-mies** : surgical excision of the navel — called also *umbilectomy*

om·phal·ic \ˌ(ˌ)äm-ˈfa-lik\ *adj* : of or relating to the navel

om·pha·li·tis \ˌäm-fə-ˈlī-təs\ *n, pl* **-lit·i·des** \-ˈli-tə-ˌdēz\ : inflammation of the navel

om·pha·lo·cele \äm-ˈfa-lə-ˌsēl, ˈäm-fə-lə-\ *n* : protrusion of abdominal contents through an opening at the navel occurring esp. as a congenital defect

om·pha·lo·mes·en·ter·ic duct \ˌäm-fə-lō-ˌmez-ᵊn-ˈter-ik-, -ˌmes-\ *n* : the duct by which the yolk sac or umbilical vesicle remains connected with the digestive tract of the vertebrate embryo — called also *vitelline duct, yolk stalk*

om·pha·lo·phle·bi·tis \-fli-ˈbī-təs\ *n, pl* **-bit·i·des** \-ˈbi-tə-ˌdēz\ : a condition (as navel ill) characterized by or resulting from inflammation and infection of the umbilical vein

onan·ism \ˈō-nə-ˌni-zəm\ *n* **1** : MASTURBATION **2** : COITUS INTERRUPTUS — **onan·is·tic** \ˌō-nə-ˈnis-tik\ *adj*

onan·ist \ˈō-nə-nist\ *n* : an individual that practices onanism

On·cho·cer·ca \ˌäŋ-kə-ˈsər-kə\ *n* : a genus of long slender filarial worms (family Dipetalonematidae) that are parasites of mammalian subcutaneous and connective tissues

on·cho·cer·ci·a·sis \ˌäŋ-kō-ˌsər-ˈkī-ə-səs\ *n, pl* **-a·ses** \-ˌsēz\ : infestation with or disease caused by filarial worms of the genus *Onchocerca; esp* : a human disease marked by subcutaneous nodules, dermatitis, and visual impairment and that is caused by a worm (*O. volvulus*) found in Africa and tropical America and transmitted by the bite of a female blackfly — called also *river blindness*

onco- *or* **oncho-** *comb form* **1** : tumor ⟨*oncology*⟩ **2** : bulk : mass ⟨*onco*sphere⟩

on·co·cyte \ˈäŋ-kō-ˌsīt\ *n* : an acidophilic granular cell esp. of the parotid gland

on·co·cy·to·ma \ˌäŋ-kō-sī-ˈtō-mə\ *n, pl* **-mas** *also* **-ma·ta** \-mə-tə\ : a tumor (as of the parotid gland) consisting chiefly or entirely of oncocytes

on·co·fe·tal \-ˈfēt-ᵊl\ *adj* : of, relating to, or occurring in both tumorous and fetal tissues

on·co·gene \ˈäŋ-kō-ˌjēn\ *n* : a gene having the potential to cause a normal cell to become cancerous

on·co·gen·e·sis \ˌäŋ-kō-ˈje-nə-səs\, *pl* **-e·ses** \-ˌsēz\ : the induction or formation of tumors

on·co·gen·ic \-ˈje-nik\ *adj* **1** : relating to tumor formation **2** : tending to cause tumors ⟨an ~ virus⟩ — **on·co·gen·i·cal·ly** *adv* — **on·co·ge·nic·i·ty** \-jə-ˈni-sə-tē\ *n*

on·col·o·gist \än-ˈkä-lə-jəst, äŋ-\ *n* : a specialist in oncology

on·col·o·gy \än-ˈkä-lə-jē, äŋ-\ *n, pl* **-gies** : the study of tumors and neoplastic diseases — **on·co·log·i·cal** \ˌäŋ-kə-ˈlä-ji-kəl\ *also* **on·co·log·ic** \-ik\ *adj*

on·col·y·sis \-ˈkä-lə-səs\ *n, pl* **-y·ses** \-ˌsēz\ : the destruction of tumor cells — **on·co·lyt·ic** \ˌäŋ-kə-ˈli-tik\ *adj* — **on·co·lyt·i·cal·ly** *adv*

on·co·pro·tein \ˌäŋ-kō-ˈprō-ˌtēn\ *n* : a protein that is coded for by a viral oncogene and that is involved in the regulation or synthesis of proteins linked to tumorigenic cell growth

on·cor·na·vi·rus \ˌäŋ-ˌkȯr-nə-ˈvī-rəs\ *n* : ONCOVIRUS

on·co·sphere *also* **on·cho·sphere** \ˈäŋ-kō-ˌsfir\ *n* : an embryo of a tapeworm (order Cyclophyllidea) that has six hooks

on·cot·ic pressure \(ˌ)äŋ-ˈkä-tik-, (ˌ)än-\ *n* : the pressure exerted by plasma proteins on the capillary wall

On·co·vin \ˈäŋ-kō-ˌvin\ *n* : a preparation of vincristine — formerly a U.S. registered trademark

on·co·vi·rus \ˈäŋ-kō-ˌvī-rəs\ *n* : any of various tumor-forming retroviruses

on·dan·se·tron \än-ˈdän-si-ˌträn\ *n* : an antiemetic drug administered orally or parenterally in the form of its hydrated hydrochloride $C_{18}H_{19}$-$N_3O\cdot HCl\cdot 2H_2O$ to prevent nausea and vomiting esp. when a consequence of chemotherapy or surgery — see ZOFRAN

one-egg *adj* : MONOZYGOTIC ⟨~ twins⟩

on·lay \ˈȯn-ˌlā, ˈän-\ *n* **1** : a metal covering attached to a tooth to restore one or more of its surfaces **2** : a graft applied to the surface of a tissue (as bone)

on·set \ˈȯn-ˌset, ˈän-\ *n* : the initial existence or symptoms of a disease

ont- *or* **onto-** *comb form* : organism ⟨*ontogeny*⟩

-ont \ˌänt\ *n comb form* : cell : organism ⟨schiz*ont*⟩

on·to·gen·e·sis \ˌän-tə-ˈje-nə-səs\ *n, pl* **-gen·e·ses** \-ˌsēz\ : ONTOGENY

on·to·ge·net·ic \-jə-ˈne-tik\ *adj* : of, relating to, or appearing in the course of ontogeny — **on·to·ge·net·i·cal·ly** *adv*

on·tog·e·ny \än-ˈtä-jə-nē\ *n, pl* **-nies** : the development or course of development of an individual organism —

called also *ontogenesis;* compare PHYLOGENY 2

onych- *or* **onycho-** *comb form* : nail of the finger or toe ⟨*onych*olysis⟩

on·ych·ec·to·my \ˌä-ni-ˈkek-tə-mē\ *n, pl* **-mies** : surgical excision of a fingernail or toenail

onych·ia \ō-ˈni-kē-ə\ *n* : inflammation of the matrix of a nail often leading to suppuration and loss of the nail

-onych·ia \ə-ˈni-kē-ə\ *n comb form* : condition of the nails of the fingers or toes ⟨leuk*onychia*⟩

-onych·i·um \ə-ˈni-kē-əm\ *n comb form* : fingernail : toenail : region of the fingernail or toenail ⟨epo*nychium*⟩

on·y·cho·gry·po·sis \ˌä-ni-kō-gri-ˈpō-səs\ *n, pl* **-po·ses** \-ˌsēz\ : an abnormal condition of the nails characterized by marked hypertrophy and increased curvature

on·y·chol·y·sis \ˌä-nə-ˈkä-lə-səs\ *n, pl* **-y·ses** \-ˌsēz\ : a loosening of a nail from the nail beginning at the free edge and proceeding to the root

on·y·cho·ma·de·sis \ˌä-ni-kō-mə-ˈdē-səs\ *n, pl* **-de·ses** \-ˌsēz\ : loosening and shedding of the nails

on·y·cho·my·co·sis \-mī-ˈkō-səs\ *n, pl* **-co·ses** \-ˌsēz\ : a fungal disease of the nails

on·y·cho·til·lo·ma·nia \ˌä-ni-kə-ˌti-lə-ˈmā-nē-ə\ *n* : an obsessive-compulsive disorder marked by the picking at or pulling out of one's nails

oo- — see O-

oo·cy·e·sis \ˌō-ə-sī-ˈē-səs\ *n, pl* **-e·ses** \-ˌsēz\ : extrauterine pregnancy in an ovary

oo·cyst \ˈō-ə-ˌsist\ *n* : ZYGOTE; *specif* : a sporozoan zygote undergoing sporogenous development

oo·cyte \ˈō-ə-ˌsīt\ *n* : an egg before maturation : a female gametocyte

oo·gen·e·sis \ˌō-ə-ˈje-nə-səs\ *n, pl* **-e·ses** \-ˌsēz\ : formation and maturation of the egg — called also *ovogenesis*

oo·go·ni·um \ˌō-ə-ˈgō-nē-əm\ *n* : a descendant of a primordial germ cell that gives rise to oocytes — **oo·go·ni·al** \-nē-əl\ *adj*

oophor- *or* **oophoro-** *comb form* : ovary ⟨*oophor*ectomy⟩

oo·pho·rec·to·my \ˌō-ə-fə-ˈrek-tə-mē\ *n, pl* **-mies** : the surgical removal of an ovary — called also *ovariectomy* — **oo·pho·rec·to·mize** \-ˌmīz\ *vb*

oo·pho·ri·tis \ˌō-ə-fə-ˈrī-təs\ *n* : inflammation of one or both ovaries

oophorus — see CUMULUS OOPHORUS

oo·plasm \ˈō-ə-ˌpla-zəm\ *n* : the cytoplasm of an egg — **oo·plas·mic** \-ˈplaz-mik\ *adj*

oo·tid \ˈō-ə-ˌtid\ *n* : an egg cell after meiosis — compare SPERMATID

opac·i·fi·ca·tion \ō-ˌpa-sə-fə-ˈkā-shən\ *n* : an act or the process of becoming or rendering opaque ⟨∼ of the cornea⟩ — **opac·i·fy** \ō-ˈpa-sə-ˌfī\ *vb*

opac·i·ty \ō-ˈpa-sə-tē\ *n, pl* **-ties** 1 : the quality or state of a body that makes it impervious to the rays of light; *broadly* : the relative capacity of matter to obstruct by absorption or reflection the transmission of radiant energy 2 : an opaque spot in a normally transparent structure (as the lens of the eye)

opaque \ō-ˈpāk\ *adj* : exhibiting opacity : not allowing passage of radiant energy

OPD *abbr* outpatient department

¹**open** \ˈō-pən\ *adj* 1 a : not covered, enclosed, or scabbed over b : not involving or encouraging a covering (as by bandages or overgrowth of tissue) or enclosure ⟨∼ treatment of burns⟩ c : relating to or being a compound fracture d : being an operation or surgical procedure in which an incision is made such that the tissues and organs are fully exposed — compare OPEN-HEART 2 : shedding the infective agent to the exterior ⟨∼ tuberculosis⟩ — compare CLOSED 2 3 a : unobstructed by congestion or occlusion ⟨∼ sinuses⟩ b : not constipated ⟨∼ bowels⟩ 4 : using a minimum of physical restrictions and custodial restraints on the freedom of movement of the patients or inmates

²**open** *vb* **opened; open·ing** 1 a : to make available for entry or passage by removing (as a cover) or clearing away (as an obstruction) b : to free (a body passage) of congestion or occlusion ⟨∼ clogged arteries⟩ 2 : to make one or more openings in ⟨∼ed the boil⟩

open–angle glaucoma *n* : a progressive form of glaucoma in which the drainage channel for the aqueous humor remains open and in which serious reduction in vision occurs only in the advanced stages of the disease due to tissue changes along the drainage channel — compare ANGLE-CLOSURE GLAUCOMA

open chain *n* : an arrangement of atoms represented by a structural formula by a chain whose ends are not joined so as to form a ring

open–heart *adj* : of, relating to, or performed on a heart temporarily stopped and relieved of circulatory function and surgically opened for repair of defects or damage ⟨∼ surgery⟩

open–label *adj* : being or relating to a clinical trial in which the treatment given to each subject is not concealed from either the researchers or the subject — compare DOUBLE-BLIND, SINGLE-BLIND

open reduction *n* : realignment of a fractured bone after incision into the fracture site

op·er·a·ble \ˈä-pə-rə-bəl\ *adj* 1 : fit, possible, or desirable to use 2 : likely to result in a favorable outcome upon surgical treatment — **op·er·a·bil·i·ty** \ˌä-pə-rə-ˈbi-lə-tē\ n

¹**op·er·ant** \ˈä-pə-rənt\ adj : of, relating to, or being an operant or operant conditioning ⟨∼ behavior⟩ — **op·er·ant·ly** adv

²**operant** n : behavior that operates on the environment to produce rewarding and reinforcing effects

operant conditioning n : conditioning in which the desired behavior or increasingly closer approximations to it are followed by a rewarding or reinforcing stimulus — compare CLASSICAL CONDITIONING

op·er·ate \ˈä-pə-ˌrāt\ vb **-at·ed; -at·ing** : to perform surgery

op·er·at·ing adj : of, relating to, or used for operations ⟨an ∼ room⟩

op·er·a·tion \ˌä-pə-ˈrā-shən\ n : a procedure performed on a living body usu. with instruments for the repair of damage or the restoration of health and esp. one that involves incision, excision, or suturing

op·er·a·tive \ˈä-pə-rə-tiv, -ˌrā-\ adj : of, relating to, involving, or resulting from an operation ⟨∼ treatment⟩

op·er·a·tor \ˈä-pə-ˌrā-tər\ n **1** : one who performs surgical operations **2** : a binding site in a DNA chain at which a genetic repressor binds to inhibit the initiation of transcription of messenger RNA by one or more nearby structural genes — called also *operator gene;* compare OPERON

op·er·a·to·ry \ˈä-pə-rə-ˌtōr-ē\ n, pl **-ries** : a working space (as of a dentist or surgeon) : SURGERY

oper·cu·lum \ō-ˈpər-kyə-ləm\ n, pl **-la** \-lə\ also **-lums** : any of several parts of the cerebrum bordering the sylvian fissure and concealing the insula

op·er·on \ˈä-pə-ˌrän\ n : a group of closely linked genes that produces a single messenger RNA molecule in transcription and that consists of structural genes and regulating elements (as an operator and promoter)

ophthalm- or **ophthalmo-** comb form : eye ⟨*ophthalmo*logy⟩ : eyeball ⟨*ophthalmo*dynamometry⟩

oph·thal·mia \äf-ˈthal-mē-ə, äp-\ n : inflammation of the conjunctiva or the eyeball

-oph·thal·mia \ˌäf-ˈthal-mē-ə, ˌäp-\ comb form : condition of having (such) eyes ⟨micr*ophthalmia*⟩

ophthalmia neo·na·to·rum \-ˌnē-ə-nə-ˈtōr-əm\ n : acute inflammation of the eyes of a newborn from infection during passage through the birth canal

oph·thal·mic \äf-ˈthal-mik, äp-\ adj **1** : of, relating to, or situated near the eye **2** : supplying or draining the eye or structures in the region of the eye

ophthalmic artery n : a branch of the internal carotid artery following the optic nerve through the optic foramen into the orbit and supplying the eye and adjacent structures

ophthalmic nerve n : the one of the three major branches or divisions of the trigeminal nerve that supply sensory fibers to the lacrimal gland, eyelids, ciliary muscle, nose, forehead, and adjoining parts — called also *ophthalmic, ophthalmic division;* compare MANDIBULAR NERVE, MAXILLARY NERVE

ophthalmic vein n : either of two veins that pass from the orbit: **a** : one that begins at the inner angle of the orbit and empties into the cavernous sinus — called also *superior ophthalmic vein* **b** : one that drains a venous network in the floor and medial wall of the orbit and divides into two parts of which one joins the pterygoid plexus of veins and the other empties into the cavernous sinus — called also *inferior ophthalmic vein*

ophthalmo- — see OPHTHALM-

oph·thal·mo·dy·na·mom·e·try \ˌäf-ˌthal-mō-ˌdī-nə-ˈmä-mə-trē, äp-\ n, pl **-tries** : measurement of the arterial blood pressure in the retina

oph·thal·mol·o·gist \ˌäf-thəl-ˈmä-lə-jist, ˌäp-, -ˌthal-\ n : a physician who specializes in ophthalmology — compare OPTICIAN 2, OPTOMETRIST

oph·thal·mol·o·gy \-jē\ n, pl **-gies** : a branch of medical science dealing with the structure, functions, and diseases of the eye — **oph·thal·mo·log·ic** \-mə-ˈlä-jik\ or **oph·thal·mo·log·i·cal** \-ji-kəl\ adj — **oph·thal·mo·log·i·cal·ly** adv

oph·thal·mom·e·ter \-ˈmä-mə-tər\ n : an instrument for measuring the eye; *specif* : KERATOMETER

oph·thal·mo·ple·gia \-ˈplē-jə, -jē-ə\ n : paralysis of some or all of the muscles of the eye — **oph·thal·mo·ple·gic** \-jik\ adj

oph·thal·mo·scope \äf-ˈthal-mə-ˌskōp\ n : an instrument for viewing the interior of the eye consisting of a concave mirror with a hole in the center through which the observer examines the eye, a source of light that is reflected into the eye by the mirror, and lenses in the mirror which can be rotated into the opening in the mirror — **oph·thal·mo·scop·ic** \ˌäf-ˌthal-mə-ˈskä-pik\ adj

oph·thal·mos·co·py \ˌäf-thal-ˈmäs-kə-pē\ n, pl **-pies** : examination of the eye with an ophthalmoscope

-o·pia \ˈō-pē-ə\ n comb form **1** : condition of having (such) vision ⟨dipl*opia*⟩ **2** : condition of having (such) a visual defect ⟨hyper*opia*⟩

¹**opi·ate** \ˈō-pē-ət, -ˌāt\ n **1** : a drug (as morphine or codeine) containing or derived from opium and tending to induce sleep and to alleviate pain; *broadly* : NARCOTIC 1 **2** : OPIOID 1

²**opiate** adj **1** : of, relating to, or containing opium or an opium derivative **2** : of, relating to, binding, or being an opiate ⟨∼ receptors⟩

opin·ion \ə-'pin-yən\ n : a formal expression of judgment or advice by an expert ⟨wanted a second ∼⟩

¹**opi·oid** \'ō-pē-ˌóid\ adj **1** : possessing some properties characteristic of opiate narcotics but not derived from opium **2** : of, involving, or induced by an opioid

²**opioid** n **1** : any of a group of endogenous neural polypeptides (as an endorphin or enkephalin) that bind esp. to opiate receptors and mimic some of the pharmacological properties of opiates — called also *opioid peptide* **2** : a synthetic drug (as methadone) possessing narcotic properties similar to opiates but not derived from opium; *broadly* : OPIATE 1

opisth- or **opistho-** comb form : dorsal : posterior ⟨*opistho*tonos⟩

opis·thor·chi·a·sis \ə-ˌpis-ˌthór-'kī-ə-səs\ n : infestation with or disease caused by trematode worms of the genus *Opisthorchis*

Op·is·thor·chis \ˌä-pəs-'thór-kəs\ n : a genus of digenetic trematode worms (family Opisthorchiidae) including several that are liver parasites of mammals including humans

op·is·thot·o·nos \ˌä-pəs-'thät-ᵊn-əs\ n : a condition of spasm of the muscles of the back, causing the head and lower limbs to bend backward and the trunk to arch forward

opi·um \'ō-pē-əm\ n : a highly addictive stimulant narcotic that consists of the dried milky juice from the seed capsules of the opium poppy, was formerly used in medicine to soothe pain, and is smoked illicitly as an intoxicant

opium poppy n : an annual Eurasian poppy (*Papaver somniferum*) that is the source of opium

op·po·nens \ə-'pō-ˌnenz\ n, pl **-nen·tes** \ˌä-pə-'nen-(ˌ)tēz\ or **-nens** : any of several muscles of the hand or foot that tend to draw one of the lateral digits across the palm or sole toward the others

opponens dig·i·ti min·i·mi \-'di-jə-ˌtī-'mi-nə-ˌmī\ n : a triangular muscle of the hand that arises from the hamate and adjacent flexor retinaculum, is inserted along the ulnar side of the metacarpal of the little finger, and functions to abduct, flex, and rotate the fifth metacarpal in opposing the little finger and thumb

opponens pol·li·cis \-'pä-lə-səs\ n : a small triangular muscle of the hand that is located below the abductor pollicis brevis, arises from the trapezium and the flexor retinaculum of the hand, is inserted along the radial side of the metacarpal of the thumb, and functions to abduct, flex, and rotate the metacarpal of the thumb in opposing the thumb and fingers

op·po·nent \ə-'pō-nənt\ n : a muscle that opposes or counteracts and limits the action of another

op·por·tun·ist \ˌä-pər-'tü-nist, -'tyü-\ n : an opportunistic microorganism

op·por·tu·nist·ic \-tü-'nis-tik, -tyü-\ adj **1** : of, relating to, or being a microorganism that is usu. harmless but can become pathogenic when the host's resistance to disease is impaired **2** : of, relating to, or being an infection or disease caused by an opportunistic organism

op·pos·able \ə-'pō-zə-bəl\ adj : capable of being placed against one or more of the remaining digits of a hand or foot ⟨an ∼ thumb⟩

oppositional defiant disorder n : a disruptive behavior pattern of childhood and adolescence characterized by defiant, disobedient, and hostile behavior esp. toward adults in positions of authority — abbr. *ODD*

-op·sia \'äp-sē-ə\ n comb form, pl **-op·sias** : vision of a (specified) kind or condition ⟨hemian*opsia*⟩

op·sin \'äp-sən\ n : any of various colorless proteins that in combination with retinal or a related prosthetic group form a visual pigment (as rhodopsin) in a reaction which is reversed by light

op·so·nin \'äp-sə-nən\ n : any of various proteins (as complement or antibodies) that bind to foreign particles and microorganisms (as bacteria) making them more susceptible to the action of phagocytes — **op·son·ic** \äp-'sä-nik\ adj

op·son·iza·tion \ˌäp-sə-nə-'zā-shən, -ˌnī-'zā-\ n : the process of modifying (as a bacterium) by the action of opsonins — **op·son·ize** \'äp-sə-ˌnīz\ vb

-op·sy \ˌäp-sē, əp-\ n comb form, pl **-op·sies** : examination ⟨bi*opsy*⟩ ⟨necr*opsy*⟩

opt abbr optician

¹**op·tic** \'äp-tik\ adj **1** : of or relating to vision ⟨∼ phenomena⟩ **2 a** : of or relating to the eye : OCULAR **b** : affecting the eye or an optic structure

²**optic** n : any of the elements (as lenses or mirrors) of an optical instrument or system — usu. used in pl.

op·ti·cal \'äp-ti-kəl\ adj **1** : of or relating to the science of optics **2 a** : of or relating to vision : VISUAL **b** : using the properties of light to aid vision **3** : of, relating to, or utilizing light ⟨∼ microscopy⟩ — **op·ti·cal·ly** adv

optical activity n : ability of a chemical substance to rotate the plane of vibration of polarized light to the right or left

optical axis n : a straight line perpendicular to the front of the cornea of the eye and extending through the center of the pupil — called also *optic axis*

optical illusion n : visual perception of a real object in such a way as to misinterpret its actual nature

optically active adj : capable of rotating the plane of vibration of polarized light to the right or left : either dextrorotatory or levorotatory — used of compounds, molecules, or atoms

optic atrophy *n* : degeneration of the optic nerve

optic axis *n* : OPTICAL AXIS

optic canal *n* : OPTIC FORAMEN

optic chiasma *n* : the X-shaped partial decussation on the undersurface of the hypothalamus through which the optic nerves are continuous with the brain — called also *optic chiasm*

optic cup *n* : the optic vesicle after invaginating to form a 2-layered cup from which the retina and pigmented layer of the eye will develop — called also *eyecup*

optic disk *n* : BLIND SPOT

optic foramen *n* : the passage through the orbit of the eye in the lesser wing of the sphenoid bone that is traversed by the optic nerve and ophthalmic artery — called also *optic canal;* see CHIASMATIC GROOVE

op·ti·cian \äp-'ti-shən\ *n* **1** : a maker of or dealer in optical items and instruments **2** : a person who reads prescriptions for visual correction, orders lenses, and dispenses eyeglasses and contact lenses — compare OPHTHALMOLOGIST, OPTOMETRIST

op·ti·cian·ry \-rē\ *n, pl* **-ries** : the profession or practice of an optician

optic lobe *n* : SUPERIOR COLLICULUS

optic nerve *n* : either of the pair of sensory nerves that comprise the second pair of cranial nerves, arise from the ventral part of the diencephalon, form an optic chiasma before passing to the eye and spreading over the anterior surface of the retina, and conduct visual stimuli to the brain — called also *second cranial nerve*

op·tics \'äp-tiks\ *n sing or pl* **1** : a science that deals with the nature and properties of light **2** : optical properties

optic stalk *n* : the constricted part of the optic vesicle by which it remains continuous with the embryonic forebrain

optic tectum *n* : SUPERIOR COLLICULUS

optic tract *n* : the portion of each optic nerve between the optic chiasma and the diencephalon proper

optic vesicle *n* : an evagination of each lateral wall of the embryonic vertebrate forebrain from which the nervous structures of the eye develop

opto- *comb form* **1** : vision ⟨*opto*metry⟩ **2** : optic : optical and ⟨*opto*kinetic⟩

op·to·ki·net·ic \äp-tō-kə-'ne-tik, -kī-\ *adj* : of, relating to, or involving movements of the eyes ⟨~ nystagmus⟩

op·tom·e·trist \äp-'tä-mə-trist\ *n* : a specialist licensed to practice optometry — compare OPHTHALMOLOGIST, OPTICIAN 2

op·tom·e·try \-trē\ *n, pl* **-tries** : the health-care profession concerned esp.

with examining the eye for defects and faults of refraction, with prescribing corrective lenses or eye exercises, with diagnosing diseases of the eye, and with treating such diseases or referring them for treatment — **op·to·met·ric** \äp-tə-'me-trik\ *adj*

OPV *abbr* oral polio vaccine

OR *abbr* operating room

ora *pl of* ²OS

orad \'ōr-ad\ *adv* : toward the mouth or oral region

orae serratae *pl of* ORA SERRATA

oral \'ōr-əl, 'är-\ *adj* **1 a** : of, relating to, or involving the mouth : BUCCAL ⟨the ~ mucous membrane⟩ **b** : given or taken through or by way of the mouth ⟨an ~ vaccine⟩ **c** : acting on the mouth **2 a** : of, relating to, or characterized by the first stage of psychosexual development in psychoanalytic theory during which libidinal gratification is derived from intake (as of food), by sucking, and later by biting **b** : of, relating to, or characterized by personality traits of passive dependence and aggressiveness — compare ANAL 2, GENITAL 3, PHALLIC 2 — **oral·ly** *adv*

oral cavity *n* : the cavity of the mouth; *esp* : the part of the mouth behind the gums and teeth that is bounded above by the hard and soft palates and below by the tongue and by the mucous membrane connecting it with the inner part of the mandible

oral contraceptive *n* : BIRTH CONTROL PILL

oral contraceptive pill *n* : BIRTH CONTROL PILL

oral hairy leukoplakia *n* : HAIRY LEUKOPLAKIA

oral sex *n* : oral stimulation of the genitals : CUNNILINGUS : FELLATIO

oral surgeon *n* : a specialist in oral surgery

oral surgery *n* **1** : a branch of dentistry that deals with the diagnosis and treatment of oral conditions requiring surgical intervention **2** : a branch of surgery that deals with conditions of the jaws and mouth structures requiring surgery

oral suspension *n* : a suspension consisting of undissolved particles of one or more medicinal agents mixed with a liquid vehicle for oral administration

ora ser·ra·ta \ōr-ə-sə-'rä-tə, -'rä-\ *n, pl* **orae ser·ra·tae** \ōr-ē-sə-'rä-tē\ : the dentate border of the retina

or·bi·cu·lar·is oculi \ōr-bi-kyə-'lar-əs-'ä-kyù-lī-lē\ *n, pl* **or·bi·cu·lar·es oculi** \-'lar-(ˌ)ēz-\ : the muscle encircling the opening of the orbit and functioning to close the eyelids

orbicularis oris \-'ōr-əs\ *n, pl* **orbiculares oris** : a muscle made up of several layers of fibers passing in different directions that encircles the mouth and controls most movements of the lips

orbiculus cil·i·ar·is \-ˌsi-lē-'er-əs\ *n* : a circular tract in the eye that extends from the ora serrata forward to the posterior part of the ciliary processes — called also *ciliary ring, pars plana*

or·bit \'òr-bət\ *n* : the bony cavity perforated for the passage of nerves and blood vessels that occupies the lateral front of the skull immediately beneath the frontal bone on each side and encloses and protects the eye and its appendages — called also *eye socket, orbital cavity* — **or·bit·al** \-²l\ *adj*

orbital fissure *n* : either of two openings transmitting nerves and blood vessels to or from the orbit: **a** : one situated superiorly between the greater wing and the lesser wing of the sphenoid bone — called also *superior orbital fissure, supraorbital fissure* **b** : one situated inferiorly between the greater wing of the sphenoid bone and the maxilla — called also *inferior orbital fissure, infraorbital fissure, sphenomaxillary fissure*

orbital plate *n* **1** : the part of the frontal bone forming most of the top of the orbit **2** : a thin plate of bone forming the lateral wall enclosing the ethmoidal air cells and forming part of the side of the orbit next to the nose

or·bi·to·fron·tal \ˌòr-bi-tə-'frən-t²l\ *adj* : located in, supplying, or being the part of the cerebral cortex in the basal region of the frontal lobe near the orbit ⟨the ∼ cortex⟩

or·bi·tot·o·my \ˌòr-bə-'tä-tə-mē\ *n, pl* **-mies** : surgical incision of the orbit

or·bi·vi·rus \'òr-bi-ˌvī-rəs\ *n* **1** *cap* : a genus of reoviruses having a genome composed of usu. 10 segments of double-stranded RNA and including the causative agents of African horse sickness and bluetongue **2** : any virus of the genus *Orbivirus*

or·chi·dec·to·my \ˌòr-kə-'dek-tə-mē\ *n, pl* **-mies** : ORCHIECTOMY

-or·chi·dism \'òr-kə-ˌdi-zəm\ *also* **-or·chism** \'òr-ˌki-zəm\ *n comb form* : a (specified) form or condition of the testes ⟨cryptorchidism⟩

or·chi·do·pexy \'òr-kə-dō-ˌpek-sē\ *n, pl* **-pex·ies** : surgical fixation of a testis — called also *orchiopexy*

or·chi·ec·to·my \ˌòr-kē-'ek-tə-mē\ *n, pl* **-mies** : surgical excision of a testis or of both testes — called also *orchidectomy*

or·chi·o·pexy \'òr-kē-ō-ˌpek-sē\ *n, pl* **-pex·ies** : ORCHIDOPEXY

or·chi·tis \òr-'kī-təs\ *n* : inflammation of a testis — **or·chit·ic** \òr-'ki-tik\ *adj*

¹or·der \'òr-dər\ *vb* **or·dered; or·der·ing** : to give a prescription for : PRESCRIBE ⟨the doctor ∼*ed* bed rest⟩

²order *n* : a category of taxonomic classification ranking above the family and below the class

or·der·ly \-lē\ *n, pl* **-lies** : a hospital attendant who does routine or heavy work (as cleaning, carrying supplies, or moving patients)

Oret·ic \ò-'re-tik\ *trademark* — used for a preparation of hydrochlorothiazide

-o·rex·ia \ə-'rek-sē-ə, ə-'rek-shə\ *n comb form* : appetite ⟨anorexia⟩

or·gan \'òr-gən\ *n* : a differentiated structure (as a heart or kidney) consisting of cells and tissues and performing some specific function in an organism

organ- *or* **organo-** *comb form* **1** : organ ⟨organelle⟩ ⟨organogenesis⟩ **2** : organic ⟨organophosphorus⟩

or·gan·elle \ˌòr-gə-'nel\ *n* : a specialized cellular part (as a mitochondrion, lysosome, or ribosome) that is analogous to an organ

or·gan·ic \òr-'ga-nik\ *adj* **1 a** : of, relating to, or arising in a bodily organ **b** : affecting the structure of the organism ⟨an ∼ disease⟩ — compare FUNCTIONAL 1b **2 a** : of, relating to, or derived from living organisms **b** (1) : of, relating to, or containing carbon compounds (2) : relating to, being, or dealt with by a branch of chemistry concerned with the carbon compounds of living beings and most other carbon compounds — **or·gan·i·cal·ly** *adv*

organic brain syndrome *n* : any mental dysfunction (as delirium or senile dementia) resulting from physical changes in brain structure and characterized esp. by impaired cognition — called also *organic brain disorder, organic mental syndrome*

or·gan·ism \'òr-gə-ˌni-zəm\ *n* : an individual constituted to carry on the activities of life by means of organs separate in function but mutually dependent : a living being — **or·gan·is·mic** \ˌòr-gə-'niz-mik\ *also* **or·gan·is·mal** \-məl\ *adj* — **or·gan·is·mi·cal·ly** *adv*

or·ga·ni·za·tion \ˌòr-gə-nə-'zā-shən\ *n* : the formation of fibrous tissue from a clot or exudate by invasion of connective tissue cells and capillaries from adjoining tissues — **or·ga·nize** \'òr-gə-ˌnīz\ *vb*

or·ga·niz·er \'òr-gə-ˌnī-zər\ *n* : a region of a developing embryo (as part of the dorsal lip of the blastopore) or a substance produced by such a region that is capable of inducing a specific type of development in undifferentiated tissue — called also *inductor*

organo- — see ORGAN-

or·gano·chlo·rine \ˌòr-ˌga-nə-ˌklòr-ˌēn, -ən\ *adj* : of, relating to, or being a chlorinated hydrocarbon and esp. one used as a pesticide (as aldrin, DDT, or dieldrin) — **organochlorine** *n*

organ of Cor·ti \-'kòr-tē\ *n* : a complex epithelial structure in the cochlea that in mammals is the chief part of the ear by which sound is directly perceived

Corti, Alfonso Giacomo Gaspare (1822–1876), Italian anatomist.

organ of Ro·sen·mül·ler \-'rō-zən-ˌmyü-lər\ *n* : EPOOPHORON

Rosenmüller, Johann Christian (1771–1820), German anatomist.

or·gan·o·gen·e·sis \ˌor-gə-nō-'je-nə-səs, ȯr-ˌga-nə-\ *n, pl* **-e·ses** \-ˌsēz\ : the origin and development of bodily organs — compare MORPHOGENESIS — **or·gan·o·ge·net·ic** \-jə-'ne-tik\ *adj*

or·gan·oid \'ȯr-gə-ˌnȯid\ *adj* : resembling an organ in structural appearance or qualities — used esp. of abnormal masses (as tumors)

or·gan·o·lep·tic \ˌȯr-gə-nō-'lep-tik, ȯr-ˌga-nə-\ *adj* **1** : being, affecting, or relating to qualities (as taste, color, and odor) of a substance (as a food) that stimulate the sense organs **2** : involving use of the sense organs

or·ga·nol·o·gy \ˌȯr-gə-'nä-lə-jē\ *n, pl* **-gies** : the study of the organs of plants and animals

or·ga·no·meg·a·ly \ˌȯr-gə-nō-'me-gə-lē\ *n, pl* **-lies** : abnormal enlargement of the viscera — called also *visceromegaly*

or·gano·mer·cu·ri·al \ˌȯr-ˌga-nō-(ˌ)mər-'kyur-ē-əl\ *n* : an organic compound or a pharmaceutical preparation containing mercury — **organomercurial** *adj*

or·gano·phos·phate \ˌȯr-ˌga-nə-'fäs-ˌfāt\ *n* : an organophosphorus pesticide — **organophosphate** *adj*

or·gano·phos·pho·rus \-'fäs-fə-rəs\ *also* **or·gano·phos·pho·rous** \-'fäs-'fȯr-əs\ *adj* : of, relating to, or being a phosphorus-containing organic pesticide (as malathion) that acts by inhibiting cholinesterase — **organophosphorus** *n*

or·gasm \'ȯr-ˌga-zəm\ *n* : the climax of sexual excitement that is usu. accompanied by ejaculation of semen in the male and by vaginal contractions in the female — **orgasm** *vb* — **or·gas·mic** \ȯr-'gaz-mik\ *also* **or·gas·tic** \-'gas-tik\ *adj*

ori- *comb form* : mouth ⟨*orifice*⟩

ori·ent \'ȯr-ē-ˌent\ *vb* : to acquaint with or adjust according to the existing situation or environment

oriental rat flea *n* : a flea of the genus *Xenopsylla* (*X. cheopis*) that is widely distributed on rodents and is a vector of plague

oriental sore *n* : a skin disease caused by a protozoan of the genus *Leishmania* (*L. tropica*) that is marked by persistent granulomatous and ulcerating lesions and occurs widely in Asia and in tropical regions

ori·en·ta·tion \ˌȯr-ē-ən-'tā-shən, -ˌen-\ *n* **1 a** : the act or process of orienting or of being oriented **b** : the state of being oriented **2** : a usu. general or lasting direction of thought, inclination, or interest — see SEXUAL ORIENTATION **3** : change of position by organs, organelles, or organisms in response to external stimulus **4** : awareness of the existing situation with reference to time, place, and identity of persons — **ori·en·ta·tion·al** \-shə-nəl\ *adj*

oriented *adj* : having psychological orientation ⟨an alert and ~ patient⟩

or·i·fice \'ȯr-ə-fəs, 'är-\ *n* : an opening through which something may pass — **or·i·fi·cial** \ˌȯr-ə-'fi-shəl, ˌär-\ *adj*

or·i·gin \'ȯr-ə-jən, 'är-\ *n* **1** : the point at which something begins or rises or from which it derives **2** : the more fixed, central, or larger attachment of a muscle — compare INSERTION 1

oris — see CANCRUM ORIS, LEVATOR ANGULI ORIS, ORBICULARIS ORIS

or·li·stat \'ȯr-li-ˌstat\ *n* : a lipase inhibitor $C_{29}H_{53}NO_5$ that prevents the absorption of dietary fat and is used to treat obesity — see XENICAL

Ormond's disease \'ȯr-ˌmändz-\ *n* : RETROPERITONEAL FIBROSIS

Ormond, John Kelso (1886–1978), American urologist.

or·ni·thine \'ȯr-nə-ˌthēn\ *n* : a crystalline amino acid $C_5H_{12}N_2O_2$ that functions esp. in urea production

ornithine car·ba·moyl·trans·fer·ase \-ˌkär-bə-ˌmȯil-'trans-fər-ˌās\ *n* : ORNITHINE TRANSCARBAMYLASE

ornithine trans·car·ba·moy·lase \-ˌtrans-ˌkär-bə-'mȯi-ˌlās\ *n* : ORNITHINE TRANSCARBAMYLASE

ornithine trans·car·ba·myl·ase \-'mi-ˌlās\ *n* : an enzyme of hepatic mitochondria that catalyzes the conversion of ornithine to citrulline as part of urea formation and that when deficient in the body results in hyperammonemia, vomiting, coma, seizures, and sometimes death

Or·ni·thod·o·ros \ˌȯr-nə-'thä-də-rəs\ *n* : a genus of ticks (family Argasidae) including some that are vectors of relapsing fever and Q fever

or·ni·tho·sis \ˌȯr-nə-'thō-səs\ *n, pl* **-tho·ses** \-ˌsēz\ : PSITTACOSIS; *esp* : a form of the disease occurring or originating in birds (as turkeys and pigeons) that are not in the family (Psittacidae) containing the parrots

oro- *comb form* **1** : mouth ⟨*oropharynx*⟩ **2** : oral and ⟨*orofacial*⟩

oro·an·tral \ˌȯr-ō-'an-trəl\ *adj* : of, relating to, or connecting the mouth and the maxillary sinus

oro·fa·cial \-'fā-shəl\ *adj* : of or relating to the mouth and face

oro·gas·tric \-'gas-trik\ *adj* : traversing or affecting the digestive tract from the mouth to the stomach

oro·man·dib·u·lar \-man-'di-byə-lər\ *adj* : of or affecting the mouth and mandible

oro·na·sal \-'nā-zəl\ *adj* : of or relating to the mouth and nose; *esp* : connecting the mouth and the nasal cavity

oro·pha·ryn·geal \-ˌfar-ən-'jē-əl, -fə-'rin-jəl, -jē-əl\ *adj* **1** : of or relating to the oropharynx **2** : of or relating to the mouth and pharynx

oropharyngeal airway *n* : a tube used to provide free passage of air between the mouth and pharynx of an unconscious person

oro·phar·ynx \-'far-iŋks\ *n, pl* **-pha·ryn·ges** \-fə-'rin-(,)jēz\ *also* **-phar·ynx·es** : the part of the pharynx that is below the soft palate and above the epiglottis and is continuous with the mouth

oro·so·mu·coid \,ȯr-ə-sō-'myü-,kȯid\ *n* : a plasma glycoprotein believed to be associated with inflammation

oro·tra·che·al \,ȯr-ō-'trā-kē-əl\ *adj* : relating to or being intubation of the trachea by way of the mouth

Oroya fever \ȯr-'ȯi-ə-\ *n* : the acute first stage of bartonellosis characterized by high fever and severe anemia

orphan disease *n* : a disease which affects a relatively small number of individuals and for which no drug therapy has been developed because the small market would make the research and the drug unprofitable

orphan drug *n* : a drug that is not developed or marketed because its extremely limited use (as in the treatment of a rare disease) makes it unprofitable

or·phen·a·drine \ȯr-'fe-nə-drən, -,drēn\ *n* : a drug used in the form of its citrate $C_{18}H_{23}NO \cdot C_6H_8O_7$ or hydrochloride $C_{18}H_{23}NO \cdot HCl$ as a muscle relaxant and antispasmodic

ORS *abbr* oral rehydration salts; oral rehydration solution

orth- *or* **ortho-** *comb form* : correct : corrective ⟨*ortho*dontia⟩

Or·tho·bun·ya·vi·rus \,ȯrthə-'bən-yə-,vī-rəs\ *n* : a genus of bunyaviruses that are transmitted by arthropods (esp. mosquitoes and ticks) and include the causative virus of La Crosse encephalitis

orth·odon·tia \,ȯr-thə-'dän-chə, -chē-ə\ *n* 1 : ORTHODONTICS 2 : dental appliances (as braces) used in orthodontic treatment

orth·odon·tics \-'dän-tiks\ *n* 1 : a branch of dentistry dealing with irregularities of the teeth and their correction (as by means of braces) 2 : the treatment provided by an orthodontist — **orth·odon·tic** \-tik\ *adj* — **or·tho·don·ti·cal·ly** *adv*

or·tho·don·tist \,ȯr-thə-'dän-tist\ *n* : a specialist in orthodontics

orthodox sleep *n* : SLOW-WAVE SLEEP

or·tho·drom·ic \,ȯr-thə-'drä-mik\ *adj* 1 : proceeding or conducting in a normal direction — used esp. of a nerve impulse or fiber 2 : characterized by orthodromic conduction

Or·tho Ev·ra \'ȯr-thō-'ev-rə\ *trademark* — used for a contraceptive transdermal patch containing norelgestromin and ethinyl estradiol

or·tho·gnath·ic \,ȯr-thag-'na-thik, -,thäg-\ *adj* : correcting deformities of the jaw and the associated malocclusion ⟨∼ surgery⟩

or·tho·myxo·vi·rus \,ȯr-thō-'mik-sə-,vī-rəs\ *n* : any of a family (*Orthomyxoviridae*) of single-stranded RNA viruses that have a spherical or filamentous virion with numerous surface glycoprotein projections and include the causative agents of influenza — see INFLUENZA VIRUS

Or·tho-No·vum \,ȯr-thō-'nō-vəm\ *trademark* — used for a preparation of norethindrone and either ethinyl estradiol or mestranol

or·tho·pae·dic, or·tho·pae·dics, or·tho·pae·dist *chiefly Brit var of* ORTHOPEDIC, ORTHOPEDICS, ORTHOPEDIST

or·tho·pe·dic \,ȯr-thə-'pē-dik\ *adj* 1 : of, relating to, or employed in orthopedics 2 : marked by or affected with a deformity, disorder, or injury of the skeleton and associated structures — **or·tho·pe·di·cal·ly** *adv*

or·tho·pe·dics \-'pē-diks\ *n sing or pl* : a branch of medicine concerned with the correction or prevention of deformities, disorders, or injuries of the skeleton and associated structures (as tendons and ligaments)

or·tho·pe·dist \-'pē-dist\ *n* : a specialist in orthopedics

or·tho·phos·pho·ric acid \,ȯr-thə-,fäs-'fȯr-ik-, -'fär-; -'fäs-fə-rik-\ *n* : PHOSPHORIC ACID 1

or·thop·nea \ȯr-'thäp-nē-ə, ,ȯr-,thäp-'nē-ə\ *n* : difficulty in breathing that occurs when lying down and is relieved upon changing to an upright position (as in congestive heart failure) — **or·thop·ne·ic** \-ik\ *adj*

or·thop·noea *chiefly Brit var of* ORTHOPNEA

or·tho·pox·vi·rus \'ȯr-thō-päks-,vī-rəs\ *n* 1 *cap* : a genus of brick-shaped poxviruses that hybridize extensively within the genus and that include the vaccinia virus and the causative agents of cowpox, monkeypox, mousepox, and smallpox 2 : any virus of the genus *Orthopoxvirus*

or·tho·psy·chi·a·trist \,ȯr-thə-sə-'kī-ə-trəst, -(,)sī-\ *n* : a specialist in orthopsychiatry

or·tho·psy·chi·a·try \-sə-'kī-ə-trē, -(,)sī-\ *n, pl* **-tries** : prophylactic psychiatry concerned esp. with incipient mental and behavioral disorders in youth — **or·tho·psy·chi·at·ric** \-,sī-kē-'a-trik\ *adj*

or·thop·tics \ȯr-'thäp-tiks\ *n sing or pl* : the treatment or the art of treating defective visual habits, defects of binocular vision, and muscle imbalance (as strabismus) by reeducation of visual habits, exercise, and visual training — **or·thop·tic** \-tik\ *adj*

or·thop·tist \-tist\ *n* : a person specializing in orthoptics

or·tho·sis \ȯr-'thō-səs\ *n, pl* **or·tho·ses** \-,sēz\ : ORTHOTIC

or·tho·stat·ic \,ȯr-thə-'sta-tik\ *adj* : of, relating to, or caused by erect posture ⟨∼ hypotension⟩

orthostatic albuminuria *n* : albuminuria that occurs only when a person is in an upright position

¹or·thot·ic \òr-'thä-tik\ *adj* **1** : of or relating to orthotics **2** : designed for the support of weak or ineffective joints or muscles ⟨∼ devices⟩

²orthotic *n* : a support or brace for weak or ineffective joints or muscles — called also *orthosis*

or·thot·ics \-tiks\ *n* : a branch of mechanical and medical science that deals with the support and bracing of weak or ineffective joints or muscles

or·thot·ist \-tist\ *n* : a person specializing in orthotics

or·tho·top·ic \,òr-thə-'tä-pik\ *adj* : of or relating to the grafting of tissue in a natural position ⟨∼ transplant⟩ — **or·tho·top·i·cal·ly** *adv*

Or·tho Tri–Cy·clen \,òr-thō-,trī-'sī-klən\ *trademark* — used for a preparation of norgestimate and ethinyl estradiol

or·tho·vol·tage \'òr-thō-,vōl-tij\ *n* : X-ray voltage of about 150 to 500 kilovolts

¹os \'äs\ *n, pl* **os·sa** \'ä-sə\ : BONE

²os \'ōs\ *n, pl* **ora** \'ōr-ə\ : ORIFICE — see PER OS

Os *symbol* osmium

OS *abbr* [Latin *oculus sinister*] left eye — used in writing prescriptions

OSA *abbr* obstructive sleep apnea

os cal·cis \-'kal-səs\ *n, pl* **ossa calcis** : CALCANEUS

os·cil·late \'ä-sə-,lāt\ *vb* **-lat·ed; -lat·ing** **1** : to swing backward and forward like a pendulum **2** : to move or travel back and forth between two points — **os·cil·la·tion** \,ä-sə-'lā-shən\ *n* — **os·cil·la·tor** \'ä-sə-,lā-tər\ *n* — **os·cil·la·to·ry** \'ä-sə-lə-,tōr-ē\ *adj*

os·cil·lo·scope \ä-'si-lə-,skōp, ə-\ *n* : an instrument in which the variations in a fluctuating electrical quantity appear temporarily as a visible waveform on the fluorescent screen of a cathode-ray tube — called also *cathode-ray oscilloscope* — **os·cil·lo·scop·ic** \ä-,si-lə-'skä-pik, ,ä-sə-lə-\ *adj*

os cox·ae \-'käk-,sē\ *n, pl* **ossa coxae** : HIP BONE

-ose \,ōs\ *n suffix* : carbohydrate; *esp* : sugar ⟨fructose⟩ ⟨pentose⟩

osel·tam·i·vir \,ō-sel-'ta-mə-,vir\ *n* : a neuraminidase inhibitor administered orally in the form of its phosphate $C_{16}H_{28}N_2O_4 \cdot H_3PO_4$ in the treatment and prevention of influenza A and B — see TAMIFLU

Os·good–Schlat·ter's disease \'äz-,gu̇d-'shlä-tərz-\ *n* : an osteochondritis of the tuberosity of the tibia that occurs esp. among adolescent males

   Osgood, Robert Bayley (1873–1956), American orthopedic surgeon.

   Schlatter, Carl (1864–1934), Swiss surgeon.

-o·side \ə-,sīd\ *n suffix* : glycoside or similar compound ⟨ganglioside⟩

-o·sis \'ō-səs\ *n suffix, pl* **-o·ses** \'ō-,sēz\ *or* **-o·sis·es** **1 a** : action : process : condition ⟨hypnosis⟩ **b** : abnormal or diseased condition ⟨leukosis⟩ **2** : increase : formation ⟨leukocytosis⟩

Os·ler's maneuver *or* **Os·ler maneuver** \'äs-lər(z)-\ *n* : a sphygmomanometric procedure of disputed usefulness in detecting false cases of hypertension in the elderly that involves inflating the cuff above the systolic blood pressure and that is held to indicate pseudohypertension if the arteries remain palpable presumably due to inelasticity and sclerosis

   W. Osler — see RENDU-OSLER-WEBER DISEASE

os·mic acid \'äz-mik-\ *n* : OSMIUM TETROXIDE

os·mi·um \'äz-mē-əm\ *n* : a hard brittle blue-gray or blue-black metallic element — symbol *Os*; see ELEMENT table

osmium tetroxide *n* : a crystalline compound OsO_4 that is an oxide of osmium used as a biological fixative and stain

osmo- *comb form* : osmosis : osmotic ⟨osmoregulation⟩

os·mol *or* **os·mole** \'äz-,mōl, 'äs-\ *n* : a standard unit of osmotic pressure based on a one molal concentration of an ion in a solution

os·mo·lal·i·ty \,äz-mō-'la-lə-tē, ,äs-\ *n, pl* **-ties** : the concentration of an osmotic solution esp. when measured in osmols or milliosmols per 1000 grams of solvent — **os·mo·lal** \äz-'mō-lal, äs-\ *adj*

os·mo·lar·i·ty \,äz-mō-'lar-ə-tē, ,äs-\ *n, pl* **-ties** : the concentration of an osmotic solution esp. when measured in osmols or milliosmols per liter of solution — **os·mo·lar** \äz-'mō-lər, äs-\ *adj*

os·mo·re·cep·tor \,äz-mō-ri-'sep-tər\ *n* : any of a group of cells sensitive to plasma osmolality that are held to exist in the brain and to regulate water balance in the body by controlling thirst and the release of vasopressin

os·mo·reg·u·la·to·ry \-'re-gyə-lə-,tōr-ē\ *adj* : of, relating to, or concerned with the maintenance of constant osmotic pressure — **os·mo·reg·u·la·tion** \,äz-mō-,re-gyə-'lā-shən, ,äs-\ *n*

os·mo·sis \äz-'mō-səs, äs-\ *n, pl* **os·mo·ses** \-,sēz\ : movement of a solvent through a semipermeable membrane (as of a living cell) into a solution of higher solute concentration that tends to equalize the concentrations of solute on the two sides of the membrane — **os·mot·ic** \-'mä-tik\ *adj* — **os·mot·i·cal·ly** *adv*

osmotic pressure *n* : the pressure produced by or associated with osmosis and dependent on molar concentration and absolute temperature: as **a** : the maximum pressure that develops in a solution separated from a solvent by a membrane permeable only to the solvent **b** : the pressure that must be applied to a solution to just prevent osmosis

ossa *pl of* 'OS

ossea — see LEONTIASIS OSSEA

os·seo·in·te·gra·tion \,ä-sē-ō,in-tə-'grā-shən\ *n* : the firm anchoring of a surgical implant (as in dentistry or in bone surgery) by the growth of bone around it without fibrous tissue formation at the interface — **os·seo·in·te·grat·ed** \-'in-tə-,grā-təd\ *adj*

os·se·ous \'ä-sē-əs\ *adj* : of, relating to, or composed of bone — **os·se·ous·ly** *adv*

osseous labyrinth *n* : BONY LABYRINTH

ossi- *comb form* : bone 〈*ossify*〉

os·si·cle \'ä-si-kəl\ *n* : a small bone or bony structure; *esp* : any of three small bones of the middle ear including the malleus, incus, and stapes — **os·sic·u·lar** \ä-'si-kyə-lər\ *adj*

ossificans — see MYOSITIS OSSIFICANS

os·si·fi·ca·tion \,ä-sə-fə-'kā-shən\ *n* **1 a** : the process of bone formation usu. beginning at particular centers in each prospective bone and involving the activities of special osteoblasts that segregate and deposit inorganic bone substance about themselves **b** : an instance of this process **2 a** : the condition of being altered into a hard bony substance 〈~ of the muscular tissue〉 **b** : a mass or particle of ossified tissue : a calcareous deposit in the tissues 〈~s in the aortic wall〉 — **os·si·fy** \'ä-sə-,fī\ *vb*

ossium — see FRAGILITAS OSSIUM

oste- *or* **osteo-** *comb form* : bone 〈*osteal*〉 〈*osteomyelitis*〉

os·te·al \'äs-tē-əl\ *adj* : of, relating to, or resembling bone; *also* : affecting or involving bone or the skeleton

os·tec·to·my \äs-'tek-tə-mē\ *n, pl* **-mies** : surgical removal of all or part of a bone

os·te·itis \,äs-tē-'ī-təs\ *n, pl* **-it·i·des** \-'i-tə-,dēz\ : inflammation of bone — called also *ostitis* — **os·te·it·ic** \-'i-tik\ *adj*

osteitis de·for·mans \-di-'for-,manz\ *n* : PAGET'S DISEASE 2

osteitis fi·bro·sa \-fī-'brō-sə\ *n* : a disease of bone that is characterized by fibrous degeneration of the bone and the formation of cystic cavities and that results in deformities of the affected bones and sometimes in fracture — called also *osteodystrophia fibrosa*

osteitis fibrosa cys·ti·ca \-'sis-tə-kə\ *n* : OSTEITIS FIBROSA

osteitis fibrosa cystica gen·er·al·is·ta \-,je-nə-rə-'lis-tə\ *n* : OSTEITIS FIBROSA

os·teo·ar·thri·tis \,äs-tē-ō-är-'thrī-təs\ *n, pl* **-thrit·i·des** \-'thri-tə-,dēz\ : arthritis typically with onset during middle age or old age that is characterized by degenerative and sometimes hypertrophic changes in the

bone and cartilage of one or more joints and a progressive wearing down of apposing joint surfaces with consequent distortion of joint position and is marked symptomatically by pain, swelling, and stiffness — abbr. *OA;* called also *degenerative arthritis, degenerative joint disease, hypertrophic arthritis;* compare RHEUMATOID ARTHRITIS — **os·teo·ar·thrit·ic** \-'thri-tik\ *adj*

os·teo·ar·throp·a·thy \-är-'thrä-pə-thē\ *n, pl* **-thies** : a disease of joints or bones; *specif* : a hypertrophic condition marked esp. by clubbing of the fingers and toes, painful swollen joints, and periostitis and subperiosteal bone formation chiefly affecting the long bones (as the radius or fibula) and that usu. occurs secondary to another disease (as bronchiectasis or cirrhosis) — called also *acropachy*

os·teo·ar·thro·sis \-är-'thrō-səs\ *n* : OSTEOARTHRITIS — **os·teo·ar·throt·ic** \-'thrä-tik\ *adj*

os·teo·ar·tic·u·lar \-är-'ti-kyə-lər\ *adj* : relating to, involving, or affecting bones and joints 〈~ diseases〉

os·teo·blast \'äs-tē-ə-,blast\ *n* : a bone-forming cell

os·teo·blas·tic \,äs-tē-ə-'blas-tik\ *adj* **1** : relating to or involving the formation of bone **2** : composed of or being osteoblasts

os·teo·blas·to·ma \-bla-'stō-mə\ *n, pl* **-mas** *also* **-ma·ta** \-mə-tə\ : a benign tumor of bone

os·teo·cal·cin \-'kal-sən\ *n* : a protein produced by osteoblasts that is found in the extracellular matrix of bone and in the serum of circulating blood and when present at excessive levels in serum may be indicative of various disorders (as postmenopausal osteoporosis) of bone metabolism

os·teo·car·ti·lag·i·nous \-,kärt-ºl-'a-jə-nəs\ *adj* : relating to or composed of bone and cartilage 〈an ~ nodule〉

osteochondr- *or* **osteochondro-** *comb form* : bone and cartilage 〈*osteochondritis*〉

os·teo·chon·dral \-'kän-drəl\ *adj* : relating to or composed of bone and cartilage

os·teo·chon·dri·tis \-,kän-'drī-təs\ *n* : inflammation of bone and cartilage

osteochondritis dis·se·cans \-'di-sə-,kanz\ *n* : partial or complete detachment of a fragment of bone and cartilage at a joint

os·teo·chon·dro·dys·pla·sia \-,kän-drō-,dis-'plā-zhə, -zhē-ə\ *n* : abnormal growth or development of cartilage and bone

os·teo·chon·dro·ma \-,kän-'drō-mə\ *n, pl* **-mas** *also* **-ma·ta** \-mə-tə\ : a benign tumor containing both bone and cartilage and usu. occurring near the end of a long bone

os·teo·chon·dro·sis \-,kän-'drō-səs\ *n, pl* **-dro·ses** \-,sēz\ : a disease esp. of children and young animals in which an ossification center esp. in the epiphyses of long bones undergoes degeneration followed by calcification — **os·teo·chon·drot·ic** \-'drä-tik\ *adj*

os·teo·clast \'äs-tē-ə-ˌklast\ *n* : any of the large multinucleate cells closely associated with areas of bone resorption (as in a healing fracture) — **os·teo·clas·tic** \ˌäs-tē-ə-'klas-tik\ *adj*

os·teo·clas·to·ma \ˌäs-tē-ō-kla-'stō-mə\ *n, pl* **-mas** *also* **-ma·ta** \-mə-tə\ : GIANT-CELL TUMOR

os·teo·cyte \'äs-tē-ə-ˌsīt\ *n* : a cell that is characteristic of adult bone, is derived from an osteoblast, and occupies a lacuna of the bone matrix

os·teo·dys·tro·phia fi·bro·sa \ˌäs-tē-ō-di-'strō-fē-ə-fī-'brō-sə\ *n* : OSTEITIS FIBROSA

os·teo·dys·tro·phy \-'dis-trə-fē\ *n, pl* **-phies** : defective ossification of bone usu. associated with disturbed calcium and phosphorus metabolism

os·teo·gen·e·sis \ˌäs-tē-ə-'je-nə-səs\ *n, pl* **-e·ses** \-ˌsēz\ : development and formation of bone

osteogenesis im·per·fec·ta \-ˌim-pər-'fek-tə\ *n* : a hereditary disease caused by defective or deficient collagen production and marked by extreme brittleness of the long bones and a bluish color of the whites of the eyes — called also *fragilitas ossium, osteopsathyrosis*

osteogenesis imperfecta con·gen·i·ta \-kən-'je-nə-tə\ *n* : a severe and often fatal form of osteogenesis imperfecta characterized by usu. multiple fractures in utero

osteogenesis imperfecta tar·da \-'tär-də\ *n* : a less severe form of osteogenesis imperfecta which is not apparent at birth

os·teo·gen·ic \ˌäs-tē-ə-'je-nik\ *also* **os·teo·ge·net·ic** \-jə-'ne-tik\ *adj* **1** : of, relating to, or functioning in osteogenesis; *esp* : producing bone **2** : originating in bone

osteogenic sarcoma *n* : OSTEOSARCOMA

¹os·te·oid \'äs-tē-ˌóid\ *adj* : resembling bone ⟨~ tissue⟩

²osteoid *n* : uncalcified bone matrix

osteoid osteoma *n* : a small benign painful tumor of bony tissue occurring esp. in the extremities of children and young adults

os·te·ol·o·gy \ˌäs-tē-'ä-lə-jē\ *n, pl* **-gies** **1** : a branch of anatomy dealing with the bones **2** : the bony structure of an organism — **os·te·o·log·i·cal** \ˌäs-tē-ə-'lä-ji-kəl\ *adj* — **os·te·ol·o·gist** \ˌäs-tē-'ä-lə-jist\ *n*

os·te·ol·y·sis \ˌäs-tē-'ä-lə-səs\ *n, pl* **-y·ses** \-ˌsēz\ : dissolution of bone esp. when associated with resorption — **os·te·o·lyt·ic** \ˌäs-tē-ə-'li-tik\ *adj*

os·te·o·ma \ˌäs-tē-'ō-mə\ *n, pl* **-mas** *also* **-ma·ta** \-mə-tə\ : a benign tumor composed of bone tissue

os·teo·ma·la·cia \ˌäs-tē-ō-mə-'lā-shə,

-shē-ə\ *n* : a disease of adults that is characterized by softening of the bones and is analogous to rickets in the young — **os·teo·ma·la·cic** \-'lā-sik\ *adj*

os·teo·my·eli·tis \-ˌmī-ə-'lī-təs\ *n, pl* **-elit·i·des** \-ə-'li-tə-ˌdēz\ : an infectious usu. painful inflammatory disease of bone that is often of bacterial origin and may result in death of bony tissue — **os·teo·my·elit·ic** \-'li-tik\ *adj*

os·te·on \'äs-tē-ˌän\ *n* : HAVERSIAN SYSTEM — **os·te·on·al** \ˌäs-tē-'än-ᵊl, -'ōn-\ *adj*

os·teo·ne·cro·sis \ˌäs-tē-ō-nə-'krō-səs\ *n, pl* **-cro·ses** \-ˌsēz\ : necrosis of bone; *esp* : AVASCULAR NECROSIS

os·teo·path \'äs-tē-ə-ˌpath\ *n* : a practitioner of osteopathy

os·te·op·a·thy \ˌäs-tē-'ä-pə-thē\ *n, pl* **-thies** **1** : a disease of bone **2** : a system of medical practice based on a theory that diseases are due chiefly to loss of structural integrity which can be restored by manipulation of the parts supplemented by therapeutic measures (as use of medicine or surgery) — **os·teo·path·ic** \ˌäs-tē-ə-'pa-thik\ *adj* — **os·teo·path·i·cal·ly** *adv*

os·teo·pe·nia \ˌäs-tē-ō-'pē-nē-ə\ *n* : reduction in bone volume to below normal levels esp. due to inadequate replacement of bone lost to normal lysis — **os·teo·pe·nic** \-nik\ *adj*

os·teo·pe·tro·sis \-pə-'trō-səs\ *n, pl* **-tro·ses** \-ˌsēz\ : a rare hereditary disease characterized by extreme density and hardness and abnormal fragility of the bones with partial or complete obliteration of the marrow cavities — called also *Albers-Schönberg disease* — **os·teo·pe·trot·ic** \-pə-'trä-tik\ *adj*

os·teo·phyte \'äs-tē-ə-ˌfīt\ *n* : an abnormal bony outgrowth or projection (as near a joint affected by osteoarthritis) : SPUR 2 — **os·teo·phyt·ic** \ˌäs-tē-ə-'fi-tik\ *adj*

os·teo·plas·tic \ˌäs-tē-ə-'plas-tik\ *adj* : of, relating to, or being osteoplasty

osteoplastic flap *n* : a surgically excised portion of the skull folded back on a hinge of skin to expose the underlying tissues (as in a craniotomy)

os·teo·plas·ty \'äs-tē-ə-ˌplas-tē\ *n, pl* **-ties** : plastic surgery on bone; *esp* : replacement of lost bone tissue or reconstruction of defective bony parts

os·teo·poi·ki·lo·sis \ˌäs-tē-ō-ˌpói-kə-'lō-səs\ *n* : an asymptomatic hereditary bone disorder characterized by numerous sclerotic foci giving bones a mottled or spotted appearance

os·teo·po·ro·sis \ˌäs-tē-ō-pə-'rō-səs\ *n, pl* **-ro·ses** \-ˌsēz\ : a condition that affects esp. older women and is characterized by decrease in bone mass with decreased density and enlargement of bone spaces producing porosity and fragility — **os·teo·po·rot·ic** \-'rä-tik\ *adj*

os·te·op·sath·y·ro·sis \ˌäs-tē-äp-ˌsa-thə-'rō-səs\ *n, pl* **-ro·ses** \-ˌsēz\ : OSTEOGENESIS IMPERFECTA

os·teo·ra·dio·ne·cro·sis \ˌäs-tē-ō-ˌrā-dē-ō-nə-'krō-səs\ *n, pl* **-cro·ses** \-ˌsēz\ : necrosis of bone following irradiation

os·teo·sar·co·ma \-sär-'kō-mə\ *n, pl* **-mas** *also* **-ma·ta** \-mə-tə\ : a sarcoma derived from bone or containing bone tissue — called also *osteogenic sarcoma*

os·teo·scle·ro·sis \-sklə-'rō-səs\ *n, pl* **-ro·ses** \-ˌsēz\ : abnormal hardening of bone or of bone marrow — **os·teo·scle·rot·ic** \-'rä-tik\ *adj*

os·teo·syn·the·sis \-'sin-thə-səs\ *n, pl* **-the·ses** \-ˌsēz\ : the operation of uniting the ends of a fractured bone by mechanical means (as a wire)

os·te·o·tome \ˈäs-tē-ə-ˌtōm\ *n* : a chisel without a bevel used for cutting bone

os·te·ot·o·my \ˌäs-tē-'ä-tə-mē\ *n, pl* **-mies** : a surgical operation in which a bone is divided or a piece of bone is excised (as to correct a deformity)

Os·ter·ta·gia \ˌäs-tər-'tā-jə, -jē-ə\ *n* : a genus of nematode worms (family Trichostrongylidae) parasitic in the abomasum of ruminants

os·ti·tis \äs-'tī-təs\ *n* : OSTEITIS

os·ti·um \ˈäs-tē-əm\ *n, pl* **os·tia** \-tē-ə\ : a mouthlike opening in a bodily part (as a fallopian tube or a blood vessel) — **os·ti·al** \ˈäs-tē-əl\ *adj*

os·to·mate \ˈäs-tə-ˌmāt\ *n* : a person who has undergone an ostomy

os·to·my \ˈäs-tə-mē\ *n, pl* **-mies** : an operation (as a colostomy, ileostomy, or urostomy) to create an artificial passage for bodily elimination

-os·to·sis \ˌäs-'tō-səs\ *n comb form, pl* **-os·to·ses** \-ˌsēz\ *or* **-os·to·sis·es** : ossification of a (specified) part or to a (specified) degree ⟨hyper*ostosis*⟩

OT *abbr* **1** occupational therapist **2** occupational therapy

ot- *or* **oto-** *comb form* **1** : ear ⟨*otitis*⟩ **2** : ear and ⟨*oto*laryngology⟩

otal·gia \ō-'tal-jə, -jē-ə\ *n* : EARACHE

other–directed *adj* : directed in thought and action primarily by external norms rather than by one's own scale of values — compare IN-NER-DIRECTED

otic \ˈō-tik\ *adj* : of, relating to, or located in the region of the ear

¹-ot·ic \ˈä-tik\ *adj suffix* **1 a** : of, relating to, or characterized by a (specified) action, process, or condition ⟨symbi*otic*⟩ **b** : having an abnormal or diseased condition of a (specified) kind ⟨epizo*otic*⟩ **2** : showing an increase or a formation of ⟨leukocy*totic*⟩

²-otic \ˈō-tik\ *adj comb form* : having (such) a relationship to the ear ⟨di*chotic*⟩

otic ganglion *n* : a small parasympathetic ganglion that is associated with the mandibular nerve and sends post-ganglionic fibers to the parotid gland by way of the auriculotemporal nerve

oti·tis \ō-'tī-təs\ *n, pl* **otit·i·des** \ō-'ti-tə-ˌdēz\ : inflammation of the ear — **otit·ic** \-'ti-tik\ *adj*

otitis ex·ter·na \-ek-'stər-nə\ *n* : inflammation of the external auditory canal; *esp* : SWIMMER'S EAR

otitis in·ter·na \-in-'tər-nə\ *n* : inflammation of the inner ear; *specif* : LABYRINTHITIS

otitis me·dia \-'mē-dē-ə\ *n* : inflammation of the middle ear; *esp* : an acute inflammation esp. in infants or young children that is caused by a virus or bacterium, usu. occurs as a complication of an upper respiratory infection, and is marked by earache, fever, hearing loss, and sometimes rupture of the tympanic membrane — see SEROUS OTITIS MEDIA

oto- — see OT-

Oto·bi·us \ō-'tō-bē-əs\ *n* : a genus of ticks (family Argasidae) that includes the spinose ear tick (*O. megnini*)

oto·co·nia \ˌō-tə-'kō-nē-ə\ *n pl* : small crystals of calcium carbonate in the saccule and utricle of the ear that under the influence of acceleration in a straight line cause stimulation of the hair cells by their movement relative to the gelatinous supporting substrate containing the embedded cilia of the hair cells — called also *statoconia*

Oto·dec·tes \ˌō-tə-'dek-ˌtēz\ *n* : a genus of mites that includes one (*O. cynotis*) causing otodectic mange — **oto·dec·tic** \-'dek-tik\ *adj*

otodectic mange *n* : ear mange caused by a mite (*O. cynotis*) of the genus *Otodectes*

oto·lar·yn·gol·o·gist \ˌō-tō-ˌlar-ən-'gä-lə-jist\ *n* : a specialist in otolaryngology — called also *otorhinolaryngologist*

oto·lar·yn·gol·o·gy \-jē\ *n, pl* **-gies** : a medical specialty concerned esp. with the ear, nose, and throat — called also *otorhinolaryngology* — **oto·lar·yn·go·log·i·cal** \-ˌlar-ən-gə-'lä-ji-kəl\ *adj*

oto·lith \ˈōt-ᵊl-ˌith\ *n* : a calcareous concretion in the internal ear composed of masses of otoconia — called also *statolith* — **oto·lith·ic** \ˌōt-ᵊl-'i-thik\ *adj*

otol·o·gist \ō-'tä-lə-jist\ *n* : a specialist in otology

otol·o·gy \-jē\ *n, pl* **-gies** : a science that deals with the ear and its diseases — **oto·log·ic** \ˌō-tə-'lä-jik\ *also* **oto·log·i·cal** \-'lä-ji-kəl\ *adj* — **oto·log·i·cal·ly** *adv*

oto·my·co·sis \ˌō-tō-mī-'kō-səs\ *n, pl* **-co·ses** \-ˌsēz\ : disease of the ear produced by the growth of fungi in the external auditory canal

oto·plas·ty \ˈō-tə-ˌplas-tē\ *n, pl* **-ties** : plastic surgery of the external ear

oto·rhi·no·lar·yn·gol·o·gist \ˌō-tō-ˌrī-nō-ˌlar-ən-'gä-lə-jist\ *n* : OTOLARYNGOLOGIST

oto·rhi·no·lar·yn·gol·o·gy \-jē\ *n, pl* **-gies** : OTOLARYNGOLOGY — **oto·rhi·no·lar·yn·go·log·i·cal** \-gə-'lä-ji-kəl\ *adj*

otor·rhea \ˌō-tə-'rē-ə\ *n* : a discharge from the external ear

otor·rhoea *chiefly Brit var of* OTOR-RHEA

oto·scle·ro·sis \ˌō-tō-sklə-'rō-səs\ *n, pl* **-ro·ses** \-ˌsēz\ : growth of spongy bone in the inner ear where it gradually obstructs the oval window or round window or both and causes progressively increasing deafness — **oto·scle·rot·ic** \-sklə-'rä-tik\ *adj*

oto·scope \'ō-tə-ˌskōp\ *n* : an instrument fitted with lighting and magnifying lens systems and used to facilitate visual examination of the auditory canal and ear drum — **oto·scop·ic** \ˌō-tə-'skä-pik\ *adj* — **otos·co·py** \ō-'täs-kə-pē\ *n*

oto·tox·ic \ˌō-tə-'täk-sik\ *adj* : producing, involving, or being adverse effects on organs or nerves involved in hearing or balance — **oto·tox·ic·i·ty** \-täk-'si-sə-tē\ *n*

OTR *abbr* registered occupational therapist

oua·bain \wä-'bā-ən, 'wä-ˌbān\ *n* : a poisonous glycoside $C_{29}H_{44}O_{12}$ used medically like digitalis

ounce \'auṅs\ *n* **1 a** : a unit of weight equal to $^1/_{12}$ troy pound or 31.103 grams   **b** : a unit of weight equal to $^1/_{16}$ avoirdupois pound or 28.350 grams   **2** : FLUID OUNCE

out·break \'aut-ˌbrāk\ *n* : a sudden rise in the incidence of a disease ⟨an ~ of measles⟩

out·breed·ing \'aut-ˌbrē-diŋ\ *n* : breeding between individuals or stocks that are relatively unrelated — compare INBREEDING — **out·bred** \-ˌbred\ *adj* — **out·breed** \-ˌbrēd\ *vb*

out·cross \'aut-ˌkrȯs\ *n* **1** : a cross between relatively unrelated individuals **2** : the progeny of an outcross — **out·cross** *vb*

out·er·course \'au-tər-ˌkȯrs\ *n* : physical sexual activity between individuals that typically includes stimulation of the genitalia but does not involve penetration of the vagina or anus with the penis

outer ear *n* : the outer visible portion of the ear that collects and directs sound waves toward the tympanic membrane by way of a canal which extends inward through the temporal bone

out·growth \'aut-ˌgrōth\ *n* **1** : the process of growing out **2** : something that grows directly out of something else ⟨an ~ of hair⟩ ⟨a bony ~⟩

out·let \'aut-ˌlet, -lət\ *n* **1** : an opening or a place through which something is let out ⟨the pelvic ~⟩ **2** : a means of release or satisfaction for an emotion or impulse

outlet forceps *n* : LOW FORCEPS

out–of–body *adj* : relating to or involving a feeling of separation from one's body and of being able to view oneself and others from an external perspective ⟨an ~ experience⟩

out·pa·tient \'aut-ˌpā-shənt\ *n* : a patient who is not hospitalized overnight but who visits a hospital, clinic, or associated facility for diagnosis or treatment — compare INPATIENT

out·pock·et·ing \'aut-ˌpä-kə-tiŋ\ *n* : EVAGINATION 2

out·pouch·ing \-ˌpau̇-chiŋ\ *n* : EVAGINATION 2

out·put \'aut-ˌpu̇t\ *n* : the amount of energy or matter discharged usu. within a specified time by a bodily system or organ ⟨renal ~⟩ ⟨urinary ~⟩ — see CARDIAC OUTPUT

ov- *or* **ovi-** *or* **ovo-** *comb form* : egg ⟨ovicide⟩ ⟨ovo- ⟨oviduct⟩

ova *pl of* OVUM

ovale — see FORAMEN OVALE

ova·le malaria \ō-'vä-lē-\ *n* : a relatively mild form of malaria caused by a protozoan of the genus *Plasmodium* (*P. ovale*) that is characterized by tertian chills and febrile paroxysms and that usu. ends spontaneously

ovalis — see FENESTRA OVALIS, FOSSA OVALIS

oval window *n* : an oval opening between the middle ear and the vestibule having the base of the stapes or columella attached to its membrane — called also *fenestra ovalis, fenestra vestibuli*

ovari- *or* **ovario-** *also* **ovar-** *comb form* **1** : ovary ⟨ovariectomy⟩ **2** : ovary and ⟨ovariohysterectomy⟩

ovar·i·an \ō-'var-ē-ən\ *also* **ovar·i·al** \-ē-əl\ *adj* : of, relating to, affecting, or involving an ovary

ovarian artery *n* : either of two arteries in the female that arise from the aorta below the renal arteries with one on each side and are distributed to the ovaries with branches supplying the ureters, the fallopian tubes, the labia majora, and the groin

ovarian follicle *n* : FOLLICLE 3

ovarian ligament *n* : LIGAMENT OF THE OVARY

ovarian vein *n* : either of two veins in the female with one on each side that drain a venous plexus in the broad ligament of the same side and empty on the right into the inferior vena cava and on the left into the left renal vein

ovar·i·ec·to·my \ˌō-ˌvar-ē-'ek-tə-mē\ *n, pl* **-mies** : OOPHORECTOMY — **ovar·i·ec·to·mize** \ˌō-ˌvar-ē-'ek-tə-ˌmīz\ *vb*

ovar·io·hys·ter·ec·to·my \ō-ˌvar-ē-ō-ˌhis-tə-'rek-tə-mē\ *n, pl* **-mies** : surgical removal of the ovaries and the uterus

ovar·i·ot·o·my \ō-ˌvar-ē-'ä-tə-mē\ *n, pl* **-mies** **1** : surgical incision of an ovary **2** : OOPHORECTOMY

ova·ry \'ō-və-rē\ *n, pl* **-ries** : one of the typically paired essential female reproductive organs that produce eggs and female sex hormones, that occur in the adult human as oval flattened bodies about one and a half inches (four centimeters) long suspended from the dorsal surface of the broad ligament of either side, that arise from the mesonephros, and that consist of a vascular fibrous stroma enclosing developing egg cells

over·achiev·er \ˌō-vər-ə-ˈchē-vər\ *n* : one who achieves success over and above the standard or expected level esp. at an early age — **over·achieve** *vb*

over·ac·tive \ˌō-vər-ˈak-tiv\ *adj* : excessively or abnormally active — **over·ac·tiv·i·ty** \-ˌak-ˈti-və-tē\ *n*

over·bite \ˈō-vər-ˌbīt\ *n* : the projection of the upper anterior teeth over the lower when the jaws are in the position they occupy in occlusion

over·breathe \ˌō-vər-ˈbrēth\ *vb* **-breathed; -breath·ing** : HYPERVENTILATE

over·com·pen·sa·tion \ˌō-vər-ˌkäm-pən-ˈsā-shən, -ˌpen-\ *n* : excessive compensation; *specif* : excessive reaction to a feeling of inferiority, guilt, or inadequacy leading to an exaggerated attempt to overcome the feeling — **over·com·pen·sate** \-ˈkäm-pən-ˌsāt\ *vb*

over·di·ag·no·sis \ˌō-vər-ˌdī-ig-ˈnō-səs, -əg-\ *n, pl* **-no·ses** \-ˌsēz\ : the diagnosis of a condition or disease more often than it is actually present — **over·di·ag·nose** \-ˈdī-ig-ˌnōs, -əg-\ *vb*

over·dis·ten·sion *or* **over·dis·ten·tion** \-dis-ˈten-chən\ *n* : excessive distension ⟨∼ of the alveoli⟩ — **over·dis·tend·ed** \-dis-ˈten-dəd\ *adj*

over·dose \ˈō-vər-ˌdōs\ *n* : too great a dose (as of a therapeutic agent); *also* : a lethal or toxic amount (as of a drug) — **over·dos·age** \ˌō-vər-ˈdō-sij\ *n* — **over·dose** \ˌō-vər-ˈdōs\ *vb*

over·eat \ˌō-vər-ˈēt\ *vb* **over·ate** \-ˈāt\; **over·eat·en** \-ˈēt-ᵊn\; **over·eat·ing** : to eat to excess — **over·eat·er** *n*

overeating disease *n* : ENTEROTOXEMIA

over·ex·ert \-ig-ˈzərt\ *vb* : to exert (oneself) too much — **over·ex·er·tion** \-ˈzər-shən\ *n*

over·ex·pose \ˌō-vər-ik-ˈspōz\ *vb* **-posed; -pos·ing** : to expose excessively ⟨skin *overexposed* to sunlight⟩ — **over·ex·po·sure** \-ˈspō-zhər\ *n*

over·ex·pres·sion \-ik-ˈspre-shən\ *n* : excessive expression of a gene (as that caused by increasing the frequency of transcription) — **over·ex·press** \-ik-ˈspres\ *vb*

over·ex·tend \-ik-ˈstend\ *vb* : to extend too far ⟨∼ the back⟩ — **over·ex·ten·sion** \-ik-ˈsten-chən\ *n*

over·fa·tigue \-fə-ˈtēg\ *n* : excessive fatigue esp. when carried beyond the recuperative capacity of the individual

over·feed \-ˈfēd\ *vb* **-fed** \-ˈfed\; **-feed·ing** : to feed or eat to excess

over·growth \ˈō-vər-ˌgrōth\ *n* **1 a** : excessive growth or increase in numbers

b : HYPERTROPHY, HYPERPLASIA **2** : something (as cells or tissue) grown over something else

over·hang \ˈō-vər-ˌhaŋ\ *n* : a portion of a filling that extends beyond the normal contour of a tooth

over·hy·dra·tion \ˌō-vər-hī-ˈdrā-shən\ *n* : a condition in which the body contains an excessive amount of fluids

over·jet \ˈō-vər-ˌjet\ *n* : displacement of the mandibular teeth sideways when the jaws are held in the position they occupy in occlusion

over·med·i·cate \-ˈme-di-ˌkāt\ *vb* **-cat·ed; -cat·ing** : to administer too much medication to : prescribe too much medication for — **over·med·i·ca·tion** \-ˌme-di-ˈkā-shən\ *n*

over·nu·tri·tion \ˌō-vər-nü-ˈtri-shən, -nyü-\ *n* : excessive food intake esp. when viewed as a factor in pathology

over·pre·scribe \-pri-ˈskrīb\ *vb* **-scribed; -scrib·ing** : to prescribe excessive or unnecessary medication — **over·pre·scrip·tion** \-pri-ˈskrip-shən\ *n*

over·pro·na·tion \-prō-ˈnā-shən\ *n* : excessive pronation of the foot in walking or running — **over·pro·nate** \-ˈprō-nāt\ *vb*

over·se·da·tion \-si-ˈdā-shən\ *n* : excessive sedation

over·shot \ˈō-vər-ˌshät\ *adj* **1** : having the upper jaw extending beyond the lower **2** : projecting beyond the lower jaw

over·stim·u·la·tion \ˌō-vər-ˌsti-myə-ˈlā-shən\ *n* : excessive stimulation — **over·stim·u·late** \-ˈsti-myə-ˌlāt\ *vb*

overt \ō-ˈvərt, ˈō-ˌvərt\ *adj* : open to view : readily perceived

over-the-coun·ter *adj* : sold lawfully without prescription ⟨∼ painkillers⟩

over·ven·ti·la·tion \ˌō-vər-ˌvent-ᵊl-ˈā-shən\ *n* : HYPERVENTILATION

over·weight \-ˈwāt\ *adj* : weighing in excess of the normal for one's age, height, and build ⟨∼ adults typically have a body mass index of 25 to 29.9⟩ — **overweight** *n*

over·work \-ˈwərk\ *vb* : to cause to work too hard, too long, or to exhaustion

ovi- — see OV-

ovi·cide \ˈō-və-ˌsīd\ *n* : an agent that kills eggs; *esp* : an insecticide effective against the egg stage — **ovi·cid·al** \ˌō-və-ˈsīd-ᵊl\ *adj*

ovi·du·cal \ˌō-və-ˈdü-kəl, -ˈdyü-\ *adj* : OVIDUCTAL

ovi·duct \ˈō-və-ˌdəkt\ *n* : a tube that serves exclusively or esp. for the passage of eggs from an ovary

ovi·duc·tal \ˌō-və-ˈdəkt-ᵊl\ *adj* : of, relating to, or affecting an oviduct

ovine \ˈō-ˌvīn\ *adj* : of, relating to, or resembling sheep ⟨∼ diseases⟩

ovine progressive pneumonia *n* : a progressive usu. fatal disease of sheep caused by a retrovirus of the genus *Lentivirus* (species *Visna/maedi virus*) — see MAEDI, VISNA

ovip·a·rous \ō-'vi-pə-rəs\ *adj* : producing eggs that develop and hatch outside the maternal body — compare OVOVIVIPAROUS, VIVIPAROUS — **ovi·par·i·ty** \ō-və-'par-ə-tē\ *n*

ovi·pos·it \'ō-və-,päz-ət, ,ō-və-'\ *vb* : to lay eggs — used esp. of insects — **ovi·po·si·tion** \,ō-və-pə-'zi-shən\ *n* — **ovi·po·si·tion·al** \-'zi-shə-nəl\ *adj*

ovi·pos·i·tor \'ō-və-,päz-ə-tər, ,ō-və-'\ *n* : a specialized organ (as of an insect) for depositing eggs

ovo- — see OV-

ovo·gen·e·sis \,ō-və-'je-nə-səs\ *n, pl* **-e·ses** \-,sēz\ : OOGENESIS

ovoid \'ō-,vȯid\ *adj* : shaped like an egg ⟨an ∼ tumor⟩

ovo–lacto vegetarian *n* : LACTO-OVO VEGETARIAN

ovo·mu·coid \-'myü-,kȯid\ *n* : a mucoprotein present in egg white

ovo·plasm \'ō-və-,pla-zəm\ *n* : the cytoplasm of an unfertilized egg

ovo·tes·tis \,ō-vō-'tes-təs\ *n, pl* **-tes** \-,tēz\ : a gonad containing both ovarian and testicular tissue

ovo·vi·tel·lin \-vī-'te-lən\ *n* : VITELLIN

ovo·vi·vip·a·rous \,ō-vō-,vī-'vi-pə-rəs\ *adj* : producing eggs that develop within the maternal body — compare OVIPAROUS, VIVIPAROUS — **ovo·vi·vi·par·i·ty** \-,vī-və-'par-ə-tē, -,vi-\ *n*

ovu·lar \'ä-vyə-lər, 'ō-\ *adj* : of or relating to an ovule or ovum

ovu·la·tion \,ä-vyə-'lā-shən, ,ō-\ *n* : the discharge of a mature ovum from the ovary — **ovu·late** \'ä-vyə-,lāt\ *vb* — **ovu·la·to·ry** \'ä-vyə-lə-,tōr-ē, 'ō-\ *adj*

ovule \'ä-,vyül, 'ō-\ *n* **1** : an outgrowth of the ovary of a seed plant that after fertilization develops into a seed **2** : a small egg; *esp* : one in an early stage of growth

ovum \'ō-vəm\ *n, pl* **ova** \-və\ : a female gamete : MACROGAMETE; *esp* : a mature egg that has undergone reduction, is ready for fertilization, and takes the form of a relatively large inactive gamete providing a comparatively great amount of reserve material and contributing most of the cytoplasm of the zygote

ox·a·cil·lin \,äk-sə-'si-lən\ *n* : a semisynthetic penicillin administered in the form of its hydrated sodium salt $C_{19}H_{18}N_3NaO_5S\cdot H_2O$ to treat infections caused by penicillin-resistant staphylococci

¹ox·a·late \'äk-sə-,lāt\ *n* : a salt or ester of oxalic acid

²oxalate *vb* **-lat·ed; -lat·ing** : to add an oxalate to (blood or plasma) to prevent coagulation

ox·al·ic acid \(,)äk-'sa-lik-\ *n* : a poisonous strong acid $(COOH)_2$ or $H_2C_2O_4$ that occurs in various plants as oxalates

ox·a·lo·ace·tic acid \,äk-sə-lō-ə-'sē-tik-\ *also* **ox·al·ace·tic acid** \,äk-sə-lə-'sē-tik-\ *n* : a crystalline acid $C_4H_4O_5$ that is formed by reversible oxidation of malic acid (as in carbohydrate me-

tabolism via the Krebs cycle) and in reversible transamination reactions (as from aspartic acid)

ox·a·lo·sis \,äk-sə-'lō-səs\ *n* : an abnormal condition characterized by hyperoxaluria and the formation of calcium oxalate deposits in tissues

ox·an·a·mide \äk-'san-ə-,mīd\ *n* : a tranquilizing drug $C_8H_{15}NO_2$

ox·an·dro·lone \äk-'san-drə-,lōn\ *n* : an anabolic steroid $C_{19}H_{30}O_3$ administered orally esp. to promote weight gain (as after chronic infection) and to relieve bone pain in osteoporosis

ox·a·pro·zin \,äk-sə-'prō-zən\ *n* : an NSAID $C_{18}H_{15}NO_3$ administered orally to treat osteoarthritis and rheumatoid arthritis — see DAYPRO

ox·az·e·pam \äk-'sa-zə-,pam\ *n* : a benzodiazepine tranquilizer $C_{15}H_{11}ClN_2O_2$

ox·a·zol·i·dine \,äk-sə-'zō-lə-,dēn, -'zä-\ *n* : the heterocyclic compound C_3H_7NO; *also* : an anticonvulsant derivative (as trimethadione) of this compound

ox·i·dase \'äk-sə-,dās, -,dāz\ *n* : any of various enzymes that catalyze oxidations; *esp* : one able to react directly with molecular oxygen

ox·i·da·tion \,äk-sə-'dā-shən\ *n* **1** : the act or process of oxidizing **2** : the state or result of being oxidized — **ox·i·da·tive** \'äk-sə-,dā-tiv\ *adj* — **ox·i·da·tive·ly** *adv*

oxidation–reduction *n* : a chemical reaction in which one or more electrons are transferred from one atom or molecule to another — called also *redox*

oxidative phosphorylation *n* : the synthesis of ATP by phosphorylation of ADP for which energy is obtained by electron transport and which takes place in the mitochondria during aerobic respiration

oxidative stress *n* : physiological stress on the body that is caused by the cumulative damage done by free radicals inadequately neutralized by antioxidants and that is held to be associated with aging

ox·ide \'äk-,sīd\ *n* : a binary compound of oxygen with an element or chemical group

ox·i·dize \'äk-sə-,dīz\ *vb* **-dized; -diz·ing** **1** : to combine with oxygen **2** : to dehydrogenate esp. by the action of oxygen **3** : to change (a compound) by increasing the proportion of the part tending to attract electrons or change (an element or ion) from a lower to a higher positive valence : remove one or more electrons from (an atom, ion, or molecule) — **ox·i·diz·able** \,äk-sə-'dī-zə-bəl\ *adj*

oxidized cellulose *n* : an acid degradation product of cellulose that is used esp. as an absorbable hemostatic agent (as in surgery)

oxidizing agent *n* : a substance that oxidizes something esp. chemically (as by accepting electrons) — compare REDUCING AGENT

ox·i·do·re·duc·tase \ˌäk-sə-dō-ri-ˈdək-ˌtās, -ˌtāz\ *n* : an enzyme that catalyzes an oxidation-reduction reaction

ox·im·e·ter \äk-ˈsi-mə-tər\ *n* : an instrument for measuring continuously the degree of oxygen saturation of the circulating blood — **ox·i·met·ric** \ˌäk-sə-ˈme-trik\ *adj* — **ox·im·e·try** \äk-ˈsi-mə-trē\ *n*

oxo·phen·ar·sine \ˌäk-sə-fe-ˈnär-ˌsēn, -sən\ *n* : an arsenical formerly used in the form of its hydrochloride $C_6H_6AsNO_2 \cdot HCl$ to treat syphilis

oxo·trem·o·rine \ˌäk-sō-ˈtre-mə-ˌrēn, -rən\ *n* : a cholinergic agent $C_{12}H_{18}N_2O$ that induces tremors

ox·pren·o·lol \ˌäks-ˈpre-nə-ˌlȯl\ *n* : a beta-adrenergic blocking agent used in the form of the hydrochloride $C_{15}H_{23}NO_3 \cdot HCl$ as a coronary vasodilator

ox·tri·phyl·line \ˌäks-ˌtri-ˈfi-ˌlēn, -ˈtri-fə-ˌlēn\ *n* : the choline salt $C_{12}H_{21}N_5O_3$ of theophylline used chiefly as a bronchodilator

ox warble *n* : the maggot of either the common cattle grub or the northern cattle grub

oxy \ˈäk-sē\ *adj* : containing oxygen or additional oxygen — often used in combination ⟨*oxy*hemoglobin⟩

oxy- *comb form* **1** : sharp : pointed : acute ⟨*oxy*cephaly⟩ **2** : quick ⟨*oxy*tocic⟩ **3** : acid ⟨*oxy*ntic⟩

oxy·ben·zone \ˌäk-sē-ˈben-ˌzōn\ *n* : a sunscreen $C_{14}H_{12}O_3$ that absorbs UVB and some UVA radiation

oxy·bu·ty·nin \ˌäk-sē-ˈbyü-tᵊn-ən\ *n* : an antispasmodic and anticholinergic drug $C_{22}H_{31}NO_3$ administered transdermally as a skin patch or orally in the form of its hydrochloride $C_{22}H_{31}NO_3 \cdot HCl$ to relax the smooth muscles of the bladder in the treatment of urge incontinence, frequent urination, and urinary urgency

oxy·bu·tyr·ic acid \-byü-ˈtir-ik-\ *n* : HYDROXYBUTYRIC ACID

oxy·ceph·a·ly \-ˈse-fə-lē\ *n, pl* **-lies** : congenital deformity of the skull due to early synostosis of the parietal and occipital bones with compensating growth in the region of the anterior fontanel resulting in a pointed or pyramidal skull — called also *acrocephaly, turricephaly* — **oxy·ce·phal·ic** \-si-ˈfa-lik\ *adj*

oxy·chlo·ro·sene \-ˈklȯr-ə-ˌsēn\ *n* : a topical antiseptic that $C_{20}H_{34}O_3S \cdot HOCl$

oxy·co·done \-ˈkō-ˌdōn\ *n* : a narcotic analgesic used esp. in the form of its hydrochloride $C_{18}H_{21}NO_4 \cdot HCl$ — see OXYCONTIN

Oxy·Con·tin \-ˈkän-tin\ *trademark* — used for a preparation of the hydrochloride of oxycodone

ox·y·gen \ˈäk-si-jən\ *n* : a colorless tasteless odorless gaseous element that constitutes 21 percent of the at-

mosphere, is active in physiological processes, and is involved esp. in combustion processes — symbol *O*; see ELEMENT table

ox·y·gen·ate \ˈäk-si-jə-ˌnāt, äk-ˈsi-jə-\ *vb* **-at·ed; -at·ing** : to impregnate, combine, or supply with oxygen ⟨*oxy*genated blood⟩ — **ox·y·gen·ation** \ˌäk-si-jə-ˈnā-shən, äk-ˌsi-jə-\ *n*

ox·y·gen·ator \ˈäk-si-jə-ˌnā-tər, äk-ˈsi-jə-\ *n* : one that oxygenates; *specif* : an apparatus that oxygenates the blood extracorporeally (as during open-heart surgery)

oxygen capacity *n* : the amount of oxygen which a quantity of blood is able to absorb

oxygen debt *n* : a cumulative deficit of oxygen available for oxidative metabolism that develops during periods of intense bodily activity and must be made good when the body returns to rest

oxygen mask *n* : a device worn over the nose and mouth through which oxygen is supplied from a storage tank

oxygen tent *n* : a canopy which can be placed over a bedridden person and within which a flow of oxygen can be maintained

oxy·he·mo·glo·bin \ˌäk-si-ˈhē-mə-ˌglō-bən\ *n* : hemoglobin loosely combined with oxygen that it releases to the tissues

oxy·me·taz·o·line \-mə-ˈta-zə-ˌlēn\ *n* : a sympathomimetic drug with vasoconstrictive activity that is used in the form of its hydrochloride $C_{16}H_{24}N_2O \cdot HCl$ chiefly as a topical nasal decongestant

oxy·mor·phone \-ˈmȯr-ˌfōn\ *n* : a semisynthetic opioid analgesic with pharmacological action similar to morphine that is used in the form of its hydrochloride $C_{17}H_{19}NO_4 \cdot HCl$

oxy·myo·glo·bin \ˌäk-si-ˈmī-ə-ˌglō-bən\ *n* : a pigment formed by the combination of myoglobin with oxygen

ox·yn·tic \äk-ˈsin-tik\ *adj* : secreting acid — used esp. of the parietal cells of the gastric glands

oxy·phen·bu·ta·zone \ˌäk-sē-ˌfen-ˈbyü-tə-ˌzōn\ *n* : a phenylbutazone derivative $C_{19}H_{20}N_2O_3$ having antiinflammatory, analgesic, and antipyretic effects

oxy·phen·cy·cli·mine \-ˈsī-klə-ˌmēn\ *n* : an anticholinergic drug with actions similar to atropine usu. used in the form of its hydrochloride $C_{20}H_{28}N_2O_3 \cdot HCl$ as an antispasmodic esp. in the treatment of peptic ulcer

oxy·quin·o·line \-ˈkwin-ᵊl-ˌēn\ *n* : 8-HYDROXYQUINOLINE

Oxy·spi·ru·ra \ˌäk-si-ˌspī-ˈrúr-ə\ *n* : a genus of nematode worms (family Thelaziidae) comprising the eye worms of birds and esp. domestic poultry

oxy·tet·ra·cy·cline \-₁te-tra-'sī-₁klēn\ *n* : a broad-spectrum antibiotic $C_{22}H_{24}N_2O_9$ produced by a soil actinomycete of the genus *Streptomyces* (*S. rimosus*) — see TERRAMYCIN

¹oxy·to·cic \₁äk-si-'tō-sik\ *adj* : hastening parturition; *also* : inducing contraction of uterine smooth muscle

²oxytocic *n* : a substance that stimulates contraction of uterine smooth muscle or hastens childbirth

oxy·to·cin \-'tōs-⁹n\ *n* **1** : a hormone $C_{43}H_{66}N_{12}O_{12}S_2$ secreted by the anterior lobe of the pituitary gland that stimulates esp. the contraction of uterine muscle and the secretion of milk **2** : a synthetic version of oxytocin used esp. to initiate or increase uterine contractions (as in the induction of labor) — see PITOCIN

oxy·uri·a·sis \₁äk-si-yù-'rī-ə-səs\ *n, pl* **-a·ses** \-₁sēz\ : infestation with or disease caused by pinworms (as of the genera *Enterobius* and *Oxyuris*)

oxy·urid \₁äk-sē-'yùr-əd\ *n* : any of a family (Oxyuridae) of nematode worms that are chiefly parasites of the vertebrate intestinal tract — see PINWORM — **oxyurid** *adj*

oxy·uris \-'yùr-əs\ *n* **1** *cap* : a genus of parasitic nematodes (family Oxyuridae) **2** : any nematode worm of the genus *Oxyuris* or a related genus (as *Enterobius*) : PINWORM

oz *abbr* ounce; ounces

oze·na \ō-'zē-nə\ *n* : a chronic disease of the nose accompanied by a fetid discharge and marked by atrophic changes in the nasal structures

ozone \'ō-₁zōn\ *n* : a very reactive form of oxygen containing three atoms per molecule that is a bluish irritating gas of pungent odor, that is a major air pollutant in the lower atmosphere but a beneficial component of the upper atmosphere, and that is used for oxidizing, bleaching, disinfecting, and deodorizing

P

P *abbr* **1** parental **2** pressure **3** pulse

P *symbol* phosphorus

p- *abbr* para- ⟨*p*-dichlorobenzene⟩

Pa *abbr* protactinium

PA \₁pē-'ā\ *n* : PHYSICIAN'S ASSISTANT

PA *abbr* pernicious anemia

PABA \'pa-bə, ₁pē-₁ā-'bē-₁ā\ *n* : PARA-AMINOBENZOIC ACID

pab·u·lum \'pa-byə-ləm\ *n* : FOOD; *esp* : a suspension or solution of nutrients in a state suitable for absorption

PAC *abbr* physician's assistant, certified

pac·chi·o·ni·an body \₁pa-kē-'ō-nē-ən-\ *n* : ARACHNOID GRANULATION

Pac·chi·o·ni \₁pä-kē-'ō-nē\, **Antonio (1665–1726)**, Italian anatomist.

pace·mak·er \'pās-₁mā-kər\ *n* **1** : a group of cells or a body part (as the sinoatrial node of the heart) that serves to establish and maintain a rhythmic activity **2** : an electrical device for stimulating or steadying the heartbeat or reestablishing the rhythm of an arrested heart — called also *pacer*

pace·mak·ing \-₁mā-kiŋ\ *n* : the act or process of serving as a pacemaker

pac·er \'pā-sər\ *n* : PACEMAKER 2

pachy- *comb form* : thick ⟨*pachy*tene⟩

pachy·men·in·gi·tis \₁pa-kē-₁me-nən-'jī-təs\ *n, pl* **-git·i·des** \-'ji-tə-₁dēz\ : inflammation of the dura mater

pachy·me·ninx \-'mē-niŋks, -'me-\ *n, pl* **-me·nin·ges** \-mə-'nin-(₁)jēz\ : DURA MATER

pachy·o·nych·ia \₁pa-kē-ō-'ni-kē-ə\ *n* : extreme usu. congenital thickness of the nails

pachy·tene \'pa-ki-₁tēn\ *n* : the stage of meiotic prophase which immediately follows the zygotene and in which the paired chromosomes are thickened and visibly divided into chromatids — **pachytene** *adj*

pac·i·fi·er \'pa-sə-₁fī-ər\ *n* **1** : a usu. nipple-shaped device for babies to suck or bite on **2** : TRANQUILIZER

pac·ing \'pā-siŋ\ *n* : the act or process of regulating or changing the timing or intensity of cardiac contractions (as by an artificial pacemaker)

Pa·cin·i·an corpuscle \pə-'si-nē-ən-\ *also* **Pa·ci·ni's corpuscle** \pə-'chē-nēz-\ *n* : a pressure-sensitive mechanoreceptor that is an oval capsule terminating some sensory nerve fibers esp. in the skin (as of the hands and feet)

Pacini, Filippo (1812–1883), Italian anatomist.

¹pack \'pak\ *n* **1** : a container shielded with lead or mercury for holding radium in large quantities esp. for therapeutic application **2 a** : absorbent material saturated with water or other liquid for therapeutic application to the body or a body part — see COLD PACK, HOT PACK; compare ICE PACK **b** : a folded square or compress of gauze or other absorbent material used esp. to maintain a clear field in surgery, to plug cavities, to check bleeding by compression, or to apply medication

²pack *vb* : to cover or surround with a pack; *specif* : to envelop (a patient) in a wet or dry sheet or blanket

packed cell volume *n* : HEMATOCRIT 2 — abbr. *PCV*

packed red blood cells *n pl* : a concentrated preparation of red blood cells that is obtained from whole blood by removing the plasma (as by centrifugation) and is used in transfusion

pack·ing \'pa-kiŋ\ *n* **1** : the therapeutic application of a pack **2** : the material used in packing

pac·li·tax·el \₁pa-kli-'tak-səl\ *n* : an antineoplastic agent $C_{47}H_{51}NO_{14}$ orig. derived from the bark of a yew tree (*Taxus brevifolia* of the family Taxaceae) of the western U.S. and Canada but now typically derived as a semisynthetic product of the English yew (*T. baccata*) and used esp. to treat ovarian cancer — see TAXOL

PaCO₂ *abbr* partial pressure of arterial carbon dioxide

PACU *abbr* postanesthesia care unit

pad \'pad\ *n* **1** : a usu. square or rectangular piece of often folded typically absorbent material (as gauze) fixed in place over some part of the body as a dressing or other protective covering **2** : a part of the body or of an appendage that resembles or is suggestive of a cushion : a thick fleshy resilient part: as **a** : the sole of the foot or underside of the toes of an animal (as a dog) that is typically thickened so as to form a cushion **b** : the underside of the extremities of the fingers; *esp* : the ball of the thumb

PAD *abbr* peripheral arterial disease

pad·dle \'pa-dᵊl\ *n* : a flat electrode that is the part of a defibrillator placed on the chest of a patient and through which a shock of electricity is discharged — called also *paddle electrode*

pad·i·mate O \'pa-di-₁māt-'ō\ *n* : a sunscreen $C_{17}H_{27}NO_2$ effective against UVB radiation

paed- *or* **paedo-** *chiefly Brit var of* PED-

pae·di·a·trics, pae·do·don·tics, paedo·phil·ia *chiefly Brit var of* PEDIATRICS, PEDODONTICS, PEDOPHILIA

PAF *abbr* platelet-activating factor

Pag·et's disease \'pa-jəts-\ *n* **1** : a rare form of breast cancer initially manifested as a scaly red rash on the nipple and areola **2** : a chronic disease of bones characterized by their great enlargement and rarefaction with bowing of the long bones and deformation of the flat bones — called also *osteitis deformans*

Pag·et \'pa-jət\, **Sir James (1814–1899)**, British surgeon.

pa·go·pha·gia \₁pā-gə-'fā-jə, -jē-ə\ *n* : the compulsive eating of ice that is a symptom of a lack of iron

-pa·gus \pə-gəs\ *n comb form, pl* **-pa·gi** \pə-₁jī, -₁gī\ : congenitally united twins with a (specified) type of fixation ⟨cranio*pagus*⟩

PAH \₁pē-(₁)ā-'āch\ *n* : POLYCYCLIC AROMATIC HYDROCARBON

PAH *abbr* **1** para-aminohippurate; para-aminohippuric acid **2** polynuclear aromatic hydrocarbon

¹pain \'pān\ *n* **1 a** : a usu. localized physical suffering associated with bodily disorder (as a disease or an injury); *also* : a basic bodily sensation that is induced by a noxious stimulus, is received by naked nerve endings, is characterized by physical discomfort (as pricking, throbbing, or aching), and typically leads to evasive action **b** : acute mental or emotional suffering or distress **2 pains** *pl* : the protracted series of involuntary contractions of the uterine musculature that constitute the major factor in parturient labor and that are often accompanied by considerable pain — **pain·ful** \-fəl\ *adj* — **pain·ful·ly** *adv* — **pain·less** \-ləs\ *adj* — **pain·less·ly** *adv*

²pain *vb* : to cause or experience pain

pain·kill·er \-₁ki-lər\ *n* : something (as a drug) that relieves pain — **pain·kill·ing** *adj*

pain spot *n* : one of many small localized areas of the skin that respond to stimulation (as by pricking or burning) by giving a sensation of pain

paint·er's colic \'pān-tərz-\ *n* : intestinal colic associated with obstinate constipation due to chronic lead poisoning

paired–associate learning *n* : the learning of items (as syllables, digits, or words) in pairs so that one member of the pair evokes recall of the other — compare ASSOCIATIVE LEARNING

palae- *or* **palaeo-** *chiefly Brit var of* PALE-

pal·aeo·cer·e·bel·lum, pal·aeo·pa·thol·ogy *chiefly Brit var of* PALEOCEREBELLUM, PALEOPATHOLOGY

pal·a·tal \'pa-lət-ᵊl\ *adj* : of, relating to, forming, or affecting the palate — **pal·a·tal·ly** *adv*

palatal bar *n* : a connector extending across the roof of the mouth to join the parts of a maxillary partial denture

palatal process *n* : PALATINE PROCESS

pal·ate \'pa-lət\ *n* : the roof of the mouth separating the mouth from the nasal cavity — see HARD PALATE, SOFT PALATE

palati — see TENSOR PALATI

¹pal·a·tine \'pa-lə-₁tīn\ *adj* : of, relating to, or lying near the palate

²palatine *n* : PALATINE BONE

palatine aponeurosis *n* : a thin fibrous lamella attached to the posterior part of the hard palate that supports the soft palate, includes the tendon of the tensor veli palatini, and supports the other muscles of the palate

palatine artery *n* **1** : either of two arteries of each side of the face: **a** : an inferior artery that arises from the facial artery and divides into two branches of which one supplies the soft palate and the palatine glands and the other supplies esp. the tonsils and the eustachian tube — called also *ascending palatine artery* **b** : a superior artery that arises from the maxillary artery and sends branches to the soft palate, the palatine glands, the mucous membrane of the hard palate, and the gums — called also *greater palatine artery* **2** : any of the branches of the palatine arteries

palatine bone *n* : a bone of extremely irregular form on each side of the skull that is situated in the posterior part of the nasal cavity between the maxilla and the pterygoid process of the sphenoid bone and that consists of a horizontal plate which joins the bone of the opposite side and forms the back part of the hard palate and a vertical plate which is extended into three processes and helps to form the floor of the orbit, the outer wall of the nasal cavity, and several adjoining parts — called also *palatine*

palatine foramen *n* : any of several foramina in the palatine bone giving passage to the palatine vessels and nerves — see GREATER PALATINE FORAMEN

palatine gland *n* : any of numerous small mucous glands in the palate opening into the mouth

palatine nerve *n* : any of several nerves arising from the pterygopalatine ganglion and supplying the roof of the mouth, parts of the nose, and adjoining parts

palatine process *n* : a process of the maxilla that projects medially, articulates posteriorly with the palatine bone, and forms with the corresponding process on the other side the anterior three-fourths of the hard palate — called also *palatal process*

palatine suture *n* : either of two sutures in the hard palate: **a** : a transverse suture lying between the horizontal plates of the palatine bones and the maxillae **b** : a median suture lying between the maxillae in front and continued posteriorly between the palatine bones

palatine tonsil *n* : TONSIL 1a

palatini — see LEVATOR VELI PALATINI, TENSOR VELI PALATINI

palato- *comb form* **1** : palate : of the palate ⟨*palato*plasty⟩ **2** : palatal and ⟨*palato*glossal arch⟩

pal·a·to·glos·sal arch \ˌpa-lə-tō-ˈglä-səl-, -ˈglō-\ *n* : the more anterior of the two ridges of soft tissue at the back of the mouth on each side that curves downward from the uvula to the side of the base of the tongue forming a recess for the palatine tonsil as it diverges from the palatopharyngeal arch and that is composed of part of the palatoglossus with its covering of mucous membrane — called also *anterior pillar of the fauces, glossopalatine arch*

pal·a·to·glos·sus \-ˈglä-səs, -ˈglȯ-\ *n, pl* **-glos·si** \-(ˌ)sī\ : a thin muscle that arises from the soft palate on each side, contributes to the structure of the palatoglossal arch, and is inserted into the side and dorsum of the tongue — called also *glossopalatinus*

pal·a·to·pha·ryn·ge·al arch \-ˌfar-ən-ˈjē-əl-, -fə-ˈrin-jəl-, -jē-əl-\ *n* : the more posterior of the two ridges of soft tissue at the back of the mouth on each side that curves downward from the uvula to the side of the pharynx forming a recess for the palatine tonsil as it diverges from the palatoglossal arch and that is composed of part of the palatopharyngeus with its covering of mucous membrane — called also *posterior pillar of the fauces, pharyngopalatine arch*

pal·a·to·pha·ryn·ge·us \-ˌfar-ən-ˈjē-əs; -fə-ˈrin-jəs, -jē-əs\ *n* : a longitudinal muscle of the pharynx that arises from the soft palate, contributes to the structure of the palatopharyngeal arch, and is inserted into the thyroid cartilage and the wall of the pharynx

pal·a·to·plas·ty \ˈpa-lə-tə-ˌplas-tē\ *n, pl* **-ties** : a plastic operation for repair of the palate (as in cleft palate)

pale \ˈpāl\ *adj* **pal·er; pal·est** : deficient in color or intensity of color ⟨a ∼ face⟩ — **pale·ness** \-nəs\ *n*

pale- *or* **paleo-** *comb form* : early : old ⟨*paleo*pathology⟩

pa·leo·cer·e·bel·lum \ˌpā-lē-ō-ˌser-ə-ˈbe-ləm\ *n, pl* **-bel·lums** *or* **-bel·la** \-ˈbe-lə\ : an evolutionarily old part of the cerebellum concerned with maintenance of normal postural relationships and made up chiefly of the anterior lobe of the vermis and of the pyramid — compare NEOCEREBELLUM

pa·leo·pa·thol·o·gy \ˌpā-lē-ō-pə-ˈthä-lə-jē\ *n, pl* **-gies** : a branch of pathology concerned with diseases of former times as determined esp. from fossil or other remains — **pa·leo·pa·thol·o·gist** \-jist\ *n*

pali- *comb form* : pathological state characterized by repetition of a (specified) act ⟨*pali*lalia⟩

pali·la·lia \ˌpa-lə-ˈlā-lē-ə\ *n* : a speech defect marked by abnormal repetition of syllables, words, or phrases

pal·in·drome \ˈpa-lən-ˌdrōm\ *n* : a palindromic sequence of DNA

pal·in·dro·mic \ˌpa-lən-ˈdrō-mik\ *adj* **1** : RECURRENT ⟨∼ rheumatism⟩ **2** : of, relating to, or consisting of a double-stranded sequence of DNA in which the order of the nucleotides is the same on each side but running in opposite directions

pal·i·sade worm \ˌpa-lə-ˈsād-\ *n* : BLOODWORM

pal·la·di·um \pə-ˈlā-dē-əm\ *n* : a silver-white malleable metallic element — symbol *Pd*; see ELEMENT table

pal·li·ate \ˈpa-lē-ˌāt\ *vb* **-at·ed; -at·ing** : to reduce the intensity or severity of (a disease); *also* : to ease (symptoms) without curing the underlying disease — **pal·li·a·tion** \ˌpa-lē-ˈā-shən\ *n*

¹**pal·lia·tive** \ˈpal-ē-ˌā-tiv, ˈpal-yə-\ *adj* : serving to palliate ⟨∼ care⟩

²**palliative** *n* : something that palliates

pal·li·dal \ˈpa-ləd-ᵊl\ *adj* : of, relating to, or involving the globus pallidus

pal·li·dum \ˈpa-lə-dəm\ *n* : GLOBUS PALLIDUS

pallidus — see GLOBUS PALLIDUS

pal·li·um \ˈpa-lē-əm\ *n, pl* **-lia** \-lē-ə\ *or* **-li·ums** : CEREBRAL CORTEX

pal·lor \ˈpa-lər\ *n* : deficiency of color esp. of the face : PALENESS

palm \ˈpälm, ˈpäm\ *n* : the somewhat concave part of the hand between the bases of the fingers and the wrist — **pal·mar** \ˈpal-mər, ˈpäl-, ˈpä-\ *adj*

palmar aponeurosis *n* : an aponeurosis of the palm of the hand that consists of a superficial longitudinal layer continuous with the tendon of the palmaris longus and of a deeper transverse layer — called also *palmar fascia*

palmar arch *n* : either of two loops of blood vessels in the palm of the hand: **a** : a deeply situated transverse artery that is composed of the terminal part of the radial artery joined to a branch of the ulnar artery and that supplies principally the deep muscles of the hand, thumb, and index finger — called also *deep palmar arch* **b** : a superficial arch that is the continuation of the ulnar artery which anastomoses with a branch derived from the radial artery and that sends branches mostly to the fingers — called also *superficial palmar arch*

palmar fascia *n* : PALMAR APONEUROSIS

palmar interosseus *n* : any of three small muscles of the palmar surface of the hand each of which arises from, extends along, and inserts on the side of the second, fourth, or fifth finger facing the middle finger and which acts to adduct its finger toward the middle finger, flex its metacarpophalangeal joint, and extend its distal two phalanges — called also *interosseus palmaris, palmar interosseous muscle*

pal·mar·is \pal-ˈmar-əs\ *n, pl* **pal·mar·es** \-ˌēz\ : either of two muscles of the palm of the hand: **a** : PALMARIS BREVIS **b** : PALMARIS LONGUS

palmaris brev·is \-ˈbrev-əs\ *n* : a short transverse superficial muscle of the ulnar side of the palm of the hand that arises from the flexor retinaculum and palmar aponeurosis, inserts into the skin on the ulnar edge of the palm, and functions to tense and stabilize the palm (as in catching a ball)

palmaris lon·gus \-ˈlòŋ-gəs\ *n* : a superficial muscle of the forearm lying on the medial side of the flexor carpi radialis that arises esp. from the medial epicondyle of the humerus, in-

serts esp. into the palmar aponeurosis, and acts to flex the hand

pal·mit·ic acid \ˌ(ˌ)pal-ˈmi-tik-, ˌ(ˌ)päl-, ˌ(ˌ)pä-\ *n* : a waxy crystalline saturated fatty acid $C_{16}H_{32}O_2$ occurring free or in the form of esters (as glycerides) in most fats and fatty oils and in several essential oils and waxes

pal·mo·plan·tar \ˌpal-mō-ˈplan-tər, ˌpäl-, ˌpä-\ *adj* : of, relating to, or affecting both the palms of the hands and the soles of the feet ⟨∼ psoriasis⟩

pal·pa·ble \ˈpal-pə-bəl\ *adj* : capable of being touched or felt; *esp* : capable of being examined by palpation

pal·pa·tion \pal-ˈpā-shən\ *n* **1** : an act of touching or feeling **2** : physical examination in medical diagnosis by pressure of the hand or fingers to the surface of the body esp. to determine the condition (as of size or consistency) of an underlying part or organ ⟨∼ of the liver⟩ — compare INSPECTION — **pal·pate** \ˈpal-ˌpāt\ *vb* — **pal·pa·to·ry** \ˈpal-pə-ˌtōr-ē\ *adj*

pal·pe·bra \ˈpal-pə-brə, pal-ˈpē-brə\ *n, pl* **pal·pe·brae** \-ˌbrē\ : EYELID — **pal·pe·bral** \pal-ˈpē-brəl\ *adj*

palpebrae — see LEVATOR PALPEBRAE SUPERIORIS

palpebral fissure *n* : the space between the margins of the eyelids — called also *rima palpebrarum*

palpebrarum — see RIMA PALPEBRARUM, XANTHELASMA PALPEBRARUM

pal·pi·tate \ˈpal-pə-ˌtāt\ *vb* **-tat·ed; -tat·ing** : to beat rapidly, irregularly, or forcibly — used esp. of the heart

pal·pi·ta·tion \ˌpal-pə-ˈtā-shən\ *n* : a rapid pulsation; *esp* : an abnormally rapid or irregular beating of the heart (as that caused by panic, arrhythmia, or strenuous physical exercise)

pal·sied \ˈpol-zēd\ *adj* : affected with palsy ⟨hands weak and ∼⟩

pal·sy \ˈpol-zē\ *n, pl* **pal·sies 1** : PARALYSIS — used chiefly in combination ⟨oculomotor ∼⟩; see BELL'S PALSY, CEREBRAL PALSY **2** : a condition that is characterized by uncontrollable tremor or quivering of the body or one or more of its parts — not used technically

pal·u·drine \ˈpa-lə-drən\ *n* : PROGUANIL

L–PAM \ˈel-ˌpam\ *n* : MELPHALAN

2–PAM \ˌtü-ˌpē-ˌā-ˈem\ *n* : PRALIDOXIME

pam·a·quine \ˈpa-mə-ˌkwin, -ˌkwēn\ *n* : a toxic antimalarial drug $C_{19}H_{29}N_3O$; *also* : PAMAQUINE NAPHTHOATE

pamaquine naph·tho·ate \-ˈnaf-thə-ˌwāt\ *n* : an insoluble salt $C_{42}H_{45}N_3O_7$ of pamaquine

pam·id·ro·nate \ˌpa-mi-ˈdrō-ˌnāt\ *n* : a disodium bisphosphonate bone-resorption inhibitor $C_3H_9NNa_2O_7P_2$ administered as an intravenous infusion esp. in the treatment of Paget's disease of bone and of hypercalcemia associated with malignancy — called also *pamidronate disodium*

Pam·ine \'pa-ˌmēn\ *trademark* — used for a preparation of the bromide salt of methscopolamine

pam·o·ate \'pa-mə-ˌwāt\ *n* : any of various salts or esters of an acid $C_{23}H_{16}O_6$ — see HYDROXYZINE

pam·pin·i·form plexus \pam-'pi-nə-ˌfórm-\ *n* : a venous plexus that is associated with each testicular vein in the male and each ovarian vein in the female — called also *pampiniform venous plexus*

PAN *abbr* peroxyacetyl nitrate

pan- *comb form* : whole : general ⟨*pan*carditis⟩ ⟨*pan*leukopenia⟩

Panadol \'pa-nə-ˌdól\ *trademark* — used for a preparation of acetaminophen

pan·car·di·tis \ˌpan-kär-'dī-təs\ *n* : general inflammation of the heart

Pan·coast's syndrome \'pan-ˌkōsts-\ *n* : a complex of symptoms associated with Pancoast's tumor which includes Horner's syndrome and neuralgia of the arm resulting from pressure on the brachial plexus

Pancoast, Henry Khunrath (1875–1939), American radiologist.

Pancoast's tumor *or* **Pancoast tumor** *n* : a malignant tumor formed at the upper extremity of the lung

pan·cre·as \'paŋ-krē-əs, 'pan-\ *n, pl* **-cre·as·es** *also* **-cre·ata** \pan-'krē-ə-tə\ : a large lobulated gland that in humans lies in front of the upper lumbar vertebrae and behind the stomach and is somewhat hammer-shaped and firmly attached anteriorly to the curve of the duodenum with which it communicates through one or more pancreatic ducts and that consists of (1) tubular acini secreting digestive enzymes which pass to the intestine and function in the breakdown of proteins, fats, and carbohydrates; (2) modified acinar cells that form islets of Langerhans between the tubules and secrete the hormones insulin and glucagon; and (3) a firm connective-tissue capsule that extends supportive strands into the organ

pancreat- *or* **pancreato-** *comb form* **1** : pancreas : pancreatic ⟨*pancreat*ectomy⟩ ⟨*pancreat*in⟩ **2** : pancreas and ⟨*pancreato*duodenectomy⟩

pan·cre·atec·to·my \ˌpaŋ-krē-ə-'tek-tə-mē, ˌpan-\ *n, pl* **-mies** : surgical excision of all or part of the pancreas — **pan·cre·atec·to·mized** \ˌpaŋ-krē-ə-'tek-tə-ˌmīzd, ˌpan-\ *adj*

pan·cre·at·ic \ˌpaŋ-krē-'a-tik, ˌpan-\ *adj* : of, relating to, or produced in the pancreas ⟨~ amylase⟩

pancreatic cholera *n* : VERNER-MORRISON SYNDROME

pancreatic duct *n* : a duct connecting the pancreas with the intestine: **a** : the chief duct of the pancreas that runs from left to right through the body of the gland, passes out its neck, and empties into the duodenum either through an opening shared with the common bile duct or through one close to it — called also *duct of Wirsung, Wirsung's duct* **b** : ACCESSORY PANCREATIC DUCT

pancreatic juice *n* : a clear alkaline secretion of pancreatic digestive enzymes (as trypsin and lipase) that flows into the duodenum

pancreatico- *comb form* : pancreatic : pancreatic and ⟨*pancreatico*duodenal⟩

pan·cre·at·i·co·du·o·de·nal \ˌpaŋ-krē-ˌa-ti-(ˌ)kō-ˌdü-ə-'dē-nəl, ˌpan-, -ˌdyü-; -dü-'äd-ᵊn-əl, -dyü-\ *adj* : of or relating to the pancreas and the duodenum

pancreaticoduodenal artery *n* : either of two arteries that supply the pancreas and duodenum forming an anastomosis giving off numerous branches to these parts: **a** : one arising from the superior mesenteric artery — called also *inferior pancreaticoduodenal artery* **b** : one arising from the gastroduodenal artery — called also *superior pancreaticoduodenal artery*

pancreaticoduodenal vein *n* : any of several veins that drain the pancreas and duodenum accompanying the inferior and superior pancreaticoduodenal arteries

pan·cre·at·i·co·du·o·de·nec·to·my \-ˌdü-ə-ˌdē-'nek-tə-mē, -ˌdyü-; -dü-ˌäd-ə-'nek-tə-mē, -dyü-\ *n, pl* **-mies** : partial or complete excision of the pancreas and the duodenum — called also *pancreatoduodenectomy*

pan·cre·at·i·co·du·o·de·nos·to·my \-'näs-tə-mē\ *n, pl* **-mies** : surgical formation of an artificial opening connecting the pancreas to the duodenum

pan·cre·at·i·co·je·ju·nos·to·my \-ji-ˌjü-'näs-tə-mē, -je-jü-\ *n, pl* **-mies** : surgical formation of an artificial passage connecting the pancreas to the jejunum

pan·cre·atin \pan-'krē-ə-tən; 'paŋ-krē-, 'pan-\ *n* : a mixture of enzymes from the pancreatic juice; *also* : a preparation containing such a mixture obtained from the pancreas of the domestic swine or ox and used as a digestant

pan·cre·ati·tis \ˌpaŋ-krē-ə-'tī-təs, ˌpan-\ *n, pl* **-atit·i·des** \-'ti-tə-ˌdēz\ : inflammation of the pancreas

pancreato- — see PANCREAT-

pan·cre·at·o·bil·i·ary \ˌpan-krē-ə-tō-'bi-lē-ˌer-ē\ *adj* : of, relating to, or affecting the pancreas and the bile ducts and gallbladder ⟨~ disease⟩

pan·cre·a·to·du·o·de·nec·to·my \'pan-krē-ə-tō-ˌdü-ə-ˌdē-'nek-tə-mē, -ˌdü-ˌäd-ə-'nek-tə-mē, -dyü-\ *n, pl* **-mies** : PANCREATICODUODENECTOMY

pan·creo·zy·min \ˌpan-krē-ō-'zī-mən\ *n* : CHOLECYSTOKININ

pan·cu·ro·ni·um bromide \,pan-kyə-'rō-nē-əm-\ *n* : a neuromuscular blocking agent $C_{35}H_{60}Br_2N_2O_4$ used as a skeletal muscle relaxant — called also *pancuronium*

pan·cy·to·pe·nia \,pan-,sī-tə-'pē-nē-ə\ *n* : an abnormal reduction in the number of red blood cells, white blood cells, and blood platelets in the blood; *also* : a disorder (as aplastic anemia) characterized by such a reduction — **pan·cy·to·pe·nic** \-'pē-nik\ *adj*

¹**pan·dem·ic** \pan-'de-mik\ *adj* : occurring over a wide geographic area and affecting an exceptionally high proportion of the population ⟨∼ malaria⟩

²**pandemic** *n* : a pandemic outbreak of a disease

pan·en·ceph·a·li·tis \,pan-in-,se-fə-'lī-təs\ *n, pl* **-lit·i·des** \-'li-tə-,dēz\ : inflammation of the brain affecting both white and gray matter — see SUBACUTE SCLEROSING PANENCEPHALITIS

pan·en·do·scope \-'en-də-,skōp\ *n* : a cystoscope fitted with an obliquely forward telescopic system that permits wide-angle viewing of the interior of the urinary bladder — **pan·en·do·scop·ic** \-,en-də-'skä-pik\ *adj* — **pan·en·dos·co·py** \-en-'däs-kə-pē\ *n*

Pa·neth cell \'pä-net-\ *n* : any of the granular epithelial cells with large acidophilic nuclei occurring at the base of the crypts of Lieberkühn in the small intestine and appendix

Paneth, Josef (1857–1890), Austrian physiologist.

pang \'paŋ\ *n* : a brief piercing spasm of pain — see BIRTH PANG, HUNGER PANGS

pan·hy·po·pi·tu·ita·rism \,pan-,hī-pō-pə-'tü-ə-tə-,ri-zəm, -'tyü-\ *n* : generalized secretory deficiency of the anterior lobe of the pituitary gland; *also* : a disorder (as Simmonds' disease) characterized by such deficiency — **pan·hy·po·pi·tu·itary** \-'tü-ə-,ter-ē, -'tyü-\ *adj*

pan·hys·ter·ec·to·my \,pan-,his-tə-'rek-tə-mē\ *n, pl* **-mies** : surgical excision of the uterus and uterine cervix — called also *total hysterectomy*

pan·ic \'pa-nik\ *n* **1** : a sudden overpowering fright; *also* : acute extreme anxiety **2** : a sudden unreasoning terror often accompanied by mass flight — **panic** *vb*

panic attack *n* : an episode of intense fear or apprehension that is of sudden onset and may occur for no apparent reason or as a reaction to an identifiable triggering stimulus (as a stressful event); *specif* : one that is accompanied by usu. four or more bodily or cognitive symptoms (as heart palpitations, dizziness, shortness of breath, or feelings of unreality) and that typically peaks within 10 minutes of onset

panic disorder *n* : an anxiety disorder characterized by recurrent unexpected panic attacks followed by a month or more of worry about their recurrence, implications, or consequences or by a change in behavior related to the panic attacks

pan·leu·ko·pe·nia \,pan-,lü-kə-'pē-nē-ə\ *n* : an acute usu. fatal epizootic disease esp. of cats that is caused by a virus of the genus *Parvovirus* (species *Feline panleukopenia virus*) and is characterized by fever, diarrhea and dehydration, and extensive destruction of white blood cells — called also *cat distemper, cat fever, feline distemper, feline enteritis, feline panleukopenia;* compare PARVOVIRUS 2

pan·nic·u·li·tis \pə-,ni-kyə-'lī-təs\ *n* **1** : inflammation of the subcutaneous layer of fat **2** : a syndrome characterized by recurring fever and usu. painful inflammatory and necrotic nodules in the subcutaneous tissues esp. of the thighs, abdomen, or buttocks — called also *relapsing febrile nodular nonsuppurative panniculitis, Weber-Christian disease*

pan·nic·u·lus \pə-'ni-kyə-ləs\ *n, pl* **-u·li** \-,lī\ : a sheet or layer of tissue; *esp* : PANNICULUS ADIPOSUS

panniculus ad·i·po·sus \-,a-də-'pō-səs\ *n* : any superficial fascia bearing deposits of fat

pan·nus \'pa-nəs\ *n, pl* **pan·ni** \-,nī\ **1** : a vascular tissue causing a superficial opacity of the cornea and occurring esp. in trachoma **2** : a sheet of inflammatory granulation tissue that spreads from the synovial membrane and invades the joint in rheumatoid arthritis ultimately leading to fibrous ankylosis

pan·oph·thal·mi·tis \(,)pan-,äf-thəl-'mī-təs, -,äp-\ *n* : inflammation involving all the tissues of the eyeball

pan·sys·tol·ic \(,)pan-sis-'tä-lik\ *adj* : persisting throughout systole ⟨a ∼ heart murmur⟩

pant \'pant\ *vb* : to breathe quickly, spasmodically, or in a labored manner

pan·to·caine \'pan-tə-,kān\ *n* : TETRACAINE

pan·to·pra·zole \pan-'tō-prə-,zōl\ *n* : a benzimidazole derivative that inhibits gastric acid secretion and is used in the form of its sodium salt $C_{16}H_{14}F_2N_3NaO_4S$ to treat erosive esophagitis and disorders (as Zollinger-Ellison syndrome) involving gastric acid hypersecretion — see PROTONIX

pan·to·the·nate \,pan-tə-'the-,nāt, pan-'tä-thə-,nāt\ *n* : a salt or ester of pantothenic acid — see CALCIUM PANTOTHENATE

pan·to·then·ic acid \,pan-tə-'the-nik-\ *n* : a viscous oily acid $C_9H_{17}NO_5$ of the vitamin B complex found in all living tissues

pan·trop·ic \(,)pan-'trä-pik\ *adj* : affecting various tissues without showing special affinity for one of them ⟨a ~ virus⟩ — compare NEUROTROPIC

pa·pa·in \pə-'pā-ən, -'pī-\ n : a protease in the juice of the green fruit of the papaya (*Carica papaya* of the family Caricaceae) used chiefly as a tenderizer for meat and in medicine as a digestant and as a topical agent in the debridement of necrotic tissue

Pa·pa·ni·co·laou smear \ˌpä-pə-'nē-kə-ˌlaὐ-, ˌpa-pə-'ni-kə-\ n : PAP SMEAR

Papanicolaou, George Nicholas (1883–1962), American anatomist and cytologist.

Papanicolaou test n : PAP SMEAR

Pa·pa·ver \pə-'pā-vər, -'pä-\ n : a genus (family Papaveraceae) of chiefly bristly hairy herbs that contains the opium poppy (*P. somniferum*)

pa·pav·er·ine \pə-'pa-və-ˌrēn, -rən\ n : a crystalline alkaloid that is used in the form of its hydrochloride $C_{20}H_{21}NO_4 \cdot HCl$ esp. as a vasodilator because of its ability to relax smooth muscle

paper chromatography n : chromatography that uses paper strips or sheets as the adsorbent stationary phase through which a solution flows and is used esp. to separate amino acids — compare COLUMN CHROMATOGRAPHY, THIN-LAYER CHROMATOGRAPHY

papill- or **papillo-** comb form 1 : papilla ⟨*papill*itis⟩ 2 : papillary ⟨*papill*oma⟩

pa·pil·la \pə-'pi-lə\ n, pl **pa·pil·lae** \-'pi-(ˌ)lē, -ˌlī\ 1 : a small projecting body part similar to a nipple in form: as **a** : a vascular process of connective tissue extending into and nourishing the root of a hair or developing tooth **b** : any of the vascular protuberances of the dermal layer of the skin extending into the epidermal layer and often containing tactile corpuscles **c** : RENAL PAPILLA **d** : any of the small protuberances on the upper surface of the tongue — see CIRCUMVALLATE PAPILLA, FILIFORM PAPILLA, FUNGIFORM PAPILLA, INTERDENTAL PAPILLA

papilla of Vater n : AMPULLA OF VATER

pap·il·lary \'pa-pə-ˌler-ē\ adj : of, relating to, or resembling a papilla : PAPILLOSE

papillary carcinoma n : a carcinoma characterized by a papillary structure

papillary layer n : the superficial layer of the dermis raised into papillae that fit into corresponding depressions on the inner surface of the epidermis

papillary muscle n : one of the small muscular columns attached at one end to the chordae tendineae and at the other to the wall of the ventricle and that maintain tension on the chordae tendineae as the ventricle contracts

pap·il·late \'pa-pə-ˌlāt, pə-'pi-lət\ adj : covered with or bearing papillae

pap·il·lec·to·my \ˌpa-pə-'lek-tə-mē\ n, pl **-mies** : the surgical removal of a papilla

pap·il·le·de·ma \ˌpa-pə-lə-'dē-mə\ n : swelling and protrusion of the blind spot of the eye caused by edema — called also *choked disk*

pap·il·li·tis \ˌpa-pə-'lī-təs\ n : inflammation of a papilla; esp : inflammation of the optic disk — see NECROTIZING PAPILLITIS

pap·il·lo·ma \ˌpa-pə-'lō-mə\ n, pl **-mas** also **-ma·ta** \-mə-tə\ : a benign tumor (as a wart or condyloma) resulting from an overgrowth of epithelial tissue on papillae of vascularized connective tissue (as of the skin) — see PAPILLOMAVIRUS

pap·il·lo·ma·to·sis \-ˌlō-mə-'tō-səs\, pl **-to·ses** \-ˌsēz\ : a condition marked by the presence of numerous papillomas

pap·il·lo·ma·tous \-'lō-mə-təs\ adj 1 : resembling or being a papilloma ⟨a ~ lesion⟩ 2 : marked or characterized by papillomas ⟨~ dermatitis⟩

pap·il·lo·ma·vi·rus \ˌpa-pə-'lō-mə-ˌvī-rəs\ n : any of a family (*Papillomaviridae*) of viruses that contain a single molecule of circular double-stranded DNA and cause papillomas in mammals — see HUMAN PAPILLOMAVIRUS

pap·il·lose \'pa-pə-ˌlōs\ adj : covered with, resembling, or bearing papillae

pa·po·va·vi·rus \pə-'pō-və-ˌvī-rəs\ n : any of a former family (Papovaviridae) that included the papillomaviruses and polyomaviruses

pap·pa·ta·ci fever also **pa·pa·ta·ci fever** \ˌpä-pə-'tä-chē-\ or **pa·pa·ta·si fever** \-'tä-sē-\ n : SANDFLY FEVER

Pap smear \'pap-\ n : a method or a test based on it for the early detection of cancer esp. of the uterine cervix that involves staining exfoliated cells by a special technique which differentiates diseased tissue — called also *Papanicolaou smear, Papanicolaou test, Pap test*

G. N. Papanicolaou — see PAPANICOLAOU SMEAR

pap·u·la \'pa-pyə-lə\ n, pl **pap·u·lae** \-ˌlē\ 1 : PAPULE 2 : a small papilla

pap·u·lar \'pa-pyə-lər\ adj : consisting of or characterized by papules

pap·u·la·tion \ˌpa-pyə-'lā-shən\ n 1 : a stage in some eruptive conditions marked by the formation of papules 2 : the formation of papules

pap·ule \'pa-(ˌ)pyül\ n : a small solid usu. conical elevation of the skin caused by inflammation, accumulated secretion, or hypertrophy of tissue elements

papulo- comb form : characterized by papules and ⟨*papulo*vesicular⟩

pap·u·lo·pus·tu·lar \ˌpa-pyə-lō-'pəs-chə-lər, -'pəs-tyü-\ adj : consisting of both papules and pustules ⟨~ acne⟩

pap·u·lo·sis \ˌpa-pyə-'lō-səs\ n : the condition of having papular lesions

pap·u·lo·ve·sic·u·lar \,pa-pyə-lō-və-'si-kyə-lər\ *adj* : marked by the presence of both papules and vesicles

pap·y·ra·ceous \,pa-pə-'rā-shəs\ *adj* : of, relating to, or being the flattened remains of one of twin fetuses which has died in the uterus and been compressed by the growth of the other

para \'par-ə\ *n, pl* **par·as** or **par·ae** \'par-ˌē\ : a woman delivered of a specified number of children — used in combination with a term or figure to indicate the number ⟨multi*para*⟩ ⟨a 36-year-old *para* 5⟩; compare GRAVIDA

para- \,par-ə, 'par-ə\ *or* **par-** *prefix* **1** : beside : alongside of : beyond : aside from ⟨*para*thyroid⟩ ⟨*par*enteral⟩ **2 a** : closely related to ⟨*para*ldehyde⟩ **b** : involving substitution at or characterized by two opposite positions in the benzene ring that are separated by two carbon atoms ⟨*para*dichlorobenzene⟩ — abbr. *p-* **3 a** : faulty : abnormal ⟨*par*esthesia⟩ **b** : associated in a subsidiary or accessory capacity ⟨*para*medical⟩ **c** : closely resembling : almost ⟨*para*typhoid⟩

para–ami·no·ben·zo·ic acid \'par-ə-ə-ˌmē-nō-ˌben-'zō-ik-, ˌpar-ə-ˌa-mə-(ˌ)nō-\ *n* : a colorless aminobenzoic acid derivative that is a growth factor of the vitamin B complex and is used as a sunscreen — called also *PABA*

para–ami·no·hip·pu·rate \-'hi-pyə-ˌrāt\ *n* : a salt of para-aminohippuric acid

para–ami·no·hip·pu·ric acid \-hi-'pyūr-ik-\ *n* : a crystalline acid administered intravenously in the form of its sodium salt $C_9H_9N_2NaO_3$ in testing kidney function

para–ami·no·sal·i·cyl·ic acid \-ˌsal-ə-'si-lik-\ *n* : the white crystalline isomer of aminosalicylic acid that is made synthetically and is used in the treatment of tuberculosis

para–aor·tic \,par-ə-ā-'ȯr-tik\ *adj* : close to the aorta ⟨~ lymph nodes⟩

para–api·cal \-'ā-pi-kəl, -'a-\ *adj* : close to the apex of the heart

para·ben \'par-ə-ben\ *n* : either of two antifungal agents used as preservatives in foods and pharmaceuticals: **a** : METHYLPARABEN **b** : PROPYLPARABEN

para·bi·o·sis \,par-ə-(ˌ)bī-'ō-səs, -bē-\ *n, pl* **-o·ses** \-ˌsēz\ : the anatomical and physiological union of two organisms either natural or artificially produced — **para·bi·ot·ic** \-'ä-tik\ *adj* — **para·bi·ot·i·cal·ly** *adv*

para·cen·te·sis \,par-ə-(ˌ)sen-'tē-səs\ *n, pl* **-te·ses** \-ˌsēz\ : a surgical puncture of a cavity of the body (as with a trocar or aspirator) usu. to draw off any abnormal effusion

para·cen·tral \,par-ə-'sen-trəl\ *adj* : lying near a center or central part

para·cen·tric \-'sen-trik\ *adj* : being an inversion that occurs in a single arm of one chromosome and does not involve the chromomere — compare PERICENTRIC

para·cer·vi·cal \-'sər-və-kəl\ *adj* **1** : located or administered next to the uterine cervix ⟨~ injection⟩ **2** : of, relating to, or occurring in the neck and esp. the back part of the neck

para·cet·a·mol \,par-ə-'sē-tə-ˌmȯl\ *n, Brit* : ACETAMINOPHEN

para·chlo·ro·phe·nol \-ˌklȯr-ə-'fē-ˌnȯl, -ˌnȯl, -fi-'nȯl\ *n* : a chlorinated phenol C_6H_5ClO used as a germicide

para·chol·era \-'kä-lə-rə\ *n* : a disease clinically resembling Asiatic cholera but caused by a different vibrio

Para·coc·cid·i·oi·des \,par-ə-(ˌ)käk-ˌsi-dē-'ȯi-ˌdēz\ *n* : a genus of imperfect fungi that includes the causative agent (*P. brasiliensis*) of South American blastomycosis

para·coc·cid·i·oi·do·my·co·sis \-(ˌ)käk-ˌsi-dē-ˌȯi-dō-(ˌ)mī-'kō-sis\ *n, pl* **-co·ses** \-ˌsēz\ : SOUTH AMERICAN BLASTOMYCOSIS

para·col·ic \-'kō-lik, -'kä-\ *adj* : adjacent to the colon ⟨~ lymph nodes⟩

para·crine \'par-ə-krən\ *adj* : of, relating to, promoted by, or being a substance secreted by cells and acting on adjacent cells — see AUTOCRINE

par·acu·sis \,par-ə-'kyü-səs, -'kü-\ *n, pl* **-acu·ses** \-ˌsēz\ : a disorder in the sense of hearing

para·den·tal \-'dent-ᵊl\ *adj* : adjacent to a tooth ⟨~ infections⟩

para·di·chlo·ro·ben·zene *also* **p-dichlorobenzene** \,par-ə-ˌdī-ˌklȯr-ə-'ben-ˌzēn, -ˌben-'\ *n* : a white crystalline compound $C_6H_4Cl_2$ used chiefly as a moth repellent and deodorizer — called also *PDB*

para·did·y·mis \-'di-də-məs\ *n, pl* **-y·mi·des** \-mə-ˌdēz\ : a group of coiled tubules situated in front of the lower end of the spermatic cord above the enlarged upper extremity of the epididymis and considered to be a remnant of tubes of the mesonephros

par·a·dox·i·cal \,par-ə-'däk-si-kəl\ *also* **par·a·dox·ic** \-sik\ *adj* : not being the normal or usual kind ⟨~ embolisms⟩

paradoxical sleep *n* : REM SLEEP

paradoxus — see PULSUS PARADOXUS

para·esoph·a·ge·al \-i-ˌsä-fə-'jē-əl\ *adj* : adjacent to the esophagus; *esp* : relating to or being a hiatal hernia in which the connection between the esophagus and the stomach remains in its normal location but part or all of the stomach herniates through the hiatus into the thorax

par·aes·the·sia *chiefly Brit var of* PARESTHESIA

par·af·fin \'par-ə-fən\ *n* **1** : a waxy crystalline substance that is a complex mixture of hydrocarbons and is used in pharmaceuticals and cosmetics **2** : ALKANE

para·fol·lic·u·lar \ˌpar-ə-fə-ˈli-kyə-lər\ *adj* : located in the vicinity of or surrounding a follicle ⟨∼ thyroid cells⟩

para·for·mal·de·hyde \-fȯr-ˈmal-də-ˌhīd, -fər-\ *n* : a white powder $(CH_2O)_x$ consisting of a polymer of formaldehyde used esp. as a fungicide

para·fo·vea \-ˈfō-vē-ə\ *n, pl* **-fo·ve·ae** \-ˈfō-vē-ˌē, -vē-ˌī\ : the area surrounding the fovea and containing both rods and cones — **para·fo·ve·al** \-ˈfō-vē-əl\ *adj*

para·gan·gli·o·ma \-ˌgaŋ-glē-ˈō-mə\ *n, pl* **-mas** *also* **-ma·ta** \-mə-tə\ : a ganglioma derived from chromaffin cells — compare PHEOCHROMOCYTOMA

para·gan·gli·on \-ˈgaŋ-glē-ən\ *n, pl* **-glia** \-glē-ə\ : one of numerous collections of chromaffin cells associated with ganglia and plexuses of the sympathetic nervous system and similar in structure to the medulla of the adrenal glands — **para·gan·gli·on·ic** \-ˌgaŋ-glē-ˈä-nik\ *adj*

par·a·gon·i·mi·a·sis \ˌpar-ə-ˌgä-nə-ˈmī-ə-səs\ *n, pl* **-a·ses** \-ˌsēz\ : infestation with or disease caused by a lung fluke of the genus *Paragonimus* (*P. westermanii*) that invades the lung

Par·a·gon·i·mus \ˌpar-ə-ˈgä-nə-məs\ *n* : a genus of digenetic trematodes (family Troglotrematidae) comprising forms normally parasitic in the lungs of mammals including humans

para·gran·u·lo·ma \-ˌgra-nyə-ˈlō-mə\ *n, pl* **-mas** *also* **-ma·ta** \-mə-tə\ **1** : a granuloma esp. of the lymph glands that is characterized by inflammation and replacement of the normal cell structure by an infiltrate **2** : a benign form of Hodgkin's disease in which paragranulomas of the lymph glands are a symptom — called also *Hodgkin's paragranuloma*

para·hip·po·cam·pal gyrus \-ˌhi-pə-ˈkam-pəl-\ *n* : a convolution on the inferior surface of the cerebral cortex of the temporal lobe that borders the hippocampus and contains elements of both the archipallium and neopallium — called also *hippocampal convolution, hippocampal gyrus*

para·in·flu·en·za \ˌpar-ə-ˌin-flü-ˈen-zə\ *n* : PARAINFLUENZA VIRUS; *also* : a respiratory illness caused by a parainfluenza virus

parainfluenza virus *n* : any of several paramyxoviruses (genera *Respirovirus* and *Rubulavirus*) that are a frequent cause of infections (as croup) in the lower respiratory tract esp. in infants and children

para·ker·a·to·sis \ˌpar-ə-ˌker-ə-ˈtō-səs\ *n, pl* **-to·ses** \-ˌsēz\ : an abnormality of the horny layer of the skin resulting in a disturbance in the process of keratinization

par·al·de·hyde \pa-ˈral-də-ˌhīd, pə-\ *n* : a colorless liquid polymer $C_6H_{12}O_3$ derived from acetaldehyde and used esp. as an anticonvulsant, hypnotic, and sedative

pa·ral·y·sis \pə-ˈra-lə-səs\ *n, pl* **-y·ses** \-ˌsēz\ : complete or partial loss of function esp. when involving the power of motion or of sensation in any part of the body — see HEMIPLEGIA, PARAPLEGIA, PARESIS 1

paralysis agi·tans \-ˈa-jə-ˌtanz\ *n* : PARKINSON'S DISEASE

¹para·lyt·ic \ˌpar-ə-ˈli-tik\ *adj* **1** : affected with or characterized by paralysis **2** : of, relating to, or resembling paralysis

²paralytic *n* : one affected with paralysis

paralytica — see DEMENTIA PARALYTICA

paralytic dementia *n* : GENERAL PARESIS

paralytic ileus *n* : ileus resulting from failure of peristalsis

paralytic rabies *n* : rabies marked by sluggishness and by early paralysis esp. of the muscles of jaw and throat — called also *dumb rabies;* compare FURIOUS RABIES

paralytic shellfish poisoning *n* : food poisoning that results from consumption of shellfish and esp. 2-shelled mollusks (as clams or mussels) contaminated with dinoflagellates causing red tide and that is characterized by paresthesia, nausea, vomiting, abdominal cramping, muscle weakness, and sometimes paralysis which may lead to respiratory failure

par·a·lyze \ˈpar-ə-ˌlīz\ *vb* **-lyzed; -lyz·ing** : to affect with paralysis — **par·a·ly·za·tion** \ˌpar-ə-lə-ˈzā-shən\ *n*

para·me·di·an \ˌpar-ə-ˈmē-dē-ən\ *adj* : situated adjacent to the midline

para·med·ic \ˌpar-ə-ˈme-dik\ *also* **para·med·i·cal** \-di-kəl\ *n* **1** : a person who works in a health field in an auxiliary capacity to a physician (as by giving injections and taking X-rays) **2** : a specially trained medical technician certified to provide a wide range of emergency medical services (as defibrillation and the intravenous administration of drugs) before or during transport to the hospital — compare EMT

para·med·i·cal \ˌpar-ə-ˈme-di-kəl\ *also* **para·med·ic** \-dik\ *adj* : concerned with supplementing the work of highly trained medical professionals

para·me·so·neph·ric duct \ˌme-zə-ˈne-frik-, -ˌmē-, -sə-\ *n* : MÜLLERIAN DUCT

para·metha·di·one \-ˌme-thə-ˈdī-ˌōn\ *n* : a liquid compound $C_7H_{11}NO_3$ that is a derivative of trimethadione and is sometimes used in the treatment of absence seizures

para·meth·a·sone \-ˈme-thə-ˌzōn\ *n* : a glucocorticoid that is used for its antiinflammatory and antiallergic actions esp. in the form of its acetate $C_{24}H_{31}FO_6$

para·me·tri·tis \-mə-ˈtrī-təs\ *n* : inflammation of the parametrium

para·me·tri·um \-'mē-trē-əm\ *n, pl* **-tria** \-trē-ə\ : the connective tissue and fat adjacent to the uterus

par·am·ne·sia \,par-,am-'nē-zhə, -əm-\ *n* : a disorder of memory: as **a** : a condition in which the proper meaning of words cannot be remembered **b** : the illusion of remembering scenes and events when experienced for the first time — called also *déjà vu;* compare JAMAIS VU

para·mo·lar \,par-ə-'mō-lər\ *adj* : of, relating to, or being a supernumerary tooth esp. on the buccal side of a permanent molar or a cusp or tubercle located esp. on the buccal aspect of a molar and representing such a tooth

par·am·y·loid·o·sis \,par-,a-mə,-ˌlȯi-'dō-səs\ *n, pl* **-oses** \-,sēz\ : amyloidosis characterized by the accumulation of an atypical form of amyloid in the tissues

para·my·oc·lo·nus mul·ti·plex \,par-ə-,mī-ə-klə-nəs-'məl-tə-,pleks\ *n* : a myoclonus characterized by tremors in corresponding muscles on two sides

para·myo·to·nia \,par-ə-,mī-ə-'tō-nē-ə\ *n* : an abnormal state characterized by tonic muscle spasm

para·myxo·vi·rus \,par-ə-'mik-sə-,vī-rəs\ *n* : any of a family (*Paramyxoviridae*) of single-stranded RNA viruses that have a helical nucleocapsid and lipid-containing envelope and that include the parainfluenza viruses, respiratory syncytial virus, and the causative agents of canine distemper, measles, mumps, Newcastle disease, and rinderpest — see MORBILLIVIRUS, RUBULAVIRUS; compare MYXOVIRUS

para·na·sal \-'nā-zəl\ *adj* : adjacent to the nasal cavities; *esp* : of, relating to, or affecting the paranasal sinuses

paranasal sinus *n* : any of various sinuses (as the maxillary sinus and frontal sinus) in the bones of the face and head that are lined with mucous membrane derived from and continuous with the lining of the nasal cavity

para·neo·plas·tic \,par-ə-,nē-ə-'plas-tik\ *adj* : caused by or resulting from the presence of cancer in the body but not the physical presence of cancerous tissue in the part or organ affected

para·noia \,par-ə-'nȯi-ə\ *n* **1** : a psychosis characterized by systematized delusions of persecution or grandeur usu. without hallucinations **2** : a tendency on the part of an individual or group toward excessive or irrational suspiciousness and distrustfulness of others

¹**para·noi·ac** \-'nȯi-,ak, -'nȯi-ik\ *also* **para·no·ic** \-'nō-ik\ *adj* : of, relating to, affected with, or characteristic of paranoia or paranoid schizophrenia

²**paranoiac** *also* **paranoic** *n* : PARANOID

¹**para·noid** \'par-ə-,nȯid\ *also* **para·noi-**

dal \,par-ə-'nȯid-ᵊl\ *adj* **1** : characterized by or resembling paranoia or paranoid schizophrenia **2** : characterized by suspiciousness, persecutory trends, or megalomania

²**paranoid** *n* : one affected with paranoia or paranoid schizophrenia — called also *paranoiac*

paranoid personality disorder *n* : a personality disorder characterized by a pervasive pattern of distrust and suspicion of others resulting in a tendency to attribute the motives of others to malevolence

paranoid schizophrenia *n* : schizophrenia characterized esp. by persecutory or grandiose delusions or hallucinations or by delusional jealousy

paranoid schizophrenic *n* : an individual affected with paranoid schizophrenia

para·nor·mal \,par-ə-'nȯr-məl\ *adj* : not understandable in terms of known scientific laws and phenomena — **para·nor·mal·ly** *adv*

para·ol·fac·to·ry \,par-ə-äl-'fak-tə-rē, -ōl-\ *n* : a small area of the cerebral cortex situated on the medial side of the frontal lobe below the corpus callosum and considered part of the limbic system

para·ox·on \-'äk-,sän\ *n* : a phosphate ester $C_{10}H_{14}NO_6P$ that is formed from parathion in the body and that is a potent anticholinesterase

para·pa·re·sis \,par-ə-pə-'rē-səs, -ə-'par-ə-səs\ *n, pl* **-re·ses** \-,sēz\ : partial paralysis affecting the lower limbs — **para·pa·ret·ic** \-pə-'re-tik\ *adj*

para·per·tus·sis \-(,)pər-'tə-sis\ *n* : a human respiratory disease closely resembling whooping cough but milder and less often fatal and caused by a different bacterium of the genus *Bordetella* (*B. parapertussis*)

para·pha·ryn·geal space \-,far-ən-'jē-əl-, -fə-'rin-jəl-, -jē-əl-\ *n* : a space bounded medially by the superior constrictor of the pharynx, laterally by the medial pterygoid muscle, posteriorly by the cervical vertebrae, and below by the muscles arising from the styloid process

par·a·pha·sia \-'fā-zhə, -zhē-ə\ *n* : aphasia in which the patient uses wrong words or uses words or sounds in senseless combinations — **para·pha·sic** \-'fā-zik\ *adj*

para·phen·yl·ene·di·amine \,fen-ᵊl-,ēn-'dī-ə-,mēn\ *n* : a benzene derivative C_6H_8N used esp. in dyeing hair and sometimes causing an allergic reaction

para·phil·ia \-'fi-lē-ə\ *n* : a pattern of recurring sexually arousing mental imagery or behavior that involves unusual and esp. socially unacceptable sexual practices (as sadism, masochism, fetishism, or pedophilia)

¹**para·phil·iac** \-'fi-lē-,ak\ *adj* : of, relating to, or characterized by paraphilia

²**paraphiliac** *n* : a person who engages in paraphilia

para·phi·mo·sis \-fī-'mō-səs, -fi-\ *n, pl* **-mo·ses** \-,sēz\ : a condition in which the foreskin is retracted behind the glans penis and cannot be brought back to its original position

para·phre·nia \-'frē-nē-ə\ *n* 1 : the group of paranoid disorders 2 : any of the paranoid disorders; *also* : SCHIZOPHRENIA — **para·phren·ic** \-'fre-nik\ *adj*

para·ple·gia \,par-ə-'plē-jə, -jē-ə\ *n* : paralysis of the lower half of the body with involvement of both legs usu. due to disease of or injury to the spinal cord

¹**para·ple·gic** \-'plē-jik\ *adj* : of, relating to, or affected with paraplegia

²**paraplegic** *n* : an individual affected with paraplegia

para·prax·is \-'prak-səs\ *n, pl* **-prax·es** \-'prak-,sēz\ : a faulty act (as a Freudian slip) of purposeful behavior

para·pro·tein \-'prō-,tēn\ *n* : any of various abnormal serum globulins with unique physical and electrophoretic characteristics

para·pro·tein·emia \-,prō-tē-'nē-mē-ə, -,prō-tē-ə-'nē-\ *n* : the presence of a paraprotein in the blood

para·pso·ri·a·sis \-sə-'rī-ə-səs\ *n, pl* **-a·ses** \-,sēz\ : a rare skin disease characterized by red scaly patches similar to those of psoriasis but causing no sensations of pain or itch

para·psy·chol·o·gy \,par-ə-(,)sī-'kä-lə-jē\ *n, pl* **-gies** : a field of study concerned with the investigation of evidence for paranormal psychological phenomena (as telepathy, clairvoyance, and psychokinesis) — **para·psy·cho·log·i·cal** \-,sī-kə-'lä-ji-kəl\ *adj* — **para·psy·chol·o·gist** \-sī-'kä-lə-jist, -sə-\ *n*

para·quat \'par-ə-,kwät\ *n* : an herbicide containing a salt of a cation $[C_{12}H_{14}N_2]^{2+}$ that is extremely toxic to the liver, kidneys, and lungs if ingested

para·re·nal \,par-ə-'rēn-ᵊl\ *adj* : adjacent to the kidney

para·ros·an·i·line \,par-ə-,rō-'zan-ᵊl-ən\ *n* : a white crystalline base $C_{19}H_{19}N_3O$ that is the parent compound of many dyes; *also* : its red chloride used esp. as a biological stain

para·sag·it·tal \-'sa-jət-ᵊl\ *adj* : situated alongside of or adjacent to a sagittal location or a sagittal plane

Par·as·ca·ris \(,)par-'as-kə-rəs\ *n* : a genus of nematode worms (family Ascaridae) including a large roundworm (*P. equorum*) that is parasitic in horses

parasit- *or* **parasito-** *also* **parasiti-** *comb form* : parasite ⟨*parasit*emia⟩

para·sit·ae·mia *chiefly Brit var of* PARASITEMIA

par·a·site \'par-ə-,sīt\ *n* : an organism living in, with, or on another organism in parasitism

par·a·sit·emia \,par-ə-,sī-'tē-mē-ə\ *n* : a condition in which parasites are present in the blood — used esp. to indicate the presence of parasites without clinical symptoms

par·a·sit·ic \,par-ə-'si-tik\ *also* **par·a·sit·i·cal** \-ti-kəl\ *adj* : relating to or having the habit of a parasite : living on another organism 2 : caused by or resulting from the effects of parasites — **par·a·sit·i·cal·ly** *adv*

par·a·sit·i·cide \-'si-tə-,sīd\ *n* : an agent that is destructive to parasites — **par·a·sit·i·cid·al** \-,si-tə-'sīd-ᵊl\ *adj*

par·a·sit·ism \'par-ə-sə-,ti-zəm, -,sī-\ *n* 1 : an intimate association between organisms of two or more kinds; *esp* : one in which a parasite obtains benefits from a host which it usu. injures 2 : PARASITOSIS

par·a·sit·ize \-sə-,tīz, -,sī-\ *vb* **-ized; -iz·ing** : to infest or live on or with as a parasite — **par·a·sit·iza·tion** \,par-ə-sə-tə-'zā-shən, -,sī-\ *n*

parasito- — *see* PARASIT-

par·a·si·tol·o·gist \-'tä-lə-jist\ *n* : a specialist in parasitology; *esp* : one who deals with the worm parasites of animals

par·a·si·tol·o·gy \,par-ə-sə-'tä-lə-jē, -,sī-\ *n, pl* **-gies** : a branch of biology dealing with parasites and parasitism esp. among animals — **par·a·si·to·log·i·cal** \-,sit-ᵊl-'ä-ji-kəl, -,sīt-\ *also* **par·a·si·to·log·ic** \-jik\ *adj* — **par·a·si·to·log·i·cal·ly** *adv*

par·a·si·to·sis \-sə-'tō-səs, -,sī-\ *n, pl* **-o·ses** \-,sēz\ : infestation with or disease caused by parasites

para·spe·cif·ic \-spi-'si-fik\ *adj* : having or being curative actions or properties in addition to the specific one considered medically useful

para·spi·nal \-'spīn-ᵊl\ *adj* : adjacent to the spinal column ⟨~ muscles⟩

para·ster·nal \-'stər-nəl\ *adj* : adjacent to the sternum — **para·ster·nal·ly** *adv*

¹**para·sym·pa·thet·ic** \,par-ə-,sim-pə-'the-tik\ *adj* : of, relating to, being, or acting on the parasympathetic nervous system ⟨~ drugs⟩

²**parasympathetic** *n* 1 : a parasympathetic nerve 2 : PARASYMPATHETIC NERVOUS SYSTEM

parasympathetic nervous system *n* : the part of the autonomic nervous system that contains chiefly cholinergic fibers, that tends to induce secretion, to increase the tone and contractility of smooth muscle, and to slow the heart rate, and that consists of a cranial part and a sacral part — called also *parasympathetic system*; compare SYMPATHETIC NERVOUS SYSTEM

¹**para·sym·pa·tho·lyt·ic** \,par-ə-,sim-pə-thō-'li-tik\ *adj* : tending to oppose the physiological results of parasympathetic nervous activity or of parasympathomimetic drugs — compare SYMPATHOLYTIC

²**parasympatholytic** *n* : a parasympatholytic substance

¹**para·sym·pa·tho·mi·met·ic** \‚par-ə-'sim-pə-(‚)thō-mī-'me-tik, -mə-\ *adj* : simulating parasympathetic nervous action in physiological effect — compare SYMPATHOMIMETIC

²**parasympathomimetic** *n* : a parasympathomimetic agent (as a drug)

para·sys·to·le \-'sis-tə-(‚)lē\ *n* : an irregularity in cardiac rhythm caused by an ectopic pacemaker in addition to the normal one

para·tax·ic \‚par-ə-'tak-sik\ *adj* : relating to or being thinking in which a cause and effect relationship is attributed to events occurring at about the same time but having no logical relationship

para·ten·on \‚par-ə-'te-nən, -(‚)nän\ *n* : the areolar tissue filling the space between a tendon and its sheath

para·thi·on \‚par-ə-'thī-ən, -‚än\ *n* : an extremely toxic sulfur-containing insecticide $C_{10}H_{14}NO_5PS$

par·a·thor·mone \‚par-ə-'thȯr-‚mōn\ *n* : PARATHYROID HORMONE

¹**para·thy·roid** \-'thī-‚rȯid\ *n* : PARATHYROID GLAND

²**parathyroid** *adj* 1 : adjacent to a thyroid gland 2 : of, relating to, or produced by the parathyroid glands

para·thy·roid·ec·to·my \-‚thī-‚rȯi-'dek-tə-mē\ *n*, *pl* **-mies** : partial or complete excision of the parathyroid glands — **para·thy·roid·ec·to·mized** \-‚mīzd\ *adj*

parathyroid gland *n* : any of usu. four small endocrine glands that are adjacent to or embedded in the thyroid gland, are composed of irregularly arranged secretory epithelial cells lying in a stroma rich in capillaries, and produce parathyroid hormone

parathyroid hormone *n* : a hormone of the parathyroid gland that regulates the metabolism of calcium and phosphorus in the body — abbr. *PTH*; called also *parathormone*

para·thy·ro·trop·ic \‚par-ə-‚thī-rō-'trä-pik\ *adj* : acting on or stimulating the parathyroid glands ⟨a ~ hormone⟩

para·tra·che·al \-'trā-kē-əl\ *adj* : adjacent to the trachea

para·tu·ber·cu·lo·sis \-tü-‚bər-kyə-'lō-səs, -tyü-\ *n*, *pl* **-lo·ses** \-‚sēz\ : JOHNE'S DISEASE

¹**para·ty·phoid** \‚par-ə-'tī-‚fȯid, -(‚)tī-'\ *adj* 1 : resembling typhoid fever 2 : of or relating to paratyphoid or its causative agent ⟨~ infection⟩

²**paratyphoid** *n* : any of numerous salmonelloses (as necrotic enteritis) resembling typhoid fever and commonly contracted by eating contaminated food — called also *paratyphoid fever*

para·um·bil·i·cal \-‚əm-'bi-li-kəl\ *adj* : adjacent to the navel ⟨~ pain⟩

para·ure·thral \-yú-'rē-thrəl\ *adj* : adjacent to the urethra

paraurethral gland *n* : any of several small glands that open into the female urethra near its opening and are homologous to glandular tissue in the prostate gland in the male — called also *Skene's gland*

para·vac·cin·ia \-vak-'si-nē-ə\ *n* : MILKER'S NODULES

para·ven·tric·u·lar nucleus \-ven-'tri-kyə-lər-, -vən-\ *n* : a discrete band of neurons in the anterior part of the hypothalamus that produce vasopressin and esp. oxytocin and that innervate the neurohypophysis

para·ver·te·bral \-(‚)vər-'tē-brəl, -'vər-tə-\ *adj* : situated, occurring, or performed beside or adjacent to the spinal column ⟨~ sympathectomy⟩

par·e·gor·ic \‚par-ə-'gȯr-ik, -'gär-\ *n* : camphorated tincture of opium used esp. to relieve pain

pa·ren·chy·ma \pə-'reŋ-kə-mə\ *n* : the essential and distinctive tissue of an organ or an abnormal growth as distinguished from its supportive framework

pa·ren·chy·mal \pə-'reŋ-kə-məl, ‚par-ən-'kī-məl\ *adj* : PARENCHYMATOUS

par·en·chy·ma·tous \‚par-ən-'kī-mə-təs, -'ki-\ *adj* : of, relating to, made up of, or affecting parenchyma

par·ent \'par-ənt\ *n* 1 : one that begets or brings forth offspring 2 : the material or source from which something is derived — **parent** *adj* — **pa·ren·tal** \pə-'rent-ᵊl\ *adj*

parental generation *n* : a generation that supplies the parents of a subsequent generation; *esp* : P_1 GENERATION — see FILIAL GENERATION

¹**par·en·ter·al** \pə-'ren-tə-rəl\ *adj* : situated or occurring outside the digestive tract; *esp* : introduced or administered otherwise than by way of the digestive tract ⟨enteric versus ~ nutrition⟩ — **par·en·ter·al·ly** *adv*

²**parenteral** *n* : an agent intended for parenteral administration

par·ent·ing \'par-ənt-iŋ\ *n* : the raising of a child by his or her parents

pa·re·sis \pə-'rē-səs, 'par-ə-səs\ *n*, *pl* **pa·re·ses** \-‚sēz\ 1 : slight or partial paralysis 2 : GENERAL PARESIS

par·es·the·sia \‚par-es-'thē-zhə, -zhē-ə\ *n* : a sensation of pricking, tingling, or creeping on the skin having no objective cause and usu. associated with injury or irritation of a sensory nerve or nerve root — **par·es·thet·ic** \-'the-tik\ *adj*

paresthetica — see MERALGIA PARESTHETICA

¹**pa·ret·ic** \pə-'re-tik\ *adj* : of, relating to, or affected with paresis

²**paretic** *n* : a person affected with paresis

par·gy·line \'pär-jə-‚lēn\ *n* : a monoamine oxidase inhibitor used in the form of its hydrochloride $C_{11}H_{13}N\cdot$HCl esp. as an antihypertensive

pa·ri·es \'par-ē-‚ēz\ *n*, *pl* **pa·ri·etes** \pə-'rī-ə-‚tēz\ : the wall of a cavity or hollow organ — usu. used in pl.

¹**pa·ri·etal** \pə-'rī-ət-ᵊl\ *adj* 1 : of or re-

lating to the walls of a part or cavity — compare VISCERAL 2 : of, relating to, or located in the upper posterior part of the head; *specif* : relating to the parietal bones

²**parietal** *n* : a parietal part (as a bone)

parietal bone *n* : either of a pair of membrane bones of the roof of the skull between the frontal and occipital bones that are large and quadrilateral in outline, meet in the sagittal suture, and form much of the top and sides of the cranium

parietal cell *n* : any of the large oval cells of the gastric mucous membrane that secrete hydrochloric acid and lie between the chief cells and the basement membrane

parietal emissary vein *n* : a vein that passes from the superior sagittal sinus inside the skull through a foramen in the parietal bone to connect with veins of the scalp

parietalis — see DECIDUA PARIETALIS

parietal lobe *n* : the middle division of each cerebral hemisphere that is situated behind the central sulcus, above the sylvian fissure, and in front of the parieto-occipital sulcus and that contains an area concerned with bodily sensations

parietal pericardium *n* : the tough thickened membranous outer layer of the pericardium that is attached to the central part of the diaphragm and the posterior part of the sternum — compare EPICARDIUM

parietal peritoneum *n* : the part of the peritoneum that lines the abdominal wall — compare VISCERAL PERITONEUM

parieto- *comb form* : parietal and ⟨*parieto*temporal⟩

pa·ri·e·to-oc·cip·i·tal \pə-ˌrī-ə-tō-äk-ˈsi-pət-ᵊl\ *adj* : of, relating to, or situated between the parietal and occipital bones or lobes

parieto–occipital sulcus *n* : a fissure near the posterior end of each cerebral hemisphere separating the parietal and occipital lobes — called also *parieto-occipital fissure*

pa·ri·e·to-tem·po·ral \-ˈtem-pə-rəl\ *adj* : of or relating to the parietal and temporal bones or lobes

Par·i·naud's oc·u·lo·glan·du·lar syn·drome \ˌpär-i-ˈnōz-ˌä-kyə-lō-ˈglan-jə-lər-\ *n* : conjunctivitis that is often unilateral, is usu. characterized by dense local infiltration by lymphoid tissue with tenderness and swelling of the preauricular lymph nodes, and is usu. associated with a bacterial infection (as in cat scratch disease and tularemia) — called also *Parinaud's conjunctivitis*

    Parinaud, Henri (1844–1905), French ophthalmologist.

Parinaud's syndrome *n* : paralysis of the upward movements of the two eyes esp. with a le-

sion or compression of the superior colliculi of the midbrain

Paris green \ˈpar-əs-\ *n* : a very poisonous copper-based bright green powder Cu(C₂H₃O₂)₂·3Cu(AsO₂)₂ that is used as an insecticide and pigment

par·i·ty \ˈpar-ə-tē\ *n, pl* **-ties** **1** : the state or fact of having borne offspring **2** : the number of times a female has given birth counting multiple births as one and usu. including stillbirths — compare GRAVIDITY 2

¹**par·kin·so·nian** \ˌpär-kən-ˈsō-nē-ən, -nyən\ *adj* **1** : of or similar to that of parkinsonism ⟨~ symptoms⟩ **2** : affected with parkinsonism and esp. Parkinson's disease ⟨~ patients⟩

    Par·kin·son \ˈpär-kən-sən\, **James (1755–1824),** British surgeon.

²**parkinsonian** *n* : an individual affected with parkinsonism and esp. Parkinson's disease

par·kin·son·ism \ˈpär-kən-sə-ˌni-zəm\ *n* **1** : PARKINSON'S DISEASE **2** : any of several neurological conditions that resemble Parkinson's disease and that result from a deficiency or blockage of dopamine caused by neurodegenerative disease, drugs, toxins, or injury to the brain

Par·kin·son's disease \ˈpär-kən-sənz-\ *also* **Parkinson disease** *n* : a chronic progressive neurological disease chiefly of later life that is linked to decreased dopamine production in the substantia nigra and is marked by tremor of resting muscles, rigidity, slowness of movement, impaired balance, and a shuffling gait — called also *paralysis agitans, parkinsonism, Parkinson's, Parkinson's syndrome*

par·odon·tal \ˌpar-ə-ˈdänt-ᵊl\ *adj* : PERIODONTAL 2 — **par·odon·tal·ly** *adv*

par·o·mo·my·cin \ˌpar-ə-mō-ˈmīs-ᵊn\ *n* : a broad-spectrum antibiotic that is obtained from a bacterium of the genus *Streptomyces* (*S. rimosus paromomycinus*) and is usu. used in the form of its sulfate C₂₃H₄₅N₁₃O₁₄·H₂SO₄ to treat intestinal amebiasis

par·o·nych·ia \ˌpar-ə-ˈni-kē-ə\ *n* : inflammation of the tissues adjacent to the nail of a finger or toe usu. accompanied by infection and pus formation — compare WHITLOW

par·ooph·o·ron \ˌpar-ō-ˈä-fə-ˌrän\ *n* : a group of rudimentary tubules in the broad ligament between the epoophoron and the uterus that constitutes a remnant of the lower part of the mesonephros in the female

par·os·mia \ˌpar-ˈäz-mē-ə\ *n* : a distortion of the sense of smell

¹**pa·rot·id** \pə-ˈrä-təd\ *adj* : of, relating to, being, produced by, or located near the parotid gland

²**parotid** *n* : PAROTID GLAND

parotid duct *n* : the duct of the parotid gland opening on the inner surface of the cheek opposite the second upper molar tooth — called also *Stensen's duct*

par·ot·id gland *n* : a serous salivary gland that is situated on each side of the face below and in front of the ear, in humans is the largest of the salivary glands, and communicates with the mouth by the parotid duct

par·o·ti·tis \ˌpar-ə-ˈtī-təs\ *n* **1** : inflammation and swelling of one or both parotid glands or other salivary glands (as in mumps) **2** : MUMPS

par·ous \ˈpar-əs\ *adj* **1** : having produced offspring **2** : of or characteristic of the parous female

-p·a·rous \p-ə-rəs\ *adj comb form* : giving birth to : producing ⟨multi*parous*⟩

par·o·var·i·um \ˌpar-ō-ˈvar-ē-əm\ *n* : EPOOPHORON — **par·o·var·i·an** \-ē-ən\ *adj*

par·ox·e·tine \par-ˈäk-sə-ˌtēn\ *n* : a drug that functions as an SSRI and is usu. administered in the form of its hydrochloride $C_{19}H_{20}FNO_3 \cdot HCl$ to treat depression, anxiety, and panic disorder — see PAXIL

par·ox·ysm \ˈpar-ək-ˌsi-zəm, pə-ˈräk-\ *n* **1** : a sudden attack or spasm (as of a disease) **2** : a sudden recurrence of symptoms or an intensification of existing symptoms — **par·ox·ys·mal** \ˌpar-ək-ˈsiz-məl, pə-ˌräk-\ *adj*

paroxysmal dyspnea *n* : CARDIAC ASTHMA

paroxysmal nocturnal hemoglobinuria *n* : a form of hemolytic anemia that is characterized by an abnormally strong response to the action of complement, by acute episodes of hemolysis esp. at night with hemoglobinuria noted upon urination after awakening, venous occlusion, and often leukopenia and thrombocytopenia — abbr. *PNH*

paroxysmal tachycardia *n* : tachycardia that begins and ends abruptly and that is initiated by a premature supraventricular beat originating in the atrium or in the atrioventricular node or bundle of His or by a premature ventricular beat

par·rot fever \ˈpar-ət-\ *n* : PSITTACOSIS

pars \ˈpärs\ *n, pl* **par·tes** \ˈpär-(ˌ)tēz\ : an anatomical part

pars com·pac·ta \-käm-ˈpak-tə\ *n* : the large dorsal part of gray matter of the substantia nigra that is next to the tegmentum

pars dis·ta·lis \-di-ˈstā-ləs\ *n* : the anterior part of the adenohypophysis that is the major secretory part of the gland

pars in·ter·me·dia \-ˌin-tər-ˈmē-dē-ə\ *n* : a thin slip of tissue fused with the neurohypophysis and representing the remains of the posterior wall of Rathke's pouch

pars ner·vo·sa \-nər-ˈvō-sə\ *n* : NEURAL LOBE

pars pla·na \-ˈplā-nə\ *n* : ORBICULUS CILIARIS

pars re·tic·u·la·ta \-ri-ˌtik-yə-ˈlä-tə, -ˈlä-\ *n* : the ventral part of gray matter of the substantia nigra continuous with the globus pallidus

pars tu·ber·a·lis \-ˌtü-bə-ˈrä-ləs, -ˌtyü-\ *n* : a thin plate of cells that is an extension of the adenohypophysis on the ventral or anterior aspect of the infundibulum

partes *pl of* PARS

parthen- *or* **partheno-** *comb form* : virgin : without fertilization ⟨*parthen*ogenesis⟩

par·the·no·gen·e·sis \ˌpär-thə-nō-ˈjenə-səs\, *n, pl* **-e·ses** \-ˌsēz\ : reproduction by development of an unfertilized usu. female gamete that occurs esp. among lower plants and invertebrate animals — **par·the·no·ge·net·ic** \-jə-ˈne-tik\ *also* **par·the·no·gen·ic** \-ˈje-nik\ *adj*

partial–birth abortion *n* : DILATION AND EXTRACTION

par·tial denture \ˈpär-shəl-\ *n* : a usu. removable artificial replacement of one or more teeth

partial epilepsy *n* : FOCAL EPILEPSY

partial mastectomy *n* : a mastectomy in which only a tumor and a wedge of surrounding healthy tissue are removed

partial pressure *n* : the pressure exerted by a (specified) component in a mixture of gases

partial seizure *n* : a seizure (as of Jacksonian epilepsy or temporal lobe epilepsy) that originates in a localized part of the cerebral cortex, that involves motor, sensory, autonomic, or psychic symptoms (as twitching of muscles, localized numbness, or auras), and that may or may not progress to a generalized seizure — called also *focal seizure;* compare GENERALIZED SEIZURE

¹par·tic·u·late \pär-ˈti-kyə-lət\ *adj* : of, relating to, or existing in the form of minute separate particles

²particulate *n* : a particulate substance

particulate inheritance *n* : MENDELIAN INHERITANCE

¹par·tu·ri·ent \pär-ˈtur-ē-ənt, -ˈtyur-\ *adj* **1** : bringing forth or about to bring forth young **2** : of or relating to parturition ⟨~ pangs⟩ **3** : typical of parturition ⟨the ~ uterus⟩

²parturient *n* : a parturient individual

parturient paresis *n* : MILK FEVER 2

par·tu·ri·tion \ˌpär-tə-ˈri-shən, ˌpärchə-, ˌpär-tyü-\ *n* : the action or process of giving birth to offspring — **par·tu·ri·tion·al** \-shə-nəl\ *adj*

pa·ru·lis \pə-ˈrü-ləs\ *n, pl* **-li·des** \-ləˌdēz\ : an abscess in the gum : GUMBOIL

par·um·bil·i·cal vein \ˌpar-ˌəm-ˈbi-li-kəl-\ *n* : any of several small veins that connect the veins of the anterior abdominal wall with the portal vein and the internal and common iliac veins

parv- *or* **parvi-** *also* **parvo-** *comb form* : small ⟨*parvo*virus⟩

par·vo \'pär-ˌvō\ *n* : PARVOVIRUS 2

par·vo·cel·lu·lar *also* **par·vi·cel·lu·lar** \ˌpär-və-'sel-yə-lər\ *adj* : of, relating to, or being small cell bodies — compare MAGNOCELLULAR

par·vo·vi·rus \'pär-vō-ˌvī-rəs\ *n* **1 a** *cap* : a genus of single-stranded DNA viruses (family *Parvoviridae*) including the causative agents of panleukopenia in cats and parvovirus in dogs **b** : any virus of the genus *Parvovirus*; *broadly* : any virus of the family (*Parvoviridae*) to which the genus *Parvovirus* belongs and which includes the causative agent of fifth disease **2** : a highly contagious febrile disease of dogs that is caused by a strain (Canine parvovirus) of a virus of the genus *Parvovirus* (species *Feline panleukopenia virus*) causing panleukopenia in cats, that is spread esp. by contact with infected feces, and that is marked by loss of appetite, lethargy, often bloody diarrhea and vomiting, and sometimes death — called also *parvo*

PAS \ˌpē-(ˌ)ā-'es\ *adj* : PERIODIC ACID-SCHIFF

PAS *abbr* para-aminosalicylic acid

PASA *abbr* para-aminosalicylic acid

pass \'pas\ *vb* : to emit or discharge from a bodily part and esp. from the bowels : EVACUATE 2, VOID

¹pas·sage \'pa-sij\ *n* **1** : the action or process of passing from one place, condition, or stage to another **2** : an anatomical channel ⟨the nasal ∼*s*⟩ **3** : a movement or an evacuation of the bowels **4 a** : an act or action of passing something or undergoing a passing ⟨∼ of a catheter through the urethra⟩ **b** : incubation of a pathogen (as a virus) in a tissue culture, a developing egg, or a living organism to increase the amount of pathogen or to alter its characteristics

²passage *vb* **pas·saged; pas·sag·ing** : to subject to passage

pas·sive \'pa-siv\ *adj* **1 a** (1) : lethargic or lacking in energy or will (2) : tending not to take an active or dominant part **b** : induced by an outside agency ⟨∼ exercise of a paralyzed leg⟩ **2 a** : of, relating to, or characterized by a state of chemical inactivity **b** : not involving expenditure of chemical energy ⟨∼ transport across a cell membrane⟩ **3** : producing passive immunity ⟨∼ immunotherapy⟩ — **pas·sive·ly** *adv* — **pas·sive·ness** *n*

¹passive–aggressive *adj* : being, marked by, or displaying behavior characterized by expression of negative feelings, resentment, and aggression in an unassertive way (as through procrastination, stubbornness, and unwillingness to communicate) — **passive–aggressively** *adv*

²passive–aggressive *n* : a passive-aggressive individual

passive congestion *n* : congestion caused by obstruction to the return flow of venous blood — called also *passive hyperemia*

passive immunity *n* : short-acting immunity acquired by transfer of antibodies (as by injection of serum from an individual with active immunity) — compare ACQUIRED IMMUNITY, NATURAL IMMUNITY — **passive immunization** *n*

passive smoke *n* : SECONDHAND SMOKE

passive smoking *n* : the involuntary inhalation of tobacco smoke (as from another's cigarette) esp. by a nonsmoker — **passive smoker** *n*

passive transfer *n* : a local transfer of skin sensitivity from an allergic to a normal individual by injection of the allergic individual's serum that is used esp. for identifying specific allergens when a high degree of sensitivity is suspected — called also *Prausnitz-Küstner reaction*

pas·siv·i·ty \pa-'si-və-tē\ *n, pl* **-ties** : the quality or state of being passive or submissive

pass out *vb* : to lose consciousness

paste \'pāst\ *n* : a soft plastic mixture or composition; *esp* : an external medicament that has a stiffer consistency than an ointment and is less greasy because of its higher percentage of powdered ingredients

pas·tern \'pas-tərn\ *n* : a part of the foot of an equine extending from the fetlock to the top of the hoof

pas·teu·rel·la \ˌpas-tə-'re-lə\ *n* **1** *cap* : a genus of gram-negative facultatively anaerobic nonmotile rod bacteria (family *Pasteurellaceae*) that include several important pathogens esp. of domestic animals — see HEMORRHAGIC SEPTICEMIA, YERSINIA **2** *pl* **-las** *or* **-lae** \-ˌlī\ : any bacterium of the genus *Pasteurella*

Pas·teur \pa-'stər, -'stœr\, **Louis** (1822–1895), French chemist and bacteriologist.

pas·teu·rel·lo·sis \ˌpas-tə-rə-'lō-səs\ *n, pl* **-lo·ses** \-ˌsēz\ : infection with or disease caused by bacteria of the genus *Pasteurella*

pas·teur·i·za·tion \ˌpas-chə-rə-'zā-shən, ˌpas-tə-\ *n* **1** : partial sterilization of a substance and esp. a liquid (as milk) at a temperature and for a period of exposure that destroys objectionable organisms **2** : partial sterilization of perishable food products with radiation — **pas·teur·ize** \'pas-chə-ˌrīz, 'pas-tə-\ *vb*

Pasteur treatment *n* : a method of aborting rabies by stimulating production of antibodies through successive inoculations with attenuated virus of gradually increasing strength

pas·tille \pas-'tēl\ *also* **pas·til** \'past-ᵊl\ *n* : LOZENGE

PAT *abbr* paroxysmal atrial tachycardia

Pa·tau syndrome \pä-'taù-\ *or* **Patau's syndrome** \-'taùz-\ *n* : TRISOMY 13

Patau, Klaus (*fl* 1960), American (German-born) geneticist.

patch \'pach\ *n* **1 a** : a piece of material used medically usu. to cover a wound or repair a defect — see PATCH GRAFT **b** : a usu. disk-shaped piece of material that is worn on the skin and contains a substance (as a drug) that is absorbed through the skin and into the bloodstream ⟨a nicotine ∼⟩ — called also *skin patch* **c** : a shield worn over the socket of an injured or missing eye **2** : a circumscribed region of tissue (as on the skin or in a section from an organ) that differs from the normal color or composition — **patch** *vb* — **patchy** \'pa-chē\ *adj*

patch graft *n* : a graft of living or synthetic material used to repair a defect in a blood vessel

patch test *n* : a test for determining allergic sensitivity that is made by applying to the unbroken skin small pads soaked with the allergen so to be tested and that indicates sensitivity when irritation develops at the point of application — compare INTRADERMAL TEST, PRICK TEST, SCRATCH TEST

pa·tel·la \pə-'te-lə\ *n, pl* **-lae** \-'te-(ˌ)lē, -ˌlī\ *or* **-las** : a thick flat triangular movable bone that forms the anterior point of the knee, protects the front of the knee joint, and increases the leverage of the quadriceps — called also *kneecap* — **pa·tel·lar** \-lər\ *adj*

patellar ligament *n* : the part of the tendon of the quadriceps that extends from the patella to the tibia — called also *patellar tendon*

patellar reflex *n* : KNEE JERK

patellar tendon *n* : PATELLAR LIGAMENT

pat·el·lec·to·my \ˌpa-tə-'lek-tə-mē\ *n, pl* **-mies** : surgical excision of the patella

pa·tel·lo·fem·o·ral \pə-ˌte-lō-'fe-mə-rəl\ *adj* : of or relating to the patella and femur ⟨the ∼ articulation⟩

pa·ten·cy \'pat-ᵊn-sē, 'pāt-\ *n, pl* **-cies** : the quality or state of being open or unobstructed

pa·tent \'pat-ᵊnt\ *adj* **1** : protected by a trademark or a trade name so as to establish proprietary rights analogous to those conveyed by a patent : PROPRIETARY ⟨∼ drugs⟩ **2** \'pāt-\ : affording free passage : being open and unobstructed

pa·tent ductus arteriosus \'pāt-ᵊnt-\ *n* : an abnormal condition in which the ductus arteriosus fails to close after birth

pat·ent medicine \'pat-ᵊnt-\ *n* : a packaged nonprescription drug which is protected by a trademark and whose contents are incompletely disclosed; *also* : any drug that is a proprietary

pa·ter·ni·ty test \pə-'tər-nə-tē-\ *n* : a test esp. of DNA or genetic traits to determine whether a given man could be the biological father of a given child — **paternity testing** *n*

path \'path\ *n, pl* **paths** \'pathz, 'paths\ : PATHWAY 1

path *abbr* pathological; pathology

path- *or* **patho-** *comb form* **1** : pathological ⟨*patho*biology⟩ **2** : pathological state : disease ⟨*patho*gen⟩

-path \ˌpath\ *n comb form* **1** : practitioner of a (specified) system of medicine that emphasizes one aspect of disease or its treatment ⟨naturo*path*⟩ **2** : one affected with a disorder (of such a part or system) ⟨psycho*path*⟩

-path·ia \'pa-thē-ə\ *n comb form* : -PATHY 2 ⟨hyper*pathia*⟩

-path·ic \'pa-thik\ *adj comb form* **1** : feeling or affected in a (specified) way ⟨tele*pathic*⟩ **2** : affected by disease of a (specified) part or kind ⟨myo*pathic*⟩ **3** : relating to therapy based on a (specified) unitary theory of disease or its treatment ⟨homeo*pathic*⟩

Path·i·lon \'pa-thə-ˌlän\ *n* : a preparation of tridihexethyl chloride — formerly a U.S. registered trademark

patho·bi·ol·o·gy \ˌpa-thō-bī-'ä-lə-jē\ *n, pl* **-gies** : PATHOLOGY 1, 2

patho·gen \'pa-thə-jən\ *n* : a specific causative agent (as a bacterium or virus) of disease

patho·gen·e·sis \ˌpa-thə-'je-nə-səs\ *n, pl* **-e·ses** \-ˌsēz\ : the origination and development of a disease

patho·ge·net·ic \-jə-'ne-tik\ *adj* **1** : of or relating to pathogenesis **2** : PATHOGENIC 2

patho·gen·ic \-'je-nik\ *adj* **1** : PATHOGENETIC 1 **2** : causing or capable of causing disease ⟨∼ microorganisms⟩ — **pa·tho·gen·i·cal·ly** *adv*

patho·ge·nic·i·ty \-jə-'ni-sə-tē\ *n, pl* **-ties** : the quality or state of being pathogenic : degree of pathogenic capacity

path·og·nom·ic \ˌpa-thəg-'nä-mik, -thə-\ *adj* : PATHOGNOMONIC

pa·tho·gno·mon·ic \ˌpa-thəg-nō-'mä-nik, -thə-\ *adj* : distinctively characteristic of a particular disease or condition

pathol *abbr* pathological; pathologist; pathology

patho·log·i·cal \ˌpa-thə-'lä-ji-kəl\ *also* **patho·log·ic** \-jik\ *adj* **1** : of or relating to pathology ⟨a ∼ laboratory⟩ **2** : altered or caused by disease ⟨∼ tissue⟩; *also* : indicative of disease — **patho·log·i·cal·ly** *adv*

pathological fracture *n* : a fracture of a bone weakened by disease

pathological liar *n* : an individual who habitually tells lies so exaggerated or bizarre that they are suggestive of mental disorder

pa·thol·o·gist \pə-'thä-lə-jist, pa-\ *n* : a specialist in pathology; *specif* : a physician who interprets and diagnoses the changes caused by disease in tissues and body fluids

pa·thol·o·gy \-jē\ *n, pl* **-gies** **1** : the study of the essential nature of diseases and esp. of the structural and functional changes produced by them **2** : the anatomic and physiological deviations from the normal that constitute disease or characterize a particular disease **3** : a treatise on or compilation of abnormalities

patho·mor·phol·o·gy \,pa-thō-mòr-'fä-lə-jē\ *n, pl* **-gies** : morphology of abnormal conditions — **patho·mor·pho·log·i·cal** \-,mòr-fə-'lä-ji-kəl\ *or* **patho·mor·pho·log·ic** \-jik\ *adj*

patho·phys·i·ol·o·gy \-,fi-zē-'ä-lə-jē\ *n, pl* **-gies** : the physiology of abnormal states; *specif* : the functional changes that accompany a particular syndrome or disease — **patho·phys·i·o·log·i·cal** \-,fi-zē-ə-'lä-ji-kəl\ *or* **patho·phys·i·o·log·ic** \-jik\ *adj*

path·way \'path-,wā\ *n* **1** : a line of communication over interconnecting neurons extending from one organ or center to another; *also* : a network of interconnecting neurons along which a nerve impulse travels **2** : the sequence of usu. enzyme-catalyzed reactions by which one substance is converted into another

-pa·thy \pə-thē\ *n comb form, pl* **-pa·thies** **1** : feeling ⟨*apathy*⟩ ⟨*telepathy*⟩ **2** : disease of a (specified) part or kind ⟨*myopathy*⟩ **3** : therapy or system of therapy based on a (specified) unitary theory of disease or its treatment ⟨*homeopathy*⟩

pa·tient \'pā-shənt\ *n* **1** : a sick individual esp. when awaiting or under the care and treatment of a physician or surgeon **2** : a client for medical service (as of a physician or dentist)

pat·ri·cide \'pa-trə-,sīd\ *n* : murder of a father by his son or daughter

pat·tern \'pa-tərn\ *n* **1** : a model for making a mold used to form a casting **2** : a reliable sample of traits, acts, tendencies, or other observable characteristics of a person, group, or institution ⟨∼*s* of behavior⟩ **3** : an established mode of behavior or cluster of mental attitudes, beliefs, and values that are held in common by members of a group

pat·tern·ing *n* : physical therapy esp. for neurological impairment based on a theory holding that repeated manipulation of body parts to simulate normal motor developmental activity (as crawling or walking) promotes neurological development or repair

pat·u·lin \'pa-chə-lən\ *n* : a very toxic colorless antibiotic $C_7H_6O_4$ produced by several molds (as *Aspergillus clavatus* and *Penicillium patulum*)

pat·u·lous \'pa-chə-ləs\ *adj* : spread widely apart : wide open or distended

Paul–Bun·nell test \'pȯl-'bə-nəl-\ *n* : a test for heterophile antibodies used in the diagnosis of infectious mononu-

cleosis — called also *Paul-Bunnell reaction*

   Paul, John Rodman (1893–1971), and Bunnell, Walls Willard (1902–1965), American physicians.

paunch \'pȯnch, 'pänch\ *n* : RUMEN

pa·vil·ion \pə-'vil-yən\ *n* : a more or less detached part of a hospital devoted to a special use

Pav·lov·ian \pav-'lò-vē-ən, -'lò-; -'lò-fē-\ *adj* : of or relating to Ivan Pavlov or to his work and theories

   Pav·lov \'pav-lòf\, **Ivan Petrovich (1849–1936),** Russian physiologist.

pav·or noc·tur·nus \'pa-,vòr-näk-'tər-nəs\ *n* : NIGHT TERRORS

Pax·il \'pak-səl\ *trademark* — used for a preparation of the hydrochloride of paroxetine

pay–bed \'pā-,bed\ *n, Brit* : hospital accommodations and services for which the patient is charged

Pb *symbol* lead

PBB \,pē-(,)bē-'bē\ *n* : POLYBROMINATED BIPHENYL

PBL *abbr* peripheral blood lymphocyte

PBMC *abbr* peripheral blood mononuclear cell

PC *abbr* **1** [Latin *post cibos*] after meals — used in writing prescriptions **2** professional corporation

PCB \,pē-(,)sē-'bē\ *n* : POLYCHLORINATED BIPHENYL

pCi *abbr* picocurie

PCL \,pē-,sē-'el\ *n* : POSTERIOR CRUCIATE LIGAMENT

PCOS *abbr* polycystic ovary syndrome

PCP \,pē-(,)sē-'pē\ *n* **1** : PHENCYCLIDINE **2** : a health-care professional and esp. a physician who is authorized (as by an HMO) to provide primary care

PCP *abbr* Pneumocystis carinii pneumonia

PCR *abbr* polymerase chain reaction

PCV *abbr* packed cell volume

PCWP *abbr* pulmonary capillary wedge pressure

Pd *symbol* palladium

PD *abbr* **1** Parkinson's disease **2** peritoneal dialysis

PDB \,pē-(,)dē-'bē\ *n* : PARADICHLOROBENZENE

PDGF *abbr* platelet-derived growth factor

PDR *abbr* *Physicians' Desk Reference*

PE *abbr* **1** physical examination **2** pulmonary embolism

peak flow meter *n* : a device that measures the maximum rate of air flow out of the lungs during forced expiration and that is used esp. for monitoring lung capacity of individuals with asthma (as to indicate bronchial narrowing) — called also *peak expiratory flow meter*

pearl \'pərl\ *n* **1** : PERLE **2** : one of the rounded concentric masses of squamous epithelial cells characteristic of certain tumors **3** : a miliary leproma of the iris **4** : a rounded abnormal mass of enamel on a tooth

pec \'pek\ *n* : PECTORALIS — usu. used in pl.

pec·tin \'pek-tən\ *n* **1** : any of various water-soluble substances that bind adjacent cell walls in plant tissues and yield a gel which is the basis of fruit jellies **2** : a product containing mostly pectin and used chiefly in making jelly and other foods, in pharmaceutical products esp. for the control of diarrhea, and in cosmetics

pectinati — see MUSCULI PECTINATI

pec·tin·e·al line \pek-'ti-nē-əl-\ *n* : a ridge on the posterior surface of the femur that runs downward from the lesser trochanter and gives attachment to the pectineus

pec·tin·e·us \pek-'ti-nē-əs\ *n, pl* **-tin·ei** \-nē-,ī, -nē-,ē\ : a flat quadrangular muscle of the upper front and inner aspect of the thigh that arises mostly from the iliopectineal line of the pubis and is inserted along the pectineal line of the femur

¹pec·to·ral \'pek-tə-rəl\ *n* **1** : a pectoral part or organ; *esp* : PECTORALIS **2** : a medicinal substance for treating diseases of the respiratory tract

²pectoral *adj* **1** : of, relating to, or occurring in or on the chest ⟨∼ arch⟩ **2** : relating to or good for diseases of the respiratory tract ⟨a ∼ syrup⟩

pectoral girdle *n* : the bony or cartilaginous arch supporting the forelimbs of a vertebrate that corresponds to the pelvic girdle of the hind limbs — called also *shoulder girdle*

pec·to·ra·lis \pek-tə-'rā-ləs\ *n, pl* **-ra·les** \-,lēz\ : either of the muscles that connect the ventral walls of the chest with the bones of the upper arm and shoulder of which in humans there are two on each side: **a** : a larger one that arises from the clavicle, the sternum, the cartilages of most or all of the ribs, and the aponeurosis of the external oblique muscle and is inserted by a strong flat tendon into the posterior bicipital ridge of the humerus — called also *pectoralis major* **b** : a smaller one that lies beneath the larger, arises from the third, fourth, and fifth ribs, and is inserted by a flat tendon into the coracoid process of the scapula — called also *pectoralis minor*

pectoralis major *n* : PECTORALIS a

pectoralis minor *n* : PECTORALIS b

pectoralis muscle *n* : PECTORALIS

pectoral muscle *n* : PECTORALIS

pectoral nerve *n* : either of two nerves that arise from the brachial plexus on each side or from the nerve trunks forming it and that supply the pectoral muscles: **a** : one lateral to the axillary artery — called also *lateral pectoral nerve, superior pectoral nerve* **b** : one medial to the axillary artery — called also *inferior pectoral nerve, medial pectoral nerve*

pec·to·ril·o·quy \,pek-tə-'ri-lə-kwē\ *n, pl* **-quies** : the sound of words heard through the chest wall and usu. indicating a cavity or consolidation of lung tissue — compare BRONCHOPHONY

pectoris — see ANGINA PECTORIS

pec·tus ex·ca·va·tum \'pek-təs-,ek-skə-'vā-təm\ *n* : FUNNEL CHEST

ped- *or* **pedo-** *comb form* : child : children ⟨*pedi*atrics⟩

ped·al \'ped-ᵊl, 'pēd-\ *adj* : of or relating to the foot

ped·er·ast \'pe-də-,rast\ *n* : one that practices anal intercourse esp. with a boy as a passive partner — **ped·er·as·tic** \,pe-də-'ras-tik\ *adj* — **ped·er·as·ty** \'ped-ə-,ras-tē\ *n*

pe·di·at·ric \,pē-dē-'a-trik\ *adj* : of or relating to pediatrics

pe·di·a·tri·cian \,pē-dē-ə-'tri-shən\ *n* : a specialist in pediatrics

pe·di·at·rics \,pē-dē-'a-triks\ *n* : a branch of medicine dealing with the development, care, and diseases of children

ped·i·cle \'pe-di-kəl\ *n* : a basal attachment: as **a** : the basal part of each side of the neural arch of a vertebra connecting the laminae with the centrum **b** : the narrow basal part by which various organs (as kidney or spleen) are continuous with other body structures **c** : the narrow base of a tumor **d** : the part of a pedicle flap left attached to the original site — **ped·i·cled** \-kəld\ *adj*

pedicle flap *n* : a flap which is left attached to the original site by a narrow base of tissue to provide a blood supply during grafting — called also *pedicle graft*

pe·dic·u·li·cide \pi-'di-kyə-lə-,sīd\ *n* : an agent for destroying lice

pe·dic·u·lo·sis \pi-,di-kyə-'lō-səs\ *n, pl* **-lo·ses** \-,sēz\ : infestation with lice

pediculosis cap·i·tis \-'ka-pi-təs\ *n* : infestation of the scalp by head lice

pediculosis cor·po·ris \-'kòr-pə-rəs\ *n* : infestation by body lice

pediculosis pubis *n* : infestation by crab lice

pe·dic·u·lus \pi-'di-kyə-ləs\ *n* **1** *cap* : a genus of lice (family Pediculidae) that includes the body louse (*P. humanus humanus*) and head louse (*P. humanus capitis*) infesting humans **2** *pl* **pe·dic·u·li** \-,lī\ *or* **pediculus** : any louse of the genus *Pediculus*

ped·i·gree \'pe-də-,grē\ *n* : a record of the ancestry of an individual

pedis — see DORSALIS PEDIS, TINEA PEDIS

pedo- — see PED-

pe·do·don·tics \,pē-də-'dän-tiks\ *n* : a branch of dentistry that is concerned with the dental care of children — **pe·do·don·tic** *adj*

pe·do·don·tist \-'dän-tist\ *n* : a specialist in pedodontics

pe·do·phile \'pē-də-,fīl\ *n* : an individual affected with pedophilia

pe·do·phil·ia \ˌpē-də-'fi-lē-ə\ n : sexual perversion in which children are the preferred sexual object — **pe·do·phil·i·ac** \ˌpē-də-'fi-lē-ˌak\ or **pe·do·phil·ic** \-'fi-lik\ adj

pe·dun·cle \'pē-ˌdəŋ-kəl, pi-'\ n 1 : a band of white matter joining different parts of the brain — see CEREBELLAR PEDUNCLE, CEREBRAL PEDUNCLE 2 : a narrow stalk by which a tumor or polyp is attached — **pe·dun·cu·lar** \pi-'dəŋ-kyə-lər\ adj

pe·dun·cu·lat·ed \pi-'dəŋ-kyə-ˌlā-təd also **pe·dun·cu·late** \-lət\ adj : having, growing on, or being attached by a peduncle ⟨a ∼ tumor⟩

pe·dun·cu·lot·o·my \pi-ˌdəŋ-kyə-'lä-tə-mē\ n, pl **-mies** : surgical incision of a cerebral peduncle for relief of involuntary movements

pe·dun·cu·lus ce·re·bel·la·ris inferior \pi-ˌdəŋ-kyə-ləs-ˌser-ə-be-'ler-əs-\ n : CEREBELLAR PEDUNCLE c

pedunculus cerebellaris me·di·us \-'mē-dē-əs\ n : CEREBELLAR PEDUNCLE b

pedunculus cerebellaris superior n : CEREBELLAR PEDUNCLE a

peel n : CHEMICAL PEEL

PEEP abbr positive end-expiratory pressure

peep·er \'pē-pər\ n : VOYEUR

Peep·ing Tom \ˌpē-piŋ-'täm\ n : VOYEUR

peer review organization n : any of a group of organizations staffed by local practicing physicians that evaluate the quality, necessity, cost, and adherence to professional standards of medical care provided to Medicare patients as a prerequisite for payment of the medical services by Medicare — abbr. PRO

Peg·a·none \'pe-gə-ˌnōn\ trademark — used for a preparation of ethotoin

Pel·i·zae·us–Merz·bach·er disease \ˌpe-lēt-'sä-əs-'merts-ˌbä-kər-\ n : a degenerative disease of the central nervous system that is inherited as an X-linked recessive trait and is characterized by slowly progressive demyelination of white matter resulting in deterioration of cognitive and motor function

Pelizaeus, Friedrich (1850–1917), and Merzbacher, Ludwig (1875–1942), German neurologists.

pe·li·o·sis hepatitis \ˌpe-lē-'ō-səs-, ˌpē-\ n : an abnormal condition characterized by the occurrence of numerous small blood-filled cystic lesions throughout the liver

pel·la·gra \pə-'la-grə, -'lä-, -'lä-\ n : a disease marked by dermatitis, gastrointestinal disorders, mental disturbance, and memory loss and associated with a diet deficient in niacin and protein — compare KWASHIORKOR — **pel·la·grous** \-grəs\ adj

pellagra–preventive factor n : NIACIN

pel·la·grin \-grən\ n : one that is affected with pellagra

pel·let \'pe-lət\ n : a usu. small rounded or spherical body; specif : a small cylindrical or ovoid compressed mass (as of a hormone) that is implanted subcutaneously for slow absorption into bodily tissues

pel·li·cle \'pe-li-kəl\ n : a thin skin or film: as a : an outer membrane of some protozoans b : a thin layer of salivary glycoproteins coating the surface of the teeth

pellucida — see SEPTUM PELLUCIDUM, ZONA PELLUCIDA

pel·oid \'pe-ˌlóid\ n : mud prepared and used for therapeutic purposes

pel·ta·tin \pel-'tā-tən\ n : either of two lactones that occur as glycosides in the rootstock of the mayapple (Podophyllum peltatum) and have some antineoplastic activity

pelv- or **pelvi-** or **pelvo-** comb form : pelvis ⟨pelvic⟩ ⟨pelvimetry⟩

pelves pl of PELVIS

¹pel·vic \'pel-vik\ adj : of, relating to, or located in or near the pelvis

²pelvic n : a pelvic part

pelvic bone n : HIP BONE

pelvic brim n : the bony ridge in the cavity of the pelvis that marks the boundary between the false pelvis and the true pelvis

pelvic cavity n : the cavity of the pelvis comprising in humans a broad upper and a more contracted lower part — compare FALSE PELVIS, TRUE PELVIS

pelvic colon n : SIGMOID COLON

pelvic diaphragm n : the muscular floor of the pelvis

pelvic fascia n : the fascia lining the pelvic cavity

pelvic girdle n : the bony or cartilaginous arch that supports the hind limbs of a vertebrate and that in humans consists of paired hip bones articulating solidly with the sacrum dorsally and with one another at the pubic symphysis

pelvic inflammatory disease n : infection of the female reproductive tract (as the fallopian tubes and ovaries) that results from microorganisms (as Neisseria gonorrhea or Chlamydia trachomatis) transmitted esp. during sexual intercourse but also by other means (as during surgery, abortion, or parturition), is marked esp. by lower abdominal pain, an abnormal vaginal discharge, and fever, and is a leading cause of infertility in women — abbr. PID

pelvic outlet n : the irregular bony opening bounded by the lower border of the pelvis and closed by muscle and other soft tissues through which the terminal parts of the excretory, reproductive, and digestive systems pass to communicate with the surface of the body

pelvic plexus n : a plexus of the autonomic nervous system that is formed by the hypogastric plexus, by branches from the sacral part of the sympathetic chain, and by the visceral branches of the second, third, and fourth sacral nerves and that is distributed to the viscera of the pelvic region

pelvic splanchnic nerve *n* : any of the groups of parasympathetic fibers that originate with cells in the second, third, and fourth sacral segments of the spinal cord, pass through the inferior portion of the hypogastric plexus, and supply the descending colon, rectum, anus, bladder, prostate gland, and external genitalia — called also *nervus erigens*

pel·vim·e·ter \pel-'vi-mə-tər\ *n* : an instrument for measuring the dimensions of the pelvis

pel·vim·e·try \pel-'vi-mə-trē\ *n, pl* **-tries** : measurement of the pelvis (as by X-ray examination)

pel·vis \'pel-vəs\ *n, pl* **pel·vis·es** \-və-səz\ *or* **pel·ves** \-,vēz\ **1** : a basin-shaped structure in the skeleton of many vertebrates that in humans is composed of the two hip bones bounding it on each side and in front while the sacrum and coccyx complete it behind **2** : PELVIC CAVITY **3** : RENAL PELVIS

pelvo- — see PELV-

pem·o·line \'pe-mə-,lēn\ *n* : a synthetic drug $C_9H_8N_2O_2$ that is a mild stimulant of the central nervous system and has been used to treat attention deficit disorder and narcolepsy

¹pem·phi·goid \'pem-fə-,gòid\ *adj* : resembling pemphigus

²pemphigoid *n* : any of several diseases that resemble pemphigus; *esp* : BULLOUS PEMPHIGOID

pem·phi·gus \'pem-fi-gəs, pem-'fī-gəs\ *n, pl* **-gus·es** *or* **-gi** \-,jī\ : any of several diseases characterized by the formation of successive eruptions of large blisters on apparently normal skin and mucous membranes often in association with sensations of itching or burning

pemphigus er·y·the·ma·to·sus \-,er-i-,thē-mə-'tō-səs\ *n* : a relatively benign form of chronic pemphigus that is characterized by the eruption esp. on the face and trunk of lesions resembling those which occur in systemic lupus erythematosus

pemphigus vul·gar·is \-vəl-'gar-əs\ *n* : a severe and often fatal form of chronic pemphigus

Pen·brit·in \pen-'bri-tən\ *n* : a preparation of ampicillin — formerly a U.S. registered trademark

pen·ci·clo·vir \,pen-'sī-klō-,vir\ *n* : an antiviral drug $C_{10}H_{15}N_5O_3$ that is applied topically esp. to treat recurrent herpes labialis

pen·cil \'pen-səl\ *n* : a small medicated or cosmetic roll or stick for local applications ⟨a menthol ∼⟩

pen·du·lar nystagmus \'pen-jə-lər-\ *n* : nystagmus marked by rhythmic side-to-side or up-and-down movements of constant speed

pe·nec·to·my \pē-'nek-tə-mē\ *n, pl* **-mies** : surgical removal of the penis

penes *pl of* PENIS

pen·e·trance \'pe-nə-trəns\ *n* : the proportion of individuals of a particular genotype that express its phenotypic effect in a given environment — compare EXPRESSIVITY

pen·e·trate \'pe-nə-,trāt\ *vb* **-trat·ed; -trat·ing 1** : to pass, extend, pierce, or diffuse into or through something **2** : to insert the penis into the vagina of in copulation — **pen·e·tra·tion** \,pe-nə-'trā-shən\ *n*

pen·flur·i·dol \,pen-'flúr-i-,dòl\ *n* : a tranquilizing drug $C_{28}H_{27}ClF_5NO$

-pe·nia \'pē-nē-ə\ *n comb form* : deficiency of ⟨*eosinopenia*⟩

pen·i·cil·la·mine \,pe-nə-'si-lə-,mēn\ *n* : an amino acid $C_5H_{11}NO_2S$ that is obtained from penicillins and is used esp. to treat cystinuria, rheumatoid arthritis, and metal poisoning (as by copper or lead)

pen·i·cil·lic acid \,pe-nə-'si-lik-\ *n* : a crystalline antibiotic $C_8H_{10}O_4$ produced by several molds of the genera *Penicillium* and *Aspergillus*

pen·i·cil·lin \,pe-nə-'si-lən\ *n* **1** : a mixture of relatively nontoxic antibiotic acids produced esp. by molds of the genus *Penicillium* (as *P. notatum* or *P. chrysogenum*) and having a powerful bacteriostatic effect against chiefly gram-positive bacteria (as staphylococci, gonococci, and pneumococci) **2** : any of numerous often hygroscopic and unstable acids (as penicillin G, penicillin O, and penicillin V) that are components of the penicillin mixture **3** : a salt or ester of a penicillin acid or a mixture of such salts or esters

pen·i·cil·lin·ase \-'si-lə-,nās, -,nāz\ *n* : BETA-LACTAMASE

penicillin F \-'ef\ *n* : a penicillin $C_{14}H_{20}N_2O_4S$ that was the first of the penicillins isolated in Great Britain

penicillin G \-'jē\ *n* : the penicillin $C_{16}H_{18}N_2O_4S$ that constitutes the principal or sole component of most commercial preparations and is used chiefly in the form of stable salts (as the sodium salt $C_{16}H_{17}N_2NaO_4S$ or the potassium salt $C_{16}H_{17}KN_2O_4S$) — called also *benzylpenicillin*; see PENICILLIN G BENZATHINE, PENICILLIN G PROCAINE

penicillin G benzathine *n* : an aqueous suspension of a relatively insoluble salt of penicillin G that provides a low but persistent serum level of penicillin G following intramuscular injection — called also *benzathine penicillin G*

penicillin G procaine *n* : an aqueous suspension of penicillin G and procaine that provides a low but persistent serum level of penicillin G following intramuscular injection — called also *procaine penicillin G*

pen·i·cil·lin O \-ʹō\ *n* : a penicillin $C_{13}H_{18}N_2O_4S_2$ that is similar to penicillin G in antibiotic activity

penicillin V \-ʹvē\ *n* : a crystalline acid that is used in the form of its potassium salt $C_{16}H_{17}KN_2O_5S$ and has antibacterial action similar to penicillin G and is more resistant to inactivation by gastric acids — called also *phenoxymethyl penicillin*

pen·i·cil·li·o·sis \ˌpe-nə-ˌsi-lē-ʹō-səs\ *n, pl* **-o·ses** \-ˌsēz\ : infection with or disease caused by molds of the genus *Penicillium*

pen·i·cil·li·um \ˌpe-nə-ʹsi-lē-əm\ *n* **1** *cap* : a genus of fungi (as the blue molds) that have been grouped with the imperfect fungi but are now often placed with the ascomycetes and that are found chiefly on moist nonliving organic matter (as decaying fruit) and including molds useful in economic fermentation and the production of antibiotics **2** *pl* **-lia** \-lē-ə\ : any mold of the genus *Penicillium*

pen·i·cil·lo·yl–poly·ly·sine \ˌpe-nə-ʹsi-lō-ˌil-ˌpä-li-ʹlī-ˌsēn\ *n* : a preparation of a penicillic acid and polylysine which is used in a skin test to determine hypersensitivity to penicillin

pen·i·cil·lus \ˌpe-nə-ʹsi-ləs\ *n, pl* **-li** \-ˌlī\ : one of the small straight arteries of the red pulp of the spleen

pe·nile \ʹpē-ˌnīl\ *adj* : of, relating to, or affecting the penis ⟨~ cancer⟩

pe·nis \ʹpē-nəs\ *n, pl* **pe·nes** \ʹpē-(ˌ)nēz\ *or* **pe·nis·es** : a male copulatory organ that in most mammals including humans usu. functions as the channel by which urine leaves the body and is typically a cylindrical organ that is suspended from the pubic arch, contains a pair of large lateral corpora cavernosa and a smaller ventromedial corpus cavernosum containing the urethra, and has a terminal glans enclosing the ends of the corpora cavernosa, covered by mucous membrane, and sheathed by a foreskin continuous with the skin covering the body of the organ

penis envy *n* : the supposed coveting of the penis by a young human female which is held in Freudian psychoanalytic theory to lead to feelings of inferiority and defensive or compensatory behavior

pen·nate \ʹpe-ˌnāt\ *adj* : having a structure like that of a feather; *esp* : being a muscle in which fibers extend obliquely from either side of a central tendon

pen·ni·form \ʹpe-ni-ˌfȯrm\ *adj* : PENNATE

pe·no·scro·tal \ˌpē-nō-ʹskrōt-ᵊl\ *adj* : of or relating to the penis and scrotum

penoscrotal raphe *n* : the ridge on the surface of the scrotum that divides it into two lateral halves and is continued forward on the underside of the penis and backward along the midline of the perineum to the anus

Pen·rose drain \ʹpen-ˌrōz-\ *n* : CIGARETTE DRAIN

Penrose, Charles Bingham (1862–1925), American gynecologist.

pen·ta·chlo·ro·phe·nol \ˌpen-tə-ˌklȯr-ə-ʹfē-ˌnȯl, -fi-ᵊl\ *n* : a crystalline compound C_6Cl_5OH used esp. as a wood preservative, insecticide, and fungicide

pen·ta·eryth·ri·tol tet·ra·ni·trate \-i-ʹri-thrə-ˌtȯl-ˌte-trə-ʹnī-ˌtrāt, -ˌtȯl-\ *n* : a crystalline ester $C_5H_8N_4O_{12}$ used in the treatment of angina pectoris

pen·ta·gas·trin \ˌpen-tə-ʹgas-trən\ *n* : a pentapeptide $C_{37}H_{49}N_7O_9S$ that stimulates gastric acid secretion

pen·ta·me·tho·ni·um \ˌpen-tə-me-ʹthō-nē-əm\ *n* : an organic ion $[C_{11}H_{28}N_2]^{2+}$ used in the form of its salts (as the bromide and iodide) for its ganglionic blocking activity in the treatment of hypertension

pent·am·i·dine \pen-ʹta-mə-ˌdēn, -dən\ *n* : a drug used chiefly in the form of its salt $C_{23}H_{36}N_4O_{10}S_2$ to treat protozoal infections (as leishmaniasis) and to prevent Pneumocystis carinii pneumonia in HIV-infected individuals

pen·ta·pep·tide \ˌpen-tə-ʹpep-ˌtīd\ *n* : a polypeptide that contains five amino acid residues

pen·ta·pip·er·ide meth·yl·sul·fate \ˌpen-tə-ʹpi-pər-ˌīd-\ *n* : PENTAPIPERIUM METHYLSULFATE

pen·ta·pi·per·i·um meth·yl·sul·fate \ˌpen-tə-pī-ʹper-ē-əm-ˌme-thəl-ʹsəl-ˌfāt\ *n* : a synthetic quaternary ammonium anticholinergic and antisecretory agent $C_{20}H_{33}NO_6S$ used esp. in the treatment of peptic ulcer

pen·ta·quine \ʹpen-tə-ˌkwēn\ *n* : an antimalarial drug used esp. in the form of its pale yellow crystalline phosphate $C_{18}H_{27}N_3O·H_3PO_4$

pen·taz·o·cine \pen-ʹta-zə-ˌsēn\ *n* : a synthetic analgesic drug $C_{19}H_{27}NO$ that is less addictive than morphine — see TALWIN

pen·to·bar·bi·tal \ˌpen-tə-ʹbär-bə-ˌtȯl\ *n* : a barbiturate used esp. in the form of its sodium salt $C_{11}H_{17}N_2NaO_3$ or calcium salt $(C_{11}H_{17}N_2O_3)_2Ca$ as a sedative, hypnotic, and antispasmodic

pen·to·bar·bi·tone \-ˌtōn\ *n, Brit* : PENTOBARBITAL

pen·to·lin·i·um tartrate \ˌpen-tə-ʹli-nē-əm-\ *n* : a ganglionic blocking agent $C_{23}H_{42}N_2O_{12}$ used as an antihypertensive drug

pen·tose \ʹpen-ˌtōs, -ˌtōz\ *n* : a monosaccharide $C_5H_{10}O_5$ that contains five carbon atoms in a molecule

pen·tos·uria \ˌpen-tō-ʹsu̇r-ē-ə, -ʹsyu̇r-\ *n* : the excretion of pentoses in the urine; *specif* : a rare hereditary anomaly characterized by regular excretion of pentoses

Pen·to·thal \'pen-tə-ˌthȯl\ *trademark* — used for a preparation of thiopental

pent·ox·i·fyl·line \ˌpen-ˌtäk-'si-fə-ˌlēn\ *n* : a methylxanthine derivative $C_{13}H_{18}N_4O_3$ that reduces blood viscosity, increases microcirculatory blood flow, and is used to treat intermittent claudication resulting from occlusive arterial disease — see TRENTAL

pen·tyl·ene·tet·ra·zol \ˌpen-ti-ˌlēn-'te-trə-ˌzȯl, -ˌzōl\ *n* : a white crystalline drug $C_6H_{10}N_4$ used as a respiratory and circulatory stimulant and for producing a state of convulsion in treating certain mental disorders — called also *leptazol*; see METRAZOL

pe·num·bra \pə-'nəm-brə\ *n, pl* **-brae** \-(ˌ)brē, -(ˌ)brī\ *or* **-bras** : a blurred area in a radiograph at the edge of an anatomical structure — **pe·num·bral** \-brəl\ *adj*

Pep·cid \'pep-səd\ *trademark* — used for a preparation of famotidine

pep pill *n* : any of various stimulant drugs (as amphetamine) in pill or tablet form

-pep·sia \'pep-shə, 'pep-sē-ə\ *n comb form* : digestion ⟨dys*pepsia*⟩

pep·sin \'pep-sən\ *n* 1 : a crystallizable protease that in an acid medium digests most proteins to polypeptides, that is secreted by glands in the mucous membrane of the stomach, and that in combination with dilute hydrochloric acid is the chief active principle of gastric juice 2 : a preparation containing pepsin obtained from the stomach esp. of the hog and used esp. as a digestant

pep·sin·o·gen \pep-'si-nə-jən\ *n* : a granular zymogen of the gastric glands that is readily converted into pepsin in a slightly acid medium

pept- *or* **pepto-** *comb form* : protein fragment or derivative ⟨*pept*ide⟩

pep·tic \'pep-tik\ *adj* 1 : relating to or promoting digestion : DIGESTIVE 2 : of, relating to, producing, or caused by pepsin ⟨~ digestion⟩

peptic ulcer *n* : an ulcer in the wall of the stomach or duodenum resulting from the digestive action of the gastric juice on the mucous membrane when the latter is rendered susceptible to its action (as from infection with the bacterium *Helicobacter pylori* or the chronic use of NSAIDs)

pep·ti·dase \'pep-tə-ˌdās, -ˌdāz\ *n* : an enzyme that hydrolyzes simple peptides or their derivatives

pep·tide \'pep-ˌtīd\ *n* : any of various amides that are derived from two or more amino acids by combination of the amino group of one acid with the carboxyl group of another and are usu. obtained by partial hydrolysis of proteins — **pep·tid·ic** \pep-'ti-dik\ *adj*

peptide bond *n* : the chemical bond between carbon and nitrogen in a peptide linkage

peptide linkage *n* : the group CONH that unites the amino acid residues in a peptide

pep·tid·er·gic \ˌpep-tī-'dər-jik\ *adj* : being, relating to, releasing, or activated by neurotransmitters that are short peptide chains ⟨~ neurons⟩

pep·ti·do·gly·can \ˌpep-tə-dō-'glī-ˌkan\ *n* : a polymer that is composed of polysaccharide and peptide chains and is found esp. in bacterial cell walls — called also *mucopeptide, murein*

Pep·to-Bis·mol \ˌpep-tō-'biz-ˌmȯl\ *trademark* — used for a preparation of bismuth subsalicylate

pep·tone \'pep-ˌtōn\ *n* 1 : any of various protein derivatives that are formed by the partial hydrolysis of proteins (as by enzymes of the gastric and pancreatic juices or by acids or alkalies) 2 : a water-soluble product containing peptones and other protein derivatives that is obtained by digesting protein with an enzyme (as pepsin or trypsin) and is used chiefly in nutrient media in bacteriology

per \'pər\ *prep* : by the means or agency of : by way of : through ⟨blood ~ rectum⟩ — see PER OS

per·acute \ˌpər-ə-'kyüt\ *adj* : very acute and violent

per·ceive \pər-'sēv\ *vb* **per·ceived; per·ceiv·ing** : to become aware of through the senses — **per·ceiv·able** \-'sē-və-bəl\ *adj*

per·cept \'pər-ˌsept\ *n* : an impression of an object obtained by use of the senses : SENSE-DATUM

per·cep·ti·ble \pər-'sep-tə-bəl\ *adj* : capable of being perceived esp. by the senses — **per·cep·ti·bly** \-blē\ *adv*

per·cep·tion \pər-'sep-shən\ *n* : awareness of the elements of environment through physical sensation ⟨color ~⟩ — compare SENSATION 1a

per·cep·tive \pər-'sep-tiv\ *adj* : responsive to sensory stimulus ⟨a ~ eye⟩ — **per·cep·tive·ly** *adv*

perceptive deafness *n* : NERVE DEAFNESS

per·cep·tu·al \(ˌ)pər-'sep-chə-wəl, -shə-\ *adj* : of, relating to, or involving perception esp. in relation to immediate sensory experience ⟨auditory ~ deficits⟩ — **per·cep·tu·al·ly** *adv*

Per·co·cet \'pər-kō-ˌset\ *trademark* — used for a preparation of acetaminophen and the hydrochloride of oxycodone

Per·co·dan \'pər-kə-ˌdan\ *trademark* — used for a preparation of aspirin and the hydrochloride of oxycodone

per·co·late \'pər-kə-ˌlāt, -lət\ *n* : a product of percolation

per·co·la·tion \ˌpər-kə-'lā-shən\ *n* 1 : the slow passage of a liquid through a filtering medium 2 : a method of extraction or purification by means of filtration **3** : the process of extracting the soluble constituents of a powdered drug by passage of a liquid through it — **per·co·late** \\'pər-kə-ˌlāt\\ *vb* — **per·co·la·tor** \\-ˌlā-tər\\ *n*

per·cus·sion \\pər-'kə-shən\\ *n* **1** : the act or technique of tapping the surface of a body part to learn the condition of the parts beneath by the resulting sound **2** : massage consisting of the striking of a body part with light rapid blows — called also *tapotement* — **per·cuss** \\pər-'kəs\\ *vb*

per·cu·ta·ne·ous \\ˌpər-kyu-'tā-nē-əs\\ *adj* : effected or performed through the skin ⟨∼ absorption⟩ — **per·cu·ta·ne·ous·ly** *adv*

percutaneous transluminal angioplasty *n* : a surgical procedure used to enlarge the lumen of a partly occluded blood vessel (as one with atherosclerotic plaques on the walls) by passing a balloon catheter through the skin into and through the vessel to the site of the lesion where the tip of the catheter is inflated to expand the lumen of the vessel

percutaneous transluminal coronary angioplasty *n* : percutaneous transluminal angioplasty of a coronary artery — called also *PTCA*

Per·di·em \\pər-'dē-ˌem\\ *trademark* — used for a laxative preparation of psyllium seed husks and senna

pe·ren·ni·al \\pə-'re-nē-əl\\ *adj* : present at all seasons of the year ⟨∼ rhinitis⟩

per·fo·rate \\'pər-fə-ˌrāt\\ *vb* **-rat·ed; -rat·ing** : to enter, penetrate, or make a hole through ⟨an ulcer ∼s the duodenal wall⟩

per·fo·rat·ed \\-ˌrā-təd\\ *adj* : characterized by perforation ⟨a ∼ eardrum⟩

per·fo·ra·tion \\ˌpər-fə-'rā-shən\\ *n* **1** : the act or process of perforating; *specif* : the penetration of a body part through accident or disease **2 a** : a rupture in a body part caused esp. by accident or disease **b** : a natural opening in an organ or body part

per·fo·ra·tor \\'pər-fə-ˌrā-tər\\ *n* : one that perforates: as **a** : an instrument used to perforate tissue (as bone) **b** : a nerve or blood vessel forming a connection between a deep system and a superficial one

per·fus·ate \\(ˌ)pər-'fyü-ˌzāt, -zət\\ *n* : a fluid (as a solution pumped through the heart) that is perfused

per·fuse \\(ˌ)pər-'fyüz\\ *vb* **-fused; -fus·ing 1** : SUFFUSE **2 a** : to cause to flow or spread : DIFFUSE **b** : to force a fluid through (an organ or tissue) esp. by way of the blood vessels

per·fu·sion \\-'fyü-zhən\\ *n* : an act or instance of perfusing; *specif* : the pumping of a fluid through an organ or tissue

per·fu·sion·ist \\pər-'fyü-zhə-nist\\ *n* : a certified medical technician responsible for extracorporeal oxygenation of the blood during open-heart surgery

and for the operation and maintenance of equipment (as a heart-lung machine) controlling it

per·go·lide \\'pər-gə-ˌlīd\\ *n* : an agonist of dopamine receptors that is used in the form of its mesylate $C_{19}H_{26}N_2S\cdot CH_4O_3S$ esp. in the treatment of Parkinson's disease

per·hex·i·line \\ˌpər-'hek-sə-ˌlēn\\ *n* : a drug $C_{19}H_{35}N$ used as a coronary vasodilator

peri- *prefix* **1** : near : around ⟨*peri*menopausal⟩ **2** : enclosing : surrounding ⟨*peri*neurium⟩

peri·anal \\ˌper-ē-'ān-ᵊl\\ *adj* : of, relating to, occurring in, or being the tissues surrounding the anus

peri·aor·tic \\-ā-'ȯr-tik\\ *adj* : of, relating to, occurring in, or being the tissues surrounding the aorta

peri·api·cal \\-'ā-pi-kəl, -'a-\\ *adj* : of, relating to, occurring in, affecting, or being the tissues surrounding the apex of the root of a tooth

peri·aq·ue·duc·tal \\-ˌa-kwə-'dəkt-ᵊl\\ *adj* : of, relating to, or being the gray matter which surrounds the aqueduct of Sylvius

peri·ar·te·ri·al \\-är-'tir-ē-əl\\ *adj* : of, relating to, occurring in, or being the tissues surrounding an artery

peri·ar·te·ri·o·lar \\-är-ˌtir-ē-'ō-lər\\ *adj* : of, relating to, occurring in, or being the tissues surrounding an arteriole

peri·ar·ter·i·tis no·do·sa \\ˌper-ē-ˌär-tə-'rī-təs-nō-'dō-sə\\ *n* : POLYARTERITIS NODOSA

peri·ar·thri·tis \\-är-'thrī-təs\\ *n, pl* **-thrit·i·des** \\-'thri-tə-ˌdēz\\ : inflammation of the structures (as the muscles, tendons, and bursa of the shoulder) around a joint

peri·ar·tic·u·lar \\-är-'ti-kyə-lər\\ *adj* : of, relating to, occurring in, or being the tissues surrounding a joint

peri·bron·chi·al \\ˌper-ə-'brän-kē-əl\\ *adj* : of, relating to, occurring in, affecting, or being the tissues surrounding a bronchus ⟨a ∼ growth⟩

peri·cap·il·lary \\-'ka-pə-ˌler-ē\\ *adj* : of, relating to, occurring in, or being the tissues surrounding a capillary

pericardi- *or* **pericardio-** *or* **pericardo-** *comb form* **1** : pericardium ⟨*pericardi*ectomy⟩ **2** : pericardial and ⟨*pericardio*phrenic artery⟩

peri·car·di·al \\ˌper-ə-'kär-dē-əl\\ *adj* : of, relating to, or affecting the pericardium; *also* : situated around the heart

pericardial cavity *n* : the fluid-filled space between the two layers of the pericardium

pericardial fluid *n* : the serous fluid that fills the pericardial cavity and protects the heart from friction

pericardial friction rub *n* : the auscultatory sound produced by the rubbing together of inflamed pericardial membranes in pericarditis — called also *pericardial rub*

peri·car·di·ec·to·my \per-ə-ˌkär-dē-'ek-tə-mē\ n, pl **-mies** : surgical excision of the pericardium

peri·car·dio·cen·te·sis \per-ə-ˌkär-dē-ō-(ˌ)sen-'tē-səs\ n, pl **-te·ses** \-ˌsēz\ : surgical puncture of the pericardium esp. to aspirate pericardial fluid

peri·car·dio·phren·ic artery \per-ə-ˌkär-dē-ə-'fre-nik-\ n : a branch of the internal thoracic artery that descends through the thorax accompanying the phrenic nerve between the pleura and the pericardium to the diaphragm

peri·car·di·os·to·my \per-ə-ˌkär-dē-'äs-tə-mē\ n, pl **-mies** : surgical formation of an opening into the pericardium

peri·car·di·ot·o·my \-'ä-tə-mē\ n, pl **-mies** : surgical incision of the pericardium

peri·car·di·tis \-ˌkär-'dī-təs\ n, pl **-dit·i·des** \-'di-tə-ˌdēz\ : inflammation of the pericardium — see ADHESIVE PERICARDITIS

peri·car·di·um \per-ə-'kär-dē-əm\ n, pl **-dia** \-dē-ə\ : the conical sac of serous membrane that encloses the heart and the roots of the great blood vessels of vertebrates and consists of an outer fibrous coat that loosely invests the heart and is prolonged on the outer surface of the great vessels except the inferior vena cava and a double inner serous coat of which one layer is closely adherent to the heart while the other lines the inner surface of the outer coat with the intervening space being filled with pericardial fluid

pericardo- — see PERICARDI-

peri·cel·lu·lar \-'sel-yə-lər\ adj : of, relating to, occurring in, or being the tissues surrounding a cell

peri·ce·men·ti·tis \-ˌsē-ˌmen-'tī-təs\ n : PERIODONTITIS

peri·ce·men·tum \-si-'men-təm\ n : PERIODONTAL LIGAMENT

peri·cen·tric \-'sen-trik\ adj : of, relating to, or involving the centromere of a chromosome 〈∼ inversion〉 — compare PARACENTRIC

peri·chol·an·gi·tis \-ˌkō-ˌlan-'jī-təs, -ˌkä-\ n : inflammation of the tissues surrounding the bile ducts

peri·chon·dri·tis \-ˌkän-'drī-təs\ n : inflammation of a perichondrium

peri·chon·dri·um \per-ə-'kän-drē-əm\ n, pl **-dria** \-drē-ə\ : the membrane of fibrous connective tissue that invests cartilage except at joints — **peri·chon·dri·al** \-drē-əl\ adj

Peri-Co·lace \per-ə-'kō-ˌlās\ trademark — used for a preparation of casanthranol and the sodium salt of docusate

peri·co·ro·nal \per-ə-'kór-ən-əl, -'kär-; -kə-'rōn-əl\ adj : occurring about or surrounding the crown of a tooth

peri·cor·o·ni·tis \-ˌkór-ə-'nī-təs, -ˌkär-\ n, pl **-nit·i·des** \-'ni-tə-ˌdēz\ : inflammation of the gum about the crown of a partially erupted tooth

peri·cyte \'per-ə-ˌsīt\ n : a cell of the connective tissue about capillaries or other small blood vessels

peri·du·ral \per-i-'dúr-əl, -'dyúr-\ adj : occurring or applied about the dura mater

peridural anesthesia n : EPIDURAL ANESTHESIA

peri·fo·cal \per-ə-'fō-kəl\ adj : of, relating to, occurring in, or being the tissues surrounding a focus (as of infection) — **peri·fo·cal·ly** adv

peri·fol·lic·u·lar \per-ə-fə-'li-kyə-lər, -fä-\ adj : of, relating to, occurring in, or being the tissues surrounding a follicle

peri·hep·a·ti·tis \-ˌhe-pə-'tī-təs\ n, pl **-tit·i·des** \-'ti-tə-ˌdēz\ : inflammation of the peritoneal capsule of the liver

peri·kary·on \-'kar-ē-ˌän, -ən\ n, pl **-karya** \-ē-ə\ : CELL BODY — **peri·kary·al** \-ē-əl\ adj

peri·lymph \'per-ə-ˌlimf\ n : the fluid between the membranous and bony labyrinths of the ear

peri·lym·phat·ic \per-ə-lim-'fa-tik\ adj : relating to or containing perilymph

peri·men·o·pause \-'me-nə-ˌpóz, -'mē-\ n : the period around the onset of menopause that is often marked by various physical signs (as hot flashes and menstrual irregularity) — **peri·men·o·paus·al** \-ˌme-nə-'pó-zəl, -ˌmē-\ adj

pe·rim·e·ter \pə-'ri-mə-tər\ n : an instrument for examining the discriminative powers of different parts of the retina

peri·me·tri·um \per-ə-'mē-trē-əm\ n, pl **-tria** \-trē-ə\ : the peritoneum covering the fundus and ventral and dorsal aspects of the uterus

pe·rim·e·try \pə-'ri-mə-trē\ n, pl **-tries** : examination of the eye by means of a perimeter — **peri·met·ric** \per-ə-'me-trik\ adj

peri·my·si·um \per-ə-'mi-zhē-əm, -zē-\ n, pl **-sia** \-zhē-ə, -zē-ə\ : the connective-tissue sheath that surrounds a muscle and forms sheaths for the bundles of muscle fibers — **peri·my·si·al** \-əl\ adj

peri·na·tal \-'nāt-əl\ adj : occurring in, concerned with, or being around the period around the time of birth 〈∼ mortality〉 — **peri·na·tal·ly** adv

peri·na·tol·o·gist \per-ə-ˌnā-'tä-lə-jist\ n : a specialist in perinatology

peri·na·tol·o·gy \-ˌnā-'tä-lə-jē\ n, pl **-gies** : a branch of medicine concerned with perinatal care

per·in·do·pril \pə-'rin-də-ˌpril\ n : an ACE inhibitor used in the form of its amine salt $C_{19}H_{32}N_2O_5 \cdot C_4H_{11}N$ to treat essential hypertension

peri·ne·al \per-ə-'nē-əl\ adj : of or relating to the perineum

perineal artery n : a branch of the internal pudendal artery that supplies the skin of the external genitalia and the superficial parts of the perineum

per·i·ne·al body *n* : a mass of muscle and fascia that separates the lower end of the vagina and the rectum in the female and the urethra and the rectum in the male

per·i·nei — see TRANSVERSUS PERINEI SUPERFICIALIS

perineo- *comb form* : perineum ⟨*perine*otomy⟩

per·i·ne·o·plas·ty \ˈper-i-ˈnē-ō-ˌplas-tē\ *n, pl* **-ties** : plastic surgery of the perineum

per·i·ne·or·rha·phy \ˌper-ə-nē-ˈȯr-ə-fē\ *n, pl* **-phies** : suture of the perineum usu. to repair a laceration occurring during labor

per·i·ne·ot·o·my \ˌper-ə-nē-ˈä-tə-mē\, *pl* **-mies** : surgical incision of the perineum

peri·neph·ric \ˌper-ə-ˈne-frik\ *adj* : PERIRENAL ⟨a ∼ abscess⟩

per·i·ne·um \ˌper-ə-ˈnē-əm\ *n, pl* **-nea** \-ˈnē-ə\ : an area of tissue that marks externally the approximate boundary of the pelvic outlet and gives passage to the urogenital ducts and rectum; *also* : the area between the anus and the posterior part of the external genitalia esp. in the female

peri·neu·ral \ˌper-ə-ˈnu̇r-əl, -ˈnyu̇r-\ *adj* : occurring about or surrounding nervous tissue or a nerve

peri·neu·ri·al \-ˈnu̇r-ē-əl, -ˈnyu̇r-\ *adj* **1** : of or relating to the perineurium **2** : PERINEURAL

peri·neu·ri·um \ˌper-ə-ˈnu̇r-ē-əm, -ˈnyu̇r-\ *n, pl* **-ria** \-ē-ə\ : the sheath of connective tissue that surrounds a bundle of nerve fibers

peri·nu·cle·ar \ˌper-i-ˈnü-klē-ər, -ˈnyü-\ *adj* : situated around or surrounding the nucleus of a cell ⟨∼ structures⟩

peri·oc·u·lar \ˌper-ē-ˈä-kyə-lər\ *adj* : surrounding the eyeball but within the orbit ⟨∼ space⟩

pe·ri·od \ˈpir-ē-əd\ *n* **1 a** : a portion of time determined by some recurring phenomenon **b** : a single cyclic occurrence of menstruation **2** : a chronological division

pe·ri·od·ic \ˌpir-ē-ˈä-dik\ *adj* : occurring or recurring at regular intervals

per·iod·ic acid \ˌpər-(ˌ)ī-ˈä-dik-\ *n* : any of the strongly oxidizing iodine-containing acids (as H_5IO_6 or HIO_4)

periodic acid–Schiff \-ˈshif\ *adj* : relating to, being, or involving a reaction testing for polysaccharides and related substances in which tissue sections are treated with periodic acid and then Schiff's reagent with a reddish violet color indicating a positive test

periodic breathing *n* : abnormal breathing characterized by an irregular respiratory rhythm; *esp* : CHEYNE=STOKES RESPIRATION

periodic ophthalmia *n* : MOON BLINDNESS

periodic table *n* : an arrangement of chemical elements based on their atomic numbers

peri·odon·tal \ˌper-ē-ō-ˈdänt-ᵊl\ *adj* **1** : investing or surrounding a tooth **2** : of or affecting the periodontium ⟨∼ infection⟩ — **peri·odon·tal·ly** *adv*

periodontal disease *n* : any disease (as gingivitis or periodontis) affecting the periodontium

periodontal ligament *n* : the fibrous connective-tissue layer covering the cementum of a tooth and holding it in place in the jawbone — called also *pericementum, periodontal membrane*

peri·odon·tics \ˌper-ə-ˈdän-tiks\ *n* : a branch of dentistry that deals with diseases of the supporting and investing structures of the teeth including the gums, cementum, periodontal ligaments, and alveolar bone — called also *periodontology*

peri·odon·tist \-ˈdän-tist\ *n* : a specialist in periodontics — called also *periodontologist*

peri·odon·ti·tis \ˌper-ē-(ˌ)dän-ˈtī-təs\ *n* : inflammation of the periodontium and esp. chronic inflammation that typically follows untreated gingivitis and that results in progressive destruction of the periodontal ligament and resorption of alveolar bone with loosening or loss of teeth — called also *pericementitis*

peri·odon·ti·um \ˌper-ē-ō-ˈdän-chē-əm, -chəm\ *n, pl* **-tia** \-chē-ə, -chə\ : the supporting structures of the teeth including the cementum, the periodontal ligament, the bone of the alveolar process, and the gums

peri·odon·to·cla·sia \-ō-ˌdän-tə-ˈklā-zhə, -zhē-ə\ *n* : any periodontal disease characterized by destruction of the periodontium

peri·odon·tol·o·gist \ˌper-ē-ō-ˌdän-ˈtä-lə-jist\ *n* : PERIODONTIST

peri·odon·tol·o·gy \-ˌdän-ˈtä-lə-jē\ *n, pl* **-gies** : PERIODONTICS

peri·odon·to·sis \ˌper-ē-ō-ˌdän-ˈtō-səs\ *n, pl* **-to·ses** \-ˌsēz\ : a severe degenerative disease of the periodontium

peri·op·er·a·tive \ˌper-ē-ˈä-pə-rə-tiv, -ˌrā-\ *adj* : relating to, occurring in, or being the period around the time of a surgical operation ⟨∼ morbidity⟩

peri·oral \-ˈȯr-əl, -ˈär-\ *adj* : of, relating to, occurring in, or being the tissues around the mouth

peri·or·bit·al \-ˈȯr-bət-ᵊl\ *adj* : of, relating to, occurring in, or being the tissues surrounding or lining the orbit of the eye ⟨∼ edema⟩

periost- *or* **perioste-** *or* **periosteo-** *comb form* : periosteum ⟨*periost*itis⟩

peri·os·te·al \ˌper-ē-ˈäs-tē-əl\ *adj* **1** : situated around or produced external to bone **2** : of, relating to, or involving the periosteum ⟨∼ cells⟩

periosteal elevator *n* : a surgical instrument used to separate the periosteum from bone

peri·os·te·um \ˌper-ē-ˈäs-tē-əm\ *n, pl* **-tea** \-tē-ə\ : the membrane of connective tissue that closely invests all bones except at the articular surfaces

peri·os·ti·tis \-ˌäs-ˈtī-təs\ *n* : inflammation of the periosteum

peri·pan·cre·at·ic \ˌper-ə-ˌpaŋ-krē-ˈa-tik, -ˌpan-\ *adj* : of, relating to, occurring in, or being the tissue surrounding the pancreas

peri·par·tum \-ˈpär-təm\ *adj* : occurring in or being the period preceding or following parturition ⟨~ cardiomyopathy⟩

pe·riph·er·al \pə-ˈri-fə-rəl\ *adj* **1** : of, relating to, involving, forming, or located near a periphery or surface part (as of the body) **2** : of, relating to, affecting, or being part of the peripheral nervous system ⟨~ nerves⟩ **3** : of, relating to, or being the outer part of the visual field ⟨good ~ vision⟩ **4** : of, relating to, or being blood in the systemic circulation ⟨~ blood⟩ — **pe·riph·er·al·ly** *adv*

peripheral arterial disease *n* : damage to or dysfunction of the arteries outside the heart resulting in reduced blood flow; *esp* : narrowing or obstruction (as from atherosclerosis) of an artery (as the iliac artery or femoral artery) supplying the legs that is marked chiefly by intermittent claudication and by numbness and tingling in the legs

peripheral nervous system *n* : the part of the nervous system that is outside the central nervous system and comprises the cranial nerves excepting the optic nerve, the spinal nerves, and the autonomic nervous system

peripheral neuropathy *n* : a disease or degenerative state (as polyneuropathy) of the peripheral nerves in which motor, sensory, or vasomotor nerve fibers may be affected and which is marked by muscle weakness and atrophy, pain, and numbness

peripheral vascular disease *n* : vascular disease (as Raynaud's disease and Buerger's disease) affecting blood vessels and esp. those supplying the extremities

peripheral vascular resistance *n* : vascular resistance to the flow of blood in peripheral arterial vessels that is typically a function of the internal vessel diameter, vessel length, and blood viscosity — called also *peripheral resistance*

Peri·pla·ne·ta \ˌper-ē-plə-ˈnē-tə\ *n* : a genus of large cockroaches that includes the American cockroach

peri·plas·mic \ˌper-ə-ˈplaz-mik\ *adj* : of, relating to, occurring in, or being the space between the cell wall and the cell membrane

peri·por·tal \ˌper-ə-ˈpȯrt-ᵊl\ *adj* : of, relating to, occurring in, or being the tissues surrounding a portal vein

peri·pro·ce·dur·al \-prə-ˈsē-jə-rəl\ *adj* : occurring soon before, during, or soon after the performance of a medical procedure ⟨~ mortality⟩

peri·rec·tal \-ˈrek-tᵊl\ *adj* : of, relating to, occurring in, or being the tissues surrounding the rectum

peri·re·nal \-ˈrēn-ᵊl\ *adj* : of, relating to, occurring in, or being the tissues surrounding the kidney ⟨~ abscesses⟩

peri·si·nu·soi·dal \-ˌsī-nə-ˈsȯid-ᵊl, -nyə-\ *adj* : of, relating to, or occurring in the tissue surrounding one or more sinusoids ⟨~ fibrosis⟩

peri·stal·sis \ˌper-ə-ˈstȯl-səs, -ˈstäl-, -ˈstal-\ *n, pl* **-stal·ses** \-ˌsēz\ : successive waves of involuntary contraction passing along the walls of a hollow muscular structure (as the esophagus or intestine) and forcing the contents onward — **peri·stal·tic** \-tik\ *adj*

peri·ten·di·ni·tis \ˌper-ə-ˌten-də-ˈnī-təs\ *n* : inflammation of the tissues around a tendon

periton- *or* **peritone-** *or* **peritoneo-** *comb form* **1** : peritoneum ⟨peritonitis⟩ **2** : peritoneal and ⟨peritoneovenous shunt⟩

peri·to·nae·um *chiefly Brit var of* PERITONEUM

peri·to·ne·al \ˌper-ə-tə-ˈnē-əl\ *adj* : of, relating to, or affecting the peritoneum — **peri·to·ne·al·ly** *adv*

peritoneal cavity *n* : a space formed when the parietal and visceral layers of the peritoneum spread apart

peritoneal dialysis *n* : DIALYSIS 2b

peri·to·neo·scope \ˌper-ə-tə-ˈnē-ə-ˌskōp\ *n* : LAPAROSCOPE — **peri·to·neo·scop·ic** \-ˌnē-ə-ˈskä-pik\ *adj*

peri·to·ne·os·co·py \ˌper-ə-ˌtō-nē-ˈäs-kə-pē\ *n, pl* **-pies** : LAPAROSCOPY 1

peri·to·ne·ve·nous shunt \ˌper-ə-tə-ˌnē-ō-ˈvē-nəs-\ *n* : a shunt between the peritoneum and the jugular vein for relief of peritoneal ascites

peri·to·ne·um \ˌper-ə-tə-ˈnē-əm\ *n, pl* **-ne·ums** *or* **-nea** \-ˈnē-ə\ : the smooth transparent serous membrane that lines the cavity of the abdomen, is folded inward over the abdominal and pelvic viscera, and consists of an outer layer closely adherent to the walls of the abdomen and an inner layer that folds to invest the viscera — *see* PARIETAL PERITONEUM, VISCERAL PERITONEUM; *compare* MESENTERY 1

peri·to·ni·tis \ˌper-ə-tə-ˈnī-təs\ *n* : inflammation of the peritoneum

peri·ton·sil·lar abscess \ˌper-ə-ˈtän-sə-lər-\ *n* : QUINSY

peri·tu·bu·lar \ˌper-ə-ˈtü-byə-lər, -ˈtyü-\ *adj* : being adjacent to or surrounding a tubule

peritubular capillary *n* : any of a network of capillaries surrounding the renal tubules

peri·um·bi·li·cal \ˌper-ē-ˌəm-ˈbi-li-kəl\ *adj* : situated or occurring adjacent to the navel ⟨~ pain⟩

peri·un·gual \-ˈəŋ-gwəl, -ˈən-\ *adj* : situated or occurring around a fingernail or toenail

peri·ure·thral \-yu̇-'rē-thrǝl\ *adj* : of, relating to, occurring in, or being the tissues surrounding the urethra

peri·vas·cu·lar \ˌper-ǝ-'vas-kyǝ-lǝr\ *adj* : of, relating to, occurring in, or being the tissues surrounding a blood vessel

peri·vas·cu·li·tis \-ˌvas-kyǝ-'lī-tǝs\ *n* : inflammation of a perivascular sheath ⟨~ in the retina⟩

peri·ve·nous \ˌper-ǝ-'vē-nǝs\ *adj* : of, relating to, occurring in, or being the tissues surrounding a vein

peri·ven·tric·u·lar \-ven-'tri-kyǝ-lǝr\ *adj* : situated or occurring around a ventricle esp. of the brain

peri·vi·tel·line space \ˌper-ǝ-vī-'te-lǝn-, -ˌlēn-, -ˌlīn\ *n* : the fluid-filled space between the fertilization membrane and the ovum after the entry of a sperm into the egg

per·i·win·kle \'per-i-ˌwiŋ-kǝl\ *n* : any of several evergreen plants of the dogbane family (Apocynaceae); *esp* : ROSY PERIWINKLE

perle \'pǝrl\ *n* **1** : a soft gelatin capsule for enclosing volatile or unpleasant tasting liquids intended to be swallowed **2** : a fragile glass vial that contains a liquid (as amyl nitrite) and that is intended to be crushed and the vapor inhaled

per·lèche \per-'lesh\ *n* : a superficial inflammatory condition of the angles of the mouth often with fissure formation that is caused esp. by infection or avitaminosis

per·ma·nent \'pǝr-mǝ-nǝnt\ *adj* : of, relating to, or being a permanent tooth ⟨~ dentition⟩

permanent tooth *n* : one of the second set of teeth of a mammal that follow the milk teeth, typically persist into old age, and in humans are 32 in number including 4 incisors, 2 canines, and 10 premolars and molars in each jaw

per·me·able \'pǝr-mē-ǝ-bǝl\ *adj* : capable of being permeated; *esp* : having pores or openings that permit liquids or gases to pass through — **per·me·abil·i·ty** \ˌpǝr-mē-ǝ-'bi-lǝ-tē\ *n*

per·me·ate \'pǝr-mē-ˌāt\ *vb* **-at·ed; -at·ing** : to diffuse through or penetrate something — **per·me·ation** \ˌpǝr-mē-'ā-shǝn\ *n*

per·mis·sive \pǝr-'mi-siv\ *adj* : supporting genetic replication (as of a virus)

per·ni·cious \pǝr-'ni-shǝs\ *adj* : highly injurious or destructive : tending to a fatal issue : DEADLY ⟨~ disease⟩

pernicious anemia *n* : a severe hyperchromic anemia marked by a progressive decrease in number and increase in size and hemoglobin content of the red blood cells and by pallor, weakness, and gastrointestinal and nervous disturbances and associated with reduced ability to absorb vitamin B_{12} due to the absence of intrinsic factor — called also *addisonian anemia*

per·nio \'pǝr-nē-ˌō\ *n, pl* **per·ni·o·nes** \ˌpǝr-nē-'ō-(ˌ)nēz\ : CHILBLAIN

pe·ro·me·lia \ˌpē-rǝ-'mē-lē-ǝ\ *n* : congenital malformation of the limbs

pe·ro·ne·al \ˌper-ō-'nē-ǝl, pǝ-'rō-nē-\ *adj* : of, relating to, or located near the fibula **2** : relating to or involving a peroneal part

peroneal artery *n* : a deeply seated artery running along the back part of the fibular side of the leg to the heel, arising from the posterior tibial artery, and ending in branches near the ankle

peroneal muscle *n* : PERONEUS

peroneal muscular atrophy *n* : a chronic inherited progressive muscular atrophy that affects the parts of the legs and feet innervated by the peroneal nerves first and later progresses to the hands and arms — called also *Charcot-Marie-Tooth disease, peroneal atrophy*

peroneal nerve *n* : COMMON PERONEAL NERVE — see DEEP PERONEAL NERVE, SUPERFICIAL PERONEAL NERVE

peroneal retinaculum *n* : either of two bands of fascia that support and bind in place the tendons of the peroneus longus and peroneus brevis muscles as they pass along the lateral aspect of the ankle: **a** : one that is situated more superiorly — called also *superior peroneal retinaculum* **b** : one that is situated more inferiorly — called also *inferior peroneal retinaculum*

peroneal vein *n* : any of several veins that drain the muscles in the lateral and posterior parts of the leg, accompany the peroneal artery, and empty into the posterior tibial veins about two-thirds of the way up the leg

pe·ro·ne·us \ˌper-ǝ-'nē-ǝs\ *n, pl* **-nei** \-'nē-ˌī\ : any of three muscles of the lower leg: **a** : PERONEUS BREVIS **b** : PERONEUS LONGUS **c** : PERONEUS TERTIUS

peroneus brev·is \-'bre-vis\ *n* : a peroneus muscle that arises esp. from the side of the lower part of the fibula, ends in a tendon that inserts on the tuberosity at the base of the fifth metatarsal bone, and assists in everting and pronating the foot

peroneus lon·gus \-'lȯŋ-gǝs\ *n* : a peroneus muscle that arises esp. from the head and side of the fibula, ends in a long tendon that inserts on the side of the first metatarsal bone and the cuneiform bone on the medial side, and aids in everting and pronating the foot

peroneus ter·ti·us \-'tǝr-shē-ǝs\ *n* : a branch of the extensor digitorum longus muscle that arises esp. from the lower portion of the fibula, inserts on the dorsal surface of the base of the fifth metatarsal bone, and flexes the foot dorsally and assists in everting it

per·oral \(ˌ)pər-ˈōr-əl, per-, -ˈär-\ *adj* : done, occurring, or obtained through or by way of the mouth ⟨∼ infection⟩ — **per·oral·ly** *adv*

per os \pər-ˈōs\ *adv* : by way of the mouth ⟨infection *per os*⟩

pe·ro·sis \pə-ˈrō-səs\ *n, pl* **pe·ro·ses** \-ˌsēz\ : a disorder of poultry that is characterized by leg deformity and is caused by a deficiency of vitamins or minerals in the diet — called also *hock disease, slipped tendon*

per·ox·i·dase \pə-ˈräk-sə-ˌdās, -ˌdāz\ *n* : an enzyme that catalyzes the oxidation of various substances by peroxides

per·ox·ide \pə-ˈräk-ˌsīd\ *n* : a compound (as hydrogen peroxide) in which oxygen is visualized as joined to oxygen

per·ox·i·some \pə-ˈräk-sə-ˌsōm\ *n* : a cytoplasmic cell organelle containing enzymes (as catalase) which act esp. in the production and decomposition of hydrogen peroxide — called also *microbody* — **per·ox·i·som·al** \-ˌräk-sə-ˈsō-məl\ *adj*

per·oxy·ace·tyl nitrate \pə-ˌräk-sē-ə-ˈsēt-ᵊl-\ *n* : a toxic compound $C_2H_3O_5N$ that is found esp. in smog and is irritating to the eyes and upper respiratory tract — abbr. *PAN*

per·pen·dic·u·lar plate \ˌpər-pən-ˈdi-kyə-lər-\ *n* 1 : a flattened bony lamina of the ethmoid bone that is the largest bony part assisting in forming the nasal septum 2 : a long thin vertical bony plate forming part of the palatine bone — compare HORIZONTAL PLATE

per·phen·a·zine \(ˌ)pər-ˈfe-nə-ˌzēn\ *n* : a phenothiazine tranquilizer $C_{21}H_{26}ClN_3OS$ that is used to control symptoms (as anxiety, agitation, and delusions) of psychotic conditions

per·rec·tal \pər-ˈrekt-ᵊl\ *adj* : done or occurring through or by way of the rectum ⟨∼ administration⟩ — **per·rec·tal·ly** *adv*

per rectum *adv* : by way of the rectum ⟨a solution injected *per rectum*⟩

Per·san·tine \pər-ˈsan-ˌtēn\ *trademark* — used for a preparation of dipyridamole

persecution complex *n* : the feeling of being persecuted esp. without basis in reality

per·se·cu·to·ry \ˈpər-sə-kyü-ˌtōr-ē, pər-ˈse-kyə-\ *adj* : of, relating to, or being feelings of persecution : PARANOID

per·sev·er·a·tion \pər-ˌse-və-ˈrā-shən\ *n* : continual involuntary repetition of a mental act usu. exhibited by speech or by some other form of overt behavior — **per·sev·er·ate** \pər-ˈse-və-ˌrāt\ *vb* — **per·sev·er·a·tive** \pər-ˈse-və-ˌrā-tiv\ *adj*

per·sis·tent \pər-ˈsis-tənt\ *adj* 1 : existing or continuing for a long time: as **a** : effective in the open for an appreciable time usu. through slow formation of a vapor ⟨mustard gas is ∼⟩ **b** : degraded only slowly by the environment ⟨∼ pesticides⟩ **c** : remaining infective for a relatively long time in a vector after an initial period of incubation ⟨∼ viruses⟩ 2 : continuing to exist despite interference or treatment ⟨a ∼ cough⟩ ⟨has been in a ∼ vegetative state for two years⟩

per·so·na \pər-ˈsō-nə, -ˌnä\ *n, pl* **per·sonas** : an individual's social facade or front that esp. in the analytic psychology of C.G. Jung reflects the role in life the individual is playing — compare ANIMA

per·son·al·i·ty \ˌpər-sə-ˈna-lə-tē\ *n, pl* **-ties** 1 : the complex of characteristics that distinguishes an individual esp. in relationships with others 2 **a** : the totality of an individual's behavioral and emotional tendencies **b** : the organization of the individual's distinguishing character traits, attitudes, or habits

personality disorder *n* : a psychopathological condition or group of conditions in which an individual's entire life pattern is considered deviant or nonadaptive although the individual shows neither neurotic symptoms nor psychotic disorganization

personality inventory *n* : any of several tests that attempt to characterize the personality of an individual by objective scoring of replies to a large number of questions concerning the individual's behavior and attitudes — see MINNESOTA MULTIPHASIC PERSONALITY INVENTORY

personality test *n* : any of several tests that consist of standardized tasks designed to determine various aspects of the personality or the emotional status of the individual examined

per·spi·ra·tion \ˌpər-spə-ˈrā-shən\ *n* 1 : the act or process of perspiring 2 : a saline fluid that is secreted by the sweat glands, that consists chiefly of water containing sodium chloride and other salts, nitrogenous substances (as urea), carbon dioxide, and other solutes, and that serves both as a means of excretion and as a regulator of body temperature through the cooling effect of its evaporation — **per·spire** \pər-ˈspīr\ *vb*

per·spi·ra·to·ry \pər-ˈspī-rə-ˌtōr-ē, ˈpər-spə-rə-\ *adj* : of, relating to, secreting, or inducing perspiration

per·sua·sion \pər-ˈswā-zhən\ *n* : a method of treating neuroses consisting essentially in rational conversation and reeducation

per·tech·ne·tate \pər-ˈtek-nə-ˌtāt\ *n* : an anion $[TcO_4]$ of technetium used esp. in the form of its sodium salt as a radiopharmaceutical in medical diagnostic scanning (as of the thyroid)

Per·thes disease \ˈpər-ˌtēz-\ *n* : LEGG-CALVÉ-PERTHES DISEASE

Per·to·frane \'pər-tə-ˌfrān\ *n* : a preparation of desipramine — formerly a U.S. registered trademark

per·tus·sis \pər-'tə-səs\ *n* : WHOOPING COUGH

peruana — see VERRUGA PERUANA

Peru balsam *n* : BALSAM OF PERU

Peruvian balsam *n* : BALSAM OF PERU

per·ver·sion \pər-'vər-zhən, -shən\ *n*
1 : the action of perverting or the condition of being perverted **2** : an aberrant sexual practice or interest esp. when habitual — **per·verse** \pər-'vərs\ *adj*

¹per·vert \pər-'vərt\ *vb* : to cause to engage in perversion or to become perverted

²per·vert \'pər-ˌvərt\ *n* : one given to some form of sexual perversion

perverted *adj* : marked by abnormality or perversion

pes an·se·ri·nus \ˌpez-ˌan-sə-'rī-nəs\ *n* : the combined tendinous insertion on the medial aspect of the tuberosity of the tibia of the sartorius, gracilis, and semitendinosus muscles

pes ca·vus \-'kā-vəs\ *n* : a foot deformity characterized by an abnormally high arch

pes·sa·ry \'pe-sə-rē\ *n, pl* **-ries 1** : a vaginal suppository **2** : a device worn in the vagina to support the uterus, remedy a malposition, or prevent conception

pest \'pest\ *n* **1** : an epidemic disease associated with high mortality; *specif* : PLAGUE 2 **2** : something resembling a pest in destructiveness; *esp* : a plant or animal detrimental to humans or human concerns

pes·ti·cide \'pes-tə-ˌsīd\ *n* : an agent used to destroy pests — **pes·ti·ci·dal** \ˌpes-tə-'sīd-ᵊl\ *adj*

pes·tif·er·ous \pes-'ti-fə-rəs\ *adj* **1** : carrying or propagating infection : PESTILENTIAL ⟨a ~ insect⟩ **2** : infected with a pestilential disease

pes·ti·lence \'pes-tə-ləns\ *n* : a contagious or infectious epidemic disease that is virulent and devastating; *specif* : BUBONIC PLAGUE — **pes·ti·len·tial** \ˌpes-tə-'len-chəl\ *adj*

pes·tis \'pes-təs\ *n* : PLAGUE 2

Pes·ti·vi·rus \'pes-tə-ˌvī-rəs\ *n* : a genus of flaviviruses that includes the causative agents of bovine viral diarrhea and hog cholera

pes·tle \'pe-səl, 'pes-təl\ *n* : a usu. club-shaped implement for pounding or grinding substances in a mortar

PET *abbr* positron-emission tomography

PetCO₂ *abbr* partial pressure of end-tidal carbon dioxide

pe·te·chia \pə-'tē-kē-ə\ *n, pl* **-chi·ae** \-kē-ˌī\ : a minute reddish or purplish spot containing blood that appears in skin or mucous membrane as a result of localized hemorrhage — **pe·te·chi·al** \-kē-əl\ *adj* — **pe·te·chi·a·tion** \pə-ˌtē-kē-'ā-shən\ *n*

peth·i·dine \'pe-thə-ˌdēn, -dən\ *n, chiefly Brit* : MEPERIDINE

pe·tit mal \'pe-tē-ˌmal, -ˌmäl\ *n* : epilepsy characterized by absence seizures; *also* : ABSENCE SEIZURE

pe·tri dish \'pē-trē-\ *n* : a small shallow dish of thin glass or plastic with a loose cover used esp. for cultures in bacteriology

Pe·tri \'pā-trē\, **Julius Richard** (1852–1921), German bacteriologist.

pe·tris·sage \ˌpā-tri-'säzh\ *n* : massage in which the muscles are kneaded

pet·ro·la·tum \ˌpe-trə-'lā-təm, -'lä-\ *n* : PETROLEUM JELLY

pe·tro·leum jelly \pə-'trō-lē-əm-'je-lē\ *n* : a neutral unctuous odorless tasteless substance obtained from petroleum and used esp. in ointments and dressings

pe·tro·sal \pə-'trō-səl\ *n* : PETROSAL BONE

petrosal bone *n* : the petrous portion of the human temporal bone

petrosal ganglion *n* : INFERIOR GANGLION 1

petrosal nerve *n* : any of several small nerves passing through foramina in the petrous portion of the temporal bone: as **a** : DEEP PETROSAL NERVE **b** : GREATER PETROSAL NERVE **c** : LESSER PETROSAL NERVE

petrosal sinus *n* : either of two venous sinuses on each side of the base of the brain: **a** : a small superior sinus that connects the cavernous and transverse sinuses of the same side — called also *superior petrosal sinus* **b** : a larger inferior sinus that extends from the posterior inferior end of the cavernous sinus through the jugular foramen to join the internal jugular vein of the same side — called also *inferior petrosal sinus*

pe·tro·tym·pan·ic fissure \ˌpe-trō-tim-'pa-nik-, ˌpē-trō-\ *n* : a narrow transverse slit dividing the glenoid fossa of the temporal bone — called also *Glaserian fissure*

pe·trous \'pe-trəs, 'pē-\ *adj* : of, relating to, or constituting the exceptionally hard and dense portion of the human temporal bone that contains the internal auditory organs and is a pyramidal process wedged in at the base of the skull between the sphenoid and occipital bones

PET scan \'pet-\ *n* : a sectional view of the body constructed by positron-emission tomography — **PET scanning** *n*

PET scanner *n* : a medical instrument consisting of integrated X-ray and computing equipment and used for positron-emission tomography

Peutz-Je·ghers syndrome \ˈpœts-'jā-gərz-\ *n* : a familial polyposis inherited as an autosomal dominant trait and characterized by numerous polyps in the stomach, small intestine, and colon and by melanin-containing spots on the skin and mucous membranes esp. of the lips and gums

Peutz, J. L. A. (1886–1957), Dutch physician.

Jeghers, Harold (1904–1990), American physician.

-pexy \ˌpek-sē\ *n comb form, pl* **-pexies** : fixation : making fast ⟨gastro*pexy*⟩

Peyer's patch \ˈpī-ərz-\ *n* : any of numerous large oval patches of closely aggregated nodules of lymphoid tissue in the walls of the small intestines esp. in the ileum that partially or entirely disappear in advanced life and in typhoid fever become the seat of ulcers which may perforate the intestines — called also *Peyer's gland*

Peyer, Johann Conrad (1653–1712), Swiss physician and anatomist.

pey·o·te \pā-ˈō-tē\ *also* **pey·otl** \-ˈōt-ᵊl\ *n* **1** : a hallucinogenic drug containing mescaline that is derived from peyote buttons **2** : a small spineless cactus (*Lophophora williamsii*) of the southwestern U.S. and Mexico — called also *mescal*

peyote button *n* : one of the dried disk-shaped tops of the peyote cactus — called also *mescal button*

Pey·ro·nie's disease \ˌpā-rə-ˈnēz-, pā-ˈrō-nēz-\ *n* : the formation of fibrous plaques in one or both corpora cavernosa of the penis resulting in distortion or deflection of the erect organ

La Peyronie \lä-pā-rô-ˈnē\, **François Gigot de (1678–1747),** French surgeon.

Pfan·nen·stiel's incision \ˈpfä-nən-ˌshtēlz-\ *n* : a long horizontal abdominal incision made below the line of the pubic hair and above the mons veneris down to and through the sheath of the rectus abdominus muscles but not the muscles themselves which are separated in the direction of their fibers — called also *bikini incision*

Pfannenstiel, Hermann Johann (1862–1909), German gynecologist.

Pfie·ster·ia \fē-ˈstir-ē-ə\ *n* : a genus of dinoflagellates including one (*Pfiesteria piscicida*) found in waters esp. along the U.S. Atlantic coast that produces a toxin which causes skin lesions in fish and may cause symptoms (as skin lesions and memory loss) in humans exposed to the toxin

p53 \ˌpē-ˌfif-tē-ˈthrē\ *n* : a tumor suppressor gene that in a defective form tends to be associated with a high risk of certain cancers (as of the colon, lung, and breast)

pg *abbr* picogram

PG *abbr* prostaglandin

PGA *abbr* pteroylglutamic acid

PGR *abbr* psychogalvanic reaction; psychogalvanic reflex; psychogalvanic response

PGY *abbr* postgraduate year

pH \ˌpē-ˈāch\ *n* : a measure of acidity and alkalinity of a solution that is a number on a scale whose values run from 0 to 14 with 7 representing neutrality, numbers less than 7 increasing acidity, and numbers greater than 7 increasing alkalinity

PHA *abbr* phytohemagglutinin

phac- *or* **phaco-** *comb form* : lens ⟨*phaco*emulsification⟩

phaco·emul·si·fi·ca·tion \ˌfa-kō-i-ˌməl-sə-fə-ˈkā-shən\ *n* : a cataract operation in which the diseased lens is reduced to a liquid by ultrasonic vibrations and drained out of the eye — **phaco·emul·si·fi·er** \-ˈməl-sə-ˌfī-ər\ *n*

phaco·ma·to·sis \ˌfa-kō-mə-ˈtō-səs\ *n, pl* **-to·ses** \-ˌsēz\ : any of a group of hereditary or congenital diseases (as neurofibromatosis) affecting the central nervous system and characterized by the development of hamartomas

phaeo·chro·mo·cy·to·ma *Brit var of* PHEOCHROMOCYTOMA

phag- *or* **phago-** *comb form* : eating : feeding ⟨*phag*edena⟩

phage \ˈfāj, ˈfäzh\ *n* : BACTERIOPHAGE

-phage \ˌfāj, ˌfäzh\ *n comb form* : one that eats ⟨bacterio*phage*⟩

phag·e·de·na \ˌfa-jə-ˈdē-nə\ *n* : rapidly spreading destructive ulceration of soft tissue — **phag·e·den·ic** \-ˈde-nik, -ˈdē-\ *adj*

phage lambda *n* : a bacteriophage (species *Enterobacteria phage λ* of the family *Siphoviridae*) of double-stranded DNA that can be integrated as a prophage into the genome of some strains of E. coli and is used as a vector to clone DNA from various organisms — called also *bacteriophage lambda, lambda, lambda phage*

phage type *n* : a set of strains of a bacterium susceptible to the same bacteriophages

phage typing *n* : determination of the phage type of a bacterium

-pha·gia \ˈfā-jə, -jē-ə\ *n comb form* : -PHAGY ⟨dys*phagia*⟩

phago·cyte \ˈfa-gə-ˌsīt\ *n* : a cell (as a macrophage or neutrophil) that engulfs and consumes foreign material (as microorganisms) and debris (as dead tissue cells) — **phago·cyt·ic** \ˌfa-gə-ˈsi-tik\ *adj*

phago·cy·tize \ˈfa-gō-ˌsī-ˌtīz, -sə-\ *vb* **-tized; -tiz·ing** : PHAGOCYTOSE

phago·cy·tose \ˌfa-gō-ˈsī-ˌtōs, -ˌtōz\ *vb* **-tosed; -tos·ing** : to consume by phagocytosis — **phago·cy·tos·able** \ˌfa-gə-sī-ˈtō-zə-bəl, -sə-, -ˌtōs-\ *adj*

phago·cy·to·sis \ˌfa-gə-sī-ˈtō-səs, -sə-\ *n, pl* **-to·ses** \-ˌsēz\ : the engulfing and usu. the destruction of particulate matter by phagocytes — **phago·cy·tot·ic** \-ˈtä-tik\ *adj*

phago·some \ˈfa-gə-ˌsōm\ *n* : a membrane-bound vesicle that encloses particulate matter taken into the cell by phagocytosis

-pha·gous \fə-gəs\ *adj comb form*
: feeding esp. on a (specified) kind of
food ⟨hemato*phagous*⟩

-ph·a·gy \f-ə-jē\ *n comb form, pl* **-pha·gies** : eating : eating of a (specified)
type or substance ⟨geo*phagy*⟩

phak- *or* **phako-** — see PHAC-

pha·lan·ge·al \ˌfā-lən-ˈjē-əl, ˌfa-; fə-ˈlan-jē-, fā-\ *adj* : of or relating to a
phalanx or the phalanges

pha·lan·gec·to·my \ˌfā-lən-ˈjek-tə-mē, ˌfa-\ *n, pl* **-mies** : surgical excision of
a phalanx of a finger or toe

pha·lanx \ˈfā-ˌlaŋks\ *n, pl* **pha·lan·ges** \fə-ˈlan-(ˌ)jēz, fā-\ : any of the digital
bones of the hand or foot distal to the
metacarpus or metatarsus that in humans are three to each finger and toe
with the exception of the thumb and
big toe which have only two each

phall- *or* **phallo-** *comb form* : penis
⟨*phallo*plasty⟩

phal·lic \ˈfa-lik\ *adj* **1** : of, relating to,
or resembling a penis **2** : of, relating
to, or characterized by the stage of
psychosexual development in psychoanalytic theory during which a child
becomes interested in his or her own
sexual organs — compare ANAL 2a,
GENITAL 3, ORAL 2a

phal·loi·din \fa-ˈlȯid-ᵊn\ *also* **phal·loi·dine** \fa-ˈlȯid-ᵊn, ˈfa-lȯi-ˌdēn\ *n* : a
very toxic crystalline peptide $C_{35}H_{46}$-
$N_8O_{10}S \cdot H_2O$ obtained from the death
cap mushroom

phal·lo·plas·ty \ˈfa-lō-ˌplas-tē\ *n, pl*
-ties : plastic surgery of the penis or
scrotum

phal·lus \ˈfa-ləs\ *n, pl* **phal·li** \ˈfa-ˌlī, -ˌlē\ *or* **phal·lus·es** **1** : PENIS **2** : the
first embryonic rudiment of the penis
or clitoris

phan·ero·zo·ite \ˌfa-nə-rō-ˈzō-ˌīt\ *n*
: an exoerythrocytic malaria parasite
found late in the course of an infection — **phan·ero·zo·it·ic** \-ˌzō-ˈi-tik\
adj

phan·tasm \ˈfan-ˌta-zəm\ *n* **1** : a fig-
ment of the imagination or disordered
mind **2** : an apparition of a living or
dead person

phantasy *var of* FANTASY

phan·tom \ˈfan-təm\ *n* **1** : a model of
the body or one of its parts **2** : a body
of material resembling a body or bodily part in mass, composition, and dimensions and used to measure
absorption of radiations

phantom limb *n* : an often painful sensation of the presence of a limb that
has been amputated — called also
phantom pain, phantom sensations

phantom tumor *n* : a swelling (as of
the abdomen) suggesting a tumor

Phar. D. *abbr* doctor of pharmacy

pharm *abbr* pharmaceutical; pharmacist; pharmacy

phar·ma \ˈfär-mə\ *n* : a pharmaceutical
company

¹phar·ma·ceu·ti·cal \ˌfär-mə-ˈsü-ti-kəl\
also **phar·ma·ceu·tic** \-tik\ *adj* : of,
relating to, or engaged in pharmacy

or the manufacture and sale of phar-
maceuticals ⟨a ~ company⟩ — **phar·ma·ceu·ti·cal·ly** *adv*

²pharmaceutical *also* **pharmaceutic** *n*
: a medicinal drug

phar·ma·ceu·tics \-tiks\ *n* : the science of preparing, using, or dispensing medicines : PHARMACY

phar·ma·cist \ˈfär-mə-sist\ *n* : a person
licensed to engage in pharmacy

pharmaco- *comb form* : medicine
: drug ⟨*pharmaco*logy⟩

phar·ma·co·dy·nam·ics \ˌfär-mə-kō-
dī-ˈna-miks, -də-\ *n* : a branch of pharmacology dealing with the reactions
between drugs and living systems —
phar·ma·co·dy·nam·ic \-mik\ *adj* —
phar·ma·co·dy·nam·i·cal·ly *adv*

phar·ma·co·ge·net·ics \-jə-ˈne-tiks\ *n*
: the study of the interrelation of
hereditary constitution and response
to drugs — **phar·ma·co·ge·net·ic**
\-tik\ *adj*

phar·ma·co·ge·no·mics \-jē-ˈnō-miks\
n : a biotechnological science that is
concerned with developing drug therapies to compensate for genetic differences in patients which cause
varied responses to a single therapeu-
tic regimen — **phar·ma·co·ge·no·mic** \-mik\ *adj*

phar·ma·cog·no·sist \ˌfär-mə-ˈkäg-nə-
sist\ *n* : a specialist in pharmacognosy

phar·ma·cog·no·sy \ˌfär-mə-ˈkäg-nə-
sē\ *n, pl* **-sies** : a branch of pharmacology dealing esp. with the composition, use, and development of
medicinal substances of biological
origin — **phar·ma·cog·nos·tic** \-ˌkäg-
ˈnäs-tik\ *or* **phar·ma·cog·nos·ti·cal**
\-ti-kəl\ *adj*

phar·ma·co·ki·net·ics \-kō-kə-ˈne-
tiks, -kō-kī-\ *n* **1** : the study of the
bodily absorption, distribution, metabolism, and excretion of drugs **2**
: the characteristic interactions of a
drug and the body in terms of its absorption, distribution, metabolism,
and excretion — **phar·ma·co·ki·net·ic** \-tik\ *adj*

phar·ma·col·o·gist \ˌfär-mə-ˈkä-lə-jist\
n : a specialist in pharmacology

phar·ma·col·o·gy \ˌfär-mə-ˈkä-lə-jē\ *n,
pl* **-gies** **1** : the science of drugs including their origin, composition,
pharmacokinetics, therapeutic use,
and toxicology **2** : the properties and
reactions of drugs esp. with relation
to their therapeutic value — **phar·ma·co·log·i·cal** \-kə-ˈlä-ji-kəl\ *also*
phar·ma·co·log·ic \-jik\ *adj* — **phar·ma·co·log·i·cal·ly** *adv*

phar·ma·co·poe·ia *or* **phar·ma·co·pe·ia** \ˌfär-mə-kə-ˈpē-ə\ *n* **1** : a book de-
scribing drugs, chemicals, and medic-
inal preparations; *esp* : one issued by
an officially recognized authority and
serving as a standard **2** : a collection
or stock of drugs — **phar·ma·co·poe·ial** *or* **phar·ma·co·pe·ial** \-əl\ *adj*

phar·ma·co·ther·a·peu·tic \-ˌther-ə-
ˈpyü-tik\ *adj* : of or relating to phar-

macotherapeutics or pharmacothera-
py ⟨a ∼ agent⟩

phar·ma·co·ther·a·peu·tics \-tiks\ *n sing or pl* : the study of the therapeutic uses and effects of drugs

phar·ma·co·ther·a·py \-ˌfär-mə-kō-ˈther-ə-pē\ *n, pl* **-pies** : the treatment of disease and esp. mental disorder with drugs

phar·ma·cy \ˈfär-mə-sē\ *n, pl* **-cies 1** : the art, practice, or profession of preparing, preserving, compounding, and dispensing medical drugs **2 a** : a place where medicines are compounded or dispensed **b** : DRUGSTORE **3** : PHARMACOPOEIA 2

Pharm. D. *abbr* doctor of pharmacy

pharyng- *or* **pharyngo-** *comb form* **1** : pharynx ⟨*pharyng*itis⟩ **2** : pharyngeal and ⟨*pharyngo*esophageal⟩

pha·ryn·ge·al \ˌfar-ən-ˈjē-əl; fə-ˈrin-jəl, -jē-əl\ *adj* **1** : relating to or located in the region of the pharynx **2 a** : innervating the pharynx esp. by contributing to the formation of the pharyngeal plexus ⟨the ∼ branch of the vagus nerve⟩ **b** : supplying or draining the pharynx ⟨the ∼ branch of the maxillary artery⟩

pharyngeal aponeurosis *n* : the middle or fibrous coat of the walls of the pharynx

pharyngeal arch *n* : BRANCHIAL ARCH

pharyngeal cavity *n* : the cavity of the pharynx that consists of a part continuous anteriorly with the nasal cavity by way of the nasopharynx, a part opening into the oral cavity by way of the isthmus of the fauces, and a part continuous posteriorly with the esophagus and opening into the larynx by way of the epiglottis

pharyngeal cleft *n* : BRANCHIAL CLEFT

pharyngeal plexus *n* : a plexus formed by branches of the glossopharyngeal, vagus, and sympathetic nerves supplying the muscles and mucous membrane of the pharynx and adjoining parts

pharyngeal pouch *n* : any of a series of evaginations of ectoderm on either side of the pharynx that meet the corresponding external furrows and give rise to the branchial clefts of the vertebrate embryo

pharyngeal tonsil *n* : a mass of lymphoid tissue at the back of the pharynx between the eustachian tubes that is usu. best developed in young children, is commonly atrophied in the adult, and is markedly subject to hypertrophy and adenoid formation esp. in children — called also *nasopharyngeal tonsil*

phar·yn·gec·to·my \ˌfar-ən-ˈjek-tə-mē\ *n, pl* **-mies** : surgical removal of a part of the pharynx

pharyngis — see CONSTRICTOR PHARYNGIS INFERIOR, CONSTRICTOR PHARYNGIS MEDIUS, CONSTRICTOR PHARYNGIS SUPERIOR

phar·yn·gi·tis \ˌfar-ən-ˈjī-təs\ *n, pl* **-git·i·des** \-ˈji-tə-ˌdēz\ : inflammation of the pharynx (as from bacterial infection)

pharyngo- — see PHARYNG-

pha·ryn·go·con·junc·ti·val fever \fə-ˌrin-gō-ˌkän-ˌjəŋk-ˈtī-vəl-\ *n* : an acute epidemic illness caused by various adenoviruses of the genus *Mastadenovirus* (esp. serotypes of species *Human adenovirus B*, *Human adenovirus C*, and *Human adenovirus E*) that usu. affects children of school age and that is typically characterized by fever, pharyngitis, and conjunctivitis

pha·ryn·go·epi·glot·tic fold \fə-ˌrin-gō-ˌe-pə-ˈglä-tik-\ *n* : either of two folds of mucous membrane extending from the base of the tongue to the epiglottis with one on each side of the midline

pha·ryn·go·esoph·a·ge·al \-i-ˌsä-fə-ˈjē-əl\ *adj* : of or relating to the pharynx and the esophagus

pharyngoesophageal diverticulum *n* : ZENKER'S DIVERTICULUM

pha·ryn·go·lar·yn·gec·to·my \fə-ˌrin-gō-ˌlar-ən-ˌjek-tə-mē\ *n, pl* **-mies** : surgical excision of the hypopharynx and larynx

pha·ryn·go·pal·a·tine arch \-ˈpa-lə-ˌtīn-\ *n* : PALATOPHARYNGEAL ARCH

pha·ryn·go·plas·ty \fə-ˈrin-gō-ˌplas-tē\ *n, pl* **-ties** : plastic surgery performed on the pharynx

phar·yn·gos·to·my \ˌfar-iŋ-ˈgäs-tə-mē\ *n, pl* **-mies** : surgical formation of an artificial opening into the pharynx

phar·yn·got·o·my \ˌfar-iŋ-ˈgä-tə-mē\ *n, pl* **-mies** : surgical incision into the pharynx

pha·ryn·go·ton·sil·li·tis \fə-ˌrin-gō-ˌtän-sə-ˈli-təs\ *n* : inflammation of the pharynx and the tonsils

pha·ryn·go·tym·pan·ic tube \-tim-ˈpa-nik-\ *n* : EUSTACHIAN TUBE

phar·ynx \ˈfar-iŋks\ *n, pl* **pha·ryn·ges** \fə-ˈrin-(ˌ)jēz\ *also* **phar·ynx·es** : the part of the digestive and respiratory tracts situated between the cavity of the mouth and the esophagus and in humans being a conical musculomembranous tube about four and a half inches (11.43 centimeters) long that is continuous above with the mouth and nasal passages, communicates through the eustachian tubes with the ears, and extends downward past the opening into the larynx to the lower border of the cricoid cartilage where it is continuous with the esophagus — see LARYNGOPHARYNX, NASOPHARYNX, OROPHARYNX

phase \ˈfāz\ *n* **1** : a particular appearance or state in a regularly recurring cycle of changes **2** : a distinguishable part in a course, development, or cycle ⟨the early ∼s of a disease⟩ **3** : a point or stage in the period of a periodic motion or process (as a light wave or a vibration) in relation to an arbitrary reference or starting point in the period **4** : a homogeneous, physically distinct, and mechanically separable portion of matter present in a nonhomogeneous physicochemical system; *esp* : one of the fundamental states of matter usu. considered to include the solid, liquid, and gaseous forms

phase–contrast microscope *n* : a microscope that translates differences in phase of the light transmitted through or reflected by the object into differences of intensity in the image — **phase–contrast microscopy** *n*

-pha·sia \'fā-zhə, -zhē-ə *also* -pha·sy \fə-sē\ *n comb form*, *pl* **-phasias** *also* **-phasies** : speech disorder (of a specified type) ⟨dys*phasia*⟩

PhD \pē-(ˌ)āch-'dē\ *abbr or n* **1** : an earned academic degree conferring the rank and title of doctor of philosophy **2** : a person who has a doctor of philosophy

Phe *abbr* phenylalanine

phe·na·caine \'fē-nə-ˌkān, 'fe-\ *n* : a crystalline base that has been used as a local anesthetic in the form of its hydrochloride $C_{18}H_{22}N_2O_2 \cdot HCl$

phen·ac·e·tin \fi-'nas-ə-tən\ *n* : a compound $C_{10}H_{13}NO_2$ formerly used to ease pain or fever but now withdrawn from use because of its link to high blood pressure, heart attacks, cancer, and kidney disease — called also *acetophenetidin*

phe·naz·o·cine \fi-'na-zə-ˌsēn\ *n* : a drug $C_{22}H_{27}NO$ related to morphine that has greater pain-relieving and slighter narcotic effect

phen·a·zone \'fe-nə-ˌzōn\ *n* : ANTIPYRINE

phen·cy·cli·dine \fen-'si-klə-ˌdēn, -'sī-, -dən\ *n* : a piperidine derivative used chiefly in the form of its hydrochloride $C_{17}H_{25}N \cdot HCl$ esp. as a veterinary anesthetic and sometimes illicitly as a psychedelic drug to induce vivid mental imagery — called also *angel dust*, *PCP*

phen·el·zine \'fen-ᵊl-ˌzēn\ *n* : a monoamine oxidase inhibitor C_8-$H_{12}N_2$ that suppresses REM sleep and is used esp. as an antidepressant drug — see NARDIL

Phen·er·gan \fe-'nər-ˌgan\ *trademark* — used for a preparation of the hydrochloride of promethazine

phe·neth·i·cil·lin \fi-ˌne-thə-'si-lən\ *n* : a semisynthetic penicillin administered orally in the form of its potassium salt $C_{17}H_{19}KN_2O_5S$ and used esp. in the treatment of less severe infections caused by bacteria that do not produce beta-lactamase

phen·eth·yl alcohol \fe-'ne-thəl-\ *n* : PHENYLETHYL ALCOHOL

phen-fen \'fen-ˌfen\ *n* : FEN-PHEN

phen·for·min \fen-'fór-mən\ *n* : a compound $C_{10}H_{15}N_5$ formerly used to treat diabetes but now withdrawn from use because of its link to lifethreatening lactic acidosis

phen·in·di·one \ˌfen-in-'dī-ˌōn\ *n* : an anticoagulant drug $C_{15}H_{10}O_2$

phen·ip·ra·zine \fe-'ni-prə-ˌzēn\ *n* : a monoamine oxidase inhibitor C_9-$H_{14}N_2$

phen·ir·amine \fe-'nir-ə-ˌmēn, -mən\ *n* : a drug used in the form of its maleate $C_{16}H_{20}N_2 \cdot C_4H_4O_4$ as an antihistamine

phen·met·ra·zine \fen-'me-trə-ˌzēn\ *n* : a sympathomimetic stimulant used in the form of its hydrochloride $C_{11}H_{15}NO \cdot HCl$ as an appetite suppressant — see PRELUDIN

phe·no·barb \'fē-nō-ˌbärb\ *n* : PHENOBARBITAL; *also* : a pill containing phenobarbital

phe·no·bar·bi·tal \ˌfē-nō-'bär-bə-ˌtól\ *n* : a crystalline barbiturate $C_{12}H_{12}$-N_2O_3 that is used orally or is administered by injection in the form of its sodium salt $C_{12}H_{11}N_2NaO_3$ as a hypnotic and sedative — see LUMINAL

phe·no·bar·bi·tone \-bə-ˌtōn\ *n*, *chiefly Brit* : PHENOBARBITAL

phe·no·copy \'fē-nə-ˌkä-pē\ *n*, *pl* **-cop·ies** : a phenotypic variation that is caused by unusual environmental conditions and resembles the normal expression of a genotype other than its own

phe·nol \'fē-ˌnōl, -ˌnól, fi-'\ *n* **1** : a corrosive poisonous crystalline acidic compound C_6H_5OH present in coal tar that is used in the manufacture of some pharmaceuticals and as a topical anesthetic in dilute solution — called also *carbolic*, *carbolic acid* **2** : any of various acidic compounds analogous to phenol — **phe·no·lic** \fi-'nō-lik, -'nä-\ *adj*

phe·nol·phtha·lein \ˌfēn-ᵊl-'tha-lē-ən, -'tha-ˌlēn, -'thā-\ *n* : a white or yellowish white crystalline compound C_{20}-$H_{14}O_4$ used in analysis as an indicator because its solution is brilliant red in alkalies and is decolorized by acids and in medicine as a laxative

phenol red *n* : PHENOLSULFONPHTHALEIN

phe·nol·sul·fon·phtha·lein \ˌfēn-ᵊl-ˌsól-fän-'tha-lē-ən, -'tha-ˌlēn, -'thā-\ *n* : a red crystalline compound $C_{19}H_{14}$-O_5S used chiefly as a test of kidney function and as an acid-base indicator

phenolsulfonphthalein test *n* : a test in which phenolsulfonphthalein is administered by injection and urine samples are subsequently taken at regular intervals to measure the rate at which it is excreted by the kidneys

phe·nom·e·non \fi-'nä-mə-ˌnän, -nən\ *n*, *pl* **-na** \-nə, -ˌnä\ **1** : an observable fact or event **2 a** : an object or aspect known through the senses rather than by thought or intuition **b** : a fact or event of scientific interest susceptible of scientific description and explanation

phe·no·thi·azine \ˌfē-nō-'thī-ə-ˌzēn\ *n* **1** : a greenish yellow crystalline compound $C_{12}H_9NS$ used as an anthelmintic and insecticide esp. in veterinary practice **2** : any of various phenothiazine derivatives (as chlorpromazine) that are used as tranquilizing agents esp. in the treatment of schizophrenia

phe·no·type \'fē-nə-ˌtīp\ *n* : the observable properties of an organism that are produced by the interaction of the genotype and the environment — compare GENOTYPE — **phe·no·typ·ic** \ˌfē-nə-'ti-pik\ *also* **phe·no·typ·i·cal** \-pi-kəl\ *adj* — **phe·no·typ·i·cal·ly** *adv*

phe·noxy·ben·za·mine \fi-ˌnäk-sē-'ben-zə-ˌmēn\ *n* : an alpha-adrenergic blocking agent used in the form of its hydrochloride $C_{18}H_{22}ClNO·HCl$ esp. to treat hypertension and sweating due to pheochromocytoma

phe·noxy·meth·yl penicillin \-'meth-ᵊl-\ *n* : PENICILLIN V

phen·pro·cou·mon \ˌfen-prō-'kü-ˌmän\ *n* : an anticoagulant drug $C_{18}H_{16}O_3$

phen·sux·i·mide \ˌfen-'sək-si-ˌmīd\ *n* : an anticonvulsant drug $C_{11}H_{11}NO_2$ sometimes used in the treatment of absence seizures

phen·ter·mine \'fen-tər-ˌmēn\ *n* : an anorectic drug administered in the form of its hydrochloride $C_{10}H_{15}N·$HCl to treat obesity

phen·tol·amine \fen-'tä-lə-ˌmēn, -mən\ *n* : an alpha-adrenergic blocking agent that is administered by injection in the form of its mesylate $C_{17}H_{19}N_3O·CH_4O_3S$ esp. in the diagnosis and treatment of hypertension due to pheochromocytoma — see REGITINE

phe·nyl \'fen-ᵊl, 'fēn-\ *n* : a monovalent chemical group C_6H_5 derived from benzene — often used in combination ⟨*phenyl*alanine⟩

phe·nyl·al·a·nine \ˌfen-ᵊl-'a-lə-ˌnēn, ˌfēn-\ *n* : an essential amino acid $C_9H_{11}NO_2$ that is obtained in its levorotatory L-form by the hydrolysis of proteins (as lactalbumin), that is essential in human nutrition, and is converted in the normal body to tyrosine — abbr. *Phe*; see PHENYLKETONURIA, PHENYLPYRUVIC ACID

phenylalanine mustard *or* **L-phenylalanine mustard** \'el-\ *n* : MELPHALAN

phen·yl·bu·ta·zone \ˌfen-ᵊl-'byü-tə-ˌzōn\ *n* : a drug $C_{19}H_{20}N_2O_2$ that is used for its analgesic and anti-inflammatory properties esp. in the treatment of arthritis, gout, and bursitis — see BUTAZOLIDIN

phen·yl·eph·rine \ˌfen-ᵊl-'e-ˌfrēn, -frən\ *n* : a sympathomimetic agent that is used in the form of its hydrochloride $C_9H_{13}NO·HCl$ esp. as a vasoconstrictor, nasal decongestant, and mydriatic and to raise blood pressure — see NEO-SYNEPHRINE

phe·nyl·eth·yl alcohol \ˌfen-ᵊl-'eth-ᵊl-, ˌfēn-\ *n* : a fragrant liquid alcohol $C_8H_{10}O$ that is used as an antibacterial preservative esp. in ophthalmic solutions with limited effectiveness

phe·nyl·eth·yl·amine \ˌfen-ᵊl-ˌeth-ᵊl-'a-ˌmēn, ˌfēn-\ *n* : a neurotransmitter $C_8H_{11}N$ that is an amine resembling amphetamine in structure and pharmacological properties; *also* : any of its derivatives

phe·nyl·ke·ton·uria \ˌfen-ᵊl-ˌkē-tə-'nu̇r-ē-ə, ˌfēn-, -'nyu̇r-\ *n* : a metabolic disorder that is caused by an enzyme deficiency resulting in the accumulation of phenylalanine and its metabolites (as phenylpyruvic acid) in the blood and their excess excretion in the urine, that is inherited as an autosomal recessive trait, and that causes usu. severe mental retardation, seizures, eczema, and abnormal body odor unless phenylalanine is restricted from the diet beginning at birth — abbr. *PKU*; called also *phenylpyruvic amentia, phenylpyruvic oligophrenia*

¹**phe·nyl·ke·ton·uric** \-'nu̇r-ik, -'nyu̇r-\ *n* : one affected with phenylketonuria

²**phenylketonuric** *adj* : of, relating to, or affected with phenylketonuria

phen·yl·mer·cu·ric \ˌfen-ᵊl-mər-'kyu̇r-ik\ *adj* : being a salt containing the positively charged ion $[C_6H_5Hg]$

phenylmercuric acetate *n* : a crystalline salt $C_8H_8HgO_2$ used chiefly as a fungicide and herbicide

phenylmercuric nitrate *n* : a crystalline basic salt that is a mixture of $C_6H_5HgNO_3$ and C_6H_5HgOH used chiefly as a fungicide and antiseptic

phen·yl·pro·pa·nol·amine \ˌfen-ᵊl-ˌprō-pə-'nó-lə-ˌmēn, -'nō-; -ˌnó-lə-ˌmēn\ *n* : a sympathomimetic drug that has been used in the form of its hydrochloride $C_9H_{13}NO·HCl$ esp. as a nasal decongestant and appetite suppressant but has been largely withdrawn from use because of its link to hemorrhagic stroke — abbr. *PPA*

phe·nyl·py·ru·vic acid \ˌfen-ᵊl-pī-ˌrü-vik-, ˌfēn-\ *n* : a crystalline keto acid $C_9H_8O_3$ found in the urine as a metabolic product of phenylalanine esp. in phenylketonuria

phenylpyruvic amentia *n* : PHENYLKETONURIA

phenylpyruvic oligophrenia *n* : PHENYLKETONURIA

phenyl salicylate *n* : a crystalline ester $C_{13}H_{10}O_3$ used as a sunscreen to absorb ultraviolet light and also as an analgesic and antipyretic — called also *salol*

phen·yl·thio·car·ba·mide \ˌfen-ᵊl-ˌthī-ō-'kär-bə-ˌmīd\ *n* : a compound $C_7H_8N_2S$ that is extremely bitter or tasteless depending on the presence or absence of a single dominant gene in the taster — called also *PTC*

phen·yl·thio·urea \-ˌthī-ō-yu̇-'rē-ə\ *n* : PHENYLTHIOCARBAMIDE

phe·nyt·o·in \fə-'ni-tə-wən\ *n* : an anticonvulsant used often in the form of its sodium salt $C_{15}H_{11}N_2NaO_2$ to prevent or treat seizures — called also *diphenylhydantoin;* see DILANTIN

pheo·chro·mo·cy·to·ma \ˌfē-ə-ˌkrō-mə-sə-ˈtō-mə, -ˌsī-\ *n, pl* **-mas** *also* **-ma·ta** \-mə-tə\ : a tumor that is derived from chromaffin cells and is usu. associated with paroxysmal or sustained hypertension

pher·e·sis \fə-ˈrē-səs\ *n, pl* **pher·e·ses** \-ˌsēz\ : APHERESIS

pher·o·mone \ˈfer-ə-ˌmōn\ *n* : a chemical substance that is produced by an animal and serves esp. as a stimulus to other individuals of the same species for one or more behavioral responses — **pher·o·mon·al** \ˌfer-ə-ˈmōn-ᵊl\ *adj*

PhG *abbr* graduate in pharmacy

phi·al \ˈfīl\ *n* : VIAL

Phi·a·loph·o·ra \ˌfī-ə-ˈlä-fə-rə\ *n* : a genus of imperfect fungi (family Dematiaceae) of which some forms are important in human mycotic infections (as chromoblastomycosis)

¹phil \ˌfil\ *or* **-phile** \ˌfil\ *n comb form* : lover : one having an affinity for or a strong attraction to ⟨acido*phil*⟩

²phil *or* **-phile** *adj comb form* : loving : having a fondness or affinity for ⟨hemo*phile*⟩

Philadelphia chromosome *n* : an abnormally short chromosome 22 that is found in the hematopoietic cells of persons affected with chronic myelogenous leukemia and lacks the major part of its long arm which has usu. undergone translocation to chromosome 9

-phil·ia \ˈfi-lē-ə\ *n comb form* **1** : tendency toward ⟨hemo*philia*⟩ **2** : abnormal appetite or liking for ⟨necro*philia*⟩

-phil·i·ac \ˈfi-lē-ˌak\ *n comb form* **1** : one having a tendency toward ⟨hemo*philiac*⟩ **2** : one having an abnormal appetite or liking for ⟨copro*philiac*⟩

-phil·ic \ˈfi-lik\ *adj comb form* : having an affinity for : loving ⟨acido*philic*⟩

phil·trum \ˈfil-trəm\ *n, pl* **phil·tra** \-trə\ : the vertical groove on the median line of the upper lip

phi·mo·sis \fī-ˈmō-səs, fi-\ *n, pl* **phi·mo·ses** \-ˌsēz\ : tightness or constriction of the orifice of the foreskin arising either congenitally or postnatally (as from balanoposthitis) and preventing retraction of the foreskin over the glans

phi phenomenon \ˈfī-\ *n* : apparent motion resulting from an orderly sequence of stimuli (as lights flashed in rapid succession a short distance apart on a sign) without any actual motion being presented to the eye

phleb- *or* **phlebo-** *comb form* : vein ⟨*phleb*itis⟩

phle·bi·tis \fli-ˈbī-təs\ *n, pl* **phle·bit·i·des** \-ˈbi-tə-ˌdēz\ : inflammation of a vein — **phle·bit·ic** \-ˈbi-tik\ *adj*

phle·bo·gram \ˈflē-bə-ˌgram\ *n* **1** : a tracing made with a sphygmograph that records the pulse in a vein **2** : a radiograph of a vein after injection of a radiopaque medium

phle·bo·graph \-ˌgraf\ *n* : a sphygmograph adapted for recording the venous pulse

phle·bog·ra·phy \fli-ˈbä-grə-fē\ *n, pl* **-phies** : the process of making phlebograms — **phle·bo·graph·ic** \ˌflē-bə-ˈgra-fik\ *adj*

phle·bo·lith \ˈflē-bə-ˌlith\ *n* : a calculus in a vein usu. resulting from the calcification of an old thrombus

phle·bol·o·gist \fli-ˈbä-lə-jist\ *n* : a specialist in phlebology

phle·bol·o·gy \fli-ˈbä-lə-jē\ *n, pl* **-gies** : a branch of medicine concerned with the veins

phle·bo·throm·bo·sis \ˌflē-bō-thräm-ˈbō-səs, *n, pl* **-bo·ses** \-ˌsēz\ : venous thrombosis accompanied by little or no inflammation — compare THROMBOPHLEBITIS

phle·bot·o·mist \fli-ˈbä-tə-mist\ *n* : one who practices phlebotomy

phle·bot·o·mize \fli-ˈbä-tə-ˌmīz\ *vb* **-mized; -miz·ing** : to draw blood from : BLEED

phle·bot·o·mus \fli-ˈbä-tə-məs\ *n* **1** *cap* : a genus of small bloodsucking sand flies (family Psychodidae) including one (*P. papatasii*) that is a vector of sandfly fever and leishmaniasis **2** *pl* **-mi** \-ˌmī\ *also* **-mus·es** : any sand fly of the genus *Phlebotomus*

phlebotomus fever *n* : SANDFLY FEVER

phle·bot·o·my \fli-ˈbä-tə-mē\ *n, pl* **-mies** : the letting of blood for transfusion, apheresis, diagnostic testing, or experimental procedures and widely used in the past to treat many types of disease but now limited to the treatment of only a few specific conditions (as hemochromatosis and polycythemia vera) — called also venesection, venotomy

Phle·bo·vi·rus \ˈflē-bə-ˌvī-rəs\ *n* : a genus of bunyaviruses including the causative agents of Rift Valley fever and sandfly fever

phlegm \ˈflem\ *n* : viscid mucus secreted in abnormal quantity in the respiratory passages

phleg·ma·sia \fleg-ˈmā-zhə, -zhē-ə\ *n, pl* **-siae** \-zhē, -zhē-ˌē\ : INFLAMMATION

phlegmasia al·ba do·lens \-ˈal-bə-ˈdō-ˌlenz\ *n* : MILK LEG

phlegmasia ce·ru·lea dolens \-sə-ˈrü-lē-ə-\ *n* : severe thrombophlebitis with extreme pain, edema, cyanosis, and possible ischemic necrosis

phleg·mon \ˈfleg-ˌmän\ *n* : purulent inflammation and infiltration of connective tissue — compare ABSCESS — **phleg·mon·ous** \ˈfleg-mə-nəs\ *adj*

phlor·e·tin \ˈflōr-ət-ən, flə-ˈrēt-ᵊn\ *n* : a crystalline phenolic ketone $C_{15}H_{14}O_5$ that is a potent inhibitor of transport systems for sugars and anions

phlo·ri·zin *or* **phlo·rhi·zin** \ˈflōr-ə-zən,

flə-'rīz-ʰ°n\ *or* phlo·rid·zin \'flȯr-əd-zən, flə-'rid-zən\ *n* : a bitter crystalline glucoside $C_{21}H_{24}O_{10}$ used chiefly in producing experimental diabetes in animals

phlyc·ten·u·lar \flik-'ten-yə-lər\ *adj* : marked by or associated with phlyctenules ⟨~ conjunctivitis⟩

phlyc·te·nule \flik-'ten-(ˌ)yül; 'flik-tə-ˌnül, -ˌnyül\ *n* : a small vesicle or pustule; *esp* : one on the conjunctiva or cornea of the eye

PHN *abbr* public health nurse

-phobe \ˌfōb\ *n comb form* : one fearing or averse to (something specified) ⟨chromo*phobe*⟩

pho·bia \'fō-bē-ə\ *n* : an exaggerated and often disabling fear usu. inexplicable to the subject and having sometimes a logical but usu. an illogical or symbolic object, class of objects, or situation — compare COMPULSION, OBSESSION

-pho·bia \'fō-bē-ə\ *n comb form* 1 : abnormal fear of ⟨acro*phobia*⟩ 2 : intolerance or aversion for ⟨photo*phobia*⟩

pho·bi·ac \'fō-bē-ˌak\ *n* : PHOBIC

¹pho·bic \'fō-bik\ *adj* : of, relating to, affected with, marked by, involving, or constituting a phobia ⟨~ disorders⟩ ⟨~ patients⟩

²phobic *n* : one who exhibits a phobia

-pho·bic \'fō-bik\ *or* -pho·bous \f-ə-bəs\ *adj comb form* 1 : having an aversion for or fear of ⟨agora*phobic*⟩ 2 : lacking affinity for ⟨hydro*phobic*⟩

phobic reaction *n* : a psychoneurosis in which the principal symptom is a phobia

pho·co·me·lia \ˌfō-kə-'mē-lē-ə\ *n* : a congenital deformity in which the limbs are extremely shortened so that the feet and hands arise close to the trunk — pho·co·me·lic \-'mē-lik\ *adj*

pho·com·e·lus \fō-'kä-mə-ləs\ *n, pl* -li \-ˌlī\ : an individual exhibiting phocomelia

phon \'fän\ *n* : the unit of loudness on a scale beginning at zero for the faintest audible sound and corresponding to the decibel scale of sound intensity with the number of phons of a given sound being equal to the decibels of a pure 1000-hertz tone judged by the average listener to be equal in loudness to the given sound

phon- *or* phono- *comb form* : sound : voice : speech : tone ⟨*phonation*⟩

pho·na·tion \fō-'nā-shən\ *n* : the production of vocal sounds and esp. speech — pho·nate \'fō-ˌnāt\ *vb*

-pho·nia \'fō-nē-ə, 'fōn-yə\ *or* -pho·ny \fə-nē\ *n comb form, pl* -phonias *or* -phonies : speech disorder (of a specified type esp. relating to phonation) ⟨dys*phonia*⟩

pho·no·car·dio·gram \ˌfō-nə-'kär-dē-ə-ˌgram\ *n* : a graphic record of heart sounds made by means of a phonocardiograph

pho·no·car·dio·graph \-ˌgraf\ *n* : an instrument used for producing a graphic record of heart sounds

pho·no·car·di·og·ra·phy \-ˌkär-dē-'ä-grə-fē\ *n, pl* -phies : the recording of heart sounds by means of a phonocardiograph — pho·no·car·dio·graph·ic \-ˌkär-dē-ə-'gra-fik\ *adj*

phor·bol \'fȯr-ˌbȯl, -ˌbōl\ *n* : an alcohol $C_{20}H_{28}O_6$ that is the parent compound of tumor-promoting esters occurring in croton oil

-pho·re·sis \fō-'rē-səs\ *n comb form, pl* -pho·re·ses \-ˌsēz\ : transmission ⟨electro*phoresis*⟩

pho·ria \'fō-rē-ə\ *n* : any of various tendencies of the lines of vision to deviate from the normal when binocular fusion of the retinal images is prevented

-pho·ria \'fȯr-ē-ə\ *n comb form* : bearing : state : tendency ⟨eu*phoria*⟩

-phor·ic \'fȯr-ik\ *adj comb form* : having (such) a bearing or tendency ⟨thanato*phoric*⟩

Phor·mia \'fȯr-mē-ə\ *n* : a genus of dipteran flies (family Calliphoridae) including one (*P. regina*) causing myiasis in sheep

phos- *comb form* : light ⟨*phosphene*⟩

phos·gene \'fäz-ˌjēn\ *n* : a colorless gas $COCl_2$ of unpleasant odor that is a severe respiratory irritant and has been used in chemical warfare

phosph- *or* phospho- *comb form* : phosphoric acid : phosphate ⟨*phospholipid*⟩

phos·pha·gen \'fäs-fə-jən, -ˌjen\ *n* : any of several phosphate compounds (as phosphocreatine) occurring esp. in muscle and releasing energy on hydrolysis of the phosphate

phos·pha·tase \'fäs-fə-ˌtās, -ˌtāz\ *n* : an enzyme that accelerates the hydrolysis and synthesis of organic esters of phosphoric acid and the transfer of phosphate groups to other compounds: **a** : ALKALINE PHOSPHATASE **b** : ACID PHOSPHATASE

phos·phate \'fäs-ˌfāt\ *n* **1 a** : a salt or ester of a phosphoric acid **b** : the negatively charged ion $PO_4{}^{3-}$ having a chemical valence of three and derived from phosphoric acid H_3PO_4 **2** : an organic compound of phosphoric acid in which the acid group is bound to nitrogen or a carboxyl group in a way that permits useful energy to be released (as in metabolism)

phos·pha·tide \'fäs-fə-ˌtīd\ *n* : PHOSPHOLIPID

phos·pha·tid·ic acid \ˌfäs-fə-'ti-dik-\ *n* : any of several acids $(RCOO)_2C_3H_5O-PO_3H_2$ that are formed from phosphatides and yield on hydrolysis two fatty-acid molecules RCOOH and one molecule each of glycerol and phosphoric acid

phos·pha·ti·dyl·cho·line \ˌfäs-fə-ˌtīd-ᵊl-'kō-ˌlēn, (ˌ)fäs-ˌfa-təd-ᵊl-\ *n* : LECITHIN

phos·pha·ti·dyl·eth·a·nol·amine \-ˌe-thə-'nä-lə-,mēn, -'nō-\ *n* : any of a group of phospholipids that occur esp. in blood plasma and in the white matter of the central nervous system — called also *cephalin*

phos·pha·ti·dyl·ser·ine \-'ser-,ēn\ *n* : a phospholipid found in mammalian cells

phos·pha·tu·ria \,fäs-fə-'tür-ē-ə, -'tyür-\ *n* : the excretion of excessive amounts of phosphates in the urine

phos·phene \'fäs-,fēn\ *n* : a sensation of light produced by stimulation of the retina (as by pressure on the eyeball when the lid is closed)

phospho- — see PHOSPH-

phos·pho·cre·atine \,fäs-(,)fō-'krē-ə-,tēn\ *n* : a compound $C_4H_{10}N_3O_5P$ of creatine and phosphoric acid that is found esp. in vertebrate muscle where it is an energy source for muscle contraction — called also *creatine phosphate*

phos·pho·di·es·ter·ase \-,dī-'es-tə-,rās, -,rāz\ *n* : a phosphatase that acts on compounds (as some nucleotides) having two ester groups to hydrolyze only one of the groups

phos·pho·di·es·ter bond \-,dī-'es-tər-\ *n* : a covalent bond in RNA or DNA that holds a polynucleotide chain together by joining a phosphate group at position 5 in the pentose sugar of one nucleotide to the hydroxyl group at position 3 in the pentose sugar of the next nucleotide — called also *phosphodiester linkage*

phos·pho·enol·pyr·uvate \'fäs-,fō-ə-,nōl-pī-'rü-,vāt, -nōl-, -,pīr-'yü-\ *n* : a salt or ester of phosphoenolpyruvic acid

phos·pho·enol·pyr·uvic acid \-pī-'rü-vik-, -,pīr-'yü-vik\ *n* : a phosphate $H_2C=C(OPO_3H_2)COOH$ formed as an intermediate in carbohydrate metabolism

phos·pho·fruc·to·ki·nase \,fäs-(,)fō-,frək-tō-'kī-,nās, -,frük-, -,frük-, -,nāz\ *n* : an enzyme that functions in carbohydrate metabolism and esp. in glycolysis by catalyzing the transfer of a second phosphate (as from ATP) to fructose

phos·pho·glu·co·mu·tase \-,glü-kō-'myü-,tās, -,tāz\ *n* : an enzyme that catalyzes the reversible isomerization of glucose-1-phosphate to glucose-6-phosphate

phos·pho·glu·co·nate \-'glü-kə-,nāt\ *n* : a compound formed by dehydrogenation of glucose-6-phosphate as the first step in a glucose degradation pathway alternative to the Krebs cycle

phosphogluconate dehydrogenase *n* : an enzyme that catalyzes the oxidative decarboxylation of phosphogluconate with the generation of NADPH

phos·pho·glyc·er·al·de·hyde \-,gli-sə-'ral-də-,hīd\ *n* : a phosphate of glyceraldehyde $C_3H_5O_3(H_2PO_3)$ that is

formed esp. in anaerobic metabolism of carbohydrates by the splitting of a diphosphate of fructose

phos·pho·ino·si·tide \-i-'nō-sə-,tīd\ *n* : any of a group of inositol-containing derivatives of phosphatidic acid that do not contain nitrogen and are found in the brain

phos·pho·ki·nase \,fäs-fō-'kī-,nās, -,nāz\ *n* : KINASE

phos·pho·li·pase \-'lī-,pās, -,pāz\ *n* : any of several enzymes that hydrolyze lecithins or phosphatidylethanolamines — called also *lecithinase*

phos·pho·lip·id \-'li-pəd\ *n* : any of numerous lipids (as lecithins and phosphatidylethanolamines) in which phosphoric acid as well as a fatty acid is esterified to glycerol and which are found in all living cells and in the bilayers of plasma membranes — called also *phosphatide*

phos·pho·lip·in \-'li-pən\ *n* : PHOSPHOLIPID

phos·pho·mono·es·ter·ase \-,mä-nō-'es-tə-,rās, -,rāz\ *n* : a phosphatase that acts on esters containing only a single ester group

phos·pho·pro·tein \,fäs-fō-'prō-,tēn\ *n* : any of various proteins (as casein) that contain combined phosphoric acid

phosphor- *or* **phosphoro-** *comb form* : phosphoric acid ⟨*phosphoro*lysis⟩

phos·pho·ri·bo·syl·py·ro·phos·phate \,fäs-fō-,rī-bə-,sil-,pī-rō-'fäs-,fāt\ *n* : a substance that is formed enzymatically from ATP and the phosphate of ribose and that plays a fundamental role in nucleotide synthesis

phosphoribosyltransferase — see HYPOXANTHINE-GUANINE PHOSPHO-RIBOSYLTRANSFERASE

phos·pho·ric \fäs-'fȯr-ik, -'fär-; 'fäs-fə-rik\ *adj* : of, relating to, or containing phosphorus esp. with a valence higher than in phosphorous compounds

phosphoric acid *n* 1 : a syrupy or deliquescent acid H_3PO_4 — called also *orthophosphoric acid* 2 : a compound consisting of phosphate groups linked directly to each other by oxygen

phos·pho·rol·y·sis \,fäs-fə-'rä-lə-səs\ *n*, *pl* **-y·ses** \-,sēz\ : a reversible reaction analogous to hydrolysis in which phosphoric acid functions in a manner similar to that of water with the formation of a phosphate (as glucose-1-phosphate in the breakdown of liver glycogen) — **phos·pho·ro·lyt·ic** \-rō-'li-tik\ *adj*

phos·pho·rous \'fäs-fə-rəs, fäs-'fȯr-əs\ *adj* : of, relating to, or containing phosphorus esp. with a valence lower than in phosphoric compounds

phos·pho·rus \'fäs-fə-rəs\ *n*, *often attrib* : a nonmetallic element that occurs widely in combined form esp. as inorganic phosphates in minerals, soils, natural waters, bones, and teeth and as organic phosphates in all living cells — symbol *P;* see ELEMENT table

phosphorus 32 *n* : a heavy radioactive isotope of phosphorus having a mass number of 32 and a half-life of 14.3 days that is produced in nuclear reactors and used chiefly in tracer studies (as in biology and in chemical analysis) and in medical diagnosis (as in location of tumors) — symbol P^{32} or ^{32}P

phos·phor·y·lase \fäs-'fôr-ə-ˌlāz\ *n* : any of a group of enzymes that catalyze phosphorolysis with the formation of organic phosphates (as glucose-1-phosphate in the breakdown and synthesis of glycogen)

phos·phor·y·la·tion \ˌfäs-ˌfôr-ə-'lā-shən\ *n* : the process by which a chemical compound takes up or combines with phosphoric acid or a phosphorus-containing group; *esp* : the enzymatic conversion of carbohydrates into their phosphoric esters in metabolic processes — **phos·phor·y·late** \fäs-'fôr-ə-ˌlāt\ *vb* — **phos·phor·y·la·tive** \fäs-'fôr-ə-ˌlā-tiv\ *adj*

phos·pho·ryl·cho·line \ˌfäs-fə-ˌril-'kō-ˌlēn\ *n* : a hapten used medicinally in the form of its chloride $C_5H_{15}ClNO_4P$ to treat hepatobiliary dysfunction

phos·pho·trans·fer·ase \ˌfäs-fō-'trans-(ˌ)fər-ˌās, -ˌāz\ *n* : any of several enzymes that catalyze the transfer of phosphorus-containing groups from one compound to another

phos·sy jaw \'fä-sē-\ *n* : a jawbone destroyed by chronic phosphorus poisoning

phot- *or* **photo-** *comb form* : light : radiant energy *photo*dermatitis\

pho·tic \'fō-tik\ *adj* : of, relating to, or involving light esp. in relation to organisms — **pho·ti·cal·ly** *adv*

pho·to·ac·ti·va·tion \ˌfō-tō-ˌak-tə-'vā-shən\ *n* : the process of activating a substance by means of radiant energy and esp. light — **pho·to·ac·ti·vate** \-'ak-tə-ˌvāt\ *vb*

photoactive \-'ak-tiv\ *adj* : physically or chemically responsive to radiant energy and esp. to light — **pho·to·ac·tiv·i·ty** \-ˌak-'ti-və-tē\ *n, pl*

pho·to·ag·ing \fō-tō-'ā-jiŋ\ *n* : the cumulative detrimental effects (as wrinkles or dark spots) on skin that result from long-term exposure to sunlight and esp. ultraviolet light — **pho·to·aged** \-'ājd\ *adj*

pho·to·al·ler·gic \ˌfō-tō-ə-'lər-jik\ *adj* : of, relating to, caused by, or affected with a photoallergy \~ dermatitis\

pho·to·al·ler·gy \-'a-lər-jē\ *n, pl* **-gies** : an allergic sensitivity to light

pho·to·bi·ol·o·gy \-(ˌ)bī-'ä-lə-jē\ *n, pl* **-gies** : a branch of biology that deals with the effects of radiant energy (as light) on living things — **pho·to·bi·o·o·gist** \ˌfō-tō-(ˌ)bī-'ä-lə-jist\ *n*

pho·to·chem·i·cal \ˌfō-tō-'ke-mi-kəl\ *adj* : of, relating to, or resulting from the chemical action of radiant energy and esp. light \~ smog\

pho·to·che·mo·ther·a·py \-ˌkē-mō-'ther-ə-pē\ *n, pl* **-pies** : treatment esp. for psoriasis in which administration of a photosensitizing drug (as psoralen) is followed by exposure to ultraviolet radiation or sunlight

¹pho·to·chro·mic \ˌfō-tə-'krō-mik\ *adj* **1** : capable of changing color on exposure to radiant energy (as light) \eyeglasses with ~ lenses\ **2** : of, relating to, or utilizing the change of color shown by a photochromic substance \a ~ process\ — **pho·to·chro·mism** \-ˌmi-zəm\ *n*

²photochromic *n* : a photochromic substance — usu. used in pl.

pho·to·co·ag·u·la·tion \-kō-ˌa·gyə-'lā-shən\ *n* : a surgical process of coagulating tissue by means of a precisely oriented high-energy light source (as a laser beam) — **pho·to·co·ag·u·la·tor** \-kō-'a·gyə-ˌlā-tər\ *n*

pho·to·con·vul·sive \ˌfō-tō-kən-'vəl-siv\ *adj* : of, relating to, being, or marked by an abnormal electroencephalographic response to a flickering light

pho·to·dam·age \-'da-mij\ *n* : damage (as to skin or DNA) caused by exposure to ultraviolet radiation — **pho·to·dam·aged** \-mijd\ *adj*

pho·to·der·ma·ti·tis \-ˌdər-mə-'tī-təs\ *n, pl* **-ti·tis·es** *or* **-tit·i·des** \'ti-tə-ˌdēz\ : any dermatitis caused or precipitated by exposure to light

pho·to·der·ma·to·sis \-ˌdər-mə-'tō-səs\ *n, pl* **-to·ses** \-ˌsēz\ : any dermatosis produced by exposure to light

pho·to·dy·nam·ic \-dī-'na-mik\ *adj* : of, relating to, or having the property of intensifying or inducing a toxic reaction to light (as the destruction of cancer cells stained with a light-sensitive dye) in a living system \~ therapy\

pho·to·flu·o·rog·ra·phy \-(ˌ)flü-ə-'rä-grə-fē\ *n, pl* **-phies** : the photography of the image produced on a fluorescent screen by X-rays — **pho·to·flu·o·ro·graph·ic** \-ˌflür-ə-'gra-fik\ *adj*

Pho·to·frin \'fō-tə-frin\ *trademark* — used for a preparation of porfimer sodium

pho·to·gen·ic \ˌfō-tə-'je-nik\ *adj* **1** : produced or precipitated by light \~ dermatitis\ **2** : producing or generating light \~ bacteria\

pho·to·ker·a·ti·tis \ˌfō-tō-ˌker-ə-'ti-təs\ *n, pl* **-tit·i·des** \-'ti-tə-ˌdēz\ : keratitis of the cornea caused by exposure to ultraviolet radiation

pho·tom·e·ter \fō-'tä-mə-tər\ *n* : an instrument for measuring the intensity of light

pho·to·mi·cro·graph \ˌfō-tə-'mī-krə-ˌgraf\ *n* : a photograph of a microscopic image — called also *microphotograph* — **pho·to·mi·cro·graph·ic** \-ˌmī-krə-'gra-fik\ *adj* — **pho·to·mi·cro·graph·i·cal·ly** *adv* — **pho·to·mi·crog·ra·phy** \-mī-'krä-grə-fē\ *n*

pho·ton \'fō-ˌtän\ *n* **1** : a unit of intensity of light at the retina equal to the illumination received per square millimeter of a pupillary area from a surface having a brightness of one candela per square meter — called also *troland* **2** : a quantum of electromagnetic radiation — **pho·ton·ic** \fō-'tä-nik\ *adj*

pho·to·patch test \'fō-tō-ˌpach-\ *n* : a test of the capability of a particular substance to photosensitize a particular human skin in which the substance is applied to the skin under a patch and the area is irradiated with ultraviolet light

pho·to·phe·re·sis \ˌfō-tō-fə-'rē-səs\ *n* : an immunomodulating therapy used esp. to treat cutaneous T-cell lymphomas that involves treating blood with a photoactive drug (as methoxsalen), obtaining a fraction rich in white blood cells, exposing the fraction to damaging ultraviolet radiation, and returning it to the body where it stimulates a therapeutic immunological response

pho·to·pho·bia \ˌfō-tə-'fō-bē-ə\ *n* **1** : intolerance to light; *esp* : painful sensitiveness to strong light **2** : an abnormal fear of light — **pho·to·pho·bic** \-'fō-bik\ *adj*

phot·oph·thal·mia \ˌfōt-ˌäf-'thal-mē-ə, -ˌäp-\ *n* : inflammation of the eye and esp. of the cornea and conjunctiva caused by exposure to light of short wavelength (as ultraviolet light)

phot·opic \fōt-'ō-pik, -'ä-\ *adj* : relating to or being vision in bright light with light-adapted eyes that is mediated by the cones of the retina

pho·to·pig·ment \'fō-tō-ˌpig-mənt\ *n* : a pigment (as a compound in the retina) that undergoes a physical or chemical change under the action of light

pho·top·sia \fō-'täp-sē-ə\ *n* : the perception of light (as luminous rays or flashes) that is purely subjective and accompanies a pathological condition esp. of the retina or brain

pho·to·re·cep·tor \ˌfō-tō-ri-'sep-tər\ *n* : a receptor for light stimuli

pho·to·re·frac·tive keratectomy \-ri-ˌfrak-tiv-\ *n* : surgical ablation of part of the corneal surface using an excimer laser in order to correct for myopia — abbr. *PRK;* compare RADIAL KERATOTOMY

pho·to·scan \'fō-tō-ˌskan\ *n* : a photographic representation of variation in tissue state (as of the kidney) determined by gamma ray emission from an injected radioactive substance — **photoscan** *vb*

pho·to·sen·si·tive \ˌfō-tō-'sen-sə-tiv\ *adj* **1** : sensitive or sensitized to the action of radiant energy **2** : being or caused by an abnormal reaction to sunlight ⟨~ rashes⟩ — **pho·to·sen·si·tiv·i·ty** \-ˌsen-sə-'ti-və-tē\ *n*

pho·to·sen·si·tize \-'sen-sə-ˌtīz\ *vb* **-tized; -tiz·ing** : to make sensitive to the influence of radiant energy and esp. light — **pho·to·sen·si·ti·za·tion** \-ˌsen-sə-tə-'zā-shən\ *n* — **pho·to·sen·si·tiz·er** *n*

pho·to·syn·the·sis \-'sin-thə-səs\ *n, pl* **-the·ses** \-ˌsēz\ : the formation of carbohydrates from carbon dioxide and a source of hydrogen (as water) in chlorophyll-containing cells (as of green plants) exposed to light — **pho·to·syn·the·size** \-ˌsīz\ *vb* — **pho·to·syn·thet·ic** \-sin-'the-tik\ *adj*

pho·to·ther·a·py \-'ther-ə-pē\ *n, pl* **-pies** : the application of light for therapeutic purposes

pho·to·tox·ic \ˌfō-tō-'täk-sik\ *adj* **1** : rendering the skin susceptible to damage (as sunburn or blisters) upon exposure to light and esp. ultraviolet light ⟨~ antibiotics⟩ **2** : induced by a phototoxic substance ⟨a ~ response⟩ — **pho·to·tox·ic·i·ty** \-täk-'si-sə-tē\ *n*

phren- *or* **phreno-** *comb form* **1** : mind ⟨*phren*ology⟩ **2** : diaphragm ⟨*phren*ic⟩

phren·em·phrax·is \ˌfren-ˌem-'frak-səs\ *n, pl* **-phrax·es** \-ˌsēz\ : crushing of the phrenic nerve for therapeutic purposes

phreni- *comb form* : phrenic nerve ⟨*phreni*cotomy⟩

-phre·nia \'frē-nē-ə, 'fre-\ *n comb form* : disordered condition of mental functions ⟨hebe*phrenia*⟩

¹phren·ic \'fre-nik\ *adj* : of or relating to the diaphragm

²phrenic *n* : PHRENIC NERVE

phrenic artery *n* : any of the several arteries supplying the diaphragm: **a** : either of two arising from the thoracic aorta and distributed over the upper surface of the diaphragm — called also *superior phrenic artery* **b** : either of two that arise from the abdominal aorta and that supply the underside of the diaphragm and the adrenal glands — called also *inferior phrenic artery*

phren·i·cec·to·my \ˌfre-nə-'sek-tə-mē\ *n, pl* **-mies** : surgical removal of part of a phrenic nerve to secure collapse of a diseased lung by paralyzing the diaphragm on one side — compare PHRENICOTOMY

phrenic nerve *n* : a nerve on each side of the body that arises chiefly from the fourth cervical nerve, passes down through the thorax to the diaphragm, and supplies or gives off branches supplying esp. the pericardium, pleura, and diaphragm — called also *phrenic*

phren·i·cot·o·my \ˌfre-ni-'kä-tə-mē\ *n, pl* **-mies** : surgical division of a phrenic nerve to secure collapse of a diseased lung by paralyzing the diaphragm on one side — compare PHRENICECTOMY

phrenic vein *n* : any of the veins that drain the diaphragm and accompany the phrenic arteries: **a** : one that accompanies the pericardiophrenic artery and usu. empties into the internal thoracic vein — called also *superior phrenic vein* **b** : any of two or three veins which follow the course of the inferior phrenic arteries and of which the one on the right empties into the inferior vena cava and the one or two on the left empty into the left renal or suprarenal vein or the inferior vena cava — called also *inferior phrenic vein*

phreno- — see PHREN-

phre·nol·o·gy \fri-'nä-lə-jē\ *n, pl* **-gies** : the study of the conformation of the skull based on the belief that it is indicative of mental faculties and character — **phre·nol·o·gist** \fri-'nä-lə-jist\ *n*

phry·no·der·ma \,frī-nə-'dər-mə\ *n* : a rough dry skin eruption marked by keratosis and usu. associated with vitamin A deficiency

PHS *abbr* Public Health Service

phthal·yl·sul·fa·thi·a·zole \,tha-,lil-,səl-fə-'thī-ə-,zōl\ *n* : a sulfonamide $C_{17}H_{13}N_3O_5S_2$ used in the treatment of intestinal infections

phthi·ri·a·sis \thə-'rī-ə-səs, thī-\ *n, pl* **-a·ses** \-,sēz\ : PEDICULOSIS; *esp* : infestation with crab lice

Phthir·i·us \'thir-ē-əs\ *n* : a genus of lice (family Phthiriidae) containing the crab louse (*P. pubis*)

Phthi·rus \'thī-rəs\ *n, syn of* PHTHIRIUS

phthi·sic \'ti-zik, 'tī-sik\ *n* : PHTHISIS — **phthisic** *or* **phthi·si·cal** \'ti-zi-kəl, 'tī-si-\ *adj*

phthisio- *comb form* : phthisis ⟨*phthisiology*⟩

phthis·i·ol·o·gy \,ti-zē-'ä-lə-jē, ,thī-\ *n, pl* **-gies** : the care, treatment, and study of tuberculosis — **phthis·i·ol·o·gist** \-jist\ *n*

phthi·sis \'tī-səs, 'thī-, 'ti-, 'thī-\ *n, pl* **phthi·ses** \-,sēz\ : a progressively wasting or consumptive condition; *esp* : pulmonary tuberculosis

phthisis bul·bi \-'bəl-,bī\ *n* : wasting and shrinkage of the eyeball following destructive diseases of the eye (as panophthalmitis)

phy·co·my·cete \,fī-kō-'mī-,sēt, -,mī-'sēt\ *n* : any of a group of lower fungi that are in many respects similar to algae and are often grouped in a class (Phycomycetes) or separated into two subdivisions (Mastigomycotina and Zygomycotina)

phy·co·my·co·sis \-,mī-'kō-səs\ *n, pl* **-co·ses** \-'kō-,sēz\ : any mycosis caused by a phycomycete (as of the genera *Rhizopus* and *Mucor*)

phyl- *or* **phylo-** *comb form* : tribe : race : phylum ⟨*phylogeny*⟩

phyl·lode \'fi-,lōd\ *adj* : having a cross section that resembles a leaf ⟨∼ tumors of the breast⟩

phyl·lo·qui·none \,fi-lō-kwi-'nōn, -'kwi-,nōn\ *n* : VITAMIN K 1a

phy·log·e·ny \fī-'lä-jə-nē\ *n, pl* **-nies** **1** : the evolutionary history of a kind of organism **2** : the evolution of a genetically related group of organisms as distinguished from the development of the individual organism — compare ONTOGENY — **phy·lo·ge·net·ic** \,fī-lō-jə-'ne-tik\ *adj* — **phy·lo·ge·net·i·cal·ly** *adv*

phy·lum \'fī-ləm\ *n, pl* **phy·la** \-lə\ : a major group of animals or in some classifications plants sharing one or more fundamental characteristics that set them apart from all other animals and plants

phys *abbr* **1** physical **2** physician **3** physiological

phy·sa·lia \fī-'sā-lē-ə\ *n* **1** *cap* : a genus of large oceanic siphonophores (family Physaliidae) including the Portuguese man-of-wars **2** : any siphonophore of the genus *Physalia*

Phy·sa·lop·tera \,fī-sə-'läp-tə-rə, ,fi-\ *n* : a large genus of nematode worms (family Physalopteridae) parasitic in the digestive tract of various vertebrates including humans

physes *pl of* PHYSIS

physi- *or* **physio-** *comb form* **1** : physical ⟨*physio*therapy⟩ **2** : physiological : physiological and ⟨*physio*pathologic⟩

phys·i·at·rics \,fi-zē-'a-triks\ *n* : PHYSICAL MEDICINE AND REHABILITATION

phys·i·at·rist \,fi-zē-'a-trist\ *n* : a physician who specializes in physical medicine and rehabilitation

phys·i·at·ry \,fi-zē-'a-trē, fə-'zī-ə-trē\ *n* : PHYSICAL MEDICINE AND REHABILITATION

¹phys·ic \'fi-zik\ *n* **1 a** : the art or practice of healing disease **b** : the practice or profession of medicine **2** : a medicinal agent or preparation; *esp* : PURGATIVE

²physic *vb* **phys·icked; phys·ick·ing** : to treat with or administer medicine to; *esp* : PURGE

¹phys·i·cal \'fi-zi-kəl\ *adj* **1** : having material existence : perceptible esp. through the senses and subject to the laws of nature **2** : of or relating to the body — **phys·i·cal·ly** *adv*

²physical *n* : PHYSICAL EXAMINATION

physical examination *n* : an examination of the bodily functions and condition of an individual

physical medicine and rehabilitation *n* : a medical specialty concerned with the prevention, diagnosis, treatment, and management of disabling diseases, disorders, and injuries typically of a musculoskeletal, cardiovascular, neuromuscular, or neurological nature by physical means (as by the use of electromyography, electrotherapy, therapeutic exercise, or pharmaceutical pain control) — called also *physiatrics, physiatry, physical medicine*

physical sign *n* : an indication of bodily condition that can be directly perceived

physical therapist *n* : a person trained and licensed to practice physical therapy — called also *physiotherapist*

physical therapy *n* : therapy for the preservation, enhancement, or restoration of movement and physical function impaired or threatened by disability, injury, or disease that utilizes therapeutic exercise, physical modalities (as massage and electrotherapy), assistive devices, and patient education and training — called also *physiotherapy*

phy·si·cian \fə-ˈzi-shən\ *n* : a skilled health-care professional trained and licensed to practice medicine; *specif* : a doctor of medicine or osteopathy

physician–assisted suicide *n* : suicide by a patient facilitated by means (as a drug prescription) or by information (as an indication of lethal dosage) provided by a physician aware of the patient's intent

physician's assistant *or* **physician assistant** *n* : a specially trained person who is certified to provide basic medical services (as the diagnosis and treatment of common ailments) usu. under the supervision of a licensed physician — called also *PA*

phys·i·co·chem·i·cal \ˌfi-zi-kō-ˈke-mi-kəl\ *adj* : being physical and chemical — **phys·i·co·chem·i·cal·ly** *adv*

physio- — see PHYSI-

phys·i·o·log·i·cal \ˌfi-zē-ə-ˈlä-ji-kəl\ *or* **phys·i·o·log·ic** \-jik\ *adj* **1** : of or relating to physiology **2** : characteristic of or appropriate to an organism's healthy or normal functioning **3** : differing in, involving, or affecting physiological factors ⟨a ~ strain of bacteria⟩ — **phys·i·o·log·i·cal·ly** *adv*

physiological chemistry *n* : a branch of science dealing with the chemical aspects of physiological and biological systems : BIOCHEMISTRY

physiological dead space *n* : the total dead space in the entire respiratory system including the alveoli — compare ANATOMICAL DEAD SPACE

physiological psychology *n* : PSYCHOPHYSIOLOGY

physiological saline *n* : a solution of a salt or salts that is essentially isotonic with tissue fluids or blood; *esp* : an approximately 0.9 percent solution of sodium chloride — called also *physiological saline solution, physiological salt solution*

phys·i·ol·o·gy \ˌfi-zē-ˈä-lə-jē\ *n, pl* **-gies 1** : a branch of biology that deals with the functions and activities of life or of living matter (as organs, tissues, or cells) and of the physical and chemical phenomena involved — compare ANATOMY 1, MORPHOLOGY 1 **2** : the organic processes and phenomena of an organism or any of its parts or of a particular bodily process **3** : a treatise on physiology — **phys·i·ol·o·gist** \-jist\ *n*

phys·io·pa·thol·o·gy \ˌfi-zē-ō-pə-ˈthä-lə-jē, -pa-\ *n, pl* **-gies** : a branch of biology or medicine that combines physiology and pathology esp. in the study of altered bodily function in disease — **phys·io·path·o·log·ic** \-ˌpa-thə-ˈlä-jik\ *or* **phys·io·path·o·log·i·cal** \-ji-kəl\ *adj*

phys·io·ther·a·peu·tic \ˌfi-zē-ō-ˌther-ə-ˈpyü-tik\ *adj* : of or relating to physical therapy

phys·io·ther·a·pist \-ˈther-ə-pist\ *n* : PHYSICAL THERAPIST

phys·io·ther·a·py \ˌfi-zē-ō-ˈther-ə-pē\ *n, pl* **-pies** : PHYSICAL THERAPY

phy·sique \fi-ˈzēk\ *n* : the form or structure of a person's body : bodily makeup ⟨a muscular ~⟩

phy·sis \ˈfī-səs\ *n, pl* **phy·ses** \-ˌsēz\ : GROWTH PLATE

Phy·so·ceph·a·lus \ˌfī-sə-ˈse-fə-ləs\ *n* : a genus of nematode worms (family Thelaziidae) including a common parasite (*P. sexalatus*) of the stomach and small intestine of swine

phy·so·stig·mine \ˌfī-sə-ˈstig-ˌmēn\ *n* : a crystalline alkaloid that is an anticholinesterase obtained from an African vine (*Physostigma venenosum*) of the legume family (Leguminosae) and is used parenterally in the form of its salicylate $C_{15}H_{21}N_3O_2 \cdot C_7H_6O_3$ esp. to reverse the toxic effects of an anticholinergic agent (as atropine) and topically in the form of its sulfate $(C_{15}H_{21}N_3O_2)_2 \cdot H_2SO_3$ as a miotic in the treatment of glaucoma — called also *eserine*

phyt- *or* **phyto-** *comb form* : plant ⟨*phyto*toxin⟩

phy·tan·ic acid \fī-ˈta-nik-\ *n* : a fatty acid that accumulates in the blood and tissues of patients affected with Refsum's disease

-phyte \ˌfīt\ *n comb form* **1** : plant having a (specified) characteristic or habitat ⟨sapro*phyte*⟩ **2** : pathological growth ⟨osteo*phyte*⟩

phy·tic acid \ˈfī-tik-\ *n* : an acid $C_6H_{18}P_6O_{24}$ that occurs in cereal grains and that when ingested interferes with the intestinal absorption of various minerals (as calcium and magnesium)

phy·to·be·zoar \ˌfī-tō-ˈbē-ˌzōr\ *n* : a concretion formed in the stomach or intestine and composed chiefly of undigested compacted vegetable fiber

phy·to·chem·i·cal \-ˈke-mi-kəl\ *n* : a chemical compound (as a carotenoid or phytosterol) occurring naturally in plants; *esp* : PHYTONUTRIENT

phy·to·es·tro·gen \-ˈes-trə-jən\ *n* : a chemical compound (as genistein) that occurs naturally in plants and has estrogenic properties

phy·to·hem·ag·glu·ti·nin \ˌfī-tō-ˌhē-mə-ˈglüt-ᵊn-ən\ *n* : a proteinaceous hemagglutinin of plant origin used esp. to induce mitosis (as in lymphocytes) — abbr. *PHA*

phy·to·na·di·one \ˌfī-tō-nə-ˈdī-ˌōn\ *n* : VITAMIN K 1a

phy·to·nu·tri·ent \-'nü-trē-ənt, -'nyü-\ *n* : a bioactive plant-derived compound (as resveratrol or sulforaphane) associated with positive health effects

phy·to·pho·to·der·ma·ti·tis \,fī-tō-,fō-tō-,dər-mə-'tī-təs\ *n, pl* **-ti·tis·es** or **-tit·i·des** \-'ti-tə-,dēz\ : an inflammatory reaction of skin that has been exposed to sunlight and esp. UVA radiation after being made hypersensitive by contact with any of various plants or plant parts and esp. those (as limes and celery) with high levels of psoralens and that is typically characterized by a burning sensation, blisters, and erythema followed by hyperpigmentation

phy·tos·ter·ol \fī-'täs-tə-,ról, -,ról\ *n* : any of various sterols derived from plants

phy·to·ther·a·py \,fī-tō-'ther-ə-pē\ *n, pl* **-pies** : the use of vegetable drugs in medicine

phy·to·tox·in \-'täk-sən\ *n* : a toxin (as ricin) produced by a plant

pia \'pī-ə, 'pē-ə\ *n* : PIA MATER

pia-arach·noid \,pī-ə-ə-'rak-,nóid, ,pē-\ *n* : LEPTOMENINGES

Pia·get·ian \,pē-ə-'je-tē-ən\ *adj* : of, relating to, or dealing with Jean Piaget or his writings, theories, or methods esp. with respect to child development

Pia·get \pē-ä-'zhä\, **Jean (1896–1980),** Swiss psychologist.

pi·al \'pī-əl, 'pē-\ *adj* : of or relating to the pia mater ⟨a ~ artery⟩

pia ma·ter \-'mä-tər, -\ *n* : the delicate and highly vascular membrane of connective tissue investing the brain and spinal cord, lying internal to the arachnoid and dura mater, dipping down between the convolutions of the brain, and sending an ingrowth into the anterior fissure of the spinal cord — called also *pia*

pi·an \pē-'an, 'pyän\ *n* : YAWS

pi·blok·to \pi-'bläk-(,)tō\ *n* : a condition among the Inuit that is characterized by attacks of disturbed behavior (as screaming and crying) and that occurs chiefly in winter

pi·ca \'pī-kə\ *n* : an abnormal craving for and eating of substances (as chalk, ashes, or bones) not normally eaten that occurs in nutritional deficiency states (as aphosphorosis) in humans or animals or in some forms of mental disorder — compare GEOPHAGY

¹Pick's disease \'piks-\ *n* : a dementia marked by progressive impairment of intellect and judgment and transitory aphasia, caused by progressive atrophic changes of the cerebral cortex, and usu. beginning in late middle age

Pick \'pik\, **Arnold (1851–1924),** Czechoslovakian psychiatrist and neurologist.

²Pick's disease *n* : pericarditis with adherent pericardium resulting in circulatory disturbances with edema and ascites

Pick, Friedel (1867–1926), Czechoslovakian physician.

Pick·wick·ian syndrome \pik-'wi-kē-ən-\ *n* : obesity accompanied by somnolence and lethargy, hypoventilation, hypoxia, and secondary polycythemia

pico-, *comb form* **1** : one trillionth (10⁻¹²) part of ⟨*pico*gram⟩ **2** : very small ⟨*pico*rnavirus⟩

pi·co·cu·rie \,pē-kō-'kyúr-ē, -kyú-'rē\ *n* : one trillionth of a curie — abbr. *pCi*

pi·co·gram \'pē-kō-,gram\ *n* : one trillionth of a gram — abbr. *pg*

pi·co·li·nate \pi-'kä-lə-,nāt\ *n* : a salt of picolinic acid

pic·o·lin·ic acid \,pi-kə-'li-nik-\ *n* : a crystalline acid $C_6H_5NO_2$ isomeric with niacin

pi·cor·na·vi·rus \pē-,kór-nə-'vī-rəs\ *n* : any of a family (*Picornaviridae*) of small single-stranded RNA viruses that include the causative agents of encephalomyocarditis, hepatitis A, poliomyelitis, foot-and-mouth disease, and hand, foot and mouth disease — see COXSACKIEVIRUS, ECHOVIRUS, ENTEROVIRUS, RHINOVIRUS

pic·ric acid \'pi-krik-\ *n* : a bitter toxic explosive yellow crystalline acid $C_6H_3N_3O_7$ — called also *trinitrophenol*

pic·ro·tox·in \,pi-krō-'täk-sən\ *n* : a poisonous bitter stimulant and convulsant substance $C_{30}H_{34}O_{13}$ obtained esp. from the berry of a southeast Asian vine (*Anamirta cocculus* of the family Menispermaceae) and administered intravenously as an antidote for barbiturate poisoning

PID *abbr* pelvic inflammatory disease

pie·dra \pē-'ā-drə\ *n* : a fungus disease of the hair marked by the formation of small stony nodules along the hair shafts

Pierre Ro·bin syndrome \,pyer-ró-'beⁿ-\ *n* : a congenital defect of the face characterized by micrognathia, abnormal smallness of the tongue, cleft palate, absence of the gag reflex, and sometimes accompanied by bilateral eye defects, glaucoma, or retinal detachment

Robin, Pierre (1867–1950), French pediatrician.

pi·geon breast \'pi-jən-\ *n* : a rachitic deformity of the chest marked by sharp projection of the sternum — **pi·geon–breast·ed** \-'bres-təd\ *adj*

pigeon chest *n* : PIGEON BREAST

pigeon-toed \-'tōd\ *adj* : having the toes turned in toward the midline of the body

pig·ment \'pig-mənt\ *n* : a coloring matter in animals and plants esp. in a cell or tissue; *also* : any of various related colorless substances — **pig·men·tary** \'pig-mən-,ter-ē\ *adj*

pigmentary retinopathy *n* : RETINITIS PIGMENTOSA

pig·men·ta·tion \,pig-mən-'tā-shən, -,men-\ n : coloration with or deposition of pigment; *esp* : an excessive deposition of bodily pigment

pigment cell n : a cell containing a deposition of coloring matter

pig·ment·ed \'pig-,men-təd\ adj : colored by a deposit of pigment

pigmentosa — see RETINITIS PIGMENTOSA

pigmentosum — see XERODERMA PIGMENTOSUM

pig·weed \'pig-,wēd\ n : any of several plants of the genus *Amaranthus* (as *A. retroflexus* and *A. hybridus*) with pollen that acts as a hay fever allergen

pil abbr [Latin *pilula*] pill — used in writing prescriptions

pil- or **pili-** or **pilo-** comb form : hair ⟨*pilomotor*⟩

pilaris — see KERATOSIS PILARIS, PITYRIASIS RUBRA PILARIS

Pi·la·tes \pə-'lä-tēz\ trademark — used for an exercise regimen typically performed with the use of specialized apparatus and designed to improve the overall condition of the body

pile \'pīl\ n 1 : a single hemorrhoid 2 **piles** pl : HEMORRHOIDS; *also* : the condition of one affected with hemorrhoids

pili pl of PILUS

pili — see ARRECTOR PILI MUSCLE

pill \'pil\ n 1 : a usu. medicinal or dietary preparation in a small rounded mass to be swallowed whole 2 *often cap* : BIRTH CONTROL PILL — usu. used with *the*

pil·lar \'pi-lər\ n : a body part likened to a pillar or column (as the margin of the external inguinal ring); *specif* : PILLAR OF THE FAUCES

pillar of the fauces n : either of two curved folds on each side that bound the fauces and enclose the tonsil — see PALATOGLOSSAL ARCH, PALATOPHARYNGEAL ARCH

pi·lo·car·pine \,pī-lə-'kär-,pēn\ n : a miotic alkaloid that is obtained from the dried crushed leaves of two So. American shrubs (*Pilocarpus jaborandi* and *P. microphyllus*) of the rue family (Rutaceae) and is used chiefly in the form of its hydrochloride $C_{11}H_{16}N_2O_2{\cdot}HCl$ or nitrate $C_{11}H_{16}N_2O_2{\cdot}HNO_3$ esp. in the treatment of glaucoma and xerostomia

pi·lo·erec·tion \,pī-lō-i-'rek-shən\ n : involuntary erection or bristling of hairs due to a sympathetic reflex usu. triggered by cold, shock, or fright or due to a sympathomimetic agent

pi·lo·mo·tor \,pī-lə-'mō-tər\ adj : moving or tending to cause movement of the hairs of the skin ⟨∼ nerves⟩

pi·lo·ni·dal \,pī-lə-'nīd-ᵊl\ adj 1 : containing hair nested in a cyst — used of congenitally anomalous cysts in the sacrococcygeal area that often become infected and discharge through a channel near the anus 2 : of, relating to, involving, or for use on pilonidal cysts, tracts, or sinuses

pi·lo·se·ba·ceous \,pī-lō-si-'bā-shəs\ adj : of or relating to hair and the sebaceous glands

pi·lus \'pī-ləs\ n, pl **pi·li** \-,lī\ : a hair or a structure (as on the surface of a bacterial cell) resembling a hair

pi·mar·i·cin \pi-'mar-ə-sən\ n : an antifungal antibiotic $C_{34}H_{49}NO_{14}$ derived from a bacterium of the genus *Streptomyces*

pim·o·zide \'pi-mə-,zīd\ n : a tranquilizer $C_{28}H_{29}F_2N_3O$

pim·ple \'pim-pəl\ n 1 : a small inflamed elevation of the skin : PAPULE; *esp* : PUSTULE 2 : a swelling or protuberance like a pimple — **pim·pled** \-pəld\ adj — **pim·ply** adj

pin \'pin\ n 1 : a metal rod driven into or through a fractured bone to immobilize it 2 : a metal rod driven into the root of a reconstructed tooth to provide support for a crown or into the jaw to provide support for an artificial tooth — **pin** vb

PIN abbr prostatic intraepithelial neoplasia

pinch \'pinch\ vb : to squeeze or compress (as part of the body) usu. in a painful or discomforting way ⟨a ∼ed nerve caused by entrapment⟩

pin·do·lol \'pin-də-,lòl, -,lōl\ n : a betablocker $C_{14}H_{20}N_2O_2$ used in the treatment of hypertension

¹pi·ne·al \'pī-nē-əl, 'pī-, pī-'\ adj : of, relating to, or being the pineal gland

²pineal n : PINEAL GLAND

pi·ne·al·ec·to·my \,pī-nē-ə-'lek-tə-mē, pī-,nē-, ,pī-\ n, pl **-mies** : surgical removal of the pineal gland — **pi·ne·alec·to·mize** \,pi-nē-ə-'lek-tə-,mīz\ vb

pineal gland n : a small body that arises from the roof of the third ventricle and is enclosed by the pia mater and that functions primarily as an endocrine gland that produces melatonin — called also *pineal, pineal body, pineal organ*

pin·e·a·lo·cyte \'pī-nē-ə-lō-,sīt\ n : the parenchymatous epithelioid cell of the pineal gland that has prominent nucleoli and long processes ending in bulbous expansions

pin·e·a·lo·ma \,pi-nē-ə-'lō-mə\ n, pl **-mas** *also* **-ma·ta** \-mə-tə\ : a tumor (as a germinoma) of the pineal gland or pineal region

pineal organ n : PINEAL GLAND

pine–needle oil n : a colorless or yellowish bitter essential oil obtained from the needles of various pines (as *Pinus sylvestris* or *P. mugo*) and used in medicine chiefly as an inhalant in treating bronchitis

pine tar n : tar obtained from the wood of pine trees (genus *Pinus* and esp. *P. palustris* of the family Pinaceae) and used in soaps and in the treatment of skin diseases

pink disease \'pink-\ n : ACRODYNIA

pink·eye \'piŋ-ˌkī\ n : an acute highly contagious conjunctivitis of humans and various domestic animals

pink spot n : the appearance of pulp through the attenuated hard tissue of the crown of a tooth affected with resorption of dentin

pin·na \'pi-nə\ n, pl **pin·nae** \'pi-ˌnē, -ˌnī\ or **pinnas** : the largely cartilaginous projecting portion of the external ear — **pin·nal** \'pin-ᵊl\ adj

pi·no·cy·to·sis \ˌpī-nə-sə-'tō-səs, ˌpī-, -ˌsī-\ n, pl **-to·ses** \-ˌsēz\ : the uptake of fluid by a cell by invagination and pinching off of the cell membrane — **pi·no·cy·tot·ic** \-'tä-tik\ or **pi·no·cyt·ic** \-'si-tik\ adj

pins and needles n pl : a pricking tingling sensation in a limb growing numb or recovering from numbness

pint \'pīnt\ n : any of various measures of liquid capacity equal to one-half quart: as **a** : a U.S. measure equal to 16 fluid ounces, 473.176 milliliters, or 28.875 cubic inches **b** : a British measure equal to 20 fluid ounces, 568.26 milliliters, or 34.678 cubic inches

pin·ta \'pin-tə, -ˌtä\ n : a chronic skin disease that is endemic in tropical America, that occurs successively as an initial papule, a generalized eruption, and a patchy loss of pigment, and that is caused by a spirochete of the genus *Treponema* (*T. careteum*) morphologically indistinguishable from the causative agent of syphilis — called also *mal del pinto*

pin·tid \'pin-təd\ n : one of many initially reddish, then brown, slate blue, or black patches on the skin characteristic of the second stage of pinta

pin·worm \'pin-ˌwərm\ n : any of numerous small oxyurid nematode worms that have the tail of the female prolonged into a sharp point and infest the intestines and esp. the cecum of various vertebrates; esp : a worm of the genus *Enterobius* (*E. vermicularis*) that is parasitic in humans

pi·o·glit·a·zone \ˌpī-ə-'gli-tə-ˌzōn\ n : a drug administered in the form of its hydrochloride $C_{19}H_{20}N_2O_3S·HCl$ to treat type 2 diabetes by decreasing insulin resistance — see ACTOS

pi·per·a·zine \pī-'per-ə-ˌzēn\ n : a crystalline heterocyclic base $C_4H_{10}N_2$ used esp. as an anthelmintic

pi·per·i·dine \pī-'per-ə-ˌdēn\ n : a liquid heterocyclic base $C_5H_{11}N$ that has a peppery ammoniacal odor

pi·per·o·caine \pī-'per-ə-ˌkān\ n : a compound derived from piperidine and benzoic acid that has been used in the form of its hydrochloride $C_{16}H_{23}NO_2·HCl$ as a local anesthetic

pi·per·o·nyl bu·tox·ide \pī-'per-ə-ˌnil-byü-'täk-ˌsīd, -nəl-\ n : an insecticide $C_{19}H_{30}O_5$; also : an oily liquid containing this compound that is used chiefly as a synergist (as for pyrethrum insecticides)

pip·er·ox·an \ˌpi-pə-'räk-ˌsan\ n : adrenolytic drug that has been used in the form of its crystalline hydrochloride $C_{14}H_{19}NO_2·HCl$ to diagnose pheochromocytoma

pi·pette also **pi·pet** \pī-'pet\ n : a small piece of apparatus which typically consists of a narrow tube into which fluid is drawn by suction (as for dispensing or measurement) and retained by closing the upper end — **pipette** also **pipet** vb

pir·ac·e·tam \pī-'ra-sə-ˌtam\ n : an amine $C_6H_{10}N_2O_2$ that has been used as a nootropic

pir·i·form or **pyr·i·form** \'pir-ə-ˌform\ adj **1** : having the form of a pear **2** : of, relating to, or being the part of the cerebral cortex of the piriform lobe that receives primary input from the olfactory bulb ⟨the ∼ cortex⟩

piriform aperture n : the anterior opening of the nasal cavities in the skull

piriform area n : PIRIFORM LOBE

piriform fossa n : PIRIFORM RECESS

pir·i·for·mis or **pyr·i·for·mis** \ˌpir-ə-'for-mis\ n : a muscle that arises from the front of the sacrum, passes out of the pelvis through the greater sciatic foramen, is inserted into the upper border of the greater trochanter of the femur, and rotates the thigh laterally

piriformis syndrome n : sciatica that is caused by compression or irritation of the sciatic nerve by the piriformis muscle and is characterized by pain, tingling, and numbness in the buttocks often extending down the leg

piriform lobe n : the lateral olfactory gyrus and the parahippocampal gyrus taken together

piriform recess n : a small cavity or pocket between the lateral walls of the pharynx on each side and the upper part of the larynx — called also *piriform fossa, piriform sinus*

Pi·ro·goff's amputation \ˌpir-ə-'gofs-\ or **Pi·ro·goff amputation** \-'gof-\ n : amputation of the foot through the articulation of the ankle with retention of part of the calcaneus — compare SYME'S AMPUTATION

Pirogoff, Nikolai Ivanovich (1810–1881), Russian surgeon.

piro·plasm \'pir-ə-ˌpla-zəm\ or **piro·plas·ma** \ˌpir-ə-'plaz-mə\ n, pl **piro·plasms** or **piro·plas·ma·ta** \ˌpir-ə-'plaz-mə-tə\ : BABESIA 2

Piro·plas·ma \ˌpir-ə-'plaz-mə\ n, syn of BABESIA

piro·plas·mo·sis \ˌpir-ə-ˌplaz-'mō-səs\ n, pl **-mo·ses** \-ˌsēz\ : infection with or disease that is caused by protozoans of a family (Babesiidae) and esp. of the genus *Babesia* and that includes Texas fever and equine piroplasmosis

pi·rox·i·cam \pi-'räk-sə-ˌkam\ n : a nonsteroidal anti-inflammatory drug

$C_{15}H_{13}N_3O_4S$ that is used to treat rheumatic diseases (as osteoarthritis)

Pir·quet test \pir-'kā-\ *n* : a tuberculin test made by applying a drop of tuberculin to a scarified spot on the skin — called also *Pirquet reaction*

Pir·quet von Ce·se·na·ti·co \pir-'kā-fŏn-,chā-se-'nä-ti-kō\, **Clemens Peter (1874–1929),** Austrian physician.

pi·si·form \'pī-sə-,fŏrm\ *n* : a bone on the little-finger side of the carpus that articulates with the triquetral bone — called also *pisiform bone*

pit \'pit\ *n* : a hollow or indentation esp. in a surface of an organism: as **a** : a natural hollow in the surface of the body **b** : one of the indented scars left in the skin by a pustular disease : POCKMARK **c** : a usu. developmental imperfection in the enamel of a tooth that takes the form of a small pointed depression — **pit** *vb*

pitch \'pich\ *n* : the property of a sound and esp. a musical tone that is determined by the frequency of the waves producing it : highness or lowness of sound

pitch·blende \'pich-,blend\ *n* : a brown to black mineral that has a distinctive luster and contains radium

Pi·to·cin \pi-'tō-sən\ *trademark* — used for a preparation of oxytocin

pi·tot tube \,pē-'tō-\ *n, often cap P* : a device that consists of a tube that is used with a manometer to measure the velocity of fluid flow (as in a blood vessel)

Pitot, Henri (1695–1771), French hydraulic engineer.

Pi·tres·sin \pi-'tres-ᵊn\ *trademark* — used for a preparation of vasopressin

pitting *n* **1** : the action or process of forming pits (as in acned skin or a tooth) **2** : the formation of a depression or indentation in living tissue that is produced by pressure with a finger or blunt instrument and disappears slowly following release of the pressure in some forms of edema

pitting edema *n* : edema in which pitting results in a depression in the edematous tissue which disappears only slowly

pi·tu·i·cyte \pə-'tü-ə-,sīt, -'tyü-\ *n* : one of the pigmented more or less fusiform cells of the stalk and posterior lobe of the pituitary gland that are derived from glial cells

¹pi·tu·i·tary \pə-'tü-ə-,ter-ē, -'tyü-\ *adj* **1** : of or relating to the pituitary gland **2** : caused or characterized by secretory disturbances of the pituitary gland ⟨a ~ dwarf⟩

²pituitary *n, pl* **-tar·ies 1** : PITUITARY GLAND **2** : the cleaned, dried, and powdered posterior lobe of the pituitary gland of cattle that is used in the treatment of uterine atony and hemorrhage, shock, and intestinal paresis

pituitary ba·soph·il·ism \-bā-'sä-fə-,li-zəm\ *n* : CUSHING'S DISEASE

pituitary gland *n* : a small oval endocrine organ that is attached to the infundibulum of the brain and occupies the sella turcica, that consists of an epithelial anterior lobe derived from a diverticulum of the oral cavity and joined to a posterior lobe of nervous origin by a pars intermedia, and that produces various hormones which directly or indirectly affect most basic bodily functions and include substances exerting a controlling and regulating influence on other endocrine organs, controlling growth and development, or modifying the contraction of smooth muscle, renal function, and reproduction — called also *hypophysis, pituitary body;* see ADENOHYPOPHYSIS, NEUROHYPOPHYSIS

pituitary portal system *n* : a portal system supplying blood to the anterior lobe of the pituitary gland through veins connecting the capillaries of the median eminence of the hypothalamus with those of the anterior lobe

pit viper *n* : any of various mostly New World venomous snakes (subfamily Crotalinae of the family Viperidae) including the rattlesnake, copperhead, and water moccasin that have a small depression on each side of the head and hollow perforated fangs

pity·ri·a·sis \,pi-tə-'rī-ə-səs\ *n, pl* **pity·ri·a·ses** \-,sēz\ **1** : any of several skin diseases marked by the formation and desquamation of fine scales **2** : a disease of domestic animals marked by dry epithelial scales or scurf

pityriasis li·che·noi·des et var·i·o·li·for·mis acu·ta \-,lī-kə-'nȯi-,dēz-et-,var-ē-,ō-lə-'fȯr-mis-ə-'kyü-tə, -'kü-\ *n* : a disease of unknown cause that is characterized by the sudden appearance of polymorphous lesions (as papules, purpuric vesicles, crusts, or ulcerations) resembling chicken pox but tending to persist from a month to as long as years — called also *PLEVA*

pityriasis ro·sea \-'rō-zē-ə\ *n* : an acute benign and self-limited skin eruption of unknown cause that consists of dry, scaly, oval, pinkish or fawn-colored papules, usu. lasts six to eight weeks, and affects esp. the trunk, arms, and thighs

pityriasis ru·bra pi·lar·is \-'rü-brə-pi-'lar-əs\ *n* : chronic dermatitis characterized by the formation of papular horny plugs in the hair follicles and pinkish macules which tend to spread and become scaly plaques

pityriasis versicolor *n* : TINEA VERSICOLOR

Pit·y·ros·po·rum \,pi-tə-'räs-pə-rəm\ *n, syn of* MALASSEZIA

piv·ot \'pi-vət\ *n* : a usu. metallic pin holding an artificial crown to the root of a tooth

pivot joint *n* : an anatomical articulation that consists of a bony pivot in a ring of bone and ligament (as that of the dens and atlas) and that permits rotatory movement only — called also *trochoid*

pivot tooth *n* : an artificial crown attached to the root of a tooth by a usu. metallic pin — called also *pivot crown*

PK \\pē-'kā\ *n* : PSYCHOKINESIS

PKC *abbr* protein kinase C

PKU *abbr* phenylketonuria

pla·ce·bo \plə-'sē-(ˌ)bō\ *n, pl* **-bos 1** : a usu. pharmacologically inert preparation prescribed more for the mental relief of the patient than for its actual effect on a disorder **2** : an inert or innocuous substance used esp. in controlled experiments testing the efficacy of another substance (as a drug)

placebo effect *n* : improvement in the condition of a patient that occurs in response to treatment but cannot be considered due to the specific treatment used

pla·cen·ta \plə-'sen-tə\ *n, pl* **-centas** or **-cen·tae** \-'sen-(ˌ)tē\ : the vascular organ that unites the fetus to the maternal uterus and mediates its metabolic exchanges through a more or less intimate association of uterine mucosal with chorionic and usu. allantoic tissues permitting exchange of material by diffusion between the maternal and fetal vascular systems but without direct contact between maternal and fetal blood and typically involving the interlocking of fingerlike vascular chorionic villi with corresponding modified areas of the uterine mucosa — see ABRUPTIO PLACENTAE — **pla·cen·tal** \-təl\ *adj*

placental barrier *n* : a semipermeable membrane made up of placental tissues and limiting the kind and amount of material exchanged between mother and fetus

placentalis — see DECIDUA PLACENTALIS

placental lactogen *n* : a somatomammotropin that is secreted by the syncytiotrophoblast and that inhibits production of maternal insulin during pregnancy — called also *chorionic somatomammotropin*

placenta pre·via \-ˈprē-vē-ə\ *n, pl* **placentae pre·vi·ae** \-vē-ˌē\ : an abnormal implantation of the placenta at or near the internal opening of the uterine cervix so that it tends to precede the child at birth usu. causing severe maternal hemorrhage

plac·en·ti·tis \ˌplas-ᵊn-'tī-təs\ *n, pl* **-tit·i·des** \-'ti-tə-ˌdēz\ : inflammation of the placenta

plac·en·tog·ra·phy \ˌplas-ᵊn-'tä-grə-fē\ *n, pl* **-phies** : radiographic visualization of the placenta after injection of a radiopaque medium

Plac·i·dyl \'pla-sə-ˌdil\ *trademark* — used for a preparation of ethchlorvynol

pla·gi·o·ceph·a·ly \ˌplā-jē-ō-'se-fə-lē\ *n, pl* **-lies** : a malformation of the head marked by an oblique slant to the main axis of the skull and usu. caused by closure of half of the coronal suture

plague \'plāg\ *n* **1** : an epidemic disease causing a high rate of mortality : PESTILENCE ⟨a ~ of cholera⟩ **2** : a virulent contagious febrile disease that is caused by a bacterium of the genus *Yersinia* (*Y. pestis* syn. *Pasteurella pestis*), that occurs in bubonic, pneumonic, and septicemic forms, and that is usu. transmitted from rats to humans by the bite of infected fleas (as in bubonic plague) or directly from person to person (as in pneumonic plague) — called also *black death*

plana — see PARS PLANA

Plan B *trademark* — used for a preparation of levonorgestrel intended to prevent pregnancy following unprotected intercourse or contraceptive failure

plane \'plān\ *n* **1 a** : a surface that contains at least three points not all in a straight line and is such that a line drawn through any two points in it lies wholly in the surface **b** : an imaginary plane used to identify parts of the body or a part of the skull — see FRANKFORT HORIZONTAL PLANE, MIDSAGITTAL PLANE **2** : a stage in surgical anesthesia ⟨a light ~ of anesthesia⟩

plane joint *n* : GLIDING JOINT

plane of polarization *n* : the plane in which electromagnetic radiation vibrates when it is polarized so as to vibrate in a single plane

plane wart *n* : FLAT WART

pla·ni·gram \'plā-nə-ˌgram, 'pla-\ *n* : TOMOGRAM

pla·nig·ra·phy \plə-'ni-grə-fē\ *n, pl* **-phies** : TOMOGRAPHY

Planned Par·ent·hood \'pland-'par-ᵊnt-ˌhůd\ *service mark* — used for services and materials promoting the accessibility of effective means of voluntary fertility control

Pla·nor·bis \plə-'nȯr-bis\ *n* : a genus of snails (family Planorbidae) that includes several intermediate hosts for schistosomes infecting humans

plantae — see QUADRATUS PLANTAE

plan·ta·go \plan-'tā-(ˌ)gō\ *n* **1** *cap* : a large genus of weeds (family Plantaginaceae) including several (*P. psyllium, P. indica,* and *P. ovata*) that have indigestible and mucilaginous seeds used as a mild cathartic — see PSYLLIUM SEED **2** : PLANTAIN

plantago seed *n* : PSYLLIUM SEED

plan·tain \'plant-ᵊn\ *n* : any plant of the genus *Plantago*

plan·tar \'plan-tər, -ˌtär\ *adj* : of, relating to, or typical of the sole of the foot ⟨the ~ aspect of the foot⟩

plantar arch *n* : an arterial arch in the

sole of the foot formed by the lateral plantar artery and a branch of the dorsalis pedis

plantar artery *n* : either of the two terminal branches into which the posterior tibial artery divides: **a** : one that is larger and passes laterally and then medially to join with a branch of the dorsalis pedis to form the plantar arch — called also *lateral plantar artery* **b** : one that is smaller and follows a more medial course as it passes distally supplying or giving off branches which supply the plantar part of the foot and the toes — called also *medial plantar artery*

plantar cal·ca·neo·na·vic·u·lar ligament \-ˌkal-ˌkā-nē-ō-nə-ˈvi-kyə-lər-\ *n* : an elastic ligament of the sole of the foot that connects the calcaneus and navicular bone and supports the head of the talus — called also *spring ligament*

plantar fascia *n* : a very strong dense fibrous membrane of the sole of the foot that lies beneath the skin and superficial layer of fat and binds together the deeper structures

plantar fasciitis *n* : inflammation involving the plantar fascia esp. in the area of its attachment to the calcaneus and causing pain under the heel in walking and running

plantar flexion *n* : movement of the foot that flexes the foot or toes downward toward the sole — compare DORSIFLEXION

plantar interosseus *n* : any of three small muscles of the plantar aspect of the foot each of which lies along the plantar side of one of the third, fourth, and fifth toes facing the second toe and acts to flex the proximal phalanx and extend the distal phalanges of its toe and to adduct its toe toward the second toe — called also *interosseus plantaris, plantar interosseus muscle*

plan·tar·is \plan-ˈtar-əs\ *n, pl* **plan·tar·es** \-ˈtar-ˌēz\ : a small muscle of the calf of the leg that arises from the lower end of the femur and the posterior ligament of the knee joint, is inserted with the Achilles tendon by a very long slender tendon into the calcaneus, and weakly flexes the leg at the knee and the foot at the ankle — see PLANTAR INTEROSSEUS, VERRUCA PLANTARIS

plantar nerve *n* : either of two nerves of the foot that are the two terminal branches into which the tibial nerve divides: **a** : a smaller one that supplies most of the deeper muscles of the foot and the skin on the lateral part of the sole and on the fifth toe as well as on the lateral part of the fourth toe — called also *lateral plantar nerve* **b** : a larger one that accompanies the medial plantar artery and supplies a number of muscles of the medial part of the foot, the skin on the medial

two-thirds of the sole, and the skin on the first to fourth toes — called also *medial plantar nerve*

plantar reflex *n* : a reflex movement of flexing the foot and toes that after the first year is the normal response to tickling of the sole — compare BABINSKI REFLEX

plantar vein *n* : either of two veins that accompany the plantar arteries: **a** : one accompanying the lateral plantar artery — called also *lateral plantar vein* **b** : one accompanying the medial plantar artery — called also *medial plantar vein*

plantar wart *n* : a wart on the sole of the foot — called also *verruca plantaris*

plan·ter's wart \ˈplan-tərz-\ *n* : PLANTAR WART

plan·ti·grade \ˈplan-tə-ˌgrād\ *adj* : walking on the sole with the heel touching the ground — **plantigrade** *n*

pla·num \ˈplā-nəm\ *n, pl* **pla·na** \-nə\ : a flat surface of bone esp. of the skull

planum tem·po·ra·le \-ˌtem-pə-ˈra-lē\ *n* : an area of the cerebral cortex between Heschl's gyrus and the sylvian fissure that is involved in speech and is usu. larger in the cerebral hemisphere on the left side of the brain

planus — see LICHEN PLANUS

plaque \ˈplak\ *n* **1 a** : a localized abnormal patch on a body part or surface and esp. on the skin ⟨psoriatic ∼⟩ **b** : a sticky usu. colorless film on teeth that is formed by and harbors bacteria **c** : an atherosclerotic lesion **d** : a histopathologic lesion of brain tissue that is characteristic of Alzheimer's disease and consists of a dense proteinaceous core composed primarily of beta-amyloid that is often surrounded and infiltrated by a cluster of degenerating axons and dendrites **2** : a visibly distinct and esp. a clear or opaque area in a bacterial culture produced by damage to or destruction of cells by a virus

Plaque·nil \ˈpla-kə-ˌnil\ *trademark* — used for a preparation of the sulfate of hydroxychloroquine

-pla·sia \ˈplā-zhə, -zhē-ə\ *or* **-pla·sy** \ˌplā-sē, -plə-sē\ *n comb form, pl* **-plasias** *or* **-plasies** : development : formation ⟨dys*plasia*⟩

plasm- *or* **plasmo-** *comb form* : plasma ⟨*plasm*apheresis⟩

-plasm \ˌpla-zəm\ *n comb form* : formative or formed material (as of a cell or tissue) ⟨cyto*plasm*⟩ ⟨endo*plasm*⟩

plas·ma \ˈplaz-mə\ *n* : the fluid part esp. of blood, lymph, or milk that is distinguished from suspended material — see BLOOD PLASMA

plasma cell *n* : a lymphocyte that is a mature antibody-secreting B cell

plasma–cell dyscrasia *n* : MONOCLONAL GAMMOPATHY

plas·ma·cy·toid \ˌplaz-mə-ˈsī-ˌtȯid\ *adj* : resembling or derived from a plasma cell

plas·ma·cy·to·ma also **plas·mo·cy·to·ma** \ˌplaz-mə-sī-ˈtō-mə\ *n, pl* -**mas** also -**ma·ta** \-mə-tə\ : a myeloma composed of plasma cells

plas·ma·cy·to·sis \ˌplaz-mə-sī-ˈtō-səs\ *n, pl* -**to·ses** \-ˌsēz\ : the presence of abnormal numbers of plasma cells in the blood

plas·ma·lem·ma \ˌplaz-mə-ˈle-mə\ *n* : PLASMA MEMBRANE

plas·mal·o·gen \plaz-ˈma-lə-jən, -ˌjen\ *n* : any of a group of phospholipids in which a fatty acid group is replaced by a fatty aldehyde and which include lecithins and phosphatidylethanolamines

plasma membrane *n* : a semipermeable limiting layer of cell protoplasm consisting of a fluid phospholipid bilayer with intercalated proteins — called also *cell membrane, plasmalemma*

plas·ma·pher·e·sis \ˌplaz-mə-fə-ˈrē-səs, -ˈfer-ə-səs\ *n, pl* -**e·ses** \-ˌsēz\ : apheresis used to remove blood plasma (as in the treatment of myasthenia gravis or in the collection of blood plasma for use in transfusion)

plasma thromboplastin an·te·ced·ent \-ˌan-tə-ˈsēd-ᵊnt\ *n* : a clotting factor whose absence is associated with a form of hemophilia — abbr. *PTA;* called also *factor XI*

plasma thromboplastin component *n* : FACTOR IX — abbr. *PTC*

plas·mat·ic \plaz-ˈma-tik\ *adj* : of, relating to, or occurring in plasma esp. of blood ⟨~ fibrils⟩

plas·mid \ˈplaz-mid\ *n* : an extrachromosomal ring of DNA that replicates independently and is found esp. in bacteria — compare EPISOME

plas·min \-min\ *n* : a proteolytic enzyme that dissolves the fibrin of blood clots

plas·min·o·gen \plaz-ˈmi-nə-jən\ *n* : the precursor of plasmin that is found in blood plasma and serum — called also *profibrinolysin*

plasminogen activator *n* : any of a group of substances (as urokinase) that convert plasminogen to plasmin — see TISSUE PLASMINOGEN ACTIVATOR

plasmo- — see PLASM-

plas·mo·di·al \plaz-ˈmō-dē-əl\ *adj* : of, relating to, or resembling a plasmodium

plas·mo·di·um \plaz-ˈmō-dē-əm\ *n* **1** *cap* : a genus of sporozoans (family Plasmodiidae) that includes all the malaria parasites affecting humans **2** *pl* -**dia** : any individual malaria parasite

-plast \ˌplast\ *n comb form* : organized particle or granule : cell ⟨chloroplast⟩

plas·ter \ˈplas-tər\ *n* : a medicated or protective dressing that consists of a film (as of cloth or plastic) spread with a usu. medicated substance

plaster cast *n* : a rigid dressing of gauze impregnated with plaster of paris

plaster of par·is \-ˈpar-is\ *n* : a white powdery slightly hydrated calcium sulfate $CaSO_4 \cdot \frac{1}{2}H_2O$ or $2CaSO_4 \cdot H_2O$ that forms a quick-setting paste with water and is used in medicine chiefly in casts and for surgical bandages

plas·tic \ˈplas-tik\ *adj* **1** : capable of being deformed continuously and permanently in any direction without breaking or tearing **2 a** : capable of growth, repair, or differentiation ⟨a ~ tissue⟩ **b** : relating to, characterized by, or exhibiting neural plasticity **3** : of, relating to, or involving plastic surgery ⟨~ repair⟩

-plas·tic \ˈplas-tik\ *adj comb form* **1** : developing : forming ⟨thromboplastic⟩ **2** : of or relating to (something designated by a term ending in -*pla-sia,* -*plasm,* or -*plasty*) ⟨neoplastic⟩

plas·tic·i·ty \pla-ˈsti-sə-tē\ *n, pl* -**ties** **1** : the quality or state of being plastic; *esp* : capacity for being molded or altered **2** : the ability to retain a shape attained by pressure deformation **3** : the capacity of organisms with the same genotype to vary in developmental pattern, in phenotype, or in behavior according to varying environmental conditions **4** : the capacity for continuous alteration of the neural pathways and synapses of the living brain and nervous system in response to experience or injury

plastic surgeon *n* : a specialist in plastic surgery

plastic surgery *n* : a branch of surgery concerned with the repair, restoration, or improvement of lost, injured, defective, or misshapen parts of the body chiefly by transfer of tissue; *also* : an operation performed for such a purpose

plas·ty \ˈplas-tē\ *n, pl* **plas·ties** : a surgical procedure for the repair, restoration, or replacement (as by a prosthesis) of a part of the body

-plas·ty \ˌplas-tē\ *n comb form, pl* -**plas·ties** : plastic surgery ⟨osteoplasty⟩

-plasy — see -PLASIA

plat- — see PLATY-

¹plate \ˈplāt\ *n* **1** : a flat thin piece or lamina (as of bone) that is part of the body **2 a** : a flat glass dish used chiefly for culturing microorganisms; *esp* : PETRI DISH **b** : a culture or culture medium contained in such a dish **3** : a supporting or reinforcing element: as **a** : the part of a denture that fits in the mouth; *broadly* : DENTURE **b** : a thin flat narrow piece of metal (as stainless steel) that is used to repair a bone defect or fracture

²plate *vb* **plat·ed; plat·ing** **1** : to inoculate and culture (microorganisms or cells) on a plate; *also* : to distribute (an inoculum) on a plate or plates for cultivation **2** : to repair (as a fractured bone) with metal plates

pla·teau \pla-'tō\ *n, pl* **plateaus** *also* **pla·teaux** \-'tōz\ : a relatively flat elevated area — see TIBIAL PLATEAU

plate·let \'plāt-lət\ *n* : a minute colorless anucleate disklike body of mammalian blood that is derived from fragments of megakaryocyte cytoplasm, that is released from the bone marrow into the blood, and that assists in blood clotting by adhering to other platelets and to damaged epithelium — called also *blood platelet, thrombocyte*

platelet–activating factor *n* : phospholipid that is produced esp. by mast cells and basophils, causes the aggregation of platelets and the release of platelet substances (as histamine or serotonin), and is a mediator of inflammation (as in asthma) — abbr. *PAF*

platelet–derived growth factor *n* : a mitogenic growth factor that is found esp. in platelets, consists of two polypeptide chains linked by bonds containing two sulfur atoms each, stimulates cell proliferation (as in connective tissue, smooth muscle, and glia), and plays a role in wound healing — abbr. *PDGF*

plate·let·phe·re·sis \,plāt-lət-'fer-ə-səs, -fə-'rē-səs\ *n, pl* **-re·ses** \-,sēz\ : apheresis used to remove blood platelets (as in the treatment of thrombocytosis or in the collection of platelets for use in transfusion)

plat·ing \'plāt-iŋ\ *n* **1** : the spreading of a sample of cells or microorganisms on a nutrient medium in a petri dish **2** : the immobilization of a fractured bone by securing a metal plate to it

Plat·i·nol \'pla-tə-,nȯl, -,nōl\ *trademark* — used for a preparation of cisplatin

plat·i·num \'plat-ᵊn-əm\ *n* : a grayish white ductile malleable metallic element used esp. as a catalyst and in alloys (as in dentistry) — symbol *Pt*; see ELEMENT table

platy- *also* **plat-** *comb form* : flat : broad ⟨*platy*pelloid⟩

platy·ba·sia \,pla-ti-'bā-sē-ə\ *n* : a developmental deformity of the base of the skull in which the lower occiput is pushed by the upper cervical spine into the cranial fossa

platy·hel·minth \,pla-ti-'hel-,minth\ *n* : FLATWORM — **platy·hel·min·thic** \-,hel-'min-thik, -tik\ *adj*

platy·pel·loid \-'pe-,lȯid\ *adj, of the pelvis* : broad and flat — compare ANDROID 1, ANTHROPOID, GYNECOID 1

pla·tys·ma \plə-'tiz-mə\ *n, pl* **-ma·ta** \-mə-tə\ *also* **-mas** : a broad thin layer of muscle that is situated on each side of the neck immediately under the superficial fascia belonging to the group of facial muscles, that is innervated by the facial nerve, and that draws the lower lip and the corner of the mouth to the side and down and when moved forcefully expands the neck and draws its skin upward

Pla·vix \'plā-viks\ *trademark* — used for a preparation of the bisulfate of clopidogrel

play therapy *n* : psychotherapy in which a child is encouraged to reveal feelings and conflicts in play rather than by verbalization

pleasure principle *n* : a tendency for individual behavior to be directed toward immediate satisfaction of instinctual drives and immediate relief from pain or discomfort — compare REALITY PRINCIPLE

pled·get \'ple-jət\ *n* : a compress or small flat mass usu. of gauze or absorbent cotton that is laid over a wound or into a cavity to apply medication, exclude air, retain dressings, or absorb the matter discharged

-ple·gia \'plē-jə, -jē-ə\ *n comb form* : paralysis ⟨diplegia⟩

pleio·tro·pic \,plī-ə-'trō-pik, -'trä-\ *adj* : producing more than one genetic effect; *specif* : having multiple phenotypic expressions ⟨a ∼ gene⟩ — **plei·ot·ro·py** \plī-'ä-trə-pē\ *n*

pleo·cy·to·sis \,plē-ō-,sī-'tō-səs, -,sēz\ *n, pl* **-to·ses** \-,sēz\ : an abnormal increase in the number of cells (as lymphocytes) in the cerebrospinal fluid

pleo·mor·phic \,plē-ə-'mȯr-fik\ *also* **pleio·mor·phic** \,plī-ə-\ *adj* : able to assume different forms : POLYMORPHIC ⟨a benign ∼ salivary adenoma of mixed cell type⟩ — **pleo·mor·phism** \,plē-ə-'mȯr-,fi-zəm\ *n*

ple·op·tics \plē-'äp-tiks\ *n* : a system of treating amblyopia by retraining visual habits using guided exercises — **ple·op·tic** \-tik\ *adj*

pleth·o·ra \'ple-thə-rə\ *n* : a bodily condition characterized by an excess of blood and marked by turgescence and a florid complexion — **ple·tho·ric** \plə-'thȯr-ik, ple-, -'thär-; 'ple-thə-rik\ *adj*

ple·thys·mo·gram \ple-'thiz-mə-,gram, plə-\ *n* : a tracing made by a plethysmograph

ple·thys·mo·graph \-,graf\ *n* : an instrument for determining and registering variations in the size of an organ or limb resulting from changes in the amount of blood present or passing through it — **ple·thys·mo·graph·ic** \-,thiz-mə-'gra-fik\ *adj* — **pleth·ys·mo·graph·i·cal·ly** *adv* — **pleth·ys·mog·ra·phy** \,ple-thiz-'mä-grə-fē\ *n*

pleur- *or* **pleuro-** *comb form* **1** : pleura ⟨*pleuro*pneumonia⟩ **2** : pleura and ⟨*pleuro*peritoneal⟩

pleu·ra \'plu̇r-ə\ *n, pl* **pleu·rae** \'plu̇r-ē\ *or* **pleu·ras** : either of a pair of two-walled sacs of serous membrane each of which lines one lateral half of the thorax, has an inner layer closely adherent to the corresponding lung, is reflected at the root of the lung to form a parietal layer that adheres to the walls of the thorax, the pericardium, the upper surface of the diaphragm, and adjacent parts, and contains a small amount of serous fluid that minimizes the friction of respiratory movements

pleu·ral \'plür-əl\ *adj* : of or relating to the pleura or the sides of the thorax

pleural cavity *n* : the space that is formed when the two layers of the pleura spread apart — called also *pleural space*

pleural effusion *n* **1** : an exudation of fluid from the blood or lymph into a pleural cavity **2** : an exudate in a pleural cavity

pleu·rec·to·my \plü-'rek-tə-mē\ *n, pl* **-mies** : surgical excision of part of the pleura

pleu·ri·sy \'plür-ə-sē\ *n, pl* **-sies** : inflammation of the pleura that is typically characterized by sudden onset, painful and difficult respiration, cough, and exudation of fluid or fibrinous material into the pleural cavity — **pleu·rit·ic** \plü-'ri-tik\ *adj*

pleu·ri·tis \plü-'rī-təs\ *n, pl* **pleu·rit·i·des** \-'ri-tə-ˌdēz\ : PLEURISY

pleu·rod·e·sis \plü-'rä-də-səs\ *n* : obliteration of the pleural cavity by inducing adherence of the visceral and parietal pleural layers (as by the use of sclerosing agents or surgical abrasion) esp. to treat pleural effusion, pneumothorax, and chylothorax

pleu·ro·dyn·ia \ˌplür-ə-'di-nē-ə\ *n* **1** : a sharp pain in the side usu. located in the intercostal muscles and believed to arise from inflammation of fibrous tissue **2** : EPIDEMIC PLEURODYNIA

pleu·ro·peri·car·di·tis \ˌplür-ō-ˌper-ə-ˌkär-'dī-təs\ *n, pl* **-dit·i·des** \-'di-tə-ˌdēz\ : inflammation of the pleura and the pericardium

pleu·ro·peri·to·ne·al \-ˌper-ə-tə-'nē-əl\ *adj* : of or relating to the pleura and the peritoneum

pleu·ro·pneu·mo·nia \ˌplür-ō-nu̇-'mō-nyə, -nyü-\ *n* **1** : pleurisy accompanied by pneumonia **2** : a highly contagious pneumonia usu. associated with pleurisy of cattle, goats, and sheep that is caused by a bacterium of the genus *Mycoplasma* (esp. *M. mycoides*) **3** : a contagious often fatal respiratory disease esp. of young pigs that is caused by a bacterium of the genus *Actinobacillus* (*A. pleuropneumoniae*) **4** : pleurisy of horses that is often accompanied by pneumonia and is caused by various bacteria

pleuropneumonia–like organism *n* : MYCOPLASMA 2

pleu·ro·pul·mo·nary \ˌplür-ō-'pu̇l-mə-ˌner-ē, -'pəl-\ *adj* : of or relating to the pleura and the lungs

PLE·VA \'plā-və\ *n* : PITYRIASIS LICHENOIDES ET VARIOLIFORMIS ACUTA

plex·ec·to·my \plek-'sek-tə-mē\ *n, pl* **-mies** : surgical removal of a plexus

plexi·form \'plek-sə-ˌfȯrm\ *adj* : of, relating to, or having the form or characteristics of a plexus 〈~ networks〉

plexiform layer *n* : either of two reticular layers of the retina consisting of nerve cell processes and situated between layers of ganglion cells and cell bodies

plex·im·e·ter \plek-'si-mə-tər\ *n* : a small hard flat plate (as of ivory) placed in contact with the body to receive the blow in percussion

plex·op·a·thy \plek-'sä-pə-thē\ *n, pl* **-thies** : an injured or diseased condition of a plexus and esp. a nerve plexus

plex·or \'plek-sər\ *n* : a small hammer with a rubber head used in medical percussion

plex·us \'plek-səs\ *n, pl* **plex·us·es** : a network of anastomosing or interlacing blood vessels or nerves

pli·ca \'plī-kə\ *n, pl* **pli·cae** \-ˌkē, -ˌsē\ : a fold or folded part; *esp* : a groove or fold of skin

plicae cir·cu·la·res \-ˌsər-kyə-'lar-(ˌ)ēz\ *n pl* : the numerous permanent crescentic folds of mucous membrane found in the small intestine esp. in the lower part of the duodenum and the jejunum — called also *valvulae conniventes*

plica fim·bri·a·ta \-ˌfim-brē-'ā-tə\ *n, pl* **plicae fim·bri·a·tae** \-'ā-tē\ : a fold resembling a fringe on the under surface of the tongue on either side of the frenulum

pli·ca·my·cin \ˌplī-kə-'mīs-ᵊn\ *n* : an antineoplastic agent $C_{52}H_{76}O_{24}$ produced by three bacteria of the genus *Streptomyces* (*S. argillaceus*, *S. tanashiensis*, and *S. plicatus*) and administered intravenously esp. in the treatment of malignant tumors of the testes or in the treatment of hypercalcemia and hypercalciuria associated with advanced neoplastic disease — called also *mithramycin*

plica semi·lu·na·ris \-ˌse-mi-ˌlü-'nar-əs\ *n, pl* **plicae semi·lu·na·res** \-(ˌ)ēz\ : the vertical fold of conjunctiva that occupies the canthus of the eye nearer the nose

pli·ca·tion \plī-'kā-shən\ *n* **1** : the tightening of stretched or weakened bodily tissues or channels by folding the excess in tucks and suturing **2** : the folding of one part on and the fastening of it to another (as areas of the bowel freed from adhesions and left without normal serosal covering) — **pli·cate** \'plī-ˌkāt\ *vb*

-ploid \ˌplȯid\ *adj comb form* : having or being a chromosome number that bears (such) a relationship to or is (so many) times the basic chromosome number characteristic of a given plant or animal group ⟨poly*ploid*⟩

ploi·dy \'plȯi-dē\ *n, pl* **ploi·dies** : degree of repetition of the basic number of chromosomes

plom·bage \'pläm-'bäzh\ *n* : the practice of inserting an inert material into the thoracic cavity to exert sustained pressure on the lungs and induce their collapse that formerly was used as a treatment for pulmonary tuberculosis

PLSS *abbr* portable life-support system

plug \'pləg\ *n* **1** : an obstructing mass of material in a bodily vessel or opening (as of the cervix or a skin lesion) **2** : a filling for a hollow tooth — **plugged** \'pləgd\ *adj*

plug·ger \'plə-gər\ *n* : a dental instrument used for packing, condensing, and consolidating filling material in a tooth cavity

plum·bism \'pləm-ˌbi-zəm\ *n* : LEAD POISONING; *esp* : chronic lead poisoning

Plum·mer–Vin·son syndrome \'pləmər-'vin-sən-\ *n* : a condition that is marked esp. by the growth of a mucous membrane across the esophageal lumen, by difficulty in swallowing, and by hypochromic anemia and that is usu. considered to be due to an iron deficiency

    Plummer, Henry Stanley (1874–1936), American physician.

    Vinson, Porter Paisley (1890–1959), American surgeon.

plu·ri·po·ten·cy \ˌplu̇r-ə-'pōt-ᵊn-sē\ *n, pl* **-cies** : PLURIPOTENTIALITY

plu·ri·po·tent \plu̇-'ri-pə-tənt\ *adj* : not fixed as to developmental potentialities; *esp* : capable of differentiating into one of many cell types ⟨∼ stem cells⟩ **2** : capable of affecting more than one organ or tissue

plu·ri·po·ten·tial \ˌplu̇r-ə-pə-'ten-chəl\ *adj* : PLURIPOTENT

plu·ri·po·ten·ti·al·i·ty \-pə-ˌten-chē-'a-lə-tē\ *n, pl* **-ties** : the quality or state of being pluripotent

plu·to·ni·um \plü-'tō-nē-əm\ *n* : a radioactive metallic element similar chemically to uranium that undergoes slow disintegration with the emission of an alpha particle to form uranium 235 — symbol *Pu;* see ELEMENT table

pm *abbr* premolar

Pm *symbol* promethium

PM *abbr* **1** [Latin *post meridiem*] after noon **2** postmortem

PMDD *abbr* premenstrual dysphoric disorder

PMN *abbr* polymorphonuclear leukocyte; polymorphonuclear neutrophil

PMNL *abbr* polymorphonuclear leukocyte

PMS \ˌpē-ˌem-'es\ *n* : PREMENSTRUAL SYNDROME

PN *abbr* psychoneurotic

-pnea \p-nē-ə\ *n comb form* : breath : breathing ⟨*ap*nea⟩

pneum- *or* **pneumo-** *comb form* **1** : air : gas ⟨*pneumo*thorax⟩ **2** : lung ⟨*pneumo*coniosis⟩ : pulmonary and ⟨*pneumo*gastric⟩ **3** : respiration ⟨*pneumo*graph⟩ **4** : pneumonia ⟨*pneumo*coccus⟩

pneumat- *or* **pneumato-** *comb form* : air : vapor : gas ⟨*pneumato*sis⟩

pneu·mat·ic \nu̇-'ma-tik, nyu̇-\ *adj* : of, relating to, or using gas (as air): as **a** : moved or worked by air pressure **b** : adapted for holding or inflated with compressed air **c** : having air-filled cavities ⟨∼ bone⟩ — **pneu·mat·i·cal·ly** *adv*

pneu·ma·ti·za·tion \ˌnu̇-mə-tə-'zā-shən, ˌnyu̇-\ *n* : the presence or development of air-filled cavities in a bone ⟨∼ of the temporal bone⟩ — **pneu·ma·tized** \'nu̇-mə-ˌtīzd, 'nyu̇-\ *adj*

pneu·ma·to·cele \'nu̇-mə-tō-ˌsēl, 'nyu̇-; nyu̇-'ma-tə-, nü-\ *n* : a gas-filled cavity or sac occurring esp. in the lung

pneu·ma·to·sis \ˌnu̇-mə-'tō-səs, ˌnyu̇-\ *n, pl* **-to·ses** \-ˌsēz\ : the presence of air or gas in abnormal places in the body

pneu·ma·tu·ria \ˌnu̇-mə-'tu̇r-ē-ə, ˌnyu̇-\ *n* : passage of gas in the urine

pneu·mo·ba·cil·lus \ˌnu̇-mō-bə-'si-ləs, ˌnyu̇-\ *n, pl* **-cil·li** \-ˌlī\ : a bacterium of the genus *Klebsiella* (*K. pneumoniae*) associated with inflammatory conditions of the respiratory tract (as pneumonia)

pneu·mo·coc·cae·mia *chiefly Brit var of* PNEUMOCOCCEMIA

pneu·mo·coc·cal \ˌnu̇-mə-'kä-kəl, ˌnyu̇-\ *adj* : of, relating to, caused by, or derived from pneumococci ⟨∼ pneumonia⟩ ⟨a ∼ vaccine⟩

pneu·mo·coc·ce·mia \ˌnu̇-mə-ˌkäk-'sē-mē-ə, ˌnyu̇-\ *n* : the presence of pneumococci in the circulating blood

pneu·mo·coc·cus \ˌnu̇-mə-'kä-kəs, ˌnyu̇-\ *n, pl* **-coc·ci** \-'kä-ˌkī, -ˌkī\ : a bacterium of the genus *Streptococcus* (*S. pneumoniae*) that causes an acute pneumonia involving one or more lobes of the lung

pneu·mo·co·lon \ˌnu̇-mə-'kō-lən, ˌnyu̇-\ *n* : the presence of air in the colon

pneu·mo·co·ni·o·sis \ˌnu̇-mō-ˌkō-nē-'ō-səs, ˌnyu̇-\ *n, pl* **-o·ses** \-ˌsēz\ : a disease of the lungs caused by the habitual inhalation of irritants (as mineral or metallic particles) — called also *miner's asthma, pneumonoconiosis;* see BLACK LUNG, SILICOSIS

pneu·mo·cys·tic pneumonia \ˌnu̇-mə-'sis-tik-, ˌnyu̇-\ *n* : PNEUMOCYSTIS CARINII PNEUMONIA

Pneu·mo·cys·tis \ˌnu̇-mə-'sis-təs, ˌnyu̇-\ *n* **1** : a genus of ascomycetous fungi that were formerly classified as protozoans and include one (*P. carinii* syn. *P. jiroveci*) causing pneumonia esp. in immunocompromised individuals **2** : PNEUMOCYSTIS CARINII PNEUMONIA

Pneumocystis ca·ri·nii pneumonia \-kə-'rī-nē-ˌē-\ *n* : a pneumonia chiefly affecting immunocompromised individuals that is caused by a fungus of the genus *Pneumocystis* (*P. carinii* syn. *P. jiroveci*), that attacks esp. the interstitial and alveolar tissues of the lungs, and that is characterized esp. by a nonproductive cough, shortness of breath, and fever — abbr. *PCP*; called also *pneumocystic pneumonia, Pneumocystis carinii pneumonitis, Pneumocystis pneumonia*

pneu·mo·cys·tog·ra·phy \ˌnü-mō-si-'stä-grə-fē, ˌnyü-\ *n, pl* **-phies** : radiography of the urinary bladder after it has been injected with air

pneu·mo·cyte \'nü-mə-ˌsīt, 'nyü-\ *n* : any of the specialized cells that occur in the alveoli of the lungs

pneu·mo·en·ceph·a·li·tis \ˌnü-mō-in-ˌse-fə-'lī-təs, ˌnyü-\ *n, pl* **-lit·i·des** \-'li-tə-ˌdēz\ : NEWCASTLE DISEASE

pneu·mo·en·ceph·a·lo·gram \-in-'se-fə-lə-ˌgram\ *n* : a radiograph made by pneumoencephalography

pneu·mo·en·ceph·a·lo·graph \-ˌgraf\ *n* : PNEUMOENCEPHALOGRAM

pneu·mo·en·ceph·a·log·ra·phy \-in-ˌse-fə-'lä-grə-fē\ *n, pl* **-phies** : radiography of the brain after the injection of air into the ventricles — **pneu·mo·en·ceph·a·lo·graph·ic** \-in-ˌse-fə-lə-'gra-fik\ *adj*

pneu·mo·en·ter·i·tis \-ˌen-tə-'rī-təs\ *n, pl* **-en·ter·it·i·des** \-'ri-tə-ˌdēz\ *or* **-en·ter·i·tis·es** : pneumonia combined with enteritis

pneu·mo·gas·tric nerve \ˌnü-mə-'gas-trik-, ˌnyü-\ *n* : VAGUS NERVE

pneu·mo·gram \'nü-mə-ˌgram, 'nyü-\ *n* : a record of respiratory movements obtained by pneumography

pneu·mo·graph \'nü-mə-ˌgraf, 'nyü-\ *n* : an instrument for recording the thoracic movements or volume change during respiration

pneu·mog·ra·phy \nü-'mä-grə-fē, nyü-\ *n, pl* **-phies** **1** : a description of the lungs **2** : radiography after the injection of air into a body cavity **3** : the process of making a pneumogram — **pneu·mo·graph·ic** \ˌnü-mə-'gra-fik, nyü-\ *adj*

pneu·mol·y·sis \-'mä-lə-səs\ *n, pl* **-y·ses** \-ˌsēz\ : PNEUMONOLYSIS

pneu·mo·me·di·as·ti·num \ˌnü-mō-ˌmē-dē-ə-'stī-nəm, ˌnyü-\ *n, pl* **-ti·na** \-nə\ **1** : an abnormal state characterized by the presence of gas (as air) in the mediastinum **2** : the induction of pneumomediastinum as an aid to radiography

pneu·mo·my·co·sis \-mī-'kō-səs\ *n, pl* **-co·ses** \-ˌsēz\ : a fungus disease of the lungs; *esp* : aspergillosis in poultry

pneumon- *or* **pneumono-** *comb form* : lung ⟨*pneumon*ectomy⟩

pneu·mo·nec·to·my \ˌnü-mə-'nek-tə-mē, ˌnyü-\ *n, pl* **-mies** : surgical excision of an entire lung or of one or more lobes of a lung — compare SEGMENTAL RESECTION

pneu·mo·nia \nü-'mō-nyə, nyü-\ *n* : a disease of the lungs that is characterized esp. by inflammation and consolidation of lung tissue followed by resolution, is accompanied by fever, chills, cough, and difficulty in breathing, and is caused chiefly by infection — see BRONCHOPNEUMONIA, LOBAR PNEUMONIA, PRIMARY ATYPICAL PNEUMONIA

pneu·mon·ic \nü-'mä-nik, nyü-\ *adj* **1** : of, relating to, or affecting the lungs : PULMONARY **2** : of, relating to, or affected with pneumonia

pneumonic plague *n* : plague of an extremely virulent form that is caused by a bacterium of the genus *Yersinia* (*Y. pestis* syn. *Pasteurella pestis*), involves chiefly the lungs, and usu. is transmitted from person to person by droplet infection — compare BUBONIC PLAGUE

pneu·mo·ni·tis \ˌnü-mə-'nī-təs, ˌnyü-\ *n, pl* **-nit·i·des** \-'ni-tə-ˌdēz\ **1** : a disease characterized by inflammation of the lungs; *esp* : PNEUMONIA **2** : FELINE PNEUMONITIS

pneu·mo·no·cen·te·sis \ˌnü-mə-(ˌ)nō-sen-'tē-səs, ˌnyü-\ *n, pl* **-te·ses** \-ˌsēz\ : surgical puncture of a lung for aspiration

pneu·mo·no·co·ni·o·sis \-ˌkō-nē-'ō-səs\ *n, pl* **-o·ses** \-ˌsēz\ : PNEUMOCONIOSIS

pneu·mo·nol·y·sis \ˌnü-mə-'nä-lə-səs, ˌnyü-\ *n, pl* **-y·ses** \-ˌsēz\ : either of two surgical procedures to permit collapse of a lung : **a** : separation of the parietal pleura from the fascia of the chest wall **b** : separation of the visceral and parietal layers of the pleura — called also *intrapleural pneumonolysis*

pneu·mo·nos·to·my \ˌnü-mə-'näs-tə-mē, ˌnyü-\ *n, pl* **-mies** : surgical formation of an artificial opening (as for drainage of an abscess) into a lung

Pneu·mo·nys·sus \ˌnü-mə-'ni-səs, ˌnyü-\ *n* : a genus of mites (family Halarachnidae) that live in the air passages of mammals and include one (*P. caninum*) found in dogs

pneu·mop·a·thy \nü-'mä-pə-thē, nyü-\ *n, pl* **-thies** : any disease of the lungs

pneu·mo·peri·car·di·um \ˌnü-mō-ˌper-ə-'kär-dē-əm, ˌnyü-\ *n, pl* **-dia** \-dē-ə\ : an abnormal state characterized by the presence of gas (as air) in the pericardium

pneu·mo·peri·to·ne·um \-ˌper-ə-tə-'nē-əm\ *n, pl* **-ne·ums** *or* **-nea** \-'nē-ə\ **1** : an abnormal state characterized by the presence of gas (as air) in the peritoneal cavity **2** : the induction of pneumoperitoneum as a therapeutic measure or as an aid to radiography

pneu·mo·scle·ro·sis \-sklə-'rō-səs\ *n, pl* **-ro·ses** \-ˌsēz\ : fibrosis of the lungs

pneu·mo·tacho·gram \'nü-mō-'tak-ə-,gram, 'nyü-\ *n* : a record of the velocity of the respiratory function obtained by use of a pneumotachograph

pneu·mo·tacho·graph \-,graf\ *n* : a device or apparatus for measuring the rate of the respiratory function

pneu·mo·tax·ic center \,nü-mə-'tak-sik-, ,nyü-\ *n* : a neural center in the upper part of the pons that provides inhibitory impulses on inspiration and thereby prevents overdistension of the lungs and helps to maintain alternately recurrent inspiration and expiration

pneu·mo·tho·rax \-'thōr-,aks\ *n, pl* **-tho·rax·es** *or* **-tho·ra·ces** \-'thōr-ə-,sēz\ : a condition in which air or other gas is present in the pleural cavity and which occurs spontaneously as a result of disease or injury of lung tissue, rupture of air-filled pulmonary cysts, or puncture of the chest wall or is induced as a therapeutic measure to collapse the lung — see TENSION PNEUMOTHORAX; compare OLEOTHORAX

pneu·mo·tro·pic \-'trō-pik, -'trä-\ *adj* : turning, directed toward, or having an affinity for lung tissues — used esp. of infective agents

PNF *abbr* proprioceptive neuromuscular facilitation

PNH *abbr* paroxysmal nocturnal hemoglobinuria

-pnoea *chiefly Brit var of* -PNEA

po *abbr* per os — used esp. in writing prescriptions

Po *symbol* polonium

pock \'päk\ *n* : a pustule in an eruptive disease (as smallpox)

pock·et \'pä-kət\ *n* : a small cavity or space; *esp* : an abnormal cavity formed in diseased tissue ⟨a gingival ~⟩ — **pocketing** *n*

pock·mark \'päk-,märk\ *n* : a mark, pit, or depressed scar caused by smallpox or acne — **pock·marked** *adj*

POD *abbr* postoperative day

pod- *or* **podo-** *comb form* **1** : foot ⟨*po·diatry*⟩ **2** : hoof ⟨*podo·dermatitis*⟩

po·dag·ra \pə-'da-grə\ *n* **1** : GOUT **2** : a painful condition of the big toe caused by gout

po·dal·ic \pō-'da-lik\ *adj* : of, relating to, or by means of the feet; *specif* : being an obstetric version in which the fetus is turned so that the feet emerge first in delivery

po·di·a·try \pə-'dī-ə-trē, pō-\ *n, pl* **-tries** : the medical care and treatment of the human foot — called also *chiropody* — **po·di·at·ric** \,pō-dē-'a-trik\ *adj* — **po·di·a·trist** \pə-'dī-ə-trist\ *n*

podo·der·ma·ti·tis \,pä-dō-,dər-mə-'tī-təs\ *n, pl* **-ti·tis·es** *or* **-tit·i·des** \-'ti-tə-,dēz\ : a condition (as foot rot) characterized by inflammation of the dermal tissue underlying the horny layers of a hoof

podo·phyl·lin \,pä-də-'fi-lən\ *n* : a resin obtained from podophyllum and used in medicine as a caustic

podo·phyl·lo·tox·in \,pä-dō-,fi-lə-'täk-sən\ *n* : a crystalline polycyclic compound $C_{22}H_{22}O_8$ constituting one of the active principles of podophyllum and podophyllin

podo·phyl·lum \-'fi-ləm\ *n* **1** *cap* : a genus of herbs (family Berberidaceae) that have poisonous rootstocks and large fleshy sometimes edible berries **2** *pl* **-phyl·li** \-'fi-,lī\ *or* **-phyllums** : the dried rhizome and rootlet of the mayapple (*Podophyllum peltatum*) that is used as a caustic or as a source of the more effective podophyllin

podophyllum resin *n* : PODOPHYLLIN

po·go·ni·on \pə-'gō-nē-ən\ *n* : the most projecting median point on the anterior surface of the chin

-poi·e·sis \(,)pȯi-'ē-səs\ *n comb form, pl* **-poi·e·ses** \-'ē-,sēz\ : production : formation ⟨lympho*poiesis*⟩

-poi·et·ic \(,)pȯi-'e-tik\ *adj comb form* : productive : formative ⟨lympho*poiet·ic*⟩

poi·ki·lo·cyte \'pȯi-ki-lə-,sīt, (,)pȯi-'ki-\ *n* : an abnormally formed red blood cell characteristic of various anemias

poi·ki·lo·cy·to·sis \,pȯi-ki-lō-sī-'tō-səs\ *n, pl* **-to·ses** \-,sēz\ : a condition characterized by the presence of poikilocytes in the blood

poi·ki·lo·der·ma \,pȯi-kə-lə-'dər-mə\ *n, pl* **-mas** *or* **-ma·ta** \-mə-tə\ : any of several disorders characterized by patchy discoloration of the skin

poi·ki·lo·ther·mic \-'thər-mik\ *adj* : COLD-BLOODED

¹point \'pȯint\ *n* **1** : a narrowly localized place or area **2** : the terminal usu. sharp or narrowly rounded part of something

²point *vb, of an abscess* : to become distended with pus prior to breaking

pointer — see HIP POINTER

point mutation *n* : a gene mutation involving the substitution, addition, or deletion of a single nucleotide base

point-of-service *adj* : of, relating to, or being a health-care insurance plan that allows enrollees to seek care from a physician affiliated with the service provider at a fixed co-payment or to choose a nonaffiliated physician and pay a larger share of the cost — abbr. *POS*

Poi·seuille's law \pwä-'zœiz-\ *n* : a statement in physics that relates the velocity of flow of a fluid (as blood) through a narrow tube (as a blood vessel or a catheter) to the pressure and viscosity of the fluid and the length and radius of the tube

    Poiseuille, Jean-Léonard-Marie (1797–1869), French physiologist and physician.

¹poi·son \'pȯiz-ᵊn\ *n* **1** : a substance that through its chemical action usu. kills, injures, or impairs an organism **2** : a substance that inhibits the activity of another substance or the course of a reaction or process

²**poison** vb **poi·soned; poi·son·ing 1** : to injure or kill with poison **2** : to treat, taint, or impregnate with poison

³**poison** adj **1** : POISONOUS ⟨a ∼ plant⟩ **2** : impregnated with poison ⟨a ∼ arrow⟩

poison dog·wood \-'dȯg-ˌwu̇d\ n : POISON SUMAC

poison gas n : a poisonous gas or a liquid or a solid giving off poisonous vapors designed (as in chemical warfare) to kill, injure, or disable by inhalation or contact

poison hemlock n : a large poisonous herb (Conium maculatum) of the carrot family (Umbelliferae) with finely divided leaves and white flowers — compare WATER HEMLOCK

poison ivy n **1 a** : a climbing plant of the genus Toxicodendron (T. radicans syn. Rhus radicans) that is esp. common in the eastern and central U.S., that has leaves in groups of three and white berries and that produces an acutely irritating oil causing a usu. intensely itching skin rash **b** : any of several plants closely related to poison ivy; esp : POISON OAK 1b **2** : a skin rash produced by poison ivy

poison oak n **1** : any of several plants related to poison ivy and producing an oil with similar irritating properties: as **a** : a bushy plant (Toxicodendron diversilobum syn. Rhus diversiloba) of the Pacific coast **b** : a bushy plant (T. toxicarium syn. R. toxicodendron) chiefly of the southeastern U.S. **2** : POISON IVY 1a **3** : a skin rash produced by poison oak

poi·son·ous \'pȯiz-ᵊn-əs\ adj : having the properties or effects of poison : VENOMOUS

poison su·mac \-'shü-ˌmak, -'sü-\ n : a swamp shrub of the genus Toxicodendron (T. vernix syn. Rhus vernix) chiefly of the eastern U.S. and Canada that has greenish white berries and produces an irritating oil — called also poison dogwood

poi·son·wood \'pȯiz-ᵊn-ˌwu̇d\ n : a caustic or poisonous tree (Metopium toxiferum) of the cashew family (Anacardiaceae) that is native to Florida and the West Indies and has compound leaves, clusters of greenish flowers, and orange-yellow fruits

poke·weed \'pōk-ˌwēd\ n : a poisonous American perennial herb (Phytolacca americana of the family Phytolaccaceae) from which is obtained a mitogen that has been used to stimulate lymphocyte proliferation

po·lar \'pō-lər\ adj **1** : of or relating to one or more poles (as of a spherical body) **2** : exhibiting polarity; esp : having a dipole or characterized by molecules having dipoles ⟨a ∼ solvent⟩ **3** : being at opposite ends of a spectrum of symptoms or manifestations ⟨∼ types of leprosy⟩

polar body n : a cell that separates from an oocyte during meiosis: **a** : one containing a nucleus produced in the first meiotic division — called also first polar body **b** : one containing a nucleus produced in the second meiotic division — called also second polar body

po·lar·i·ty \pō-'lar-ə-tē, pə-\ n, pl **-ties 1** : the quality or condition inherent in a body that exhibits contrasting properties or powers in contrasting parts or directions **2** : attraction toward a particular object or in a specific direction **3** : the particular state either positive or negative with reference to the two poles or to electrification

po·lar·ize \'pō-lə-ˌrīz\ vb **-ized; -iz·ing 1** : to vibrate or cause (as light waves) to vibrate in a definite pattern **2** : to give physical polarity to — **po·lar·i·za·tion** \ˌpō-lə-rə-'zā-shən\ n

polarizing microscope n : a microscope equipped to produce polarized light for examination of a specimen

pole \'pōl\ n **1 a** : either of the two terminals of an electric cell or battery **b** : one of two or more regions in a magnetized body at which the magnetism is concentrated **2** : either of two morphologically or physiologically differentiated areas at opposite ends of an axis in an organism, organ, or cell

poli- or **polio-** comb form : of or relating to the gray matter of the brain or spinal cord ⟨poliomyelitis⟩

pol·i·co·sa·nol also **poly·co·sa·nol** \ˌpä-lē-'kō-sə-ˌnȯl\ n : a mixture of alcohols derived chiefly from the waxy coating of sugarcane and used esp. as a dietary supplement to lower cholesterol levels

pol·i·clin·ic \ˌpä-lē-'kli-nik\ n : a dispensary or department of a hospital at which outpatients are treated — compare POLYCLINIC

po·lio \'pō-lē-ˌō\ n : POLIOMYELITIS

po·lio·dys·tro·phy \ˌpō-lē-ō-'dis-trə-fē\ n, pl **-phies** : atrophy of the gray matter esp. of the cerebrum

po·lio·en·ceph·a·li·tis \ˌpō-lē-(ˌ)ō-in-ˌse-fə-'lī-təs\ n, pl **-lit·i·des** \-'li-tə-ˌdēz\ : inflammation of the gray matter of the brain

po·lio·en·ceph·a·lo·my·eli·tis \-in-ˌse-fə-lō-ˌmī-ə-'lī-təs\ n, pl **-elit·i·des** \-'li-tə-ˌdēz\ : inflammation of the gray matter of the brain and the spinal cord

po·lio·my·eli·tis \ˌpō-lē-(ˌ)ō-ˌmī-ə-'lī-təs\ n, pl **-elit·i·des** \-'li-tə-ˌdēz\ : an acute infectious virus disease caused by the poliovirus, characterized by fever, motor paralysis, and atrophy of skeletal muscles often with permanent disability and deformity, and marked by inflammation of nerve cells in the ventral horns of the spinal cord — called also infantile paralysis, polio — **po·lio·my·elit·ic** \-'li-tik\ adj

po·li·o·sis \ˌpō-lē-'ō-səs\ *n, pl* **-o·ses** \-ˌsēz\ : loss of color from the hair

polio vaccine *n* : a vaccine intended to confer immunity to poliomyelitis

po·lio·vi·rus \'pō-lē-(ˌ)ō-ˌvī-rəs\ *n* : a picornavirus of the genus *Enterovirus* (species *Poliovirus*) occurring in three distinct serotypes that cause poliomyelitis — see SABIN VACCINE, SALK VACCINE

po·litz·er bag \'pō-lit-sər-, 'pä-\ *n* : a soft rubber bulb used to inflate the middle ear by increasing air pressure in the nasopharynx

Politzer, Adam (1835–1920), Austrian otologist.

pol·len \'pä-lən\ *n* : a mass of male spores in a seed plant appearing usu. as a fine dust

pol·lex \'pä-ˌleks\ *n, pl* **pol·li·ces** \'pä-lə-ˌsēz\ : the first digit of the forelimb : THUMB

pollicis — see ABDUCTOR POLLICIS BREVIS, ABDUCTOR POLLICIS LONGUS, ADDUCTOR POLLICIS, EXTENSOR POLLICIS BREVIS, EXTENSOR POLLICIS LONGUS, FLEXOR POLLICIS BREVIS, FLEXOR POLLICIS LONGUS, OPPONENS POLLICIS, PRINCEPS POLLICIS

pol·li·ci·za·tion \ˌpä-lə-sə-'zā-shən\ *n* : the reconstruction or replacement of the thumb esp. from part of the index finger

pol·li·no·sis *or* **pol·le·no·sis** \ˌpä-lə-'nō-səs\ *n, pl* **-no·ses** \-ˌsēz\ : HAY FEVER

pol·lut·ant \pə-'lüt-ᵊnt\ *n* : something that pollutes

pol·lute \pə-'lüt\ *vb* **pol·lut·ed; pol·lut·ing** : to contaminate (an environment) esp. with man-made waste — **pol·lut·er** *n* — **pol·lut·ive** \-'lü-tiv\ *adj*

pol·lu·tion \pə-'lü-shən\ *n* **1** : the action of polluting or the condition of being polluted **2** : POLLUTANT

po·lo·ni·um \pə-'lō-nē-əm\ *n* : a radioactive metallic element that emits an alpha particle to form an isotope of lead — symbol *Po*; see ELEMENT table

poly- *comb form* **1** : many : several : much : MULTI- ⟨*poly*arthritis⟩ **2** : excessive : abnormal : HYPER- ⟨*poly*dactyly⟩

poly(A) \ˌpä-lē-'ā\ *n* : RNA or a segment of RNA that is composed of a polynucleotide chain consisting entirely of adenine-containing nucleotides and that codes for polylysine when functioning as messenger RNA in protein synthesis — called also *polyadenylate, polyadenylic acid*

poly·acryl·amide \ˌpä-lē-ə-'kri-lə-ˌmid\ *n* : a polymer (–CH₂CHCONH₂–)ₓ derived from acrylic acid

polyacrylamide gel *n* : hydrated polyacrylamide that is used esp. to provide a medium for the suspension of a substance to be subjected to gel electrophoresis

poly·ad·e·nyl·ate \ˌpä-lē-ˌad-ᵊn-'i-ˌlāt\ *n* : POLY(A) — **poly·ad·e·nyl·at·ed** \-ˌā-təd\ *adj* — **poly·ad·e·nyl·a·tion** \-i-'lā-shən\ *n*

poly·ad·e·nyl·ic acid \-'i-lik-\ *n* : POLY(A)

poly·an·dry \'pä-lē-ˌan-drē\ *n, pl* **-dries** : the state or practice of having more than one husband or male mate at one time — compare POLYGAMY, POLYGYNY — **poly·an·drous** \ˌpä-lē-'an-drəs\ *adj*

poly·ar·ter·i·tis \ˌpä-lē-ˌär-tə-'rī-təs\ *n* : POLYARTERITIS NODOSA

polyarteritis nodosa *n* : an acute inflammatory disease involving all layers of the arterial wall and characterized by degeneration, necrosis, exudation, and the formation of inflammatory nodules along the outer layer — called also *periarteritis nodosa*

poly·ar·thral·gia \-är-'thral-jē-ə\ *n* : pain in two or more joints

poly·ar·thri·tis \-är-'thrī-təs\ *n, pl* **-thrit·i·des** \-'thri-tə-ˌdēz\ : arthritis involving two or more joints

poly·ar·tic·u·lar \-är-'ti-kyə-lər\ *adj* : having or affecting many joints ⟨~ arthritis⟩ — compare MONOARTICULAR, OLIGOARTICULAR

poly·bro·mi·nat·ed biphenyl \ˌpä-lē-'brō-mə-ˌnā-təd-\ *n* : any of several compounds that are similar to polychlorinated biphenyls in environmental toxicity and in structure except that various hydrogen atoms are replaced by bromine rather than chlorine — called also *PBB*

poly(C) \ˌpä-lē-'sē\ *n* : POLYCYTIDYLIC ACID

poly·chlo·ri·nat·ed biphenyl \ˌpä-lē-'klōr-ə-ˌnā-təd-\ *n* : any of several compounds that are produced by replacing hydrogen atoms in biphenyl with chlorine, have various industrial applications, and are toxic environmental pollutants which tend to accumulate in animal tissues — called also *PCB*

poly·chon·dri·tis \-kän-'drī-təs\ *n* : inflammation of cartilage at multiple sites in the body — see RELAPSING POLYCHONDRITIS

poly·chro·ma·sia \-krō-'mā-zhə, -zhē-ə\ *n* : the quality of being polychromatic; *specif* : POLYCHROMATOPHILIA

poly·chro·mat·ic \-krō-'ma-tik\ *adj* **1** : showing a variety or a change of colors **2** of a cell or tissue : exhibiting polychromatophilia

¹**poly·chro·ma·to·phil** \-krō-'ma-tə-ˌfil, -'krō-mə-tə-\ *n* : a young or degenerated red blood cell staining with both acid and basic dyes

²**polychromatophil** *adj* : exhibiting polychromatophilia; *esp* : staining with both acid and basic dyes

poly·chro·mato·phil·ia \-krō-ˌma-tə-'fi-lē-ə\ *n* : the quality of being stain-able with more than one type of stain and esp. with both acid and basic dyes — **poly·chro·mato·phil·ic** \-krō-,ma-tə-'fi-lik\ *adj*

poly·clin·ic \,pä-lē-'kli-nik\ *n* : a clinic or hospital treating diseases of many sorts — compare POLICLINIC

poly·clo·nal \,pä-lē-'klōn-ə¹\ *adj* : produced by or being cells derived from two or more cells of different ancestry or genetic constitution ⟨~ antibody synthesis⟩

polycosanol *var of* POLICOSANOL

poly·cy·clic \,pä-lē-'sī-klik, -'si-\ *adj* : having more than one cyclic component; *esp* : having two or more usu. fused rings in a molecule

polycyclic aromatic hydrocarbon *n* : any of a class of hydrocarbon molecules with multiple carbon rings that include numerous carcinogenic substances and environmental pollutants — called also *PAH, polynuclear aromatic hydrocarbon*

poly·cys·tic \-'sis-tik\ *adj* : having or involving more than one cyst

polycystic kidney disease *n* : either of two hereditary diseases characterized by gradually enlarging bilateral cysts of the kidney which lead to reduced renal functioning: **a** : a disease that is inherited as an autosomal dominant trait, is usu. asymptomatic until middle age, and is marked by side or back pain, hematuria, urinary tract infections, and nephrolithiasis **b** : a disease that is inherited as an autosomal recessive trait, usu. affects infants or children, and results in renal failure

polycystic ovary syndrome *n* : a variable disorder that is marked esp. by amenorrhea, hirsutism, obesity, infertility, and ovarian enlargement and is usu. initiated by an elevated level of luteinizing hormone, androgen, or estrogen which results in an abnormal cycle of gonadotropin release by the pituitary gland — called also *polycystic ovarian disease, polycystic ovarian syndrome, polycystic ovary disease, Stein-Leventhal syndrome*

poly·cy·thae·mia, poly·cy·thae·mic *chiefly Brit var of* POLYCYTHEMIA, POLYCYTHEMIC

poly·cy·the·mia \-(,)sī-'thē-mē-ə\ *n* : a condition marked by an abnormal increase in the number of circulating red blood cells; *esp* : POLYCYTHEMIA VERA

polycythemia ve·ra \-'vir-ə\ *n* : chronic polycythemia that is a myeloproliferative disorder of unknown cause characterized by an increase in total blood volume and viscosity and typically accompanied by nosebleed, headache, dizziness, weakness, itchy skin, reddish complexion, distension of the circulatory vessels, and splenomegaly — called also *erythremia, Vaquez's disease*

poly·cy·the·mic \,pä-lē-(,)sī-'thē-mik\ *adj* : relating to or involving polycythemia or polycythemia vera

poly·cyt·i·dyl·ic acid \-,si-tə-'di-lik-\ *n* : RNA or a segment of RNA that is composed of a polynucleotide chain consisting entirely of cytosine-containing nucleotides, and that codes for a polypeptide chain consisting of proline residues when functioning as messenger RNA in protein synthesis — called also *poly(C)*; see POLY I:C

poly·dac·tyl \-'dak-t²l\ *adj* : characterized by polydactyly; *also* : being a gene that determines polydactyly

poly·dac·tyl·ia \-,dak-'ti-lē-ə\ *n* : POLYDACTYLY

poly·dac·tyl·ism \-'dakt-²l-,i-zəm\ *n* : POLYDACTYLY

poly·dac·ty·ly \-'dak-tə-lē\ *n, pl* **-lies** : the condition of having more than the normal number of toes or fingers

poly·dip·sia \-'dip-sē-ə\ *n* : excessive or abnormal thirst — **poly·dip·sic** \-sik\ *adj*

poly·drug \'pä-lē-'drəg\ *adj* : of, relating to, or being the abuse of more than one drug esp. when illicit; *also* : engaging in polydrug abuse

poly·em·bry·o·ny \,pä-lē-'em-brē-ə-nē, -(,)em-'brī-\ *n, pl* **-nies** : the production of two or more embryos from one ovule or egg

poly·en·do·crine \-'en-də-krən, -,krīn, -,krēn\ *adj* : relating to or affecting more than one endocrine gland

po·lyg·a·my \pə-'li-gə-mē\ *n, pl* **-mies** : marriage in which a spouse of either sex may have more than one mate at the same time — compare POLYANDRY, POLYGYNY — **po·lyg·a·mous** \-məs\ *adj*

poly·gene \'pä-lē-,jēn\ *n* : any of a group of nonallelic genes that collectively control the inheritance of a quantitative character or modify the expression of a qualitative character — called also *multiple factor*

poly·ge·nic \,pä-lē-'jē-nik, -'je-\ *adj* : of, relating to, or resulting from polygenes : MULTIFACTORIAL

poly·glan·du·lar \-'glan-jə-lər\ *adj* : of, relating to, or involving several glands

poly·graph \'pä-lē-,graf\ *n* : an instrument for simultaneously recording variations of several different pulsations (as of the pulse, blood pressure, and respiration) — see LIE DETECTOR — **poly·graph·ic** \,pä-lē-'gra-fik\ *adj*

po·lyg·y·ny \pə-'li-jə-nē\ *n, pl* **-nies** : the state or practice of having more than one wife or female mate at one time — compare POLYANDRY, POLYGAMY — **po·lyg·y·nous** \-nəs\ *adj*

poly·hy·dram·ni·os \,pä-lē-hī-'dram-nē-,äs\ *n* : HYDRAMNIOS

poly I:C \,pä-lē-,ī-'sē\ *n* : a synthetic 2-stranded RNA composed of one strand of polyinosinic acid and one strand of polycytidylic acid that induces interferon formation and has been used experimentally as an anticancer and antiviral agent — called also *poly I:poly C*

poly·ino·sin·ic acid \,pä-lē-,i-nə-'sin-ik-, -,ī-nə-\ *n* : RNA or a segment of RNA that is composed of a polynucleotide chain consisting entirely of inosinic acid residues — see POLY I:C

poly I:poly C \,pä-lē-'ī-,pä-lē-'sē\ *n* : POLY I:C

poly·ke·tide \,pä-lē-'kē-,tīd\ *n* : any of a large class of diverse compounds that are characterized by more than two CO groups connected by single intervening carbon atoms, that are produced esp. by certain bacteria and fungi, and that include various substances (as erythromycin and lovastatin) having antibiotic, anticancer, cholesterol-lowering, or immunosuppressive effects

poly·ly·sine \,pä-lē-'lī-,sēn\ *n* : a protein whose polypeptide chain consists entirely of lysine residues

poly·mer \'pä-lə-mər\ *n* : a chemical compound or mixture of compounds formed by polymerization and consisting essentially of repeating structural units — **poly·mer·ic** \,pä-lə-'mer-ik\ *adj* — **po·ly·mer·ism** \pə-'li-mə-,ri-zəm, 'pä-lə-mə-\ *n*

poly·mer·ase \-mə-,rās, -,rāz\ *n* : any of several enzymes that catalyze the formation of DNA or RNA from precursor substances in the presence of preexisting DNA or RNA acting as a template

polymerase chain reaction *n* : an in vitro technique for rapidly synthesizing large quantities of a given DNA segment that involves separating the DNA into its two complementary strands, binding a primer to each single strand at the end of the given DNA segment where synthesis will start, using DNA polymerase to synthesize two-stranded DNA from each single strand, and repeating the process — abbr. *PCR*

po·ly·mer·iza·tion \pə-,li-mə-rə-'zā-shən, ,pä-lə-mə-rə-\ *n* : a chemical reaction in which two or more small molecules combine to form larger molecules that contain repeating structural units of the original molecules — compare ASSOCIATION 3 — **po·ly·mer·ize** \pə-'li-mə-,rīz, 'pä-lə-mə-\ *vb*

poly·meth·yl meth·ac·ry·late \,pä-lē-'me-thəl-me-'tha-krə-,lāt\ *n* : a thermoplastic polymeric resin that is used esp. in hard contact lenses and in prostheses to replace bone

poly·mi·cro·bi·al \,pä-lē-mī-'krō-bē-əl\ *adj* : of, relating to, or caused by several types of microorganisms

poly·mod·al \,pä-lē-'mō-d³l\ *adj* : responding to several different forms of sensory stimulation

poly·morph \'pä-lē-,mȯrf\ *n* **1** : a polymorphic organism; *also* : one of the several forms of such an organism **2** : a polymorphonuclear leukocyte

poly·mor·phic \,pä-lē-'mȯr-fik\ *adj* : of, relating to, or having polymorphism — **poly·mor·phi·cal·ly** \-fi-k(ə-)lē\ *adv*

polymorphic light eruption *n* : POLYMORPHOUS LIGHT ERUPTION

poly·mor·phism \-'mȯr-,fi-zəm\ *n* : the quality or state of existing in or assuming several different forms: as **a** : existence of a species in several forms independent of the variations of sex **b** : existence of a gene in several allelic forms; *also* : a variation in a specific DNA sequence **c** : existence of a molecule (as an enzyme) in several forms in a single species

¹poly·mor·pho·nu·cle·ar \-,mȯr-fō-'nü-klē-ər, -'nyü-\ *adj, of a leukocyte* : having the nucleus complexly lobed; *specif* : being a mature neutrophil with a characteristic distinctly lobed nucleus

²polymorphonuclear *n* : POLYMORPH 2

poly·mor·phous \-'mȯr-fəs\ *adj* : having, assuming, or occurring in various forms — **poly·mor·phous·ly** *adv*

polymorphous light eruption *n* : photodermatosis that is marked esp. by red papules or blisters often accompanied by itching or a burning sensation

polymorphous perverse *adj* : relating to or exhibiting infantile sexual tendencies in which the genitals are not yet identified as the sole or principal sexual organs nor coitus as the goal of erotic activity

poly·my·al·gia \,pä-li-mī-'al-jē-ə\ *n* : myalgia affecting several muscle groups; *specif* : POLYMYALGIA RHEUMATICA

polymyalgia rheu·mat·i·ca \-rü-'ma-ti-kə\ *n* : a disorder of the elderly characterized by muscular pain and stiffness in the shoulders and neck and in the pelvic area

poly·myo·si·tis \-,mī-ə-'sī-təs\ *n* : inflammation of several muscles at once; *specif* : an inflammatory muscle disease of unknown cause that affects skeletal muscles and is characterized esp. by weakness of muscles (as of the shoulder or hip) closest to the trunk — see DERMATOMYOSITIS

poly·myx·in \,pä-lē-'mik-sən\ *n* : any of several toxic antibiotics obtained from a soil bacterium of the genus *Bacillus* (*B. polymyxa*) and active against gram-negative bacteria

polymyxin B *n* : the least toxic of the polymyxins used in the form of its sulfate chiefly in the treatment of some localized, gastrointestinal, or systemic infections

polymyxin E *n* : COLISTIN

poly·neu·ri·tis \,pä-lē-nù-'rī-təs, -nyù-\ *n, pl* **-rit·i·des** \-'ri-tə-,dēz\ *or* **-ri·tis·es** : neuritis of several peripheral nerves at the same time — see GUILLAIN-BARRÉ SYNDROME — **poly·neu·rit·ic** \-'ri-tik\ *adj*

poly·neu·ro·pa·thy \-nù-'rä-pə-thē,

-nyü-\ *n, pl* **-thies** : a disease of nerves; *esp* : a noninflammatory degenerative disease of nerves usu. caused by toxins (as of lead)

poly·nu·cle·ar \-'nü-klē-ər, -'nyü-\ *adj* : chemically polycyclic esp. with respect to the benzene ring

polynuclear aromatic hydrocarbon *n* : POLYCYCLIC AROMATIC HYDROCARBON

poly·nu·cle·o·tide \-'nü-klē-ə-ˌtīd, -'nyü-\ *n* : a polymeric chain of nucleotides

poly·oma·vi·rus \ˌpä-lē-'ō-mə-ˌvī-rəs\ *n* **1** *cap* : a genus of double-stranded DNA viruses (family *Polyomaviridae*) that induce tumors usu. in specific mammals and that include simian virus 40 and the causative agent of progressive multifocal leukoencephalopathy **2** : any virus of the genus *Polyomavirus* or of the family (*Polyomaviridae*) to which it belongs

poly·opia \ˌpä-lē-'ō-pē-ə\ *n* : perception of more than one image of a single object esp. with one eye

poly·os·tot·ic \ˌpä-lē-ä-'stä-tik\ *adj* : involving or relating to many bones

pol·yp \'pä-ləp\ *n* : a projecting mass of swollen and hypertrophied or tumorous membrane

pol·yp·ec·to·my \ˌpä-li-'pek-tə-mē\ *n, pl* **-mies** : the surgical excision of a polyp

poly·pep·tide \ˌpä-lē-'pep-ˌtīd\ *n* : a molecular chain of amino acids — **poly·pep·tid·ic** \-(ˌ)pep-'ti-dik\ *adj*

poly·pha·gia \-'fā-jə, -jē-ə\ *n* : excessive appetite or eating — compare HYPERPHAGIA

poly·phar·ma·cy \-'fär-mə-sē\ *n, pl* **-cies** : the practice of administering many different medicines esp. concurrently for the treatment of the same disease

poly·pha·sic \-'fā-zik\ *adj* **1** : of, relating to, or having more than one phase — compare DIPHASIC b, MONOPHASIC 1 **2** : having several periods of activity interrupted by intervening periods of rest in each 24 hours ⟨an infant is essentially ∼⟩

poly·phe·nol \ˌpä-li-'fē-ˌnōl, -ˌnȯl\ *n* : a phenol containing more than one hydroxyl group in a molecule; *esp* : an antioxidant phytochemical that tends to prevent or neutralize the damaging effects of free radicals — **poly·phe·no·lic** \-fi-'nō-lik, -'nä-\ *adj*

poly·ploid \'pä-lē-ˌplȯid\ *adj* : having or being a chromosome number that is a multiple greater than two of the monoploid number — **poly·ploi·dy** \-ˌplȯi-dē\ *n*

po·lyp·nea \pä-'lip-nē-ə, pə-\ *n* : rapid or panting respiration — **po·lyp·ne·ic** \-nē-ik\ *adj*

po·lyp·noea *chiefly Brit var of* POLYPNEA

pol·yp·oid \'pä-lə-ˌpȯid\ *adj* **1** : resembling a polyp ⟨a ∼ intestinal growth⟩

2 : marked by the formation of lesions suggesting polyps ⟨∼ disease⟩

pol·yp·o·sis \ˌpä-li-'pō-səs\ *n, pl* **-o·ses** \-ˌsēz\ : a condition characterized by the presence of numerous polyps — see FAMILIAL ADENOMATOUS POLYPOSIS

poly·ra·dic·u·lo·neu·rop·a·thy \ˌpä-li-rə-ˌdi-kyə-lō-nü-'rä-pə-thē, -nyü-\ *n, pl* **-thies** : an inflammatory disorder (as Guillain-Barré syndrome) affecting peripheral nerves and the nerve roots of the spinal nerves and marked by demyelination or axon degeneration

poly·ri·bo·some \ˌpä-lē-'rī-bə-ˌsōm\ *n* : a cluster of ribosomes linked together by a molecule of messenger RNA and forming the site of protein synthesis — called also *polysome* — **poly·ri·bo·som·al** \-ˌrī-bə-'sō-məl\ *adj*

poly·sac·cha·ride \-'sa-kə-ˌrīd\ *n* : a carbohydrate that can be decomposed by hydrolysis into two or more molecules of monosaccharides; *esp* : one (as cellulose, starch, or glycogen) containing many monosaccharide units and marked by complexity — called also *glycan*

poly·se·ro·si·tis \-ˌsir-ə-'sī-təs\ *n* : inflammation of several serous membranes (as the pleura, pericardium, and peritoneum) at the same time

poly·some \'pä-lē-ˌsōm\ *n* : POLYRIBOSOME

poly·som·no·gram \ˌpä-lē-'säm-nə-ˌgram\ *n* : a record of physiological variables during sleep obtained by polysomnography

poly·som·no·graph \ˌpä-lē-'säm-nə-ˌgraf\ *n* : a polygraph used for polysomnography

poly·som·nog·ra·phy \ˌpä-lē-ˌsäm-'nä-grə-fē\ *n, pl* **-phies** : the technique or process of using a polygraph to make a continuous record during sleep of multiple physiological variables (as breathing, heart rate, and muscle activity) — **poly·som·nog·ra·pher** \-ˌsäm-'nä-grə-fər\ *n* — **poly·som·no·graph·ic** \-nə-'gra-fik\ *adj*

poly·sor·bate \ˌpä-lē-'sȯr-ˌbāt\ *n* : any of several emulsifiers used in the preparation of some pharmaceuticals and foods — see TWEEN

poly·sper·my \'pä-lē-ˌspər-mē\ *n, pl* **-mies** : the entrance of several spermatozoa into one egg — compare MONOSPERMY — **poly·sper·mic** \ˌpä-lē-'spər-mik\ *adj*

poly·sub·stance \'pä-lē-'səb-stəns\ *n, often attrib* : a group of substances used often indiscriminately by a substance abuser

poly·syn·ap·tic \ˌpä-lē-sə-'nap-tik\ *adj* : involving two or more synapses in the central nervous system — **poly·syn·ap·ti·cal·ly** *adv*

poly·tene \'pä-lē-ˌtēn\ *adj* : relating to, being, or having chromosomes each of which consists of many strands with the corresponding chromomeres in contact — **poly·te·ny** \-ˌte-nē\ *n*

poly·tet·ra·flu·o·ro·eth·yl·ene \ˌpä-lē-ˌte-trə-ˌflu̇r-ō-ˈe-thə-ˌlēn\ *n* : a polymer $(CF_2-CF_2)_n$ that is a resin used to fabricate prostheses — abbr. *PTFE*; see TEFLON

poly·the·lia \ˌpä-lē-ˈthē-lē-ə\ *n* : the condition of having more than the normal number of nipples

poly·thi·a·zide \-ˈthī-ə-ˌzīd, -zəd\ *n* : an antihypertensive and diuretic drug $C_{11}H_{13}ClF_3N_3O_4S_3$ — see RENESE

poly(U) \ˌpä-lē-ˈyü\ *n* : POLYURIDYLIC ACID

poly·un·sat·u·rate \ˌpä-lē-ˌən-ˈsa-chə-ˌrät\ *n* : a polyunsaturated oil or fatty acid

poly·un·sat·u·rat·ed \-ˌən-ˈsa-chə-ˌrā-təd\ *adj, of an oil, fat, or fatty acid* : having in each molecule many chemical bonds in which two or three pairs of electrons are shared by two atoms — compare MONOUNSATURATED

poly·uria \-ˈyu̇r-ē-ə\ *n* : excessive secretion of urine

poly·uri·dyl·ic acid \-ˌyu̇r-ə-ˌdi-lik-\ *n* : RNA or a segment of RNA that is composed of a polynucleotide chain consisting entirely of uracil-containing nucleotides and that codes for a polypeptide chain consisting of phenylalanine residues when functioning as messenger RNA in protein synthesis — called also *poly(U)*

poly·va·lent \ˌpä-lē-ˈvā-lənt\ *adj* : effective against, sensitive toward, or counteracting more than one exciting agent (as a toxin or antigen) ⟨a ∼ vaccine⟩ — **poly·va·lence** \-ləns\ *n*

poly·vi·nyl·pyr·rol·i·done \-ˌvīn-ᵊl-pi-ˈrä-lə-ˌdōn\ *n* : a water-soluble chemically inert polymer $(C_6H_9NO)_n$ used in medicine as a vehicle for drugs (as iodine) and esp. formerly as a plasma expander — called also *povidone*

Pompe's disease \ˈpämps-\ *n* : an often fatal glycogen storage disease that results from an enzyme deficiency, is characterized by abnormal accumulation of glycogen esp. in the liver, heart, and muscle, and usu. appears during infancy — called also *acid maltase deficiency*

Pompe, Johann Cassianius *(fl 1932)*, Dutch physician.

pom·pho·lyx \ˈpäm-fə-ˌliks\ *n* : a skin disease marked by an eruption of vesicles esp. on the palms and soles

pon·der·al index \ˈpän-də-rəl-\ *n* : a measure of relative body mass expressed as the ratio of the cube root of body weight to height multiplied by 100

P_1 generation \ˈpē-ˈwən-\ *n* : a generation consisting of stocks which are usu. homozygous for one or more traits and from which the parents used in the first cross of a genetic experiment are selected — compare F_1 GENERATION

pons \ˈpänz\ *n, pl* **pon·tes** \ˈpän-ˌtēz\ : a broad mass of chiefly transverse nerve fibers in the mammalian brain stem lying ventral to the cerebellum at the anterior end of the medulla oblongata

pons Va·ro·lii \-və-ˈrō-lē-ˌī, -lē-ˌē\ *n, pl* **pontes Varolii** : PONS

Va·ro·lio \vä-ˈrō-lē-ō\, Costanzo (1543–1575), Italian anatomist.

Pon·ti·ac fever \ˈpän-tē-ˌak-\ *n* : an illness caused by a bacterium of the genus *Legionella* (*L. pneumophila*) that is a less severe form of Legionnaires' disease in which pneumonia does not develop

pon·tic \ˈpän-tik\ *n* : an artificial tooth on a dental bridge

pon·tile \ˈpän-ˌtīl, -təl\ *adj* : PONTINE

pon·tine \ˈpän-ˌtīn\ *adj* : of or relating to the pons ⟨a study of ∼ lesions⟩

pontine flexure *n* : a flexure of the embryonic hindbrain that serves to delimit the developing cerebellum and medulla oblongata

pontine nucleus *n* : any of various large groups of nerve cells in the basal part of the pons that receive fibers from the cerebral cortex and send fibers to the cerebellum by way of the middle cerebellar peduncles

pontis — see BRACHIUM PONTIS

Pon·to·caine \ˈpän-tə-ˌkān\ *trademark* — used for a preparation of the hydrochloride of tetracaine

¹**pool** \ˈpu̇l\ *vb, of blood* : to accumulate or become static (as in the veins of a bodily part) ⟨blood ∼ed in his legs⟩

²**pool** *n* : a readily available supply: as **a** : the whole quantity of a particular material present in the body and available for function or the satisfying of metabolic demands — see GENE POOL **b** : a body product (as blood) collected from many donors and stored for later use

pop·li·te·al \ˌpä-plə-ˈtē-əl, päp-ˈli-tē-\ *adj* : of or relating to the back part of the leg behind the knee joint

popliteal artery *n* : the continuation of the femoral artery that after passing through the thigh crosses the popliteal space and soon divides into the anterior and posterior tibial arteries

popliteal fossa *n* : POPLITEAL SPACE

popliteal ligament — see ARCUATE POPLITEAL LIGAMENT, OBLIQUE POPLITEAL LIGAMENT

popliteal nerve — see LATERAL POPLITEAL NERVE, MEDIAL POPLITEAL NERVE

popliteal space *n* : a lozenge-shaped space at the back of the knee joint — called also *popliteal fossa*

popliteal vein *n* : a vein formed by the union of the anterior and posterior tibial veins and ascending through the popliteal space to the thigh where it becomes the femoral vein

pop·li·te·us \ˌpä-plə-ˈtē-əs, päp-ˈli-tē-əs\ *n, pl* **-li·tei** \-tē-ˌī\ : a flat muscle that originates from the lateral condyle of the femur, forms part of the floor of the popliteal space, and functions to flex the leg and rotate the femur medially

pop·per \'pä-pər\ *n, slang* : a vial of amyl nitrite or butyl nitrite esp. when used illicitly as an aphrodisiac

pop·py \'pä-pē\ *n, pl* **poppies** : any herb of the genus *Papaver* (family Papaveraceae); *esp* : OPIUM POPPY

pop·u·la·tion \ˌpä-pyə-'lā-shən\ *n* 1 : the organisms inhabiting a particular locality 2 : a group of individual persons, objects, or items from which samples are taken for statistical measurement

population genetics *n* : a branch of genetics concerned with gene and genotype frequencies in populations — see HARDY-WEINBERG LAW

por·ce·lain \'pōr-sə-lən\ *n* : a hard, fine-grained, nonporous, and usu. translucent and white ceramic ware that has many uses in dentistry

por·cine \'pōr-ˌsīn\ *adj* : of or derived from swine ⟨~ heterografts⟩

pore \'pōr\ *n* : a minute opening esp. in an animal or plant; *esp* : one by which matter passes through a membrane

-pore \ˌpōr\ *n comb form* : opening ⟨blasto*pore*⟩

por·en·ceph·a·ly \ˌpōr-in-'se-fə-lē\ *n, pl* **-lies** : the presence of cavities in the brain — **por·en·ce·phal·ic** \-ˌen-sə-'fa-lik\ *adj*

por·fi·mer sodium \'pōr-fə-mər-\ *n* : a photosensitizing mixture of porphyrin polymers that is administered by intravenous injection to induce photosensitivity in tumor cells (as of esophageal carcinoma) before subjecting them to laser light in photodynamic therapy — see PHOTOFRIN

pork tapeworm \'pōrk-\ *n* : a tapeworm of the genus *Taenia* (*T. solium*) that infests the human intestine as an adult, has a cysticercus larva that typically develops in swine, and is contracted by humans through ingestion of the larva in raw or imperfectly cooked pork

po·ro·ceph·a·li·a·sis \ˌpō-rō-ˌse-fə-'lī-ə-səs\ *n, pl* **-a·ses** \-ˌsēz\ : infestation with or disease caused by a tongue worm of the genus *Porocephalus*

Po·ro·ceph·a·lus \-'se-fə-ləs\ *n* : a genus of tongue worms (family Porocephalidae) occurring as adults in the lungs of reptiles and as young in various vertebrates including humans

po·ro·ker·a·to·sis \-ˌker-ə-'tō-səs\ *n* : any of several uncommon inherited skin disorders characterized by hypertrophy of the stratum corneum

po·ro·sis \pə-'rō-səs\ *n, pl* **po·ro·ses** \-ˌsēz\ *or* **porosises** : a condition (as of a bone) characterized by porosity; *specif* : rarefaction (as of bone) with increased translucency to X-rays

po·ros·i·ty \pə-'rä-sə-tē, pō-, pò-\ *n, pl*

-ties 1 **a** : the quality or state of being porous **b** : the ratio of the volume of interstices of a material to the volume of its mass 2 : PORE

po·rot·ic \pə-'rä-tik\ *adj* : exhibiting or marked by porous structure or osteoporosis ⟨~ bone⟩

po·rous \'pōr-əs\ *adj* 1 : possessing or full of pores ⟨~ bones⟩ 2 : permeable to fluids

por·pho·bi·lin·o·gen \ˌpōr-fō-bī-'li-nə-jən\ *n* : an acid $C_{10}H_{14}N_2O_4$ having two carboxyl groups per molecule that is derived from pyrrole and is found in the urine in acute porphyria

por·phyr·ia \pōr-'fir-ē-ə\ *n* : any of several usu. hereditary abnormalities of porphyrin metabolism characterized by excretion of excess porphyrins in the urine

porphyria cu·ta·nea tar·da \-kyü-'tā-nē-ə-'tär-də\ *n* : a common porphyria that is marked by an excess of uroporphyrin caused by an enzyme deficiency chiefly of the liver and that is characterized esp. by skin lesions upon exposure to light, scarring, hyperpigmentation, and hypertrichosis

por·phy·rin \'pōr-fə-rən\ *n* : any of various compounds with a structure that consists essentially of four pyrrole rings joined by four =CH– groups; *esp* : one (as hemoglobin) containing a central metal atom and usu. having biological activity

por·phy·rin·uria \ˌpōr-fə-rə-'nür-ē-ə, -'nyùr-\ *n* : the presence of porphyrin in the urine

port \'pōrt\ *n* : an opening, passage, or channel through which something can be introduced into the body: as **a** : a small medical device (as of plastic or titanium) that is implanted below the skin, is attached to a catheter typically inserted into a blood vessel, and has a small opening through which a needle can be inserted to administer fluids or drugs or withdraw blood **b** : an incision (as one made between intercostal spaces) for passing a medical instrument (as an endoscope) into the body

por·ta \'pōr-tə\ *n, pl* **por·tae** \-ˌtē\ : an opening in a bodily part where the blood vessels, nerves, or ducts leave and enter : HILUM

por·ta·ca·val \ˌpōr-tə-'kā-vəl\ *adj* : extending from the portal vein to the vena cava ⟨~ anastomosis⟩

portacaval shunt *n* : a surgical shunt by which the portal vein is made to empty into the inferior vena cava in order to bypass a damaged liver

porta hep·a·tis \-'he-pə-təs\ *n* : the fissure running transversely on the underside of the liver where most of the vessels enter or leave — called also *transverse fissure*

¹**por·tal** \'pōrt-ᵊl\ *n* : a communicating part or area of an organism: as **a** : PORTAL VEIN **b** : the point at which something enters the body

²**portal** *adj* **1** : of or relating to the porta hepatis **2** : of, relating to, or being a portal vein or a portal system

portal cirrhosis *n* : LAENNEC'S CIRRHOSIS

portal hypertension *n* : hypertension in the hepatic portal system caused by venous obstruction or occlusion that produces splenomegaly and ascites in its later stages

portal system *n* : a system of veins that begins and ends in capillaries — see HEPATIC PORTAL SYSTEM, PITUITARY PORTAL SYSTEM

portal vein *n* : a large vein that is formed by fusion of other veins, that terminates in a capillary network, and that delivers blood to some area of the body other than the heart; *esp* : HEPATIC PORTAL VEIN

por·tio \'pȯr-tē-ˌō, 'pȯr-tē-ˌō\ *n, pl* **-ti·o·nes** \ˌpȯr-shē-'ō-ˌnēz\ : a part, segment, or branch (as of an organ or nerve) ⟨the visible ~ of the cervix⟩

por·to·sys·tem·ic \ˌpȯr-tō-sis-'te-mik\ *adj* : connecting the hepatic portal system and the venous part of the systemic circulation ⟨a ~ shunt⟩

Por·tu·guese man–of–war \'pȯr-chə-ˌgēz-ˌman-əv-'wȯr\ *n, pl* **Portuguese man–of–wars** *also* **Portuguese men–of–war** : any siphonophore of the genus *Physalia* including tropical and subtropical oceanic forms having a large crested bladderlike float and long tentacles capable of inflicting a painful sting

port–wine stain \'pȯrt-ˌwīn-\ *n* : a reddish purple superficial hemangioma of the skin commonly occurring as a birthmark — called also *nevus flammeus, port-wine mark*

POS *abbr* point-of-service

¹**po·si·tion** \pə-'zi-shən\ *n* : a particular arrangement or location; *specif* : an arrangement of the parts of the body considered particularly desirable for some medical or surgical procedure ⟨knee-chest ~⟩ ⟨lithotomy ~⟩ — **po·si·tion·al** \pə-'zi-shə-nəl\ *adj*

²**position** *vb* : to put in proper position

pos·i·tive \'pä-zə-tiv\ *adj* **1** : being, relating to, or charged with electricity of which the proton is the elementary unit **2** : affirming the presence of that sought or suspected to be present ⟨a ~ test for blood⟩ — **positive** *n* — **pos·i·tive·ly** *adv* — **pos·i·tive·ness** *n*

positive electron *n* : POSITRON

positive end–expiratory pressure *n* : a technique of assisting breathing by increasing the air pressure in the lungs and air passages near the end of expiration so that an increased amount of air remains in the lungs following expiration — abbr. *PEEP*

positive pressure *n* : pressure that is greater than atmospheric pressure

pos·i·tron \'pä-zə-ˌträn\ *n* : a positively charged particle having the same mass and magnitude of charge as the electron

positron–emission tomography *n* : tomography in which an in vivo, noninvasive, cross-sectional image of regional metabolism is obtained by a usu. color-coded cathode-ray tube representation of the distribution of gamma radiation given off in the collision of electrons in cells with positrons emitted by radionuclides incorporated into metabolic substances — abbr. *PET*

post- *prefix* **1** : after : later than ⟨*post*operative⟩ ⟨*post*coronary⟩ **2** : behind : posterior to ⟨*post*auricular⟩

post·abor·tion \ˌpōst-ə-'bȯr-shən\ *adj* : occurring after an abortion

post·ab·sorp·tive \-əb-'sȯrp-tiv\ *adj* : being in or typical of the period following absorption of nutrients from the digestive tract

post·ad·o·les·cence \-ˌad-ᵊl-'es-ᵊns\ *n* : the period following adolescence and preceding adulthood — **post·ad·o·les·cent** \-ᵊnt\ *adj or n*

post·an·es·the·sia \-ˌa-nəs-'thē-zhə\ *adj* : POSTANESTHETIC

postanesthesia care unit *n* : RECOVERY ROOM

post·an·es·thet·ic \-'the-tik\ *adj* : occurring in, used in, or being the period following administration of an anesthetic ⟨~ encephalopathy⟩

post·an·ox·ic \-ə-'näk-sik\ *adj* : occurring or being after a period of anoxia

post·au·ric·u·lar \-ō-'ri-kyə-lər\ *adj* : located or occurring behind the auricle of the ear ⟨a ~ incision⟩

post·ax·i·al \-'ak-sē-əl\ *adj* : of or relating to the ulnar side of the vertebrate forelimb or the fibular side of the hind limb; *also* : of or relating to the side of an animal or side of one of its limbs that is posterior to the axis of its body or limbs

post·cap·il·lary \-'ka-pə-ˌler-ē\ *adj* : of, relating to, affecting, or being a venule of the circulatory system

post·car·di·ot·o·my \-ˌkär-dē-'ä-tə-mē\ *adj* : occurring or being in the period following open-heart surgery

post·cen·tral \-'sen-trəl\ *adj* : located behind a center or central structure; *esp* : located behind the central sulcus of the cerebral cortex

postcentral gyrus *n* : a gyrus of the parietal lobe located just posterior to the central sulcus, lying parallel to the precentral gyrus of the temporal lobe, and comprising the somatosensory cortex

post·cho·le·cys·tec·to·my syndrome \-ˌkō-lə-ˌ(ˌ)sis-'tek-tə-mē-\ *n* : persistent pain and associated symptoms (as indigestion and nausea) following a cholecystectomy

post·co·i·tal \-'kō-ət-ᵊl, -'ēt-ᵊl; -'kȯit-ᵊl\ *adj* : occurring, existing, or being administered after coitus

post·cor·o·nary \-'kȯr-ə-ˌner-ē, -'kär-\ *adj* **1** : relating to, occurring in, or being the period following a heart attack ⟨∼ exercise⟩ **2** : having suffered a heart attack ⟨a ∼ patient⟩

post·dam \ˌpōst-'dam\ *n* : a posterior extension of a full denture to accomplish a complete seal between denture and tissues

post·en·ceph·a·lit·ic \-in-ˌse-fə-'li-tik\ *adj* : occurring after and presumably as a result of encephalitis ⟨∼ parkinsonism⟩

¹**pos·te·ri·or** \pō-'stir-ē-ər, pä-\ *adj* : situated behind: as **a** : situated at or toward the hind part of the body : CAUDAL **b** : DORSAL — used of human anatomy in which the upright posture makes dorsal and caudal identical

²**pos·te·ri·or** \pä-'stir-ē-ər, pō-\ *n* : the posterior bodily parts; *esp* : BUTTOCKS

posterior auricular artery *n* : a small branch of the external carotid artery that supplies or gives off branches supplying the back of the ear and the adjacent region of the scalp, the middle ear, tympanic membrane, and mastoid cells — called also *posterior auricular*

posterior auricular vein *n* : a vein formed from venous tributaries in the region behind the ear that joins with the posterior facial vein to form the external jugular vein

posterior brachial cutaneous nerve *n* : a branch of the radial nerve that arises on the medial side of the arm in the axilla and supplies the skin on the dorsal surface almost to the olecranon

posterior cerebral artery *n* : CEREBRAL ARTERY c

posterior chamber *n* : a narrow space in the eye behind the peripheral part of the iris and in front of the suspensory ligament of the lens and the ciliary processes — compare ANTERIOR CHAMBER

posterior column *n* : DORSAL HORN

posterior commissure *n* : a bundle of white matter crossing from one side of the brain to the other just rostral to the superior colliculi and above the opening of the aqueduct of Sylvius into the third ventricle

posterior communicating artery *n* : COMMUNICATING ARTERY b

posterior cord *n* : a cord of nerve tissue that is formed from the posterior divisions of the three trunks of the brachial plexus and that divides into the axillary and radial nerves — compare LATERAL CORD, MEDIAL CORD

posterior cricoarytenoid *n* : CRICO-ARYTENOID 2

posterior cruciate ligament *n* : a cruciate ligament of each knee that attaches the back of the tibia with the front of the femur and functions esp. to limit the backward motion of the tibia — called also *PCL*

posterior elastic lamina *n* : DESCEMET'S MEMBRANE

posterior facial vein *n* : a vein that is

formed in the upper part of the parotid gland behind the mandible by the union of several tributaries and joins with the posterior auricular vein to form the external jugular vein

posterior femoral cutaneous nerve *n* : a nerve that arises from the sacral plexus and is distributed to the skin of the perineum and of the back of the thigh and leg — compare LATERAL FEMORAL CUTANEOUS NERVE

posterior funiculus *n* : a longitudinal division on each side of the spinal cord comprising white matter between the dorsal root and the posterior median sulcus — compare ANTERIOR FUNICULUS, LATERAL FUNICULUS

posterior gray column *n* : DORSAL HORN

posterior horn *n* **1** : DORSAL HORN **2** : the cornu of the lateral ventricle of each cerebral hemisphere that curves backward into the occipital lobe — compare ANTERIOR HORN 2, INFERIOR HORN

posterior humeral circumflex artery *n* : an artery that branches from the axillary artery in the shoulder, curves around the back of the humerus, and is distributed esp. to the deltoid muscle and shoulder joint — compare ANTERIOR HUMERAL CIRCUMFLEX ARTERY

posterior inferior cerebellar artery *n* : an artery that usu. branches from the vertebral artery and supplies much of the medulla oblongata, the inferior portion of the cerebellum, and part of the floor of the fourth ventricle

posterior inferior iliac spine *n* : a projection on the posterior margin of the ilium that is situated below the posterior superior iliac spine and is separated from it by a notch — called also *posterior inferior spine*

posterior intercostal artery *n* : INTERCOSTAL ARTERY b

posterior lobe *n* **1** : NEUROHYPOPHYSIS **2** : the part of the cerebellum between the primary fissure and the flocculonodular lobe

pos·te·ri·or·ly *adv* : in a posterior direction

posterior median septum *n* : a sheet of glial tissue in the midsagittal plane of the spinal cord that partitions the posterior part of the spinal cord into right and left halves

posterior median sulcus *n* : a shallow groove along the midline of the posterior part of the spinal cord that separates the two posterior funiculi

posterior naris *n* : CHOANA

posterior nasal spine *n* : the nasal spine that is formed by the union of processes of the two palatine bones

posterior pillar of the fauces *n* : PALATOPHARYNGEAL ARCH

posterior pituitary *n* **1** : NEUROHY-

POPHYSIS **2** : an extract of the neuro-hypophysis of domesticated animals for medicinal use — called also *posterior pituitary extract*

posterior pituitary gland *n* : NEURO-HYPOPHYSIS

posterior root *n* : DORSAL ROOT

posterior sacrococcygeal muscle *n* : SACROCOCCYGEUS DORSALIS

posterior spinal artery *n* : SPINAL ARTERY b

posterior spinocerebellar tract *n* : SPINOCEREBELLAR TRACT a

posterior superior alveolar artery *n* : a branch of the maxillary artery that supplies the upper molar and bicuspid teeth

posterior superior alveolar vein *n* : any of several tributaries of the pterygoid plexus that drain the upper posterior teeth and gums

posterior superior iliac spine *n* : a projection at the posterior end of the iliac crest — called also *posterior superior spine*

posterior synechia *n* : SYNECHIA b

posterior temporal artery *n* : TEMPORAL ARTERY 3c

posterior tibial artery *n* : TIBIAL ARTERY a

posterior tibial vein *n* : TIBIAL VEIN a

posterior triangle *n* : a triangular region that is a landmark in the neck and has its apex above at the occipital bone — compare ANTERIOR TRIANGLE

posterior ulnar recurrent artery *n* : ULNAR RECURRENT ARTERY b

posterior vein of the left ventricle *n* : a vein that ascends on the surface of the left ventricle facing the diaphragm and that usu. empties into the coronary sinus — called also *posterior vein*

posterior vitreous detachment *n* : VITREOUS DETACHMENT

postero- *comb form* : posterior and ⟨*postero*anterior⟩ ⟨*postero*lateral⟩

pos·tero·an·te·ri·or \ˌpäs-tə-rō-an-'tir-ē-ər\ *adj* : involving or produced in a direction from the back toward the front (as of the body or an organ)

pos·tero·lat·er·al \ˌpäs-tə-rō-'la-tə-rəl\ *adj* : posterior and lateral in position or direction ⟨the ∼ aspect of the leg⟩ — **pos·tero·lat·er·al·ly** *adv*

pos·tero·me·di·al \-'mē-dē-əl\ *adj* : located on or near the dorsal midline of the body or a body part

post·ex·po·sure \ˌpōst-ik-'spō-zhər\ *adj* : occurring after exposure (as to a virus) — **postexposure** *adv*

¹**post·fer·til·i·za·tion** \-ˌfər-tᵊl-ə-'zā-shən\ *adj* : occurring in the period following fertilization

²**postfertilization** *adv* : after fertilization ⟨occurred 48 hours ∼⟩

post·gan·gli·on·ic \ˌgaŋ-glē-'ä-nik\ *adj* : distal to a ganglion; *specif* : of, relating to, or being an axon arising from a cell body within an autonomic ganglion — compare PREGANGLIONIC

post·gas·trec·to·my \-ga-'strek-tə-mē\ *adj* : occurring in, being in, or characteristic of the period following a gastrectomy

postgastrectomy syndrome *n* : dumping syndrome following a gastrectomy

post·hem·or·rhag·ic \-ˌhe-mə-'ra-jik\ *adj* : occurring after and as the result of a hemorrhage ⟨∼ shock⟩

post·he·pat·ic \-hi-'pa-tik\ *adj* : occurring or located behind the liver

post·hep·a·tit·ic \-ˌhe-pə-'ti-tik\ *adj* : occurring after and esp. as a result of hepatitis ⟨∼ cirrhosis⟩

post·her·pet·ic \-hər-'pe-tik\ *adj* : occurring after and esp. as a result of herpes ⟨∼ scars⟩

pos·thi·tis \(ˌ)päs-'thī-təs\ *n, pl* **pos·thit·i·des** \-'thi-tə-ˌdēz\ : inflammation of the prepuce

post·hyp·not·ic \ˌpōst-hip-'nä-tik\ *adj* : of, relating to, or characteristic of the period following a hypnotic trance during which the subject will still carry out suggestions made by the operator during the trance state

post·ic·tal \-'ikt-ᵊl\ *adj* : occurring after a sudden attack (as of epilepsy)

posticus — see TIBIALIS POSTICUS

post·im·mu·ni·za·tion \-ˌi-myə-nə-'zā-shən\ *adj* : occurring or existing after immunization ⟨∼ symptoms⟩

post·in·farc·tion \-in-'färk-shən\ *adj* **1** : occurring after and esp. as a result of myocardial infarction ⟨∼ ventricular septal defect⟩ **2** : having suffered myocardial infarction

post·in·fec·tion \-in-'fek-shən\ *adj* : relating to, occurring in, or being the period following infection — **postinfection** *adv*

post·ir·ra·di·a·tion \-i-ˌrā-dē-'ā-shən\ *adj* : occurring after irradiation — **postirradiation** *adv*

post·isch·emic \-is-'kē-mik\ *adj* : occurring after and esp. as a result of ischemia ⟨∼ renal failure⟩

post·junc·tion·al \-'jəŋk-shə-nəl\ *adj* : of, relating to, occurring on, or located on the muscle fiber side of a neuromuscular junction

post·mas·tec·to·my \-ma-'stek-tə-mē\ *adj* **1** : occurring after and esp. as a result of a mastectomy **2** : having undergone mastectomy

post·ma·ture \-mə-'chúr, -'tyúr, -'túr\ *adj* : remaining in the uterus for longer than the normal period of gestation ⟨a ∼ fetus⟩

post·meno·paus·al \ˌpōst-ˌme-nə-'pó-zəl\ *adj* **1** : having undergone menopause ⟨∼ women⟩ **2** : occurring after menopause ⟨∼ osteoporosis⟩ — **post·meno·paus·al·ly** *adv*

¹**post·mor·tem** \-'mór-təm\ *adj* : done, occurring, or collected after death ⟨∼ tissue specimens⟩

²**postmortem** *n* : AUTOPSY

post–mortem *adv* : after death

postmortem examination *n* : AUTOPSY

postmortem lividity *n* : LIVOR MORTIS

post·na·sal \-'nā-zəl\ *adj* : lying or occurring posterior to the nose

postnasal drip *n* : flow of mucous secretion from the posterior part of the nasal cavity onto the wall of the pharynx occurring usu. as a chronic accompaniment of an allergic state or a viral infection

post·na·tal \-'nāt-ᵊl\ *adj* : occurring or being after birth; *specif* : of or relating to an infant immediately after birth ⟨~ care⟩ — compare NEONATAL, PRENATAL — **post·na·tal·ly** *adv*

post·ne·crot·ic cirrhosis \-nə-'krä-tik-\ *n* : cirrhosis of the liver following widespread necrosis of liver cells esp. as a result of hepatitis

post·neo·na·tal \-,nē-ō-'nāt-ᵊl\ *adj* : of, relating to, or affecting the infant usu. from the end of the first month to a year after birth ⟨~ mortality⟩

post·nor·mal \-'nȯr-məl\ *adj* : having, characterized by, or resulting from a position (as of the mandible) that is distal to the normal position ⟨~ occlusion⟩ — compare PRENORMAL — **post·nor·mal·i·ty** \-nȯr-'ma-lə-tē\ *n*

post·op \'pōst-'äp\ *adj* : POSTOPERATIVE — **post-op** *adv*

post·op·er·a·tive \,pōst-'ä-pə-rə-tiv\ *adj* **1** : relating to, occurring in, or being the period following a surgical operation ⟨~ care⟩ **2** : having undergone a surgical operation ⟨a ~ patient⟩ — **post·op·er·a·tive·ly** *adv*

post·or·bit·al \-'ȯr-bət-ᵊl\ *adj* : situated or occurring behind the orbit of the eye

post·ovu·la·to·ry \-'ä-vyə-lə-,tōr-ē, -'ō-\ *adj* : occurring, being, or used in the period following ovulation

post·par·tum \-'pär-təm\ *adj* **1** : occurring in or being the period following parturition ⟨~ depression⟩ **2** : being in the postpartum period ⟨~ mothers⟩ — **postpartum** *adv*

post·phle·bit·ic \-flə-'bi-tik\ *adj* : occurring after and esp. as the result of phlebitis ⟨~ edema⟩

postphlebitic syndrome *n* : CHRONIC VENOUS INSUFFICIENCY

post·pi·tu·i·tary \-pə-'tü-ə-,ter-ē, -'tyü-\ *adj* : arising in or derived from the posterior lobe of the pituitary gland

post·po·lio \-'pō-lē-,ō\ *adj* : recovered from poliomyelitis; *also* : affected with post-polio syndrome

post–polio syndrome *n* : a condition that affects former poliomyelitis patients long after recovery from the disease and that is characterized by muscle weakness, joint and muscle pain, and fatigue

post·pran·di·al \-'pran-dē-əl\ *adj* : occurring after a meal ⟨~ hypoglycemia⟩ — **post·pran·di·al·ly** *adv*

post·pu·ber·tal \-'pyü-bərt-ᵊl\ *adj* : occurring after puberty

post·pu·bes·cent \-pyü-'bes-ᵊnt\ *adj* : occurring or being in the period following puberty : POSTPUBERTAL

post·ra·di·a·tion \-,rā-dē-'ā-shən\ *adj* : occurring after exposure to radiation

postrema — see AREA POSTREMA

post·res·i·den·cy \-'rez-ə-dən-sē\ *adj* : occurring or obtained in the period following medical residency ⟨~ training⟩

post·sple·nec·to·my \-spli-'nek-tə-mē\ *adj* : occurring after and esp. as a result of a splenectomy ⟨~ sepsis⟩

post·stroke \-'strōk\ *adj* : occurring in or being in the period following a stroke ⟨~ depression⟩ ⟨a ~ patient⟩

post·sur·gi·cal \-'sər-ji-kəl\ *adj* : POSTOPERATIVE ⟨~ swelling⟩

post·syn·ap·tic \,pōst-sə-'nap-tik\ *adj* **1** : occurring after synapsis ⟨a ~ chromosome⟩ **2** : of, occurring in, or being a neuron by which a nerve impulse is conveyed away from a synapse ⟨~ dopamine receptors⟩ — **post·syn·ap·ti·cal·ly** *adv*

post·tran·scrip·tion·al \-trans-'krip-shə-nəl\ *adj* : occurring, acting, or existing after genetic transcription — **post·tran·scrip·tion·al·ly** *adv*

post·trans·fu·sion \-trans-'fyü-zhən\ *adj* **1** : caused by transfused blood ⟨~ hepatitis⟩ **2** : occurring after blood transfusion ⟨~ shock⟩

post·trans·la·tion·al \-trans-'lā-shə-nəl, -shən-ᵊl\ *adj* : occurring or existing after genetic translation — **post·trans·la·tion·al·ly** *adv*

post·trans·plant \-'trans-,plant\ *adj* : occurring or being in the period following transplant surgery

post·trans·plan·ta·tion \-,trans-,plan-'tā-shən\ *adj* : POSTTRANSPLANT

post·trau·mat·ic \,pōst-trə-'ma-tik, -trȯ-, -traȯ-\ *adj* : occurring after or as a result of trauma ⟨~ epilepsy⟩

post–traumatic stress disorder *n* : a psychological reaction that occurs after experiencing a highly stressing event (as wartime combat, physical violence, or a natural disaster) outside the range of normal human experience and that is usu. characterized by depression, anxiety, flashbacks, recurrent nightmares, and avoidance of reminders of the event — abbr. *PTSD*; called also *delayed-stress disorder*, *delayed-stress syndrome*, *posttraumatic stress syndrome*; compare COMBAT FATIGUE

post·treat·ment \-'trēt-mənt\ *adj* : relating to, typical of, or occurring in the period following treatment ⟨~ examinations⟩ — **posttreatment** *adv*

pos·tur·al \'päs-chə-rəl\ *adj* : of, relating to, or involving posture; *also* : ORTHOSTATIC ⟨~ hypotension⟩

postural drainage *n* : drainage of the lungs by placing the patient in an inverted position so that fluids are drawn by gravity toward the trachea

pos·ture \'päs-chər\ *n* : the position or

bearing of the body whether characteristic or assumed for a special purpose ⟨erect ∼⟩

post·vac·ci·nal \-'vak-sən-°l\ *adj* : occurring after and esp. as a result of vaccination ⟨∼ dermatosis⟩

post·vac·ci·na·tion \-₁vak-sə-'nā-shən\ *adj* : POSTVACCINAL

post·wean·ing \-'wē-niŋ\ *adj* : relating to, occurring in, or being the period following weaning

pot \'pät\ *n* : MARIJUANA

po·ta·ble \'pō-tə-bəl\ *adj* : suitable for drinking ⟨∼ water⟩

po·tas·si·um \pə-'ta-sē-əm\ *n* : a silver-white soft low-melting metallic element that occurs abundantly in nature esp. combined in minerals — symbol *K;* see ELEMENT table

potassium alum *n* : ALUM

potassium aluminum sulfate *n* : ALUM

potassium an·ti·mo·nyl·tar·trate \-₁an-tə-mə-₁nil-'tär-₁trāt, -₁nēl-\ *n* : TARTAR EMETIC

potassium bicarbonate *n* : a crystalline water-soluble salt KHCO₃ that is sometimes used as an antacid and urinary alkalizer and to treat potassium deficiency — see KLOR-CON

potassium bromide *n* : a crystalline salt KBr that is used as a sedative

potassium chlorate *n* : a crystalline salt KClO₃ used esp. in veterinary medicine as a mild astringent

potassium chloride *n* : a crystalline salt KCl that is used esp. in the treatment of potassium deficiency — see K-DUR, KLOR-CON

potassium citrate *n* : a crystalline salt K₃C₆H₅O₇ used chiefly as a systemic and urinary alkalizer and in the treatment of hypokalemia

potassium cyanide *n* : a very poisonous crystalline salt KCN

potassium hydroxide *n* : a white solid KOH that dissolves in water to form a strongly alkaline liquid and that is used as a powerful caustic and in the making of pharmaceuticals

potassium iodide *n* : a crystalline salt KI that is very soluble in water and is used medically chiefly in the treatment of hyperthyroidism, to block thyroidal uptake of radioactive iodine, and as an expectorant

potassium nitrate *n* : a crystalline salt KNO₃ that is a strong oxidizing agent and has been used in medicine chiefly as a diuretic — called also *saltpeter*

potassium perchlorate *n* : a crystalline salt KClO₄ that is sometimes used as a thyroid inhibitor

potassium permanganate *n* : a dark purple salt KMnO₄ used as a disinfectant

potassium phosphate *n* : any of various phosphates of potassium; *esp* : a salt K₂HPO₄ used as a saline cathartic

potassium sodium tartrate *n* : ROCHELLE SALT

potassium thiocyanate *n* : a crystalline salt KSCN that has been used as an antihypertensive agent

pot·bel·ly \'pät-₁be-lē\ *n, pl* **-lies** : an enlarged, swollen, or protruding abdomen; *also* : a condition characterized by such an abdomen that is symptomatic of disease or malnourishment

po·ten·cy \'pōt-°n-sē\ *n, pl* **-cies** : the quality or state of being potent : as **a** : chemical or medicinal strength or efficacy ⟨a drug's ∼⟩ **b** : the ability to copulate — usu. used of the male **c** : initial inherent capacity for development of a particular kind

po·tent \'pōt-°nt\ *adj* **1** : having force or power **2** : chemically or medicinally effective ⟨a ∼ vaccine⟩ **3** : able to copulate — usu. used of the male — **po·tent·ly** *adv*

¹**po·ten·tial** \pə-'ten-chəl\ *adj* : existing in possibility : capable of development into actuality — **po·ten·tial·ly** *adv*

²**potential** *n* **1** : something that can develop or become actual **2 a** : any of various functions from which the intensity or the velocity at any point in a field may be readily calculated; *specif* : ELECTRICAL POTENTIAL **b** : POTENTIAL DIFFERENCE

potential difference *n* : the difference in electrical potential between two points that represents the work involved or the energy released in the transfer of a unit quantity of electricity from one point to the other

potential energy *n* : the energy that a piece of matter has because of its position or because of the arrangement of parts

po·ten·ti·ate \pə-'ten-chē-₁āt\ *vb* **-at·ed; -at·ing** : to make effective or active or more effective or more active; *also* : to augment the activity of (as a drug) synergistically — **po·ten·ti·a·tion** \-₁ten-chē-'ā-shən\ *n* — **po·ten·ti·a·tor** \-'ten-chē-₁ā-tər\ *n*

Po·to·mac horse fever \pə-'tō-mək-\ *n* : an often fatal disease of horses that is marked by fever, loss of appetite, diarrhea, and laminitis and is caused by a rickettsial bacterium (*Neorickettsia risticii* syn. *Ehrlichia risticii*) — called also *Potomac fever*

Pott's disease \'päts-\ *n* : tuberculosis of the spine with destruction of bone resulting in curvature of the spine and occas. in paralysis of the lower extremities

Pott, Percivall (1714–1788), British surgeon.

Pott's fracture *n* : a fracture of the lower part of the fibula often accompanied with injury to the tibial articulation so that the foot is dislocated outward

pouch \'paùch\ *n* : an anatomical structure resembling a bag or pocket

pouch of Doug·las \-'də-gləs\ *n* : a

deep peritoneal recess between the uterus and the upper vaginal wall anteriorly and the rectum posteriorly — called also **cul-de-sac**, **cul-de-sac of Douglas**, **Douglas's cul-de-sac**, **Douglas's pouch**

Douglas, James (1675–1742), British anatomist.

poul·tice \'pōl-təs\ n : a soft usu. heated and sometimes medicated mass spread on cloth and applied to sores or other lesions to supply moist warmth, relieve pain, or act as a counterirritant or antiseptic — called also *cataplasm* — **poultice** vb

pound \'paùnd\ n, pl **pounds** also **pound** : any of various units of mass and weight; *specif* : a unit now in general use among English-speaking peoples equal to 16 avoirdupois ounces or 7000 grains or 0.4536 kilogram — called also *avoirdupois pound*

Pou·part's ligament \pü-'pärz-\ n : INGUINAL LIGAMENT

Poupart, François (1661–1709), French surgeon and naturalist.

po·vi·done \'pō-və-ˌdōn\ n : POLYVINYLPYRROLIDONE

povidone–iodine n : a solution of polyvinylpyrrolidone and iodine used as an antibacterial agent in topical application (as in preoperative prepping or a surgical scrub) — see BETADINE

pow·der \'paù-dər\ n : a product in the form of discrete usu. fine particles; *specif* : a medicine or medicated preparation in the form of a powder

pow·er \'paù-ər\ n : MAGNIFICATION

pox \'päks\ n, pl **pox** or **pox·es** 1 : a virus disease (as chicken pox) characterized by pustules or eruptions 2 *archaic* : SMALLPOX 3 : SYPHILIS

pox·vi·rus \'päks-ˌvī-rəs\ n : any of a family (*Poxviridae*) of large brick-shaped or ovoid double-stranded DNA viruses that include the vaccinia virus, the orthopoxviruses, and the causative agents of fowl pox, molluscum contagiosum, myxomatosis of rabbits, sheep pox, sore mouth of sheep, and swinepox

PPA abbr phenylpropanolamine

ppb abbr parts per billion

PPD abbr purified protein derivative

PPI abbr proton pump inhibitor

PPLO \ˌpē-(ˌ)pē-(ˌ)el-'ō\ n, pl **PPLO** : MYCOPLASMA

ppm abbr parts per million

PPO \ˌpē-(ˌ)pē-'ō\ n, pl **PPOs** : an organization providing health care that gives economic incentives to the individual purchaser of a health-care contract to patronize certain physicians, laboratories, and hospitals which agree to supervision and reduced fees — called also *preferred provider organization*; compare HMO

Pr symbol praseodymium

practical nurse n : a nurse who cares for the sick professionally without having the training or experience required of a registered nurse; *esp* : LICENSED PRACTICAL NURSE

prac·tice also **prac·tise** \'prak-təs\ n 1 : the continuous exercise of a profession 2 a : a professional business; *esp* : one constituting an incorporeal property ⟨the doctor sold his ~ and retired⟩ — **practice** also **practise** vb

prac·ti·tio·ner \prak-'ti-shə-nər\ n : one who practices a profession and esp. medicine

prac·to·lol \'prak-tə-ˌlȯl\ n : a beta-blocker C₁₄H₂₂N₂O₃ used in the control of arrhythmia

Pra·der–Wil·li syndrome \'prä-dər-'vi-lē-\ n : a genetic disorder characterized by short stature, mental retardation, hypotonia, abnormally small hands and feet, hypogonadism, and uncontrolled appetite leading to extreme obesity

Prader, Andrea (1919–2001), and **Willi, Heinrich (1900–1971),** Swiss pediatricians.

praecox — see DEMENTIA PRAECOX, EJACULATIO PRAECOX

pra·li·dox·ime \ˌpra-li-'däk-ˌsēm\ n : a substance that restores the reactivity of cholinesterase and is used in the form of its chloride C₇H₉ClN₂O to counteract phosphorylation (as by an organophosphate pesticide) — called also *2-PAM, pralidoxime chloride*; see PROTOPAM

pram·i·pex·ole \ˌpra-mi-'pek-ˌsōl\ n : a dopamine agonist administered in the form of its dihydrochloride C₁₀H₁₇N₃S·2HCl to treat the symptoms of Parkinson's disease

pran·di·al \'pran-dē-əl\ adj : of or relating to a meal

pra·seo·dym·i·um \ˌprä-zē-ō-'di-mē-əm, ˌprä-sē-\ n : a yellowish white trivalent metallic element — symbol *Pr*; see ELEMENT table

Praus·nitz–Küst·ner reaction \'praùs-nits-'küst-nər-\ n : PASSIVE TRANSFER

Prausnitz, Carl Willy (1876–1963), German bacteriologist.

Küstner, Heinz (1897–1963), German gynecologist.

Prav·a·chol \'pra-və-ˌkȯl\ trademark — used for a preparation of pravastatin

prav·a·stat·in \'pra-və-ˌsta-t⁰n\ n : a statin C₂₃H₃₅NaO₇ that is administered orally to treat hypercholesterolemia — called also *pravastatin sodium*; see PRAVACHOL

-prax·ia \'prak-sē-ə\ n comb form : performance of movements ⟨apraxia⟩

pra·ze·pam \'prä-zə-ˌpam\ n : a benzodiazepine derivative C₁₉H₁₇ClN₂O used as a tranquilizer

praz·i·quan·tel \ˌpra-zi-'kwän-ˌtel\ n : an anthelmintic drug C₁₉H₂₄N₂O₂ — see BILTRICIDE

pra·zo·sin \'prä-zə-ˌsin\ n : an antihypertensive peripheral vasodilator usu. used in the form of its hydrochloride C₁₉H₂₁N₅O₄·HCl — see MINIPRESS

pre- *prefix* **1** : earlier than : prior to : before ⟨*prenatal*⟩ ⟨*precancerous*⟩ **2** : in front of : before ⟨*premolar*⟩

pre·ad·mis·sion \ˌprē-əd-ˈmi-shən\ *adj* : occurring in or relating to the period prior to admission (as to a hospital)

pre·ad·o·les·cence \ˌprē-ˌad-ᵊl-ˈes-ᵊns\ *n* : the period of human development just preceding adolescence; *specif* : the period between the approximate ages of 9 and 12 — **pre·ad·o·les·cent** \-ˌad-ᵊl-ˈes-ᵊnt\ *adj or n*

pre·adult \-ə-ˈdəlt, -ˈā-ˌdəlt\ *adj* : occurring or existing prior to adulthood

pre·al·bu·min \-al-ˈbyü-mən, -ˈal-ˌbyü-\ *n* : TRANSTHYRETIN

¹**pre·an·es·thet·ic** \-ˌa-nəs-ˈthe-tik\ *adj* : used or occurring before administration of an anesthetic ⟨∼ medication⟩

²**preanesthetic** *n* : a substance used to induce an initial light state of anesthesia

pre·au·ric·u·lar \-ȯ-ˈri-kyə-lər\ *adj* : situated or occurring anterior to the auricle of the ear ⟨∼ lymph nodes⟩

pre·ax·i·al \-ˈak-sē-əl\ *adj* : situated in front of an axis of the body

pre·can·cer \-ˈkan-sər\ *n* : a precancerous lesion or condition

pre·can·cer·ous \-ˈkan-sə-rəs\ *adj* : tending to become cancerous

¹**pre·cap·il·lary** \-ˈka-pə-ˌler-ē\ *adj* : being on the arterial side of and immediately adjacent to a capillary

²**precapillary** *n, pl* **-lar·ies** : METARTERIOLE

precapillary sphincter *n* : a sphincter of smooth muscle tissue located at the arterial end of a capillary and serving to control blood flow to the tissues

pre·cen·tral \-ˈsen-trəl\ *adj* : situated in front of the central sulcus of the brain

precentral gyrus *n* : the gyrus containing the motor area immediately anterior to the central sulcus

pre·cep·tee \ˌprē-ˌsep-ˈtē\ *n* : a person who works for and studies under a preceptor ⟨a ∼ in urology⟩

pre·cep·tor \prī-ˈsep-tər, ˈprē-ˌ\ *n* : a practicing physician who gives personal instruction, training, and supervision to a medical student or young physician

pre·cep·tor·ship \prī-ˈsep-tər-ˌship, ˈprē-ˌ\ *n* : the state of being a preceptee : a period of training under a preceptor

¹**pre·cip·i·tate** \prī-ˈsi-pə-ˌtāt\ *vb* **-tat·ed; -tat·ing** **1** : to bring about esp. abruptly **2 a** : to separate or cause to separate from solution or suspension **b** : to cause (vapor) to condense and fall or deposit

²**pre·cip·i·tate** \prī-ˈsi-pə-tət, -ˌtāt\ *n* : a substance separated from a solution or suspension by chemical or physical change usu. as an insoluble amorphous or crystalline solid

precipitated chalk *n* : precipitated calcium carbonate used esp. as an ingredient of toothpastes and tooth powders for its polishing qualities

precipitated sulfur *n* : sulfur obtained as a pale yellowish or grayish powder by precipitation and used chiefly in treating skin diseases

pre·cip·i·ta·tion \prī-ˌsi-pə-ˈtā-shən\ *n* **1 a** : the process of forming a precipitate from a solution **b** : the process of precipitating or removing solid or liquid particles from a smoke or gas by electrical means **2** : PRECIPITATE

pre·cip·i·tin \prī-ˈsi-pə-tən\ *n* : any of various antibodies which form insoluble precipitates with specific antigens

precipitin test *n* : a serological test using precipitins to detect the presence of a specific antigen; *specif* : a test used in criminology for determining the human or other source of a blood stain

pre·clin·i·cal \ˌprē-ˈkli-ni-kəl\ *adj* **1 a** : of, relating to, concerned with, or being the period preceding clinical manifestations ⟨the ∼ stage of diabetes mellitus⟩ **b** : occurring prior to a clinical trial ⟨∼ animal testing⟩ **2** : of, relating to, or being the period in medical or dental education preceding the clinical study of medicine or dentistry

pre·co·cious \prī-ˈkō-shəs\ *adj* **1** : exceptionally early in development or occurrence ⟨∼ puberty⟩ **2** : exhibiting mature qualities at an unusually early age — **pre·co·cious·ly** *adv* — **pre·co·cious·ness** *n* — **pre·coc·i·ty** \prī-ˈkä-sə-tē\ *n*

pre·cog·ni·tion \ˌprē-(ˌ)käg-ˈni-shən\ *n* : clairvoyance relating to an event or state not yet experienced — compare PSYCHOKINESIS, TELEKINESIS — **pre·cog·ni·tive** \-ˈkäg-nə-tiv\ *adj*

pre·co·i·tal \-ˈkō-ət-ᵊl, -kō-ˈēt-\ *adj* : used or occurring before coitus

pre·co·ma \-ˈkō-mə\ *n* : a stuporous condition preceding coma ⟨diabetic ∼⟩

pre·con·cep·tion \-kən-ˈsep-shən\ *adj* : occurring prior to conception

¹**pre·con·scious** \ˌprē-ˈkän-chəs\ *adj* : not present in consciousness but capable of being recalled without encountering any inner resistance or repression — **pre·con·scious·ly** *adv*

²**preconscious** *n* : the preconscious part of the psyche esp. in psychoanalysis

pre·cor·di·al \-ˈkȯr-dē-əl, -ˈkȯr-jəl\ *adj* **1** : situated or occurring in front of the heart **2** : of or relating to the precordium

pre·cor·di·um \-ˈkȯr-dē-əm\ *n, pl* **-dia** \-dē-ə\ : the part of the ventral surface of the body overlying the heart and stomach and comprising the epigastrium and the lower median part of the thorax

pre·cu·ne·us \-ˈkyü-nē-əs\ *n, pl* **-nei** \-nē-ˌī\ : a somewhat rectangular convolution bounding the mesial aspect of the parietal lobe of the cerebrum and lying immediately in front of the cuneus

pre·cur·sor \pri-'kər-sər, 'prē-\ n **1** : one that precedes and indicates the onset of another **2** : a substance, cell, or cellular component from which another substance, cell, or cellular component is formed esp. by natural processes

pre·den·tin \,prē-'dent-ᵊn\ or **pre·den·tine** \-'den-,tēn, -den-'\ n : immature uncalcified dentin consisting chiefly of fibrils

pre·di·a·be·tes \,prē-,dī-ə-'bē-tēz, -'bē-təs\ n : an inapparent abnormal state that precedes the development of clinically evident diabetes

¹**pre·di·a·bet·ic** \-'be-tik\ n : a prediabetic individual

²**prediabetic** adj : of, relating to, or affected with prediabetes ⟨~ patients⟩

pre·dic·tor \pri-'dik-tər\ n : a preliminary symptom or indication (as of the development of a disease)

pre·di·ges·tion \,prē-dī-'jes-chən, -də-\ n : artificial or natural digestion of food — **pre·di·gest** \-'jest\ vb

pre·dis·pose \,prē-di-'spōz\ vb **-posed; -pos·ing** : to make susceptible — **pre·dis·po·si·tion** \,prē-,dis-pə-'zi-shən\ n

pred·nis·o·lone \pred-'ni-sə-,lōn\ n : a glucocorticoid $C_{21}H_{28}O_5$ used often in the form of an ester or methyl derivative esp. as an anti-inflammatory drug in the treatment of arthritis

pred·ni·sone \'pred-nə-,sōn, -,zōn\ n : a glucocorticoid $C_{21}H_{26}O_5$ that is used as an anti-inflammatory agent, as an antineoplastic agent, and as an immunosuppressant

pre·drug \,prē-'drəg\ adj : existing or occurring prior to the administration of a drug ⟨~ baseline values⟩

pre·ec·lamp·sia \,prē-i-'klamp-sē-ə\ n : a serious condition developing in late pregnancy that is characterized by a sudden rise in blood pressure, excessive weight gain, generalized edema, proteinuria, severe headache, and visual disturbances and that may result in eclampsia if untreated — compare ECLAMPSIA a, TOXEMIA OF PREGNANCY

¹**pre·eclamp·tic** \-tik\ adj : relating to or affected with preeclampsia ⟨a ~ patient⟩

²**preeclamptic** n : a woman affected with preeclampsia

pree·mie also **pre·mie** \'prē-mē\ n : a baby born prematurely

pre·erup·tive \,prē-i-'rəp-tiv\ adj : occurring or existing prior to an eruption ⟨a ~ tooth position⟩

pre·ex·ci·ta·tion \-,ek-,sī-'tā-shən, -sə-\ n : premature activation of part or all of the cardiac ventricle by an electrical impulse from the atrium that typically is conducted along an anomalous pathway (as muscle fibers on the heart surface) bypassing the atrioventricular node, that may pro-

duce arrhythmias, and that is characteristic of Lown-Ganong-Levine syndrome and Wolff-Parkinson-White syndrome — **pre·ex·cit·ed** \-ik-'sī-təd\ adj

pre·ex·po·sure \-ik-'spō-zhər\ adj : of, relating to, occurring in, or being the period preceding exposure (as to a stimulus or a pathogen)

preferred provider organization n : PPO

pre·fron·tal \,prē-'frənt-ᵊl\ adj **1** : situated or occurring anterior to a frontal structure ⟨a ~ bone⟩ **2** : of, relating to, or constituting the prefrontal cortex or prefrontal cortex of the brain

prefrontal cortex n : the gray matter of the anterior part of the frontal lobe that is highly developed in humans and plays a role in the regulation of complex cognitive, emotional, and behavioral functioning

prefrontal lobe : the anterior part of the frontal lobe that is bounded posteriorly by the ascending frontal convolution, is made up chiefly of association areas, and mediates various inhibitory controls

prefrontal lobotomy n : lobotomy of the white matter in the frontal lobe of the brain — called also frontal lobotomy

pre·gan·gli·on·ic \,prē-,gaŋ-glē-'ä-nik\ adj : anterior or proximal to a ganglion; specif : being, affecting, involving, or relating to a usu. myelinated efferent nerve fiber arising from a cell body in the central nervous system and terminating in an autonomic ganglion — compare POSTGANGLIONIC

pre·gen·i·tal \-'jen-ət-ᵊl\ adj : of, relating to, or characteristic of the oral, anal, and phallic phases of psychosexual development

preg·nan·cy \'preg-nən-sē\ n, pl **-cies** **1** : the condition of being pregnant **2** : an instance of being pregnant

pregnancy disease n : a form of ketosis affecting pregnant ewes that is marked by listlessness, staggering, and collapse and is esp. frequent in ewes carrying twins or triplets

pregnancy test n : a physiological test to determine the existence of pregnancy in an individual

preg·nane \'preg-,nān\ n : a crystalline steroid $C_{21}H_{36}$ that is the parent compound of the corticosteroid and progestational hormones

preg·nane·di·ol \,preg-,nān-'dī-,ȯl\ n : a crystalline biologically inactive derivative $C_{21}H_{36}O_2$ of pregnane found esp. in the urine of pregnant women

preg·nant \'preg-nənt\ adj : containing a developing embryo, fetus, or unborn offspring within the body : GESTATING : GRAVID

preg·nen·o·lone \preg-'nen-ᵊl-,ōn\ n : a steroid ketone $C_{21}H_{32}O_2$ that is formed by the oxidation of steroids (as cholesterol) and yields progesterone on dehydrogenation

pre·hos·pi·tal \ˌprē-ˈhäs-(ˌ)pit-ᵊl\ *adj* : occurring before or during transportation (as of a trauma victim) to a hospital ⟨~ emergency care⟩

pre·hy·per·ten·sion \ˌhī-pər-ˈten-chən\ *n* : slightly to moderately elevated arterial blood pressure that in adults is usu. indicated by a systolic blood pressure of 120 to 139 mm Hg or a diastolic blood pressure of 80 to 89 mm Hg and that is considered a risk factor for hypertension — **pre·hy·per·ten·sive** \-ˈhī-pər-ˌten-siv\ *adj*

pre·im·mu·ni·za·tion \-ˌi-myə-nə-ˈzā-shən\ *adj* : existing or occurring in the period before immunization

pre·im·plan·ta·tion \-ˌim-ˌplan-ˈtā-shən\ *adj* : of, involving, or being an embryo before uterine implantation

pre·in·cu·ba·tion \ˌprē-ˌiŋ-kyə-ˈbā-shən\ *n* : incubation (as of a cell or culture) prior to a treatment or process — **pre·in·cu·bate** \-ˈiŋ-kyə-ˌbāt\ *vb*

pre·in·va·sive \-in-ˈvā-siv\ *adj* : not yet having become invasive — used of malignant cells or lesions remaining in their original focus

pre·leu·ke·mia \-lü-ˈkē-mē-ə\ *n* : MYELODYSPLASTIC SYNDROME — **pre·leu·ke·mic** \-mik\ *adj*

pre·load \ˌprē-ˈlōd\ *n* : the stretched condition of the heart muscle at the end of diastole just before contraction

Pre·lu·din \pri-ˈlüd-ᵊn\ *n* : a preparation of the hydrochloride of phenmetrazine — formerly a U.S. registered trademark

pre·ma·lig·nant \ˌprē-mə-ˈlig-nənt\ *adj* : PRECANCEROUS

Prem·a·rin \ˈpre-mə-rən\ *trademark* — used for a preparation of conjugated estrogens

¹**pre·ma·ture** \ˌprē-mə-ˈchu̇r, -ˈtyu̇r, -ˈtu̇r-\ *adj* : happening, arriving, existing, or performed before the proper, usual, or intended time; *esp* : born after a gestation period of less than 37 weeks ⟨~ babies⟩ — **pre·ma·ture·ly** *adv*

²**premature** *n* : PREEMIE

premature beat *n* : EXTRASYSTOLE

premature delivery *n* : expulsion of the human fetus after the 28th week of gestation but before the normal time

premature ejaculation *n* : ejaculation of semen that occurs prior to or immediately after penetration of the vagina by the penis — called also *ejaculatio praecox*

premature ejaculator *n* : a man who experiences premature ejaculation

pre·ma·tu·ri·ty \ˌprē-mə-ˈtu̇r-ə-tē, -ˈtyu̇r-, -ˈchu̇r-\ *n, pl* **-ties** : the condition of an infant born viable but before its proper time

pre·max·il·la \ˌprē-mak-ˈsi-lə\ *n, pl* **-lae** \-ˌlē\ : either member of a pair of bones of the upper jaw situated between and in front of the maxilla

that in humans form the median anterior part of the superior maxillary bones

pre·max·il·lary \-ˈmak-sə-ˌler-ē\ *adj* **1** : situated in front of the maxillary bones **2** : relating to or being the premaxillae

¹**pre·med** \ˈprē-ˈmed\ *n* : a premedical student or course of study

²**premed** *adj* : PREMEDICAL

pre·med·i·cal \-ˈme-di-kəl\ *adj* : preceding and preparing for the professional study of medicine

pre·med·i·ca·tion \ˌme-də-ˈkā-shən\ *n* : preliminary medication; *esp* : medication to induce a relaxed state preparatory to the administration of an anesthetic — **pre·med·i·cate** \ˈme-də-ˌkāt\ *vb*

pre·mei·ot·ic \ˌprē-mī-ˈä-tik\ *adj* : of, occurring in, or typical of a stage prior to meiosis ⟨~ DNA synthesis⟩

pre·me·nar·chal \ˌprē-me-ˈnär-kəl\ *or* **pre·me·nar·che·al** \-kē-əl\ *adj* : of, relating to, or being in the period of life of a female before the first menstrual period occurs

pre·meno·paus·al \ˌme-nə-ˈpȯ-zəl, -ˌmē-\ *adj* : of, relating to, or being in the period preceding menopause and esp. the perimenopausal period

pre·meno·pause \ˈme-nə-ˌpȯz, -ˈmē-\ *n* : the premenopausal period of a woman's life; *esp* : PERIMENOPAUSE

pre·men·stru·al \-ˈmen-strə-wəl\ *adj* : of, relating to, occurring, or being in the period just preceding menstruation — **pre·men·stru·al·ly** *adv*

premenstrual dysphoric disorder *n* : severe premenstrual syndrome marked esp. by depression, anxiety, cyclical mood shifts, and lethargy — abbr. *PMDD*

premenstrual syndrome *n* : a varying constellation of symptoms manifested by some women prior to menstruation that may include emotional instability, irritability, insomnia, fatigue, anxiety, depression, headache, edema, and abdominal pain — called also *PMS*

premenstrual tension *n* : tension occurring as a part of the premenstrual syndrome

pre·men·stru·um \-ˈmen-strə-wəm\ *n, pl* **-stru·ums** *or* **-strua** \-strə-wə\ : the period or physiological state that immediately precedes menstruation

premie *var of* PREEMIE

¹**pre·mo·lar** \ˌprē-ˈmō-lər\ *adj* : situated in front of or preceding the molar teeth; *esp* : being or relating to those teeth in front of the true molars and behind the canines

²**premolar** *n* : a premolar tooth that in humans is one of two on each side of each jaw — called also *bicuspid*

pre·mon·i·to·ry \pri-ˈmä-nə-ˌtōr-ē\ *adj* : giving warning ⟨a ~ symptom⟩

pre·mor·bid \ˌprē-ˈmȯr-bəd\ *adj* : occurring or existing before the occurrence of physical disease or emotional illness ⟨∼ personality⟩

pre·mor·tem \-'mȯrt-°m\ *adj* : existing or taking place immediately before death — **premortem** *adv*

pre·mo·tor \-'mō-tər\ *adj* : of, relating to, or being the area of the cortex of the frontal lobe lying immediately in front of the motor area of the precentral gyrus

Prem·pro \'prem-ˌprō\ *trademark* — used for a preparation of conjugated estrogens and medroxyprogesterone acetate

pre·my·cot·ic \ˌprē-mī-'kä-tik\ *adj* : of, relating to, or being the earliest and nonspecific stage of eczematoid eruptions of mycosis fungoides

pre·na·tal \-'nāt-°l\ *adj* **1** : occurring, existing, or performed before birth ⟨∼ care⟩ ⟨the ∼ period⟩ ⟨∼ testing⟩ **2** : providing or receiving prenatal medical care ⟨a ∼ clinic⟩ ⟨a ∼ patient⟩ — compare NEONATAL, POSTNATAL — **pre·na·tal·ly** *adv*

pre·neo·plas·tic \-ˌnē-ə-'plas-tik\ *adj* : existing or occurring prior to the formation of a neoplasm ⟨∼ cells⟩

pre·nor·mal \-'nȯr-məl\ *adj* : having, characterized by, or resulting from a position (as of the mandible) that is proximal to the normal position — compare POSTNORMAL — **pre·nor·mal·i·ty** \-ˌnȯr-'ma-lə-tē\ *n*

pre·op \'prē-ˌäp\ *adj* : PREOPERATIVE

pre·op·er·a·tive \ˌprē-'ä-pə-rə-tiv, -ˌrāt-\ *adj* **1** : occurring, performed, or administered before and usu. close to a surgical operation ⟨∼ care⟩ **2** : having not yet undergone a surgical operation ⟨∼ patients⟩ — **pre·op·er·a·tive·ly** *adv*

pre·op·tic \-'äp-tik\ *adj* : situated in front of an optic part or region

preoptic area *n* : a region of the brain that is situated immediately below the anterior commissure, above the optic chiasma, and anterior to the hypothalamus and that regulates certain autonomic activities often with the hypothalamus

preoptic nucleus *n* : any of several groups of nerve cells located in the preoptic area esp. in the lateral and the medial portions

preoptic region *n* : PREOPTIC AREA

pre·ovu·la·to·ry \ˌprē-'ä-vyə-lə-ˌtȯr-ē, -'ō-\ *adj* : occurring in, being in, existing in, or typical of the period immediately preceding ovulation ⟨∼ ovarian follicles⟩

¹prep \'prep\ *n* : the act or an instance of preparing a patient for a surgical operation

²prep *vb* **prepped; prep·ping** : to prepare for a surgical operation or examination ⟨nurses *prepped* the patient⟩

prep·a·ra·tion \ˌpre-pə-'rā-shən\ *n* : a medicinal substance made ready for use ⟨a ∼ for colds⟩

prepared chalk *n* : finely ground calcium carbonate that is freed of most of its impurities and used esp. in dentistry for polishing

pre·par·tum \ˌprē-'pär-təm\ *adj* : ANTEPARTUM

pre·pa·tel·lar bursa \-pə-'te-lər-\ *n* : a synovial bursa situated between the patella and the skin

pre·pa·tent period \-'pāt-°nt-\ *n* : the period between infection with a parasite and the demonstration of the parasite in the body

pre·po·ten·cy \-'pōt-°n-sē\ *n, pl* **-cies** : unusual ability of an individual or strain to transmit its characters to offspring because of homozygosity for numerous dominant genes — **pre·po·tent** \-'pōt-°nt\ *adj*

pre·pran·di·al \-'pran-dē-əl\ *adj* : of, relating to, or suitable for the time just before a meal ⟨∼ blood glucose⟩

pre·preg·nan·cy \-'preg-nən-sē\ *adj* : existing or occurring prior to pregnancy ⟨∼ obesity⟩

pre·psy·chot·ic \-sī-'kä-tik\ *adj* : preceding or predisposing to psychosis : possessing recognizable features prognostic of psychosis

pre·pu·ber·al \-'pyü-bə-rəl\ *adj* : PREPUBERTAL

pre·pu·ber·tal \-'pyü-bərt-°l\ *adj* : of, relating to, occurring in, or being in the period immediately preceding puberty — **pre·pu·ber·ty** \-bər-tē\ *n*

pre·pu·bes·cent \-pyü-'bes-°nt\ *adj* : PREPUBERTAL

pre·puce \'prē-ˌpyüs\ *n* : FORESKIN; *also* : a similar fold investing the clitoris

pre·pu·tial \prē-'pyü-shəl\ *adj* : of, relating to, or being a prepuce

preputial gland *n* : any of the small glands at the base of the glans penis that secrete smegma — called also *gland of Tyson, Tyson's gland*

pre·pu·tium cli·tor·i·dis \prē-'pyü-shəm-kli-'tȯr-ə-dəs\ *n* : the prepuce which invests the clitoris

pre·py·lo·ric \ˌprē-pī-'lȯr-ik\ *adj* : situated or occurring anterior to the pylorus ⟨∼ ulcers⟩

pre·re·nal \-'rēn-°l\ *adj* : occurring in the circulatory system before the kidney is reached ⟨∼ disorders⟩

prerenal azotemia *n* : uremia caused by extrarenal factors

pre·rep·li·ca·tive \ˌprē-'re-pli-ˌkā-tiv\ *adj* : relating to or being the G₁ phase of the cell cycle

pre·ret·i·nal \-'ret-°n-əl\ *adj* : situated or occurring anterior to the retina

pre·sa·cral \-'sā-krəl, -'sä-\ *adj* : done or effected by way of the anterior aspect of the sacrum ⟨∼ nerve block⟩

presby- *or* **presbyo-** *comb form* : old age ⟨*presby*opia⟩

pres·by·cu·sis \ˌprez-bi-'kyü-səs, ˌpres-\ *n, pl* **-cu·ses** \-ˌsēz\ : a lessening of hearing acuteness resulting from degenerative changes in the ear that occur esp. in old age

pres·by·ope \'prez-bē-ˌōp; 'pres-\ *n* : one affected with presbyopia

pres·by·opia \,prez-bē-'ō-pē-ə, ,pres-\ *n* : a visual condition which becomes apparent esp. in middle age and in which loss of elasticity of the lens of the eye causes defective accommodation and inability to focus sharply for near vision — **pres·by·opic** \-'ō-pik, -'ä-\ *adj*

pre·scribe \pri-'skrīb\ *vb* **pre·scribed; pre·scrib·ing** : to designate the use of as a remedy ⟨~ a drug⟩

pre·scrip·tion \pri-'skrip-shən\ *n* 1 : a written direction for the preparation, compounding, and administration of a medicine 2 : a prescribed remedy 3 : a written formula for the grinding of corrective lenses for eyeglasses 4 : a written direction for the application of physical therapy measures (as directed exercise or electrotherapy) in cases of injury or disability

prescription drug *n* : a drug that can be obtained only by means of a physician's prescription

pre·se·nile \,prē-'sē-,nīl\ *adj* 1 : of, relating to, occurring in, or being the period immediately preceding the development of senility in an organism or person 2 : prematurely displaying symptoms of senile dementia

presenile dementia *n* : dementia beginning in middle age and progressing rapidly — compare ALZHEIMER'S DISEASE

pre·sen·il·in \prē-,se-'ni-lən\ *n* : any of several proteins of cell membranes that are believed to contribute to the development of Alzheimer's disease

pre·sent \pri-'zent\ *vb* 1 a : to show or manifest ⟨patients who ~ symptoms of malaria⟩ b : to become manifest ⟨Lyme disease often ~s with erythema migrans, fatigue, fever, and chills⟩ c : to come forward as a patient ⟨he ~ed with fever and abdominal pain⟩ 2 : to become directed toward the opening of the uterus — used of a fetus or a part of a fetus

pre·sen·ta·tion \,prē-,zen-'tā-shən, ,prez-ᵊn-\ *n* 1 : the position in which the fetus lies in the uterus in labor with respect to the mouth of the uterus ⟨face ~⟩ 2 : appearance in conscious experience either as a sensory product or as a memory image 3 : a presenting symptom or group of symptoms 4 : a formal oral report of a patient's medical history

pre·sent·ing \pri-'zen-tiŋ\ *adj* : of, relating to, or being a symptom, condition, or sign which is patent upon initial examination of a patient or which the patient discloses to the physician ⟨~ symptoms⟩

pre·ser·va·tive \pri-'zər-və-tiv\ *n* : something that preserves or has the power of preserving; *specif* : an additive used to protect against decay, discoloration, or spoilage ⟨a food ~⟩

pre·sphe·noid \,prē-'sfē-,nòid\ *n* : a bone or cartilage usu. united with the basisphenoid in the adult and in hu-

mans forming the anterior part of the body of the sphenoid — **presphenoid** *also* **pre·sphe·noi·dal** \-sfi-'nòid-ᵊl\ *adj*

pres·sor \'pre-,sòr, -sər\ *adj* : raising or tending to raise blood pressure ⟨~ substances⟩; *also* : involving or producing an effect of vasoconstriction

pres·so·re·cep·tor \,pre-sō-ri-'sep-tər\ *n* : BARORECEPTOR

pres·sure \'pre-shər\ *n* 1 : the application of force to something by something else in direct contact with it : COMPRESSION 2 : ATMOSPHERIC PRESSURE 3 : a touch sensation aroused by moderate compression of the skin

pressure bandage *n* : a thick pad of gauze or other material placed over a wound and attached firmly so that it will exert pressure — called also *pressure dressing*

pressure point *n* 1 : a region of the body in which the distribution of soft and skeletal parts is such that a static position (as of a part in a cast or of a bedridden person) tends to cause circulatory deficiency and necrosis due to local compression of blood vessels — compare BEDSORE 2 : a discrete point on the body to which pressure is applied (as in acupressure or reflexology) for therapeutic purposes 3 : a point where a blood vessel runs near a bone and can be compressed (as to check bleeding) by the application of pressure against the bone

pressure sore *n* : BEDSORE

pressure suit *n* : an inflatable suit for high-altitude or space flight to protect the body from low pressure

pre·sump·tive \pri-'zəmp-tiv\ *adj* 1 : expected to develop in a particular direction under normal conditions 2 : being the embryonic precursor of ⟨~ neural tissue⟩

pre·sur·gi·cal \,prē-'sər-ji-kəl\ *adj* : occurring before, performed before, or preliminary to surgery ⟨~ care⟩

pre·symp·to·mat·ic \-,simp-tə-'ma-tik\ *adj* : relating to, being, or occurring before symptoms appear ⟨~ diagnosis of a hereditary disease⟩

pre·syn·ap·tic \-sə-'nap-tik\ *adj* : of, occurring in, or being a neuron by which a nerve impulse is conveyed to a synapse ⟨a ~ neuron⟩ ⟨~ inhibition⟩ — **pre·syn·ap·ti·cal·ly** *adv*

pre·sys·tol·ic \-sis-'tä-lik\ *adj* : of, relating to, or occurring just before cardiac systole ⟨a ~ murmur⟩

pre·tec·tal \-'tekt-ᵊl\ *adj* : occurring in or being the transitional zone of the brain stem between the midbrain and the diencephalon that is associated esp. with the analysis and distribution of light impulses

pre·term \-'tərm\ *adj* : of, relating to, being, or born by premature birth ⟨~ infants⟩ ⟨~ labor⟩

pre·ter·mi·nal \-'tər-mə-nəl\ *adj* 1 : occurring or being in the period

prior to death ⟨∼ cancer⟩ ⟨a ∼ patient⟩ **2** : situated or occurring anterior to an end (as of a nerve)
pre·tib·i·al \-'ti-bē-əl\ *adj* : lying or occurring anterior to the tibia
pretibial fever *n* : a rare infectious disease that is characterized by an eruption in the pretibial region, headache, backache, malaise, chills, and fever and that is caused by a spirochete of the genus *Leptospira* (*L. interrogans autumnalis*)
pretibial myxedema *n* : myxedema characterized primarily by a mucoid edema in the pretibial area
pre·trans·plan·ta·tion \-ˌtrans-ˌplan-'tā-shən\ *adj* : occurring or being in the period before transplant surgery ⟨∼ hospitalization⟩
pre·treat·ment \ˌprē-'trēt-mənt\ *n* : preliminary or preparatory treatment — **pre·treat** \-'trēt\ *vb* — **pretreatment** *adj*
Prev·a·cid \'pre-və-ˌsid\ *trademark* — used for a preparation of lansoprazole
prev·a·lence \'pre-və-ləns\ *n* : the percentage of a population that is affected with a particular disease at a given time — compare INCIDENCE
pre·ven·ta·tive \pri-'ven-tə-tiv\ *adj or n* : PREVENTIVE ⟨a ∼ drug⟩
¹**pre·ven·tive** \pri-'ven-tiv\ *n* : something (as a drug) used to prevent disease
²**preventive** *adj* : devoted to or concerned with the prevention of disease
preventive medicine *n* : a branch of medical science dealing with methods (as vaccination) of preventing the occurrence of disease
pre·ver·te·bral \ˌprē-'vər-tə-brəl, -ˌ)vər-'tē-brəl\ *adj* : situated or occurring anterior to a vertebra or the spinal column ⟨∼ muscles⟩
pre·ves·i·cal space \ˌprē-'ve-si-kəl\ *n* : RETROPUBIC SPACE
previa — see PLACENTA PREVIA
pre·vi·able \-'vī-ə-bəl\ *adj* : not sufficiently developed to survive outside the uterus ⟨a ∼ fetus⟩
pre·vil·lous \-'vi-ləs\ *adj* : relating to, being in, or being the stage of embryonic development before the formation of villi ⟨a ∼ human embryo⟩
pri·a·pism \'prī-ə-ˌpi-zəm\ *n* : an abnormal, more or less persistent, and often painful erection of the penis; *esp* : one caused by disease rather than sexual desire
Price–Jones curve \'prīs-'jōnz-\ *n* : a graph of the frequency distribution of the diameters of red blood cells in a sample that has been smeared, stained, and magnified for direct observation and counting
 Price–Jones, Cecil (1863–1943), British hematologist.
prick·le cell \'pri-kəl-\ *n* : a cell of the stratum spinosum of the skin having numerous intercellular bridges which give the separated cells a prickly appearance in microscopic preparations

prickle cell layer *n* : STRATUM SPINOSUM
prick·ly heat \'pri-klē-\ *n* : a noncontagious cutaneous eruption of red pimples with intense itching and tingling caused by inflammation around the sweat ducts — called also *heat rash*; see MILIARIA
prick test *n* : a test for allergic susceptibility made by placing a drop of the allergy-producing substance on the skin and making breaks in the skin by lightly pricking the surface — compare INTRADERMAL TEST, PATCH TEST, SCRATCH TEST
pril·o·caine \'pri-lə-ˌkān\ *n* : a local anesthetic related to lidocaine and used in the form of its hydrochloride $C_{13}H_{20}N_2O·HCl$ as a nerve block for pain esp. in surgery and dentistry
Pril·o·sec \'pri-lə-ˌsek\ *trademark* — used for a preparation of omeprazole
pri·mal scream therapy \'prī-məl-\ *n* : psychotherapy in which the patient recalls and reenacts a particularly disturbing past experience usu. occurring early in life and expresses normally repressed anger or frustration esp. through spontaneous and unrestrained screams, hysteria, or violence — called also *primal scream, primal therapy*
pri·ma·quine \'prī-mə-ˌkwēn, 'pri-, -kwin\ *n* : an antimalarial drug used in the form of its diphosphate $C_{15}H_{21}N_3O·2H_3PO_4$
pri·ma·ry \'prī-ˌmer-ē, 'prī-mə-rē\ *adj* **1 a** (1) : first in order of time or development (2) : relating to or being the milk teeth and esp. the 20 milk teeth in the human set **b** (1) : arising spontaneously : IDIOPATHIC ⟨∼ insomnia⟩ (2) : being an initial tumor or site esp. of cancer **c** : providing primary care ⟨a ∼ physician⟩ **2** : belonging to the first group or order in successive divisions, combinations, or ramifications ⟨∼ nerves⟩ **3** : of, relating to, or being the amino acid sequence in proteins — compare SECONDARY 3, TERTIARY 2
primary aldosteronism *n* : aldosteronism caused by an adrenal tumor — called also *Conn's syndrome*
primary amenorrhea *n* : amenorrhea in which menstruation has not yet occurred by age 16
primary atypical pneumonia *n* : any of a group of pneumonias (as Q fever and psittacosis) caused esp. by a virus, mycoplasma, rickettsia, or chlamydia
primary care *n* : health care provided by a medical professional (as a general practitioner or a pediatrician) with whom a patient has initial contact and by whom the patient may be referred to a specialist for further treatment — often used attributively ⟨*primary care* physicians⟩; called also *primary health care*; compare SECONDARY CARE, TERTIARY CARE
primary fissure *n* : a fissure of the

cerebellum that is situated between the culmen and declive and that marks the boundary between the anterior lobe and the posterior lobe

primary health care n : PRIMARY CARE

primary host n : DEFINITIVE HOST

primary hypertension n : ESSENTIAL HYPERTENSION

primary oocyte n : a diploid oocyte that has not yet undergone meiosis

primary spermatocyte n : a diploid spermatocyte that has not yet undergone meiosis

primary syphilis n : the first stage of syphilis that is marked by the development of a chancre and the spread of the causative spirochete in the tissues of the body

primary thrombocythemia n : THROMBOCYTHEMIA

primary tooth n : MILK TOOTH

pri·mate \'prī-ˌmāt\ n : any of an order (Primates) of mammals including humans, apes, monkeys, lemurs, and living and extinct related forms

prime mover \'prīm-\ n : AGONIST 1

prim·er \'prī-mər\ n : a molecule (as a short strand of RNA or DNA) whose presence is required for formation of another molecule (as a longer chain of DNA)

pri·mi·done \'prī-mə-ˌdōn\ n : an anticonvulsant phenobarbital derivative $C_{12}H_{14}N_2O_2$ used esp. to control epileptic seizures

pri·mi·grav·id \ˌprī-mə-'gra-vid\ adj : pregnant for the first time

pri·mi·grav·i·da \-'gra-vi-də\ n, pl **-i·das** or **-i·dae** \-ˌdē\ : an individual pregnant for the first time

pri·mip·a·ra \prī-'mi-pə-rə\ n, pl **-ras** or **-rae** \-ˌrē\ 1 : an individual bearing a first offspring 2 : an individual that has borne only one offspring

pri·mip·a·rous \-rəs\ adj : of, relating to, or being a primipara : bearing young for the first time — compare MULTIPAROUS 2

prim·i·tive \'pri-mə-tiv\ adj 1 : closely approximating an early ancestral type : little evolved 2 : belonging to or characteristic of an early stage of development 〈∼ cells〉

primitive streak n : an elongated band of cells that forms along the axis of an embryo early in gastrulation by the movement of lateral cells toward the axis and that develops a groove along its midline through which cells move to the interior of the embryo to form the mesoderm

pri·mor·di·al \prī-'mȯr-dē-əl\ adj : earliest formed in the growth of an individual or organ : PRIMITIVE

pri·mor·di·um \-dē-əm\ n, pl **-dia** \-dē-ə\ : the rudiment or commencement of a part or organ : ANLAGE

prin·ceps pol·li·cis \'prin-ˌseps-'pä-lə-səs\ n : a branch of the radial artery that passes along the ulnar side of the first metacarpal and divides into branches running along the palmar side of the thumb

prin·ci·ple \'prin-sə-pəl\ n : an ingredient (as a chemical) that exhibits or imparts a characteristic quality 〈the active ∼ of a drug〉

Prin·i·vil \'pri-nə-ˌvil\ trademark — used for a preparation of lisinopril

P–R interval \ˌpē-'är-\ n : the interval between the beginning of the P wave and the beginning of the QRS complex of an electrocardiogram that represents the time between the beginning of the contraction of the atria and the beginning of the contraction of the ventricles

Prinz·met·al's angina \'prinz-ˌme-t⁰lz-\ n : angina pectoris of a variant form that is characterized by chest pain during rest and by an elevated ST segment during pain and that is typically caused by an obstructive lesion in the coronary artery

Prinzmetal, Myron (1908–1987), American cardiologist.

pri·on \'prē-ˌän\ n : any of various infectious proteins that are abnormal forms of normal cellular proteins, that proliferate by inducing the normal protein to convert to the abnormal form, and that in mammals include pathogenic forms which arise sporadically, as a result of genetic mutation, or by transmission (as by ingestion of infected tissue) and which upon accumulation in the brain cause a prion disease

prion disease n : any of a group of spongiform encephalopathies that are caused and transmitted by prions and that include bovine spongiform encephalopathy, Creutzfeldt-Jakob disease, fatal familial insomnia, Gerstmann-Sträussler-Scheinker syndrome, kuru, scrapie, and variant Creutzfeldt-Jakob disease — called also transmissible spongiform encephalopathy

pri·vate \'prī-vət\ adj 1 : of, relating to, or receiving hospital service in which the patient has more privileges than a semiprivate or ward patient 2 : of, relating to, or being private practice 〈a ∼ practitioner〉

private–duty adj : caring for a single patient either in the home or in a hospital 〈a ∼ nurse〉

private practice n 1 : practice of a profession (as medicine) independently and not as an employee 2 : the patients depending on and using the services of a physician in private practice

privileged communication n : a communication between parties to a confidential relation (as between physician and patient) such that the recipient cannot be legally compelled to disclose it as a witness

PRK abbr photorefractive keratectomy

PRL abbr prolactin

prn *abbr* [Latin *pro re nata*] as needed; as the circumstances require — used in writing prescriptions

PRO *abbr* peer review organization

pro- *prefix* **1 a** : PRE- 1 ⟨*proestrus*⟩ **b** : rudimentary : PROT- ⟨*pronucleus*⟩ **c** : being a precursor of ⟨*proinsulin*⟩ **2** : front : anterior ⟨*pronephros*⟩ **3** : projecting ⟨*prognathous*⟩

pro·abor·tion \ˌprō-ə-ˈbȯr-shən\ *adj* : favoring the legalization of abortion — **pro·abor·tion·ist** \-shə-nist\ *n*

pro·ac·cel·er·in \ˌprō-ak-ˈse-lə-rən\ *n* : FACTOR V

pro·ac·tive \-ˈak-tiv\ *adj* : relating to, caused by, or being interference between previous learning and the recall or performance of later learning ⟨∼ inhibition of memory⟩

pro·band \ˈprō-ˌband\ *n* : an individual affected with a disorder who is the first subject in a study (as of a genetic character in a family lineage) — called also *propositus*

Pro–Ban·thine \ˌprō-ˈban-ˌthēn\ *n* : a preparation of propantheline bromide — formerly a U.S. registered trademark

probe \ˈprōb\ *n* **1** : a surgical instrument that consists typically of a light slender fairly flexible pointed metal instrument like a small rod that is used typically for locating a foreign body, for exploring a wound or suppurative tract by prodding or piercing, or for penetrating and exploring bodily passages and cavities **2** : a device (as an ultrasound generator) or a substance (as radioactively labeled DNA) used to obtain specific information for diagnostic or experimental purposes — **probe** *vb*

pro·ben·e·cid \ˌprō-ˈbe-nə-səd\ *n* : a drug $C_{13}H_{19}NO_4S$ that acts on renal tubular function and is used to increase the concentration of some drugs (as penicillin) in the blood by inhibiting their excretion and to increase the excretion of urates in gout

pro·bi·ot·ic \ˌprō-bī-ˈä-tik\ *n* : a preparation (as a dietary supplement) containing live bacteria (as lactobacilli) that is taken orally to restore beneficial bacteria to the body; *also* : a bacterium in such a preparation — **probiotic** *adj*

pro·bos·cis \prə-ˈbä-səs, -ˈbäs-kəs\ *n, pl* **-bos·cis·es** *also* **-bos·ci·des** \-ˈbä-sə-ˌdēz\ : any of various elongated or extensible tubular organs or processes of the oral region of an invertebrate

pro·bu·col \ˈprō-byə-ˌkȯl\ *n* : an antioxidant drug $C_{31}H_{48}O_2S_2$ that is used to reduce levels of serum cholesterol

pro·cain·amide \prō-ˈkā-nə-ˌmīd, -məd; -ˌkā-ˈna-məd\ *n* : a base of an amide related to procaine that is used in the form of its hydrochloride $C_{13}H_{21}N_3O·HCl$ as a cardiac depressant esp. in the treatment of ventricu-

lar and atrial arrhythmias — see PRONESTYL

pro·caine \ˈprō-ˌkān\ *n* : a basic ester $C_{13}H_{20}N_2O_2$ of para-aminobenzoic acid used in the form of its hydrochloride $C_{13}H_{20}N_2O_2·HCl$ as a local anesthetic — see NOVOCAIN, NOVOCAINE

procaine penicillin G *n* : PENICILLIN G PROCAINE

pro·car·ba·zine \prō-ˈkär-bə-ˌzēn, -zən\ *n* : an antineoplastic drug that is a monoamine oxidase inhibitor and is used in the form of its hydrochloride $C_{12}H_{19}N_3O·HCl$ esp. in the palliative treatment of Hodgkin's disease

Pro·car·dia \prō-ˈkär-dē-ə\ *trademark* — used for a preparation of nifedipine

procaryote *var of* PROKARYOTE

pro·ce·dure \prə-ˈsē-jər\ *n* **1** : a particular way of accomplishing something or of acting **2** : a step in a procedure; *esp* : a series of steps followed in a regular definite order

pro·ce·rus \prō-ˈsir-əs\ *n, pl* **-ri** \-ˌrī\ *or* **-rus·es** : a facial muscle that arises from the nasal bone and a cartilage in the side of the nose and that inserts into the skin of the forehead between the eyebrows

pro·cess \ˈprä-ˌses, ˈprō-, -səs\ *n* **1 a** : a natural progressively continuing operation or development marked by a series of gradual changes that succeed one another in a relatively fixed way and lead toward a particular result or end ⟨the ∼ of growth⟩ **b** : a natural continuing activity or function ⟨such life ∼es as breathing⟩ **2** : a part of the mass of an organism or organic structure that projects outward from the main mass ⟨a bone ∼⟩

pro·ces·sus \prō-ˈse-səs\ *n, pl* **processus** : PROCESS 2

processus vag·i·na·lis \-ˌva-jə-ˈnā-ləs\ *n* : a pouch of peritoneum that is carried into the scrotum by the descent of the testicle and which in the scrotum forms the tunica vaginalis

pro·chlor·per·azine \ˌprō-ˌklȯr-ˈper-ə-ˌzēn\ *n* : a tranquilizing and antiemetic drug $C_{20}H_{24}ClN_3S$ — see COMPAZINE

pro–choice \ˌprō-ˈchȯis\ *adj* : favoring the legalization of abortion — **pro·choic·er** \-ˈchȯi-sər\ *n*

pro·ci·den·tia \ˌprō-sə-ˈden-chə, ˌprä-, -chē-ə\ *n* : PROLAPSE; *esp* : severe prolapse of the uterus in which the cervix projects from the vaginal opening

proc·li·na·tion \ˌprä-klə-ˈnā-shən\ *n* : the condition of being inclined forward ⟨∼ of the upper incisors⟩

¹pro·co·ag·u·lant \ˌprō-kō-ˈa-gyə-lənt\ *n* : a procoagulant substance

²procoagulant *adj* : promoting the coagulation of blood ⟨∼ activity⟩

pro·col·la·gen \-ˈkä-lə-jən\ *n* : a molecular precursor of collagen

pro·con·ver·tin \-kən-ˈvərt-ᵊn\ *n* : FACTOR VII

pro·cre·ate \'prō-krē-‚āt\ *vb* **-at·ed;** **-at·ing** : to beget or bring forth offspring : PROPAGATE, REPRODUCE — **pro·cre·ation** \‚prō-krē-'ā-shən\ *n* — **pro·cre·ative** \'prō-krē-‚ā-tiv\ *adj*

proct- or **procto-** *comb form* **1 a** : rectum ⟨*procto*scope⟩ **b** : rectum and ⟨*procto*sigmoidectomy⟩ **2** : anus and rectum ⟨*procto*logy⟩

proct·al·gia fu·gax \‚präk-'tal-jə-'fyü-‚gaks, -jē-ə-\ *n* : a condition characterized by the intermittent occurrence of sudden sharp pain in the rectal area

proc·tec·to·my \präk-'tek-tə-mē\ *n, pl* **-mies** : surgical excision of the rectum

proc·ti·tis \präk-'tī-təs\ *n* : inflammation of the anus and rectum

proc·toc·ly·sis \präk-'tä-klə-səs\ *n, pl* **-ly·ses** \-‚sēz\ : slow injection of large quantities of a fluid (as a solution of salt) into the rectum in supplementing the liquid intake of the body

proc·to·co·li·tis \‚präk-tō-kə-'lī-təs\ *n* : inflammation of the rectum and colon

proc·tol·o·gy \präk-'tä-lə-jē\ *n, pl* **-gies** : a branch of medicine dealing with the structure and diseases of the anus, rectum, and sigmoid colon — **proc·to·log·ic** \‚präk-tə-'lä-jik\ or **proc·to·log·i·cal** \-ji-kəl\ *adj* — **proc·tol·o·gist** \-jist\ *n*

proc·to·pexy \'präk-tə-‚pek-sē\ *n, pl* **-pex·ies** : the suturing of the rectum to an adjacent structure (as the sacrum)

proc·to·plas·ty \'präk-tə-‚plas-tē\ *n, pl* **-ties** : plastic surgery of the rectum and anus

proc·to·scope \'präk-tə-‚skōp\ *n* : an instrument used for dilating and visually inspecting the rectum — **proc·to·scop·ic** \‚präk-tə-'skä-pik\ *adj* — **proc·to·scop·i·cal·ly** *adv* — **proc·tos·co·py** \präk-'täs-kə-pē\ *n*

proc·to·sig·moid·ec·to·my \‚präk-tō-‚sig-‚mòi-'dek-tə-mē\ *n, pl* **-mies** : complete or partial surgical excision of the rectum and sigmoid colon

proc·to·sig·moid·itis \-‚sig-mòi-'dī-təs\ *n* : inflammation of the rectum and sigmoid colon

proc·to·sig·moid·o·scope \-sig-'mòi-də-‚skōp\ *n* : SIGMOIDOSCOPE

proc·to·sig·moid·os·co·py \-‚sig-‚mòi-'däs-kə-pē\ *n, pl* **-pies** : SIGMOIDOSCOPY — **proc·to·sig·moid·o·scop·ic** \-‚mòi-də-'skä-pik\ *adj*

proc·tot·o·my \präk-'tä-tə-mē\ *n, pl* **-mies** : surgical incision into the rectum

prod·ro·ma \'prä-drə-mə\ *n, pl* **-mas** or **-ma·ta** \prō-'drō-mə-tə\ : PRODROME

pro·drome \'prō-‚drōm\ *n* : a premonitory symptom of disease — **pro·dro·mal** \‚prō-'drō-məl\ *also* **pro·dro·mic** \-mik\ *adj*

pro·drug \'prō-‚drəg\ *n* : a pharmacologically inactive substance that is the modified form of a pharmacologically

active drug to which it is converted (as by enzymatic action) in the body

pro·duc·tive \prə-'dək-tiv, prō-\ *adj* : raising mucus or sputum (as from the bronchi) ⟨a ~ cough⟩

pro·en·zyme \‚prō-'en-‚zīm\ *n* : ZYMOGEN

pro·eryth·ro·blast \-i-'ri-thrə-‚blast\ *n* : a hemocytoblast that gives rise to erythroblasts

pro·es·trus \-'es-trəs\ *n* : a preparatory period immediately preceding estrus and characterized by growth of graafian follicles, increased estrogenic activity, and alteration of uterine and vaginal mucosa

professional corporation *n* : a corporation organized by one or more licensed individuals (as a doctor or dentist) esp. for the purpose of providing professional services and obtaining tax advantages — abbr. *PC*

pro·fi·bri·no·ly·sin \‚prō-‚fī-brə-nə-'lis-ᵊn\ *n* : PLASMINOGEN

pro·file \'prō-‚fil\ *n* **1** : a set of data exhibiting the significant features of something and often obtained by multiple tests **2** : a graphic representation of the extent to which an individual or group exhibits traits or abilities as determined by tests or ratings ⟨a personality ~⟩

pro·fla·vine \‚prō-'flā-‚vēn\ *also* **pro·fla·vin** \-vin\ *n* : a yellow crystalline mutagenic acridine dye $C_{13}H_{11}N_3$; *also* : the orange to brownish red hygroscopic crystalline sulfate used as an antiseptic esp. for wounds — see ACRIFLAVINE

pro·found·ly \prə-'faund-lē, prō-\ *adv* **1** : totally or completely ⟨~ deaf persons⟩ **2** : to the greatest possible degree ⟨~ mentally retarded persons⟩

pro·fun·da artery \prə-'fən-də-\ *n* **1** : DEEP BRACHIAL ARTERY **2** : DEEP FEMORAL ARTERY

profunda fem·o·ris \-'fe-mə-rəs\ *n* : DEEP FEMORAL ARTERY

profunda femoris artery *n* : DEEP FEMORAL ARTERY

profundus — see FLEXOR DIGITORUM PROFUNDUS

pro·gen·i·tor \prō-'je-nə-tər, prə-\ *n* **1** : an ancestor of an individual in a direct line of descent along which some or all of the ancestral genes could theoretically have passed **2** : a biologically ancestral form

prog·e·ny \'prä-jə-nē\ *n, pl* **-nies** : offspring of animals or plants

pro·ge·ria \prō-'jir-ē-ə\ *n* : a rare genetic disorder of childhood marked by slowed physical growth and characteristic signs (as baldness, wrinkled skin, and atherosclerosis) of rapid aging with death usu. occurring during puberty

pro·ges·ta·tion·al \‚prō-‚jes-'tā-shə-nəl\ *adj* : preceding pregnancy or gestation; *esp* : of, relating to, inducing, or constituting the modifications of the female mammalian system associated with ovulation and corpus luteum formation ⟨∼ hormones⟩

pro·ges·ter·one \prō-'jes-tə-ˌrōn\ *n* : a female steroid sex hormone $C_{21}H_{30}O_2$ that is secreted by the corpus luteum to prepare the endometrium for implantation and later by the placenta during pregnancy to prevent rejection of the developing embryo or fetus; *also* : a synthetic steroid resembling progesterone in action

pro·ges·tin \prō-'jes-tən\ *n* : PROGESTERONE; *esp* : a synthetic progesterone (as levonorgestrel)

pro·ges·to·gen *also* **pro·ges·ta·gen** \-'jes-tə-jən\ *n* : a naturally occurring or synthetic progestational steroid — **pro·ges·to·gen·ic** *also* **pro·ges·ta·gen·ic** \prə-ˌjes-tə-'je-nik\ *adj*

pro·glot·tid \prō-'glä-tid\ *n* : a segment of a tapeworm containing both male and female reproductive organs

pro·glot·tis \-'glä-tis\ *n, pl* **-glot·ti·des** \-'glä-tə-ˌdēz\ : PROGLOTTID

prog·nath·ic \präg-'na-thik, -'nā-\ *adj* : PROGNATHOUS

prog·na·thous \'präg-nə-thəs\ *adj* : having the jaws projecting beyond the upper part of the face — **prog·na·thism** \'präg-nə-ˌthi-zəm, präg-'nā-\ *n*

prog·no·sis \präg-'nō-səs\ *n, pl* **-no·ses** \-ˌsēz\ **1** : the act or art of foretelling the course of a disease **2** : the prospect of survival and recovery from a disease as anticipated from the usual course of that disease or indicated by special features of the case — **prog·nos·tic** \präg-'näs-tik\ *adj*

prog·nos·ti·cate \präg-'näs-tə-ˌkāt\ *vb* **-cat·ed; -cat·ing** : to make a prognosis about the probable outcome of — **prog·nos·ti·ca·tion** \-ˌnäs-tə-'kā-shən\ *n*

programmed cell death *n* : APOPTOSIS

pro·gres·sive \prə-'gre-siv\ *adj* **1** : increasing in extent or severity ⟨a ∼ disease⟩ **2** : of, relating to, or being a multifocal lens with a gradual transition between focal lengths ⟨∼ bifocals⟩ — **pro·gres·sive·ly** *adv*

progressive multifocal leukoencephalopathy *n* : a progressive and fatal demyelinating disease of the central nervous system that typically occurs in immunosuppressed individuals due to loss of childhood immunity to a virus of the genus *Polyomavirus* (species *JC polyomavirus*) ubiquitous in human populations and that is characterized by hemianopia, hemiplegia, alterations in mental state, and eventually coma

progressive supranuclear palsy *n* : an uncommon neurological disorder that is of unknown etiology, typically occurs from late middle age onward, and is marked by loss of voluntary vertical eye movement, muscular rigidity and dystonia of the neck and trunk, pseudobulbar paralysis, bradykinesia, and dementia — called also *supranuclear palsy*

pro·guan·il \prō-'gwän-ᵊl\ *n* : an antimalarial drug used in the form of its hydrochloride $C_{11}H_{16}ClN_5 \cdot HCl$ — called also *chloroguanide*

pro·hor·mone \prō-'hȯr-ˌmōn\ *n* : a physiologically inactive precursor of a hormone

pro·in·su·lin \-'in-sə-lən\ *n* : a single-chain pancreatic polypeptide precursor of insulin that gives rise to the double chain of insulin by loss of the middle part of the molecule

pro·ject \prə-'jekt\ *vb* **1** : to attribute or assign (something in one's own mind or a personal characteristic) to a person, group, or object **2** : to connect by sending nerve fibers or processes

pro·jec·tile vomiting \prə-'jek-təl-, -ˌtīl-\ *n* : vomiting that is sudden, usu. without nausea, and so sufficiently vigorous that the vomit is forcefully projected to a distance

pro·jec·tion \prə-'jek-shən\ *n* **1 a** : the act of referring a mental image constructed by the brain from bits of data collected by the sense organs to the actual source of stimulation outside the body **b** : the attribution of one's own ideas, feelings, or attitudes to other people or to objects; *esp* : the externalization of blame, guilt, or responsibility as a defense against anxiety **2** : the functional correspondence and connection of parts of the cerebral cortex with other parts of the organism

projection area *n* : an area of the cerebral cortex having connection through projection fibers with subcortical centers that in turn are linked with peripheral sense or motor organs

projection fiber *n* : a nerve fiber connecting some part of the cerebral cortex with lower sensory or motor centers — compare ASSOCIATION FIBER

pro·jec·tive \prə-'jek-tiv\ *adj* : of, relating to, or being a technique, device, or test (as the Rorschach test) designed to analyze the psychodynamic constitution of an individual by presenting unstructured or ambiguous material (as blots of ink, pictures, and sentence elements) that will elicit interpretive responses revealing personality structure

pro·kary·ote *also* **pro·cary·ote** \prō-'kar-ē-ˌōt\ *n* : a typically unicellular organism (as a bacterium) that lacks a distinct nucleus and membrane-bound organelles — compare EUKARYOTE — **pro·kary·ot·ic** *also* **pro·cary·ot·ic** \-ˌkar-ē-'ä-tik\ *adj*

pro·ki·net·ic \prō-kə-'ne-tik, -kī-\ *adj* : stimulating motility of the esophageal and gastrointestinal muscles — **prokinetic** *n*

pro·lac·tin \prō-'lak-tən\ *n* : a protein hormone of the adenohypophysis of the pituitary gland that induces and maintains lactation in the postpartum mammalian female — abbr. *PRL*; called also *luteotropic hormone, luteotropin, mammotropin*

pro·la·min *or* **pro·la·mine** \'prō-lə-mən, -ˌmēn\ *n* : any of various simple proteins that are found esp. in the seeds of grasses and are soluble in alcohol

pro·lapse \prō-'laps, 'prō-ˌ\ *n* : the falling down or slipping of a body part from its usual position or relations ⟨uterine ∼⟩ — **pro·lapse** \prō-'laps\ *vb*

pro–life \ˌprō-'līf\ *adj* : ANTIABORTION

pro–lif·er \-'lī-fər\ *n* : a person who opposes the legalization of abortion

proliferans — see RETINITIS PROLIFERANS

pro·lif·er·a·tion \prə-ˌli-fə-'rā-shən\ *n* **1 a** : rapid and repeated production of new parts or of offspring (as in a mass of cells by a rapid succession of cell divisions) **b** : a growth so formed **2** : the action, process, or result of increasing by proliferation — **pro·lif·er·ate** \-'li-fə-ˌrāt\ *vb* — **pro·lif·er·a·tive** \-'li-fə-ˌrā-tiv\ *adj*

proligerus — see DISCUS PROLIGERUS

pro·line \'prō-ˌlēn\ *n* : an amino acid $C_5H_9NO_2$ that can be synthesized by animals from glutamate

Pro·lix·in \prō-'lik-sən\ *trademark* — used for a preparation of fluphenazine

pro·lo·ther·a·py \ˌprō-lō-'ther-ə-pē\ *n* : an alternative therapy for treating musculoskeletal pain that involves injecting an irritant substance (as dextrose) into a ligament or tendon to promote the growth of new tissue

pro·mas·ti·gote \prō-'mas-ti-ˌgōt\ *n* : a protozoan (family Trypanosomatidae and esp. genus *Leishmania*) that is in a flagellated usu. extracellular stage characterized by a single anterior flagellum and no undulating membrane — **promastigote** *adj*

pro·ma·zine \'prō-mə-ˌzēn\ *n* : a tranquilizer derived from phenothiazine that is used in the form of its hydrochloride $C_{17}H_{20}N_2S\cdot HCl$ similarly to chlorpromazine — see SPARINE

pro·mega·kary·o·cyte \ˌprō-ˌme-gə-'kar-ē-ō-ˌsīt\ *n* : a cell in an intermediate stage of development between a megakaryoblast and a megakaryocyte

pro·meth·a·zine \prō-'me-thə-ˌzēn\ *n* : an antihistamine drug derived from phenothiazine and used chiefly in the form of its hydrochloride $C_{17}H_{20}N_2S\cdot HCl$ — see PHENERGAN

pro·meth·es·trol \-me-'thes-ˌtrȯl\ *n* : a synthetic estrogen $C_{20}H_{26}O_2$

pro·me·thi·um \prō-'mē-thē-əm\ *n* : a radioactive metallic element obtained as a fission product of uranium or from neutron-irradiated neodymium — symbol *Pm;* see ELEMENT table

prom·i·nence \'prä-mə-nəns\ *n* : an elevation or projection on an anatomical structure (as a bone)

prominens — see VERTEBRA PROMINENS

pro·mis·cu·ous \prə-'mis-kyə-wəs\ *adj* : not restricted to one sexual partner — **pro·mis·cu·i·ty** \ˌprä-məs-'kyü-ə-tē, prə-ˌmis-\ *n*

pro·mono·cyte \prə-'mä-nə-ˌsīt\ *n* : a cell in an intermediate stage of development between a monoblast and a monocyte

prom·on·to·ry \'prä-mən-ˌtȯr-ē\ *n, pl* **-ries** : a bodily prominence: as **a** : the angle of the ventral side of the sacrum where it joins the vertebra **b** : a prominence on the inner wall of the tympanum of the ear

pro·mot·er \prə-'mōt-ər\ *n* **1** : a substance that in very small amounts is able to increase the activity of a catalyst **2** : a binding site in a DNA chain at which RNA polymerase binds to initiate transcription of messenger RNA by one or more nearby structural genes **3** : a chemical believed to promote carcinogenicity or mutagenicity

pro·my·elo·cyte \prō-'mī-ə-lə-ˌsīt\ *n* : a cell in bone marrow that is in an intermediate stage of development between a myeloblast and a myelocyte and has the characteristic granulations but lacks the specific staining reactions of a mature granulocyte of the blood — **pro·my·elo·cyt·ic** \-ˌmī-ə-lə-'si-tik\ *adj*

promyelocytic leukemia *n* : a leukemia in which the predominant blood cell type is the promyelocyte

pro·na·tion \prō-'nā-shən\ *n* : rotation of an anatomical part towards the midline: as **a** : rotation of the hand and forearm so that the palm faces backwards or downwards **b** : rotation of the medial bones in the midtarsal region of the foot inward and downward so that in walking the foot tends to come down on its inner margin — **pro·nate** \'prō-ˌnāt\ *vb*

pro·na·tor \'prō-ˌnā-tər\ *n* : a muscle that produces pronation

pronator qua·dra·tus \-kwä-'drā-təs\ *n* : a deep muscle of the forearm passing transversely from the ulna to the radius and serving to pronate the forearm

pronator te·res \-'tir-ˌēz\ *n* : a muscle of the forearm arising from the medial epicondyle of the humerus and the coronoid process of the ulna, inserting into the lateral surface of the middle third of the radius, and serving to pronate and flex the forearm

prone \'prōn\ *adj* : having the front or ventral surface downward; *esp* : lying facedown — **prone** *adv*

pro·neph·ros \prō-'ne-frəs, -ˌfräs\ *n, pl* **-neph·roi** \-'ne-ˌfrȯi\ : either member of the first and most anterior pair of the three paired vertebrate renal organs present but nonfunctional in embryos of reptiles, birds, and mammals — compare MESONEPHROS, META-

NEPHROS — **pro·neph·ric** \prō-'ne-frik\ *adj*

Pro·nes·tyl \prō-'nes-til\ *trademark* — used for a preparation of the hydrochloride of procainamide

pron·to·sil \'prän-tə-ˌsil\ *n* : any of three sulfonamide drugs: **a** : a red azo dye $C_{12}H_{13}N_5O_2S$ that was the first sulfa drug tested clinically **b** : SULFANILAMIDE **c** : AZOSULFAMIDE

pro·nu·cle·us \prō-'nü-klē-əs, -'nyü-\ *n, pl* **-clei** \-klē-ˌī\ *also* **-cle·us·es** : the haploid nucleus of a male or female gamete (as an egg or sperm) up to the time of fusion with that of another gamete in fertilization — **pro·nu·cle·ar** \-klē-ər\ *adj*

prop·a·gate \'prä-pə-ˌgāt\ *vb* **-gat·ed; -gat·ing** **1** : to reproduce or cause to reproduce sexually or asexually **2** : to cause to spread or to be transmitted — **prop·a·ga·tion** \ˌprä-pə-'gā-shən\ *n* — **prop·a·ga·tive** \'prä-pə-ˌgā-tiv\ *adj*

pro·pam·i·dine \prō-'pa-mə-ˌdēn, -dən\ *n* : an antiseptic drug $C_{17}H_{20}N_4O_2$

pro·pan·o·lol \prō-'pa-nə-ˌlȯl, -ˌlōl\ *n* : PROPRANOLOL

pro·pan·the·line bromide \prō-'panthə-ˌlēn-\ *n* : an anticholinergic drug $C_{23}H_{30}BrNO_3$ used esp. in the treatment of peptic ulcer — called also *propantheline*; see PRO-BANTHINE

pro·par·a·caine \prō-'par-ə-ˌkān\ *n* : a drug used in the form of its hydrochloride $C_{16}H_{26}N_2O_3 \cdot HCl$ as a topical anesthetic

Pro·pe·cia \prō-'pē-shə\ *trademark* — used for a preparation of finasteride

pro·per·din \prō-'pərd-ᵊn\ *n* : a blood serum protein that participates in the activation of complement in a pathway which does not involve the presence of antibodies

pro·peri·to·ne·al \prō-ˌper-ə-tə-'nē-əl\ *adj* : lying between the parietal peritoneum and the ventral musculature of the body cavity ⟨∼ fat⟩

pro·phage \'prō-ˌfāj, -ˌfäzh\ *n* : an intracellular form of a bacteriophage in which it is harmless to the host, is usu. integrated into the hereditary material of the host, and reproduces when the host does

pro·phase \-ˌfāz\ *n* **1** : the initial stage of mitosis and of the mitotic division of meiosis characterized by the condensation of chromosomes consisting of two chromatids, disappearance of the nucleolus and nuclear membrane, and formation of the mitotic spindle **2** : the initial stage of the first division of meiosis in which the chromosomes become visible, homologous pairs of chromosomes undergo synapsis and crossing-over, chiasmata appear, chromosomes condense with homologues visible as tetrads, and the nuclear membrane and nucleolus disappear — see DIAKINESIS, DIPLOTENE,

LEPTOTENE, PACHYTENE, ZYGOTENE — **pro·pha·sic** \prō-'fā-zik\ *adj*

¹pro·phy·lac·tic \ˌprō-fə-'lak-tik, ˌprä-\ *adj* **1** : guarding from or preventing the spread or occurrence of disease or infection ⟨∼ therapy⟩ **2** : tending to prevent or ward off : PREVENTIVE — **pro·phy·lac·ti·cal·ly** *adv*

²prophylactic *n* : something (as a drug) that is prophylactic; *esp* : a device and esp. a condom for preventing venereal infection or conception

pro·phy·lax·is \-'lak-səs\ *n, pl* **-lax·es** \-'lak-ˌsēz\ : measures designed to preserve health and prevent the spread of disease : protective or preventive treatment

pro·pio·lac·tone \ˌprō-pē-ō-'lak-ˌtōn\ *or* β-**pro·pio·lac·tone** \ˌbā-tə-\ *n* : a liquid disinfectant $C_3H_4O_2$

pro·pi·o·ma·zine \ˌprō-pē-'ō-mə-ˌzēn\ *n* : a phenothiazine used esp. in the form of its hydrochloride $C_{20}H_{24}N_2OS \cdot HCl$ as a sedative

pro·pi·o·nate \'prō-pē-ə-ˌnāt\ *n* : a salt or ester of propionic acid

pro·pi·oni·bac·te·ri·um \ˌprō-pē-ˌä-nə-bak-'tir-ē-əm\ *n* **1** *cap* : a genus of gram-positive nonmotile usu. anaerobic bacteria (family Propionibacteriaceae) including forms found esp. on human skin and in dairy products **2** *pl* **-ria** \-ē-ə\ : any bacterium of the genus *Propionibacterium*

pro·pi·on·ic acid \ˌprō-pē-'ä-nik-\ *n* : a liquid sharp-odored fatty acid $C_3H_6O_2$

pro·po·fol \'prō-pō-ˌfȯl\ *n* : a sedating and hypnotic agent $C_{12}H_{18}O$ administered in the form of an injectable emulsion to induce and maintain anesthesia or sedation

pro·pos·i·ta \prō-'pä-zə-tə\ *n, pl* **-i·tae** \-ˌtē\ : a female proband

pro·pos·i·tus \prō-'pä-zə-təs\ *n, pl* **-i·ti** \-ˌtī\ : PROBAND

pro·poxy·phene \prō-'päk-sə-ˌfēn\ *n* : a narcotic analgesic structurally related to methadone but less addicting that is administered in the form of its hydrochloride $C_{22}H_{29}NO_2 \cdot HCl$ or hydrated napsylate $C_{22}H_{29}NO_2 \cdot C_{10}H_8SO_3 \cdot H_2O$ — called also *dextropropoxyphene*; see DARVOCET-N, DARVON

pro·pran·o·lol \prō-'pra-nə-ˌlȯl, -ˌlōl\ *n* : a beta-blocker used in the form of its hydrochloride $C_{16}H_{21}NO_2 \cdot HCl$ esp. in the treatment of hypertension, cardiac arrhythmias, and angina pectoris and in the prevention of migraine headache — called also *propanolol*; see INDERAL

propria — see LAMINA PROPRIA, SUBSTANTIA PROPRIA, TUNICA PROPRIA

¹pro·pri·e·tary \prə-'prī-ə-ˌter-ē\ *n, pl* **-tar·ies** : something that is used, produced, or marketed under exclusive legal right of the inventor or maker; *specif* : a drug (as a patent medicine) that is protected by secrecy, patent, or copyright against free competition as to name, product, composition, or process of manufacture

²**pro·pri·e·tary** *adj* **1** : used, made, or marketed by one having the exclusive legal right ⟨a ∼ drug⟩ **2** : privately owned and managed and run as a profit-making organization ⟨a ∼ clinic⟩

pro·prio·cep·tion \ˌprō-prē-ō-ˈsep-shən\ *n* : the reception of stimuli produced within the organism — **pro·prio·cep·tive** \-ˈsep-tiv\ *adj*

proprioceptive neuromuscular facilitation *n* : a method of stretching muscles to maximize their flexibility that is often performed with a partner or trainer and that involves a series of contractions and relaxations with enforced stretching during the relaxation phase — abbr. PNF

pro·prio·cep·tor \-ˈsep-tər\ *n* : a sensory receptor located deep in the tissues (as in skeletal or heart muscle) that functions in proprioception

pro·prio·spi·nal \-ˈspīn-ᵊl\ *adj* : distinctively or exclusively spinal ⟨a ∼ neuron⟩

proprius — see EXTENSOR DIGITI QUINTI PROPRIUS, EXTENSOR INDICIS PROPRIUS

pro·pto·sis \präp-ˈtō-səs, prō-ˈtō-\ *n*, *pl* **-pto·ses** \-ˌsēz\ : forward projection or displacement esp. of the eyeball

pro·pyl·ene glycol \ˈprō-pə-ˌlēn-\ *n* : a sweet viscous liquid $C_3H_8O_2$ used esp. as an antifreeze and solvent, in brake fluids, and as a food preservative

pro·pyl gallate \ˈprō-pəl-\ *n* : a white crystalline antioxidant $C_{10}H_{12}O_5$ that is used as a preservative

pro·pyl·hex·e·drine \ˌprō-pəl-ˈhek-sə-ˌdrēn\ *n* : a sympathomimetic drug $C_{10}H_{21}N$ used chiefly as a nasal decongestant

pro·pyl·par·a·ben \-ˈpar-ə-ˌben\ *n* : an ester $C_{10}H_{12}O_3$ used as a preservative in pharmaceutical preparations

pro·pyl·thio·ura·cil \-ˌthī-ō-ˈyùr-ə-ˌsil\ *n* : a crystalline compound C_7H_{10}-N_2OS used as an antithyroid drug in the treatment of goiter

pro·re·nin \prō-ˈrē-nən, -ˈre-\ *n* : the precursor of the kidney enzyme renin

pros- *prefix* : in front ⟨*pros*encephalon⟩

Pros·car \ˈpräs-ˌkär\ *trademark* — used for a preparation of finasteride

pro·sec·tor \prō-ˈsek-tər\ *n* : a person who makes dissections for anatomic demonstrations

pros·en·ceph·a·lon \ˌprä-sen-ˈse-fə-ˌlän, -lən\ *n* : FOREBRAIN

prosop- *or* **prosopo-** *comb form* : face ⟨*prosop*agnosia⟩

pros·op·ag·no·sia \ˌprä-sə-pag-ˈnō-zhə\ *n* : a form of visual agnosia characterized by an inability to recognize faces

pro·spec·tive \prə-ˈspek-tiv\ *adj* : relating to or being a study (as of the incidence of disease) that starts with the present condition of a population of individuals and follows them into the future — compare RETROSPECTIVE

pros·ta·cy·clin \ˌpräs-tə-ˈsī-klən\ *n* : a prostaglandin that is a metabolite of arachidonic acid, inhibits aggregation of platelets, and dilates blood vessels

pros·ta·glan·din \ˌpräs-tə-ˈglan-dən\ *n* : any of various oxygenated unsaturated cyclic fatty acids of animals that have a variety of hormonelike actions (as in controlling blood pressure or smooth muscle contraction)

prostaglandin E₁ \-ˈē-ˈwən\ *n* : ALPROSTADIL

prostat- *or* **prostato-** *comb form* : prostate gland ⟨*prostat*itis⟩

prostatae — see LEVATOR PROSTATAE

pros·tate \ˈpräs-ˌtāt\ *n* : PROSTATE GLAND

pros·ta·tec·to·my \ˌpräs-tə-ˈtek-tə-mē\ *n*, *pl* **-mies** : surgical removal or resection of the prostate gland

prostate gland *n* : a firm partly muscular partly glandular body that is situated about the base of the mammalian male urethra and secretes an alkaline viscid fluid which is a major constituent of the ejaculatory fluid — called also *prostate*

prostate–specific antigen *n* : a protease that is secreted by the epithelial cells of the prostate and is used in the diagnosis of prostate cancer since its concentration in the blood serum tends to be proportional to the clinical stage of the disease — abbr. PSA

pros·tat·ic \prä-ˈsta-tik\ *adj* : of, relating to, or affecting the prostate gland

prostatic intraepithelial neoplasia *n* : the formation of atypical epithelial cells in the prostate gland that are believed to be early precursors of adenocarcinoma — abbr. PIN

prostatic urethra *n* : the part of the male urethra from the base of the prostate gland where the urethra begins as the outlet of the bladder to the point where it emerges from the apex of the prostate gland

prostatic utricle *n* : a small blind pouch that projects from the wall of the prostatic urethra into the prostate gland

pros·ta·tism \ˈpräs-tə-ˌti-zəm\ *n* : disease of the prostate gland; *esp* : a disorder resulting from obstruction of the bladder neck by an enlarged prostate gland

pros·ta·ti·tis \ˌpräs-tə-ˈtī-təs\ *n* : inflammation of the prostate gland

pros·the·sis \präs-ˈthē-səs, ˈpräs-thə-\ *n*, *pl* **-the·ses** \-ˌsēz\ : an artificial device to replace a missing part of the body ⟨a dental ∼⟩

pros·thet·ic \präs-ˈthe-tik\ *adj* **1** : of, relating to, or being a prosthesis ⟨a ∼ device⟩; *also* : of or relating to prosthetics ⟨∼ research⟩ **2** : of, relating to, or constituting a nonprotein group of a conjugated protein — **pros·thet·i·cal·ly** *adv*

prosthetic dentistry n : PROSTH-ODONTICS

pros·thet·ics \-tiks\ n sing or pl : the surgical and dental specialty concerned with the design, construction, and fitting of prostheses

prosthetic valve endocarditis n : endocarditis caused by or involving a surgically implanted prosthetic heart valve — abbr. PVE

pros·the·tist \'präs-thə-tist\ n : a specialist in prosthetics

pros·thi·on \'präs-thē-ˌän\ n : a point on the alveolar arch midway between the median upper incisor teeth

prosth·odon·tics \ˌpräs-thə-'dän-tiks\ n sing or pl : the dental specialty concerned with the making of artificial replacements for missing parts of the mouth and jaw — called also *prosthetic dentistry* — **prosth·odon·tic** \-tik\ adj

prosth·odon·tist \-'dän-tist\ n : a specialist in prosthodontics

Pro·stig·min \prō-'stig-mən\ trademark — used for a preparation of neostigmine

[1]**pros·trate** \'präs-ˌtrāt\ adj : completely overcome ⟨was ~ from the heat⟩

[2]**prostrate** vb **pros·trat·ed; pros·trat·ing** : to put into a state of extreme bodily exhaustion ⟨*prostrated* by fever⟩

pros·tra·tion \prä-'strā-shən\ n : complete physical or mental exhaustion — see HEAT EXHAUSTION

prot·ac·tin·i·um \ˌprō-ˌtak-'ti-nē-əm\ n : a shiny metallic radioelement — symbol *Pa;* see ELEMENT table

prot·amine \'prō-tə-ˌmēn\ n : any of various strongly basic proteins of relatively low molecular weight that are rich in arginine and are found associated esp. with DNA in place of histone in the sperm cells of various animals (as fish)

protamine zinc insulin n : a suspension of insulin and salts of protamine and zinc in a buffered aqueous solution that is used for subcutaneous injection and has a slow onset and long duration — abbr. PZI

prot·anom·a·ly \ˌprō-tə-'nä-mə-lē\ n, pl **-lies** : deficient color vision in which an abnormally large proportion of red is required to match the spectrum — compare DEUTERANOMALY, TRICHROMAT — **prot·anom·a·lous** \-ləs\ adj

pro·ta·nope \'prō-tə-ˌnōp\ n : an individual affected with protanopia

prot·an·opia \ˌprō-tə-'nō-pē-ə\ n : a dichromatism in which the spectrum is seen in tones of yellow and blue with confusion of red and green and reduced sensitivity to monochromatic lights from the red end of the spectrum

prote- or **proteo-** comb form : protein ⟨*proteo*lysis⟩

pro·te·ase \'prō-tē-ˌās, -ˌāz\ n : any of numerous enzymes that hydrolyze proteins and are classified according to the most prominent functional group (as serine or cysteine) at the active site — called also *proteinase*

protease inhibitor n : a substance that inhibits the action of a protease; *specif* : any of various drugs (as indinavir or saquinavir) that inhibit the action of HIV protease so that cleavage of viral proteins into mature infectious particles is prevented and that are used esp. in combination with other antiretroviral agents in the treatment of HIV infection

[1]**pro·tec·tive** \prə-'tek-tiv\ adj : serving to protect the body or one of its parts from disease or injury

[2]**protective** n : a protective agent (as a medicine or a dressing)

pro·tein \'prō-ˌtēn\ n, often attrib **1** : any of numerous naturally occurring extremely complex substances that consist of amino acid residues joined by peptide bonds, contain the elements carbon, hydrogen, nitrogen, oxygen, usu. sulfur, and occas. other elements (as phosphorus or iron), and include many essential biological compounds (as enzymes, hormones, or antibodies) **2** : the total nitrogenous material in plant or animal substances; *esp* : CRUDE PROTEIN

pro·tein·aceous \ˌprō-tə-'nā-shəs, -ˌtē-\ adj : of, relating to, resembling, or being protein

pro·tein·ase \'prō-tə-ˌnās, -ˌtē-, -ˌnāz\ n : PROTEASE

protein C n : a vitamin K-dependent proteolytic glycoprotein synthesized in the liver that circulates in the blood plasma in an inactive form and when activated forms a complex with protein S to cleave factors V and VIII and inhibit the formation of thrombin

protein kinase n : any of a class of allosteric enzymes that possess a catalytic subunit which transfers a phosphate from ATP to one or more amino acid residues in a protein's side chain resulting in a conformational change affecting protein function and that include many which are activated by the binding of a second messenger (as cyclic AMP)

protein kinase C n : any of a group of isoenzymes of protein kinase that modify the conformation and activity of various intracellular proteins by catalyzing the phosphorylation of specific serine or threonine amino acid residues — abbr. PKC

pro·tein·osis \ˌprō-ˌtē-'nō-səs\ n, pl **-o·ses** \-ˌsēz\ or **-o·sis·es** : the accumulation of abnormal amounts of protein in bodily tissues — see PULMONARY ALVEOLAR PROTEINOSIS

protein S n : a vitamin K-dependent glycoprotein synthesized in the liver that circulates in the blood plasma and in its free form functions as a cofactor to facilitate the action of activated protein C

pro·tein·uria \ˌprō-tə-'n(y)ur-ē-ə, -ˌtē-, -'nyur-\ *n* : the presence of excess protein in the urine — **pro·tein·uric** \-'nur-ik, -'nyur-\ *adj*

pro·teo·gly·can \ˌprō-tē-ə-'glī-ˌkan\ *n* : any of a class of glycoproteins of high molecular weight that are found in the extracellular matrix of connective tissue

pro·teo·lip·id \-'li-pəd\ *n* : any of a class of proteins that have a high lipid content and are soluble in lipids and insoluble in water

pro·te·ol·y·sis \ˌprō-tē-'ä-lə-səs\ *n, pl* **-y·ses** \-ˌsēz\ : the hydrolysis of proteins or peptides with formation of simpler and soluble products (as in digestion) — **pro·teo·lyt·ic** \ˌprō-tē-ə-'li-tik\ *adj* — **pro·teo·lyt·i·cal·ly** *adv*

pro·te·ome \'prō-tē-ˌōm\ *n* : the complement of proteins expressed in a cell, tissue, or organism by a genome

pro·te·o·mics \ˌprō-tē-'ō-miks\ *n* : a branch of biotechnology concerned with applying the techniques of molecular biology, biochemistry, and genetics to analyzing the structure, function, and interactions of the proteins produced by the genes of a particular cell, tissue, or organism, with organizing the information in databases, and with applications of the data — compare GENOMICS — **pro·te·o·mic** \-mik\ *adj*

pro·te·us \'prō-tē-əs\ *n* **1** *cap* : a genus of aerobic usu. motile enterobacteria that are often found in decaying organic matter and include a common causative agent (*P. mirabilis*) of urinary tract infections **2** *pl* **-tei** \-ˌī\ : any bacterium of the genus *Proteus*

pro·throm·bin \prō-'thräm-bən\ *n* : a plasma protein produced in the liver in the presence of vitamin K and converted into thrombin by the action of various activators (as thromboplastin) in the clotting of blood — **pro·throm·bic** \-bik\ *adj*

prothrombin time *n* : the time required for a particular specimen of prothrombin to induce blood-plasma clotting under standardized conditions in comparison with a time of between 11.5 and 12 seconds for normal human blood

pro·ti·re·lin \prō-'tī-rə-lən\ *n* : THYROTROPIN-RELEASING HORMONE

pro·tist \'prō-ˌtist\ *n* : any of a diverse taxonomic group and esp. a kingdom (Protista syn. Protoctista) of eukaryotic organisms that are unicellular and sometimes colonial or less often multicellular and that typically include the protozoans, most algae, and often some fungi (as slime molds) — **pro·tis·tan** \prō-'tis-tən\ *adj or n*

pro·to·col \'prō-tə-ˌkȯl, -ˌkäl\ *n* **1** : an official account of a proceeding; *esp* : the notes or records relating to a case, an experiment, or an autopsy **2** : a detailed plan of a scientific or medical experiment, treatment, or procedure

pro·to·di·as·to·le \ˌprō-tō-dī-'as-tə-lē\ *n* **1** : the period just before aortic valve closure **2** : the period just after aortic valve closure — **pro·to·di·a·stol·ic** \-ˌdī-ə-'stä-lik\ *adj*

pro·ton \'prō-ˌtän\ *n* : an elementary particle that is identical with the nucleus of the hydrogen atom, that along with neutrons is a constituent of all other atomic nuclei, that carries a positive charge numerically equal to the charge of an electron, and that has a mass of $1.673{\times}10^{-24}$ gram — **pro·ton·ic** \prō-'tä-nik\ *adj*

Pro·to·nix \'prō-tə-ˌniks\ *trademark* — used for a preparation of the sodium salt of pantoprazole

proton pump *n* : a molecular mechanism that transports hydrogen ions across cell membranes

proton pump inhibitor *n* : any of a group of drugs (as omeprazole) that inhibit the activity of proton pumps and are used to inhibit gastric acid secretion in the treatment of ulcers and gastroesophageal reflux disease — abbr. *PPI*

pro·to–on·co·gene \ˌprō-tō-'än-kə-ˌjēn\ *n* : a gene having the potential for change into an active oncogene

Pro·to·pam \'prō-tə-ˌpam\ *trademark* — used for a preparation of pralidoxime

pro·to·path·ic \ˌprō-tə-'pa-thik\ *adj* : of, relating to, being, or mediating cutaneous sensory reception that is responsive only to rather gross stimuli — compare EPICRITIC

pro·to·plasm \'prō-tə-ˌpla-zəm\ *n* **1** : the organized colloidal complex of organic and inorganic substances (as proteins and water) that constitutes esp. the living nucleus, cytoplasm, and mitochondria of the cell **2** : CYTOPLASM — **pro·to·plas·mic** \ˌprō-tə-'plaz-mik\ *adj*

pro·to·plast \'prō-tə-ˌplast\ *n* : the nucleus, cytoplasm, and plasma membrane of a cell as distinguished from inert walls and inclusions

pro·to·por·phyr·ia \ˌprō-tō-pȯr-'fir-ē-ə\ *n* : the presence of protoporphyrin in the blood — see ERYTHROPOIETIC PROTOPORPHYRIA

pro·to·por·phy·rin \ˌprō-tō-'pȯr-fə-rən\ *n* : a purple porphyrin acid $C_{34}H_{34}N_4O_4$ obtained from hemin or heme by removal of bound iron

Pro·to·stron·gy·lus \-'strän-jə-ləs\ *n* : a genus of lungworms (family Metastrongylidae) including one (*P. rufescens*) parasitic esp. in sheep and goats

Pro·to·the·ca \ˌprō-tə-'thē-kə\ *n* : a genus of unicellular algae including two (*P. zopfii* and *P. wickerhamii*) that cause mastitis in cows and sometimes localized infection in humans

pro·to·the·co·sis \-thē-'kō-səs\ *n, pl* **-co·ses** \-ˌsēz\ : an infection produced by an alga of the genus *Prototheca*

protozoa *pl of* PROTOZOON

pro·to·zo·a·ci·dal \ˌprō-tə-ˌzō-ə-ˈsīd-ə̇l\ *adj* : destroying protozoans

pro·to·zo·al \-ˈzō-əl\ *adj* : of or relating to protozoans

pro·to·zo·an \-ˈzō-ən\ *n* : any of a phylum or subkingdom (Protozoa) of chiefly motile unicellular protists (as amoebas, trypanosomes, sporozoans, and paramecia) that are represented in almost every kind of habitat and include some pathogenic parasites of humans and domestic animals — **protozoan** *adj*

pro·to·zo·ol·o·gy \-zō-ˈä-lə-jē\ *n, pl* **-gies** : a branch of zoology dealing with protozoans — **pro·to·zo·ol·o·gist** \-jist\ *n*

pro·to·zo·on \ˌprō-tə-ˈzō-ˌän\ *n, pl* **pro·to·zoa** : PROTOZOAN

pro·tract \prō-ˈtrakt\ *vb* : to extend forward or outward — compare RETRACT

pro·trac·tion \-ˈtrak-shən\ *n* **1** : the act of moving an anatomical part forward **2** : the state of being protracted; *esp* : protrusion of the jaws

pro·trip·ty·line \prō-ˈtrip-tə-ˌlēn\ *n* : a tricyclic antidepressant drug $C_{19}H_{21}N$ — see VIVACTIL

pro·trude \prō-ˈtrüd\ *vb* **pro·trud·ed**; **pro·trud·ing** : to project or cause to project : jut out — **pro·tru·sion** \prō-ˈtrü-zhən\ *n*

pro·tru·sive \-ˈtrü-siv, -ziv\ *adj* **1** : thrusting forward **2** : PROTUBERANT

pro·tu·ber·ance \prō-ˈtü-bə-rəns, -ˈtyü-\ *n* **1** : something that is protuberant ⟨a bony ∼⟩ **2** : the quality or state of being protuberant

protuberans — see DERMATOFIBROSARCOMA PROTUBERANS

pro·tu·ber·ant \-rənt\ *adj* : bulging beyond the surrounding or adjacent surface ⟨a ∼ joint⟩ ⟨∼ eyes⟩

proud flesh *n* : an excessive growth of granulation tissue (as in an ulcer)

pro·ven·tric·u·lus \ˌprō-ven-ˈtri-kyə-ləs\ *n, pl* **-li** \-ˌlī, -ˌlē\ : the glandular or true stomach of a bird that is situated between the crop and gizzard

Pro·ven·til \prō-ˈven-til\ *trademark* — used for a preparation of the sulfate of albuterol

pro·vi·rus \-ˈvī-rəs\ *n* : a form of a virus that is integrated into the genetic material of a host cell and by replicating with it can be transmitted from one cell generation to the next without causing lysis — **pro·vi·ral** \prō-ˈvī-rəl\ *adj*

pro·vi·ta·min \-ˈvī-tə-mən\ *n* : a precursor of a vitamin convertible into the vitamin in an organism

provitamin A *n* : a provitamin of vitamin A; *esp* : CAROTENE

Pro·vo·cho·line \ˌprō-və-ˈkō-ˌlēn\ *trademark* — used for a preparation of the chloride of methacholine

pro·voke \prə-ˈvōk\ *vb* **pro·voked**; **pro·vok·ing** : to call forth or induce (a physical reaction) — **prov·o·ca·tion** \ˌprä-və-ˈkā-shən\ *n* — **pro·voc·a·tive** \prə-ˈvä-kə-tiv\ *adj*

prox·e·mics \präk-ˈsē-miks\ *n sing or pl* : the study of the nature, degree, and effect of the spatial separation individuals naturally maintain (as in various social and interpersonal situations) and of how this separation relates to environmental and cultural factors — **prox·e·mic** \-mik\ *adj*

prox·i·mad \ˈpräk-sə-ˌmad\ *adv* : PROXIMALLY

prox·i·mal \ˈpräk-sə-məl\ *adj* **1 a** : situated next to or near the point of attachment or origin or a central point; *esp* : located toward the center of the body ⟨the ∼ end of a bone⟩ — compare DISTAL 1a **b** : of, relating to, or being the mesial and distal surfaces of a tooth **2** : sensory rather than physical or social ⟨∼ stimuli⟩ — compare DISTAL 2 — **prox·i·mal·ly** *adv*

proximal convoluted tubule *n* : the convoluted portion of the vertebrate nephron that lies between Bowman's capsule and the loop of Henle and functions esp. in the resorption of sugar, sodium and chloride ions, and water from the glomerular filtrate — called also *proximal tubule*

proximal radioulnar joint *n* : a pivot joint between the upper end of the radius and the ring formed by the radial notch of the ulna and its annular ligament that permits rotation of the proximal head of the radius

proximal tubule *n* : PROXIMAL CONVOLUTED TUBULE

prox·i·mate cause \ˈpräk-sə-mət-\ *n* : a cause that directly or with no intervening agency produces an effect

Pro·zac \ˈprō-ˌzak\ *trademark* — used for a preparation of the hydrochloride of fluoxetine

PrP *abbr* prion protein

pru·rig·i·nous \prü-ˈri-jə-nəs\ *adj* : resembling, caused by, affected with, or being prurigo ⟨∼ dermatosis⟩

pru·ri·go \prü-ˈrī-(ˌ)gō\ *n* : a chronic inflammatory skin disease marked by a general eruption of small itching papules

pru·rit·ic \prü-ˈri-tik\ *adj* : of, relating to, or marked by itching

pru·ri·tus \prü-ˈrī-təs\ *n* : localized or generalized itching due to irritation of sensory nerve endings : ITCH

pruritus ani \-ˈā-ˌnī\ *n* : pruritus of the anal region

pruritus vul·vae \-ˈvəl-vē\ *n* : pruritus of the vulva

Prus·sian blue \ˈprə-shən-ˈblü\ *n* : a dark blue iron-containing dye $Fe_4[Fe(CN)_6]_3 \cdot xH_2O$ used as a test for ferric iron

prus·sic acid \ˈprə-sik-\ *n* : HYDROCYANIC ACID

PSA *abbr* prostate-specific antigen

psal·te·ri·um \sol-'tir-ē-əm\ n, pl **-ria** \-ē-ə\ **1** : OMASUM **2** : HIPPOCAMPAL COMMISSURE

psam·mo·ma \sa-'mō-mə\ n, pl **-mas** or **-ma·ta** \-mə-tə\ : a hard fibrous tumor of the meninges of the brain and spinal cord containing calcareous matter — **psam·mo·ma·tous** \sa-'mō-mə-təs, -'mä-\ adj

pseud- or **pseudo-** comb form : false : spurious ⟨pseudarthrosis⟩

pseud·ar·thro·sis \,süd-är-'thrō-səs\ also **pseu·do·ar·thro·sis** \,sü-dō-\ n, pl **-thro·ses** \-'thrō-,sēz\ : an abnormal union formed by fibrous tissue between parts of a bone that has fractured usu. spontaneously due to congenital weakness — called also false joint

pseu·do·an·eu·rysm \,sü-dō-'an-yə-,ri-zəm\ n : a vascular abnormality (as a bulging of the aorta) that resembles an aneurysm in radiography

pseu·do·bul·bar \-'bəl-bər\ adj : simulating that (as bulbar paralysis) which is caused by lesions of the medulla oblongata ⟨∼ paralysis⟩

pseu·do·cho·lin·es·ter·ase \-,kō-lə-'nes-tə-,rās, -,rāz\ n : CHOLINESTERASE 2

pseu·do·cow·pox \-'kau̇-,päks\ n : MILKER'S NODULES

pseu·do·cy·e·sis \-sī-'ē-səs\ n, pl **-e·ses** \-,sēz\ : a psychosomatic state that occurs without conception and is marked by some of the physical symptoms (as cessation of menses, enlargement of the abdomen, and apparent fetal movements) and changes in hormonal balance of pregnancy

pseu·do·cyst \'sü-dō-,sist\ n : a cluster of toxoplasmas in an enucleate host cell

pseu·do·de·men·tia \,sü-dō-di-'men-chə\ n : a condition of extreme apathy which outwardly resembles dementia but is not the result of actual mental deterioration

pseu·do·ephed·rine \-i-'fe-drən\ n : an alkaloid $C_{10}H_{15}NO$ that is isomeric with ephedrine and is used chiefly in the form of its hydrochloride $C_{10}H_{15}NO·HCl$ or sulfate $(C_{10}H_{15}NO)_2·H_2SO_4$ esp. to relieve nasal congestion

pseu·do·gout \-'gaut\ n : an arthritic condition which resembles gout but is characterized by the deposition of crystalline salts other than urates in and around the joints

pseu·do·her·maph·ro·dite \-(,)hər-'ma-frə-,dīt\ n : an individual exhibiting pseudohermaphroditism — **pseu·do·her·maph·ro·dit·ic** \-(,)hər-,ma-frə-'di-tik\ adj

pseu·do·her·maph·ro·dit·ism \-rə-,dī-,ti-zəm\ n : the condition of having the gonads of one sex and the external genitalia and other sex organs so variably developed that the sex of the individual is uncertain

pseu·do·hy·per·ten·sion \-,hī-pər-

'ten-chən\ n : a condition esp. of some elderly, diabetic, and uremic individuals in which an erroneously high blood pressure reading is given by sphygmomanometry usu. due to loss of flexibility of the arterial walls

pseu·do·hy·per·tro·phic \,sü-dō-,hī-pər-'trō-fik\ adj : falsely hypertrophic; specif : being a form of muscular dystrophy in which the muscles become swollen with deposits of fat and fibrous tissue — **pseu·do·hy·per·tro·phy** \-hī-'pər-trə-fē\ n

pseu·do·hy·po·para·thy·roid·ism \-,hī-pō-,par-ə-'thī-,rȯi-,di-zəm\ n : a usu. inherited disorder that clinically resembles hypoparathyroidism but results from the body's inability to respond normally to parathyroid hormone rather than from a deficiency of the hormone itself

pseu·do·mem·brane \,sü-dō-'mem-,brān\ n : FALSE MEMBRANE

pseu·do·mem·bra·nous \-'mem-brə-nəs\ adj : characterized by the presence or formation of a false membrane ⟨∼ colitis⟩

pseu·do·mo·nad \-'mō-,nad, -nəd\ n : any bacterium of the genus Pseudomonas

pseu·do·mo·nal \-'mō-nəl\ adj : of, relating to, or caused by bacteria of the genus Pseudomonas ⟨∼ infection⟩

pseu·do·mo·nas \,sü-dō-'mō-nəs, sü-'dä-mə-nəs\ n **1** cap : a genus of gram-negative rod-shaped motile bacteria (family Pseudomonadaceae) including some that are saprophytes or plant or animal pathogens — see BURKHOLDERIA **2** pl **pseu·do·mo·na·des** \,sü-dō-'mō-nə-,dēz, -'mä-\ : PSEUDOMONAD

pseu·do·neu·rot·ic \-nu̇-'rä-tik, -nyu̇-\ adj : having or characterized by neurotic symptoms which mask an underlying psychosis ⟨∼ schizophrenia⟩

pseu·do·pa·ral·y·sis \-pə-'ra-lə-səs\ n, pl **-y·ses** \-,sēz\ : apparent lack or loss of muscular power (as that produced by pain) that is not accompanied by true paralysis

pseu·do·par·kin·son·ism \-'pär-kən-sə-,ni-zəm\ n : a condition (as one induced by a drug) characterized by symptoms like those of parkinsonism

pseu·do·phyl·lid·ean \,sü-dō-fi-'li-dē-ən\ n : any of an order (Pseudophyllidea) of tapeworms (as the fish tapeworm of humans) including numerous parasites of fish-eating vertebrates — **pseudophyllidean** adj

pseu·do·pod \'sü-də-,päd\ n **1** : PSEUDOPODIUM 2 **a** : a slender extension from the edge of a wheal at the site of injection of an allergen **b** : one of the slender processes of some tumor cells extending out from the main mass of a tumor

pseu·do·po·di·um \,sü-də-'pō-dē-əm\ n, pl **-dia** \-dē-ə\ : a temporary protrusion or retractile process of the cytoplasm of a cell (as an amoeba or a white blood cell) that functions esp. as an organ of locomotion or in taking up food or other particulate matter

pseu·do·pol·yp \'sü-dō-ˌpä-ləp\ n : a projecting mass of hypertrophied mucous membrane (as in the colon) resulting from local inflammation

pseu·do·preg·nan·cy \ˌsü-dō-'preg-nən-sē\ n, pl **-cies** : a condition which resembles pregnancy: as **a** : PSEUDOCYESIS **b** : an anestrous state resembling pregnancy that occurs in various mammals usu. after an infertile copulation — **pseu·do·preg·nant** \-nənt\ adj

pseu·do·ra·bies \-ˈrā-bēz\ n : an acute febrile virus disease of domestic animals (as cattle and swine) that is caused by a herpesvirus of the genus *Varicellovirus* (species *Suid herpesvirus 1*) and is marked by cutaneous irritation and intense itching followed by encephalomyelitis and pharyngeal paralysis and commonly terminating in death within 48 hours — called also *mad itch*

pseu·do·sar·co·ma·tous \ˌsü-dō-sär-ˈkō-mə-təs\ adj : resembling but not being a true sarcoma ⟨a ~ polyp⟩

pseu·do·strat·i·fied \-ˈstra-tə-ˌfīd\ adj : of, relating to, or being an epithelium consisting of closely packed cells which appear to be arranged in layers but all of which are in fact attached to the basement membrane — **pseu·do·strat·i·fi·ca·tion** \-ˌstra-tə-fə-ˈkā-shən\ n

pseu·do·tu·ber·cle \-ˈtü-bər-kəl, -ˈtyü-\ n : a nodule or granuloma resembling a tubercle of tuberculosis but due to other causes

pseu·do·tu·ber·cu·lo·sis \-ˌtü-ˌbər-kyə-ˈlō-səs, -tyü-\ n, pl **-lo·ses** \-ˌsēz\ **1** : any of several diseases that are characterized by the formation of granulomas resembling tubercular nodules and are caused by a bacterium (as *Yersinia pseudotuberculosis*) other than the tubercle bacillus **2** : CASEOUS LYMPHADENITIS

pseu·do·tu·mor \-ˈtü-mər, -ˈtyü-\ n : an abnormality (as a temporary swelling) that resembles a tumor — **pseu·do·tu·mor·al** \-mə-rəl\ adj

pseudotumor cer·e·bri \-ˈser-ə-ˌbrī\ n : an abnormal condition that is characterized by increased intracranial pressure, headache, and papilledema without any demonstrable intracranial lesion and that tends to occur in overweight women from 20 to 50 years of age — called also *benign intracranial hypertension*

pseu·do·uri·dine \-ˈyur-ə-ˌdēn\ n : a nucleoside $C_9H_{12}O_6N_2$ that is a uracil derivative incorporated as a structural component into transfer RNA

pseu·do·xan·tho·ma elas·ti·cum \ˌsü-dō-zan-ˈthō-mə-i-ˈlas-ti-kəm\ n : a chronic degenerative disease of elastic tissues that is marked by the occurrence of small yellowish papules and plaques on areas of abnormally loose skin

¹psi \ˈsī\ adj : relating to, concerned with, or being parapsychological psychic events or powers

²psi n : psi events or phenomena

psi·lo·cin \ˈsī-lə-sən\ n : a hallucinogenic tertiary amine $C_{12}H_{16}N_2O$ obtained from a basidiomycetous fungus (*Psilocybe mexicana*)

psi·lo·cy·bin \ˌsī-lə-ˈsī-bən\ n : a hallucinogenic indole $C_{12}H_{17}N_2O_4P$ obtained from a basidiomycetous fungus (*Psilocybe mexicana* or *P. cubensis* syn. *Stropharia cubensis*)

psit·ta·co·sis \ˌsi-tə-ˈkō-səs\ n, pl **-co·ses** \-ˌsēz\ : an infectious disease of birds caused by a bacterium of the genus *Chlamydia* (*C. psittaci*), marked by diarrhea and wasting, and transmissible to humans in whom it usu. occurs as an atypical pneumonia accompanied by high fever — called also *parrot fever*; compare ORNITHOSIS — **psit·ta·co·tic** \-ˈkä-tik, -ˈkō-\ adj

pso·as \ˈsō-əs\ n, pl **pso·ai** \ˈsō-ˌī\ or **pso·ae** \-ˌē\ : either of two internal muscles of the loin: **a** : PSOAS MAJOR **b** : PSOAS MINOR

psoas major n : the larger of the two psoas muscles that arises from the anterolateral surfaces of the lumbar vertebrae, passes beneath the inguinal ligament to insert with the iliacus into the lesser trochanter of the femur, and serves esp. to flex the thigh

psoas minor n : the smaller of the two psoas muscles that arises from the last dorsal and first lumbar vertebrae and inserts into the brim of the pelvis, that functions to flex the trunk and the lumbar spinal column, and that is often absent

psoas muscle n : PSOAS

pso·ra·len \ˈsōr-ə-lən\ n : a substance $C_{11}H_6O_3$ found in some plants that photosensitizes mammalian skin and is used in conjunction with ultraviolet light to treat psoriasis; also : any of various derivatives of psoralen having similar properties — see PUVA

pso·ri·a·si·form \sə-ˈrī-ə-si-ˌfórm\ adj : resembling psoriasis or a psoriatic lesion

pso·ri·a·sis \sə-ˈrī-ə-səs\ n, pl **-a·ses** \-ˌsēz\ : a chronic skin disease characterized by circumscribed red patches covered with white scales — **pso·ri·at·ic** \ˌsōr-ē-ˈa-tik\ adj

psoriatic arthritis n : a severe form of arthritis accompanied by inflammation, psoriasis of the skin or nails, and a negative test for rheumatoid factor — called also *psoriatic arthropathy*

Pso·rop·tes \sō-ˈräp-(ˌ)tēz\ n : a genus of mites (family Psoroptidae) living on and irritating the skin of various mammals and resulting in the development of inflammatory skin diseases (as mange)

pso·rop·tic \sə-'räp-tik\ *adj* : of, relating to, caused by, or being mites of the genus *Psoroptes* ⟨~ mange⟩

PSRO *abbr* professional standards review organization

PSVT *abbr* paroxysmal supraventricular tachycardia

psych *abbr* psychology

psych- or **psycho-** *comb form* **1** : mind : mental processes and activities ⟨*psycho*dynamic⟩ ⟨*psycho*logy⟩ **2** : psychological methods ⟨*psycho*therapy⟩ **3** : brain ⟨*psycho*surgery⟩ **4** : mental and ⟨*psycho*somatic⟩

psych·as·the·nia \,sī-kəs-'thē-nē-ə\ *n* : a neurotic state characterized esp. by phobias, obsessions, or compulsions that one knows are irrational

psy·che \'sī-(,)kē\ *n* : the specialized cognitive, conative, and affective aspects of a psychosomatic unity : MIND; *specif* : the totality of the id, ego, and superego including both conscious and unconscious components

¹**psy·che·del·ic** \,si-kə-'de-lik\ *n* : a psychedelic drug (as LSD)

²**psychedelic** *adj* **1** : of, relating to, or being drugs (as LSD) capable of producing abnormal psychic effects (as hallucinations) and sometimes psychotic states **2** : produced by or associated with the use of psychedelic drugs — **psy·che·del·i·cal·ly** *adv*

psy·chi·at·ric \,sī-kē-'a-trik\ *adj* **1** : relating to or employed in psychiatry ⟨~ disorders⟩ **2** : engaged in the practice of psychiatry : dealing with cases of mental disorder ⟨~ nursing⟩ — **psy·chi·at·ri·cal·ly** *adv*

psy·chi·a·trist \sə-'kī-ə-trist, sī-\ *n* : a physician specializing in psychiatry

psy·chi·a·try \-trē\ *n, pl* **-tries** : a branch of medicine that deals with the science and practice of treating mental, emotional, or behavioral disorders esp. as originating in endogenous causes or resulting from faulty interpersonal relationships

¹**psy·chic** \'sī-kik\ *also* **psy·chi·cal** \-ki-kəl\ *adj* **1** : of or relating to the psyche : PSYCHOGENIC **2** : sensitive to nonphysical or supernatural forces and influences — **psy·chi·cal·ly** *adv*

²**psychic** *n* : a person apparently sensitive to nonphysical forces

psychic energizer *n* : ANTIDEPRESSANT

psychic energy *n* : the force driving and sustaining mental activity

psy·cho \'sī-(,)kō\ *n, pl* **psychos** : a deranged or psychopathic individual — not used technically — **psycho** *adj*

psycho- see PSYCH-

psy·cho·acous·tics \,sī-kō-ə-'kü-stiks\ *n* : a branch of science dealing with hearing, the sensations produced by sounds, and the problems of communication — **psy·cho·acous·tic** \-stik\ *adj*

psy·cho·ac·tive \,sī-kō-'ak-tiv\ *adj* : affecting the mind or behavior ⟨~ drugs⟩

psy·cho·anal·y·sis \,sī-kō-ə-'na-lə-səs\ *n, pl* **-y·ses** \-,sēz\ **1** : a method of analyzing psychic phenomena and treating mental and emotional disorders that is based on the concepts and theories of Sigmund Freud, that emphasizes the importance of free association and dream analysis, and that involves treatment sessions during which the patient is encouraged to talk freely about personal experiences and esp. about early childhood and dreams **2** : a body of empirical findings and a set of theories on human motivation, behavior, and personality development that developed esp. with the aid of psychoanalysis **3** : a school of psychology, psychiatry, and psychotherapy founded by Sigmund Freud and rooted in and applying psychoanalysis — **psy·cho·an·a·lyt·ic** \-,an-ᵊl-'i-tik\ *also* **psy·cho·an·a·lyt·i·cal** \-ti-kəl\ *adj* — **psy·cho·an·a·lyt·i·cal·ly** *adv* — **psy·cho·an·a·lyze** \-'an-ᵊl-,īz\ *vb*

psy·cho·an·a·lyst \-'an-ᵊl-ist\ *n* : one who practices or adheres to the principles of psychoanalysis; *specif* : a psychotherapist trained at an established psychoanalytic institute

psy·cho·bi·ol·o·gy \-bī-'ä-lə-jē\ *n, pl* **-gies** : the study of mental functioning and behavior in relation to other biological processes — **psy·cho·bi·o·log·i·cal** \-,bī-ə-'lä-ji-kəl\ *also* **psy·cho·bi·o·log·ic** \-jik\ *adj* — **psy·cho·bi·ol·o·gist** \-bī-'ä-lə-jist\ *n*

psy·cho·di·ag·nos·tics \-,dī-ig-'näs-tiks\ *n* : a branch of psychology concerned with the use of tests in the evaluation of personality and the determination of factors underlying human behavior — **psy·cho·di·ag·nos·tic** \-tik\ *adj*

psy·cho·dra·ma \,sī-kō-'drä-mə, -'dra-\ *n* : an extemporized dramatization designed to afford catharsis and social relearning for one or more of the participants from whose life history the plot is abstracted — **psy·cho·dra·mat·ic** \-kō-drə-'ma-tik\ *adj*

psy·cho·dy·nam·ics \,sī-kō-dī-'na-miks, -də-\ *n sing or pl* **1** : the psychology of mental or emotional forces or processes developing esp. in early childhood and their effects on behavior and mental states **2** : explanation or interpretation (as of behavior or mental states) in terms of mental or emotional forces or processes **3** : motivational forces acting esp. at the unconscious level — **psy·cho·dy·nam·ic** \-mik\ *adj* — **psy·cho·dy·nam·i·cal·ly** *adv*

psy·cho·ed·u·ca·tion·al \-,e-jə-'kā-shə-nəl\ *adj* : of or relating to the psychological aspects of education; *specif*

: relating to or used in the education of children with behavioral disorders or learning disabilities

psy·cho·gal·van·ic reflex \-gal-'va-nik-\ *n* : a momentary decrease in the apparent electrical resistance of the skin resulting from activity of the sweat glands in response to mental or emotional stimulation — called also *psychogalvanic reaction, psychogalvanic response*

psy·cho·gen·e·sis \ˌsī-kō-'je-nə-səs\ *n, pl* **-e·ses** \-ˌsēz\ **1** : the origin and development of mental functions, traits, or states **2** : development from mental as distinguished from physical origins

psy·cho·gen·ic \-'je-nik\ *adj* : originating in the mind or in mental or emotional conflict ⟨∼ impotence⟩ ⟨a ∼ disorder⟩ — **psy·cho·gen·i·cal·ly** *adv*

psy·cho·ge·ri·at·rics \-ˌjer-ē-'a-triks, -ˌji-\ *n* : a branch of psychiatry concerned with behavioral and emotional disorders among the elderly — **psy·cho·ge·ri·at·ric** \-trik\ *adj*

psy·cho·ki·ne·sis \-kə-'nē-səs, -kī-\ *n, pl* **-ne·ses** \-ˌsēz\ : movement of physical objects by the mind without use of physical means — called also *PK;* compare PRECOGNITION, TELEKINESIS — **psy·cho·ki·net·ic** \-'ne-tik\ *adj*

psy·cho·ki·net·ics \-kə-'ne-tiks, -kī-\ *n* : a branch of parapsychology that deals with psychokinesis

psychol *abbr* psychologist; psychology

psy·cho·lin·guis·tics \ˌsī-kō-liŋ-'gwis-tiks\ *n* : the study of the mental faculties involved in the perception, production, and acquisition of language — **psy·cho·lin·guist** \-'liŋ-gwist\ *n* — **psy·cho·lin·guis·tic** \-liŋ-'gwis-tik\ *adj*

psy·cho·log·i·cal \ˌsī-kə-'lä-ji-kəl\ *also* **psy·cho·log·ic** \-jik\ *adj* **1 a** : relating to, characteristic of, directed toward, influencing, arising in, or acting through the mind esp. in its affective or cognitive functions ⟨∼ phenomena⟩ **b** : directed toward the mind or toward the mind specif. in its conative function ⟨∼ warfare⟩ **2** : relating to, concerned with, deriving from, or used in psychology ⟨∼ tests⟩ ⟨a ∼ clinic⟩ — **psy·cho·log·i·cal·ly** *adv*

psy·chol·o·gist \sī-'kä-lə-jist\ *n* : a specialist in psychology

psy·chol·o·gize \-ˌjīz\ *vb* **-gized; -giz·ing** : to explain, interpret, or speculate in psychological terms

psy·chol·o·gy \-jē\ *n, pl* **-gies 1** : the science of mind and behavior **2 a** : the mental or behavioral characteristics typical of an individual or group or a particular form of behavior ⟨mob ∼⟩ ⟨the ∼ of arson⟩ **b** : the study of mind and behavior in relation to a particular field of knowledge or activity ⟨the ∼ of learning⟩ **3** : a

theory, system, or branch of psychology ⟨Freudian ∼⟩

psy·cho·met·ric \ˌsī-kə-'me-trik\ *adj* : of or relating to psychometrics — **psy·cho·met·ri·cal·ly** *adv*

psy·cho·me·tri·cian \-mə-'tri-shən\ *n* **1** : a person (as a clinical psychologist) who is skilled in the administration and interpretation of objective psychological tests **2** : a psychologist who devises, constructs, and standardizes psychometric tests

psy·cho·met·rics \-'me-triks\ *n* **1** : a branch of clinical or applied psychology dealing with the use and application of mental measurement **2** : the technique of mental measurements : the use of quantitative devices for assessing psychological trends

psy·chom·e·trist \sī-'kä-mə-trist\ *n* : PSYCHOMETRICIAN

psy·chom·e·try \sī-'kä-mə-trē\ *n, pl* **-tries** : PSYCHOMETRICS

psy·cho·mo·tor \ˌsī-kō-'mō-tər\ *adj* **1** : of or relating to motor action directly proceeding from mental activity **2** : of or relating to temporal lobe epilepsy ⟨∼ seizures⟩

psychomotor epilepsy *n* : TEMPORAL LOBE EPILEPSY

psy·cho·neu·ro·im·mu·nol·o·gy \-ˌnür-ō-ˌi-myü-'nä-lə-jē, -ˌnyür-\ *n* : a field of medicine that deals with the influence of emotional states (as stress) and nervous system activity on immune function esp. in relation to their role in affecting the onset and progression of disease — **psy·cho·neu·ro·im·mu·nol·o·gist** \-jəst\ *n*

psy·cho·neu·ro·sis \ˌsī-kō-nü-'rō-səs, -nyü-\ *n, pl* **-ro·ses** \-ˌsēz\ : NEUROSIS; *esp* : a neurosis based on emotional conflict in which an impulse that has been blocked seeks expression in a disguised response or symptom

¹**psy·cho·neu·rot·ic** \-'rä-tik\ *adj* : of, relating to, being, or affected with a psychoneurosis ⟨a ∼ disorder⟩

²**psychoneurotic** *n* : a psychoneurotic individual

psy·cho·path \'sī-kō-ˌpath\ *n* : a mentally ill or unstable individual; *esp* : one having an antisocial personality

psy·cho·path·ic \ˌsī-kō-'pa-thik\ *adj* : of, relating to, or characterized by psychopathy — **psy·cho·path·i·cal·ly** *adv*

psychopathic personality *n* **1** : ANTISOCIAL PERSONALITY **2** : an individual having an antisocial personality

psychopathic personality disorder *n* : ANTISOCIAL PERSONALITY DISORDER

psy·cho·pa·thol·o·gist \ˌsī-kō-pə-'thä-lə-jist, -pa-\ *n* : a specialist in psychopathology

psy·cho·pa·thol·o·gy \ˌsī-kō-pə-'thä-lə-jē, -pa-\ *n, pl* **-gies 1** : the study of psychological and behavioral dysfunction occurring in mental disorder or in social disorganization **2** : disordered psychological and behavioral functioning (as in mental disorder) — **psy·cho·patho·log·i·cal** \-ˌpa-thə-ˈlä-ji-kəl\ *also* **psy·cho·patho·log·ic** \-jik\ *adj* — **psy·cho·patho·log·i·cal·ly** *adv*

psy·chop·a·thy \sī-ˈkä-pə-thē\ *n, pl* **-thies 1** : mental disorder **2** : ANTI-SOCIAL PERSONALITY

psy·cho·phar·ma·ceu·ti·cal \ˌsī-kō-ˌfär-mə-ˈsü-ti-kəl\ *n* : a drug having an effect on the mental state of the user

psy·cho·phar·ma·col·o·gy \ˌsī-kō-ˌfär-mə-ˈkä-lə-jē\ *n, pl* **-gies** : the study of the effect of drugs on the mind and behavior — **psy·cho·phar·ma·co·log·i·cal** \-ˌfär-mə-kə-ˈlä-ji-kəl\ *also* **psy·cho·phar·ma·co·log·ic** \-ˈlä-jik\ *adj* — **psy·cho·phar·ma·col·o·gist** \-ˌfär-mə-ˈkä-lə-jist\ *n*

psy·cho·phys·ics \-ˈfi-ziks\ *n* : a branch of psychology concerned with the effect of physical processes (as intensity of stimulation) on mental processes and esp. sensations of an organism — **psy·cho·phys·i·cal** \ˌsī-kō-ˈfi-zi-kəl\ *adj* — **psy·cho·phys·i·cal·ly** *adv* — **psy·cho·phys·i·cist** \-ˈfi-zə-sist\ *n*

psy·cho·phys·i·o·log·i·cal \ˌsī-kō-ˌfi-zē-ə-ˈlä-ji-kəl\ *also* **psy·cho·phys·i·o·log·ic** \-jik\ *adj* **1** : of or relating to psychophysiology **2** : combining or involving mental and bodily processes

psy·cho·phys·i·ol·o·gy \-ˌfi-zē-ˈä-lə-jē\ *n, pl* **-gies** : a branch of psychology that deals with the effects of normal and pathological physiological processes on mental functioning — called also *physiological psychology* — **psy·cho·phys·i·ol·o·gist** \-jist\ *n*

psy·cho·sex·u·al \ˌsī-kō-ˈsek-shə-wəl\ *adj* **1** : of or relating to the mental, emotional, and behavioral aspects of sexual development **2** : of or relating to mental or emotional attitudes concerning sexual activity **3** : of or relating to the psychophysiology of sex

psy·cho·sis \sī-ˈkō-səs\ *n, pl* **-cho·ses** \-ˌsēz\ : a serious mental disorder (as schizophrenia) characterized by defective or lost contact with reality often with hallucinations or delusions

psy·cho·so·cial \ˌsī-kō-ˈsō-shəl\ *adj* **1** : involving both psychological and social aspects **2** : relating to social conditions relating to mental health ⟨~ medicine⟩ — **psy·cho·so·cial·ly** *adv*

psy·cho·so·mat·ic \ˌsī-kō-sə-ˈma-tik\ *adj* **1** : of, relating to, concerned with, or involving both mind and body **2 a** : of, relating to, involving, or concerned with bodily symptoms caused by mental or emotional disturbance **b** : exhibiting psychosomatic symptoms — **psy·cho·so·mat·i·cal·ly** *adv*

psy·cho·so·mat·ics \-tiks\ *n* : a branch of medical science dealing with interrelationships between the mind or emotions and the body and esp. with the relation of psychological conflict to somatic symptomatology

psy·cho·sur·geon \-ˈsər-jən\ *n* : a surgeon specializing in psychosurgery

psy·cho·sur·gery \-ˈsər-jə-rē\ *n, pl* **-ger·ies** : cerebral surgery employed in treating psychic symptoms — **psy·cho·sur·gi·cal** \-ˈsər-ji-kəl\ *adj*

psy·cho·syn·the·sis \ˌsī-kō-ˈsin-thə-səs\ *n, pl* **-the·ses** \-ˌsēz\ : a form of psychotherapy combining psychoanalytic techniques with meditation and exercise

psy·cho·ther·a·peu·tics \-tiks\ *n sing or pl* : PSYCHOTHERAPY

psy·cho·ther·a·pist \-ˈther-ə-pist\ *n* : an individual (as a psychiatrist, clinical psychologist, or psychiatric social worker) who is a practitioner of psychotherapy

psy·cho·ther·a·py \ˌsī-kō-ˈther-ə-pē\ *n, pl* **-pies 1** : treatment of mental or emotional disorder or maladjustment by psychological means esp. involving verbal communication (as in psychoanalysis, nondirective psychotherapy, reeducation, or hypnosis) **2** : any alteration in an individual's interpersonal environment, relationships, or life situation brought about esp. by a qualified therapist and intended to have the effect of alleviating symptoms of mental or emotional disturbance — **psy·cho·ther·a·peu·tic** \-ˌther-ə-ˈpyü-tik\ *adj* — **psy·cho·ther·a·peu·ti·cal·ly** *adv*

¹**psy·chot·ic** \sī-ˈkä-tik\ *adj* : of, relating to, marked by, or affected with psychosis — **psy·chot·i·cal·ly** *adv*

²**psychotic** *n* : a psychotic individual

¹**psy·choto·mi·met·ic** \sī-ˌkä-tō-mə-ˈme-tik, -mī-\ *adj* : of, relating to, involving, or inducing psychotic alteration of behavior and personality ⟨~ drugs⟩ — **psy·choto·mi·met·i·cal·ly** *adv*

²**psychotomimetic** *n* : a psychotomimetic agent (as a drug)

¹**psy·cho·tro·pic** \ˌsī-kə-ˈtrō-pik\ *adj* : acting on the mind ⟨~ drugs⟩

²**psychotropic** *n* : a psychotropic substance (as a drug)

psyl·li·um \ˈsi-lē-əm\ *n* **1** : FLEAWORT **2** : PSYLLIUM SEED

psyllium seed *n* : the seed of a fleawort (esp. *Plantago psyllium*) that has the property of swelling and becoming gelatinous when moist and is used as a mild laxative — called also *plantago seed, psyllium*; see METAMUCIL

pt *abbr* **1** patient **2** pint

Pt *symbol* platinum

PT *abbr* **1** physical therapist **2** physical therapy

PTA *abbr* plasma thromboplastin antecedent

PTC \ˌpē-(ˌ)tē-ˈsē\ *n* : PHENYLTHIO-CARBAMIDE

PTC *abbr* plasma thromboplastin component

PTCA \ˌpē-(ˌ)tē-(ˌ)sē-ˈā\ *n* : PERCUTA-NEOUS TRANSLUMINAL CORONARY ANGIOPLASTY

pter·o·yl·glu·tam·ic acid \ˌter-ō-il-glü-
ˈta-mik-\ *n* : FOLIC ACID — abbr. *PGA*

pteryg- *or* **pterygo-** *comb form* : pterygoid and ⟨*pterygo*maxillary⟩

pte·ryg·i·um \te-ˈri-jē-əm\ *n, pl* **-iums**
or **-ia** \-jē-ə\ **1** : a triangular fleshy
mass of thickened conjunctiva occurring usu. at the inner side of the eyeball, covering part of the cornea, and
causing a disturbance of vision **2** : a
forward growth of the cuticle over
the nail

¹pter·y·goid \ˈter-ə-ˌgȯid\ *adj* : of, relating to, being, or lying in the region of
the inferior part of the sphenoid bone

²pterygoid *n* : a pterygoid part (as a
pterygoid muscle or nerve)

pterygoid canal *n* : an anteroposterior
canal in the base of each medial
pterygoid plate of the sphenoid bone
that gives passage to the Vidian artery
and the Vidian nerve — called also
Vidian canal

pter·y·goi·de·us \ˌter-ə-ˈgȯi-dē-əs\ *n,
pl* **-dei** \-dē-ˌī\ : PTERYGOID MUSCLE

pterygoid fossa *n* : a V-shaped depression on the posterior part of each
pterygoid process that contains the
medial pterygoid muscle and the tensor veli palatini

pterygoid hamulus *n* : a hook-shaped
process forming the inferior extremity of each medial pterygoid plate of
the sphenoid bone and providing a
support around which the tendon of
the tensor veli palatini moves

pterygoid muscle *n* : either of two
muscles extending from the sphenoid
bone to the lower jaw: **a** : a muscle
that arises from the greater wing of
the sphenoid bone and from the outer
surface of the lateral pterygoid plate,
is inserted into the condyle of the
mandible and the articular disk of the
temporomandibular joint, and acts as
an antagonist of the masseter, temporalis, and medial pterygoid muscles
— called also *external pterygoid muscle, lateral pterygoid muscle* **b** : a muscle that arises from the inner surface
of the lateral pterygoid plate and
from the palatine and maxillary
bones, is inserted into the ramus and
the gonial angle, cooperates with the
masseter and temporalis in elevating
the lower jaw, and controls certain
lateral and rotary movements of the
jaw — called also *internal pterygoid
muscle, medial pterygoid muscle*

pterygoid nerve *n* : either of two
branches of the mandibular nerve: **a**
: one that is distributed to the lateral
pterygoid muscle — called also *lateral
pterygoid nerve* **b** : one that is distributed to the medial pterygoid muscle,
tensor tympani, and tensor veli palatini — called also *medial pterygoid
nerve*

pterygoid plate *n* : either of two vertical plates making up a pterygoid
process of the sphenoid bone: **a** : a
broad thin plate that forms the lateral

part of the pterygoid process and
gives attachment to the lateral pterygoid muscle on its lateral surface and
to the medial pterygoid muscle on its
medial surface — called also *lateral
pterygoid plate* **b** : a long narrow plate
that forms the medial part of the
pterygoid process and terminates in
the pterygoid hamulus — called also
medial pterygoid plate

pterygoid plexus *n* : a plexus of veins
draining the region of the pterygoid
muscles and emptying chiefly into the
facial vein by way of the deep facial
vein and into the maxillary vein

pterygoid process *n* : a process that
extends downward from each side of
the sphenoid bone, that consists of
the medial and lateral pterygoid
plates which are fused above anteriorly and separated below by a fissure
whose edges articulate with a process
of the palatine bone, and that contains on its posterior aspect the pterygoid and scaphoid fossae which give
attachment to muscles

pter·y·go·man·dib·u·lar raphe \ˌter-ə-
gō-man-ˈdi-byə-lər-\ *n* : a fibrous
seam that descends from the pterygoid hamulus of the medial pterygoid
plate to the mylohyoid line of the
mandible and that separates and gives
rise to the superior constrictor of the
pharynx and the buccinator

pter·y·go·max·il·lary \ˌter-ə-gō-ˈmak-
sə-ˌler-ē\ *adj* : of, relating to, or connecting the pterygoid process of the
sphenoid bone and the maxilla

pterygomaxillary fissure *n* : a vertical
gap between the lateral pterygoid
plate of the pterygoid process and the
maxilla that gives passage to part of
the maxillary artery and vein

pter·y·go·pal·a·tine fossa \ˌter-ə-gō-
ˈpa-lə-ˌtīn-\ *n* : a small triangular
space beneath the apex of the orbit
that contains among other structures
the pterygopalatine ganglion —
called also *pterygomaxillary fossa*

pterygopalatine ganglion *n* : an autonomic ganglion of the maxillary nerve
that is situated in the pterygopalatine
fossa and that receives preganglionic
parasympathetic fibers from the facial nerve and sends postganglionic
fibers to the nasal mucosa, palate,
pharynx, and orbit — called also
*Meckel's ganglion, sphenopalatine
ganglion*

PTFE *abbr* polytetrafluoroethylene

PTH *abbr* parathyroid hormone

Pthir·us \ˈthir-əs\ *n, syn of* PHTHIRUS

pto·maine \ˈtō-ˌmān, tō-ˈ\ *n* : any of
various organic bases formed by the
action of putrefactive bacteria on nitrogenous matter and including some
which are poisonous

ptomaine poisoning *n* : food poisoning caused by bacteria or bacterial
products — not used technically

pto·sis \ˈtō-səs\ *n, pl* **pto·ses** \-ˌsēz\ : a
sagging or prolapse of an organ or

part; *esp* : a drooping of the upper eyelid (as from paralysis of the oculomotor nerve) — **ptot·ic** \'tä-tik\ *adj*

PTSD *abbr* post-traumatic stress disorder

ptyal- *or* **ptyalo-** *comb form* : saliva ⟨*ptyal*ism⟩

pty·a·lin \'tī-ə-lən\ *n* : an amylase found in saliva that converts starch into sugar

pty·a·lism \-,li-zəm\ *n* : an excessive flow of saliva

-p·ty·sis \p-tə-səs\ *n comb form, pl* **-pty·ses** \p-tə-,sēz\ : spewing : expectoration ⟨hemo*ptysis*⟩

Pu *symbol* plutonium

pub·ar·che \'pyü-,bär-kē\ *n* : the beginning of puberty marked by the first growth of pubic hair

pu·ber·al \'pyü-bər-əl\ *adj* : PUBERTAL

pu·ber·tal \'pyü-bərt-ᵊl\ *adj* : of, relating to, or occurring in puberty

pu·ber·ty \'pyü-bər-tē\ *n, pl* **-ties** 1 : the condition of being or the period of becoming first capable of reproducing sexually marked by maturing of the genital organs, development of secondary sex characteristics, and in humans and the higher primates by the first occurrence of menstruation in the female 2 : the age at which puberty occurs being typically between 13 and 16 years in boys and 11 and 14 in girls

¹**pu·bes** \'pyü-(,)bēz\ *n, pl* **pubes** 1 : the hair that appears on the lower part of the hypogastric region at puberty — called also *pubic hair* 2 : the lower part of the hypogastric region : the pubic region

²**pubes** *pl of* PUBIS

pu·bes·cent \pyü-'bes-ᵊnt\ *adj* 1 : arriving at or having reached puberty 2 : of or relating to puberty

pu·bic \'pyü-bik\ *adj* : of, relating to, or situated in or near the region of the pubes or the pubis

pubic arch *n* : the notch formed by the inferior rami of the two conjoined pubic bones as they diverge from the midline

pubic bone *n* : PUBIS

pubic crest *n* : the border of a pubis between its pubic tubercle and the pubic symphysis

pubic hair *n* : PUBES 1

pubic louse *n* : CRAB LOUSE

pubic symphysis *n* : the rather rigid articulation of the two pubic bones in the midline of the lower anterior part of the abdomen — called also *symphysis pubis*

pubic tubercle *n* : a rounded eminence on the upper margin of each pubis near the pubic symphysis

pu·bis \'pyü-bəs\ *n, pl* **pu·bes** \-(,)bēz\ : the ventral and anterior of the three principal bones composing either half of the pelvis that in humans consists of two rami diverging posteriorly from the region of the pubic symphysis with the superior ramus ex-

tending to the acetabulum of which it forms a part and uniting there with the ilium and ischium and the inferior ramus extending below the obturator foramen where it unites with the ischium — called also *pubic bone*

public health *n* : the art and science dealing with the protection and improvement of community health by organized community effort and including preventive medicine and sanitary and social science

public health nurse *n* : VISITING NURSE

pu·bo·cap·su·lar ligament \,pyü-bō-'kap-sə-lər-\ *n* : PUBOFEMORAL LIGAMENT

pu·bo·coc·cy·geus \-käk-'si-jəs, -jē-əs\ *n, pl* **-cy·gei** \-'si-jē-,ī\ : the inferior subdivision of the levator ani that arises from the dorsal surface of the pubis, that inserts esp. into the coccyx, and that acts to help support the pelvic viscera, to draw the lower end of the rectum toward the pubis, and to constrict the rectum and in the female the vagina — compare ILIOCOCCYGEUS — **pu·bo·coc·cy·geal** \,pyü-bō-käk-'si-jəl, -jē-əl\ *adj*

pu·bo·fem·o·ral ligament \,pyü-bō-'fe-mə-rəl-\ *n* : a ligament of the hip joint that extends from the superior ramus of the pubis to the capsule of the hip joint near the neck of the femur and that acts to prevent excessive extension and abduction of the thigh

pu·bo·pros·tat·ic ligament \,pyü-bō-präs-'ta-tik-\ *n* : any of three strands of pelvic fascia in the male that correspond to the pubovesical ligament in the female and that support the prostate gland and indirectly the bladder

pu·bo·rec·ta·lis \,pyü-bō-rek-'tä-ləs\ *n* : a band of muscle fibers that is part of the pubococcygeus and acts to hold the rectum and anal canal at right angles to each other except during defecation

pu·bo·vag·i·na·lis \,pyü-bō-,va-jə-'nä-ləs\ *n* : the most medial and anterior fasciculi of the pubococcygeal part of the levator ani in the female that correspond to the levator prostatae in the male, pass along the sides of the vagina, insert into the coccyx, and act to constrict the vagina

pu·bo·ves·i·cal ligament \,pyü-bō-'ve-si-kəl-\ *n* : any of three strands of pelvic fascia in the female that correspond to the puboprostatic ligament in the male and that support the bladder

¹**pu·den·dal** \pyü-'dend-ᵊl\ *adj* : of, relating to, occurring in, or lying in the region of the external genital organs

²**pudendal** *n* : a pudendal anatomical part (as the pudendal nerve)

pudendal artery — see EXTERNAL PUDENDAL ARTERY, INTERNAL PUDENDAL ARTERY

pudendal nerve *n* : a nerve that arises from the second, third, and fourth sacral nerves and that supplies the external genitalia, the skin of the perineum, and the anal sphincters

pudendal vein — see INTERNAL PUDENDAL VEIN

pu·den·dum \pyù-'den-dəm\ *n, pl* **-da** \-də\ : the external genital organs of a human; *esp* : the external genitalia of a woman — usu. used in pl.

pu·er·ile \'pyü-ər-əl, -ī̇l\ *adj* **1** : marked by or suggesting childishness and immaturity **2** : being respiration that is like that of a child in being louder than normal ⟨∼ breathing⟩

pu·er·per·al \pyü-'ər-pə-rəl\ *adj* : of, relating to, or occurring during childbirth or the period immediately following ⟨∼ infection⟩

puerperal fever *n* : an abnormal condition that results from infection (as by streptococci) of the placental site following delivery or abortion and is characterized in mild form by fever of not over 100.4°F (38.0°C) but may progress to a localized endometritis or spread through the uterine wall and develop into peritonitis or pass into the bloodstream and produce sepsis — called also *childbed fever, puerperal sepsis*

pu·er·pe·ri·um \,pyü-ər-'pir-ē-əm\ *n, pl* **-ria** \-ē-ə\ : the period between childbirth and the return of the uterus to its normal size

PUFA \'pə-fə\ *n* : a polyunsaturated fatty acid

puff·er *n* : PUFFER FISH

puffer fish *n* : any of a family (Tetraodontidae) of chiefly tropical marine bony fishes which can distend themselves to a globular form and most of which are highly poisonous — called also *blowfish, globefish;* see FUGU

Pu·lex \'pyü-,leks\ *n* : a genus of fleas (family Pulicidae) that includes the most common flea (*P. irritans*) that regularly attacks human beings

¹pull \'pùl\ *vb* **1** : EXTRACT 1 **2** : to strain or stretch abnormally ⟨∼ a muscle⟩

²pull *n* : an injury resulting from abnormal straining or stretching esp. of a muscle — see GROIN PULL

pul·lo·rum disease \pə-'lōr-əm-\ *n* : a destructive typically diarrheic salmonellosis esp. of the domestic chicken caused by a bacterium of the genus *Salmonella* (*S. pullorum*) — called also *pullorum*

pulmon- *also* **pulmoni-** *or* **pulmono-** *comb form* : lung ⟨*pulmono*logist⟩

pulmonale, pulmonalia — see COR PULMONALE

pul·mo·nary \'pùl-mə-,ner-ē, 'pəl-\ *adj* : relating to, functioning like, associated with, or carried on by the lungs

pulmonary adenomatosis *n* : JAAGSIEKTE

pulmonary alveolar proteinosis *n* : a chronic disease of the lungs characterized by the filling of the alveoli with proteinaceous material and by the progressive loss of lung function

pulmonary artery *n* : an arterial trunk or either of its two main branches that carry venous blood to the lungs: **a** : a large arterial trunk that arises from the conus arteriosus of the right ventricle and branches into the right and left pulmonary arteries — called also *pulmonary trunk* **b** : a branch of the pulmonary trunk that passes to the right lung where it divides into branches — called also *right pulmonary artery* **c** : a branch of the pulmonary trunk that passes to the left lung where it divides into branches — called also *left pulmonary artery*

pulmonary capillary wedge pressure *n* : WEDGE PRESSURE — abbr. *PCWP*

pulmonary circulation *n* : the passage of venous blood from the right atrium of the heart through the right ventricle and pulmonary arteries to the lungs where it is oxygenated and its return via the pulmonary veins to enter the left auricle and participate in the systemic circulation

pulmonary edema *n* : abnormal accumulation of fluid in the lungs

pulmonary embolism *n* : embolism of a pulmonary artery or one of its branches that is produced by foreign matter and most often a blood clot originating in a vein of the leg or pelvis and that is marked by labored breathing, chest pain, fainting, rapid heart rate, cyanosis, shock, and sometimes death — abbr. *PE*

pulmonary ligament *n* : a supporting fold of pleura that extends from the lower part of the lung to the pericardium

pulmonary plexus *n* : either of two nerve plexuses associated with each lung that lie on the dorsal and ventral aspects of the bronchi of each lung

pulmonary stenosis *n* : abnormal narrowing of the orifice between the pulmonary artery and the right ventricle

pulmonary trunk *n* : PULMONARY ARTERY a

pulmonary valve *n* : a valve consisting of three semilunar cusps separating the pulmonary trunk from the right ventricle

pulmonary vein *n* : any of usu. four veins comprising two from each lung that return oxygenated blood from the lungs to the superior part of the left atrium

pulmonary wedge pressure *n* : WEDGE PRESSURE

pulmoni- *or* **pulmono-** — see PULMON-

pul·mon·ic \pùl-'mä-nik, ,pəl-\ *adj* : PULMONARY ⟨∼ lesions⟩

pulmonic stenosis *n* : PULMONARY STENOSIS

pul·mo·nol·o·gist \ˌpu̇l-mə-ˈnä-lə-jist, ˌpəl-\ *n* : a specialist in pulmonology

pul·mo·nol·o·gy \-jē\ *n, pl* **-gies** : a branch of medicine concerned with the anatomy, physiology, and pathology of the lungs

pulp \ˈpəlp\ *n* : a mass of soft tissue: as **a** : DENTAL PULP **b** : the characteristic somewhat spongy tissue of the spleen **c** : the fleshy portion of the fingertip — **pulp·al** \ˈpəl-pəl\ *adj* — **pulp·less** *adj*

pulp canal *n* : ROOT CANAL 1

pulp cavity *n* : the central cavity of a tooth containing the dental pulp and made up of the root canal and the pulp chamber

pulp chamber *n* : the part of the pulp cavity lying in the crown of a tooth

pulp·ec·to·my \ˌpəl-ˈpek-tə-mē\ *n, pl* **-mies** : the removal of the pulp of a tooth

pulp·i·tis \ˌpəl-ˈpī-təs\ *n, pl* **pulp·it·i·des** \-ˈpi-tə-ˌdēz\ : inflammation of the pulp of a tooth

pulposi, pulposus — see NUCLEUS PULPOSUS

pulp·ot·o·my \ˌpəl-ˈpä-tə-mē\ *n, pl* **-mies** : removal in a dental procedure of the coronal portion of the pulp of a tooth in such a manner that the pulp of the root remains intact and viable

pulp stone *n* : a lump of calcified tissue within the dental pulp — called also *denticle*

pulpy kidney \ˈpəl-pē-\ *n* : a destructive enterotoxemia of lambs caused by a bacterium of the genus *Clostridium* (*C. perfringens*) — called also *pulpy kidney disease*

pul·sate \ˈpəl-ˌsāt\ *vb* **pul·sat·ed; pul·sat·ing** : to exhibit a pulse or pulsation ⟨a *pulsating* artery⟩

pul·sa·tion \ˌpəl-ˈsā-shən\ *n* : rhythmic throbbing or vibrating (as of an artery); *also* : a single beat or throb — **pul·sa·tile** \ˈpəl-sət-ᵊl, -sə-ˌtīl\ *adj*

pulse \ˈpəls\ *n* **1 a** : a regularly recurrent wave of distension in arteries that results from the progress through an artery of blood injected into the arterial system at each contraction of the ventricles of the heart **b** : the palpable beat resulting from such pulse as detected in a superficial artery (as the radial artery); *also* : the number of such beats in a specified period of time (as one minute) ⟨a resting ∼ of 70⟩ **2** : PULSATION **3** : a dose of a substance esp. when applied over a short period of time ⟨∼s of intravenous methylprednisolone⟩ — **pulse** *vb* — **pulse·less** \ˈpəls-ləs\ *adj*

pulse–chase *adj* : involving the exposure of cells to a substrate bearing a radioactive label for a predetermined time followed by exposure to a high concentration of unlabeled substrate in order to stop uptake of the labeled substrate and follow its metabolic course

pulse–field gel electrophoresis *n* : gel electrophoresis that is used esp. to separate large fragments of DNA and that involves changing the direction of the electric current periodically in order to minimize overlap of the separated molecules due to diffusion — called also *pulsed-field electrophoresis*

pulsed light *n* : high intensity white light that is emitted in a series of flashes of brief duration (as 10 to 20 milliseconds in length) ⟨*pulsed light* therapy to treat rosacea⟩

pulse–la·bel \ˈpəls-ˌlā-bəl\ *vb* **-la·beled** *or* **-la·belled; -la·bel·ing** *or* **-la·bel·ling** : to cause a pulse of a radiolabeled atom or substance to become incorporated into (as a molecule or cell component) ⟨∼*ed* DNA⟩

pulseless disease *n* : TAKAYASU'S ARTERITIS

pulse oximeter *n* : a device that measures the oxygen saturation of arterial blood in a subject by utilizing a sensor attached typically to a finger, toe, or ear to determine the percentage of oxyhemoglobin in blood pulsating through a network of capillaries — **pulse oximetry** *n*

pulse pressure *n* : the pressure that is characteristic of the arterial pulse and represents the difference between diastolic and systolic pressures of the heart cycle

pulse rate *n* : the rate of the arterial pulse usu. observed at the wrist and stated in beats per minute

pul·sus al·ter·nans \ˈpəl-səs-ˈȯl-tər-ˌnanz\ *n* : alternation of strong and weak beats of the arterial pulse due to alternate strong and weak ventricular contractions

pulsus par·a·dox·us \-ˌpar-ə-ˈdäk-səs\ *n* : a pulse that weakens abnormally during inspiration and is symptomatic of various abnormalities (as pericarditis)

pulv *abbr* [Latin *pulvis*] powder — used in writing prescriptions

pul·vi·nar \ˌpəl-ˈvī-nər\ *n* : a rounded prominence on the back of the thalamus

Pul·vule \ˈpəl-ˌvyül\ *trademark* — used for a gelatin-based medicinal capsule

¹pump \ˈpəmp\ *n* **1** : a device that raises, transfers, or compresses fluids or that attenuates gases esp. by suction or pressure or both **2** : HEART **3** : an act or the process of pumping **4** : a mechanism by which atoms, ions, or molecules are transported across cell membranes — see PROTON PUMP, SODIUM PUMP

²pump *vb* **1** : to raise (as water) with a pump **2** : to draw fluid from with a pump **3** : to transport (as ions) against a concentration gradient by the expenditure of energy

punch–drunk \'pənch-ˌdrəŋk\ *adj*
: suffering from cerebral injury usu.
resulting from minute brain hemorrhages caused by repeated head blows
received in boxing and marked esp.
by mental confusion, incoordination,
and slurred speech

puncta *pl of* PUNCTUM

punctata — see KERATITIS PUNCTATA

punc·tate \'pəŋk-ˌtāt\ *adj* : characterized by dots or points ⟨∼ skin le-
sions⟩

punc·tum \'pəŋk-təm\ *n, pl* **punc·ta**
\-tə\ : a small area marked off from a
surrounding surface — see LACRIMAL
PUNCTUM

¹punc·ture \'pəŋk-chər\ *n* **1** : an act of
puncturing **2** : a hole, wound, or perforation made by puncturing

²puncture *vb* **punc·tured; punc·tur-
ing** : to pierce with or as if with a
pointed instrument or object

pu·pa \'pyü-pə\ *n, pl* **pu·pae** \-(ˌ)pē,
-ˌpī\ *or* **pupas** : an intermediate usu.
quiescent stage of an insect that occurs between the larva and the adult
in forms (as a moth or beetle) which
undergo complete metamorphosis
and that is characterized by internal
changes by which larval structures
are replaced by those typical of the
adult — **pu·pal** \'pyü-pəl\ *adj*

pu·pil \'pyü-pəl\ *n* : the contractile
usu. round aperture in the iris of the
eye — **pu·pil·lary** *also* **pu·pil·ary**
\'pyü-pə-ˌler-ē\ *adj*

pupillae — see SPHINCTER PUPILLAE

pupillary reflex *n* : the contraction of
the pupil in response to light entering
the eye

pupillo- *comb form* : pupil ⟨*pupillo*me-
ter⟩

pu·pil·log·ra·phy \ˌpyü-pə-'lä-grə-fē\
n, pl **-phies** : the measurement of the
reactions of the pupil

pu·pil·lom·e·ter \ˌpyü-pə-'lä-mə-tər\ *n*
: an instrument for measuring the diameter of the pupil of the eye — **pu·
pil·lom·e·try** \-mə-trē\ *n*

pur·ga·tion \ˌpər-'gā-shən\ *n* **1** : the
act of purging; *specif* : vigorous evacuation of the bowels (as from the action of a cathartic) **2** : administration
of or treatment with a purgative

¹pur·ga·tive \'pər-gə-tiv\ *adj* : purging
or tending to purge : CATHARTIC —
pur·ga·tive·ly *adv*

²purgative *n* : a purging medicine
: CATHARTIC

¹purge \'pərj\ *vb* **purged; purg·ing** : to
have or cause strong and usu. re-
peated emptying of the bowels

²purge *n* **1** : something that purges; *esp*
: PURGATIVE **2** : an act or instance of
purging

purified protein derivative *n* : a purified preparation of tuberculin used in
skin tests (as the Mantoux test) to detect tuberculous infection — *abbr.*
PPD

pu·rine \'pyu̇r-ˌēn\ *n* **1** : a crystalline
base $C_5H_4N_4$ that is the parent of

compounds of the uric-acid group **2**
: a derivative of purine; *esp* : a base (as
adenine or guanine) that is a constituent of DNA or RNA

purine base *n* : any of a group of crystalline bases comprising purine and
bases derived from it (as adenine)
some of which are components of nucleosides and nucleotides

Pur·kin·je cell \pər-'kin-jē-\ *n* : any of
numerous nerve cells that occupy the
middle layer of the cerebellar cortex
and are characterized by a large
globe-shaped body with massive dendrites directed outward and a single
slender axon directed inward —
called also *Purkinje neuron*

Pur·ky·ně, *or* **Purkinje** \'pùr-kin-ye,
-yä\ **Jan Evangelista (1787–1869),**
Bohemian physiologist.

Purkinje fiber *n* : any of the modified
cardiac muscle fibers with few nuclei,
granulated central cytoplasm, and
sparse peripheral striations that make
up Purkinje's network

Purkinje's network *n* : a network of
intracardiac conducting tissue made
up of syncytial Purkinje fibers that lie
in the myocardium and constitute the
bundle of His and other conducting
tracts which spread out from the
sinoatrial node — called also *Purkinje's system, Purkinje's tissue*

pu·ro·my·cin \ˌpyür-ə-'mīs-ᵊn\ *n* : an
antibiotic $C_{22}H_{29}N_7O_5$ that is obtained
from an actinomycete (*Streptomyces
alboniger*) and is a potent inhibitor of
protein synthesis

pur·pu·ra \'pər-pü-rə, -pyü-\ *n* : any of
several hemorrhagic states characterized by patches of purplish discoloration resulting from extravasation
of blood into the skin and mucous
membranes — see THROMBOCY-
TOPENIC PURPURA — **pur·pu·ric**
\ˌpər-'pyür-ik\ *adj*

purpura ful·mi·nans \-'fúl-mə-ˌnanz,
-'fòl-\ *n* : purpura of an often severe
progressive form esp. of children that
is characterized by widespread necrosis of the skin and that occurs chiefly
in conjunction with acute infection
(as by meningococci) esp. as a manifestation of disseminated intravascular coagulation and that in neonates is
typically associated with deficiency of
protein C or protein S

purpura hem·or·rhag·i·ca \-ˌhe-mə-
'ra-jə-kə\ *n* : THROMBOCYTOPENIC
PURPURA

purse–string suture *n* : a surgical suture passed as a running stitch in and
out along the edge of a circular
wound in such a way that when the
ends of the suture are drawn tight the
wound is closed like a purse

pu·ru·lence \'pyúr-ə-ləns, 'pyúr-yə-\ *n*
: the quality or state of being purulent; *also* : PUS

pu·ru·lent \-lənt\ *adj* **1** : containing,
consisting of, or being pus **2** : accompanied by suppuration

pus \'pəs\ *n* : thick opaque usu. yellowish white fluid matter formed by suppuration and composed of exudate containing white blood cells, tissue debris, and microorganisms — **pus·sy** \'pə-sē\ *adj*

pus·tu·lar \'pəs-chə-lər, 'pəs-tyə-\ *adj* 1 : of, relating to, or resembling pustules ⟨~ eruptions⟩ 2 : covered with pustules

pus·tule \'pəs-ˌchül, -ˌ(ˌ)tyül, -ˌ(ˌ)tül\ *n* 1 : a small circumscribed elevation of the skin containing pus and having an inflamed base 2 : a small often distinctively colored elevation or spot resembling a blister or pimple

pu·ta·men \pyü-'tā-mən\ *n, pl* **pu·tam·i·na** \-'ta-mə-nə\ : an outer reddish layer of gray matter in the lentiform nucleus

pu·tre·fac·tion \ˌpyü-trə-'fak-shən\ *n* 1 : the decomposition of organic matter; *esp* : the typically anaerobic splitting of proteins by bacteria and fungi with the formation of foul-smelling incompletely oxidized products 2 : the state of being putrefied — **pu·tre·fac·tive** \-tiv\ *adj* — **pu·tre·fy** \'pyü-trə-ˌfī\ *vb*

pu·tres·cine \pyü-'tre-ˌsēn\ *n* : a crystalline slightly poisonous ptomaine $C_4H_{12}N_2$ that is formed by decarboxylation of ornithine, occurs widely but in small amounts in living things, and is found esp. in putrid flesh

pu·trid \'pyü-trəd\ *adj* 1 : being in a state of putrefaction 2 : of, relating to, or characteristic of putrefaction

PUVA \ˌpē-ˌyü-ˌvē-'ā\ *n* [psoralen ultraviolet *A*] : photochemotherapy for psoriasis using psoralen and UVA

PVD *abbr* peripheral vascular disease

PVE *abbr* prosthetic valve endocarditis

PVP *abbr* polyvinylpyrrolidone

PWA \ˌpē-ˌdə-bəl-ˌyü-'ā\ *n* : a person affected with AIDS

P wave \'pē-ˌwāv\ *n* : a deflection in an electrocardiographic tracing that represents atrial activity of the heart — compare QRS COMPLEX, T WAVE

Px *abbr* 1 pneumothorax 2 prognosis

py- *or* **pyo-** *comb form* : pus ⟨*py*emia⟩

py·ae·mia *chiefly Brit var of* PYEMIA

py·ar·thro·sis \ˌpī- är-'thrō-səs\ *n, pl* **-thro·ses** \-ˌsēz\ : the formation or presence of pus within a joint

pycn- *or* **pycno-** — *see* PYKN-

pycnic, pycnosis *var of* PYKNIC, PYKNOSIS

pyc·no·dys·os·to·sis *or* **pyk·no·dys·os·to·sis** \ˌpik-nō-ˌdis-ä-'stō-səs\ *n, pl* **-to·ses** \-ˌsēz\ : a rare condition inherited as an autosomal recessive trait and characterized esp. by short stature, fragile bones, shortness of the fingers and toes, failure of the anterior fontanel to close properly, and a receding chin

pyel- *or* **pyelo-** *comb form* : renal pelvis ⟨*pyelo*graphy⟩

py·eli·tis \ˌpī-ə-'lī-təs\ *n* : inflammation of the lining of the renal pelvis

py·elo·gram \'pī-ə-lə-ˌgram\ *n* : a radiograph made by pyelography

py·elog·ra·phy \ˌpī-ə-'lä-grə-fē\ *n, pl* **-phies** : radiographic visualization of the renal pelvis after injection of a radiopaque substance through the ureter or into a vein — *see* RETROGRADE PYELOGRAPHY — **py·elo·graph·ic** \ˌpī-ə-lə-'gra-fik\ *adj*

py·elo·li·thot·o·my \ˌpī-ə-lō-li-'thä-tə-mē\ *n, pl* **-mies** : surgical incision of the renal pelvis of a kidney for removal of a kidney stone

py·elo·ne·phri·tis \ˌpī-ə-lō-ni-'frī-təs\ *n, pl* **-phrit·i·des** \-'fri-tə-ˌdēz\ : inflammation of both the parenchyma of a kidney and the lining of its renal pelvis esp. due to bacterial infection — **py·elo·ne·phrit·ic** \-'fri-tik\ *adj*

py·elo·plas·ty \'pī-ə-lə-ˌplas-tē\ *n, pl* **-ties** : plastic surgery of the renal pelvis of a kidney

py·emia \pī-'ē-mē-ə\ *n* : septicemia accompanied by multiple abscesses and secondary toxemic symptoms and caused by pus-forming microorganisms (as the bacterium *Staphylococcus aureus*) — **py·emic** \-mik\ *adj*

Py·emo·tes \ˌpī-ə-'mō-tēz\ *n* : a genus of mites that are usu. ectoparasites of insects that include one (*P. ventricosus*) which causes grain itch in humans

py·gop·a·gus \pī-'gä-pə-gəs\ *n, pl* **-gi** \-ˌgī, -ˌjī\ : a twin fetus joined in the sacral region

pykn- *or* **pykno-** *also* **pycn-** *or* **pycno-** *comb form* 1 : close : compact : dense : bulky ⟨*pykn*ic⟩ 2 : marked by short stature or shortness of digits ⟨*pycno*dysostosis⟩

¹pyk·nic *also* **pyc·nic** \'pik-nik\ *adj* : characterized by shortness of stature, broadness of girth, and powerful muscularity : ENDOMORPHIC 2

²pyknic *also* **pycnic** *n* : a person of pyknic build

pyknodysostosis *var of* PYCNODYSOSTOSIS

pyk·no·lep·sy \'pik-nə-ˌlep-sē\ *n, pl* **-sies** : a condition marked by epileptiform attacks resembling those of petit mal epilepsy

pyk·no·sis *also* **pyc·no·sis** \pik-'nō-səs\ *n, pl* **pyk·no·ses** *also* **pyc·no·ses** \-ˌsēz\ : a degenerative condition of a cell nucleus marked by clumping of the chromosomes, hyperchromatism, and shrinking of the nucleus — **pyk·not·ic** *also* **pyc·not·ic** \-'nä-tik\ *adj*

pyl- *or* **pyle-** *or* **pylo-** *comb form* : portal vein ⟨*pyle*phlebitis⟩

py·le·phle·bi·tis \ˌpī-lə-fli-'bī-təs\ *n, pl* **-bit·i·des** \-'bi-tə-ˌdēz\ : inflammation of the renal portal vein usu. secondary to intestinal disease and with suppuration

py·lon \'pī-ˌlän, -lən\ *n* : a simple temporary artificial leg

pylor- *or* **pyloro-** *comb form* : pylorus ⟨*pyloro*plasty⟩

py·lo·ric \pī-'lȯr-ik, pə-\ *adj* : of or relating to the pylorus; *also* : of, relating to, or situated in or near the posterior part of the stomach

pyloric glands *n pl* : the short coiled tubular glands of the mucous coat of the stomach occurring chiefly near the pyloric end

pyloric sphincter *n* : the circular fold of mucous membrane containing a ring of muscle fibers that closes the pylorus — called also *pyloric valve*

pyloric stenosis *n* : narrowing of the pyloric opening (as from congenital malformation)

py·lo·ro·my·ot·o·my \pī-lȯr-ō-mī-'ä-tə-mē, pə-lȯr-ə-\ *n, pl* **-mies** : surgical incision of the muscle fibers of the pyloric sphincter for relief of stenosis caused by muscular hypertrophy

py·lo·ro·plas·ty \pī-'lȯr-ə-plas-tē\ *n, pl* **-ties** : plastic surgery on the pylorus (as to enlarge a stricture)

py·lo·ro·spasm \pī-'lȯr-ə-spa-zəm\ *n* : spasm of the pyloric sphincter often marked by pain and vomiting

py·lo·rus \pī-'lȯr-əs, pə-\ *n, pl* **py·lo·ri** \-'lȯr-ī, -(ˌ)ē\ : the opening from the stomach into the intestine — see PYLORIC SPHINCTER

pyo- — see PY-

pyo·der·ma \ˌpī-ə-'dər-mə\ *n* : a bacterial skin inflammation marked by pus-filled lesions

pyoderma gan·gre·no·sum \-ˌgaŋ-gri-'nō-səm\ *n* : a chronic noninfectious condition that is marked by the formation of purplish nodules and pustules which tend to coalesce and form ulcers and that is associated with various underlying systemic or malignant diseases (as ulcerative colitis, rheumatoid arthritis, or leukemia)

pyo·gen·ic \ˌpī-ə-'je-nik\ *adj* : producing pus ⟨∼ bacteria⟩; *also* : marked by pus production ⟨∼ meningitis⟩

pyo·me·tra \ˌpī-ə-'mē-trə\ *n* : an accumulation of pus in the uterine cavity

pyo·myo·si·tis \ˌpī-ō-ˌmī-ə-'sī-təs\ *n* : infiltrative bacterial inflammation of muscles leading to the formation of abscesses

pyo·ne·phro·sis \-ni-'frō-səs\ *n, pl* **-phro·ses** \-ˌsēz\ : a collection of pus in the kidney

py·or·rhea \ˌpī-ə-'rē-ə\ *n* **1** : a discharge of pus **2** : an advanced form of chronic periodontis marked esp. by the discharge of pus from the alveoli — **py·or·rhe·ic** \-'rē-ik\ *adj*

py·or·rhoea chiefly Brit var of PYORRHEA

pyo·sal·pinx \ˌpī-ō-'sal-(ˌ)piŋks\ *n, pl* **-sal·pin·ges** \-sal-'pin-(ˌ)jēz\ : a collection of pus in an oviduct

pyo·tho·rax \-'thȯr-ˌaks\ *n, pl* **-tho·rax·es** or **-tho·ra·ces** \-'thȯr-ə-(ˌ)sēz\ : EMPYEMA

pyr- or **pyro-** *comb form* **1** : fire : heat ⟨*pyro*mania⟩ **2** : fever ⟨*pyro*gen⟩

pyr·a·mid \'pir-ə-ˌmid\ *n* **1** : a polyhedron having for its base a polygon and for faces triangles with a common vertex **2** : an anatomical structure resembling a pyramid: as **a** : RENAL PYRAMID **b** : either of two large bundles of motor fibers from the cerebral cortex that reach the medulla oblongata and are continuous with the corticospinal tracts of the spinal cord **c** : a conical projection making up the central part of the inferior vermis of the cerebellum — **py·ram·i·dal** \pə-'ra-məd-ʔl\ *adj*

pyramidal cell *n* : any of numerous large multipolar pyramid-shaped cells in the cerebral cortex

pyramidal decussation *n* : DECUSSATION OF PYRAMIDS

py·ram·i·da·lis \pə-ˌra-mə-'dā-ləs\ *n, pl* **-da·les** \-(ˌ)lēz\ or **-dalises** : a small triangular muscle of the lower front part of the abdomen that is situated in front of and in the same sheath with the rectus and functions to tense the linea alba

pyramidal tract *n* : CORTICOSPINAL TRACT

py·ram·i·dot·o·my \pə-ˌra-mə-'dä-tə-mē\ *n, pl* **-mies** : a surgical procedure in which a corticospinal tract is severed (as for relief of parkinsonism)

py·ra·mis \'pir-ə-məs\ *n, pl* **py·ram·i·des** \pə-'ra-mə-ˌdēz\ : PYRAMID 2

py·ran·tel \pə-'ran-ˌtel\ *n* : an anthelmintic drug used in the form of its pamoate $C_{11}H_{14}N_2S \cdot C_{23}H_{16}O_6$ or tartrate $C_{11}H_{14}N_2S \cdot C_4H_6O_6$

pyr·a·zin·amide \ˌpir-ə-'zi-nə-ˌmīd, -məd\ *n* : a tuberculostatic drug $C_5H_5N_3O$

py·re·thrin \pī-'rē-thrən, -'re-\ *n* : either of two oily liquid esters $C_{21}H_{28}O_3$ and $C_{22}H_{28}O_5$ that have insecticidal properties and are the active components of pyrethrum

py·re·thrum \pī-'rē-thrəm, -'re-\ *n* : an insecticide made from the dried heads of any of several Old World chrysanthemums (genus *Chrysanthemum* of the family Compositae)

py·rex·ia \pī-'rek-sē-ə\ *n* : abnormal elevation of body temperature : FEVER — **py·rex·i·al** \-sē-əl\ *adj*

py·rex·ic \-sik\ *adj* : PYREXIAL

pyr·i·dine \'pir-ə-ˌdēn\ *n* : a toxic water-soluble flammable liquid base C_5H_5N of pungent odor

pyridine nucleotide *n* : a nucleotide characterized by a pyridine derivative as a nitrogen base; *esp* : NAD

pyr·i·do·stig·mine \ˌpir-ə-dō-'stig-ˌmēn\ *n* : a drug that is an anticholinesterase administered in the form of its bromide $C_9H_{13}BrN_2O_2$ esp. in the treatment of myasthenia gravis — see MESTINON

pyr·i·dox·al \ˌpir-ə-'däk-ˌsal\ *n* : a crystalline aldehyde $C_8H_9NO_3$ of the vitamin B_6 group that in the form of its phosphate is active as a coenzyme

pyr·i·dox·amine \ˌpir-ə-'däk-sə-ˌmēn\

n : an amine $C_8H_{12}N_2O_2$ of the vitamin B_6 group that in the form of its phosphate is active as a coenzyme

pyr·i·dox·ine \ˌpir-ə-ˈdäk-ˌsēn, -sən\ *n* : a crystalline phenolic alcohol $C_8H_{11}NO_3$ of the vitamin B_6 group found esp. in cereals and convertible in the body into pyridoxal and pyridoxamine

pyridoxine hydrochloride *n* : the hydrochloride salt $C_8H_{11}NO_3 \cdot HCl$ of pyridoxine that is used therapeutically (as in the treatment of pyridoxine deficiency)

pyriform, pyriformis *var of* PIRIFORM, PIRIFORMIS

py·ril·amine \pī-ˈri-lə-ˌmēn\ *n* : an oily liquid base $C_{17}H_{23}N_3O$ or its bitter crystalline maleate $C_{21}H_{27}N_3O_5$ used as an antihistamine drug in the treatment of various allergies

py·ri·meth·amine \ˌpī-rə-ˈme-thə-ˌmēn\ *n* : a folic acid antagonist $C_{12}H_{13}ClN_4$ that is used in the treatment of toxoplasmosis and the prevention of malaria

py·rim·i·dine \pī-ˈri-mə-ˌdēn, pə-\ *n* **1** : a weakly basic organic compound $C_4H_4N_2$ of penetrating odor that is composed of a single six-membered ring having four carbon atoms with nitrogen atoms in positions one and three **2** : a derivative of pyrimidine having its characteristic ring structure; *esp* : a base (as cytosine, thymine, or uracil) that is a constituent of DNA or RNA

pyrithione zinc *n* : ZINC PYRITHIONE

pyro- see PYR-

py·ro·gal·lic acid \ˌpī-rō-ˈga-lik-\ *n* : PYROGALLOL

py·ro·gal·lol \-ˈga-ˌlȯl, -ˈgȯ-, -ˌlōl\ *n* : a poisonous crystalline phenol $C_6H_6O_3$

formerly used as a topical antimicrobial (as in the treatment of psoriasis)

py·ro·gen \ˈpī-rə-jən\ *n* : a fever-producing substance

py·ro·gen·ic \ˌpī-rō-ˈje-nik\ *adj* : producing or produced by fever — **py·ro·ge·nic·i·ty** \-jə-ˈni-sə-tē\ *n*

py·ro·ma·nia \ˌpī-rō-ˈmā-nē-ə, -nyə\ *n* : an irresistible impulse to start fires — **py·ro·ma·ni·a·cal** \-mə-ˈnī-ə-kəl\ *adj*

py·ro·ma·ni·ac \-nē-ˌak\ *n* : an individual affected with pyromania

py·ro·sis \pī-ˈrō-səs\ *n* : HEARTBURN

py·rox·y·lin \pī-ˈräk-sə-lin\ *n* : a flammable mixture of nitrates of cellulose — see COLLODION

pyr·role \ˈpir-ˌōl\ *n* : a toxic liquid heterocyclic compound C_4H_5N that has a ring consisting of four carbon atoms and one nitrogen atom, and is the parent compound of many biologically important substances (as bile pigments, porphyrins, and chlorophyll); *broadly* : a derivative of pyrrole

py·ru·vate \pī-ˈrü-ˌvāt\ *n* : a salt or ester of pyruvic acid

pyruvate kinase *n* : an enzyme that functions in glycolysis by catalyzing esp. the transfer of phosphate from phosphoenolpyruvate to ADP forming pyruvate and ATP

py·ru·vic acid \pī-ˈrü-vik-\ *n* : a 3-carbon acid $C_3H_4O_3$ that is an intermediate in carbohydrate metabolism and can be formed either from glucose after phosphorylation or from glycogen by glycolysis

py·uria \pī-ˈyür-ē-ə\ *n* : the presence of pus in the urine; *also* : a condition (as pyelonephritis) characterized by pus in the urine

PZI *abbr* protamine zinc insulin

qd *abbr* [Latin *quaque die*] every day — used in writing prescriptions

Q fever *n* : a disease that is characterized by high fever, chills, muscular pains, headache, and sometimes pneumonia, is caused by a rickettsial bacterium of the genus *Coxiella* (*C. burnetii*) of which domestic animals serve as reservoirs, and that is transmitted to humans esp. by inhalation of infective airborne bacteria (as in contaminated dust)

qh *or* **qhr** *abbr* [Latin *quaque hora*] every hour — used in writing prescriptions often used with a number indicating the hours between doses ⟨*q4h* means every 4 hours⟩

qid *abbr* [Latin *quater in die*] four times a day — used in writing prescriptions

qi·gong \ˈchē-ˈgŭŋ\ *n, often cap* : an ancient Chinese healing art involving

meditation, controlled breathing, and movement exercises designed to improve physical and mental well-being and prevent disease — called also *chi kung, ch'i kung*

QRS \ˌkyü-(ˌ)är-ˈes\ *n* : QRS COMPLEX

QRS complex *n* : the series of deflections in an electrocardiogram that represent electrical activity generated by ventricular depolarization prior to contraction of the ventricles — compare P WAVE, T WAVE

qt *abbr* quart

QT interval \ˌkyü-ˈtē-\ *n* : the interval from the beginning of the QRS complex to the end of the T wave on an electrocardiogram that represents the time during which contraction of the ventricles occurs

quaa·lude \ˈkwā-ˌlüd\ *n* : a tablet or capsule of methaqualone

quack \'kwak\ *n* : an ignorant or dishonest practitioner of medicine — **quack** *adj* — **quack·ery** \'kwa-kə-rē\ *n*

quad \'kwäd\ *n* : QUADRICEPS — usu. used in pl.

quad·rant \'kwä-drənt\ *n* : any of the four more or less equivalent segments into which an anatomic structure may be divided by vertical and horizontal partitioning through its midpoint ⟨pain in the lower right ∼ of the abdomen⟩

quad·rant·ec·to·my \ˌkwä-drən-'tek-tə-mē\ *n* : a partial mastectomy involving excision of a tumor along with the involved quadrant of the breast including the skin and underlying fascia — compare LUMPECTOMY

quad·rate lobe \'kwä-ˌdrāt-\ *n* : a small lobe of the liver on the underside of the right lobe to the left of the fissure for the gallbladder

qua·dra·tus fem·o·ris \kwä-'drā-təs-'fe-mə-rəs\ *n* : a small flat muscle of the gluteal region that arises from the ischial tuberosity, inserts into the greater trochanter and adjacent region of the femur, and serves to rotate the thigh laterally

quadratus la·bii su·pe·ri·or·is \-'lā-bē-ˌī-sü-ˌpir-ē-'ôr-əs\ *n* : LEVATOR LABII SUPERIORIS

quadratus lum·bor·um \-ləm-'bôr-əm\ *n* : a quadrilateral-shaped muscle of the abdomen that arises from the iliac crest and the iliolumbar ligament, inserts into the lowest rib and the upper four lumbar vertebrae, and functions esp. to flex the trunk laterally

quadratus plan·tae \-'plan-ˌtē\ *n* : a muscle of the sole of the foot that arises by two heads from the calcaneus, inserts into the lateral side of the tendons of the flexor digitorum longus, and aids in flexing the toes

quad·ri·ceps \'kwä-drə-ˌseps\ *n* : a large extensor muscle of the front of the thigh divided above into four parts which include the rectus femoris, vastus lateralis, vastus intermedius, and vastus medialis, and which unite in a single tendon to enclose the patella as a sesamoid bone at the knee and insert as the patellar ligament into the tuberosity of the tibia — called also *quadriceps muscle*

quadriceps fem·o·ris \-'fe-mə-rəs\ *n* : QUADRICEPS

quadrigemina — see CORPORA QUADRIGEMINA

quad·ri·pa·re·sis \ˌkwä-drə-pə-'rē-səs\ *n, pl* -**re·ses** \-ˌsēz\ : muscle weakness affecting all four limbs — called also *tetraparesis*

quad·ri·pa·ret·ic \-pə-'re-tik\ *adj* : of, relating to, or affected with quadriparesis ⟨a ∼ patient⟩

quad·ri·ple·gia \ˌkwä-drə-'plē-jə, -jē-ə\ *n* : paralysis of all four limbs — called also *tetraplegia*

¹**quad·ri·ple·gic** \ˌkwä-drə-'plē-jik\ *adj* : of, relating to, or affected with quadriplegia ⟨∼ patients⟩

²**quadriplegic** *n* : one affected with quadriplegia

quad·ru·ped \'kwä-drə-ˌped\ *n* : an animal having four feet — **qua·dru·pe·dal** \kwä-'drü-pəd-ᵊl, ˌkwä-drə-'ped-\ *adj*

qua·dru·plet \kwä-'drü-plət, -'drü-; 'kwä-drə-\ *n* **1** : one of four offspring born at one birth **2 quadruplets** *pl* : a group of four offspring born at one birth

quads *pl of* QUAD

qual·i·ty \'kwä-lə-tē\ *n, pl* -**ties** : the character of an X-ray beam that determines its penetrating power and is dependent upon its wavelength distribution

quality assurance *n* : a program for the systematic monitoring and evaluation of the various aspects of a project, service, or facility to ensure that standards of quality are being met

quan·ti·ta·tive analysis \'kwän-tə-ˌtā-tiv-\ *n* : chemical analysis designed to determine the amounts or proportions of the components of a substance

quantitative character *n* : an inherited character that is phenotypically in all degrees of variation between one often indefinite extreme and another : a character determined by polygenes

quantitative inheritance *n* : genetic inheritance of a character (as human skin color) controlled by polygenes

quan·tum \'kwän-təm\ *n, pl* **quan·ta** \'kwän-tə\ **1** : one of the very small increments or parcels into which many forms of energy are subdivided **2** : one of the small molecular packets of a neurotransmitter (as acetylcholine) released into the synaptic cleft in the transmission of a nerve impulse across a synapse — **quan·tal** \-tᵊl\ *adj*

quar·an·tine \'kwȯr-ən-ˌtēn, 'kwär-\ *n* **1 a** : a term during which a ship arriving in port and suspected of carrying contagious disease is held in isolation from the shore **b** : a regulation placing a ship in quarantine **c** : a place where a ship is detained during quarantine **2 a** : a restraint upon the activities or communication of persons or the transport of goods designed to prevent the spread of disease or pests **b** : a place in which those under quarantine are kept — **quar·an·tin·able** *adj* — **quarantine** *vb*

quart \'kwȯrt\ *n* **1** : a British unit of liquid or dry capacity equal to ¼ gallon or 69.355 cubic inches or 1.136 liters **2** : a U.S. unit of liquid capacity equal to ¼ gallon or 57.75 cubic inches or 0.946 liters

quar·tan \'kwȯrt-ᵊn\ *adj* : recurring at approximately 72-hour intervals ⟨∼ chills and fever⟩ — compare TERTIAN

quartan malaria n : MALARIAE MALARIA

quartz \'kwȯrts\ n : a silica-containing mineral SiO₂

quas·sia \'kwä-shə, -shē-ə, -sē-ə\ n : a drug derived from the heartwood and bark of various tropical trees (family Simaroubaceae) and used esp. as a remedy for roundworms

qua·ter·na·ry \'kwä-tər-₁ner-ē, kwə-'tər-nə-rē\ adj : consisting of, containing, or being an atom bonded to four other atoms

quaternary ammonium compound n : any of numerous strong bases and their salts derived from ammonium by replacement of the hydrogen atoms with organic radicals and important esp. as surface-active agents, disinfectants, and drugs

que·bra·cho \kā-'brä-₍₎chō, ki-\ n : a tree (Aspidosperma quebracho) of the dogbane family (Apocynaceae) which occurs in Argentina and Chile and whose dried bark has been used medicinally esp. to relieve dyspnea

Queck·en·stedt test \'kvek-ᵊn-₁shtet-\ n : a test for spinal blockage of the subarachnoid space in which manual pressure is applied to the jugular vein to elevate venous pressure, which indicates the absence of a block when there is a simultaneous increase in cerebrospinal fluid pressure, and which indicates the presence of a block when cerebrospinal fluid pressure remains the same or almost the same — called also Queckenstedt sign

Queckenstedt, Hans Heinrich Georg (1876–1918), German physician.

quer·ce·tin \'kwər-sə-tən\ n : a yellow crystalline pigment C₁₅H₁₀O₇ occurring usu. in the form of glycosides in various plants

Quete·let index \ke-tə-'lā-\ or Quetelet's index \-'läz-\ n : BODY MASS INDEX

Qué·te·let \kā-tə-lā\, Lambert Adolphe Jacques (1796–1874), Belgian astronomer and statistician.

quick \'kwik\ n : a painfully sensitive spot or area of flesh (as that underlying a fingernail or toenail)

quick·en \'kwi-kən\ vb **quick·ened**; **quick·en·ing** : to reach the stage of gestation at which fetal motion is felt

quickening n : the first motion of a fetus in the uterus felt by the mother usu. somewhat before the middle of the period of gestation

quick·sil·ver \'kwik-₁sil-vər\ n : MERCURY 1

qui·es·cent \kwī-'es-ᵊnt, kwē-\ adj 1 : being in a state of arrest ⟨~ tuberculosis⟩ 2 : causing no symptoms ⟨~ gallstones⟩ — **qui·es·cence** \-ᵊns\ n

quin- or **quino-** comb form 1 : quina : cinchona bark ⟨quinine⟩ ⟨quinoline⟩ 2 : quinoline ⟨quinethazone⟩

qui·na \'kē-nə\ n : CINCHONA 2, 3

quin·a·crine \'kwi-nə-₁krēn\ n : an antimalarial drug derived from acridine and used esp. in the form of its dihydrochloride C₂₃H₃₀ClN₃O·2HCl·2H₂O — called also mepacrine; see ATABRINE

quin·al·bar·bi·tone \₁kwi-nal-'bär-bi-₁tōn\ n, chiefly Brit : SECOBARBITAL

quin·a·pril \'kwi-nə-₁pril\ n : an ACE inhibitor used orally in the form of its hydrochloride C₂₅H₃₀N₂O₅·HCl to treat hypertension — see ACCUPRIL

Quin·cke's disease \'kviŋ-kəz-\ n : ANGIOEDEMA

Quincke, Heinrich Irenaeus (1842–1922), German physician.

Quincke's edema n : ANGIOEDEMA

quin·eth·a·zone \₁kwi-'ne-thə-₁zōn\ n : a diuretic C₁₀H₁₂ClN₃O₃S used in the treatment of edema and hypertension

quin·i·dine \'kwi-nə-₁dēn, -dən\ n : a dextrorotatory stereoisomer of quinine found in some species of cinchona and used chiefly in the form of its hydrated sulfate (C₂₀H₂₄N₂O₂)₂·H₂SO₄·2H₂O to treat irregularities of cardiac rhythm and sometimes in place of quinine as an antimalarial

qui·nine \'kwī-₁nīn, 'kwi-, -₁nēn\ n 1 : a bitter crystalline alkaloid C₂₀H₂₄N₂O₂ obtained from cinchona bark that is administered orally in the form of its salts (as the hydrated sulfate (C₂₀H₂₄N₂O₂)₂·H₂SO₄·2H₂O) as an antimalarial

quin·o·line \'kwin-ᵊl-₁ēn\ n 1 : a pungent oily nitrogenous base C₉H₇N that is the parent compound of many alkaloids, drugs, and dyes 2 : a derivative of quinoline

quin·o·lone \'kwi-nə-₁lōn\ n : any of a class of synthetic antibacterial drugs that are derivatives of quinolines and inhibit the replication of bacterial DNA; esp : FLUOROQUINOLONE

qui·none \kwi-'nōn, 'kwi-₁\ n 1 : either of two isomeric cyclic crystalline compounds C₆H₄O₂ that are irritating to the skin and mucous membranes 2 : any of various usu. yellow, orange, or red compounds structurally related to the quinones and including several that are biologically important as coenzymes, hydrogen acceptors, or vitamins

quin·sy \'kwin-zē\ n, pl **quin·sies** : an abscess in the connective tissue around a tonsil usu. resulting from bacterial infection and often accompanied by fever, pain, and swelling — called also peritonsillar abscess

quint \'kwint\ n : QUINTUPLET

quinti — see EXTENSOR DIGITI QUINTI PROPRIUS

quin·tu·plet \kwin-'tə-plət, -'tü-, -'tyü-; 'kwin-tə-\ n 1 : one of five children or offspring born at one birth 2 **quintuplets** pl : a group of five such offspring

qui·nu·cli·di·nyl ben·zi·late \kwi-'nü-klə-ˌdēn-ᵊl-'ben-zə-ˌlāt, -'nyü-\ *n* : BZ

quit·tor \'kwi-tər\ *n* : a purulent inflammation (as a necrobacillosis) of the feet esp. of horses and donkeys

quo·tid·i·an \kwō-'ti-dē-ən\ *adj* : occurring every day ⟨∼ fever⟩

quo·tient \'kwō-shənt\ *n* : the numerical ratio usu. multiplied by 100 between a test score and a measurement

on which that score might be expected largely to depend

qv *abbr* [Latin *quantum vis*] as much as you will — used in writing prescriptions

Q wave \'kyü-ˌ\ *n* : the short initial downward stroke of the QRS complex in an electrocardiogram formed during the beginning of ventricular depolarization

r *abbr* roentgen

R *symbol* chemical group and esp. an organic chemical group

Ra *symbol* radium

RA *abbr* rheumatoid arthritis

rabbit fever *n* : TULAREMIA

ra·bep·ra·zole \rə-'be-prə-ˌzōl\ *n* : a benzimidazole derivative that inhibits gastric acid secretion and is administered in the form of its sodium salt $C_{18}H_{20}N_3O_3S$ esp. to treat gastroesophageal reflux disease, duodenal ulcers, and disorders (as Zollinger=Ellison syndrome) involving gastric acid hypersecretion — see ACIPHEX

ra·bid \'ra-bəd\ *adj* : affected with rabies ⟨a ∼ dog⟩

ra·bies \'rā-bēz\ *n, pl* **rabies** : an acute virus disease of the nervous system of warm-blooded animals that is caused by a rhabdovirus (species *Rabies virus* of the genus *Lyssavirus*) transmitted in infected saliva usu. through the bite of a rabid animal and that is characterized typically by increased salivation, abnormal behavior, and eventual paralysis and death when untreated — called also *hydrophobia*

race \'rās\ *n* **1** : an actually or potentially interbreeding group within a species; *also* : a taxonomic category (as a subspecies) representing such a group **2** : a category of humankind that shares certain distinctive physical traits

ra·ce·mic \rā-'sē-mik, rə-\ *adj* : of, relating to, or constituting a compound or mixture that is composed of equal amounts of dextrorotatory and levorotatory forms of the same compound and is not optically active

ra·ce·mose \'ra-sə-ˌmōs; rā-'sē-, rə-\ *adj* : having or growing in a form like that of a cluster of grapes ⟨∼ glands⟩

rachi- *or* **rachio-** *comb form* : spine ⟨*rachi*schisis⟩

ra·chis·chi·sis \rə-'kis-kə-səs\ *n, pl* **-chi·ses** \-ˌsēz\ : a congenital abnormality (as spina bifida) characterized by a cleft of the spinal column

ra·chit·ic \rə-'ki-tik\ *adj* : of, relating to, or affected by rickets ⟨∼ lesions⟩

rachitic rosary *n* : BEADING

ra·chi·tis \rə-'kī-təs\ *n, pl* **-chit·i·des** \-'ki-tə-ˌdēz\ : RICKETS

¹rad \'rad\ *n* : a unit of absorbed dose of ionizing radiation equal to an energy of 100 ergs per gram of irradiated material

²rad *abbr* [Latin *radix*] root — used in writing prescriptions

radi- — see RADIO-

¹ra·di·al \'rā-dē-əl\ *adj* **1** : arranged or having parts arranged like rays **2** : of, relating to, or situated near the radius or the thumb side of the hand or forearm **3** : developing uniformly around a central axis ⟨∼ cleavage of an egg⟩ — **ra·di·al·ly** *adv*

²radial *n* : a body part (as an artery) lying near or following the course of the radius

radial artery *n* : the smaller of the two branches into which the brachial artery divides just below the bend of the elbow and which passes along the radial side of the forearm to the wrist then winds backward around the outer side of the carpus and enters the palm between the first and second metacarpal bones to form the deep palmar arch

radial collateral ligament *n* : a ligament of the elbow that connects the lateral epicondyle with the lateral side of the annular ligament and helps to stabilize the elbow joint — called also *lateral collateral ligament*; compare ULNAR COLLATERAL LIGAMENT

radialis — see EXTENSOR CARPI RADIALIS BREVIS, EXTENSOR CARPI RADIALIS LONGUS, FLEXOR CARPI RADIALIS, NERVUS RADIALIS

radial keratotomy *n* : a surgical operation on the cornea for the correction of myopia that involves flattening the cornea by making a series of incisions in a radial pattern resembling the spokes of a wheel — abbr. *RK;* compare PHOTOREFRACTIVE KERATECTOMY

radial nerve *n* : a large nerve that arises from the posterior cord of the brachial plexus and passes spirally down the humerus to the front of the lateral epicondyle where it divides into a superficial branch distributed to the skin of the back of the hand and arm and a deep branch to the underlying extensor muscles — called also *nervus radialis*

radial notch *n* : a narrow depression on the lateral side of the coronoid process of the ulna that articulates with the head of the radius and gives attachment to the annular ligament of the radius

radial tuberosity *n* : an oval eminence on the medial side of the radius distal to the neck where the tendon of the biceps brachii muscle inserts

radial vein *n* : any of several deep veins of the forearm that unite at the elbow with the ulnar veins to form the brachial veins

ra·di·ant energy \'rā-dē-ənt-\ *n* : energy traveling as electromagnetic waves

radiata — see CORONA RADIATA

ra·di·ate \'rā-dē-ˌāt\ *vb* **-at·ed; -at·ing** **1** : to issue in or as if in rays : spread from a central point **2** : IRRADIATE

ra·di·ate ligament \'rā-dē-ət-, -ˌāt-\ *n* : a branching ligament uniting the front of the head of a rib with the bodies of the two vertebrae and the intervertebral disk between them — called also *stellate ligament*

ra·di·a·tion \ˌrā-dē-'ā-shən\ *n* **1** : energy radiated in the form of waves or particles **2 a** : the action or process of radiating **b** (1) : the process of emitting radiant energy in the form of waves or particles (2) : the combined processes of emission, transmission, and absorption of radiant energy **3** : a tract of nerve fibers within the brain; *esp* : one concerned with the distribution of impulses arising from sensory stimuli to the relevant coordinating centers and nuclei

radiation sickness *n* : sickness that results from exposure to radiation and is commonly marked by fatigue, nausea, vomiting, loss of teeth and hair, and in more severe cases by damage to blood-forming tissue with decrease in red and white blood cells and with bleeding — called also *radiation syndrome*

radiation therapist *n* : RADIOTHERAPIST

radiation therapy *n* : RADIOTHERAPY

¹rad·i·cal \'ra-di-kəl\ *adj* **1** : designed to remove the root of a disease or all diseased tissue ⟨~ surgery⟩ **2** : involving complete removal of an organ ⟨~ prostatectomy⟩ — compare CONSERVATIVE — **rad·i·cal·ly** *adv*

²radical *n* : FREE RADICAL; *also* : a group of atoms bonded together that is considered an entity in various kinds of reactions

radical hysterectomy *n* : the surgical removal of the uterus, parametrium, and uterine cervix along with the partial removal of the pelvic lymph nodes that is typically performed to treat cervical or endometrial cancer — see WERTHEIM OPERATION

radical mastectomy *n* : a mastectomy in which the breast tissue, associated skin, nipple, areola, axillary lymph nodes, and pectoral muscles are removed — called also *Halsted radical mastectomy*; compare MODIFIED RADICAL MASTECTOMY, TOTAL MASTECTOMY

ra·dic·u·lar \rə-'di-kyə-lər, ra-\ *adj* **1** : of, relating to, or involving a nerve root **2** : of, relating to, or occurring at the root of a tooth ⟨a ~ cyst⟩

ra·dic·u·li·tis \rə-ˌdi-kyə-'lī-təs\ *n* : inflammation of a nerve root

ra·dic·u·lop·a·thy \-'lä-pə-thē\ *n, pl* **-thies** : any pathological condition of the nerve roots

radii *pl of* RADIUS

radio- *also* **radi-** *comb form* **1** : radiant energy : radiation ⟨*radio*active⟩ ⟨*ra*diopaque⟩ **2** : radioactive ⟨*radio*element⟩ **3** : radium : X-rays ⟨*radio*therapy⟩ **4** : radioactive isotopes esp. as produced artificially ⟨*radio*cobalt⟩

ra·dio·ac·tiv·i·ty \ˌrā-dē-ō-ak-'ti-və-tē\ *n, pl* **-ties** : the property possessed by some elements (as uranium) or isotopes (as carbon 14) of spontaneously emitting alpha or beta rays and sometimes also gamma rays by the disintegration of their atomic nuclei — **ra·dio·ac·tive** \-'ak-tiv\ *adj* — **ra·dio·ac·tive·ly** *adv*

ra·dio·al·ler·go·sor·bent \ˌrā-dē-ō-ə-ˌlər-gō-'sȯr-bənt\ *adj* : relating to, involving, or being a radioallergosorbent test ⟨~ testing⟩

radioallergosorbent test *n* : a radioimmunoassay for specific antibodies of immunoglobulin class IgE in which an insoluble matrix containing allergenic antigens is reacted with a sample of antibody-containing serum and then reacted again with antihuman antibodies against individual IgE antibodies to make specific determinations — abbr. RAST

ra·dio·as·say \ˌrā-dō-'a-ˌsā, -a-'sā\ *n* : an assay based on examination of the sample in terms of radiation components

ra·dio·au·to·gram \-'ȯ-tə-ˌgram\ *n* : AUTORADIOGRAPH

ra·dio·au·to·graph \-'ȯ-tə-ˌgraf\ *n* : AUTORADIOGRAPH — **radioautograph** *vb* — **ra·dio·au·to·graph·ic** \-ˌȯ-tə-'gra-fik\ *adj* — **ra·dio·au·tog·ra·phy** \-ȯ-'tä-grə-fē\ *n*

ra·dio·bi·ol·o·gy \ˌrā-dē-ō-bī-'ä-lə-jē\ *n, pl* **-gies** : a branch of biology dealing with the effects of radiation or radioactive materials on biological systems — **ra·dio·bi·o·log·i·cal** \-ˌbī-ə-'lä-ji-kəl\ *also* **ra·dio·bi·o·log·ic** \-jik\ *adj* — **ra·dio·bi·o·log·i·cal·ly** *adv* — **ra·dio·bi·ol·o·gist** \-bī-'ä-lə-jist\ *n*

¹ra·dio·chem·i·cal \-'ke-mi-kəl\ *adj* : of, relating to, being, or using radiochemicals or the methods of radiochemistry ⟨∼ analysis⟩ ⟨∼ purity⟩

²**ra·dio·chem·i·cal** n : a chemical prepared with radioactive elements esp. for medical research or application (as for use as a tracer)

ra·dio·chem·is·try \ˌrā-dē-ō-'ke-mə-strē\ n, pl **-tries** : a branch of chemistry dealing with radioactive substances and phenomena including tracer studies — **ra·dio·chem·ist** \-'ke-mist\ n

ra·dio·chro·mato·gram \-krō-'ma-tə-ˌgram\ n : a chromatogram revealing one or more radioactive substances

ra·dio·chro·ma·tog·ra·phy \-ˌkrō-mə-'tä-grə-fē\ n, pl **-phies** : the process of making a quantitative or qualitative determination of a radioisotope-labeled substance by measuring the radioactivity of the appropriate zone or spot in the chromatogram — **ra·dio·chro·ma·to·graph·ic** \-krə-ˌma-tə-'gra-fik, -ˌkrō-mə-\ adj

ra·dio·co·balt \-'kō-ˌbólt\ n : radioactive cobalt; esp : COBALT 60

ra·dio·con·trast \-'kän-ˌtrast\ adj : relating to or being a radioactive contrast medium

ra·dio·den·si·ty \-'den-sə-tē\ n, pl **-ties** : RADIOPACITY

ra·dio·der·ma·ti·tis \-ˌdər-mə-'tī-təs\ n, pl **-ti·tis·es** or **-tit·i·des** \-'ti-tə-ˌdēz\ : dermatitis resulting from overexposure to sources of radiant energy (as X-rays or radium)

ra·dio·di·ag·no·sis \-ˌdī-ig-'nō-səs\ n, pl **-no·ses** \-ˌsēz\ : diagnosis by means of radiology — compare RADIOTHERAPY

ra·dio·el·e·ment \-'e-lə-mənt\ n : a radioactive element whether formed naturally or produced artificially

ra·dio·en·zy·mat·ic \-ˌen-zə-'ma-tik\ adj : of, relating to, or produced by a radioactive enzyme

radio frequency n, pl **-cies** : any of the electromagnetic wave frequencies that lie in the range extending from below 3000 hertz to about 300 billion hertz and that include the frequencies used for communications signals (as for radio and television broadcasting and cell-phone transmissions) or radio signals — **radiofrequency** adj

ra·dio·gen·ic \ˌrā-dē-ō-'je-nik\ adj : produced or caused by radioactivity

ra·dio·gram \'rā-dē-ō-ˌgram\ n : RADIOGRAPH

ra·dio·graph \-ˌgraf\ n : an X-ray or gamma-ray photograph — **radiograph** vb — **ra·dio·graph·ic** \ˌrā-dē-ō-'gra-fik\ adj

ra·di·og·ra·pher \ˌrā-dē-'ä-grə-fər\ n : a person who makes radiographs; specif : an X-ray technician

ra·di·og·ra·phy \ˌrā-dē-'ä-grə-fē\ n, pl **-phies** : the art, act, or process of making radiographs

ra·dio·im·mu·no·as·say \ˌrā-dē-ō-i-myə-nō-'a-ˌsā, -i-ˌmyü-, -a-'sā\ n : immunoassay of a substance (as insulin)

that has been radiolabeled — abbr. *RIA* — **ra·dio·im·mu·no·as·say·able** adj

ra·dio·im·mu·no·elec·tro·pho·re·sis \-i-ˌlek-trə-fə-'rē-səs\ n, pl **-re·ses** \-ˌsēs\ : immunoelectrophoresis in which the substances separated in the electrophoretic system are identified by radioactive labels on antigens or antibodies

ra·dio·im·mu·no·log·i·cal \-ˌi-myə-nə-'lä-ji-kəl\ also **ra·dio·im·mu·no·log·ic** \-'lä-jik\ adj : of, relating to, or involving a radioimmunoassay

ra·dio·io·dide \-'ī-ə-ˌdīd\ n : an iodide containing radioactive iodine

ra·dio·io·din·ate \-'ī-ə-də-ˌnāt\ vb **-at·ed; -at·ing** : to treat or label with radioactive iodine — **ra·dio·io·din·ation** \-ˌī-ə-də-'nā-shən\ n

ra·dio·io·dine \-'ī-ə-ˌdīn, -dən, -ˌdēn\ n : radioactive iodine; esp : IODINE-131

ra·dio·iron \-'ī(-ə)rn\ n : radioactive iron; esp : a heavy isotope having the mass number 59 that is produced in nuclear reactors or cyclotrons and is used in biochemical tracer studies

ra·dio·iso·tope \ˌrā-dē-ō-'ī-sə-ˌtōp\ n : a radioactive isotope — **ra·dio·iso·to·pic** \-ˌī-sə-'tä-pik, -'tō-\ adj

ra·dio·la·bel \-'lā-bəl\ vb **-la·beled** or **-la·belled; -la·bel·ing** or **-la·bel·ling** : to label with a radioactive atom or substance — **radiolabel** n

ra·di·ol·o·gist \ˌrā-dē-'ä-lə-jist\ n : a physician specializing in the use of radiant energy for diagnostic and therapeutic purposes

ra·di·ol·o·gy \-jē\ n, pl **-gies** 1 : the science of radioactive substances and high-energy radiations 2 : a branch of medicine concerned with the use of radiant energy (as X-rays or ultrasound) in the diagnosis and treatment of disease — **ra·dio·log·i·cal** \ˌrā-dē-ə-'lä-ji-kəl\ or **ra·dio·log·ic** \-jik\ adj — **ra·dio·log·i·cal·ly** adv

ra·dio·lu·cent \ˌrā-dē-ō-'lüs-ᵊnt\ adj : partly or wholly permeable to radiation and esp. X-rays — compare RADIOPAQUE — **ra·dio·lu·cen·cy** \-'lüs-ᵊn-sē\ n

ra·dio·mi·met·ic \-mə-'me-tik, -mī-\ adj : producing effects similar to those of radiation ⟨∼ agents⟩

ra·dio·ne·cro·sis \-nə-'krō-səs, -ne-\ n, pl **-cro·ses** \-ˌsēz\ : ulceration or destruction of tissue resulting from irradiation — **ra·dio·ne·crot·ic** \-'krä-tik\ adj

ra·dio·nu·clide \-'nü-ˌklīd, -'nyü-\ n : a radioactive nuclide

ra·dio·opac·i·ty \ˌrā-dē-ō-ō-'pa-sə-tē\ n, pl **-ties** : the quality or state of being radiopaque

ra·dio·paque \-ō-'pāk\ adj : being opaque to radiation and esp. X-rays — compare RADIOLUCENT

ra·dio·phar·ma·ceu·ti·cal \ˌrā-dē-ō-ˌfär-mə-'sü-ti-kəl\ n : a radioactive drug used for diagnostic or therapeutic purposes — **radiopharmaceutical** *adj*

ra·dio·phar·ma·cy \-'fär-mə-sē\ *n, pl* **-cies** : a branch of pharmacy concerned with radiopharmaceuticals; *also* : a pharmacy that supplies radiopharmaceuticals — **ra·dio·phar·ma·cist** \-sist\ *n*

ra·dio·phos·pho·rus \-'fäs-fə-rəs\ *n* : radioactive phosphorus; *esp* : PHOSPHORUS 32

ra·dio·pro·tec·tive \-prə-'tek-tiv\ *adj* : serving to protect or aiding in protecting against the injurious effect of radiations ⟨∼ drugs⟩ — **ra·dio·pro·tec·tion** \-'tek-shən\ *n*

ra·dio·pro·tec·tor \-'tek-tər\ *also* **ra·dio·pro·tec·tor·ant** \-'tek-tə-rənt\ *n* : a radioprotective chemical agent

ra·dio·re·cep·tor assay \-ri-'sep-tər-\ *n* : an assay for a substance and esp. a hormone in which a mixture of the test sample and a known amount of the radiolabeled substance under test is exposed to a measured quantity of receptors for the substance and the amount in the test sample is determined from the proportion of receptors occupied by radiolabeled molecules of the substance

ra·dio·re·sis·tant \-ri-'zis-tənt\ *adj* : resistant to the effects of radiant energy ⟨∼ cancer cells⟩ — **ra·dio·re·sis·tance** \-təns\ *n*

ra·dio·sen·si·tive \rā-dē-ō-'sen-sə-tiv\ *adj* : sensitive to the effects of radiant energy ⟨∼ cancer cells⟩ — **ra·dio·sen·si·tiv·i·ty** \-sen-sə-'ti-və-tē\ *n*

ra·dio·sen·si·tiz·er \-'sen-sə-,tī-zər\ *n* : a substance or condition capable of increasing the radiosensitivity of a cell or tissue — **ra·dio·sen·si·ti·za·tion** \-sen-sə-tə-'zā-shən\ *n* — **ra·dio·sen·si·tiz·ing** \-'sen-sə-,tī-zin\ *adj*

ra·dio·so·di·um \-'sō-dē-əm\ *n* : radioactive sodium; *esp* : a heavy isotope having the mass number 24 that is produced in nuclear reactors and is used in the form of a salt (as sodium chloride) chiefly in biochemical tracer studies

ra·dio·stron·tium \-'strän-chē-əm, -chəm, -tē-əm\ *n* : radioactive strontium; *esp* : STRONTIUM 90

ra·dio·sur·gery \-'sər-jə-rē\ *n, pl* **-ger·ies** : STEREOTACTIC RADIOSURGERY — **ra·dio·sur·gi·cal** \-'sər-ji-kəl\ *adj*

ra·dio·te·lem·e·try \-tə-'le-mə-trē\ *n, pl* **-tries** **1** : TELEMETRY **2** : BIOTELEMETRY — **ra·dio·tele·met·ric** \-,te-lə-'me-trik\ *adj*

ra·dio·ther·a·py \rā-dē-ō-'ther-ə-pē\ *n, pl* **-pies** : the treatment of disease by means of radiation (as X-rays) — called also *radiation therapy;* compare RADIODIAGNOSIS — **ra·dio·ther·a·peu·tic** \-,ther-ə-'pyü-tik\ *adj* — **ra·dio·ther·a·pist** \-'ther-ə-pist\ *n*

ra·dio·tox·ic·i·ty \-täk-'si-sə-tē\ *n, pl* **-ties** : the toxicity of radioactive substances

ra·dio·trac·er \'rā-dē-ō-,trā-sər\ *n* : a radioactive tracer

ra·dio·ul·nar \,rā-dē-ō-'əl-nər\ *adj* : of, relating to, or connecting the radius and ulna

radioulnar joint *n* : any of three joints connecting the radius and ulna at their proximal and distal ends and along their shafts — see DISTAL RADIOULNAR JOINT

radio wave *n* : an electromagnetic wave with radio frequency

ra·di·um \'rā-dē-əm\ *n, often attrib* : an intensely radioactive shining white metallic element that emits alpha particles and gamma rays to form radon and is used in the treatment of cancer — symbol *Ra;* see ELEMENT table

ra·di·us \'rā-dē-əs\ *n, pl* **ra·dii** \-dē-,ī\ *also* **ra·di·us·es** : the bone on the thumb side of the forearm that is articulated with the ulna at both ends so as to permit partial rotation about that bone, that bears on its inner aspect somewhat distal to the head a prominence for the insertion of the biceps tendon, and that has the lower end broadened for articulation with the proximal bones of the carpus so that rotation of the radius involves also that of the hand

ra·don \'rā-dän\ *n* : a heavy radioactive gaseous element of the group of inert gases formed by disintegration of radium and used similarly to radium in medicine — symbol *Rn;* see ELEMENT table

rag·weed \'rag-,wēd\ *n* : any of various chiefly No. American weedy herbaceous plants comprising the genus *Ambrosia* and producing highly allergenic pollen: as **a** : an annual weed (*A. artemisiifolia*) with finely divided foliage that is common on open or cultivated ground in much of No. America **b** : a coarse annual (*A. trifida*) with some or all of the leaves usu. deeply 3-cleft or 5-cleft — called also *great ragweed*

Rail·lie·ti·na \,rāl-yə-'tī-nə\ *n* : a large genus of tapeworms (family Davaineidae of the order Cyclophyllidea) of which the adults are parasitic in birds, rodents, or rarely humans and the larvae are parasitic in various insects

Rail·liet \rī-'yā\, **Louis–Joseph Alcide** (1852–1930), French veterinarian.

rain·bow \'rān-,bō\ *n, slang* : a combination of the sodium derivatives of amobarbital and secobarbital in a blue and red capsule

rale \'ral, 'räl\ *n* : an abnormal sound heard accompanying the normal respiratory sounds on auscultation of the chest — compare RATTLE, RHONCHUS

ral·ox·i·fene \ra-'läk-sə-,fēn\ *n* : a selective estrogen receptor modulator used orally in the form of its hydrochloride $C_{28}H_{27}NO_4S\cdot HCl$ esp. to prevent or treat postmenopausal osteoporosis — see EVISTA

ram·i·fi·ca·tion \ˌra-mə-fə-ˈkā-shən\ *n* **1** : the act or process of branching; *specif* : the mode of arrangement of branches **2** : a branch or offshoot from a main stock or channel ⟨the ∼ of an artery⟩; *also* : the resulting branched structure — **ram·i·fy** \ˈra-mə-ˌfī\ *vb*

ra·mip·ril \rə-ˈmi-prəl\ *n* : an ACE inhibitor $C_{23}H_{32}N_2O_5$ used esp. to treat hypertension — see ALTACE

ra·mus \ˈrā-məs\ *n, pl* **ra·mi** \-ˌmī\ : a projecting part, elongated process, or branch: as **a** : the posterior more or less vertical part of the lower jaw on each side which articulates with the skull **b** (1) : the upper more cranial branch of the pubis that extends from the pubic symphysis to the body of the pubis at the acetabulum and forms the cranial part of the obturator foramen — called also *superior ramus* (2) : the thin flat lower branch of the pubis that extends from the pubic symphysis to unite with the ramus of the ischium in forming the inferior rim of the obturator foramen — called also *inferior ramus* **c** : a branch of the ischium that extends down and forward from the ischial tuberosity to unite with the inferior ramus of the pubis in forming the inferior rim of the obturator foramen — called also *inferior ramus* **d** : a branch of a nerve — see RAMUS COMMUNICANS

ramus com·mu·ni·cans \-kə-ˈmyü-nə-ˌkanz\ *n, pl* **rami com·mu·ni·can·tes** \-kə-ˌmyü-nə-ˈkan-ˌtēz\ : any of the bundles of nerve fibers connecting a sympathetic ganglion with a spinal nerve and being divided into two kinds: **a** : one consisting of myelinated preganglionic fibers — called also *white ramus, white ramus communicans* **b** : one consisting of unmyelinated postganglionic fibers — called also *gray ramus*

ran *past of* RUN

randomized controlled trial *n* : a clinical trial in which the subjects are randomly distributed into groups which are either subjected to the experimental procedure (as use of a drug) or which serve as controls — called also *randomized clinical trial*

rang *past of* RING

ra·nit·i·dine \rə-ˈni-tə-ˌdēn\ *n* : an antihistamine used in the form of its hydrochloride $C_{13}H_{22}N_4O_3S \cdot HCl$ to inhibit gastric acid secretion (as in the treatment of duodenal ulcers or Zollinger-Ellison syndrome) — see ZANTAC

ran·u·la \ˈran-yə-lə\ *n* : a cyst formed under the tongue by obstruction of a gland duct

rap·a·my·cin \ˌra-pə-ˈmī-sᵊn\ *n* : an immunosuppressive agent $C_{51}H_{79}NO_{13}$

rape \ˈrāp\ *n* : unlawful sexual activity and usu. sexual intercourse carried out forcibly or under threat of injury against the will usu. of a female or with a person who is beneath a certain age or incapable of valid consent — compare SEXUAL ASSAULT, STATUTORY RAPE — **rape** *vb*

ra·phe \ˈrā-fē\ *n* : the seamlike union of the two lateral halves of a part or organ (as of the tongue, perineum, or scrotum) having externally a ridge or furrow and internally usu. a fibrous connective tissue septum

raphe nucleus *n* : any of several groups of nerve cells situated along or near the median plane of the tegmentum of the midbrain

rapid eye movement *n* : a rapid movement of the eyes associated esp. with REM sleep — called also *REM*

rapid eye movement sleep *n* : REM SLEEP

rapid plasma reagin test *n* : a flocculation test for syphilis employing the antigen used in the VDRL test with charcoal particles added so that the flocculation can be seen without the aid of a microscope — called also *RPR card test*

rap·ist \ˈrā-pist\ *n* : an individual who commits rape

rap·port \ra-ˈpȯr, rə-\ *n* : harmonious accord or relation that fosters cooperation, communication, or trust ⟨∼ between a patient and psychotherapist⟩

rapture of the deep *n* : NITROGEN NARCOSIS

rap·tus \ˈrap-təs\ *n* : a pathological paroxysm of activity giving vent to impulse or tension (as in an act of violence)

rar·efy *also* **rar·i·fy** \ˈrar-ə-ˌfī\ *vb* **-efied** *also* **-i·fied; -efy·ing** *also* **-i·fy·ing** : to make or become rare, thin, porous, or less dense : to expand without the addition of matter — **rar·efac·tion** \ˌrar-ə-ˈfak-shən\ *n*

ras \ˈras\ *n, often attrib* [*rat sarcoma*] : any of a family of genes that undergo mutation to oncogenes and esp. to some commonly linked to human cancers (as of the colon, lung, and pancreas) ⟨∼ oncogenes⟩

rash \ˈrash\ *n* : an eruption on the body typically with little or no elevation above the surface

RAST *abbr* radioallergosorbent test

rat \ˈrat\ *n* : any of the numerous rodents (family Muridae) of *Rattus* and related genera that include forms (as the brown rat and the black rat) which live in and about human habitations and are destructive pests and vectors of various diseases (as bubonic plague)

rat–bite fever *n* : either of two febrile human diseases usu. transmitted by the bite of a rat: **a** : a septicemia marked by irregular relapsing fever, rashes esp. on the hands and feet, muscular pain and arthritis, and nausea and caused by a bacterium of the genus *Streptobacillus* (*S. moniliformis*) **b** : a disease that is marked by sharp elevation of temperature, swelling of lymph glands, eruption, recurrent inflammation of the bite wound, and muscular pains in the part where the bite wound occurred and that is caused by a bacterium of the genus *Spirillum* (*S. minor* syn. *S. minus*) — called also *sodoku*

rate \\'rāt\\ *n* **1** : a fixed ratio between two things **2** : a quantity, amount, or degree of something measured per unit of something else — see DEATH RATE, HEART RATE, METABOLIC RATE, PULSE RATE, SEDIMENTATION RATE

rat flea *n* : any of various fleas that occur on rats: as **a** : NORTHERN RAT FLEA **b** : ORIENTAL RAT FLEA

Rath·ke's pouch \\'rät-kəz-\\ *n* : a pouch of ectoderm that grows out from the upper surface of the embryonic stomodeum and gives rise to the adenohypophysis of the pituitary gland — called also *Rathke's pocket*
Rathke, Martin Heinrich (1793–1860), German anatomist.

rat·i·cide \\'rat-ə-ˌsīd\\ *n* : a substance used to kill rats

ra·tio \\'rā-(ˌ)shō, -shē-ˌō\\ *n, pl* **ra·tios** : the relationship in quantity, amount, or size between two or more things — see SEX RATIO

ra·tion \\'ra-shən, 'rā-\\ *n* : a food allowance for one day — **ration** *vb*

ra·tio·nal—emo·tive therapy \\'ra-shə-nᵊl-i-ˈmō-tiv-\\ *n* : cognitive therapy based on a theory of Albert Ellis that a patient can be taught to effect emotional well-being by changing negative and irrational thoughts to positive and rational ones

ra·tio·nal·ize \\'ra-shə-nə-ˌlīz\\ *vb* **-ized; -iz·ing** : to attribute (one's actions) to rational and creditable motives without analysis of true and esp. unconscious motives; *also* : to provide plausible but untrue reasons for conduct — **ra·tio·nal·i·za·tion** \\ˌra-shə-nə-lə-ˈzā-shən\\ *n*

rational therapy *n* : RATIONAL-EMOTIVE THERAPY

rat louse *n* : a sucking louse (*Polyplax spinulosa*) that is a widely distributed parasite of rats and transmits murine typhus from rat to rat

rat mite *n* : a widely distributed mite of the genus *Ornithonyssus* (*O. bacoti*) that usu. feeds on rodents but may cause dermatitis in and transmit typhus to humans

rat·tle \\'rat-ᵊl\\ *n* : a throat noise caused by air passing through mucus; *specif* : DEATH RATTLE — compare RALE, RHONCHUS

rat·tle·box \\-ˌbäks\\ *n* : CROTALARIA 2; *esp* : one (*Crotalaria spectabilis*) that is highly toxic to farm animals

rat·tle·snake \\-ˌsnāk\\ *n* : any of the American pit vipers that have a series of horny interlocking joints at the

end of the tail which make a sharp rattling sound when vibrated and that comprise the genera *Sistrurus* and *Crotalus* — see DIAMONDBACK RATTLESNAKE, TIGER RATTLESNAKE, TIMBER RATTLESNAKE

Rat·tus \\'ra-təs\\ *n* : a genus of rodents (family Muridae) that comprise the common rats

Rau·dix·in \\raù-ˈdiks-ən, rò-\\ *trademark* — used for a preparation of reserpine

rau·wol·fia \\raù-ˈwùl-fē-ə, rò-\\ **1** : any of a genus (*Rauwolfia* syn. *Rauwolfia*) of tropical trees and shrubs of the dogbane family (Apocynaceae) that yield medicinal alkaloids (as reserpine) **2** : the dried root or an extract from the root of a rauwolfia (esp. *Rauwolfia serpentina* of Asia) used chiefly in the treatment of hypertension
Rauwolf, Leonhard (1535–1596), German botanist.

ray·less goldenrod \\'rā-ləs-\\ *n* : a shrubby or herbaceous plant (*Haplopappus heterophyllus* syn. *Isocoma wrightii* of the family Compositae) esp. of open saline ground from Texas to Arizona and northern Mexico that causes trembles in cattle

Ray·naud's disease \\rā-ˈnōz-\\ *n* : a vascular disorder marked by recurrent spasm of the capillaries and esp. those of the fingers and toes upon exposure to cold, characterized by pallor, cyanosis and redness in succession, usu. accompanied by pain, and in severe cases progressing to local gangrene — called also *Raynaud's*
Raynaud, Maurice (1834–1881), French physician.

Raynaud's phenomenon *n* : the symptoms associated with Raynaud's disease — called also *Raynaud's syndrome*

Rb *symbol* rubidium

RBC *abbr* **1** red blood cells **2** red blood count

RBE *abbr* relative biological effectiveness

rBGH *abbr* recombinant bovine growth hormone

RBRVS *abbr* resource-based relative value scale

rBST *abbr* recombinant bovine somatotropin

RCT *abbr* randomized clinical trial; randomized controlled trial

rd *abbr* rutherford

RD *abbr* registered dietitian

RDA *abbr* recommended daily allowance; recommended dietary allowance

RDH *abbr* registered dental hygienist

RDS *abbr* respiratory distress syndrome

Re *symbol* rhenium

re·ab·sorb \\ˌrē-əb-ˈsòrb, -ˈzòrb\\ *vb* : to take up (something previously secreted or emitted) ⟨sugars *~ed* in the kidney\; *also* : RESORB — **re·ab·sorp·tion** \-'sorp-shən, -'zorp-\ *n*

re·act \rē-'akt\ *vb* 1 : to respond to a stimulus 2 : to undergo or cause to undergo chemical reaction

re·ac·tion \rē-'ak-shən\ *n* 1 : the act or process or an instance of reacting 2 : bodily response to or activity aroused by a stimulus : **a** : an action induced by vital resistance to another action; *esp* : the response of tissues to a foreign substance (as an antigen or infective agent) **b** : depression or exhaustion due to excessive exertion or stimulation **c** : abnormally heightened activity succeeding depression or shock **d** : a mental or emotional disorder forming an individual's response to his or her life situation 3 **a** (1) : chemical transformation or change : the interaction of chemical entities (2) : the state resulting from such a reaction **b** : a process involving change in atomic nuclei

reaction formation *n* : a psychological defense mechanism in which one form of behavior substitutes for or conceals a diametrically opposed repressed impulse in order to protect against it

reaction time *n* : the time elapsing between the beginning of the application of a stimulus and the beginning of an organism's reaction to it

re·ac·ti·vate \rē-'ak-tə-ˌvāt\ *vb* **-vat·ed;** **-vat·ing** : to cause to be again active or more active: as **a** : to cause (as a repressed complex) to reappear in consciousness or behavior **b** : to cause (a quiescent disease) to become active again in an individual — **re·ac·ti·va·tion** \-ˌak-tə-'vā-shən\ *n*

re·ac·tive \rē-'ak-tiv\ *adj* 1 **a** : of, relating to, or marked by reaction (∼ symptoms) **b** : capable of reacting chemically 2 **a** : readily responsive to a stimulus **b** : occurring as a result of stress or emotional upset esp. from factors outside the organism (∼ depression) — **re·ac·tiv·i·ty** \rē-ˌak-'ti-və-tē\ *n*

reactive arthritis *n* : acute arthritis that sometimes develops following a bacterial infection (as with the bacteria of the genera *Shigella, Salmonella,* or *Chlamydia*)

re·ac·tor \rē-'ak-tər\ *n* 1 : one that reacts: as **a** : a chemical reagent **b** : an individual reacting to a stimulus **c** : an individual reacting positively to a foreign substance (as in a test for disease) 2 : a device for the controlled release of nuclear energy

re·agent \rē-'ā-jənt\ *n* : a substance used (as in detecting a component or in preparing a product) because of its chemical or biological activity

re·agin \rē-'ā-jən, -gən\ *n* 1 : a substance that is in the blood of individuals with syphilis and is responsible for positive serological reactions for syphilis 2 : an antibody (as IgE in hu-mans) that mediates hypersensitive allergic reactions of rapid onset — **re·agin·ic** \ˌrē-ə-'ji-nik, -'gi-\ *adj*

reality principle *n* : the tendency to defer immediate instinctual gratification so as to achieve longer-range goals or so as to meet external demands — compare PLEASURE PRINCIPLE

reality testing *n* : the psychological process in which acts are explored and their outcomes determined so that the individual will be aware of these consequences when the stimulus to act in a given fashion recurs

ream·er \'rē-mər\ *n* : an instrument used in dentistry to enlarge and clean out a root canal

re·am·pu·ta·tion \ˌrē-ˌam-pyə-'tā-shən\ *n* : the second of two amputations performed upon the same member

re·anas·to·mo·sis \ˌrē-ə-ˌnas-tə-'mō-səs\ *n, pl* **-mo·ses** \-ˌsēz\ : the reuniting (as by surgery or healing) of a divided vessel

re·at·tach \ˌrē-ə-'tach\ *vb* : to attach again (∼ a severed finger) — **re·at·tach·ment** \-mənt\ *n*

re·base \rē-'bās\ *vb* **re·based;** **re·bas·ing** : to modify the base of (a denture) after an initial period of wear in order to produce a good fit

re·bleed \'rē-ˌblēd\ *vb* **re·bled** \-ˌbled\; **re·bleed·ing** 1 : to bleed or hemorrhage again (identify patients at risk of ∼*ing*) 2 *of a hemorrhage* : to occur again — **rebleed** *n*

re·bound \'rē-ˌbaund, ri-'\ *n* : a return to a previous state or condition following removal of a stimulus or cessation of treatment

rebound tenderness *n* : a sensation of pain felt when pressure (as to the abdomen) is suddenly removed

re·breathe \ˌrē-'brēth\ *vb* **re·breathed;** **re·breath·ing** 1 : to breathe (as reconstituted air) again 2 : to inhale previously exhaled air or gases

re·cal·ci·fi·ca·tion \ˌrē-ˌkal-sə-fə-'kā-shən\ *n* : the restoration of calcium or calcium compounds to decalcified tissue (as bone or blood) — **re·cal·ci·fied** \-'kal-sə-ˌfīd\ *adj*

recalcification time *n* : a measure of the time taken for clot formation in recalcified blood

re·cal·ci·trant \ri-'kal-sə-trənt\ *adj* : not responsive to treatment (∼ warts)

re·call \ri-'kól, 'rē-ˌ\ *n* : remembrance of what has been previously learned or experienced — **recall** \ri-'kól\ *vb*

re·can·a·li·za·tion \ˌrē-ˌkan-°l-ə-'zā-shən\ *n* : the process of restoring flow to or reuniting an interrupted channel of a bodily tube (as an artery or vas deferens) — **re·can·a·lize** \-kə-'na-ˌlīz, -'kan-°l-ˌīz\ *vb*

re·cep·tive \ri-'sep-tiv\ *adj* 1 : open and responsive to ideas, impressions, or suggestions **2 a** *of a sensory end organ* : fit to receive and transmit stimuli **b** : SENSORY 1 — **re·cep·tive·ness** *n* — **re·cep·tiv·i·ty** \ˌrē-ˌsep-'ti-və-tē, ri-\ *n*

re·cep·tor \ri-'sep-tər\ *n* **1** : a cell or group of cells that receives stimuli : SENSE ORGAN **2** : a chemical group or molecule (as a protein) on the cell surface or in the cell interior that has an affinity for a specific chemical group, molecule, or virus **3** : a cellular entity (as a beta-receptor) that is a postulated intermediary between a chemical agent (as a neurohormone) acting on nervous tissue and the physiological or pharmacological response

re·cess \'rē-ˌses, ri-'\ *n* : an anatomical depression or cleft : FOSSA

re·ces·sion \ri-'se-shən\ *n* : pathological withdrawal of tissue from its normal position ⟨advanced gum ~⟩

¹re·ces·sive \ri-'se-siv\ *adj* **1** : producing little or no phenotypic effect when occurring in heterozygous condition with a contrasting allele ⟨~ genes⟩ **2** : expressed only when the determining gene is in the homozygous condition ⟨~ traits⟩ — **re·ces·sive·ly** *adv* — **re·ces·sive·ness** *n*

²recessive *n* **1** : a recessive character or gene **2** : an organism possessing one or more recessive characters

re·cid·i·vism \ri-'si-də-ˌvi-zəm\ *n* : a tendency to relapse into a previous condition or mode of behavior ⟨~ among former cigarette smokers⟩ — **re·cid·i·vist** \-vist\ *n*

rec·i·pe \'re-sə-(ˌ)pē\ *n* : PRESCRIPTION 1

re·cip·i·ent \ri-'si-pē-ənt\ *n* : one who receives biological material (as blood or an organ) from a donor

reciprocal inhibition *n* **1** : RECIPROCAL INNERVATION **2** : behavior modification in which the patient is exposed to anxiety-producing stimuli while in a controlled state of relaxation so that the anxiety response is gradually inhibited

reciprocal innervation *n* : innervation so that the contraction of a muscle or set of muscles (as of a joint) is accompanied by the simultaneous inhibition of an antagonistic muscle or set of muscles

reciprocal translocation *n* : exchange of parts between nonhomologous chromosomes

Reck·ling·hau·sen's disease \'rek-kliŋ-ˌhau-zənz-\ *n* : NEUROFIBROMATOSIS

Recklinghausen, Friedrich Daniel von (1833–1910), German pathologist.

rec·og·ni·tion \ˌre-kəg-'ni-shən\ *n* : the form of memory that consists in knowing or feeling that a present object has been met before

¹re·com·bi·nant \ˌrē-'käm-bə-nənt\ *adj* **1** : relating to or exhibiting genetic recombination **2 a** : relating to or con-

taining genetically engineered DNA **b** : produced by genetic engineering ⟨~ bovine growth hormone⟩

²recombinant *n* : an individual exhibiting recombination

recombinant DNA *n* : genetically engineered DNA usu. incorporating DNA from more than one species of organism

re·com·bi·na·tion \ˌrē-ˌkäm-bə-'nā-shən\ *n* : the formation by the processes of crossing-over and independent assortment of new combinations of genes in progeny that did not occur in the parents — **re·com·bi·na·tion·al** *adj*

recommended daily allowance *n, often cap R&D&A* : the amount of a nutriment (as a vitamin or mineral) that is recommended for daily consumption by the Food and Nutrition Board of the National Academy of Sciences — abbr. *RDA;* called also *recommended dietary allowance*

re·com·pres·sion \ˌrē-kəm-'pre-shən\ *n* : a renewed heightening of atmospheric pressure esp. as treatment for decompression sickness

re·con·sti·tute \rē-'kän-stə-ˌtüt, -ˌtyüt\ *vb* **-tut·ed; -tut·ing** : to constitute again or anew; *esp* : to restore to a former condition by adding liquid ⟨*reconstituted* blood⟩ — **re·con·sti·tu·tion** \-ˌkän-stə-'tü-shən, -'tyü-\ *n*

re·con·struc·tion \ˌrē-kən-'strək-shən\ *n* : repair of an organ or part by reconstructive surgery ⟨breast ~⟩ — **re·con·struct** \ˌrē-kən-'strəkt\ *vb* — **re·con·struc·tive** \-'strək-tiv\ *adj*

reconstructive surgery *n* : surgery to restore function or normal appearance by remaking defective organs or parts

re·cov·er \ri-'kə-vər\ *vb* **re·cov·ered; re·cov·er·ing** : to regain a normal position or condition (as of health) — **re·cov·er·able** \ri-'kə-və-rə-bəl\ *adj*

recovered memory *n* : a forgotten memory of a traumatic event (as sexual abuse) experienced typically during childhood and recalled many years later that is sometimes held to be an invalid or false remembrance generated by outside influence

re·cov·ery \ri-'kə-və-rē\ *n, pl* **-er·ies** : the act of regaining or returning toward a normal or healthy state

recovery room *n* : a hospital room which is equipped with apparatus for meeting postoperative emergencies and in which surgical patients are kept during the immediate postoperative period for care and recovery from anesthesia — abbr. *RR*

rec·re·a·tion·al drug \ˌre-krē-'ā-shə-nəl-\ *n* : a drug (as cocaine, marijuana, or methamphetamine) used without medical justification for its psychoactive effects often in the belief that occasional use of such a substance is not habit-forming or addictive

recreational therapy *n* : therapy

based on engagement in recreational activities (as sports or music) esp. to enhance the functioning, independence, and well-being of individuals affected with a disabling condition — **recreational therapist** *n*

re·cru·des·cence \ˌrē-krü-ˈdes-ᵊns\ *n* : increased severity of a disease after a remission; *also* : recurrence of a disease after a brief intermission — **re·cru·desce** \ˌrē-krü-ˈdes\ *vb* — **re·cru·des·cent** \-ˈdes-ᵊnt\ *adj*

re·cruit·ment \ri-ˈkrüt-mənt\ *n* **1** : the increase in intensity of a reflex when the initiating stimulus is prolonged without alteration of intensity due to the activation of increasing numbers of motor neurons **2** : an abnormally rapid increase in the sensation of loudness with increasing sound intensity that occurs in deafness of neural origin

rect- *or* **recto-** *comb form* **1** : rectum ⟨*recta*l⟩ **2** : rectal and ⟨*recto*vaginal⟩

recta *pl of* RECTUM

recta — see VASA RECTA

rec·tal \ˈrekt-ᵊl\ *adj* : relating to, affecting, or being near the rectum ⟨∼ bleeding⟩ — **rec·tal·ly** *adv*

rectal artery *n* : any of three arteries supplying esp. the rectum: **a** : one arising from the internal pudendal artery and supplying the lower part of the rectum and the perineal region — called also *inferior hemorrhoidal artery, inferior rectal artery* **b** : one arising from the internal iliac artery and supplying the middle part of the rectum — called also *middle hemorrhoidal artery, middle rectal artery* **c** : one that is a continuation of the inferior mesenteric artery and that supplies the upper part of the rectum — called also *superior hemorrhoidal artery, superior rectal artery*

rectal vein *n* : any of three veins that receive blood from the rectal venous plexus: **a** : one draining the lower part of the rectal venous plexus and emptying into the internal pudendal vein — called also *inferior hemorrhoidal vein, inferior rectal vein* **b** : one draining the bladder, prostate, and seminal vesicle by way of the middle part of the rectal venous plexus and emptying into the internal iliac vein — called also *middle hemorrhoidal vein, middle rectal vein* **c** : one draining the upper part of the rectal venous plexus and forming the first part of the inferior mesenteric vein — called also *superior hemorrhoidal vein, superior rectal vein*

rectal venous plexus *n* : a plexus of veins that surrounds the rectum and empties esp. into the rectal veins — called also *rectal plexus*

recti *pl of* RECTUS

recto- — see RECT-

rec·to·cele \ˈrek-tə-ˌsēl\ *n* : herniation of the rectum through a defect in the intervening fascia into the vagina

rec·to·sig·moid \ˌrek-tō-ˈsig-ˌmȯid\ *n* : the distal part of the sigmoid colon and the proximal part of the rectum

rec·to·uter·ine pouch \ˌrek-tō-ˈyü-tə-ˌrīn-, -rən-\ *n* : a sac between the rectum and the uterus that is formed by a folding of the peritoneum — compare RECTOVESICAL POUCH

rec·to·vag·i·nal \-ˈvaj-ən-ᵊl\ *adj* : of, relating to, or connecting the rectum and the vagina ⟨a ∼ fistula⟩

rec·to·ves·i·cal fascia \ˌrek-tō-ˈve-si-kəl-\ *n* : a membrane derived from the pelvic fascia and investing the rectum, bladder, and adjacent parts

rectovesical pouch *n* : a sac between the rectum and the urinary bladder in males that is formed by a folding of the peritoneum — compare RECTOUTERINE POUCH

rec·tum \ˈrek-təm\ *n, pl* **rectums** *or* **rec·ta** \-tə\ : the terminal part of the intestine from the sigmoid colon to the anus

rec·tus \ˈrek-təs\ *n, pl* **rec·ti** \-ˌtī\ **1** : any of several straight muscles (as the rectus femoris) **2** : any of four muscles of the eyeball that arise from the border of the optic foramen and run forward to insert into the sclera of the eyeball: **a** : one that inserts into the superior aspect of the sclera — called also *rectus superior, superior rectus* **b** : one that inserts into the lateral aspect of the sclera — called also *lateral rectus, rectus lateralis* **c** : one that inserts into the medial aspect of the sclera — called also *medial rectus, rectus medialis* **d** : one that inserts into the inferior aspect of the sclera — called also *inferior rectus, rectus inferior*

rectus ab·do·mi·nis \-ab-ˈdä-mə-nəs\ *n* : a long flat muscle on either side of the linea alba extending along the whole length of the front of the abdomen, arising from the pubic crest and symphysis, inserted into the cartilages of the fifth, sixth, and seventh ribs, and acting to flex the spinal column, tense the anterior wall of the abdomen, and assist in compressing the contents of the abdomen

rectus ca·pi·tis posterior major \-ˈka-pə-təs-\ *n* : a muscle on each side of the back of the neck that arises from the spinous process of the axis, inserts into the lateral aspect of the inferior nuchal line and the adjacent inferior area of the occipital bone, and acts to extend and rotate the head

rectus capitis posterior minor *n* : a muscle on each side of the back of the neck that arises from the posterior arch of the atlas, inserts esp. into the medial aspect of the inferior nuchal line, and acts to extend the head

rectus fe·mo·ris \-ˈfe-mə-rəs\ *n* : a division of the quadriceps muscle lying in the anterior middle region of the thigh, arising from the ilium by two heads, inserted into the tuberosity of the tibia by a narrow flattened tendon, and acting to flex the thigh at the hip and with the rest of the quadriceps to extend the leg at the knee

rectus inferior *n* : RECTUS 2d

rectus lat·e·ra·lis \-ˌla-tə-ˈrā-ləs, -ˈra-\ *n* : RECTUS 2b

rectus me·di·a·lis \-ˌmē-dē-ˈā-ləs, -ˈa-\ *n* : RECTUS 2c

rectus oc·u·li \-ˈä-kyù-ˌlī, -ˌlē\ *n* : RECTUS 2

rectus superior *n* : RECTUS 2a

re·cum·bent \ri-ˈkəm-bənt\ *adj* : lying down ⟨a patient ∼ on a stretcher⟩ — **re·cum·ben·cy** \-bən-sē\ *n*

re·cu·per·a·tion \rē-ˌkü-pə-ˈrā-shən, -ˌkyü-\ *n* : restoration to health or strength — **re·cu·per·ate** \ri-ˈkü-pə-ˌrāt\ *vb*

re·cu·per·a·tive \-ˈkü-pə-ˌrā-tiv, -ˈkyü-\ *adj* **1** : of or relating to recuperation ⟨∼ powers⟩ **2** : aiding in recuperation : RESTORATIVE

re·cur·rence \ri-ˈkər-əns\ *n* **1** : return of symptoms of a disease after a remission **2** : reappearance of a tumor after previous removal — **re·cur** \ri-ˈkər\ *vb*

re·cur·rent \-ˈkər-ənt\ *adj* **1** : running or turning back in a direction opposite to a former course — used of various nerves and branches of vessels in the arms and legs **2** : returning or happening time after time ⟨∼ pain⟩ — **re·cur·rent·ly** *adv*

recurrent fever *n* : RELAPSING FEVER

recurrent laryngeal nerve *n* : LARYNGEAL NERVE b — called also *recurrent laryngeal*

red alga \ˈred-\ *n* : any of a division (Rhodophyta) of chiefly marine algae with mostly red pigmentation

red–blind *adj* : affected with protanopia

red blindness *n* : PROTANOPIA

red blood cell *n* : any of the hemoglobin-containing cells that carry oxygen to the tissues and are responsible for the red color of blood — called also *erythrocyte, red blood corpuscle, red cell, red corpuscle;* compare WHITE BLOOD CELL

red blood count *n* : a blood count of the red blood cells — abbr. *RBC*

red bone marrow *n* : BONE MARROW b

red bug \-ˌbəg\ *n, Southern & Midland* : CHIGGER 2

red cell *n* : RED BLOOD CELL

red corpuscle *n* : RED BLOOD CELL

red devils *n pl, slang* : REDS

red–green color blindness *n* : deficiency of color vision ranging from imperfect perception of red and green to an ability to see only tones of yellow, blue, and gray — called also *red-green blindness*

re·dia \ˈrē-dē-ə\ *n, pl* **re·di·ae** \-dē-ˌē\ *also* **re·di·as** : a larva produced within the sporocyst of many trematodes that produces another generation of larvae like itself or develops into a cercaria — **re·di·al** \-dē-əl\ *adj*

red·in·te·gra·tion \ri-ˌdin-tə-ˈgrā-shən, rē-\ *n* **1** : revival of the whole of a previous mental state when a phase of it recurs **2** : arousal of any response by a part of the complex of stimuli that orig. aroused that response — **red·in·te·gra·tive** \-ˈdin-tə-ˌgrā-tiv\ *adj*

red marrow *n* : BONE MARROW b

red nucleus *n* : a nucleus of gray matter in the tegmentum of the midbrain on each side of the middle line that receives fibers from the cerebellum of the opposite side by way of the superior cerebellar peduncle and gives rise to fibers of the rubrospinal tract of the opposite side

red·out \ˈred-ˌaùt\ *n* : a condition in which centripetal acceleration (as that created when an aircraft abruptly enters a dive) drives blood to the head and causes reddening of the visual field and headache — compare BLACKOUT, GRAYOUT

re·dox \ˈrē-ˌdäks\ *n* : OXIDATION-REDUCTION — **redox** *adj*

red pulp *n* : a parenchymatous tissue of the spleen that consists of loose plates or cords infiltrated with red blood cells — compare WHITE PULP

reds *n pl, slang* : red drug capsules containing the sodium salt of secobarbital — called also *red devils*

red tide *n* : seawater discolored by the presence of large numbers of dinoflagellates esp. of the genera *Gonyaulax* and *Gymnodinium* which produce a toxin poisonous esp. to many forms of marine vertebrate life and to humans who consume contaminated shellfish — see PARALYTIC SHELLFISH POISONING; compare SAXITOXIN

re·duce \ri-ˈdüs, -ˈdyüs\ *vb* **re·duced; re·duc·ing** **1** : to correct (as a fracture or a herniated mass) by bringing displaced or broken parts back into their normal positions **2 a** : to combine with or subject to the action of hydrogen **b** (1) : to change (an element or ion) from a higher to a lower oxidation state (2) : to add one or more electrons to (an atom or ion or molecule) **3** : to lose weight by dieting — **re·duc·ible** \-ˈdü-sə-bəl, -ˈdyü-\ *adj*

reducing *adj* : causing or facilitating reduction

reducing agent *n* : a substance (as hydrogen) that donates electrons or a share in its electrons to another substance — compare OXIDIZING AGENT

reducing sugar *n* : a sugar (as glucose or lactose) that is capable of reducing a mild oxidizing agent (as Fehling solution) — see BENEDICT'S TEST

re·duc·tase \ri-ˈdək-ˌtās, -ˌtāz\ *n* : an enzyme that catalyzes chemical reduction

re·duc·tion \ri-ˈdək-shən\ *n* **1** : the replacement or realignment of a body part in normal position or restoration of a bodily condition to normal **2** : the process of reducing by chemical or electrochemical means **3** : MEIOSIS; *specif* : production of the gametic chromosome number in the first meiotic division

reduction division *n* : the usu. first division of meiosis in which chromosome reduction occurs; *also* : MEIOSIS

re·dun·dant \ri-'dən-dənt\ *adj* : characterized by or containing an excess or superfluous amount

re·du·pli·ca·tion \ri-ˌdü-pli-'kā-shən, ˌrē-, -ˌdyü-\ *n* : an act or instance of doubling ⟨~ of the chromosomes⟩

red water *n* : any of several cattle diseases characterized by hematuria; *esp* : any of several babesioses (as Texas fever) in which hemoglobin liberated by the destruction of red blood cells appears in the urine

red worm *n* : BLOODWORM

Reed–Stern·berg cell \'rēd-'stərn-bərg-\ *n* : a binucleate or multinucleate acidophilic giant cell of B cell orgin found in the tissues in Hodgkin's disease

   Reed, Dorothy (1874–1964), American pathologist.

   Sternberg, Carl (1872–1935), Austrian pathologist.

re·ed·u·ca·tion \ˌrē-ˌe-jə-'kā-shən\ *n* **1** : training in the use of muscles in new functions or of prosthetic devices in old functions in order to replace or restore lost functions ⟨neuromuscular ~⟩ **2** : training to develop new behaviors (as habits) to replace others that are considered undesirable — **re·ed·u·cate** \-'e-jə-ˌkāt\ *vb*

reef·er \'rē-fər\ *n* : a marijuana cigarette; *also* : MARIJUANA 2

re·en·try \ˌrē-'en-trē\ *n, pl* **-tries** : a cardiac mechanism that is held to explain certain abnormal heart actions (as tachycardia) and that involves the transmission of a wave of depolarization along an alternate pathway when the original pathway is blocked with return of the impulse along the blocked pathway when the alternate pathway is refractory and then transmission along the open pathway resulting in an abnormality

re·ep·i·the·li·al·i·za·tion \ˌrē-ˌe-pə-ˌthē-lē-ə-li-'zā-shən\ *n* : restoration of epithelium over a denuded area (as a burn site) by natural growth or plastic surgery

re·fer \ri-'fər\ *vb* **re·ferred; re·fer·ring** **1** : to regard as coming from or localized in a certain portion of the body or of space **2** : to send or direct for diagnosis or treatment

re·fer·able *also* **re·fer·rable** \'re-fə-rə-bəl, ri-'fər-ə-\ *adj* : capable of being considered in relation to something else ⟨complaints ~ to the upper left abdominal quadrant⟩

ref·er·ence \'re-frəns, -fə-rəns\ *adj* : of known potency and used as a standard in the biological assay of a sample of the same drug of unknown strength

reference — see IDEA OF REFERENCE

re·fer·ral \ri-'fər-əl\ *n* **1** : the process of directing or redirecting (as a medical case or a patient) to an appropriate specialist or agency for definitive treatment **2** : one that is referred

referred pain *n* : a pain subjectively localized in one region though due to irritation in another region

¹re·fill \'rē-'fil\ *vb* : to fill (a prescription) a second or subsequent time — **re·fill·able** *adj*

²re·fill \'rē-ˌfil\ *n* : a prescription compounded and dispensed for a second or subsequent time without an order from the physician

re·flect \ri-'flekt\ *vb* **1** : to bend or fold back : impart a backward curve, bend, or fold to **2** : to push or lay aside (as tissue or an organ) during surgery in order to gain access to the part to be operated on **3** : to throw back light or sound — **re·flec·tion** \ri-'flek-shən\ *n*

¹re·flex \'rē-ˌfleks\ *n* **1** : an automatic and often inborn response to a stimulus that involves a nerve impulse passing inward from a receptor to the spinal cord and thence outward to an effector (as a muscle or gland) without reaching the level of consciousness and often without passing to the brain ⟨the knee-jerk ~⟩ **2** : the process that culminates in a reflex and comprises reception, transmission, and reaction **3 reflexes** *pl* : the power of acting or responding with adequate speed

²reflex *adj* **1** : bent, turned, or directed back : REFLECTED **2** : of, relating to, or produced by a reflex without intervention of consciousness

reflex arc *n* : the complete nervous path that is involved in a reflex

re·flex·ion *Brit var of* REFLECTION

re·flex·ive \ri-'flek-siv\ *adj* : characterized by habitual and unthinking behavior; *also* : relating to or consisting of a reflex

re·flex·ly *adv* : in a reflex manner : by means of reflexes

re·flexo·gen·ic \ri-ˌflek-sə-'je-nik\ *adj* **1** : causing or being the point of origin of reflexes ⟨a ~ zone⟩ **2** : originating reflexly

re·flex·ol·o·gy \ˌrē-ˌflek-'sä-lə-jē\ *n, pl* **-gies 1** : the study and interpretation of behavior in terms of simple and complex reflexes **2** : massage of the feet or hands based on the belief that pressure applied to specific points on these extremities benefits other parts of the body — **re·flex·ol·o·gist** \-jist\ *n*

reflex sympathetic dystrophy *n* : a painful disorder that usu. follows a localized injury, that is marked by burning pain, swelling, and motor and sensory disturbances esp. of an extremity, and that is associated with sympathetic nervous system dysfunction — abbr. *RSD;* see SHOULDER–HAND SYNDROME

re·flux \'rē-ˌfləks\ n 1 : a flowing back : REGURGITATION ⟨~ of gastric acid⟩ ⟨mitral valve ~⟩ 2 : GASTROESOPHAGEAL REFLUX — **reflux** adj — **reflux** vb

re·frac·tile \ri-'frak-təl, -ˌtīl\ adj : REFRACTIVE ⟨~ cells⟩

re·frac·tion \ri-'frak-shən\ n 1 : the deflection from a straight path undergone by a light ray or a wave of energy in passing obliquely from one medium (as air) into another (as glass) in which its velocity is different 2 a : the refractive power of the eye b : the act or technique of determining ocular refraction and identifying abnormalities as a basis for the prescription of corrective lenses — **re·fract** \ri-'frakt\ vb

re·frac·tion·ist \-shə-nist\ n : a person (as an optometrist) skilled esp. in the determination of errors of refraction in the eye

re·frac·tive \ri-'frak-tiv\ adj 1 : having power to refract ⟨a ~ lens⟩ 2 : relating to or due to refraction — **re·fractive·ly** adv

refractive index n : INDEX OF REFRACTION

re·frac·to·ri·ness \ri-'frak-tə-rē-nəs\ n : the insensitivity to further immediate stimulation that develops in irritable and esp. nervous tissue as a result of intense or prolonged stimulation

re·frac·to·ry \ri-'frak-tə-rē\ adj 1 : resistant to treatment or cure ⟨a ~ fulminant lesion⟩ 2 : unresponsive to stimulus 3 : resistant or not responding to an infectious agent : IMMUNE

refractory period n : the brief period immediately following the response esp. of a muscle or nerve before it recovers the capacity to make a second response — called also *refractory phase*; see ABSOLUTE REFRACTORY PERIOD, RELATIVE REFRACTORY PERIOD

re·frac·ture \ˌrē-'frak-chər\ vb **-tured; -tur·ing** : to break along the line of a previous fracture — **refracture** n

Ref·sum's disease \'ref-səmz-\ n : an autosomal recessive lipidosis characterized by faulty metabolism of phytanic acid resulting in its accumulation in the blood, retinitis pigmentosa, ataxia, deafness, and mental retardation

  Refsum, Sigvold Bernhard (1907–1991), Norwegian physician.

re·gen·er·a·tion \ri-ˌje-nə-'rā-shən, ˌrē-\ n : the renewal, regrowth, or restoration of a body or a bodily part, tissue, or substance after injury or as a normal bodily process ⟨continual ~ of epithelial cells⟩ — compare REGULATION 2a — **re·gen·er·ate** \ri-'je-nə-ˌrāt\ vb — **re·gen·er·a·tive** \ri-'je-nə-ˌrā-tiv, -rə-\ adj

re·gime \rā-'zhēm, ri-'jēm\ n : REGIMEN

reg·i·men \'re-jə-mən\ n : a systematic plan (as of diet, therapy, or medication) esp. when designed to improve and maintain the health of a patient

re·gion \'rē-jən\ n 1 : any of the major subdivisions into which the body or one of its parts is divisible 2 : an indefinite area surrounding a specified body part ⟨pain in the ~ of the heart⟩

re·gion·al \'rēj-ən-əl\ adj : of, relating to, or affecting a particular bodily region : LOCALIZED

regional anatomy n : a branch of anatomy dealing with regions of the body esp. with reference to diagnosis and treatment of disease or injury — called also *topographic anatomy*

regional anesthesia n : anesthesia of a region of the body accomplished by a series of encircling injections of an anesthetic — compare BLOCK ANESTHESIA

regional enteritis n : CROHN'S DISEASE

regional ileitis n : CROHN'S DISEASE

reg·is·tered \'re-ji-stərd\ adj : qualified by formal, official, or legal certification or authentication

registered nurse n : a graduate trained nurse who has been licensed by a state authority after passing qualifying examinations for registration — called also *RN*

reg·is·trar \'re-ji-ˌsträr\ n 1 : an admitting officer at a hospital 2 *Brit* : RESIDENT

reg·is·try \'re-ji-strē\ n, pl **-tries** 1 : a place where data, records, or laboratory samples are kept and usu. are made available for research or comparative study ⟨a cancer ~⟩ 2 : an establishment at which nurses available for employment are listed and through which they are hired

Reg·i·tine \'re-jə-ˌtēn\ n : a preparation of the mesylate of phentolamine — formerly a U.S. registered trademark

re·gres·sion \ri-'gre-shən\ n : a trend or shift toward a lower, less severe, or less perfect state: as a : progressive decline (as in size or severity) of a manifestation of disease ⟨tumor ~⟩ b (1) : a gradual loss of differentiation and function by a body part esp. as a physiological change accompanying aging ⟨menopausal ~ of the ovaries⟩ (2) : gradual loss (as in old age) of memories and acquired skills c : reversion to an earlier mental or behavioral level or to an earlier stage of psychosexual development (as in response to stress or to suggestion) — **re·gress** \ri-'gres\ vb — **re·gres·sive** \ri-'gre-siv\ adj

re·grow \ˌrē-'grō\ vb **re·grew** \-'grü\; **re·grown** \-'grōn\; **re·grow·ing** : to continue growth after interruption or injury — **re·growth** \-'grōth\ n

reg·u·lar \'re-gyə-lər\ adj : conforming to what is usual or normal: as a : recurring or functioning at fixed or normal intervals ⟨~ bowel movements⟩ b : having menstrual periods or bowel

movements at normal intervals —
reg·u·lar·i·ty \ˌre-gyə-'lar-ə-tē\ n —
reg·u·lar·ly adv

reg·u·la·tion \ˌre-gyə-'lā-shən, -gə-\ n
1 : the act of fixing or adjusting the time, amount, degree, or rate of something; also : the resulting state or condition **2 a** : the process of redistributing material (as in an embryo) to restore a damaged or lost part independent of new tissue growth — compare REGENERATION **b** : the mechanism by which an early embryo maintains normal development **3** : the control of the kind and rate of cellular processes by controlling the activity of individual genes — **reg·u·late** \-ˌlāt\ vb — **reg·u·la·to·ry** \-lə-ˌtōr-ē\ adj

reg·u·la·tive \'re-gyə-ˌlā-tiv, -lə\ adj : INDETERMINATE ⟨∼ eggs⟩

reg·u·la·tor \'re-gyə-ˌlā-tər\ n : REGULATORY GENE

regulatory gene or **regulator gene** n : a gene that regulates the expression of one or more structural genes by controlling the production of a protein (as a genetic repressor) which regulates their rate of transcription

re·gur·gi·tant \rē-'gər-jə-tənt\ adj : characterized by, allowing, or being a backward flow (as of blood) ⟨∼ cardiac valves⟩

re·gur·gi·ta·tion \rē-ˌgər-jə-'tā-shən\ n
1 : an act of bringing swallowed food back up into the mouth **2** : the backward flow of blood through a defective heart valve — see AORTIC REGURGITATION, MITRAL REGURGITATION — **re·gur·gi·tate** \rə-'gər-jə-ˌtāt\ vb

re·hab \'rē-ˌhab\ n, often attrib : REHABILITATION; esp : a program for rehabilitating esp. drug or alcohol abusers

re·ha·bil·i·tant \ˌrē-hə-'bi-lə-tənt, ˌrē-ə-\ n : an individual undergoing rehabilitation

re·ha·bil·i·ta·tion \ˌrē-hə-ˌbi-lə-'tā-shən, ˌrē-ə-\ n, often attrib **1 a** : the physical restoration of a sick or disabled person by therapeutic measures and reeducation **b** : the process of restoring an individual (as a drug addict) to a useful and constructive place in society through some form of vocational, correctional, or therapeutic retraining **2** : the result of rehabilitation : the state of undergoing or of having undergone rehabilitation — **re·ha·bil·i·tate** \-'bi-lə-ˌtāt\ vb — **re·ha·bil·i·ta·tive** \-'bi-lə-ˌtā-tiv\ adj

re·hears·al \ri-'hər-səl\ n **1** : a method for improving memory by mentally or verbally repeating over and over the information to be remembered **2** : the repeated mental review of a desired action or behavioral response

Reh·fuss tube \'rā-fəs-\ n : a flexible tube that is used esp. for withdrawing gastric juice from the stomach for analysis

Rehfuss, Martin Emil (1887–1964), American physician.

re·hy·drate \rē-'hī-ˌdrāt\ vb **-drat·ed; -drat·ing** : to restore fluid to (something dehydrated); esp : to restore body fluid lost in dehydration to ⟨∼ a patient⟩ — **re·hy·dra·tion** \ˌrē-hī-'drā-shən\ n

Rei·ki \'rā-ˌkē\ n : a system of hands-on touching based on the belief that such touching by an experienced practitioner produces beneficial effects by strengthening and normalizing certain vital energy fields held to exist within the body

re·im·plan·ta·tion \ˌrē-ˌim-plan-'tā-shən\ n **1** : the restoration of a bodily tissue or part (as a tooth) to the site from which it was removed **2** : the implantation of a fertilized egg in the uterus after it has been removed from the body and fertilized in vitro — **re·im·plant** \-im-'plant\ vb

re·in·farc·tion \ˌrē-in-'färk-shən\ n : an infarction occurring subsequent to a previous infarction

re·in·fec·tion \ˌrē-in-'fek-shən\ n : infection following recovery from or superimposed on a previous infection of the same type

re·in·force·ment \ˌrē-ən-'fōrs-mənt\ n : the action of causing a subject (as a student or an experimental animal) to learn to give or to increase the frequency of a desired response that in classical conditioning involves the repeated presentation of an unconditioned stimulus (as the sight of food) paired with a conditioned stimulus (as the sound of a bell) and that in operant conditioning involves the use of a reward following a correct response or a punishment following an incorrect response; also : the reward, punishment, or unconditioned stimulus used in reinforcement — **re·in·force** \-'fōrs\ vb

re·in·forc·er \-'fōr-sər\ n : a stimulus (as a reward or removal of an electric shock) that increases the probability of a desired response in operant conditioning by being applied or removed following the desired response

re·in·fuse \ˌrē-in-'fyüz\ vb **-fused; -fus·ing** : to return (as blood or lymphocytes) to the body by infusion after having been previously withdrawn — **re·in·fu·sion** \-'fyü-zhən\ n

re·in·jec·tion \ˌrē-in-'jek-shən\ n : an injection made subsequent to a previous injection — **re·in·ject** \-'jekt\ vb

re·in·ner·va·tion \ˌrē-ˌi-nər-'vā-shən, -in-ˌər-\ n : restoration of function esp. to a denervated muscle by supplying it with nerves by regrowth or by grafting — **re·in·ner·vate** \-i-'nər-ˌvāt, -'i-nər-\ vb

re·in·oc·u·la·tion \ˌrē-i-ˌnä-kyə-'lā-shən\ n : inoculation a second or subsequent time with the same organism as the original inoculation — **re·in·oc·u·late** \-'nä-kyə-ˌlāt\ vb

re·in·te·gra·tion \rē-ˌin-tə-ˈgrā-shən\ n
: repeated and renewed integration (as of the personality and mental activity after mental disorder) — **re·in·te·grate** \-ˈin-tə-ˌgrāt\ vb

Reiss·ner's membrane \ˈrīs-nərz-\ n
: VESTIBULAR MEMBRANE

Reissner, Ernst (1824–1878), German anatomist.

Rei·ter's syndrome \ˈrī-tərz-\ n : a disease that is usu. initiated by infection in genetically predisposed individuals and is characterized usu. by recurrence of arthritis, conjunctivitis, and urethritis — called also *Reiter's disease*

Reiter, Hans Conrad Julius (1881–1969), German bacteriologist.

re·jec·tion \ri-ˈjek-shən\ n **1** : the action of rebuffing, repelling, refusing to hear, or withholding love from another esp. by communicating negative feelings toward and a wish to be free of the other person **2** : an immune response in which foreign tissue (as of a skin graft or transplanted organ) is attacked by immune system components (as antibodies, T cells, and macrophages) of the recipient organism — **re·ject** \-ˈjekt\ vb — **re·jec·tive** \-ˈjek-tiv\ adj

re·lapse \ri-ˈlaps, ˈrē-\ n : a recurrence of illness; esp : a recurrence of symptoms of a disease after a period of improvement — **re·lapse** \ri-ˈlaps\ vb

relapsing febrile nodular non·sup·pu·ra·tive panniculitis \-ˌnän-ˈsə-pyə-rə-tiv-, -ˌrā-\ n : PANNICULITIS 2

relapsing fever n : a variable acute infectious disease that is marked by sudden recurring episodes of high fever which usu. last from three to seven days, are typically accompanied by myalgia, arthralgia, headache, nausea, and chills, and often end in a crisis stage and that is caused by a spirochete of the genus *Borrelia* transmitted by the bite of a body louse (*Pediculus humanus humanus*) or a tick of the genus *Ornithodoros* and found in the circulating blood

relapsing polychondritis n : a connective tissue disease esp. of cartilage that is characterized usu. by recurrent progressively destructive episodes of tissue inflammation (as of the ears, nose, larynx, and trachea)

re·late \ri-ˈlāt\ vb **re·lat·ed; re·lat·ing**
: to have meaningful social relationships : interact realistically ⟨an inability to ∼ to other people⟩

re·la·tion \ri-ˈlā-shən\ n **1** : the attitude or stance which two or more persons or groups assume toward one another ⟨race ∼s⟩ **2 a** : the state of being mutually or reciprocally interested (as in social matters) **b** relations pl : SEXUAL INTERCOURSE — **re·la·tion·al** \-shə-nəl\ adj

re·la·tion·ship \-shən-ˌship\ n **1** : the state of being related or interrelated

⟨the ∼ between diet and health⟩ **2 a**
: a state of affairs existing between those having relations or dealings ⟨doctor-patient ∼s⟩ **b** : an emotional attachment between individuals

relative biological effectiveness n
: the relative capacity of a particular ionizing radiation to produce a response in a biological system — abbr. *RBE*

relative humidity n : the ratio of the amount of water vapor actually present in the air to the greatest amount possible at the same temperature — compare ABSOLUTE HUMIDITY

relative refractory period n : the period shortly after the firing of a nerve fiber when partial repolarization has occurred and a greater than normal stimulus can stimulate a second response — called also *relative refractory phase;* compare ABSOLUTE REFRACTORY PERIOD

re·lax \ri-ˈlaks\ vb **1** : to slacken or make less tense or rigid ⟨alternately contracting and ∼ing their muscles⟩ **2** : to relieve from nervous tension **3** of a muscle or muscle fiber : to return to an inactive or resting state; esp : to become inactive and lengthen **4** : to relieve from constipation — **re·lax·ation** \ˌrē-ˌlak-ˈsā-shən, ri-ˌlak-\ n

re·lax·ant \ri-ˈlak-sənt\ n : a substance (as a drug) that relaxes; specif : one that relieves muscular tension — **relaxant** adj

re·lax·in \ri-ˈlak-sən\ n : a polypeptide sex hormone of the corpus luteum that facilitates birth by causing relaxation of the pelvic ligaments

re·leas·er \ri-ˈlē-sər\ n : a stimulus that serves as the initiator of complex reflex behavior

releasing factor n : HYPOTHALAMIC RELEASING FACTOR

Re·len·za \rə-ˈlen-zə\ trademark — used for a preparation of zanamivir

re·li·abil·i·ty \ri-ˌlī-ə-ˈbi-lə-tē\ n, pl -ties : the extent to which an experiment, test, or measuring procedure yields the same results on repeated trials — **re·li·able** \ri-ˈlī-ə-bəl\ adj

re·lief \ri-ˈlēf\ n : removal or lightening of something oppressive or distressing ⟨∼ of pain⟩

re·lieve \ri-ˈlēv\ vb **re·lieved; re·liev·ing 1** : to bring about the removal or alleviation of (pain or discomfort) **2** : to emit the contents of the bladder or bowels of (oneself) — **re·liev·er** n

rem \ˈrem\ n : the dosage of an ionizing radiation that will cause the same biological effect as one roentgen of X-ray or gamma-ray dosage — compare REP

REM \ˈrem\ n : RAPID EYE MOVEMENT

re·me·di·a·ble \ri-ˈmē-dē-ə-bəl\ adj
: capable of being remedied

re·me·di·al \ri-ˈmē-dē-əl\ adj : affording a remedy : intended as a remedy ⟨∼ surgery⟩

re·me·di·a·tion \ri-,mē-dē-'ā-shən\ *n* : the act or process of remedying

rem·e·dy \'re-mə-dē\ *n, pl* **-dies** : a medicine, application, or treatment that relieves or cures a disease — **remedy** *vb*

re·min·er·al·i·za·tion \,rē-,mi-nə-rə-lə-'zā-shən\ *n* : the restoring of minerals to demineralized structures or substances ⟨∼ of bone⟩ — **re·min·er·al·ize** \-'mi-nə-rə-,līz\ *vb*

re·mis·sion \ri-'mi-shən\ *n* : a state or period during which the symptoms of a disease are abated

re·mit \ri-'mit\ *vb* **re·mit·ted; re·mit·ting** : to abate symptoms for a period : go into or be in remission

re·mit·tent \ri-'mit-ᵊnt\ *adj* : marked by alternating periods of abatement and increase of symptoms ⟨∼ fever⟩

REM latency *n* : the time span between the start of sleeping and the start of REM sleep

re·mod·el·ing \rē-'mä-dᵊl-iŋ\ *n* : the process of bone resorption and formation that involves the activity of osteoclasts and osteoblasts — **re·mod·el** \-'mä-dᵊl\ *vb*

REM sleep *n* : a state of sleep that recurs cyclically several times during a normal period of sleep and that is characterized by increased neuronal activity of the forebrain and midbrain, by depressed muscle tone, and esp. in humans by dreaming, rapid eye movements, and vascular congestion of the sex organs — called also *paradoxical sleep, rapid eye movement sleep;* compare SLOW-WAVE SLEEP

re·nal \'rēn-ᵊl\ *adj* : relating to, involving, affecting, or located in the region of the kidneys : NEPHRIC

renal artery *n* : either of two branches of the abdominal aorta of which each supplies one of the kidneys and gives off smaller branches to the ureter, adrenal gland, and adjoining structures

renal calculus *n* : KIDNEY STONE

renal cast *n* : a cast of a renal tubule consisting of granular, hyaline, albuminoid, or other material formed in and discharged from the kidney in renal disease

renal clearance *n* : CLEARANCE

renal colic *n* : the severe pain produced by the passage of a calculus from the kidney through the ureter

renal column *n* : any of the masses of cortical tissue extending between the sides of the renal pyramids of the kidney as far as the renal pelvis — called also *Bertin's column, column of Bertin*

renal corpuscle *n* : the part of a nephron that consists of Bowman's capsule with its included glomerulus — called also *Malpighian body, Malpighian corpuscle*

renal diabetes *n* : RENAL GLYCOSURIA

renal glycosuria *n* : excretion of glucose associated with increased permeability of the kidneys without increased sugar concentration in the blood

renal hypertension *n* : hypertension that is associated with disease of the kidneys and is caused by kidney damage or malfunctioning

renal osteodystrophy *n* : a painful rachitic condition of abnormal bone growth that is associated with chronic acidosis, hypocalcemia, hyperplasia of the parathyroid glands, and hyperphosphatemia caused by chronic renal insufficiency — called also *renal rickets*

renal papilla *n* : the apex of a renal pyramid which projects into the lumen of a calyx of the kidney and through which collecting tubules discharge urine

renal pelvis *n* : a funnel-shaped structure in each kidney that is formed at one end by the expanded upper portion of the ureter lying in the renal sinus and at the other end by the union of the calyxes of the kidney

renal plexus *n* : a plexus of the autonomic nervous system that arises esp. from the celiac plexus, surrounds the renal artery, and accompanies it into the kidney which it innervates

renal pyramid *n* : any of the conical masses that form the medullary substance of the kidney, project as the renal papillae into the renal pelvis, and are made up of bundles of straight uriniferous tubules opening at the apex of the conical mass — called also *Malpighian pyramid*

renal rickets *n* : RENAL OSTEODYSTROPHY

renal sinus *n* : the main cavity of the kidney that is an expansion behind the hilum and contains the renal pelvis, calyxes, and the major renal vessels

renal syndrome — see HEMORRHAGIC FEVER WITH RENAL SYNDROME

renal threshold *n* : the concentration level up to which a substance (as glucose) in the blood is prevented from passing through the kidneys into the urine

renal tubular acidosis *n* : decreased ability of the kidneys to excrete hydrogen ions that is associated with a defect in the renal tubules without a defect in the glomeruli and that results in the production of urine deficient in acidity

renal tubule *n* : the part of a nephron that leads away from a glomerulus, that is made up of a proximal convoluted tubule, loop of Henle, and distal convoluted tubule, and that empties into a collecting tubule

renal vein *n* : a short thick vein that is formed in each kidney by the convergence of the interlobar veins, leaves the kidney through the hilum, and empties into the inferior vena cava

Ren·du–Os·ler–We·ber   disease

\rän-'dü-'äs-lər-'we-bər-, ˌrän-'dyü-\ *n* : HEREDITARY HEMORRHAGIC TELANGIECTASIA

Ren·du \rän-'dǖ\, **Henry–Jules–Louis–Marie (1844–1902),** French physician.

Osler, Sir William (1849–1919), American physician.

F. P. Weber — see WEBER-CHRISTIAN DISEASE

Ren·ese \'re-ˌnēz\ *trademark* — used for a preparation of polythiazide

reni- or **reno-** *comb form* **1** : kidney ⟨*reni*form⟩ **2** : renal and ⟨*reno*vascular⟩

re·ni·form \'rē-nə-ˌfôrm, 're-\ *adj* : suggesting a kidney in outline

re·nin \'rē-nən, 're-\ *n* : a proteolytic enzyme of the blood that is produced and secreted by the juxtaglomerular cells of the kidney and hydrolyzes angiotensinogen to angiotensin I

ren·nin \'re-nən\ *n* : an enzyme that coagulates milk, occurs esp. with pepsin in the gastric juice of young animals, and is used chiefly in making cheese

re·no·gram \'rē-nə-ˌgram\ *n* : a radiograph made by renography

re·nog·ra·phy \rē-'nä-grə-fē\ *n, pl* **-phies** : the radiographic visualization of the kidneys and ureters after administration of a radiolabeled substance — **re·no·graph·ic** \ˌrē-nə-'gra-fik\ *adj*

re·no·vas·cu·lar \ˌrē-nō-'vas-kyə-lər\ *adj* : of, relating to, or involving the blood vessels of the kidneys ⟨~ hypertension⟩

Ren·shaw cell \'ren-ˌshò-\ *n* : an interneuron in the ventral horn of gray matter of the spinal cord that has an inhibitory effect on motor neurons

Renshaw, Birdsey (1911–1948), American neurologist.

re·oc·clu·sion \ˌrē-ə-'klü-zhən\ *n* : the reoccurrence of occlusion in an artery after it has been treated (as by balloon angioplasty) with apparent success — **re·oc·clude** \-ə-'klüd\ *vb*

re·op·er·a·tion \ˌrē-ˌä-pə-'rā-shən\ *n* : an operation to correct a condition not corrected by a previous operation or to correct the complications of a previous operation — **re·op·er·ate** \-'ä-pə-ˌrāt\ *vb*

Reo·Pro \rē-ō-ˌprō\ *trademark* — used for a preparation of abciximab

reo·vi·rus \ˌrē-ō-'vī-rəs\ *n* : any of a family (*Reoviridae*) of double-stranded RNA viruses that have a capsid with one to three concentric protein layers and include the rotaviruses and the causative agents of bluetongue and Colorado tick fever — **reo·vi·ral** \-rəl\ *adj*

rep \'rep\ *n, pl* **rep** or **reps** : the dosage of an ionizing radiation that will develop the same amount of energy upon absorption in human tissues as one roentgen of X-ray or gamma-ray exposure — compare REM

rep *abbr* [Latin *repetatur*] let it be repeated — used in writing prescriptions

re·peat \ri-'pēt, 'rē-ˌ\ *n* : a genetic duplication in which the duplicated parts are adjacent to each other along the chromosome

re·per·fu·sion \ˌrē-pər-'fyü-zhən\ *n* : restoration of the flow of blood to a previously ischemic tissue or organ (as the heart) ⟨~ following heart attack⟩ — **re·per·fuse** \-'fyüz\ *vb*

repetition compulsion *n* : an irresistible tendency to repeat an emotional experience or to return to a previous psychological state

repetitive strain injury *n* : any of various musculoskeletal disorders (as carpal tunnel syndrome or tendinitis) that are caused by cumulative damage to muscles, tendons, ligaments, nerves, or joints (as of the hand or arm) from highly repetitive movements and that are characterized esp. by pain, weakness, and loss of feeling — called also *cumulative trauma disorder, repetitive motion injury, repetitive stress injury, repetitive stress syndrome, RSI*

replacement therapy *n* : therapy involving the supplying of something (as hormones or blood) lacking from or lost to the system — see ESTROGEN REPLACEMENT THERAPY, HORMONE REPLACEMENT THERAPY

re·plan·ta·tion \ˌrē-ˌplan-'tā-shən\ *n* : reattachment or reinsertion of a bodily part (as a limb or tooth) after separation from the body — **re·plant** \rē-'plant\ *vb*

rep·li·case \'re-pli-ˌkās, -ˌkāz\ *n* : a polymerase that promotes synthesis of a particular RNA in the presence of a template of RNA — called also *RNA replicase, RNA synthetase*

rep·li·ca·tion \ˌre-plə-'kā-shən\ *n* **1** : the action or process of reproducing or duplicating ⟨~ of DNA⟩ **2** : performance of an experiment or procedure more than once — **rep·li·cate** \'re-pli-ˌkāt\ *vb* — **rep·li·cate** \-kət\ *n* — **rep·li·ca·tive** \'re-pli-ˌkā-tiv\ *adj*

rep·li·con \'re-pli-ˌkän\ *n* : a linear or circular section of DNA or RNA which replicates sequentially as a unit

re·po·lar·i·za·tion \ˌrē-pō-lə-rə-'zā-shən\ *n* : restoration of the difference in charge between the inside and outside of the plasma membrane of a muscle fiber or cell following depolarization — **re·po·lar·ize** \-'pō-lə-ˌrīz\ *vb*

re·port·able \ri-'pōr-tə-bəl\ *adj* : required by law to be reported ⟨~ diseases⟩

re·po·si·tion \ˌrē-pə-'zi-shən\ *vb* : to return to or place in a normal or proper position ⟨~ a dislocated shoulder⟩

re·pos·i·to·ry \ri-'pä-zə-ˌtōr-ē\ *adj, of a drug* : designed to act over a prolonged period ⟨~ penicillin⟩

re·press \ri-'pres\ *vb* **1** : to exclude from consciousness ⟨∼ conflicts⟩ **2** : to inactivate (a gene or formation of a gene product) by allosteric combination at a DNA binding site

re·pressed \ri-'prest\ *adj* : subjected to or marked by repression ⟨∼ anger⟩

re·press·ible \ri-'pre-sə-bəl\ *adj* : capable of being repressed

re·pres·sion \ri-'pre-shən\ *n* **1** : the action or process of repressing ⟨gene ∼⟩ **2 a** : a process by which unacceptable desires or impulses are excluded from consciousness and left to operate in the unconscious — compare SUPPRESSION c **b** : an item so excluded

re·pres·sive \ri-'pre-siv\ *adj* : tending to repress or to cause repression

re·pres·sor \ri-'pre-sər\ *n* : one that represses; *esp* : a protein that is determined by a regulatory gene, binds to a genetic operator, and inhibits the initiation of transcription of messenger RNA

re·pro·duce \ˌrē-prə-'düs, -'dyüs\ *vb* **-duced; -duc·ing 1** : to produce (new individuals of the same kind) by a sexual or asexual process **2** : to achieve (an original result or score) again or anew by repeating an experiment or test

re·pro·duc·tion \ˌrē-prə-'dək-shən\ *n* : the act or process of reproducing; *specif* : the process by which plants and animals give rise to offspring — **re·pro·duc·tive** \ˌrē-prə-'dək-tiv\ *adj* — **re·pro·duc·tive·ly** *adv*

reproductive system *n* : the system of organs and parts which function in reproduction consisting in the male esp. of the testes, penis, seminal vesicles, prostate, and urethra and in the female esp. of the ovaries, fallopian tubes, uterus, vagina, and vulva

RES *abbr* reticuloendothelial system

res·cin·na·mine \re-'si-nə-ˌmēn, -mən\ *n* : an antihypertensive, tranquilizing, and sedative drug $C_{35}H_{42}N_2O_9$

re·sect \ri-'sekt\ *vb* : to perform resection on ⟨∼ an ulcer⟩ — **re·sect·abil·i·ty** \ri-ˌsek-tə-'bi-lə-tē\ *n* — **re·sect·able** \ri-'sek-tə-bəl\ *adj*

re·sec·tion \ri-'sek-shən\ *n* : the surgical removal of part of an organ or structure ⟨∼ of the lower bowel⟩

re·sec·to·scope \ri-'sek-tə-ˌskōp\ *n* : an instrument consisting of a tubular fenestrated sheath with a sliding knife within it that is used for surgery within cavities (as of the prostate through the urethra)

re·ser·pine \ri-'sər-ˌpēn, 're-sər-pən\ *n* : an alkaloid $C_{33}H_{40}N_2O_9$ extracted esp. from the root of rauwolfias and used in the treatment of hypertension, mental disorders, and tension states — see RAUDIXIN, SERPASIL

reservatus — see COITUS RESERVATUS

re·serve \ri-'zərv\ *n* **1** : something stored or kept available for future use or need ⟨oxygen ∼⟩ — see CARDIAC RESERVE **2** : the capacity of a solution to neutralize alkali or acid when its reaction is shifted from one hydrogen-ion concentration to another — **reserve** *adj*

res·er·voir \'re-zər-ˌvwär, -ˌvwòr\ *n* **1** : a space (as the cavity of a glandular acinus) in which a body fluid is stored **2** : an organism in which a parasite that is pathogenic for some other species lives and multiplies without damaging its host; *also* : a noneconomic organism within which a pathogen of economic or medical importance flourishes without regard to its pathogenicity for the reservoir ⟨rats are ∼s of plague⟩ — compare CARRIER

reservoir host *n* : RESERVOIR 2

res·i·den·cy \'re-zəd-ən-sē\ *n, pl* **-cies** : a period of advanced medical training and education that normally follows graduation from medical school and licensing to practice medicine and that consists of supervised practice of a specialty in a hospital and in its outpatient department and instruction from specialists on the hospital staff

res·i·dent \'re-zə-dənt\ *n* : a physician serving a residency

res·i·den·tial \ˌre-zə-'den-shəl\ *adj* : provided to patients residing in a facility ⟨∼ drug treatment⟩

¹re·sid·u·al \ri-'zi-jə-wəl\ *adj* **1** : of, relating to, or being something that remains: as **a** : remaining after a disease or operation ⟨∼ paralysis⟩ **b** : remaining in a body cavity after maximum normal expulsion has occurred ⟨∼ urine⟩ — see RESIDUAL VOLUME **2 a** : leaving a residue that remains effective for some time after application ⟨∼ insecticides⟩ **b** : of or relating to a residual insecticide

²residual *n* **1** : an internal aftereffect of experience or activity that influences later behavior **2** : a residual abnormality (as a scar or limp)

residual air *n* : RESIDUAL VOLUME

residual volume *n* : the volume of air still remaining in the lungs after the most forcible expiration possible and amounting usu. to 60 to 100 cubic inches (980 to 1640 cubic centimeters) — called also *residual air;* compare SUPPLEMENTAL AIR

res·i·due \'re-zə-ˌdü, -ˌdyü\ *n* : something that remains after a part is taken, separated, or designated; *specif* : a constituent structural unit of a usu. complex molecule ⟨amino acid ∼s in a protein⟩

res·in \'rez-ⁿn\ *n* : any of various substances obtained from the gum or sap of some trees and used esp. in various varnishes and plastics and in medicine; *also* : a comparable synthetic product — **res·in·ous** \'rez-ⁿn-əs\ *adj*

re·sis·tance \ri-'zis-təns\ *n* **1 a** : the

inherent ability of an organism to resist harmful influences (as infection) **b** : the capacity of a species or strain of microorganism to survive exposure to a toxic agent (as a drug) formerly effective against it   **2 a** : the opposition offered by a body to the passage through it of a steady electric current **b** : opposition or impediment to the flow of a fluid (as blood or respiratory gases) through one or more passages — see VASCULAR RESISTANCE   **3 a** : psychological defense mechanism wherein a psychoanalysis patient rejects, denies, or otherwise resists therapeutic efforts by the analyst — **re·sis·tant** \-tənt\ *adj*

re·so·cial·i·za·tion \‚rē-‚sō-shə-lə-'zā-shən\ *n* : readjustment of an individual to life in society

res·o·lu·tion \‚re-zə-'lü-shən\ *n* **1** : the separating of a chemical compound or mixture into its constituents   **2** : the process or capability of making distinguishable the individual parts of an object, closely adjacent optical images, or sources of light   **3** : the subsidence of a pathological state (as inflammation) — **re·solve** \ri-'zälv, -'zȯlv\ *vb*

res·o·nance \'rez-ᵊn-əns\ *n* **1** : a quality imparted to voiced sounds by vibration in anatomical resonating chambers or cavities (as the mouth or the nasal cavity)   **2** : the sound elicited on percussion of the chest   **3** : the enhancement of an atomic, nuclear, or particle reaction or a scattering event by excitation of internal motion in the system   **b** : MAGNETIC RESONANCE

re·sorb \rē-'sȯrb, -'zȯrb\ *vb* : to break down and assimilate (something previously differentiated) ⟨∼ed bone⟩ — **re·sorb·able** \-ə-bəl\ *adj*

res·or·cin \rə-'zȯrs-ᵊn\ *n* : RESORCINOL

res·or·cin·ol \-‚ȯl, -‚ōl\ *n* : a crystalline phenol $C_6H_6O_2$ used in medicine as a fungicidal, bactericidal, and keratolytic agent

resorcinol monoacetate *n* : a liquid compound $C_8H_8O_3$ that slowly liberates resorcinol and that is used esp. to treat diseases of the scalp

re·sorp·tion \rē-'sȯrp-shən, -'zȯrp-\ *n* : the action or process of resorbing something — **re·sorp·tive** \-tiv\ *adj*

re·spi·ra·ble \'res-pə-rə-bəl, ri-'spī-rə-\ *adj* : fit for breathing; *also* : capable of being taken in by breathing

res·pi·ra·tion \‚res-pə-'rā-shən\ *n* **1 a** : the movement of respiratory gases (as oxygen and carbon dioxide) into and out of the lungs   **b** : a single complete act of breathing ⟨30 ∼s per minute⟩   **2** : the physical and chemical processes by which an organism supplies its cells and tissues with the oxygen needed for metabolism and relieves them of the carbon dioxide formed in energy-producing reactions   **3** : CELLULAR RESPIRATION

res·pi·ra·tor \'res-pə-‚rā-tər\ *n* **1** : a device (as a gas mask) worn over the mouth or nose to protect the respiratory system by filtering out dangerous substances (as dust or fumes)   **2** : a device for maintaining artificial respiration — called also *ventilator*

res·pi·ra·to·ry \'res-pə-rə-‚tōr-ē, ri-'spī-rə-\ *adj* **1** : of or relating to respiration ⟨∼ diseases⟩   **2** : serving for or functioning in respiration ⟨∼ organs⟩

respiratory acidosis *n* : acidosis caused by excessive retention of carbon dioxide due to a respiratory abnormality (as obstructive lung disease)

respiratory alkalosis *n* : alkalosis that is caused by excessive elimination of carbon dioxide due to a respiratory abnormality (as hyperventilation)

respiratory center *n* : a region in the medulla oblongata that regulates respiratory movements

respiratory chain *n* : the metabolic pathway along which electron transport occurs in cellular respiration; *also* : the series of enzymes involved in this pathway

respiratory distress syndrome *n* : a respiratory disorder occurring in newborn premature infants that is characterized by deficiency of the surfactant coating the inner surface of the lungs resulting in failure of the lungs to expand and contract properly during breathing — abbr. *RDS;* called also *hyaline membrane disease;* see ACUTE RESPIRATORY DISTRESS SYNDROME

respiratory pigment *n* : any of various permanently or intermittently colored conjugated proteins and esp. hemoglobin that function in the transfer of oxygen in cellular respiration

respiratory quotient *n* : the ratio of the volume of carbon dioxide given off in respiration to that of the oxygen consumed — abbr. *RQ*

respiratory syncytial virus *n* : a paramyxovirus (species *Human respiratory syncytial virus* of the genus *Pneumovirus*) that forms syncytia in tissue culture and is responsible for severe respiratory diseases (as bronchopneumonia and bronchiolitis) in children and esp. in infants — abbr. *RSV*

respiratory system *n* : a system of organs functioning in respiration and consisting esp. of the nose, nasal passages, nasopharynx, larynx, trachea, bronchi, and lungs — called also *respiratory tract;* see LOWER RESPIRATORY TRACT, UPPER RESPIRATORY TRACT

respiratory therapist *n* : a specialist in respiratory therapy

respiratory therapy *n* : therapy concerned with the maintenance or improvement of respiratory functioning

res·pi·ra·to·ry tract *n* : RESPIRATORY SYSTEM

res·pi·ra·to·ry tree *n* : the trachea, bronchi, and bronchioles

re·spire \ri-ˈspīr\ *vb* **re·spired; re·spir·ing** 1 : BREATHE; *specif* : to inhale and exhale air successively 2 *of a cell or tissue* : to take up oxygen and produce carbon dioxide through oxidation

res·pi·rom·e·ter \ˌres-pə-ˈrä-mə-tər\ *n* : an instrument for studying the character and extent of respiration — **res·pi·ro·met·ric** \ˌres-pə-rō-ˈme-trik\ *adj* — **res·pi·rom·e·try** \ˌres-pə-ˈrä-mə-trē\ *n*

re·spond \ri-ˈspänd\ *vb* 1 : to react in response 2 : to show favorable reaction ⟨∼ to chemotherapy⟩

re·spon·dent \ri-ˈspän-dənt\ *adj* : relating to or being behavior or responses to a stimulus that are followed by a reward ⟨∼ conditioning⟩

re·spond·er \ri-ˈspän-dər\ *n* : one that responds (as to treatment)

re·sponse \ri-ˈspäns\ *n* : the activity or inhibition of previous activity of an organism or any of its parts resulting from stimulation ⟨a conditioned ∼⟩

re·spon·sive \ri-ˈspän-siv\ *adj* : making a response; *esp* : responding to treatment — **re·spon·sive·ness** *n*

rest \ˈrest\ *n* 1 : a state of repose or sleep; *also* : a state of inactivity or motionlessness — see BED REST 2 : the part of a partial denture that rests on an abutment tooth, distributes stresses, and holds the clasp in position 3 : a firm cushion used to raise or support a portion of the body during surgery ⟨a kidney ∼⟩ — **rest** *vb*

re·ste·no·sis \ˌres-tə-ˈnō-səs\ *n, pl* **-no·ses** \-ˌsēz\ : the reoccurrence of stenosis in a blood vessel or heart valve following apparently successful treatment (as by balloon angioplasty)

rest home *n* : an establishment that provides housing and general care for the aged or the convalescent

res·ti·form body \ˈres-tə-ˌfȯrm-\ *n* : CEREBELLAR PEDUNCLE c

rest·ing *adj* 1 : not physiologically active 2 : occurring in or performed on a subject at rest ⟨a ∼ tremor⟩

resting cell *n* : a living cell with a nucleus that is not undergoing division (as by mitosis)

resting potential *n* : the membrane potential of a cell that is not exhibiting the activity resulting from a stimulus — compare ACTION POTENTIAL

resting stage *n* : INTERPHASE

rest·less \ˈrest-ləs\ *adj* 1 : deprived of rest or sleep 2 : providing no rest

restless legs syndrome *n* : a neurological disorder of uncertain pathophysiology that is characterized by aching, burning, crawling, or creeping sensations of the legs that occur esp. at night usu. when lying down (as

before sleep) — called also *restless legs*

res·to·ra·tion \ˌres-tə-ˈrā-shən\ *n* : the act of restoring or the condition of being restored: as **a** : a returning to a normal or healthy condition **b** : the replacing of missing teeth or crowns; *also* : a dental replacement (as a denture) used for restoration — **re·stor·ative** \ri-ˈstȯr-ə-tiv\ *adj or n*

re·store \ri-ˈstȯr\ *vb* **re·stored; re·stor·ing** : to bring back to or put back into a former or original state

Res·to·ril \ˈres-tə-ˌril\ *trademark* — used for a preparation of temazepam

re·straint \ri-ˈstränt\ *n* : a device (as a straitjacket) that restricts movement

re·stric·tion \ri-ˈstrik-shən\ *n, often attrib* : the breaking of double-stranded DNA into fragments by restriction enzymes ⟨∼ sites⟩

restriction endonuclease *n* : RESTRICTION ENZYME

restriction enzyme *n* : any of various enzymes that break DNA into fragments at specific sites in the interior of the molecule and are often used as tools in molecular analysis

restriction fragment *n* : a segment of DNA produced by the action of a restriction enzyme on a molecule of DNA

restriction fragment length polymorphism *n* : variation in the length of a restriction fragment produced by a specific restriction enzyme acting on DNA from different individuals that usu. results from a genetic mutation (as an insertion or deletion) and that may be used as a genetic marker — called also *RFLP*

rest seat *n* : an area on the surface of a tooth that is specially prepared (as by grinding) for the attachment of a dental rest

re·sus·ci·ta·tion \ri-ˌsə-sə-ˈtā-shən, rē-\ *n* : the act of reviving from apparent death or from unconsciousness — see CARDIOPULMONARY RESUSCITATION — **re·sus·ci·tate** \-ˈsə-sə-ˌtāt\ *vb* — **re·sus·ci·ta·tive** \ri-ˈsə-sə-ˌtā-tiv\ *adj*

re·sus·ci·ta·tor \ri-ˈsə-sə-ˌtā-tər\ *n* : an apparatus used to restore respiration (as of a partially asphyxiated person)

res·ver·a·trol \rez-ˈvir-ə-ˌtrȯl\ *n* : a compound $C_{14}H_{12}O_3$ found esp. in the skin of grapes and certain grape-derived products (as red wine) that has been linked to a reduced risk of coronary artery disease and cancer

re·tain·er \ri-ˈtā-nər\ *n* 1 : the part of a dental replacement (as a bridge) by which it is made fast to adjacent natural teeth 2 : a dental appliance used to hold teeth in their correct position esp. following orthodontic treatment

re·tar·da·tion \ˌrē-ˌtär-ˈdā-shən, ri-\ *n* 1 : an abnormal slowness of thought or action; *esp* : MENTAL RETARDATION 2 : slowness in development or progress

re·tard·ed \ri-'tär-dəd\ *adj, sometimes offensive* : slow or limited in intellectual or emotional development : characterized by mental retardation

retch \'rech\ *vb* : to make an effort to vomit; *also* : VOMIT — **retch** *n*

re·te \'rē-tē, 'rā-\ *n, pl* **re·tia** \-tē-ə\ **1** : a network esp. of blood vessels or nerves : PLEXUS **2** : an anatomical part resembling or including a network

re·ten·tion \ri-'ten-chən\ *n* **1** : the act of retaining: as **a** : abnormal retaining of a fluid or secretion in a body cavity ⟨~ of urine⟩ **b** : the holding in place of a tooth or dental replacement by means of a retainer **2** : a preservation of the aftereffects of experience and learning that makes recall or recognition possible

re·ten·tive \ri-'ten-tiv\ *adj* : tending to retain: as **a** : having a good memory ⟨a ~ mind⟩ **b** : of, relating to, or being a dental retainer

rete peg *n* : any of the inwardly directed prolongations of the Malpighian layer of the epidermis that mesh with the dermal papillae of the skin

rete testis *n, pl* **retia tes·ti·um** \-'tes-tē-əm\ : the network of tubules in the mediastinum testis

retia *pl of* RETE

reticul- *or* **reticulo-** *comb form* : reticulum ⟨*reticulo*cyte⟩

reticula *pl of* RETICULUM

re·tic·u·lar \ri-'ti-kyə-lər\ *adj* : of, relating to, or forming a network

reticular activating system *n* : a part of the reticular formation that extends from the brain stem to the midbrain and thalamus with connections distributed throughout the cerebral cortex and that controls the degree of activity of the central nervous system (as in maintaining sleep and wakefulness)

reticular cell *n* : RETICULUM CELL; *esp* : RETICULOCYTE

reticular fiber *n* : any of the thin branching fibers of connective tissue that form an intricate interstitial network ramifying through other tissues and organs

reticular formation *n* : a mass of nerve cells and fibers situated primarily in the brain stem and functioning upon stimulation esp. in arousal of the organism — called also *reticular substance*

reticularis — see LIVEDO RETICULARIS, ZONA RETICULARIS

reticular lamina *n* : a thin extracellular layer that sometimes lies below the basal lamina, is composed chiefly of collagenous fibers, and serves to anchor the basal lamina to underlying connective tissue

reticular layer *n* : the deeper layer of the dermis formed of interlacing fasciculi of white fibrous tissue

reticular tissue *n* : RETICULUM 2a

re·tic·u·late body \ri-'ti-kyə-lət-\ *n* : a chlamydial cell of a spherical intracellular form that is larger than an elementary body and reproduces by binary fission

re·tic·u·lin \ri-'ti-kyə-lən\ *n* : a protein substance similar to collagen that is a constituent of reticular tissue

re·tic·u·lo·cyte \ri-'ti-kyə-lō-ˌsīt\ *n* : an immature red blood cell that appears esp. during regeneration of lost blood and that has a fine basophilic reticulum formed of the remains of ribosomes — **re·tic·u·lo·cyt·ic** \ri-ˌti-kyə-lō-'si-tik\ *adj*

re·tic·u·lo·cy·to·pe·nia \ri-ˌti-kyə-lō-ˌsī-tə-'pē-nē-ə\ *n* : an abnormal decrease in the number of reticulocytes in the blood

re·tic·u·lo·cy·to·sis \-ˌsī-'tō-səs\ *n, pl* **-to·ses** \-ˌsēz\ : an increase in the number of reticulocytes in the blood

re·tic·u·lo·en·do·the·li·al \ri-ˌti-kyə-lō-ˌen-də-'thē-lē-əl\ *adj* : of, relating to, or being the reticuloendothelial system ⟨~ tissue⟩ ⟨~ cells⟩

reticuloendothelial system *n* : MONONUCLEAR PHAGOCYTE SYSTEM; *broadly* : the mononuclear phagocyte system plus certain other cells now known to be pinocytic or only weakly phagocytic

re·tic·u·lo·en·do·the·li·o·sis \-ˌthē-lē-'ō-səs\ *n, pl* **-o·ses** \-ˌsēz\ : any of several disorders characterized by proliferation of phagocytic cells (as macrophages) — called also *reticulosis*

re·tic·u·lo·sar·co·ma \-ˌsär-'kō-mə\ *n, pl* **-mas** *or* **-ma·ta** \-mə-tə\ : HISTIOCYTIC LYMPHOMA

re·tic·u·lo·sis \ri-ˌti-kyə-'lō-səs\ *n, pl* **-lo·ses** \-ˌsēz\ : RETICULOENDOTHELIOSIS

re·tic·u·lo·spi·nal tract \ri-ˌti-kyə-lō-'spī-nᵊl-\ *n* : a tract of nerve fibers that originates in the reticular formation of the pons and medulla oblongata and descends to the spinal cord

re·tic·u·lum \ri-'ti-kyə-ləm\ *n, pl* **-la** \-lə\ **1** : the second compartment of the stomach of a ruminant in which folds of the mucous membrane form hexagonal cells — called also *honeycomb*; compare ABOMASUM, OMASUM, RUMEN **2** : a reticular structure: as **a** : the network of interstitial tissue composed of reticular fibers — called also *reticular tissue* **b** : the network often visible in fixed protoplasm both of the cell body and the nucleus of many cells

reticulum cell *n* : any of the branched anastomosing cells of the mononuclear phagocyte system that form the reticular fibers

reticulum cell sarcoma *n* : HISTIOCYTIC LYMPHOMA

retin- *or* **retino-** *comb form* : retina ⟨*retin*itis⟩ ⟨*retino*scopy⟩

ret·i·na \'ret-ᵊn-ə\ *n, pl* **retinas** *or* **ret·i·nae** \-ᵊn-ˌē\ : the sensory membrane that lines most of the large posterior chamber of the eye, is composed of several layers including one containing the rods and cones, and functions as the immediate instrument of vision by receiving the image formed by the lens and converting it into chemical and nervous signals which reach the brain by way of the optic nerve

Retin-A \ˌret-ᵊn-ˈā\ *trademark* — used for a preparation of tretinoin

ret·i·nac·u·lar \ˌre-tᵊn-ˈak-yə-lər\ *adj* : of, relating to, or being a retinaculum

ret·i·nac·u·lum \ˌret-ᵊn-ˈa-kyə-ləm\ *n, pl* **-la** \-lə\ : a connecting or retaining band esp. of fibrous tissue — see EXTENSOR RETINACULUM, FLEXOR RETINACULUM, INFERIOR EXTENSOR RETINACULUM, INFERIOR PERONEAL RETINACULUM, PERONEAL RETINACULUM, SUPERIOR EXTENSOR RETINACULUM, SUPERIOR PERONEAL RETINACULUM

¹**ret·i·nal** \ˈret-ᵊn-əl\ *adj* : of, relating to, involving, or being a retina ⟨~ rods⟩

²**ret·i·nal** \ˈret-ᵊn-ˌal, -ˌȯl\ *n* : a yellowish to orange aldehyde $C_{20}H_{28}O$ derived from vitamin A that in combination with proteins forms the visual pigments of the retinal rods and cones — called also *retinene, retinene₁, vitamin A aldehyde*

retinal artery — see CENTRAL ARTERY OF THE RETINA

retinal detachment *n* : a condition of the eye in which the retina has separated from the choroid — called also *detached retina, detachment of the retina*

retinal disparity *n* : the slight difference in the two retinal images due to the angle from which each eye views an object

retinal vein — see CENTRAL RETINAL VEIN

ret·i·nene \ˈret-ᵊn-ˌēn\ *n* : either of two aldehydes derived from vitamin A: **a** : RETINAL **b** : an orange-red crystalline compound $C_{20}H_{26}O$ related to vitamin A_2

retinene₁ \-ˈwən\ *n* : RETINAL

retinene₂ \-ˈtü\ *n* : RETINENE b

ret·i·ni·tis \ˌret-ᵊn-ˈī-təs\ *n, pl* **-nit·i·des** \-ˈi-tə-ˌdēz\ : inflammation of the retina

retinitis pig·men·to·sa \-ˌpig-mən-ˈtō-sə, -(ˌ)men-, -zə\ *n* : any of several hereditary progressive degenerative diseases of the eye marked by night blindness in the early stages, atrophy and pigment changes in the retina, constriction of the visual field, and eventual blindness — abbr. *RP;* called also *pigmentary retinopathy*

retinitis pro·lif·er·ans \-prə-ˈli-fə-ˌranz\ *n* : neovascularization of the retina associated esp. with diabetic retinopathy

retino- — see RETIN-

ret·i·no·blas·to·ma \ˌret-ᵊn-ō-ˌblas-ˈtō-mə\ *n, pl* **-mas** *also* **-ma·ta** \-mə-tə\ : a hereditary malignant tumor of the retina that develops during childhood, is derived from retinal germ cells, and is associated with a chromosomal abnormality

ret·i·no·cho·roid·i·tis \-ˌkōr-ˌȯi-ˈdī-təs\ *n* : inflammation of the retina and the choroid

ret·i·no·ic acid \ˌret-ᵊn-ˈō-ik-\ *n* : either of two isomers of an acid $C_{20}H_{28}O_2$ derived from vitamin A and used esp. in the treatment of acne: **a** *or* **all-trans-retinoic acid** : TRETINOIN **b** *or* **13-cis-retinoic acid** : ISOTRETINOIN

ret·i·noid \ˈret-ᵊn-ˌȯid\ *n* : any of various synthetic or naturally occurring analogs of vitamin A — **retinoid** *adj*

ret·i·nol \ˈret-ᵊn-ˌȯl, -ˌōl\ *n* : VITAMIN A a

retinol palmitate *n* : RETINYL PALMITATE

ret·i·nop·a·thy \ˌret-ᵊn-ˈä-pə-thē\ *n, pl* **-thies** : any of various noninflammatory disorders of the retina including some that cause blindness ⟨diabetic ~⟩

retinopathy of prematurity *n* : an ocular disorder of premature infants that is characterized by the presence of an opaque fibrous membrane behind the lens of each eye — abbr. *ROP;* called also *retrolental fibroplasia*

ret·i·no·scope \ˈret-ᵊn-ə-ˌskōp\ *n* : an apparatus used in retinoscopy

ret·i·nos·co·py \ˌret-ᵊn-ˈäs-kə-pē\ *n, pl* **-pies** : a method of determining the state of refraction of the eye by illuminating the retina with a mirror and observing the direction of movement of the retinal illumination and adjacent shadow when the mirror is turned

ret·i·no·tec·tal \ˌret-ᵊn-ō-ˈtek-təl\ *adj* : of, relating to, or being the nerve fibers connecting the retina and the tectum of the midbrain ⟨~ pathways⟩

ret·i·nyl palmitate \ˈret-ᵊn-əl-\ *n* : a light yellow to red oil $C_{36}H_{60}O_2$ that is a derivative of vitamin A — called also *retinol palmitate, vitamin A palmitate*

re·tract \ri-ˈtrakt\ *vb* **1** : to draw back or in ⟨~ the lower jaw⟩ — compare PROTRACT **2** : to use a retractor

re·trac·tion \ri-ˈtrak-shən\ *n* : an act or instance of retracting; *specif* : backward or inward movement of an organ or part

re·trac·tor \ri-ˈtrak-tər\ *n* : one that retracts: as **a** : any of various surgical instruments for holding tissues away from the field of operation **b** : a muscle that draws in an organ or part

retro- *prefix* **1** : backward : back ⟨*retro*flexion⟩ **2** : situated behind ⟨*retro*pubic⟩

ret·ro·bul·bar \ˌre-trō-ˈbəl-bər, -ˌbär\ *adj* : situated, occurring, or administered behind the eyeball ⟨a ~ injection⟩

retrobulbar neuritis *n* : inflammation of the part of the optic nerve lying immediately behind the eyeball

ret·ro·cli·na·tion \-kli-'nā-shən\ *n* : the condition of being inclined backward

ret·ro·flex·ion \re-trō-'flek-shən\ *n* : the state of being bent back; *specif* : the bending back of the body of the uterus upon the cervix — compare RETROVERSION

ret·ro·gnath·ia \-'na-thē-ə\ *n* : RETROGNATHISM

ret·ro·gnath·ism \re-trō-'na-ˌthi-zəm\ *n* : a condition characterized by recession of one or both of the jaws

ret·ro·grade \'re-trō-ˌgrād\ *adj* **1** : characterized by retrogression **2** : occurring or performed in a direction opposite to the normal or forward direction of conduction or flow: as **a** : occurring along nerve cell processes toward the cell body ⟨~ axonal transport⟩ **b** : occurring opposite to the normal direction or path of blood circulation ⟨~ blood flow⟩ — compare ANTEROGRADE 1 **3** : affecting memories of a period prior to a shock or seizure ⟨~ amnesia⟩ — **ret·ro·grade·ly** *adv*

retrograde pyelogram *n* : a radiograph of the kidney made by retrograde pyelography

retrograde pyelography *n* : pyelography performed by injection of radiopaque material through the ureter

ret·ro·gres·sion \ˌre-trō-'gre-shən\ *n* : a reversal in development or condition: as **a** : return to a former and less complex level of development or organization **b** : subsidence or decline of symptoms or manifestations of a disease — **ret·ro·gres·sive** \-'gre-siv\ *adj*

ret·ro·len·tal fibroplasia \ˌre-trō-'lent-ᵊl-\ *n* : RETINOPATHY OF PREMATURITY

ret·ro·mo·lar \-'mō-lər\ *adj* : situated or occurring behind the last molar

ret·ro·per·i·to·ne·al \ˌ-per-ə-tə-'nē-əl\ *adj* : situated or occurring behind the peritoneum ⟨~ bleeding⟩ ⟨a ~ tumor⟩ — **ret·ro·per·i·to·ne·al·ly** *adv*

retroperitoneal fibrosis *n* : proliferation of fibrous tissue behind the peritoneum often leading to blockage of the ureters — called also *Ormond's disease*

retroperitoneal space *n* : RETROPERITONEUM

ret·ro·per·i·to·ne·um \ˌ-per-ə-tə-'nē-əm\ *n*, *pl* **-ne·ums** *or* **-nea** \-'nē-ə\ : the space between the peritoneum and the posterior abdominal wall that contains esp. the kidneys and associated structures, the pancreas, and part of the aorta and inferior vena cava

ret·ro·pha·ryn·geal \-ˌfar-ən-'jē-əl, -fə-'rin-jəl, -jē-əl\ *adj* : situated or occurring behind the pharynx

ret·ro·pu·bic \ˌre-trō-'pyü-bik\ *adj* **1** : situated or occurring behind the pubis **2** : performed by way of the retropubic space ⟨~ prostatectomy⟩

retropubic space *n* : the potential space occurring between the pubic symphysis and the urinary bladder

ret·ro·rec·tal \-'rekt-ᵊl\ *adj* : situated or occurring behind the rectum

ret·ro·spec·tive \-'spek-tiv\ *adj* : relating to or being a study (as of a disease) that starts with the present condition of a population of individuals and collects data about their past history to explain their present condition — compare PROSPECTIVE

ret·ro·ster·nal \-'stər-nəl\ *adj* : situated or occurring behind the sternum

ret·ro·ver·sion \-'vər-zhən, -shən\ *n* : the bending backward of the uterus and cervix out of the normal axis so that the fundus points toward the sacrum and the cervix toward the pubic symphysis — compare RETROFLEXION

Ret·ro·vir \'re-trō-ˌvir\ *trademark* — used for a preparation of AZT

ret·ro·vi·rol·o·gy \ˌre-trō-vī-'rä-lə-jē\ *n*, *pl* **-gies** : a branch of virology concerned with the study of retroviruses — **ret·ro·vi·rol·o·gist** \-jist\ *n*

ret·ro·vi·rus \'re-trō-ˌvī-rəs\ *n* : any of a family (*Retroviridae*) of single-stranded RNA viruses that produce reverse transcriptase by means of which DNA is synthesized using their RNA as a template and incorporated into the genome of infected cells, that are often tumorigenic, and that include the lentiviruses (as HIV), HTLV-I, and Rous sarcoma virus — called also *RNA tumor virus* — **ret·ro·vi·ral** \-ˌvī-rəl\ *adj* — **ret·ro·vi·ral·ly** \-ē\ *adv*

re·tru·sion \ri-'trü-zhən\ *n* : backward displacement; *specif* : a condition in which a tooth or the jaw is posterior to its proper occlusal position — **re·trude** \-'trüd\ *vb* — **re·tru·sive** \-'trü-siv\ *adj*

Rett's syndrome *or* **Rett syndrome** \ˌret(s)-\ *n* : a progressive neurodevelopmental disorder that affects females usu. during infancy, that is characterized by cognitive and psychomotor deterioration, slowed head and brain growth, stereotyped hand movements, seizures, and mental retardation

Rett, Andreas (*fl* 1966–1968), Austrian physician.

reuniens — see DUCTUS REUNIENS

re·up·take \rē-'əp-ˌtāk\ *n* : the reabsorption by a neuron of a neurotransmitter following the transmission of a nerve impulse across a synapse

re·vac·ci·na·tion \ˌrē-ˌvak-sə-'nā-shən\ *n* : vaccination administered some period after an initial vaccination esp. to strengthen or renew immunity — **re·vac·ci·nate** \-'vak-sə-ˌnāt\ *vb*

re·vas·cu·lar·iza·tion \ˌrē-ˌvas-kyə-lə-rə-'zā-shən\ *n* : a surgical procedure for the provision of a new, augmented, or restored blood supply to a body part or organ ⟨myocardial ∼⟩

reverse genetics *n* : genetics that is concerned with genetic material whose nucleotide sequence is known and that analyzes its contribution to the phenotype of the organism by modifying the nucleotide sequence and observing the resulting change in phenotype — **reverse-genetic** *adj*

reverse transcriptase *n* : a polymerase esp. of retroviruses that catalyzes the formation of DNA using RNA as a template

reverse transcriptase inhibitor *n* : a drug (as AZT) that inhibits the activity of retroviral reverse transcriptase

reverse transcription *n* : the process of synthesizing DNA using RNA as a template and reverse transcriptase as a catalyst

re·vers·ible \ri-'vər-sə-bəl\ *adj* **1** : capable of going through a series of actions (as changes) either backward or forward **2** : capable of being corrected or undone : not permanent or irrevocable — **re·vers·ibly** *adv*

re·ver·sion \ri-'vər-zhən, -shən\ *n* **1** : an act or the process of returning (as to a former condition) **2** : a return toward an ancestral type or condition : reappearance of an ancestral character — **re·vert** \ri-'vərt\ *vb*

re·ver·tant \ri-'vərt-ənt\ *n* : a mutant gene, individual, or strain that regains a former capability (as the production of a particular protein) by undergoing further mutation ⟨yeast ∼s⟩ — **revertant** *adj*

revision surgery *n* : surgery performed to replace or compensate for a failed implant (as in a hip replacement) or to correct undesirable sequelae (as scar tissue) of previous surgery

re·vive \ri-'vīv\ *vb* **re·vived**; **re·viv·ing** **1** : to return or restore to consciousness or life **2** : to restore from a depressed, inactive, or unused state — **re·viv·able** \-'vī-və-bəl\ *adj*

re·ward \ri-'wörd\ *n* : a stimulus (as food) that serves to reinforce a desired response — **reward** *vb*

Reye's syndrome \'rīz-, 'rāz-\ *also* **Reye syndrome** \'rī-, 'rā-\ *n* : an often fatal encephalopathy esp. of childhood characterized by fever, vomiting, fatty infiltration of the liver, and swelling of the kidneys and brain

Reye, Ralph Douglas Kenneth (1912–1977), Australian pathologist.

Rf *symbol* rutherfordium

RF *abbr* rheumatic fever

R factor \'är-\ *n* : a group of genes present in some bacteria that provide a basis for resistance to antibiotics and can be transferred from cell to cell by conjugation

RFLP \är-(,)ef-(,)el-'pē\ *n* : RESTRICTION FRAGMENT LENGTH POLYMORPHISM

Rh \är-'āch\ *adj* : of, relating to, or being an Rh factor ⟨∼ antigens⟩

Rh *symbol* rhodium

rhabd- *or* **rhabdo-** *comb form* : rodlike structure ⟨*rhabdovirus*⟩

rhab·do·my·ol·y·sis \,rab-dō-mī-'ä-lə-səs\ *n, pl* **-y·ses** \-,sēz\ : the destruction or degeneration of skeletal muscle tissue (as from traumatic injury, excessive exertion, or stroke) that is accompanied by the release of muscle cell contents (as myoglobin and potassium) into the bloodstream resulting in hypovolemia, hyperkalemia, and sometimes acute renal failure

rhab·do·my·o·ma \,rab-dō-mī-'ō-mə\ *n, pl* **-mas** *also* **-ma·ta** \-mə-tə\ : a benign tumor composed of striated muscle fibers ⟨a cardiac ∼⟩

rhab·do·myo·sar·co·ma \,rab-(,)dō-,mī-ə-sär-'kō-mə\ *n, pl* **-mas** *also* **-ma·ta** \-mə-tə\ : a malignant tumor composed of striated muscle fibers

rhab·do·virus \-,vī-rəs\ *n* : any of a family (*Rhabdoviridae*) of single-stranded RNA viruses that are rod- or bullet-shaped, are found in plants and animals, and include the causative agents of rabies and vesicular stomatitis

rhachitis *var of* RACHITIS

rhag·a·des \'ra-gə-,dēz\ *n pl* : linear cracks or fissures in the skin occurring esp. at the angles of the mouth or about the anus

rhaphe *var of* RAPHE

Rh disease *n* : ERYTHROBLASTOSIS FETALIS

rhe·ni·um \'rē-nē-əm\ *n* : a rare heavy metallic element — symbol *Re;* see ELEMENT table

rheo- *comb form* : flow : current ⟨*rheo*base⟩

rheo·base \'rē-ō-,bās\ *n* : the minimal electrical current required to excite a tissue (as nerve or muscle) given an indefinitely long time during which the current is applied — compare CHRONAXIE

rhe·sus factor \'rē-səs-\ *n* : RH FACTOR

rheum \'rüm\ *n* : a watery discharge from the mucous membranes esp. of the eyes or nose; *also* : a condition (as a cold) marked by such discharge — **rheumy** \'rü-mē\ *adj*

¹**rheu·mat·ic** \rù-'ma-tik\ *adj* : of, relating to, characteristic of, or affected with rheumatism ⟨∼ pain⟩

²**rheumatic** *n* : a person affected with rheumatism

rheumatica — see POLYMYALGIA RHEUMATICA

rheumatic disease *n* : any of several diseases (as rheumatic fever or fibrositis) characterized by inflammation and pain in muscles or joints : RHEUMATISM

rheumatic fever *n* : an acute often recurrent disease that occurs chiefly in children and young adults following group A streptococcal infection of the upper respiratory tract (as in strep throat) and is characterized by fever, inflammation, pain, and swelling in and around the joints, inflammatory involvement of the pericardium and valves of the heart, and often the formation of small nodules chiefly in the subcutaneous tissues and the heart

rheumatic heart disease *n* : active or inactive disease of the heart that results from rheumatic fever and is characterized by inflammatory changes in the myocardium or scarring of the valves causing reduced functional capacity of the heart

rheu·ma·tism \'rü-mə-ˌti-zəm, 'rü-mə-\ *n* **1** : any of various conditions characterized by inflammation or pain in muscles, joints, or fibrous tissue ⟨muscular ~⟩ **2** : RHEUMATOID ARTHRITIS

rheu·ma·toid \-ˌtȯid\ *adj* : characteristic of or affected with rheumatoid arthritis

rheumatoid arthritis *n* : a usu. chronic disease that is considered an autoimmune disease and is characterized esp. by pain, stiffness, inflammation, swelling, and sometimes destruction of joints — abbr. *RA*; compare OSTEOARTHRITIS

rheumatoid factor *n* : an autoantibody of high molecular weight that reacts against immunoglobulins of the class IgG and is often present in rheumatoid arthritis

rheumatoid spondylitis *n* : ANKYLOSING SPONDYLITIS

rheu·ma·tol·o·gist \ˌrü-mə-ˈtä-lə-jist, ˌrü-\ *n* : a specialist in rheumatology

rheu·ma·tol·o·gy \-jē\ *n, pl* **-gies** : a medical science dealing with rheumatic diseases — **rheu·ma·to·log·ic** \-tə-ˈlä-jik\ *or* **rheu·ma·to·log·i·cal** \-ji-kəl\ *adj*

Rh factor \ˌär-ˈāch-\ *n* : a genetically determined protein on the red blood cells of some people that is one of the substances used to classify human blood as to compatibility for transfusion and that when present in a fetus but not in the mother causes a serious immunogenic reaction in which the mother produces antibodies that cross the placenta and attack the red blood cells of the fetus — called also *rhesus factor*

rhin- *or* **rhino-** *comb form* **1 a** : nose ⟨*rhin*itis⟩ **b** : nose and ⟨*rhino*tracheitis⟩ **2** : nasal ⟨*rhino*virus⟩

rhi·nal \'rīn-ᵊl\ *adj* : of or relating to the nose : NASAL

rhin·en·ceph·a·lon \ˌrī-(ˌ)nen-ˈse-fə-ˌlän, -lən\ *n, pl* **-la** \-lä\ : the anterior inferior part of the forebrain that is chiefly concerned with olfaction and that is considered to include the olfactory bulb together with the forebrain olfactory structures receiving fibers directly from it and often esp. formerly the limbic system which is now known to be concerned with emotional states and affect — called also *smell brain* — **rhin·en·ce·pha·lic** \ˌrī-ˌnen-sə-ˈfa-lik\ *adj*

rhi·ni·tis \rī-ˈnī-təs\ *n, pl* **-nit·i·des** \-ˈni-tə-ˌdēz\ : inflammation of the mucous membrane of the nose marked esp. by rhinorrhea, nasal congestion and itching, and sneezing; *also* : any of various conditions characterized by rhinitis — see ALLERGIC RHINITIS, RHINITIS MEDICAMENTOSA, VASOMOTOR RHINITIS

rhinitis me·dic·a·men·to·sa \-mə-ˌdi-kə-men-ˈtō-sə\ *n* : an increase in the severity or duration of rhinitis that results from prolonged use of decongestant nasal spray

rhi·no·log·ic \ˌrī-nə-ˈlä-jik\ *or* **rhi·no·log·i·cal** \-ji-kəl\ *adj* : of or relating to the nose ⟨~ disease⟩

rhi·nol·o·gist \rī-ˈnä-lə-jist\ *n* : a physician who specializes in rhinology

rhi·nol·o·gy \-jē\ *n, pl* **-gies** : a branch of medicine that deals with the nose and its diseases

rhi·no·phar·yn·gi·tis \ˌrī-nō-ˌfar-ən-ˈjī-təs\ *n, pl* **-git·i·des** \-ˈji-tə-ˌdēz\ : inflammation of the mucous membrane of the nose and pharynx

rhi·no·phy·ma \-ˈfī-mə\ *n, pl* **-mas** *or* **-ma·ta** \-mə-tə\ : a nodular swelling and congestion of the nose in an advanced stage of rosacea

rhi·no·plas·ty \'rī-nō-ˌplas-tē\ *n, pl* **-ties** : plastic surgery on the nose usu. for cosmetic purposes — called also *nose job* — **rhi·no·plas·tic** \ˌrī-nō-ˈplas-tik\ *adj*

rhi·no·pneu·mo·ni·tis \ˌrī-nō-ˌnü-mə-ˈnī-təs, -ˌnyü-\ *n* : an acute febrile respiratory disease of horses that is caused by two herpesviruses of the genus *Varicellovirus* (species *Equid herpesvirus 1* and *Equid herpesvirus 4*) and is characterized esp. by rhinopharyngitis and tracheobronchitis

rhi·nor·rhea \ˌrī-nə-ˈrē-ə\ *n* : excessive mucous secretion from the nose

rhi·nor·rhoea *chiefly Brit var of* RHINORRHEA

rhi·no·scope \'rī-nə-ˌskōp\ *n* : an instrument (as an endoscope) for examining the cavities and passages of the nose

rhi·nos·co·py \rī-ˈnäs-kə-pē\ *n, pl* **-pies** : examination of the nasal passages — **rhi·no·scop·ic** \ˌrī-nə-ˈskä-pik\ *adj*

rhi·no·si·nus·itis \ˌrī-nō-ˌsī-nə-ˈsī-təs, -nyə-\ *n* : inflammation of the mucous membranes of the nose and one or more paranasal sinuses

rhi·no·spo·rid·i·o·sis \ˌrī-nō-spə-ˌri-dē-ˈō-səs\ *n, pl* **-o·ses** \-ˌsēz\ : a fungal disease of the external mucous membranes (as of the nose) that is characterized by the formation of pinkish red, friable, sessile, or pedunculated polyps and is caused by an ascomycetous fungus (*Rhinosporidium seeberi*)

rhi·not·o·my \rī-'nä-tə-mē\ n, pl **-mies** : surgical incision of the nose

rhi·no·tra·che·itis \ˌrī-nō-ˌträ-kē-'ī-təs\ n : inflammation of the nasal cavities and trachea; *esp* : a disease of the upper respiratory system in cats and esp. young kittens that is characterized by sneezing, conjunctivitis with discharge, and nasal discharges — see INFECTIOUS BOVINE RHINOTRACHEITIS

rhi·no·vi·rus \ˌrī-nō-'vī-rəs\ n **1** *cap* : a genus of picornaviruses including two species (*Human rhinovirus A* and *Human rhinovirus B*) having numerous serotypes causing respiratory infections (as the common cold) in humans **2** : any virus of the genus *Rhinovirus*

Rhipi·ceph·a·lus \ˌri-pə-'se-fə-ləs\ n : a genus of ixodid ticks that are parasitic on many mammals and some birds and include vectors of serious diseases (as east coast fever)

rhi·zo·me·lic \ˌrī-zə-'mē-lik\ adj : of or relating to the hip and shoulder joints

rhi·zot·o·my \rī-'zä-tə-mē\ n, pl **-mies** : the operation of cutting the anterior or posterior spinal nerve roots

Rh–neg·a·tive \ˌär-ˌāch-'ne-gə-tiv\ adj : lacking Rh factor in the blood

rhod- or **rhodo-** comb form : rose : red ⟨*rhodopsin*⟩

rho·di·um \'rō-dē-əm\ n : a white hard ductile metallic element — symbol *Rh;* see ELEMENT table

rho·dop·sin \rō-'däp-sən\ n : a red photosensitive pigment in the retinal rods that is important in vision in dim light, is quickly bleached by light to a mixture of opsin and retinal, and is regenerated in the dark — called also *visual purple*

Rho·do·tor·u·la \ˌrō-də-'tȯr-yə-lə\ n : a genus of yeasts (family Cryptococcaceae) including one (*R. rubra* syn. *R. mucilaginosa*) sometimes present in the blood or involved in endocarditis prob. as a secondary infection

rhomb·en·ceph·a·lon \ˌräm-(ˌ)ben-'se-fə-ˌlän, -lən\ n, pl **-la** \-lə\ : HINDBRAIN — **rhomb·en·ce·phal·ic** \-sə-'fa-lik\ adj

rhom·boi·de·us \räm-'bȯi-dē-əs\ n, pl **-dei** \-dē-ˌī\ : either of two muscles that lie beneath the trapezius muscle and connect the spinous processes of various vertebrae with the medial border of the scapula: **a** : RHOMBOIDEUS MINOR **b** : RHOMBOIDEUS MAJOR

rhomboideus major n : a muscle arising from the spinous processes of the second through fifth thoracic vertebrae, inserted into the vertebral border of the scapula, and acting to adduct and laterally rotate the scapula — called also *rhomboid major*

rhomboideus minor n : a muscle arising from the inferior part of the ligamentum nuchae and from the spinous processes of the seventh cervical and first thoracic vertebrae, inserted into the vertebral border of the scapula at the base of the bony process terminating in the acromion, and acting to adduct and laterally rotate the scapula — called also *rhomboid minor*

rhomboid fossa n : the floor of the fourth ventricle of the brain formed by the dorsal surfaces of the pons and medulla oblongata

rhomboid major n : RHOMBOIDEUS MAJOR

rhomboid minor n : RHOMBOIDEUS MINOR

rhon·chus \'rän-kəs\ n, pl **rhon·chi** \'rän-ˌkī\ : a whistling or snoring sound heard on auscultation of the chest when the air channels are partly obstructed — compare RALE, RATTLE

rho·ta·cism \'rō-tə-ˌsi-zəm\ n : a defective pronunciation of *r*; *esp* : substitution of some other sound for that of *r*

Rh–pos·i·tive \ˌär-ˌāch-'pä-zə-tiv\ adj : containing Rh factor in the red blood cells

rhus \'rüs\ n **1** *cap* : a genus of shrubs and trees of the cashew family (Anacardiaceae) native to temperate and warm regions — see TOXICODENDRON **2** pl **rhuses** or **rhus** : any shrub or tree of the genus *Rhus* : SUMAC

rhus dermatitis n : dermatitis caused by contact with various plants (as poison ivy) of the genus *Rhus* or *Toxicodendron*

rhythm \'ri-thəm\ n **1** : a regularly recurrent quantitative change in a variable biological process: as **a** : the pattern of recurrence of the cardiac cycle ⟨an irregular ∼⟩ **b** : the recurring pattern of physical and functional changes associated with the mammalian and esp. human sexual cycle **2** : RHYTHM METHOD — **rhyth·mic** \'rith-mik\ or **rhyth·mi·cal** \-mi-kəl\ adj — **rhyth·mi·cal·ly** adv — **rhyth·mic·i·ty** \rith-'mi-sə-tē\ n

rhythm method n : a method of birth control involving abstinence during the period in which ovulation is most likely to occur

rhyt·i·dec·to·my \ˌri-tə-'dek-tə-mē\ n, pl **-mies** : FACE-LIFT

RIA abbr radioimmunoassay

rib \'rib\ n : any of the paired curved bony or partly cartilaginous rods that stiffen the lateral walls of the body and protect the viscera and that in humans normally include 12 pairs of which all are articulated with the spinal column at the dorsal end and the first 10 are connected also at the ventral end with the sternum by costal cartilages — see FALSE RIB, FLOATING RIB, TRUE RIB

rib- or **ribo-** comb form : related to ribose ⟨*ribo*flavin⟩

ri·ba·vi·rin \ˌrī-bə-'vī-rən\ n : a synthetic broad-spectrum antiviral drug $C_9H_{12}N_4O_5$ that is a nucleoside resembling guanosine

rib cage *n* : the bony enclosing wall of the chest consisting chiefly of the ribs and the structures connecting them — called also *thoracic cage*

ri·bo·fla·vin \ˌrī-bə-ˈflā-vən, ˈrī-bə-ˌ\ *also* **ri·bo·fla·vine** \-ˌvēn\ *n* : a yellow crystalline compound $C_{17}H_{20}N_4O_6$ that is a growth-promoting member of the vitamin B complex and occurs both free (as in milk) and combined (as in liver) — called also *lactoflavin, vitamin B₂*

riboflavin phosphate *or* **riboflavin 5′–phosphate** \-ˈfīv-ˌprīm-\ *n* : FMN

ri·bo·nu·cle·ase \ˌrī-bō-ˈnü-klē-ˌās, -ˈnyü-, -ˌāz\ *n* : an enzyme that catalyzes the hydrolysis of RNA — called also *RNase*

ri·bo·nu·cle·ic acid \ˌrī-bō-nü-ˌklē-ik-, -nyü-, -ˌklā-\ *n* : RNA

ri·bo·nu·cleo·pro·tein \-ˌnü-klē-ō-ˈprō-ˌtēn, -ˌnyü-\ *n* : a nucleoprotein that contains RNA

ri·bo·nu·cle·o·side \-ˈnü-klē-ə-ˌsīd, -ˈnyü-\ *n* : a nucleoside that contains ribose

ri·bo·nu·cle·o·tide \-ˌtīd\ *n* : a nucleotide that contains ribose and occurs esp. as a constituent of RNA

ri·bose \ˈrī-ˌbōs, -ˌbōz\ *n* : a pentose $C_5H_{10}O_5$ found esp. in the levorotatory D-form as a constituent of a number of nucleosides (as adenosine, cytidine, and guanosine) esp. in RNA

ribosomal RNA *n* : RNA that is a fundamental structural element of ribosomes — called also *rRNA*

ri·bo·some \ˈrī-bə-ˌsōm\ *n* : any of the RNA- and protein-rich cytoplasmic organelles that are sites of protein synthesis — **ri·bo·som·al** \ˌrī-bə-ˈsō-məl\ *adj*

ri·bo·zyme \-ˌzīm\ *n* : a molecule of RNA that functions as an enzyme (as by catalyzing the cleavage of other RNA molecules)

RICE *abbr* rest, ice, compression, elevation — used esp. for the initial treatment of many usu. minor sports-related injuries (as sprains)

rice–water stool *n* : a watery stool containing white flecks of mucus, epithelial cells, and bacteria that is characteristic of severe forms of diarrhea (as in Asiatic cholera)

ri·cin \ˈrīs-ᵊn, ˈris-\ *n* : a poisonous protein in the castor bean

rick·ets \ˈri-kəts\ *n* : a deficiency disease that affects the young during the period of skeletal growth, is characterized esp. by soft and deformed bones, and is caused by failure to assimilate and use calcium and phosphorus normally due to inadequate sunlight or vitamin D — called also *rachitis;* see OSTEOMALACIA

rick·etts·ae·mia *chiefly Brit var of* RICKETTSEMIA

rick·etts·emia \ˌri-kət-ˈsē-mē-ə\ *n* : an abnormal presence of rickettsiae in the blood

Rick·etts, Howard Taylor (1871–1910), American pathologist.

rick·ett·sia \ri-ˈket-sē-ə\ *n* **1** *cap* : a genus of rod-shaped, coccoid, or diplococcus-shaped bacteria (family Rickettsiaceae) that are transmitted by biting arthropods (as lice or ticks) and cause a number of serious diseases (as Rocky Mountain spotted fever and typhus) **2** *pl* **-si·ae** \-sē-ˌē\ *also* **-sias** *or* **-sia** : any bacterium of the genus *Rickettsia* or of the family (Rickettsiaceae) to which it belongs — **rick·ett·si·al** \-sē-əl\ *adj*

rick·ett·si·al·pox \ri-ˌket-sē-əl-ˈpäks\ *n* : a disease characterized by fever, chills, headache, backache, and a spotty rash and caused by a bacterium of the genus *Rickettsia* (*R. akari*) transmitted to humans by the bite of a mite of the genus *Allodermanyssus* (*A. sanguineus*) living on rodents (as the house mouse)

rick·ett·si·o·sis \ri-ˌket-sē-ˈō-səs\ *n, pl* **-o·ses** \-ˌsēz\ : infection with or disease caused by a rickettsia

ridge·ling *or* **ridg·ling** \ˈrij-liŋ\ *n* **1** : a partially castrated male animal **2** : a male animal having one or both testes retained in the inguinal canal

Rie·del's disease \ˈrēd-ᵊlz-\ *n* : chronic thyroiditis in which the thyroid gland becomes hard and stony and firmly attached to surrounding tissues

Riedel, Bernhard Moritz Karl Ludwig (1846–1916), German surgeon.

Riedel's struma *n* : RIEDEL'S DISEASE

rif·a·bu·tin \ˈri-fə-ˌbyü-tᵊn\ *n* : a semisynthetic antibacterial drug $C_{46}H_{62}N_4O_{11}$ used esp. to prevent and treat infection with bacteria of the Mycobacterium avium complex

ri·fam·pin \rī-ˈfam-pən\ *or* **ri·fam·pi·cin** \rī-ˈfam-pə-sən\ *n* : a semisynthetic antibiotic $C_{43}H_{58}N_4O_{12}$ that is used esp. in the treatment of tuberculosis and to treat asymptomatic carriers of meningococci

rif·a·my·cin \ˌri-fə-ˈmīs-ᵊn\ *n* : any of several antibiotics that are derived from a bacterium of the genus *Streptomyces* (*S. mediterranei*)

Rift Valley fever *n* : an acute usu. epizootic mosquito-borne disease of domestic animals (as sheep and cattle) chiefly of eastern and southern Africa that is caused by a bunyavirus of the genus *Phlebovirus* (species *Rift Valley fever virus*), is marked esp. by fever, abortion, death of newborns, diarrhea, and jaundice, and is sometimes transmitted to humans usu. in a milder form marked by flulike symptoms

right atrioventricular valve *n* : TRICUSPID VALVE

right brain *n* : the right cerebral hemisphere of the human brain esp. when viewed in terms of its predominant thought processes (as creativity and intuitive thinking) • — **right–brained** *adj*

right colic flexure *n* : HEPATIC FLEX-URE

right–eyed *adj* : using the right eye in preference (as in using a monocular microscope)

right gastric artery *n* : an artery that arises from the hepatic artery, passes to the left along the lesser curvature of the stomach while giving off a number of branches, and eventually joins a branch of the left gastric artery

right gastroepiploic artery *n* : GAS-TROEPIPLOIC ARTERY a

right–hand·ed \-'han-dəd\ *adj* **1** : using the right hand habitually or more easily than the left **2** : relating to, designed for, or done with the right hand **3** : having the same direction or course as the movement of the hands of a watch viewed from in front **4** : DEXTROROTATORY — **right–hand·ed** *adv* — **right–hand·ed·ness** *n*

right heart *n* : the right atrium and ventricle : the half of the heart that receives blood from the systemic circulation and passes it into the pulmonary arteries

right lymphatic duct *n* : a short vessel that receives lymph from the right side of the head, neck, and thorax, the right arm, right lung, right side of the heart, and convex surface of the liver and that discharges it into the right subclavian vein at its junction with the right internal jugular vein

right pulmonary artery *n* : PUL-MONARY ARTERY b

right subcostal vein *n* : SUBCOSTAL VEIN a

right–to–life *adj* : ANTIABORTION

right–to–lif·er \ˌrīt-tə-'lī-fər\ *n* : AN-TIABORTIONIST

ri·gid·i·ty \rə-'ji-də-tē\ *n, pl* **-ties** : the quality or state of being stiff or devoid of or deficient in flexibility: as **a** : abnormal stiffness of muscle **b** : emotional inflexibility and resistance to change — **rig·id** \'ri-jəd\ *adj*

rigidus — see HALLUX RIGIDUS

rig·or \'ri-gər\ *n* **1 a** : CHILL 1 **b** : a tremor caused by a chill **2 a** : rigidity or torpor of organs or tissue that prevents response to stimuli **b** : RIGOR MORTIS

rig·or mor·tis \'ri-gər-'mȯr-təs\ *n* : temporary rigidity of muscles occurring after death

Ri·ley–Day syndrome \ˌrī-lē-'dā-\ *n* : FAMILIAL DYSAUTONOMIA
  Riley, Conrad Milton (1913–2005), and Day, Richard Lawrence (1905–1989), American pediatricians.

ri·ma \'rī-mə\ *n, pl* **ri·mae** \-ˌmē\ : an anatomical fissure or cleft

rima glot·ti·dis \-'glä-tə-dəs\ *n* : the passage in the glottis between the true vocal cords

ri·man·ta·dine \rə-'man-tə-ˌdēn\ *n* : a synthetic antiviral drug that is chemically related to amantadine and is administered orally in the form of its

hydrochloride $C_{12}H_{21}N \cdot HCl$ to prevent and treat influenza

rima pal·pe·bra·rum \-ˌpal-pē-'brer-əm\ *n* : PALPEBRAL FISSURE

rin·der·pest \'rin-dər-ˌpest\ *n* : an acute infectious disease of ruminant animals (as cattle) that is caused by a paramyxovirus of the genus *Morbillivirus* (species *Rinderpest virus*) and is marked by fever, diarrhea, and inflammation of mucous membranes and by high mortality in epidemics

¹**ring** \'rin\ *n* **1 a** : a circular band **b** : an anatomical structure having a circular opening : ANNULUS **2** : an arrangement of atoms represented in formulas or models in a cyclic manner as a closed chain

²**ring** *vb* **rang** \'ran\; **rung** \'rən\; **ring·ing** : to have the sensation of being filled with a humming sound ⟨his ears *rang*⟩

ring·bone \-ˌbōn\ *n* : a bony outgrowth on the phalangeal bones of a horse's foot that usu. produces lameness

Ring·er's fluid \'rin-ərz-\ *n* : RINGER'S SOLUTION
  Ringer, Sidney (1835–1910), British physiologist.

Ringer's lactate *or* **Ringer's lactate solution** *n* : LACTATED RINGER'S SO-LUTION

Ring·er's solution \'rin-ərz-\ *also* **Ring·er solution** \'rin-ər-\ *n* : a sterile aqueous solution of calcium chloride, sodium chloride, and potassium chloride that provides a medium essentially isotonic to many animal tissues and that is used esp. to replenish fluids and electrolytes by intravenous infusion or to irrigate tissues by topical application — compare LACTATED RINGER'S SOLUTION

ring·hals \'rin-ˌhals\ *n* : a venomous African elapid snake (*Haemachatus haemachatus*) that rarely bites but when threatened spits a venom that is harmless to intact skin but may cause severe damage to eyes upon contact

ring·worm \'rin-ˌwərm\ *n* : any of several contagious diseases of the skin, hair, or nails of humans and domestic animals caused by fungi (as of the genus *Trichophyton*) and characterized by ring-shaped discolored patches on the skin that are covered with vesicles and scales — called also *tinea*

Rin·ne's test \'ri-nəs-\ *or* **Rin·ne test** \'ri-nə-\ *n* : a test for determining a subject's ability to hear a vibrating tuning fork when it is held next to the ear and when it is placed on the mastoid process with diminished hearing acuity through air and somewhat heightened hearing acuity through bone being symptomatic of conduction deafness
  Rinne, Heinrich Adolf R. (1819–1868), German otologist.

ris·ed·ro·nate \ri-'se-drə-ˌnāt\ *n* : a sodium bisphosphonate salt $C_7H_{10}N$-

NaO₇P₂ used esp. to prevent or treat osteoporosis in postmenopausal women — see ACTONEL

risk \'risk\ *n* **1** : possibility of loss, injury, disease, or death ⟨hypertension increases the ∼ of stroke⟩ **2** : a person considered in terms of the possible bad effects of a particular course of treatment ⟨a poor surgical ∼⟩ — **at risk** : in a state or condition marked by a high level of risk or susceptibility ⟨patients *at risk* of developing infections⟩

risk factor *n* : something that increases risk or susceptibility ⟨a fatty diet is a *risk factor* for heart disease⟩

ri·so·ri·us \ri-'sōr-ē-əs, -'zōr-\ *n, pl* **-ri·i** \-ē-ˌī\ : a narrow band of muscle fibers arising from the fascia over the masseter muscle, inserted into the tissues at the corner of the mouth, and acting to retract the angle of the mouth

Ris·per·dal \'ris-pər-ˌdal\ *trademark* — used for a preparation of risperidone

ris·per·i·done \ri-'sper-ə-ˌdōn\ *n* : an antipsychotic drug C₂₃H₂₇FN₄O₂ used esp. to treat schizophrenia and acute manic episodes of bipolar disorder — see RISPERDAL

ris·to·ce·tin \ˌris-tə-'sēt-ᵊn\ *n* : either of two antibiotics or a mixture of both produced by an actinomycete of the genus *Nocardia* (*N. lurida*)

ri·sus sar·do·ni·cus \'rī-səs-ˌsär-'dä-ni-kəs, 'rē-\ *n* : a facial expression characterized by raised eyebrows and grinning distortion of the face resulting from spasm of facial muscles esp. in tetanus

Rit·a·lin \'ri-tə-lən\ *trademark* — used for a preparation of the hydrochloride of methylphenidate

rit·o·drine \'ri-tə-ˌdrēn, -drən\ *n* : a drug administered intravenously in the form of its hydrochloride C₁₇H₂₁-NO₃·HCl as a smooth muscle relaxant esp. to inhibit premature labor

ri·to·na·vir \ˌri-'tō-nə-ˌvir\ *n* : an antiviral protease inhibitor C₃₇H₄₈N₆O₅S₂ administered orally to treat HIV infection and AIDS — see NORVIR

Rit·ter's disease \'ri-tərz-\ *n* : STAPHYLOCOCCAL SCALDED SKIN SYNDROME

Ritter von Rittershain, Gottfried (1820–1883), German physician.

rit·u·al \'ri-chə-wəl\ *n* : any act or practice regularly repeated in a set precise manner for relief of anxiety ⟨obsessive-compulsive ∼s⟩

river blindness *n* : ONCHOCERCIASIS

RK *abbr* radial keratotomy

RLF *abbr* retrolental fibroplasia

RLQ *abbr* right lower quadrant (abdomen)

RLS *abbr* restless legs syndrome

Rn *symbol* radon

RN \ˌär-'en\ *n* : REGISTERED NURSE

RNA \ˌär-(ˌ)en-'ā\ *n* : any of various nucleic acids that contain ribose and uracil as structural components and are associated with the control of cellular chemical activities — called also *ribonucleic acid;* see MESSENGER RNA, RIBOSOMAL RNA, TRANSFER RNA

RNAi *n* : RNA INTERFERENCE

RNA interference *n* : a posttranscriptional genetic mechanism which suppresses gene expression and in which double-stranded RNA cleaved into small fragments initiates the degradation of a complementary messenger RNA; *also* : a technique (as the introduction of double-stranded RNA into an organism) that artificially induces RNA interference and is used for studying or regulating gene expression

RNA polymerase *n* : any of a group of enzymes that promote the synthesis of RNA using DNA or RNA as a template

RNA replicase *n* : REPLICASE

RNase *or* **RNAase** \ˌär-ˌen-'ā-ˌās, -'ā-ˌāz\ *n* : RIBONUCLEASE

RNA syn·the·tase \-'sin-thə-ˌtās, -ˌtāz\ *n* : REPLICASE

RNA tumor virus *n* : RETROVIRUS

RNA virus *n* : a virus (as a retrovirus) whose genome consists of RNA

roach \'rōch\ *n* : COCKROACH

roar·ing \'rōr-iŋ\ *n* : noisy inhalation in a horse caused by paralysis and muscular atrophy of part of the larynx

Rob·ert·so·ni·an \ˌrä-bərt-'sō-nē-ən\ *adj* : relating to or being a reciprocal translocation that takes place between two acrocentric chromosomes and that yields one nonfunctional chromosome having two short arms and one functional chromosome having two long arms of which one arm is derived from each parent chromosome

Rob·ert·son \'rä-bərt-sən\, **William Rees Brebner** (1881–1941), American biologist.

Ro·bi·nul \'rō-bi-ˌnůl\ *trademark* — used for a preparation of glycopyrrolate

Ro·cha·li·maea \ˌrō-kə-li-'mē-ə\ *n, syn of* BARTONELLA

Ro·chelle salt \rō-'shel-\ *n* : a crystalline salt C₄H₄KNaO₆·4H₂O that is a mild purgative — called also *potassium sodium tartrate, Seignette salt, sodium potassium tartrate*

rock \'räk\ *n* **1** : a small crystallized mass of crack cocaine **2** : CRACK — called also *rock cocaine*

Rocky Mountain spotted fever *n* : an acute bacterial disease that is characterized by chills, fever, prostration, pains in muscles and joints, and a red purple eruption and that is caused by a bacterium of the genus *Rickettsia* (*R. rickettii*) usu. transmitted by ixodid ticks and esp. by the American dog tick and Rocky Mountain wood tick

Rocky Mountain wood tick *n* : a widely distributed wood tick of the genus *Dermacentor* (*D. andersoni*) of western No. America that is a vector of Rocky Mountain spotted fever and sometimes causes tick paralysis

rod \ˈräd\ *n* **1** : any of the long rod-shaped photosensitive receptors in the retina responsive to faint light — compare CONE 1 **2** : a bacterium shaped like a rod

ro·dent \ˈrōd-ᵊnt\ *n* : any of an order (Rodentia) of relatively small mammals (as a mouse or a rat) that have in both jaws a single pair of incisors with a chisel-shaped edge — **rodent** *adj*

ro·den·ti·cide \rō-ˈden-tə-ˌsīd\ *n* : an agent that kills, repels, or controls rodents

rodent ulcer *n* : a chronic persistent ulcer of the exposed skin and esp. of the face that is destructive locally, spreads slowly, and is usu. a carcinoma derived from basal cells

rod·like \ˈräd-ˌlīk\ *adj* : resembling a rod < ~ bacteria>

rod of Cor·ti \-ˈkȯr-tē\ *n* : any of the minute modified epithelial elements that rise from the basilar membrane of the organ of Corti in two spirally arranged rows so that the free ends of the members incline toward and interlock with corresponding members of the opposite row and enclose the tunnel of Corti

A. G. G. Corti — see ORGAN OF CORTI

¹**roent·gen** *also* **rönt·gen** \ˈrent-gən, ˈrənt-, -jən, -shən\ *adj* : of, relating to, or using X-rays

Rönt·gen, *or* **Roent·gen** \ˈrœnt-gən\, **Wilhelm Conrad** (1845–1923), German physicist.

²**roentgen** *also* **röntgen** *n* : the international unit of x-radiation or gamma radiation equal to the amount of radiation that produces in one cubic centimeter of dry air at 0°C (32°F) and standard atmospheric pressure ionization of either sign equal to one electrostatic unit of charge

roent·gen·o·gram \ˈrent-gə-nə-ˌgram, ˈrənt-, -jə-, -shə-\ *n* : RADIOGRAPH

roent·gen·og·ra·phy \ˌrent-gə-ˈnä-grə-fē, ˌrənt-, -jə-, -shə-\ *n, pl* **-phies** : RADIOGRAPHY — **roent·gen·o·graph·ic** \-nə-ˈgra-fik\ *adj* — **roent·gen·o·graph·i·cal·ly** *adv*

roent·gen·ol·o·gist \-ˈnä-lə-jist\ *n* : RADIOLOGIST

roent·gen·ol·o·gy \-ˈnä-lə-jē\ *n, pl* **-gies** : RADIOLOGY 2 — **roent·gen·o·log·ic** \-nə-ˈlä-jik\ *or* **roent·gen·o·log·i·cal** \-ji-kəl\ *adj* — **roent·gen·o·log·i·cal·ly** *adv*

roent·gen·os·co·py \-ˈnäs-kə-pē\ *n, pl* **-pies** : observation or examination by means of a fluoroscope : FLUOROSCOPY — **roent·gen·o·scop·ic** \-nə-ˈskä-pik\ *adj*

roentgen ray *n* : X-RAY 1

ro·fe·cox·ib \ˌrō-fe-ˈkäk-sib\ *n* : a COX-2 inhibitor $C_{17}H_{14}O_4S$ used to relieve the signs and symptoms of osteoarthritis and rheumatoid arthritis, to manage acute pain in adults, and to treat primary dysmenorrhea but withdrawn from sale by the manufacturer because of its link to cardiovascular events (as heart attack and stroke) — see VIOXX

Ro·gaine \ˈrō-ˌgān\ *trademark* — used for a preparation of minoxidil

Rog·er·i·an \rä-ˈjer-ē-ən\ *adj* : of or relating to the system of therapy or the theory of personality of Carl Rogers

Rog·ers \ˈrä-jərz\, **Carl Ransom** (1902–1987), American psychologist.

Ro·hyp·nol \rō-ˈhip-ˌnȯl\ *n* : a preparation of flunitrazepam — formerly a U.S. registered trademark

Ro·lan·dic area \rō-ˈlan-dik-\ *n* : the motor area of the cerebral cortex lying just anterior to the central sulcus and comprising part of the precentral gyrus

L. Rolando — see FISSURE OF ROLANDO

Rolandic fissure *n* : CENTRAL SULCUS

role *also* **rôle** \ˈrōl\ *n* : a socially prescribed pattern of behavior usu. determined by an individual's status in a particular society

role model *n* : a person whose behavior in a particular role is imitated by others

role–play \ˈrōl-ˌplā\ *vb* **1** : ACT OUT **2** : to play a role

rolf \ˈrȯlf, ˈrälf\ *vb, often cap* : to practice Rolfing on — **rolf·er** *n, often cap*

Rolf, Ida P. (1896–1979), American biochemist and physiotherapist.

Rolf·ing \ˈrȯl-fiŋ, ˈräl-\ *service mark* — used for a system of deep muscle massage intended to serve as both physical and emotional therapy

ro·li·tet·ra·cy·cline \ˌrō-li-ˌte-trə-ˈsī-ˌklēn\ *n* : a semisynthetic broad-spectrum tetracycline antibiotic $C_{27}H_{33}N_3O_8$ usu. administered intravenously or intramuscularly

roller — see TONGUE ROLLER

roll·er bandage \ˈrō-lər-\ *n* : a long rolled bandage

Rom·berg's sign \ˈräm-ˌbərgz-\ *or* **Rom·berg sign** \-ˌbərg-\ *n* : a diagnostic sign of tabes dorsalis and other diseases of the nervous system consisting of a swaying of the body when the feet are placed close together and the eyes are closed

Romberg, Moritz Heinrich (1795–1873), German pathologist.

Romberg's test *or* **Romberg test** *n* : a test for the presence of Romberg's sign by placing the feet close together and closing the eyes

ron·geur \rōⁿ-ˈzhər\ *n* : a heavy-duty forceps for removing small pieces of bone or tough tissue

ron·nel \ˈrän-ᵊl\ *n* : an organophosphate $C_8H_8Cl_3O_3PS$ that is used esp. as a systemic insecticide to protect cattle from pests

röntgen *var of* ROENTGEN

roof \'rüf, 'rúf\ *n, pl* **roofs** \'rüfs, 'rúfs, 'rüvz, 'rúvz\ **1** : the vaulted upper boundary of the mouth supported largely by the palatine bones and limited anteriorly by the dental lamina and posteriorly by the uvula and upper part of the fauces **2** : a covering structure of any of various parts of the body other than the mouth ⟨∼ of the skull⟩

roof•ie \'rü-fē\ *n, pl* **roof•ies** *slang* : a tablet of flunitrazepam used illicitly

room•ing–in \'rü-miŋ-'in, 'rú-\ *n* : an arrangement whereby a newborn infant is kept in the mother's hospital room instead of in a nursery

room temperature *n* : a temperature of from 59° to 77°F (15° to 25°C) that is suitable for human occupancy

root \'rüt, 'rút\ *n* **1** : the part of a tooth within the socket; *also* : the part of the processes into which the root of a tooth is often divided **2** : the enlarged basal part of a hair within the skin — called also *hair root* **3** : the proximal end of a nerve; *esp* : one or more bundles of nerve fibers joining the cranial and spinal nerves with their respective nuclei and columns of gray matter — see DORSAL ROOT, VENTRAL ROOT **4** : the part of an organ or physical structure by which it is attached to the body ⟨the ∼ of the tongue⟩ — **root•less** \-ləs\ *adj*

root canal *n* **1** : the part of the pulp cavity lying in the root of a tooth — called also *pulp canal* **2** : a dental operation to save a tooth by removing the contents of its root canal and filling the cavity with a protective substance (as gutta-percha)

root•ed \'rü-təd, 'rú-\ *adj* **1** : having such or so many roots ⟨single-*rooted* premolars⟩ **2** : having a contracted root nearly closing the pulp cavity and preventing further growth

root•let \'rüt-lət, 'rút-\ *n* : a small root; *also* : one of the ultimate divisions of a nerve root

root planing *n* : the scraping of a bacteria-impregnated layer of cementum from the surface of a tooth root to prevent or treat periodontitis

ROP *abbr* retinopathy of prematurity

Ror•schach \'rór-,shäk\ *adj* : of, relating to, used in connection with, or resulting from the Rorschach test

Rorschach test *n* : a projective personality test that uses a subject's interpretation of 10 standard black or colored inkblot designs to assess personality traits and emotional tendencies — called also *Rorschach, Rorschach inkblot test*

    Rorschach, Hermann (1884–1922), Swiss psychiatrist.

ro•sa•cea \rō-'zā-shə, -shē-ə\ *n* : a chronic inflammatory disorder involving esp. the skin of the nose, forehead, and cheeks that is characterized by congestion, flushing, telangiecta-

sia, and marked nodular swelling of tissues esp. of the nose — called also *acne rosacea*

rosary pea *n* **1** : a tropical leguminous twining herb (*Abrus precatorius*) that bears jequirity beans and has a root used as a substitute for licorice **2** : JEQUIRITY BEAN 1

rosea — see PITYRIASIS ROSEA

rose ben•gal \-ben-'gól, -beŋ-\ *n* : either of two bluish red acid dyes that are derivatives of fluorescein

rose bengal test *n* : a test of liver function by determining the time taken for an injected quantity of rose bengal to be absorbed from the bloodstream

rose cold *n* : ROSE FEVER

rose fever *n* : hay fever occurring in the spring or early summer

ro•se•o•la \,rō-zē-'ō-lə, rō-'zē-ə-lə\ *n* : a rose-colored eruption in spots or a disease marked by such an eruption; *esp* : ROSEOLA INFANTUM — **ro•se•o•lar** \-lər\ *adj*

roseola in•fan•tum \-in-'fan-təm\ *n* : a mild virus disease of infants and children that is characterized by fever lasting three days followed by an eruption of rose-colored spots and is caused by a herpesvirus (species *Human herpesvirus 6* of the genus *Roseolovirus*) — called also *exanthema subitum, exanthem subitum*

ro•sette \rō-'zet\ *n* : a rose-shaped cluster of cells

ro•si•glit•a•zone \,rō-sə-'gli-tə-,zōn\ *n* : a drug that is used in the form of its maleate $C_{18}H_{19}N_3O_3S \cdot C_4H_4O_4$ to treat type 2 diabetes by decreasing insulin resistance — see AVANDIA

ros•tral \'räs-trəl, 'rós-\ *adj* **1** : of or relating to a rostrum **2** : situated toward the oral or nasal region: as **a** *of a part of the spinal cord* : SUPERIOR 1 **b** *of a part of the brain* : anterior or ventral ⟨the ∼ pons⟩ — **ros•tral•ly** *adv*

ros•trum \'räs-trəm, 'rós-\ *n, pl* **ros•trums** *or* **ros•tra** \-trə\ : a bodily part or process suggesting a bird's bill: as **a** : the reflected anterior portion of the corpus callosum below the genu **b** : the interior median spine of the body of the basisphenoid bone articulating with the vomer

ro•su•va•stat•in \rō-'sü-və-,sta-t°n\ *n* : a statin that is administered orally in the form of its calcium salt $(C_{22}H_{27}FN_3O_6S)_2Ca$ esp. to treat hypercholesterolemia — see CRESTOR

rosy periwinkle *n* : an Old World tropical shrub (*Catharanthus roseus* syn. *Vinca rosea*) of the dogbane family (Apocynaceae) that is the source of several antineoplastic drugs (as vinblastine and vincristine) — called also *Madagascar periwinkle, periwinkle*

¹rot \'rät\ *vb* **rot•ted; rot•ting** : to undergo decomposition from the action of bacteria or fungi

²rot *n* **1** : the process of rotting : the state of being rotten **2** : any of several parasitic diseases esp. of sheep marked by necrosis and wasting

ro·ta·tor \'rō-ˌtā-tər, rō-'\ *n, pl* **rotators** *or* **ro·ta·to·res** \ˌrō-tə-'tōr-ēz\ : a muscle that partially rotates a part on its axis; *specif* : any of several small muscles in the dorsal region of the spine arising from the back part and back part of a transverse process and inserted into the lamina of the vertebra above

rotator cuff \-ˌkəf\ *n* : a supporting and strengthening structure of the shoulder joint that is made up of part of its capsule blended with tendons of the subscapularis, infraspinatus, supraspinatus, and teres minor muscles as they pass to the capsule or across it to insert on the humerus — called also *musculotendinous cuff*

ro·ta·vi·rus \'rō-tə-ˌvī-rəs\ *n* **1** *cap* : a genus of reoviruses that have a virion with a three-layered protein capsid, no lipid envelope, and a core of 11 discrete segments of double-stranded RNA and that include one (species *Rotavirus A*) causing epidemics of severe and sometimes fatal diarrhea in infants and young children worldwide **2** : any virus of the genus *Rotavirus* — **ro·ta·vi·ral** \-rəl\ *adj*

ro·te·none \'rōt-ᵊn-ˌōn\ *n* : a crystalline insecticide $C_{23}H_{22}O_6$ that is of low toxicity for warm-blooded animals and is used esp. in home gardens

rotunda — see FENESTRA ROTUNDA

rotundum — see FORAMEN ROTUNDUM

Rou·get cell \rü-'zhā\ *n* : any of numerous branching cells adhering to the endothelium of capillaries and regarded as a contractile element in the capillary wall

Rouget, Charles–Marie–Benjamin (1824–1904), French physiologist and anatomist.

rough \'rəf\ *adj* : having a broken, uneven, or bumpy surface; *specif* : forming or being rough colonies usu. made up of organisms that form chains or filaments and tend to marked decrease in capsule formation and virulence — used of dissociated strains of bacteria; compare SMOOTH

rough·age \'rə-fij\ *n* : FIBER 2; *also* : food (as bran) containing much indigestible material acting as fiber

rough endoplasmic reticulum *n* : endoplasmic reticulum that is studded with ribosomes

rou·leau \rü-'lō\ *n, pl* **rou·leaux** \same *or* -'lōz\ *or* **rouleaus** : a group of red blood corpuscles resembling a stack of coins

round \'raund\ *vb* : to go on rounds

round cell *n* : a small lymphocyte or a closely related cell esp. occurring in an area of chronic infection or as the typical cell of some sarcomas

round ligament *n* **1** : a fibrous cord resulting from the obliteration of the umbilical vein of the fetus and passing from the navel to the notch in the anterior border of the liver and along the undersurface of that organ **2** : either of a pair of rounded cords arising from each side of the uterus and traceable through the inguinal canal to the tissue of the labia majora into which they merge

rounds *n pl* : a series of professional calls on hospital patients made by a doctor or nurse — see GRAND ROUNDS

round–shouldered *adj* : having the shoulders stooping or rounded

round window *n* : a round opening between the middle ear and the cochlea that is closed over by a membrane — called also *fenestra cochleae, fenestra rotunda*

round·worm \'raund-ˌwərm\ *n* : NEMATODE; *also* : a related round-bodied unsegmented worm (as an acanthocephalan) as distinguished from a flatworm

roup \'rüp, 'raup\ *n* : TRICHOMONIASIS c

Rous sarcoma \'raus-\ *n* : a readily transplantable malignant fibrosarcoma of chickens that is caused by the Rous sarcoma virus

Rous, Francis Peyton (1879–1970), American pathologist.

Rous sarcoma virus *n* : a retrovirus (species *Rous sarcoma virus* of the genus *Alpharetrovirus*) that contains an oncogene causing Rous sarcoma

route \'rüt, 'raut\ *n* : a method of transmitting a disease or of administering a remedy

Roux–en–Y gastric bypass \ˌrü-ˌen-'wī-, ˌrü-ˌän-ˌē-'grek\ *n* : a gastric bypass surgical procedure in the treatment of severe obesity that involves partitioning off part of the upper stomach to form a small pouch, dividing the jejunum into upper and lower parts, and forming a Y-shaped anastomosis by attaching the free end of the lower part of the jejunum to a new outlet on the upper stomach pouch and attaching the free end of what was the upper jejunum to a new opening on the small intestine — called also *Roux-en-Y*

Roux, César (1857–1934), Swiss surgeon.

RP *abbr* retinitis pigmentosa

RPh *abbr* registered pharmacist

RPR card test \ˌär-ˌpē-ˌär-'kärd-\ *n* : RAPID PLASMA REAGIN TEST

RPT *abbr* registered physical therapist

RQ *abbr* respiratory quotient

RR *abbr* recovery room

RRA *abbr* registered records administrator

-r·rha·gia \'rā-jə, 'rä-, -jē-ə, -zhə, -zhē-ə\ *n comb form* : abnormal or excessive discharge or flow ⟨metrorrhagia⟩ — **-r·rha·gic** \'rä-jik\ *adj comb form*

-r·rha·phy \r-ə-fē\ *n comb form, pl* **-r·rha·phies** : suture : sewing ⟨nephrorrhaphy⟩

-r·rhea \'rē-ə\ *n comb form* : flow : discharge ⟨logorrhea⟩ ⟨leukorrhea⟩

-r·rhex·is \'rek-səs\ *n comb form, pl* **-r·rhex·es** \'rek-,sēz\ : rupture ⟨erythrocytorrhexis⟩

-r·rhoea *chiefly Brit var of* -RRHEA

RRL *abbr* registered records librarian

rRNA \'är-,är-,en-'ā\ *n* : RIBOSOMAL RNA

RRT *abbr* registered respiratory therapist

RSD *abbr* reflex sympathetic dystrophy

RSI \,är-,es-'ī\ *n* : repetitive strain injury

RS–T segment \,är-,es-'tē-\ *n* : ST SEGMENT

RSV *abbr* 1 respiratory syncytial virus 2 Rous sarcoma virus

RT *abbr* 1 reaction time 2 recreational therapy 3 respiratory therapist

Ru *symbol* ruthenium

rub \'rəb\ *n* 1 : the application of friction with pressure ⟨an alcohol ∼⟩ 2 : a sound heard in auscultation that is produced by the friction of one structure moving against another

rub·ber \'rə-bər\ *n* : CONDOM 1

rubber dam *n* : a thin sheet of rubber that is stretched around a tooth to keep it dry during dental work or is used in strips to provide drainage in surgical wounds

rubbing alcohol *n* : a cooling and soothing liquid for external application that contains approximately 70 percent denatured ethanol or isopropyl alcohol

¹ru·be·fa·cient \,rü-bə-'fā-shənt\ *adj* : causing redness of the skin

²rubefacient *n* : a substance (as capsaicin) for external application that produces redness of the skin

ru·bel·la \rü-'be-lə\ *n* : GERMAN MEASLES — see MATERNAL RUBELLA

ru·be·o·la \,rü-bē-'ō-lə, rü-'bē-ə-lə\ *n* : MEASLES 1a — **ru·be·o·lar** \-lər\ *adj*

ru·be·o·sis \,rü-bē-'ō-səs\ *n, pl* **-o·ses** \-'ō-,sēz\ *or* **-osises** : a condition characterized by abnormal redness; *esp* : RUBEOSIS IRIDIS

rubeosis iri·dis \-'ī-rə-dəs\ *n* : abnormal redness of the iris resulting from neovascularization and often associated with diabetes

ru·bid·i·um \rü-'bi-dē-əm\ *n* : a soft silvery metallic element — symbol *Rb*; see ELEMENT table

Rubin test \'rü-bən-\ *n* : a test to determine the patency or occlusion of the fallopian tubes by insufflating them with carbon dioxide

 Rubin, Isidor Clinton (1883–1958), American gynecologist.

ru·bor \'rü-,bȯr\ *n* : redness of the skin (as from inflammation)

rubra — see PITYRIASIS RUBRA PILARIS

ru·bri·cyte \'rü-bri-,sīt\ *n* : an immature red blood cell that has a nucleus, is about half the size of developing

red blood cells in preceding stages, and has cytoplasm that stains erratically blue, purplish, and gray due to the presence of hemoglobin : a polychromatic normoblast

ru·bro·spi·nal \,rü-brō-'spī-nəl\ *adj* 1 : of, relating to, or connecting the red nucleus and the spinal cord 2 : of, relating to, or constituting a tract of crossed nerve fibers passing from the red nucleus to the spinal cord and relaying impulses from the cerebellum and corpora striata to the motor neurons of the spinal cord

Ru·bu·la·vi·rus \,rü-byə-lə-'vī-rəs\ *n* : a genus of paramyxoviruses that includes two of the parainfluenza viruses and the causative agent of mumps

ru·di·ment \'rü-də-mənt\ *n* : an incompletely developed organ or part; *esp* : an organ or part just beginning to develop : ANLAGE

ru·di·men·ta·ry \,rü-də-'men-tə-rē\ *adj* : very imperfectly developed or represented only by a vestige

Ruf·fi·ni's corpuscle \rü-'fē-nēz-\ *or* **Ruf·fi·ni corpuscle** \-nē-\ *n* : any of numerous oval sensory end organs occurring in the subcutaneous tissue of the fingers — called also *Ruffini's brush, Ruffini's end organ*

 Ruffini, Angelo (1864–1929), Italian histologist and embryologist.

RU–486 \,är-(,)yü-,fȯr-,ā-tē-'siks\ *n* : a drug $C_{29}H_{35}NO_2$ taken orally to induce abortion esp. early in pregnancy by blocking the body's use of progesterone — called also *mifepristone*

ru·ga \'rü-gə\ *n, pl* **ru·gae** \-,gī, -,gē, -,jē\ : an anatomical fold or wrinkle esp. of the viscera — usu. used in pl. ⟨the *rugae* of an empty stomach⟩

ru·men \'rü-mən\ *n, pl* **ru·mi·na** \-mə-nə\ *or* **rumens** : the large first compartment of the stomach of a ruminant from which food is regurgitated for rumination and in which cellulose is broken down by the action of symbiotic microorganisms — called also *paunch;* compare ABOMASUM, OMASUM, RETICULUM

ru·men·ot·o·my \,rü-mə-'nä-tə-mē\ *n, pl* **-mies** : surgical incision into the rumen

ru·mi·nant \'rü-mə-nənt\ *adj* : of or relating to two suborders (Ruminantia and Tylopoda) of even-toed hoofed mammals (as sheep and oxen) that chew the cud and have a complex 3- or 4-chambered stomach — **ruminant** *n*

ru·mi·na·tion \,rü-mə-'nā-shən\ *n* : the act or process of regurgitating and chewing again previously swallowed food — **ru·mi·nate** \'rü-mə-,nāt\ *vb*

rump \'rəmp\ *n* 1 : the upper rounded part of the hindquarters of a quadruped mammal 2 : the seat of the body : BUTTOCKS

Rum·pel–Leede test \'rům-pel-'lēd-\ *n* : a test in which the increased bleeding tendency characteristic of various disorders (as scarlet fever and thrombocytopenia) is indicated by the formation of multiple petechiae on the forearm following application of a tourniquet to the upper arm

Rumpel, Theodor (1862–1923), German physician.

Leede, Carl Stockbridge (1882–1964), American physician.

run \'rən\ *vb* **ran** \'ran\; **run; run·ning** : to discharge fluid (as pus or serum) ⟨a *running* sore⟩ — **run a fever** *or* **run a temperature** : to have a fever

rung *past part of* RING

runner's high *n* : a feeling of euphoria that is experienced by some individuals engaged in strenuous running and that is held to be associated with the release of endorphins by the brain

runner's knee *n* : pain in the region of the knee esp. when related to running that may have a simple anatomical basis (as tightness of a muscle) or may be a symptom of iliotibial band friction syndrome or an indication of chondromalacia patellae

run·ny \'rə-nē\ *adj* : secreting a thin flow of mucus ⟨a ∼ nose⟩

runs \'rənz\ *n sing or pl* : DIARRHEA — used with *the*

ru·pia \'rü-pē-ə\ *n* : an eruption occurring esp. in tertiary syphilis consisting of vesicles having an inflamed base and filled with serous purulent or bloody fluid which dries up and forms large blackish conical crusts — **ru·pi·al** \-əl\ *adj*

rup·ture \'rəp-chər\ *n* **1** : the tearing apart of a tissue ⟨∼ of an intervertebral disk⟩ **2** : HERNIA — **rupture** *vb*

RUQ *abbr* right upper quadrant (abdomen)

rush \'rəsh\ *n* **1** : a rapid and extensive wave of peristalsis along the walls of the intestine ⟨peristaltic ∼⟩ **2** : the immediate pleasurable feeling produced by a drug (as heroin or amphetamine) — called also *flash*

Russian spring–summer encephalitis *n* : a tick-borne encephalitis of Europe and Asia caused by a strain (Far Eastern subtype) of the tick-borne encephalitis virus and transmitted by ticks of the genus *Ixodes*

¹rut \'rət\ *n* **1** : an annually recurrent state of sexual excitement in the male deer; *broadly* : sexual excitement in a mammal esp. when periodic **2** : the period during which rut normally occurs — often used with *the*

²rut *vb* **rut·ted; rut·ting** : to be in or enter into a state of rut

ru·the·ni·um \rü-'thē-nē-əm\ *n* : a hard brittle grayish rare metallic element — symbol *Ru;* see ELEMENT table

ruth·er·ford \'rə-thər-fərd\ *n* : a unit strength of a radioactive source corresponding to one million disintegrations per second — abbr. *rd*

Rutherford, Ernest (Baron Rutherford of Nelson) (1871–1937), British physicist.

ruth·er·ford·ium \rə-thər-'fòr-dē-əm\ *n* : a short-lived radioactive element that is artificially produced — symbol *Rf;* see ELEMENT table

ru·tin \'rüt-ᵊn\ *n* : a yellow crystalline glycoside $C_{27}H_{30}O_{16}$ that occurs in various plants (as tobacco) and that is used chiefly for strengthening capillary blood vessels (as in cases of hypertension and radiation injury)

R wave \'är-ˌwāv\ *n* : the positive upward deflection in the QRS complex of an electrocardiogram that follows the Q wave

Rx \ˌär-'eks\ *n* : a medical prescription

S *abbr* **1** sacral — used esp. with a number from 1 to 5 to indicate a vertebra or segment of the spinal cord in the sacral region **2** signa — used to introduce the signature in writing a prescription **3** subject **4** svedberg

S *symbol* sulfur

sa *abbr* [Latin *secundum artem*] according to art — used in writing prescriptions

S–A *abbr* sinoatrial

sa·bal \'sā-ˌbal\ *n* : SAW PALMETTO

sa·ber shin \'sā-bər-\ *n* : a tibia that has a pronounced anterior convexity caused by disease (as congenital syphilis or rickets)

Sa·bin vaccine \'sā-bin-\ *n* : a polio vaccine that is taken by mouth and contains the three serotypes of poliovirus in a weakened live state — called also *Sabin oral vaccine*

Sabin, Albert Bruce (1906–1993), American immunologist.

sac \'sak\ *n* : a soft-walled anatomical cavity usu. having a narrow opening or none at all and often containing a special fluid ⟨a synovial ∼⟩ — see AIR SAC, AMNIOTIC SAC, LACRIMAL SAC

sac·cade \sa-'käd\ *n* : a small rapid jerky movement of the eye as it jumps from fixation on one point to another (as in reading) — **sac·cad·ic** \-'kä-dik\ *adj*

saccharo- *or* **saccharo-** *comb form* : sugar ⟨*sacchar*ide⟩

sac·cha·rase \'sa-kə-ˌrās, -ˌrāz\ *n* : INVERTASE

sac·cha·ride \'sa-kə-ˌrīd, -rid\ *n* : a simple sugar, combination of sugars, or polymerized sugar

sac·cha·rin \'sa-kə-rin\ *n* : a crystalline compound $C_7H_5NO_3S$ that is unrelated to the carbohydrates, is many times sweeter than sucrose, and is used as a calorie-free sweetener

sac·cha·ro·my·ces \ˌsa-kə-rō-'mī-(ˌ)sēz\ *n* **1** *cap* : a genus of usu. unicellular yeasts (family Saccharomycetaceae) distinguished by their sparse or absent mycelium and by their facility in reproducing asexually by budding **2** *pl* **saccharomyces** : any yeast of the genus *Saccharomyces*

sac·cu·lar \'sa-kyə-lər\ *adj* : resembling a sac ⟨a ~ aneurysm⟩

sac·cu·lat·ed \-ˌlā-təd\ *also* **sac·cu·late** \-ˌlāt, -lət\ *adj* : having or formed of a series of saccular expansions

sac·cu·la·tion \ˌsa-kyə-'lā-shən\ *n* **1** : the quality or state of being sacculated **2** : the process of developing or segmenting into sacculated structures **3** : a sac or sacculated structure; *esp* : one of a linear series of such structures ⟨the ~s of the colon⟩

sac·cule \'sa-(ˌ)kyül\ *n* : a little sac; *specif* : the smaller chamber of the membranous labyrinth of the ear that contains the macula sacculi

sac·cu·lus \'sa-kyə-ləs\ *n, pl* **-li** \-ˌlī, -ˌlē\ : SACCULE

sac·like \'sak-ˌlīk\ *adj* : having the form of or suggesting a sac

sacr- *or* **sacro-** *comb form* **1** : sacrum ⟨*sacral*⟩ **2** : sacral and ⟨*sacroiliac*⟩

sacra *pl of* SACRUM

¹sa·cral \'sa-krəl, 'sā-\ *adj* : of, relating to, or lying near the sacrum

²sacral *n* : a sacral vertebra or sacral nerve

sacral artery — see LATERAL SACRAL ARTERY, MIDDLE SACRAL ARTERY

sacral canal *n* : the part of the vertebral canal lying in the sacrum

sacral cornu *n* : a rounded process on each side of the fifth sacral vertebra

sacral crest *n* : any of several crests or tubercles on the sacrum: as **a** : one on the midline of the dorsal surface — called also *median sacral crest* **b** : any of a series of tubercles on each side of the dorsal surface lateral to the sacral foramina that represent the transverse processes of the sacral vertebrae and serve as attachments for ligaments — called also *lateral sacral crest*

sacral foramen *n* : any of 16 openings in the sacrum of which there are four on each side of the dorsal surface giving passage to the posterior branches of the sacral nerves and four on each side of the pelvic surface giving passage to the anterior branches of the sacral nerves

sacral hiatus *n* : the opening into the vertebral canal in the midline of the dorsal surface of the sacrum between the laminae of the fifth sacral vertebra

sa·cral·i·za·tion \ˌsa-krə-lə-'zā-shən\ *n* : a congenital anomaly in which the fifth lumbar vertebra is fused to the sacrum in varying degrees

sacral nerve *n* : any of the spinal nerves of the sacral region of which there are five pairs and which have anterior and posterior branches passing out through the sacral foramina

sacral plexus *n* : a nerve plexus that lies against the posterior and lateral walls of the pelvis, is formed by the union of the lumbosacral trunk and the first, second, and third sacral nerves, and continues into the thigh as the sciatic nerve

sacral promontory *n* : the inwardly projecting anterior part of the body of the first sacral vertebra

sacral vein — see LATERAL SACRAL VEIN, MEDIAN SACRAL VEIN

sacral vertebra *n* : any of the five fused vertebrae that make up the sacrum

sacro- — see SACR-

sa·cro·coc·cy·geal \ˌsā-krō-käk-'si-jəl, ˌsa-, -jē-əl\ *adj* : of, relating to, affecting, or performed by way of the region of the sacrum and coccyx

sa·cro·coc·cy·geus dor·sa·lis \-käk-'si-jē-əs-ˌdȯr-'sā-ləs\ *n* : an inconstant muscle that sometimes extends from the dorsal part of the sacrum to the coccyx — called also *posterior sacrococcygeal muscle*

sacrococcygeus ven·tra·lis \-ven-'trā-ləs\ *n* : an inconstant muscle that sometimes extends from the ventral surface of the lower sacral vertebrae to the coccyx — called also *anterior sacrococcygeal muscle*

¹sa·cro·il·i·ac \ˌsā-krō-'i-lē-ˌak, ˌsā-\ *adj* : of, relating to, affecting, or being the region of the joint between the sacrum and the ilium ⟨~ distress⟩

²sacroiliac *n* : SACROILIAC JOINT

sacroiliac joint *n* : the joint or articulation between the sacrum and ilium — called also *sacroiliac, sacroiliac articulation*

sa·cro·il·i·i·tis \ˌsā-krō-ˌi-lē-'ī-təs, ˌsa-\ *n* : inflammation of the sacroiliac joint or region

sa·cro·spi·na·lis \ˌsā-krō-spī-'nā-ləs, ˌsa-krō-spī-'na-ləs\ *n* : a muscle that extends the length of the back and neck, that arises from the iliac crest, the sacrum, and the lumbar and two lower thoracic vertebrae, and that splits in the upper lumbar region into the iliocostalis muscles, the longissimus muscles, and the spinalis muscles — called also *erector spinae*

sa·cro·spi·nous ligament \ˌsā-krō-'spī-nəs-, ˌsa-\ *n* : a ligament on each side of the body that is attached by a broad base to the lateral margins of the sacrum and coccyx and passes to the ischial spine and that closes off the greater sciatic notch to form the greater sciatic foramen and with the sacrotuberous ligament closes off the lesser sciatic notch to form the lesser sciatic foramen

sa·cro·tu·ber·ous ligament \ˌsā-krō-ˈtü-bə-rəs-, ˌsa-, -ˈtyü-\ n : a thin fan-shaped ligament on each side of the body that is attached above to the posterior superior and posterior inferior iliac spines and to the sacrum and coccyx, that passes obliquely downward to insert into the inner margin of the ischial tuberosity, and that with the sacrospinous ligament closes off the lesser sciatic notch to form the lesser sciatic foramen

sa·cro·uter·ine ligament \-ˈyü-tə-ˌrīn-, -rən-\ n : UTEROSACRAL LIGAMENT

sa·crum \ˈsa-krəm, ˈsā-\ n, pl **sa·cra** \ˈsa-krə, ˈsā-\ : the part of the spinal column that is directly connected with or forms a part of the pelvis by articulation with the ilia and that in humans forms the dorsal wall of the pelvis and consists of five fused vertebrae diminishing in size to the apex at the lower end which bears the coccyx

SAD abbr seasonal affective disorder

sad·dle \ˈsad-ᵊl\ n : the part of a partial denture that carries an artificial tooth and has connectors for adjacent teeth attached to its ends

sad·dle·bag \ˈsa-dᵊl-ˌbag\ n : a bulge of lumpy fat in the outer area of the upper thighs

saddle block anesthesia n : spinal anesthesia confined to the perineum, the buttocks, and the inner aspect of the thighs — called also *saddle block*

saddle joint n : a joint (as the carpometacarpal joint of the thumb) with saddle-shaped articular surfaces that are convex in one direction and concave in another and that permit movements in all directions except axial rotation

sad·dle-nose \ˈsad-ᵊl-ˌnōz\ n : a nose marked by depression of the bridge resulting from injury or disease

sa·dism \ˈsā-ˌdiz-əm, ˈsa-\ n : a sexual perversion in which gratification is obtained by the infliction of physical or mental pain on others (as on a love object) — compare ALGOLAGNIA, MASOCHISM — **sa·dis·tic** \sə-ˈdis-tik, sā-, sa-\ adj — **sa·dis·ti·cal·ly** adv

Sade \ˈsäd\, **Marquis de (Comte Donatien–Alphonse–François) (1740–1814),** French soldier and writer.

sa·dist \ˈsā-dist, ˈsa-\ n : an individual who practices sadism

sa·do·mas·och·ism \ˌsā-dō-ˈma-sə-ˌki-zəm, ˌsa-, -zō-ˌki-\ n : the derivation of pleasure from the infliction of physical or mental pain either on others or on oneself — **sa·do·mas·och·ist·ic** \-ˌma-sə-ˈkist-ik\ also **sado·masochist** adj

L. von Sacher–Masoch — see MASOCHISM

sa·do·mas·och·ist \-kist\ n : an individual who practices sadomasochism

safe \ˈsāf\ adj **saf·er; saf·est** : not causing harm or injury; esp : having a low incidence of adverse reactions and significant side effects when adequate instructions for use are given and having a low potential for harm under conditions of widespread availability — **safe·ty** \ˈsāf-tē\ n

safe period n : a portion of the menstrual cycle of the human female during which conception is least likely to occur and which usu. includes several days immediately before and after the menstrual period and the period itself

safe sex n : sexual activity and esp. sexual intercourse in which various measures (as the use of latex condoms or the practice of monogamy) are taken to avoid disease (as AIDS) transmitted by sexual contact — called also *safer sex*

saf·flow·er oil \ˈsa-ˌflaü-ər-\ n : an edible oil that is low in saturated fatty acids and is obtained from the seeds of the safflower (*Carthamus tinctorius* of the family Compositae)

sag·it·tal \ˈsa-jət-ᵊl\ adj **1** : of, relating to, or being the sagittal suture of the skull **2** : of, relating to, situated in, or being the median plane of the body or any plane parallel to it ⟨a ~ section⟩ — **sag·it·tal·ly** adv

sagittal plane n : MIDSAGITTAL PLANE; also : any plane parallel to a midsagittal plane : a parasagittal plane

sagittal sinus n : either of two venous sinuses of the dura mater: **a** : one passing backward in the convex attached superior margin of the falx cerebri and ending at the internal occipital protuberance by fusion with the transverse sinus — called also *superior sagittal sinus* **b** : one lying in the posterior two thirds of the concave free inferior margin of the falx cerebri and ending posteriorly by joining the great cerebral vein to form the straight sinus — called also *inferior sagittal sinus*

sagittal suture n : the deeply serrated articulation between the two parietal bones in the median plane of the top of the head

sa·go spleen \ˈsā-(ˌ)gō-\ n : a spleen which is affected with amyloid degeneration and in which the amyloid is deposited in the Malpighian corpuscles which appear in cross section as gray translucent bodies

sagrada — see CASCARA SAGRADA

Saint An·tho·ny's fire \ˌsānt-ˈan-thə-nēz-\ n : any of several inflammations or gangrenous conditions (as erysipelas or ergotism) of the skin

Anthony, Saint (ca 250–350), Egyptian monk.

Saint–John's-wort \ˌsānt-ˈjänz-ˌwərt, -ˌwòrt\ n **1** : any of a genus (*Hypericum* of the family Guttiferae) of yellow-flowered herbs and shrubs; esp : one (*H. perforatum*) causing photosensitization in sheep, cattle, horses, and goats when ingested **2** *usu* **Saint John's wort** : the dried aerial parts of a Saint-John's-wort (*Hypericum perforatum*) that are held to relieve depression and are used in herbal remedies and dietary supplements

John the Baptist, Saint (*fl* first century AD), Jewish prophet.

Saint Lou·is encephalitis \ˌsänt-ˈlü-is-\ *n* : a No. American encephalitis that is caused by a virus of the genus *Flavivirus* (species *St. Louis encephalitis virus*) transmitted by several mosquitoes of the genus *Culex*

Saint Vi·tus' dance \-ˈvī-təs-\ *also* **Saint Vitus's dance** \-ˈvī-tə-səz-\ *n* : CHOREA; *esp* : SYDENHAM'S CHOREA

Vitus, Saint (*d ca* 300), Italian martyr.

sal·abra·sion \ˌsal-ə-ˈbrā-zhən\ *n* : a method of removing tattoos from skin in which moist gauze pads saturated with sodium chloride are used to abrade the tattooed area by rubbing

sal am·mo·ni·ac \ˌsal-ə-ˈmō-nē-ˌak\ *n* : AMMONIUM CHLORIDE

sal·bu·ta·mol \sal-ˈbyü-tə-ˌmȯl, -ˌmōl\ *n* : ALBUTEROL

salicyl- *or* **salicylo-** *comb form* : related to salicylic acid ⟨*salicyl*amide⟩

sal·i·cyl·amide \ˌsa-lə-ˈsil-ə-ˌmīd\ *n* : the crystalline amide $C_7H_7NO_2$ of salicylic acid used chiefly as an analgesic, antipyretic, and antirheumatic

sal·i·cyl·an·il·ide \ˌsa-lə-sə-ˈlan-ᵊl-ˌīd\ *n* : a fungicidal agent $C_{13}H_{11}NO_2$ used esp. in the external treatment of tinea capitis caused by a fungus of the genus *Microsporum* (*M. audouini*)

sa·lic·y·late \sə-ˈlis-ə-ˌlāt\ *n* : a salt or ester of salicylic acid; *also* : SALICYLIC ACID

sal·i·cyl·azo·sul·fa·pyr·i·dine \ˌsa-lə-si-ˌlā-zō-ˌsəl-fə-ˈpir-ə-ˌdēn\ *n* : SULFASALAZINE

sal·i·cyl·ic acid \ˌsa-lə-ˈsil-ik-\ *n* : a crystalline phenolic acid $C_7H_6O_3$ that is used esp. in making pharmaceuticals and dyes, as an antiseptic and disinfectant esp. in treating skin diseases, and in the form of salts and other derivatives as an analgesic and antipyretic — see ASPIRIN

sal·i·cyl·ism \ˈsa-lə-si-ˌli-zəm\ *n* : a toxic condition produced by the excessive intake of salicylic acid or salicylates and marked by ringing in the ears, nausea, and vomiting

¹sa·line \ˈsā-ˌlēn, -ˌlīn\ *adj* **1** : consisting of or containing salt ⟨a ∼ solution⟩ **2** : of, relating to, or resembling salt : SALTY ⟨a ∼ taste⟩ **3** : consisting of or relating to the salts esp. of lithium, sodium, potassium, and magnesium ⟨a ∼ cathartic⟩ **4** : relating to or being abortion induced by the injection of a highly concentrated saline solution into the amniotic sac ⟨∼ amniocentesis⟩ — **sa·lin·i·ty** \sā-ˈlin-ət-ē, sə-\ *n*

²saline *n* **1 a** : a metallic salt; *esp* : a salt of potassium, sodium, or magnesium with a cathartic action **b** : an aqueous solution of one or more such salts **2** : a saline solution used in physiology; *esp* : PHYSIOLOGICAL SALINE

sa·li·va \sə-ˈlī-və\ *n* : a slightly alkaline secretion of water, mucin, protein, salts, and often a starch-splitting enzyme (as ptyalin) that is secreted into the mouth by salivary glands, lubricates ingested food, and often begins the breakdown of starches

saliva ejector *n* : a narrow tubular device providing suction to draw saliva, blood, and debris from the mouth of a dental patient in order to maintain a clear operative field

sal·i·vary \ˈsa-lə-ˌver-ē\ *adj* : of or relating to saliva or the glands that secrete it; *esp* : producing or carrying saliva

salivary gland *n* : any of various glands that discharge a fluid secretion and esp. saliva into the mouth cavity and that in humans comprise large compound racemose glands including the parotid glands, the sublingual glands, and the submandibular glands

sal·i·va·tion \ˌsa-lə-ˈvā-shən\ *n* : the act or process of producing a flow of saliva; *esp* : excessive secretion of saliva often accompanied by soreness of the mouth and gums — **sal·i·vate** \ˈsa-lə-ˌvāt\ *vb*

sal·i·va·to·ry \ˈsa-lə-və-ˌtōr-ē\ *adj* : inducing salivation

Salk vaccine \ˈsȯk-, ˈsȯlk-\ *n* : a polio vaccine which contains the three serotypes of poliovirus in which the serotypes have been inactivated by treatment with formaldehyde

Salk, Jonas Edward (1914–1995), American immunologist.

sal·met·er·ol \sal-ˈme-tə-ˌrȯl, -ˌrōl\ *n* : a bronchodilator administered by oral inhalation in the form of a salt $C_{25}H_{37}NO_4 \cdot C_{11}H_8O_3$ to treat asthma and bronchospasm — see ADVAIR DISKUS

sal·mo·nel·la \ˌsal-mə-ˈne-lə\ *n* **1** *cap* : a genus of aerobic gram-negative rod-shaped usu. motile enterobacteria that are pathogenic for humans and other warm-blooded animals and cause food poisoning, acute gastrointestinal inflammation, typhoid fever, or septicemia **2** *pl* **-nel·lae** \-ˈne-lē\ *or* **-nellas** *or* **-nella** : any bacterium of the genus *Salmonella*

Salm·on \ˈsa-mən\, **Daniel Elmer** (1850–1914), American veterinarian.

sal·mo·nel·lo·sis \ˌsal-mə-ˌne-ˈlō-səs\ *n*, *pl* **-lo·ses** \-ˌsēz\ : infection with or disease caused by bacteria of the genus *Salmonella* typically marked by gastroenteritis but often complicated by septicemia, meningitis, endocarditis, and various focal lesions (as in the kidneys)

salmon poisoning *n* : a highly fatal febrile disease of dogs and other canines that resembles canine distemper and is caused by a rickettsial bacterium (*Neorickettsia helminthoeca*) transmitted by encysted larvae of a fluke (*Nanophyetus salmincola*) ingested with the raw flesh of infested salmon, trout, or salamanders

sal·ol \'sa-ˌlȯl, -ˌōl\ *n* : PHENYL SALICYLATE

salping- *or* **salpingo-** *comb form* 1 : fallopian tube ⟨*salpingo*plasty⟩ 2 : eustachian tube ⟨*salpingo*pharyngeus⟩

sal·pin·gec·to·my \ˌsal-pən-ˈjek-tə-mē\ *n, pl* **-mies** : surgical excision of a fallopian tube

sal·pin·gi·tis \ˌsal-pən-ˈjī-təs\ *n, pl* **-git·i·des** \-ˈji-tə-ˌdēz\ : inflammation of a fallopian or eustachian tube

salpingitis isth·mi·ca no·do·sa \-ˈis-mə-kə-nə-ˈdō-sə\ *n* : salpingitis of the fallopian tubes marked by nodular thickening of the muscular coat

sal·pin·gog·ra·phy \ˌsal-piŋ-ˈgä-grə-fē\ *n, pl* **-phies** : visualization of a fallopian tube by radiography following injection of an opaque medium

sal·pin·gol·y·sis \ˌsal-piŋ-ˈgä-lə-səs\ *n, pl* **-y·ses** : surgical correction of adhesions in a fallopian tube

sal·pin·go—oo·pho·rec·to·my \ˌsal-ˌpiŋ-gō-ˌō-ə-fə-ˈrek-tə-mē\ *n, pl* **-mies** : surgical excision of a fallopian tube and an ovary

sal·pin·go—oo·pho·ri·tis \-ˌō-ə-fə-ˈrī-təs\ *n* : inflammation of a fallopian tube and an ovary

sal·pin·go·pha·ryn·ge·us \-fə-ˈrin-jē-əs\ *n* : a muscle of the pharynx that arises from the inferior part of the eustachian tube near its opening and passes downward to join the posterior part of the palatopharyngeus

sal·pin·go·plas·ty \sal-ˈpiŋ-gə-ˌplas-tē\ *n, pl* **-ties** : plastic surgery of a fallopian tube

sal·pin·gos·to·my \ˌsal-piŋ-ˈgäs-tə-mē\ *n, pl* **-mies** : a surgical opening of a fallopian tube (as to establish patency)

¹salt \'sȯlt\ *n* 1 a : a crystalline compound NaCl that is the chloride of sodium, is abundant in nature, and is used esp. to season or preserve food — called also *sodium chloride* b : any of numerous compounds that result from replacement of part or all of the acid hydrogen of an acid by a metal or a group acting like a metal : an ionic crystalline compound 2 **salts** *pl* a : a mineral or saline mixture (as Epsom salts) used as an aperient or cathartic b : SMELLING SALTS — **salty** \'sȯl-tē\ *adj*

²salt *adj* 1 : SALINE 2 : being or inducing the one of the four basic taste sensations that is suggestive of seawater — compare BITTER, SOUR, SWEET

sal·ta·to·ry \'sal-tə-ˌtȯr-ē, 'sȯl-\ *adj* : proceeding by leaps rather than by gradual transitions ⟨∼ conduction of nerve impulses⟩

salt·pe·ter \'sȯlt-ˈpē-tər\ *n* 1 : POTASSIUM NITRATE 2 : SODIUM NITRATE

¹sal·uret·ic \ˌsal-yə-ˈre-tik\ *adj* : facilitating the urinary excretion of salt and esp. of sodium ion ⟨a ∼ drug⟩

²saluretic *n* : a saluretic agent

sal·vage \'sal-vij\ *vb* **sal·vaged; sal·vag·ing** : to save (an organ, tissue, or patient) by preventive or therapeutic measures ⟨*salvaged* lung tissue⟩ — **salvage** *n*

sal·var·san \'sal-vər-ˌsan\ *n* : ARSPHENAMINE

salve \'sav, 'säv, 'salv, 'sälv\ *n* : an unctuous adhesive substance for application to wounds or sores

sal vo·la·ti·le \ˌsal-və-ˈlat-ᵊl-ē\ *n* 1 : AMMONIUM CARBONATE 2 : SMELLING SALTS

sa·mar·i·um \sə-ˈmar-ē-əm\ *n* : a pale gray lustrous metallic element — symbol *Sm;* see ELEMENT table

SAMe \'sa-mē\ *n* : S-adenosylmethionine esp. when used as a dietary supplement (as to relieve depression or arthritic pain and inflammation)

san·a·to·ri·um \ˌsa-nə-ˈtȯr-ē-əm\ *n, pl* **-riums** *or* **-ria** \-ē-ə\ 1 : an establishment that provides therapy combined with a regimen (as of diet and exercise) for treatment or rehabilitation 2 a : an institution for rest and recuperation (as of convalescents) b : an establishment for the treatment of the chronically ill ⟨a tuberculosis ∼⟩

sand \'sand\ *n* : gritty particles in various body tissues or fluids

sand crack *n* : a fissure in the wall of a horse's hoof often causing lameness

sand flea *n* : CHIGOE 1

sand fly *n* : any of various small biting dipteran flies (families Psychodidae, Simuliidae, and Ceratopogonidae); *esp* : any fly of the genus *Phlebotomus*

sand·fly fever \'sand-ˌflī-\ *n* : a virus disease of brief duration that is characterized by fever, headache, pain in the eyes, malaise, and leukopenia and is caused by either of two bunyaviruses assigned or tentatively assigned to the genus *Phlebovirus* (species *Sandfly fever Naples virus* and species *Sandfly fever Sicilian virus*) transmitted by the bite of a sand fly of the genus *Phlebotomus* (esp. *P. papatasii*) — called also *pappataci fever, phlebotomus fever*

Sand·hoff—Jatz·ke·witz disease \-ˈjats-kə-ˌvits-\ *n* : SANDHOFF'S DISEASE

Sand·hoff's disease \'sand-ˌhȯfs-\ *or* **Sand·hoff disease** \-ˌhȯf-\ *n* : a hereditary disorder of lipid metabolism that is closely related to or is a variant of Tay-Sachs disease, typically affects individuals of non-Jewish ancestry, and is characterized by great reduction in or absence of both hexosaminidase A and hexosaminidase B
  Sandhoff, K., An·dreae \än-ˈdrā-ə\, **U., and Jatzkewitz, H.,** German medical scientists.

sane \ˈsān\ *adj* **san·er; san·est** **1** : free from hurt or disease : HEALTHY **2** : mentally sound; *esp* : able to anticipate and appraise the effect of one's actions **3** : proceeding from a sound mind ⟨∼ behavior⟩ — **sane·ly** *adv*

san·guin·e·ous \saŋ-ˈgwi-nē-əs, san-\ *adj* : of, relating to, or containing blood

san·guin·ous \ˈsaŋ-gwə-nəs\ *adj* : SANGUINEOUS

san·i·tar·i·an \ˌsa-nə-ˈter-ē-ən\ *n* : a specialist in sanitary science and public health ⟨a milk ∼⟩

san·i·tar·i·um \ˌsa-nə-ˈter-ē-əm\ *n, pl* **-i·ums** *or* **-ia** \-ē-ə\ : SANATORIUM

san·i·tary \ˈsa-nə-ˌter-ē\ *adj* **1** : of or relating to health ⟨∼ measures⟩ **2** : of, relating to, or used in the disposal esp. of domestic waterborne waste **3** : characterized by or readily kept in cleanliness ⟨∼ food handling⟩ — **san·i·tari·ly** \ˌsa-nə-ˈter-ə-lē\ *adv*

sanitary napkin *n* : a disposable absorbent pad used (as during menstruation) to absorb the flow from the uterus

san·i·ta·tion \ˌsa-nə-ˈtā-shən\ *n* **1** : the act or process of making sanitary **2** : the promotion of hygiene and prevention of disease by maintenance of sanitary conditions ⟨mouth ∼⟩

san·i·tize \ˈsa-nə-ˌtīz\ *vb* **-tized; -tiz·ing** : to make sanitary (as by cleaning or sterilizing) — **san·i·ti·za·tion** \ˌsa-nə-tə-ˈzā-shən\ *n*

san·i·to·ri·um \ˌsa-nə-ˈtōr-ē-əm\ *n, pl* **-ri·ums** *or* **-ria** \-ē-ə\ : SANATORIUM

san·i·ty \ˈsa-nə-tē\ *n, pl* **-ties** : the quality or state of being sane; *esp* : soundness or health of mind

San Joa·quin fever \ˌsan-ˌwä-ˈkēn-\ *n* : COCCIDIOIDOMYCOSIS

San Joaquin valley fever *n* : COCCIDIOIDOMYCOSIS

S–A node \ˌes-ˈā-\ *n* : SINOATRIAL NODE

santa — see YERBA SANTA

sap — see CELL SAP, NUCLEAR SAP

sa·phe·no·fem·o·ral \sə-ˌfē-nō-ˈfe-mə-rəl\ *adj* : of or relating to the saphenous and the femoral veins

sa·phe·nous \sə-ˈfē-nəs, ˈsa-fə-nəs\ *adj* : of, relating to, associated with, or being either of the saphenous veins

saphenous nerve *n* : a nerve that is the largest and longest branch of the femoral nerve and supplies the skin over the medial side of the leg

saphenous opening *n* : a passage for the great saphenous vein in the fascia lata of the thigh — called also *fossa ovalis*

saphenous vein *n* : either of two chief superficial veins of the leg: **a** : one originating in the foot and passing up the medial side of the leg and through the saphenous opening to join the femoral vein — called also *great saphenous vein, long saphenous vein* **b** : one originating similarly and passing up the back of the leg to join the

popliteal vein at the knee — called also *short saphenous vein, small saphenous vein*

sa·pon·i·fi·ca·tion \sə-ˌpä-nə-fə-ˈkā-shən\ *n* **1** : the hydrolysis of a fat by an alkali with the formation of a soap and glycerol **2** : the hydrolysis esp. by an alkali of an ester into the corresponding alcohol and acid; *broadly* : HYDROLYSIS — **sa·pon·i·fy** \sə-ˈpä-nə-ˌfī\ *vb*

sap·phic \ˈsa-fik\ *adj or n* : LESBIAN **Sap·pho** \ˈsa-(ˌ)fō\ *(fl ca* 610 BC*–ca* 580 BC), Greek lyric poet.

sap·phism \ˈsa-ˌfi-zəm\ *n* : LESBIANISM

sap·phist \-fist\ *n* : LESBIAN

sapr- *or* **sapro-** *comb form* : dead or decaying organic matter ⟨*sapro*phyte⟩

sap·ro·phyte \ˈsa-prə-ˌfīt\ *n* : a saprophytic organism

sap·ro·phyt·ic \ˌsa-prə-ˈfi-tik\ *adj* : obtaining food by absorbing dissolved organic material; *esp* : obtaining nourishment from the products of organic breakdown and decay ⟨∼ fungi⟩ — **sap·ro·phyt·i·cal·ly** *adv*

sap·ro·zo·ic \-ˈzō-ik\ *adj* : SAPROPHYTIC — used of animals (as protozoans)

sa·quin·a·vir \sə-ˈkwi-nə-ˌvir\ *n* : a protease inhibitor $C_{38}H_{50}N_6O_5$ or its mesylate $C_{38}H_{50}N_6O_5 \cdot CH_4O_3S$ administered orally often in combination with other antiretroviral drugs to treat HIV infection

sar·al·a·sin \sä-ˈra-lə-sən\ *n* : an antihypertensive polypeptide used esp. in the form of its hydrated acetate $C_{42}H_{65}N_{13}O_{10} \cdot nC_2H_4O_2 \cdot nH_2O$ to treat and diagnose hypertension

sarc- *or* **sarco-** *comb form* **1** : flesh ⟨*sarc*oid⟩ **2** : striated muscle ⟨*sarc*olemma⟩

sar·co·cyst \ˈsär-kə-ˌsist\ *n* : the large intramuscular cyst of a protozoan of the genus *Sarcocystis*

Sar·co·cys·tis \ˌsär-kə-ˈsis-təs\ *n* : a genus of sporozoan protozoans (order Sarcosporidia) that form cysts in vertebrate muscle

sar·co·cys·to·sis \ˌsär-kə-ˌsis-ˈtō-səs\ *n* : infestation with or disease caused by sporozoan protozoans of the genus *Sarcocystis* — called also *sarcosporidiosis*

¹**sar·coid** \ˈsär-ˌkȯid\ *adj* : of, relating to, resembling, or being sarcoid or sarcoidosis ⟨∼ fibroblastic tissue⟩

²**sarcoid** *n* **1** : any of various diseases characterized esp. by the formation of nodules in the skin **2** : a nodule characteristic of sarcoid or of sarcoidosis

sar·coid·o·sis \ˌsär-ˌkȯi-ˈdō-səs\ *n, pl* **-o·ses** \-ˌsēz\ : a chronic disease of unknown cause that is characterized by the formation of nodules resembling true tubercles esp. in the lymph nodes, lungs, bones, and skin — called also *Boeck's sarcoid*

sar·co·lem·ma \ˌsär-kə-ˈle-mə\ *n* : the thin transparent homogeneous sheath enclosing a striated muscle fiber — **sar·co·lem·mal** \-məl\ *adj*

sar·co·ly·sine \ˌsär-kə-ˈlī-sən\ *or* **sar·co·ly·sin** \-sēn\ *also* L—**sar·co·ly·sin** \ˈel-\ *or* L—**sar·co·ly·sine** \ *n* : MELPHALAN

sar·co·ma \sär-ˈkō-mə\ *n, pl* **-mas** *also* **-ma·ta** \-mə-tə\ : a malignant tumor arising in tissue of mesodermal origin (as connective tissue, bone, cartilage, or striated muscle) that spreads by extension into neighboring tissue or by way of the bloodstream — compare CARCINOMA

sarcoma bot·ry·oi·des \-ˌbä-trē-ˈòi-ˌdēz\ *n* : a malignant tumor of striated muscle that resembles a bunch of grapes and occurs esp. in the urogenital tract of young children

sar·co·ma·to·sis \(ˌ)sär-ˌkō-mə-ˈtō-səs\ *n, pl* **-to·ses** \-ˌsēz\ : a disease characterized by the presence and spread of sarcomas

sar·co·ma·tous \sär-ˈkō-mə-təs\ *adj* : of, relating to, or resembling sarcoma

sar·co·mere \ˈsär-kə-ˌmir\ *n* : any of the repeating structural units of striated muscle fibrils — **sar·co·mer·ic** \ˌsär-kə-ˈmer-ik\ *adj*

Sar·coph·a·ga \sär-ˈkä-fə-gə\ *n* : a genus of dipteran flies (family Sarcophagidae) comprising typical flesh flies

sar·co·plasm \ˈsär-kə-ˌpla-zəm\ *n* : the cytoplasm of a striated muscle fiber — compare MYOPLASM — **sar·co·plas·mic** \ˌsär-kə-ˈplaz-mik\ *adj*

sarcoplasmic reticulum *n* : the endoplasmic reticulum of cardiac muscle and skeletal striated muscle fiber that functions esp. as a storage and release area for calcium

Sar·cop·tes \sär-ˈkäp-(ˌ)tēz\ *n* : a genus of whitish itch mites (family Sarcoptidae)

sar·cop·tic \sär-ˈkäp-tik\ *adj* : of, relating to, caused by, or being itch mites of the genus *Sarcoptes*

sarcoptic mange *n* : mange caused by mites of the genus *Sarcoptes* that burrow in the skin esp. of the head and face — compare CHORIOPTIC MANGE, DEMODECTIC MANGE

sar·co·sine \ˈsär-kə-ˌsēn, -sən\ *n* : a sweetish crystalline amino acid $C_3H_7NO_2$ formed by the decomposition of creatine or made synthetically

sar·co·some \ˈsär-kə-ˌsōm\ *n* : a mitochondrion of a striated muscle fiber — **sar·co·som·al** \ˌsär-kə-ˈsō-məl\ *adj*

sar·co·spo·rid·i·o·sis \ˌsär-kō-spə-ˌri-dē-ˈō-səs\ *n, pl* **-o·ses** \-ˌsēz\ : SARCOCYSTOSIS

sardonicus — see RISUS SARDONICUS

sar·gram·o·stim \sär-ˈgra-məs-təm\ *n* : a granulocyte-macrophage colony-stimulating factor produced by recombinant DNA technology that is used esp. following autologous bone marrow transplantation to accelerate the division and differentiation of the transplanted bone marrow cells

sa·rin \ˈsär-ən, zä-ˈrēn\ *n* : an extremely toxic chemical warfare agent $C_4H_{10}FO_2P$ — called also *GB*

SARS \ˈsärz\ *n* : a severe respiratory illness that is transmitted esp. by contact with infectious material (as respiratory droplets or body fluids), is caused by a virus of the genus *Coronavirus* (species *Severe acute respiratory syndrome virus*), is characterized by fever, headache, body aches, a dry cough, and hypoxia and usu. by pneumonia — called also *severe acute respiratory syndrome*

sar·to·ri·us \sär-ˈtòr-ē-əs\ *n, pl* **-rii** \-ē-ˌī\ : a muscle that arises from the anterior superior iliac spine, crosses the front of the thigh obliquely to insert on the upper part of the inner surface of the tibia, is the longest muscle in the human body, and acts to flex, abduct, and rotate the thigh laterally at the hip joint and to flex the leg at the knee joint and to rotate it medially in a way that enables one to sit with the heel of one leg on the knee of the opposite leg

sas·sa·fras \ˈsa-sə-ˌfras\ *n* **1** : a tall eastern No. American tree (*Sassafras albidum*) of the laurel family (Lauraceae) with mucilaginous twigs and leaves **2** : the carcinogenic dried root bark of the sassafras formerly used as a diaphoretic and flavoring agent

sat·el·lite \ˈsat-ᵊl-ˌīt\ *n* **1** : a short segment separated from the main body of a chromosome by a constriction **2** : a bodily structure lying near or associated with another (as a vein accompanying an artery) **3** : a smaller lesion accompanying a main one and situated nearby — **satellite** *adj*

satellite cell *n* **1** : a cell surrounding a ganglion cell **2** : a stem cell that lies adjacent to a skeletal muscle fiber and plays a role in muscle growth, repair, and regeneration

satellite DNA *n* : a fraction of a eukaryotic organism's DNA that differs in density from most of its DNA as determined by centrifugation, that apparently consists of short repetitive nucleotide sequences, that does not undergo transcription, and that is often found esp. in centromeric regions

sat·el·li·to·sis \ˌsat-ᵊl-ī-ˈtō-səs\ *n, pl* **-o·ses** \-ˌsēz\ : the usu. abnormal clustering of one type of cell around another; *esp* : the clustering of glial cells around neurons in the brain that is associated with certain pathological states (as oligodendroglioma)

sa·ti·ety \sə-ˈtī-ə-tē\ *n, pl* **-ties** : the quality or state of being fed or gratified to or beyond capacity

¹sat·u·rate \ˈsa-chə-ˌrāt\ *vb* **-rat·ed; -rat·ing** **1** : to treat, furnish, or charge with something to the point where no more can be absorbed, dissolved, or retained **2** : to cause to combine until there is no further tendency to combine

²**sat·u·rate** \-rət\ *n* : a saturated chemical compound

sat·u·rat·ed \'sa-chə-ˌrā-təd\ *adj* **1** : being a solution that is unable to absorb or dissolve any more of a solute at a given temperature and pressure **2** : being an organic compound having no double or triple bonds between carbon atoms

sat·u·ra·tion \ˌsa-chə-ˈrā-shən\ *n* **1** : the act of saturating : the state of being saturated **2** : conversion of an unsaturated to a saturated chemical compound (as by hydrogenation) **3** : a state of maximum impregnation; *esp* : the presence in air of the most water possible under existent pressure and temperature **4** : the one of the three psychological dimensions of color perception that is related to the purity of the color and that decreases as the amount of white present in the stimulus increases — called also *intensity*; compare BRIGHTNESS, HUE

sat·ur·nine \'sa-tər-ˌnīn\ *adj* **1** : of or relating to lead **2** : of, relating to, or produced by the absorption of lead into the system ⟨∼ poisoning⟩

sat·urn·ism \'sa-tər-ˌni-zəm\ *n* : LEAD POISONING

sa·ty·ri·a·sis \ˌsā-tə-ˈrī-ə-səs, ˌsa-\ *n, pl* **-a·ses** \-ˌsēz\ : excessive or abnormal sexual desire in the male — compare NYMPHOMANIA

sau·cer·ize \'sȯ-sər-ˌīz\ *vb* **-ized; -iz·ing** : to form a shallow depression by excavation of tissue to promote granulation and healing of (a wound) — **sau·cer·iza·tion** \ˌsȯ-sər-ə-ˈzā-shən\ *n*

sau·na \'saů-nə, 'sȯ-nə\ *n* **1** : a Finnish steam bath in which the steam is provided by water thrown on hot stones; *also* : a bathhouse or room used for such a bath **2** : a dry heat bath; *also* : a room or cabinet used for such a bath

sa·vant \sə-ˈvänt\ *n* : IDIOT SAVANT

saw \'sȯ\ *n* : a hand or power tool used to cut hard material (as bone) and equipped usu. with a toothed blade or disk

saw pal·met·to \-pal-ˈme-tō\ *n* : a preparation derived from the berry-like fruit of a shrubby palm (*Serenoa repens*) of the southeastern U.S. that is held to have a therapeutic effect on the prostate gland and is used in herbal remedies and dietary supplements — called also *sabal*

saxi·tox·in \ˌsak-sə-ˈtäk-sən\ *n* : a potent nonprotein neurotoxin $C_{10}H_{17}$-N_7O_4·2HCl that originates esp. in dinoflagellates of the genus *Gonyaulax* found in red tides and that sometimes occurs in and renders toxic normally edible mollusks which feed on them

Sb *symbol* [Latin *stibium*] antimony

SBS *abbr* sick building syndrome

Sc *symbol* scandium

SCA *abbr* **1** sickle-cell anemia **2** spinocerebellar ataxia **3** sudden cardiac arrest

scab \'skab\ *n* **1** : scabies of domestic animals **2** : a hardened covering of dried secretions (as blood, serum, or pus) that forms over a wound — called also *crust* — **scab** *vb* — **scab·by** \'ska-bē\ *adj*

scabby mouth *n* : SORE MOUTH 1

sca·bi·cide \'skā-bə-ˌsīd\ *n* : a drug that destroys the itch mite causing scabies

sca·bies \'skā-bēz\ *n, pl* **scabies** : contagious itch or mange esp. with exudative crusts that is caused by parasitic mites and esp. by a mite of the genus *Sarcoptes* (*S. scabiei*) — **sca·bi·et·ic** \ˌskā-bē-ˈe-tik\ *adj*

scab mite *n* : any of several small mites that cause mange, scabies, or scab; *esp* : one of the genus *Psoroptes*

sca·la \'skā-lə\ *n, pl* **sca·lae** \-ˌlē\ : any of the three spirally arranged canals into which the bony canal of the cochlea is partitioned by the vestibular and basilar membranes and which comprise the cochlear duct, scala tympani, and scala vestibuli

scala me·dia \-ˈmē-dē-ə\ *n, pl* **scalae me·di·ae** \-dē-ˌē\ : COCHLEAR DUCT

scala tym·pa·ni \-ˈtim-pə-ˌnī, -ˌnē\ *n, pl* **scalae tym·pa·no·rum** \-ˌtim-pə-ˈnōr-əm\ : the lymph-filled spirally arranged canal in the bony canal of the cochlea that is separated from the cochlear duct by the basilar membrane, communicates at its upper end with the scala vestibuli, and abuts at its lower end upon the membrane that separates the round window from the middle ear

scala ves·tib·u·li \-ve-ˈsti-byə-ˌlī\ *n, pl* **scalae ves·tib·u·lo·rum** \-ve-ˌsti-byə-ˈlō-rəm\ : the lymph-filled spirally arranged canal in the bony canal of the cochlea that is separated from the cochlear duct below by the vestibular membrane, is connected with the oval window, and receives vibrations from the stapes

¹**scald** \'skȯld\ *vb* : to burn with hot liquid or steam ⟨∼ed skin⟩

²**scald** *n* : an injury to the body caused by scalding

scalded–skin syndrome *n* : TOXIC EPIDERMAL NECROLYSIS — see STAPHYLOCOCCAL SCALDED SKIN SYNDROME

¹**scale** \'skāl\ *n* **1** : a small thin dry lamina shed (as in many skin diseases) from the skin **2** : a film of tartar encrusting the teeth

²**scale** *vb* **scaled; scal·ing 1** : to take off or come off in thin layers or scales ⟨∼ tartar from the teeth⟩ **2** : to shed scales or fragmentary surface matter : EXFOLIATE ⟨*scaling* skin⟩

³**scale** *n* **1** : a series of marks or points at known intervals used to measure distances (as the height of the mer-

cury in a thermometer) **2** : a graduated series or scheme of rank or order **3** : a graded series of tests or of performances used in rating individual intelligence or achievement

sca·lene \'skā-ˌlēn, skā-'\ *n* : SCALENUS — called also *scalene muscle*

sca·le·not·o·my \ˌskā-lə-'nä-tə-mē\ *n, pl* **-mies** : surgical severing of one or more scalenus muscles near their insertion on the ribs

sca·le·nus \skā-'lē-nəs\ *n, pl* **sca·le·ni** \-ˌnī\ : any of usu. three deeply situated muscles on each side of the neck of which each extends from the transverse processes of two or more cervical vertebrae to the first or second rib: **a** : one arising from the transverse processes of the third to sixth cervical vertebrae, inserting on the scalene tubercle of the first rib, and functioning to bend the neck forward and laterally and to rotate it to the side — called also *scalenus anterior, scalenus anticus* **b** : one arising from the transverse processes of the lower six cervical vertebrae, inserting on the upper surface of the first rib, and functioning similarly to the scalenus anterior — called also *scalenus medius* **c** : one arising from the transverse processes of the fourth to sixth cervical vertebrae, inserting on the outer surface of the second rib, and functioning to raise the second rib and to bend and slightly rotate the neck — called also *scalenus posterior*

scalenus anterior *n* : SCALENUS a

scalenus an·ti·cus \-an-'tī-kəs\ *n* : SCALENUS a

scalenus anticus syndrome *n* : a complex of symptoms including pain and numbness in the region of the shoulder, arm, and neck that is caused by compression of the brachial plexus or subclavian artery or both by the scalenus anticus muscle

scalenus me·di·us \-'mē-dē-əs\ *n* : SCALENUS b

scalenus posterior *n* : SCALENUS c

scal·er \'skā-lər\ *n* : any of various dental instruments for removing tartar from teeth

scalp \'skalp\ *n* : the part of the integument of the head usu. covered with hair in both sexes

scal·pel \'skal-pəl\ *n* : a small straight thin-bladed knife used esp. in surgery

scalp ringworm *n* : TINEA CAPITIS

scaly \'skā-lē\ *adj* **scal·i·er; -est** : covered with or composed of scale or scales ⟨∼ skin⟩ — **scal·i·ness** *n*

¹**scan** \'skan\ *vb* **scanned; scan·ning** **1 a** : to examine esp. systematically with a sensing device (as a beam of radiation) **b** : to pass an electron beam over and convert (an image) into variations of electrical properties (as voltage) that convey information electronically **2** : to make a scan of (as the human body) in order to detect the presence or localization of radioactive material

²**scan** *n* **1** : the act or process of scanning **2 a** : a depiction (as a photograph) of the distribution of a radioactive material in something (as a bodily organ) **b** : an image of a bodily part produced (as by computer) by combining ultrasonic or radiographic data obtained from several angles or sections

scan·di·um \'skan-dē-əm\ *n* : a white metallic element — symbol *Sc*; see ELEMENT table

scan·ner \'ska-nər\ *n* : a device for making scans of a living body — see CAT SCANNER, PET SCANNER

scanning electron micrograph *n* : a micrograph made by scanning electron microscopy

scanning electron microscope *n* : an electron microscope in which a beam of focused electrons moves across the object with the secondary electrons produced by the object and the electrons scattered by the object being collected to form a three-dimensional image on a display screen — called also *scanning microscope* — **scanning electron microscopy** *n*

scanning speech *n* : speech characterized by regularly recurring pauses between words or syllables

Scan·zo·ni maneuver \skänt-'sō-nē-\ *also* **Scan·zo·ni's maneuver** \-nēz-\ *n* : rotation of an abnormally positioned fetus by means of forceps with subsequent reapplication of forceps for delivery

Scanzoni, Friedrich Wilhelm (1821–1891), German obstetrician.

scaph- *or* **scapho-** *comb form* : scaphoid ⟨*scapho*cephaly⟩

sca·pha \'ska-fə\ *n* : an elongated depression of the ear that separates the helix and antihelix

scaph·o·ceph·a·ly \ˌska-fə-'se-fə-lē\ *n, pl* **-lies** : a congenital deformity of the skull in which the vault is narrow, elongated, and boat-shaped because of premature ossification of the sagittal suture

¹**scaph·oid** \'ska-ˌföid\ *adj* **1** : shaped like a boat : NAVICULAR **2** : characterized by concavity ⟨a ∼ abdomen⟩

²**scaphoid** *n* **1** : NAVICULAR a **2** : the largest carpal bone of the proximal row of the wrist that occupies the most lateral position on the thumb side — called also *navicular*

scaphoid bone *n* : SCAPHOID

scaphoid fossa *n* : a shallow oval depression that is situated above the pterygoid fossa on the pterygoid process of the sphenoid bone and that provides attachment for the origin of the tensor veli palatini muscle

scapul- *or* **scapulo-** *comb form* : scapular and ⟨*scapulo*humeral⟩

scap·u·la \'ska-pyə-lə\ *n, pl* **-lae** \-ˌlē, -ˌlī\ *or* **-las** : either of a pair of large essentially flat and triangular bones lying one in each dorsolateral part of the thorax, being the principal bone of the corresponding half of the pectoral girdle, providing articulation for the humerus, and articulating with the corresponding clavicle — called also *shoulder blade*

scapulae — see LEVATOR SCAPULAE

scap·u·lar \'ska-pyə-lər\ *adj* : of, relating to, or affecting the shoulder or scapula ⟨a ∼ fracture⟩

scapular notch *n* : a semicircular notch on the superior border of the scapula next to the coracoid process that gives passage to the suprascapular nerve and is converted to a foramen by the suprascapular ligament

scap·u·lo·hu·mer·al \,ska-pyə-lō-'hyü-mə-rəl\ *adj* : of or relating to the scapula and the humerus

scap·u·lo·tho·rac·ic \,ska-pyə-lō-thə-'ra-sik\ *adj* : of or relating to the scapula and the thorax ⟨∼ pain⟩

scar \'skär\ *n* 1 : a mark left (as in the skin) by the healing of injured tissue 2 : a lasting emotional injury — **scar** *vb*

scar·i·fy \'skar-ə-ˌfī\ *vb* **-fied; -fy·ing** : to make scratches or small cuts in (as the skin) ⟨∼ an area for vaccination⟩ — **scar·i·fi·ca·tion** \,skar-ə-fə-'kā-shən\ *n*

scar·la·ti·na \,skär-lə-'tē-nə\ *n* : SCARLET FEVER — **scar·la·ti·nal** \-'tēn-ᵊl\ *adj*

scar·la·ti·ni·form \-'tē-nə-ˌfȯrm\ *adj* : resembling the rash of scarlet fever

scar·let fever \'skär-lət-\ *n* : an acute contagious febrile disease caused by Group A bacteria of the genus *Streptococcus* (esp. various strains of *S. pyogenes*) and characterized by inflammation of the nose, throat, and mouth, generalized toxemia, and a red rash — called also *scarlatina*

scarlet red *n* : SUDAN IV

Scar·pa's fascia \'skär-pəz-\ *n* : the deep layer of the superficial fascia of the anterior abdominal wall

Scarpa, Antonio (1752–1832), Italian anatomist and surgeon.

Scarpa's triangle *n* : FEMORAL TRIANGLE

scar tissue *n* : the connective tissue forming a scar and composed chiefly of fibroblasts in recent scars and largely of dense collagenous fibers in old scars

ScD *abbr* doctor of science

Schatz·ki ring \'shats-kē-\ *or* **Schatz·ki's ring** \-kēz-\ *n* : a local narrowing in the lower part of the esophagus that may cause dysphagia

Schatzki, Richard (1901–1992), American radiologist.

sched·ule \'ske-ˌjül, -jəl; 'she-jü-wəl\ *n* 1 : a program or plan that indicates the sequence of each step or procedure; *esp* : REGIMEN 2 *often cap* : an official list of drugs that are subject to the same legal controls and restrictions — usu. used with a Roman nu-

meral from I to V indicating decreasing potential for abuse or addiction ⟨the Drug Enforcement Administration classifies heroin as a ∼ I drug while diazepam is on ∼ IV⟩

Scheie syndrome \'shī-\ *n* : an autosomal recessive mucopolysaccharidosis similar to Hurler's syndrome but less severe that is characterized by clouding of the cornea, slight deformity of the extremities, and disease of the aorta but not by mental retardation

Scheie, Harold Glendon (1909–1990), American ophthalmologist.

sche·ma \'skē-mə\ *n, pl* **sche·ma·ta** \-mə-tə\ *also* **sche·mas** 1 : a nonconscious adjustment of the brain to the afferent impulses indicative of bodily posture that is a prerequisite of appropriate bodily movement and of spatial perception 2 : a mental codification of experience that includes a particular organized way of perceiving cognitively and responding to a complex situation or set of stimuli — **sche·mat·ic** \ski-'ma-tik\ *adj*

scheme \'skēm\ *n* : SCHEMA

Scheuer·mann's disease \'shȯi-ər-ˌmänz-\ *n* : osteochondrosis of the vertebrae associated in the active state with pain and kyphosis

Scheuermann, Holger Werfel (1877–1960), Danish orthopedist.

Schick test \'shik-\ *n* : a serological test for susceptibility to diphtheria by cutaneous injection of a diluted diphtheria toxin that causes an area of reddening and induration in susceptible individuals

Schick, Béla (1877–1967), American pediatrician.

Schiff's reagent \'shifs-\ *or* **Schiff reagent** \'shif-\ *n* : a solution of fuchsin decolorized by treatment with sulfur dioxide that gives a useful test for aldehydes because they restore the reddish violet color of the dye — compare FEULGEN REACTION

Schiff, Hugo Josef (1834–1915), German chemist.

Schil·der's disease \'shil-dərz-\ *n* : ADRENOLEUKODYSTROPHY

Schilder, Paul Ferdinand (1886–1940), Austrian psychiatrist.

Schil·ler's test \'shil-ərz-\ *n* : a preliminary test for cancer of the uterine cervix in which the cervix is painted with an aqueous solution of iodine and potassium iodide and which shows up healthy tissue by staining it brown and possibly cancerous tissue as white or yellow

Schiller, Walter (1887–1960), American pathologist.

Schilling test *n* : a test for gastrointestinal absorption of vitamin B$_{12}$ in which a dose of the radioactive vitamin is taken orally, a dose of the nonradioactive vitamin is given by injection to impede uptake of the absorbed radioactive dose by the liver, and the proportion of the radioactive dose absorbed is determined by measuring the radioactivity of the urine

Schilling, Robert Frederick (*b* 1919), American hematologist.

schin·dy·le·sis \ˌskin-də-'lē-səs\ *n, pl* **-le·ses** \-ˌsēz\ : an articulation in which one bone is received into a groove or slit in another

Schiøtz tonometer \'shyüts-, 'shyərts-\ *n* : a tonometer used to measure intraocular pressure in millimeters of mercury

Schiøtz, Hjalmar (1850–1927), Norwegian physician.

-schi·sis \skə-səs\ *n comb form, pl* **-schi·ses** \skə-ˌsēz\ *also* **-schi·sis·es** : breaking up of attachments or adhesions : fissure ⟨gastro*schisis*⟩ ⟨cranio*schisis*⟩

schisto- *comb form* : cleft : divided ⟨*schisto*cyte⟩

schis·to·cyte \'shis-tə-ˌsīt, 'skis-\ *n* : a hemoglobin-containing fragment of a red blood cell

schis·to·so·ma \ˌshis-tə-'sō-mə, ˌskis-\ *n* **1** *cap* : a genus of elongated digenetic trematode worms (family Schistosomatidae) that parasitize the blood vessels of birds and mammals and include species (as *S. haematobium, S. japonicum,* and *S. mansoni*) causing human schistosomiasis **2** : any trematode of the genus *Schistosoma* : SCHISTOSOME

schis·to·some \'shis-tə-ˌsōm, 'skis-\ *n* : any trematode worm of the genus *Schistosoma* or of the family (Schistosomatidae) to which it belongs — called also *blood fluke* — **schis·to·so·mal** \ˌshis-tə-'sō-məl, ˌskis-\ *adj*

schistosome dermatitis *n* : SWIMMER'S ITCH

schis·to·so·mi·a·sis \ˌshis-tə-sō-'mī-ə-səs, ˌskis-\ *n, pl* **-a·ses** \-ˌsēz\ : infestation with or disease caused by schistosomes; *specif* : a severe endemic disease of humans in much of Asia, Africa, and So. America that is caused by any of three trematode worms of the genus *Schistosoma* (*S. haematobium, S. mansoni,* and *S. japonicum*) which multiply in snail intermediate hosts and are disseminated into freshwaters as cercariae that bore into the body, migrate through the tissues to the visceral venous plexuses (as of the bladder or intestine) where they attain maturity, and cause much of their injury through hemorrhage and damage to tissues resulting from the passage of the usu. spiny eggs to the intestine and bladder — called also *bilharzia, bilharziasis, snail fever;* compare SWIMMER'S ITCH

schistosomiasis hae·ma·to·bi·um \-ˌhē-mə-'tō-bē-əm\ *n* : schistosomiasis caused by a schistosome (*Schistosoma haematobium*) occurring over most of Africa and in Asia Minor and predominantly involving infestation of the veins of the urinary bladder

schistosomiasis ja·pon·i·ca \-jə-'pä-ni-kə\ *n* : schistosomiasis caused by a schistosome (*Schistosoma japonicum*) occurring chiefly in eastern Asia and the Pacific islands and predominantly involving infestation of the portal and mesenteric veins — see KATAYAMA SYNDROME

schistosomiasis man·so·ni \-'man-sə-ˌnī\ *n* : schistosomiasis caused by a schistosome (*Schistosoma mansoni*) occurring chiefly in central Africa and eastern So. America and predominantly involving infestation of the mesenteric and portal veins — called also *Manson's disease*

P. Manson — see MANSONELLA

schis·to·som·u·lum \ˌshis-tə-'säm-yə-ləm, ˌskis-\ *n, pl* **-la** \-lə\ : an immature schistosome in the body of the definitive host

schiz- *or* **schizo-** *comb form* **1** : characterized by or involving cleavage ⟨*schizo*gony⟩ **2** : schizophrenia ⟨*schizo*id⟩

schizo \'skit-(ˌ)sō\ *n, pl* **schiz·os** : SCHIZOPHRENIC

schizo–af·fec·tive \-ə-'fek-tiv\ *adj* : relating to, characterized by, or exhibiting symptoms of both schizophrenia and bipolar disorder

schi·zog·o·ny \ski-'zä-gə-nē, skit-'sä-\ *n, pl* **-nies** : asexual reproduction by multiple segmentation characteristic of sporozoans (as the malaria parasite) — **schizo·gon·ic** \ˌskit-sə-'gä-nik\ *or* **schi·zog·o·nous** \ski-'zä-gə-nəs, skit-'sä-\ *adj*

¹**schiz·oid** \'skit-ˌsóid\ *adj* : characterized by, resulting from, tending toward, or suggestive of schizophrenia

²**schizoid** *n* : a schizoid individual

schizoid personality *n* **1** : a personality disorder characterized by shyness, withdrawal, inhibition of emotional expression, and apparent diminution of affect — called also *schizoid personality disorder* **2** : an individual with a schizoid personality

schiz·ont \'ski-ˌzänt, 'skit-ˌsänt\ *n* : a multinucleate sporozoan (as a malaria parasite) that reproduces by schizogony

schi·zon·ti·cide \ski-'zän-tə-ˌsīd, skit-'sän-\ *n* : an agent selectively destructive of the schizont of a sporozoan parasite — **schi·zon·ti·ci·dal** \ski-ˌzän-tə-'sīd-ᵊl, skit-ˌsän-\ *adj*

schizo·phrene \'skit-sə-ˌfrēn\ *n* : SCHIZOPHRENIC

schizo·phre·nia \ˌskit-sə-'frē-nē-ə\ *n* : a psychotic disorder characterized by loss of contact with the environment, by noticeable deterioration in the level of functioning in everyday life, and by disintegration of personality expressed as disorder of feeling, thought (as in delusions), perception (as in hallucinations), and behavior — called also *dementia praecox;* see PARANOID SCHIZOPHRENIA

¹schizo·phren·ic \-'fre-nik\ *adj* : relating to, characteristic of, or affected with schizophrenia ⟨~ behavior⟩

²schizophrenic *n* : an individual affected with schizophrenia

schizophrenic reaction *n* : SCHIZOPHRENIA

schiz·o·phren·i·form \,skit-sə-'fre-nə-,förm\ *adj* : resembling schizophrenia in appearance or manifestations but tending to last less than six months but more than one month ⟨~ disorder⟩

schiz·o·phreno·gen·ic \,skit-sə-,fre-nə-'je-nik\ *adj* : tending to produce schizophrenia ⟨~ factors⟩

schizos *pl of* SCHIZO

schizo·ty·pal \,skit-sə-'tī-pəl\ *adj* : characterized by, exhibiting, or being patterns of thought, perception, communication, and behavior suggestive of schizophrenia but not of sufficient severity to warrant a diagnosis of schizophrenia ⟨~ personality disorder⟩

Schlemm's canal \'shlemz-\ *n* : CANAL OF SCHLEMM

Schön·lein–Hen·och \'shœn-līn-'he-nək\ *adj* : being a form of purpura that is characterized by swelling and pain of the joints in association with gastrointestinal bleeding and pain

> **Schönlein, Johann Lucas (1793–1864),** German physician.
> **Henoch, Eduard Heinrich (1820–1910),** German pediatrician.

Schönlein's disease *n* : Schönlein-Henoch purpura that is characterized esp. by swelling and pain of the joints — compare HENOCH'S PURPURA

Schuff·ner's dots \'shúf-nərz-\ *n pl* : punctate granulations present in red blood cells invaded by the tertian malaria parasite

> **Schüff·ner** \'shuef-nər\, **Wilhelm August Paul (1867–1949),** German pathologist.

Schüller–Christian disease *n* : HAND-SCHÜLLER-CHRISTIAN DISEASE

Schwann cell \'shwän-\ *n* : a myelin-secreting glial cell that spirally wraps around an axon of the peripheral nervous system to form the myelin sheath

> **Schwann** \'shvän\, **Theodor Ambrose Hubert (1810–1882),** German anatomist and physiologist.

schwan·no·ma \shwä-'nō-mə\ *n, pl* **-mas** \-məz\ *or* **-ma·ta** \-mə-tə\ : NEURILEMMOMA

Schwann's sheath *n* : NEURILEMMA

sci·at·ic \sī-'a-tik\ *adj* **1** : of, relating to, or situated near the hip **2** : of, relating to, or caused by sciatica ⟨~ pains⟩

sci·at·i·ca \sī-'a-ti-kə\ *n* : pain along the course of a sciatic nerve esp. in the back of the thigh caused by compression, inflammation, or reflex mechanisms; *broadly* : pain in the lower back, buttocks, hips, or adjacent parts

sciatic foramen *n* : either of two foramina on each side of the pelvis that are formed by the hip bone, the sacrospinous ligament, and the sacrotuberous ligament: **a** : one giving passage to the piriformis muscle and to the sciatic, superior and inferior gluteal, and pudendal nerves together with their associated arteries and veins — called also *greater sciatic foramen* **b** : one giving passage to the tendon of the obturator internus muscle and its nerve, to the internal pudendal artery and veins, and to the pudendal nerve — called also *lesser sciatic foramen*

sciatic nerve *n* : either of the pair of largest nerves in the body that arise one on each side from the sacral plexus and that pass out of the pelvis through the greater sciatic foramen and down the back of the thigh to its lower third where division into the tibial and common peroneal nerves occurs

sciatic notch *n* : either of two notches on the dorsal border of the hip bone on each side that when closed off by ligaments form the corresponding sciatic foramina: **a** : a relatively large notch just above the ischial spine that is converted into the greater sciatic foramen by the sacrospinous ligament — called also *greater sciatic notch* **b** : a smaller notch just below the ischial spine that is converted to the lesser sciatic foramen by the sacrospinous ligament and the sacrotuberous ligament — called also *lesser sciatic notch*

SCID *abbr* severe combined immunodeficiency

sci·ence \'sī-əns\ *n* : knowledge or a system of knowledge covering general truths or the operation of general laws esp. as obtained and tested through the scientific method and concerned with the physical world and its phenomena — **sci·en·tif·ic** \,sī-ən-'ti-fik\ *adj* — **sci·en·tif·i·cal·ly** *adv*

scientific method *n* : principles and procedures for the systematic pursuit of knowledge involving the recognition and formulation of a problem, the collection of data through observation and experiment, and the formulation and testing of hypotheses

sci·en·tist \'sī-ən-tist\ *n* : one learned in science and esp. natural science : a scientific investigator

scin·ti·gram \'sin-tə-,gram\ *n* : a picture produced by scintigraphy

scin·tig·ra·phy \sin-'ti-grə-fē\ *n, pl* **-phies** : a diagnostic technique in which a two-dimensional picture of internal body tissue is produced through the detection of radiation emitted by a radioactive substance administered into the body — **scin·ti·graph·ic** \,sin-tə-'gra-fik\ *adj*

scintillating scotoma *n* : a blind spot in the visual field that is bordered by shimmering or flashing light and that is often a premonitory symptom of migraine attack

scin·til·la·tion \ˌsint-ᵊl-ˈā-shən\ *n*, *often attrib* : a flash of light produced in a phosphorescent substance by an ionizing event — **scin·til·late** \ˈsint-ᵊl-ˌāt\ *vb*

scintillation counter *n* : a device for detecting and registering individual scintillations (as in radioactive emission) — called also *scintillometer*

scin·til·la·tor \ˈsint-ᵊl-ˌā-tər\ *n* **1** : a phosphorescent substance in which scintillations occur (as in a scintillation counter) **2** : a device for sending out scintillations of light **3** : SCINTILLATION COUNTER

scin·til·lom·e·ter \ˌsint-ᵊl-ˈä-mə-tər\ *n* : SCINTILLATION COUNTER

scin·ti·scan \ˈsin-ti-ˌskan\ *n* : a two-dimensional representation of radioisotope radiation from a bodily organ (as the spleen or kidney)

scirrhi *pl of* SCIRRHUS

scir·rhous \ˈsir-əs, ˈskir-\ *adj* : of, relating to, or being a scirrhous carcinoma ⟨∼ infiltration⟩

scirrhous carcinoma *n* : a hard slow-growing malignant tumor having a preponderance of fibrous tissue

scir·rhus \ˈsir-əs, ˈskir-\ *n*, *pl* **scir·rhi** \ˈsir-ˌī, ˈskir-, -ˌē\ : SCIRRHOUS CARCINOMA

scler- or **sclero-** *comb form* **1** : hard ⟨*sclero*derma⟩ **2** : sclera ⟨*scler*itis⟩

sclera \ˈskler-ə\ *n* : the dense fibrous opaque white outer coat enclosing the eyeball except the part covered by the cornea — called also *sclerotic coat*, *sclerotic coat* — **scler·al** \ˈskler-əl\ *adj*

sclerae — see SINUS VENOSUS SCLERAE

scle·rec·to·my \sklə-ˈrek-tə-mē\ *n*, *pl* **-mies** : surgical removal of a part of the sclera

scle·re·ma neo·na·to·rum \sklə-ˈrē-mə-ˌnē-ə-nə-ˈtōr-əm\ *n* : hardening of the cutaneous and subcutaneous tissues in newborn infants

scle·ri·tis \sklə-ˈrī-təs\ *n* : inflammation of the sclera

scle·ro·cor·ne·al \ˌskler-ō-ˈkȯr-nē-əl\ *adj* : of or involving both sclera and cornea

sclero·dac·ty·ly \-ˈdak-tə-lē\ *n*, *pl* **-lies** : scleroderma of the fingers and toes

sclero·der·ma \ˌskler-ə-ˈdər-mə\ *n*, *pl* **-mas** *or* **-ma·ta** \-mə-tə\ : a usu. slowly progressive disease marked by the deposition of fibrous connective tissue in the skin and often in internal organs and structures, by hand and foot pain upon exposure to cold, and by tightening and thickening of the skin — **sclero·der·ma·tous** \-təs\ *adj*

scle·ro·ma \sklə-ˈrō-mə\ *n*, *pl* **-mas** *or* **-ma·ta** \-mə-tə\ : hardening of tissues

sclero·pro·tein \ˌskler-ō-ˈprō-ˌtēn\ *n* : any of various proteins (as collagen and keratin) that occur esp. in connective and skeletal tissues, are usu.

insoluble in aqueous solvents, and are resistant to chemical reagents — called also *albuminoid*

scle·rose \sklə-ˈrōs, -ˈrōz\ *vb* **-rosed; -ros·ing** **1** : to cause sclerosis in **2** : to undergo or become affected with sclerosis

scle·ros·ing *adj* : causing or characterized by sclerosis ⟨∼ agents⟩ — see SUBACUTE SCLEROSING PANENCEPHALITIS

scle·ro·sis \sklə-ˈrō-səs\ *n*, *pl* **-ro·ses** \-ˌsēz\ **1** : a pathological condition in which a tissue has become hard and which is produced by overgrowth of fibrous tissue and other changes (as in arteriosclerosis) or by increase in interstitial tissue and other changes (as in multiple sclerosis) — called also *hardening* **2** : any of various diseases characterized by sclerosis — usu. used in combination; see ARTERIOSCLEROSIS, MULTIPLE SCLEROSIS

scle·ro·stome \ˈskler-ə-ˌstōm\ *n* : STRONGYLE

sclerosus — see LICHEN SCLEROSUS ET ATROPHICUS

sclero·ther·a·py \ˌskler-ō-ˈther-ə-pē\ *n*, *pl* **-pies** : the injection of a sclerosing agent (as saline) into a varicose vein to produce inflammation and scarring which closes the lumen and is followed by shrinkage; *also* : PROLOTHERAPY

¹scle·rot·ic \sklə-ˈrä-tik\ *adj* **1** : being or relating to the sclera ⟨the ∼ layer of the eye⟩ **2** : of, relating to, or affected with sclerosis ⟨∼ arteries⟩

²sclerotic *n* : SCLERA

sclerotic coat *n* : SCLERA

scle·ro·tium \sklə-ˈrō-shəm, -shē-əm\ *n*, *pl* **-tia** \-shə, -shē-ə\ : a compact mass of hardened mycelium of a fungus that is stored with reserve food material — **scle·ro·tial** \-shəl\ *adj*

sclero·tome \ˈskler-ə-ˌtōm\ *n* : the ventral and mesial portion of a somite that proliferates mesenchyme which migrates about the notochord to form the axial skeleton and ribs — **sclero·tom·ic** \ˌskler-ə-ˈtō-mik, -ˈtä-\ *adj*

scle·rot·o·my \sklə-ˈrä-tə-mē\ *n*, *pl* **-mies** : surgical cutting of the sclera

ScM *abbr* master of science

SCM *abbr* state certified midwife

SCN *abbr* suprachiasmatic nucleus

sco·lex \ˈskō-ˌleks\ *n*, *pl* **sco·li·ces** \ˈskō-lə-ˌsēz\ *also* **scol·e·ces** \skä-lə-ˌsēz, ˈskō-\ *or* **scolexes** : the head of a tapeworm from which the proglottids are produced by budding

sco·li·o·sis \ˌskō-lē-ˈō-səs\ *n*, *pl* **-o·ses** \-ˌsēz\ : a lateral curvature of the spine — compare KYPHOSIS, LORDOSIS — **sco·li·ot·ic** \-ˈä-tik\ *adj*

scoop \ˈsküp\ *n* : a spoon-shaped surgical instrument used in extracting various materials (as debris and pus)

scope \ˈskōp\ *n* : any of various instruments (as an endoscope or microscope) for viewing or observing

-scope \ˌskōp\ *n comb form* : means (as an instrument) for viewing or observing ⟨micro*scope*⟩ ⟨laparo*scope*⟩

-scop·ic \ˈskä-pik\ *adj comb form* : viewing or observing ⟨laparo*scopic*⟩

sco·pol·amine \skō-ˈpä-lə-ˌmēn, -mən\ *n* : a poisonous alkaloid $C_{17}H_{21}NO_4$ similar to atropine that is found in various plants (as jimsonweed) of the nightshade family (Solanaceae) and is used chiefly in the form of its hydrated hydrobromide $C_{17}H_{21}NO_4$·HBr·3H_2O for its anticholinergic effects (as preventing nausea and in motion sickness and inducing mydriasis) — called also *hyoscine*

sco·po·phil·ia \ˌskō-pə-ˈfi-lē-ə\ *also* **scop·to·phil·ia** \ˌskäp-tə-ˈfi-lē-ə\ *n* : a desire to look at sexually stimulating scenes esp. as a substitute for actual sexual participation — **sco·po·phil·ic** *or* **scop·to·phil·ic** \-ˈfi-lik\ *adj*

sco·po·phil·i·ac *also* **scop·to·phil·i·ac** \-ˈfi-lē-ˌak\ *n* : an individual affected with scopophilia — **scopophiliac** *also* **scoptophiliac** *adj*

-s·co·py \s-kə-pē\ *n comb form, pl* **-s·co·pies** : viewing : observation ⟨laparo*scopy*⟩

scor·bu·tic \skȯr-ˈbyü-tik\ *adj* : of, relating to, producing, or affected with scurvy ⟨a ~ diet⟩

scor·pi·on \ˈskȯr-pē-ən\ *n* : any of an order (Scorpionida) of arachnids that have an elongated body and a narrow segmented tail bearing a venomous stinger at the tip

sco·to·ma \skə-ˈtō-mə\ *n, pl* **-mas** *or* **-ma·ta** \-mə-tə\ : a spot in the visual field in which vision is absent or deficient

sco·to·pic \skə-ˈtō-pik, -ˈtä-\ *adj* : of, relating to, being, or suitable for scotopic vision ⟨~ sensitivity⟩

scotopic vision *n* : vision in dim light with dark-adapted eyes that involves only the retinal rods as light receptors

¹**scour** \ˈskau̇r\ *vb, of a domestic animal* : to suffer from diarrhea or dysentery

²**scour** *n sing or pl* : diarrhea or dysentery occurring esp. in young domestic animals

scra·pie \ˈskrā-pē\ *n* : a usu. fatal prion disease of sheep and goats that is characterized by twitching, excitability, intense itching, excessive thirst, emaciation, weakness, and finally paralysis

scrap·ing \ˈskrā-piŋ\ *n* : material scraped esp. from diseased tissue for microscopic examination

scratch test *n* : a test for allergic susceptibility made by rubbing an extract of an allergy-producing substance into small breaks or scratches in the skin — compare INTRADERMAL TEST, PATCH TEST, PRICK TEST

screen \ˈskrēn\ *vb* : to test or examine for the presence of something (as a disease) ⟨~ patients for cancer⟩

screen — see INTENSIFYING SCREEN, SUNSCREEN

screen memory *n* : a recollection of early childhood that may be falsely recalled or magnified in importance and that masks another memory of deep emotional significance

screw·fly \ˈskrü-ˌflī\ *n, pl* **-flies** : SCREWWORM FLY

screw·worm \ˈskrü-ˌwərm\ *n* **1** : either of two dipteran flies of the genus *Cochliomyia* : **a** : one (*C. hominivorax*) of the warmer parts of America whose larva develops in sores or wounds or in the nostrils of mammals including humans; *esp* : its larva **b** : SECONDARY SCREWWORM **2** : an Old World dipteran fly (*Chrysomyia bezziana*) that causes myiasis chiefly in Africa and southern Asia

screwworm fly *n* : the adult of a screwworm — called also *screwfly*

scrip \ˈskrip\ *n* : PRESCRIPTION 1

script \ˈskript\ *n* : PRESCRIPTION 1

scroful- *or* **scrofulo-** *comb form* : scrofula ⟨*scrofulo*derma⟩

scrof·u·la \ˈskrō-fyə-lə, ˈskrä-\ *n* : tuberculosis of lymph nodes esp. in the neck — called also *king's evil*

scrof·u·lo·der·ma \ˌskrō-fyə-lō-ˈdər-mə, ˌskrä-\ *n* : a disease of the skin of tuberculous origin

scrot- *or* **scroti-** *or* **scroto-** *comb form* : scrotum ⟨*scroto*plasty⟩

scro·tal \ˈskrōt-ᵊl\ *adj* **1** : of or relating to the scrotum **2** : lying in or having descended into the scrotum ⟨~ testes⟩

scro·to·plas·ty \ˈskrō-tə-ˌplas-tē\ *n, pl* **-ties** : plastic surgery performed on the scrotum

scro·tum \ˈskrō-təm\ *n, pl* **scro·ta** \-tə\ *or* **scrotums** : the external pouch that in most mammals contains the testes

scrub \ˈskrəb\ *vb* **scrubbed; scrubbing** : to clean and disinfect (the hands and forearms) before participating in surgery — **scrub** *n*

scrub nurse *n* : a nurse who assists the surgeon in an operating room

scrub typhus *n* : an acute febrile disease that is caused by a rickettsial bacterium (*Orientia tsutsugamushi* syn. *Rickettsia tsutsugamushi*) transmitted by mite larvae, resembles louse-borne typhus, and is widespread in the western Pacific area — called also *tsutsugamushi disease*

scru·ple \ˈskrü-pəl\ *n* : a unit of apothecaries' weight equal to 20 grains or ⅓ dram or 1.296 grams

scurf \ˈskərf\ *n* : thin dry scales detached from the epidermis esp. in an abnormal skin condition; *specif* : DANDRUFF — **scurfy** \ˈskər-fē\ *adj*

scur·vy \ˈskər-vē\ *n, pl* **scur·vies** : a disease that is characterized by spongy gums, loosening of the teeth, and a bleeding into the skin and mucous membranes and that is caused by a lack of vitamin C

Se *symbol* selenium

sea·bath·er's eruption \\'sē-ˌbā-thərz-\\ *n* : acute pruritic dermatitis that occurs on parts of the body covered by a swimsuit within 24 hours after exposure to seawater containing certain tiny coelenterate larvae (as of thimble jellyfishes or sea anemones)

sea·borg·i·um \\sē-'bȯr-gē-əm\\ *n* : a short-lived radioactive element that is artificially produced — symbol *Sg*; see ELEMENT table

seal \\'sēl\\ *vb* : to apply dental sealant to

seal·ant \\'sē-lənt\\ *n* : a plastic material that is applied to parts of teeth with imperfections (as pits and fissures) usu. to prevent dental decay

seal finger *n* : a finger rendered swollen and painful by erysipeloid or a similar infection and occurring esp. in individuals handling seals or sealskins

sea lice *n pl* : tiny coelenterate larvae that cause seabather's eruption; *also* : SEABATHER'S ERUPTION

sea·sick·ness \\'sē-ˌsik-nəs\\ *n* : motion sickness experienced on the water — called also *mal de mer* — **seasick** *adj*

sea snake *n* : any of a family (Hydrophidae) of numerous venomous snakes inhabiting the tropical parts of the Pacific and Indian oceans

seasonal affective disorder *n* : depression that tends to recur as the days grow shorter during the fall and winter — abbr. *SAD*

¹seat \\'sēt\\ *n* : a part or surface esp. in dentistry on or in which another part or surface rests — see REST SEAT

²seat *vb* : to provide with or position on a dental seat

seat·worm \\-ˌwərm\\ *n* : a pinworm of the genus *Enterobius* (*E. vermicularis*) that is parasitic in humans

sea wasp *n* : any of various jellyfishes (order or suborder Cubomedusae of the class Scyphozoa) of tropical waters that inflict a painful and sometimes fatal sting — called also *box jellyfish*

se·ba·ceous \\si-'bā-shəs\\ *adj* **1** : secreting sebum **2** : of, relating to, or being fatty material ⟨a ∼ exudate⟩

sebaceous cyst *n* : a cyst filled with sebaceous matter and formed by distension of a sebaceous gland as a result of obstruction of its excretory duct

sebaceous gland *n* : any of the small sacculated glands that are lodged in the substance of the dermis, usu. open into the hair follicles, and secrete sebum

sebi- *or* **sebo-** *comb form* : fat : grease : sebum ⟨*sebo*rrhea⟩

seb·or·rhea \\ˌse-bə-'rē-ə\\ *n* : abnormally increased secretion and discharge of sebum producing an oily appearance of the skin and the formation of greasy scales

seb·or·rhe·al \\ˌse-bə-'rē-əl\\ *adj* : SEBORRHEIC

seb·or·rhe·ic \\-'rē-ik\\ *adj* : of, relating to, or characterized by seborrhea

seborrheic dermatitis *n* : a red, scaly, itchy dermatitis chiefly affecting areas (as of the face, scalp, or chest) with many large sebaceous glands

seborrheic keratosis *n* : a benign hyperkeratotic tumor that occurs singly or in clusters on the surface of the skin, is usu. brown or black in color, and typically has a warty texture often with a waxy appearance

se·bor·rhoea, se·bor·rhoe·al, se·bor·rhoe·ic *chiefly Brit var of* SEBORRHEA, SEBORRHEAL, SEBORRHEIC

se·bum \\'sē-bəm\\ *n* : fatty lubricant matter that is secreted by sebaceous glands of the skin and acts to soften and protectively coat the hair and skin

seco·bar·bi·tal \\ˌse-kō-'bär-bə-ˌtȯl\\ *n* : a barbiturate used chiefly in the form of its sodium salt $C_{12}H_{17}N_2NaO_3$ as a hypnotic and sedative — called also *quinalbarbitone*; see SECONAL

Sec·o·nal \\'se-kə-ˌnȯl, -ˌnal, -nəl\\ *trademark* — used for a preparation of the sodium salt of secobarbital

sec·ond·ary \\'se-kən-ˌder-ē\\ *adj* **1** : not first in order of occurrence or development: as **a** : dependent or consequent on another disease ⟨∼ diabetes⟩ **b** : occurring or being in the second stage ⟨∼ symptoms of syphilis⟩ **c** : occurring some time after the original injury ⟨a ∼ hemorrhage⟩ **2** : characterized by or resulting from the substitution of two atoms or groups in a molecule ⟨a ∼ salt⟩ **3** : relating to or being the three-dimensional coiling of the polypeptide chain of a protein esp. in the form of an alpha-helix — compare PRIMARY 3, TERTIARY 2 — **sec·ond·ari·ly** \\ˌse-kən-'der-ə-lē\\ *adv*

secondary amenorrhea *n* : the temporary or permanent cessation of menstruation in a woman who has previously experienced normal menses

secondary care *n* : medical care provided by a specialist or facility upon referral by a primary care physician that requires more specialized knowledge, skill, or equipment than the primary care physician has — compare PRIMARY CARE, TERTIARY CARE

secondary dentin *n* : dentin formed following the loss (as by erosion or abrasion) of original dentin

secondary gain *n* : a benefit (as sympathetic attention) associated with a mental disorder

secondary hypertension *n* : hypertension that results from an underlying identifiable cause

secondary infection *n* : infection occurring at the site of a preexisting infection

secondary oocyte *n* : an oocyte that is produced by division of a primary oocyte in the first meiotic division

secondary screwworm n : a screwworm of the genus *Cochliomyia* (*C. macellaria*) chiefly of warmer parts of America whose larva develops in dead tissue (as of wounds); *esp* : its larva

secondary sex characteristic n : a physical characteristic (as the breasts of a female) that appears in members of one sex at puberty or in seasonal breeders at the breeding season and is not directly concerned with reproduction — called also *secondary sex character, secondary sexual characteristic*

secondary spermatocyte n : a spermatocyte that is produced by division of a primary spermatocyte in the first meiotic division and that divides in the second meiotic division to give spermatids

secondary syphilis n : the second stage of syphilis that appears from 2 to 6 months after primary infection, that is marked by lesions esp. in the skin but also in organs and tissues, and that lasts from 3 to 12 weeks

secondary tympanic membrane n : a membrane closing the round window and separating the scala tympani from the middle ear

second cranial nerve n : OPTIC NERVE

second–degree burn n : a burn marked by pain, blistering, and superficial destruction of dermis with edema and hyperemia of the tissues beneath the burn

secondhand smoke n : tobacco smoke that is exhaled by a smoker or given off by burning tobacco (as of a cigarette) and is inhaled by persons nearby — called also *passive smoke*

second in·ten·tion \-in-ˈten-chən\ n : the healing of an incised wound by granulations that bridge the gap between skin edges — compare FIRST INTENTION

sec·ond–line \ˈse-kənd-ˈlīn\ adj : being or using a drug that is not the usual or preferred choice — compare FIRST-LINE

second messenger n : an intracellular substance (as cyclic AMP) that mediates cell activity by relaying a signal from an extracellular molecule (as of a hormone or neurotransmitter) bound to the cell's surface

second polar body n : POLAR BODY b

second wind n : recovered full power of respiration after the first exhaustion during exertion due to improved heart action

secret- or **secreto-** comb form : secretion ⟨*secretin*⟩

se·cre·ta·gogue \si-ˈkrē-tə-ˌgäg\ n : a substance that stimulates secretion

se·cre·tase \si-ˈkrē-ˌtās\ n : any of several transmembrane proteases that are capable of cleaving amyloid precursor protein and include two forms that function in the generation of beta-amyloid

se·cre·tin \si-ˈkrēt-ᵊn\ n : an intestinal proteinaceous hormone capable of stimulating secretion by the pancreas and liver

se·cre·tion \si-ˈkrē-shən\ n **1** : the process of segregating, elaborating, and releasing some material either functionally specialized (as saliva) or isolated for excretion (as urine) **2** : a product of secretion formed by an animal or plant; *esp* : one performing a specific useful function in the organism — **se·crete** \si-ˈkrēt\ vb — **se·cre·to·ry** \ˈsē-krə-ˌtōr-ē, si-ˈkrē-tə-rē\ adj

se·cre·tor \si-ˈkrē-tər\ n : an individual of blood group A, B, or AB who secretes the antigens characteristic of these blood groups in bodily fluids (as saliva)

secretory otitis media n : SEROUS OTITIS MEDIA

-sect \ˌsekt\ vb comb form : cut : divide ⟨hemi*sect*⟩ ⟨tran*sect*⟩

sec·tion \ˈsek-shən\ n **1** : the action or an instance of cutting or separating by cutting; *esp* : the action of dividing (as tissues) surgically ⟨abdominal ∼⟩ — see CESAREAN SECTION **2** : a very thin slice (as of tissue) suitable for microscopic examination — **section** vb

se·cun·di·grav·id \si-ˌkən-dē-ˈgra-vəd\ adj : pregnant for the second time

se·cun·di·grav·i·da \-ˈgra-vi-də\ n, pl **-dae** \-ˌdē, -ˌdī\ also **-das** : a woman in her second pregnancy

sec·un·dines \ˈse-kən-ˌdēnz, -ˌdīnz; se-ˈkən-dənz\ n pl : AFTERBIRTH

sec·un·dip·a·ra \ˌse-kən-ˈdi-pə-rə\ n, pl **-ras** or **-rae** \-ˌrē, -ˌrī\ : a woman who has borne children in two separate pregnancies

security blanket n : a blanket carried by a child as a protection against anxiety

se·date \si-ˈdāt\ vb **se·dat·ed; se·dat·ing** : to dose with sedatives

se·da·tion \si-ˈdā-shən\ n **1** : the inducing of a relaxed easy state esp. by the use of sedatives **2** : a state resulting from sedation — see CONSCIOUS SEDATION, DEEP SEDATION

¹sed·a·tive \ˈse-də-tiv\ adj : tending to calm, moderate, or tranquilize nervousness or excitement

²sedative n : a sedative agent or drug

¹sed·i·ment \ˈse-də-mənt\ n : the matter that settles to the bottom of a liquid

²sed·i·ment \-ˌment\ vb : to deposit as sediment

sed·i·men·ta·tion \ˌse-də-(ˌ)men-ˈtā-shən\ n **1** : the action or process of depositing sediment **2** : the depositing esp. by mechanical means of matter suspended in a liquid

sedimentation rate n : the speed at which red blood cells settle to the bottom of a column of citrated blood measured in millimeters deposited per hour and which is used esp. in diagnosing the progress of various abnormal conditions

sed rate \'sed-\ n : SEDIMENTATION RATE

¹**seed** \'sēd\ n, pl **seed** or **seeds** 1 a : the fertilized ripened ovule of a flowering plant **b** : a propagative animal structure; esp : SEMEN 2 : a small usu. glass and gold or platinum capsule used as a container for a radioactive substance (as radium or radon) to be applied usu. interstitially in the treatment of cancer — **seed•ed** \'sē-dəd\ adj

²**seed** adj : selected or used to produce a new crop or stock ⟨∼ virus⟩

Seeing Eye trademark — used for a guide dog trained to lead the blind

¹**seg•ment** \'seg-mənt\ n : one of the constituent parts into which a body, entity, or quantity is divided or marked off by or as if by natural boundaries — **seg•men•tal** \seg-'ment-ᵊl\ adj — **seg•men•tal•ly** adv

²**seg•ment** \'seg-ˌment\ vb 1 : to cause to undergo segmentation by division or multiplication of cells 2 : to separate into segments

segmental resection n : excision of a segment of an organ; specif : excision of a portion of a lobe of a lung — called also segmentectomy; compare PNEUMONECTOMY

seg•men•ta•tion \ˌseg-(ˌ)men-'tā-shən\ n 1 : the act or process of dividing into segments; esp : the formation of many cells from a single cell (as in a developing egg) 2 : annular contraction of smooth muscle (as of the intestine) that seems to cut the part affected into segments

segmentation cavity n : BLASTOCOEL

seg•men•tec•to•my \ˌseg-mən-'tek-tə-mē\ n, pl **-mies** : SEGMENTAL RESECTION

seg•ment•ed \'seg-ˌmen-təd, seg-'\ adj 1 : having or made up of segments 2 : being a cell in which the nucleus is divided into lobes connected by a fine filament ⟨∼ neutrophils⟩

seg•re•gant \'se-gri-gənt\ n : SEGREGATE

¹**seg•re•gate** \'se-gri-ˌgāt\ vb **-gat•ed; -gat•ing** : to undergo genetic segregation

²**seg•re•gate** \-gət\ n : an individual or class of individuals differing in one or more genetic characters from the parental line usu. because of segregation of genes

seg•re•ga•tion \ˌse-gri-'gā-shən\ n : the separation of allelic genes that occurs typically during meiosis

Sei•gnette's salt \sen-'yet-\ or **Sei•gnette's salt** \-'yets-\ n : ROCHELLE SALT

    Seignette, Pierre (1660–1719), French pharmacist.

sei•zure \'sē-zhər\ n 1 : a sudden attack (as of disease); esp : the physical manifestations (as convulsions, sensory disturbances, or loss of consciousness) resulting from abnormal electrical discharges in the brain (as in epilepsy) 2 : an abnormal electrical discharge in the brain

Sel•dane \'sel-ˌdān\ n : a preparation of terfenadine — formerly a U.S. registered trademark

se•lec•tin \sə-'lek-tin\ n : any of a family of sugar-binding lectins that are found on the surface of cells (as endothelial cells and white blood cells) and that promote their adhesion to other cells and mediate their migration to sites of inflammation

se•lec•tion \sə-'lek-shən\ n : a natural or artificial process that results or tends to result in the survival and propagation of some individuals or organisms but not of others with the result that the inherited traits of the survivors are perpetuated — compare DARWINISM

se•lec•tive \sə-'lek-tiv\ adj 1 : of, relating to, or characterized by selection : selecting or tending to select 2 : highly specific in activity or effect — **se•lec•tive•ly** adv — **se•lec•tiv•i•ty** \sə-ˌlek-'ti-və-tē, ˌsē-\ n

selective estrogen receptor modulator n : any of a class of drugs (as raloxifene or tamoxifen) that bind with estrogen receptors and act as estrogen agonists in some tissues and estrogen antagonists in other tissues — abbr. SERM

selective mutism n : an anxiety disorder of childhood characterized by consistent failure to speak in specific social settings (as at school) despite having the ability to speak normally in other settings (as at home) — called also elective mutism

selective reduction n : abortion of one or more but not all embryos in a pregnancy with multiple embryos — called also selective termination

selective serotonin reuptake inhibitor n : SSRI

se•leg•i•line \si-'le-jə-ˌlēn\ n : the levorotatory form of deprenyl that is administered in the form of its hydrochloride $C_{13}H_{17}N·HCl$ esp. as an adjuvant to therapy using the combination of L-dopa and carbidopa in the treatment of Parkinson's disease

sel•e•nif•er•ous \ˌse-lə-'ni-fə-rəs\ adj : containing or yielding selenium

se•le•ni•um \sə-'lē-nē-əm\ n : a nonmetallic element that is an essential trace element found esp. in grains and meat — symbol Se; see ELEMENT table, SELENOSIS

selenium sulfide n : the sulfide SeS_2 of selenium usu. in the form of an orange powder that is used in preparations for treating dandruff and seborrheic dermatitis of the scalp

sel•e•no•me•thi•o•nine \ˌse-lə-nō-mə-'thī-ə-ˌnēn\ n : a selenium analog $C_5H_{11}NO_2Se$ of methionine that is used as a diagnostic aid in scintigraphy esp. of the pancreas and as a dietary supplement

sel·e·no·sis \,se-lə-'nō-səs\ *n* : poisoning due to excessive intake of selenium; *esp* : poisoning of livestock by high levels of selenium consumed in plants grown in seleniferous soils — called also *alkali disease;* see BLIND STAGGERS

self \'self\ *n, pl* **selves** \'selvz\ **1** : the union of elements (as body, emotions, thoughts, and sensations) that constitute the individuality and identity of a person **2** : material that is part of an individual organism 〈the immune system distinguishes ~ from nonself〉

self–abuse \,self-ə-'byüs\ *n* : MASTURBATION

self–ac·tu·al·ize \'self-'ak-chə-wə-,līz\ *vb* **-ized; -iz·ing** : to realize fully one's potential — **self–ac·tu·al·iza·tion** \-,ak-chə-wə-lə-'zā-shən\ *n*

self–ad·min·is·ter \-əd-'mi-nə-stər\ *vb* : to administer to oneself 〈~ed an analgesic〉 — **self–ad·min·is·tra·tion** \-,mi-nə-'strā-shən\ *n*

self–anal·y·sis \-ə-'na-lə-səs\ *n, pl* **-y·ses** \-,sēz\ : a systematic attempt by an individual to understand his or her own personality without the aid of another person — **self–an·a·lyt·i·cal** \-,a-nə-'li-ti-kəl\ *also* **self–an·a·lyt·ic** \-tik\ *adj*

self–an·ti·gen \-'an-ti-jən\ *n* : any molecule or chemical group of an organism which acts as an antigen in inducing antibody formation in another organism but to which the healthy immune system of the parent organism is tolerant

self–as·sem·bly \-ə-'sem-blē\ *n, pl* **-blies** : the process by which a complex macromolecule (as collagen) or a supramolecular system (as a virus) spontaneously assembles itself from its components — **self–as·sem·ble** \-bəl\ *vb*

self–aware·ness \-ə-'wer-nəs\ *n* : an awareness of one's own personality or individuality — **self–aware** *adj*

self–care \-'ker\ *n* : care for oneself : SELF-TREATMENT

self–con·cept \'self-'kän-,sept\ *n* : the mental image one has of oneself

self–de·struc·tion \-di-'strək-shən\ *n* : destruction of oneself; *esp* : SUICIDE

self–de·struc·tive \-'strək-tiv\ *adj* : acting or tending to harm or destroy oneself 〈~ behavior〉; *also* : SUICIDAL — **self–de·struc·tive·ly** *adv* — **self–de·struc·tive·ness** *n*

self–ex·am·i·na·tion \-ig-,za-mə-'nā-shən\ *n* : examination of one's body esp. for evidence of disease 〈~ for detection of breast cancer〉

self–hyp·no·sis \,self-hip-'nō-səs\ *n, pl* **-no·ses** \-,sēz\ : hypnosis of oneself : AUTOHYPNOSIS

self–im·age \-'i-mij\ *n* : one's conception of oneself or of one's role

self–in·duced \-in-'düst, -'dyüst\ *adj* : induced by oneself 〈a ~ abortion〉

self–in·flict·ed \-in-'flik-təd\ *adj* : inflicted by oneself 〈~ vomiting〉

self–in·ject \-in-'jekt\ *vb* : to inject oneself with a drug or other substance — **self–in·ject·able** \-'jek-tə-bəl\ *adj* — **self–in·jec·tion** \-'jek-shən\ *n*

self·ish \'sel-fish\ *adj* : being an actively replicating repetitive sequence of nucleic acid that serves no known function 〈~ DNA〉; *also* : being genetic material solely concerned with its own replication 〈~ genes〉

self–lim·it·ed \-'li-mə-təd\ *adj* : limited by one's or its own nature; *specif* : running a definite and limited course

self–lim·it·ing *adj* : SELF-LIMITED

self–med·i·ca·tion \-,me-də-'kā-shən\ *n* : medication of oneself esp. without the advice of a physician : SELF-TREATMENT — **self–med·i·cate** \-'me-də-,kāt\ *vb*

self–mu·ti·la·tion \-,myü-tə-'lā-shən\ *n* : injury or disfigurement of oneself

self–re·ac·tive \-rē-'ak-tiv\ *adj* : capable of participating in an autoimmune response 〈~ T cells〉

self–rec·og·ni·tion \-,re-kəg-'ni-shən\ *n* : the process by which the immune system of an organism distinguishes between the body's own chemicals, cells, and tissues and those of foreign organisms or agents — compare SELF-TOLERANCE

self–re·fer·ral \-ri-'fər-əl\ *n* : the referral of a patient to a specialized medical facility (as a medical imaging center) in which the referring physician has a financial interest — **self–re·fer** \-ri-'fər\ *vb*

self–rep·li·cat·ing \-'re-plə-,kā-tiŋ\ *adj* : reproducing itself autonomously 〈DNA is a ~ molecule〉 — **self–rep·li·ca·tion** \-,re-plə-'kā-shən\ *n*

self–stim·u·la·tion \-,stim-yə-'lā-shən\ *n* : stimulation of oneself as a result of one's own activity or behavior; *esp* : MASTURBATION — **self–stim·u·la·to·ry** \-'stim-yə-lə-,tōr-ē\ *adj*

self–tan·ner \-'ta-nər\ *n* : a product (as one containing dihydroxyacetone) that when applied to the skin reacts chemically with its surface layer to give the appearance of a tan

self–tol·er·ance \-'tä-lə-rəns\ *n* : the physiological state that exists in a developing organism when its immune system has proceeded far enough in the process of self-recognition to lose the capacity to attack and destroy its own bodily constituents — called also *horror autotoxicus*

self–treat·ment \-'trēt-mənt\ *n* : medication of oneself or treatment of one's own disease without medical supervision or prescription

sel·la \'se-lə\ *n, pl* **sellas** *or* **sel·lae** \-,lē\ : SELLA TURCICA

sellae — see DIAPHRAGMA SELLAE

sel·lar \'se-lər, -,lär\ *adj* : of, relating to, or involving the sella turcica

sella tur·ci·ca \-'tər-ki-kə, -si-\ *n, pl* **sellae tur·ci·cae** \-ki-,kī, -si-,sē\ : a depression in the middle line of the upper surface of the sphenoid bone in which the pituitary gland is lodged

SEM *abbr* scanning electron microscope; scanning electron microscopy

se·men \'sē-mən\ *n* : a viscid whitish fluid of the male reproductive tract consisting of spermatozoa suspended in secretions of the accessory glands (as of the prostate and Cowper's glands)

semi·cir·cu·lar canal \ˌse-mē-'sər-kyə-lər-, ˌse-ˌmī-\ *n* : any of the loop-shaped tubular parts of the labyrinth of the ear that together constitute a sensory organ associated with the maintenance of bodily equilibrium, that consist of an inner membranous canal of the membranous labyrinth and a corresponding outer bony canal of the bony labyrinth, and that form a group of three in each ear usu. in planes nearly at right angles to each other — see SEMICIRCULAR DUCT

semicircular duct *n* : any of the three loop-shaped membranous inner tubular parts of the semicircular canals that are about one-fourth the diameter of the corresponding outer bony canals, that communicate at each end with the utricle, and that have near one end an expanded ampulla containing the crista

semi·co·ma \-'kō-mə\ *n* : a semicomatose state from which a person can be aroused

semi·co·ma·tose \-'kō-mə-ˌtōs\ *adj* : marked by or affected with stupor and disorientation but not complete coma ⟨a ∼ state⟩ ⟨∼ patients⟩

semi·con·scious \-'kän-chəs\ *adj* : incompletely conscious : imperfectly aware or responsive — **semi·con·scious·ness** *n*

semi·con·ser·va·tive \-kən-'sər-və-tiv\ *adj* : relating to or being genetic replication in which a double-stranded molecule of nucleic acid separates into two single strands each of which serves as a template for the formation of a complementary strand that together with the template forms a complete molecule — **semi·con·ser·va·tive·ly** *adv*

semi·dom·i·nant \-'dä-mi-nənt\ *adj* : producing an intermediate phenotype in the heterozygous condition

semi·flu·id \-'flü-əd\ *adj* : having the qualities of both a fluid and a solid : VISCOUS — **semifluid** *n*

semi·lu·nar \-'lü-nər\ *adj* : shaped like a crescent

semilunar bone *n* : LUNATE BONE

semilunar cartilage *n* : MENISCUS a(2)

semilunar cusp *n* : any of the crescentic cusps making up the semilunar valves

semilunares — see LINEA SEMILUNARIS, PLICA SEMILUNARIS

semilunar ganglion *n* : TRIGEMINAL GANGLION

semilunaris — see HIATUS SEMILUNARIS, LINEA SEMILUNARIS, PLICA SEMILUNARIS

semilunar line *n* : LINEA SEMILUNARIS

semilunar lobule *n* : either of a pair of crescent-shaped lobules situated one on each side in the posterior and ventral part of the cerebellum

semilunar notch *n* : TROCHLEAR NOTCH

semilunar valve *n* **1** : either of two valves of which one is situated at the opening between the heart and the aorta and the other at the opening between the heart and the pulmonary artery, which prevent regurgitation of blood into the ventricles, and each of which is made up of three crescent-shaped cusps **2** : SEMILUNAR CUSP

semi·mem·bra·no·sus \ˌse-mē-ˌmem-brə-'nō-səs, ˌse-ˌmī-\ *n, pl* **-no·si** \-ˌsī\ : a large muscle of the inner part and back of the thigh that arises by a thick tendon from the back part of the tuberosity of the ischium, is inserted into the medial condyle of the tibia, and acts to flex the leg and rotate it medially and to extend the thigh

sem·i·nal \'se-mən-ᵊl\ *adj* : of, relating to, or consisting of semen

seminal duct *n* : a tube or passage serving esp. or exclusively as an efferent duct of the testis and in humans being made up of the tubules of the epididymis, the vas deferens, and the ejaculatory duct

seminal fluid *n* **1** : SEMEN **2** : the part of the semen that is produced by various accessory glands (as the prostate gland and seminal vesicles) : semen excepting the spermatozoa

seminal vesicle *n* : either of a pair of glandular pouches that lie one on either side of the male reproductive tract and that in human males secrete a sugar- and protein-containing fluid into the ejaculatory duct

sem·i·nif·er·ous \ˌse-mə-'ni-fə-rəs\ *adj* : producing or bearing semen

seminiferous tubule *n* : any of the coiled threadlike tubules that make up the bulk of the testis and are lined with a layer of epithelial cells from which the spermatozoa are produced

sem·i·no·ma \ˌse-mi-'nō-mə\ *n, pl* **-mas** *also* **-ma·ta** \-mə-tə\ : a germinoma of the testis

semi·per·me·able \ˌse-mē-'pər-mē-ə-bəl, ˌse-ˌmī-\ *adj* : partially but not freely or wholly permeable; *specif* : permeable to some usu. small molecules but not to other usu. larger particles ⟨∼ membranes⟩ — **semi·per·me·abil·i·ty** \-ˌpər-mē-ə-'bi-lə-tē\ *n*

semi·pri·vate \-'prī-vət\ *adj* : of, receiving, or associated with hospital service giving a patient more privileges than a ward patient but fewer than a private patient ⟨a ∼ room⟩

semi·spi·na·lis \-ˌspī-'nä-ləs\ *n, pl* **-les**

\-ˌlēz\ : any of three muscles of the cervical and thoracic parts of the spinal column: **a** : SEMISPINALIS THORACIS **b** : SEMISPINALIS CERVICIS **c** : SEMISPINALIS CAPITIS

semispinalis cap·i·tis \-ˈkā-pi-təs\ *n* : a deep longitudinal muscle of the back that arises esp. from the transverse processes of the upper six or seven thoracic and the seventh cervical vertebrae, is inserted on the outer surface of the occipital bone between two ridges behind the foramen magnum, and acts to extend and rotate the head — called also *complexus*

semispinalis cer·vi·cis \-ˈsər-vi-sis\ *n* : a deep longitudinal muscle of the back that arises from the transverse processes of the upper five or six thoracic vertebrae, is inserted into the cervical spinous processes from the axis to the fifth cervical vertebra, and with the semispinalis thoracis acts to extend the spinal column and rotate it toward the opposite side

semispinalis tho·ra·cis \-thō-ˈrā-səs\ *n* : a deep longitudinal muscle of the back that arises from the transverse processes of the lower five thoracic vertebrae, is inserted into the spinous processes of the upper four thoracic and lower two cervical vertebrae, and with the semispinalis cervicis acts to extend the spinal column and rotate it toward the opposite side

semi·syn·thet·ic \-sin-ˈthe-tik\ *adj* **1** : produced by chemical alteration of a natural starting material ⟨~ penicillins⟩ **2** : containing both chemically identified and complex natural ingredients ⟨a ~ diet⟩ — **semi·syn·thet·i·cal·ly** \-ti-k(ə-)lē\ *adv*

sem·i·ten·di·no·sus \-ˌten-də-ˈnō-səs\ *n, pl* **-no·si** \-ˌsī\ : a fusiform muscle of the posterior and inner part of the thigh that arises from the ischial tuberosity along with the biceps femoris, that is inserted by a long round tendon into the inner surface of the upper part of the shaft of the tibia, and that acts to flex the leg and rotate it medially and to extend the thigh

Sem·li·ki For·est virus \ˈsem-lē-kē-ˈfôr-əst-\ *n* : a togavirus of the genus *Alphavirus* (species *Semliki Forest virus*) isolated from mosquitoes in a Ugandan forest and capable of infecting humans and laboratory animals

Sen·dai virus \ˈsen-ˌdī-\ *n* : a paramyxovirus (species *Sendai virus* of the genus *Respirovirus*) first reported in Japan that infects swine, mice, and humans

se·ne·cio \si-ˈnē-shē-ˌō, -shō\ *n, pl* **-cios** **1** *cap* : a genus of widely distributed plants (family Compositae) including some containing various alkaloids which are poisonous to livestock **2** *pl* **-cios** : any plant of the genus *Senecio*

se·ne·ci·o·sis \se-ˌnē-sē-ˈō-səs\ *n, pl* **-o·ses** \-ˌsēz\ : a frequently fatal intoxication esp. of livestock feeding on plants of the genus *Senecio*

se·nes·cence \si-ˈnes-ᵊns\ *n* : the state of being old : the process of becoming old — **se·nes·cent** \-ᵊnt\ *adj*

se·nile \ˈsē-ˌnīl\ *adj* **1** : of, relating to, exhibiting, or characteristic of old age; *esp* : exhibiting a loss of cognitive abilities (as memory) associated with old age **2** : being a cell that cannot undergo mitosis and is in a stage of declining function prior to the time of death ⟨~ red blood cells⟩

senile cataract *n* : a cataract of a type that occurs in the aged and is characterized by an initial opacity in the lens, subsequent swelling of the lens, and final shrinkage with complete loss of transparency

senile dementia *n* : a mental disorder of old age esp. of the degenerative type associated with Alzheimer's disease — called also *senile psychosis*

senile psychosis *n* : SENILE DEMENTIA

senilis — see ARCUS SENILIS, LENTIGO SENILIS

se·nil·i·ty \si-ˈni-lə-tē, se-\ *n, pl* **-ties** : the quality or state of being senile

se·ni·um \ˈsē-nē-əm\ *n* : the final period in the normal life span

sen·na \ˈse-nə\ *n* **1** : any of a genus (*Cassia* syn. *Senna*) of leguminous plants; *esp* : one used medicinally **2** : the dried leaflets or pods of various sennas (esp. *Cassia angustifolia* syn. *Senna alexandrina*) used as a purgative

sen·sa·tion \sen-ˈsā-shən, sən-\ *n* **1 a** : a mental process (as hearing or smelling) due to immediate bodily stimulation often as distinguished from awareness of the process — compare PERCEPTION **b** : awareness (as of pain) due to stimulation of a sense organ **c** : a state of consciousness of a kind usu. due to physical objects or internal bodily changes ⟨a ~ of hunger⟩ **2** : something (as a physical object or pain) that causes or is the object of sensation

¹**sense** \ˈsens\ *n* **1 a** : the faculty of perceiving by means of sense organs **b** : a specialized animal function or mechanism (as sight, hearing, smell, taste, or touch) basically involving a stimulus and a sense organ **c** : the sensory mechanisms constituting a unit distinct from other functions (as movement or thought) **2** : a particular sensation or kind or quality of sensation ⟨a good ~ of balance⟩

²**sense** *vb* **sensed; sens·ing** : to perceive by the senses

sense–da·tum \ˈsens-ˈdā-təm, -ˈda-, -ˈdä-\ *n, pl* **sense–da·ta** \-tə\ : the immediate private perceived object of sensation as distinguished from the objective material object itself

sense organ *n* : a bodily structure that receives a stimulus (as heat or sound waves) and is affected in such a manner as to initiate a wave of excitation in associated sensory nerve fibers : RECEPTOR

sen·si·bil·i·ty \ˌsen-sə-'bi-lə-tē\ *n, pl* **-ties** **1** : ability to receive sensations ⟨tactile ∼⟩ **2** : awareness of and responsiveness toward something

sen·si·ble \'sen-sə-bəl\ *adj* **1** : perceptible to the senses or to reason or understanding **2** : capable of receiving sensory impressions ⟨∼ to pain⟩

sen·si·tive \'sen-sə-tiv\ *adj* **1** : SENSORY 2 ⟨∼ nerves⟩ **2 a** : receptive to sense impressions **b** : capable of being stimulated or excited by external agents **3** : highly responsive or susceptible: as **a** : easily hurt or damaged ⟨∼ skin⟩; *esp* : easily hurt emotionally **b** : excessively or abnormally susceptible : HYPERSENSITIVE **c** : capable of indicating minute differences — **sen·si·tive·ness** *n* — **sen·si·tiv·i·ty** \ˌsen-sə-'ti-və-tē\ *n*

sensitivity training *n* : training in a small interacting group that is designed to increase each individual's awareness of his or her own feelings and the feelings of others and to enhance interpersonal relations

sen·si·ti·za·tion \ˌsen-sə-tə-'zā-shən\ *n* **1** : the action or process of making sensitive or hypersensitive ⟨allergic ∼ of the skin⟩ **2** : the process of becoming sensitive or hypersensitive (as to an antigen); *also* : the resulting state **3** : a form of nonassociative learning characterized by an increase in responsiveness upon repeated exposure to a stimulus — compare HABITUATION 3 — **sen·si·tize** \'sen-sə-ˌtīz\ *vb*

sen·si·tiz·er \-ˌtī-zər\ *n* : a substance that sensitizes the skin on first contact so that subsequent contact causes inflammation

sen·sor \'sen-ˌsȯr, -sər\ *n* : a device that responds to a physical stimulus (as heat, light, sound, or motion) and transmits a resulting impulse; *also* : SENSE ORGAN

sensori- *or* **senso-** *comb form* : sensory : sensory and ⟨*sensori*motor⟩

sen·so·ri·al \sen-'sȯr-ē-əl\ *adj* : SENSORY

sen·so·ri·mo·tor \ˌsen-sə-rē-'mō-tər\ *adj* : of, relating to, or functioning in both sensory and motor aspects of bodily activity ⟨∼ disturbances⟩

sen·so·ri·neu·ral \-'nu̇r-əl, -'nyu̇r-\ *adj* : of, relating to, or involving the aspects of sense perception mediated by nerves ⟨∼ hearing loss⟩

sen·so·ri·um \sen-'sȯr-ē-əm\ *n, pl* **-ri·ums** *or* **-ria** \-ē-ə\ **1** : the parts of the brain or the mind concerned with the reception and interpretation of sensory stimuli; *broadly* : the entire sensory apparatus **2 a** : ability of the brain to receive and interpret sensory stimuli **b** : the state of consciousness judged in terms of this ability

sen·so·ry \'sen-sə-rē\ *adj* **1** : of or relating to sensation or the senses **2** : conveying nerve impulses from the sense organs to the nerve centers : AFFERENT ⟨∼ nerve fibers⟩

sensory aphasia *n* : inability to understand spoken, written, or tactile speech symbols that results from damage (as by a brain lesion) to an area of the brain (as Wernicke's area) concerned with language — called also *Wernicke's aphasia*

sensory area *n* : an area of the cerebral cortex that receives afferent nerve fibers from lower sensory or motor areas

sensory cell *n* **1** : a peripheral nerve cell (as an olfactory cell) located at a sensory receiving surface and being the primary receptor of a sensory impulse **2** : a nerve cell (as a spinal ganglion cell) transmitting sensory impulses

sensory neuron *n* : a neuron that transmits nerve impulses from a sense organ towards the central nervous system — compare INTERNEURON, MOTOR NEURON

sensory root *n* : a nerve root containing only sensory fibers; *specif* : DORSAL ROOT — compare MOTOR ROOT

sen·ti·nel \'sent-ᵊn-əl\ *adj* : being an individual or part of a population potentially susceptible to an infection or infestation that is being monitored for the appearance or recurrence of the causative pathogen or parasite

sentinel node *n* : the first lymph node to receive lymphatic drainage from the site of a primary tumor — called also *sentinel lymph node*

sep·a·ra·tion \ˌse-pə-'rā-shən\ *n* **1** : the process of isolating or extracting from or of becoming isolated from a mixture; *also* : the resulting state **2** : DISLOCATION — see SHOULDER SEPARATION — **sep·a·rate** \'se-pə-ˌrāt\ *vb*

separation anxiety *n* : a form of anxiety experienced by a child or adolescent that is caused by separation from a significant nurturant figure and typically a parent or from familiar surroundings

sep·a·ra·tor \'se-pə-ˌrā-tər\ *n* : a dental appliance for separating adjoining teeth to give access to their surfaces

sep·sis \'sep-səs\ *n, pl* **sep·ses** \'sep-ˌsēz\ : a systemic response typically to a serious usu. localized infection (as of the abdomen or lungs) esp. of bacterial origin that is usu. marked by abnormal body temperature and white blood cell count, tachycardia, and tachypnea; *specif* : systemic inflammatory response syndrome induced by a documented infection — see MULTIPLE ORGAN DYSFUNCTION SYNDROME, SEPTIC SHOCK

sept- *or* **septo-** *also* **septi-** *comb form* : septum ⟨*septal*⟩ ⟨*septo*plasty⟩

septa *pl of* SEPTUM

sep·tal \'sept-ᵊl\ *adj* : of or relating to a septum ⟨∼ defects⟩

sep·tal cartilage *n* : the cartilage of the nasal septum

septa pel·lu·ci·da *pl of* SEPTUM PELLU- CIDUM

sep·tate \'sep-ˌtāt\ *adj* : divided by or having a septum — **sep·ta·tion** \sep- 'tā-shən\ *n*

septa trans·ver·sa *pl of* SEPTUM TRANS- VERSUM

sep·tec·to·my \sep-'tek-tə-mē\ *n, pl* **-mies** : surgical excision of a septum

sep·tic \'sep-tik\ *adj* 1 : of, relating to, or causing putrefaction 2 : relating to, involving, caused by, or affected with sepsis ⟨∼ arthritis⟩ ⟨∼ pa- tients⟩

septic abortion *n* : spontaneous or in- duced abortion associated with bacte- rial infection (as by E. coli, beta- hemolytic streptococci, or *Clostridi- um perfringens*)

sep·ti·cae·mia *chiefly Brit var of* SEP- TICEMIA

sep·ti·ce·mia \ˌsep-tə-'sē-mē-ə\ *n* : in- vasion of the bloodstream by viru- lent microorganisms from a focus of infection that is accompanied by acute systemic illness — called also *blood poisoning*; see PYEMIA; com- pare SEPSIS — **sep·ti·ce·mic** \-'sē- mik\ *adj*

septic shock *n* : a life-threatening se- vere form of sepsis that usu. results from the presence of bacteria and their toxins in the bloodstream and is characterized esp. by persistent hy- potension with reduced blood flow to organs and tissues and often organ dysfunction

septic sore throat *n* : STREP THROAT

septo- — see SEPT-

sep·to·plas·ty \'sep-tə-ˌplas-tē\ *n, pl* **-ties** : surgical repair of the nasal sep- tum

sep·tos·to·my \sep-'täs-tə-mē\ *n, pl* **-mies** : the surgical creation of an opening through the interatrial sep- tum

Sep·tra \'sep-trə\ *trademark* — used for a preparation of sulfamethoxazole and trimethoprim

sep·tum \'sep-təm\ *n, pl* **sep·ta** \-tə\ : a dividing wall or membrane esp. be- tween bodily spaces or masses of soft tissue; *esp* : NASAL SEPTUM

septum pel·lu·ci·dum \-pə-'lü-sə-dəm\ *n, pl* **septa pel·lu·ci·da** \-də\ : the thin double partition extending vertically from the lower surface of the corpus callosum to the fornix and neighbor- ing parts and separating the lateral ventricles of the brain

septum trans·ver·sum \-tranz-'vər- səm\ *n, pl* **septa trans·ver·sa** \-sə\ : the diaphragm or the embryonic structure from which it in part devel- ops

sep·tup·let \sep-'tə-plət, -'tü-plət, -'tyü-; 'sep-tə-\ *n* 1 : one of seven off- spring born at one birth 2 **septuplets** *pl* : a group of seven such offspring

se·quel \'sē-kwəl, -ˌkwel\ *n* : SEQUELA

se·quela \si-'kwe-lə\ *n, pl* **se·quel·ae** \-(ˌ)lē\ : a negative aftereffect ⟨neuro- logical *sequelae* of bacterial meningi- tis⟩

¹se·quence \'sē-kwəns, -ˌkwens\ *n* 1 : a continuous or connected series; *specif* : the exact order of bases in a nucleic acid or of amino acids in a protein 2 : a consequence, result, or subsequent development (as of a disease)

²sequence *vb* **se·quenced; se·quenc- ing** : to determine the sequence of chemical constituents (as amino acid residues in a protein or bases in a strand of DNA)

se·quenc·er \'sē-kwən-sər, -ˌkwen-\ *n* : one that sequences; *esp* : a device for determining the order of occurrence of amino acids in a protein or of bases in a nucleic acid

se·quen·tial \si-'kwen-chəl\ *adj* 1 : oc- curring as a sequela of disease or in- jury 2 : of, relating to, forming, or taken or administered in a sequence ⟨∼ chemotherapy⟩ — **sequential** *n*

se·ques·ter \si-'kwes-tər\ *vb* : to hold (as a metallic ion) in solution esp. for the purpose of suppressing undesired chemical or biological activity

se·ques·trant \-trənt\ *n* : a sequester- ing agent (as citric acid)

se·ques·tra·tion \ˌsē-kwəs-'trā-shən, ˌse-, si-ˌkwes-\ *n* 1 : the formation of a sequestrum 2 : the process of se- questering or result of being se- questered

se·ques·trec·to·my \ˌsē-ˌkwe-'strek- tə-mē\ *n, pl* **-mies** : the surgical re- moval of a sequestrum

se·ques·trum \si-'kwes-trəm\ *n, pl* **-trums** *also* **-tra** \-trə\ : a fragment of dead bone detached from adjoining sound bone

Ser *abbr* serine; seryl

sera *pl of* SERUM

serial section *n* : any of a series of sec- tions cut in sequence by a microtome from a prepared specimen — **serially sectioned** *adj* — **serial sectioning** *n*

ser·ine \'ser-ˌēn\ *n* : a nonessential amino acid $C_3H_7NO_3$ that occurs esp. as a structural part of many proteins and phosphatidylethanolamines and is a precursor of glycine — abbr. Ser

se·ri·ous \'sir-ē-əs\ *adj* : having impor- tant or dangerous possible conse- quences ⟨a ∼ injury⟩

SERM *abbr* selective estrogen receptor modulator

sero- *comb form* 1 : serum ⟨*serology*⟩ ⟨*sero*diagnosis⟩ 2 : serous and ⟨*sero*- purulent⟩

se·ro·con·ver·sion \ˌsir-ō-kən-'vər- zhən, ˌser-\ *n* : the production of anti- bodies in response to an antigen — **se·ro·con·vert** \-'vərt\ *vb*

se·ro·con·vert·er \-kən-'vər-tər\ *n* : one that is undergoing or has under- gone seroconversion

se·ro·di·ag·no·sis \-ˌdī-ig-'nō-səs\ *n, pl* **-no·ses** \-ˌsēz\ : diagnosis by the use of serum (as in the Wassermann test) — **se·ro·di·ag·nos·tic** \-'näs-tik\ *adj*

se·ro·ep·i·de·mi·o·log·ic \-ˌe-pə-ˌdē-mē-ə-ə-'lä-jik\ *or* **se·ro·ep·i·de·mi·o·log·i·cal** \-ji-kəl\ *adj* : of, relating to, or being epidemiological investigations involving the identification of antibodies to specific antigens in populations of individuals — **se·ro·ep·i·de·mi·ol·o·gy** \-mē-'ä-lə-jē\ *n*

se·ro·group \'sir-ō-ˌgrüp\ *n* : a group of serotypes having one or more antigens in common

se·rol·o·gist \si-'rä-lə-jist\ *n* : a specialist in serology

se·rol·o·gy \si-'rä-lə-jē\ *n, pl* **-gies** : a medical science dealing with blood serum esp. in regard to its immunological reactions and properties; *also* : the testing of blood serum to detect the presence of antibodies against a specific antigen — **se·ro·log·i·cal** \ˌsir-ə-'lä-ji-kəl\ *or* **se·ro·log·ic** \-jik\ *adj* — **se·ro·log·i·cal·ly** *adv*

se·ro·neg·a·tive \ˌsir-ō-'ne-gə-tiv, ˌser-ō-\ *adj* : having or being a negative serum reaction esp. in a test for the presence of an antibody ⟨a ∼ patient⟩ — **se·ro·neg·a·tiv·i·ty** \-ˌne-gə-'ti-və-tē\ *n*

se·ro·pos·i·tive \-'pä-zə-tiv\ *adj* : having or being a positive serum reaction esp. in a test for the presence of an antibody ⟨a ∼ donor⟩ — **se·ro·pos·i·tiv·i·ty** \-ˌpä-zə-'ti-və-tē\ *n*

se·ro·prev·a·lence \-'pre-və-ləns\ *n* : the frequency of individuals in a population that have a particular element (as antibodies to HIV) in their blood serum

se·ro·pu·ru·lent \-'pyùr-ə-lənt, -'pyùr-yə-\ *adj* : consisting of a mixture of serum and pus ⟨a ∼ exudate⟩

se·ro·re·ac·tiv·i·ty \-(ˌ)rē-ˌak-'ti-və-tē\ *n, pl* **-ties** : reactivity of blood serum — **se·ro·re·ac·tion** \-rē-'ak-shən, ˌser-\ *n* — **se·ro·re·ac·tive** \-rē-'ak-tiv\ *adj*

se·ro·sa \sə-'rō-zə\ *n, pl* **-sas** *also* **-sae** \-zē\ : a usu. enclosing serous membrane — **se·ro·sal** \-zəl\ *adj*

se·ro·san·guin·e·ous \ˌsir-ō-san-'gwi-nē-əs, ˌser-ō-, -saŋ-\ *adj* : containing or consisting of both blood and serous fluid ⟨a ∼ discharge⟩

se·ro·si·tis \ˌsir-ō-'sī-təs, ˌser-\ *n* : inflammation of one or more serous membranes ⟨peritoneal ∼⟩

se·ro·sta·tus \'sir-ə-ˌstā-təs, 'ser-, -ˌsta-\ *n* : status with respect to being seropositive or seronegative for a particular antibody ⟨HIV ∼⟩

se·ro·sur·vey \'sir-ō-ˌsər-ˌvā, 'ser-\ *n* : a test of blood serum from a group of individuals to determine seroprevalence (as of antibodies to HIV)

se·ro·ther·a·py \ˌsir-ō-'ther-ə-pē, ˌser-ō-\ *n, pl* **-pies** : the treatment of a disease with specific immune serum

se·ro·to·ner·gic \ˌsir-ə-tə-'nər-jik\ *or* **se·ro·to·nin·er·gic** \ˌsir-ə-ˌtō-nə-'nər-jik\ *adj* : liberating, activated by, or

involving serotonin in the transmission of nerve impulses

se·ro·to·nin \ˌsir-ə-'tō-nən, ˌser-\ *n* : a phenolic amine neurotransmitter $C_{10}H_{12}N_2O$ that is a powerful vasoconstrictor and is found esp. in the brain, blood serum, and gastric mucous membrane of mammals — called also *5-HT, 5-hydroxytryptamine*

¹se·ro·type \'sir-ə-ˌtīp, 'ser-\ *n* **1** : a group of intimately related microorganisms distinguished by a common set of antigens **2** : the set of antigens characteristic of a serotype — **se·ro·typ·ic** \ˌsir-ə-'ti-pik\ *adj*

²serotype *vb* **-typed; -typ·ing** : to determine the serotype of ⟨∼ streptococci⟩

se·rous \'sir-əs\ *adj* : of, relating to, producing, or resembling serum; *esp* : having a thin watery constitution

serous cavity *n* : a cavity (as the peritoneal cavity, pleural cavity, or pericardial cavity) that is lined with a serous membrane

serous cell *n* : a cell (as of the parotid gland) that secretes a serous fluid

serous gland *n* : a gland secreting a serous fluid

serous membrane *n* : any of various thin membranes (as the peritoneum, pericardium, or pleurae) that consist of a single layer of thin flat mesothelial cells resting on a connective-tissue stroma, secrete a serous fluid, and usu. line bodily cavities or enclose the organs contained in such cavities — compare MUCOUS MEMBRANE

serous otitis media *n* : a form of otitis media that is characterized by the accumulation of serous exudate in the middle ear and that typically results from an unresolved attack of acute otitis media — called also *secretory otitis media*

ser·o·var \'sir-ə-ˌvär, 'ser-, -ˌvar\ *n* : SEROTYPE 1

Ser·pa·sil \'sər-pə-ˌsil\ *n* : a preparation of reserpine — formerly a U.S. registered trademark

ser·pig·i·nous \(ˌ)sər-'pi-jə-nəs\ *adj* : slowly spreading; *esp* : healing over in one portion while continuing to advance in another ⟨∼ ulcer⟩

ser·pin \'sir-pən, 'ser-\ *n* [*serine proteinase inhibitor*] : any of a group of structurally related proteins (as antithrombin and antitrypsin) that are typically inhibitors of proteases having serine as the main functional group and that include some (as angiotensinogen) which have lost their inhibitory action

serrata — see ORA SERRATA

ser·rat·ed \sə-'rā-təd, 'ser-ˌā-\ *or* **ser·rate** \'ser-ˌāt, sə-'rāt\ *adj* : notched or toothed on the edge

Ser·ra·tia \se-'rā-shə, -shē-ə\ *n* : a genus of aerobic saprophytic flagellated rod-shaped bacteria (family Enterobacteriaceae) including one (*S.*

marcescens) associated with some human opportunistic infections

Ser·ra·ti \se-ˈrä-tē\, **Serafino**, Italian boatman.

ser·ra·tus \se-ˈrä-təs\ *n, pl* **ser·ra·ti** \-ˈrä-ˌtī\ : any of three muscles of the thorax that have complex origins but arise chiefly from the ribs or vertebrae: **a** : SERRATUS ANTERIOR **b** : SERRATUS POSTERIOR INFERIOR **c** : SERRATUS POSTERIOR SUPERIOR

serratus anterior *n* : a thin muscular sheet of the thorax that arises from the first eight or nine ribs and from the intercostal muscles between them, is inserted into the ventral side of the medial margin of the scapula, and acts to stabilize the scapula by holding it against the chest wall and to rotate it in raising the arm

serratus posterior inferior *n* : a thin quadrilateral muscle at the junction of the thoracic and lumbar regions that arises chiefly from the spinous processes of the lowest two thoracic and first two or three lumbar vertebrae, is inserted into the lowest four ribs, and acts to counteract the pull of the diaphragm on the ribs to which it is attached

serratus posterior superior *n* : a thin quadrilateral muscle of the upper and dorsal part of the thorax that arises chiefly from the spinous processes of the lowest two cervical and the first two or three thoracic vertebrae, is inserted into the second to fifth ribs, and acts to elevate the upper ribs

Ser·to·li cell \ˈsər-tə-lē-, ser-ˈtō-lē-\ *also* **Ser·to·li's cell** \-lēz-\ *n* : any of the elongated striated cells in the seminiferous tubules of the testis to which the spermatids become attached and from which they apparently derive nourishment

Sertoli, Enrico (1842–1910), Italian physiologist.

ser·tra·line \ˈsər-trə-ˌlēn\ *n* : a drug that functions as an SSRI and is administered orally in the form of its hydrochloride $C_{17}H_{17}NCl_2 \cdot HCl$ used to treat depression, anxiety, panic disorder, and obsessive-compulsive disorder — see ZOLOFT

¹**se·rum** \ˈsir-əm\ *n, pl* **se·ra** \-ə\ *or* **serums** : the watery portion of an animal fluid remaining after coagulation: **a** (1) : the clear yellowish fluid that remains from blood plasma after fibrinogen, prothrombin, and other clotting factors have been removed by clot formation — called also *blood serum* (2) : ANTISERUM **b** : a normal or pathological serous fluid (as in a blister)

²**serum** *adj* : occurring or found in the serum of the blood ⟨a ∼ cholesterol⟩

serum albumin *n* : a crystallizable albumin or mixture of albumins that normally constitutes more than half of the protein in blood serum, serves to maintain the osmotic pressure of the blood, and is used in transfusions esp. for the treatment of shock

serum globulin *n* : a globulin or mixture of globulins occurring in blood serum and containing most of the antibodies of the blood

serum hepatitis *n* : HEPATITIS B

serum sickness *n* : an allergic reaction to the injection of foreign serum manifested by hives, swelling, eruption, arthritis, and fever

ser·vice \ˈsər-vis\ *n* : a branch of a hospital medical staff devoted to a particular specialty ⟨pediatric ∼⟩

service mark *n* : a mark or device used to identify a service (as transportation or insurance) offered to customers — compare TRADEMARK

se·ryl \ˈsir-əl, ˈser-\ *n* : the amino acid radical or residue $HOCH_2CH$- $(NH_2)CO$- of serine — abbr. *Ser*

¹**ses·a·moid** \ˈse-sə-ˌmȯid\ *adj* : of, relating to, or being a nodular mass of bone or cartilage in a tendon esp. at a joint or bony prominence

²**sesamoid** *n* : a sesamoid bone (as the patella) or cartilage

ses·a·moid·itis \ˌse-sə-ˌmȯi-ˈdī-təs\ *n* : inflammation of the navicular bone and adjacent structures in the horse

ses·sile \ˈse-sil, -ˌsīl\ *adj* **1** : attached directly by a broad base : not pedunculated ⟨a ∼ tumor⟩ **2** : firmly attached : not free to move about

¹**set** \ˈset\ *vb* **set; set·ting** : to restore to normal position or connection when dislocated or fractured ⟨∼ a broken bone⟩

²**set** *n* : a state of psychological preparedness usu. of limited duration for action in response to an anticipated stimulus or situation

Se·tar·ia \se-ˈtar-ē-ə\ *n* : a genus of filarial worms parasitic as adults in the body cavity of various ungulate mammals (as cattle and deer)

se·ton \ˈsēt-ᵊn\ *n* : one or more threads or horsehairs or a strip of linen introduced beneath the skin by a knife or needle to provide drainage

set·tle \ˈset-ᵊl\ *vb* **set·tled; set·tling** *of an animal* **1** : IMPREGNATE 1a **2** : CONCEIVE

seventh cranial nerve *n* : FACIAL NERVE

seventh nerve *n* : FACIAL NERVE

severe acute respiratory syndrome *n* : SARS

severe combined immunodeficiency *n* : a rare congenital disorder of the immune system that is characterized by inability to produce a normal complement of antibodies and T cells and that results usu. in early death — abbr. *SCID;* called also *severe combined immune deficiency, severe combined immunodeficiency disease;* see ADENOSINE DEAMINASE

¹**sex** \ˈseks\ *n* **1** : either of the two major forms of individuals that occur in many species and that are distinguished respectively as male or fe-

male   **2** : the sum of the structural, functional, and behavioral characteristics of living things that are involved in reproduction by two interacting parents and that distinguish males and females   **3 a** : sexually motivated phenomena or behavior   **b** : SEXUAL INTERCOURSE

²sex *vb* : to identify the sex of

sex cell *n* : GAMETE; *also* : its cellular precursor

sex chromatin *n* : BARR BODY

sex chromosome *n* : a chromosome (as the X chromosome or the Y chromosome in humans) that is directly concerned with the inheritance of sex and that contains the genes governing the inheritance of various sex-linked and sex-limited characters

sex gland *n* : GONAD

sex hormone *n* : a steroid hormone (as estradiol, progesterone, androstenedione, or testosterone) that is produced esp. by the ovaries, testes, or adrenal cortex and that exerts estrogenic, progestational, or androgenic activity on the growth or function of the reproductive organs or the development of secondary sex characteristics

sex-limited *adj* : expressed in the phenotype of only one sex ⟨∼ traits⟩

sex-linked *adj*   **1** : located in a sex chromosome ⟨a ∼ gene⟩   **2** : mediated by a sex-linked gene ⟨a ∼ character⟩ — **sex-linkage** *n*

sex object *n* : a person regarded esp. exclusively as an object of sexual interest

sex·ol·o·gy \sek-ˈsä-lə-jē\ *n, pl* **-gies** : the study of sex or of the interaction of the sexes esp. among human beings — **sex·ol·o·gist** \-jist\ *n*

sex ratio *n* : the proportion of males to females in a population esp. as expressed by the number of males per hundred females

sex·tu·plet \sek-ˈstə-plət, -ˈstü-, -ˈstyü-; ˈsek-stə-\ *n*   **1** : any of six offspring born at one birth   **2** **sextuplets** *pl* : a group of six offspring born at one birth

sex·u·al \ˈsek-shə-wəl\ *adj*   **1** : of, relating to, or associated with sex or the sexes ⟨∼ differentiation⟩ ⟨∼ conflict⟩   **2** : having or involving sex ⟨∼ reproduction⟩ — **sex·u·al·ly** *adv*

sexual assault *n* : illegal sexual contact that usu. involves force upon a person without consent or is inflicted upon a person who is incapable of giving consent (as because of age or mental incapacity) or who places the assailant (as a family friend) in a position of trust or authority

sexual intercourse *n*   **1** : heterosexual intercourse involving penetration of the vagina by the penis : COITUS   **2** : intercourse (as anal or oral intercourse) that does not involve penetration of the vagina by the penis

sex·u·al·i·ty \sek-shə-ˈwa-lə-tē\ *n, pl*

-ties : the quality or state of being sexual: **a** : the condition of having sex   **b** : sexual activity   **c** : expression of sexual receptivity or interest esp. when excessive

sexually transmitted disease *n* : any of various diseases or infections that can be transmitted by direct sexual contact including some (as syphilis, gonorrhea, chlamydia, and genital herpes) chiefly spread by sexual means and others (as hepatitis B and AIDS) often contracted by nonsexual means — called also *STD*

sexual orientation *n* : the inclination of an individual with respect to heterosexual, homosexual, and bisexual behavior — called also *sexual preference*

sexual relations *n pl* : COITUS

Se·za·ry syndrome \ˌsā-zä-ˈrē-\ *or* **Se·za·ry's syndrome** \-ˈrēz-\ *n* : cutaneous T-cell lymphoma characterized by exfoliative dermatitis with intense itching and by the presence in the peripheral blood and in the skin of numerous large malignant mononuclear T cells with irregularly shaped nuclei

   Sézary, Albert (1880–1956), French physician.

SFA \ˌes-ˌef-ˈā\ *n* : a saturated fatty acid

Sg *symbol* seaborgium

SGOT *abbr* serum glutamic-oxaloacetic transaminase

SGPT *abbr* serum glutamic pyruvic transaminase

SH *abbr* serum hepatitis

shad·ow \ˈsha-(ˌ)dō\ *n*   **1** : a dark outline or image on an X-ray photograph where the X-rays have been blocked by a radiopaque mass (as a tumor)   **2** : a colorless or slightly pigmented or stained body (as a degenerate cell or empty membrane) only faintly visible under the microscope

shaft \ˈshaft\ *n* : a long slender cylindrical body or part: as   **a** : the cylindrical part of a long bone between the enlarged ends   **b** : HAIR SHAFT

shaft louse *n* : a biting louse of the genus *Menopon* (*M. gallinae*) that commonly infests domestic fowls

shaken baby syndrome *n* : one or more of a group of symptoms (as limb paralysis, lethargy, seizures, or loss of consciousness) that tend to occur in an infant which has been severely shaken but that may also result from other actions (as tossing) causing internal trauma (as hemorrhage, hematoma, or contusions) esp. to the brain region, and that may ultimately result in permanent brain damage or death — called also *shaken infant syndrome*

shakes \ˈshāks\ *n sing or pl*   **1** : a condition of trembling; *specif* : DELIRIUM TREMENS   **2** : MALARIA 1

shaking palsy *n* : PARKINSON'S DISEASE

shal·low \ˈsha-(ˌ)lō\ *adj* : displacing comparatively little air ⟨∼ breathing⟩

sham \ˈsham\ *adj* : being a treatment or procedure that is performed as a control and that is similar to but omits a key therapeutic element of the treatment or procedure under investigation ⟨a ∼ injection of saline solution⟩

shank \'shaŋk\ n : the part of the leg between the knee and the ankle in humans or a corresponding part in other vertebrates

shape \'shāp\ vb **shaped; shap·ing** : to modify (behavior) by rewarding changes that tend toward a desired response

sharp \'shärp\ n : a medical instrument that is sharp or may produce sharp pieces by shattering — usu. used in pl.

Shar·pey's fiber \'shär-pēz-\ n : any of the thready processes of the periosteum that penetrate the tissue of the superficial lamellae of bones
   Sharpey,   William   (1802–1880), British anatomist and physiologist.

sheath \'shēth\ n, pl **sheaths** \'shēthz, 'shēths\ **1** : an investing cover or case of a plant or animal body or body part: as **a** : the tubular fold of skin into which the penis of many mammals is retracted **b** : the connective tissue of an organ or part that binds together its component elements and holds it in place **2** : CONDOM 1 — **sheathed** adj

sheath of Schwann \-'shwän\ n : NEURILEMMA
   T. A. H. Schwann — see SCHWANN CELL

shed \'shed\ vb **shed; shed·ding** : to give off or out: as **a** : to lose as part of a natural process ⟨∼ the milk teeth⟩ **b** : to discharge usu. gradually from the body ⟨∼ a virus in the urine⟩

Shee·han's syndrome \'shē-ənz-\ also **Shee·han syndrome** \-ən-\ n : necrosis of the pituitary gland with associated hypopituitarism resulting from postpartum hemorrhage
   Sheehan, Harold Leeming (1900–1988), British pathologist.

sheep botfly n : a dipteran fly of the genus Oestrus (O. ovis) whose larvae parasitize sheep and lodge esp. in the nasal passages and frontal sinuses

sheep ked n : a wingless bloodsucking dipteran fly of the genus Melophagus (M. ovinus) that feeds chiefly on sheep and is a vector of sheep trypanosomiasis — called also ked, sheep tick

sheep pox n : a disease of sheep that is caused by a poxvirus (species Sheeppox virus of the genus Capripoxvirus) and was formerly epizootic in warmer Old World areas

sheep tick n : SHEEP KED

shellfish poisoning — see PARALYTIC SHELLFISH POISONING

shell shock n : COMBAT FATIGUE — **shell–shocked** \'shel-,shäkt\ adj

shi·at·su also **shi·at·zu** \shē-'ät-sü\ n, often cap : acupressure esp. of a form that originated in Japan

Shi·ga bacillus \'shē-gə-\ n : a widely distributed but chiefly tropical bacterium of the genus Shigella (S. dysenteriae) that causes dysentery

Shiga, Kiyoshi (1870–1957), Japanese bacteriologist.

shi·gel·la \shi-'ge-lə\ n **1** cap : a genus of nonmotile aerobic enterobacteria that form acid but no gas on many carbohydrates and that cause dysenteries in animals and esp. humans **2** pl **-gel·lae** \-,lē\ also **-gellas** : any bacterium of the genus Shigella **3** : SHIGELLOSIS

shig·el·lo·sis \,shig-ə-'lō-səs\ n, pl **-lo·ses** \-'lō-,sēz\ : infection with or dysentery caused by bacteria of the genus Shigella

shin \'shin\ n : the front part of the leg below the knee

shin·bone \'shin-,bōn\ n : TIBIA

shin·er \'shī-nər\ n : BLACK EYE

shin·gles \'shiŋ-gəlz\ n : an acute viral inflammation of the sensory ganglia of spinal and cranial nerves associated with a vesicular eruption and neuralgic pain and caused by reactivation of the herpesvirus causing chicken pox — called also herpes zoster, zona, zoster

shin splints n sing or pl : painful injury to and inflammation of the tibial and toe extensor muscles or their fasciae that is caused by repeated minimal traumas (as by running on a hard surface)

shipping fever n : an often fatal febrile disease esp. of young cattle and sheep that occurs under highly stressful conditions (as crowding in feedlots), is marked by high fever and pneumonia, and is caused by a bacterium (esp. Mannheimia haemolytica syn. Pasteurella haemolytica) usu. in association with a virus

shiv·er \'shi-vər\ vb : to undergo trembling : experience rapid involuntary muscular twitching esp. in response to cold — **shiver** n

shivering n **1** : an act or action of one that shivers **2** : a constant abnormal twitching of various muscles in the horse that is prob. due to sensory nerve derangement

shock \'shäk\ n **1** : a sudden or violent disturbance in the mental or emotional faculties **2** : a state of profound depression of the vital processes of the body that is characterized by pallor, rapid but weak pulse, rapid and shallow respiration, reduced total blood volume, and low blood pressure and that is caused usu. by severe esp. crushing injuries, hemorrhage, burns, or major surgery **3** : sudden stimulation of the nerves or convulsive contraction of the muscles accompanied by a feeling of concussion that is caused by the discharge of electricity through the body — compare ELECTROCONVULSIVE THERAPY — **shock** vb

shock lung *n* : a condition of severe pulmonary edema associated with shock

shock therapy *n* : the treatment of mental disorder by the artificial induction of coma or convulsions through use of drugs or electric current — called also *convulsive therapy*, *shock treatment*; see ELECTROCONVULSIVE THERAPY

shoot \'shüt\ *vb* **shot** \'shät\; **shooting 1** : to give an injection to **2** : to take or administer (as a drug) by hypodermic needle

shoot·ing *adj* : characterized by sudden sharp piercing sensations ⟨~ pains⟩

short bone *n* : a bone (as of the tarsus or carpus) that is of approximately equal length in all dimensions

short bowel syndrome *n* : malabsorption from the small intestine that is marked by diarrhea, malnutrition, and steatorrhea and that results from resection of the small intestine — called also *short gut syndrome*

short ciliary nerve *n* : any of 6 to 10 delicate nerve filaments of parasympathetic, sympathetic, and general sensory function that arise in the ciliary ganglion and innervate the smooth muscles and tunics of the eye — compare LONG CILIARY NERVE

shortness of breath *n* : difficulty in drawing sufficient breath : labored breathing

short–nosed cattle louse *n* : a large bluish sucking louse of the genus *Haematopinus* (*H. eurysternus*) that attacks domestic cattle

short posterior ciliary artery *n* : any of 6 to 10 arteries that arise from the ophthalmic artery or its branches and supply the choroid and the ciliary processes — compare LONG POSTERIOR CILIARY ARTERY

short saphenous vein *n* : SAPHENOUS VEIN b

short–sight·ed \'short-'sī-təd\ *adj* : NEARSIGHTED

short–sight·ed·ness *n* : MYOPIA

short–term memory *n* : memory that involves recall of information for a relatively short time (as a few seconds) — abbr. STM

shot \'shät\ *n* : an injection of a drug, immunizing substance, nutrient, or medicament ⟨a flu ~⟩

shoul·der \'shōl-dər\ *n* **1** : the laterally projecting part of the body formed of the bones and joints with their covering tissue by which the arm is connected with the trunk **2** : the two shoulders and the upper part of the back — usu. used in pl.

shoulder blade *n* : SCAPULA

shoulder girdle *n* : PECTORAL GIRDLE

shoulder–hand syndrome *n* : reflex sympathetic dystrophy affecting the upper extremities and characterized by pain in and stiffening of the shoulder followed by swelling and stiffening of the hand and fingers

shoulder joint *n* : the ball-and-socket joint of the humerus and the scapula

shoulder separation *n* : a dislocation of the shoulder at the acromioclavicular joint

show \'shō\ *n* **1** : a discharge of mucus streaked with blood from the vagina at the onset of labor **2** : the first appearance of blood in a menstrual period

shrink \'shrink\ *n* : a clinical psychiatrist or psychologist — called also *headshrinker*

shud·der \'shə-dər\ *vb* **shud·dered; shud·der·ing** : to tremble convulsively : SHIVER — **shudder** *n*

shunt \'shənt\ *n* **1** : a passage by which a bodily fluid (as blood) is diverted from one channel, circulatory path, or part to another; *esp* : such a passage established by surgery or occurring as an abnormality ⟨an arteriovenous ~⟩ **2 a** : a surgical procedure for the establishment of an artificial shunt — see PORTACAVAL SHUNT **b** : a device (as a narrow tube) used to establish an artificial shunt — **shunt** *vb*

¹shut–in \'shət-ˌin\ *n* : a person who is confined to home, a room, or bed because of illness or incapacity

²shut–in \'shət-'in\ *adj* **1** : confined to one's home or an institution by illness or incapacity **2** : tending to avoid social contact : WITHDRAWN

Shy–Dra·ger syndrome \'shī-'drā-gər-\ *n* : multiple system atrophy in which autonomic dysfunction predominates — called also *Shy-Drager disease*

Shy, George Milton (1919–1967), and Drager, Glenn Albert (1917–1967), American neurologists.

Si *symbol* silicon

SI *abbr* [French *Système International d'Unités*] International System of Units

sial- *or* **sialo-** *comb form* : saliva ⟨*sial*olith⟩ ⟨*sialo*rrhea⟩

si·al·ad·e·ni·tis \ˌsī-ə-ˌlad-ən-'ī-təs\ *n* : inflammation of a salivary gland

si·al·a·gogue \sī-'al-ə-ˌgäg\ *n* : an agent that promotes the flow of saliva — called also *sialogogue*

si·al·ic acid \sī-'a-lik-\ *n* : any of a group of reducing amido acids that are essentially carbohydrates and are found esp. as components of blood glycoproteins and mucoproteins

si·alo·ad·e·nec·to·my \ˌsī-ə-lō-ˌad-ən-'ek-tə-mē\ *n, pl* **-mies** : surgical excision of a salivary gland

si·alo·gly·co·pro·tein \-ˌglī-kō-'prō-ˌtēn\ *n* : a glycoprotein (as of blood) having sialic acid as a component

si·al·o·gogue \sī-'a-lə-ˌgäg\ *n* : SIALAGOGUE

si·al·o·gram \sī-'a-lə-ˌgram\ *n* : a radiograph of the salivary tract made by sialography

si·a·log·ra·phy \ˌsī-ə-'lä-grə-fē\ *n, pl*

-phies : radiography of the salivary tract after injection of a radiopaque substance

si·al·o·lith \sī-'a-lə-ˌlith\ *n* : a calculus occurring in a salivary gland

si·al·o·li·thi·a·sis \ˌsī-ə-lō-li-'thī-ə-səs\ *n, pl* **-a·ses** \-ˌsēz\ : the formation or presence of a calculus or calculi in a salivary gland

si·al·or·rhea \ˌsī-ə-lə-'rē-ə\ *n* : excessive salivation

si·al·or·rhoea *chiefly Brit var of* SIALORRHEA

Si·a·mese twin \'sī-ə-ˌmēz, -ˌmēs-\ *n* : either of a pair of conjoined twins

sib \'sib\ *n* : a brother or sister considered irrespective of sex

sib·i·lant \'si-bə-lənt\ *adj* : having, containing, or producing the sound of or a sound resembling that of the *s* or *sh* in *sash* ⟨~ breathing⟩

sib·ling \'si-bliŋ\ *n* : SIB; *also* : one of two or more individuals having one common parent

sibling rivalry *n* : competition between siblings esp. for the attention, affection, and approval of their parents

si·bu·tra·mine \sə-'byü-trə-ˌmēn\ *n* : an appetite suppressant that is used orally in the form of its hydrated hydrochloride $C_{17}H_{26}ClN \cdot HCl \cdot H_2O$ in the treatment of obesity and that exerts its therapeutic effect by inhibiting the reuptake of norepinephrine, serotonin, and dopamine

sicca — *see* KERATOCONJUNCTIVITIS SICCA

sic·ca syndrome \'si-kə-\ *n* : SJÖGREN'S SYNDROME

sick \'sik\ *adj* **1 a** : affected with disease or ill health **b** : of, relating to, or intended for use in sickness **c** : affected with nausea : inclined to vomit or being in the act of vomiting **2** : mentally or emotionally unsound or disordered

sick bay *n* : a compartment in a ship used as a dispensary and hospital; *broadly* : a place for the care of the sick or injured

sick·bed \'sik-ˌbed\ *n* : the bed upon which one lies sick

sick building syndrome *n* : a set of symptoms (as headache, fatigue, eye irritation, and breathing difficulties) that typically affect workers in modern airtight office buildings, that are believed to be caused by indoor pollutants (as formaldehyde fumes, particulate matter, or microorganisms), and that tend to disappear when affected individuals leave the building — *abbr.* SBS

sick call *n* : a scheduled time at which individuals (as soldiers) may report as sick to a medical officer

sick·en \'si-kən\ *vb* : to make or become sick

sick·en·ing *adj* : causing sickness or nausea ⟨a ~ odor⟩

sick headache *n* : MIGRAINE

sick·lae·mia *chiefly Brit var of* SICKLEMIA

¹sick·le \'si-kəl\ *n* : a dental scaler with a curved 3-sided point

²sickle *adj* : of, relating to, or characteristic of sickle-cell anemia or sickle-cell trait ⟨~ hemoglobin⟩

³sickle *vb* **sick·led; sick·ling** : to change (a red blood cell) into a sickle cell

sick leave *n* **1** : an absence from work permitted because of illness **2** : the number of days per year for which an employer agrees to pay employees who are sick

sickle cell *n* **1** : an abnormal red blood cell of crescent shape **2** : a condition characterized by sickle cells : SICKLE-CELL ANEMIA, SICKLE-CELL TRAIT

sickle-cell anemia *n* : a chronic anemia that occurs in individuals (as those of African or Mediterranean descent) who are homozygous for the gene controlling hemoglobin S and that is characterized by destruction of red blood cells and by episodic blocking of blood vessels by the adherence of sickle cells to the vascular endothelium which causes the serious complications of the disease (as organ failure) — *abbr.* SCA

sickle-cell disease *n* : SICKLE-CELL ANEMIA

sickle-cell trait *n* : a usu. asymptomatic blood condition in which some red blood cells tend to sickle but usu. not enough to produce anemia and which occurs in individuals (as those of African or Mediterranean descent) who are heterozygous for the gene controlling hemoglobin S

sick·le·mia \si-'klē-mē-ə\ *n* : SICKLE-CELL TRAIT — **sick·le·mic** \-mik\ *adj*

sick·ler \'si-klər\ *n* : a person with sickle-cell trait or sickle-cell anemia

sick·ly \'si-klē\ *adj* **1** : somewhat unwell; *also* : habitually ailing **2** : produced by or associated with sickness **3** : producing or tending to produce disease **4** : tending to produce nausea

sick·ness \'sik-nəs\ *n* **1** : the condition of being ill : ill health **2** : a specific disease **3** : NAUSEA

sick·room \'sik-ˌrüm, -ˌrüm\ *n* : a room in which a person is confined by sickness

sick sinus syndrome *n* : a cardiac disorder typically characterized by alternating tachycardia and bradycardia

side \'sīd\ *n* **1** : the right or left part of the wall or trunk of the body ⟨a pain in the ~⟩ **2** : a lateral half or part of an organ or structure ⟨the right ~ of one leg⟩

side·bone \-ˌbōn\ *n* **1** *or* **sidebones** : abnormal ossification of the cartilages in the lateral posterior part of a horse's hoof (as of a forefoot) often causing lameness — used with a sing. verb **2** : one of the bony structures characteristic of sidebone

side chain *n* : a branched chain of atoms attached to the principal chain or to a ring in a molecule

side effect *n* : a secondary and usu. adverse effect (as of a drug) — called also *side reaction*

sider- *or* **sidero-** *comb form* : iron ⟨*sidero*penia⟩

sid·ero·blast \'si-də-rə-ˌblast\ *n* : an erythroblast containing cytoplasmic iron granules — **sid·ero·blas·tic** \ˌsi-də-rə-'blas-tik\ *adj*

sid·ero·cyte \'si-də-rə-ˌsīt\ *n* : an atypical red blood cell containing iron not bound in hemoglobin

sid·er·o·pe·nia \ˌsi-də-rə-'pē-nē-ə\ *n* : iron deficiency in the blood serum — **sid·ero·pe·nic** \-'pē-nik\ *adj*

sid·er·o·sis \ˌsi-də-'rō-səs\ *n, pl* **-o·ses** \-ˌsēz\ *also* **-o·sis·es** 1 : pneumoconiosis occurring in iron workers from inhalation of particles of iron 2 : deposit of iron pigment in a bodily tissue — **sid·er·ot·ic** \ˌsi-də-'rä-tik\ *adj*

side·stream \'sīd-ˌstrēm\ *adj* : relating to or being tobacco smoke that is emitted from the lit end of a cigarette or cigar — compare MAINSTREAM

side·wind·er \'sīd-ˌwīn-dər\ *n* : a small pale-colored rattlesnake of the genus *Crotalus* (*C. cerastes*) of the southwestern U.S. that moves by thrusting its body diagonally forward in a series of S-shaped curves — called also *horned rattlesnake*

SIDS *abbr* sudden infant death syndrome

sie·vert \'sē-vərt\ *n* : an SI unit for the dosage of ionizing radiation equal to 100 rems — abbr. *Sv*
    Sievert, Rolf Maximilian (1896–1966), Swedish physicist.

Sig *abbr* signa — used to introduce the signature in writing a prescription

sight \'sīt\ *n* 1 : something that is seen 2 : the process, power, or function of seeing; *specif* : the sense by which light stimuli received by the eye are interpreted by the brain in the construction of a representation of the position, shape, brightness, and usu. color of objects in space 3 a : a perception of an object by the eye b : the range of vision

sight·ed \'sī-təd\ *adj* : having sight : not blind

sight·less \'sīt-ləs\ *adj* : lacking sight : BLIND — **sight·less·ness** *n*

¹sig·moid \'sig-ˌmȯid\ *adj* 1 a : curved like the letter C b : curved in two directions like the letter S 2 : of, relating to, or being the sigmoid colon of the intestine ⟨~ lesions⟩

²sigmoid *n* : SIGMOID COLON

sigmoid artery *n* : any of several branches of the inferior mesenteric artery that supply the sigmoid colon

sigmoid colon *n* : the contracted and crooked part of the colon immediately above the rectum — called also *pelvic colon, sigmoid flexure*

sig·moid·ec·to·my \ˌsig-ˌmȯi-'dek-tə-mē\ *n, pl* **-mies** : surgical excision of part of the sigmoid colon

sigmoid flexure *n* : SIGMOID COLON

sigmoid notch *n* 1 : MANDIBULAR NOTCH 2 : TROCHLEAR NOTCH

sig·moid·o·scope \sig-'mȯi-də-ˌskōp\ *n* : an endoscope designed to be passed through the anus in order to permit inspection, diagnosis, treatment, and photography esp. of the sigmoid colon — called also *proctosigmoidoscope*

sig·moid·os·co·py \ˌsig-ˌmȯi-'däs-kə-pē\ *n, pl* **-pies** : the process of using a sigmoidoscope — called also *proctosigmoidoscopy* — **sig·moid·o·scop·ic** \-də-'skä-pik\ *adj*

sigmoid sinus *n* : a sinus on each side of the brain that is a continuation of the transverse sinus on the same side, follows an S-shaped course to the jugular foramen, and empties into the internal jugular vein

sigmoid vein *n* : any of several veins that drain the sigmoid colon and empty into the superior rectal vein

sign \'sīn\ *n* 1 : one of a set of gestures used to represent language 2 : an objective evidence of disease esp. as observed and interpreted by the physician — compare SYMPTOM

sig·na \'sig-nə\ *vb* : write on label — used to introduce the signature in writing a prescription; abbr. *S, Sig*

signal node *n* : a supraclavicular lymph node which when tumorous is often a secondary sign of gastrointestinal cancer — called also *Virchow's node*

sig·na·ture \'sig-nə-ˌchu̇r, -chər, -ˌtyu̇r, -ˌtu̇r\ *n* : the part of a medical prescription which contains the directions to the patient

sig·net ring cell \'sig-nət-\ *n* : a cell that has its nucleus shifted to one side by a large cytoplasmic vacuole and that occurs esp. in mucin-producing adenocarcinomas esp. of the stomach — called also *signet cell*

sign language *n* : a formal language employing a system of hand gestures for communication (as by the deaf) — compare FINGER SPELLING

Si·las·tic \si-'las-tik\ *trademark* — used for a soft pliable plastic

sil·den·a·fil \sil-'de-nə-ˌfil\ *n* : a drug that is used in the form of its citrate $C_{22}H_{30}N_6O_4S·C_6H_8O_7$ to treat erectile dysfunction — see VIAGRA

si·lence \'sī-ləns\ *vb* **si·lenced; si·lenc·ing** : to block the genetic expression of : SUPPRESS

si·lent \'sī-lənt\ *adj* 1 : not exhibiting the usual signs or symptoms of presence ⟨a ~ infection⟩ ⟨~ ischemia⟩ 2 : yielding no detectable response to stimulation — used esp. of an association area of the brain ⟨~ cortex⟩ 3 : having no detectable function or effect ⟨~ genes⟩ — **si·lent·ly** *adv*

silic- *or* **silico-** *comb form* 1 : relating

to or containing silicon or its compounds ⟨*silicone*⟩ **2** : silicosis and ⟨*silico*tuberculosis⟩

sil·i·ca \'si-li-kə\ *n* : the dioxide of silicon SiO_2

silica gel *n* : colloidal silica possessing many fine pores and therefore extremely adsorbent

silicate cement *n* : a dental cement used in restorations

sil·i·con \'si-li-kən, -ˌkän\ *n* : a nonmetallic element that occurs combined as the most abundant element next to oxygen in the earth's crust — symbol *Si;* see ELEMENT table

silicon dioxide *n* : SILICA

sil·i·cone \'si-lə-ˌkōn\ *n* : any of various polymeric organic silicon compounds some of which have been used as surgical implants

sil·i·co·sis \ˌsi-lə-'kō-səs\ *n, pl* **-co·ses** \-ˌsēz\ : pneumoconiosis characterized by massive fibrosis of the lungs resulting in shortness of breath and caused by prolonged inhalation of silica dusts

¹**sil·i·cot·ic** \ˌsi-lə-'kä-tik\ *adj* : relating to, caused by, or affected with silicosis ⟨~ patients⟩ ⟨~ lungs⟩

²**silicotic** *n* : an individual affected with silicosis

sil·i·co·tu·ber·cu·lo·sis \ˌsi-li-kō-tu̇-ˌbər-kyə-'lō-səs, -tyü-\ *n, pl* **-lo·ses** \-ˌsēz\ : silicosis and tuberculosis in the same lung

silk \'silk\ *n* **1** : a lustrous tough elastic fiber produced by silkworms **2** : strands of silk thread of various thicknesses used as suture material in surgery ⟨surgical ~⟩

sil·ver \'sil-vər\ *n* : a white metallic element that has the highest thermal and electric conductivity of any substance — symbol *Ag;* see ELEMENT table

silver iodide *n* : a compound AgI that darkens on exposure to light and is used in medicine as a local antiseptic

silver nitrate *n* : an irritant compound $AgNO_3$ used in medicine esp. as an antiseptic and caustic

silver protein *n* : any of several colloidal light-sensitive preparations of silver and protein used in aqueous solution on mucous membranes as antiseptics and classified by their efficacy and irritant properties: as **a** : a preparation containing 19 to 23 percent of silver — called also *mild silver protein* **b** : a more irritant preparation containing 7.5 to 8.5 percent of silver — called also *strong silver protein*

sil·y·marin \ˌsil-li-'mar-ən\ *n* : an antioxidant flavonoid $C_{25}H_{22}O_{10}$ isolated from seeds of the milk thistle that is held to protect the liver from or clear it of toxins and is used in dietary supplements and herbal remedies

si·meth·i·cone \si-'me-thi-ˌkōn\ *n* : a liquid mixture of silicone polymers used as an antiflatulent — see MYLICON

sim·i·an crease \'si-mē-ən-\ *n* : a deep crease extending across the palm that results from the fusion of the two normally occurring horizontal palmar creases and is found esp. in individuals with Down syndrome

simian immunodeficiency virus *n* : SIV

simian virus 40 \-'fȯr-tē\ *n* : a virus of the genus *Polyomavirus* (species *Simian virus 40*) that infects monkeys and has been shown experimentally to cause tumors in laboratory animals (as newborn hamsters) — called also *SV40*

Sim·monds' disease \'si-məndz-\ *n* : a disease characterized by panhypopituitarism that causes progressive emaciation, atrophy of the gonads, thyroid, and adrenal cortex, and loss of body hair and that results from atrophy or destruction of the anterior lobe of the pituitary gland

   Simmonds, Morris (1855–1925), German physician.

¹**sim·ple** \'sim-pəl\ *adj* **sim·pler; simplest** **1** : free from complexity or difficulty: as **a** : easily treated or cured **b** : controlled by a single gene ⟨~ inherited characters⟩ **2** : of, relating to, or being an epithelium in which the cells are arranged in a single layer

²**simple** *n* : a medicinal plant **2** : a vegetable drug having only one ingredient

simple fracture *n* : a bone fracture that does not form an open wound in the skin — compare COMPOUND FRACTURE

simple mastectomy *n* : TOTAL MASTECTOMY

simple ointment *n* : WHITE OINTMENT

simple sugar *n* : MONOSACCHARIDE

simplex — see EPIDERMOLYSIS BULLOSA SIMPLEX, GENITAL HERPES SIMPLEX, HERPES SIMPLEX, LICHEN SIMPLEX CHRONICUS

Sim·plex·vi·rus \'sim-ˌpleks-ˌvī-rəs\ *n* : a genus of herpesviruses that usu. infect primates and that includes two (HSV-1 and HSV-2) which are specific for humans and tend to persist in the human host as latent infections in neurons

sim·u·late \'sim-yə-ˌlāt\ *vb* **-lat·ed; -lat·ing** : to have or produce a symptomatic resemblance to — **sim·u·la·tion** \ˌsim-yə-'lā-shən\ *n*

Si·mu·li·um \si-'myü-lē-əm\ *n* : a genus of dark-colored bloodsucking dipteran flies (family Simuliidae) of which some are vectors of onchocerciasis or of protozoan diseases of birds — see BLACKFLY

sim·va·stat·in \'sim-və-ˌsta-t³n\ *n* : a statin $C_{25}H_{38}O_5$ that inhibits the synthesis of cholesterol and is used orally to treat hypercholesterolemia — see VYTORIN, ZOCOR

si·nal \'sī-n³l\ *adj* : of, relating to, or coming from a sinus ⟨a ~ discharge⟩

Sind·bis virus \'sind-bis-\ *n* : a togavirus of the genus *Alphavirus* (species *Sindbis virus*) transmitted by mosquitoes and causing a febrile disease marked by joint pain, a rash, and malaise in parts of Africa, the Middle East, Europe, Asia, and Australia

Sin·e·met \'si-nə-ˌmet\ *trademark* — used for a preparation containing carbidopa and L-dopa

Sin·e·quan \'si-nə-ˌkwan\ *trademark* — used for a preparation of the hydrochloride of doxepin

sin·ew \'sin-yü\ *n* : TENDON

single–blind *adj* : of, relating to, or being an experimental procedure in which the experimenters but not the subjects know the makeup of the test and control groups during the actual course of the experiments — compare DOUBLE-BLIND, OPEN-LABEL

single bond *n* : a chemical bond in which one pair of electrons is shared by two atoms in a molecule and which is usu. represented in chemical formulas by a single line

single nucleotide polymorphism *n* : SNP

single photon absorptiometry *n* : a scanning technique using photons of a single energy to measure the density of a material and esp. bone

single photon emission computed tomography *n* : a medical imaging technique that is used esp. for mapping brain function and that is similar to positron-emission tomography in using the photons emitted by the agency of a radioactive tracer to create an image but that differs in being able to detect only a single photon for each nuclear disintegration and in generating a lower-quality image — abbr. *SPECT*

sin·gle·ton \'sin-gəl-tən\ *n* : an offspring born singly

Sin·gu·lair \ˌsin-gyə-'ler\ *trademark* — used for a preparation of the sodium salt of montelukast

¹**si·nis·tral** \'si-nəs-trəl, sə-'nis-\ *adj* : of, relating to, or inclined to the left; *esp* : LEFT-HANDED

²**sinistral** *n* : a person exhibiting dominance of the left hand and eye : a left-handed person

sin·is·tral·i·ty \ˌsi-nə-'stra-lə-tē\ *n, pl* **-ties** : the quality or state of having the left side or one or more of its parts (as the hand or eye) different from and usu. more efficient than the right or its corresponding parts; *also* : LEFT-HANDEDNESS

sino- *also* **sinu-** *comb form* : relating to a sinus or sinuses *or* ⟨*sino*atrial node⟩

si·no·atri·al \ˌsī-nō-'ā-trē-əl\ *or* **si·nu·atri·al** \ˌsī-n(y)ü-\ *adj* : of, involving, or being the sinoatrial node

sinoatrial node *n* : a small mass of tissue that is made up of Purkinje fibers, ganglion cells, and nerve fibers, that is embedded in the musculature of the right atrium, and that originates the impulses stimulating the heartbeat — called also *S-A node, sinus node*

si·no·au·ric·u·lar \-ò-'ri-kyə-lər\ *adj* : SINOATRIAL

si·no·pul·mo·nary \ˌsī-nō-'pùl-mə-ˌner-ē, -'pəl-\ *adj* : of, relating to, involving, or affecting the paranasal sinuses and the airway of the lungs

sin·se·mil·la \ˌsin-sə-'mē-lə, -'mi-, -yə, -lyə\ *n* : highly potent marijuana from female plants having a high resin content; *also* : a female hemp plant grown to produce sinsemilla

si·nus \'sī-nəs\ *n* : a cavity or hollow in the body: as **a** : a narrow elongated tract extending from a focus of suppuration and serving for the discharge of pus ⟨a tuberculous ∼⟩ **b** (1) : a cavity in the substance of a bone of the skull that usu. communicates with the nostrils and contains air (2) : a channel for venous blood (3) : a dilatation in a bodily canal or vessel

sinus bradycardia *n* : abnormally slow sinus rhythm; *specif* : sinus rhythm at a rate lower than 60 beats per minute

si·nus·itis \ˌsī-nə-'sī-təs, -nyə-\ *n* : inflammation of a sinus of the skull

sinus node *n* : SINOATRIAL NODE

sinus of the dura mater *n* : any of numerous venous channels (as the sagittal sinuses) that are situated between the two layers of the dura mater and drain blood from the brain and the bones forming the cranium and empty it into the internal jugular vein — called also *dural sinus*

sinus of Val·sal·va \-väl-'säl-və\ *n* : any one of the pouches of the aorta and pulmonary artery which are located behind the flaps of the semilunar valves and into which the blood in its regurgitation toward the heart enters and thereby closes the valves — called also *aortic sinus*

Valsalva, Antonio Maria (1666–1723), Italian anatomist.

si·nu·soid \'sī-nə-ˌsòid, -nyə-\ *n* : a minute endothelium-lined space or passage for blood in the tissues of an organ (as the liver) — **si·nu·soi·dal** \ˌsī-nə-'sòid-ᵊl, -nyə-\ *adj* — **si·nu·soi·dal·ly** *adv*

si·nus·ot·o·my \ˌsī-nə-'sä-tə-mē, -nyə-\ *n, pl* **-mies** : surgical incision into a sinus of the skull

sinus rhythm *n* : the rhythm of the heart produced by impulses from the sinoatrial node

sinus tachycardia *n* : abnormally rapid sinus rhythm; *specif* : sinus rhythm at a rate greater than 100 beats per minute

si·nus ve·no·sus \ˌsī-nəs-vi-'nō-səs\ *n* : an enlarged pouch that adjoins the heart, is formed by the union of the large systemic veins, and is the passage through which venous blood enters the embryonic heart

sinus venosus scle·rae \-'sklē-rē\ *n* : CANAL OF SCHLEMM

si·pho·no·phore \sī-ˈfä-nə-ˌfōr, ˈsī-fə-nə-\ n : any of an order (Siphonophora) of compound free-swimming or floating oceanic coelenterates — see PORTUGUESE MAN-OF-WAR

si·re·no·me·lia \ˌsī-rə-nō-ˈmē-lē-ə\ n : a congenital malformation in which the lower limbs are fused

SIRS abbr systemic inflammatory response syndrome

sirup var of SYRUP

sis·ter \ˈsis-tər\ n, chiefly Brit : a head nurse in a hospital ward or clinic; broadly : NURSE

sister chromatid n : any of the chromatids formed by replication of one chromosome during interphase of the cell cycle esp. while they are still joined by a centromere

Sis·tru·rus \si-ˈstrür-əs\ n : a genus of small rattlesnakes having the top of the head covered with scales

site \ˈsīt\ n : the place, scene, or point of something — see ACTIVE SITE

si·to·sta·nol \ˌsī-tō-ˈsta-nᵒl\ n : a plant sterol $C_{29}H_{52}O$ that is derived from sitosterol and has been shown to reduce serum cholesterol by inhibiting cholesterol absorption

si·tos·ter·ol \sī-ˈtäs-tə-ˌrȯl, sə-, -ˌrōl\ n : any of several sterols that occur widely in plant products (as wheat germ) and are used in the synthesis of steroid hormones; esp : BETA-SITOSTEROL

situ — see IN SITU

sit·u·a·tion·al \ˌsi-chə-ˈwā-shə-nəl\ adj : of, relating to, or occurring in a particular set of circumstances ⟨∼ impotence⟩ ⟨∼ hypertension⟩

si·tus \ˈsī-təs\ n : the place where something exists or originates : SITE

situs in·ver·sus \-in-ˈv�érater-səs\ n : a congenital abnormality characterized by lateral transposition of the viscera (as of the heart or the liver)

sitz bath \ˈsits-\ n 1 : a tub in which one bathes in a sitting posture 2 : a bath in which the hips and buttocks are immersed in hot water for the therapeutic effect of moist heat in the perineal and anal regions

SIV \ˌes-ˌī-ˈvē\ n : a retrovirus of the genus Lentivirus (species Simian immunodeficiency virus) that causes a disease in monkeys similar to AIDS and that is closely related to HIV-2 of humans — called also simian immunodeficiency virus

six–o–six or **606** \ˌsiks-ˌō-ˈsiks\ n : ARSPHENAMINE

sixth cranial nerve n : ABDUCENS NERVE

six–year molar n : one of the first permanent molar teeth of which there are four including one on each side of the upper and lower jaws and which erupt at about six years of age — called also sixth-year molar; compare TWELVE-YEAR MOLAR

Sjö·gren's syndrome \ˈshȫ-ˌgrenz-\ also **Sjögren syndrome** \-ˌgren-\ n : a chronic inflammatory autoimmune disease that affects esp. older women, that is characterized by dryness of mucous membranes esp. of the eyes and mouth and by infiltration of the affected tissues by lymphocytes, and that is often associated with rheumatoid arthritis — called also sicca syndrome, Sjögren's, Sjögren's disease

    Sjögren, Henrik Samuel Conrad (1899–1986), Swedish ophthalmologist.

skelet- or **skeleto-** comb form 1 : skeleton ⟨skeletal⟩ 2 : skeletal and ⟨skeletomuscular⟩

skel·e·tal \ˈske-lət-ᵒl\ adj : of, relating to, forming, attached to, or resembling a skeleton ⟨∼ structures⟩

skeletal muscle n : striated muscle that is usu. attached to the skeleton and is usu. under voluntary control

skel·e·to·mus·cu·lar \ˌske-lə-tō-ˈməs-kyə-lər\ adj : constituting, belonging to, or dependent upon the skeleton and the muscles that move it

skel·e·ton \ˈske-lət-ᵒn\ n : a usu. rigid supportive or protective structure or framework of an organism; esp : the bony or more or less cartilaginous framework supporting the soft tissues and protecting the internal organs of a vertebrate

Skene's gland \ˈskēnz-\ n : PARAURETHRAL GLAND

    Skene, Alexander Johnston Chalmers (1838–1900), American gynecologist.

skia·gram \ˈskī-ə-ˌgram\ n : RADIOGRAPH

skia·graph \-ˌgraf\ n : RADIOGRAPH

skilled nursing facility n : a health-care institution that meets specific federal criteria (as the supervision of the care of every patient by a physician and the employment full-time of at least one registered nurse) for Medicaid and Medicare reimbursement for nursing care

skim milk n : milk from which the cream has been taken — called also skimmed milk

¹**skin** \ˈskin\ n : the 2-layered covering of the body consisting of an outer ectodermal epidermis that is more or less cornified and penetrated by the openings of sweat and sebaceous glands and an inner mesodermal dermis that is composed largely of connective tissue and is richly supplied with blood vessels and nerves

²**skin** vb **skinned; skin·ning** : to cut or scrape the skin of ⟨skinned his knee⟩

skin·fold \ˈskin-ˌfōld\ n, often attrib : a fold of skin formed by pinching or compressing the skin and subcutaneous layers esp. in order to estimate the amount of body fat

skinfold caliper n : a pair of calipers used to form and measure the thickness of skinfolds in order to estimate the amount of body fat — usu. used in pl.

skin graft *n* : a piece of skin that is taken from a donor area to replace skin in a defective or denuded area (as one that has been burned); *also* : the procedure by which such a piece of skin is removed and transferred to a new area

skinned \'skind\ *adj* : having skin esp. of a specified kind — usu. used in combination ⟨dark-*skinned*⟩

Skin·ner box \'ski-nər-ˌbäks\ *n* : a laboratory apparatus in which an animal is caged for experiments in operant conditioning and which typically contains a lever that must be pressed by the animal to gain reward or avoid punishment

    Skinner, Burrhus Frederic (1904–1990), American psychologist.

Skin·ner·ian \ski-'nir-ē-ən, -'ner-\ *adj* : of, relating to, or suggestive of the behavioristic theories of B. F. Skinner

skin patch *n* : PATCH 1b

skin tag \-ˌtag\ *n* : a small soft pendulous growth on the skin esp. around the eyes or on the neck, armpits, or groin — called also *acrochordon*

skin test *n* : a test (as a scratch test or a tuberculin test) for an allergic or immune response to a substance that is performed by administering the substance to or through the skin and is used esp. in detecting allergic hypersensitivity — **skin testing** *n*

skull \'skəl\ *n* : the skeleton of the head forming a bony case that encloses and protects the brain and chief sense organs and supports the jaws

skull·cap \'skəl-ˌkap\ *n* : the upper portion of the skull : CALVARIUM

SLE *abbr* systemic lupus erythematosus

sleep \'slēp\ *n* **1** : the natural periodic suspension of consciousness during which the powers of the body are restored — compare REM SLEEP, SLOW-WAVE SLEEP **2** : a state resembling sleep: as **a** : DEATH 1 ⟨put a pet cat to ∼⟩ **b** : a state marked by a diminution of feeling followed by tingling ⟨his foot went to ∼⟩ — **sleep** *vb* — **sleep·i·ness** \'slē-pē-nəs\ *n* — **sleepy** *adj*

sleep apnea *n* : brief periods of recurrent cessation of breathing during sleep that is caused esp. by obstruction of the airway or a disturbance in the brain's respiratory center and is associated esp. with excessive daytime sleepiness

sleeping pill *n* : a drug and esp. a barbiturate that is taken as a tablet or capsule to induce sleep — called also *sleeping tablet*

sleeping sickness *n* **1** : a serious disease that is prevalent in much of tropical Africa, is marked by fever, headache, protracted lethargy, confusion, sleep disturbances, tremors, and loss of weight, and is caused by either of two trypanosomes (*Trypanosoma brucei gambiense* and *T. b. rhodesiense*) transmitted by tsetse flies — called also *African sleeping sickness* **2** : any of various viral encephalitides or encephalomyelitides of which lethargy or somnolence is a prominent feature; *esp* : EQUINE ENCEPHALITIS

sleep·less \'slē-pləs\ *adj* : not able to sleep : INSOMNIAC — **sleep·less·ness** *n*

sleep spindle *n* : a burst of synchronous alpha waves that occurs during light sleep

sleep·walk·er \'slēp-ˌwȯ-kər\ *n* : one who is subject to somnambulism : one who walks while sleeping — called also *somnambulist* — **sleep·walk** \-ˌwȯk\ *vb*

sleepy sickness *n*, *Brit* : ENCEPHALITIS LETHARGICA

slide \'slīd\ *n* : a flat piece of glass or plastic on which an object is mounted for microscopic examination

sliding filament hypothesis *n* : a theory in physiology holding that muscle contraction occurs when the actin filaments next to the Z line at each end of a sarcomere are drawn toward each other between the thicker myosin filaments more centrally located in the sarcomere by the projecting globular heads of myosin molecules that form temporary attachments to the actin filaments — called also *sliding filament theory;* see CROSSBRIDGE

slim disease \'slim-\ *n* : AIDS; *also* : severe wasting of the body in the later stages of AIDS

sling \'sliŋ\ *n* : a hanging bandage suspended from the neck to support an arm or hand

slipped disk *n* : a protrusion of an intervertebral disk and its nucleus pulposus that produces pressure upon spinal nerves resulting in low-back pain and often sciatic pain

slipped tendon *n* : PEROSIS

slit lamp \'slit-ˌlamp\ *n* : a lamp for projecting a narrow beam of intense light that is used in conjunction with a biomicroscope for examining the anterior parts (as of the conjunctiva or cornea) of an eye; *also* : a unit consisting of both the lamp and biomicroscope

¹slough \'sləf\ *n* : dead tissue separating from living tissue; *esp* : a mass of dead tissue separating from an ulcer

²slough \'sləf\ *vb* : to separate in the form of dead tissue from living tissue

slow infection *n* : a degenerative disease caused by a slow virus

slow–reacting substance *n* : SLOW-REACTING SUBSTANCE OF ANAPHYLAXIS — abbr. *SRS*

slow–reacting substance of anaphylaxis *n* : a mixture of three leukotrienes produced in anaphylaxis that causes contraction of smooth muscle after minutes in contrast to histamine which acts in seconds and that is prob. responsible for the bronchoconstriction occurring in anaphylaxis — abbr. *SRS-A*

slow-release \ˌslō-ri-ˈlēs\ *adj* : SUSTAINED-RELEASE

slow-twitch \ˈslō-ˌtwich\ *adj* : of, relating to, or being muscle fiber that contracts slowly esp. during sustained physical activity requiring endurance — compare FAST-TWITCH

slow virus *n* : any of various infectious agents now usu. considered to be prions that have a long period between infection and the clinical appearance of a serious or fatal disease (as scrapie or Creutzfeldt-Jakob disease) associated with it

slow wave *n* : DELTA WAVE

slow-wave sleep *n* : a state of deep usu. dreamless sleep that occurs regularly during a normal period of sleep with intervening periods of REM sleep and that is characterized by delta waves and a low level of autonomic physiological activity — called also *non-REM sleep, NREM sleep, orthodox sleep, S sleep, synchronized sleep*

slug·gish \ˈslə-gish\ *adj* : markedly slow in movement, progression, or response ⟨~ healing⟩ — **slug·gish·ly** *adv* — **slug·gish·ness** *n*

Sm *symbol* samarium

small bowel *n* : SMALL INTESTINE

small calorie *n* : CALORIE 1a

small-cell lung cancer *n* : cancer of a highly malignant form that affects the lungs, tends to metastasize to other parts of the body, and is characterized by small round or oval cells which resemble oat grains and have little cytoplasm — called also *oat-cell cancer, oat-cell carcinoma, small-cell carcinoma, small-cell lung carcinoma*

small intestine *n* : the part of the intestine that lies between the stomach and colon, consists of duodenum, jejunum, and ileum, secretes digestive enzymes, and is the chief site of the absorption of digested nutrients — called also *small bowel*

small·pox \ˈsmȯl-ˌpäks\ *n* : an acute contagious febrile disease of humans that is caused by a poxvirus of the genus *Orthopoxvirus* (species *Variola virus*), is characterized by skin eruption with pustules, sloughing, and scar formation, and is believed to have been eradicated globally by widespread vaccination — called also *variola;* see VARIOLA MAJOR, VARIOLA MINOR

small saphenous vein *n* : SAPHENOUS VEIN b

smart \ˈsmärt\ *vb* : to cause or be the cause or seat of a sharp poignant pain; *also* : to feel or have such a pain

smart drug *n* : NOOTROPIC

smear \ˈsmir\ *n* : material spread on a surface (as of a microscopic slide); *also* : a preparation made by spreading material on a surface — see PAP SMEAR, VAGINAL SMEAR — **smear** *vb*

smeg·ma \ˈsmeg-mə\ *n* : the secretion of a sebaceous gland; *specif* : the cheesy sebaceous matter that collects between the glans penis and the foreskin or around the clitoris and labia minora

¹**smell** \ˈsmel\ *vb* **smelled** \ˈsmeld\ *or* **smelt** \ˈsmelt\; **smell·ing** : to perceive the odor or scent of through stimuli affecting the olfactory nerves : get the odor or scent of with the nose

²**smell** *n* **1** : the property of a thing that affects the olfactory organs : ODOR **2** : the special sense concerned with the perception of odor

smell brain *n* : RHINENCEPHALON

smelling salts *n pl* : a usu. scented aromatic preparation of ammonium carbonate and ammonia water used as a stimulant and restorative

Smith fracture \ˈsmith-\ *or* **Smith's fracture** \ˈsmiths-\ *n* : a fracture of the lower portion of the radius with forward displacement of the lower fragment — compare COLLES' FRACTURE

  Smith, Robert William (1807–1873), British surgeon.

Smith-Pe·ter·sen nail \ˈsmith-ˈpē-tər-sən-\ *n* : a metal nail used to fix the femoral head in fractures of the neck of the femur

  Smith-Petersen, Marius Nygaard (1886–1953), American orthopedic surgeon.

smog \ˈsmäg, ˈsmȯg\ *n* : a fog made heavier and darker by smoke and chemical fumes; *also* : a photochemical haze caused by the action of solar ultraviolet radiation on atmosphere polluted with hydrocarbons and oxides of nitrogen esp. from automobile exhaust

smoke \ˈsmōk\ *vb* **smoked; smok·ing** : to inhale and exhale the fumes of burning plant material and esp. tobacco; *esp* : to smoke tobacco habitually

smok·er \ˈsmō-kər\ *n* : a person who smokes habitually

smooth \ˈsmüth\ *adj* : forming or being a colony with a flat shiny surface usu. made up of organisms that form no chains or filaments, show characteristic internal changes, and tend toward marked increase in capsule formation and virulence — used of dissociated strains of bacteria; compare ROUGH

smooth muscle *n* : muscle tissue that lacks cross striations, that is made up of elongated spindle-shaped cells having a central nucleus, and that is found esp. in hollow organs and structures (as the small intestine and bladder) as thin sheets performing functions not subject to direct voluntary control — called also *nonstriated muscle, unstriated muscle;* compare CARDIAC MUSCLE, STRIATED MUSCLE

Sn *symbol* tin

snail \ˈsnāl\ *n* : any of various gastropod mollusks and esp. those having an external enclosing spiral shell including some which serve as intermediate hosts of trematodes

snail fever n : SCHISTOSOMIASIS

snake \'snāk\ n : any of numerous limbless scaled reptiles (suborder Serpentes syn. Ophidia) with a long tapering body and with salivary glands often modified to produce venom which is injected through grooved or tubular fangs

snake·bite \-ˌbīt\ n : the bite of a snake; *also* : the condition resulting from the bite of a venomous snake characterized by variable symptoms (as pain and swelling at the puncture site, blurred vision, difficulty in breathing, or internal bleeding)

snare \'snar\ n : a surgical instrument consisting usu. of a wire loop constricted by a mechanism in the handle and used for removing tissue masses (as tonsils or polyps)

sneeze \'snēz\ vb sneezed; sneez·ing : to make a sudden violent spasmodic audible expiration of breath through the nose and mouth esp. as a reflex act following irritation of the nasal mucous membrane — **sneeze** n

Snel·len chart \'sne-lən-\ n : the chart used in the Snellen test with black letters of various sizes against a white background

Snellen, Hermann (1834–1908), Dutch ophthalmologist.

Snellen test n : a test for visual acuity presenting letters of graduated sizes to determine the smallest size that can be read at a standard distance

SNF abbr skilled nursing facility

snif·fles \'sni-fəlz\ n pl 1 : a head cold marked by nasal discharge 2 : BULLNOSE — usu. used with a sing. verb

snore \'snȯr\ vb snored; snor·ing : to breathe during sleep with a rough hoarse noise due to vibration of the soft palate — **snore** n — **snor·er** n

snort \'snȯrt\ vb : to inhale (a narcotic drug in powdered form) through the nostrils ⟨~ cocaine⟩

snow \'snō\ n, slang 1 : COCAINE 2 : HEROIN

snow blindness n : inflammation and photophobia caused by exposure of the eyes to ultraviolet rays reflected from snow or ice — **snow–blind** \-ˌblīnd\ or **snow–blind·ed** \-ˌblīn-dəd\ adj

SNP \'snip\ n : a variant DNA sequence in which the purine or pyrimidine base (as cytosine) of a single nucleotide has been replaced by another such base (as thymine) — called also *single nucleotide polymorphism*

snuff \'snəf\ n : a preparation of pulverized tobacco to be inhaled through the nostrils, chewed, or placed against the gums; *also* : a preparation of a powdered drug to be inhaled through the nostrils

snuf·fles \'snə-fəlz\ n pl 1 : SNIFFLES

1 2 : a respiratory disorder (as bullnose) in animals marked esp. by catarrhal inflammation and sniffling — usu. used with a sing. verb

soak \'sōk\ n : an often hot medicated solution with which a body part is soaked usu. long or repeatedly esp. to promote healing, relieve pain, or stimulate local circulation

soap \'sōp\ n 1 : a cleansing and emulsifying agent made usu. by action of alkali on fat or fatty acids and consisting essentially of sodium or potassium salts of such acids 2 : a salt of a fatty acid and a metal

SOB abbr short of breath

so·cial \'sō-shəl\ adj 1 : tending to form cooperative and interdependent relationships with others of one's kind 2 : of or relating to human society, the interaction of the individual and the group, or the welfare of human beings as members of society ⟨immature ~ behavior⟩ — **so·cial·ly** adv

social disease n 1 : VENEREAL DISEASE 2 : a disease (as tuberculosis) whose incidence is directly related to social and economic factors

so·cial·i·za·tion \ˌsō-shə-lə-'zā-shən\ n : the process by which a human being beginning at infancy acquires the habits, beliefs, and accumulated knowledge of society through education and training for adult status — **so·cial·ize** \'sō-shə-ˌlīz\ vb

socialized medicine n : medical and hospital services for the members of a class or population administered by an organized group (as a state agency) and paid for from funds obtained usu. by assessments, philanthropy, or taxation

social psychiatry n 1 : a branch of psychiatry that deals in collaboration with related specialties (as sociology and anthropology) with the influence of social and cultural factors on the causation, course, and outcome of mental disorder 2 : the application of psychodynamic principles to the solution of social problems

social psychology n : the study of the manner in which the personality, attitudes, motivations, and behavior of the individual influence are influenced by social groups — **social psychologist** n

social recovery n : a return to effective social functioning (as following stroke, a traumatic event, or treatment for mental disorder)

social work n : any of various professional services, activities, or methods concretely concerned with the investigation, treatment, and material aid of the economically, physically, mentally, or socially disadvantaged — **social worker** n

socio- comb form 1 : society : social ⟨*socio*path⟩ 2 : social and ⟨*socio*psychological⟩

so·cio·cul·tur·al \ˌsō-sē-ō-'kəl-chə-rəl, ˌsō-shē-\ adj : of, relating to, or involving a combination of social and cultural factors — **so·ci·o·cul·tur·al·ly** *adv*

so·ci·ol·o·gy \ˌsō-sē-'ä-lə-jē, ˌsō-shē-\ *n, pl* **-gies** : the science of society, social institutions, and social relationships; *specif* : the systematic study of the development, structure, interaction, and collective behavior of organized groups of human beings — **so·cio·log·i·cal** \ˌsō-sē-ə-'lä-ji-kəl, ˌsō-shē-ə-\ *also* **so·cio·log·ic** \-jik\ *adj* — **so·cio·log·i·cal·ly** *adv* — **so·ci·ol·o·gist** \ˌsō-sē-'ä-lə-jist, -shē-\ *n*

so·cio·med·i·cal \ˌsō-sē-ō-'me-di-kəl, ˌsō-shē-\ *adj* : of or relating to the interrelations of medicine and social welfare

so·cio·path \'sō-sē-ə-ˌpath, 'sō-shē-ə-\ *n* : a sociopathic person : PSYCHOPATH

so·cio·path·ic \ˌsō-sē-ə-'pa-thik, ˌsō-shē-ə-\ *adj* : of, relating to, or characterized by antisocial behavior or an antisocial personality — **so·ci·op·a·thy** \ˌsō-sē-'ä-pə-thē, ˌsō-shē-\ *n*

so·cio·psy·cho·log·i·cal \ˌsō-sē-ō-ˌsī-kə-'lä-ji-kəl, ˌsō-shē-\ *adj* **1** : of, relating to, or involving a combination of social and psychological factors **2** : of or relating to social psychology

so·cio·sex·u·al \-'sek-shə-wəl\ *adj* : of or relating to the interpersonal aspects of sexuality

sock·et \'sä-kət\ *n* : an opening or hollow that forms a holder for something: as **a** : any of various hollows in body structures in which some other part normally lodges ⟨the bony ~ of the eye⟩ ⟨an inflamed tooth ~⟩; *esp* : the depression in a bone with which the rounded head of another bone fits in a ball-and-socket joint **b** : a cavity terminating an artificial limb into which the bodily stump fits

SOD *abbr* superoxide dismutase

so·da \'sō-də\ *n* : SODIUM CARBONATE; *also* : SODIUM BICARBONATE

soda lime *n* : a granular mixture of calcium hydroxide with sodium hydroxide or potassium hydroxide or both used to absorb moisture and acid gases and esp. carbon dioxide (as in gas masks and in oxygen therapy)

sod disease \'säd-\ *n* : VESICULAR DERMATITIS

so·di·um \'sō-dē-əm\ *n* : a silver white soft waxy ductile element — symbol *Na;* see ELEMENT table

sodium ascorbate *n* : the sodium salt $C_6H_7NaO_6$ of vitamin C

sodium benzoate *n* : a crystalline or granular salt $C_7H_5O_2Na$ used chiefly as a food preservative

sodium bicarbonate *n* : a white crystalline weakly alkaline salt $NaHCO_3$ used in medicine esp. as an antacid — called also *baking soda, bicarb, bicarbonate of soda*

sodium bromide *n* : a crystalline salt $NaBr$ having a biting saline taste that

is used in medicine as a sedative, hypnotic, and anticonvulsant

sodium caprylate *n* : the sodium salt $C_8H_{15}O_2Na$ of caprylic acid used esp. in the topical treatment of fungal infections

sodium carbonate *n* : any of several salts (as Na_2CO_3) of carbonic acid

sodium chloride *n* : SALT 1a

sodium citrate *n* : a crystalline salt $C_6H_5Na_3O_7$ used chiefly as an expectorant, a systemic and urinary alkalizer, and in combination as an anticoagulant (as in stored blood)

sodium cro·mo·gly·cate \-ˌkrō-mō-'glī-ˌkāt\ *n* : CROMOLYN SODIUM

sodium di·hy·dro·gen phosphate \-ˌdī-'hī-drə-jən-\ *n* : SODIUM PHOSPHATE 1

sodium fluoride *n* : a poisonous crystalline salt NaF that is used in trace amounts in the fluoridation of water, toothpastes, and oral rinses and as an antiseptic — see LURIDE

sodium glutamate *n* : MONOSODIUM GLUTAMATE

sodium hydroxide *n* : a white brittle solid $NaOH$ that dissolves readily in water to form a strongly alkaline and caustic solution and that is used in pharmacy as an alkalizing agent

sodium hypochlorite *n* : an unstable salt $NaOCl$ produced usu. in aqueous solution and used as a bleaching and disinfecting agent

sodium iodide *n* : a crystalline salt NaI used as an iodine supplement and expectorant

sodium io·do·hip·pu·rate \-ˌī-,ō-dō-'hi-pyə-,rāt\ *n* : HIPPURAN

sodium lactate *n* : a hygroscopic syrupy salt $C_3H_5NaO_3$ used chiefly as an antacid in medicine and as a substitute for glycerol

sodium lau·ryl sulfate \-'lȯ-ril-\ *n* : a crystalline sodium salt $C_{12}H_{25}NaO_4S$; *also* : a mixture of sulfates of sodium consisting principally of this salt and used as a detergent, wetting, and emulsifying agent (as in toothpastes, ointments, and shampoos)

sodium mor·rhu·ate \-'mȯr-ü-ˌāt\ *n* : MORRHUATE SODIUM

sodium nitrate *n* : a crystalline salt $NaNO_3$ used in curing meat — called also *saltpeter*

sodium nitrite *n* : salt $NaNO_2$ that is used as a meat preservative and in medicine as a vasodilator and an antidote for cyanide poisoning

sodium ni·tro·prus·side \-ˌnī-trō-'prə-ˌsīd\ *n* : a red crystalline salt $C_5Fe-N_6Na_2O$ administered intravenously as a vasodilator esp. in hypertensive emergencies — see NIPRIDE

sodium pentobarbital *n* : the sodium salt of pentobarbital

sodium pentobarbitone *n, Brit* : SODIUM PENTOBARBITAL

sodium per·bor·ate \-pər-'bȯr-ˌāt\ *n* : a white crystalline powder $NaBO_3$·$4H_2O$ used as an oral antiseptic

sodium phosphate n **1** : a phosphate NaH_2PO_4 of sodium containing one sodium atom per molecule that with the phosphate containing two sodium atoms per molecule constitutes the principal buffer system of the urine — called also *sodium dihydrogen phosphate* **2** : a phosphate Na_2HPO_4 of sodium containing two sodium atoms per molecule that is used in medicine as a laxative and antacid

sodium potassium tartrate n : RO-CHELLE SALT

sodium pump n **1** : a molecular mechanism by which sodium ions move across a plasma membrane by active transport; *esp* : one that is controlled by a specialized plasma membrane protein by which a high concentration of potassium ions and a low concentration of sodium ions are maintained within a cell **2** : the specialized plasma membrane protein that controls the sodium pump mechanism

sodium salicylate n : a crystalline salt $NaC_7H_5O_3$ that has a sweetish saline taste and is used chiefly as an analgesic, antipyretic, and antirheumatic

sodium secobarbital n : the sodium salt $C_{12}H_{17}N_2NaO_3$ of secobarbital

sodium stearate n : a white powdery water-soluble salt $C_{18}H_{35}NaO_2$ used esp. in glycerin suppositories, cosmetics, and some toothpastes

sodium sulfate n : a bitter salt Na_2SO_4 used in its hydrated form as a cathartic — see GLAUBER'S SALT

sodium thiosulfate n : a hygroscopic crystalline salt $Na_2O_3S_2$ used as an antidote in poisoning esp. by cyanides and as an antifungal agent

sodium valproate n : the sodium salt $C_8H_{15}NaO_2$ of valproic acid used as an anticonvulsant

so·do·ku \'sō-də-ˌkü\ n : RAT-BITE FEVER b

sod·om·ist \'sä-də-mist\ n : SODOMITE

sod·om·ite \-ˌmīt\ n : one who practices sodomy

sod·omy \'sä-də-mē\ n, pl **-om·ies** : anal or oral copulation with a member of the same or opposite sex; *also* : copulation with an animal — **sod·om·it·ic** \ˌsä-də-'mi-tik\ or **sod·om·it·i·cal** \-ti-kəl\ adj — **sod·om·ize** \'sä-də-ˌmīz\ vb

soft \'soft\ adj **1** : yielding to physical pressure **2** : deficient in or free from substances (as calcium and magnesium salts) that prevent lathering of soap ⟨~ water⟩ **3** : having relatively low energy ⟨~ X-rays⟩ **4** : BIODEGRADABLE **5** of a drug : considered less detrimental than a hard narcotic ⟨marijuana is usually regarded as a ~ drug⟩ **6** : being or based on interpretive or speculative data ⟨~ evidence⟩

soft chancre n : CHANCROID

soft contact lens n : a contact lens made of soft water-absorbing plastic that adheres closely and with minimal discomfort to the eye

soft-gel \'soft-ˌjel\ n : a pliable soft gelatin capsule containing a liquid preparation (as a medicine)

soft lens n : SOFT CONTACT LENS

soft palate n : the membranous and muscular fold suspended from the posterior margin of the hard palate and partially separating the mouth cavity from the pharynx

soft spot n : a fontanel of a fetal or young skull

sol \'säl, 'sōl\ n : a fluid colloidal system; *esp* : one in which the medium is a liquid

so·la·nine or **so·la·nin** \'sō-lə-ˌnēn, -nən\ n : a bitter poisonous crystalline alkaloid $C_{45}H_{72}NO_{15}$ from several plants (as some potatoes or tomatoes) of the nightshade family (Solanaceae)

so·la·num \sə-'lā-nəm, -'lä-, -'la-\ n **1** cap : a genus of often spiny herbs, shrubs, and trees of the nightshade family (Solanaceae) that have white, purple, or yellow flowers and a fruit that is a berry **2** : any plant of the genus *Solanum*

so·lar·i·um \sō-'lar-ē-əm, sə-\ n, pl **-ia** \-ē-ə\ also **-ums** : a room (as in a hospital) used esp. for sunbathing or therapeutic exposure to light

so·lar plex·us \'sō-lər-'plek-səs\ n **1** : CELIAC PLEXUS **2** : the part of the abdomen including the stomach and celiac plexus that is particularly vulnerable to the effects of a blow to the body wall in front of it — not used technically

soldier's heart n : NEUROCIRCULATORY ASTHENIA

sole \'sōl\ n : the undersurface of a foot

So·le·nop·sis \ˌsō-lə-'näp-səs\ n : a genus of small stinging ants including several tropical and subtropical forms (as the imported fire ants)

so·le·us \'sō-lē-əs\ n, pl **so·lei** \-lē-ˌī\ also **soleuses** : a broad flat muscle of the calf of the leg that lies deep to the gastrocnemius, arises from the back and upper part of the tibia and fibula and from a tendinous arch between them, inserts by a tendon that unites with that of the gastrocnemius to form the Achilles tendon, and acts to flex the foot

¹sol·id \'sä-ləd\ adj **1** : being without an internal cavity : not hollow ⟨~ tumors⟩ **2** : possessing or characterized by the properties of a solid

²solid n **1** : a substance that does not flow perceptibly under moderate stress and under ordinary conditions retains a definite size and shape **2** : the part of a solution or suspension that when freed from solvent or suspending medium has the qualities of a solid — usu. used in pl. ⟨milk ~s⟩

solitarius — see TRACTUS SOLITARIUS

sol·i·tary \'sä-lə-ˌter-ē\ adj : occurring singly and not as part of a group

sol·u·bil·i·ty \ˌsäl-yə-'bi-lə-tē\ n, pl

-ties 1 : the quality or state of being soluble **2** : the amount of a substance that will dissolve in a given amount of another substance

sol·u·ble \'säl-yə-bəl\ *adj* **1** : susceptible of being dissolved in or as if in a fluid **2** : capable of being emulsified

soluble RNA *n* : TRANSFER RNA

sol·ute \'säl-ˌyüt\ *n* : a dissolved substance

so·lu·tion \sə-'lü-shən\ *n* **1 a** : an act or the process by which a solid, liquid, or gaseous substance is homogeneously mixed with a liquid or sometimes a gas or solid **b** : the homogeneous mixture formed by this process **2 a** : a liquid containing a dissolved substance ⟨an aqueous ∼⟩ **b** : a liquid and usu. aqueous medicinal preparation with the solid ingredients soluble **c** : the condition of being dissolved ⟨a substance in ∼⟩

¹**sol·vent** \'säl-vənt, 'sȯl-\ *adj* : that dissolves or can dissolve ⟨∼ fluids⟩ ⟨∼ action of water⟩

²**solvent** *n* : a usu. liquid substance capable of dissolving or dispersing one or more other substances

so·ma \'sō-mə\ *n, pl* **so·ma·ta** \'sō-mə-tə\ *or* **somas 1** : the body of an organism **2** : all of an organism except the germ cells **3** : CELL BODY

som·aes·thet·ic *chiefly Brit var of* SOMESTHETIC

somat- *or* **somato-** *comb form* **1** : body ⟨*somato*sensory⟩ **2** : somatic and ⟨*somato*psychic⟩

so·mat·ic \sō-'ma-tik, sə-\ *adj* **1 a** : of, relating to, or affecting the body esp. as distinguished from the germ plasm or psyche : PHYSICAL **b** : of, relating to, supplying, or involving skeletal muscles ⟨the ∼ nervous system⟩ **2** : of or relating to the wall of the body as distinguished from the viscera : PARIETAL — **so·mat·i·cal·ly** *adv*

somatic cell *n* : any of the cells of the body that compose the tissues, organs, and parts of that individual other than the germ cells

somatic mutation *n* : a mutation occurring in a somatic cell

so·ma·ti·za·tion \ˌsō-mə-tə-'zā-shən\ *n* : conversion of a mental state (as depression or anxiety) into physical symptoms; *also* : the existence of physical bodily complaints in the absence of a known medical condition

somatization disorder *n* : a somatoform disorder characterized by multiple and recurring physical complaints for which the patient has sought medical treatment over several years without any organic or physiological basis for the symptoms being found

so·ma·to·form disorder \'sō-mə-tə-ˌfȯrm-, sə-'ma-tə-\ *n* : any of a group of psychological disorders (as body dysmorphic disorder or hypochondriasis) marked by physical complaints for which no organic or physiological explanation is found and for which

there is a strong likelihood that psychological factors are involved

so·ma·to·mam·mo·tro·pin \ˌsō-mə-tə-ˌma-mə-'trō-pᵊn, sə-ˌma-tə-\ *n* : any of several hormones (as growth hormone and prolactin) having lactogenic and somatotropic properties; *esp* : PLACENTAL LACTOGEN

so·ma·to·me·din \sō-ˌma-tə-'mēd-ᵊn, ˌsō-mə-tə-\ *n* : any of several endogenous peptides produced esp. in the liver that are dependent on and mediate growth hormone activity; *specif* : INSULIN-LIKE GROWTH FACTOR

so·ma·to·pause \sō-'ma-tə-ˌpȯz, 'sō-mə-tə-\ *n* : a gradual and progressive decrease in growth hormone secretion that occurs normally with increasing age during adult life and is associated with an increase in adipose tissue and LDL levels and a decrease in lean body mass

so·ma·to·plasm \sō-'ma-tə-ˌpla-zəm, 'sō-mət-ə-\ *n* **1** : protoplasm of somatic cells as distinguished from that of germ cells **2** : somatic cells as distinguished from germ cells

so·ma·to·pleure \sō-'ma-tə-ˌplu̇r, 'sō-mə-tə-\ *n* : a complex fold of tissue in the embryo that consists of an outer layer of mesoderm together with the ectoderm ensheathing it and that gives rise to the amnion and chorion — compare SPLANCHNOPLEURE

so·ma·to·psy·chic \ˌsō-mə-tə-'sī-kik, sō-ˌma-tə-\ *adj* : of or relating to the body and the mind

so·ma·to·sen·so·ry \sō-ˌma-tə-'sens-ə-rē, ˌsō-mə-tə-\ *adj* : of, relating to, or being sensory activity having its origin elsewhere than in the special sense organs (as eyes and ears) and conveying information about the state of the body proper and its immediate environment ⟨∼ pathways⟩

somatosensory cortex *n* : either of two regions in the postcentral gyrus that receive and process somatosensory stimuli — called also *somatosensory area*

so·ma·to·stat·in \sō-ˌma-tə-'stat-ᵊn\ *n* : a polypeptide neurohormone that is found esp. in the hypothalamus, is composed of a chain of 14 amino acid residues, and inhibits the secretion of several other hormones (as growth hormone, insulin, and gastrin)

so·ma·to·ther·a·py \ˌsō-mə-tə-'ther-ə-pē, sō-ˌma-tə-\ *n, pl* **-pies** : therapy for psychological problems that uses physiological intervention (as by drugs or surgery) to modify behavior — **so·ma·to·ther·a·peu·tic** \-ˌther-ə-'pyü-tik\ *adj*

so·ma·to·top·ic \-'tä-pik\ *adj* : of, relating to, or mediating the orderly and specific relation between particular body regions (as a hand or the face) and corresponding motor areas of the brain — **so·ma·to·top·i·cal·ly** *adv*

so·ma·to·trope \sō-'ma-tə-ˌtrōp, 'sō-mə-tə-\ *n* : SOMATOTROPH

so·ma·to·troph \-ˌtrȯf, -ˌträf\ *n* : any of various cells of the adenohypophysis of the pituitary gland that secrete growth hormone — called also *somatotrope*

so·ma·to·trop·ic \-ˈtrō-pik, -ˈträ-\ *or* **so·ma·to·tro·phic** \-ˈtrō-fik\ *adj* : promoting growth ⟨∼ activity⟩

somatotropic hormone *n* : GROWTH HORMONE

so·ma·to·tro·pin \-ˈtrō-pən\ *also* **so·ma·to·tro·phin** \-fən\ *n* : GROWTH HORMONE

-some \ˌsōm\ *n comb form* **1** : body ⟨chromo*some*⟩ **2** : chromosome ⟨mono*some*⟩

som·es·thet·ic \ˌsō-mes-ˈthe-tik\ *adj* : of, relating to, or concerned with bodily sensations ⟨the ∼ area of the brain⟩

-so·mia \ˈsō-mē-ə\ *n comb form* : condition of having (such) a body ⟨micro*somia*⟩

-som·ic \ˌsō-mik\ *adj comb form* : having or being a chromosome complement of which one or more but not all chromosomes or genomes exhibit (such) a degree of reduplication ⟨mono*somic*⟩

so·mite \ˈsō-ˌmīt\ *n* : one of the longitudinal series of segments into which the body of many animals is divided : METAMERE

somnambul- *comb form* : sleep in which motor acts are performed ⟨somnambul*ist*⟩

som·nam·bu·lant \säm-ˈnam-byə-lənt\ *adj* : walking or tending to walk while asleep

som·nam·bu·late \-ˌlāt\ *vb* **-lat·ed; -lat·ing** : to walk while asleep — **som·nam·bu·la·tion** \-ˌnam-byə-ˈlā-shən\ *n*

som·nam·bu·lism \säm-ˈnam-byə-ˌli-zəm\ *n* **1** : an abnormal condition of sleep in which motor acts (as walking) are performed **2** : actions characteristic of somnambulism — **som·nam·bu·lis·tic** \-ˌnam-byə-ˈlis-tik\ *adj*

som·nam·bu·list \säm-ˈnam-byə-list\ *n* : SLEEPWALKER

somni- *comb form* : sleep ⟨somni*facient*⟩

¹som·ni·fa·cient \ˌsäm-nə-ˈfā-shənt\ *adj* : inducing sleep : HYPNOTIC 1

²somnifacient *n* : a somnifacient agent (as a drug) : HYPNOTIC 1

som·nif·er·ous \säm-ˈni-fə-rəs\ *adj* : SOPORIFIC

som·no·lence \ˈsäm-nə-ləns\ *n* : the quality or state of being drowsy — **som·no·lent** \-lənt\ *adj*

So·mo·gyi effect \ˈsō-mō-jē-ə\ *n* : hyperglycemia following an episode of hypoglycemia; *esp* : hyperglycemia that occurs after breakfast following nocturnal hypoglycemia and that may occur in type 1 diabetes esp. when too much insulin has been taken the day before — called also *Somogyi phenomenon;* compare DAWN PHENOMENON

Somogyi, Michael (1883–1971), American biochemist.

son- *or* **sono-** *comb form* : sound ⟨sono*gram*⟩

So·na·ta \sō-ˈnä-tə\ *trademark* — used for a preparation of zaleplon

sono·gram \ˈsä-nə-ˌgram\ *n* : an image produced by ultrasound — called also *echogram, ultrasonogram*

so·nog·ra·pher \sō-ˈnä-grə-fər\ *n* : a person trained in the use of ultrasound — called also *ultrasonographer*

so·nog·ra·phy \sō-ˈnä-grə-fē\ *n, pl* **-phies** : ULTRASOUND 2 — **sono·graph·ic** \ˌsä-nə-ˈgra-fik\ *adj* — **sono·graph·i·cal·ly** \-fi-k(ə-)lē\ *adv*

so·po·rif·er·ous \ˌsä-pə-ˈri-fə-rəs, ˌsō-\ *adj* : SOPORIFIC

¹so·po·rif·ic \-ˈri-fik\ *adj* : causing or tending to cause sleep

²soporific *n* : a soporific agent (as a drug)

sorb \ˈsȯrb\ *vb* : to take up and hold by either adsorption or absorption

sor·bic acid \ˈsȯr-bik-\ *n* : a crystalline acid $C_6H_8O_2$ obtained from the unripe fruits of the mountain ash (genus *Sorbus*) or synthesized and used esp. as a fungicide and food preservative

sor·bi·nil \ˈsȯr-bə-ˌnil\ *n* : a drug $C_{11}H_{19}FN_2O_3$ that has been used experimentally in the treatment of diabetic neuropathy

sor·bi·tol \ˈsȯr-bə-ˌtȯl, -ˌtōl\ *n* : a faintly sweet alcohol $C_6H_{14}O_6$ that occurs esp. in fruits of the mountain ash (genus *Sorbus*), is made synthetically, and is used esp. as a humectant, a softener, and a sweetener and in making ascorbic acid

sor·des \ˈsȯr-(ˌ)dēz\ *n, pl* **sordes** : the crusts that collect on the teeth and lips in debilitating diseases with protracted low fever

¹sore \ˈsȯr\ *adj* **sor·er; sor·est** **1** : causing pain or distress ⟨a ∼ wound⟩ **2** : painful esp. from overuse, injury, or inflammation ⟨∼ muscles⟩ — **sore·ly** *adv* — **sore·ness** *n*

²sore *n* : a localized sore spot on the body; *esp* : one (as an ulcer) with the tissues ruptured or abraded and usu. with infection

sore mouth *n* **1** : a highly contagious disease of sheep and goats that is caused by a poxvirus (species *Orf virus* of the genus *Parapoxvirus*), occurs esp. in young animals, and is characterized by extensive vesiculation and subsequent ulceration about the lips, gums, and tongue — called also *scabby mouth* **2** : necrobacillosis affecting the mouth; *esp* : CALF DIPHTHERIA

sore·muz·zle \-\,məz-ᵊl\ *n* : BLUE-TONGUE

sore throat *n* : painful throat due to inflammation of the fauces and pharynx

SOS *abbr* [Latin *si opus sit*] if occasion require; if necessary — used in writing prescriptions

so·ta·lol \'sō-tə-\,lōl, -\,lōl\ *n* : a beta-adrenergic blocking agent administered in the form of its hydrochloride $C_{12}H_{20}N_2O_3S·HCl$ to treat ventricular arrhythmias

souf·fle \'sü-fəl\ *n* : a blowing sound heard on auscultation ⟨the uterine ∼ heard in pregnancy⟩

¹**sound** \'saúnd\ *adj* 1 : free from injury or disease : exhibiting normal health 2 : deep and undisturbed ⟨a ∼ sleep⟩ — **sound·ness** *n*

²**sound** *n* 1 : a particular auditory impression ⟨heart ∼s heard by auscultation⟩ 2 : the sensation perceived by the sense of hearing 3 : mechanical radiant energy that is transmitted by waves of pressure in a material medium (as air) and is the objective cause of hearing

³**sound** *vb* : to explore or examine (a body cavity) with a sound

⁴**sound** *n* : an elongated instrument for exploring or examining body cavities ⟨a uterine ∼⟩

sound pollution *n* : NOISE POLLUTION

sound wave *n* 1 : SOUND 1 2 *pl* : longitudinal pressure waves esp. when transmitting audible sound

sour \'saúr\ *adj* : causing, characterized by, or being the one of the four basic taste sensations that is produced chiefly by acids — compare BITTER, SALT, SWEET — **sour·ness** *n*

South American blastomycosis *n* : blastomycosis caused by a fungus of the genus *Paracoccidioides* (*P. brasiliensis* syn. *Blastomyces brasiliensis*) and characterized by formation of ulcers on the mucosal surfaces of the mouth that spread to lips, nose, and cheeks, by great enlargement of lymph nodes esp. of the throat and chest, and by involvement of the gastrointestinal tract — called also *paracoccidioidomycosis*

South·ern blot \'sə-thərn-\ *n* : a blot consisting of a sheet of a cellulose derivative or nylon that contains spots of DNA for identification by a suitable molecular probe — compare NORTHERN BLOT, WESTERN BLOT — **Southern blotting** *n*

Southern, Edwin M. (*fl* 1975), British biologist.

spa \'spä, 'spó\ *n* 1 a : a mineral spring b : a resort with mineral springs 2 : a commercial establishment (as a resort) providing facilities devoted esp. to health, fitness, weight loss, beauty, and relaxation

space maintainer *n* : a temporary orthodontic appliance used following the loss or extraction of a tooth (as a milk tooth) to prevent the shifting of

adjacent teeth into the resulting space — called also *space retainer*

space medicine *n* : a branch of medicine concerned with the physiological and biological effects on the human body of spaceflight

space perception *n* : the perception of the properties and relationships of objects in space esp. with respect to direction, size, distance, and orientation

spac·er \'spā-sər\ *n* : a region of chromosomal DNA between genes that is not transcribed into messenger RNA and is of uncertain function

space retainer *n* : SPACE MAINTAINER

space sickness *n* : sickness and esp. nausea and dizziness that occurs under the conditions of sustained spaceflight — **space·sick** \'späs-\,sik\ *adj*

Spanish flu *n* : influenza that is caused by a subtype (H1N1) of the orthomyxovirus causing influenza A and that was responsible for about 500,000 deaths in the U.S. in the influenza pandemic of 1918–1919 — called also *Spanish influenza*; compare ASIAN FLU, HONG KONG FLU

Spanish fly *n* 1 : a green beetle (*Lytta vesicatoria* of the family Meloidae) of southern Europe that is the source of cantharides 2 : CANTHARIS 2

spar·ga·no·sis \,spär-gə-'nō-səs\ *n, pl* **-no·ses** \-\,sēz\ : the condition of being infected with sparganum

spar·ga·num \'spär-gə-nəm\ *n, pl* **-na** \-nə\ *also* **-nums** : an intramuscular or subcutaneous vermiform parasite that is the larva of a tapeworm (as *Spirometra mansoni*)

Spar·ine \'spär-\,ēn\ *n* : a preparation of promazine — formerly a U.S. registered trademark

spar·te·ine \'spär-tē-ən, 'spär-\,tēn\ *n* : a liquid alkaloid used esp. formerly in medicine in the form of its hydrated sulfate $C_{15}H_{26}N_2·H_2SO_4·5H_2O$

spasm \'spa-zəm\ *n* 1 : an involuntary and abnormal contraction of muscle or muscle fibers or of a hollow organ (as the esophagus) that consists largely of involuntary muscle fibers 2 : the state or condition of a muscle or organ affected with spasms — **spas·mod·ic** \spaz-'mä-dik\ *adj* — **spas·mod·i·cal·ly** *adv*

spasmodic dysmenorrhea *n* : dysmenorrhea associated with painful contractions of the uterus

spas·mo·gen·ic \,spaz-mə-'je-nik\ *adj* : inducing spasm ⟨a ∼ drug⟩

spas·mo·lyt·ic \,spaz-mə-'li-tik\ *adj* : ANTISPASMODIC ⟨∼ drugs⟩ — **spasmolytic** *n*

spas·mo·phil·ia \,spaz-mə-'fi-lē-ə\ *n* : an abnormal tendency to convulsions, tetany, or spasms from even slight mechanical or electrical stimulation ⟨∼ associated with rickets⟩

¹**spas·tic** \'spas-tik\ *adj* 1 : of, relating to, or characterized by spasm 2 : affected with or marked by spasticity or

spastic paralysis ⟨a ∼ patient⟩ ⟨∼ hemiplegia⟩ — **spas·ti·cal·ly** *adv*

²**spastic** *n* : an individual affected with spastic paralysis

spastic cerebral palsy *n* : the most common form of cerebral palsy marked by hypertonic muscles and stiff and jerky movements

spastic colon *n* : IRRITABLE BOWEL SYNDROME

spas·tic·i·ty \spa-'sti-sə-tē\ *n, pl* **-ties** : a spastic state or condition; *esp* : muscular hypertonicity with increased tendon reflexes

spastic paralysis *n* : paralysis with tonic spasm of the affected muscles and with increased tendon reflexes

spat *past and past part of* SPIT

spa·tial \'spā-shəl\ *adj* **1** : relating to, occupying, or having the character of space ⟨∼ disorientation⟩ **2** : of or relating to facility in perceiving relations (as of objects) in space ⟨∼ ability⟩ — **spa·tial·ly** \-sh(ə-)lē\ *adv*

spatial summation *n* : sensory summation that involves stimulation of several spatially separated neurons at the same time

spat·u·la \'spa-chə-lə\ *n* : a flat thin instrument used for spreading or mixing soft substances, scooping, lifting, or scraping

spav·in \'spa-vən\ *n* : a bony enlargement of the hock of a horse associated with strain — **spav·ined** \-vənd\ *adj*

spay \'spā\ *vb* **spayed; spay·ing** : to remove the ovaries and uterus of (a female animal)

SPCA *abbr* Society for the Prevention of Cruelty to Animals

spe·cial·ist \'spe-shə-list\ *n* : a medical practitioner whose practice is limited to a particular class of patients (as children) or of diseases (as skin diseases) or of technique (as surgery); *esp* : a physician who is qualified by advanced training and certification by a specialty examining board to so limit his or her practice

Spe·cial K \'spe-shəl-'kā\ *n, slang* : the anesthetic ketamine used illicitly usu. by being inhaled in powdered form esp. for the dreamlike or hallucinogenic state it produces

special sense *n* : any of the senses of sight, hearing, equilibrium, smell, taste, or touch

spe·cial·ty \'spe-shəl-tē\ *n, pl* **-ties** : something (as a branch of medicine) in which one specializes

spe·cies \'spē-(,)shēz, -(,)sēz\ *n, pl* **species 1 a** : a category of biological classification ranking immediately below the genus or subgenus, comprising related organisms or populations potentially capable of interbreeding, and being designated by a binomial that consists of the name of the genus followed by an uncapitalized noun or adjective that is Latin or has a Latin form and agrees grammatically with the genus name **b** : an individual or kind belonging to a biological species **2** : a particular kind of atomic nucleus, atom, molecule, or ion

¹**spe·cif·ic** \spi-'si-fik\ *adj* **1 a** : restricted by nature to a particular individual, situation, relation, or effect **b** : exerting a distinctive influence (as on a body part or a disease) ⟨∼ antibodies⟩ **2** : of, relating to, or constituting a species and esp. a biological species

²**specific** *n* : a drug or remedy having a specific mitigating effect on a disease

specific epithet *n* : a noun or adjective that is Latin or has a Latin form and follows the genus name in a taxonomic binomial

specific gravity *n* : the ratio of the density of a substance to the density of some substance (as pure water) taken as a standard when both densities are obtained by weighing in air

spec·i·fic·i·ty \,spe-sə-'fi-sə-tē\ *n, pl* **-ties** : the quality or condition of being specific: as **a** : the condition of being peculiar to a particular individual or group of organisms ⟨host ∼ of a parasite⟩ **b** : the condition of participating in or catalyzing only one or a few chemical reactions ⟨enzyme ∼⟩

spec·i·men \'spe-sə-mən\ *n* **1** : an individual, item, or part typical of a group, class, or whole **2** : a portion or quantity of material for use in testing, examination, or study ⟨a urine ∼⟩

SPECT *abbr* single photon emission computed tomography

spec·ta·cles \'spek-ti-kəlz\ *n pl* : GLASSES

spec·ti·no·my·cin \,spek-tə-nō-'mīs-ᵊn\ *n* : a white crystalline broad-spectrum antibiotic derived from a bacterium of the genus *Streptomyces* (*S. spectabilis*) that is used clinically esp. in the form of its hydrated dihydrochloride $C_{14}H_{24}N_2O_7 \cdot 2HCl \cdot 5H_2O$ to treat gonorrhea — called also *actinospectacin*; see TROBICIN

spec·tral \'spek-trəl\ *adj* : of, relating to, or made by a spectrum

spec·trin \'spek-trən\ *n* : a large cytoskeletal protein that is found on the inner cell membrane of red blood cells and that functions esp. in maintaining cell shape

spec·trom·e·ter \spek-'trä-mə-tər\ *n* **1** : an instrument used for measuring wavelengths of light spectra **2** : any of various analytical instruments in which an emission (as of particles or radiation) is dispersed according to some property (as mass or energy) of the emission and the amount of dispersion is measured ⟨nuclear magnetic resonance ∼⟩ — **spec·tro·met·ric** \,spek-trə-'me-trik\ *adj* — **spec·trom·e·try** \spek-'trä-mə-trē\ *n*

spec·tro·pho·tom·e·ter \,spek-trō-fə-'tä-mə-tər\ *n* : a photometer for measuring the relative intensities of the light in different parts of a spectrum — **spec·tro·pho·to·met·ric** \-trə-ˌfō-tə-ˈme-trik\ *adj* — **spec·tro·pho·to·met·ri·cal·ly** *adv* — **spec·tro·pho·tom·e·try** \ˌspek-(ˌ)trō-fə-ˈtä-mə-trē\ *n*

spec·tro·scope \ˈspek-trə-ˌskōp\ *n* : an instrument for forming and examining optical spectra — **spec·tro·scop·ic** \ˌspek-trə-ˈskä-pik\ *adj* — **spec·tro·scop·i·cal·ly** *adv* — **spec·tros·co·pist** \spek-ˈträs-kə-pist\ *n* — **spec·tros·co·py** \spek-ˈträs-kə-pē\ *n*

spec·trum \ˈspek-trəm\ *n, pl* **spec·tra** \-trə\ *or* **spectrums** 1 : an array of the components of an emission or wave separated and arranged in the order of some varying characteristic (as wavelength, mass, or energy) 2 : a continuous sequence or range; *specif* : a range of effectiveness against pathogenic organisms — see BROAD-SPECTRUM, NARROW-SPECTRUM

spec·u·lum \ˈspe-kyə-ləm\ *n, pl* **-la** \-lə\ *also* **-lums** : any of various instruments for insertion into a body passage to facilitate visual inspection or medication ⟨a vaginal ∼⟩ ⟨a nasal ∼⟩ — **spec·u·lar** \-lər\ *adj*

speech \ˈspēch\ *n* : the communication or expression of thoughts in spoken words

speech center *n* : a brain center exerting control over speech : BROCA'S AREA

speech therapist *n* : a person specially trained in speech therapy

speech therapy *n* : therapeutic treatment of speech defects (as lisping and stuttering)

speed \ˈspēd\ *n* : METHAMPHETAMINE; *also* : a related stimulant drug and esp. an amphetamine

spell \ˈspel\ *n* : a period of bodily or mental distress or disorder ⟨a ∼ of coughing⟩ ⟨fainting ∼s⟩

sperm \ˈspərm\ *n, pl* **sperm** *or* **sperms** 1 : SEMEN 2 : a male gamete : SPERMATOZOON — **sper·mat·ic** \(ˌ)spər-ˈma-tik\ *adj*

sperm- *or* **spermo-** *or* **sperma-** *or* **spermi-** *comb form* : seed : germ : sperm ⟨*spermi*cidal⟩

spermat- *or* **spermato-** *comb form* : seed : spermatozoa ⟨*spermatid*⟩

spermatic artery — see INTERNAL SPERMATIC ARTERY

spermatic cord *n* : a cord that suspends the testis within the scrotum, contains the vas deferens and vessels and nerves of the testis, and extends from the deep inguinal ring through the inguinal canal and superficial inguinal ring downward into the scrotum

spermatic duct *n* : VAS DEFERENS

spermatic plexus *n* : a nerve plexus that receives fibers from the renal plexus and a plexus associated with the aorta and that passes with the testicular artery to the testis

spermatic vein *n* : TESTICULAR VEIN

sper·ma·tid \ˈspər-mə-tid\ *n* : one of the haploid cells that are formed by division of the secondary spermatocytes and that differentiate into spermatozoa — compare OOTID

sper·ma·to·cele \(ˌ)spər-ˈma-tə-ˌsēl\ *n* : a cystic swelling of the ducts in the epididymis or in the rete testis usu. containing spermatozoa

sper·ma·to·cide \(ˌ)spər-ˈma-tə-ˌsīd\ *n* : SPERMICIDE — **sper·ma·to·cid·al** \-ˌma-tə-ˈsīd-ᵊl\ *adj*

sper·ma·to·cyte \(ˌ)spər-ˈma-tə-ˌsīt\ *n* : a cell giving rise to sperm; *esp* : a cell that is derived from a spermatogonium and ultimately gives rise to four haploid spermatids

sper·ma·to·gen·e·sis \(ˌ)spər-ˌma-tə-ˈje-nə-səs\ *n, pl* **-e·ses** \-ˌsēz\ : the process of male gamete formation including formation of a primary spermatocyte from a spermatogonium, meiotic division of the spermatocyte, and transformation of the four resulting spermatids into spermatozoa — **sper·ma·to·gen·ic** \-ˈje-nik\ *adj*

sper·ma·to·go·ni·um \-ˈgō-nē-əm\ *n, pl* **-nia** \-nē-ə\ : a primitive male germ cell that gives rise to primary spermatocytes in spermatogenesis — **sper·ma·to·go·ni·al** \-nē-əl\ *adj*

sper·ma·tor·rhea \ˌspər-mə-tə-ˈrē-ə, (ˌ)spər-ˌma-\ *n* : abnormally frequent or excessive emission of semen without orgasm

sper·ma·tor·rhoea *chiefly Brit var of* SPERMATORRHEA

spermatozoa *pl of* SPERMATOZOON

sper·ma·to·zo·al \ˌspər-mə-tə-ˈzō-əl, (ˌ)spər-ˌma-\ *adj* : of or relating to spermatozoa

sper·ma·to·zo·an \(ˌ)spər-ˌma-tə-ˈzō-ən, ˌspər-mə-\ *n* : SPERMATOZOON — **spermatozoan** *adj*

sper·ma·to·zo·on \-ˈzō-ˌän, -ˈzō-ən\ *n, pl* **-zoa** \-ˈzō-ə\ : a motile male gamete of an animal usu. with rounded or elongate head and a long posterior flagellum

sperm cell *n* : SPERM 2

sperm duct *n* : VAS DEFERENS

spermi- *or* **spermo-** — see SPERM-

-sper·mia \ˈspər-mē-ə\ *n comb form* : condition of having or producing (such) sperm or semen ⟨a*spermia*⟩

-sper·mic \ˈspər-mik\ *adj comb form* : being the product of (such) a number of spermatozoa : resulting from (such) a multiple fertilization ⟨poly*spermic*⟩

sper·mi·cide \ˈspər-mə-ˌsīd\ *n* : a preparation or substance (as nonoxynol-9) used to kill sperm — called also *spermatocide* — **sper·mi·cid·al** \ˌspər-mə-ˈsīd-ᵊl\ *adj* — **sper·mi·cid·al·ly** *adv*

sper·mio·gen·e·sis \ˌspər-mē-ō-ˈje-nə-səs\ *n, pl* **-e·ses** \-ˌsēz\ 1 : SPERMATOGENESIS 2 : transformation of a spermatid into a spermatozoon

-sper·my \ˈspər-mē\ *n comb form, pl* **-sper·mies** : state of exhibiting or resulting from (such) a fertilization ⟨poly*spermy*⟩

SPF \ˌes-(ˌ)pē-'ef\ *n* : a number assigned to a sunscreen that is the factor by which the time required for unprotected skin to become sunburned is increased when the sunscreen is used — called also *sun protection factor*

S phase *n* : the period in the cell cycle during which DNA replication takes place — compare G₁ PHASE, G₂ PHASE, M PHASE

sphen- *or* **spheno-** *comb form* : sphenoid and ⟨*spheno*palatine⟩

sphe·no·eth·moid recess \ˌsfē-nō-'eth-ˌmȯid-\ *n* : a small space between the sphenoid bone and the superior nasal concha into which the sphenoid sinus opens

¹**sphe·noid** \'sfē-ˌnȯid\ *or* **sphe·noi·dal** \sfē-'nȯid-ᵊl\ *adj* : of, relating to, or being a compound bone of the base of the cranium formed by the fusion of several bony elements with the basisphenoid and in humans consisting of a median body from whose sides extend a pair of broad curved winglike expansions in front of which is another pair of much smaller triangular lateral processes while ventrally two large deeply cleft processes extend downward — see GREATER WING, LESSER WING

²**sphenoid** *n* : a sphenoid bone

sphenoid sinus *or* **sphenoidal sinus** *n* : either of two irregular cavities in the body of the sphenoid bone that communicate with the nasal cavities

sphe·no·man·dib·u·lar ligament \ˌsfē-nō-man-'di-byə-lər-\ *n* : a flat thin band of fibrous tissue derived from Meckel's cartilage which extends downward from the sphenoid bone to the lingula of the mandibular foramen

sphe·no·max·il·lary fissure \ˌsfē-nō-'mak-sə-ˌler-ē-, -mak-'si-lə-re-\ *n* : ORBITAL FISSURE b

¹**sphe·no·pal·a·tine** \ˌsfē-nō-'pa-lə-ˌtīn\ *adj* : of, relating to, lying in, or distributed to the vicinity of the sphenoid and palatine bones

²**sphenopalatine** *n* : a sphenopalatine part; *specif* : PTERYGOPALATINE GANGLION

sphenopalatine foramen *n* : a foramen between the sphenoidal and orbital parts of the vertical plate of the palatine bone; *also* : a deep notch between these parts that by articulation with the sphenoid bone is converted into a foramen

sphenopalatine ganglion *n* : PTERYGOPALATINE GANGLION

sphe·no·pa·ri·e·tal sinus \ˌsfē-nō-pə-'rī-ət-ᵊl-\ *n* : a venous sinus of the dura mater on each side of the cranium arising at a meningeal vein near the apex of the lesser wing of the sphenoid bone and draining into the anterior part of the cavernous sinus

spher- *or* **sphero-** *comb form* : spherical ⟨*spherocyte*⟩

sphe·ro·cyte \'sfir-ə-ˌsīt, 'sfer-\ *n* : a more or less globular red blood cell that is characteristic of some hemolytic anemias — **sphe·ro·cyt·ic** \ˌsfir-ə-'si-tik, ˌsfer-\ *adj*

sphe·ro·cy·to·sis \ˌsfir-ō-sī-'tō-səs, ˌsfer-\ *n* : the presence of spherocytes in the blood; *esp* : HEREDITARY SPHEROCYTOSIS

sphinc·ter \'sfiŋk-tər\ *n* : an annular muscle surrounding and able to contract or close a bodily opening — see ANAL SPHINCTER, CARDIAC SPHINCTER, PRECAPILLARY SPHINCTER, PYLORIC SPHINCTER — **sphinc·ter·al** \-tə-rəl\ *adj*

sphincter ani ex·ter·nus \-'ā-,nī-ik-'stər-nəs\ *n* : ANAL SPHINCTER a

sphincter ani in·ter·nus \-in-'tər-nəs\ *n* : ANAL SPHINCTER b

sphinc·ter·ic \sfiŋk-'ter-ik\ *adj* : of, relating to, or being a sphincter

sphincter of Od·di \-'ä-dē\ *n* : a complex sphincter closing the duodenal orifice of the common bile duct

Oddi, Ruggero (1864–1913), Italian physician.

sphinc·tero·plas·ty \'sfiŋk-tər-ə-ˌplas-tē\ *n, pl* **-ties** : plastic surgery of a sphincter ⟨anal ∼⟩

sphinc·ter·ot·o·my \ˌsfiŋk-tər-'ä-tə-mē\ *n, pl* **-mies** : surgical incision of a sphincter

sphincter pu·pil·lae \-pyü-'pi-lē\ *n* : a broad flat band of smooth muscle in the iris that surrounds the pupil of the eye

sphincter ure·thrae \-yù-'rē-thrē\ *n* : a muscle composed of fibers that arise from the inferior ramus of the ischium and that interdigitate with those from the opposite side of the body to form in the male a narrow ring of muscle around the urethra — called also *urethral sphincter*

sphincter va·gi·nae \-və-'jī-nē\ *n* : the bulbocavernosus of the female

sphingo- *comb form* : sphingomyelin ⟨*sphingo*sine⟩

sphin·go·lip·id \ˌsfiŋ-gō-'li-pəd\ *n* : any of a group of lipids (as sphingomyelins and cerebrosides) that yield sphingosine or one of its derivatives as one product of hydrolysis

sphin·go·lip·i·do·sis \-ˌli-pə-'dō-səs\ *n, pl* **-do·ses** \-ˌsēz\ : any of various usu. hereditary disorders (as Gaucher's disease and Tay-Sachs disease) characterized by abnormal metabolism and storage of sphingolipids

sphin·go·my·elin \ˌsfiŋ-gō-'mī-ə-lən\ *n* : any of a group of crystalline phosphatides that are obtained esp. from nerve tissue and that on hydrolysis yield a fatty acid, sphingosine, choline, and phosphoric acid

sphin·go·my·elin·ase \-'mī-ə-lə-ˌnās, -ˌnāz\ *n* : any of several enzymes that catalyze the hydrolysis of sphingomyelin and are lacking in some metabolic deficiency diseases (as Niemann-Pick disease)

sphin·go·sine \'sfiŋ-gə-ˌsēn, -sən\ *n* : an unsaturated amino alcohol $C_{18}H_{37}NO_2$ containing two hydroxyl groups and obtained by hydrolysis of various sphingomyelins, cerebrosides, and gangliosides

sphygmo- *comb form* : pulse ⟨*sphygmogram*⟩

sphyg·mo·gram \'sfig-mə-ˌgram\ *n* : a tracing made by a sphygmograph and consisting of a series of curves that correspond to the beats of the heart

sphyg·mo·graph \'sfig-mə-ˌgraf\ *n* : an instrument that records graphically the movements or character of the pulse — **sphyg·mo·graph·ic** \ˌsfig-mə-'graf-ik\ *adj*

sphyg·mo·ma·nom·e·ter \ˌsfig-mō-mə-'nä-mə-tər\ *n* : an instrument for measuring blood pressure and esp. arterial blood pressure — **sphyg·mo·mano·met·ric** \-ˌma-nə-'me-trik\ *adj* — **sphyg·mo·ma·nom·e·try** \-mə-trē\ *n*

spi·ca \'spī-kə\ *n, pl* **spi·cae** \-ˌkē\ *or* **spicas** : a bandage that is applied in successive V-shaped crossings and is used to immobilize a limb esp. at a joint; *also* : such a bandage impregnated with plaster of paris

spic·ule \'spi-(ˌ)kyül\ *n* : a minute slender pointed usu. hard body (as of bone)

spi·der \'spī-dər\ *n* **1** : any of an order (Araneae syn. Araneida) of arachnids having a body with two main divisions, four pairs of walking legs, and two or more pairs of abdominal organs for spinning threads of silk used esp. in making webs for catching prey **2** : SPIDER NEVUS ⟨an arterial ∼⟩

spider nevus *n* : a pigmented area on the skin formed of dilated capillaries or arterioles radiating from a central point like the legs of a spider — called also *spider angioma*

spider vein *n* : a telangiectasia (as on the legs or face) often appearing as a central area with outward radiations resembling the legs of a spider

Spiel·mey·er–Vogt disease \'shpēl-ˌmī-ər-'fōkt-\ *n* : BATTEN DISEASE
Spielmeyer, Walter (1879–1935), and **Vogt, Heinrich (1875–1957),** German neurologists.

spi·ge·lian hernia \spī-'jē-lē-ən-\ *n, often cap S* : a hernia occurring along the linea semilunaris
Spie·ghel \'spē-gəl\, **Adriaan van den (1578–1625),** Flemish anatomist.

spigelian lobe *n, often cap S* : CAUDATE LOBE

¹spike \'spīk\ *n* **1** : the pointed element in the wave tracing in an electroencephalogram **2** : a sharp increase in body temperature followed by a rapid fall **3** : a momentary sharp increase and fall in the record of an action potential; *also* : ACTION POTENTIAL

²spike *vb* **spiked; spik·ing** : to undergo a sudden sharp increase in (temperature or fever) usu. up to an indicated level ⟨her fever *spiked* to 103°⟩

spike potential *n* **1** : SPIKE 3 **2** : ACTION POTENTIAL

spik·ing *adj* : characterized by recurrent sharp rises in body temperature ⟨a ∼ fever⟩; *also* : resulting from a sharp rise in body temperature ⟨a ∼ temperature of 105°⟩

spin- *or* **spini-** *or* **spino-** *comb form* **1** : spinal column : spinal cord ⟨*spinotectal tract*⟩ **2** : of, relating to, or involving the spinal cord and ⟨*spinocerebellar*⟩

spi·na \'spī-nə\ *n, pl* **spi·nae** \-ˌnē\ : an anatomical spine or spinelike process

spina bi·fi·da \-'bi-fə-də, -'bī-\ *n* : a neural tube defect marked by congenital cleft of the spinal column usu. with hernial protrusion of the meninges and sometimes the spinal cord — see MENINGOCELE, MYELOCELE, MYELOMENINGOCELE

spina bifida oc·cul·ta \-ˌə-'kəl-tə\ *n* : a mild often asymptomatic form of spina bifida in which there is no hernial protrusion of the meninges of the spinal cord

spinae — see ERECTOR SPINAE

¹spi·nal \'spīn-ᵊl\ *adj* **1** : of, relating to, or situated near the spinal column **2 a** : of, relating to, or affecting the spinal cord ⟨∼ reflexes⟩ **b** : having the spinal cord functionally isolated (as by surgical section) from the brain ⟨experiments on ∼ animals⟩ **c** : used for spinal anesthesia ⟨a ∼ anesthetic⟩ **3** : made for or fitted to the spinal column ⟨a ∼ brace⟩ — **spi·nal·ly** *adv*

²spinal *n* : a spinal anesthetic

spinal accessory nerve *n* : ACCESSORY NERVE

spinal and bulbar muscular atrophy *n* : KENNEDY'S DISEASE

spinal anesthesia *n* : anesthesia produced by injection of an anesthetic into the subarachnoid space of the spine

spinal artery *n* : any of three arteries that supply the spinal cord and its membranes and adjacent structures: **a** : a single unpaired artery that is formed by the anastomosis of a branch of the vertebral artery on each side — called also *anterior spinal artery* **b** : either of two arteries of which one arises from a vertebral artery on each side below the level at which the corresponding branch of the anterior spinal artery arises — called also *posterior spinal artery*

spinal canal *n* : VERTEBRAL CANAL

spinal column *n* : the articulated series of vertebrae connected by ligaments and separated by more or less elastic intervertebral fibrocartilages that forms the supporting axis of the body and a protection for the spinal cord and that extends from the hind end of the skull through the median dorsal part of the body to the coccyx

— called also *backbone, spine, vertebral column*

spinal cord *n* : the thick longitudinal cord of nervous tissue that in vertebrates extends along the back dorsal to the bodies of the vertebrae and is enclosed in the vertebral canal formed by their neural arches, is continuous anteriorly with the medulla oblongata, gives off at intervals pairs of spinal nerves to the various parts of the trunk and limbs, serves not only as a pathway for nervous impulses to and from the brain but as a center for carrying out and coordinating many reflex actions independently of the brain, and is composed largely of white matter arranged in columns and tracts of longitudinal fibers about a large central core of gray matter — called also *medulla spinalis*

spinales *pl of* SPINALIS

spinal fluid *n* : CEREBROSPINAL FLUID

spinal fusion *n* : surgical fusion of two or more vertebrae for remedial immobilization of the spine

spinal ganglion *n* : a ganglion on the dorsal root of each spinal nerve that is one of a series of ganglia containing cell bodies of sensory neurons — called also *dorsal root ganglion*

spi·na·lis \spī-ˈnā-ləs, spi-ˈna-lis\ *n, pl* **spi·na·les** \-(ˌ)lēz\ : the most medial division of the sacrospinalis situated next to the spinal column and acting to extend it or any of the three muscles making up this division: **a** : SPINALIS THORACIS **b** : SPINALIS CERVICIS **c** : SPINALIS CAPITIS

spinalis ca·pi·tis \-ˈka-pə-təs\ *n* : a muscle that arises with, inserts with, and is intimately associated with the semispinalis capitis

spinalis cer·vi·cis \-ˈsər-və-səs\ *n* : an inconstant muscle that arises esp. from the spinous processes of the lower cervical and upper thoracic vertebrae and inserts esp. into the spinous process of the axis

spinalis tho·ra·cis \-thō-ˈrā-səs\ *n* : an upward continuation of the sacrospinalis that is situated medially and blends with the longissimus thoracis, arises from the spinous processes of the first two lumbar and last two thoracic vertebrae, and inserts into the spinous processes of the upper thoracic vertebrae

spinal meningitis *n* : inflammation of the meninges of the spinal cord; *also* : CEREBROSPINAL MENINGITIS

spinal muscular atrophy *n* : any of several inherited disorders (as Kugelberg-Welander disease) that are characterized by the degeneration of motor neurons in the spinal cord resulting in muscular weakness and atrophy and that in some forms (as Werdnig-Hoffmann disease) are fatal

spinal nerve *n* : any of the paired nerves which leave the spinal cord, supply muscles of the trunk and limbs, and connect with the nerves of the sympathetic nervous system, which arise by a short motor ventral root and a short sensory dorsal root, and of which there are 31 pairs in humans classified according to the part of the spinal cord from which they arise into 8 pairs of cervical nerves, 12 pairs of thoracic nerves, 5 pairs of lumbar nerves, 5 pairs of sacral nerves, and one pair of coccygeal nerves

spinal puncture *n* : LUMBAR PUNCTURE

spinal shock *n* : a temporary condition following transection of the spinal cord that is characterized by muscular flaccidity and loss of motor reflexes in all parts of the body below the point of transection

spinal stenosis *n* : narrowing of the lumbar spinal column that produces pressure on the nerve roots resulting in sciatica and a condition resembling intermittent claudication and that usu. occurs in middle or old age

spinal tap *n* : LUMBAR PUNCTURE

spin·dle \ˈspind-ᵊl\ *n* **1** : something shaped like a round stick or pin with tapered ends: as **a** : a network of chiefly microtubular fibers along which the chromosomes are distributed during mitosis and meiosis **b** : MUSCLE SPINDLE **2** : SLEEP SPINDLE

spindle cell *n* : a spindle-shaped cell (as in some tumors)

spindle–cell sarcoma *n* : a sarcoma (as a fibrosarcoma) composed chiefly or entirely of spindle cells

spindle fiber *n* : any of the filaments constituting a mitotic spindle

spine \ˈspīn\ *n* **1** : SPINAL COLUMN **2** : a pointed prominence or process (as on a bone)

spin echo *n* : a signal that is detected in a nuclear magnetic resonance spectrometer and is produced by a planned series of radio-frequency pulses — usu. used attributively; compare GRADIENT ECHO

spine of the scapula *n* : a projecting triangular bony process on the dorsal surface of the scapula that divides it obliquely into the area of origin of parts of the supraspinatus and infraspinatus muscles and that terminates in the acromion

spini- *or* **spino-** — see SPIN-

spinn·bar·keit \ˈspin-ˌbär-ˌkīt, ˈshpin-\ *n* : the elastic quality that is characteristic of mucus of the uterine cervix esp. shortly before ovulation

spi·no·cer·e·bel·lar \ˌspī-nō-ˌser-ə-ˈbe-lər\ *adj* : of or relating to the spinal cord and cerebellum ⟨~ pathways⟩

spinocerebellar ataxia *n* : any of a group of inherited neurodegenerative disorders that are characterized by cerebellar dysfunction manifested esp. by progressive ataxia — abbr. *SCA*

spinocerebellar tract *n* : any of four nerve tracts which pass from the spinal cord to the cerebellum and of which two are situated on each side external to the crossed corticospinal tracts: **a** : a posterior tract on each side that begins at the level of the attachments of the second or third lumbar spinal nerves and ascends to the inferior cerebellar peduncle and vermis of the cerebellum — called also *dorsal spinocerebellar tract, posterior spinocerebellar tract* **b** : an anterior tract on each side that arises from cells mostly in the dorsal horn of gray matter on the same or opposite side and passes through the medulla oblongata and pons to the superior cerebellar peduncle and vermis — called also *ventral spinocerebellar tract*

spi·no·ol·i·vary \-ˈä-lə-ˌver-ē\ *adj* : connecting the spinal cord with the olivary nuclei ⟨~ fibers⟩

spi·nose ear tick \ˈspī-ˌnōs-\ *n* : an ear tick of the genus *Otobius* (*O. megnini*) of the southwestern U.S. and Mexico that is a serious pest of cattle, horses, sheep, and goats

spinosum — see FORAMEN SPINOSUM, STRATUM SPINOSUM

spi·no·tec·tal tract \ˌspī-nō-ˈtekt-ᵊl-\ *n* : an ascending tract of nerve fibers in each lateral funiculus of white matter of the spinal cord that passes upward and terminates in the superior colliculus of the opposite side

spi·no·tha·lam·ic \ˌspī-nō-thə-ˈla-mik\ *adj* : of, relating to, comprising, or associated with the spinothalamic tracts ⟨the ~ system⟩

spinothalamic tract *n* : any of four tracts of nerve fibers of the spinal cord that are arranged in pairs with one member of a pair on each side and that ascend to the thalamus by way of the brain stem: **a** : one on each side of the anterior median fissure that carries nerve impulses relating to the sense of touch — called also *anterior spinothalamic tract, ventral spinothalamic tract* **b** : one on each lateral part of the spinal cord that carries nerve impulses relating to the senses of touch, pain, and temperature — called also *lateral spinothalamic tract*

spi·nous \ˈspī-nəs\ *adj* : slender and pointed like a spine

spinous process *n* : SPINE 2; *specif* : the median spinelike or platelike dorsal process of the neural arch of a vertebra

spiny–headed worm *n* : ACANTHOCEPHALAN

spi·ral \ˈspī-rəl\ *adj* **1 a** : winding around a center or pole and gradually receding from or approaching another **b** : HELICAL ⟨the ~ structure of DNA⟩ **2** : being a fracture in which the break is produced by twisting apart the bone — **spiral** *n* — **spi·ral·ly** *adv*

spiral ganglion *n* : a mass of bipolar cell bodies occurring in the modiolus

of the organ of Corti and giving off axons which comprise the cochlear nerve

spiralis — see LAMINA SPIRALIS

spiral lamina *n* : a twisting shelf of bone which projects from the modiolus into the canal of the cochlea — called also *lamina spiralis*

spiral ligament *n* : the thick periosteum that forms the outer wall of the cochlear duct

spiral organ *n* : ORGAN OF CORTI

spiral valve *n* : a series of crescentic folds of mucous membrane somewhat spirally arranged on the interior of the gallbladder and continuing into the cystic duct

spi·ra·my·cin \ˌspī-rə-ˈmīs-ᵊn\ *n* : a mixture of macrolide antibiotics produced by a soil bacterium of the genus *Streptomyces* (*S. ambofaciens*) and having antibacterial activity

spi·ril·lum \spī-ˈri-ləm\ *n* **1** *cap* : a genus of gram-negative bacteria having tufts of flagella at both poles and usu. living in stagnant water rich in organic matter — see RAT-BITE FEVER b **2** *pl* **-ril·la** \-ˈri-lə\ : any bacterium of the genus *Spirillum*

spir·it \ˈspir-ət\ *n* **1 a** : the liquid containing ethyl alcohol and water that is distilled from an alcoholic liquid or mash — often used in pl. **b** : a usu. volatile organic solvent (as an alcohol, ester, or hydrocarbon) **2** : an alcoholic solution of a volatile substance ⟨~ of camphor⟩

spirit of hartshorn *or* **spirits of hartshorn** \-ˈhärts-ˌhȯrn\ *n* : AMMONIA WATER

spiro- *comb form* : respiration ⟨*spirometer*⟩

Spi·ro·cer·ca \ˌspī-rō-ˈsər-kə\ *n* : a genus of red filarial worms (family Thelaziidae) forming nodules in the walls of the digestive tract and sometimes the aorta of canines esp. in warm regions

spi·ro·chaet·ae·mia, **spi·ro·chaete,** **spi·ro·chae·ti·ci·dal,** **spi·ro·chaet·osis** *chiefly Brit var of* SPIROCHETEMIA, SPIROCHETE, SPIROCHETICIDAL, SPIROCHETOSIS

spi·ro·chete \ˈspī-rə-ˌkēt\ *n* : any of an order (Spirochaetales) of slender spirally undulating bacteria including those causing syphilis, yaws, Lyme disease, and relapsing fever — **spi·ro·chet·al** \ˌspī-rə-ˈkēt-ᵊl\ *adj*

spi·ro·chet·emia \ˌspī-rə-ˌkē-ˈtē-mē-ə\ *n* : the abnormal presence of spirochetes in the circulating blood

spi·ro·che·ti·ci·dal \ˌspī-rə-ˌkē-tə-ˈsīd-ᵊl\ *adj* : destructive to spirochetes ⟨a ~ drug⟩ — **spi·ro·che·ti·cide** \ˌspī-rə-ˈkē-tə-ˌsīd\ *n*

spi·ro·chet·osis \ˌspī-rə-ˌkē-ˈtō-səs\ *n,* *pl* **-oses** \-ˌsēz\ : infection with or a disease caused by spirochetes

spi·ro·gram \ˈspī-rə-ˌgram\ *n* : a graphic record of respiratory movements traced on a revolving drum

spi·ro·graph \ˈspī-rə-ˌgraf\ *n* : an instrument for recording respiratory movements — **spi·ro·graph·ic** \ˌspī-rə-ˈgra-fik\ *adj* — **spi·rog·ra·phy** \spī-ˈrä-grə-fē\ *n*

spi·rom·e·ter \spī-ˈrä-mə-tər\ *n* : an instrument for measuring the air entering and leaving the lungs — **spi·ro·met·ric** \ˌspī-rə-ˈme-trik\ *adj* — **spi·rom·e·try** \-ˈrä-mə-trē\ *n*

Spi·rom·e·tra \spī-ˈrä-mə-trə, spi-\ *n* : a genus of pseudophyllidean tapeworms including several (as *S. mansoni* of Asia and *S. mansonoides* of the southern U.S.) which sometimes cause sparganosis in humans

spi·ro·no·lac·tone \ˌspī-rə-nō-ˈlak-ˌtōn, spi-ˌrō-nə-\ *n* : an aldosterone antagonist $C_{24}H_{32}O_4$ that promotes diuresis and sodium excretion and is used to treat essential hypertension, edema with congestive heart failure, hepatic cirrhosis with ascites, nephrotic syndrome, and idiopathic edema

¹**spit** \ˈspit\ *vb* **spit** *or* **spat** \ˈspat\; **spit·ting** : to eject (as saliva) from the mouth

²**spit** *n* : SALIVA

spitting cobra *n* : any of several cobras (as *Naja nigrocollis* and *Hemachatus haemachatus* of Africa) that in defense typically eject their venom toward the victim without striking

spit·tle \ˈspit-ᵊl\ *n* : SALIVA

splanch·nic \ˈsplaŋk-nik\ *adj* : of or relating to the viscera : VISCERAL

splanch·ni·cec·to·my \ˌsplaŋk-nə-ˈsek-tə-mē\ *n, pl* **-mies** : surgical excision of a segment of one or more splanchnic nerves to relieve hypertension

splanchnic ganglion *n* : a small ganglion on the greater splanchnic nerve that is usu. located near the eleventh or twelfth thoracic vertebra

splanchnic nerve *n* : any of three nerves situated on each side of the body and formed by the union of branches from the six or seven lower thoracic and first lumbar ganglia of the sympathetic system: **a** : a superior one ending in the celiac ganglion — called also *greater splanchnic nerve* **b** : a middle one ending in a detached ganglionic mass of the celiac ganglion — called also *lesser splanchnic nerve* **c** : an inferior one ending in the renal plexus — called also *least splanchnic nerve, lowest splanchnic nerve*

splanchno- *comb form* : viscera ⟨*splanchno*logy⟩

splanch·nol·o·gy \ˌsplaŋk-ˈnä-lə-jē\ *n, pl* **-gies** : a branch of anatomy concerned with the viscera

splanch·no·pleure \ˈsplaŋk-nə-ˌplu̇r\ *n* : a layer of tissue that consists of the inner of the two layers into which the unsegmented sheet of mesoderm splits in the embryo together with the endoderm internal to it and that forms most of the walls and substance of the visceral organs — compare SOMATOPLEURE

splay·foot \ˈsplā-ˌfu̇t, -ˈfu̇t\ *n* : a foot abnormally flattened and spread out; *specif* : FLATFOOT — **splay·foot·ed** \-ˈfu̇-təd\ *adj*

spleen \ˈsplēn\ *n* : a highly vascular ductless organ that plays a role in the final destruction of red blood cells, filtration and storage of blood, and production of lymphocytes, and that in humans is a dark purplish flattened oblong object of a soft fragile consistency lying in the upper left part of the abdominal cavity near the cardiac end of the stomach and which is divisible into a loose friable red pulp in intimate connection with the blood supply and with red blood cells free in its interstices and a denser white pulp chiefly of lymphoid tissue condensed in masses about the small arteries

splen- *or* **spleno-** *comb form* : spleen ⟨*splen*ectomy⟩ ⟨*spleno*megaly⟩

sple·nec·to·my \spli-ˈnek-tə-mē\ *n, pl* **-mies** : surgical excision of the spleen — **sple·nec·to·mize** \spli-ˈnek-tə-ˌmīz\ *vb*

splen·ic \ˈsple-nik\ *adj* : of, relating to, or located in the spleen

splenic artery *n* : the branch of the celiac artery that carries blood to the spleen and sends branches also to the pancreas and the cardiac end of the stomach

splenic fever *n* : ANTHRAX

splenic flexure *n* : the sharp bend of the colon under the spleen where the transverse colon joins the descending colon — called also *left colic flexure*

splenic flexure syndrome *n* : pain in the upper left quadrant of the abdomen that may radiate upward to the left shoulder and inner aspect of the left arm and that sometimes mimics angina pectoris but is caused by bloating and gas in the colon

splenic pulp *n* : the characteristic tissue of the spleen

splenic vein *n* : the vein that carries blood away from the spleen and that joins the superior mesenteric vein to form the portal vein — called also *lienal vein*

sple·ni·um \ˈsplē-nē-əm\ *n, pl* **-nia** \-nē-ə\ : the thick rounded fold that forms the posterior border of the corpus callosum and is continuous by its undersurface with the fornix

sple·ni·us \-nē-əs\ *n, pl* **-nii** \-nē-ˌī\ : either of two flat oblique muscles on each side of the back of the neck and upper thoracic region: **a** : SPLENIUS CAPITIS **b** : SPLENIUS CERVICIS

splenius cap·i·tis \-ˈka-pi-təs\ *n* : a flat muscle on each side of the back of the neck and the upper thoracic region that arises from the caudal half of the ligamentum nuchae and the spinous processes of the seventh cervical and the first three or four thoracic vertebrae, that is inserted into the occipital bone and the mastoid process of the temporal bone, and that rotates the head to the side on which it is located and with the help of the muscle on the opposite side extends it

sple·ni·us cer·vi·cis \-'sər-vi-kəs\ *n* : a flat narrow muscle on each side of the back of the neck and the upper thoracic region that arises from the spinous processes of the third to sixth thoracic vertebrae, is inserted into the transverse processes of the first two or three cervical vertebrae, and acts to rotate the head to the side on which it is located and with the help of the muscle on the opposite side to extend and arch the neck

spleno- — see SPLEN-

sple·no·cyte \'splē-nə-ˌsīt, 'splen-\ *n* : a macrophage of the spleen

sple·no·meg·a·ly \ˌsple-nō-'me-gə-lē\ *n, pl* **-lies** : abnormal enlargement of the spleen

sple·no·re·nal \ˌsple-nō-'rēn-ᵊl\ *adj* : of, relating to, or joining the splenic and renal veins or arteries

sple·no·sis \splē-'nō-səs\ *n, pl* **-no·ses** \-ˌsēz\ *or* **-no·sis·es** : a rare condition in which fragments of tissue from a ruptured spleen become implanted throughout the peritoneal cavity and often undergo regeneration and vascularization

splice \'splīs\ *vb* **spliced; splic·ing** : to combine or insert (as genes) by genetic engineering ⟨~ a gene into a bacterium⟩ — see GENE-SPLICING

spli·ceo·some \'splī-sē-ə-ˌsōm\ *n* : a ribonucleoprotein complex that is the site in the cell nucleus where introns are excised from precursor messenger RNA and exons are joined together to form functional messenger RNA — **spli·ceo·som·al** \ˌsplī-sē-ə-'sō-məl\ *adj*

¹splint \'splint\ *n* **1** : material or a device used to protect and immobilize a body part **2** : a bony enlargement on the upper part of the cannon bone of a horse usu. on the inside of the leg

²splint *vb* **1** : to support and immobilize (as a broken bone) with a splint **2** : to protect against pain by reducing the motion of

splin·ter \'splin-tər\ *n* : a thin piece (as of wood) split or broken off lengthwise; *esp* : such a piece embedded in the skin — **splinter** *vb*

split \'split\ *vb* **split; split·ting** : to divide or break down (a chemical compound) into constituents; *also* : to remove by such separation

split–brain \'split-ˌbrān\ *adj* : of, relating to, concerned with, or having undergone separation of the two cerebral hemispheres by surgical division of the optic chiasma and corpus callosum ⟨~ patients⟩

split personality *n* **1** : SCHIZOPHRENIA — not used technically **2** : MUL-

TIPLE PERSONALITY DISORDER — not used technically

spondyl- *or* **spondylo-** *comb form* : vertebra : vertebrae ⟨*spondylosis*⟩

spon·dyl·ar·thri·tis \ˌspän-di-lär-'thrī-təs\ *n, pl* **-thrit·i·des** \-'thrit-ə-ˌdēz\ : arthritis of the spine

spon·dy·li·tis \ˌspän-də-'lī-təs\ *n* : inflammation of the vertebrae ⟨tuberculous ~⟩ — see ANKYLOSING SPONDYLITIS — **spon·dy·lit·ic** \-'li-tik\ *adj*

spon·dy·lo·ar·throp·a·thy \ˌspän-də-lō-är-'thrä-pə-thē\ *also* **spon·dyl·ar·throp·a·thy** \ˌspän-də-lär-'thrä-\ *n, pl* **-thies** : any of several diseases (as ankylosing spondylitis) affecting the joints of the spine

spon·dy·lo·lis·the·sis \ˌspän-də-lō-lis-'thē-səs\ *n* : forward displacement of a lumbar vertebra on the one below it and esp. of the fifth lumbar vertebra on the sacrum producing pain by compression of nerve roots

spon·dy·lol·y·sis \ˌspän-də-'lä-lə-səs\ *n, pl* **-y·ses** \-ˌsēz\ : disintegration or dissolution of a vertebra

spon·dy·lop·a·thy \ˌspän-də-'lä-pə-thē\ *n, pl* **-thies** : any disease or disorder of the vertebrae

spon·dy·lo·sis \ˌspän-də-'lō-səs\ *n, pl* **-lo·ses** \-ˌsēz\ *or* **-lo·sis·es** : any of various degenerative diseases of the spine

sponge \'spənj\ *n* **1 a** : a pad (as of folded gauze) used in surgery and medicine (as to remove discharge or apply medication) **b** : a porous dressing (as of fibrin or gelatin) applied to promote wound healing **c** : a plastic prosthesis used in chest cavities following lung surgery **2** : an absorbent contraceptive device impregnated with spermicide that is inserted into the vagina before sexual intercourse to cover the cervix and act as a barrier to sperm — **sponge** *vb*

sponge bath *n* : a bath in which water is applied to the body without actual immersion

spongi- *or* **spongio-** *comb form* : spongy ⟨*spongioblast*⟩

spon·gi·form \'spən-ji-ˌfȯrm\ *adj* : of, relating to, or being a spongiform encephalopathy ⟨~ lesions⟩

spongiform encephalopathy *n* : any of various degenerative diseases of the brain characterized by the development of porous spongelike lesions in brain tissue and by deterioration in neurological functioning; *specif* : PRION DISEASE

spon·gi·o·blast \'spən-jē-ō-ˌblast, 'spän-\ *n* : any of the ectodermal cells of the embryonic spinal cord or other nerve center that are at first columnar but become branched at one end and that give rise to the glial cells

spon·gi·o·blas·to·ma \ˌspən-jē-ō-(ˌ)bla-'stō-mə, ˌspän-\ *n, pl* **-mas** *also* **-ma·ta** \-mə-tə\ : GLIOBLASTOMA

spon·gi·o·cyte \'spən-jē-ō-ˌsīt, 'spän-\ *n* : any of the cells of the adrenal cortex that have a spongy appearance due to lipid vacuoles the contents of which have been dissolved out

spon·gi·o·sa \ˌspən-jē-ˈō-sə, ˌspän-\ *n* : the part of a bone (as much of the epiphyseal area of long bones) made up of spongy cancellous bone

spon·gi·o·sis \ˌspən-jē-ˈō-səs, ˌspän-\ *n* : swelling localized in the epidermis and often occurring in eczema

spongiosum — see CORPUS SPONGIOSUM, STRATUM SPONGIOSUM

spongy \ˈspən-jē\ *adj* **spong·i·er; -est** : resembling a sponge; *esp* : full of cavities ⟨CANCELLOUS ⟨~ bone⟩⟩

spon·ta·ne·ous \spän-ˈtā-nē-əs\ *adj* **1** : proceeding from natural feeling or native tendency without external constraint **2** : developing without apparent external influence, force, cause, or treatment ⟨a ~ nosebleed⟩ — **spon·ta·ne·ous·ly** *adv*

spontaneous abortion *n* : naturally occurring expulsion of a nonviable fetus

spontaneous recovery *n* : reappearance of an extinguished conditioned response without positive reinforcement

spoon nails \ˈspün-\ *n* : KOILONYCHIA

spor- *or* **spori-** *or* **sporo-** *comb form* : seed : spore ⟨*sporo*cyst⟩

spo·rad·ic \spə-ˈra-dik\ *adj* **1** : occurring occasionally, singly, or in scattered instances ⟨~ diseases⟩ — compare ENDEMIC, EPIDEMIC 1 **2** : arising or occurring randomly with no known cause ⟨~ CreutzfeldtJakob disease⟩ — **spo·rad·i·cal·ly** *adv*

Spor·a·nox \ˈspȯr-ə-ˌnäks\ *trademark* — used for a preparation of itraconazole

spore \ˈspȯr\ *n* : a primitive usu. unicellular often environmentally resistant dormant or reproductive body produced by plants, fungi, and some microorganisms and capable of development into a new individual either directly or after fusion with another spore — **spore** *vb*

spo·ro·blast \ˈspō-rə-ˌblast\ *n* : a cell of a sporozoan resulting from sexual reproduction and producing spores and sporozoites

spo·ro·cyst \-ˌsist\ *n* **1** : a case or cyst secreted by some sporozoans preliminary to sporogony; *also* : a sporozoan encysted in such a case **2** : a saccular body that is the first asexual reproductive form of a digenetic trematode, develops from a miracidium, and buds off cells from its inner surface which develop into rediae

spo·ro·gen·e·sis \ˌspōr-ə-ˈje-nə-səs\ *n, pl* **-e·ses** \-ˌsēz\ **1** : reproduction by spores **2** : spore formation — **spo·rog·e·nous** \spə-ˈrä-jə-nəs, spȯ-\ *also* **spo·ro·gen·ic** \ˌspȯr-ə-ˈje-nik\ *adj*

spo·rog·o·ny \spə-ˈrä-gə-nē\ *n, pl* **-nies** : reproduction by spores; *specif* : formation of spores containing sporozoites that is characteristic of some sporozoans and that results

from the encystment and subsequent division of a zygote — **spo·ro·gon·ic** \ˌspȯr-ə-ˈgä-nik\ *adj*

spo·ront \ˈspȯr-ˌänt\ *n* : a sporozoan that engages in sporogony

spo·ro·phore \ˈspȯr-ə-ˌfȯr\ *n* : the spore-producing organ esp. of a fungus

spo·ro·thrix \-ˌthriks\ *n* **1** *cap* : a genus of imperfect fungi (family Moniliaceae) that includes the causative agent (*S. schenckii*) of sporotrichosis **2** : any fungus of the genus *Sporothrix*

spo·ro·tri·cho·sis \ˌspə-ˌrä-tri-ˈkō-səs, ˌspȯr-ə-tri-\ *n, pl* **-cho·ses** \-ˌsēz\ : infection with or disease caused by a fungus of the genus *Sporothrix* (*S. schenckii* syn. *Sporotrichum schenckii*) that is characterized by often ulcerating or suppurating nodules in the skin, subcutaneous tissues, and nearby lymph nodes and that is usu. transmitted by entry of the fungus through a skin abrasion or wound

spo·ro·zo·an \ˌspȯr-ə-ˈzō-ən\ *n* : any of a class (Sporozoa) of strictly parasitic protozoans that have a complex life cycle usu. involving both asexual and sexual generations often in different hosts and that include many serious pathogens (as malaria parasites and babesias) — **sporozoan** *adj*

spo·ro·zo·ite \-ˈzō-ˌīt\ *n* : a usu. motile infective form of some sporozoans (as the malaria parasite) that is a product of sporogony and initiates an asexual cycle in the new host

sport \ˈspȯrt\ *n* : an individual exhibiting a sudden deviation from type beyond the normal limits of individual variation usu. as a result of mutation esp. of somatic tissue

sports medicine *n* : a medical specialty concerned with the prevention and treatment of injuries and disorders that are related to participation in sports

spor·u·la·tion \ˌspȯr-ə-ˈlā-shən, ˌspȯr-yə-\ *n* : the formation of spores; *esp* : division into many small spores (as after encystment) — **spor·u·late** \ˈspȯr-ə-ˌlāt, ˈspȯr-yə-\ *vb*

¹spot \ˈspät\ *n* : a circumscribed mark or area: as **a** : a circumscribed surface lesion of disease (as measles) **b** : a circumscribed abnormality in an organ seen by means of X-rays or an instrument ⟨a ~ on the lung⟩

²spot *vb* **spot·ted; spot·ting** : to experience abnormal and sporadic bleeding in small amounts from the uterus

spot film *n* : a radiograph of a restricted area in the body

spotted cow·bane \-ˈkau̇-ˌbān\ *n* : a tall biennial No. American herb (*Cicuta maculata*) of the carrot family (Umbelliferae) with clusters of tuberous roots that resemble small sweet potatoes and are extremely poisonous — called also *spotted hemlock*

spotted fever *n* : any of various eruptive fevers; *esp* : ROCKY MOUNTAIN SPOTTED FEVER

¹sprain \'sprān\ *n* : a sudden or violent twist or wrench of a joint causing the stretching or tearing of ligaments and often rupture of blood vessels with hemorrhage into the tissues; *also* : the condition resulting from a sprain that is usu. marked by swelling, inflammation, hemorrhage, and discoloration — compare ³STRAIN b — **sprain** *vb*

sprain fracture *n* : AVULSION FRACTURE

¹spray \'sprā\ *n* : a jet of vapor or finely divided liquid; *specif* : a jet of fine medicated vapor used as an application to a diseased part or to charge the air of a room with a disinfectant or deodorant

²spray *vb* : to emit a stream or spray of urine ⟨a cat ∼s to mark its territory⟩

spreading factor *n* : HYALURONIDASE

Spreng·el's deformity \'shpreŋ-əlz-, -gəlz-\ *n* : a congenital elevation of the scapula

    Sprengel, Otto Gerhard Karl (1852–1915), German surgeon.

spring \'spriŋ\ *n* : any of various elastic orthodontic devices used esp. to apply constant pressure to misaligned teeth

spring ligament *n* : PLANTAR CALCANEONAVICULAR LIGAMENT

¹sprout \'spraůt\ *vb* : to send out new growth : produce sprouts

²sprout *n* : a new outgrowth (as of nerve tissue)

sprue \'sprü\ *n* 1 : CELIAC DISEASE 2 : a disease of tropical regions that is of unknown cause and is characterized by fatty diarrhea and malabsorption of nutrients — called also *tropical sprue*

spud \'spəd\ *n* : any of various small surgical instruments with a shape resembling that of a spade

spu·ma·vi·rus \'spü-mə-₁vī-rəs\ *n* : FOAMY VIRUS

spur \'spər\ *n* 1 : a projection from an anatomical part : CALCAR 2 : a bony outgrowth : OSTEOPHYTE ⟨heel ∼s⟩ — **spurred** \'spərd\ *adj*

spu·ri·ous \'spyür-ē-əs\ *adj* : simulating a symptom or condition without being pathologically or morphologically genuine ⟨∼ labor pains⟩

spu·tum \'spü-təm, 'spyü-\ *n*, *pl* **spu·ta** \-tə\ : matter expectorated from the respiratory system and esp. the lungs and bronchi that is composed chiefly of mucus but may contain pus, blood, fibrin, or microorganisms (as bacteria) in diseased states

squa·la·mine \'skwä-lə-₁mēn\ *n* : a steroid broad-spectrum antibiotic $C_{34}H_{67}N_3O_5S$ that has been shown to inhibit angiogenesis in tumors

squa·ma \'skwä-mə, 'skwä-\ *n*, *pl* **squa·mae** \'skwä-₁mē, 'skwä-₁mī\ : a structure resembling a scale or plate: as **a** : the curved platelike posterior portion of the occipital bone **b** : the vertical portion of the frontal bone that forms the forehead **c** : the thin anterior upper portion of the temporal bone

squame \'skwām\ *n* : a scale or flake (as of skin)

squa·mous \'skwā-məs\ *adj* **1 a** : covered with or consisting of scales **b** : of, relating to, or being a stratified epithelium that consists at least in its outer layers of small scalelike cells **2** : resembling a scale or plate; *esp* : of, relating to, or being the thin anterior upper portion of the temporal bone

squamous carcinoma *n* : SQUAMOUS CELL CARCINOMA

squamous cell *n* : a cell of or derived from squamous epithelium

squamous cell carcinoma *n* : a carcinoma made up of or arising from squamous cells and usu. occurring in areas of the body exposed to strong sunlight over a period of many years

squash bite \'skwäsh-, 'skwȯsh-\ *n* : an impression of the teeth and mouth made by closing the teeth on modeling composition or wax

squill \'skwil\ *n* **1** : a Mediterranean bulbous herb of the genus Urginea (esp. *U. maritima*) **2** : the dried sliced bulb of a white-bulbed form of the squill (*Urginea maritima*) used esp. formerly as an expectorant, cardiac stimulant, and diuretic — called also *white squill*

¹squint \'skwint\ *vb* **1** : to be cross-eyed **2** : to look or peer with eyes partly closed

²squint *n* **1** : STRABISMUS **2** : an instance or habit of squinting

squir·rel corn \'skwər-əl-\ *n* : a poisonous No. American herb (*Dicentra canadensis* of the family Fumariaceae)

Sr *symbol* strontium

SR *abbr* slow-release; sustained-release

sRNA \'es-₁är-(₁)en-'ā\ *n* : TRANSFER RNA

SRS *abbr* slow-reacting substance

SRS–A *abbr* slow-reacting substance of anaphylaxis

ss *abbr* [Latin *semis*] one half — used in writing prescriptions

S sleep *n* : SLOW-WAVE SLEEP

SSPE *abbr* subacute sclerosing panencephalitis

SSRI \₁es-₁es-₁är-'ī\ *n* : any of a class of antidepressants (as fluoxetine or sertraline) that inhibit the inactivation of serotonin by blocking its reuptake by presynaptic nerve cell endings — called also *selective serotonin reuptake inhibitor*

SSSS *abbr* staphylococcal scalded skin syndrome

ST \₁es-'tē\ *n* : ST SEGMENT

stab \'stab\ *n* : a wound produced by a pointed weapon — **stab** *vb*

stab·bing *adj* : having a sharp piercing quality ⟨∼ pain⟩

stab cell *n* : BAND FORM

sta·bil·i·ty \stə-'bi-lə-tē\ *n, pl* **-ties** : the quality, state, or degree of being stable ⟨emotional ∼⟩

sta·bi·lize \'stā-bə-ˌlīz\ *vb* **-lized; -liz·ing** : to make or become stable ⟨∼ a patient's condition⟩ — **sta·bi·li·za·tion** \ˌstā-bə-lə-'zā-shən\ *n* — **sta·bi·liz·er** \'stā-bə-ˌlī-zər\ *n*

sta·ble \'stā-bəl\ *adj* **sta·bler; sta·blest** 1 : not changing or fluctuating ⟨∼ condition⟩ 2 : not subject to insecurity or emotional illness ⟨a ∼ personality⟩ 3 a : not readily altering in chemical makeup or physical state b : not spontaneously radioactive

stable factor *n* : FACTOR VII

stable fly *n* : a biting dipteran fly of the genus *Stomoxys* (*S. calcitrans*) that is abundant about stables and often enters dwellings esp. in autumn

stachy·bot·ryo·tox·i·co·sis \ˌsta-ki-ˌbä-trē-ō-ˌtäk-sə-'kō-səs\ *n, pl* **-co·ses** \-ˌsēz\ : a serious and sometimes fatal intoxication chiefly affecting domestic animals (as horses) that is due to ingestion of a toxin produced by a mold (*Stachybotrys chartarum*)

sta·di·om·e·ter \ˌstā-dē-'ä-mə-tər\ *n* : a device for measuring height that typically consists of a vertical ruler with a sliding horizontal rod or paddle which is adjusted to rest on the top of the head

Sta·dol \'stā-ˌdȯl\ *trademark* — used for a preparation of the tartrate of butorphanol

staff \'staf\ *n* : the doctors and surgeons regularly attached to a hospital and helping to determine its policies and guide its activities

staff nurse *n* : a registered nurse employed by a medical facility who does not assist in surgery

staff of Aes·cu·la·pi·us \-ˌes-kyə-'lā-pē-əs\ *n* : a conventionalized representation of a staff branched at the top with a single snake twined around it that is used as a symbol of medicine and as the official insignia of the American Medical Association — called also *Aesculapian staff*

¹**stage** \'stāj\ *n* 1 : a period or step in a process, activity, or development: as a : one of the distinguishable periods of growth and development of a plant or animal b : a period or phase in the course of a disease; *also* : the degree of involvement or severity of a disease c : one of two or more operations performed at different times but constituting a single procedure ⟨a two-*stage* thoracoplasty⟩ d : any of the four degrees indicating depth of general anesthesia 2 : the small platform of a microscope on which an object is placed for examination

²**stage** *vb* **staged; stag·ing** : to determine the phase or severity of (a disease) based on a classification of established symptomatic criteria; *also* : to evaluate (a patient) to determine the phase, severity, or progression of a disease

stag·gers \'sta-gərz\ *n pl* 1 : any of various abnormal conditions of domestic animals associated with damage to the central nervous system and marked by incoordination and a reeling unsteady gait — used with a sing. or pl. verb; see BLIND STAGGERS 2 : vertigo occurring as a symptom of decompression sickness

stag·horn calculus \'stag-ˌhȯrn-\ *n* : a large renal calculus with multiple irregular branches

stag·ing \'stā-jiŋ\ *n* : the classification of the severity of a disease in distinct stages on the basis of established symptomatic criteria

¹**stain** \'stān\ *vb* 1 a : to cause discoloration of b : to color by processes affecting chemically or otherwise the material itself ⟨∼ bacteria with a fluorescent dye⟩ 2 : to receive a stain

²**stain** *n* 1 : a discolored spot or area (as on the skin or teeth) — see PORT-WINE STAIN 2 : a dye or mixture of dyes used in microscopy to make minute and transparent structures visible, to differentiate tissue elements, or to produce specific chemical reactions

stair·case effect \'star-ˌkās-\ *n* : TREPPE

stalk \'stȯk\ *n* : a slender supporting or connecting part : PEDUNCLE ⟨the pituitary ∼⟩ — **stalked** \'stȯkt\ *adj* — **stalk·less** *adj*

stam·i·na \'sta-mi-nə\ *n* : the strength or vigor of bodily constitution : capacity for standing fatigue or resisting disease

stam·mer \'sta-mər\ *vb* **stam·mered; stam·mer·ing** : to make involuntary stops and repetitions in speaking : STUTTER — **stammer** *n* — **stam·mer·er** \'sta-mər-ər\ *n*

stammering *n* 1 : the act of one who stammers 2 : a speech disorder characterized by involuntary stops and repetitions or blocking of utterance : STUTTERING

stanch *also* **staunch** \'stȯnch, 'stänch\ *vb* : to check or stop the flowing of ⟨∼ bleeding⟩; *also* : to stop the flow of blood from ⟨∼ a wound⟩

stand·still \'stand-ˌstil\ *n* : a state characterized by absence of motion or of progress : ARREST ⟨cardiac ∼⟩

Stan·ford–Bi·net test \'stan-fərd-bi-'nā-\ *n* : an intelligence test prepared at Stanford University as a revision of the Binet-Simon scale and commonly employed with children — called also *Stanford-Binet*

A. Binet — see BINET AGE

stan·nous fluoride \'sta-nəs-\ *n* : a white compound SnF_2 of tin and fluorine used in toothpastes and oral rinses to combat tooth decay

sta·nol \'sta-ˌnȯl, 'stā-\ *n* : any of the fully saturated phytosterols — see SITOSTANOL

stan·o·lone \'sta-nə-ˌlōn\ *n* : a semisynthetic dihydrotestosterone derivative $C_{19}H_{30}O_2$ used esp. in the treatment of breast cancer

stan·o·zo·lol \'sta-nə-zō-ˌlȯl\ *n* : an anabolic steroid $C_{21}H_{32}N_2O$

sta·pe·dec·to·my \ˌstā-pi-'dek-tə-mē\ *n, pl* **-mies** : surgical removal and prosthetic replacement of part or all of the stapes to relieve deafness

sta·pe·di·al \stā-'pē-dē-əl, stə-\ *adj* : of, relating to, or located near the stapes

sta·pe·di·us \stə-'pē-dē-əs\ *n, pl* **-dii** \-dē-ˌī\ : a small muscle of the middle ear that arises from the wall of the tympanum, is inserted into the neck of the stapes by a tendon that sometimes contains a slender spine of bone, and serves to check and dampen vibration of the stapes — called also *stapedius muscle*

sta·pes \'stā-(ˌ)pēz\ *n, pl* **stapes** or **sta·pe·des** \stə-'pē-ˌdēz\ : the innermost of the chain of three ossicles in the middle ear which has the form of a stirrup, a base occupying the oval window of the tympanum, and a head connected with the incus — called also *stirrup*

staph \'staf\ *n* : STAPHYLOCOCCUS 2; *also* : an infection with staphylococci

staphyl- or **staphylo-** *comb form* : staphylococcus ⟨*staphylotoxin*⟩

staph·y·lo·coc·cal \ˌsta-fə-lō-'kä-kəl\ *also* **staph·y·lo·coc·cic** \-'kä-kik, -'käk-sik\ *adj* : of, relating to, caused by, or being a staphylococcus

staphylococcal scalded skin syndrome *n* : an acute skin disorder esp. of infants and immunocompromised individuals that is characterized by widespread erythema, peeling, and necrosis of the skin, that is caused by a toxin produced by a bacterium of the genus *Staphylococcus* (*S. aureus*), and that exposes the affected individual to serious infections but is rarely fatal if diagnosed and treated promptly — abbr. *SSSS;* compare TOXIC EPIDERMAL NECROLYSIS

staph·y·lo·coc·co·sis \ˌsta-fə-lō-kä-'kō-səs\ *n* : infection with or disease caused by staphylococci

staph·y·lo·coc·cus \ˌsta-fə-lō-'kä-kəs\ *n* **1** *cap* : a genus of nonmotile gram-positive spherical bacteria that is placed in either of two families (Staphylococcaceae or Micrococcaceae), contains forms occurring singly, in pairs or tetrads, or in irregular clusters, and includes causative agents of various diseases (as skin infections, food poisoning, and endocarditis) **2** *pl* **-coc·ci** \-'käk-ˌsī\ : any bacterium of the genus *Staphylococcus; broadly* : MICROCOCCUS 2

staph·y·lo·ki·nase \-'kī-ˌnās, -ˌnāz\ *n* : a protease from some pathogenic staphylococci that converts plasminogen to plasmin

staph·y·lo·ma \ˌsta-fə-'lō-mə\ *n* : a protrusion of the cornea or sclera of the eye

staph·y·lo·tox·in \ˌsta-fə-lō-'täk-sən\ : a toxin produced by staphylococci

sta·ple \'stā-pəl\ *n* : a usu. U-shaped and typically metal surgical fastener used to hold layers of tissue together (as in the closure of an incision) — **staple** *vb* — **sta·pler** \-plər\ *n*

starch \'stärch\ *n* : a white odorless tasteless granular or powdery complex carbohydrate $(C_6H_{10}O_5)_x$ that is the chief storage form of carbohydrate in plants, is an important foodstuff, has demulcent and absorbent properties, and is used in pharmacy esp. as a dusting powder and as a constituent of ointments and pastes — **starchy** \'stär-chē\ *adj*

Star·ling's hypothesis \'stär-linz-\ *also* **Star·ling hypothesis** \-liŋ-\ *n* : a hypothesis in physiology: the flow of fluids across capillary walls depends on the balance between the force of blood pressure on the walls and the osmotic pressure across the walls so that the declining gradient in blood pressure from the arterial to the venous end of the capillary results in an outflow of fluids at its arterial end with an increasing inflow toward its venous end

E. H. Starling — see FRANK-STARLING LAW

Starling's law of the heart *n* : a statement in physiology: the strength of the heart's systolic contraction is directly proportional to its diastolic expansion with the result that under normal physiological conditions the heart pumps out of the right atrium all the blood returned to it without letting any back up in the veins — called also *Frank-Starling law, Frank-Starling law of the heart, Starling's law*

starve \'stärv\ *vb* **starved; starv·ing** **1 a** : to perish from lack of food **b** : to suffer extreme hunger **2** : to deprive of nourishment — **star·va·tion** \stär-'vā-shən\ *n*

sta·sis \'stā-səs, 'sta-\ *n, pl* **sta·ses** \'stā-ˌsēz, 'sta-\ : a slowing or stoppage of the normal flow of a bodily fluid or semifluid ⟨biliary ∼⟩: as **a** : slowing of the current of circulating blood **b** : reduced motility of the intestines with retention of feces

stasis ulcer *n* : an ulcer (as on the lower leg) caused by localized slowing or stoppage of blood flow

stat \'stat\ *adv* : STATIM

-stat \ˌstat\ *n comb form* : agent causing inhibition of growth without destruction ⟨bacterio*stat*⟩

state \'stāt\ *n* : mode or condition of being: as **a** : condition of mind or temperament ⟨a manic ∼⟩ **b** : a condition or stage in the physical being of something ⟨the gaseous ∼ of water⟩

state hospital *n* : a hospital for the mentally ill that is run by a state

stat·im \'sta-tim\ *adv* : immediately or without delay

stat·in \'sta-tᵊn\ *n* : any of a group of lipid-lowering drugs (as lovastatin and simvastatin) that function by inhibiting a liver enzyme which controls the synthesis of cholesterol and by promoting the production of LDL= binding receptors in the liver resulting in usu. marked decrease in the level of LDL and a modest increase in the level of HDL circulating in blood plasma

sta·tion \'stā-shən\ *n* **1** : the place at which someone is positioned or is assigned to remain ⟨the nurse's ∼ on a hospital ward⟩ **2** : the act or manner of standing : POSTURE

sta·tion·ary \'stā-shə-,ner-ē\ *adj* **1** : fixed in position : not moving **2** : characterized by a lack of change

stato- *comb form* : balance : equilibrium ⟨*stato*lith⟩

stato·co·nia \,sta-tə-tə'kō-nē-ə\ *n pl* : OTOLITHIA

stato·lith \'stat-ᵊl-,ith\ *n* : OTOLITH

sta·tus \'stā-təs, 'sta-\ *n, pl* **sta·tus·es** : a particular state or condition

status asth·mat·i·cus \-az-'ma-ti-kəs\ *n* : a prolonged severe attack of asthma that is unresponsive to initial standard therapy, is characterized esp. by dyspnea, dry cough, wheezing, and hypoxemia, and that may lead to respiratory failure

status ep·i·lep·ti·cus \-,e-pə-'lep-ti-kəs\ *n* : a state in epilepsy in which the attacks occur in rapid succession without recovery of consciousness

stat·u·to·ry rape \'sta-chə-,tōr-ē-\ *n* : sexual intercourse with a person who is below the age of consent as defined by law

staunch *var of* STANCH

stav·u·dine \'sta-vyü-,dēn\ *n* : D4T

STD \,es-(,)tē-'dē\ *n* : SEXUALLY TRANSMITTED DISEASE

steady state *n* : a state of physiological equilibrium esp. in connection with a specified metabolic relation or activity

steal \'stēl\ *n* : abnormal circulation characterized by deviation (as through collateral vessels or by backward flow) of blood to tissues where the normal flow of blood has been cut off by occlusion of an artery

ste·ap·sin \stē-'ap-sən\ *n* : the lipase in pancreatic juice

stea·rate \'stē-ə-,rāt, 'stir-,āt\ *n* : a salt or ester of stearic acid

stea·ric acid \stē-'ar-ik-, 'stir-ik-\ *n* : a white crystalline fatty acid $C_{18}H_{36}O_2$ obtained from tallow and some other hard fats; *also* : a commercial mixture of stearic and palmitic acids

stea·rin \'stē-ə-rən, 'stir-ən\ *n* : an ester of glycerol and stearic acid

$C_3H_5(C_{18}H_{35}O_2)_3$ that is a predominant constituent of many hard fats

steat- or **steato-** *comb form* : fat ⟨*steatoma*⟩

ste·a·ti·tis \,stē-ə-'tī-təs\ *n* : inflammation of fatty tissue; *esp* : YELLOW FAT DISEASE

ste·a·to·ma \,stē-ə-'tō-mə\ *n, pl* **-mas** or **-ma·ta** \-mə-tə\ : SEBACEOUS CYST

ste·ato·py·gia \,stē-ə-tə-'pi-jē-ə, stē-,a-tō-, -'pī-\ *n* : an accumulation of a large amount of fat on the buttocks — **ste·ato·py·gous** \-'pī-gəs\ or **ste·ato·py·gic** \-'pi-jik, -'pī-\ *adj*

ste·at·or·rhea \,(,)stē-ə-tə-'rē-ə\ *n* : an excess of fat in the stools

ste·at·or·rhoea *chiefly Brit var of* STEATORRHEA

ste·a·to·sis \,stē-ə-'tō-səs\ *n, pl* **-to·ses** \-,sēz\ : FATTY DEGENERATION

Stein–Lev·en·thal syndrome \'stīn-'lev-ᵊn-,thäl-\ *n* : POLYCYSTIC OVARY SYNDROME

Stein, Irving Freiler (1887–1976), and Leventhal, Michael Leo (1901–1971), American gynecologists.

Stein·mann pin \'stīn-mən-\ *n* : a stainless steel spike used for the internal fixation of fractures of long bones

Steinmann, Fritz (1872–1932), Swiss surgeon.

Stel·a·zine \'ste-lə-,zēn\ *trademark* — used for a preparation of the hydrochloride of trifluoperazine

stel·late \'ste-,lāt\ *adj* : shaped like a star ⟨a ∼ ulcer⟩

stellate cell *n* : a cell (as a Kupffer cell) with radiating cytoplasmic processes

stellate ganglion *n* : a composite ganglion formed by fusion of the most inferior of the three cervical ganglia with the first thoracic ganglion of the sympathetic chain

stellate ligament *n* : RADIATE LIGAMENT

stellate reticulum *n* : a loosely-connected mass of stellate epithelial cells that in early developmental stages makes up a large portion of the enamel organ

stem cell *n* : an unspecialized cell that gives rise to differentiated cells ⟨hematopoietic *stem cells*⟩

ste·nosed \ste-'nōst, -'nōzd\ *adj* : affected with stenosis : abnormally constricted ⟨a ∼ eustachian tube⟩

ste·nos·ing \ste-'nō-siŋ, -ziŋ\ *adj* : causing or characterized by stenosis (as of a tendon sheath)

ste·no·sis \stə-'nō-səs\ *n, pl* **-no·ses** \-,sēz\ : a narrowing or constriction of the diameter of a bodily passage or orifice ⟨esophageal ∼⟩ — see AORTIC STENOSIS, MITRAL STENOSIS, PULMONARY STENOSIS, SPINAL STENOSIS, SUBAORTIC STENOSIS

ste·not·ic \stə-'nä-tik\ *adj* : of, relating to, characterized by, or causing stenosis ⟨∼ lesions⟩

Sten·sen's duct *also* **Sten·son's duct** \'sten-sənz-\ *n* : PAROTID DUCT

Sten·sen *or* **Steen·sen** \'stän-sən\, **Niels** (*Latin* **Nicolaus Steno**) (1638–1686), Danish anatomist and geologist.

stent \'stent\ *also* **stint** \'stint\ *n* **1** : a mold formed from a resinous compound and used for holding a surgical graft in place; *also* : something (as a pad of gauze immobilized by sutures) used like a stent **2** : a short narrow metal or plastic tube often in the form of a mesh that is inserted into the lumen of an antomical vessel (as an artery or bile duct) esp. to keep a previously blocked passageway open

Stent, Charles R. (1845–1901), British dentist.

stent·ing \'sten-tiŋ\ *n* : a surgical procedure or operation for inserting a stent into an anatomical vessel — **stent** *vb*

Steph·a·no·fi·lar·ia \,ste-fə-,nō-fi-'lar-ē-ə\ *n* : a genus of filarial worms parasitic in the skin and subcutaneous tissues of ruminants and horses where they may cause dermatitis and extensive degenerative lesions

Steph·a·nu·rus \,ste-fə-'nùr-əs, -'nyùr-\ *n* : a genus of strongylid nematode worms that includes the kidney worm (*S. dentatus*) of swine

ster·co·ra·ceous \,stər-kə-'rā-shəs\ *adj* : of, relating to, containing, produced by, or being feces : FECAL

ster·cu·lia gum \stər-'kül-yə-, -'kyül-\ *n* : KARAYA GUM

stere- *or* **stereo-** *comb form* **1** : stereoscopic 〈*stereo*psis〉 **2** : having or dealing with three dimensions of space 〈*stereo*taxic〉

ste·reo·acu·i·ty \,ster-ē-ō-ə-'kyü-ə-tē, ,stir-\ *n, pl* **-ties** : the ability to detect differences in distance using stereoscopic cues that is measured by the smallest difference in the images presented to the two eyes that can be detected reliably

ste·reo·cil·i·um \,ster-ē-ō-'si-lē-əm, ,stir-\ *n, pl* **-cil·ia** \-lē-ə\ : a microvillus that resembles cilia and projects from the surface of certain cells (as the auditory hair cells) — see KINOCILIUM

ste·re·og·no·sis \,ster-ē-äg-'nō-səs, ,stir-\ *n* : ability to perceive or the perception of material qualities (as shape) of an object by handling or lifting it : tactile recognition

ste·reo·iso·mer \,ster-ē-ō-'ī-sə-mər, ,stir-\ *n* : any of a group of isomers in which atoms are linked in the same order but differ in their spatial arrangement — **ste·reo·iso·mer·ic** \-,ī-sə-'mer-ik\ *adj* — **ste·reo·isom·er·ism** \-ī-'sä-mə-,ri-zəm\ *n*

ste·re·op·sis \,ster-ē-'äp-səs, ,stir-\ *n* : stereoscopic vision

ste·reo·scope \'ster-ē-ə-,skōp, 'stir-\ *n* : an optical instrument with two eyepieces for helping the observer to combine the images of two pictures taken from points of view a little way

apart and thus to get the effect of solidity or depth

ste·reo·scop·ic \,ster-ē-ə-'skä-pik, ,stir-\ *adj* **1** : of or relating to the stereoscope or the production of three-dimensional images **2** : characterized by the seeing of objects in three dimensions 〈~ vision〉 — **ste·reo·scop·i·cal·ly** *adv* — **ste·re·os·co·py** \,ster-ē-'äs-kə-pē, ,stir-; 'ster-ē-ə-,skō-pē, 'stir-\ *n*

ste·reo·tac·tic \,ster-ē-ə-'tak-tik, ,stir-\ *adj* : involving, being, utilizing, or used in a surgical technique for precisely directing the tip of a delicate instrument (as a needle) or beam of radiation in three planes using coordinates provided by medical imaging (as computed tomography) in order to reach a specific locus in the body — **ste·reo·tac·ti·cal·ly** *adv*

stereotactic radiosurgery *n* : a surgical technique involving the use of narrow beams of radiation (as gamma rays) that are precisely targeted by stereotactic methods to destroy tumors or lesions esp. of the brain

ste·reo·tax·ic \,ster-ē-ə-'tak-sik, ,stir-\ *adj* : STEREOTACTIC — **ste·reo·tax·i·cal·ly** *adv*

ste·reo·tax·is \-'tak-səs\ *n, pl* **-tax·es** \-,sēz\ : a stereotactic technique or procedure

¹**ste·reo·type** \'ster-ē-ə-,tīp, 'stir-\ *vb* **-typed; -typ·ing** **1** : to repeat without variation 〈*stereotyped* behavior〉 **2** : to develop a mental stereotype about

²**stereotype** *n* : something conforming to a fixed or general pattern; *esp* : an often oversimplified or biased mental picture held to characterize the typical individual of a group — **ste·reo·typ·i·cal** \,ster-ē-ə-'ti-pi-kəl\ *also* **ste·reo·typ·ic** \-'pik\ *adj*

ste·reo·ty·py \'ster-ē-ə-,tī-pē, 'stir-\ *n, pl* **-pies** : frequent almost mechanical repetition of the same posture, movement, or form of speech (as in schizophrenia or autism)

ster·il·ant \'ster-ə-lənt\ *n* : a sterilizing agent

ster·ile \'ster-əl\ *adj* **1** : failing to produce or incapable of producing offspring 〈a ~ hybrid〉 **2** : free from living organisms and esp. microorganisms 〈a ~ cyst〉 — **ster·ile·ly** *adv* — **ste·ril·i·ty** \stə-'ri-lə-tē\ *n*

ster·il·ize \'ster-ə-,līz\ *vb* **-ized; -iz·ing** : to make sterile: **a** : to deprive of the power of reproducing **b** : to free from living microorganisms (as by the use of physical or chemical agents) — **ster·il·i·za·tion** \,ster-ə-lə-'zā-shən\ *n* — **ster·il·iz·er** \'ster-ə-,lī-zər\ *n*

stern- *or* **sterno-** *comb form* **1** : breast : sternum : breastbone 〈*sterno*tomy〉 **2** : sternal and 〈*sterno*costal〉

ster·nal \'stərn-ᵊl\ *adj* : of or relating to the sternum

ster·ne·bra \'stər-nə-brə\ *n, pl* **-brae** \-,brē, -,brī\ : any of the four segments into which the body of the sternum is divided in childhood and which fuse to form the gladiolus

ster·no·cla·vic·u·lar \ˌstər-nō-kla-ˈvi-kyə-lər\ *adj* : of, relating to, or being articulation of the sternum and the clavicle ⟨∼ dislocation⟩

ster·no·clei·do·mas·toid \ˌstər-nō-ˌklī-də-ˈmas-ˌtȯid\ *n* : a thick superficial muscle on each side that arises by one head from the first segment of the sternum and by a second from the inner part of the clavicle, that inserts into the mastoid process and occipital bone, and that acts esp. to bend, rotate, flex, and extend the head — **sternocleidomastoid** *adj*

ster·no·clei·do·mas·toi·de·us \-ˌmas-ˈtȯi-dē-əs\ *n, pl* **-dei** \-dē-ˌī\ : STERNOCLEIDOMASTOID

ster·no·cos·tal \ˌstər-nō-ˈkäst-ᵊl\ *adj* : of, relating to, or situated between the sternum and ribs

ster·no·hy·oid \ˌstər-nō-ˈhī-ˌȯid\ *n* : an infrahyoid muscle on each side of the midline that arises from the medial end of the clavicle and the first segment of the sternum, inserts into the body of the hyoid bone, and acts to depress the hyoid bone and the larynx — **sternohyoid** *adj*

ster·no·hy·oi·de·us \-hī-ˈȯi-dē-əs\ *n, pl* **-dei** \-dē-ˌī\ : STERNOHYOID

ster·no·mas·toid muscle \-ˈmas-ˌtȯid-\ *n* : STERNOCLEIDOMASTOID

ster·no·thy·roid \ˌstər-nō-ˈthī-ˌrȯid\ *n* : an infrahyoid muscle on each side of the body below the sternohyoid that arises from the sternum and from the cartilage of the first and sometimes of the second ribs, inserts into the thyroid cartilage, and acts to draw the larynx downward by depressing the thyroid cartilage — **sternothyroid** *adj*

ster·no·thy·roi·de·us \-thī-ˈrȯi-dē-əs\ *n, pl* **-dei** \-dē-ˌī\ : STERNOTHYROID

ster·not·o·my \stər-ˈnä-tə-mē\ *n, pl* **-mies** : surgical incision through the sternum

ster·num \ˈstər-nəm\ *n, pl* **-nums** or **-na** \-nə\ : a compound ventral bone or cartilage that lies in the median central part of the body of most vertebrates other than fishes and that in humans is about seven inches (18 centimeters) long, consists in the adult of three parts, and connects with the clavicles and the cartilages of the upper seven pairs of ribs — called also *breastbone*

ster·nu·ta·tion \ˌstər-nyə-ˈtā-shən\ *n* : the act, fact, or noise of sneezing

ster·nu·ta·tor \ˈstər-nyə-ˌtā-tər\ *n* : an agent that induces sneezing and often lacrimation and vomiting

ste·roid \ˈster-ˌȯid, ˈstir-\ *n* : any of numerous natural or synthetic compounds containing a 17-carbon 4-ring system and including the sterols and various hormones and glycosides — see ANABOLIC STEROID — **steroid** or **ste·roi·dal** \stə-ˈrȯid-ᵊl\ *adj*

steroid hormone *n* : any of numerous hormones (as estrogen, testosterone, cortisone, and aldosterone) having the characteristic ring structure of steroids and formed in the body from cholesterol

ste·roido·gen·e·sis \stə-ˌrȯi-də-ˈje-nə-səs; ˌstir-ˌȯi-, ˌster-\ *n, pl* **-e·ses** \-ˌsēz\ : synthesis of steroids ⟨adrenal ∼⟩ — **ste·roido·gen·ic** \-ˈje-nik\ *adj*

ste·rol \ˈstir-ˌȯl, ˈster-, -ˌōl\ *n* : any of various solid steroid alcohols (as cholesterol) widely distributed in animal and plant lipids

ster·to·rous \ˈstər-tə-rəs\ *adj* : characterized by a harsh snoring or gasping sound — **ster·to·rous·ly** *adv*

stetho·scope \ˈste-thə-ˌskōp\ *n* : an instrument used to detect and study sounds produced in the body that are conveyed to the ears of the listener through rubber tubing connected with a usu. cup-shaped piece placed upon the area to be examined — **stetho·scop·ic** \ˌste-thə-ˈskä-pik\ *adj* — **stetho·scop·i·cal·ly** *adv*

Ste·vens–John·son syndrome \ˈstē-vənz-ˈjän-sən-\ *n* : a severe and sometimes fatal form of erythema multiforme that is characterized esp. by extensive erosive lesions of mucous membranes (as of the mouth, nose, esophagus, anus, and genitalia) and by purulent conjunctivitis which sometimes results in blindness

    Stevens, Albert Mason (1884–1945), and Johnson, Frank Chambliss (1894–1934), American pediatricians.

ste·via \ˈstē-vē-ə\ *n* : a very sweet noncaloric glycoside-containing substance that is obtained from the leaves of a So. American shrub (*Stevia rebaudiana* of the family Compositae) and is approved in the U.S. as a dietary supplement

STH *abbr* somatotropic hormone

sthen·ic \ˈsthe-nik\ *adj* **1** : notably or excessively vigorous or active ⟨∼ fever⟩ ⟨∼ emotions⟩ **2** : PYKNIC

stib·o·phen \ˈsti-bə-ˌfen\ *n* : a crystalline antimony compound $C_{12}H_4$-$Na_5O_{16}S_4Sb·7H_2O$ used in the treatment of various tropical diseases

Stick·ler syndrome \ˈstik-lər-\ *n* : a variable disorder of connective tissue that is charcterized by myopia, retinal detachment, cleft palate, micrognathia, flat facies, premature arthritis, hip deformity, and hyperextensibility of the large joints and is inherited as an autosomal dominant trait

    Stickler, Gunnar B. (fl 1965–67), American pediatrician.

stick·tight flea \ˈstik-ˌtīt-\ *n* : a flea of the genus *Echidnophaga* (*E. gallinacea*) that is parasitic esp. on the heads of chickens

sties *pl of* STY

stiff \ˈstif\ *adj* : lacking in suppleness ⟨∼ muscles⟩ — **stiff·ness** *n*

stiff–lamb disease \\'stif-,lam-\ *n* : white muscle disease occurring in lambs

stiff–man syndrome *n* : a chronic progressive disorder of uncertain etiology that is characterized by painful spasms and increasing stiffness of the muscles

sti·fle \\'stī-fəl\ *n* : the joint next above the hock in the hind leg of a quadruped (as a horse or a dog) corresponding to the human knee

stig·ma \\'stig-mə\ *n, pl* **stig·ma·ta** \stig-'mä-tə, 'stig-mə-tə\ *or* **stigmas** 1 : an identifying mark or characteristic; *specif* : a specific diagnostic sign of a disease ⟨the *stigmata* of syphilis⟩ 2 : PETECHIA 3 : a small spot, scar, or opening on a plant or animal

stilb·am·i·dine \stil-'ba-mə-,dēn\ *n* : a drug used chiefly in the form of one of its salts $C_{20}H_{28}N_4O_8S_2$ in treating various fungal infections

stil·bes·trol \stil-'bes-,trōl, -,trōl\ *n* : DIETHYLSTILBESTROL

sti·let \\'stī-lət\ *or* **sti·lette** \sti-'let\ *n* : STYLET

still·birth \\'stil-,bərth\ *n* : the birth of a dead fetus — compare LIVE BIRTH

still·born \-,bórn\ *adj* : dead at birth — compare LIVE-BORN — **stillborn** *n*

Still's disease \\'stilz-\ *n* : rheumatoid arthritis esp. in children

    Still, Sir George Frederic (1868–1941), British pediatrician.

stim·u·lant \\'stim-yə-lənt\ *n* 1 : an agent (as a drug) that produces a temporary increase of the functional activity or efficiency of an organism or any of its parts 2 : STIMULUS

stim·u·late \-,lāt\ *vb* **-lat·ed; -lat·ing** 1 : to excite to activity or growth or to greater activity 2 a : to function as a physiological stimulus to (as a nerve or muscle) b : to arouse or affect by a stimulant (as a drug) — **stim·u·la·tion** \,stim-yə-'lā-shən\ *n* — **stim·u·la·tive** \'stim-yə-,lā-tiv\ *adj* — **stim·u·la·to·ry** \-lə-,tōr-ē\ *adj*

stim·u·la·tor \\'stim-yə-,lā-tər\ *n* : one that stimulates or provides a stimulus

stim·u·lus \\'stim-yə-ləs\ *n, pl* **-li** \-,lī, -,lē\ 1 : STIMULANT 1 2 : an agent (as an environmental change) that directly influences the activity of living protoplasm (as by exciting a sensory organ or evoking muscular contraction or glandular secretion)

stimulus–response *adj* : of, relating to, or being a reaction to a stimulus; *also* : representing the activity of an organism as composed of such reactions ⟨~ psychology⟩

sting \\'stiŋ\ *vb* **stung** \'stəŋ\; **sting·ing** 1 : to prick painfully: as a : to pierce or wound with a poisonous or irritating process b : to affect with sharp quick pain 2 : to feel or cause a keen burning pain or smart — **sting** *n*

sting·er \\'stiŋ-ər\ *n* 1 : a sharp organ (as of a bee or scorpion) that is usu. connected with a poison gland or otherwise adapted to wound by piercing and injecting a poison 2 : a usu. sports-related injury of the brachial plexus marked by a painful burning sensation that radiates from the neck down the arm and is often accompanied by weakness or numbness of the affected area — called also *burner*

stinging nettle *n* : NETTLE 1; *esp* : a Eurasian nettle (*Urtica dioica*) widely naturalized in No. America and having numerous hairs that are extremely irritating to the skin

sting·ray \\'stiŋ-,rā\ *n* : any of numerous large flat cartilaginous fishes (order Rajiformes and esp. family Dasyatidae) with one or more large sharp barbed dorsal spines near the base of the whiplike tail capable of inflicting severe wounds

stint *var of* STENT

stip·pling \\'stip-liŋ\ *n* : the appearance of spots : a spotted condition (as in basophilic red blood cells)

stir·rup \\'stər-əp, 'stir-əp\ *n* 1 : STAPES 2 : an attachment to an examining or operating table designed to raise and spread the legs of a patient

stitch \\'stich\ *n* 1 : a local sharp and sudden pain esp. in the side 2 a : one in-and-out movement of a threaded needle in suturing b : a portion of a suture left in the tissue after one stitch ⟨removal of ~*es*⟩ — **stitch** *vb*

STM *abbr* short-term memory

stock \\'stäk\ *n* : a population, colony, or culture of organisms used for scientific research or medical purposes

Stock·holm syndrome \'stäk-,hō(l)m-\ *n* : the psychological tendency of a hostage to bond with, identify with, or sympathize with his or her captor

stock·ing \\'stäk-iŋ\ — see ELASTIC STOCKING

Stokes–Ad·ams syndrome \'stōks-'a-dəmz-\ *n* : fainting and convulsions induced by complete heart block with a pulse rate of 40 beats per minute or less — called also *Adams-Stokes syndrome, Stokes-Adams attack, Stokes-Adams disease*

    W. Stokes — see CHEYNE-STOKES RESPIRATION

    Adams, Robert (1791–1875), British physician.

sto·ma \\'stō-mə\ *n, pl* **-mas** : an artificial permanent opening esp. in the abdominal wall made in surgical procedures ⟨a colostomy ~⟩

stom·ach \\'stə-mik\ *n* 1 a : a saclike expansion of the digestive tract communicating anteriorly with the esophagus and posteriorly with the duodenum and being typically a simple often curved sac with an outer serous coat, a strong complex muscular wall that contracts rhythmically, and a mucous lining membrane that contains gastric glands b : one of the compartments of a ruminant stomach

2 : the part of the body that contains the stomach : BELLY, ABDOMEN

stom·ach·ache \-ˌāk\ *n* : pain in or in the region of the stomach

sto·mach·ic \stə-ˈma-kik\ *n* : a stimulant or tonic for the stomach

stomach pump *n* : a suction pump with a flexible tube for removing the contents of the stomach

stomach tube *n* : a flexible tube passed into the stomach (as by way of the nasal passages and esophagus or through a surgical opening in the abdominal wall) for introduction of material (as food) or removal of gastric contents

stomach worm *n* : any of various nematode worms parasitic in the stomach of mammals or birds; *esp* : a worm of the genus *Haemonchus* (*H. contortus*) common in ruminants (as sheep) but rare in humans

sto·mal \ˈstō-məl\ *adj* : of, relating to, or situated near a surgical stoma

stomat- *or* **stomato-** *comb form* : mouth ⟨*stomatitis*⟩ ⟨*stomatology*⟩

sto·ma·ti·tis \ˌstō-mə-ˈtī-təs\ *n, pl* **-ti·ti·des** \-ˈti-tə-ˌdēz\ *or* **-ti·tis·es** \ˌtī-tə-səz\ : any of numerous inflammatory diseases of the mouth — see APHTHOUS STOMATITIS, GANGRENOUS STOMATITIS, VESICULAR STOMATITIS

sto·ma·to·gnath·ic \ˌstō-mə-(ˌ)täg-ˈna-thik\ *adj* : of or relating to the jaws and the mouth

sto·ma·tol·o·gist \ˌstō-mə-ˈtä-lə-jist\ *n* : a specialist in stomatology

sto·ma·tol·o·gy \ˌstō-mə-ˈtä-lə-jē\ *n, pl* **-gies** : a branch of medical science dealing with the mouth and its disorders — **sto·ma·to·log·i·cal** \ˌstō-mət-ᵊl-ˈä-ji-kəl\ *also* **sto·ma·to·log·ic** \-jik\ *adj*

-sto·mia \ˈstō-mē-ə\ *n comb form* : mouth exhibiting (such) a condition ⟨*xerostomia*⟩

sto·mo·de·um *or* **sto·mo·dae·um** \ˌstō-mə-ˈdē-əm\ *n, pl* **-dea** *or* **-daea** \-ˈdē-ə\ *also* **-deums** *or* **-daeums** : the embryonic anterior ectodermal part of the digestive tract — **sto·mo·de·al** *or* **sto·mo·dae·al** \-ˈdē-əl\ *adj*

Sto·mox·ys \stə-ˈmäk-səs\ *n* : a genus of bloodsucking dipteran flies (family Muscidae) that includes the stable fly

-s·to·my \s-tə-mē\ *n comb form, pl* **-s·to·mies** : surgical operation establishing a usu. permanent opening into (such) a part ⟨entero*stomy*⟩

stone \ˈstōn\ *n* : CALCULUS 1

stoned \ˈstōnd\ *adj* : being drunk or under the influence of a drug (as marijuana) taken esp. for pleasure : HIGH

stool \ˈstül\ *n* : a discharge of fecal matter

stop codon *n* : a genetic codon in messenger RNA that signals the termination of protein synthesis during translation

storage disease *n* : the abnormal accumulation in the body of one or more specific substances and esp.

metabolic substances (as cerebrosides in Gaucher's disease) — see GLYCOGEN STORAGE DISEASE

sto·rax \ˈstōr-ˌaks\ *n* **1** : a fragrant balsam obtained from the bark of an Asian tree of the genus *Liquidambar* (*L. orientalis*) that is used as an expectorant — called also *Levant storax* **2** : a balsam similar to storax that is obtained from a No. American tree of the genus *Liquidambar* (*L. styraciflua*) — called also *liquidambar*

storm \ˈstorm\ *n* : a crisis or sudden increase in the symptoms of a disease — see THYROID STORM

stormy \ˈstor-mē\ *adj* **storm·i·er; -est** : having alternating exacerbations and remissions of symptoms

STP \ˌes-(ˌ)tē-ˈpē\ *n* : a hallucinogenic drug chemically related to mescaline and amphetamine — called also *DOM*

stra·bis·mus \strə-ˈbiz-məs\ *n* : inability of one eye to attain binocular vision with the other because of imbalance of the muscles of the eyeball — called also *heterotropia, squint*; compare CROSS-EYE — **stra·bis·mic** \strə-ˈbiz-mik\ *adj*

straightjacket *var of* STRAITJACKET

straight sinus *n* : a venous sinus of the brain that is located along the line of junction of the falx cerebri and tentorium cerebelli and passes posteriorly to terminate in the confluence of sinuses

¹strain \ˈstrān\ *n* : a group of presumed common ancestry with clear-cut physiological but usu. not morphological distinctions ⟨a ∼ of bacteria⟩

²strain *vb* **1 a** : to exert (as oneself) to the utmost **b** : to injure by overuse, misuse, or excessive pressure **2** : to contract the muscles forcefully in attempting to defecate — often used in the phrase *strain at stool*

³strain *n* : an act of straining or the condition of being strained: as **a** : excessive physical or mental tension; *also* : a force, influence, or factor causing such tension **b** : bodily injury from excessive tension, effort, or use ⟨heart ∼⟩; *esp* : one resulting from a wrench or twist and involving undue stretching of muscles or ligaments ⟨back ∼⟩ — compare SPRAIN

strait·jack·et *also* **straight·jack·et** \ˈstrāt-ja-kət\ *n* : a cover or garment of strong material (as canvas) used to bind the body and esp. the arms closely in restraining a violent prisoner or patient

stra·mo·ni·um \strə-ˈmō-nē-əm\ *n* **1** : the dried leaves of the jimsonweed (*Datura stramonium*) or of a related plant of the genus *Datura* containing the alkaloids atropine, hyoscyamine, and scopolamine and used esp. formerly in medicine (as to treat asthma) **2** : JIMSONWEED

strand \ˈstrand\ *n* : something (as a molecular chain) resembling a thread

strand·ed \ˈstran-dəd\ *adj* : having a

strand or strands esp. of a specified kind or number — usu. used in combination <double-*stranded* DNA> — **strand·ed·ness** *n*

stran·gle \'straŋ-gəl\ *vb* **stran·gled; stran·gling 1** : to choke to death **2** : to obstruct seriously or fatally the normal breathing of

stran·gles \-gəlz\ *n sing or pl* : an infectious febrile disease of horses and other equines that is caused by a bacterium of the genus *Streptococcus* (*S. equi*)

stran·gu·lat·ed hernia \'straŋ-gyə-ˌlā-təd-\ *n* : a hernia in which the blood supply of the herniated viscus is so constricted by swelling and congestion as to arrest its circulation

stran·gu·la·tion \ˌstraŋ-gyə-'lā-shən\ *n* **1** : the action or process of strangling or of becoming constricted so as to stop circulation **2** : the state or condition resulting from strangulation; *esp* : excessive or pathological constriction or compression of a bodily tube (as a blood vessel or a loop of intestine) that interrupts its ability to act as a passage — **stran·gu·late** \'straŋ-gyə-ˌlāt\ *vb*

stran·gu·ry \'straŋ-gyə-rē, -ˌgyùr-ē\ *n, pl* **-ries** : a slow and painful discharge of urine drop by drop produced by spasmodic muscular contraction of the urethra and bladder

¹strap \'strap\ *n* : a flexible band or strip

²strap *vb* **strapped; strap·ping 1** : to secure or attach by means of a strap **2** : to support (as a sprained joint) with overlapping strips of adhesive plaster

strapping *n* : the application of adhesive plaster in overlapping strips upon or around a part (as a sprained ankle) to serve as a splint or to hold surgical dressings in place; *also* : material so used

strat·i·fied \'stra-tə-ˌfīd\ *adj* : arranged in layers; *esp* : of, relating to, or being an epithelium consisting of more than one layer of cells — **strat·i·fi·ca·tion** \ˌstra-tə-fə-'kā-shən\ *n*

stra·tum \'strā-təm, 'stra-\ *n, pl* **stra·ta** \'strā-tə, 'stra-\ : a layer of tissue

stratum ba·sa·le \-bā-'sā-lē\ *n, pl* **strata ba·sa·lia** \-lē-ə\ **1** : the basal layer of the epidermis consisting of a single row of columnar or cuboidal epithelial cells that continually divide and replace the rest of the epidermis as it wears away — called also *stratum germinativum;* see MALPIGHIAN LAYER **2** : the deep layer of the endometrium between the stratum spongiosum and the myometrium that is retained during menstruation

stratum com·pac·tum \-kəm-'pak-təm\ *n, pl* **strata com·pac·ta** \-'pak-tə\ : the relatively dense superficial layer of the endometrium

stratum corneum *n, pl* **strata cornea** : the outer more or less horny part of the epidermis

stratum ger·mi·na·ti·vum \-ˌjər-mə-nə-'tī-vəm\ *n, pl* **strata ger·mi·na·ti·va** \-və\ : STRATUM BASALE 1

stratum gran·u·lo·sum \-ˌgran-yə-'lō-səm\ *n, pl* **strata gran·u·lo·sa** \-sə\ : a layer of granular cells lying immediately above the stratum basale in most parts of the epidermis

stratum in·ter·me·di·um \-ˌin-tər-'mē-dē-əm\ *n, pl* **strata in·ter·me·dia** \-dē-ə\ : the cell layer of the enamel organ next to the layer of ameloblasts

stratum lu·ci·dum \-'lü-si-dəm\ *n, pl* **strata lu·ci·da** \-də\ : a thin somewhat translucent layer of cells lying under the stratum corneum esp. in thickened epidermis

stratum spi·no·sum \-spi-'nō-səm\ *n, pl* **strata spi·no·sa** \-sə\ : the layers of prickle cells over the layer of the stratum basale capable of undergoing mitosis — called also *prickle cell layer;* see MALPIGHIAN LAYER

stratum spon·gi·o·sum \-ˌspən-jē-'ō-səm\ *n, pl* **strata spon·gi·o·sa** \-sə\ : the middle layer of the endometrium between the stratum basale and stratum compactum that contains dilated and tortuous portions of the uterine glands

strawberry gallbladder *n* : an abnormal condition characterized by the deposition of cholesterol in the lining of the gallbladder in a pattern resembling the surface of a strawberry

strawberry mark *n* : a tumor of the skin filled with small blood vessels and appearing usu. as a red and elevated birthmark

strawberry tongue *n* : a tongue that is red from swollen congested papillae and that occurs esp. in scarlet fever and Kawasaki disease

¹streak \'strēk\ *n* **1** : a usu. irregular line or stripe — see PRIMITIVE STREAK **2** : inoculum implanted in a line on a solid medium

²streak *vb* : to implant (inoculum) in a line on a solid medium

stream \'strēm\ *n* : an unbroken current or flow (as of a bodily fluid) — see BLOODSTREAM, MIDSTREAM

stream of consciousness *n* : the continuous unedited flow of conscious experience through the mind

street virus *n* : a naturally occurring rabies virus as distinguished from virus attenuated in the laboratory

strength \'streŋth, 'strenth\ *n, pl* **strengths 1** : the quality or state of being strong : capacity for exertion or endurance **2** : degree of potency of effect or of concentration **3** : degree of ionization of a solution — used of acids and bases

strep \'strep\ *n, often attrib* : STREPTOCOCCUS <a ~ infection>

strepho·sym·bo·lia \ˌstre-fō-sim-'bō-lē-ə\ *n* : a learning disorder in which symbols and esp. phrases, words, or letters appear to be reversed or transposed in reading

strep throat *n* : an inflammatory sore throat caused by hemolytic Group A streptococci and marked by fever, prostration, and toxemia — called also *septic sore throat, strep sore throat*

strepto- *comb form* **1** : twisted : twisted chain ⟨*strepto*coccus⟩ **2** : *strepto*coccus ⟨*strepto*kinase⟩

strep·to·ba·cil·lus \ˌstrep-tō-bə-ˈsil-ləs\ *n* **1** *cap* : a genus of facultatively anaerobic gram-negative rod-shaped bacteria (family Fusobacteriaceae) in which the individual cells are often joined in a chain **2** *pl* **-li** \-ˌlī\ : any bacterium of the genus *Streptobacillus; esp* : one (*S. moniliformis*) that is the causative agent of one form of rat-bite fever — **strep·to·ba·cil·la·ry** \-ˈba-sə-ˌler-ē, -bə-ˈsi-lə-rē\ *adj*

strep·to·coc·cal \ˌstrep-tə-ˈkä-kəl\ *also* **strep·to·coc·cic** \-ˈkä-kik, -ˈkäk-sik\ *adj* : of, relating to, caused by, or being streptococci ⟨∼ gingivitis⟩

strep·to·coc·cus \-ˈkä-kəs\ *n* **1** *cap* : a genus of spherical or ovoid chiefly nonmotile and parasitic gram-positive bacteria (family Streptococcaceae) that divide only in one plane, occur in pairs or chains, and include important pathogens of humans and domestic animals **2** *pl* **-coc·ci** \-ˈkä-ˌkī, -ˈkäk-ˌsī\ : any bacterium of the genus *Streptococcus; broadly* : a coccus occurring in chains

strep·to·dor·nase \ˌstrep-tō-ˈdor-ˌnās, -ˌnāz\ *n* : a deoxyribonuclease from hemolytic streptococci that dissolves pus and is usu. administered in a mixture with streptokinase — see VARIDASE

strep·to·gram·in \ˌstrep-tō-ˈgra-mən\ *n* : an antibiotic complex produced by a bacterium of the genus *Streptomyces* (*S. graminofaciens*)

strep·to·ki·nase \ˌstrep-tō-ˈki-ˌnās, -ˌnāz\ *n* : a proteolytic enzyme produced by hemolytic streptococci that promotes the dissolution of blood clots by activating plasminogen to produce plasmin — see VARIDASE

strep·to·ly·sin \ˌstrep-tə-ˈlīs-ᵊn\ *n* : any of various antigenic hemolysins produced by streptococci

strep·to·my·ces \-ˈmī-ˌsēz\ *n* **1** *cap* : a genus of mostly soil streptomycetes including some that form antibiotics as by-products of their metabolism **2** *pl* **streptomyces** : any bacterium of the genus *Streptomyces*

strep·to·my·cete \-ˈmī-ˌsēt, -mī-ˈsēt\ *n* : any of a family (Streptomycetaceae) of actinomycetes that are typically aerobic soil saprophytes but include a few parasites of plants and animals

strep·to·my·cin \-ˈmīs-ᵊn\ *n* : an antibiotic $C_{21}H_{39}N_7O_{12}$ that is produced by a soil actinomycete of the genus *Streptomyces* (*S. griseus*), is active against bacteria, and is used esp. in the treatment of infections (as tuberculosis) by gram-negative bacteria

strep·to·ni·grin \-ˈnī-grən\ *n* : a toxic antibiotic $C_{25}H_{22}N_4O_8$ from an actinomycete of the genus *Streptomyces* (*S. flocculus*) that is used as an antineoplastic agent

strep·to·zo·cin \ˌstrep-tə-ˈzō-sən\ *n* : STREPTOZOTOCIN

strep·to·zot·o·cin \ˌstrep-tə-ˈzä-tə-sən\ *n* : a broad-spectrum antibiotic $C_8H_{15}N_3O_7$ with antineoplastic and diabetogenic properties that has been isolated from a bacterium of the genus *Streptomyces* (*S. achromogenes*)

stress \ˈstres\ *n* **1 a** : a force exerted when one body or body part presses on, pulls on, pushes against, or tends to compress or twist another body or body part **b** : the deformation caused in a body by such a force **2 a** : a physical, chemical, or emotional factor that causes bodily or mental tension and may be a factor in disease causation **b** : a state of bodily or mental tension resulting from factors that tend to alter an existent equilibrium **3** : the force exerted between teeth of the upper and lower jaws during mastication — **stress** *vb* — **stress·ful** \ˈstres-fəl\ *adj* — **stress·ful·ly** *adv*

stress breaker *n* : a flexible dental device used to lessen the occlusal forces exerted on teeth to which a partial denture is attached

stress fracture *n* : a usu. hairline fracture of a bone (as of the foot) that has been subjected to repeated stress

stress incontinence *n* : involuntary leakage of urine from the bladder accompanying physical activity (as in laughing or coughing) which places increased pressure on the abdomen — compare URGE INCONTINENCE

stress·or \ˈstre-sər, -ˌsor\ *n* : a stimulus that causes stress

stress test *n* : an electrocardiographic test of heart function before, during, and after a controlled period of increasingly strenuous exercise (as on a treadmill)

¹**stretch** \ˈstrech\ *vb* **1** : to extend or become extended in length or breadth **2** : to enlarge or distend esp. by force

²**stretch** *n* : the act of stretching : the state of being stretched

stretch·er \ˈstre-chər\ *n* : a device for carrying a sick, injured, or dead person

stretch·er–bear·er \-ˌbar-ər\ *n* : a person who carries one end of a stretcher

stretch marks *n pl* : striae on the skin (as of the hips, abdomen, and breasts) from excessive stretching and rupture of elastic fibers esp. due to pregnancy or obesity

stretch receptor *n* : MUSCLE SPINDLE

stretch reflex *n* : a spinal reflex involving reflex contraction of a muscle in response to stretching — called also *myotatic reflex*

stria \ˈstrī-ə\ *n, pl* **stri·ae** \ˈstrī-ˌē\ **1** : STRIATION 2 **2** : a narrow structural band esp. of nerve fibers **3** : a stripe or line (as in the skin) distinguished from surrounding tissue by color, texture, or elevation — see STRETCH MARKS

striata *pl of* STRIATUM

stri·a·tal \strī-'āt-ºl\ *adj* : of or relating to the corpus striatum ⟨∼ neurons⟩

striate cortex \'strī-ət-, -ˌāt-\ *n* : an area of the brain that receives visual impulses, contains a conspicuous band of myelinated fibers, and is located mostly in the walls and along the edges of the calcarine sulcus of the occipital lobe — called also *visual projection area*

stri·at·ed \'strī-ˌā-təd\ *adj* 1 : marked with striae 2 : of, relating to, or being striated muscle

striated muscle *n* : muscle tissue that is marked by transverse dark and light bands, that is made up of elongated fibers, and that includes skeletal and usu. cardiac muscle — compare SMOOTH MUSCLE, VOLUNTARY MUSCLE

stria ter·mi·na·lis \-ˌtər-mə-'nā-ləs\ : a bundle of nerve fibers that passes from the amygdala mostly to the anterior part of the hypothalamus with a few fibers crossing the anterior commissure to the amygdala on the opposite side

stri·a·tion \strī-'ā-shən\ *n* 1 : the fact or state of being striated 2 : a minute groove, scratch, or channel esp. when one of a parallel series 3 : any of the alternate dark and light cross bands of a myofibril of striated muscle

stri·a·to·ni·gral \strī-ˌā-tə-'nī-grəl\ *adj* : connecting the corpus striatum and substantia nigra ⟨∼ axons⟩

stri·a·tum \strī-'ā-təm\ *n, pl* **stri·a·ta** \-'ā-tə\ 1 : CORPUS STRIATUM 2 : NEOSTRIATUM

stria vas·cu·la·ris \-ˌvas-kyə-'ler-əs\ : the upper part of the spiral ligament of the cochlear duct that contains numerous small blood vessels

stric·ture \'strik-chər\ *n* : an abnormal narrowing of a bodily passage (as from inflammation or the formation of scar tissue); *also* : the narrowed part

stri·dor \'strī-dər, -ˌdȯr\ *n* : a harsh vibrating sound heard during respiration in cases of obstruction of the air passages ⟨laryngeal ∼⟩ — **strid·u·lous** \'stri-jə-ləs\ *adj*

stridulus — see LARYNGISMUS STRIDULUS

strike \'strīk\ *n* : cutaneous myiasis (as of sheep) ⟨body ∼⟩ ⟨blowfly ∼⟩

string·halt \'striŋ-ˌhȯlt\ *n* : a condition of lameness in the hind legs of a horse caused by muscular spasms — **string-halt·ed** \-ˌhȯl-təd\ *adj*

strip \'strip\ *vb* **stripped** \'stript\ *also* **stript**; **strip·ping** : to remove (a vein) by means of a stripper

strip·per \'strip-pər\ *n* : a surgical instrument used for removal of a vein

stroke \'strōk\ *n* : sudden diminution or loss of consciousness, sensation, and voluntary motion caused by rupture or obstruction (as by a clot) of a blood vessel of the brain — called also *apoplexy, brain attack, cerebral accident, cerebrovascular accident;* see HEMORRHAGIC STROKE, ISCHEMIC STROKE

stroke volume *n* : the volume of blood pumped from a ventricle of the heart in one beat

stro·ma \'strō-mə\ *n, pl* **stro·ma·ta** \-mə-tə\ 1 : the supporting framework of an animal organ typically consisting of connective tissue 2 : the spongy protoplasmic framework of some cells (as a red blood cell) — **stro·mal** \-məl\ *adj*

strong silver protein *n* : SILVER PROTEIN b

stron·gyle \'strän-ˌjīl\ *n* : STRONGYLID; *esp* : a worm of the genus *Strongylus* or closely related genera that is parasitic esp. in the intestines and tissues of the horse

stron·gy·lid \'strän-jə-lid\ *n* : any of a family (Strongylidae) of nematode worms that are parasites of vertebrates — **strongylid** *adj*

stron·gy·li·do·sis \ˌsträn-jə-lə-'dō-səs\ *n* : STRONGYLOSIS

stron·gy·loid \'strän-jə-ˌlȯid\ *n* : any of a superfamily (Strongyloidea) of nematode worms including the hookworms, strongyles, and related forms — **strongyloid** *adj*

Stron·gy·loi·des \ˌsträn-jə-'lȯi-ˌdēz\ *n* : a genus of nematode worms (family Strongyloididae) having both free-living males and females and parthenogenetic females parasitic in the intestine of various vertebrates and including some medically and economically important pests of humans

stron·gy·loi·di·a·sis \ˌsträn-jə-ˌlȯi-'dī-ə-səs\ *n, pl* **-a·ses** \-ə-ˌsēz\ : infestation with or disease caused by nematodes of the genus *Strongyloides*

stron·gy·loi·do·sis \-'dō-səs\ : STRONGYLOIDIASIS

stron·gy·lo·sis \ˌsträn-jə-'lō-səs\ *n* : infestation with or disease caused by strongyles — called also *strongylidosis*

Stron·gy·lus \'strän-jə-ləs\ *n* : a genus of strongylid nematode worms including gastrointestinal parasites of the horse

stron·tium \'strän-chəm, -chē-əm, -tē-əm\ *n* : a soft malleable ductile bivalent metallic element — symbol *Sr;* see ELEMENT table

strontium 90 *n* : a heavy radioactive isotope of strontium having the mass number 90 that is present in the fallout from nuclear explosions and is hazardous because like calcium it can be assimilated in biological processes and deposited in the bones — called also *radiostrontium*

stro·phan·thin \strō-'fan-thən\ *n* : a bitter toxic glycoside $C_{36}H_{54}O_{14}$ from a woody vine of the genus *Strophanthus* (*S. kombé*) used similarly to digitalis; *also* : a related glycoside (as ouabain)

stro·phan·thus \-thəs\ *n* **1** *cap* : a genus of Asian and African trees, shrubs, or woody vines of the dogbane family (Apocynaceae) including one (*S. kombé*) that yields strophanthin **2** : the dried seeds of any of several plants of the genus *Strophanthus* (as *S. kombé* and *S. hispidus*) that contain strophanthin and are in moderate doses a cardiac stimulant but in larger doses a violent poison

struck \'strək\ *n* : enterotoxemia esp. of adult sheep

struc·tur·al \'strək-chə-rəl\ *adj* **1** : of or relating to the physical makeup of a plant or animal body ⟨~ defects of the heart⟩ — compare FUNCTIONAL 1a **2** : of, relating to, or affecting structure ⟨~ stability⟩ — **struc·tur·al·ly** *adv*

structural formula *n* : an expanded molecular formula (as H-O-H for water) showing the arrangement within the molecule of atoms and of bonds

structural gene *n* : a gene that codes for the amino acid sequence of a protein (as an enzyme) or for a ribosomal RNA or transfer RNA

struc·tur·al·ism \'strək-chə-rə-ˌli-zəm\ *n* : psychology concerned esp. with resolution of the mind into structural elements

struc·ture \'strək-chər\ *n* **1** : something (as an anatomical part) arranged in a definite pattern of organization **2 a** : the arrangement of particles or parts in a substance or body ⟨molecular ~⟩ **b** : organization of parts as dominated by the general character of the whole ⟨personality ~⟩ **3** : the aggregate of elements of an entity in their relationships to each other

stru·ma \'strü-mə\ *n, pl* **-mae** \-(ˌ)mē\ *or* **-mas** : GOITER

struma lym·pho·ma·to·sa \-ˌlim-ˌfō-mə-'tō-sə\ *n* : HASHIMOTO'S THYROIDITIS

stru·vite \'strü-ˌvīt\ *n* : a hydrated magnesium-containing mineral Mg(NH₄)(PO₄)·6H₂O which is found in kidney stones associated with bacteria that cleave urea

strych·nine \'strik-ˌnīn, -nən, -ˌnēn\ *n* : a bitter poisonous alkaloid $C_{21}H_{22}N_2O_2$ that is obtained from nux vomica and related plants of the genus *Strychnos* and is used as a poison (as for rodents) and medicinally as a stimulant of the central nervous system

Strych·nos \'strik-nəs, -ˌnäs\ *n* : a large genus of tropical trees and woody vines (family Loganiaceae) — see CURARE, NUX VOMICA, STRYCHNINE

STS *abbr* serologic test for syphilis

ST segment *or* **S–T segment** \ˌes-'tē-\ *n* : the part of an electrocardiogram between the QRS complex and the T wave

Stu·art–Prow·er factor \'stü-ərt-'prau̇-ər-, -'styü-\ *n* : FACTOR X

  Stuart and Prower, 20th-century hospital patients.

stuff \'stəf\ *vb* : to choke or block up (as nasal passages) ⟨a ~ed up nose⟩ — **stuff·i·ness** \'stə-fē-nəs\ *n* — **stuffy** \'stəf-ē\ *adj*

stump \'stəmp\ *n* **1** : the basal portion of a bodily part (as a limb) remaining after the rest is removed **2** : a rudimentary or vestigial bodily part

stung *past and past part of* STING

stunt \'stənt\ *vb* : to hinder the normal growth, development, or progress of

stupe \'stüp, 'styüp\ *n* : a hot wet often medicated cloth applied externally (as to stimulate circulation)

stu·pe·fy \'stü-pə-ˌfī, 'styü-\ *vb* **-fied; -fy·ing** : to make stupid, groggy, or insensible — **stu·pe·fac·tion** \ˌstü-pə-'fak-shən, ˌstyü-\ *n*

stu·por \'stü-pər, 'styü-\ *n* : a condition of greatly dulled or completely suspended sense or sensibility ⟨a drunken ~⟩; *specif* : a chiefly mental condition marked by absence of spontaneous movement, greatly diminished responsiveness to stimulation, and usu. impaired consciousness — **stu·por·ous** \'stü-pə-rəs, 'styü-\ *adj*

stur·dy \'stər-dē\ *n, pl* **sturdies** : GID

Sturge–Web·er syndrome \'stərj-'we-bər-\ *n* : a rare congenital condition that is characterized by a port-wine stain affecting the facial skin on one side in the area innervated by the first branch of the trigeminal nerve and by malformed blood vessels in the brain that may cause progressive mental retardation, epilepsy, and glaucoma in the eye on the affected side — called also *Sturge-Weber disease*

  Sturge, William Allen (1850–1919), and Weber, Frederick Parkes (1863–1962), British physicians.

stut·ter \'stə-tər\ *vb* : to speak with involuntary disruption or blocking of speech (as by repetition or prolongation of vocal sounds) — **stutter** *n* — **stut·ter·er** \'stə-tər-ər\ *n*

stuttering *n* **1** : the act of one who stutters **2** : a disorder of vocal communication that is marked esp. by involuntary disruption or blocking of speech (as by repetition or prolongation of vocal sounds or inability to start a word) and that is typically accompanied by fear and anxiety and by a struggle to avoid speech errors

sty *or* **stye** \'stī\ *n, pl* **sties** *or* **styes** : an inflamed swelling of a sebaceous gland at the margin of an eyelid — called also *hordeolum*

styl- *or* **stylo-** *comb form* : styloid process ⟨*stylo*glossus⟩

sty·let \stī-'let, 'stī-lət\ *also* **sty·lette** \stī-'let\ *n* **1** : a slender surgical probe **2** : a thin wire inserted into a catheter to maintain rigidity or into a hollow needle to maintain patency

sty·lo·glos·sus \ˌstī-lō-ˈglä-səs, -ˈglȯ-\ *n, pl* **-glos·si** \-ˈglä-ˌsī, -ˈglȯ-\ : a muscle that arises from the styloid process of the temporal bone, inserts along the side and underpart of the tongue, and functions to draw the tongue upwards

sty·lo·hy·oid \ˌstī-lō-ˈhī-ˌȯid\ *n* : STYLOHYOID MUSCLE

sty·lo·hy·oi·de·us \-ˈhī-ˈȯi-dē-əs\ *n, pl* **-dei** \-dē-ˌī\ : STYLOHYOID MUSCLE

stylohyoid ligament *n* : a band of fibrous tissue connecting the tip of the styloid process of the temporal bone to the ceratohyal of the hyoid bone

stylohyoid muscle *n* : a slender muscle that arises from the posterior surface of the styloid process of the temporal bone, inserts into the body of the hyoid bone, and acts to elevate and retract the hyoid bone resulting in elongation of the floor of the mouth — called also *stylohyoid, stylohyoideus*

sty·loid \ˈstī-ˌlȯid\ *adj* : having a slender pointed shape

styloid process *n* : any of several long slender pointed bony processes: as **a** : a sharp spine that projects downward and forward from the inferior surface of the temporal bone just in front of the stylomastoid foramen **b** : an eminence on the distal extremity of the ulna giving attachment to a ligament of the wrist joint **c** : a conical prolongation of the lateral surface of the distal extremity of the radius that gives attachment to several tendons and ligaments

sty·lo·man·dib·u·lar ligament \ˌstī-lō-man-ˈdi-byə-lər\ *n* : a band of deep fascia that connects the styloid process of the temporal bone to the gonial angle

sty·lo·mas·toid foramen \-ˈmas-ˌtȯid-\ *n* : a foramen that occurs on the lower surface of the temporal bone between the styloid and mastoid processes

sty·lo·pha·ryn·ge·us \ˌstī-lō-fə-ˈrin-jē-əs, -ˌfar-ən-ˈjē-əs\ *n, pl* **-gei** \-jē-ˌī\ : a slender muscle that arises from the base of the styloid process of the temporal bone, inserts into the side of the pharynx, and acts with the contralateral muscle in swallowing to increase the transverse diameter of the pharynx by drawing its sides upward and laterally

¹**styp·tic** \ˈstip-tik\ *adj* : tending to check bleeding; *esp* : having the property of arresting oozing of blood (as from a shallow surface injury) when applied to a bleeding part ⟨~ agent⟩

²**styptic** *n* : an agent (as a drug) having a styptic effect

styptic pencil *n* : a cylindrical stick of a medicated styptic substance used esp. in shaving to stop the bleeding from small cuts

sub- *prefix* **1** : under : beneath : below ⟨*sub*coastal⟩ **2** : subordinate portion of : subdivision of ⟨*sub*species⟩ **3**

: less than completely or perfectly ⟨*sub*normal⟩

sub·acro·mi·al \ˌsəb-ə-ˈkrō-mē-əl\ *adj* : of, relating to, or affecting the subacromial bursa ⟨~ bursitis⟩

subacromial bursa *n* : a bursa lying between the acromion and the capsule of the shoulder joint

sub·acute \ˌsəb-ə-ˈkyüt\ *adj* **1** : falling between acute and chronic in character esp. when closer to acute ⟨~ endocarditis⟩ **2** : less marked in severity or duration than a corresponding acute state ⟨~ pain⟩ — **sub·acute·ly** *adv*

subacute sclerosing panencephalitis *n* : a usu. fatal neurological disease of children and young adults that is caused by infection of the brain by a previously latent morbillivirus causing measles and that is marked esp. by behavioral changes, myoclonic seizures, progressive deterioration of motor and mental functioning, and coma — abbr. *SSPE*

sub·aor·tic stenosis \ˌsəb-ā-ˈȯr-tik-\ *n* : aortic stenosis produced by an obstruction in the left ventricle below the aortic valve

sub·arach·noid \ˌsəb-ə-ˈrak-ˌnȯid\ *also* **sub·arach·noi·dal** \-rak-ˈnȯid-ᵊl\ *adj* **1** : situated or occurring under the arachnoid membrane ⟨~ hemorrhage⟩ **2** : of, relating to, or involving the subarachnoid space and the fluid within it ⟨~ meningitis⟩

subarachnoid space *n* : the space between the arachnoid and the pia mater through which the cerebrospinal fluid circulates

sub·cal·lo·sal \ˌsəb-ka-ˈlō-səl\ *adj* : situated below the corpus callosum

subcallosal area *n* : a small area of cortex in each cerebral hemisphere below the genu of the corpus callosum

sub·cap·su·lar \ˌsəb-ˈkap-sə-lər\ *adj* : situated or occurring beneath or within a capsule ⟨~ cataracts⟩

subcarbonate — see BISMUTH SUBCARBONATE

sub·cel·lu·lar \ˌsəb-ˈsel-yə-lər\ *adj* **1** : of less than cellular scope or level of organization **2** : relating to or being local or restricted area within a cell

sub·chon·dral \-ˈkän-drəl\ *adj* : situated beneath cartilage ⟨~ bone⟩

sub·cho·roi·dal \ˌsəb-kə-ˈrȯid-ᵊl\ *adj* : situated or occurring between the choroid and the retina ⟨~ fluid⟩

sub·class \ˈsəb-ˌklas\ *n* : a category in biological classification ranking below a class and above an order

subclavia — see ANSA SUBCLAVIA

¹**sub·cla·vi·an** \ˌsəb-ˈklā-vē-ən\ *adj* : of, relating to, being, performed on, or inserted into a part (as an artery or vein) located under the clavicle ⟨a ~ catheter⟩

²**subclavian** *n* : a subclavian part

subclavian artery *n* : the proximal part of the main artery of the arm that arises on the right side from the brachiocephalic artery and on the left side from the arch of the aorta and that supplies or gives off branches supplying the brain, neck, anterior wall of the thorax, and shoulder

subclavian trunk *n* : a large lymphatic vessel on each side of the body that receives lymph from the axilla and arms and that on the right side empties into the right lymphatic duct and on the left side into the thoracic duct

subclavian vein *n* : the proximal part of the main vein of the arm that is a continuation of the axillary vein and extends from the level of the first rib to the sternal end of the clavicle where it unites with the internal jugular vein to form the brachiocephalic vein

sub·cla·vi·us \ˌsəb-ˈklā-vē-əs\ *n, pl* **-vii** \-vē-ˌī\ : a small muscle on each side of the body that arises from the junction of the first rib and its cartilage, inserts into the inferior surface of the clavicle, and acts to stabilize the clavicle by depressing and drawing forward its lateral end during movements of the shoulder joint

sub·clin·i·cal \ˈkli-ni-kəl\ *adj* : not detectable or producing effects that are not detectable by the usual clinical tests ⟨a ~ infection⟩ ⟨~ cancer⟩ — **sub·clin·i·cal·ly** *adv*

sub·con·junc·ti·val \ˌsəb-ˌkän-jəŋk-ˈti-vəl\ *adj* : situated or occurring beneath the conjunctiva ⟨~ hemorrhage⟩ — **sub·con·junc·ti·val·ly** *adv*

¹sub·con·scious \ˌsəb-ˈkän-chəs\ *adj* **1** : existing in the mind but not immediately available to consciousness : affecting thought, feeling, and behavior without entering awareness **2** : imperfectly conscious : partially but not fully aware — **sub·con·scious·ly** *adv* — **sub·con·scious·ness** *n*

²subconscious *n* : the mental activities just below the threshold of consciousness; *also* : the aspect of the mind concerned with such activities — compare UNCONSCIOUS

sub·cor·a·coid \-ˈkōr-ə-ˌkȯid\ *adj* : situated or occurring under the coracoid process of the scapula

sub·cor·ti·cal \-ˈkȯr-ti-kəl\ *adj* : of, relating to, involving, or being nerve centers below the cerebral cortex ⟨~ lesions⟩ — **sub·cor·ti·cal·ly** *adv*

sub·cos·tal \-ˈkäs-təl, -ˈkȯs-\ *adj* : situated or performed below a rib

subcostal artery *n* : either of a pair of arteries that are the most posterior branches of the thoracic aorta and follow a course beneath the last pair of ribs

sub·cos·ta·lis \-käs-ˈtā-ləs, -kȯs-\ *n, pl* **-ta·les** \-ˌlēz\ : any of a variable number of small muscles that arise on the inner surface of a rib, are inserted into the inner surface of the second or third rib below, and prob. function to draw adjacent ribs together

subcostal vein *n* : either of two veins: **a** : one that arises on the right side of the anterior abdominal wall and joins in the formation of the azygos vein — called also *right subcostal vein* **b** : one on the left side of the body that usu. empties into the hemiazygos vein — called also *left subcostal vein*

sub·cul·ture \ˈsəb-ˌkəl-chər\ *n* **1** : a culture (as of bacteria) derived from another culture **2** : an act or instance of producing a subculture — **subculture** *vb*

subcutanea — see TELA SUBCUTANEA

sub·cu·ta·ne·ous \ˌsəb-kyü-ˈtā-nē-əs\ *adj* : being, living, used, or made under the skin ⟨~ parasites⟩ — **sub·cu·ta·ne·ous·ly** *adv*

subcutaneous bursa *n* : a bursa lying between the skin and a bony process or a ligament

subcutaneous emphysema *n* : the presence of a gas and esp. air in the subcutaneous tissue

sub·cu·tic·u·lar \-kyü-ˈti-kyə-lər\ *adj* : situated or occurring beneath a cuticle ⟨~ sutures⟩ ⟨~ tissues⟩

sub·cu·tis \ˌsəb-ˈkyü-təs\ *n* : the deeper part of the dermis

sub·del·toid \ˌsəb-ˈdel-ˌtȯid\ *adj* : situated underneath or inferior to the deltoid muscle ⟨~ calcareous deposits⟩

subdeltoid bursa *n* : the bursa that lies beneath the deltoid muscle

sub·der·mal \-ˈdər-məl\ *adj* : SUBCUTANEOUS — **sub·der·mal·ly** *adv*

sub·di·a·phrag·mat·ic \ˌsəb-ˌdī-ə-fra-ˈma-tik, -ˌfrag-\ *adj* : situated, occurring, or performed below the diaphragm ⟨a ~ abscess⟩

subdivision *n* : a category in botanical classification ranking below a division and above a class

sub·du·ral \ˌsəb-ˈdu̇r-əl, -ˈdyu̇r-\ *adj* : situated, occurring, or performed under the dura mater or between the dura mater and the arachnoid ⟨~ empyema⟩ — **sub·du·ral·ly** *adv*

subdural hematoma *n* : a hematoma that occurs between the dura mater and arachnoid in the subdural space

subdural space *n* : a fluid-filled space or potential space between the dura mater and the arachnoid

sub·en·do·car·di·al \ˌsəb-ˌen-dō-ˈkär-dē-əl\ *adj* : situated or occurring beneath the endocardium or between the endocardium and myocardium

sub·en·do·the·li·al \-ˌen-dō-ˈthē-lē-əl\ *adj* : situated under an endothelium

sub·ep·en·dy·mal \-e-ˈpen-də-məl\ *adj* : situated under the ependyma

sub·epi·der·mal \ˌsəb-ˌe-pə-ˈdər-məl\ *adj* : lying beneath or constituting the innermost part of the epidermis

sub·epi·the·li·al \-ˌe-pə-ˈthē-lē-əl\ *adj* : situated or occurring beneath an epithelial layer; *also* : SUBCUTANEOUS

sub·fam·i·ly \ˈsəb-ˌfam-lē\ *n* : a category in biological classification ranking below a family and above a genus

sub·fas·cial \-ˈfa-shəl, -shē-əl\ *adj* : situated, occurring, or performed below a fascia ⟨∼ tumor⟩ ⟨∼ suturing⟩

sub·fe·brile \-ˈfe-ˌbrīl, -ˈfē-\ *adj* : of, relating to, or constituting a body temperature very slightly above normal but not febrile

sub·fer·til·i·ty \-fər-ˈti-lə-tē\ *n, pl* **-ties** : the condition of being less than normally fertile though still capable of effecting fertilization — **sub·fer·tile** \-ˈfərt-ᵊl\ *adj*

sub·ge·nus \ˈsəb-ˌjē-nəs\ *n, pl* **-gen·e·ra** \-ˌje-nər-ə\ : a category in biological classification ranking below a genus and above a species

sub·gin·gi·val \ˌsəb-ˈjin-jə-vəl\ *adj* : situated, performed, or occurring beneath the gums and esp. between the gums and the basal part of the crowns of the teeth — **sub·gin·gi·val·ly** *adv*

sub·glot·tic \-ˈglä-tik\ *adj* : situated or occurring below the glottis

su·bic·u·lum \sə-ˈbi-kyə-ləm\ *n, pl* **-la** \-lə\ : a part of the parahippocampal gyrus that is a ventral continuation of the hippocampus and is situated ventrally and medially to the dentate gyrus; *also* : a section of this that borders the hippocampal sulcus — **su·bic·u·lar** \-lər\ *adj*

sub·in·tern \-ˈin-ˌtərn\ *n* : a medical student in the last year of medical school who performs work supervised by interns and residents in a hospital

sub·in·ti·mal \-ˈin-tə-məl\ *adj* : situated beneath an intima and esp. between the intima and media of an artery

sub·in·vo·lu·tion \-ˌin-və-ˈlü-shən\ *n* : partial or incomplete involution

sub·ja·cent \ˌsəb-ˈjās-ᵊnt\ *adj* : lying immediately under or below ⟨∼ tissue⟩

sub·ject \ˈsəb-jikt\ *n* **1** : an individual whose reactions or responses are studied **2** : a dead body for anatomical study and dissection

sub·jec·tive \(ˌ)səb-ˈjek-tiv\ *adj* **1 a** : relating to or determined by the mind as the subject of experience ⟨∼ reality⟩ **b** : characteristic of or belonging to reality as perceived rather than as independent of mind **c** : relating to or being experience or knowledge as conditioned by personal mental characteristics or states **2 a** : arising from conditions within the brain or sense organs and not directly caused by external stimuli ⟨∼ sensations⟩ **b** : arising out of or identified by means of one's perception of one's own states and processes and not observable by an examiner ⟨a ∼ symptom of disease⟩ — compare OBJECTIVE 2 — **sub·jec·tive·ly** *adv*

subjective vertigo *n* : vertigo characterized by a sensation that one's body is revolving in space

sub·le·thal \ˌsəb-ˈlē-thəl\ *adj* : less than but usu. only slightly less than lethal ⟨a ∼ dose⟩

sub·li·ma·tion \ˌsə-blə-ˈmā-shən\ *n* : the process of converting and expressing a primitive instinctual desire or impulse to a form that is socially or culturally acceptable — **sub·li·mate** \ˈsə-blə-ˌmāt\ *vb*

sub·lim·i·nal \(ˌ)səb-ˈli-mə-nəl\ *adj* **1** : inadequate to produce a sensation or a perception **2** : existing or functioning below the threshold of consciousness ⟨the ∼ mind⟩ ⟨∼ advertising⟩ — **sub·lim·i·nal·ly** *adv*

¹sub·lin·gual \ˌsəb-ˈliŋ-gwəl, -gyə-wəl\ *adj* **1** : situated or administered under the tongue ⟨∼ tablets⟩ **2** : of or relating to the sublingual glands — **sub·lin·gual·ly** *adv*

²sublingual *n* : SUBLINGUAL GLAND

sublingual gland *n* : a small salivary gland on each side of the mouth lying beneath the mucous membrane in a fossa in the mandible near the symphysis — called also *sublingual salivary gland*

sub·lob·u·lar vein \ˌsəb-ˈlä-byə-lər-\ *n* : one of several veins in the liver into which the central veins empty and which in turn empty into the hepatic veins

sub·lux·a·tion \ˌsəb-ˌlək-ˈsā-shən\ *n* : partial dislocation (as of one of the bones in a joint) — **sub·lux·at·ed** \ˈsəb-ˌlək-ˌsā-təd\ *adj*

¹sub·man·dib·u·lar \ˌsəb-man-ˈdi-byə-lər\ *adj* **1** : of, relating to, situated, or performed in the region below the lower jaw **2** : of, relating to, or associated with the submandibular glands

²submandibular *n* : a submandibular part (as an artery or bone)

submandibular ganglion *n* : an autonomic ganglion that is situated on the hyoglossus muscle above the deep part of the submandibular gland, receives preganglionic fibers from the facial nerve, and sends postganglionic fibers to the submandibular and sublingual glands — called also *submaxillary ganglion*

submandibular gland *n* : a salivary gland inside of and near the lower edge of the mandible on each side and discharging by Wharton's duct into the mouth under the tongue — called also *submandibular salivary gland, submaxillary gland, submaxillary salivary gland*

sub·max·il·lary \ˌsəb-ˈmak-sə-ˌler-ē\ *adj or n* : SUBMANDIBULAR

submaxillary ganglion *n* : SUBMANDIBULAR GANGLION

submaxillary gland *n* : SUBMANDIBULAR GLAND

submaxillary salivary gland *n* : SUBMANDIBULAR GLAND

sub·max·i·mal \ˌsəb-ˈmak-sə-məl\ *adj* : being less than the maximum of which an individual is capable

sub·men·tal \-ˈment-ᵊl\ *adj* : located in, affecting, or performed on the area under the chin

submental artery *n* : a branch of the

facial artery that branches off near the submandibular gland and is distributed to the muscles of the jaw

sub·meta·cen·tric \,səb-,me-tə-'sen-trik\ *adj* : having the centromere situated so that one chromosome arm is somewhat shorter than the other — **submetacentric** *n*

sub·mi·cro·scop·ic \,səb-,mī-krə-'skä-pik\ *adj* : too small to be seen in an ordinary light microscope ⟨∼ particles⟩ — compare MICROSCOPIC 2 — **sub·mi·cro·scop·i·cal·ly** *adv*

sub·mis·sion \səb-'mi-shən\ *n* : the condition of being submissive

sub·mis·sive \-'mi-səv\ *adj* : characterized by tendencies to yield to the will or authority of others ⟨a ∼ personality⟩ — **sub·mis·sive·ness** *n*

sub·mu·co·sa \,səb-myü-'kō-sə\ *n* : a supporting layer of loose connective tissue directly under a mucous membrane — **sub·mu·co·sal** \-zəl\ *adj*

sub·mu·cous \,səb-'myü-kəs\ *adj* : lying under or involving the tissues under a mucous membrane

subnitrate — see BISMUTH SUBNITRATE

sub·nor·mal \,səb-'nȯr-məl\ *adj* **1** : lower or smaller than normal ⟨a ∼ temperature⟩ **2** : having less of something and esp. of intelligence than is normal — **sub·nor·mal·i·ty** \,səb-nȯr-'ma-lə-tē\ *n*

sub·oc·cip·i·tal \-äk-'si-pət-ᵊl\ *adj* **1** : situated or performed below the occipital bone **2** : situated or performed below the occipital lobe of the brain

suboccipital nerve *n* : the first cervical nerve that supplies muscles around the suboccipital triangle and that sends branches to the rectus capitis posterior minor and semispinalis capitis

suboccipital triangle *n* : a space of the suboccipital region on each side of the dorsal cervical region that is bounded superiorly and medially by a muscle arising by a tendon from a spinous process of the axis and inserting into the inferior nuchal line and the adjacent inferior region of the occipital bone, that is bounded superiorly and laterally by the obliquus capitis superior, and that is bounded inferiorly and laterally by the obliquus capitis inferior

sub·op·ti·mal \,səb-'äp-tə-məl\ *adj* : less than optimal ⟨a ∼ dose⟩

sub·or·der \'səb-,ȯr-dər\ *n* : a category in biological classification ranking below an order and above a family

sub·peri·os·te·al \-,per-ē-'äs-tē-əl\ *adj* : situated or occurring beneath the periosteum — **sub·peri·os·te·al·ly** *adv*

sub·phren·ic \,səb-'fre-nik\ *adj* : situated or occurring below the diaphragm

subphrenic space *n* : a space on each side of the falciform ligament be-

tween the underside of the diaphragm and the upper side of the liver

sub·phy·lum \'səb-,fī-ləm\ *n, pl* **-la** \-lə\ : a category in biological classification ranking below a phylum and above a class

sub·pleu·ral \,səb-'plu̇r-əl\ *adj* : situated or occurring between the pleura and the body wall — **sub·pleu·ral·ly** *adv*

sub·pop·u·la·tion \,səb-,pä-pyə-'lā-shən\ *n* : an identifiable fraction or subdivision of a population

sub·po·tent \,səb-'pōt-ᵊnt\ *adj* : less potent than normal ⟨∼ drugs⟩ — **sub·po·ten·cy** \-'pōt-ᵊn-sē\ *n*

sub·pu·bic angle \,səb-'pyü-bik-\ *n* : the angle that is formed just below the pubic symphysis by the meeting of the inferior ramus of the pubis on one side with the corresponding part on the other side

sub·ret·i·nal \-'ret-ᵊn-əl\ *adj* : situated or occurring beneath the retina

sub·sa·lic·y·late \-sə-'li-sə-,lāt\ *n* : a basic salicylate (as bismuth subsalicylate)

sub·sar·co·lem·mal \-,sär-kə-'le-məl\ *adj* : situated or occurring beneath a sarcolemma ⟨∼ mitochondria⟩

sub·scap·u·lar \,səb-'ska-pyə-lər\ *adj* : situated under the scapula

subscapular artery *n* : an artery that is usu. the largest branch of the axillary artery, that arises opposite the lower border of the subscapularis muscle, and that passes down and back to the lower part of the scapula where it forms branches and anastomoses with arteries in that region

subscapular fossa *n* : the concave depression of the anterior surface of the scapula

sub·scap·u·lar·is \,səb-,ska-pyə-'lar-əs\ *n* : a large triangular muscle that fills up the subscapular fossa, that arises from the surface of the scapula, that is inserted into the lesser tubercle of the humerus, and that stabilizes the shoulder joint as part of the rotator cuff and rotates the humerus medially when the arm is held by the side of the body

sub·scrip·tion \səb-'skrip-shən\ *n* : a part of a prescription that contains directions to the pharmacist

sub·se·rous \,səb-'sir-əs\ *or* **sub·se·ro·sal** \-sə-'rō-zəl\ *adj* : situated or occurring under a serous membrane

sub·side \səb-'sīd\ *vb* **sub·sid·ed; sub·sid·ing** : to lessen in severity : become diminished — **sub·si·dence** \səb-'sīd-ᵊns, 'səb-səd-əns\ *n*

sub·spe·cial·ist \,səb-'spe-shə-list\ *n* : a physician having a subspecialty

sub·spe·cial·ty \,səb-'spe-shəl-tē\ *n, pl* **-ties** : a subordinate field of specialization

sub·spe·cies \'səb-,spē-shēz, -sēz\ *n* : a subdivision of a species: as **a** : a category in biological classification that ranks immediately below a species and designates a population of a particular geographical region genetically distinguishable from other such populations of the same species and capable of interbreeding successfully with them where its range overlaps theirs **b** : a named subdivision (as a race or variety) of a species — **sub·spe·cif·ic** \ˌsəb-spi-ˈsi-fik\ adj

sub·stage \ˈsəb-ˌstāj\ n : an attachment to a microscope by means of which accessories (as mirrors or condensers) are held in place beneath the stage of the instrument

sub·stance \ˈsəb-stəns\ n : something (as alcohol, cocaine, or marijuana) deemed harmful and usu. subject to legal restriction 〈heroin is a controlled ∼〉 〈∼ abuse〉

substance P n : a neuropeptide that consists of 11 amino acid residues, that is widely distributed in the brain, spinal cord, and peripheral nervous system, and that acts across nerve synapses to produce prolonged postsynaptic excitation

sub·stan·tia gel·a·ti·no·sa \ˌsəb-ˈstan-chə-ˌje-lə-tə-ˈnō-sə\ n : a mass of gelatinous gray matter that lies on the dorsal surface of the dorsal horn and extends the entire length of the spinal cord into the medulla oblongata and that functions in the transmission of painful sensory information

substantia in·nom·i·na·ta \-ˌi-ˌnä-mə-ˈnä-tə\ n : a band of large cells of indeterminate function that lie just under the surface of the globus pallidus

sub·stan·tia ni·gra \ˌsəb-ˈstan-chə-ˈnī-grə, -ˈni-\ n, pl **sub·stan·ti·ae ni·grae** \-chē-ˌē-ˈnī-ˌgrē, -ˈni-\ : a layer of deeply pigmented gray matter situated in the midbrain and containing the cell bodies of a tract of dopamine-producing nerve cells whose secretion tends to be deficient in Parkinson's disease

substantia pro·pria \-ˈprō-prē-ə\ n, pl **substantiae pro·pri·ae** \-prē-ˌē\ : the layer of lamellated transparent fibrous connective tissue that makes up the bulk of the cornea of the eye

sub·ster·nal \ˌsəb-ˈstər-nəl\ adj : situated or perceived behind or below the sternum 〈∼ pain〉

sub·stit·u·ent \ˌsəb-ˈsti-chə-wənt\ n : an atom or group that replaces another atom or group in a molecule — **substituent** adj

sub·sti·tute \ˈsəb-stə-ˌtüt, -ˌtyüt\ n : a person or thing that takes the place or function of another — **substitute** adj

sub·sti·tu·tion \ˌsəb-stə-ˈtü-shən, -ˈtyü-\ n **1** : the turning from an obstructed desire to another desire whose gratification is socially acceptable **2** : the turning from an obstructed form of behavior to a different and often more primitive expression of the same tendency

sub·strate \ˈsəb-ˌstrāt\ n **1** : the base on which an organism lives **2** : a substance acted upon (as by an enzyme)

sub·stra·tum \ˈsəb-ˌstrā-təm, -ˌstra-\ n, pl **-stra·ta** \-tə\ : SUBSTRATE 1

sub·struc·ture \ˈsəb-ˌstrək-chər\ n : an underlying or supporting structure — **sub·struc·tur·al** \-chə-rəl\ adj

sub·syn·dro·mal \ˌsəb-sin-ˈdrō-məl\ adj : characterized by or exhibiting symptoms that are not severe enough for diagnosis as a clinically recognized syndrome 〈∼ depression〉

sub·ta·lar \ˌsəb-ˈtā-lər\ adj : situated or occurring beneath the talus; specif : of, relating to, or being the articulation formed between the posterior facet of the inferior surface of the talus and the posterior facet of the superior surface of the calcaneus

sub·tem·po·ral decompression \-ˈtem-pə-rəl-\ n : relief of intracranial pressure by excision of a portion of the temporal bone

sub·tha·lam·ic \ˌsəb-thə-ˈla-mik\ adj : of or relating to the subthalamus

subthalamic nucleus n : an oval mass of gray matter that is located in the caudal part of the subthalamus and when affected with lesions is associated with hemiballismus of the contralateral side of the body

sub·thal·a·mus \ˌsəb-ˈtha-lə-məs\ n, pl **-mi** \-ˌmī\ : the ventral part of the thalamus

sub·ther·a·peu·tic \-ˌther-ə-ˈpyü-tik\ adj : not producing a therapeutic effect 〈∼ doses of penicillin〉

sub·thresh·old \ˌsəb-ˈthresh-ˌhōld\ adj : inadequate to produce a response 〈∼ dosages〉 〈a ∼ stimulus〉

sub·to·tal \ˌsəb-ˈtōt-ᵊl\ adj : somewhat less than complete : nearly total 〈∼ thyroidectomy〉

sub·tro·chan·ter·ic \ˌsəb-ˌtrō-kən-ˈter-ik, -ˌkan-\ adj : situated or occurring below a trochanter

sub·un·gual \ˌsəb-ˈəŋ-gwəl, -ˈən-\ adj : situated or occurring under a fingernail or toenail 〈a ∼ abscess〉

sub·val·vu·lar \ˌsəb-ˈval-vyə-lər\ adj : situated or occurring below a valve (as a semilunar valve) 〈∼ stenosis〉

sub·vi·ral \ˌsəb-ˈvī-rəl\ adj : relating to, being, or caused by a piece or a structural part (as a protein) of a virus

sub·xi·phoid \ˌsəb-ˈzī-ˌfȯid, -ˈzi-\ adj : situated, occurring, or performed below the xiphoid process

succedaneum — see CAPUT SUCCEDANEUM

suc·ci·nate \ˈsək-sə-ˌnāt\ n : a salt or ester of succinic acid

succinate dehydrogenase n : an iron-containing flavoprotein enzyme that catalyzes often reversibly the dehydrogenation of succinic acid to fumaric acid — called also succinic dehydrogenase

suc·cin·ic acid \(ˌ)sək-ˈsi-nik-\ n : a crystalline acid $C_4H_6O_4$ containing two carboxyl groups that is formed in the Krebs cycle and in various fermentation processes

suc·ci·nyl·cho·line \ˌsək-sə-nəl-ˈkō-ˌlēn, -ˌnil-\ *n* : a basic compound that acts similarly to curare and is used intravenously chiefly in the form of its chloride salt as a short-term relaxant of skeletal muscle in surgery — called also *suxamethonium*; see ANECTINE

suc·ci·nyl·sul·fa·thi·a·zole \ˌsək-sə-nəl-ˌsəl-fə-ˈthī-ə-ˌzōl, -ˌnil-\ *n* : a sulfa drug $C_{13}H_{13}N_3O_5S_2$ used esp. for treating gastrointestinal infections

suc·cus en·ter·i·cus \ˌsə-kəs-en-ˈter-i-kəs\ *n* : INTESTINAL JUICE

suc·cus·sion \sə-ˈkə-shən\ *n* : the action or process of shaking or the condition of being shaken esp. with violence: **a** : a shaking of the body to ascertain if fluid is present in a cavity and esp. in the thorax **b** : the splashing sound made by succussion

suck \ˈsək\ *vb* **1** : to draw (as liquid) into the mouth through a suction force produced by movements of the lips and tongue **2** : to draw out by suction

suck·er \ˈsə-kər\ *n* **1** : an organ in various animals (as a trematode or tapeworm) used for adhering or holding **2** : a mouth (as of a leech) adapted for sucking or adhering

sucking louse *n* : any of an order (Anoplura) of wingless insects comprising the true lice with mouthparts adapted for sucking body fluids

suck·le \ˈsə-kəl\ *vb* **suck·led; suck·ling** **1** : to give milk to from the breast or udder **2** : to draw milk from the breast or udder of

su·cral·fate \sü-ˈkral-ˌfāt\ *n* : an aluminum complex $C_{12}H_mAl_{16}O_nS_8$ where *m* and *n* are approximately 54 and 75 that is used in the treatment of duodenal ulcers — see CARAFATE

su·cra·lose \ˈsü-krə-ˌlōs\ *n* : a white crystalline powder $C_{12}H_{19}Cl_3O_8$ that is derived from sucrose and is used as a low-calorie sweetener

su·crase \ˈsü-ˌkrās, -ˌkrāz\ *n* : INVERTASE

su·crose \ˈsü-ˌkrōs, -ˌkrōz\ *n* : a sweet crystalline dextrorotatory disaccharide sugar $C_{12}H_{22}O_{11}$ that occurs naturally in most plants and is obtained commercially esp. from sugarcane or sugar beets

¹suc·tion \ˈsək-shən\ *n* **1** : the act or process of sucking **2 a** : the act or process of exerting a force upon a solid, liquid, or gaseous body by reason of reduced air pressure over part of its surface **b** : force so exerted **3** : the act or process of removing secretions or fluids from hollow or tubular organs or cavities by means of a tube and a device (as a suction pump) that operates on negative pressure

²suction *vb* : to remove (as from a body cavity or passage) by suction

suction lipectomy *n* : LIPOSUCTION

suction pump *n* : a common pump in which the liquid to be raised is pushed by atmospheric pressure into the partial vacuum under a retreating valved piston on the upstroke and reflux is prevented by a valve in the pipe that permits flow in only one direction — see STOMACH PUMP

su·dam·i·na \sü-ˈda-mə-nə\ *n pl* : a transient eruption of minute translucent vesicles caused by retention of sweat in the sweat glands and in the corneous layer of the skin and occurring after profuse perspiration — called also *miliaria crystallina* — **su·dam·i·nal** \-nəl\ *adj*

Su·dan \sü-ˈdan\ *n* : any of several azo solvent dyes including some which have a specific affinity for fatty substances

Sudan IV \-ˈfȯr\ *n* : a red dye used chiefly as a biological stain and in ointments for promoting the growth of epithelium (as in the treatment of burns, wounds, or ulcers) — called also *scarlet red*

su·dan·o·phil·ia \sü-ˌda-nə-ˈfi-lē-ə\ *n* : the quality or state of being sudanophilic

su·dan·o·phil·ic \sü-ˌda-nə-ˈfi-lik\ *also* **su·dan·o·phil** \sü-ˈda-nə-ˌfil\ *adj* : staining selectively with Sudan dyes; *also* : containing lipids

sudden cardiac arrest *n* : CARDIAC ARREST — abbr. *SCA*

sudden cardiac death *n* : death occurring within minutes or hours following onset of acute symptoms of cardiac arrest resulting from an arrhythmia

sudden death *n* : unexpected death that is instantaneous or occurs within minutes from any cause other than violence; *esp* : SUDDEN CARDIAC DEATH

sudden infant death syndrome *n* : death of an apparently healthy infant usu. before one year of age that is of unknown cause and occurs esp. during sleep — abbr. *SIDS;* called also *cot death, crib death*

su·do·mo·tor \ˈsü-də-ˌmō-tər\ *adj* : of, relating to, or being nerve fibers controlling the activity of sweat glands

su·do·rif·er·ous gland \ˌsü-də-ˈri-fə-rəs-\ *n* : SWEAT GLAND

¹su·do·rif·ic \-ˈri-fik\ *adj* : causing or inducing sweat : DIAPHORETIC

²sudorific *n* : a sudorific agent or medicine

su·fen·ta·nil \sü-ˈfen-tə-ˌnil\ *n* : an opioid analgesic that is administered intravenously in the form of its citrate $C_{22}H_{30}N_2O_2S \cdot C_6H_8O_7$ as an anesthetic or an anesthetic adjuvant

suf·fo·cate \ˈsə-fə-ˌkāt\ *vb* **-cat·ed; -cat·ing** **1** : to stop the respiration of (as by strangling or asphyxiation) **2** : to deprive of oxygen **3** : to die from being unable to breathe — **suf·fo·ca·tion** \ˌsə-fə-ˈkā-shən\ *n* — **suf·fo·ca·tive** \ˈsə-fə-ˌkā-tiv\ *adj*

suf·fuse \sə-ˈfyüz\ *vb* **suf·fused; suf·fus·ing** : to flush or spread over or through in the manner of a fluid and esp. blood — **suf·fu·sion** \sə-'fyü-zhən\ n

sug·ar \'shu̇-gər\ n **1** : a sweet substance that is colorless or white when pure, consists chiefly of sucrose, and is obtained esp. from sugarcane or sugar beets **2** : any of various water-soluble compounds that vary widely in sweetness and comprise the saccharides of smaller molecular size including sucrose

sugar diabetes n : DIABETES MELLITUS

sugar pill n : a pharmacologically inert pill : PLACEBO

sui·cide \'sü-ə-ˌsīd\ n **1** : the act or an instance of taking one's own life voluntarily and intentionally **2** : a person who commits or attempts suicide — **sui·cid·al** \ˌsü-ə-'sīd-ᵊl\ adj — **sui·cid·al·ly** \-ᵊl-ē\ adv — **suicide** vb

sui·cid·ol·o·gy \ˌsü-ə-ˌsī-'dä-lə-jē\ n, pl **-gies** : the study of suicide and suicide prevention — **sui·cid·ol·o·gist** \-jist\ n

suit — see G SUIT, PRESSURE SUIT

suite \'swēt\ n : a group of rooms in a medical facility dedicated to a specified function or specialty ⟨surgical ~⟩

sul·bac·tam \səl-'bak-ˌtam, -təm\ n : a beta-lactamase inhibitor that is usu. administered in the form of its sodium salt $C_8H_{10}NNaO_5S$ in combination with a beta-lactam antibiotic (as ampicillin)

sul·cus \'səl-kəs\ n, pl **sul·ci** \-ˌkī, -ˌsī\ : FURROW, GROOVE; esp : a shallow furrow on the surface of the brain separating adjacent convolutions — compare FISSURE 1c — **sul·cal** \'səl-kəl\ adj

sulcus ter·mi·na·lis \-ˌtər-mə-'nä-ləs\ n, pl **sulci ter·mi·na·les** \-ˌlēz\ **1** : a V-shaped groove separating the anterior two thirds of the tongue from the posterior third and containing the circumvallate papillae **2** : a shallow groove on the outside of the right atrium of the heart

sulf- or **sulfo-** comb form : sulfur : containing sulfur ⟨sulfarsphenamine⟩

¹sul·fa \'səl-fə\ adj **1** : related chemically to sulfanilamide **2** : of, relating to, employing, or containing sulfa drugs ⟨~ therapy⟩

²sulfa n : SULFA DRUG

sul·fa·cet·a·mide also **sul·fa·cet·i·mide** \ˌsəl-fə-'se-tə-ˌmīd, -məd\ n : a sulfa drug $C_8H_{10}N_2O_3S$ that is used chiefly for treating infections of the urinary tract and in the form of its sodium salt $C_8H_9N_2NaO_3S$ to treat infections of the eye and acne vulgaris

sul·fa·di·a·zine \ˌsəl-fə-'dī-ə-ˌzēn\ n : a sulfa drug $C_{10}H_{10}N_4O_2S$ used esp. in the treatment of toxoplasmosis

sulfa drug n : any of various synthetic organic bacteria-inhibiting drugs that are sulfonamides closely related chemically to sulfanilamide — called also **sulfa**

sul·fa·gua·ni·dine \ˌsəl-fə-'gwä-nə-ˌdēn\ n : a sulfa drug $C_7H_{10}N_4O_2S$ used esp. in veterinary medicine — called also **sulfanilylguanidine**

sul·fa·mer·a·zine \ˌsəl-fə-'mer-ə-ˌzēn\ n : a sulfa drug $C_{11}H_{12}N_4O_2S$ that is a derivative of sulfadiazine and is used similarly

sul·fa·meth·a·zine \-'me-thə-ˌzēn\ n : a sulfa drug $C_{12}H_{14}N_4O_2S$ that is a derivative of sulfadiazine and is used similarly

sul·fa·meth·ox·a·zole \-ˌme-'thäk-sə-ˌzōl\ n : an antibacterial sulfonamide $C_{10}H_{11}N_3O_3S$ used alone or in combination with trimethoprim (as in the treatment of urinary tract infections or acute otitis media) — see BACTRIM, SEPTRA

sul·fa·mez·a·thine \-'me-zə-ˌthēn\ n : SULFAMETHAZINE

Sul·fa·my·lon \ˌsəl-fə-'mī-ˌlän\ trademark — used for a preparation of the acetate of mafenide

sul·fa·nil·amide \ˌsəl-fə-'ni-lə-ˌmīd, -məd\ n : a crystalline sulfonamide $C_6H_8N_2O_3S$ that is the amide of sulfanilic acid and the parent compound of most of the sulfa drugs

sul·fan·i·lyl·gua·ni·dine \ˌsəl-ˌfa-ni-ˌlil-'gwä-nə-ˌdēn\ n : SULFAGUANIDINE

sul·fa·pyr·i·dine \ˌsəl-fə-'pir-ə-ˌdēn\ n : a sulfa drug $C_{11}H_{11}N_3O_2S$ that is derived from pyridine and sulfanilamide and is used in small doses in the treatment of dermatitis herpetiformis and esp. formerly against pneumococcal and gonococcal infections

sul·fa·qui·nox·a·line \-kwi-'näk-sə-ˌlēn\ n : a sulfa drug $C_{14}H_{12}N_4O_2S$ used esp. in veterinary medicine

sulf·ars·phen·a·mine \ˌsəl-ˌfärs-'fe-nə-ˌmēn, -mən\ n : an orange-yellow powder $C_{14}H_{14}As_2N_2Na_2O_8S_2$ formerly used to treat syphilis

sul·fa·sal·a·zine \ˌsəl-fə-'sa-lə-ˌzēn\ n : a sulfonamide $C_{18}H_{14}N_4O_5S$ used in the treatment of chronic ulcerative colitis — called also **salicylazosulfapyridine**

¹sul·fate \'səl-ˌfāt\ n **1** : a salt or ester of sulfuric acid **2** : a bivalent group or anion SO_4 characteristic of sulfuric acid and the sulfates

²sulfate vb **sul·fat·ed; sul·fat·ing** : to treat or combine with sulfuric acid or a sulfate

sul·fa·thi·a·zole \ˌsəl-fə-'thī-ə-ˌzōl\ n : a sulfa drug $C_9H_9N_3O_2S_2$ derived from thiazole and sulfanilamide but seldom prescribed due to its toxicity

sul·fa·tide \'səl-fə-ˌtīd\ n : any of the sulfates of cerebrosides that often accumulate in the central nervous systems of individuals affected with metachromatic leukodystrophy

sulf·he·mo·glo·bin \ˌsəlf-'hē-mə-ˌglō-bən\ n : a green pigment formed from hemoglobin and found in putrefied organs and cadavers

sulf·he·mo·glo·bi·ne·mia \ˌsəlf-ˌhē-mə-ˌglō-bə-'nē-mē-ə\ n : the presence of sulfhemoglobin in the blood

sulf·hy·dryl \ˌsəlf-ˈhī-drəl\ n : THIOL 2 — used chiefly in molecular biology

sul·fide \ˈsəl-ˌfīd\ n 1 : any of various organic compounds characterized by a sulfur atom attached to two carbon atoms 2 : a binary compound (as CuS) of sulfur usu. with a more electrically positive element or group

sul·fin·py·ra·zone \ˌsəl-fən-ˈpī-rə-ˌzōn\ n : a uricosuric drug C₂₃H₂₀N₂O₃S used in the treatment of chronic gout

sul·fi·sox·a·zole \ˌsəl-fə-ˈsäk-sə-ˌzōl\ n : a sulfa drug C₁₁H₁₃N₃O₃S derived from sulfanilamide that is less likely than other sulfanilamide derivatives to produce renal damage because of its greater solubility

sulfo- — see SULF-

sul·fo·bro·mo·phthal·ein \ˌsəl-fə-ˌbrō-mō-ˈtha-lē-ən, -ˈthā-ˌlēn\ n : a diagnostic material used in the form of its disodium salt C₂₀H₈Br₄Na₂O₁₀S₂ in a liver function test

sul·fon·amide \ˌsəl-ˈfä-nə-ˌmīd, -məd; -ˈfō-nə-ˌmīd\ n : any of various amides (as sulfanilamide) of a sulfonic acid; also : SULFA DRUG

sul·fon·eth·yl·meth·ane \ˌsəl-ˌfō-ˌne-thəl-ˈme-ˌthān\ n : a crystalline hypnotic C₈H₁₈O₄S₂ that is an ethyl analog of sulfonmethane

sul·fon·ic acid \ˌsəl-ˈfä-nik-, -ˈfō-\ n : any of numerous acids that contain the SO₃H group

sul·fon·meth·ane \ˌsəl-ˌfōn-ˈme-ˌthān\ n : a crystalline hypnotic C₅H₁₀O₄S₂

sul·fo·nyl·urea \ˌsəl-fə-ˌnil-ˈyùr-ē-ə, -ˌni-ˈlùr-\ n : any of several hypoglycemic compounds related to the sulfonamides and used in the oral treatment of type 2 diabetes

sul·fo·raph·ane \ˌsəl-fō-ˈra-ˌfān\ n : a compound C₆H₁₁NOS₂ found in vegetables (as broccoli and cauliflower) of the mustard family that stimulates the production of enzymes in the body which initiate antioxidant activity

sul·fo·sal·i·cyl·ic acid \ˌsəl-fō-ˌsa-lə-ˈsi-lik-\ n : a sulfonic acid derivative C₇H₆O₆S₃ used esp. to detect and precipitate proteins (as albumin) from urine

sulf·ox·one sodium \ˌsəl-ˈfäk-ˌsōn-\ n : a crystalline salt C₁₄H₁₄N₂N₂O₆S₃ used in the treatment of leprosy

sul·fur \ˈsəl-fər\ n : a nonmetallic element that occurs either free or combined esp. in sulfides and sulfates — symbol S; see ELEMENT table — **sul·fur** adj

sulfurated potash n : a mixture composed principally of sulfurated potassium compounds that is used in treating skin diseases

sulfur dioxide n : a heavy pungent toxic gas SO₂ that is a major air pollutant esp. in industrial areas

sul·fu·ric \ˌsəl-ˈfyùr-ik\ adj : of, relating to, or containing sulfur esp. with a higher valence than sulfurous compounds

sulfuric acid n : a heavy corrosive oily strong acid H₂SO₄ having two replaceable hydrogen atoms

sulfur mustard n : MUSTARD GAS

sul·fu·rous \ˈsəl-fə-rəs, -fyə-; ˌsəl-ˈfyùr-əs\ adj 1 : of, relating to, or containing sulfur esp. with a lower valence than sulfuric compounds 2 : resembling or emanating from sulfur and esp. burning sulfur

sulfurous acid n : a weak unstable acid H₂SO₃ used in medicine as an antiseptic

su·lin·dac \sə-ˈlin-ˌdak\ n : an NSAID C₂₀H₁₇FO₃S used esp. in the treatment of rheumatoid arthritis

sul·i·so·ben·zone \ˌsəl-i-sō-ˈben-ˌzōn\ n : a sunscreening agent C₁₄H₁₂O₆S

sulph- or **sulpho-** chiefly Brit var of SULF-

sul·pha, sul·phate, sul·phide, sul·phur, sul·phu·ric chiefly Brit var of SULFA, SULFATE, SULFIDE, SULFUR, SULFURIC

sul·pir·ide \ˈsəl-(ˌ)pir-ˌīd\ n : an antipsychotic drug C₁₅H₂₃N₃O₄S used esp in the treatment of schizophrenia

su·mac also **su·mach** \ˈsü-ˌmak, ˈshü-\ n 1 : any plant of the genus Rhus 2 : POISON SUMAC

su·ma·trip·tan \ˌsü-mə-ˈtrip-ˌtan, -tən\ n : a triptan C₁₄H₂₁N₃O₂S administered as a nasal spray or in the form of its succinate C₁₄H₂₁N₃O₂S·C₄H₆O₄ either as an oral tablet or by injection to treat migraine attacks — see IMITREX

sum·ma·tion \(ˌ)sə-ˈmā-shən\ n : cumulative action or effect; esp : the process by which a sequence of stimuli that are individually inadequate to produce a response are cumulatively able to induce a nerve impulse — see SPATIAL SUMMATION, TEMPORAL SUMMATION

summer complaint n : SUMMER DIARRHEA

summer diarrhea n : diarrhea esp. of children that is prevalent in hot weather and is usu. caused by ingestion of food contaminated by various microorganisms

summer sores n sing or pl : a skin disease of the horse caused by larval roundworms of the genus Habronema

sun·block \ˈsən-ˌbläk\ n : a preparation (as a lotion) applied to the skin to prevent sunburn (as by physically blocking out ultraviolet radiation); also : its active ingredient (as titanium dioxide) — compare SUNSCREEN

sun·burn \ˈsən-ˌbərn\ n : inflammation of the skin caused by overexposure to ultraviolet radiation esp. from sunlight — **sunburn** vb

sun·down·ing \ˈsən-ˌdaù-niŋ\ n : a state of increased agitation, confusion, disorientation, and anxiety that typically occurs in the late afternoon or evening in some individuals affected with dementia

sun·glass·es \-ˌgla-səs\ *n pl* : glasses used to protect the eyes from the sun

sun·lamp \'sən-ˌlamp\ *n* : an electric lamp designed to emit radiation of wavelengths from ultraviolet to infrared and used esp. for therapeutic purposes or for producing tan artificially

sun protection factor *n* : SPF

sun·screen \-ˌskrēn\ *n* : a preparation (as a lotion) applied to the skin to prevent sunburn (as by chemically absorbing ultraviolet radiation); *also* : its active ingredient (as benzophenone) — compare SUNBLOCK — **sun·screen·ing** *adj*

sunshine vitamin *n* : VITAMIN D

sun·stroke \-ˌstrōk\ *n* : heatstroke caused by direct exposure to the sun

sun·tan \-ˌtan\ *n* : a browning of the skin from exposure to the rays of the sun — **sun·tanned** \-ˌtand\ *adj*

super- *prefix* 1 : greater than normal : excessive ⟨*super*ovulation⟩ 2 : situated or placed above, on, or at the top of ⟨*super*cilary⟩; *specif* : situated on the dorsal side

su·per·cil·i·ary \ˌsü-pər-'si-lē-ˌer-ē\ *adj* : of, relating to, or adjoining the eyebrow : SUPRAORBITAL

superciliary ridge *n* : a prominence of the frontal bone above the eye caused by the projection of the frontal sinuses — called also *browridge, superciliary arch, supraorbital ridge*

su·per·coil \'sü-pər-ˌkȯil\ *n* : a double helix (as of DNA) that has undergone additional twisting in the same or in the opposite direction as the turns in the original helix — **supercoil** *vb*

su·per·ego \ˌsü-pər-'ē-(ˌ)gō, 'sü-pər-ˌ, -'e-(ˌ)gō\ *n* : the one of the three divisions of the psyche in psychoanalytic theory that is only partly conscious, represents internalization of parental conscience and the rules of society, and functions to reward and punish through a system of moral attitudes, conscience, and a sense of guilt — compare EGO, ¹ID

su·per·fam·i·ly \'sü-pər-ˌfam-lē\ *n, pl* **-lies** : a category of taxonomic classification between a family and an order

su·per·fat·ted \'sü-pər-ˌfa-təd\ *adj* : containing extra oil or fat ⟨~ soap⟩

su·per·fe·cun·da·tion \ˌsü-pər-ˌfe-kən-'dā-shən, -ˌfē-\ *n* : successive fertilization of two or more ova from the same ovulation esp. by different mates

su·per·fe·ta·tion \ˌsü-pər-fē-'tā-shən\ *n* : successive fertilization of two or more ova of different ovulations resulting in the presence of embryos of unlike ages in the same uterus

su·per·fi·cial \ˌsü-pər-'fi-shəl\ *adj* 1 : of, relating to, or located near the surface ⟨~ blood vessels⟩ 2 : lying on, not penetrating below, or affecting only the surface ⟨~ wounds⟩ — **su·per·fi·cial·ly** *adv*

superficial external pudendal artery *n* : EXTERNAL PUDENDAL ARTERY a

superficial fascia *n* : the thin layer of loose fatty connective tissue underlying the skin and binding it to the parts beneath — called also *hypodermis, tela subcutanea;* compare DEEP FASCIA

superficial inguinal ring *n* : the inguinal ring that is the external opening of the inguinal canal — called also *external inguinal ring;* compare DEEP INGUINAL RING

superficialis — see FLEXOR DIGITORUM SUPERFICIALIS, TRANSVERSUS PERINEI SUPERFICIALIS

superficial palmar arch *n* : PALMAR ARCH b

superficial peroneal nerve *n* : a nerve that arises as a branch of the common peroneal nerve and that innervates or supplies branches innervating the muscles of the anterior part of the leg and the skin on the lower anterior part of the leg, on the dorsum of the foot, on the lateral and medial sides of the foot, and between the toes — called also *musculocutaneous nerve;* compare DEEP PERONEAL NERVE

superficial temporal artery *n* : the one of the two terminal branches of each external carotid artery that arises in the substance of the parotid gland, passes upward over the zygomatic process of the temporal bone, and is distributed by way of branches esp. to the more superficial parts of the side of the face and head

superficial temporal vein *n* : TEMPORAL VEIN a(1)

superficial transverse metacarpal ligament *n* : a transverse ligamentous band across the palm of the hand in the superficial fascia at the base of the fingers — called also *superficial transverse ligament*

superficial transverse perineal muscle *n* : TRANSVERSUS PERINEI SUPERFICIALIS

su·per·fuse \ˌsü-pər-'fyüz\ *vb* **-fused; -fus·ing** : to maintain the metabolic or physiological activity of (as an isolated organ) by submitting to a continuous flow of a sustaining medium over the outside — **su·per·fu·sion** \-'fyü-zhən\ *n*

su·per·gene \'sü-pər-ˌjēn\ *n* : a group of linked genes acting as an allelic unit esp. when due to the suppression of crossing-over

su·per·he·lix \'sü-pər-ˌhē-liks\ *n* : SUPERCOIL — **su·per·he·li·cal** \ˌsü-pər-'he-li-kəl, -'hē-\ *adj*

su·per·in·fec·tion \ˌsü-pər-in-'fek-shən\ *n* : a second infection superimposed on an earlier one esp. by a different microbial agent of exogenous or endogenous origin that is resistant to the treatment used against the first infection — **su·per·in·fect** \-in-'fekt\ *vb*

su·pe·ri·or \su̇-'pir-ē-ər\ *adj* 1 : situated toward the head and further away from the feet than another and esp. another similar part — compare INFERIOR 1 **2** : situated in a more anterior or dorsal position in the body of a quadruped — compare INFERIOR 2

superior alveolar nerve *n* : any of the branches of the maxillary nerve or of the infraorbital nerve that supply the teeth and gums of the upper jaw

superior articular process *n* : ARTICULAR PROCESS a

superior carotid triangle *n* : a space in each lateral half of the neck that is bounded in back by the sternocleidomastoid muscle, below by the omohyoid muscle, and above by the stylohyoid and digastric muscles

superior cerebellar artery *n* : an artery that arises from the basilar artery just before it divides to form the posterior cerebral arteries and supplies or gives off branches supplying the superior part of the cerebellum, midbrain, pineal gland, and choroid plexus of the third ventricle

superior cerebellar peduncle *n* : CEREBELLAR PEDUNCLE a

superior colliculus *n* : either member of the anterior and higher pair of corpora quadrigemina that together constitute a primitive center for vision — called also *optic lobe, optic tectum;* compare INFERIOR COLLICULUS

superior concha *n* : NASAL CONCHA c

superior constrictor *n* : a 4-sided muscle of the pharynx that acts to constrict part of the pharynx in swallowing — called also *constrictor pharyngis superior, superior pharyngeal constrictor muscle;* compare INFERIOR CONSTRICTOR, MIDDLE CONSTRICTOR

superior extensor retinaculum *n* : EXTENSOR RETINACULUM 1b

superior ganglion *n* **1** : the upper and smaller of the two sensory ganglia of the glossopharyngeal nerve that may be absent but when present is situated in a groove in which the nerve passes through the jugular foramen — called also *jugular ganglion;* compare INFERIOR GANGLION 1 **2** : the upper of the two ganglia of the vagus nerve that is situated at the point where it exits through the jugular foramen — called also *jugular ganglion, superior vagal ganglion;* compare INFERIOR GANGLION 2

superior gluteal artery *n* : GLUTEAL ARTERY a

superior gluteal nerve *n* : GLUTEAL NERVE a

superior gluteal vein *n* : any of several veins that accompany the superior gluteal artery and empty into the internal iliac vein

superior hemorrhoidal artery *n* : RECTAL ARTERY c

superior hemorrhoidal vein *n* : RECTAL VEIN c

superior intercostal vein *n* : a vein on each side formed by the union of the veins draining the first two or three intercostal spaces of which the one on the right usu. empties into the azygos vein but sometimes into the right brachiocephalic vein and the one on the left empties into the left innominate vein after crossing the arch of the aorta

superioris — see LEVATOR LABII SUPERIORIS, LEVATOR LABII SUPERIORIS ALAEQUE NASI, LEVATOR PALPEBRAE SUPERIORIS, QUADRATUS LABII SUPERIORIS

superiority complex *n* : an excessive striving for or pretense of superiority to compensate for supposed inferiority

superior laryngeal artery *n* : LARYNGEAL ARTERY b

superior laryngeal nerve *n* : LARYNGEAL NERVE a — called also *superior laryngeal*

superior longitudinal fasciculus *n* : a large bundle of association fibers in the white matter of each cerebral hemisphere that extends above the insula from the frontal lobe to the occipital lobe where it curves downward and forward into the temporal lobe

su·pe·ri·or·ly \sù-ˈpir-ē-ər-lē\ *adv* : in or to a more superior position or direction

superior meatus *n* : a curved relatively short anteroposterior passage on each side of the nose that occupies the middle third of the lateral wall of a nasal cavity between the superior and middle nasal conchae — compare INFERIOR MEATUS, MIDDLE MEATUS

superior mesenteric artery *n* : MESENTERIC ARTERY b

superior mesenteric ganglion *n* : MESENTERIC GANGLION b

superior mesenteric plexus *n* : MESENTERIC PLEXUS b

superior mesenteric vein *n* : MESENTERIC VEIN b

superior nasal concha *n* : NASAL CONCHA c

superior nuchal line *n* : NUCHAL LINE a

superior oblique *n* : OBLIQUE b(1)

superior olive *n* : a small gray nucleus situated on the dorsolateral aspect of the trapezoid body — called also *superior olivary nucleus;* compare INFERIOR OLIVE

superior ophthalmic vein *n* : OPHTHALMIC VEIN a

superior orbital fissure *n* : ORBITAL FISSURE a

superior pancreaticoduodenal artery *n* : PANCREATICODUODENAL ARTERY b

superior pectoral nerve *n* : PECTORAL NERVE a

superior peroneal retinaculum *n* : PERONEAL RETINACULUM a

superior petrosal sinus *n* : PETROSAL SINUS a

superior pharyngeal constrictor muscle *n* : SUPERIOR CONSTRICTOR

superior phrenic artery *n* : PHRENIC ARTERY a

superior phrenic vein *n* : PHRENIC VEIN a

superior ramus *n* : RAMUS b(1)

superior rectal artery *n* : RECTAL ARTERY c

superior rectal vein *n* : RECTAL VEIN c

superior rectus *n* : RECTUS 2a

superior sagittal sinus *n* : SAGITTAL SINUS a

superior temporal gyrus *n* : TEMPORAL GYRUS a

superior thyroid artery *n* : THYROID ARTERY a

superior turbinate *n* : NASAL CONCHA c

superior turbinate bone *n* : NASAL CONCHA c

superior ulnar collateral artery *n* : a long slender artery that arises from the brachial artery or one of its branches just below the middle of the upper arm, descends to the elbow following the course of the ulnar nerve, and terminates under the flexor carpi ulnaris — compare INFERIOR ULNAR COLLATERAL ARTERY

superior vagal ganglion *n* : SUPERIOR GANGLION 2

superior vena cava *n* : a vein that is the second largest vein in the human body, is formed by the union of the two brachiocephalic veins at the level of the space between the first two ribs, and returns blood to the right atrium of the heart from the upper half of the body

superior vena cava syndrome *n* : a condition characterized by elevated venous pressure of the upper extremities with accompanying distension of the affected veins and swelling of the face and neck and caused by blockage (as by a thrombus) or compression (as by a tumor) of the superior vena cava

superior vermis *n* : VERMIS 1a

superior vesical *n* : VESICAL ARTERY a

superior vesical artery *n* : VESICAL ARTERY a

superior vestibular nucleus *n* : the one of the four vestibular nuclei on each side of the medulla oblongata that sends ascending fibers to the oculomotor and trochlear nuclei in the cerebrum on the same side of the brain

superior vocal cords *n pl* : FALSE VOCAL CORDS

su·per·na·tant \ˌsü-pər-ˈnāt-ᵊnt\ *n* : the usu. clear liquid overlying material deposited by settling, precipitation, or centrifugation — **supernatant** *adj*

su·per·nu·mer·ary \ˌsü-pər-ˈnü-mə-ˌrer-ē, -ˈnyü-\ *adj* : exceeding the usual or normal number ⟨∼ teeth⟩

supero- *comb form* : situated above ⟨*supero*lateral⟩

su·pero·lat·er·al \ˌsü-pə-rō-ˈla-tə-rəl\ *adj* : situated above and toward the side

su·per·ovu·la·tion \-ˌä-vyə-ˈlā-shən\ *n* : ovulation marked by the production of more than the normal number of mature eggs at one time — **su·per·ovu·late** \-ˈä-vyə-ˌlāt\ *vb*

su·per·ox·ide \-ˈäk-ˌsīd\ *n* : the monovalent anion O_2^- or a compound containing it ⟨potassium ∼ KO_2⟩

superoxide dis·mu·tase \-dis-ˈmyü-ˌtās, -ˌtāz\ *n* : a metal-containing antioxidant enzyme that reduces potentially harmful free radicals of oxygen formed during normal metabolic cell processes to oxygen and hydrogen peroxide — abbr. *SOD*

su·per·po·tent \ˌsü-pər-ˈpōt-ᵊnt\ *adj* : of greater than normal or acceptable potency ⟨∼ topical corticosteroids⟩ — **su·per·po·ten·cy** \-ᵊn-sē\ *n*

su·per·scrip·tion \ˌsü-pər-ˈskrip-shən\ *n* : the part of a pharmaceutical prescription which contains or consists of the Latin word *recipe* or the sign ℞

su·per·son·ic \-ˈsä-nik\ *adj* : ULTRASONIC 1 — **su·per·son·i·cal·ly** *adv*

su·per·vene \ˌsü-pər-ˈvēn\ *vb* **-vened; -ven·ing** : to follow or result as an additional, adventitious, or unlooked-for development (as in the course of a disease)

su·pi·na·tion \ˌsü-pə-ˈnā-shən\ *n* **1** : rotation of the forearm and hand so that the palm faces forward or upward and the radius lies parallel to the ulna; *also* : a corresponding movement of the foot and leg **2** : the position resulting from supination — **su·pi·nate** \ˈsü-pə-ˌnāt\ *vb*

su·pi·na·tor \ˈsü-pə-ˌnā-tər\ *n* : a muscle that produces the motion of supination; *specif* : a deeply situated muscle of the forearm that arises in two layers from the lateral epicondyle of the humerus and adjacent parts of the ligaments and bones of the elbow and that passes over the head of the radius to insert into its neck and the lateral surface of its shaft

supinator crest *n* : a bony ridge on the upper lateral surface of the shaft of the ulna that is the origin for part of the supinator muscle

su·pine \sù-ˈpīn, ˈsü-ˌpīn\ *adj* **1** : lying on the back or with the face upward **2** : marked by supination

¹**sup·ple·ment** \ˈsə-plə-mənt\ *n* **1** : something that completes or makes an addition **2** : DIETARY SUPPLEMENT

²**sup·ple·ment** \-ˌment\ *vb* : to add a supplement to : serve as a supplement for — **sup·ple·men·ta·tion** \ˌsə-plə-ˌmen-ˈtā-shən, -mən-\ *n*

sup·ple·men·tal \ˌsə-plə-ˈment-ᵊl\ *adj* : serving to supplement : SUPPLEMENTARY

supplemental air *n* : the air that can still be expelled from the lungs after an ordinary expiration — compare RESIDUAL AIR

sup·ple·men·ta·ry \ˌsə-plə-ˈmen-tə-rē\ adj : added or serving as a supplement ⟨~ vitamins⟩

sup·ply \sə-ˈplī\ vb sup·plied; sup·ply·ing : to furnish (organs, tissues, or cells) with a vital element (as blood or nerve fibers) — used of nerves and blood vessels

¹sup·port \sə-ˈpōrt\ vb 1 : to hold up or serve as a foundation or prop for 2 : to maintain in condition, action, or existence ⟨~ life⟩ — sup·por·tive \-ˈpōr-tiv\ adj

²support n 1 : the act or process of supporting : the condition of being supported ⟨respiratory ~⟩ 2 : SUPPORTER

sup·port·er n : a woven or knitted band or elastic device supporting a part; esp : ATHLETIC SUPPORTER

support group n : a group of people with common experiences and concerns who provide emotional and moral support for one another

support hose n : stockings (as elastic stockings) worn to supply mild compression to assist the veins of the legs — usu. used with a pl. verb; called also support hosiery

sup·pos·i·to·ry \sə-ˈpä-zə-ˌtōr-ē\ n, pl -ries : a solid but readily melting cone or cylinder of usu. medicated material for insertion into a bodily passage or cavity (as the rectum)

sup·press \sə-ˈpres\ vb 1 : to exclude from consciousness ⟨~ed anxiety⟩ 2 : to restrain from a usual course or action ⟨~ a cough⟩ 3 : INHIBIT 2; esp : to inhibit the genetic expression of ⟨~ a mutation⟩ — sup·press·ible \-ˈpre-sə-bəl\ adj

¹sup·press·ant \sə-ˈpres-ᵊnt\ adj : SUPPRESSIVE

²suppressant n : an agent (as a drug) that tends to suppress or reduce in intensity rather than eliminate something

sup·pres·sion \sə-ˈpre-shən\ n : an act or instance of suppressing: as **a** : stoppage of a bodily function or an act or symptom **b** : the failure of development of a bodily part or organ **c** : the conscious intentional exclusion from consciousness of a thought or feeling — compare REPRESSION 2a

sup·pres·sive \sə-ˈpre-siv\ adj : tending or serving to suppress something (as the symptoms of a disease) ⟨~ drugs⟩

sup·pres·sor \sə-ˈpre-sər\ n : one that suppresses; esp : a mutant gene that suppresses the expression of another nonallelic mutant gene when both are present

suppressor T cell n : a T cell that suppresses the immune response of B cells and other T cells to an antigen — called also suppressor cell, suppressor lymphocyte, suppressor T lymphocyte; compare CYTOTOXIC T CELL, HELPER T CELL

sup·pu·ra·tion \ˌsə-pyə-ˈrā-shən\ n : the formation of, conversion into, or process of discharging pus — **sup·pu·rate** \ˈsə-pyə-ˌrāt\ vb — **sup·pu·ra·tive** \ˈsə-pyə-ˌrā-tiv\ adj

suppurativa — see HIDRADENITIS SUPPURATIVA

supra- prefix **1** : SUPER- 2 ⟨supraorbital⟩ **2** : transcending ⟨supramolecular⟩

su·pra·cer·vi·cal hysterectomy \ˌsü-prə-ˈsər-vi-kəl-\ n : a hysterectomy in which the uterine cervix is not removed

su·pra·chi·as·mat·ic \-ˌkī-əz-ˈma-tik\ adj : SUPRAOPTIC

suprachiasmatic nucleus n : either of a pair of neuron clusters in the hypothalamus directly above the optic chiasma that receive photic input from the retina via the optic nerve and that regulate the body's circadian rhythms — abbr. SCN

su·pra·cla·vic·u·lar \-kla-ˈvi-kyə-lər, -klə-\ adj : situated or occurring above the clavicle ⟨~ lymph nodes⟩

supraclavicular nerve n : any of three nerves that are descending branches of the cervical plexus arising from the third and fourth cervical nerves and that supply the skin over the upper chest and shoulder

su·pra·clu·sion \ˌsü-prə-ˈklü-zhən\ n : SUPRAOCCLUSION

su·pra·con·dy·lar \ˌsü-prə-ˈkän-də-lər, -ˌprä-\ adj : of, relating to, affecting, or being the part of a bone situated above a condyle ⟨a ~ fracture⟩

supracondylar ridge n : either of two ridges above the condyle of the humerus of which one is situated laterally and the other medially and which give attachment to muscles

su·pra·gin·gi·val \-ˈjin-jə-vəl\ adj : located on the surface of a tooth not surrounded by gingiva ⟨~ calculus⟩

su·pra·gle·noid \-ˈgle-ˌnȯid, -ˈglē-\ adj : situated or occurring superior to the glenoid cavity

su·pra·glot·tic \-ˈglä-tik\ adj : situated or occurring above the glottis

su·pra·hy·oid \-ˈhī-ˌȯid\ adj : situated or occurring superior to the hyoid bone ⟨~ lymphadenectomy⟩

suprahyoid muscle n : any of several muscles (as the mylohyoid and geniohyoid) passing upward to the jaw and face from the hyoid bone

su·pra·mar·gi·nal gyrus \-ˈmär-jən-ᵊl-\ n : a gyrus of the inferior part of the parietal lobe that is continuous in front with the postcentral gyrus and posteriorly and inferiorly with the superior temporal gyrus

su·pra·mo·lec·u·lar \-mə-ˈle-kyə-lər\ adj : more complex than a molecule; also : composed of many molecules

su·pra·nu·cle·ar \-ˈnü-klē-ər, -ˈnyü-\ adj : situated, occurring, or produced by a lesion superior or cortical to a nucleus esp. of the brain

supranuclear palsy *n* : PROGRESSIVE SUPRANUCLEAR PALSY

su·pra·oc·clu·sion \-ə-'klü-zhən\ *n* : the projection of a tooth beyond the plane of occlusion

su·pra·op·tic \-'äp-tik\ *adj* : situated or occurring above the optic chiasma

supraoptic nucleus *n* : a small nucleus of closely packed neurons that overlies the optic chiasma and is intimately connected with the neurohypophysis

su·pra·or·bit·al \-'ȯr-bət-ᵊl\ *adj* : situated or occurring above the orbit of the eye

supraorbital artery *n* : a branch of the ophthalmic artery supplying the orbit and parts of the forehead

supraorbital fissure *n* : ORBITAL FISSURE a

supraorbital foramen *n* : SUPRAORBITAL NOTCH

supraorbital nerve *n* : a branch of the frontal nerve supplying the forehead, scalp, cranial periosteum, and adjacent parts

supraorbital notch *n* : a notch or foramen in the bony border of the upper inner part of the orbit serving for the passage of the supraorbital nerve, artery, and vein

supraorbital ridge *n* : SUPERCILIARY RIDGE

supraorbital vein *n* : a vein that drains the supraorbital region and unites with the frontal vein to form the angular vein

su·pra·phys·i·o·log·i·cal \-ˌfi-zē-ə-'lä-ji-kəl\ *also* **su·pra·phys·i·o·log·ic** \-'lä-jik\ *adj* : greater than normally present in the body

su·pra·pu·bic \-'pyü-bik\ *adj* : situated, occurring, or performed from above the pubis ⟨∼ prostatectomy⟩ — **su·pra·pu·bi·cal·ly** *adv*

¹**su·pra·re·nal** \-'rēn-ᵊl\ *adj* : situated above or anterior to the kidneys; *specif* : ADRENAL

²**suprarenal** *n* : a suprarenal part; *esp* : ADRENAL GLAND

suprarenal artery *n* : any of three arteries on each side of the body that supply the adrenal gland located on the same side and that arise from the inferior phrenic artery, the abdominal aorta, and the renal artery

suprarenal gland *n* : ADRENAL GLAND

suprarenal vein *n* : either of two veins of which one arises from the right adrenal gland and empties directly into the inferior vena cava while the other arises from the left adrenal gland, passes behind the pancreas, and empties into the renal vein on the left side

su·pra·scap·u·lar \ˌsü-prə-'ska-pyə-lər, -ˌprä-\ *adj* : situated or occurring superior to the scapula

suprascapular artery *n* : a branch of the thyrocervical trunk that passes over the suprascapular ligament to the back of the scapula

suprascapular ligament *n* : a thin flat ligament that is attached at one end to the coracoid process and at the other end to the upper margin of the scapula on its dorsal surface

suprascapular nerve *n* : a branch of the brachial plexus that supplies the supraspinatus and infraspinatus muscles

suprascapular notch *n* : a deep notch in the upper border of the scapula at the base of the coracoid process giving passage to the suprascapular nerve

su·pra·sel·lar \-'se-lər\ *adj* : situated or rising above the sella turcica — used chiefly of tumors of the pituitary gland

su·pra·spi·nal \-'spī-nəl\ *adj* : situated or occurring above a spine

supraspinal ligament *n* : a fibrous cord that joins the tips of the spinous processes of the vertebrae from the seventh cervical vertebra to the sacrum and that continues forward to the skull as the ligamentum nuchae — called also *supraspinous ligament*

su·pra·spi·na·tus \-ˌspī-'nā-təs\ *n* : a muscle of the back of the shoulder that arises from the supraspinous fossa of the scapula, that inserts into the top of the greater tubercle of the humerus, that is one of the muscles making up the rotator cuff of the shoulder, and that rotates the humerus laterally and helps to abduct the arm

su·pra·spi·nous fossa \ˌsü-prə-'spī-nəs-\ *n* : a smooth concavity above the spine on the dorsal surface of the scapula that gives origin to the supraspinatus muscle

supraspinous ligament *n* : SUPRASPINAL LIGAMENT

su·pra·ster·nal \-'stərn-ᵊl\ *adj* : situated above or measured from the top of the sternum ⟨∼ height⟩

suprasternal notch *n* : the depression in the top of the sternum between its articulations with the two clavicles

suprasternal space *n* : a long narrow space in the lower part of the deep fascia of the cervical region containing areolar tissue, the sternal part of the sternocleidomastoid muscles, and the lower part of the anterior jugular veins

su·pra·ten·to·ri·al \-ten-'tȯr-ē-əl\ *adj* : relating to, occurring in, affecting, or being the tissues overlying the tentorium cerebelli ⟨a ∼ glioma⟩

su·pra·thresh·old \-'thresh-ˌhōld\ *adj* : of sufficient strength or quantity to produce a perceptible physiological effect ⟨∼ stimuli⟩

su·pra·troch·le·ar artery \-'trä-klē-ər-\ *n* : one of the terminal branches of the ophthalmic artery that ascends upon the forehead from the inner angle of the orbit

supratrochlear nerve *n* : a branch of the frontal nerve supplying the skin of the forehead and the upper eyelid

su·pra·val·vu·lar \-'val-vyə-lər\ *adj* : situated or occurring above a valve ⟨∼ aortic stenosis⟩

su·pra·ven·tric·u·lar \-ven-'tri-kyə-lər\ *adj* : relating to or being a rhythmic abnormality of the heart caused by impulses originating above the ventricles (as in the atrioventricular node) ⟨∼ tachycardia⟩

su·pra·vi·tal \-'vīt-ᵊl\ *adj* : constituting or relating to the staining of living tissues or cells surviving after removal from a living body by dyes that penetrate living substance but induce more or less rapid degenerative changes — compare INTRAVITAL 2 — **su·pra·vi·tal·ly** *adv*

supreme thoracic artery *n* : THORACIC ARTERY 1a

su·ral nerve \'sur-əl-\ *n* : any of several nerves in the region of the calf of the leg; *esp* : one formed by the union of a branch of the tibial nerve with a branch of the common peroneal nerve that supplies branches to the skin of the back of the leg and sends a continuation to the little toe by way of the lateral side of the foot

sur·a·min \'sur-ə-mən\ *n* : a trypanocidal drug $C_{51}H_{34}N_6Na_6O_{23}S_6$ administered intravenously in the early stages of African sleeping sickness — called also *germanin, suramin sodium*

surface–active *adj* : altering the properties and esp. lowering the tension at the surface of contact between phases ⟨soaps are typical ∼ substances⟩

surface tension *n* : the attractive force exerted upon the surface molecules of a liquid by the molecules beneath that tends to draw the surface molecules into the bulk of the liquid and makes the liquid assume the shape having the least surface area

sur·fac·tant \(ˌ)sər-'fak-tənt, 'sər-ˌ\ *n* : a surface-active substance; *specif* : a surface-active lipoprotein mixture which coats the alveoli and which prevents collapse of the lungs by reducing the surface tension of pulmonary fluids — **surfactant** *adj*

surg *abbr* 1 surgeon 2 surgery 3 surgical

sur·geon \'sər-jən\ *n* 1 : a medical specialist who performs surgery : a physician qualified to treat those diseases that are amenable to or require surgery — compare INTERNIST 2 : the senior medical officer of a military unit

surgeon general *n, pl* **surgeons general** : the chief medical officer of a branch of the armed services or of a public health service

sur·gery \'sər-jə-rē\ *n, pl* **-ger·ies** 1 : a branch of medicine concerned with diseases and conditions requiring or amenable to operative or manual procedures 2 a *Brit* : a physician's or dentist's office b : a room or area where surgery is performed 3 a : the

work done by a surgeon b : OPERATION

sur·gi·cal \'sər-ji-kəl\ *adj* 1 : of, relating to, or concerned with surgeons or surgery 2 : requiring surgical treatment ⟨a ∼ appendix⟩ 3 : used in or in connection with surgery ⟨∼ gauze⟩ 4 : following or resulting from surgery ⟨∼ fevers⟩

sur·gi·cal·ly \'sər-ji-klē, -kə-lē\ *adv* : by means of surgery

surgical neck *n* : a slightly narrowed part of the humerus below the greater and lesser tubercles that is frequently the site of fractures

sur·gi·cen·ter \'sər-jə-ˌsen-tər\ *n* : a medical facility that performs minor surgery on an outpatient basis

sur·ra \'sur-ə\ *n* : a severe febrile and hemorrhagic disease of tropical or subtropical domestic animals that is caused by a protozoan of the genus *Trypanosoma* (T. evansi)

sur·ro·ga·cy \'sər-ə-gə-sē\ *n, pl* **-cies** : the practice of serving as a surrogate mother

sur·ro·gate \-gət\ *n* : one that serves as a substitute: as a : a representation of a person substituted through symbolizing (as in a dream) for conscious recognition of the person b : a drug substituted for another drug c : SURROGATE MOTHER

surrogate mother *n* : a woman who becomes pregnant usu. by artificial insemination or surgical implantation of a fertilized egg for the purpose of carrying the fetus to term for another woman — **surrogate motherhood** *n*

sur·veil·lance \sər-'vā-ləns, -lyəns\ *n* : close and continuous observation or testing ⟨serological ∼⟩ — see IMMUNOLOGICAL SURVEILLANCE

sur·vi·vor·ship \sər-'vī-vər-ˌship\ *n* 1 : the state of being a survivor 2 : the probability of surviving to a particular age; *also* : the number or proportion of survivors (as of an age group)

¹**sus·cep·ti·ble** \sə-'sep-tə-bəl\ *adj* 1 : having little resistance to a specific infectious disease : capable of being infected 2 : predisposed to develop a noninfectious disease ⟨∼ to diabetes⟩ 3 : abnormally reactive to various drugs — **sus·cep·ti·bil·i·ty** \sə-ˌsep-tə-'bi-lə-tē\ *n*

²**susceptible** *n* : one that is susceptible (as to a disease)

suspended animation *n* : temporary suspension of the vital functions

sus·pen·sion \sə-'spen-chən\ *n* 1 a : the state of a substance when its particles are mixed with but undissolved in a fluid or solid b : a substance in this state — see ORAL SUSPENSION 2 : a system consisting of a solid dispersed in a solid, liquid, or gas usu. in particles of larger than colloidal size

¹**sus·pen·so·ry** \sə-'spen-sə-rē\ *adj* : serving to suspend : providing support

²**suspensory** n, pl **-ries** : something that suspends or holds up; esp : a fabric supporter for the scrotum

suspensory ligament n : a ligament or fibrous membrane suspending an organ or part: as **a** : a ringlike fibrous membrane connecting the ciliary body and the lens of the eye and holding the lens in place **b** : FALCIFORM LIGAMENT

suspensory ligament of the ovary n : a fold of peritoneum that consists of a part of the broad ligament that is attached to the ovary near the end joining the fallopian tube and that contains blood and lymph vessels passing to and from the ovary — called also infundibulopelvic ligament; compare LIGAMENT OF THE OVARY

sustained–release adj : designed to slowly release a drug in the body over an extended period of time ⟨∼ capsules⟩ — compare TIMED-RELEASE

sus·ten·tac·u·lar cell \ˌsəs-tən-ˈta-kyə-lər-\ n : a supporting epithelial cell (as of the olfactory epithelium) that lacks a specialized function

sustentacular fiber of Müller n : FIBER OF MÜLLER

sus·ten·tac·u·lum ta·li \ˌsəs-tən-ˈta-kyə-ləm-ˈtā-ˌlī\ n : a medial process of the calcaneus supporting part of the talus

su·ture \ˈsü-chər\ n **1 a** : a stitch made with a suture **b** : a strand or fiber used to sew parts of the living body **c** : the act or process of sewing with sutures **2 a** : the line of union in an immovable articulation (as between the bones of the skull); also : such an articulation **b** : a furrow at the junction of adjacent bodily parts — **su·tur·al** \ˈsü-chə-rəl\ adj — **suture** vb

suxa·me·tho·ni·um \ˌsük-sə-mə-ˈthō-nē-əm\ n, chiefly Brit : SUCCINYLCHOLINE

Sv abbr sievert

sved·berg \ˈsfed-ˌbərg, -ˌber-ē\ n : a unit of time amounting to 10⁻¹³ second that is used to measure the sedimentation velocity of a colloidal solution (as of a protein) in an ultracentrifuge and to determine molecular weight by substitution in an equation — called also svedberg unit

Svedberg, Theodor (1884–1971), Swedish chemist.

SV40 \ˌes-ˌvē-ˈfȯr-tē\ n : SIMIAN VIRUS 40

SVT abbr supraventricular tachycardia

swab \ˈswäb\ n **1** : a wad of absorbent material usu. wound around one end of a small stick and used for applying medication or for removing material from an area **2** : a specimen taken with a swab ⟨a throat ∼⟩ — **swab** vb

swamp fever n : EQUINE INFECTIOUS ANEMIA

Swan–Ganz catheter \ˈswän-ˈganz-\ n : a soft catheter with a balloon tip that is used for measuring blood pressure in the pulmonary artery

Swan, Harold James Charles (b 1922), and Ganz, William (b 1919), American cardiologists.

S wave \ˈes-\ n : the negative downward deflection in the QRS complex of an electrocardiogram that follows the R wave

sway·back \ˈswā-ˌbak\ n **1** : an abnormally hollow condition or sagging of the back found esp. in horses; also : a back so shaped **2** : LORDOSIS **3** : a copper-deficiency disease of young or newborn lambs that is marked by demyelination of the brain — **sway·backed** \-ˌbakt\ adj

¹**sweat** \ˈswet\ vb **sweat** or **sweat·ed**; **sweat·ing** : to excrete moisture in visible quantities through the opening of the sweat glands : PERSPIRE

²**sweat** n **1** : the fluid excreted from the sweat glands of the skin : PERSPIRATION **2** : abnormally profuse sweating — often used in pl. ⟨soaking ∼s⟩ — **sweaty** \-ē\ adj

sweat duct n : the part of a sweat gland which extends through the dermis to the surface of the skin

sweat gland n : a simple tubular gland of the skin that secretes perspiration and in humans is widely distributed in nearly all parts of the skin — called also sudoriferous gland

sweat test n : a test for cystic fibrosis that involves measuring the subject's sweat for abnormally high sodium chloride content

swee·ny \ˈswē-nē\ n, pl **sweenies** : an atrophy of the shoulder muscles of a horse; broadly : any muscular atrophy of a horse

sweet \ˈswēt\ adj : being or inducing the one of the four basic taste sensations that is typically induced by disaccharides and is mediated esp. by receptors in taste buds at the front of the tongue — compare BITTER, SALT 2, SOUR — **sweet·ness** n

Sweet's syndrome \ˈswēts-\ n : a disease that occurs esp. in middle-aged women, that is characterized by red raised often painful patches on the skin, fever, and neutrophilia in the peripheral blood, that responds to treatment with corticosteroids but not antibiotics, and that is of unknown cause but is sometimes associated with an underlying malignant disorder — called also acute febrile neutrophilic dermatosis

Sweet, Robert Douglas (1917–2001), British dermatologist.

swell \ˈswel\ vb **swelled**; **swelled** or **swol·len** \ˈswō-lən\; **swell·ing** : to become distended or puffed up

swell·ing \ˈswel-iŋ\ n : an abnormal bodily protuberance or localized enlargement ⟨an inflammatory ∼⟩

Swift's disease \ˈswifts-\ n : ACRODYNIA

Swift, H. (fl 1918), Australian physician.

swimmer's ear n : inflammation of

the canal in the outer ear that is characterized by itching, redness, swelling, pain, discharge, and sometimes hearing loss and that typically occurs when water trapped in the outer ear during swimming becomes infected usu. with a bacterium

swimmer's itch n : an itching inflammation that is a reaction to the invasion of the skin by schistosomes that are not normally parasites of humans — called also *schistosome dermatitis*

swine \'swīn\ n : any of various stout-bodied short-legged mammals (family Suidae) with a thick bristly skin and a long flexible snout; *esp* : one domesticated from a species (*Sus scrofa*) that occurs wild in the Old World

swine dysentery n : an acute infectious hemorrhagic dysentery of swine

swine erysipelas n : a destructive contagious disease of various mammals and birds that is caused by a bacterium of the genus *Erysipelothrix* (*E. rhusiopathiae*) — called also *erysipelas*

swine fever n 1 : HOG CHOLERA 2 : AFRICAN SWINE FEVER

swineherd's disease n : a form of leptospirosis contracted from swine

swine influenza n : an acute contagious febrile but seldom fatal disease of swine that is marked by severe coughing and inflammation of the upper respiratory tract, that is caused by infection with a subtype (esp. H1N1 or N3N2) of the orthomyxovirus causing influenza A, and that is often complicated by infection with another pathogen (as the pseudorabies virus) — called also *swine flu*

swine·pox \'swīn-ˌpäks\ n : a mild virus disease of young pigs that is marked by fever, loss of appetite, relative indifference to normal stimuli, and production of skin lesions and that is caused by a poxvirus (species *Swinepox virus* of the genus *Suipoxvirus*) transmitted esp. by the hog louse

swol·len adj : protuberant or abnormally distended (as by injury or disease)

sy·co·sis \sī-'kō-səs\ n, pl **sy·co·ses** \-ˌsēz\ : a chronic inflammatory disease involving the hair follicles esp. of the bearded part of the face and marked by papules, pustules, and tubercles perforated by hairs with crusting

sycosis bar·bae \-'bär-bē\ n : sycosis of the bearded part of the face

Syd·en·ham's chorea \'sid-ᵊn-əmz-\ n : chorea following infection (as rheumatic fever) and occurring usu. in children and adolescents — called also *Saint Vitus' dance*
  Sydenham, Thomas (1624–1689), British physician.

syl·vat·ic \sil-'va-tik\ adj : occurring in, affecting, or transmitted by wild animals ⟨∼ diseases⟩

sylvatic plague n : a form of plague of which wild rodents and their fleas are the reservoirs and vectors and which is widely distributed in western No. and So. America though rarely affecting humans

syl·vi·an \'sil-vē-ən\ adj, often cap : of or relating to the sylvian fissure
  Du·bois \dē-'bwä\ or **De Le Boë** \dä-lä-'bō-ā\, **François** or **Franz** (*Latin* **Franciscus Sylvius**) (1614–1672), Dutch anatomist, physician, and chemist.

sylvian fissure n, often cap 1st S : a deep fissure of the lateral aspect of each cerebral hemisphere that divides the temporal from the parietal and frontal lobes — called also *fissure of Sylvius, lateral fissure, lateral sulcus*

sym- — see SYN-

sym·bi·ont \'sim-ˌbī-ˌänt, -bē-\ n : an organism living in symbiosis; *esp* : the smaller member of a symbiotic pair — called also *symbiote*

sym·bi·o·sis \ˌsim-ˌbī-'ō-səs, -bē-\ n, pl **-bi·o·ses** \-ˌsēz\ 1 : the living together in more or less intimate association or close union of two dissimilar organisms 2 : the intimate living together of two dissimilar organisms in a mutually beneficial relationship — **sym·bi·ot·ic** \ˌsim-ˌbī-'ä-tik, -bē-\ adj — **sym·bi·ot·i·cal·ly** \-i-k(ə-)lē\ adv

sym·bi·ote \'sim-ˌbī-ˌōt, -bē-\ n : SYMBIONT

sym·bleph·a·ron \sim-'ble-fə-ˌrän\ n : adhesion between an eyelid and the eyeball

sym·bol \'sim-bəl\ n : something that stands for or suggests something else; *esp* : an object or act representing something in the unconscious mind that has been repressed ⟨phallic ∼s⟩ — **sym·bol·ic** \sim-'bä-lik\ adj — **sym·bol·i·cal·ly** adv

Syme's amputation \'sīmz-\ or **Syme amputation** \'sīm-\ n : amputation of the foot through the articulation of the ankle with removal of the malleoli of the tibia and fibula — compare PIROGOFF'S AMPUTATION
  Syme, James (1799–1870), British surgeon.

Sym·me·trel \'si-mə-ˌtrel\ *trademark* — used for a preparation of the hydrochloride of amantadine

sym·me·try \'si-mə-trē\ n, pl **-tries** : correspondence in size, shape, and relative position of parts on opposite sides of a dividing line or median plane or about a center or axis — see BILATERAL SYMMETRY, RADIAL SYMMETRY — **sym·met·ri·cal** \sə-'me-tri-kəl\ or **sym·met·ric** \-trik\ adj — **sym·met·ri·cal·ly** adv

sympath- or **sympatho-** comb form : sympathetic nerve : sympathetic nervous system ⟨*sympatho*lytic⟩

sym·pa·thec·to·my \ˌsim-pə-'thek-tə-mē\ n, pl **-mies** : surgical interruption of sympathetic nerve pathways — **sym·pa·thec·to·mized** \-ˌmīzd\ adj

¹**sym·pa·thet·ic** \ˌsim-pə-ˈthe-tik\ adj **1** : of or relating to the sympathetic nervous system **2** : mediated by or acting on the sympathetic nerves — **sym·pa·thet·i·cal·ly** adv

²**sympathetic** n : a sympathetic structure; esp : SYMPATHETIC NERVOUS SYSTEM

sympathetic chain n : either of the pair of ganglionated longitudinal cords of the sympathetic nervous system of which one is situated on each side of the spinal column — called also *sympathetic trunk;* compare VERTEBRAL GANGLION

sympathetic nerve n : a nerve of the sympathetic nervous system

sympathetic nervous system n : the part of the autonomic nervous system that contains chiefly adrenergic fibers and tends to depress secretion, decrease the tone and contractility of smooth muscle, and increase heart rate and that consists of preganglionic fibers arising in the thoracic and upper lumbar parts of the spinal cord and passing through white rami communicantes to ganglia located in a pair of sympathetic chains situated one on each side of the spinal column or to more peripheral ganglia or ganglionated plexuses and postganglionic fibers passing typically through gray rami communicantes to spinal nerves with which they are distributed to various end organs — called also *sympathetic system;* compare PARASYMPATHETIC NERVOUS SYSTEM

sympathetico- comb form : SYMPATH- ⟨*sympathetico*mimetic⟩

sym·pa·thet·i·co·mi·met·ic \ˌsim-pə-ˈthe-ti-kō-mə-ˈme-tik\ adj or n : SYMPATHOMIMETIC

sympathetic ophthalmia n : inflammation in an uninjured eye as a result of injury and inflammation of the other

sym·pa·thet·i·co·to·nia \ˌsim-pə-ˌthe-ti-kə-ˈtō-nē-ə\ n : SYMPATHICOTONIA

sympathetic system n : SYMPATHETIC NERVOUS SYSTEM

sympathetic trunk n : SYMPATHETIC CHAIN

sympathico- comb form : SYMPATH- ⟨*sympathico*tonia⟩

sym·path·i·co·lyt·ic \sim-ˌpa-thi-kō-ˈli-tik\ adj or n : SYMPATHOLYTIC

sym·path·i·co·mi·met·ic \-mə-ˈme-tik, -mī-\ adj or n : SYMPATHOMIMETIC

sym·path·i·co·to·nia \sim-ˌpa-thi-kō-ˈtō-nē-ə\ n : a condition produced by relatively great activity or stimulation of the sympathetic nervous system and characterized by goose bumps, vascular spasm, and abnormally high blood pressure — called also *sympatheticotonia* — **sym·path·i·co·ton·ic** \-ˈtä-nik\ adj

sym·pa·thin \ˈsim-pə-thən\ n : a substance (as norepinephrine) that is secreted by sympathetic nerve endings and acts as a chemical mediator

sym·pa·tho·ad·re·nal \ˌsim-pə-thō-ə-ˈdrē-nəl\ adj : relating to or involving the sympathetic nervous system and the adrenal medulla

sym·pa·tho·go·nia \ˌsim-pə-thō-ˈgō-nē-ə\ n : precursor cells of the sympathetic nervous system

sym·pa·tho·go·ni·o·ma \-ˌgō-nē-ˈō-mə\ n, pl **-ma·ta** \-mə-tə\ or **-mas** : a tumor derived from sympathogonia; also : NEUROBLASTOMA

¹**sym·pa·tho·lyt·ic** \ˌsim-pə-thō-ˈli-tik\ adj : tending to oppose the physiological results of sympathetic nervous activity or of sympathomimetic drugs — compare PARASYMPATHOLYTIC

²**sympatholytic** n : a sympatholytic agent

¹**sym·pa·tho·mi·met·ic** \-mə-ˈme-tik, -(ˌ)mī-\ adj : simulating sympathetic nervous action in physiological effect — compare PARASYMPATHOMIMETIC

²**sympathomimetic** n : a sympathomimetic agent

sym·phal·an·gism \(ˌ)sim-ˈfa-lən-ˌji-zəm\ n : ankylosis of the joints of one or more digits

sym·phy·se·al \ˌsim-fə-ˈsē-əl\ adj : of, relating to, or constituting a symphysis

sym·phys·i·ot·o·my \ˌsim-fə-zē-ˈä-tə-mē, sim-ˌfi-zē-\ n, pl **-mies** : the operation of dividing the pubic symphysis

sym·phy·sis \ˈsim-fə-səs\ n, pl **-phy·ses** \-ˌsēz\ **1** : an immovable or more or less movable articulation of various bones in the median plane of the body **2** : an articulation (as between the bodies of vertebrae) in which the bony surfaces are connected by pads of fibrous cartilage without a synovial membrane

symphysis pubis n : PUBIC SYMPHYSIS

symp·tom \ˈsimp-təm\ n : subjective evidence of disease or physical disturbance observed by the patient; broadly : something that indicates the presence of a physical disorder — compare SIGN 2

symp·tom·at·ic \ˌsimp-tə-ˈma-tik\ adj **1 a** : being a symptom of a disease **b** : having the characteristics of a particular disease but arising from another cause ⟨∼ epilepsy resulting from brain damage⟩ **2** : concerned with or affecting symptoms ⟨∼ treatment⟩ **3** : having symptoms ⟨a ∼ patient⟩ — **symp·tom·at·i·cal·ly** adv

symp·tom·atol·o·gy \ˌsimp-tə-mə-ˈtä-lə-jē\ n, pl **-gies 1** : SYMPTOM COMPLEX **2** : a branch of medical science concerned with symptoms of diseases — **symp·tom·at·o·log·i·cal** \-ˌmat-ᵊl-ˈä-ji-kəl\ or **symp·tom·at·o·log·ic** \-ˈä-jik\ adj — **symp·tom·at·o·log·i·cal·ly** adv

symptom complex n : a group of symptoms occurring together and characterizing a particular disease

symp·tom·less \'simp-təm-ləs\ *adj*
: exhibiting no symptoms

syn- *or* **sym-** *prefix* **1** : with : together with ⟨*sym*biosis⟩ **2** : at the same time ⟨*syn*esthesia⟩

syn·aes·the·sia *chiefly Brit var of* SYNESTHESIA

syn·an·throp·ic \si-nan-'thrä-pik\ *adj* : ecologically associated with humans ⟨~ flies⟩ — **syn·an·thro·py** \sin-'an-thrə-pē\ *n*

¹**syn·apse** \'si-,naps, sə-'naps\ *n* **1** : the place at which a nervous impulse passes from one neuron to another **2** : SYNAPSIS

²**synapse** *vb* **syn·apsed; syn·aps·ing** : to form a synapse or come together in synapsis

syn·ap·sis \sə-'nap-səs\ *n, pl* **-ap·ses** \-,sēz\ : the association of homologous chromosomes with chiasma formation that is characteristic of the first meiotic prophase and is held to be the mechanism for genetic crossing-over

syn·ap·tic \si-'nap-tik\ *adj* **1** : of, relating to, or participating in synapsis ⟨~ chromosomes⟩ **2** : of or relating to a synapse ⟨~ transmission⟩ — **syn·ap·ti·cal·ly** *adv*

synaptic cleft *n* : the space between neurons at a nerve synapse across which a nerve impulse is transmitted by a neurotransmitter — called also *synaptic gap*

synaptic vesicle *n* : a small secretory vesicle that contains a neurotransmitter, is found inside an axon near the presynaptic membrane, and releases its contents into the synaptic cleft after fusing with the membrane

syn·ap·to·gen·e·sis \si-,nap-tə-'je-nə-səs\ *n, pl* **-e·ses** \-,sēz\ : the formation of nerve synapses

syn·ap·tol·o·gy \si-nap-'tä-lə-jē\ *n, pl* **-gies** : the scientific study of nerve synapses

syn·ap·to·phy·sin \si-'nap-tə-,fī-sⁿn\ *n* : a transmembrane glycoprotein found chiefly in presynaptic vesicles of neurons and neurosecretory granules of neuroendocrine cells

syn·ap·to·some \sə-'nap-tə-,sōm\ *n* : a nerve ending that is isolated from homogenized nerve tissue — **syn·ap·to·som·al** \-,nap-tə-'sō-məl\ *adj*

syn·ar·thro·sis \,si-när-'thrō-səs\ *n, pl* **-thro·ses** \-,sēz\ : an immovable articulation in which the bones are united by intervening fibrous connective tissues

syn·chon·dro·sis \,sin-,kän-'drō-səs\ *n, pl* **-dro·ses** \-,sēz\ : an immovable skeletal articulation in which the union is cartilaginous

syn·cho·ri·al \,sin-'kōr-ē-əl, siŋ-\ *adj* : having a common placenta — used of multiple fetuses

syn·chro·nic·i·ty \,sin-krə-'ni-sə-tē\ *n, pl* **-ties** : the coincidental occurrence of events and esp. psychic events (as similar thoughts in widely separated persons) that seem related but are not explained by conventional mechanisms of causality — used esp. in the psychology of C. G. Jung

syn·chro·nized sleep \'sin-krə-,nīzd-, -sin-\ *n* : SLOW-WAVE SLEEP

syn·co·pe \'sin-kə-pē, 'sin-\ *n* : loss of consciousness resulting from insufficient blood flow to the brain : FAINT — **syn·co·pal** \'sin-kə-pəl, 'sin-\ *adj*

syn·cy·tial \sin-'si-shəl, -shē-əl\ *adj* : of, relating to, or constituting syncytium

syn·cy·tio·tro·pho·blast \sin-,si-shē-ō-'trō-fə-,blast\ *n* : the outer syncytial layer of the trophoblast that actively invades the uterine wall forming the outermost fetal component of the placenta — called also *syntrophoblast;* compare CYTOTROPHOBLAST

syn·cy·tium \sin-'si-shəm, -shē-əm\ *n, pl* **-tia** \-shə, -shē-ə\ : a multinucleate mass of protoplasm resulting from fusion of cells

syn·dac·tyl \sin-'dakt-ᵊl\ *adj* : having two or more digits wholly or partly united

syn·dac·ty·lism \sin-'dak-tə-,li-zəm\ *n* : SYNDACTYLY

syn·dac·ty·lous \sin-'dak-tə-ləs\ *adj* : SYNDACTYL

syn·dac·ty·ly \-lē\ *n, pl* **-lies** : a union of two or more digits that occurs in humans often as a hereditary disorder marked by the joining or webbing of two or more fingers or toes

syndesm- *or* **syndesmo-** *comb form* : ligament ⟨*syndesm*osis⟩

syn·des·mo·sis \,sin-,dez-'mō-səs, -,des-\ *n, pl* **-mo·ses** \-,sēz\ : an articulation in which the contiguous surfaces of the bones are rough and are bound together by a ligament

syn·drome \'sin-,drōm\ *n* : a group of signs and symptoms that occur together and characterize a particular abnormality

syndrome X *n* **1** : angina pectoris of a usu. benign form in which the coronary arteriogram is normal **2** : METABOLIC SYNDROME

syn·drom·ic \sin-'drō-mik, -'drä-\ *adj* : occurring as a syndrome or part of a syndrome ⟨~ deafness⟩

syn·e·chia \si-'ne-kē-ə, -'nē-\ *n, pl* **-chiae** \-kē-,ē, -,ī\ : an adhesion of parts and esp. one involving the iris of the eye: as **a** : adhesion of the iris to the cornea — called also *anterior synechia* **b** : adhesion of the iris to the crystalline lens — called also *posterior synechia*

syn·eph·rine \sə-'ne-frən\ *n* : a crystalline sympathomimetic amine $C_9H_{13}NO_2$ isomeric with phenylephrine

syn·er·gic \si-'nər-jik\ *adj* : working together ⟨~ muscle contraction⟩ — **syn·er·gi·cal·ly** *adv*

syn·er·gism \'si-nər-ji-zəm\ *n* : interaction of discrete agents (as drugs) such that the total effect is greater than the sum of the individual effects — called also *synergy;* compare ANTAGONISM b — **syn·er·gis·tic** \ˌsi-nər-ˈjis-tik\ *adj* — **syn·er·gis·ti·cal·ly** *adv*

syn·er·gist \-jist\ *n* **1** : an agent that increases the effectiveness of another agent when combined with it; *esp* : a drug that acts in synergism with another **2** : an organ (as a muscle) that acts in concert with another to enhance its effect — compare AGONIST 1, ANTAGONIST a

syn·er·gize \ˈsi-nər-ˌjīz\ *vb* **-gized; -giz·ing 1** : to act as synergists : exhibit synergism **2** : to increase the activity of (a substance)

syn·er·gy \-jē\ *n, pl* **-gies** : SYNERGISM

syn·es·the·sia \ˌsi-nəs-ˈthē-zhə, -zhē-ə\ *n* : a concomitant sensation and esp. a subjective sensation or image of a sense (as of color) other than the one (as of sound) that is being stimulated; *also* : the condition marked by the experience of such sensations — **syn·es·thet·ic** \-ˈthe-tik\ *adj*

Syn·ga·mus \ˈsiŋ-gə-məs\ *n* : a genus (family Syngamidae) of nematode worms that are parasitic in the trachea or esophagus of various birds and mammals and include the gapeworm (*S. trachea*)

syn·ga·my \ˈsiŋ-gə-mē\ *n, pl* **-mies** : sexual reproduction by union of gametes

syn·ge·ne·ic \ˌsin-jə-ˈnē-ik\ *adj* : genetically identical esp. with respect to antigens or immunological reactions ⟨~ tumor cells⟩ — compare ALLOGENEIC, XENOGENEIC

syn·kary·on \sin-ˈkar-ē-ˌän, -ē-ən\ *n* : a cell nucleus formed by the fusion of two preexisting nuclei

syn·ki·ne·sia \ˌsin-kə-ˈnē-zhə, -ˌkī-, -zhē-ə\ *n* : SYNKINESIS

syn·ki·ne·sis \-ˈnē-səs\ *n, pl* **-ne·ses** \-ˌsēz\ : involuntary movement in one part when another part is moved : an associated movement — **syn·ki·net·ic** \-ˈne-tik\ *adj*

syn·os·to·sis \ˌsi-ˌnäs-ˈtō-səs\ *n, pl* **-to·ses** \-ˌsēz\ : union of two or more separate bones to form a single bone; *also* : the union so formed — **syn·os·tot·ic** \-ˈtä-tik\ *adj*

syn·o·vec·to·my \ˌsi-nə-ˈvek-tə-mē\ *n, pl* **-mies** : surgical removal of a synovial membrane

sy·no·via \sə-ˈnō-vē-ə, sī-\ *n* : SYNOVIAL FLUID

sy·no·vi·al \-vē-əl\ *adj* : of, relating to, or secreting synovial fluid ⟨~ effusion⟩; *also* : lined with synovial membrane ⟨a ~ bursa⟩

synovial cyst *n* : a cyst (as a Baker's cyst) containing synovial fluid

synovial fluid *n* : a transparent viscid lubricating fluid secreted by a membrane of an articulation, bursa, or tendon sheath — called also *joint fluid, synovia*

synovial joint *n* : DIARTHROSIS

synovial membrane *n* : the dense connective-tissue membrane that secretes synovial fluid and that lines the ligamentous surfaces of joint capsules, tendon sheaths where free movement is necessary, and bursae

sy·no·vi·tis \ˌsī-nə-ˈvī-təs\ *n* : inflammation of a synovial membrane usu. with pain and swelling of the joint

sy·no·vi·um \sə-ˈnō-vē-əm, sī-\ *n* : SYNOVIAL MEMBRANE

syn·the·sis \ˈsin-thə-səs\ *n, pl* **-the·ses** \-ˌsēz\ **1** : the composition or combination of parts or elements so as to form a whole **2** : the production of a substance by the union of chemical elements, groups, or simpler compounds or by the degradation of a complex compound ⟨protein ~⟩ — **syn·the·size** \-ˌsīz\ *vb*

syn·the·tase \ˈsin-thə-ˌtās, -ˌtāz\ *n* : an enzyme that catalyzes the linking together of two molecules esp. by using the energy derived from the concurrent splitting off of a group from a triphosphate (as ATP) — called also *ligase*

¹syn·thet·ic \sin-ˈthe-tik\ *adj* : of, relating to, or produced by chemical or biochemical synthesis; *esp* : produced artificially ⟨~ drugs⟩ — **syn·thet·i·cal·ly** *adv*

²synthetic *n* : a product (as a drug) of chemical synthesis

Syn·throid \ˈsin-ˌthrȯid\ *trademark* — used for a preparation of the sodium salt of levothyroxine

syn·tro·pho·blast \sin-ˈtrō-fə-ˌblast\ *n* : SYNCYTIOTROPHOBLAST

syphil- *or* **syphilo-** *comb form* : syphilis ⟨*syphiloma*⟩

syph·i·lid \ˈsi-fə-lid\ *n* : a skin eruption caused by syphilis

syph·i·lis \ˈsi-fə-ləs\ *n* : a chronic contagious usu. venereal and often congenital disease that is caused by a spirochete of the genus *Treponema* (*T. pallidum*) and if left untreated produces chancres, rashes, and systemic lesions in a clinical course with three stages continued over many years — called also *lues;* see PRIMARY SYPHILIS, SECONDARY SYPHILIS, TERTIARY SYPHILIS

¹syph·i·lit·ic \ˌsi-fə-ˈli-tik\ *adj* : of, relating to, or infected with syphilis — **syph·i·lit·i·cal·ly** *adv*

²syphilitic *n* : a person infected with syphilis

syph·i·lo·ma \ˌsi-fə-ˈlō-mə\ *n, pl* **-mas** *or* **-ma·ta** \-mə-tə\ : a syphilitic tumor : GUMMA ⟨a testicular ~⟩

sy·rette \sə-ˈret\ *n, often cap* : a small collapsible tube fitted with a hypodermic needle for injecting a single dose of a medicinal agent

syring- *or* **syringo-** *comb form* : tube : fistula ⟨*syringo*bulbia⟩

sy·ringe \sə-ˈrinj, ˈsir-inj\ *n* : a device used to inject fluids into or withdraw them from something (as the body or its cavities): as **a** : a device that consists of a nozzle of varying length and a compressible rubber bulb and is used for injection or irrigation ⟨an ear ∼⟩ **b** : an instrument (as for the injection of medicine or the withdrawal of bodily fluids) that consists of a hollow barrel fitted with a plunger and a hollow needle **c** : a gravity device consisting of a reservoir fitted with a long rubber tube ending with an exchangeable nozzle that is used for irrigation of the vagina or bowel — **syringe** *vb*

sy·rin·go·bul·bia \sə-ˌriŋ-gō-ˈbəl-bē-ə\ *n* : the presence of abnormal cavities in the medulla oblongata

sy·rin·go·my·elia \sə-ˌriŋ-gō-mī-ˈē-lē-ə\ *n* : a chronic progressive disease of the spinal cord associated with sensory disturbances, muscle atrophy, and spasticity

syr·inx \ˈsir-iŋks\ *n, pl* **sy·rin·ges** \sə-ˈriŋ-ˌgēz, -ˈrin-ˌjēz\ *or* **syr·inx·es** : a pathological cavity in the brain or spinal cord esp. in syringomyelia

syr·o·sin·go·pine \ˌsir-ō-ˈsiŋ-gə-ˌpēn, -ˌpin\ *n* : an antihypertensive agent $C_{35}H_{42}N_2O_{11}$ that is closely related to reserpine

syr·up *also* **sir·up** \ˈsər-əp, ˈsir-əp\ *n* : a thick sticky liquid consisting of a concentrated solution of sugar and water with or without the addition of a flavoring agent or medicinal substance — **syr·upy** \-ə-pē\ *adj*

syrup of ipecac *n* : IPECAC SYRUP

sys·tem \ˈsis-təm\ *n* **1** : a group of body organs that together perform one or more vital functions — see CIRCULATORY SYSTEM, DIGESTIVE SYSTEM, ENDOCRINE SYSTEM, LIMBIC SYSTEM, NERVOUS SYSTEM, REPRODUCTIVE SYSTEM, RESPIRATORY SYSTEM **2** : the body considered as a functional unit

¹sys·tem·ic \sis-ˈte-mik\ *adj* : of, relating to, or common to a system: as **a** : affecting the body generally — compare LOCAL **b** : supplying those parts of the body that receive blood through the aorta rather than through the pulmonary artery **c** : being a pesticide that as used is harmless to a higher animal or a plant but when absorbed into the bloodstream or the sap makes the whole organism toxic to pests (as an insect or fungus) — **sys·tem·i·cal·ly** *adv*

²systemic *n* : a systemic pesticide

systemic circulation *n* : the passage of arterial blood from the left atrium of the heart through the left ventricle, the systemic arteries, and the capillaries to the organs and tissues that receive much of its oxygen in exchange for carbon dioxide and the return of the carbon-dioxide carrying blood via the systemic veins to enter the right atrium of the heart and to participate in the pulmonary circulation

systemic inflammatory response syndrome *n* : a severe systemic response to a condition (as trauma, an infection, or a burn) that provokes an acute inflammatory reaction indicated by the presence of two or more of a group of symptoms including abnormally increased or decreased body temperature, heart rate greater than 90 beats per minute, respiratory rate greater than 20 breaths per minute or a reduced concentration of carbon dioxide in the arterial blood, and the white blood cell count greatly decreased or increased or consisting of more than ten percent immature neutrophils — abbr. *SIRS;* see SEPSIS

systemic lupus erythematosus *n* : an inflammatory connective tissue disease of unknown cause that occurs chiefly in women and is characterized esp. by fever, skin rash, and arthritis, often by acute hemolytic anemia, by small hemorrhages in the skin and mucous membranes, by inflammation of the pericardium, and in serious cases by involvement of the kidneys and central nervous system — called also *systemic lupus*

systemic necrotizing vasculitis *n* : NECROTIZING VASCULITIS

sys·to·le \ˈsis-tə-(ˌ)lē\ *n* : the contraction of the heart by which the blood is forced onward and the circulation kept up — compare DIASTOLE — **sys·tol·ic** \sis-ˈtä-lik\ *adj*

systolic blood pressure *n* : the highest arterial blood pressure of a cardiac cycle occurring immediately after systole of the left ventricle of the heart — called also *systolic pressure;* compare DIASTOLIC BLOOD PRESSURE

T

T *abbr* **1** thoracic — used with a number from 1 to 12 to indicate a vertebra or segment of the spinal cord ⟨a fracture of *T-12*⟩ **2** thymine

T *symbol* tritium

2,4,5–T — see entry alphabetized as TWO, FOUR, FIVE-T in the letter *t*

Ta *symbol* tantalum

TA *abbr* transactional analysis

tab \ˈtab\ *n* : TABLET

ta·bar·dil·lo \ˌtä-bär-ˈdē-yō\ *n* : murine typhus occurring esp. in Mexico

ta·bel·la \tə-ˈbe-lə\ *n, pl* **-lae** \-ˌlē\ : a medicated lozenge or tablet

ta·bes \'tā-(ₐ)bēz\ *n, pl* **tabes** **1** : wasting accompanying a chronic disease **2** : TABES DORSALIS

tabes dor·sa·lis \-dór-'sā-ləs, -'sa-\ *n* : a syphilitic disorder that involves the dorsal horns of the spinal cord and the sensory nerve trunks and that is marked by wasting, pain, lack of coordination of voluntary movements and reflexes, and disorders of sensation, nutrition, and vision — called also *locomotor ataxia*

ta·bet·ic \tə-'be-tik\ *adj* : of, relating to, or affected with tabes and esp. tabes dorsalis ⟨~ pains⟩ ⟨a ~ joint⟩

ta·ble·spoon \'tā-bəl-ˌspün\ *n* : a unit of measure equal to 4 fluid drams or ¹/₂ fluid ounce or 15 milliliters

ta·ble·spoon·ful \ˌtā-bəl-'spün-ˌfül, 'tā-bəl-ₐ\ *n, pl* **tablespoonfuls** \-ₐfülz\ *also* **ta·ble·spoons·ful** \-'spünz-ˌfül,-ˌspünz-\ : TABLESPOON

tab·let \'ta-blət\ *n* : a small mass of medicated material (as in the shape of a disk) ⟨an aspirin ~⟩

tabo- *comb form* : progressive wasting : tabes ⟨*tabo*paresis⟩

ta·bo·pa·re·sis \ˌtā-bō-pə-'rē-səs, -'par-ə-səs\ *n, pl* **-re·ses** \-ˌsēz\ : paresis occurring with tabes and esp. with tabes dorsalis

tache noire \'täsh-'nwär\ *n, pl* **taches noires** *same or* -'nwärz\ : a small dark-centered ulcer that appears at the site of a tick bite and is the primary lesion of boutonneuse fever

ta·chis·to·scope \tə-'kis-tə-ˌskōp-, ta-\ *n* : an apparatus for the brief exposure of visual stimuli that is used in the study of learning, attention, and perception — **ta·chis·to·scop·ic** \-ˌkis-tə-'skä-pik\ *adj* — **ta·chis·to·scop·i·cal·ly** *adv*

tachy- *comb form* : rapid : accelerated ⟨*tachy*cardia⟩

tachy·ar·rhyth·mia \ˌta-kē-ā-'rith-mē-ə\ *n* : arrhythmia characterized by a rapid irregular heartbeat

tachy·car·dia \ˌta-ki-'kär-dē-ə\ *n* : relatively rapid heart action whether physiological (as after exercise) or pathological — see JUNCTIONAL TACHYCARDIA, PAROXYSMAL TACHYCARDIA, SINUS TACHYCARDIA, VENTRICULAR TACHYCARDIA; compare BRADYCARDIA — **tachy·car·di·ac** \-dē-ˌak\ *adj*

tachy·phy·lax·is \ˌta-ki-fi-'lak-səs\ *n, pl* **-lax·es** \-ˌsēz\ : diminished response to later increments in a sequence of applications of a physiologically active substance — **tachy·phy·lac·tic** \-fi-'lak-tik\ *adj*

tachy·pnea \ˌta-kip-'nē-ə\ *n* : increased rate of respiration — **tachy·pne·ic** \-'nē-ik\ *adj*

tachy·pnoea *chiefly Brit var of* TACHYPNEA

tac·rine \'ta-ˌkrēn, ˌ-krīn\ *n* : an anticholinesterase used in the form of its hydrochloride C₁₃H₁₄N₂·HCl esp. in the palliative treatment of cognitive deficits in learning, memory, and mood associated with Alzheimer's disease — called also *tetrahydroaminoacridine, THA*; see COGNEX

¹tac·tile \'tak-təl, -ˌtīl\ *adj* **1** : of, relating to, mediated by, or affecting the sense of touch **2** : having or being organs or receptors for the sense of touch — **tac·tile·ly** *adv*

²tactile *n* : a person whose prevailing mental imagery is tactile rather than visual, auditory, or motor — compare AUDILE, VISUALIZER

tactile corpuscle *n* : one of the numerous minute bodies (as a Meissner's corpuscle) in the skin and some mucous membranes that usu. consist of a group of cells enclosed in a capsule, contain nerve terminations, and are held to be end organs of touch

tactile receptor *n* : an end organ (as a Meissner's corpuscle or a Pacinian corpuscle) that responds to light touch

tac·toid \'tak-ˌtóid\ *n* : an elongated particle (as in a sickle cell) that appears as a spindle-shaped body under a polarizing microscope

tac·tu·al \'tak-chə-wəl\ *adj* : of or relating to the sense or the organs of touch : derived from or producing the sensation of touch : TACTILE ⟨a ~ sense⟩

ta·da·la·fil \tə-'da-lə-ˌfil\ *n* : a drug C₂₂H₁₉N₃O₄ that is used to treat erectile dysfunction — see CIALIS

taen- *or* **taeni-** *also* **ten-** *or* **teni-** *comb form* : tapeworm ⟨*taenia*sis⟩

tae·nia \'tē-nē-ə\ *n* **1 a** *also* **te·nia** \'tē-nē-ə\ *pl* **taenias** *also* **tenias** : TAPEWORM **b** *cap* : a genus of taeniid tapeworms that comprises forms usu. occurring as adults in the intestines of carnivores and as larvae in various ruminants, and that includes the beef tapeworm (*T. saginata*) and the pork tapeworm (*T. solium*) — compare ECHINOCOCCUS **2** *also* **tenia** *pl* **tae·ni·ae** \-nē-ˌē, -ˌī\ *or* **taenias** *also* **te·ni·ae** *or* **tenias** : a band of nervous tissue or of muscle

taenia co·li *also* **tenia coli** \-'kō-ˌlī\ *n, pl* **taeniae coli** *also* **teniae coli** : any of three external longitudinal muscle bands of the large intestine

tae·ni·a·sis *also* **te·ni·a·sis** \tē-'nī-ə-səs\ *n, pl* **-a·ses** : infestation with or disease caused by tapeworms

tae·ni·id \'tē-nē-əd\ *n* : any of a family (Taeniidae) of tapeworms that includes numerous forms of medical or veterinary importance — **taeniid** *adj*

tae·ni·oid \'tē-nē-ˌóid\ *adj* : resembling or related to the taeniid tapeworms

¹tag \'tag\ *n* **1 a** : a shred of flesh or muscle **b** : a small abnormal projecting piece of tissue esp. when potentially or actually neoplastic in character **2** : LABEL

²tag *vb* **tagged; tag·ging** : LABEL

Tag·a·met \'ta-gə-ˌmet\ *trademark* — used for a preparation of cimetidine

tai chi *also* **t'ai chi** \'tī-'jē, -'chē\ *n, often cap T&C* : an ancient Chinese discipline involving a continuous series of controlled usu. slow movements designed to improve physical and mental well-being — called also *t'ai chi ch'uan, tai chi chuan* \-chü-ˈän\

tail \ˈtāl\ *n, often attrib* **1** : the rear end or a process or prolongation of the rear end of the body of an animal **2** : any of various parts of bodily structures that are terminal: as **a** : the distal tendon of a muscle **b** : the slender left end of the human pancreas **c** : the common convoluted tube that forms the lower part of the epididymis **3** : the motile part of a sperm that extends from the middle portion to the end and that comprises the flagellum

tail-bone \-ˈbōn\ *n* **1** : a caudal vertebra **2** : COCCYX

tail bud *n* : a knob of embryonic tissue that contributes to the formation of the posterior part of the vertebrate body — called also *end bud*

Ta·ka·ya·su's arteritis \ˌtä-kə-ˈyä-süz-\ *n* : a chronic inflammatory disease esp. of the aorta and its major branches that results in progressive stenosis, occlusion, and aneurysm formation and is marked esp. by diminution or loss of the pulse (as in the arm) and by ischemic symptoms (as visual disturbances or pain or weakness of the extremities) — called also *pulseless disease, Takayasu's disease*

   Takayasu, Michishige (1872–1938), Japanese physician.

¹take \ˈtāk\ *vb* **took** \ˈtùk\; **tak·en** \ˈtā-kən\; **tak·ing** **1** : to establish a take esp. by uniting or growing **2** *of a vaccine or vaccination* : to produce a take

²take *n* **1** : a local or systemic reaction indicative of successful vaccination **2** : a successful union (as of a graft)

take up *vb* : to absorb or incorporate into itself — **take–up** *n*

tali *pl of* TALUS

tali·pes \ˈta-lə-ˌpēz\ *n* : CLUBFOOT 1

talipes equi·no·var·us \-ˌe-kwi-nō-ˈvar-əs\ *n* : a congenital deformity of the foot in which both talipes equinus and talipes varus occur so that walking is done on the toes and outer side of the sole

talipes equi·nus \-ˈe-kwi-nəs\ *n* : a congenital deformity of the foot in which the sole is permanently flexed so that walking is done on the toes without touching the heel to the ground

talipes valgus *n* : a congenital deformity of the foot in which it is rotated inward so that walking is done on the inner side of the sole

talipes varus *n* : a congenital deformity of the foot in which it is rotated outward so that walking is done on the outer side of the sole

talk therapy *n* : psychotherapy emphasizing conversation between therapist and patient

talo- *comb form* : astragalar and ⟨*talo*tibial⟩

ta·lo·cru·ral \ˌtä-lō-ˈkrùr-əl\ *adj* : relating to or being the ankle joint

ta·lo·na·vic·u·lar \ˌtä-lō-nə-ˈvi-kyə-lər\ *adj* : of or relating to the talus and the navicular of the tarsus

ta·lo·tib·i·al \ˌtä-lō-ˈti-bē-əl\ *adj* : of or relating to the talus and the tibia

ta·lus \ˈtā-ləs\ *n, pl* **ta·li** \ˈtā-ˌlī\ **1** : the human astragalus that bears the weight of the body and together with the tibia and fibula forms the ankle joint — called also *anklebone* **2** : the entire ankle

Tal·win \ˈtal-ˌwin\ *trademark* — used for a preparation of pentazocine

Tam·i·flu \ˈta-mi-ˌflü\ *trademark* — used for a preparation of the phosphate of oseltamivir

ta·mox·i·fen \ta-ˈmäk-si-ˌfen\ *n* : a selective estrogen receptor modulator that acts as an estrogen antagonist in breast tissue and is administered orally in the form of its citrate $C_{26}H_{29}NO\cdot C_6H_8O_7$ esp. to treat breast cancer — see NOLVADEX

¹tam·pon \ˈtam-ˌpän\ *n* : a wad of absorbent material (as of cotton) introduced into a body cavity or canal usu. to absorb secretions (as from menstruation) or to arrest hemorrhaging

²tampon *vb* : to place or insert a tampon into

tam·pon·ade \ˌtam-pə-ˈnād\ *n* **1** : the closure or blockage (as of a wound) by or as if by a tampon esp. to stop bleeding **2** : CARDIAC TAMPONADE

tam·su·lo·sin \tam-ˈsü-lə-sən\ *n* : an alpha-adrenergic blocking agent administered orally in the form of its hydrochloride $C_{20}H_{28}N_2O_5S\cdot HCl$ to treat benign prostatic hyperplasia — see FLOMAX

tan \ˈtan\ *n* : a brown color imparted to the skin by exposure to the sun or wind — **tan** *vb*

T and A *abbr* tonsillectomy and adenoidectomy

tan·dem repeat \ˈtan-dəm-\ *n* : any of several identical DNA segments lying one after the other in a sequence

tan·gle \ˈtaŋ-gəl\ *n* : NEUROFIBRILLARY TANGLE

tan·ta·lum \ˈtant-ᵊl-əm\ *n* : a hard ductile gray-white acid-resisting metallic element sometimes used in surgical implants and sutures — symbol *Ta;* see ELEMENT table

T antigen \ˈtē-\ *n* : any of several proteins produced by some DNA viruses (as simian virus 40) that induce tumor formation and play a role in viral replication

tap \ˈtap\ *n* : the procedure of removing fluid (as from a body cavity) — see LUMBAR PUNCTURE — **tap** *vb*

¹tape \ˈtāp\ *n* : a narrow band of woven fabric; *esp* : ADHESIVE TAPE

²tape *vb* **taped; tap·ing** : to fasten, tie, bind, cover, or support with tape and esp. adhesive tape

ta·pe·tum \tə-'pē-təm\ *n, pl* **ta·pe·ta** \-'pē-tə\ **1** : any of various membranous layers or areas esp. of the choroid and retina of the eye **2** : a layer of nerve fibers derived from the corpus callosum and forming part of the roof of each lateral ventricle of the brain — **ta·pe·tal** \-təl\ *adj*

tape·worm \'tāp-ˌwərm\ *n* : any of a class (Cestoda) of flatworms that are parasitic esp. in the digestive tract of vertebrates and that typically consist of a head bearing an attachment organ usu. with suckers or hooks for adhering to the host's intestine followed by an undifferentiated growth region from which buds off a chain of proglottids — called also *cestode;* see BEEF TAPEWORM, CAT TAPEWORM, DOG TAPEWORM, FISH TAPEWORM, FRINGED TAPEWORM, PORK TAPEWORM

ta·pote·ment \tə-'pōt-mənt\ *n* : PERCUSSION 2

tar \'tär\ *n* **1** : any of various dark brown or black viscous liquids obtained by distillation of organic material (as wood or coal); *esp* : one used medicinally (as to treat skin diseases) **2** : a substance in some respects resembling tar; *esp* : a residue present in smoke from burning tobacco that contains combustion by-products (as resins and phenols)

ta·ran·tu·la \tə-'ran-chə-lə, -tə-lə\ *n, pl* **-las** *also* **-lae** \-ˌlē\ : any of a family (Theraphosidae) of large hairy American spiders that are typically rather sluggish and capable of biting sharply though most forms are not significantly poisonous to humans

tarda — see OSTEOGENESIS IMPERFECTA TARDA

tar·dive \'tär-div\ *adj* : tending to or characterized by lateness esp. in development or maturity

tardive dyskinesia *n* : a neurological disorder characterized by involuntary uncontrollable movements esp. of the mouth, tongue, trunk, and limbs and occurring esp. as a side effect of prolonged use of antipsychotic drugs (as phenothiazine) — abbr. *TD*

tar·get \'tär-gət\ *n* **1** : something to be affected by an action or development; *specif* : an organ, part, or tissue that is affected by the action of a hormone **2** : a body, surface, or material bombarded with nuclear particles or electrons **3** : the thought or object that is to be recognized (as by telepathy) or affected (as by psychokinesis) in a parapsychological experiment

target cell *n* : a cell that is acted on selectively by a specific agent (as a virus, drug, or hormone)

tar·ry stool \'tär-ē-\ *n* : an evacuation from the bowels having the color of tar caused esp. by hemorrhage in the stomach or upper intestines

¹tar·sal \'tär-səl\ *adj* **1** : of or relating to the tarsus **2** : being or relating to

plates of dense connective tissue that serve to stiffen the eyelids

²tarsal *n* : a tarsal part (as a bone)

tarsal gland *n* : MEIBOMIAN GLAND

tarsal plate *n* : the plate of strong dense fibrous connective tissue that forms the supporting structure of the eyelid

tarso- *comb form* **1** : tarsus ⟨*tar*sometatarsal⟩ **2** : tarsal plate ⟨*tarsor*rhaphy⟩

tar·so·meta·tar·sal \ˌtär-sō-ˌme-tə-'tär-səl\ *adj* : of or relating to the tarsus and metatarsus ⟨∼ articulations⟩

tar·sor·rha·phy \tär-'sôr-ə-fē\ *n, pl* **-phies** : the operation of suturing the eyelids together entirely or in part

tar·sus \'tär-səs\ *n, pl* **tar·si** \-ˌsī, -ˌsē\ **1** : the part of the foot between the metatarsus and the leg; *also* : the small bones that support this part of the limb **2** : TARSAL PLATE

tar·tar \'tär-tər\ *n* : an incrustation on the teeth consisting of plaque that has become hardened by the deposition of mineral salts (as calcium carbonate)

tartar emetic *n* : a poisonous crystalline salt $KSbOC_4H_4O_6 \cdot \frac{1}{2}H_2O$ of sweetish metallic taste used esp. formerly in medicine as an expectorant, anthelmintic, and emetic — called also *antimony potassium tartrate, potassium antimonyltartrate*

tar·tar·ic acid \ˌ(ˌ)tär-ˈtar-ik-\ *n* : a strong acid $C_4H_6O_6$ of plant origin that contains two carboxyl groups and occurs in three isomeric forms

tar·trate \'tär-ˌtrāt\ *n* : a salt or ester of tartaric acid

tar·tra·zine \'tär-trə-ˌzēn, -zən\ *n* : a yellow azo dye used in coloring foods and drugs that sometimes causes bronchoconstriction in individuals with asthma

¹taste \'tāst\ *vb* **tast·ed; tast·ing** **1** : to ascertain the flavor of by taking a little into the mouth **2** : to have a specific flavor

²taste *n* **1** : the special sense that is concerned with distinguishing the sweet, sour, bitter, or salty quality of a dissolved substance and is mediated by taste buds on the tongue **2** : the objective sweet, sour, bitter, or salty quality of a dissolved substance as perceived by the sense of taste **3** : a sensation obtained from a substance in the mouth that is typically produced by the stimulation of the sense of taste combined with those of touch and smell

taste bud *n* : an end organ mediating the sensation of taste and lying chiefly in the epithelium of the tongue and esp. in the walls of the circumvallate papillae

taste cell *n* : a neuroepithelial cell that is located in a taste bud and is the actual receptor of the sensation of taste

taste hair *n* : the hairlike free end of a taste cell

taster • tear gas

748

tast·er \'tās-tər\ *n* : a person able to taste the chemical phenylthiocarbamide

tat \'tat\ *n, often cap* **1** : a protein produced by a lentivirus (as HIV) that greatly increases the rate of viral transcription and replication and enhances the susceptibility of T cells to infection — called also *tat protein* **2** : the viral gene that codes for the tat protein

TAT *abbr* thematic apperception test

tat·too \ta-'tü\ *n, pl* **tattoos** : an indelible mark or figure fixed upon the body by insertion of pigment under the skin or by production of scars — **tattoo** *vb*

tau \'taů, 'tȯ\ *n* : a protein that binds to and regulates the assembly and stability of neuronal microtubules and that is found in an abnormal form as the major component of neurofibrillary tangles — called also *tau protein*

tau·rine \'tȯ-ˌrēn\ *n* : a colorless crystalline acid $C_2H_7NO_3S$ that is synthesized in the body from cysteine and methionine, is similar to amino acids but is not a component of proteins, and is involved in various physiological functions (as bile conjugation and cell membrane stabilization)

tau·ro·cho·lic acid \ˌtȯr-ə-ˈkō-lik-, -ˈkä-\ *n* : a deliquescent acid occurring in the form of its sodium salt $C_{26}H_{44}NNaO_7S$ in bile

tax·is \'tak-səs\ *n, pl* **tax·es** \-ˌsēz\ **1** : the manual restoration of a displaced body part; *specif* : the reduction of a hernia manually **2 a** : reflex movement by a freely moving and usu. simple organism in relation to a source of stimulation (as a light) **b** : a reflex reaction involving a taxis

Tax·ol \'tak-ˌsȯl\ *trademark* — used for a preparation of paclitaxel

tax·on \'tak-ˌsän\ *n, pl* **taxa** \-sə\ *also* **tax·ons** **1** : a taxonomic group or entity **2** : the name applied to a taxonomic group in a formal system of nomenclature

tax·on·o·my \tak-'sä-nə-mē\ *n, pl* **-mies** **1** : the study of the general principles of scientific classification **2** : orderly classification of plants and animals according to their presumed natural relationships — **tax·o·nom·ic** \ˌtak-sə-ˈnä-mik\ *adj* — **tax·o·nom·i·cal·ly** \-k(ə-)lē\ *adv* — **tax·on·o·mist** \-mist\ *n*

Tax·o·tere \'tak-sə-ˌter, -ˌtir\ *trademark* — used for a preparation of docetaxel

Tay–Sachs disease \'tā-'saks-\ *n* : a hereditary disorder of lipid metabolism typically affecting individuals of eastern European Jewish ancestry that is marked by the accumulation of lipids esp. in nervous tissue due to a deficiency of hexosaminidase A, that is characterized by weakness, macrocephaly, red retinal spots, hyperacusis, retarded development, blindness, convulsions, paralysis, and death in early childhood, and that is

inherited as an autosomal recessive trait — called also *Tay-Sachs;* see SANDHOFF'S DISEASE

Tay, Warren (1843–1927), British physician.
Sachs, Bernard (1858–1944), American neurologist.

Tb *symbol* terbium

TB \ˌtē-'bē\ *n* : TUBERCULOSIS

TB *abbr* tubercle bacillus

TBE *abbr* tick-borne encephalitis

TBG *abbr* thyroid-binding globulin; thyroxine-binding globulin

TBI *abbr* traumatic brain injury

Tc *symbol* technetium

TCA *abbr* tricyclic antidepressant

TCDD \ˌtē-(ˌ)sē-(ˌ)dē-'dē\ *n* : a carcinogenic dioxin $C_{12}H_4O_2Cl_4$ found esp. as a contaminant in 2,4,5-T — called also *2,3,7,8-tetrachlorodibenzo-para-dioxin, 2,3,7,8-tetrachlorodibenzo-p-dioxin*

TCE *abbr* trichloroethylene

T cell *n* : any of several lymphocytes (as a helper T cell) that differentiate in the thymus, possess highly specific cell-surface antigen receptors, and include some that control the initiation or suppression of cell-mediated and humoral immunity (as by the regulation of T and B cell maturation and proliferation) and others that lyse antigen-bearing cells — called also *T lymphocyte;* see CYTOTOXIC T CELL, HELPER T CELL, KILLER CELL, SUPPRESSOR T CELL, T4 CELL

T–cell leukemia — see ADULT T-CELL LEUKEMIA

TCR *abbr* T cell (antigen) receptor — used for the receptor on an immunoreactive T cell that enables it to bind and react with a specific antigen

Td *abbr* tetanus diphtheria — used for a vaccine containing toxoids of the bacteria causing tetanus and diphtheria

TD *abbr* tardive dyskinesia

tds *abbr* [Latin *ter die sumendum*] to be taken three times a day — used in writing prescriptions

Te *symbol* tellurium

TEA *abbr* tetraethylammonium

teaching hospital *n* : a hospital that is affiliated with a medical school and provides the means for medical education to students, interns, residents, and sometimes postgraduates

¹tear \'tir\ *n* **1** : a drop of clear saline fluid secreted by the lacrimal gland and diffused between the eye and eyelids to moisten the parts and facilitate their motion **2** *pl* : a secretion of profuse tears that overflow the eyelids and dampen the face

²tear *vb* : to fill with tears : shed tears

³tear \'tar\ *vb* **tore** \'tōr\; **torn** \'tōrn\; **tear·ing** : to wound by or as if by pulling apart by force ⟨∼ the skin⟩

⁴tear *n* : a wound made by tearing a bodily part ⟨a muscle ∼⟩

tear duct *n* : LACRIMAL DUCT

tear gas *n* : a solid, liquid, or gaseous

substance that on dispersion in the atmosphere irritates mucous membranes resulting esp. in blinding of the eyes with tears

tear gland *n* : LACRIMAL GLAND

tease \'tēz\ *vb* **teased; teas·ing** : to tear in pieces; *esp* : to shred (a tissue or specimen) for microscopic examination

tea·spoon \'tē-ˌspün\ *n* : a unit of measure equal to ⅙ fluid ounce or ⅓ tablespoon or 5 milliliters

tea·spoon·ful \-ˌfúl\ *n, pl* **teaspoonfuls** \-ˌfúlz\ *also* **tea·spoons·ful** \-ˌspünz-ˌfúl\ : TEASPOON

teat \'tit, 'tēt\ *n* : the protuberance through which milk is drawn from an udder or breast : NIPPLE

tech *abbr* technician

tech·ne·tium \tek-'nē-shəm, -shē-əm\ *n* : a radioactive metallic element obtained esp. from nuclear fuel as a product of uranium fission and used in medicine in the preparation of radiopharmaceuticals — symbol *Tc*; see ELEMENT table, PERTECHNETATE

tech·nic \'tek-nik\ *n* : TECHNIQUE

tech·ni·cian \tek-'ni-shən\ *n* : a specialist in the technical details of a subject or occupation ⟨a medical ∼⟩

tech·nique \tek-'nēk\ *n* : a method or body of methods for accomplishing a desired end ⟨new surgical ∼s⟩

tecta *pl of* TECTUM

tec·tal \'tek-təl\ *adj* : of or relating to a tectum

tec·to·ri·al membrane \tek-'tōr-ē-əl-\ *n* : a membrane having the consistency of jelly that covers the surface of the organ of Corti

tec·to·spi·nal \ˌtek-tō-'spīn-ᵊl\ *adj* : of, relating to, or being a tract of myelinated nerve fibers that mediate various visual and auditory reflexes and that originate in the superior colliculus, cross to the opposite side, and terminate in the ventral horn of gray matter in the cervical region of the spinal cord

tec·tum \'tek-təm\ *n, pl* **tec·ta** \-tə\ **1** : a bodily structure resembling or serving as a roof **2** : the dorsal part of the midbrain including the corpora quadrigemina

teeth *pl of* TOOTH

teethe \'tēth\ *vb* **teethed; teeth·ing** : to cut one's teeth : grow teeth

teeth·ing \'tē-thin\ *n* **1** : the first growth of teeth **2** : the phenomena accompanying the growth of teeth through the gums

teg·men \'teg-mən\ *n, pl* **teg·mi·na** \-mə-nə\ : an anatomical layer or cover; *specif* : TEGMEN TYMPANI

teg·men·tum \teg-'men-təm\ *n, pl* **-men·ta** \-tə\ : an anatomical covering : TEGMEN; *esp* : the part of the ventral midbrain above the substantia nigra — **teg·men·tal** \-təl\ *adj*

tegmen tym·pa·ni \-'tim-pə-ˌnī\ *n* : a thin plate of bone that covers the middle ear

tegmina *pl of* TEGMEN

Teg·o·pen \'te-gə-ˌpen\ *trademark* — used for a preparation of cloxacillin

Teg·re·tol \'te-grə-ˌtól\ *trademark* — used for a preparation of carbamazepine

tel- *or* **telo-** *also* **tele-** *comb form* : end ⟨*tel*angiectasia⟩

te·la \'tē-lə\ *n, pl* **te·lae** \-ˌlē\ : an anatomical tissue or layer of tissue

tela cho·roi·dea \-kō-'rói-dē-ə\ *n* : a fold of pia mater roofing a ventricle of the brain

tel·an·gi·ec·ta·sia \ˌte-ˌlan-jē-ˌek-'tā-zhə, ˌtē-, tə-, -zhē-ə\ *or* **tel·an·gi·ec·ta·sis** \-'ek-tə-səs\ *n, pl* **-ta·sias** *or* **-ta·ses** \-tə-ˌsēz\ **1** : an abnormal dilation of red, blue, or purple superficial capillaries, arterioles, or venules typically located just below the skin's surface (as on the face) — see SPIDER VEIN **2** : HEREDITARY HEMORRHAGIC TELANGIECTASIA — **tel·an·gi·ec·tat·ic** \-ˌek-'ta-tik\ *adj*

te·la sub·cu·ta·nea \ˌtē-lə-ˌsəb-kyü-'tā-nē-ə\ *n* : SUPERFICIAL FASCIA

tele·di·ag·no·sis \ˌte-lə-ˌdī-əg-'nō-səs\ *n, pl* **-no·ses** \-ˌsēz\ : medical diagnosis made by means of telemedicine

tele·ki·ne·sis \ˌte-lə-kə-'nē-səs, -kī-\ *n, pl* **-ne·ses** \-ˌsēz\ : the apparent production of motion in objects (as by a spiritualistic medium) without contact or other physical means — compare PRECOGNITION, PSYCHOKINESIS — **tele·ki·net·ic** \-'ne-tik\ *adj* — **tele·ki·net·i·cal·ly** *adv*

tele·med·i·cine \-'me-də-sən\ *n* : the practice of medicine when the doctor and patient are widely separated using two-way voice and visual communication (as by satellite, computer, or closed-circuit television) — **tele·med·i·cal** \-di-kəl\ *adj*

¹**tele·me·ter** \'te-lə-ˌmē-tər\ *n* : an electrical apparatus for measuring a quantity (as pressure or temperature), transmitting the result esp. by radio to a distant station, and there indicating or recording the quantity measured

²**telemeter** *vb* : to transmit by telemeter

te·lem·e·try \tə-'le-mə-trē\ *n, pl* **-tries** **1** : the science or process of telemetering data **2** : data transmitted by telemetry **3** : BIOTELEMETRY — **tele·met·ric** \ˌte-lə-'me-trik\ *adj*

tel·en·ceph·a·lon \ˌte-len-'se-fə-ˌlän, -lən\ *n, pl* **-la** \-lə\ *or* **-lons** : the anterior subdivision of the embryonic forebrain or the corresponding part of the adult forebrain that includes the cerebral hemispheres and associated structures — **tel·en·ce·phal·ic** \-ˌen-sə-'fa-lik\ *adj*

te·lep·a·thy \tə-'le-pə-thē\ *n, pl* **-thies** : apparent communication from one mind to another by extrasensory means — **tele·path·ic** \ˌte-lə-'pa-thik\ *adj* — **tele·path·i·cal·ly** *adv*

tele·ra·di·ol·o·gy \ˌte-lə-ˌrā-dē-'ä-lə-jē\ *n* : radiology concerned with the transmission of digitized medical images over electronic networks and with the interpretation of the transmitted images for diagnostic purposes

tele·ther·a·py \-'ther-ə-pē\ *n, pl* **-pies** : the treatment of diseased tissue with high-intensity radiation (as gamma rays from radioactive cobalt)

tel·lu·ri·um \tə-'lür-ē-əm, te-\ *n* : a semimetallic element related to selenium and sulfur — symbol *Te;* see ELEMENT table

telo- *see* TEL-

telo·cen·tric \ˌte-lə-'sen-trik, ˌtē-\ *adj* : having the centromere terminally situated so that there is only one chromosomal arm ⟨a ~ chromosome⟩ — compare ACROCENTRIC, METACENTRIC — **telocentric** *n*

te·lo·gen \'tē-lə-ˌjen\ *n* : the resting phase of the hair growth cycle following anagen and preceding shedding

te·lo·me·rase \te-'lō-mə-ˌrās, -ˌrāz\ *n* : a DNA polymerase that is a ribonucleoprotein catalyzing the elongation of chromosomal telomeres in eukaryotic cell division and is particularly active in cancer cells

telo·mere \'te-lə-ˌmir, 'tē-\ *n* : the natural end of a eukaryotic chromosome composed of a usu. repetitive DNA sequence and serving to stabilize the chromosome — **telo·mer·ic** \ˌte-lə-'mer-ik\ *adj*

telo·phase \'te-lə-ˌfāz, 'tē-\ *n* **1** : the final stage of mitosis and of the second division of meiosis in which the spindle disappears and the nuclear envelope reforms around each set of chromosomes **2** : the final stage in the first division of meiosis that may be missing in some organisms and that is characterized by the gathering at opposite poles of the cell of half the original number of chromosomes including one from each homologous pair

TEM \ˌtē-(ˌ)ē-'em\ *n* : TRIETHYLENE-MELAMINE

TEM *abbr* transmission electron microscope; transmission electron microscopy

te·maz·e·pam \tə-'maz-ə-ˌpam\ *n* : a benzodiazepine $C_{16}H_{13}ClN_2O_2$ used for its sedative and tranquilizing effects in the treatment of insomnia — see RESTORIL

temp \'temp\ *n* : TEMPERATURE

tem·per·ate \'tem-pə-rət\ *adj* : existing as a prophage in infected cells and rarely causing lysis ⟨~ bacteriophages⟩

tem·per·a·ture \'tem-pər-ˌchür, -pə-rə-, -chər, -ˌtyùr\ *n* **1** : degree of hotness or coldness measured on a definite scale — see THERMOMETER **2 a** : the degree of heat that is natural to a living body **b** : a condition of abnormally high body heat

tem·plate \'tem-plət\ *n* : a molecule (as of DNA) that serves as a pattern for the synthesis of another macromolecule (as messenger RNA)

tem·ple \'tem-pəl\ *n* **1** : the flattened space on each side of the forehead **2** : one of the side supports of a pair of glasses jointed to the bows and passing on each side of the head

¹tem·po·ral \'tem-pə-rəl\ *n* : a temporal part (as a bone or muscle)

²temporal *adj* : of or relating to the temples or the sides of the skull behind the orbits

temporal arteritis *n* : GIANT CELL ARTERITIS

temporal artery *n* **1** : either of two branches of the maxillary artery that supply the temporalis and anastomose with the middle temporal artery — called also *deep temporal artery* **2 a** : SUPERFICIAL TEMPORAL ARTERY **b** : a branch of the superficial temporal artery that arises just above the zygomatic arch and sends branches to the temporalis — called also *middle temporal artery* **3** : any of three branches of the middle cerebral artery: **a** : one that supplies the anterior parts of the superior, middle, and inferior temporal gyri — called also *anterior temporal artery* **b** : one that supplies the middle parts of the superior and middle temporal gyri — called also *intermediate temporal artery* **c** : one that supplies the middle and posterior parts of the superior temporal gyrus and the posterior parts of the middle and inferior temporal gyri — called also *posterior temporal artery*

temporal bone *n* : a compound bone of the side of the skull that has four principal parts including the squamous, petrous, and tympanic portions and the mastoid process

temporal fossa *n* : a broad fossa on the side of the skull behind the orbit that contains muscles for raising the lower jaw and that in humans is occupied by the temporalis muscle

temporal gyrus *n* : any of three major convolutions of the external surface of the temporal lobe: **a** : the one that is uppermost and borders the sylvian fissure — called also *superior temporal gyrus* **b** : one lying in the middle between the other two — called also *middle temporal gyrus* **c** : the lowest of the three — called also *inferior temporal gyrus*

tem·po·ral·is \ˌtem-pə-'rā-ləs\ *n* : a large muscle in the temporal fossa that serves to raise the lower jaw — called also *temporalis muscle, temporal muscle*

temporal line *n* : either of two nearly parallel ridges or lines on each side of the skull

temporal lobe *n* : a large lobe of each cerebral hemisphere that is situated in front of the occipital lobe and contains a sensory area associated with the organ of hearing

temporal lobe epilepsy *n* : epilepsy characterized by partial rather than generalized seizures that typically originate in the temporal lobe and are marked by impairment of consciousness, automatisms, unusual changes in behavior, and hallucinations (as of odors) — abbr. *TLE;* called also *psychomotor epilepsy*

temporal muscle *n* : TEMPORALIS

temporal nerve — see AURICULOTEMPORAL NERVE, DEEP TEMPORAL NERVE

temporal process *n* : a process of the zygomatic bone that forms part of the zygomatic arch

temporal summation *n* : sensory summation that involves the addition of single stimuli over a short period of time

temporal vein *n* : any of several veins draining the temporal region: as **a** (1) : a large vein on each side of the head that unites with the maxillary vein to form a vein that contributes to the formation of the external jugular vein (2) : a vein that drains the lateral orbital region and empties into the superficial temporal vein just above the zygomatic arch — called also *middle temporal vein* **b** : any of several veins arising from behind the temporalis and emptying into the pterygoid plexus — called also *deep temporal vein*

temporo- *comb form* : temporal and ⟨*temporo*mandibular⟩

tem·po·ro·man·dib·u·lar \'tem-pə-rō-man-'di-byə-lər\ *adj* : of, relating to, or affecting the temporomandibular joint ⟨∼ dysfunction⟩

temporomandibular disorder *n* : TEMPOROMANDIBULAR JOINT SYNDROME — abbr. *TMD*

temporomandibular joint *n* : the diarthrosis between the temporal bone and mandible that includes the condyloid process below separated by an articular disk from the glenoid fossa above and that allows for the opening, closing, protrusion, retraction, and lateral movement of the mandible — abbr. *TMJ*

temporomandibular joint syndrome *n* : a group of symptoms that may include pain or tenderness in the temporomandibular joint or surrounding muscles, headache, earache, neck, back, or shoulder pain, limited jaw movement, or a clicking or popping sound in the jaw and that are caused either by dysfunction of the temporomandibular joint or another problem affecting the region of the temporomandibular joint — called also *temporomandibular disorder, temporomandibular joint disorder, temporomandibular joint dysfunction, TMJ syndrome*

tem·po·ro·pa·ri·etal \-pə-'rī-ət-ᵊl\ *adj* : of or relating to the temporal and parietal bones or lobes

ten- — see TAEN-

te·na·cious \tə-'nā-shəs\ *adj* : tending to adhere or cling esp. to another substance : VISCOUS ⟨∼ sputum⟩

te·nac·u·lum \tə-'na-kyə-ləm\ *n, pl* **-la** \-lə\ *or* **-lums** : a slender sharp‑pointed hook attached to a handle and used mainly in surgery for seizing and holding parts (as arteries)

ten·der \'ten-dər\ *adj* : sensitive to touch or palpation ⟨∼ skin⟩ — **ten·der·ness** *n*

ten·di·ni·tis *or* **ten·don·itis** \,ten-də-'nī-təs\ *n* : inflammation of a tendon

ten·di·nous *also* **ten·do·nous** \'ten-də-nəs\ *adj* **1** : consisting of tendons ⟨∼ tissue⟩ **2** : of, relating to, or resembling a tendon

tendinous arch *n* : a thickened arch of fascia which gives origin to muscles or ligaments or through which pass vessels or nerves; *esp* : a thickening in the pelvic fascia that gives attachment to supporting ligaments

ten·do cal·ca·ne·us \'ten-dō-kal-'kā-nē-əs\ *n* : ACHILLES TENDON

ten·don \'ten-dən\ *n* : a tough cord or band of dense white fibrous connective tissue that unites a muscle with some other part, transmits the force which the muscle exerts, and is continuous with the connective-tissue epimysium and perimysium of the muscle and when inserted into a bone with the periosteum of the bone

tendonitis *var of* TENDINITIS

tendon of Achil·les \-ə-'ki-lēz\ *n* : ACHILLES TENDON

tendon of Zinn \-'tsin\ *n* : LIGAMENT OF ZINN

tendon organ *n* : GOLGI TENDON ORGAN

tendon reflex *n* : a reflex act (as a knee jerk) in which a muscle is made to contract by a blow upon its tendon

tendon sheath *n* : a synovial sheath covering a tendon (as in the hand)

¹-tene \,tēn\ *adj comb form* : having (such or so many) chromosomal filaments ⟨poly*tene*⟩ ⟨pachy*tene*⟩

²-tene *n comb form* : stage of meiotic prophase characterized by (such) chromosomal filaments ⟨diplo*tene*⟩

tenens, tenentes — see LOCUM TENENS

te·nes·mus \tə-'nez-məs\ *n* : a distressing but ineffectual urge to evacuate the rectum or urinary bladder

teni- — see TAEN-

tenia, tenia coli, teniasis *var of* TAENIA, TAENIA COLI, TAENIASIS

te·nip·o·side \tə-'ni-pə-ˌsīd\ *n* : an antineoplastic agent $C_{32}H_{32}O_{13}S$ that is a semisynthetic derivative of podophyllotoxin

tennis elbow *n* : inflammation and pain over the outer side of the elbow involving the lateral epicondyle of the humerus and usu. resulting from excessive strain on and twisting of the forearm — called also *lateral humeral epicondylitis*

teno- *comb form* : tendon ⟨*teno*synovitis⟩

te·no·de·sis \te-nə-'dē-səs\ *n, pl* **-de·ses** \-sēz\ : the operation of suturing the end of a tendon to a bone

te·nol·y·sis \ti-'nä-lə-səs\ *n, pl* **-y·ses** \-sēz\ : a surgical procedure to free a tendon from surrounding adhesions

teno·my·ot·o·my \te-nō-mī-'ä-tə-mē\ *n, pl* **-mies** : surgical excision of a portion of a tendon and muscle

Te·non's capsule \tə-'nōnz-, 'te-nənz-\ *n* : a thin connective-tissue membrane ensheathing the eyeball behind the conjunctiva

Te·non \tə-'nō"\, **Jacques René** (1724–1816), French surgeon.

Ten·or·min \'te-nər-ˌmin\ *trademark* — used for preparation of atenolol

teno·syn·o·vi·tis \te-nō-ˌsi-nə-'vī-təs\ *n* : inflammation of a tendon sheath

te·not·o·my \te-'nä-tə-mē\ *n, pl* **-mies** : surgical division of a tendon

TENS *abbr* transcutaneous electrical nerve stimulation; transcutaneous electrical nerve stimulator

tense \'tens\ *adj* **tens·er; tens·est 1** : stretched tight : made taut or rigid **2** : feeling or showing nervous tension — **tense** *vb* — **tense·ness** *n*

Ten·si·lon \'ten-si-ˌlän\ *trademark* — used for a preparation of edrophonium

ten·sion \'ten-chən\ *n* **1 a** : the act or action of stretching or the condition or degree of being stretched to stiffness ⟨muscular ∼⟩ : STRESS 1b **2 a** : either of two balancing forces causing or tending to cause extension **b** : the stress resulting from the elongation of an elastic body **3** : inner striving, unrest, or imbalance often with physiological indication of emotion **4** : PARTIAL PRESSURE — **ten·sion·al** \'ten-chə-nəl\ *adj* — **ten·sion·less** *adj*

tension headache *n* : headache marked by mild to moderate pain of variable duration that affects both sides of the head and is typically accompanied by contraction of the neck and scalp muscles

tension pneumothorax *n* : pneumothorax resulting from a wound in the chest wall which acts as a valve that permits air to enter the pleural cavity but prevents its escape

tension–time index *n* : a measure of ventricular work and oxygen demand that is found by multiplying the average pressure in the ventricle during the period in which it ejects blood by the time it takes to do this

ten·sor \'ten(t)-sər, 'ten-ˌsó(ə)r\ *n* : a muscle that stretches a part or makes it tense — called also *tensor muscle*

tensor fas·ci·ae la·tae \-'fa-shē-ē-'lā-tē\ *or* **tensor fas·cia la·ta** \-'fa-shē-ə-'lā-tə\ *n* : a muscle that arises esp. from the anterior part of the iliac crest and from the anterior superior iliac spine, is inserted into the iliotib-

ial band of the fascia lata, and acts to flex and abduct the thigh

tensor pa·la·ti \-'pa-lə-ˌtī\ *n* : TENSOR VELI PALATINI

tensor tym·pa·ni \-'tim-pə-ˌnī\ *n* : a small muscle of the middle ear that is located in the bony canal just above the bony part of the eustachian tube and that serves to adjust the tension of the tympanic membrane — called also *tensor tympani muscle*

tensor ve·li pa·la·ti·ni \-'vē-ˌlī-ˌpa-lə-'tī-ˌnī\ *n* : a ribbonlike muscle of the palate that acts esp. to tense the soft palate

tent \'tent\ *n* : a canopy or enclosure placed over the head and shoulders to retain vapors or oxygen during medical administration

tenth cranial nerve *n* : VAGUS NERVE

ten·to·ri·al \ten-'tōr-ē-əl\ *adj* : of, relating to, or involving the tentorium cerebelli ⟨a ∼ meningioma⟩

tentorial notch *n* : an oval opening that is bounded by the anterior border of the tentorium cerebelli, that surrounds the midbrain, and that gives passage to the posterior cerebral arteries — called also *tentorial incisure*

ten·to·ri·um \-ē-əm\ *n, pl* **-ria** \-ē-ə\ : TENTORIUM CEREBELLI

tentorium ce·re·bel·li \-ˌser-ə-'be-ˌlī\ *n* : an arched fold of dura mater that covers the upper surface of the cerebellum and supports the occipital lobes of the cerebrum

Ten·u·ate \'ten-yə-ˌwāt\ *trademark* — used for a preparation of the hydrochloride of diethylpropion

te·pa \'tē-pə\ *n* : a soluble crystalline compound $C_6H_{12}N_3OP$ used esp. as a chemical sterilizing agent of insects and in medicine as a palliative in some kinds of cancer — see THIOTEPA

TEPP \ˌtē-ˌē-ˌpē-'pē\ *n* : a liquid organophosphate $C_8H_{20}O_7P_2$ that is a powerful anticholinesterase and is used esp. as an insecticide — called also *tetraethyl pyrophosphate*

terat- *or* **terato-** *comb form* : developmental malformation ⟨*terato*genic⟩

te·rato·car·ci·no·ma \ˌter-ə-tō-ˌkärs-ᵊn-'ō-mə\ *n, pl* **-mas** *also* **-ma·ta** \-mə-tə\ : a malignant teratoma; *esp* : one involving germinal cells of the testis or ovary

te·rato·gen \tə-'ra-tə-jən\ *n* : a teratogenic agent (as a drug or virus)

ter·a·to·gen·e·sis \ˌter-ə-tə-'je-nə-səs\ *n, pl* **-e·ses** \-ˌsēz\ : production of developmental malformations

ter·a·to·gen·ic \-'je-nik\ *adj* : of, relating to, or causing developmental malformations ⟨a ∼ agent⟩ ⟨∼ effects⟩ — **ter·a·to·ge·nic·i·ty** \-jə-'ni-sə-tē\ *n*

ter·a·to·log·i·cal \ter-ət-ᵊl-'ä-ji-kəl\ *or* **ter·a·to·log·ic** \-jik\ *adj* **1** : abnormal in growth or structure **2** : of or relating to teratology

ter·a·tol·o·gy \ˌter-ə-'tä-lə-jē\ *n, pl* **-gies** : the study of malformations or serious deviations from the normal type in organisms — **ter·a·tol·o·gist** \-jist\ *n*

ter·a·to·ma \ₜter-ə-'tō-mə\ *n, pl* **-mas** *also* **-ma·ta** \-mə-tə\ : a tumor derived from more than one embryonic layer and made up of a heterogeneous mixture of tissues (as epithelium, bone, cartilage, or muscle)

te·ra·zo·sin \tə-'rā-zə-ˌsin\ *n* : an alpha-adrenergic blocking agent administered orally in the form of its hydrated hydrochloride $C_{19}H_{25}N_5$-$O_4 \cdot HCl \cdot 2H_2O$ esp. in the treatment of benign prostatic hyperplasia and hypertension — see HYTRIN

ter·bin·a·fine \tər-'bi-nə-ˌfēn\ *n* : an antifungal agent used in the form of its hydrochloride $C_{21}H_{25}N \cdot HCl$ orally in the treatment of onychomycosis and topically in the treatment of tinea corporis, tinea cruris, and athlete's foot — see LAMISIL

ter·bi·um \'tər-bē-əm\ *n* : a usu. trivalent metallic element — symbol *Tb;* see ELEMENT table

ter·bu·ta·line \tər-'byü-tə-ˌlēn\ *n* : a bronchodilator used esp. in the form of its sulfate $(C_{12}H_{19}NO_3)_2 \cdot H_2SO_4$

ter·e·bene \'ter-ə-ˌbēn\ *n* : a mixture of terpenes that has been used as an expectorant

teres — see LIGAMENTUM TERES, PRONATOR TERES

te·res major \'ter-ēz-, 'tir-\ *n* : a thick somewhat flattened muscle that arises from the lower axillary border of the scapula, inserts on the medial border of the bicipital groove of the humerus, and functions in opposition to the muscles comprising the rotator cuff by extending the arm when it is in the flexed position and by rotating it medially

teres minor *n* : a long cylindrical muscle that arises from the upper axillary border of the scapula, inserts chiefly on the greater tubercle of the humerus, contributes to the formation of the rotator cuff of the shoulder, and acts to rotate the arm laterally and draw the humerus toward the glenoid fossa

ter·fen·a·dine \(ˌ)tər-'fe-nə-ˌdēn\ *n* : a drug $C_{32}H_{41}NO_2$ formerly used as a nonsedating antihistamine but now withdrawn from U.S. markets because of its link to cardiac arrhythmias — see SELDANE

¹term \'tərm\ *n* : the time at which a pregnancy of normal length terminates ⟨had her baby at full ∼⟩

²term *adj* : carried to, occurring at, or associated with full term

¹ter·mi·nal \'tər-mə-nəl\ *adj* **1** : of, relating to, or being at an end, extremity, boundary, or terminus ⟨the ∼ phalanx of a finger⟩ **2 a** : leading ultimately to death : FATAL ⟨∼ cancer⟩ **b** : approaching or close to death : being in the final stages of a fatal disease ⟨a ∼ patient⟩ **3** : being at or near the

end of a chain of atoms making up a molecule — **ter·mi·nal·ly** *adv*

²terminal *n* : a part that forms an end; *esp* : NERVE ENDING

terminale — see FILUM TERMINALE

terminal ganglion *n* : a usu. parasympathetic ganglion situated on or close to an innervated organ and being the site where preganglionic nerve fibers terminate

terminalis — see LAMINA TERMINALIS, NERVUS TERMINALIS, STRIA TERMINALIS, SULCUS TERMINALIS

terminal nerve *n* : NERVUS TERMINALIS

ter·mi·na·tor \'tər-mə-ˌnā-tər\ *n* : a codon that stops protein synthesis since it does not code for a transfer RNA — called also *termination codon, terminator codon*

ter·pene \'tər-ˌpēn\ *n* : any of various isomeric hydrocarbons $C_{10}H_{16}$ found in essential oils; *broadly* : any of numerous hydrocarbons $(C_5H_8)_n$ found esp. in essential oils, resins, and balsams

ter·pin hydrate \'tər-pin-\ *n* : a crystalline or powdery compound $C_{10}H_{18}(OH)_2 \cdot H_2O$ used as an expectorant for coughs

Ter·ra·my·cin \ₜter-ə-'mīs-ᵊn\ *trademark* — used for a preparation of oxytetracycline

¹ter·tian \'tər-shən\ *adj* : recurring at approximately 48-hour intervals — used chiefly of vivax malaria; compare QUARTAN

²tertian *n* : a tertian fever; *specif* : VIVAX MALARIA

ter·tia·ry \'tər-shē-ˌer-ē, -shə-rē\ *adj* **1** : of third rank, importance, or value **2 a** : involving or resulting from the substitution of three atoms or groups ⟨∼ amines⟩ **b** : of, relating to, or being the normal folded structure of the coiled chain of a protein or of a DNA or RNA — compare PRIMARY 3, SECONDARY 3 **3** : occurring in or being a third stage **4** : providing tertiary care

tertiary care *n* : highly specialized health care usu. over an extended period of time that involves advanced and complex procedures and treatments performed by medical specialists in state-of-the-art facilities — compare PRIMARY CARE, SECONDARY CARE

tertiary syphilis *n* : the third stage of syphilis that develops after the disappearance of the secondary symptoms and is marked by ulcers in and gummas under the skin and commonly by involvement of the skeletal, cardiovascular, and nervous systems

tertius — see PERONEUS TERTIUS

Tesch·en disease \'te-shən-\ *n* : a mild to severe encephalomyelitis of swine caused by a picornavirus (species *Porcine teschovirus* of the genus *Teschovirus*)

test \'test\ *n* **1** : a critical examination, observation, evaluation, or trial **2** : a means of testing: as **a** (1) : a procedure or reaction used to identify or characterize a substance or constituent (2) : a reagent used in such a test **b** : a diagnostic procedure for determining the nature of a condition or disease or for revealing a change in function **c** : something (as a series of questions) for measuring the skill, knowledge, intelligence, capacities, or aptitudes of an individual or group **3** : a result or value determined by testing — **test** *adj or vb*

test·cross \'test-ˌkròs\ *n* : a genetic cross between a homozygous recessive individual and a corresponding suspected heterozygote to determine the genotype of the latter — **test·cross** *vb*

testes *pl of* TESTIS

tes·ti·cle \'tes-ti-kəl\ *n* : TESTIS; *esp* : one usu. with its enclosing structures

tes·tic·u·lar \tes-'ti-kyə-lər\ *adj* : of, relating to, or derived from the testes

testicular artery *n* : either of a pair of arteries which supply blood to the testes and of which one arises on each side from the front of the aorta a little below the corresponding renal artery and passes downward to the spermatic cord of the same side and along it to the testis — called also *internal spermatic artery*

testicular feminization *n* : a genetic disorder that is marked by the presence in a phenotypically female individual of the normal X and Y chromosomes of a male, usu. normal but undescended testes, and external genitalia that is female or slightly virilized, that results from complete or partial insensitivity to androgens in the body, and that is inherited as an X-linked recessive trait — called also *androgen insensitivity syndrome, testicular feminization syndrome*

testicular vein *n* : any of the veins leading from the testes, forming with tributaries from the epididymis the pampiniform plexus in the spermatic cord, and thence accompanying the testicular artery and eventually uniting to form a single trunk which on the right side opens into the vena cava and on the left into the renal vein — called also *spermatic vein*

tes·tis \'tes-təs\ *n, pl* **tes·tes** \'tes-ˌtēz\ : a typically paired male reproductive gland that usu. consists largely of seminiferous tubules from the epithelium of which spermatozoa develop and that descends into the scrotum before the attainment of sexual maturity and in many cases before birth

tes·tos·ter·one \te-'stäs-tə-ˌrōn\ *n* : a hormone that is a hydroxy steroid ketone $C_{19}H_{28}O_2$ produced by the testes or made synthetically and that is responsible for inducing and maintaining male secondary sex characteristics

testosterone enan·thate \-ē-'nan-ˌthāt\ *n* : a white or whitish crystalline ester $C_{26}H_{40}O_3$ of testosterone that is administered chiefly by intramuscular injection esp. in the treatment of conditions (as hypogonadism) associated with deficient or absent endogenous testosterone or in the palliative treatment of metastatic breast cancer

testosterone propionate *n* : a white or whitish crystalline ester $C_{22}H_{32}O_3$ of testosterone that is administered and used similarly to testosterone enanthate

test–tube *adj* **1** : IN VITRO ⟨∼ experiments⟩ **2** : produced by in vitro fertilization ⟨∼ babies⟩

test tube *n* : a plain or lipped tube usu. of thin glass closed at one end

te·tan·ic \te-'ta-nik\ *adj* : of, relating to, being, or tending to produce tetany or tetanus ⟨a ∼ condition⟩

tet·a·nize \'tet-ᵊn-ˌīz\ *vb* **-nized; -niz·ing** : to induce tetanus in

tet·a·nus \'tet-ᵊn-əs, 'tet-nəs\ *n* **1 a** : an acute infectious disease characterized by tonic spasm of voluntary muscles and esp. of the muscles of the jaw and caused by an exotoxin produced by a bacterium of the genus *Clostridium* (*C. tetani*) which is usu. introduced through a wound — compare LOCKJAW **b** : TETANUS BACILLUS **2** : prolonged contraction of a muscle resulting from a series of motor impulses following one another too rapidly to permit intervening relaxation of the muscle

tetanus bacillus *n* : the bacterium of the genus *Clostridium* (*C. tetani*) that causes tetanus

tet·a·ny \'tet-ᵊn-ē, 'tet-nē\ *n, pl* **-nies** : a condition of physiological calcium imbalance that is marked by intermittent tonic spasm of the voluntary muscles and is associated with deficiencies of parathyroid secretion or other disturbances (as vitamin D deficiency)

tet·ra·ben·a·zine \ˌte-trə-'be-nə-ˌzēn\ *n* : a serotonin antagonist $C_{19}H_{27}NO_3$ that is used esp. in the treatment of psychosis and anxiety

tet·ra·caine \'te-trə-ˌkān\ *n* : a crystalline basic ester that is closely related chemically to procaine and is used chiefly in the form of its hydrochloride $C_{15}H_{24}N_2O_2 \cdot HCl$ as a local anesthetic — called also *amethocaine, pantocaine;* see PONTOCAINE

tet·ra·chlo·ride \ˌte-trə-'klōr-ˌīd\ *n* : a chloride containing four atoms of chlorine

2,3,7,8–tet·ra·chlo·ro·di·ben·zo–para–di·ox·in \ˌtü-ˌthrē-ˌse-vən-ˌāt-ˌte-trə-ˌklōr-ō-dī-ˌben-zō-ˌpar-ə-dī-'äk-sən\ *n* : TCDD

2,3,7,8–tet·ra·chlo·ro·di·ben·zo–p–di·ox·in \-ˌpē-dī-'äk-sən\ *n* : TCDD

tet·ra·cy·cline \ˌte-trə-'sī-ˌklēn\ *n* : a yellow crystalline broad-spectrum antibiotic that is produced by a soil actinomycete of the genus *Streptomyces* (*S. viridifaciens*) or made synthetically and that is administered chiefly in the form of its hydrochloride $C_{22}H_{24}N_2O_8$·HCl; *also* : any of several chemically related antibiotics

tet·rad \'te-ˌtrad\ *n* : a group or arrangement of four: as **a** : a group of four cells produced by the successive divisions of a mother cell **b** : a group of four synapsed chromatids that become visibly evident in the pachytene stage of meiotic prophase

tet·ra·eth·yl·am·mo·ni·um \ˌte-trə-ˌe-thə-lə-'mō-nē-əm\ *n* : a quaternary ammonium ion $(C_2H_5)_4N^+$ containing four ethyl groups; *also* : a salt of this ion (as the crystalline chloride used as a ganglionic blocking agent) — abbr. *TEA*

tet·ra·eth·yl py·ro·phos·phate \ˌte-trə-ˌe-thəl-ˌpī-rō-'fäs-ˌfāt\ *n* : TEPP

tet·ra·eth·yl·thi·u·ram di·sul·fide \ˌte-trə-ˌe-thəl-'thī-yu̇-ˌram-ˌdī-'səl-ˌfīd\ *n* : DISULFIRAM

tet·ra·hy·dro·ami·no·ac·ri·dine \ˌte-trə-ˌhī-drə-ə-mē-nō-'a-krə-ˌdēn\ *n* : TACRINE

tet·ra·hy·dro·can·nab·i·nol \-ˌhī-drə-kə-'na-bə-ˌnȯl, -ˌnōl\ *n* : THC; *esp* : THC a

te·tral·o·gy of Fal·lot \te-ˌtra-lə-jē-əv-fä-'lō\ *n* : a congenital abnormality of the heart characterized by pulmonary stenosis, an opening in the interventricular septum, malposition of the aorta over both ventricles, and hypertrophy of the right ventricle

  Fallot, Étienne–Louis–Arthur (1850–1911), French physician.

tetranitrate — see ERYTHRITYL TETRANITRATE, PENTAERYTHRITOL TETRANITRATE

tet·ra·pa·re·sis \ˌte-trə-pə-'rē-səs\ *n, pl* **-re·ses** \-ˌsēz\ : QUADRIPARESIS

tet·ra·pa·ret·ic \-pə-'re-tik\ *adj* : QUADRIPARETIC

tet·ra·ple·gia \ˌte-trə-'plē-jə, -jē-ə\ *n* : QUADRIPLEGIA

tet·ra·ple·gic \-'plē-jik\ *adj or n* : QUADRIPLEGIC

tet·ra·ploid \'te-trə-ˌplȯid\ *adj* : having or being a chromosome number four times the monoploid number ⟨a ∼ cell⟩ — **tet·ra·ploi·dy** \-ˌplȯi-dē\ *n*

tet·ra·zo·li·um \ˌte-trə-'zō-lē-əm\ *n* : a cation or group CH_3N_4 that is analogous to ammonium; *also* : any of several derivatives used esp. as electron acceptors to test for metabolic activity in living cells

te·tro·do·tox·in \te-ˌtrō-də-'täk-sən\ *n* : a neurotoxin $C_{11}H_{17}N_3O_8$ that is found esp. in puffer fishes and that blocks nerve conduction by suppressing permeability of the nerve fiber to sodium ions

te·trox·ide \te-'träk-ˌsīd\ *n* : a compound of an element or group with four atoms of oxygen — see OSMIUM TETROXIDE

Texas fever *n* : an infectious disease of cattle transmitted by the cattle tick and caused by a sporozoan of the genus *Babesia* (*B. bigemina*) that destroys red blood cells — called also *Texas cattle fever*

T4 *or* **T₄** \ˌtē-'fȯr\ *n* : THYROXINE

T4 cell *n* : any of the T cells (as a helper T cell) that bear the CD4 molecule on their surface and become severely depleted in AIDS — called also *helper/inducer T cell*, *T4 lymphocyte*

TGF *abbr* transforming growth factor

T–group \'tē-ˌgrüp\ *n* : a group of people under the leadership of a trainer who seek to develop self-awareness and sensitivity to others by verbalizing feelings uninhibitedly at group sessions — compare ENCOUNTER GROUP

Th *symbol* thorium

THA \ˌtē-ˌāch-'ā\ *n* : TACRINE

thalam- *or* **thalamo-** *comb form* **1** : thalamus ⟨*thalam*otomy⟩ **2** : thalamic and ⟨*thalamo*cortical⟩

tha·lam·ic \thə-'la-mik\ *adj* : of, relating to, or involving the thalamus

thal·a·mo·cor·ti·cal \ˌtha-lə-mō-'kȯr-ti-kəl\ *adj* : of, relating to, or connecting the thalamus and the cerebral cortex

thal·a·mot·o·my \ˌtha-lə-'mä-tə-mē\ *n, pl* **-mies** : a surgical operation involving electrocoagulation of areas of the thalamus to interrupt pathways of nervous transmission through the thalamus for relief of certain mental and psychomotor disorders

thal·a·mus \'tha-lə-məs\ *n, pl* **-mi** \-ˌmī, -ˌmē\ : the largest subdivision of the diencephalon that consists chiefly of an ovoid mass of nuclei in each lateral wall of the third ventricle and serves to relay impulses to and from the cerebral cortex

thal·as·sae·mia, thal·as·sae·mic *chiefly Brit var of* THALASSEMIA, THALASSEMIC

thal·as·se·mia \ˌtha-lə-'sē-mē-ə\ *n* : any of a group of inherited hypochromic anemias and esp. Cooley's anemia controlled by a series of allelic genes that cause reduction in or failure of synthesis of one of the globin chains making up hemoglobin and that tend to occur esp. in individuals of Mediterranean, African, or southeastern Asian ancestry — sometimes used with a prefix (as alpha-, beta-, or delta-) to indicate the hemoglobin chain affected; called also *Mediterranean anemia;* see BETA= THALASSEMIA

thalassemia major *n* : COOLEY'S ANEMIA

thalassemia minor *n* : a mild form of thalassemia associated with the heterozygous condition for the gene involved

¹**thal·as·se·mic** \ˌtha-lə-'sē-mik\ *adj* : of, relating to, or affected with thalassemia

²**thalassemic** *n* : an individual affected with thalassemia

tha·las·so·ther·a·py \thə-ˌla-sō-'ther-ə-pē\ *n, pl* **-pies** : exposure to seawater (as in a hot tub) or application of sea products (as seaweed or sea salt) to the body for health or beauty benefits

tha·lid·o·mide \thə-'li-də-ˌmīd, -məd\ *n* : a sedative, hypnotic, and antiemetic drug $C_{13}H_{10}N_2O_4$ that was used chiefly in Europe during the late 1950s and early 1960s esp. to treat morning sickness but was withdrawn after being shown to cause serious malformations (as missing or severely shortened arms or legs) in infants born to mothers using it during the first trimester of pregnancy and is now used as a treatment for the cutaneous complications of leprosy

thal·li·um \'tha-lē-əm\ *n* : a sparsely but widely distributed poisonous metallic element — symbol *Tl*; see ELEMENT table

thanat- *or* **thanato-** *comb form* : death ⟨*thanato*logy⟩

than·a·tol·o·gy \ˌtha-nə-'tä-lə-jē\ *n, pl* **-gies** : the description or study of the phenomena of death and of psychological mechanisms for coping with them — **than·a·to·log·i·cal** \ˌtha-nə-tə-'lä-ji-kəl\ *adj* — **than·a·tol·o·gist** \ˌtha-nə-'tä-lə-jist\ *n*

than·a·to·phor·ic \ˌtha-nə-tə-'för-ik\ *adj* : relating to, affected with, or being a severe form of congenital dwarfism which results in early death

Than·a·tos \'tha-nə-ˌtäs\ *n* : DEATH INSTINCT

THC \ˌtē-(ˌ)āch-'sē\ *n* : either of two physiologically active isomers $C_{21}H_{30}O_2$ that occur naturally in hemp plant resin or are synthetically prepared: **a** : one that is the chief intoxicant in marijuana and is used medicinally — called also *delta-9= tetrahydrocannabinol, delta-9-THC*; see DRONABINOL **b** : one that is present in marijuana only in minute quantities

the·ater *or* **the·atre** \'thē-ə-tər\ *n* **1** : a room often with rising tiers of seats for assemblies (as for lectures or surgical demonstrations) **2** *usu* **theatre**, *Brit* : a hospital operating room

the·ba·ine \thə-'bā-ˌēn\ *n* : a poisonous crystalline alkaloid $C_{19}H_{21}NO_3$ found in opium in small quantities

The·be·sian vein \thə-'bē-zhən-\ *n* : any of the minute veins of the heart wall that drain directly into the cavity of the heart — called also *Thebesian vessel*

The·be·si·us \te-'bā-zē-əs\, **Adam Christian** (1686–1732), German anatomist.

the·ca \'thē-kə\ *n, pl* **the·cae** \'thē-ˌsē, -ˌkē\ : an enveloping case or sheath of an anatomical part — **the·cal** \-kəl\ *adj*

theca cell *n* **1** : THECA LUTEIN CELL **2** : a cell of the columnar epithelium lining the gastric pits of the stomach

theca ex·ter·na \-ek-'stər-nə\ *n* : the outer layer of the theca folliculi that is composed of fibrous and muscular tissue

theca fol·lic·u·li \-fə-'li-kyə-ˌlī\ *n* : the outer covering of a graafian follicle that is made up of the theca externa and theca interna

theca in·ter·na \-in-'tər-nə\ *n* : the inner layer of the theca folliculi that is highly vascular and that contributes theca lutein cells to the formation of the corpus luteum

theca lutein cell *n* : a cell of the corpus luteum that is derived from cells of the theca interna and secretes estrone and estradiol as well as progesterone — called also *theca cell*

thei·le·ria \thī-'lir-ē-ə\ *n* **1** *cap* : a genus of protozoans (family Theileriidae) that includes a parasite (*T. parva*) causing east coast fever of cattle **2** *pl* **-ri·ae** \-ē-ˌē\ *also* **-rias** : any organism of the genus *Theileria* — **thei·le·ri·al** \-ē-əl\ *adj*

Thei·ler \'tī-lər\, **Sir Arnold** (1867–1936), South African veterinary bacteriologist.

thei·le·ri·a·sis \thī-lə-'rī-ə-səs\ *n, pl* **-a·ses** \-ˌsēz\ : THEILERIOSIS

thei·le·ri·o·sis \thī-ˌlir-ē-'ō-səs\ *n, pl* **-o·ses** \-ˌsēz\ *or* **-osises** : infection with or disease caused by a protozoan of the genus *Theileria*; *esp* : EAST COAST FEVER

the·lar·che \thē-'lär-kē\ *n* : the beginning of breast development at the onset of puberty ⟨premature ∼⟩

The·la·zia \thə-'lā-zē-ə\ *n* : a genus of nematode worms (family Thelaziidae) that includes various eye worms

T–help·er cell \ˌtē-'hel-pər-\ *n* : HELPER T CELL

T–helper lymphocyte *n* : HELPER T CELL

thematic apperception test *n* : a projective psychological test that is used in clinical psychology to make personality, psychodynamic, and diagnostic assessments based on the subject's verbal responses to a series of black and white pictures — abbr. TAT

the·nar \'thē-ˌnär, -nər\ *adj* : of, relating to, involving, or constituting the thenar eminence or the thenar muscles

thenar eminence *n* : the ball of the thumb

thenar muscle *n* : any of the muscles that comprise the intrinsic musculature of the thumb and include the abductor pollicis brevis, adductor pollicis, flexor pollicis brevis, and opponens pollicis

the·o·bro·ma oil \ˌthē-ə-'brō-mə-\ *n* : COCOA BUTTER — used esp. in pharmacy

theo·bro·mine \ˌthē-ə-'brō-ˌmēn, -mən\ *n* : a bitter alkaloid $C_7H_8N_4O_2$ closely related to caffeine that is used as a diuretic, myocardial stimulant, and vasodilator

the·oph·yl·line \thē-'ä-fə-lən\ *n* : a feebly basic bitter crystalline compound $C_7H_8N_4O_2$ that is present in small amounts in tea, is isomeric with theobromine, and is used in medicine esp. as a bronchodilator

theophylline ethylenediamine *n* : AMINOPHYLLINE

the·o·ry \'thir-ē\ *n, pl* **-ries** **1** : the general or abstract principles of a body of fact, a science, or an art **2** : a plausible or scientifically acceptable general principle or body of principles offered to explain natural phenomena **3** : a working hypothesis that is considered probable based on experimental evidence of factual or conceptual analysis and is accepted as a basis for experimentation — **the·o·ret·i·cal** \,thē-ə-'re-ti-kəl\ *also* **the·o·ret·ic** \-tik\ *adj* — **the·o·ret·i·cal·ly** *adv*

ther·a·peu·sis \,ther-ə-'pyü-səs\ *n, pl* **-peu·ses** \-,sēz\ : THERAPEUTICS

ther·a·peu·tic \-'pyü-tik\ *adj* **1** : of or relating to the treatment of disease or disorders by remedial agents or methods **2** : CURATIVE, MEDICINAL — **ther·a·peu·ti·cal·ly** *adv*

therapeutic abortion *n* : abortion induced when pregnancy constitutes a threat to the physical or mental health of the mother

therapeutic index *n* : a measure of the relative desirability of a drug for the attaining of a particular medical end that is usu. expressed as the ratio of the largest dose producing no toxic symptoms to the smallest dose routinely producing cures

ther·a·peu·tics \,ther-ə-'pyü-tiks\ *n sing or pl* : a branch of medical science dealing with the application of remedies to diseases ⟨cancer ∼⟩ — called also *therapeusis*

therapeutic touch *n* : a technique often included in alternative medicine in which the practitioner passes his or her hands over the body of the person being treated and that is held to induce relaxation, reduce pain, and promote healing

therapeutic window *n* **1** : the range of dosage of a drug or of its concentration in a bodily system that provides safe effective therapy **2** : a usu. short time interval (as after clinical onset of stroke) during which a particular therapy can be given safely and effectively

ther·a·peu·tist \-'pyü-tist\ *n* : a person skilled in therapeutics

ther·a·py \'ther-ə-pē\ *n, pl* **-pies** : therapeutic treatment esp. of bodily, mental, or behavioral disorder — **ther·a·pist** \'ther-ə-pist\ *n*

the·rio·ge·nol·o·gy \,thir-ē-ō-jə-'nä-lə-jē\ *n, pl* **-gies** : a branch of veterinary medicine concerned with veterinary obstetrics and with the diseases and physiology of animal reproductive systems — **the·rio·gen·o·log·i·cal** \,thir-ē-ō-,je-nə-'lä-ji-kəl\ *adj* — **the·**

rio·ge·nol·o·gist \,thir-ē-ō-jə-'nä-lə-jist\ *n*

therm- *or* **thermo-** *comb form* : heat ⟨*thermo*receptor⟩

ther·mal \'thər-məl\ *adj* **1** : of, relating to, or caused by heat **2** : being or involving a state of matter dependent upon temperature — **ther·mal·ly** *adv*

-ther·mia \'thər-mē-ə\ *or* **-ther·my** \,thər-mē\ *n comb form, pl* **-thermias** *or* **-thermies** : state of heat : generation of heat ⟨hypo*thermia*⟩

ther·mo·co·ag·u·la·tion \,thər-mō-kō-,a-gyə-'lā-shən\ *n* : surgical coagulation of tissue by the application of heat

ther·mo·di·lu·tion \,thər-mō-dī-'lü-shən\ *adj* : relating to or being a method of determining cardiac output by measurement of the change in temperature in the bloodstream after injecting a measured amount of cool fluid (as saline)

ther·mo·gen·e·sis \,thər-mō-'je-nə-səs\ *n, pl* **-e·ses** \-,sēz\ : the production of heat esp. in the body — **ther·mo·gen·ic** \-'je-nik\ *adj*

ther·mo·gram \'thər-mə-,gram\ *n* **1** : the record made by a thermograph **2** : a photographic record made by thermography

ther·mo·graph \-,graf\ *n* **1** : THERMOGRAM **2** : the apparatus used in thermography **3** : a thermometer that produces an automatic record

ther·mog·ra·phy \(,)thər-'mä-grə-fē\ *n, pl* **-phies** : a technique for detecting and measuring variations in the heat emitted by various regions of the body and transforming them into visible signals that can be recorded photographically — **ther·mo·graph·ic** \,thər-mə-'gra-fik\ *adj* — **ther·mo·graph·i·cal·ly** *adv*

ther·mo·la·bile \,thər-mō-'lā-,bīl, -bəl\ *adj* : unstable when heated — **ther·mo·la·bil·i·ty** \-lā-'bi-lə-tē\ *n*

ther·mol·y·sis \(,)thər-'mä-lə-səs\ *n, pl* **-y·ses** \-,sēz\ **1** : the dissipation of heat from the living body **2** : decomposition by heat

ther·mom·e·ter \thər-'mä-mə-tər\ *n* : an instrument for determining temperature

ther·mo·met·ric \,thər-mə-'me-trik\ *adj* : of or relating to a thermometer or to thermometry

ther·mom·e·try \thər-'mä-mə-trē\ *n, pl* **-tries** : the measurement of temperature

ther·mo·plas·tic \,thər-mə-'plas-tik\ *adj* : capable of softening or fusing when heated and of hardening again when cooled ⟨∼ resins⟩ — **thermoplastic** *n*

ther·mo·re·cep·tor \,thər-mō-ri-'sep-tər\ *n* : a sensory end organ that is stimulated by heat or cold

ther·mo·reg·u·la·tion \-,re-gyə-'lā-shən\ *n* : the maintenance or regulation of temperature; *specif* : the maintenance of a particular temperature of the living body — **ther·mo·reg·u·late** \-'re-gyə-ˌlāt\ *vb* — **ther·mo·reg·u·la·to·ry** \-'re-gyə-lə-ˌtōr-ē\ *adj*

ther·mo·sta·ble \ˌthər-mō-'stā-bəl\ *adj* : stable when heated — **ther·mo·sta·bil·i·ty** \-stə-'bi-lə-tē\ *n*

ther·mo·ther·a·py \ˌthər-mō-'ther-ə-pē\ *n, pl* **-pies** : treatment of disease by heat (as by hot air or hot baths)

-thermy — see **-THERMIA**

the·ta rhythm \'thā-tə-ˌrith-əm\ *n* : a relatively high amplitude brain wave pattern between approximately 4 and 9 hertz that is characteristic esp. of the hippocampus but occurs in many regions of the brain including the cortex — called also *theta, theta wave*

thi- or **thio-** *comb form* : containing sulfur ⟨*thia*mine⟩ ⟨*thio*pental⟩

thia·ben·da·zole \ˌthī-ə-'ben-də-ˌzōl\ *n* : a drug $C_{10}H_7N_3S$ used in the control of parasitic nematodes and in the treatment of fungus infections

thi·acet·azone \ˌthī-ə-'se-tə-ˌzōn\ *n* : a bitter pale yellow crystalline tuberculostatic drug $C_{10}H_{12}N_4OS$

thi·ami·nase \thī-'a-mə-ˌnās, 'thī-ə-mə-, -ˌnāz\ *n* : an enzyme that catalyzes the breakdown of thiamine

thi·a·mine \'thī-ə-mən, -ˌmēn\ *also* **thi·a·min** \-mən\ *n* : a vitamin $C_{12}H_{17}N_4OSCl$ of the vitamin B complex that is a water-soluble salt occurring widely both in plants and animals and that is essential for carbohydrate metabolism and for normal functioning of the nervous system — called also *vitamin B₁*

Thi·ara \thī-'ar-ə\ *n* : a genus of freshwater snails (family Thiaridae) that includes several forms (as *T. granifera*) which are intermediate hosts of medically important trematodes

thi·a·zide \'thī-ə-ˌzīd, -zəd\ *n* : any of a group of drugs used as oral diuretics esp. in the control of hypertension

thi·a·zine \'thī-ə-ˌzēn\ *n* : any of various compounds that are characterized by a ring composed of four carbon atoms, one sulfur atom, and one nitrogen atom and include some that are important as tranquilizers — see **PHENOTHIAZINE**

thi·a·zol·i·dine·di·one \ˌthī-ə-ˌzō-lə-ˌdēn-'dī-ˌōn\ *n* : any of a class of drugs (as pioglitazone and rosiglitazone) used to reduce insulin resistance in the treatment of type 2 diabetes

thi·a·zole \'thī-ə-ˌzōl\ *n* **1** : a colorless basic liquid C_3H_3NS; *also* : any of various thiazole derivatives

thick filament *n* : a myofilament of one of the two types making up myofibrils that is 10 to 12 nanometers (100 to 120 angstroms) in width and is composed of the protein myosin — compare **THIN FILAMENT**

Thiersch graft \'tirsh-\ *n* : a skin graft that consists of thin strips or sheets of epithelium with the tops of the der-

mal papillae and that is split off with a sharp knife

Thiersch, Carl (1822–1895), German surgeon.

thigh \'thī\ *n* : the proximal segment of the leg extending from the hip to the knee and supported by a single large bone — compare **FEMUR**

thigh bone *n* : **FEMUR**

thimble jellyfish *n* : a small jellyfish (*Linuche unguiculata*) whose tiny larvae cause seabather's eruption esp. in coastal waters of southern Florida and the Caribbean

thi·mer·o·sal \thī-'mer-ə-ˌsal\ *n* : a crystalline mercurial antiseptic $C_9H_9HgNaO_2S$ used esp. for its antifungal and bacteriostatic properties — see **MERTHIOLATE**

thin filament *n* : a myofilament of the one of the two types making up myofibrils that is about 5 nanometers (50 angstroms) in width and is composed chiefly of the protein actin — compare **THICK FILAMENT**

thin–layer chromatography *n* : chromatography in which the stationary phase is an absorbent medium (as silica gel) arranged as a thin layer on a rigid support (as a glass plate) — abbr. *TLC*; compare **COLUMN CHROMATOGRAPHY, PAPER CHROMATOGRAPHY** — **thin–layer chromatogram** *n* — **thin–layer chromatographic** *adj*

thio \'thī-ō\ *adj* : relating to or containing sulfur esp. in place of oxygen

thio- — see **THI-**

thio acid *n* : an acid in which oxygen is partly or wholly replaced by sulfur

thio·amide \ˌthī-ō-'a-ˌmīd, -məd\ *n* : an amide of a thio acid

thio·car·ba·mide \ˌthī-ō-'kär-bə-ˌmīd, -ˌkär-'ba-ˌmīd\ *n* : **THIOUREA**

thio·oc·tic acid *also* **6,8–thi·oc·tic acid** \ˌ(ˌ)siks-ˌāt-)thī-'äk-tik-\ *n* : a lipoic acid $C_8H_{14}O_2S_2$ that has been reported to ameliorate the effects of poisoning by mushrooms (as the death cap) of the genus *Amanita*

thio·cy·a·nate \ˌthī-ō-'sī-ə-ˌnāt, -nət\ *n* : a compound that consists of the chemical group SCN bonded by the sulfur atom to a group or an atom other than a hydrogen atom

thiocyanoacetate — see **ISOBORNYL THIOCYANOACETATE**

thio·es·ter \ˌthī-ō-'es-tər\ *n* : an ester formed by uniting a carboxyl group of one compound (as acetic acid) with a sulfhydryl group of another (as coenzyme A)

thio·gua·nine \-'gwä-ˌnēn\ *n* : a crystalline compound $C_5H_5N_5S$ that is an antimetabolite and has been used in the treatment of leukemia

thi·ol \'thī-ˌōl, -ˌōl\ *n* **1** : any of various compounds having the general formula RSH which are analogous to alcohols but in which sulfur replaces the oxygen of the hydroxyl group and which have disagreeable odors **2** : the functional group –SH characteristic of thiols — **thi·o·lic** \thī-'ō-lik\ *adj*

thio·pen·tal \ˌthī-ō-'pen-ˌtal, -ˌtȯl\ *n* : a barbiturate used in the form of its sodium salt $C_{11}H_{17}N_2NaO_2S$ esp. as an intravenous anesthetic — see PENTOTHAL

thio·pen·tone \-ˌtōn\ *n, Brit* : THIOPENTAL

thio·rid·a·zine \ˌthī-ə-'ri-də-ˌzēn, -zən\ *n* : a phenothiazine tranquilizer used in the form of its hydrochloride $C_{21}H_{26}N_2S_2 \cdot HCl$ for relief of anxiety states and in the treatment of psychotic disorders and severe childhood behavioral problems — see MELLARIL

thio·te·pa \ˌthī-ə-'tē-pə\ *n* : a sulfur analog $C_6H_{12}N_3PS$ of tepa that is used esp. as an antineoplastic agent and is less toxic than tepa

thio·thix·ene \ˌthī-ō-'thik-ˌsēn\ *n* : an antipsychotic drug $C_{23}H_{29}N_3O_2S_2$ used esp. in the treatment of schizophrenia — see NAVANE

thio·ura·cil \ˌthī-ō-'yu̇r-ə-ˌsil\ *n* : a bitter crystalline compound $C_4H_4N_2OS$ that depresses the function of the thyroid gland

thio·urea \-yu̇-'rē-ə\ *n* : a colorless bitter compound $CS(NH_2)_2$ analogous to and resembling urea that is used esp. in medicine as an antithyroid drug — called also *thiocarbamide*

thio·xan·thene \ˌthī-ō-'zan-ˌthēn\ *n* : a compound $C_{13}H_{10}S$ that is the parent compound of various antipsychotic drugs (as thiothixene); *also* : a derivative of thioxanthene

third cranial nerve *n* : OCULOMOTOR NERVE

third–degree burn *n* : a severe burn characterized by destruction of the skin through the depth of the dermis and possibly into underlying tissues, loss of fluid, and sometimes shock

third eyelid *n* : NICTITATING MEMBRANE

third ventricle *n* : the median unpaired ventricle of the brain bounded by parts of the telencephalon and diencephalon

thirst \'thərst\ *n* : a sensation of dryness in the mouth and throat associated with a desire for liquids; *also* : the bodily condition (as of dehydration) that induces this sensation — **thirsty** \'thər-stē\ *adj*

Thom·as splint \'tä-məs-\ *n* : a metal splint for fractures of the arm or leg that consists of a ring at one end to fit around the upper arm or leg and two metal shafts extending down the sides of the limb in a long U with a crosspiece at the bottom where traction is applied

Thomas, Hugh Owen (1834–1891), British orthopedic surgeon.

Thom·sen's disease \'tȯm-sənz-, 'täm-\ *n* : MYOTONIA CONGENITA

Thomsen, Asmus Julius Thomas (1815–1896), Danish physician.

thon·zyl·a·mine \thän-'zi-lə-ˌmēn, -mən\ *n* : an antihistamine derived from pyrimidine and used in the form of its hydrochloride $C_{16}H_{22}N_4O \cdot HCl$

thorac- *or* **thoraci-** *or* **thoraco-** *comb form* **1** : chest : thorax ⟨*thoraco*plasty⟩ **2** : thoracic and ⟨*thoraco*lumbar⟩

tho·ra·cen·te·sis \ˌthō-rə-sen-'tē-səs\ *n, pl* **-te·ses** \-ˌsēz\ : aspiration of fluid from the chest (as in empyema) — called also *thoracocentesis*

thoraces *pl of* THORAX

tho·rac·ic \thə-'ra-sik\ *adj* : of, relating to, located within, or involving the thorax — **tho·rac·i·cal·ly** *adv*

thoracic aorta *n* : the part of the aorta that lies in the thorax and extends from the arch to the diaphragm

thoracic artery *n* : either of two arteries that branch from the axillary artery or from one of its branches: **a** : a small artery that supplies or sends branches to the two pectoralis muscles and the walls of the chest — called also *supreme thoracic artery* **b** : an artery that supplies both pectoralis muscles and the serratus anterior and sends branches to the lymph nodes of the axilla and to the subscapularis muscle — called also *lateral thoracic artery*; compare INTERNAL THORACIC ARTERY

thoracic cage *n* : RIB CAGE

thoracic cavity *n* : the division of the body cavity that lies above the diaphragm, is bounded peripherally by the wall of the chest, and contains the heart and lungs

thoracic duct *n* : the main trunk of the system of lymphatic vessels that lies along the front of the spinal column and receives chyle from the intestine and lymph from the abdomen, the lower limbs, and the entire left side of the body — called also *left lymphatic duct*

thoracic ganglion *n* : any of the ganglia of the sympathetic chain in the thoracic region that occur in 12 or fewer pairs

thoracic nerve *n* : any of the spinal nerves of the thoracic region that consist of 12 pairs of which one pair emerges just below each thoracic vertebra

thoracic vertebra *n* : any of the 12 vertebrae dorsal to the thoracic region and characterized by articulation with the ribs

thoracis — see ILIOCOSTALIS THORACIS, LONGISSIMUS THORACIS, SEMISPINALIS THORACIS, SPINALIS THORACIS, TRANSVERSUS THORACIS

thoraco- — see THORAC-

tho·ra·co·ab·dom·i·nal \ˌthō-rə-ˌkō-ab-'dä-mə-nəl\ *also* **tho·rac·i·co·ab·dom·i·nal** \thə-ˌra-si-ˌkō-\ *adj* : of, relating to, involving, or affecting the thorax and the abdomen

tho·ra·co·acro·mi·al artery \ˌthō-rə-ˌkō-ə-'krō-mē-əl-\ *n* : a short branch of the axillary artery that divides into four branches supplying the region of the pectoralis muscles, deltoid, subclavius, and sternoclavicular joint

tho·ra·co·cen·te·sis \-sen-'tē-səs\ *n, pl* **-te·ses** \-,sēz\ : THORACENTESIS

tho·ra·co·dor·sal artery \,thō-rə-kō-'dòr-səl-\ *n* : an artery that is continuous with the axillary artery and supplies or gives off branches supplying the subscapularis muscle, latissimus dorsi, serratus anterior, and the intercostal muscles

thoracodorsal nerve *n* : a branch of the posterior cord of the brachial plexus that supplies the latissimus dorsi

tho·ra·co·lum·bar \-'ləm-bər, -,bär\ *adj* **1** : of, relating to, arising in, or involving the thoracic and lumbar regions ⟨∼ spine fractures⟩ **2** : SYMPATHETIC ⟨∼ nerve fibers⟩

tho·ra·co·plas·ty \'thòr-ə-kō-,plas-tē\ *n, pl* **-ties** : the surgical operation of removing or resecting one or more ribs so as to obliterate the pleural cavity and collapse a diseased lung

tho·ra·co·scope \thə-'rā-kə-,skōp, -'ra-\ *n* : an endoscope that is inserted through a puncture in the chest wall in an intercostal space (as for visual examination of the chest cavity) — **tho·ra·co·scop·ic** \thə-,rā-kə-'skä-pik\ *adj*

tho·ra·cos·co·py \,thōr-ə-'käs-kə-pē\ *n, pl* **-pies** : examination of the chest and esp. the pleural cavity by means of a thoracoscope

tho·ra·cos·to·my \,thōr-ə-'käs-tə-mē\ *n, pl* **-mies** : surgical opening of the chest (as for drainage)

tho·ra·cot·o·my \,thōr-ə-'kä-tə-mē\ *n, pl* **-mies** : surgical incision of the chest wall

tho·rax \'thòr-,aks\ *n, pl* **tho·rax·es** or **tho·ra·ces** \'thòr-ə-,sēz\ **1** : the part of the body that is situated between the neck and the abdomen and is supported by the ribs, costal cartilages, and sternum; *also* : THORACIC CAVITY **2** : the middle of the three chief divisions of the body of an insect; *also* : the corresponding part of a crustacean or an arachnid

Tho·ra·zine \'thòr-ə-,zēn\ *trademark* — used for a preparation of the hydrochloride of chlorpromazine

tho·ri·um \'thòr-ē-əm\ *n* : a radioactive metallic element — symbol *Th;* see ELEMENT table

thorn–headed worm or **thorny–headed worm** *n* : ACANTHOCEPHALAN

thor·ough·pin \'thər-ō-,pin\ *n* : a synovial swelling just above the hock of a horse that is often associated with lameness

Thr *abbr* threonine

thread lungworm *n* : a slender nematode worm of the genus *Dictyocaulus* (*D. filaria*) that parasitizes the air passages of the lungs of sheep

thread·worm \'thred-,wərm\ *n* : any long slender nematode worm

thready pulse \'thre-dē-\ *n* : a scarcely perceptible and commonly rapid pulse that feels like a fine mobile thread under a palpating finger

three–day fever *n* : a fever or febrile state lasting three days: as **a** : SANDFLY FEVER **b** : ROSEOLA INFANTUM

3TC \,thrē-(,)tē-'sē\ *trademark* — used for a preparation of lamivudine

thre·o·nine \'thrē-ə-,nēn\ *n* : a colorless crystalline essential amino acid $C_4H_9NO_3$ — abbr. *Thr*

thresh·old \'thresh-,hōld\ *n* : the point at which a physiological or psychological effect begins to be produced (as the degree of stimulation of a nerve which just produces a response) — called also *limen*

thrill \'thril\ *n* : an abnormal fine tremor or vibration in the respiratory or circulatory systems felt on palpation

throat \'thrōt\ *n* **1** : the part of the neck in front of the spinal column **2** : the passage through the throat to the stomach and lungs containing the pharynx and upper part of the esophagus, the larynx, and the trachea

throat botfly *n* : a botfly of the genus *Gasterophilus* (*G. nasalis*) that lays its eggs on the hairs about the mouth and throat of the horse from where the larvae migrate to the stomach and intestine — called also *throat fly*

¹throb \'thräb\ *vb* **throbbed; throbbing** : to pulsate or pound esp. with abnormal force or rapidity

²throb *n* : a single pulse of a pulsating movement or sensation

throe \'thrō\ *n* : PANG, SPASM — usu. used in pl. ⟨death ∼s⟩

thromb- or **thrombo-** *comb form* **1** : blood clot : clotting of blood ⟨*thrombin*⟩ **2** : marked by or associated with thrombosis ⟨*thromboangiitis*⟩

throm·base \'thräm-,bās\ *n* : THROMBIN

throm·bas·the·nia \,thräm-bəs-'thē-nē-ə\ *n* : an inherited abnormality of the blood platelets characterized esp. by defective clot retraction and often prolonged bleeding time

throm·bec·to·my \thräm-'bek-tə-mē\ *n, pl* **-mies** : surgical excision of a thrombus

thrombi *pl of* THROMBUS

throm·bin \'thräm-bən\ *n* : a proteolytic enzyme formed from prothrombin that facilitates the clotting of blood by catalyzing conversion of fibrinogen to fibrin — called also *thrombase*

throm·bo·an·gi·i·tis \,thräm-bō-,an-jē-'ī-təs\ *n, pl* **-it·i·des** \-'ī-tə-,dēz\ : inflammation of the lining of a blood vessel with thrombus formation

thromboangiitis ob·lit·er·ans \-ə-'bli-tə-,ranz\ *n* : BUERGER'S DISEASE

throm·bo·cyte \'thräm-bə-,sīt\ *n* : PLATELET — **throm·bo·cyt·ic** \,thräm-bə-'si-tik\ *adj*

throm·bo·cy·the·mia \ˌthräm-bō-sī-ˈthē-mē-ə\ *n* : a myeloproliferative disorder marked esp. by an abnormal chronic increase in the number of circulating platelets

throm·bo·cy·top·a·thy \ˌthräm-bə-ˌsī-ˈtä-pə-thē\ *n, pl* **-thies** : any of various functional disorders of platelets

throm·bo·cy·to·pe·nia \ˌthräm-bə-ˌsī-tə-ˈpē-nē-ə, -nyə\ *n* : persistent decrease in the number of blood platelets that is often associated with hemorrhagic conditions — called also *thrombopenia* — **throm·bo·cy·to·pe·nic** \-nik\ *adj*

thrombocytopenic purpura *n* : purpura that is characterized by bleeding into the skin with the production of petechiae or ecchymoses and by hemorrhages into mucous membranes and that is associated with a reduction in circulating blood platelets and prolonged bleeding time ⟨idiopathic *thrombocytopenic purpura*⟩ — called also *purpura hemorrhagica, Werlhof's disease*

throm·bo·cy·to·sis \ˌthräm-bə-ˌsī-ˈtō-səs\ *n, pl* **-to·ses** \-ˈtō-ˌsēz\ : increase and esp. abnormal increase in the number of platelets in the blood that typically occurs in association with a myeloproliferative disorder (as thrombocythemia or chronic myelogenous leukemia) or as a nonspecific response to an underlying disorder or disease (as a systemic infection); *also* : THROMBOCYTHEMIA

throm·bo·em·bo·lism \ˌthräm-bō-ˈem-bə-ˌli-zəm\ *n* : the blocking of a blood vessel by a particle that breaks away from a blood clot at its site of formation — **throm·bo·em·bol·ic** \-em-ˈbä-lik\ *adj*

throm·bo·end·ar·te·rec·to·my \ˌthräm-bō-ˌen-ˌdär-tə-ˈrek-tə-mē\ *n, pl* **-mies** : surgical excision of a thrombus and the adjacent arterial lining

throm·bo·gen·e·sis \ˌthräm-bō-ˈje-nə-səs\ *n, pl* **-e·ses** \-ˌsēz\ : the formation of a thrombus

throm·bo·gen·ic \ˌthräm-bə-ˈje-nik\ *adj* : tending to produce a thrombus — **throm·bo·ge·nic·i·ty** \-jə-ˈni-sə-tē\ *n*

throm·bo·ki·nase \ˌthräm-bō-ˈkī-ˌnās, -ˌnāz\ *n* : THROMBOPLASTIN

¹**throm·bo·lyt·ic** \ˌthräm-bə-ˈli-tik\ *adj* : destroying or breaking up a thrombus ⟨a ∼ agent⟩ ⟨∼ therapy⟩ — **throm·bol·y·sis** \ˌthräm-ˈbä-lə-səs\ *n*

²**thrombolytic** *n* : a thrombolytic drug (as streptokinase or urokinase) : CLOT-BUSTER

throm·bo·pe·nia \ˌthräm-bō-ˈpē-nē-ə\ *n* : THROMBOCYTOPENIA — **throm·bo·pe·nic** \-ˈpē-nik\ *adj*

throm·bo·phil·ia \-ˈfi-lē-ə\ *n* : a hereditary or acquired predisposition to thrombosis

throm·bo·phle·bi·tis \-fli-ˈbī-təs\ *n, pl* **-bit·i·des** \-ˈbi-tə-ˌdēz\ : inflammation of a vein with formation of a thrombus — compare PHLEBOTHROMBOSIS

throm·bo·plas·tic \ˌthräm-bō-ˈplas-tik\ *adj* : initiating or accelerating the clotting of blood ⟨a ∼ substance⟩

throm·bo·plas·tin \ˌthräm-bō-ˈplas-tən\ *n* : a complex enzyme that is found esp. in blood platelets and functions in the conversion of prothrombin to thrombin in the clotting of blood — called also *thrombokinase*

throm·bo·plas·tin·o·gen \-plas-ˈti-nə-jən\ *n* : FACTOR VIII

throm·bo·poi·e·tin \-ˈpȯi-ə-tən\ *n* : a hormone that regulates blood platelet production by promoting the proliferation and maturation of megakaryocyte progenitor cells and the development of megakaryocytes into blood platelets

throm·bo·sis \thräm-ˈbō-səs, thrəm-\ *n, pl* **-bo·ses** \-ˌsēz\ : the formation or presence of a blood clot within a blood vessel — see CORONARY THROMBOSIS, DEEP VEIN THROMBOSIS — **throm·bose** \ˈthräm-ˌbōs, -ˌbōz\ *vb* — **throm·bot·ic** \thräm-ˈbä-tik\ *adj*

thrombotic thrombocytopenic purpura *n* : a rare disease that is marked by the systemic formation of thrombi in the capillaries and arterioles, that primarily affects adult females, and that is similar clinically to hemolytic uremic syndrome but is usu. distinguished by only mild renal dysfunction and significant neurological deficits and by the presence of large aggregates of von Willebrand factor — called also *TTP*

throm·box·ane \thräm-ˈbäk-ˌsān\ *n* : any of several substances that are produced esp. by platelets, are formed from endoperoxides, cause constriction of vascular and bronchial smooth muscle, and promote blood clotting

throm·bus \ˈthräm-bəs\ *n, pl* **throm·bi** \-ˌbī, -ˌbē\ : a clot of blood formed within a blood vessel and remaining attached to its place of origin — compare EMBOLUS

throw·back \ˈthrō-ˌbak\ *n* **1** : reversion to an earlier type or phase : ATAVISM **2** : an instance or product of atavistic reversion

throw up *vb* : VOMIT

thrush \ˈthrəsh\ *n* **1** : a disease that is caused by a fungus of the genus *Candida* (*C. albicans*), occurs esp. in infants and children, and is marked by white patches in the oral cavity; *broadly* : CANDIDIASIS ⟨vaginal ∼⟩ **2** : a suppurative disorder of the feet in various animals (as the horse)

thu·li·um \ˈthü-lē-əm, ˈthyü-\ *n* : a metallic element — symbol *Tm;* see ELEMENT table

thumb \ˈthəm\ *n* : the short and thick first or most preaxial digit of the human hand that differs from the other fingers in having only two phalanges, in having greater freedom of movement, and in being opposable to the other fingers

thumb–suck·ing \-ˌsə-kiŋ\ *n* : the habit esp. of infants and young children of sucking a thumb — **thumb–suck·er** *n*

thym- *or* **thymo-** *comb form* : thymus ⟨*thym*ic⟩ ⟨*thymo*cyte⟩

thy·mec·to·my \thī-ˈmek-tə-mē\ *n, pl* **-mies** : surgical excision of the thymus — **thy·mec·to·mize** \-ˌmīz\ *vb*

thyme oil \ˈtīm-, ˈthīm-\ *n* : a fragrant essential oil that is obtained from various thymes (genus *Thymus* of the mint family, Labiatae) and is used chiefly as an antiseptic in pharmaceutical and dental preparations

-thy·mia \ˈthī-mē-ə\ *n comb form* : condition of mind and will ⟨dys*thymia*⟩

thy·mic \ˈthī-mik\ *adj* : of or relating to the thymus ⟨a ∼ tumor⟩

thymic corpuscle *n* : HASSALL'S CORPUSCLE

thy·mi·co·lym·phat·ic \ˌthī-mi-(ˌ)kō-lim-ˈfa-tik\ *adj* : of, relating to, or affecting both the thymus and the lymphatic system ⟨∼ involution⟩

thy·mi·dine \ˈthī-mə-ˌdēn\ *n* : a nucleoside $C_{10}H_{14}N_2O_5$ that is composed of thymine and deoxyribose and occurs as a structural part of DNA

thymidine kinase *n* : an enzyme that catalyzes the phosphorylation of thymidine in a pathway leading to DNA synthesis, that is active esp. in tissues undergoing growth or regeneration, and that is the key enzyme mediating replication in certain viruses (as the herpesvirus causing herpes simplex)

thy·mine \ˈthī-ˌmēn\ *n* : a pyrimidine base $C_5H_6N_2O_2$ that is one of the four bases coding genetic information in the polynucleotide chain of DNA — compare ADENINE, CYTOSINE, GUANINE, URACIL

thy·mo·cyte \ˈthī-mə-ˌsīt\ *n* : a cell of the thymus; *esp* : a thymic lymphocyte

thy·mol \ˈthī-ˌmȯl, -ˌmōl\ *n* : a crystalline phenol $C_{10}H_{14}O$ of aromatic odor and antiseptic properties found esp. in thyme oil or made synthetically and used chiefly as a fungicide and preservative

thy·mo·ma \thī-ˈmō-mə\ *n, pl* **-mas** *also* **-ma·ta** \-mə-tə\ : a tumor that arises from the tissue elements of the thymus

thy·mo·sin \ˈthī-mə-sən\ *n* : a mixture of polypeptides isolated from the thymus; *also* : any of these polypeptides

thy·mus \ˈthī-məs\ *n, pl* **thy·mus·es** *also* **thy·mi** \-ˌmī\ : a glandular structure of largely lymphoid tissue that functions in cell-mediated immunity by being the site where T cells develop, that is present in the young of most vertebrates typically in the upper anterior chest or at the base of the neck, and that gradually decreases in size and activity after puberty — called also *thymus gland*

thyr- *or* **thyro-** *comb form* **1** : thyroid ⟨*thyro*globulin⟩ **2** : thyroid and ⟨*thyro*arytenoid⟩

thy·ro·ac·tive \ˌthī-rō-ˈak-tiv\ *adj* **1** : capable of entering into the thyroid metabolism and of being incorporated into the thyroid hormone ⟨∼ iodine⟩ **2** : simulating the action of the thyroid hormone ⟨∼ iodinated casein⟩

thy·ro·ar·y·te·noid \-ˌar-ə-ˈtē-ˌnȯid, -ə-ˈrit-ᵊn-ˌȯid\ *n* : a broad thin muscle that arises esp. from the thyroid cartilage, inserts into the arytenoid cartilage, and that functions to relax and shorten the vocal cords — called also *thyroarytenoid muscle;* see INFERIOR THYROARYTENOID LIGAMENT

thy·ro·ar·y·te·noi·de·us \-ˌar-ə-tə-ˈnȯi-dē-əs\ *n* : THYROARYTENOID

thy·ro·cal·ci·to·nin \ˌthī-rō-ˌkal-sə-ˈtō-nən\ *n* : CALCITONIN

thy·ro·cer·vi·cal \-ˈsər-vi-kəl\ *adj* : of, relating to, or being the thyrocervical trunk ⟨the ∼ artery⟩

thyrocervical trunk *n* : a short thick branch of the subclavian artery that divides into the inferior thyroid, suprascapular, and transverse cervical arteries

thy·ro·epi·glot·tic ligament \ˌthī-rō-ˌe-pə-ˈglä-tik-\ *n* : a long narrow ligamentous cord connecting the thyroid cartilage and epiglottis

thy·ro·glob·u·lin \ˌthī-rō-ˈglä-byə-lən\ *n* : an iodine-containing protein of the thyroid gland that on proteolysis yields thyroxine and triiodothyronine

thy·ro·glos·sal \ˌthī-rō-ˈglä-səl\ *adj* : of, relating to, or originating in the thyroglossal duct ⟨∼ cysts⟩

thyroglossal duct *n* : a temporary duct connecting the embryonic thyroid gland and the tongue

thy·ro·hy·al \ˌthī-rō-ˈhī-əl\ *n* : the larger and more lateral of the two lateral projections on each side of the human hyoid bone — called also *greater cornu;* compare CERATOHYAL

¹thy·ro·hy·oid \-ˈhī-ˌȯid\ *adj* : of, relating to, or supplying the thyrohyoid muscle

²thyrohyoid *n* : a thyrohyoid part; *esp* : THYROHYOID MUSCLE

thyrohyoid membrane *n* : a broad fibroelastic sheet that connects the upper margin of the thyroid cartilage and the upper margin of the back of the hyoid bone

thyrohyoid muscle *n* : a small quadrilateral muscle that arises from the thyroid cartilage, inserts into the thyrohyal of the hyoid bone, and functions to depress the hyoid bone and to elevate the thyroid cartilage — called also *thyrohyoid*

¹thy·roid \ˈthī-ˌrȯid\ *also* **thy·roi·dal** \thī-ˈrȯid-ᵊl\ *adj* **1** : of, relating to, or being the thyroid gland ⟨∼ disorders⟩ **2** : of, relating to, or being the thyroid cartilage

²**thyroid** *n* **1** : a large bilobed endocrine gland that arises as a median ventral outgrowth of the pharynx, lies in the anterior base of the neck, and produces esp. the hormones thyroxine and triiodothyronine — called also *thyroid gland* **2** : a preparation of the thyroid gland of various domestic animals (as pigs) used in treating thyroid disorders — called also *thyroid extract*

thyroid artery *n* : either of two arteries supplying the thyroid gland and nearby structures at the front of the neck: **a** : one that branches from the external carotid artery or sometimes from the common carotid artery — called also *superior thyroid artery* **b** : one that branches from the thyrocervical trunk — called also *inferior thyroid artery*

thyroid–binding globulin *n* : THYROXINE-BINDING GLOBULIN

thyroid cartilage *n* : the chief cartilage of the larynx that consists of two broad lamellae joined at an angle and that forms the Adam's apple

thy·roid·ec·to·my \ˌthī-ˌroi-'dek-tə-mē\ *n, pl* **-mies** : surgical excision of thyroid gland tissue — **thy·roid·ec·to·mize** \-ˌmīz\ *vb*

thyroid extract *n* : THYROID 2

thyroid gland *n* : THYROID 1

thyroid hormone *n* : any of several closely related metabolically active compounds (as triiodothyronine) that are stored in the thyroid gland in the form of thyroglobulin or circulate in the blood usu. bound to plasma protein; *esp* : THYROXINE

thy·roid·itis \ˌthī-ˌroi-'dī-təs\ *n* : inflammation of the thyroid gland

thy·roid·ol·o·gy \-'dä-lə-jē\ *n, pl* **-gies** : the study of the thyroid gland — **thy·roid·ol·o·gist** \-jəst\ *n*

thyroid–stimulating hormone *n* : a hormone secreted by the adenohypophysis of the pituitary gland that regulates the formation and secretion of thyroid hormone — called also *thyrotropic hormone, thyrotropin, TSH*

thyroid storm *n* : a sudden life-threatening exacerbation of the symptoms (as high fever, tachycardia, weakness, or extreme restlessness) of hyperthyroidism that is brought on by various causes (as infection, surgery, or stress)

thyroid vein *n* : any of several small veins draining blood from the thyroid gland and nearby structures in the front of the neck

thy·ro·nine \'thī-rə-ˌnēn, -nən\ *n* : a phenolic amino acid $C_9H_{11}NO_4$ of which thyroxine is a derivative; *also* : any of various derivatives and esp. iodine-containing derivatives of this

thy·rot·o·my \thī-'rä-tə-mē\ *n, pl* **-mies** : surgical incision or division of the thyroid cartilage

thy·ro·tox·ic \ˌthī-rō-'täk-sik\ *adj* : of, relating to, induced by, or affected with hyperthyroidism

thy·ro·tox·i·co·sis \ˌthī-rō-ˌtäk-sə-'kō-səs\ *n, pl* **-co·ses** \-ˌsēz\ : HYPERTHYROIDISM

thy·ro·tro·pic \ˌthī-rə-'trō-pik, -'trä-\ *also* **thy·ro·tro·phic** \-'trō-fik\ *adj* : exerting or characterized by a direct influence on the secretory activity of the thyroid gland ⟨∼ functions⟩

thyrotropic hormone *n* : THYROID-STIMULATING HORMONE

thy·ro·tro·pin \ˌthī-rə-'trō-pən\ *also* **thy·ro·tro·phin** \-fən\ *n* **1** : THYROID-STIMULATING HORMONE **2** : a recombinant form of thyroid-stimulating hormone used esp. as a diagnostic agent (as in the detection of thyroid cancer) — called also *thyrotropin alfa*

thyrotropin–releasing hormone *n* : a tripeptide hormone synthesized in the hypothalamus that stimulates secretion of thyrotropin by the anterior lobe of the pituitary gland — abbr. *TRH;* called also *protirelin, thyrotropin-releasing factor*

thy·rox·ine *or* **thy·rox·in** \thī-'räk-ˌsēn, -sən\ *n* : an iodine-containing hormone $C_{15}H_{11}I_4NO_4$ that is an amino acid produced by the thyroid gland as a product of the cleavage of thyroglobulin, that increases metabolic rate, and that is used to treat thyroid disorders — called also *T4*

thyroxine–binding globulin *n* : a blood serum glycoprotein that is synthesized in the liver and that binds tightly to thyroxine and less firmly to triiodothyronine preventing their removal from the blood by the kidneys and releasing them as needed at sites of activity — abbr. *TBG;* called also *thyroid-binding globulin*

Thysa·no·so·ma \ˌthī-sə-nō-'sō-mə\ *n* : a genus of tapeworms (family Anoplocephalidae) including the common fringed tapeworm of ruminants

Ti *symbol* titanium

TIA *abbr* transient ischemic attack

tib·ia \'ti-bē-ə\ *n, pl* **-i·ae** \-bē-ˌē, -bē-ˌī\ *also* **-i·as** : the inner and usu. larger of the two bones of the leg between the knee and ankle that articulates above with the femur and below with the talus — called also *shinbone* — **tib·i·al** \-bē-əl\ *adj*

tibial artery *n* : either of the two arteries of the lower leg formed by the bifurcation of the popliteal artery: **a** : a larger posterior artery that divides into the lateral and medial plantar arteries — called also *posterior tibial artery* **b** : a smaller anterior artery that continues beyond the ankle joint into the foot as the dorsalis pedis artery — called also *anterior tibial artery*

tibial collateral ligament *n* : MEDIAL COLLATERAL LIGAMENT 1

tib·i·a·lis \ˌti-bē-'ā-ləs\ *n, pl* **tib·i·a·les** \-(ˌ)lēz\ : either of two muscles of the calf of the leg: **a** : a muscle arising chiefly from the lateral condyle and part of the shaft of the tibia, inserting by a long tendon into the first cuneiform and first metatarsal bones, and acting to flex the foot dorsally and to invert it — called also *tibialis anterior, tibialis anticus* **b** : a deeply situated muscle that arises from the tibia and fibula, interosseous membrane, and intermuscular septa, that is inserted by a tendon passing under the medial malleolus into the navicular and first cuneiform bones, and that flexes the foot in the direction of the sole and tends to invert it — called also *tibialis posterior, tibialis posticus*

tibialis anterior *n* : TIBIALIS a

tibialis an·ti·cus \-an-'tī-kəs\ *n* : TIBIALIS a

tibialis pos·ti·cus \-pōs-'tī-kəs\ *n* : TIBIALIS b

tibial nerve *n* : the large nerve in the back of the leg that is a continuation of the sciatic nerve and terminates at the medial malleolus in the lateral and medial plantar nerves — called also *medial popliteal nerve*

tibial plateau *n* : the smooth bony surface of either the lateral condyle or the medial condyle of the tibia that articulates with the corresponding condylar surface of the femur

tibial vein *n* : any of several veins that accompany the corresponding tibial arteries and that unite to form the popliteal vein: **a** : one accompanying the posterior tibial artery — called also *posterior tibial vein* **b** : one accompanying the anterior tibial artery — called also *anterior tibial vein*

tibio- *comb form* : tibial and ⟨*tibiofemoral*⟩

tib·io·fem·o·ral \ˌti-bē-ō-'fe-mə-rəl\ *adj* : relating to or being the articulation occurring between the tibia and the femur ⟨the ~ joint⟩

tib·io·fib·u·lar \-'fi-byə-lər\ *adj* : of, relating to, or connecting the tibia and fibula ⟨the proximal ~ joint⟩

tib·io·tar·sal \-'tar-səl\ *adj* : of, relating to, or affecting the tibia and the tarsus

tic \'tik\ *n* **1** : local and habitual spasmodic motion of particular muscles esp. of the face : TWITCHING **2** : a habitual usu. unconscious quirk of behavior or speech

ti·car·cil·lin \ˌtī-kär-'si-lən\ *n* : a semisynthetic antibiotic used esp. in the form of its disodium salt $C_{15}H_{14}$-$N_2Na_2O_6S$

tic dou·lou·reux \'tik-ˌdü-lə-'rü, -'rœ\ *n* : TRIGEMINAL NEURALGIA

tick \'tik\ *n* **1** : any of a superfamily (Ixodoidea of the order Acarina) of bloodsucking arachnids that are larger than the closely related mites, attach themselves to warm-blooded vertebrates to feed, and include important vectors of various infectious diseases **2** : any of various usu. wing-

less parasitic dipteran flies (as the sheep ked)

tick–bite fever *n* : boutonneuse fever esp. as it occurs in South Africa

tick–borne *adj* : capable of being transmitted by the bites of ticks

tick–borne encephalitis *n* : any encephalitis transmitted by ticks; *specif* : a mild to fatal virus disease of humans of Europe and Asia that is characterized most often by meningitis or encephalitis or both or sometimes only by a mild fever and that is caused by the tick-borne encephalitis virus — abbr. *TBE*; see RUSSIAN SPRING-SUMMER ENCEPHALITIS

tick–borne encephalitis virus *n* : a virus of the genus *Flavivirus* (species *Tick-borne encephalitis virus*) that causes tick-borne encephalitis in Europe and Asia

tick–borne fever *n* : a usu. mild rickettsial disease of ruminant mammals (as sheep and cattle) esp. in Europe that is caused by a bacterium of the genus *Anaplasma* (*A. phagocytophilum* syn. *Ehrlichia phagocytophila*) which is transmitted by a tick of the genus *Ixodes* and that is marked by fever, listlessness, and anorexia

tick fever *n* **1** : TEXAS FEVER **2** : a febrile disease (as Rocky Mountain spotted fever or relapsing fever) transmitted by the bites of ticks

tick paralysis *n* : a progressive spinal paralysis that moves upward toward the brain and is caused by a neurotoxin secreted by some ticks (as *Dermacentor andersoni*)

tick typhus *n* : any of various tick=borne rickettsial spotted fevers (as Rocky Mountain spotted fever or boutonneuse fever)

ti·cryn·a·fen \tī-'kri-nə-ˌfen\ *n* : a diuretic, uricosuric, and antihypertensive agent $C_{13}H_8Cl_2O_4S$ withdrawn from use because of its link to hepatic disorders

tid *abbr* [Latin *ter in die*] three times a day — used in writing prescriptions

tid·al \'tīd-ᵊl\ *adj* : of, relating to, or constituting tidal air

tidal air *n* : the air that passes in and out of the lungs in an ordinary breath

tidal volume *n* : the volume of the tidal air

tide \'tīd\ *n* : a temporary increase or decrease in a specified substance or quality in the body or one of its systems ⟨an acid ~ during fasting⟩

tie off *vb* **tied off; ty·ing off** *or* **tie·ing off** : to close by means of an encircling or enveloping ligature ⟨*tie off* a bleeding vessel⟩

Tie·tze's syndrome \'tēt-səz-\ *n* : a condition of unknown origin that is characterized by inflammation of costochondral cartilage — called also *costochondritis, Tietze's syndrome*

Tietze, Alexander (1864–1927), German surgeon.

tiger mosquito *n* **1** : YELLOW-FEVER

MOSQUITO **2** : ASIAN TIGER MOSQUITO

tiger rattlesnake *n* : a rather small rattlesnake of the genus *Crotalus* (*C. tigris*) that occurs in mountainous deserts of western No. America

ti·groid substance \'tī-ˌgroid-\ *n* : NISSL BODIES

TIL \ˌtē-(ˌ)ī-'el\ *n* : TUMOR-INFILTRATING LYMPHOCYTE

timber rattlesnake *n* : a moderate-sized rattlesnake of the genus *Crotalus* (*C. horridus*) widely distributed through the eastern half of the U.S.

time \'tīm\ *n* : the measured or measurable period during which an action, process, or condition exists or continues — see BLEEDING TIME, COAGULATION TIME, PROTHROMBIN TIME, REACTION TIME

timed–release *or* **time–release** *adj* : consisting of or containing a drug that is released in small amounts over time (as by dissolution of a coating) usu. in the gastrointestinal tract ⟨∼ capsules⟩ — compare SUSTAINED-RELEASE

ti·mo·lol \'tī-mə-ˌlol\ *n* : a beta-blocker used esp. in the form of its maleate $C_{13}H_{24}N_4O_3S \cdot C_4H_4O_4$ to treat hypertension, to reduce the risk of reinfarction, and to lower intraocular pressure associated esp. with open-angle glaucoma — see TIMOPTIC

Ti·mop·tic \tə-'mäp-tik\ *trademark* — used for a preparation of the maleate of timolol

tin \'tin\ *n* : a soft white crystalline metallic element malleable at ordinary temperatures — symbol *Sn;* see ELEMENT table

Ti·nac·tin \ti-'nak-tən\ *trademark* — used for a preparation of tolnaftate

tinc·to·ri·al \tiŋk-'tōr-ē-əl\ *adj* : of or relating to dyeing or staining

tinc·tu·ra \tiŋk-'tur-ə, -'tyur-\ *n, pl* **-rae** \-rē\ : TINCTURE

tinc·ture \'tiŋk-chər\ *n* : a solution of a medicinal substance in an alcoholic menstruum — compare LIQUOR

tin·ea \'ti-nē-ə\ *n* : any of several fungal diseases of the skin; *esp* : RINGWORM

tinea ca·pi·tis \-'ka-pə-təs\ *n* : an infection of the scalp caused by fungi of the genera *Trichophyton* and *Microsporum* and characterized by scaly patches penetrated by a few dry brittle hairs

tinea cor·po·ris \-'kor-pə-rəs\ *n* : a fungal infection involving parts of the body not covered with hair — called also *body ringworm*

tinea cru·ris \-'krur-əs\ *n* : a fungal infection involving esp. the groin and perineum

tinea pe·dis \-'pe-dəs\ *n* : ATHLETE'S FOOT

tinea ver·si·col·or \-'vər-si-ˌkə-lər\ *n* : a chronic noninflammatory infection of the skin esp. of the trunk that is caused by a lipophilic fungus (*Pity-*

rosporum orbiculare syn. *Melassezia furfur*) and is marked by the formation of irregular macular patches — called also *pityriasis versicolor*

Ti·nel's sign \ti-'nelz-\ *n* : a tingling sensation felt in the distal portion of a limb upon percussion of the skin over a regenerating nerve in the limb

Tinel, Jules (1879–1952), French neurologist.

tine test \'tin-\ *n* : a tuberculin test in which the tuberculin is introduced intradermally by means of four tines on a stainless steel disk

tin·ni·tus \'ti-nə-təs, ti-'nī-təs\ *n* : a sensation of noise (as a ringing or roaring) that is caused by a bodily condition (as a disturbance of the auditory nerve or wax in the ear) and typically is of subjective form which can only be heard by the one affected

tis·sue \'ti-(ˌ)shü\ *n* : an aggregate of cells usu. of a particular kind together with their intercellular substance that form one of the structural materials of a plant or an animal and that in animals include connective tissue, epithelium, muscle tissue, and nerve tissue

tissue culture *n* : the process or technique of making body tissue grow in a culture medium outside the organism; *also* : a culture of tissue

tissue fluid *n* : a fluid that permeates the spaces between individual cells, is in osmotic contact with the blood and lymph, and serves in interstitial transport of nutrients and waste

tissue plasminogen activator *n* : a clot-dissolving enzyme that has an affinity for fibrin, that catalyzes the conversion of plasminogen to plasmin, that is produced naturally in blood vessel linings, and that is used in a genetically engineered form to prevent damage to heart muscle following a heart attack and to reduce neurological damage following ischemic stroke — abbr. *TPA*

tissue typing *n* : the determination of the degree of compatibility of tissues or organs from different individuals based on the similarity of histocompatibility antigens esp. on lymphocytes and used esp. as a measure of potential rejection in an organ transplant procedure

tis·su·lar \'ti-shyə-lər\ *adj* : of, relating to, or affecting organismic tissue

ti·ta·ni·um \tī-'tā-nē-əm, -'ta-\ *n* : a silvery gray metallic element — symbol *Ti;* see ELEMENT table

titanium dioxide *n* : an oxide TiO_2 of titanium that is used in sunblocks

ti·ter \'tī-tər\ *n* **1** : the strength of a solution or the concentration of a substance in solution as determined by titration **2** : the dilution of a serum containing a specific antibody at which the solution just retains a specific activity (as neutralizing an antigen) which it loses at any greater dilution — **ti·tered** \-tərd\ *adj*

ti·tra·tion \tī-'trā-shən\ n : a method or the process of determining the concentration of a dissolved substance in terms of the smallest amount of a reagent of known concentration required to bring about a given effect in reaction with a known volume of the test solution — **ti·trate** \'tī-,trāt\ vb

ti·tre chiefly Brit var of TITER

tit·u·ba·tion \,ti-chə-'bā-shən\ n : a staggering gait observed in some nervous disturbances

Tl symbol thallium

TLC abbr thin-layer chromatography

TLE abbr temporal lobe epilepsy

T lymphocyte \'tē-\ n : T CELL

Tm symbol thulium

TMD abbr temporomandibular disorder

TMJ abbr temporomandibular joint

TMJ syndrome \,tē-,em-'jā-\ n : TEMPOROMANDIBULAR JOINT SYNDROME

TNF abbr tumor necrosis factor

toad·stool \'tōd-,stül\ n : a fungus having an umbrella-shaped spore-bearing structure : MUSHROOM; esp : a poisonous or inedible one as distinguished from an edible mushroom

to·bac·co \tə-'ba-(,)kō\ n, pl **-cos** 1 : any of a genus (Nicotiana) of plants of the nightshade family (Solanaceae); esp : an annual So. American herb (N. tabacum) cultivated for its leaves 2 : the leaves of cultivated tobacco prepared for use in smoking or chewing or as snuff 3 : manufactured products of tobacco; also : the use of tobacco as a practice

to·bra·my·cin \,tō-brə-'mī-sᵊn\ n : a colorless water-soluble antibiotic $C_{18}H_{37}N_5O_9$ isolated from a soil bacterium of the genus Streptomyces (S. tenebrarius) and effective esp. against gram-negative bacteria

tocodynamometer var of TOKODYNAMOMETER

to·col·y·sis \tō-'kä-lə-səs\ n, pl **-y·ses** \-,sēz\ : inhibition of uterine contractions

¹**to·co·lyt·ic** \,tō-kə-'li-tik\ adj : inhibiting uterine contractions

²**tocolytic** n : a tocolytic drug

to·coph·er·ol \tō-'kä-fə-,rȯl, -,rōl\ n : any of several fat-soluble oily phenolic compounds with varying degrees of antioxidant vitamin E activity; esp : ALPHA-TOCOPHEROL

to·co·tri·en·ol \,tō-kō-'trī-ə-,nȯl, -nōl\ n : any of several compounds that are structurally similar to the tocopherols

Todd's paralysis \'tädz-\ n : temporary weakness or paralysis of one limb or one side of the body that occurs following a seizure

    Todd, Robert Bentley (1809–1860), British physician.

toe \'tō\ n : one of the terminal members of a foot

toed \'tōd\ adj : having a toe or toes esp. of a specified kind or number — usu. used in combination ⟨five-toed⟩

toe·nail \'tō-,nāl\ n : a nail of a toe

To·fra·nil \tō-'frā-nil\ trademark — used for a preparation of imipramine

to·ga·vi·rus \'tō-gə-,vī-rəs\ n : any of a family (Togaviridae) of single-stranded RNA viruses that have a spherical virion and include the causative agents of German measles and the three equine encephalitides — see ALPHAVIRUS

toi·let \'tȯi-lət\ n : cleansing in preparation for or in association with a medical or surgical procedure ⟨pulmonary ~⟩

toilet training n : the process of training a child to control bladder and bowel movements and to use the toilet — **toilet train** \-,trān\ vb

token economy n : a system of operant conditioning used for behavior modification that involves rewarding desirable behaviors with tokens which can be exchanged for items or privileges and punishing undesirable behaviors by taking away tokens

to·ko·dy·na·mom·e·ter or **to·co·dy·na·mom·e·ter** \,tō-kō-,dī-nə-'mä-mə-tər\ n : an instrument by means of which the force of uterine puerperal contractions can be measured

to·laz·amide \tō-'la-zə-,mīd\ n : a sulfonylurea $C_{14}H_{21}N_3O_3S$ used orally to lower blood sugar in the treatment of type 2 diabetes mellitus — see TOLINASE

to·laz·o·line \tō-'la-zə-,lēn\ n : a weak alpha-adrenergic blocking agent used in the form of its hydrochloride $C_{10}H_{12}N_2 \cdot HCl$ to produce peripheral vasodilation

tol·bu·ta·mide \täl-'byü-tə-,mīd\ n : a sulfonylurea $C_{12}H_{18}N_2O_3S$ used orally to lower blood sugar in the treatment of type 2 diabetes

Tol·ec·tin \'tä-lek-tin\ trademark — used for a preparation of the hydrated sodium salt of tolmetin

tol·er·ance \'tä-lə-rəns\ n 1 : the capacity of the body to endure or become less responsive to a substance (as a drug) or a physiological insult with repeated use or exposure ⟨developed a ~ to painkillers⟩ 2 : the immunological state marked by unresponsiveness to a specific antigen — **tol·er·ant** \-rənt\ adj — **tol·er·ate** \-,rāt\ vb

tol·er·a·tion \,tä-lə-'rā-shən\ n : TOLERANCE

tol·ero·gen \'tä-lə-rə-jən\ n : a tolerogenic antigen

tol·ero·gen·ic \,tä-lə-rə-'je-nik\ adj : capable of producing immunological tolerance ⟨~ antigens⟩

To·li·nase \'tō-lə-,nās, 'tä-lə-,nāz\ n : a preparation of tolazamide — formerly U.S. registered trademark

tol·met·in \'täl-mə-tən\ n : an anti-inflammatory drug administered esp. in the form of its hydrated sodium salt $C_{15}H_{14}NNaO_3 \cdot 2H_2O$ — see TOLECTIN

767

tolnaftate • tonometer

tol·naf·tate \\ˈtäl-ˈnaf-ˌtāt\\ *n* : a topical antifungal drug $C_{19}H_{17}NOS$ — see TINACTIN

tol·ter·o·dine \\ˈtäl-ˈter-ə-ˌdēn\\ *n* : an anticholinergic drug administered in the form of its tartrate $C_{22}H_{31}NO\cdot C_4H_6O_6$ to treat urge incontinence, frequent urination, and urinary urgency associated with an overactive bladder

to·lu \\tə-ˈlü, tō-\\ *n* : BALSAM OF TOLU

tolu balsam *n* : BALSAM OF TOLU

tol·u·ene·sul·fon·ic acid \\ˌtäl-yə-ˌwēn-səl-ˈfä-nik-\\ *n* : any of three isomeric crystalline oily liquid strong acids $CH_3C_6H_4SO_3H$

-tome \\ˌtōm\\ *n comb form* **1** : part : segment ⟨myo*tome*⟩ **2** : cutting instrument ⟨micro*tome*⟩

Tomes' fiber \\ˈtōmz-\\ *n* : any of the fibers extending from the odontoblasts into the alveolar canals : a dentinal fiber — called also *Tomes' process*

Tomes, Sir John (1815–1895), British dental surgeon.

Tom·my John surgery \\ˈtä-mē-ˈjän-\\ *n* : ULNAR COLLATERAL LIGAMENT RECONSTRUCTION

John, Thomas Edward (b 1943), American baseball player.

to·mo·gram \\ˈtō-mə-ˌgram\\ *n* : a radiograph made by tomography

to·mo·graph \\-ˌgraf\\ *n* : an X-ray machine used for tomography

to·mog·ra·phy \\tō-ˈmä-grə-fē\\ *n, pl* **-phies** : a method of producing a three-dimensional image of the internal structures of a solid object (as the human body) by the observation and recording of the differences in the effects on the passage of waves of energy impinging on those structures — see COMPUTED TOMOGRAPHY, POSITRON-EMISSION TOMOGRAPHY — **to·mo·graph·ic** \\ˌtō-mə-ˈgra-fik\\ *adj*

-t·o·my \\t-ə-mē\\ *n comb form,* pl **-t·o·mies** : incision : section ⟨laparo*tomy*⟩

¹tone \\ˈtōn\\ *n* **1** : a sound of definite pitch and vibration **2 a** : the state of a living body or of any of its organs or parts in which the functions are healthy and performed with due vigor **b** : normal tension or responsiveness to stimuli; *specif* : TONUS 2

²tone *vb* **toned; ton·ing** : to impart tone to

tone–deaf \\ˈtōn-ˌdef\\ *adj* : relatively insensitive to differences in musical pitch — **tone deafness** *n*

ton·er \\ˈtō-nər\\ *n* : one that tones; *esp* : a liquid cosmetic for cleansing the skin and contracting the pores

tongue \\ˈtəŋ\\ *n* : a process of the floor of the mouth that is attached basally to the hyoid bone, that consists essentially of a mass of extrinsic muscle attaching its base to other parts, intrinsic muscle by which parts of the structure move in relation to each other, and an epithelial covering rich in sensory end organs and small

glands, and that functions esp. in taking and swallowing food and as a speech organ

tongue depressor *n* : a thin wooden blade rounded at both ends that is used to depress the tongue to allow for inspection of the mouth and throat — called also *tongue blade*

tongue roll·er \\-ˌrō-lər\\ *n* : a person who carries a dominant gene which confers the capacity to roll the tongue into the shape of a U

tongue thrust \\-ˌthrəst\\ *n* : the thrusting of the tongue against or between the incisors during the act of swallowing which if persistent in early childhood can lead to various dental abnormalities

tongue–tie *n* : a congenital defect characterized by limited mobility of the tongue due to shortness of its frenulum — **tongue–tied** *adj*

tongue worm *n* : any of a phylum or arthropod class (Pentastomida) of parasitic invertebrates that live as adults in the respiratory passages of reptiles, birds, or mammals — see HALZOUN

-to·nia \\ˈtō-nē-ə\\ *n comb form* : condition or degree of tonus ⟨myo*tonia*⟩

¹ton·ic \\ˈtä-nik\\ *adj* **1 a** : characterized by tonus ⟨∼ contraction of muscle⟩; *also* : marked by or being prolonged muscular contraction ⟨∼ convulsions⟩ **b** : producing or adapted to produce healthy muscular condition and reaction of organs (as muscles) **2 a** : increasing or restoring physical or mental tone **b** : yielding a tonic substance — **ton·i·cal·ly** *adv*

²tonic *n* : an agent (as a drug) that increases body tone

tonic–clonic *adj* : relating to, marked by, or being a generalized seizure that is initially tonic and then becomes clonic and is characterized by the abrupt loss of consciousness ⟨∼ epilepsy⟩

to·nic·i·ty \\tō-ˈni-sə-tē\\ *n, pl* **-ties 1** : the property of possessing tone; *esp* : healthy vigor of body or mind **2** : TONUS 2

ton·i·co·clon·ic \\ˌtä-ni-kō-ˈklä-nik\\ *adj* : TONIC-CLONIC

tono- *comb form* **1** : tone ⟨*tono*topic⟩ **2** : pressure ⟨*tono*meter⟩

tono–clon·ic \\ˌtä-nō-ˈklä-nik\\ *adj* : TONIC-CLONIC

tono·fi·bril \\-ˈfī-brəl, -ˈfi-\\ *n* : a thin fibril made up of tonofilaments

tono·fil·a·ment \\-ˈfi-lə-mənt\\ *n* : a slender cytoplasmic organelle found esp. in some epithelial cells

to·nog·ra·phy \\tō-ˈnä-grə-fē\\ *n, pl* **-phies** : the procedure of recording measurements (as of intraocular pressure) with a tonometer — **to·no·graph·ic** \\ˌtō-nə-ˈgra-fik, ˌtä-\\ *adj*

to·nom·e·ter \\tō-ˈnä-mə-tər\\ *n* : an instrument for measuring tension or pressure and esp. intraocular pressure

— to·no·met·ric \ˌtō-nə-ˈme-trik, ˌtä-\ adj — to·nom·e·try \tō-ˈnä-mə-trē\ n

to·no·top·ic \ˌtō-nə-ˈtä-pik\ adj : relating to or being the anatomic organization by which specific sound frequencies are received by specific receptors in the inner ear with nerve impulses traveling along selected pathways to specific sites in the brain

ton·sil \ˈtän-səl\ n 1 a : either of a pair of prominent masses of lymphoid tissue that lie one on each side of the throat between the anterior and posterior pillars of the fauces and are composed of lymph follicles grouped around one or more deep crypts — called also *palatine tonsil* b : PHARYNGEAL TONSIL c : LINGUAL TONSIL 2 : a rounded prominence situated medially on the lower surface of each lateral hemisphere of the cerebellum — ton·sil·lar \ˈtän-sə-lar\ adj

tonsill- or tonsillo- comb form : tonsil ⟨*tonsill*ectomy⟩

tonsillar crypt n : any of the deep invaginations occurring on the surface of the palatine and pharyngeal tonsils

ton·sil·lec·to·my \ˌtän-sə-ˈlek-tə-mē\ n, pl -mies : surgical excision of the tonsils

ton·sil·li·tis \ˌtän-sə-ˈlī-təs\ n : inflammation of the tonsils and esp. the palatine tonsils typically due to viral or bacterial infection and marked by red enlarged tonsils usu. with sore throat, fever, difficult swallowing, hoarseness or loss of voice, and tender or swollen lymph nodes

ton·sil·lo·phar·yn·geal \ˌtän-sə-lō-ˌfar-ən-ˈjē-əl; -fə-ˈrin-jəl, -jē-əl\ adj : of, relating to, or involving the tonsils and pharynx ⟨the ~ area⟩

ton·sil·lo·phar·yn·gi·tis \-ˌfar-ən-ˈjī-təs\ n, pl -git·i·des \-ˈji-tə-ˌdēz\ : inflammation of the tonsils and pharynx

to·nus \ˈtō-nəs\ n 1 : TONE 2a 2 : a state of partial contraction that is characteristic of normal muscle, is maintained at least in part by a continuous bombardment of motor impulses originating reflexly, and serves to maintain body posture — called also *muscle tone;* compare CLONUS

-to·ny \ˌtō-nē, tⁿn-ē\ n comb form, pl -to·nies -TONIA ⟨hypo*tony*⟩

tooth \ˈtüth\ n, pl teeth \ˈtēth\ : any of the hard bony appendages that are borne on the jaws and serve esp. for the prehension and mastication of food — see MILK TOOTH, PERMANENT TOOTH

tooth·ache \ˈtüth-ˌāk\ n : pain in or about a tooth — called also *odontalgia*

tooth·brush \-ˌbrəsh\ n : a brush for cleaning the teeth — tooth·brush·ing n

tooth bud n : a mass of tissue having the potentiality of differentiating into a tooth

tooth germ n : TOOTH BUD

tooth·less \ˈtüth-ləs\ adj : having no teeth

tooth·paste \ˈtüth-ˌpāst\ n : a paste for cleaning the teeth

tooth·pick \-ˌpik\ n : a pointed instrument (as a slender tapering piece of wood) used for removing food particles lodged between the teeth

top- or topo- comb form : local ⟨*topec*tomy⟩ ⟨*topo*gnosia⟩

to·pec·to·my \tə-ˈpek-tə-mē\ n, pl -mies : surgical excision of selected portions of the frontal cortex of the brain esp. for the relief of medically intractable epilepsy

to·pha·ceous \tə-ˈfā-shəs\ adj : relating to, being, or characterized by the occurrence of tophi ⟨~ gout⟩

to·phus \ˈtō-fəs\ n, pl to·phi \ˈtō-ˌfī, -ˌfē\ : a deposit of urates in tissues (as cartilage) characteristic of gout

top·i·cal \ˈtä-pi-kəl\ adj : designed for or involving application to or action on the surface of a part of the body ⟨applied a ~ anesthetic to numb the skin⟩ — top·i·cal·ly adv

top·og·no·sia \ˌtä-ˌpäg-ˈnō-zhə, ˌtō-, -zhē-ə\ n : recognition of the location of a stimulus on the skin or elsewhere in the body

topo·graph·i·cal \ˌtä-pə-ˈgra-fi-kəl\ or topo·graph·ic \-fik\ adj 1 : of, relating to, or concerned with topography 2 : of or relating to a mind made up of different strata and esp. of the conscious, preconscious, and unconscious — topo·graph·i·cal·ly adv

topographic anatomy n : REGIONAL ANATOMY

to·pog·ra·phy \tə-ˈpä-grə-fē\ n, pl -phies 1 : the physical or natural features of an object or entity and their structural relationships ⟨the ~ of the abdomen⟩ 2 : REGIONAL ANATOMY

topo·isom·er·ase \ˌtō-pō-ī-ˈsä-mə-ˌrās\ n : any of a class of enzymes that reduce supercoiling in DNA by breaking and rejoining one or both strands of the DNA molecule

Top·rol \ˈtäp-ˌról\ trademark — used for a preparation of the succinate of metoprolol

TORCH \ˈtórch\ n [*toxoplasma, rubella virus, cytomegalovirus, herpes simplex virus*] : a group of pathological agents that cause similar symptoms in newborns and that include esp. a toxoplasma (*Toxoplasma gonii*), cytomegalovirus, herpes simplex virus, and the togavirus causing German measles

TORCH infection n : a group of symptoms esp. of newborn infants that include hepatosplenomegaly, jaundice, and thrombocytopenia, and are caused by infection with one or more of the TORCH agents — called also *TORCH syndrome*

tori pl of TORUS

to·ric \ˈtōr-ik\ adj : of, relating to, or shaped like a torus or segment of a torus; *specif* : being a simple lens having for one of its surfaces a segment of an equilateral zone of a torus and consequently having different refracting power in different meridians

tor·pid \'tór-pəd\ *adj* : sluggish in functioning or acting : characterized by torpor — **tor·pid·i·ty** \tór-'pi-də-tē\ *n*

tor·por \'tór-pər\ *n* : a state of mental and motor inactivity with partial or total insensibility : extreme sluggishness or stagnation of function

¹**torque** \'tórk\ *n* : a force that produces or tends to produce rotation or torsion; *also* : a measure of the effectiveness of such a force

²**torque** *vb* **torqued; torqu·ing** : to impart torque to : cause to twist

torr \'tór\ *n, pl* **torr** : a unit of pressure equal to ¹/₇₆₀ of an atmosphere or about 0.019 pounds per square inch

tor·sades de pointes \tór-ˌsäd(z)-də-'pwant\ *or* **tor·sade de pointes** \-ˌsäd-\ *n* : ventricular tachycardia that is characterized by fluctuation of the QRS complexes around the electrocardiographic baseline and is typically caused by a long QT interval

tor·sion \'tór-shən\ *n* **1** : the twisting of a bodily organ or part on its own axis ⟨intestinal ∼⟩ **2** : the twisting or wrenching of a body by the exertion of forces tending to turn one end or part about a longitudinal axis while the other is held fast or turned in the opposite direction; *also* : the state of being twisted — **tor·sion·al** \'tór-shə-nəl\ *adj*

torsion dystonia *n* : DYSTONIA MUSCULORUM DEFORMANS

tor·so \'tór-(ˌ)sō\ *n, pl* **torsos** *or* **tor·si** \'tór-ˌsē\ : the human trunk

tort·ed \'tór-təd\ *adj, chiefly Brit* : marked by torsion

tor·ti·col·lis \ˌtór-tə-'kä-ləs\ *n* : a twisting of the neck to one side that results in abnormal carriage of the head and is usu. caused by muscle spasms — called also *wryneck*

tor·tu·ous \'tór-chə-wəs\ *adj* : marked by repeated twists, bends, or turns ⟨a ∼ blood vessel⟩ — **tor·tu·os·i·ty** \ˌtór-chə-'wä-sə-tē\ *n*

tor·u·la \'tór-yə-lə, 'tär-\ *n* **1** *pl* **-lae** \-ˌlē, -ˌlī\ *also* **-las** : CRYPTOCOCCOSIS **2** *cap* : a genus of yeasts including pathogens (as *T. histolytica* syn. *Cryptococcus neoformans* that causes cryptococcosis) usu. placed in the genus *Cryptococcus*

Tor·u·lop·sis \ˌtór-yə-'läp-səs, ˌtär-\ *n* : a genus of round, oval, or cylindrical yeasts that include forms which in other classifications are placed either in the genus *Torula* or *Cryptococcus*

tor·u·lo·sis \ˌtór-yə-'lō-səs, ˌtär-\ *n* : CRYPTOCOCCOSIS

to·rus \'tór-əs\ *n, pl* **to·ri** \'tór-ˌī, -ˌē\ : a smooth rounded anatomical protuberance (as a bony ridge on the skull)

torus tu·ba·ri·us \-ˌtü-'ber-ē-əs, -tyü-\ *n* : a protrusion on the lateral wall of the nasopharynx marking the pharyngeal end of the cartilaginous part of the eustachian tube

torus ure·ter·i·cus \-ˌyúr-ə-'ter-i-kəs\ *n* : a band of smooth muscle joining the orifices of the ureter and forming the base of the trigone of the bladder

tos·yl·ate \'tä-sə-ˌlāt\ *n* : an ester of the para isomer of toluenesulfonic acid

total hysterectomy *n* : PANHYSTERECTOMY

total mastectomy *n* : a mastectomy in which the breast tissue, associated skin, nipple, and areola are removed — called also *simple mastectomy*

to·ti·po·ten·cy \ˌtō-tə-'pōt-ᵊn-sē\ *n, pl* **-cies** : ability of a cell or bodily part to generate or regenerate the whole organism

to·ti·po·tent \tō-'ti-pə-tənt\ *adj* : capable of developing into a complete organism or differentiating into any of its cells or tissues ⟨∼ blastomeres⟩

touch \'təch\ *n* **1** : the special sense by which pressure or traction exerted on the skin or mucous membrane is perceived **2** : a light attack ⟨a ∼ of fever⟩

Tou·rette's syndrome \tùr-'ets-\ *or* **Tou·rette syndrome** \-'et-\ *n* : a familial neurological disorder of variable expression that is characterized by recurrent involuntary tics involving body movements (as eye blinks or grimaces) and vocalizations (as grunts or utterance of inappropriate words), often has one or more associated conditions (as obsessive-compulsive disorder), is more common in males than females, and usu. has an onset in childhood and often stabilizes or ameliorates in adulthood — abbr. *TS;* called also *Gilles de la Tourette syndrome, Tourette's disease, Tourette's disorder*

Gilles de la Tourette \'zhēl-də-lä-'tür-et\, **Georges** (1857–1904), French physician.

tour·ni·quet \'tùr-ni-kət, 'tər-\ *n* : a device (as a bandage twisted tight with a stick) to check bleeding or blood flow

tower head *n* : OXYCEPHALY

tower skull *n* : OXYCEPHALY

tox- *or* **toxi-** *or* **toxo-** *comb form* **1** : toxic : poisonous ⟨*tox*in⟩ **2** : toxin : poison ⟨*toxi*genic⟩

tox·ae·mia *chiefly Brit var of* TOXEMIA

Tox·as·ca·ris \täk-'sas-kə-rəs\ *n* : a genus of ascarid roundworms that infest the small intestine of the dog and cat and related wild animals

tox·e·mia \täk-'sē-mē-ə\ *n* : an abnormal condition associated with the presence of toxic substances in the blood: as **a** : a generalized intoxication due to absorption and systemic dissemination of bacterial toxins from a focus of infection **b** : intoxication due to dissemination of toxic substances (as some by-products of protein metabolism) that cause functional or organic disturbances (as in the kidneys) — **tox·e·mic** \-ˈmik\ *adj*

toxemia of pregnancy *n* : a disorder of unknown cause that is peculiar to pregnancy, is usu. of sudden onset, is marked by hypertension, albuminuria, edema, headache, and visual disturbances, and may or may not be accompanied by convulsions

toxi- — see TOX-

¹**tox·ic** \ˈtäk-sik\ *adj* **1** : of, relating to, or caused by a poison or toxin **2 a** : affected by a poison or toxin **b** : affected with toxemia of pregnancy **3** : POISONOUS ⟨~ drugs⟩ — **tox·ic·i·ty** \täk-ˈsis-ə-tē\ *n*

²**toxic** *n* : a toxic substance

toxic- or **toxico-** *comb form* : poison ⟨toxicology⟩ ⟨toxicosis⟩

toxic epidermal necrolysis *n* : a skin disorder characterized by widespread erythema and the formation of flaccid bullae and later by skin that is scalded in appearance and separates from the body in large sheets — called also *epidermal necrolysis, Lyell's syndrome, scalded-skin syndrome;* compare STAPHYLOCOCCAL SCALDED SKIN SYNDROME

Tox·i·co·den·dron \ˌtäk-si-kō-ˈden-ˌdrän\ *n* : a genus of shrubs and trees of the cashew family (Anacardiaceae) that was split off from the genus *Rhus* and includes some plants (as poison ivy, poison oak, and poison sumac) producing irritating oils that cause dermatitis

tox·i·co·gen·ic \ˌtäk-si-kō-ˈje-nik\ *adj* : producing toxins or poisons

tox·i·co·log·i·cal \ˌtäk-si-kə-ˈlä-ji-kəl\ or **tox·i·co·log·ic** \-ˈjik\ *adj* : of or relating to toxicology or toxins — **tox·i·co·log·i·cal·ly** *adv*

tox·i·col·o·gy \ˌtäk-si-ˈkä-lə-jē\ *n, pl* **-gies** : a science that deals with poisons and their effect and with the problems involved (as clinical, industrial, or legal) — **tox·i·col·o·gist** *n*

tox·i·co·sis \ˌtäk-sə-ˈkō-səs\ *n, pl* **-co·ses** \-ˌsēz\ : a pathological condition caused by the action of a poison or toxin

toxic shock *n* : TOXIC SHOCK SYNDROME

toxic shock syndrome *n* : an acute and sometimes fatal disease that is characterized by fever, nausea, diarrhea, diffuse erythema, and shock, is associated esp. with the presence of a bacterium of the genus *Staphylococcus* (*S. aureus*), and occurs esp. in menstruating females using tampons — called also *toxic shock*

toxi·gen·ic \ˌtäk-sə-ˈje-nik\ *adj* : producing toxin ⟨~ bacteria⟩ — **toxi·ge·nic·i·ty** \ˌtäk-si-jə-ˈni-sə-tē\ *n*

tox·in \ˈtäk-sən\ *n* : a poisonous substance that is a specific product of the metabolic activities of a living organism and is usu. very unstable, notably toxic when introduced into the tissues, and typically capable of inducing antibody formation

toxin–antitoxin *n* : a mixture of toxin and antitoxin used esp. formerly in immunizing against a disease (as diphtheria) for which they are specific

toxo- — see TOX-

Tox·o·ca·ra \ˌtäk-sə-ˈkar-ə\ *n* : a genus of nematode worms including the common ascarids (*T. canis* and *T. cati*) of the dog and cat

tox·o·ca·ri·a·sis \ˌtäk-sə-kə-ˈrī-ə-səs\ *n, pl* **-a·ses** \-ˌsēz\ : infection with or disease caused by nematode worms of the genus *Toxocara*

tox·oid \ˈtäk-ˌsȯid\ *n* : a toxin of a pathogenic organism treated so as to destroy its toxicity but leave it capable of inducing the formation of antibodies on injection ⟨diphtheria ~⟩ — called also *anatoxin*

toxo·plas·ma \ˌtäk-sə-ˈplaz-mə\ *n* **1** *cap* : a genus of sporozoans that are typically serious pathogens of vertebrates **2** *pl* **-mas** or **-ma·ta** \-mə-tə\ *also* **-ma** : any sporozoan of the genus *Toxoplasma* — **toxo·plas·mic** \-mik\ *adj*

toxo·plas·mo·sis \-ˌplaz-ˈmō-səs\ *n, pl* **-mo·ses** \-ˌsēz\ : infection with or disease caused by a sporozoan of the genus *Toxoplasma* (*T. gondii*) that invades the tissues and may seriously damage the central nervous system esp. of infants

tPA *abbr* tissue plasminogen activator

TPI *abbr* Treponema pallidum immobilization (test)

TPN \ˌtē-(ˌ)pē-ˈen\ *n* : NADP

TPN *abbr* total parenteral nutrition

TPR *abbr* temperature, pulse, respiration

tra·bec·u·la \trə-ˈbe-kyə-lə\ *n, pl* **-lae** \-ˌlē\ *also* **-las** **1** : a small bar, rod, bundle of fibers, or septal membrane in the framework of a bodily organ or part (as the spleen) **2** : any of the intersecting osseous bars occurring in cancellous bone — **tra·bec·u·lar** \-lar\ *adj* — **tra·bec·u·la·tion** \trə-ˌbe-kyə-ˈlā-shən\ *n*

trabecular meshwork *n* : trabecular tissue that separates the angle of the anterior chamber from the canal of Schlemm and that contains spaces through which aqueous humor normally drains from the anterior chamber into the canal of Schlemm

tra·bec·u·lec·to·my \trə-ˌbe-kyə-ˈlek-tə-mē\ *n, pl* **-mies** : surgical excision of a small portion of the trabecular meshwork in order to facilitate drainage of aqueous humor for the relief of glaucoma

tra·bec·u·lo·plas·ty \trə-ˈbe-kyə-lō-ˌplas-tē\ *n, pl* **-ties** : plastic surgery of a trabecula; *specif* : laser surgery to create small openings in the trabecular meshwork of the eye from which the aqueous humor can drain to reduce intraocular pressure caused by open-angle glaucoma

trace \'trās\ *n* **1** : the marking made by a recording instrument (as a kymograph) **2** : an amount of a chemical constituent not always quantitatively determinable because of minuteness **3** : ENGRAM — **trace** *vb* — **trace·able** \'trā-sə-bəl\ *adj*

trace element *n* : a chemical element present in minute quantities; *esp* : one used by organisms and held essential to their physiology — compare MICRONUTRIENT 2

trac·er \'trā-sər\ *n* : a substance used to trace the course of a process; *specif* : a labeled element or atom that can be traced throughout chemical or biological processes by its radioactivity or its unusual isotopic mass

trache- *or* **tracheo-** *comb form* **1** : trachea ⟨*tracheo*scopy⟩ **2** : tracheal and ⟨*tracheo*bronchial⟩

tra·chea \'trā-kē-ə\ *n, pl* **tra·che·ae** \-kē-ͺē\ *also* **tra·che·as** : the main trunk of the system of tubes by which air passes to and from the lungs that is about four inches (10 centimeters) long and somewhat less than an inch (2.5 centimeters) in diameter, extends down the front of the neck from the larynx, divides in two to form the bronchi, has walls of fibrous and muscular tissue stiffened by incomplete cartilaginous rings which keep it from collapsing, and is lined with mucous membrane whose epithelium is composed of columnar ciliated mucus=secreting cells — called also *windpipe* — **tra·che·al** \-əl\ *adj*

tracheal node *n* : any of a group of lymph nodes arranged along each side of the thoracic part of the trachea

tracheal ring *n* : any of the 16 to 20 C=shaped bands of highly elastic cartilage which are found as incomplete rings in the anterior two-thirds of the tracheal wall and of which there are usu. 6 to 8 in the right bronchus and 9 to 12 in the left

tra·che·itis \ͺtrā-kē-'ī-təs\ *n* : inflammation of the trachea

trachel- *or* **trachelo-** *comb form* **1** : neck ⟨*trachelo*mastoid muscle⟩ **2** : uterine cervix ⟨*trachelo*plasty⟩

trach·e·lec·to·my \ͺtra-kə-'lek-tə-mē\ *n, pl* **-mies** : CERVICECTOMY

trach·e·lo·mas·toid muscle \ͺtra-kə-lō-'mas-ͺtȯid-\ *n* : LONGISSIMUS CAPITIS

trach·e·lo·plas·ty \'tra-kə-lō-ͺplas-tē\ *n, pl* **-ties** : a plastic operation on the neck of the uterus

trach·e·lor·rha·phy \ͺtra-kə-'lȯr-ə-fē\ *n, pl* **-phies** : the operation of sewing up a laceration of the uterine cervix

tra·cheo·bron·chi·al \ͺtrā-kē-ō-'brän-kē-əl\ *adj* : of, relating to, affecting, or produced in the trachea and bronchi ⟨~ secretion⟩ ⟨~ lesions⟩

tracheobronchial node *n* : any of the lymph nodes arranged in four or five groups along the trachea and bronchi

— called also *tracheobronchial lymph node*

tracheobronchial tree *n* : the trachea and bronchial tree considered together

tra·cheo·bron·chi·tis \ͺtrā-kē-ō-brän-'kī-təs\ *n, pl* **-chit·i·des** \-'ki-tə-ͺdēz\ : inflammation of the trachea and bronchi

tra·cheo·esoph·a·ge·al \-i-ͺsä-fə-'jē-əl\ *adj* : relating to or connecting the trachea and the esophagus ⟨a ~ fistula⟩

tra·cheo·plas·ty \'trā-kē-ə-ͺplas-tē\ *n, pl* **-ties** : plastic surgery on the trachea

tra·che·os·co·py \ͺtrā-kē-'äs-kə-pē\ *n, pl* **-pies** : inspection of the interior of the trachea (as by a bronchoscope)

tra·cheo·sto·ma \ͺtrā-kē-'äs-tə-mə\ *n* : an opening into the trachea created by tracheostomy

tra·che·os·to·my \ͺtrā-kē-'äs-tə-mē\ *n, pl* **-mies** : the surgical formation of an opening into the trachea through the neck esp. to allow the passage of air; *also* : the opening itself

tra·che·ot·o·my \ͺtrā-kē-'ä-tə-mē\ *n, pl* **-mies** **1** : the surgical operation of cutting into the trachea esp. through the skin **2** : the opening created by a tracheotomy

tra·cho·ma \trə-'kō-mə\ *n* : a chronic contagious conjunctivitis marked by inflammatory granulations on the conjunctival surfaces, caused by a bacterium of the genus *Chlamydia* (*C. trachomatis*), and commonly resulting in blindness if left untreated — **tra·cho·ma·tous** \trə-'kō-mə-təs, -'kä-\ *adj*

trac·ing \'trā-siŋ\ *n* : a graphic record made by an instrument (as an electrocardiograph) that registers some movement

tract \'trakt\ *n* **1** : a system of body parts or organs that act together to perform some function ⟨the digestive ~⟩ — see GASTROINTESTINAL TRACT, LOWER RESPIRATORY TRACT, UPPER RESPIRATORY TRACT **2** : a bundle of nerve fibers having a common origin, termination, and function and esp. one within the spinal cord or brain — called also *fiber tract*; see CORTICOSPINAL TRACT, OLFACTORY TRACT, OPTIC TRACT, SPINOTHALAMIC TRACT; compare FASCICULUS b

trac·tion \'trak-shən\ *n* **1** : the pulling of or tension established in one body part by another **2** : a pulling force exerted on a skeletal structure (as in a fracture) by means of a special device or apparatus ⟨a ~ splint⟩; *also* : a state of tension created by such a pulling force ⟨a leg in ~⟩

tract of Burdach *n* : FASCICULUS CUNEATUS

K. F. Burdach — see COLUMN OF BURDACH

tract of Lissauer *n* : DORSOLATERAL TRACT

Lissauer, Heinrich (1861—1891), German neurologist.

trac·tot·o·my \trak-ˈtä-tə-mē\ *n, pl* **-mies** : surgical division of a nerve tract

trac·tus \ˈtrak-təs\ *n, pl* **tractus** : TRACT 2

tractus sol·i·ta·ri·us \-ˌsä-li-ˈtar-ē-əs\ *n* : a descending tract of nerve fibers that is situated near the dorsal surface of the medulla oblongata, mediates esp. the sense of taste, and includes fibers from the facial, glossopharyngeal, and vagus nerves

trade·mark \ˈtrād-ˌmärk\ *n* : a device (as a word or mark) that points distinctly to the origin or ownership of merchandise to which it is applied and that is legally reserved for the exclusive use of the owner — compare SERVICE MARK

trag·a·canth \ˈtra-jə-ˌkanth, -gə-, -kənth; ˈtra-gə-ˌsanth\ *n* : a gum obtained from various Asian or East European plants (genus *Astragalus* and esp. *A. gummifer*) of the legume family (Leguminosae) and is used as an emulsifying, suspending, and thickening agent and as a demulcent — called also *gum tragacanth*

tra·gus \ˈtrā-gəs\ *n, pl* **tra·gi** \-ˌgī, -ˌjī\ : a small projection in front of the external opening of the ear

train·able \ˈtrā-nə-bəl\ *adj* : affected with moderate mental retardation and capable of being trained in self-care and in simple social and work skills in a sheltered environment — compare EDUCABLE

trained nurse *n* : GRADUATE NURSE

trait \ˈtrāt\ *n* : an inherited characteristic

tram·a·dol \ˈtra-mə-ˌdȯl\ *n* : a synthetic opioid analgesic administered orally in the form of its hydrochloride $C_{16}H_{25}NO_2 \cdot HCl$ to treat moderate to severe pain — see ULTRAM

trance \ˈtrans\ *n* **1** : a sleeplike altered state of consciousness (as of deep hypnosis) usu. characterized by partly suspended animation with diminished or absent sensory and motor activity and subsequent lack of recall **2** : a state of profound abstraction or absorption

tran·ex·am·ic acid \ˌtra-nek-ˈsa-mik-\ *n* : an antifibrinolytic drug $C_8H_{15}NO_2$

tran·quil·ize *also* **tran·quil·lize** \ˈtraŋ-kwə-ˌlīz, ˈtran-\ *vb* **-ized** *also* **-lized**; **-iz·ing** *also* **-liz·ing** : to relieve of mental tension and anxiety by means of drugs — **tran·quil·i·za·tion** \ˌtraŋ-kwə-lə-ˈzā-shən, ˌtran-\ *n*

tran·quil·iz·er *also* **tran·quil·liz·er** \-ˌlī-zər\ *n* : a drug used to reduce mental disturbance (as anxiety and tension) — see ANTIPSYCHOTIC

trans \ˈtrans, ˈtranz\ *n* : characterized by or having certain groups of atoms on opposite sides of the longitudinal axis of a double bond or of the plane of a ring in a molecule

trans·ab·dom·i·nal \ˌtrans-ab-ˈdä-mə-nəl, ˌtranz-\ *adj* : passing through or performed by passing through the abdomen or the abdominal wall ⟨~ amniocentesis⟩

trans·ac·tion·al analysis \-ˈak-shə-nəl-\ *n* : a system of psychotherapy involving analysis of individual episodes of social interaction for insight that will aid communication — abbr. *TA*

trans·am·i·nase \-ˈa-mə-ˌnās, -ˌnāz\ *n* : an enzyme promoting transamination

trans·am·i·na·tion \-ˌa-mə-ˈnā-shən\ *n* : a reversible oxidation-reduction reaction in which an amino group is transferred typically from an alpha-amino acid to an alpha-keto acid

trans·bron·chi·al \-ˈbräŋ-kē-əl\ *adj* : occurring or performed by way of a bronchus; *specif* : involving the passage of a bronchoscope through the lumen of a bronchus

trans·cap·il·lary \-ˈka-pə-ˌler-ē\ *adj* : existing or taking place across the capillary walls

trans·cath·e·ter \-ˈka-thə-tər\ *adj* : performed through the lumen of a catheter ⟨~ embolization⟩

trans·cer·vi·cal \-ˈsər-vi-kəl\ *adj* : performed by way of the uterine cervix

trans·con·dy·lar \-ˈkän-də-lər\ *adj* : passing through a pair of condyles ⟨a ~ fracture of the humerus⟩

trans·cor·ti·cal \-ˈkȯr-ti-kəl\ *adj* : crossing the cortex of the brain; *esp* : passing from the cortex of one hemisphere to that of the other

trans·cor·tin \-ˈkȯrt-ᵊn\ *n* : an alpha globulin produced in the liver that binds with and transports cortisol in the blood

trans·cra·ni·al \-ˈkrā-nē-əl\ *adj* : passing or performed through the skull ⟨~ Doppler ultrasound⟩

tran·scribe \trans-ˈkrīb\ *vb* **tran·scribed; tran·scrib·ing** : to cause (as DNA) to undergo genetic transcription

tran·script \ˈtrans-ˌkript\ *n* : a sequence of RNA produced by transcription from a DNA template

tran·scrip·tase \tran-ˈskrip-ˌtās, -ˌtāz\ *n* : RNA POLYMERASE; *also* : REVERSE TRANSCRIPTASE

tran·scrip·tion \trans-ˈkrip-shən\ *n* : the process of constructing a messenger RNA molecule using a DNA molecule as a template with resulting transfer of genetic information to the messenger RNA — compare REVERSE TRANSCRIPTION, TRANSLATION — **tran·scrip·tion·al** \-shə-nəl\ *adj* — **tran·scrip·tion·al·ly** *adv*

transcription factor *n* : any of various proteins that bind to DNA and play a role in the regulation of gene expression by promoting transcription

tran·scrip·tion·ist \-shə-nist\ *n* : one that transcribes; *esp* : MEDICAL TRANSCRIPTIONIST

trans·cu·ta·ne·ous \ˌtrans-kyü-ˈtā-nē-əs\ *adj* : passing, entering, or made by penetration through the skin

transcutaneous electrical nerve stimulation *n* : electrical stimulation of the skin to relieve pain by interfering with the neural transmission of signals from underlying pain receptors — abbr. *TENS;* called also *transcutaneous nerve stimulation* — **transcutaneous electrical nerve stimulator** *n*

trans·der·mal \ˌtrans-ˈdər-məl, ˌtranz-\ *adj* : relating to, being, or supplying a medication in a form for absorption through the skin into the bloodstream ⟨∼ drug delivery⟩ ⟨a ∼ nicotine patch⟩ ⟨∼ nitroglycerin⟩ — **trans·der·mal·ly** *adv*

trans·dia·phrag·mat·ic \ˌdī-ə-frag-ˈma-tik, -ˌfrag-\ *adj* : occurring, passing, or performed through the diaphragm ⟨∼ hernia⟩

trans·duce \ˈdüs, -ˈdyüs\ *vb* **trans·duced; trans·duc·ing 1** : to convert (as energy) into another form **2** : to cause (genetic material) to undergo transduction; *also* : to introduce genetic material into (a cell) by transduction

trans·duc·tion \-ˈdek-shən\ *n* : the action or process of transducing; *esp* : the transfer of genetic material from one organism (as a bacterium) to another by a genetic vector and esp. a bacteriophage — compare TRANSFORMATION 2 — **trans·duc·tion·al** \-shə-nəl\ *adj*

trans·duo·de·nal \ˌdü-ə-ˈdē-nəl, -ˌdyü-; -dü-ˈäd-ᵊn-əl, -dyü-\ *adj* : performed by cutting across or through the duodenum

tran·sect \tran-ˈsekt\ *vb* : to cut transversely — **tran·sec·tion** \-ˈsek-shən\ *n*

trans·epi·the·li·al \ˌtrans-ˌe-pə-ˈthē-lē-əl, ˌtranz-\ *adj* : existing or taking place across an epithelium

transeptal *var of* TRANSSEPTAL

trans·esoph·a·ge·al \-i-ˌsä-fə-ˈjē-əl\ *adj* : passing through or performed by way of the esophagus ⟨∼ echocardiography⟩

transexual *var of* TRANSSEXUAL

trans fat *n* : a fat containing trans-fatty acids

trans–fat·ty acid \ˈtrans-ˈfa-tē, ˈtranz-\ *n* : an unsaturated fatty acid characterized by a trans arrangement of alkyl chains that is formed esp. during the hydrogenation of vegetable oils and has been linked to an increase in blood cholesterol

trans·fec·tant \trans-ˈfek-tənt\ *n* : a cell that has incorporated foreign nucleic acid and esp. DNA through a process of transfection

trans·fec·tion \trans-ˈfek-shən\ *n* : infection of a cell with isolated viral nucleic acid followed by production of the complete virus in the cell; *also* : the incorporation of exogenous DNA into a cell — **trans·fect** \-ˈfekt\ *vb*

trans·fem·o·ral \-ˈfe-mə-rəl\ *adj* **1** : passing through or performed by way of the femoral artery ⟨∼ angiography⟩ **2 a** : occurring across or involving the femur ⟨∼ amputation⟩ **b** : having undergone transfemoral amputation; *also* : suitable for use following transfemoral amputation

trans·fer \ˈtrans-ˌfər\ *n* **1** : TRANSFERENCE **2** : the carryover or generalization of learned responses from one type of situation to another — see NEGATIVE TRANSFER

trans·fer·ase \ˈtrans-(ˌ)fər-ˌās, -ˌāz\ *n* : an enzyme that promotes transfer of a group from one molecule to another

trans·fer·ence \trans-ˈfər-əns, ˈtrans-(ˌ)\ *n* : the redirection of feelings and desires and esp. of those unconsciously retained from childhood toward a new object (as a psychoanalyst conducting therapy)

transference neurosis *n* : a neurosis developed in the course of psychoanalytic treatment and manifested by the reliving of infantile experiences in the presence of the analyst

transfer factor *n* : a substance that is produced and secreted by a lymphocyte functioning in cell-mediated immunity and that upon incorporation into a lymphocyte which has not been sensitized confers on it the same immunological specificity as the sensitized cell

trans·fer·rin \trans-ˈfer-ən\ *n* : a beta globulin in blood plasma capable of combining with ferric ions and transporting iron in the blood

transfer RNA *n* : a relatively small RNA that transfers a particular amino acid to a growing polypeptide chain at the ribosomal site of protein synthesis during translation — called also *soluble RNA, tRNA;* compare MESSENGER RNA

trans·fix·ion \trans-ˈfik-shən\ *n* : a piercing of a part of the body (as by a suture or pin) in order to fix it in position — **trans·fix** \-ˈfiks\ *vb*

trans·form \trans-ˈfȯrm\ *vb* **1** : to change or become changed in structure, appearance, or character **2** : to cause (a cell) to undergo genetic transformation

trans·for·ma·tion \ˌtrans-fər-ˈmā-shən, -fȯr-\ *n* **1** : an act, process, or instance of transforming or being transformed **2 a** : genetic modification of a bacterium by incorporation of free DNA from another ruptured bacterial cell — compare TRANSDUCTION **b** : genetic modification of a cell by the uptake and incorporation of exogenous DNA

transforming growth factor *n* : any of a group of polypeptides that are secreted by a variety of cells (as monocytes, T cells, or blood platelets) and have diverse effects (as inducing angiogenesis, stimulating fibroblast proliferation, or inhibiting T cell proliferation) on the division and activity of cells — abbr. *TGF*

trans·fuse \trans-'fyüz\ *vb* **transfused; trans·fus·ing 1** : to transfer (as blood) into a vein or artery of a human being or an animal **2** : to subject (a patient) to transfusion — **trans·fus·able** *or* **trans·fus·ible** \trans-'fyü-zə-bəl\ *adj*

trans·fu·sion \trans-'fyü-zhən\ *n* **1** : the process of transfusing fluid (as blood) into a vein or artery **2** : something transfused — **trans·fu·sion·al** \-zhə-nəl\ *adj*

trans·fu·sion·ist \-zhə-nist\ *n* : one skilled in performing transfusions

trans·gen·der \-'jen-dər\ *or* **trans·gen·dered** \-dərd\ *adj* : of, relating to, or being a person (as a transsexual or a transvestite) who identifies with or expresses a gender identity that differs from the one which corresponds to the person's sex at birth — **transgen·der·ism** \-də-,ri-zəm\ *n*

trans·gene \'trans-,jēn, 'tranz\ *n* : a gene that is taken from the genome of one organism and introduced into the genome of another organism by artificial techniques

¹**trans·gen·ic** \,trans-'je-nik, ,tranz-\ *adj* : being or used to produce an organism or cell of one species into which one or more genes of another species have been incorporated ⟨~ crops⟩; *also* : produced by or composed of transgenic plants or animals

²**transgenic** *n* **1 transgenics** *pl* : a branch of biotechnology concerned with the production of transgenic plants, animals, and foods **2** : a transgenic plant or animal

trans·glu·ta·min·ase \-'glü-tə-mə,nās, -glü-'ta-mə-,nāz\ *n* : a clotting factor that is a variant of factor XIII and that promotes the formation of links between strands of fibrin

trans·he·pat·ic \-hi-'pa-tik\ *adj* : passing through or performed by way of the bile ducts; *specif* : involving direct injection (as of a radiopaque medium) into the bile ducts

tran·sient \'tran-zē-ənt, -shənt, -chənt\ *adj* : passing away in time : existing temporarily ⟨~ symptoms⟩

transient global amnesia *n* : temporary amnesia of short duration (as several hours) that is marked by sudden onset, by loss of past memories, and by an inability to form new memories

transient ischemic attack *n* : a brief episode of cerebral ischemia that is usu. characterized by temporary blurring of vision, slurring of speech, numbness, paralysis, or syncope and that is often predictive of a serious stroke — abbr. *TIA;* called also *ministroke*

trans·il·lu·mi·nate \,trans-ə-'lü-mə,nāt, ,tranz-\ *vb* **-nat·ed; -nat·ing** : to pass light through (a body part) for medical examination — **trans·il·lu·mi·na·tion** \-ə-,lü-mə-'nā-shən\ *n*

tran·si·tion·al \tran-'si-shə-nəl, -'zi-\ *adj* : of, relating to, or being an epithelium (as in the urinary bladder) that consists of several layers of soft cuboidal cells which become flattened when stretched

trans·la·tion \trans-'lā-shən, tranz-\ *n* : the process of forming a protein molecule at a ribosomal site of protein synthesis from information contained in messenger RNA — compare TRANSCRIPTION — **trans·late** \-'lāt\ *vb* — **trans·la·tion·al** \-'lā-shə-nəl\ *adj*

trans·lo·ca·tion \,trans-lō-'kā-shən, ,tranz-\ *n* **1** : transfer of part of a chromosome to a different position esp. on a nonhomologous chromosome; *esp* : the exchange of parts between nonhomologous chromosomes **2** : a chromosome or part of a chromosome that has undergone translocation — **trans·lo·cate** \-'lō-,kāt\ *vb*

trans·lum·bar \,trans-'ləm-bər, ,tranz-, -,bär\ *adj* : passing through or performed by way of the lumbar region; *specif* : involving the injection of a radiopaque medium through the lumbar region ⟨~ aortography⟩

trans·lu·mi·nal \-'lü-mə-nəl\ *adj* : passing across or performed by way of a lumen; *specif* : involving the passage of an inflatable catheter along the lumen of a blood vessel ⟨~ angioplasty⟩

trans·mem·brane \-'mem-,brān\ *adj* : taking place, existing, or arranged from one side to the other of a membrane ⟨~ proteins⟩ ⟨a ~ potential⟩

trans·mis·si·ble \trans-'mi-sə-bəl, tranz-\ *adj* : capable of being transmitted ⟨~ diseases⟩ — **trans·mis·si·bil·i·ty** \-,mi-sə-'bi-lə-tē\ *n*

transmissible mink encephalopathy *n* : a prion disease of mink that resembles scrapie

transmissible spongiform encephalopathy *n* : PRION DISEASE — abbr. *TSE*

trans·mis·sion \trans-'mi-shən, tranz-\ *n* : an act, process, or instance of transmitting ⟨~ of HIV⟩

transmission deafness *n* : CONDUCTION DEAFNESS

transmission electron microscope *n* : a conventional electron microscope which produces an image of a cross-sectional slice of a specimen all points of which are illuminated by the electron beam at the same time — **transmission electron microscopy** *n*

trans·mit \trans-'mit, tranz-\ *vb* **transmit·ted; trans·mit·ting** : to pass, transfer, or convey from one person or place to another: as **a** : to pass or convey by heredity ⟨~ a genetic abnormality⟩ **b** : to convey (infection) abroad or to another ⟨mosquitoes ~

malaria⟩ **c** : to cause (energy) to be conveyed through space or a medium ⟨substances that ~ nerve impulses⟩

trans·mit·ta·ble \-ˈmi-tə-bəl\ *adj* : TRANSMISSIBLE

trans·mit·ter \-ˈmi-tər\ *n* : one that transmits; *specif* : NEUROTRANSMITTER

trans·mu·ral \ˌtrans-ˈmyu̇r-əl, ˌtranz-\ *adj* : passing or administered through an anatomical wall ⟨~ stimulation of the ileum⟩; *also* : involving the whole thickness of a wall ⟨~ myocardial infarction⟩ — **trans·mu·ral·ly** *adv*

trans·neu·ro·nal \-nu̇-ˈrōn-ᵊl, -nyu̇-, -ˈnu̇r-ən-ᵊl, -ˈnyu̇r-\ *adj* : TRANSSYNAPTIC ⟨~ cell atrophy⟩

trans·or·bit·al \-ˈȯr-bət-ᵊl\ *adj* : passing through or performed by way of the eye socket

trans·ovar·i·al \-ō-ˈvar-ē-əl\ *adj* : relating to or being transmission of a pathogen from an organism (as a tick) to its offspring by infection of eggs in its ovary — **trans·ovar·i·al·ly** *adv*

trans·ovar·i·an \-ē-ən\ *adj* : TRANSOVARIAL

trans·par·ent \trans-ˈpar-ənt\ *adj* **1** : having the property of transmitting light so that bodies lying beyond are seen clearly **2** : allowing the passage of a specified form of radiation (as X-rays)

trans·pep·ti·dase \trans-ˈpep-tə-ˌdās, tranz-, -ˌdāz\ *n* : an enzyme that catalyzes the transfer of an amino acid residue or a peptide residue from one amino compound to another

trans·peri·to·ne·al \-ˌper-ə-tə-ˈnē-əl\ *adj* : passing or performed through the peritoneum

trans·per·son·al \-ˈpərs-nəl\ *adj* : of, relating to, or being psychology or psychotherapy concerned esp. with esoteric mental experience (as mysticism and altered states of consciousness) beyond the usual limits of ego and personality

trans·pla·cen·tal \ˌtrans-plə-ˈsent-ᵊl\ *adj* : relating to, involving, or being passage (as of an antibody) between mother and fetus through the placenta — **trans·pla·cen·tal·ly** *adv*

¹**trans·plant** \trans-ˈplant\ *vb* : to transfer from one place to another; *esp* : to transfer (an organ or tissue) from one part or individual to another — **trans·plant·abil·i·ty** \-ˌplan-tə-ˈbi-lə-tē\ *n* — **trans·plant·able** \-ˈplan-tə-bəl\ *adj* — **trans·plan·ta·tion** \ˌtrans-ˌplan-ˈtā-shən\ *n*

²**trans·plant** \ˈtrans-ˌplant\ *n* **1** : something (as an organ or part) that is transplanted **2** : the act or process of transplanting ⟨a liver ~⟩

trans·pleu·ral \-ˈplu̇r-əl\ *adj* : passing through or requiring passage through the pleura ⟨a ~ surgical procedure⟩

¹**trans·port** \trans-ˈpȯrt, ˈtrans-ˌ\ *vb* : to transfer or convey from one place to another

²**trans·port** \ˈtrans-ˌpȯrt\ *n* : an act or process of transporting; *specif* : ACTIVE TRANSPORT

transposable element *n* : a segment of genetic material that is capable of changing its location in the genome or in some bacteria of undergoing transfer between an extrachromosomal plasmid and a chromosome — called also *transposable genetic element*

trans·pose \trans-ˈpōz\ *vb* **transposed; trans·pos·ing** : to transfer from one place or period to another; *specif* : to subject to or undergo genetic transposition — **trans·pos·able** \-ˈpō-zə-bəl\ *adj*

trans·po·si·tion \ˌtrans-pə-ˈzi-shən\ *n* : an act, process, or instance of transposing or being transposed: as **a** : the displacement of a viscus to a side opposite from that which it normally occupies ⟨~ of the heart⟩ **b** : the transfer of a segment of DNA from one site to another in the genome either between chromosomal sites or between an extrachromosomal site (as on a plasmid) and a chromosome — **trans·po·si·tion·al** \-ˈzi-shə-nəl\ *adj*

trans·po·son \ˌtrans-ˈpō-ˌzän\ *n* : a transposable element esp. when it contains genetic material controlling functions other than those related to its relocation

trans·py·lor·ic \-pī-ˈlȯr-ik\ *adj* : relating to or being the transverse plane or the line marking its intersection with the surface of the abdomen that passes below the rib cage cutting the pylorus of the stomach and the first lumbar vertebra and that is one of the four planes marking off the nine abdominal regions

trans·rec·tal \-ˈrekt-ᵊl\ *adj* : passing through or performed by way of the rectum ⟨~ prostatic biopsy⟩

trans·sep·tal *also* **tran·sep·tal** \-ˈsept-ᵊl\ *adj* **1** : passing across a septum ⟨~ fibers between teeth⟩ **2** : passing or performed through a septum ⟨~ cardiac catheterization⟩

trans·sex·u·al *also* **tran·sex·u·al** \-ˈsek-shə-wəl\ *n* : a person who psychologically identifies with the opposite sex and may seek to live as a member of this sex esp. by undergoing surgery and hormone therapy to obtain the necessary physical appearance (as by changing the external sex organs) — **transsexual** *also* **transexual** *adj* — **trans·sex·u·al·ism** *also* **tran·sex·u·al·ism** \-wə-ˌli-zəm\ *n* — **trans·sex·u·al·i·ty** *also* **tran·sex·u·al·ity** \-ˌsek-shə-ˈwa-lə-tē\ *n*

trans·sphe·noi·dal \-sfi-ˈnȯid-ᵊl\ *adj* : performed by entry through the sphenoid bone ⟨~ hypophysectomy⟩

trans·syn·ap·tic \-sə-ˈnap-tik\ *adj* : occurring or taking place across nerve synapses ⟨~ degeneration⟩

trans·tho·rac·ic \-thə-ˈra-sik\ *adj* **1** : performed or made by way of the thoracic cavity **2** : crossing or having connections that cross the thoracic cavity ⟨a ~ pacemaker⟩ — **trans·tho·rac·i·cal·ly** *adv*

trans·thy·re·tin \-'thī-rə-tin\ *n* : a protein component of blood serum that functions esp. in the transport of thyroxine — called also *prealbumin*

trans·tib·i·al \-'ti-bē-əl\ *adj* **1** : occurring across or involving the tibia ⟨~ amputation⟩ **2** : having undergone transtibial amputation; *also* : suitable for use following transtibial amputation ⟨a ~ prosthesis⟩

trans·tra·che·al \-'trā-kē-əl\ *adj* : passing through or administered by way of the trachea ⟨~ anesthesia⟩

tran·su·date \,tran-'sü-dət, -'syü-, -'zü-, -'zyü-, -,dāt\ *n* : a transuded substance

tran·su·da·tion \,tran-sü-'dā-shən, -syü-, -zü-, -zyü-\ *n* **1** : the act or process of transuding or being transuded **2** : TRANSUDATE

tran·sude \tran-'süd, -'syüd, -'züd, -'zyüd\ *vb* **tran·sud·ed; tran·sud·ing** : to pass or permit passage of through a membrane or permeable substance

trans·ure·tero·ure·ter·os·to·my \,trans-yù-,rē-tə-,rō-yù-,rē-tə-'räs-tə-mē\ *n, pl* **-mies** : anastomosis of a ureter to the contralateral ureter

trans·ure·thral \-yù-'rē-thrəl\ *adj* : passing through or performed by way of the urethra ⟨~ prostatectomy⟩

trans·vag·i·nal \-'va-jən-ᵊl\ *adj* : passing through or performed by way of the vagina ⟨~ laparoscopy⟩

trans·ve·nous \-'vē-nəs\ *adj* : relating to or involving the use of an intravenous catheter containing an electrode carrying electrical impulses from an extracorporeal source to the heart

trans·ven·tric·u·lar \-ven-'tri-kyə-lər, -vən-\ *adj* : passing through or performed by way of a ventricle

transversa, transversum — see SEPTUM TRANSVERSUM

trans·ver·sa·lis cer·vi·cis \,trans-vər-'sā-ləs-'sər-vi-səs\ *n* : LONGISSIMUS CERVICIS

transversalis fascia *n* : the whole deep layer of fascia lining the abdominal wall; *also* : the part of this covering the inner surface of the transversus abdominis and separating it from the peritoneum

trans·verse \trans-'vərs, tranz-, 'trans-, 'tranz-\ *adj* **1** : acting, lying, or being across : set crosswise **2** : made at right angles to the long axis of the body ⟨a ~ section⟩ — **trans·verse·ly** *adv*

transverse carpal ligament *n* : FLEXOR RETINACULUM 2

transverse cervical artery *n* : an inconstant branch of the thyrocervical trunk or of the subclavian artery that supplies the region at the base of the neck and the muscles of the scapula

transverse colon *n* : the part of the large intestine that extends across the abdominal cavity joining the ascending colon to the descending colon

transverse crural ligament *n* : EXTENSOR RETINACULUM 1b

transverse facial artery *n* : a large branch of the superficial temporal artery that arises in the parotid gland and supplies the parotid gland, masseter muscle, and adjacent parts

transverse fissure *n* : PORTA HEPATIS

transverse foramen *n* : a foramen in each transverse process of a cervical vertebra through which the vertebral artery and vertebral vein pass in each cervical vertebra except the seventh

transverse ligament *n* : any of various ligaments situated transversely with respect to a bodily axis or part: as **a** : the transverse part of the cruciate ligament of the atlas **b** : one in the anterior part of the knee connecting the anterior margins of the lateral and medial menisci

transverse process *n* : a process that projects on the dorsolateral aspect of each side of the neural arch of a vertebra

transverse sinus *n* : either of two large venous sinuses of the cranium that begin at the bony protuberance on the middle of the inner surface of the occipital bone at the intersection of its bony ridges and that terminate at the jugular foramen on either side to become the internal jugular vein

transverse thoracic muscle *n* : TRANSVERSUS THORACIS

transverse tubule *n* : T TUBULE

trans·ver·sion \trans-'vər-zhən, tranz-\ *n* : the eruption of a tooth in an abnormal position on the jaw

transversum — see SEPTUM TRANSVERSUM

trans·ver·sus ab·dom·i·nis \trans-'vər-səs-əb-'dä-mə-nəs\ *n* : a flat muscle with transverse fibers that forms the innermost layer of the anterolateral wall of the abdomen and that acts to constrict the abdominal viscera and assist in expulsion of the contents of various abdominal organs (as in defecation, vomiting, and parturition)

transversus pe·rin·ei su·per·fi·ci·a·lis \-pe-'ri-nē-,ī-,sü-pər-,fi-shē-'ā-ləs\ *n* : a small band of muscle of the urogenital region of the perineum that arises from the ischial tuberosity and that with the contralateral muscle inserts into and acts to stabilize the mass of tissue in the midline between the anus and the penis or vagina — called also *superficial transverse perineal muscle*

transversus tho·ra·cis \-thə-'rā-səs\ *n* : a thin flat sheet of muscle and tendon fibers of the anterior wall of the chest that arises esp. from the xiphoid process and lower third of the sternum, inserts into the costal cartilages of the second to sixth ribs, and acts to draw the ribs downward — called also *transverse thoracic muscle*

trans·ves·i·cal \trans-'ve-si-kəl, tranz-\ *adj* : passing through or performed by way of the urinary bladder

trans·ves·tism \trans-'ves-ˌti-zəm, tranz-\ *n* : adoption of the dress and often the behavior of the opposite sex — called also *eonism*

trans·ves·tite \trans-'ves-ˌtīt, tranz-\ *n* : a person and esp. a male who adopts the dress and often the behavior typical of the opposite sex esp. for purposes of emotional or sexual gratification — **transvestite** *adj*

Tran·xene \'tran-ˌzēn\ *trademark* — used for a preparation of clorazepate

tran·yl·cy·pro·mine \ˌtran-əl-'sī-prə-ˌmēn\ *n* : an antidepressant drug that is an inhibitor of monoamine oxidase and is administered in the form of its sulfate $(C_9H_{13}N)_2 \cdot H_2SO_4$

tra·pe·zi·um \trə-'pē-zē-əm, tra-\ *n, pl* **-zi·ums** *or* **-zia** \-zē-ə\ : a bone in the distal row of the carpus at the base of the thumb — called also *greater multangular*

tra·pe·zi·us \trə-'pē-zē-əs, tra-\ *n, pl* **-zii** \-zē-ˌī\ *also* **-zi·us·es** : a large flat triangular superficial muscle of each side of the upper back that arises from the occipital bone, the ligamentum nuchae, and the spinous processes of the last cervical and all the thoracic vertebrae, is inserted into the outer part of the clavicle, the acromion, and the spine of the scapula, and serves chiefly to rotate the scapula so as to present the glenoid cavity upward

trap·e·zoid \'tra-pə-ˌzòid\ *n* : a bone in the distal row of the carpus at the base of the index finger — called also *lesser multangular*, *trapezoid bone*, *trapezoideum*

trapezoid body *n* : a bundle of transverse fibers in the dorsal part of the pons

trap·e·zoi·de·um \ˌtra-pə-'zòi-dē-əm\ *n* : TRAPEZOID

tras·tu·zu·mab \ˌtras-'tü-zü-ˌmab\ *n* : a genetically engineered monoclonal antibody administered by injection to slow or inhibit tumor growth in some advanced breast cancers — see HERCEPTIN

Tras·y·lol \'tra-sə-ˌlòl\ *trademark* — used for a preparation of aprotinin

trau·ma \'traù-mə, 'trò-\ *n, pl* **traumas** *also* **trau·ma·ta** \-mə-tə\ **1 a** : an injury (as a wound) to living tissue caused by an extrinsic agent ⟨surgical ∼⟩ — see BLUNT TRAUMA **b** : a disordered psychological or behavioral state resulting from mental or emotional stress or physical injury **2** : an agent, force, or mechanism that causes trauma — **trau·mat·ic** \trə-'ma-tik, trò-, traù-\ *adj* — **trau·mat·i·cal·ly** *adv*

trauma center *n* : a hospital unit specializing in the treatment of patients with acute and esp. life-threatening traumatic injuries

traumat- *or* **traumato-** *comb form* : wound : trauma ⟨*traumatism*⟩

trau·ma·tism \'traù-mə-ˌti-zəm, 'trò-\ *n* : the development or occurrence of trauma; *also* : TRAUMA

trau·ma·tize \-ˌtīz\ *vb* **-tized; -tiz·ing** : to inflict a trauma upon ⟨*traumatized* tissues⟩ ⟨children *traumatized* by physical abuse⟩ — **trau·ma·ti·za·tion** \ˌtraù-mə-tə-'zā-shən, ˌtrò-\ *n*

trau·ma·tol·o·gist \ˌtraù-mə-'tä-lə-jəst, ˌtrò-\ *n* : a surgeon who practices traumatology or who is on duty at a trauma center

trau·ma·tol·o·gy \ˌtraù-mə-'tä-lə-jē, ˌtrò-\ *n, pl* **-gies** : the surgical treatment of wounds ⟨pediatric ∼⟩

tra·vail \trə-'vāl, 'tra-ˌvāl\ *n* : LABOR, PARTURITION

traveler's diarrhea *n* : intestinal sickness and diarrhea affecting a traveler and typically caused by ingestion of pathogenic microorganisms (as some E. coli) — compare MONTEZUMA'S REVENGE

travel sickness *n* : MOTION SICKNESS

tray \'trā\ *n* : an appliance consisting of a rimmed body and a handle for use in holding plastic material against the gums or teeth in making negative impressions for dentures

traz·o·done \'tra-zə-ˌdōn\ *n* : an antidepressant drug that is administered in the form of its hydrochloride $C_{19}H_{22}ClN_5O \cdot HCl$ and inhibits the uptake of serotonin by the brain

Trea·cher Col·lins syndrome \'trē-chər-'kä-lənz-\ *n* : MANDIBULOFACIAL DYSOSTOSIS

Collins, Edward Treacher (1862–1932), British ophthalmologist.

tread·mill \'tred-ˌmil\ *n* : a device having an endless belt on which an individual walks or runs in place that is used for exercise and in tests of physiological functions — see STRESS TEST

treat \'trēt\ *vb* : to care for or deal with medically or surgically : deal with by medical or surgical means ⟨∼*ed* their diseases⟩ — **treat·abil·i·ty** \ˌtrē-tə-'bi-lə-tē\ *n* — **treat·able** \'trē-tə-bəl\ *adj* — **treat·ment** \'trēt-mənt\ *n*

tree \'trē\ *n* : an anatomical system or structure having many branches — see BILIARY TREE, BRONCHIAL TREE, TRACHEOBRONCHIAL TREE

-tre·ma \'trē-mə\ *n comb form, pl* **-tremas** *or* **-tre·ma·ta** \'trē-mə-tə\ : hole : orifice : opening ⟨helicotrema⟩

trem·a·tode \'tre-mə-ˌtōd\ *n* : any of a class (Trematoda) of parasitic flatworms including the flukes — **trematode** *adj*

trem·bles \'trem-bəlz\ *n* : severe poisoning of livestock and esp. cattle by a toxic alcohol present in white snakeroot and rayless goldenrod that is characterized esp. by muscular tremors, weakness, and constipation

tremens — see DELIRIUM TREMENS

trem·or \'tre-mər\ n : a trembling or shaking usu. from physical weakness, emotional stress, or disease

trem·u·lous \'trem-yə-ləs\ adj : characterized by or affected with trembling or tremors — **trem·u·lous·ness** n

trench fever n : a disease that is marked by fever and pain in muscles, bones, and joints and that is caused by a bacterium (*Bartonella quintana* syn. *Rochalimaea quintana*) transmitted by the human body louse (*Pediculus humanus humanus*)

trench foot n : a painful foot disorder resembling frostbite and resulting from exposure to cold and wet

trench mouth n : ACUTE NECROTIZING ULCERATIVE GINGIVITIS; *also* : VINCENT'S ANGINA

Tren·de·len·burg position \'trend-ᵊl-ən-ˌbərg-\ n : a position of the body for medical examination or operation in which the patient is placed head down on a table inclined at about 45 degrees from the floor with the knees uppermost and the legs hanging over the end of the table

Trendelenburg, Friedrich (1844–1924), German surgeon.

Tren·tal \'tren-ˌtal\ *trademark* — used for a preparation of pentoxifylline

treph·i·na·tion \ˌtre-fə-'nā-shən\ n : an act or instance of using a trephine (as to perforate the skull)

tre·phine \'trē-ˌfīn\ n : a surgical instrument for cutting out circular sections (as of bone or corneal tissue) — **tre·phine** \'trē-ˌfīn, tri-'\ vb

trep·o·ne·ma \ˌtre-pə-'nē-mə\ n 1 cap : a genus of anaerobic spirochetes (family Spirochaetaceae) that are pathogenic in humans and other warm-blooded animals and include one (*T. pallidum*) causing syphilis and another (*T. pertenue*) causing yaws 2 pl **-ma·ta** \-mə-tə\ *or* **-mas** : any spirochete of the genus *Treponema* — **trep·o·ne·mal** \-'nē-məl\ adj

Treponema pal·li·dum immobilization test \-'pa-lə-dəm-\ n : a serological test for syphilis — abbr. TPI

trep·o·ne·ma·to·sis \ˌtre-pə-ˌnē-mə-'tō-səs, -ˌne-\ n, pl **-to·ses** \-ˌsēz\ : infection with or disease caused by spirochetes of the genus *Treponema*

trep·o·neme \'tre-pə-ˌnēm\ n : TREPONEMA 2

trep·pe \'tre-pə\ n : the graduated series of increasingly vigorous contractions that results when a corresponding series of identical stimuli is applied to a rested muscle — called also *staircase effect*

tre·tin·o·in \tre-'ti-nō-ən, 'tre-tə-ˌnòin\ n : a trans isomer of retinoic acid that is used chiefly as a topical agent applied to the skin to treat acne vulgaris and to reduce facial wrinkles, roughness, and pigmented spots — called

also *all-trans-retinoic acid, retinoic acid*; see ISOTRETINOIN, RETIN-A

TRF *abbr* thyrotropin-releasing factor

TRH *abbr* thyrotropin-releasing hormone

tri·ac·e·tyl·ole·an·do·my·cin \(ˌ)trī-ˌa-sət-ᵊl-ˌō-lē-ˌan-dō-'mīs-ᵊn\ n : TROLEANDOMYCIN

tri·ad \'trī-ˌad\ n : a union or group of three ⟨a ~ of symptoms⟩

tri·age \trē-'äzh, 'trē-ˌ\ n 1 : the sorting of and allocation of treatment to patients and esp. battle and disaster victims according to a system of priorities designed to maximize the number of survivors 2 : the sorting of patients (as in an emergency room) according to the urgency of their need for care — **triage** vb

tri·al \'trī-əl\ n 1 : a tryout or experiment to test quality, value, or usefulness — see CLINICAL TRIAL 2 : one of a number of repetitions of an experiment

tri·am·cin·o·lone \ˌtrī-ˌam-'sin-ᵊl-ˌōn\ n : a glucocorticoid drug $C_{21}H_{27}FO_6$ that has anti-inflammatory and immunosuppressant effects and is used chiefly in the treatment of skin disorders, asthma, and allergic rhinitis — see AZMACORT, NASACORT

tri·am·ter·ene \trī-'am-tər-ˌēn\ n : a diuretic drug $C_{12}H_{11}N_7$ that promotes potassium retention — see DYAZIDE, MAXZIDE

tri·an·gle \'trī-ˌaŋ-gəl\ n : a three-sided region or space and esp. an anatomical one — see ANTERIOR TRIANGLE, FEMORAL TRIANGLE, POSTERIOR TRIANGLE, SUBOCCIPITAL TRIANGLE, SUPERIOR CAROTID TRIANGLE

tri·an·gu·lar \trī-'aŋ-gyə-lər\ n : TRIQUETRAL BONE

triangular bone n : TRIQUETRAL BONE

triangular fossa n : a shallow depression in the anterior part of the top of the ear's auricle between the two crura into which the antihelix divides

tri·an·gu·la·ris \trī-ˌaŋ-gyə-'lar-əs\ n, pl **-la·res** \-'lar-ˌēz\ 1 : a flat triangular muscle that extends from the base of the mandible to the angle formed by the joining of the upper and lower lips and that acts to depress this angle 2 : TRIQUETRAL BONE

triangular ridge n : a triangular surface that slopes downward from the tip of a cusp of a molar or premolar toward the center of its occlusal surface

tri·at·o·ma \trī-'a-tə-mə\ n 1 cap : a genus of large blood-sucking bugs (family Reduviidae) that feed on mammals and sometimes transmit Chagas' disease to their hosts — see CONENOSE 2 : any bug of the genus *Triatoma*

¹tri·at·o·mid \trī-'a-tə-mid\ adj : belonging to the genus *Triatoma*

²triatomid n : TRIATOMA 2

tri·az·i·quone \trī-'a-zə-ˌkwōn\ n : an antineoplastic drug $C_{12}H_{13}N_3O_2$

tri·azo·lam \trī-'a-zə-ˌlam\ *n* : a benzodiazepine $C_{17}H_{12}Cl_2N_4$ used as a sleep-inducing agent in the short-term treatment of insomnia — see HALCION

tri·azole \'trī-ə-ˌzōl\ *n* : any of a group of compounds that are characterized by a ring composed of two carbon atoms and three nitrogen atoms and that include a number of antifungal agents (as fluconazole)

trib·a·dism \'tri-bə-ˌdi-zəm\ *n* : a homosexual practice among women in which the external genitalia are rubbed together

tri·bro·mo·eth·a·nol \ˌtrī-ˌbrō-mō-'e-thə-ˌnȯl, -ˌnōl\ *n* : a crystalline bromine derivative $C_2H_3Br_3O$ of ethyl alcohol used as a basal anesthetic

trib·u·tary \'tri-byə-ˌter-ē\ *n, pl* **-tar·ies** : a vein that empties into a larger vein

tri·car·box·yl·ic acid cycle \ˌtrī-ˌkär-ˌbäk-'si-lik-\ *n* : KREBS CYCLE

tri·ceps \'trī-ˌseps\ *n, pl* **triceps** : a muscle that arises from three heads: **a** : the large extensor muscle that is situated along the back of the upper arm, arises by the long head from the infraglenoid tubercle of the scapula and by two heads from the shaft of the humerus, is inserted into the olecranon at the elbow, and extends the forearm at the elbow joint — called also *triceps brachii* **b** : the gastrocnemius and soleus muscles viewed as constituting together one muscle

triceps bra·chii \-'brā-kē-ˌī\ *n* : TRICEPS a

trich- *or* **tricho-** *comb form* : hair : filament ⟨*trichobezoar*⟩

-trich·ia \'tri-kē-ə\ *n comb form* : condition of having (such) hair ⟨*atrichia*⟩

tri·chi·a·sis \tri-'kī-ə-səs\ *n* : a turning inward of the eyelashes often causing irritation of the eyeball

tri·chi·na \tri-'kī-nə\ *n, pl* **-nae** \-ˌ(ˌ)nē\ *also* **-nas** : a small slender nematode worm of the genus *Trichinella* (*T. spiralis*) that as an adult is a short-lived parasite of the intestines of a flesh-eating mammal where it produces immense numbers of larvae which migrate to the muscles, become encysted, may persist for years, and if consumed by a new host in raw or insufficiently cooked meat are liberated by the digestive processes and rapidly become adult to initiate a new parasitic cycle — see TRICHINOSIS

Trichina *n, syn of* TRICHINELLA

trich·i·nel·la \ˌtri-kə-'ne-lə\ *n* **1** *cap* : a genus of nematode worms (family Trichinellidae) comprising the trichinae **2** *pl* **-lae** \-ˌlē\ : TRICHINA

trich·i·ni·a·sis \ˌtri-kə-'nī-ə-səs\ *n, pl* **-a·ses** \-ˌsēz\ : TRICHINOSIS

trich·i·no·sis \ˌtri-kə-'nō-səs\ *n, pl* **-no·ses** \-ˌsēz\ : infestation with or disease caused by trichinae contracted by eating raw or insufficiently cooked infested food and esp. pork and marked initially by abdominal pain,

nausea, and diarrhea and later by muscular pain, dyspnea, fever, and edema — called also *trichiniasis*

tri·chlor·fon *also* **tri·chlor·phon** \(ˌ)trī-'klȯr-ˌfän\ *n* : an organophosphate $C_4H_8Cl_3O_4P$ used as a parasiticide in veterinary medicine

tri·chlor·me·thi·a·zide \ˌtrī-ˌklȯr-me-'thī-ə-ˌzīd\ *n* : a diuretic and antihypertensive drug $C_8H_8Cl_3N_3O_4S_2$ — see METAHYDRIN, NAQUA

tri·chlo·ro·ace·tic acid \ˌtrī-ˌklȯr-ō-ə-'sē-tik-\ *also* **tri·chlor·ace·tic** \-ˌklȯr-ə-'sē-tik\ *n* : a strong acid $C_2Cl_3HO_2$ used in medicine as a caustic and astringent

tri·chlo·ro·eth·y·lene \-'e-thə-ˌlēn\ *also* **tri·chlor·eth·y·lene** \-ˌklȯr-'e-thə-ˌlēn\ *n* : a nonflammable liquid C_2HCl_3 used in medicine as an anesthetic and analgesic — abbr. *TCE*

tri·chlo·ro·meth·ane \-'me-ˌthān\ *n* : CHLOROFORM

tri·chlo·ro·phe·nol \-'fē-ˌnȯl, -ˌnōl, -fi-\ *n* : a bactericide and fungicide $C_6H_3Cl_3O$ that is a major constituent of hexachlorophene

tri·chlo·ro·phen·oxy·ace·tic acid \(ˌ)tri-ˌklȯr-ō-fə-ˌnäk-sē-ə-'sē-tik-\ *n* : 2,4,5-T

tricho·be·zoar \ˌtri-kō-'bē-ˌzȯr\ *n* : HAIR BALL

Tricho·bil·har·zia \ˌtri-kō-bil-'här-zē-ə, -'härt-sē-ə\ *n* : a genus of digenetic trematode worms (family Schistosomatidae) including forms that normally parasitize aquatic birds and cause swimmer's itch in humans

Tricho·dec·tes \ˌtri-kə-'dek-ˌtēz\ *n* : a genus of biting lice (family Trichodectidae) of domesticated mammals

tricho·epi·the·li·o·ma \ˌtri-kō-ˌe-pə-ˌthē-lē-'ō-mə\ *n, pl* **-mas** *also* **-ma·ta** \-mə-tə\ : a benign epithelial tumor developing from the hair follicles esp. on the face

tri·chol·o·gy \tri-'kä-lə-jē\ *n, pl* **-gies** : scientific study of hair and its diseases

tricho·mo·na·cide \ˌtri-kə-'mō-nə-ˌsīd\ *n* : an agent used to destroy trichomonads — **tricho·mo·na·cid·al** \-ˌmō-nə-'sīd-ᵊl\ *adj*

¹tricho·mo·nad \ˌtri-kə-'mō-ˌnad, -nəd\ *n* : any protozoan of the genus *Trichomonas*

²trichomonad *adj* : TRICHOMONAL

tricho·mo·nal \ˌtri-kə-'mō-nəl\ *adj* : of, relating to, or caused by flagellated protozoans of the genus *Trichomonas*

trich·o·mo·nas \ˌtri-kə-'mō-nəs\ *n* **1** *cap* : a genus of flagellated protozoans (family Trichomonadidae) that are parasites of the digestive or genitourinary tracts of numerous vertebrate and invertebrate hosts including one (*T. vaginalis*) causing human vaginitis **2** : a protozoan of the genus *Trichomanas* : TRICHOMONAD

tricho·mo·ni·a·sis \ˌtri-kə-mə-'nī-ə-səs\ *n, pl* **-a·ses** \-ˌsēz\ : infection with or disease caused by trichomonads: as **a** : a human sexually transmitted disease occurring esp. as vaginitis with a persistent discharge and caused by a trichomonad (*Trichomonas vaginalis*) that may also invade the male urethra and bladder **b** : a venereal disease of domestic cattle caused by a trichomonad (*T. foetus*) and marked by abortion and sterility **c** : one or more diseases of various birds caused by trichomonads (esp. *T. gallinae*) and resembling blackhead — called also *roup*

tricho·phy·ton \ˌtri-kə-ˈfī-ˌtän, tri-ˈkä-fə-ˌtän\ *n* **1** *cap* : a genus of dermatophytic fungi (family Moniliaceae) including several causing ringworm — see EPIDERMOPHYTON **2** : any fungus of the genus *Trichophyton*

Tricho·spo·ron \ˌtri-kə-ˈspōr-ˌän, tri-ˈkäs-pə-ˌrän\ *n* : a genus of parasitic imperfect fungi (order Moniliales) that includes the causative agent (*T. beigelii*) of white piedra

tricho·stron·gyle \ˌtri-kə-ˈsträn-ˌjīl\ *n* : any worm of the genus *Trichostrongylus*

tricho·stron·gy·lo·sis \ˌtri-kō-ˌsträn-jə-ˈlō-səs\ *n* : infestation with or disease caused by roundworms of the genus *Trichostrongylus* chiefly in young sheep and cattle

Tricho·stron·gy·lus \ˌtri-kō-ˈsträn-jə-ləs\ *n* : a genus of nematode worms (family Trichostrongylidae) parasitic in birds and mammals including humans that comprises forms formerly placed in the genus *Strongylus*

tricho·til·lo·ma·nia \ˌti-lə-ˈmā-nē-ə\ *n* : abnormal desire to pull out one's hair — called also *hairpulling* — **tricho·til·lo·man·ic** \-ˈma-nik\ *adj*

tri·chro·mat \ˈtrī-krō-ˌmat, (ˌ)trī-ˈ\ *n* : an individual with trichromatism

tri·chro·mat·ic \ˌtrī-krō-ˈma-tik\ *adj* **1** : of, relating to, or consisting of three colors (~ light) **2 a** : relating to or being the theory that human color vision involves three types of retinal sensory receptors **b** : characterized by trichromatism (~ vision)

tri·chro·ma·tism \(ˌ)trī-ˈkrō-mə-ˌti-zəm\ *n* : color vision based on the perception of three primary colors and esp. red, green, and blue — compare DEUTERANOMALY, PROTANOMALY

trich·u·ri·a·sis \ˌtri-kyə-ˈrī-ə-səs\ *n, pl* **-a·ses** \-ˌsēz\ : infestation with or disease caused by nematode worms of the genus *Trichuris*

Trich·u·ris \tri-ˈkyu̇r-əs\ *n* : a genus of nematode worms (family Trichuridae) comprising the whipworms

tri·clo·car·ban \ˌtri-klō-ˈkär-ˌban\ *n* : an antiseptic $C_{13}H_9Cl_3N_2O$ used esp. in soaps

tri·clo·san \trī-ˈklō-ˌsan\ *n* : a whitish crystalline powder $C_{12}H_7Cl_3O_2$ used esp. as a broad-spectrum antibacterial agent (as in soaps, deodorants, and mouthwash)

Tri·Cor \ˈtrī-ˌkȯr\ *trademark* — used for a preparation of fenofibrate

tri·cus·pid \(ˌ)trī-ˈkəs-pəd\ *adj* **1** : having three cusps (~ molars) **2** : of, relating to, or involving the tricuspid valve of the heart (~ disease)

tricuspid valve *n* : a valve that is situated at the opening of the right atrium of the heart into the right ventricle and that resembles the mitral valve in structure but consists of three triangular membranous flaps — called also *right atrioventricular valve*

¹tri·cy·clic \(ˌ)trī-ˈsī-klik, -ˈsi-\ *adj* : being a chemical with three usu. fused rings in the molecular structure and esp. a tricyclic antidepressant

²tricyclic *n* : TRICYCLIC ANTIDEPRESSANT

tricyclic antidepressant *n* : any of a group of antidepressant drugs (as imipramine and amitriptyline) that contain three fused benzene rings, potentiate the action of catecholamines (as norepinephrine and serotonin) by inhibiting their uptake by nerve endings, and do not inhibit the action of monoamine oxidase

tri·di·hex·eth·yl chloride \ˌtrī-ˌdī-ˌheks-ˈeth-ᵊl-\ *n* : a quaternary ammonium compound $C_{21}H_{36}ClNO$ used as an anticholinergic drug — see PATHILON

Tri·di·one \trī-ˈdī-ˌōn\ *trademark* — used for a preparation of trimethadione

triethiodide — see GALLAMINE TRIETHIODIDE

tri·eth·yl·ene gly·col \(ˌ)trī-ˈe-thə-ˌlēn-ˈglī-ˌkȯl, -ˌkōl\ *n* : a hygroscopic liquid alcohol $C_6H_{14}O_4$ that is used in medicine as an air disinfectant

tri·eth·yl·ene·mel·amine \(ˌ)trī-ˌe-thə-ˌlēn-ˈme-lə-ˌmēn, -mən\ *n* : a cytotoxic crystalline compound $C_9H_{12}N_6$ used as an antineoplastic drug — called also *TEM*

tri·fa·cial nerve \ˌtrī-ˈfā-shəl-\ *n* : TRIGEMINAL NERVE

trifacial neuralgia *n* : TRIGEMINAL NEURALGIA

tri·fluo·per·a·zine \ˌtrī-ˌflü-ō-ˈper-ə-ˌzēn, -zən\ *n* : a phenothiazine tranquilizer used in the form of its hydrochloride $C_{21}H_{24}F_3N_3S\cdot HCl$ to treat psychotic disorders and esp. schizophrenia — see STELAZINE

tri·flu·pro·ma·zine \ˌtrī-ˌflü-ˈprō-mə-ˌzēn, -zən\ *n* : a phenothiazine tranquilizer used in the form of its hydrochloride $C_{18}H_{19}F_3N_3S\cdot HCl$ esp. in the treatment of psychotic disorders and as an antiemetic — see VESPRIN

¹tri·fo·cal \(ˌ)trī-ˈfō-kəl\ *adj, of an eyeglass lens* : having one part that corrects for near vision, one for intermediate vision (as at arm's length), and one for distant vision

²tri·fo·cal \ˈtrī-ˌfō-kəl\ *n* **1** : a trifocal glass or lens **2** *pl* : eyeglasses with trifocal lenses

¹tri·gem·i·nal \trī-'je-mə-nəl\ *adj* : of or relating to the trigeminal nerve

²trigeminal *n* : TRIGEMINAL NERVE

trigeminal ganglion *n* : the large flattened sensory root ganglion of the trigeminal nerve that lies within the skull and behind the orbit — called also *gasserian ganglion, semilunar ganglion*

trigeminal nerve *n* : either of the fifth pair of cranial nerves that are mixed nerves and in humans are the largest of the cranial nerves and that arise by a small motor root and a larger sensory root which both emerge from the side of the pons with the sensory root bearing the trigeminal ganglion and dividing into ophthalmic, maxillary, and mandibular nerves and the motor root supplying fibers to the mandibular nerve and through this to the muscles of mastication — called also *fifth cranial nerve, trifacial nerve, trigeminus*

trigeminal neuralgia *n* : an intense paroxysmal neuralgia involving one or more branches of the trigeminal nerve — called also *tic douloureux*

trigger finger *n* : an abnormal condition in which flexion or extension of a finger may be momentarily obstructed by spasm followed by a snapping into place

trigger point *n* : a sensitive area of the body which when stimulated gives rise to reaction elsewhere in the body; *esp* : a localized usu. tender or painful area of the body and esp. of a muscle that when stimulated gives rise to pain elsewhere in the body — called also *trigger zone*

tri·glyc·er·ide \(ˌ)trī-'gli-sə-ˌrīd\ *n* : any of a group of lipids that are esters formed from one molecule of glycerol and three molecules of one or more fatty acids, are widespread in adipose tissue, and commonly circulate in the blood in the form of lipoproteins — called also *neutral fat*

tri·gone \'trī-ˌgōn\ *also* **tri·gon** \-ˌgän\ *n* : a triangular body part; *specif* : a smooth triangular area on the inner surface of the bladder limited by the apertures of the ureters and urethra

tri·go·ni·tis \ˌtrī-gə-'nī-təs\ *n* : inflammation of the trigone of the bladder

tri·go·no·ceph·a·ly \ˌtri-gə-nə-'se-fə-lē, ˌtrī-gō-nō-\ *n, pl* **-lies** : a congenital deformity in which the head is somewhat triangular and flat

tri·go·num \trī-'gō-nəm\ *n, pl* **-nums** *or* **-na** \-nə\ : a triangular anatomical part : TRIGONE

trigonum ha·ben·u·lae \-hə-'ben-yə-ˌlē\ *n* : a triangular area on the dorsomedial surface of the lateral geniculate body rostral to the pineal gland

trigonum ves·i·cae \-'ve-si-kē\ *n* : the trigone of the urinary bladder

tri·halo·meth·ane \ˌtrī-ˌhā-lə-'me-ˌthān\ *n* : any of various derivatives CHX_3 of methane (as chloroform) having three halogen atoms per molecule and formed esp. during the chlorination of drinking water

tri·io·do·thy·ro·nine \ˌtrī-ˌī-ə-dō-'thī-rə-ˌnēn\ *n* : a crystalline iodine-containing hormone $C_{15}H_{12}I_3NO_4$ that is an amino acid derived from thyroxine and is used esp. in the form of its soluble sodium salt $C_{15}H_{11}I_3NNaO_4$ in the treatment of hypothyroidism and metabolic insufficiency — called also *liothyronine, T3*

tri·mep·ra·zine \trī-'me-prə-ˌzēn\ *n* : a phenothiazine used esp. in the form of its tartrate $(C_{18}H_{22}N_2S)_2 \cdot C_4H_6O_6$ as an antipruritic

tri·mes·ter \(ˌ)trī-'mes-tər, 'trī-ˌ\ *n* : a period of three or about three months; *esp* : any of three periods of approximately three months each into which a human pregnancy is divided

tri·metha·di·one \ˌtrī-ˌme-thə-'dī-ˌōn\ *n* : a crystalline anticonvulsant $C_6H_9NO_3$ used chiefly in the treatment of absence seizures — see TRIDIONE

tri·meth·a·phan \trī-'me-thə-ˌfan\ *n* : a ganglionic blocking agent used as a salt $C_{32}H_{40}N_2O_5S_2$ to lower blood pressure esp. in hypertensive emergencies

tri·metho·ben·za·mide \ˌtrī-ˌme-thə-'ben-zə-ˌmīd\ *n* : an antiemetic drug used esp. in the form of its hydrochloride $C_{21}H_{28}N_2O_5 \cdot HCl$

tri·meth·o·prim \trī-'me-thə-ˌprim\ *n* : a synthetic antibacterial drug $C_{14}H_{18}N_4O_3$ used alone esp. to treat urinary tract infections and Pneumocystis carinii pneumonia and in combination with sulfamethoxazole to treat these as well as other infections (as shigellosis or acute otitis media) — see BACTRIM, SEPTRA

tri·me·trex·ate \ˌtrī-mi-'trek-ˌsāt\ *n* : a toxic drug structurally related to methotrexate that is administered intravenously in the form of its salt $C_{19}H_{23}N_5O_3 \cdot C_6H_{10}O_7$ with concurrent administration of leucovorin to reduce toxicity and is used esp. in the treatment of Pneumocystis carinii pneumonia and certain carcinomas

Tri·mox \'trī-ˌmäks\ *trademark* — used for a preparation of amoxicillin

tri·ni·tro·phe·nol \(ˌ)trī-ˌnī-trō-'fē-ˌnōl, -ˌnōl, -fi-'nōl\ *or* **2,4,6–trinitrophenol** \ˌtü-ˌfōr-ˌsiks-\ *n* : PICRIC ACID

tri·no·mi·al \trī-'nō-mē-əl\ *n* : a biological taxonomic name of three terms of which the first designates the genus, the second the species, and the third the subspecies or variety

tri·nu·cle·o·tide \(ˌ)trī-'nü-klē-ə-ˌtīd, -'nyü-\ *n* : a nucleotide consisting of three mononucleotides in combination : CODON

tri·or·tho·cre·syl phosphate \ˌtrī-ˌor-thō-ˌkre-səl-, -ˌkrē-\ *n* : a usu. colorless, odorless, tasteless neurotoxin $C_{21}H_{21}O_2P$

trioxsalen • Trobicin 782

tri·ox·sa·len \ˌtrī-ˈäk-sə-lən\ *n* : a synthetic psoralen $C_{14}H_{12}O_3$ that promotes tanning of the skin

tri·par·a·nol \trī-ˈpar-ə-ˌnȯl, -ˌnōl\ *n* : a drug $C_{27}H_{32}ClNO_2$ formerly used to inhibit the formation of cholesterol but now withdrawn from use because of its links to numerous toxic side effects

tri·pel·en·na·mine \ˌtrī-pe-ˈlnə-ˌmēn, -mən\ *n* : an antihistamine drug used in the form of its citrate $C_{16}H_{21}N_3 \cdot C_6H_8O_7$ or hydrochloride $C_{16}H_{21}N_3 \cdot HCl$

tri·pep·tide \(ˌ)trī-ˈpep-ˌtīd\ *n* : a peptide that yields three amino acid residues on hydrolysis

tri·phen·yl·meth·ane \ˌtrī-ˌfen-əl-ˈme-ˌthān, -ˌfēn-\ *n* : a crystalline hydrocarbon $CH(C_6H_5)_3$ from which various dyes are derived

tri·phos·pha·tase \(ˌ)trī-ˈfäs-fə-ˌtās, -ˌtāz\ *n* : an enzyme that catalyzes hydrolysis of a triphosphate — see ATPASE

tri·phos·phate \(ˌ)trī-ˈfäs-ˌfāt\ *n* : a salt or acid that contains three phosphate groups — see ATP, GTP

tri·phos·pho·pyr·i·dine nucleotide \ˌtrī-ˌfäs-fō-ˈpir-ə-ˌdēn-\ *n* : NADP

triple bond *n* : a chemical bond in which three pairs of electrons are shared by two atoms in a molecule and which is usu. represented in chemical formulas by three lines

triple E *n* : EASTERN EQUINE ENCEPHALITIS

tri·ple·gia \(ˌ)trī-ˈplē-jə, -jē-ə\ *n* : hemiplegia plus paralysis of a limb on the opposite side

triple point *n* : the condition of temperature and pressure under which the gaseous, liquid, and solid phases of a substance can exist in equilibrium

triple screen *n* : a blood test for pregnant women for alpha-fetoprotein, human chorionic gonadotropin, and estriol in order to assess the risk of fetal abnormality (as Down syndrome, anencephaly, and spina bifida) — called also *triple test*

trip·let \ˈtri-plət\ *n* **1 a** : a combination, set, or group of three **b** : CODON **2 a** : one of three children or offspring born at one birth **b** triplets *pl* : a group of three offspring born at one birth

¹trip·loid \ˈtri-ˌplȯid\ *adj* : having or being a chromosome number three times the monoploid number — **trip·loi·dy** \-ˌplȯi-dē\ *n*

²triploid *n* : a triploid individual

trip·tan \ˈtrip-ˌtan, -tən\ *n* : any of a class of drugs (as sumatriptan) that bind to and are agonists of serotonin receptors and are used to treat migraine attacks

tri·que·tral bone \trī-ˈkwē-trel-\ *n* : the bone in the proximal row of the carpus that is third counting from the thumb side of the wrist, has a pyramidal shape, and is situated between the

lunate and pisiform bones — called also *triangular, triangular bone, triangularis, triquetral*

tri·que·trum \trī-ˈkwē-trəm\ *n, pl* **tri·que·tra** \-trə\ : TRIQUETRAL BONE

tris \ˈtris\ *n, often cap* : a white crystalline powder $C_4H_{11}NO_3$ used as a buffer (as in the treatment of acidosis) — called also *tris buffer, tromethamine*

tri·sac·cha·ride \(ˌ)trī-ˈsa-kə-ˌrīd\ *n* : a sugar that yields on complete hydrolysis three monosaccharide molecules

tris·kai·deka·pho·bia \ˌtris-ˌkī-ˌde-kə-ˈfō-bē-ə, ˌtris-kə-\ *n* : fear of the number 13

tris·mus \ˈtriz-məs\ *n* : spasm of the muscles of mastication resulting from any of various abnormal conditions or diseases (as tetanus)

¹tri·so·mic \(ˌ)trī-ˈsō-mik\ *adj* : relating to, caused by, or characterized by trisomy ⟨~ cells⟩

²trisomic *n* : a trisomic individual

tri·so·my \ˈtrī-ˌsō-mē\ *n, pl* **-mies** : the condition (as in Down syndrome) of having one or a few chromosomes triploid in an otherwise diploid set

trisomy 18 *n* : a congenital condition that is characterized esp. by mental retardation and by craniofacial, cardiac, gastrointestinal, and genitourinary abnormalities, is caused by trisomy of the human chromosome numbered 18, and is typically fatal esp. within the first year of life — called also *Edwards syndrome*

trisomy 13 *n* : a congenital condition that is characterized esp. by usu. severe mental retardation and by craniofacial, cardiac, ocular, and cerebral abnormalities, is caused by trisomy of the human chromosome numbered 13, and is typically fatal esp. within the first six months of life — called also *Patau syndrome*

trisomy 21 *n* : DOWN SYNDROME

¹trit·an·ope \ˈtrīt-ᵊn-ˌōp, ˈtrit-\ *n* : an individual affected with tritanopia

trit·an·opia \ˌtrīt-ᵊn-ˈō-pē-ə, ˌtrit-\ *n* : dichromatism in which the spectrum is seen in tones of red and green — **trit·an·opic** \ˌtrīt-ᵊn-ˈō-pik, ˌtrit-ᵊn-ˈä-\ *adj*

tri·ti·um \ˈtri-tē-əm, -shəm, -shē-əm\ *n* : a radioactive isotope of hydrogen that has three times the mass of ordinary hydrogen — symbol T

¹trit·u·rate \ˈtri-chə-ˌrāt\ *vb* **-rat·ed; -rat·ing** : to pulverize thoroughly by rubbing or grinding — **trit·u·ra·tion** \ˌtri-chə-ˈrā-shən\ *n*

²trit·u·rate \-rət\ *n* : a triturated substance

tri·va·lent \(ˌ)trī-ˈvā-lənt\ *adj* : conferring immunity to three different pathogenic strains or species ⟨a ~ influenza vaccine⟩

tRNA \ˌtē-ˌär-ˌen-ˈā\ *n* : TRANSFER RNA

Tro·bi·cin \trō-ˈbīs-ᵊn\ *trademark* — used for a preparation of the hydrated dihydrochloride of spectinomycin

tro·car *also* **tro·char** \'trō-ˌkär\ *n* : a sharp-pointed surgical instrument fitted with a cannula and used esp. to insert the cannula into a body cavity as a drainage outlet

tro·chan·ter \trō-'kan-tər\ *n* : a rough prominence or process at the upper part of the femur serving usu. for the attachment of muscles and being usu. two on each femur: **a** : a larger one situated on the outer part of the upper end of the shaft at its junction with the neck — called also *greater trochanter* **b** : a smaller one situated at the lower back part of the junction of the shaft and neck — called also *lesser trochanter* — **tro·chan·ter·ic** \ˌtrō-kən-'ter-ik, -ˌkan-\ *adj*

trochanteric fossa *n* : a depression at the base of the internal surface of the greater trochanter of the femur for the attachment of the tendon of the obturator externus

tro·che \'trō-kē\ *n* : LOZENGE

troch·lea \'trä-klē-ə\ *n* : an anatomical structure resembling a pulley: as **a** : the articular surface on the medial condyle of the humerus that articulates with the ulna **b** : the fibrous ring in the inner upper part of the orbit through which the tendon of the superior oblique muscle of the eye passes

troch·le·ar \-ər\ *adj* **1** : of, relating to, or being a trochlea **2** : of, relating to, or being a trochlear nerve ⟨~ fibers⟩

trochlear fovea *n* : a depression located in the orbital surface of each bony plate of the frontal bone and forming a point of attachment for the superior oblique muscle of the eye

trochlear nerve *n* : either of the fourth pair of cranial nerves that arise from the dorsal aspect of the brainstem just below the inferior colliculus and supply the superior oblique muscle of the eye with motor fibers

trochlear notch *n* : the deep depression in the proximal end of the ulna by which the ulna articulates with the trochlea of the humerus at the elbow — called also *semilunar notch, sigmoid notch*

trochlear nucleus *n* : a nucleus that is situated behind the oculomotor nucleus and is the source of the motor fibers of the trochlear nerve

tro·choid \'trō-ˌkȯid\ *n* : PIVOT JOINT

tro·glit·a·zone \trō-'gli-tə-ˌzōn\ *n* : a drug $C_{24}H_{27}NO_5S$ formerly used to treat type 2 diabetes but now withdrawn from use because of its link to serious hepatic reactions

tro·land \'trō-lənd\ *n* : PHOTON 1

Troland, Leonard Thompson (1889–1932), American psychologist and physicist.

tro·le·an·do·my·cin \ˌtrō-lē-ˌan-də-'mīs-ᵊn\ *n* : an antibacterial drug $C_{41}H_{67}NO_{15}$ used chiefly against bacteria of the genus *Streptococcus* (esp. *S. pneumoniae* and *S. pyogenes*) — called also *triacetyloleandomycin*

trol·ley *also* **trol·ly** \'trä-lē\ *n, pl* **trolleys** *also* **trollies** *Brit* : GURNEY

trol·ni·trate \ˌträl-'nī-ˌtrāt\ *n* : an organic nitrate with vasodilator activity that is used in the form of its diphosphate salt $C_6H_{12}N_4O_9 \cdot 2H_3PO_4$ to prevent attacks of angina pectoris

Trom·bic·u·la \träm-'bi-kyə-lə\ *n* : a genus of mites (family Trombiculidae) including some forms that in Asia transmit scrub typhus

tro·meth·a·mine \trō-'me-thə-ˌmēn\ *n* : TRIS

troph- *or* **tropho-** *comb form* : nutritive ⟨*tropho*blast⟩

troph·ec·to·derm \ˌtrō-'fek-tə-ˌdərm\ *n* : TROPHOBLAST; *esp* : the outer layer of the blastocyst after differentiation of the ectoderm, mesoderm, and endoderm when the outer layer is continuous with the embryonic ectoderm

tro·phic \'trō-fik\ *adj* **1** : of or relating to nutrition : NUTRITIONAL ⟨~ disorders⟩ **2** : TROPIC **3** : promoting cellular growth, differentiation, and survival — **tro·phi·cal·ly** *adv*

-tro·phic \'trō-fik\ *adj comb form* **1** : of, relating to, or characterized by (such) nutrition or growth ⟨hyper*trophic*⟩ **2** : -TROPIC ⟨gonado*trophic*⟩

trophic ulcer *n* : an ulcer (as a bedsore) caused by faulty nutrition in the affected part

tro·pho·blast \'trō-fə-ˌblast\ *n* : the outer layer of the blastocyst that supplies nutrition to the embryo, facilitates implantation by eroding away the tissues of the uterus with which it comes in contact, and differentiates into the extraembryonic membranes surrounding the embryo — called also *trophoderm* — **tro·pho·blas·tic** \ˌtrō-fə-'blas-tik\ *adj*

troph·o·derm \'trō-fə-ˌdərm\ *n* : TROPHOBLAST

tro·pho·zo·ite \ˌtrō-fə-'zō-ˌīt\ *n* : a protozoan of a vegetative form as distinguished from one of a reproductive or resting form

-tro·phy \trə-fē\ *n comb form, pl* **-trophies** : nutrition : nurture : growth ⟨hypo*trophy*⟩

tro·pia \'trō-pē-ə\ *n* : deviation of an eye from the normal position with respect to the line of vision when the eyes are open : STRABISMUS — see ESOTROPIA, HYPERTROPIA

tro·pic \'trō-pik\ *adj* **1** : of, relating to, or characteristic of tropism or of a tropism **2** *of a hormone* : influencing the activity of a specified gland

-tro·pic \'trō-pik\ *adj comb form* : attracted to or acting upon (something specified) ⟨neuro*tropic*⟩

tropical medicine *n* : a branch of medicine dealing with tropical diseases and other medical problems of tropical regions

tropical oil *n* : any of several oils (as coconut oil) that are high in saturated fatty acids

tropical sprue *n* : SPRUE 2

tropical ulcer *n* : a chronic sloughing sore of unknown cause occurring usu. on the legs and prevalent in wet tropical regions

tro·pic·amide \trə-'pi-kə-ˌmīd\ *n* : a synthetic anticholinergic $C_{17}H_{20}N_2O_2$ used esp. to dilate pupils in ophthalmological examinations — see MYDRIACYL

-tro·pin \'trō-pən\ *or* **-tro·phin** \-fən\ *n comb form* : hormone ⟨lipo*tropin*⟩

tro·pism \'trō-ˌpi-zəm\ *n* : involuntary orientation by an organism or one of its parts (as by differential growth) toward or away from a source of stimulation; *also* : a reflex reaction involving a tropism

tro·po·col·la·gen \ˌträ-pə-'kä-lə-jən, ˌtrō-\ *n* : a subunit of collagen fibrils consisting of three polypeptide strands arranged in a helix

tro·po·my·o·sin \ˌträ-pə-'mī-ə-sən, ˌtrō-\ *n* : a protein of muscle that forms a complex with troponin regulating the interaction of actin and myosin in muscular contraction

tro·po·nin \'trō-pə-nən, 'trä-, -ˌnin\ *n* : a protein of muscle that together with tropomyosin forms a regulatory protein complex controlling the interaction of actin and myosin and that when combined with calcium ions permits muscular contraction

trough — see GINGIVAL TROUGH

troy \'troi\ *adj* : expressed in troy weight ⟨a ∼ ounce⟩

troy weight *n* : a series of units of weight based on a pound of 12 ounces and an ounce of 480 grains or 31.103 grams

Trp *abbr* tryptophan

true bug \'trü-\ *n* : BUG 1c

true conjugate *n* : CONJUGATE DIAMETER

true pelvis *n* : the lower more contracted part of the pelvic cavity — called also *true pelvic cavity;* compare FALSE PELVIS

true rib *n* : any of the ribs having costal cartilages connected directly with the sternum and in humans constituting the first seven pairs — called also *vertebrosternal rib*

true vocal cords *n pl* : the lower pair of vocal cords each of which encloses a vocal ligament, extends from the inner surface of one side of the thyroid cartilage near the median line to a process of the corresponding arytenoid cartilage on the same side of the larynx, and when drawn taut, approximated to the contralateral member of the pair, and subjected to a flow of breath produces the voice — called also *inferior vocal cords, vocal folds*

trun·cal \'trəŋ-kəl\ *adj* : of or relating to the trunk of the body or of a bodily part (as a nerve) ⟨∼ obesity⟩

trun·cus \'trəŋ-kəs\ *n* : TRUNK 2

truncus bra·chio·ce·phal·i·cus \-ˌbrä-kē-(ˌ)ō-se-'fa-li-kəs\ *n* : BRACHIOCEPHALIC ARTERY

truncus ce·li·a·cus \-se-'lī-ə-kəs\ *n* : CELIAC ARTERY

trunk \'trəŋk\ *n* **1** : the human body apart from the head and appendages : TORSO **2** : the main body of an anatomical part (as a nerve or blood vessel) that divides into branches

truss \'trəs\ *n* : a device worn to reduce a hernia by pressure

truth serum *n* : a hypnotic or anesthetic (as thiopental) held to induce a subject under questioning to talk freely

trypan- *or* **trypano-** *comb form* : trypanosome ⟨*trypano*cidal⟩

try·pano·ci·dal \tri-ˌpa-nə-'sīd-əl\ *adj* : destroying trypanosomes ⟨a ∼ drug⟩ — **try·pano·cide** \tri-'pa-nə-ˌsīd\ *n*

try·pano·so·ma \tri-ˌpa-nə-'sō-mə\ *n* **1** *cap* : a genus of parasitic flagellate protozoans (family Trypanosomatidae) that infest the blood of various vertebrates including humans, are usu. transmitted by the bite of an insect, and include some that cause serious diseases (as Chagas' disease, African sleeping sickness, and surra) **2** *pl* **-mas** *or* **-ma·ta** \-mə-tə\ : TRYPANOSOME

try·pano·some \tri-'pa-nə-ˌsōm\ *n* : any flagellate of the genus *Trypanosoma* — **try·pano·so·mal** \-ˌpa-nə-'sō-məl\ *adj*

try·pano·so·mi·a·sis \tri-ˌpa-nə-sə-'mī-ə-səs\ *n, pl* **-a·ses** \-ˌsēz\ : infection with or disease caused by flagellates of the genus *Trypanosoma*

tryp·ars·amide \tri-'pär-sə-ˌmīd\ *n* : an arsenical $C_8H_{10}AsN_2O_4Na \cdot \frac{1}{2}H_2O$ used esp. formerly to treat African sleeping sickness and syphilis

tryp·sin \'trip-sən\ *n* **1** : a crystallizable proteolytic enzyme that is produced and secreted in the pancreatic juice in the form of inactive trypsinogen and activated in the intestine — compare CHYMOTRYPSIN **2** : a preparation from the pancreatic juice containing principally proteolytic enzymes and used chiefly as a digestive and lytic agent

tryp·sin·ize \'trip-sə-ˌnīz\ *vb* **-ized; -iz·ing** : to subject to the action of trypsin ⟨*trypsinized* tissue cells⟩ — **tryp·sin·i·za·tion** \ˌtrip-sə-nə-'zā-shən\ *n*

tryp·sin·o·gen \trip-'si-nə-jən\ *n* : the inactive substance released by the pancreas into the duodenum to form trypsin

tryp·tase \'trip-ˌtās, -ˌtāz\ *n* : a protease of human mast cells that has been implicated as a pathological mediator of numerous allergic and inflammatory conditions (as asthma, rhinitis, and conjunctivitis)

tryp·tic \'trip-tik\ *adj* : of, relating to, or produced by trypsin or its action

tryp·to·phan \'trip-tə-ˌfan\ *also* **tryp·to·phane** \-ˌfān\ *n* : a crystalline essential amino acid $C_{11}H_{12}N_2O_2$ that is widely distributed in proteins — abbr. *Trp*

L–tryptophan — see entry alphabetized in the letter *l*

TS *abbr* Tourette's syndrome; Tourette syndrome

TSE *abbr* transmissible spongiform encephalopathy

tset·se \'tset-sē, 'tsēt-, 'tet-, 'tēt-\ *n, pl* **tsetse** *or* **tsetses** : TSETSE FLY

tsetse fly *n* : any of several dipteran flies of the genus *Glossina* that occur in sub-Saharan Africa and include vectors of human and animal trypanosomes (as those causing sleeping sickness) — called also *tsetse*

TSH \ˌtē-ˌ(ˌ)es-'āch\ *n* : THYROID-STIM-ULATING HORMONE

TSS *abbr* toxic shock syndrome

T suppressor cell *n* : SUPPRESSOR T CELL

tsu·tsu·ga·mu·shi disease \ˌtsüt-sə-gə-'mü-shē-, ˌtüt-, ˌsüt-, -'gä-mü-shē-\ *n* : SCRUB TYPHUS

T system *n* : the system of T tubules in striated muscle

T3 *or* **T₃** \ˌtē-'thrē\ *n* : TRIIODOTHYRO-NINE

TTP \ˌtē-ˌtē-'pē\ *n* : THROMBOTIC THROMBOCYTOPENIC PURPURA

T–tube *n* : a narrow flexible tube in the form of a T that is used for drainage esp. of the common bile duct

T tubule *n* : any of the small tubules which run transversely through a striated muscle fiber and through which electrical impulses are transmitted from the sarcoplasm to the fiber's interior

tub·al \'tü-bəl, 'tyü-\ *adj* : of, relating to, or involving a tube and esp. a fallopian tube ⟨a ∼ infection⟩

tubal abortion *n* : an aborted tubal pregnancy

tubal ligation *n* : ligation of the fallopian tubes that by preventing passage of ova from the ovaries to the uterus serves as a method of female sterilization

tubal pregnancy *n* : ectopic pregnancy in a fallopian tube

tubarius — see TORUS TUBARIUS

¹tube \'tüb, 'tyüb\ *n* **1** : a slender channel within a plant or animal body : DUCT — see BRONCHIAL TUBE, EUSTACHIAN TUBE, FALLOPIAN TUBE **2 a** : a piece of laboratory or technical apparatus usu. serving to isolate or convey a product of reaction **b** : TEST TUBE **3** : a hollow cylindrical device (as a cannula) used for insertion into bodily passages or hollow organs for removal or injection of materials

²tube *vb* **tubed; tub·ing** : to furnish with, enclose in, or pass through a tube

tubed *adj* : having the sides sewn together so as to form a tube

tuberalis — see PARS TUBERALIS

tu·ber ci·ne·re·um \'tü-bər-si-'nir-ē-əm, 'tyü-\ *n* : an eminence of gray matter which lies on the lower surface of the brain of which the upper surface forms part of the floor of the third ventricle and the lower surface bears the infundibulum to which the pituitary gland is attached

tu·ber·cle \'tü-bər-kəl, 'tyü-\ *n* **1** : a small knobby prominence or excrescence: as **a** : a prominence on the crown of a molar tooth **b** : a small rough prominence (as the greater tubercle or adductor tubercle) on a bone usu. being smaller than a tuberosity and serving for the attachment of one or more muscles or ligaments **c** : an eminence near the head of a rib that articulates with the transverse process of a vertebra **d** : any of several prominences (as the acoustic tubercle) in the central nervous system that mark the nuclei of various nerves **2** : a small discrete lump in the substance of an organ or in the skin; *esp* : the specific lesion of tuberculosis consisting of a packed mass of epithelioid cells, giant cells, disintegration products of white blood cells and bacilli, and usu. a necrotic center

tubercle bacillus *n* : a bacterium of the genus *Mycobacterium* (*M. tuberculosis*) that is a causative agent of tuberculosis; *also* : a related mycobacterium (*M. bovis*) that causes tuberculosis in cattle and sometimes humans esp. in underdeveloped countries

tubercul- *or* **tuberculo-** *comb form* **1** : tubercle ⟨*tubercular*⟩ **2** : tubercle bacillus ⟨*tuberculin*⟩ **3** : tuberculosis ⟨*tuberculoid*⟩

¹tu·ber·cu·lar \tù-'bər-kyə-lər, tyü-\ *adj* **1 a** : of, relating to, or affected with tuberculosis : TUBERCULOUS **b** : caused by the tubercle bacillus ⟨∼ meningitis⟩ **2** : characterized by lesions that are or resemble tubercles ⟨∼ leprosy⟩ **3** : relating to, resembling, or constituting a tubercle

²tubercular *n* : an individual affected with tuberculosis

tu·ber·cu·lid \tù-'bər-kyə-lid, tyü-\ *n* : a tuberculous lesion of the skin; *esp* : one that is an id

tu·ber·cu·lin \tù-'bər-kyə-lən, tyü-\ *n* : a sterile solution containing the growth products of or specific substances extracted from the tubercle bacillus and used in the diagnosis of tuberculosis — see PURIFIED PROTEIN DERIVATIVE

tuberculin reaction *n* : a skin reaction that occurs at the site of a tuberculin test

tuberculin test *n* : a test (as the Mantoux test or tine test) for hypersensitivity to tuberculin in which tuberculin is introduced (as by injection) usu.

into the skin of the individual tested and the appearance of inflammation or induration at the site of introduction is construed as indicating past or present tubercular infection — called also *tuberculin skin test*

tu·ber·cu·loid \tü-ˈbər-kyə-ˌlȯid, tyü-\ *adj* **1** : resembling tuberculosis and esp. the tubercles characteristic of it **2** : of, relating to, characterized by, or affected with tuberculoid leprosy

tuberculoid leprosy *n* : the one of the two major forms of leprosy that is characterized by the presence of few or no Hansen's bacilli in the lesions and by the loss of sensation in affected areas of the skin — compare LEPROMATOUS LEPROSY

tu·ber·cu·lo·ma \tü-ˌbər-kyə-ˈlō-mə, tyü-\ *n, pl* **-mas** \-məz\ *also* **-ma·ta** \-mə-tə\ : a large solitary caseous tubercle of tuberculous character occurring esp. in the brain

tu·ber·cu·lo·sis \tü-ˌbər-kyə-ˈlō-səs, tyü-\ *n, pl* **-lo·ses** \-ˌsēz\ : a usu. chronic highly variable disease that is caused by a bacterium of the genus *Mycobacterium* (*Mycobacterium tuberculosis*) and rarely in the U.S. by a related mycobacterium (*M. bovis*), is usu. communicated by inhalation of the airborne causative agent, affects esp. the lungs but may spread to other areas (as the kidney or spinal column) from local lesions or by way of the lymph or blood vessels, and is characterized by fever, cough, difficulty in breathing, inflammatory infiltrations, formation of tubercles, caseation, pleural effusion, and fibrosis — called also *TB*

¹tu·ber·cu·lo·stat·ic \tü-ˌbər-kyə-lō-ˈsta-tik, tyü-\ *adj* : inhibiting the growth of the tubercle bacillus

²tuberculostatic *n* : a tuberculostatic agent

tu·ber·cu·lous \tü-ˈbər-kyə-ləs, tyü-\ *adj* **1** : constituting or affected with tuberculosis **2** : caused by or resulting from the presence or products of the tubercle bacillus ⟨~ peritonitis⟩

tu·ber·os·i·ty \ˌtü-bə-ˈrä-sə-tē, ˌtyü-\ *n, pl* **-ties** : a rounded prominence; *esp* : a large prominence on a bone usu. serving for the attachment of muscles or ligaments ⟨ischial *tuberosities*⟩

tuberous sclerosis *n* : a genetic disorder of the skin and nervous system that is typically characterized by epilepsy and mental retardation, by a facial rash resembling acne, and by multiple hamartomas of the brain, kidney, retina, skin, and heart and that is inherited as an autosomal dominant trait or results from spontaneous mutation — called also *epiloia*

tu·bo·cu·ra·rine \ˌtü-bō-kyü-ˈrär-ən, -ˌēn, ˌtyü-\ *n* : a toxic alkaloid that is obtained chiefly from the bark and stems of a So. American vine (*Chondrodendron tomentosum* of the family Menispermaceae), that in its dextro-

rotatory form constitutes the chief active constituent of curare, and that is used in the form of its hydrated hydrochloride $C_{37}H_{41}ClN_2O_6 \cdot HCl \cdot 5H_2O$ esp. as a skeletal muscle relaxant

tu·bo–ovar·i·an \ˌtü-bō-ō-ˈvar-ē-ən, ˌtyü-\ *adj* : of, relating to, or affecting a fallopian tube and ovary

tu·bu·lar \ˈtü-byə-lər, ˈtyü-\ *adj* **1** : having the form of or consisting of a tube **2** : of, relating to, or sounding as if produced through a tube or tubule

tu·bule \ˈtü-(ˌ)byül, ˈtyü-\ *n* : a small tube; *esp* : a slender elongated anatomical channel

tu·bu·lin \ˈtü-byə-lən, ˈtyü-\ *n* : a globular protein that polymerizes to form microtubules

tu·bu·lo·ac·i·nar \ˌtü-byə-lō-ˈa-sə-nər, ˌtyü-\ *or* **tu·bu·lo·ac·i·nous** \-nəs\ *adj* : TUBULOALVEOLAR

tu·bu·lo·al·ve·o·lar \ˌtü-byə-lō-al-ˈvē-ə-lər, ˌtyü-\ *adj* : of, relating to, or being a gland having branching tubules which end in secretory alveoli

tu·bu·lo·in·ter·sti·tial \ˌtü-byə-lō-ˌin-tər-ˈsti-shəl, ˌtyü-\ *adj* : affecting or involving the tubules and interstitial tissue of the kidney ⟨~ disease⟩

tu·bu·lus \ˈtü-byə-ləs, ˈtyü-\ *n, pl* **tu·bu·li** \-ˌlī\ : TUBULE

tuck \ˈtək\ *n* : a cosmetic surgical operation for the removal of excess skin or fat from a body part — see TUMMY TUCK

Tu·i·nal \ˈtü-i-ˌnäl\ *trademark* — used for a preparation of amobarbital and secobarbital

tu·lar·ae·mia *chiefly Brit var of* TULAREMIA

tu·la·re·mia \ˌtü-lə-ˈrē-mē-ə, ˌtyü-\ *n* : an infectious disease esp. of wild rabbits, rodents, some domestic animals, and humans that is caused by a bacterium (*Francisella tularensis*), is transmitted esp. by the bites of insects, and in humans is marked by symptoms (as fever) of toxemia — called also *rabbit fever* — **tu·la·re·mic** \-mik\ *adj*

tulle gras \ˌtül-ˈgrä\ *n* : fine-meshed gauze impregnated with a fatty substance (as soft paraffin)

tu·me·fa·cient \ˌtü-mə-ˈfā-shənt, ˌtyü-\ *adj* : producing swelling

tu·me·fac·tion \-ˈfak-shən\ *n* **1** : an action or process of swelling or becoming tumorous **2** : SWELLING

tu·me·fac·tive \-ˈfak-tiv\ *adj* : producing swelling ⟨~ lesions⟩

tu·mes·cence \tü-ˈmes-ᵊns, tyü-\ *n* : the quality or state of being tumescent; *esp* : readiness for sexual activity marked esp. by vascular congestion of the sex organs

tu·mes·cent \-ˈmes-ᵊnt\ *adj* : somewhat swollen ⟨~ tissue⟩

tummy tuck *n* : ABDOMINOPLASTY

tu·mor \ˈtü-mər, ˈtyü-\ *n* : an abnormal benign or malignant new growth of tissue that possesses no physiological function and arises from uncontrolled usu. rapid cellular proliferation — see CANCER 1, CARCINOMA, SARCOMA — **tu·mor·al** \'tü-mə-rəl\ *adj* — **tu·mor·like** \-ˌlīk\ *adj*

tu·mor·i·cid·al \ˌtü-mə-rə-'sīd-ᵊl, ˌtyü-\ *adj* : destroying tumor cells

tu·mor·i·gen·ic \-'je-nik\ *adj* : producing or tending to produce tumors; *also* : CARCINOGENIC — **tu·mor·i·gen·e·sis** \-ˈje-nə-səs\ *n* — **tu·mor·i·ge·nic·i·ty** \-jə-'ni-sə-tē\ *n*

tumor–infiltrating lymphocyte *n* : a T cell that infiltrates a malignant tumor and when cultured with interleukin-2 in adoptive immunotherapy possesses greater cytotoxicity than a lymphokine-activated killer cell — called also *TIL*

tumor necrosis factor *n* : a protein that is produced chiefly by monocytes and macrophages in response esp. to endotoxins, that mediates inflammation, and that induces the destruction of some tumor cells and the activation of white blood cells — abbr. *TNF*

tumor suppressor gene *n* : any of a class of genes (as p53) that act in normal cells to inhibit unrestrained cell division and that when inactivated (as by mutation) place the cell at increased risk for malignant proliferation — called also *anti-oncogene*

tu·mor·ous \'tü-mə-rəs, 'tyü-\ *adj* : of, relating to, or resembling a tumor

tumor virus *n* : a virus (as Rous sarcoma virus) that causes neoplastic or cancerous growth

tu·mour *chiefly Brit var of* TUMOR

Tums \'təmz\ *trademark* — used for a preparation of calcium carbonate

Tun·ga \'təŋ-gə\ *n* : a genus of fleas (family Tungidae) that include the chigoe (*T. penetrans*)

tung·sten \'təŋ-stən\ *n* : a gray-white high-melting ductile metallic element — symbol *W*; called also *wolfram*; see ELEMENT table

tu·nic \'tü-nik, 'tyü-\ *n* : an enclosing or covering membrane or tissue : TUNICA ⟨the ∼*s* of the eye⟩

tu·ni·ca \'tü-ni-kə, 'tyü-\ *n, pl* **tu·ni·cae** \-nə-ˌkē, -ˌkī, -ˌsē\ : an enveloping membrane or layer of body tissue

tunica adventitia *n* : ADVENTITIA

tunica al·bu·gin·ea \-ˌal-bù-'ji-nē-ə, -byù-\ *n, pl* **tunicae al·bu·gin·e·ae** \-'ji-nē-ˌē, -ˌī\ : a white fibrous capsule esp. of the testis

tunica intima *n* : INTIMA

tunica media *n* : MEDIA

tunica mucosa *n* : mucous membrane and esp. that lining the digestive tract

tunica muscularis *n* : MUSCULAR COAT

tunica pro·pria \-'prō-prē-ə\ *n* : LAMINA PROPRIA

tunica va·gi·na·lis \-ˌva-jə-'nā-ləs, -'na-\ *n, pl* **tunicae va·gi·na·les** \-(ˌ)lez\ : a pouch of serous membrane covering the testis and derived from the peritoneum

tuning fork *n* : a 2-pronged metal implement that gives a fixed tone when struck

tun·nel \'tən-ᵊl\ *n* : a bodily channel — see CARPAL TUNNEL

tunnel of Cor·ti \-'kór-tē\ *n* : a spiral passage in the organ of Corti

tunnel vision *n* : constriction of the visual field resulting in loss of peripheral vision

tur·bel·lar·i·an \ˌtər-bə-'lar-ē-ən\ *n* : any of a class (Turbellaria) of mostly aquatic and free-living flatworms — **turbellarian** *adj*

tur·bid \'tər-bəd\ *adj* : thick or opaque with matter in suspension : cloudy or muddy in appearance ⟨∼ urine⟩ — **tur·bid·i·ty** \ˌtər-'bi-də-tē\ *n*

tur·bi·dim·e·ter \ˌtər-bə-'di-mə-tər\ *n* 1 : an instrument for measuring and comparing the turbidity of liquids by viewing light through them and determining how much light is transmitted 2 : NEPHELOMETER — **tur·bi·di·met·ric** \ˌtər-bə-də-'me-trik, ˌtər-ˌbi-\ *adj* — **tur·bi·dim·e·try** \ˌtər-bə-'di-mə-trē\ *n*

¹tur·bi·nate \'tər-bə-nət, -ˌnāt\ *adj* : of, relating to, or being a nasal concha

²turbinate *n* : NASAL CONCHA

turbinate bone *also* **tur·bi·nat·ed bone** \'tər-bə-ˌnā-təd-\ *n* : NASAL CONCHA

turcica — see SELLA TURCICA

turf toe *n* : a minor but painful usu. sports-related injury involving hyperextension of the big toe that results in spraining or tearing of the ligament of the metatarsophalangeal joint

tur·ges·cent \ˌtər-'jes-ᵊnt\ *adj* : becoming turgid, distended, or swollen — **tur·ges·cence** \-'jes-ᵊns\ *n*

tur·gid \'tər-jəd\ *adj* : being in a normal or abnormal state of distension : SWOLLEN ⟨∼ limbs⟩ ⟨∼ living cells⟩ — **tur·gid·i·ty** \ˌtər-'ji-də-tē\ *n*

tur·gor \'tər-gər, -ˌgór\ *n* : the normal state of turgidity and tension in living cells

tu·ris·ta \tù-'rē-stə\ *n* : TRAVELER'S DIARRHEA

turn \'tərn\ *vb* : to injure by twisting or wrenching ⟨∼*ed* his ankle⟩

Tur·ner's syndrome \'tər-nərz-\ *or* **Tur·ner syndrome** \-nər-\ *n* : a genetically determined condition that is typically associated with the presence of only one complete X chromosome and no Y chromosome and is characterized esp. by a female phenotype, underdeveloped and usu. infertile ovaries, absence of menstrual onset, and short stature

Turner, Henry Hubert (1892–1970), American endocrinologist.

turn·over \'tərn-ˌō-vər\ *n* : the continuous process of loss and replacement of a constituent (as a neurotransmitter, cell, or tissue) of a living system

tur·ri·ceph·a·ly \ˌtər-ə-'se-fə-lē\ *n, pl* **-lies** : OXYCEPHALY

tus·sive \'tə-siv\ *adj* : of, relating to, or involved in coughing ⟨∼ force⟩

T wave \'tē-,wāv\ *n* : the deflection in an electrocardiogram that represents the electrical activity produced by ventricular repolarization — compare P WAVE, QRS COMPLEX

Tween \'twēn\ *trademark* — used for any of several preparations of polysorbates

twee·zers \'twē-zərz\ *n sing or pl* : any of various small metal instruments that are usu. held between the thumb and index finger, are used for plucking, holding, or manipulating, and consist of two legs joined at one end

twelfth cranial nerve *n* : HYPOGLOSSAL NERVE

12–step \'twelv-,step\ *adj* : of, relating to, or characteristic of a program that is designed esp. to help an individual overcome an addiction, compulsion, serious shortcoming, or traumatic experience by adherence to 12 tenets emphasizing personal growth and dependence on a higher spiritual being

twelve–year molar *n* : any of the second permanent molar teeth which erupt at about 12 years of age and include four of which one is located on each side of the upper and lower jaws — compare SIX-YEAR MOLAR

twenty–twenty *or* **20/20** *adj* : having the normal visual acuity of the human eye that according to some common scale can distinguish at a distance of 20 feet characters one-third inch in diameter ⟨∼ vision⟩

twig \'twig\ *n* : a minute branch of a nerve or artery

twi·light sleep \'twī-,līt-\ *n* : a state in which awareness of pain is dulled and memory of pain is dimmed or effaced and which is produced by hypodermic injection of morphine and scopolamine and used esp. formerly chiefly in childbirth

twilight state *n* : a dreamy state lacking touch with present reality, occurring in epilepsy, hysteria, and schizophrenia, and sometimes induced with narcotics

¹**twin** \'twin\ *adj* : born with one other or as a pair at one birth ⟨∼ girls⟩

²**twin** *n* **1** : either of two offspring produced at a birth **2 twins** *pl* : a group of two offspring born at one birth — **twin·ship** \-,ship\ *n*

twinge \'twinj\ *n* : a sudden sharp stab of pain

twin·ning \'twi-niŋ\ *n* : the bearing of twins

twitch \'twich\ *n* : a brief spasmodic contraction of muscle fibers; *also* : a slight jerk of a body part caused by such a contraction — **twitch** *vb*

two–egg *adj* : DIZYGOTIC ⟨∼ twins⟩

2,4–D \,tü-,fȯr-'dē\ *n* : a white crystalline irritant compound $C_8H_6Cl_2O_3$ used as a weed killer — called also *2,4-dichlorophenoxyacetic acid;* see AGENT ORANGE

2,4,5–T \-,fīv-'tē\ *n* : an irritant compound $C_8H_5Cl_3O_3$ used esp. formerly as a herbicide and defoliant — called also *trichlorophenoxyacetic acid;* see AGENT ORANGE

two–winged fly *n* : FLY 1

Tx *abbr* treatment

ty·ba·mate \'tī-bə-,māt\ *n* : a tranquilizing drug $C_{13}H_{26}N_2O_4$

ty·lec·to·my \tī-'lek-tə-mē\ *n, pl* **-mies** : LUMPECTOMY

Ty·le·nol \'tī-lə-,nȯl\ *trademark* — used for a preparation of acetaminophen

ty·lo·sin \'tī-lə-sən\ *n* : an antibacterial antibiotic $C_{45}H_{77}NO_{17}$ from an actinomycete of the genus *Streptomyces* (*S. fradiae*) used in veterinary medicine and as a feed additive

ty·lo·sis \tī-'lō-səs\ *n, pl* **ty·lo·ses** \-'lō-sēz\ : a thickening and hardening of the skin : CALLOSITY

tympani — see CHORDA TYMPANI, SCALA TYMPANI, TEGMEN TYMPANI, TENSOR TYMPANI

tym·pan·ic \tim-'pa-nik\ *adj* : of, relating to, or being a tympanum

tympanic antrum *n* : a large air-containing cavity in the mastoid process communicating with the tympanum and often being the location of dangerous inflammation — called also *mastoid antrum*

tympanic canal *n* : SCALA TYMPANI

tympanic cavity *n* : MIDDLE EAR

tympanic membrane *n* : a thin membrane separating the middle ear from the inner part of the external auditory canal that vibrates in response to sound waves and transmits the resulting mechanical vibrations to the ossicles of the middle ear — called also *eardrum, tympanum*

tympanic nerve *n* : a branch of the glossopharyngeal nerve arising from the petrosal ganglion and entering the middle ear where it takes part in forming the tympanic plexus — called also *Jacobson's nerve*

tympanic plate *n* : a curved platelike bone that is part of the temporal bone and forms the floor and anterior wall of the external auditory canal

tympanic plexus *n* : a nerve plexus of the middle ear that is formed by the tympanic nerve and two or three filaments from the carotid plexus, sends fibers to the mucous membranes of the middle ear, the eustachian tube, and the mastoid cells, and gives off the lesser petrosal nerve to the otic ganglion

tym·pa·ni·tes \,tim-pə-'nī-tēz\ *n* : a distension of the abdomen caused by accumulation of gas in the intestinal tract or peritoneal cavity

tym·pa·nit·ic \,tim-pə-'ni-tik\ *adj* **1** : of, relating to, or affected with tympanites ⟨a ∼ abdomen⟩ **2** : resonant on percussion : hollow-sounding

tym·pa·no·plas·ty \'tim-pə-nō-,plas-tē\ *n, pl* **-ties** : a reparative surgical operation performed on the middle ear

tym·pa·nos·to·my \ˌtim-pə-ˈnäs-tə-mē\ *n, pl* **-mies** : MYRINGOTOMY

tym·pa·not·o·my \ˌtim-pə-ˈnä-tə-mē\ *n, pl* **-mies** : MYRINGOTOMY

tym·pa·num \ˈtim-pə-nəm\ *n, pl* **-na** \-nə\ *also* **-nums 1** : TYMPANIC MEMBRANE **2** : MIDDLE EAR

tym·pa·ny \-nē\ *n, pl* **-nies 1** : TYMPANITES **2** : a resonant sound heard in percussion (as of the abdomen)

¹type \ˈtīp\ *n* : a particular kind, class, or group ⟨cell ∼*s*⟩; *specif* : a group distinguishable on physiological or serological bases ⟨salmonella ∼*s*⟩

²type *vb* **typed; typ·ing** : to determine the type of (as a sample of blood or a culture of bacteria)

type A *adj* : relating to, characteristic of, having, or being a personality that is marked by impatience, aggressiveness, and competitiveness and that is held to be associated with increased risk of cardiovascular disease

type B *adj* : relating to, characteristic of, having, or being a personality that is marked by a lack of excessive aggressiveness and tension and that is held to be associated with reduced risk of cardiovascular disease

type 1 diabetes *n* : diabetes of a form that usu. develops during childhood or adolescence and is characterized by a severe deficiency of insulin secretion resulting from atrophy of the islets of Langerhans and causing hyperglycemia and a marked tendency toward ketoacidosis — called also *insulin-dependent diabetes, insulin-dependent diabetes mellitus, juvenile diabetes, juvenile-onset diabetes, type 1 diabetes mellitus*

type 2 diabetes *n* : diabetes mellitus of a common form that develops esp. in adults and most often in obese individuals and that is characterized by hyperglycemia resulting from impaired insulin utilization coupled with the body's inability to compensate with increased insulin production — called also *adult-onset diabetes, late-onset diabetes, maturity-onset diabetes, non-insulin-dependent diabetes, non-insulin-dependent diabetes mellitus, type 2 diabetes mellitus*

¹typhoid \ˈtī-ˌfȯid, (ˌ)tī-ˈ\ *adj* **1** : of, relating to, or suggestive of typhus **2** : of, relating to, affected with, or constituting typhoid fever

²typhoid *n* **1** : TYPHOID FEVER **2** : any of several diseases of domestic animals resembling human typhus or typhoid fever

ty·phoi·dal \tī-ˈfȯid-ᵊl\ *adj* : of, relating to, or resembling typhoid fever

typhoid fever *n* : a communicable disease marked by fever, diarrhea, prostration, headache, splenomegaly, eruption of rose-colored spots, leukopenia, and intestinal inflammation

and caused by a bacterium of the genus *Salmonella* (*S. typhi*)

ty·phus \ˈtī-fəs\ *n* : any of various bacterial diseases caused by rickettsiae: as **a** : a severe human febrile disease that is caused by one (*Rickettsia prowazekii*) transmitted esp. by body lice and is marked by high fever, stupor alternating with delirium, intense headache, and a dark red rash — called also *louse-borne typhus* **b** : MURINE TYPHUS **c** : SCRUB TYPHUS

typhus fever *n* : TYPHUS

Tyr *abbr* tyrosine

ty·ra·mine \ˈtī-rə-ˌmēn\ *n* : a phenolic amine $C_8H_{11}NO$ that is found in various foods and beverages (as cheese and red wine), has a sympathomimetic action, and is derived from tyrosine

ty·ro·ci·dine *also* **ty·ro·ci·din** \ˌtī-rə-ˈsīd-ᵊn\ *n* : a basic polypeptide antibiotic produced by a soil bacterium of the genus *Bacillus* (*B. brevis*) — see TYROTHRICIN

Ty·rode solution \ˈtī-ˌrōd-\ *or* **Ty·rode's solution** \-ˌrōdz-\ *n* : physiological saline containing sodium chloride 0.8, potassium chloride 0.02, calcium chloride 0.02, magnesium chloride 0.01, sodium bicarbonate 0.1, and sodium dihydrogen phosphate 0.005 percent

Tyrode, Maurice Vejux (1878–1930), American pharmacologist.

ty·ro·sin·ae·mia *chiefly Brit var of* TYROSINEMIA

ty·ro·sine \ˈtī-rə-ˌsēn\ *n* : a phenolic amino acid $C_9H_{11}NO_3$ that is a precursor of several important substances (as epinephrine and melanin) — *abbr. Tyr*

tyrosine hydroxylase *n* : an enzyme that catalyzes the first step in the biosynthesis of catecholamines (as dopamine and norepinephrine)

ty·ro·sin·emia \ˌtī-rō-si-ˈnē-mē-ə\ *n* : a rare inherited disorder of tyrosine metabolism that is characterized by abnormally high concentrations of tyrosine in the blood and urine with associated abnormalities esp. of the liver and kidneys

ty·ro·sin·osis \ˌtī-rō-si-ˈnō-səs\ *n* : a condition of faulty metabolism of tyrosine marked by the excretion of unusual amounts of tyrosine in the urine

ty·ro·sin·uria \ˌtī-rō-si-ˈnu̇r-ē-ə, -ˈnyu̇r-\ *n* : the excretion of tyrosine in the urine

ty·ro·thri·cin \ˌtī-rə-ˈthrīs-ᵊn\ *n* : an antibiotic mixture that consists chiefly of tyrocidine and gramicidin, is obtained from a soil bacterium of the genus *Bacillus* (*B. brevis*), and is used in the topical treatment of infections esp. of the skin and mouth caused by gram-positive bacteria

Ty·son's gland \ˈtī-sᵊnz-\ *n* : PREPUTIAL GLAND

E. Tyson — see GLAND OF TYSON

U *abbr* uracil

U *symbol* uranium

ubi·qui·none \yü-'bi-kwə-ˌnōn, ˌyü-bi-kwi-'nōn\ *n* : any of a group of lipid-soluble quinones that are found esp. in mitochondria and function in oxidative phosphorylation as electron-carrying coenzymes in electron transport; *esp* : COENZYME Q10

ubiq·ui·tin \yü-'bi-kwə-tən\ *n* : a chiefly eukaryotic protein that when bound to other cellular proteins marks them for proteolytic degradation

UCL \ˌyü-ˌsē-'el\ *n* : ULNAR COLLATERAL LIGAMENT

ud·der \'ə-dər\ *n* : a large pendulous organ (as of a cow) consisting of two or more mammary glands enclosed in a common envelope and each provided with a single nipple

¹**ul·cer** \'əl-sər\ *n* : a break in skin or mucous membrane with loss of surface tissue, disintegration and necrosis of epithelial tissue, and often pus ⟨a stomach ~⟩

²**ulcer** *vb* **ul·cered; ul·cer·ing** : ULCERATE

ul·cer·ate \'əl-sə-ˌrāt\ *vb* **-at·ed; -at·ing** : to become affected with or as if with an ulcer — **ul·cer·ation** \ˌəl-sə-'rā-shən\ *n*

ul·cer·a·tive \'əl-sə-ˌrā-tiv, -rə-\ *adj* : of, relating to, or characterized by an ulcer or by ulceration ⟨~ gingivitis⟩

ulcerative colitis *n* : a chronic inflammatory disease of the colon that is of unknown cause and is characterized by diarrhea with discharge of mucus and blood, cramping abdominal pain, and inflammation and edema of the mucous membrane with patches of ulceration

ulcero- *comb form* **1** : ulcer ⟨*ulcero*genic⟩ **2** : ulcerous and ⟨*ulcero*glandular⟩

ul·cero·gen·ic \ˌəl-sə-rō-'je-nik\ *adj* : tending to produce or develop into ulcers or ulceration ⟨an ~ drug⟩

ul·cero·glan·du·lar \ˌəl-sə-rō-'glan-jə-lər\ *adj* : being a type of tularemia in which the place of infection is the skin where a papule and then an ulcer develops with enlargement of the lymph nodes in the associated region

ul·cer·ous \'əl-sə-rəs\ *adj* **1** : characterized or caused by ulceration **2** : affected with an ulcer

ul·cus \'əl-kəs\ *n, pl* **ul·cera** \'əl-sə-rə\ : ULCER

ul·na \'əl-nə\ *n, pl* **ul·nae** \-nē\ *or* **ul·nas** : the bone on the little-finger side of the forearm that forms with the humerus the elbow joint and serves as a pivot in rotation of the hand

¹**ul·nar** \'əl-nər\ *adj* **1** : of or relating to the ulna **2** : located on the same side of the forearm as the ulna

²**ulnar** *n* : an ulnar anatomical part

ulnar artery *n* : an artery that is the larger of the two terminal branches of the brachial artery, runs along the ulnar side of the forearm, and gives off near its origin the anterior and posterior ulnar recurrent arteries

ulnar collateral artery — see INFERIOR ULNAR COLLATERAL ARTERY, SUPERIOR ULNAR COLLATERAL ARTERY

ulnar collateral ligament *n* : a triangular ligament of the elbow that connects the medial epicondyle with the medial edge of the coronoid process and the olecranon, that helps to stabilize the elbow joint, and that is often injured in sports (as baseball) which involve repeated overhand throwing — called also *medial collateral ligament,* UCL; compare RADIAL COLLATERAL LIGAMENT

ulnar collateral ligament reconstruction *n* : a surgical procedure in which a torn ulnar collateral ligament is replaced with a tendon graft typically obtained from the palmaris longus — called also *Tommy John surgery*

ulnaris — see EXTENSOR CARPI ULNARIS, FLEXOR CARPI ULNARIS

ulnar nerve *n* : a large superficial nerve of the arm that is a continuation of the medial cord of the brachial plexus, passes around the elbow superficially in a groove between the olecranon and the medial epicondyle of the humerus, and continues down the inner side of the forearm to supply the skin and muscles of the little-finger side of the forearm and hand — see FUNNY BONE

ulnar notch *n* : the narrow medial concave surface on the lower end of the radius that articulates with the ulna

ulnar recurrent artery *n* : either of the two small branches of the ulnar artery arising from its medial side: **a** : one that arises just below the elbow and supplies the brachialis muscle and the pronator teres — called also *anterior ulnar recurrent artery* **b** : one that is larger, arises lower on the arm, and supplies the elbow and associated muscles — called also *posterior ulnar recurrent artery*

ulnar vein *n* : any of several deep veins of the forearm that accompany the ulnar artery and unite at the elbow with the radial veins to form the brachial veins

ul·tra·cen·tri·fuge \ˌəl-trə-'sen-trə-ˌfyüj\ *n* : a high-speed centrifuge able to sediment colloidal and other very small particles (as proteins or nucleic acids) — **ul·tra·cen·trif·u·gal** \ˌəl-'tri-fyə-gəl, -fi-\ *adj* — **ul·tra·cen·trif·u·ga·tion** \-ˌsen-trə-fyü-'gā-shən\ *n* — **ultracentrifuge** *vb*

ul·tra·fil·tra·tion \ˌəl-trə-fil-ˈtrā-shən\ *n* : filtration through a medium (as a semipermeable capillary wall) which allows small molecules (as of water) to pass but holds back larger ones (as of protein) — **ul·tra·fil·tra·ble** \-ˈfil-trə-bəl\ *adj* — **ul·tra·fil·trate** \-ˈfil-ˌtrāt\ *n*

Ul·tram \ˈəl-ˌtram\ *trademark* — used for a preparation of the hydrochloride of tramadol

ul·tra·mi·cro·scope \ˌəl-trə-ˈmī-krə-ˌskōp\ *n* : an apparatus for making visible by scattered light particles too small to be perceived by the ordinary microscope — called also *dark-field microscope* — **ul·tra·mi·cros·co·py** \-mī-ˈkräs-kə-pē\ *n*

ul·tra·mi·cro·scop·ic \-ˌmī-krə-ˈskä-pik\ *also* **ul·tra·mi·cro·scop·i·cal** \-pi-kəl\ *adj* **1** : SUBMICROSCOPIC **2** : of or relating to an ultramicroscope — **ul·tra·mi·cro·scop·i·cal·ly** *adv*

ul·tra·mi·cro·tome \-ˈmī-krə-ˌtōm\ *n* : a microtome for cutting extremely thin sections for electron microscopy — **ul·tra·mi·crot·o·my** \-mī-ˈkrä-tə-mē\ *n*

ul·tra·son·ic \-ˈsä-nik\ *adj* **1 a** : having a frequency above the human ear's audibility limit of about 20,000 hertz — used of waves and vibrations **b** : utilizing, produced by, or relating to ultrasonic waves or vibrations ⟨an ∼ scaler for tartar removal⟩ **2** : ULTRASOUND — **ul·tra·son·i·cal·ly** *adv*

ul·tra·sono·gram \-ˈsä-nə-ˌgram\ *n* : SONOGRAM

ul·tra·so·nog·ra·pher \ˌəl-trə-sə-ˈnä-grə-fər\ *n* : SONOGRAPHER

ul·tra·so·nog·ra·phy \-fē\ *n, pl* **-phies** : ULTRASOUND **2** — **ul·tra·so·no·graph·ic** \-ˌsä-nə-ˈgra-fik, -ˌsō-\ *adj*

¹ul·tra·sound \ˈəl-trə-ˌsaùnd\ *n* **1** : vibrations of the same physical nature as sound but with frequencies above the range of human hearing **2** : the diagnostic or therapeutic use of ultrasound and esp. a noninvasive technique involving the formation of a two-dimensional image used for the examination and measurement of internal body structures and the detection of bodily abnormalities — called also *echography, sonography, ultrasonography* **3** : a diagnostic examination using ultrasound

²ultrasound *adj* : of, relating to, performed by, using, or specializing in ultrasound ⟨an ∼ technician⟩

ul·tra·vi·o·let \ˌəl-trə-ˈvī-ə-lət\ *adj* **1** : situated beyond the visible spectrum at its violet end — used of radiation having a wavelength shorter than wavelengths of visible light and longer than those of X-rays **2** : relating to, producing, or employing ultraviolet radiation — **ultraviolet** *n*

ultraviolet A *n* : UVA

ultraviolet B *n* : UVB

ultraviolet microscope *n* : a microscope equipped to irradiate material under examination with ultraviolet radiation in order to detect or study fluorescent components — called also *fluorescence microscope*

uma·mi \ù-ˈmä-mē\ *n* : a taste sensation that is meaty or savory and is produced by several amino acids and nucleotides (as aspartate, inosinate, and glutamate) — **umani** *adj*

um·bi·lec·to·my \ˌəm-bi-ˈlek-tə-mē\ *n, pl* **-mies** : OMPHALECTOMY

um·bil·i·cal \ˌəm-ˈbi-li-kəl\ *adj* **1** : of, relating to, or used at the navel **2** : of or relating to the central abdominal region that is situated between the right and left lumbar regions and between the epigastric region above and the hypogastric region below

umbilical artery *n* : either of a pair of arteries that arise from the fetal hypogastric arteries and pass through the umbilical cord to the placenta to which they carry the deoxygenated blood from the fetus

umbilical cord *n* : a cord arising from the navel that connects the fetus with the placenta and contains the two umbilical arteries and the umbilical vein

umbilical hernia *n* : a hernia of abdominal viscera at the navel

umbilical ligament *n* — see MEDIAL UMBILICAL LIGAMENT, MEDIAN UMBILICAL LIGAMENT

umbilical vein *n* : a vein that passes through the umbilical cord to the fetus and returns the oxygenated and nutrient blood from the placenta to the fetus

umbilical vesicle *n* : the yolk sac of a mammalian embryo having a transitory connection with the digestive tract by way of the omphalomesenteric duct

um·bil·i·cat·ed \ˌəm-ˈbi-lə-ˌkā-təd\ *or* **um·bil·i·cate** \-kət\ *adj* : having a small depression that resembles a navel ⟨∼ vesicles⟩ — **um·bil·i·cate** \-ˌkāt\ *vb*

um·bi·li·cus \ˌəm-bə-ˈlī-kəs, ˌəm-ˈbi-li-\ *n, pl* **um·bi·li·ci** \ˌəm-bə-ˈlī-ˌkī, -ˌsī; ˌəm-ˈbi-lə-ˌkī, -ˌkē\ *or* **um·bi·li·cus·es** : NAVEL

um·bo \ˈəm-(ˌ)bō\ *n, pl* **um·bo·nes** \ˌəm-ˈbō-(ˌ)nēz\ *or* **um·bos** : an elevation in the tympanic membrane of the ear

un·anes·the·tized \ˌən-ə-ˈnes-thə-ˌtīzd\ *adj* : not having been subjected to an anesthetic ⟨an ∼ patient⟩

un·bal·anced \ˌən-ˈba-lənst\ *adj* : mentally disordered or deranged

un·blind·ed \-ˈblīn-dəd\ *adj* : made or done with knowledge of significant facts by the participants : not blind ⟨∼ studies of a drug's effectiveness⟩

un·born \-ˈbȯrn\ *adj* : not yet born : existing in utero ⟨∼ children⟩

un·bro·ken \-ˈbrō-kən\ *adj* : not broken ⟨∼ skin⟩ ⟨an ∼ blister⟩

un·cal \ˈən-kəl\ *adj* : of or relating to the uncus ⟨the ∼ region⟩

un·cal·ci·fied \ˌən-ˈkal-sə-ˌfīd\ *adj* : not calcified ⟨∼ osteoid tissue⟩

uncal herniation *n* : downward displacement of the uncus and adjacent structures into the tentorial notch

unci *pl of* UNCUS

un·ci·form \ˈən-sə-ˌfȯrm\ *n* : HAMATE

unciform bone *n* : HAMATE

Un·ci·nar·ia \ˌən-sə-ˈnar-ē-ə\ *n* : a genus of hookworms (family Ancylostomatidae) now usu. restricted to a few parasites of carnivorous mammals but formerly often including most of the common hookworms

un·ci·nate fasciculus \ˈən-sə-ˌnāt-\ *n* : a hook-shaped bundle of long association fibers connecting the frontal lobe with the anterior portion of the temporal lobe

uncinate fit *n* : a seizure of a form of temporal lobe epilepsy that originates in the region of the uncus and is characterized by hallucinations of taste and odor and disturbances of consciousness

uncinate process *n* : a hooklike body part: as **a** : an irregular downwardly and backwardly directed process of each lateral mass of the ethmoid bone that articulates with the inferior nasal conchae **b** : a bony upward projection arising from each side of the upper surface of any of the cervical vertebrae numbered three to seven and forming a raised lateral margin **c** : the portion of the pancreas that wraps behind the superior mesenteric artery and superior mesenteric vein

un·cir·cum·cised \ˌən-ˈsər-kəm-ˌsīzd\ *adj* : not circumcised

un·com·pen·sat·ed \-ˈkäm-pən-ˌsā-təd, -ˌpen-\ *adj* **1** : accompanied by a change in the pH of the blood ⟨∼ acidosis⟩ ⟨∼ alkalosis⟩ — compare COMPENSATED **2** : not corrected or affected by physiological compensation ⟨∼ congestive heart failure⟩

un·com·pli·cat·ed \ˌən-ˈkäm-plə-ˌkā-təd\ *adj* : not involving or marked by complications ⟨∼ peptic ulcer⟩

un·con·di·tion·al \ˌən-kən-ˈdi-shə-nəl\ *adj* : UNCONDITIONED 2

un·con·di·tioned \-ˈdi-shənd\ *adj* **1** : not dependent on or subjected to conditioning or learning **2** : producing an unconditioned response

¹un·con·scious \ˌən-ˈkän-chəs\ *adj* **1** : not marked by conscious thought, sensation, or feeling ⟨∼ motivation⟩ **2** : of or relating to the unconscious **3** : having lost consciousness ⟨was ∼ for three days⟩ — **un·con·scious·ly** *adv* — **un·con·scious·ness** *n*

²unconscious *n* : the part of mental life that is not ordinarily integrated or available to consciousness yet may be manifested as a motive force in overt behavior (as in neurosis) and is often revealed (as through dreams, slips of the tongue, or dissociated acts) — compare SUBCONSCIOUS

un·con·trolled \ˌən-kən-ˈtrōld\ *adj* **1**

: not being under control ⟨∼ hypertension⟩ **2** : not incorporating suitable experimental controls ⟨∼ drug trials⟩

un·co·or·di·nat·ed \-kō-ˈȯrd-ᵊn-ˌā-təd\ *adj* : not coordinated : lacking proper or effective coordination ⟨∼ muscles⟩

un·crossed \-ˈkrȯst\ *adj* : not forming a decussation ⟨∼ nerve fibers⟩

unc·tu·ous \ˈəŋk-chə-wəs, -shə-\ *adj* : rich in oil or fat : FATTY

un·cur·able \ˌən-ˈkyúr-ə-bəl\ *adj* : INCURABLE

un·cus \ˈəŋ-kəs\ *n, pl* **un·ci** \ˈən-ˌsī\ : a hooked anatomical part or process; *specif* : the anterior curved end of the parahippocampal gyrus

un·dec·y·le·nic acid \ˌən-ˌde-sə-ˈle-nik-, -ˌlē-\ *n* : an acid $C_{11}H_{20}O_2$ used in the treatment of fungus infections (as ringworm) of the skin

¹un·der \ˈən-dər\ *adv* : in or into a condition of unconsciousness ⟨put the patient ∼ prior to surgery⟩

²under *prep* : receiving or using the action or application of ⟨an operation performed ∼ local anesthesia⟩

³under *adj* : being in an induced state of unconsciousness

un·der·achiev·er \ˌən-dər-ə-ˈchē-vər\ *n* : a person and esp. a student who fails to achieve his or her potential or does not do as well as expected — **un·der·achieve** \-ˈchēv\ *vb* — **un·der·achieve·ment** \-mənt\ *n*

un·der·ac·tive \-ˈak-tiv\ *adj* : characterized by an abnormally low level of activity ⟨an ∼ thyroid gland⟩ — **un·der·ac·tiv·i·ty** \-ak-ˈti-və-tē\ *n*

un·der·arm \ˈən-dər-ˌärm\ *n* : ARMPIT

un·der·cut \ˈən-dər-ˌkət\ *n* : the part of a tooth lying between the gum and the points of maximum outward bulge on the tooth's surfaces

un·der·de·vel·oped \ˌən-dər-di-ˈve-ləpt\ *adj* : not normally or adequately developed ⟨∼ muscles⟩ — **un·der·de·vel·op·ment** \-əp-mənt\ *n*

un·der·di·ag·nose \-ˈdī-ig-ˌnōs, -ˌnōz\ *vb* **-nosed; -nos·ing** : to diagnose (a condition or disease) less often than it is actually present

un·der·dos·age \-ˈdō-sij\ *n* : the administration or taking of an underdose

¹un·der·dose \-ˈdōs\ *vb* **-dosed; -dos·ing** : to take or administer an insufficient dose

²un·der·dose \-ˌdōs\ *n* : an insufficient dose

un·der·feed \ˌən-dər-ˈfēd\ *vb* **-fed** \-ˈfed\; **-feed·ing** : to feed with too little food

un·der·nour·ished \ˌən-dər-ˈnər-isht\ *adj* : supplied with less than the minimum amount of the foods essential for sound health and growth — **un·der·nour·ish·ment** \-ˈnər-ish-mənt\ *n*

un·der·nu·tri·tion \-nü-ˈtri-shən, -nyü-\ *n* : deficient bodily nutrition due to inadequate food intake or faulty assimilation — **un·der·nu·tri·tion·al** \-shə-nəl\ *adj*

un·der·sexed \-'sekst\ *adj* : deficient in sexual desire

un·der·shot \'ən-dər-ˌshät\ *adj* : having the lower incisor teeth or lower jaw projecting beyond the upper when the mouth is closed — used chiefly of animals

un·der·tak·er \'ən-dər-ˌtā-kər\ *n* : one whose business is to prepare the dead for burial and to arrange and manage funerals — called also *mortician*

un·der·treat \-'trēt\ *vb* : to treat inadequately or inappropriately ⟨∼ a disease⟩ — **un·der·treat·ment** \-mənt\ *n*

un·der·ven·ti·la·tion \ˌən-dər-ˌven-ti-'lā-shən\ *n* : HYPOVENTILATION

un·der·weight \-'wāt\ *adj* : weighing less than the normal amount for one's age, height, and build

un·de·scend·ed \ˌən-di-'sen-dəd\ *adj* : retained within the iliac region rather than descending into the scrotum ⟨an ∼ testis⟩

un·de·vel·oped \ˌən-di-'ve-ləpt\ *adj* : lacking in development : not developed ⟨physiologically ∼⟩

un·di·ag·nos·able \-ˌdī-ig-'nō-sə-bəl\ *adj* : not capable of being diagnosed

un·di·ag·nosed \-'nōst\ *adj* : not diagnosed : eluding diagnosis ⟨∼ disease⟩

un·dif·fer·en·ti·at·ed \-ˌdi-fə-'ren-chē-ˌā-təd\ *adj* : not differentiated ⟨an ∼ sarcoma⟩

un·di·gest·ed \ˌən-dī-'jes-təd\ *adj* : not digested ⟨∼ food⟩

un·di·gest·ible \-dī-'jes-tə-bəl\ *adj* : not capable of being digested

un·du·lant fever \'ən-jə-lənt-, -dyə-\ *n* : BRUCELLOSIS

un·erupt·ed \ˌən-i-'rəp-təd\ *adj, of a tooth* : not yet having emerged through the gum

un·fer·til·ized \-'fərt-ᵊl-ˌīzd\ *adj* : not fertilized ⟨an ∼ egg⟩

ung *abbr* [Latin *unguentum*] ointment — used in writing prescriptions

un·gual \'əŋ-gwəl, 'ən-\ *adj* : of or relating to a fingernail or toenail

un·guent \'əŋ-gwənt, 'ən-jənt\ *n* : a soothing or healing salve : OINTMENT

un·guis \'əŋ-gwəs, 'ən-\ *n, pl* **un·gues** \-ˌgwēz\ : a fingernail or toenail

un·gu·late \'əŋ-gyə-lət, 'ən-, -ˌlāt\ *n* : a hoofed typically herbivorous quadruped mammal (as a ruminant, swine, camel, or horse) of a group formerly considered a major mammalian taxon (Ungulata) — **ungulate** *adj*

Unh *symbol* unnilhexium

un·healed \ˌən-'hēld\ *adj* : not healed

un·health·ful \-'helth-fəl\ *adj* : detrimental to good health ⟨∼ working conditions⟩ — **un·health·ful·ness** *n*

un·healthy \-'hel-thē\ *adj* **un·health·i·er; -est** 1 : not conducive to health ⟨an ∼ climate⟩ 2 : not in good health : SICKLY — **un·health·i·ness** *n*

un·hy·gi·en·ic \ˌən-ˌhī-'je-nik, -'jē-, -jē-'e-\ *adj* : not healthful or sanitary — **un·hy·gi·en·i·cal·ly** \-ni-k(ə-)lē\ *adv*

uni·cel·lu·lar \ˌyü-ni-'sel-yə-lər\ *adj* : having or consisting of a single cell ⟨∼ microorganisms⟩ — **uni·cel·lu·lar·i·ty** \-ˌsel-yə-'lar-ə-tē\ *n*

uni·fo·cal \ˌyü-ni-'fō-kəl\ *adj* : arising from or occurring in a single focus or location ⟨∼ infection⟩

uni·la·mel·lar \ˌyü-ni-lə-'me-lər\ *adj* : having only one lamella or layer

uni·lat·er·al \ˌyü-ni-'la-tə-rəl\ *adj* : occurring on, performed on, or affecting one side of the body or one of its parts ⟨∼ exophthalmos⟩ — **uni·lat·er·al·ly** *adv*

uni·loc·u·lar \ˌyü-ni-'lä-kyə-lər\ *adj* : containing a single cavity

un·im·mu·nized \(ˌ)ən-'i-myə-ˌnīzd\ *adj* : not immunized

un·in·fect·ed \ˌən-in-'fek-təd\ *adj* : free from infection ⟨an ∼ fracture⟩

uni·nu·cle·ate \ˌyü-ni-'nü-klē-ət, -'nyü-\ *also* **uni·nu·cle·at·ed** \-ˌā-təd\ *adj* : having a single nucleus : MONONUCLEAR

union \'yü-nyən\ *n* : an act or instance of uniting or joining two or more things into one: as **a** : the growing together of severed parts ⟨∼ of a fractured bone⟩ **b** : the joining of two germ cells in the process of fertilization

uni·ovu·lar \ˌyü-nē-'ä-vyə-lər\ *adj* : MONOZYGOTIC ⟨∼ twins⟩

unip·a·ra \yü-'ni-pə-rə\ *n, pl* **-ras** or **-rae** \-ˌrē\ : a woman who has borne one child

uni·pa·ren·tal \ˌyü-ni-pə-'ren-tᵊl\ *adj* : having, involving, or derived from a single parent; *specif* : involving or being inheritance in which an offspring's complete genotype or all copies of one or more genes, chromosome parts, or whole chromosomes are derived from a single parent ⟨∼ disomy⟩ — **uni·pa·ren·tal·ly** \-ē\ *adv*

uni·pen·nate \ˌyü-ni-'pe-ˌnāt\ *adj* : having the fibers arranged obliquely and inserting into a tendon only on one side ⟨a ∼ muscle⟩

uni·po·lar \ˌyü-ni-'pō-lər\ *adj* 1 : involving or being an electrode or lead attached to the surface of a bodily site (as the chest) for recording the difference in electrical potential between the site and that of another electrode or lead having zero potential 2 : having but one process ⟨a ∼ neuron⟩ 3 : relating to or being a manic-depressive disorder in which there is a depressive phase only ⟨∼ depression⟩ — compare BIPOLAR 3

un·ir·ra·di·at·ed \ˌun-ir-'ā-dē-ˌā-təd\ *adj* : not having been exposed to radiation ⟨∼ lymphocytes⟩

unit \'yü-nət\ *n* 1 : an amount of a biologically active agent (as a drug or antigen) required to produce a specific result under strictly controlled conditions ⟨a ∼ of penicillin⟩ 2 : a small molecule esp. when combined in a larger molecule 3 : an area in a medical facility and esp. a hospital that is specially staffed and equipped to provide a particular type of care

unit·age \'yü-nə-tij\ *n* **1** : specification of the amount constituting a unit (as of a vitamin) **2** : amount in units ⟨a ~ of 50,000 per capsule⟩

unit membrane *n* : the limiting membrane of cells and various organelles viewed formerly as a 3-layered structure with an inner lipid layer and two outer protein layers and currently as a fluid phospholipid bilayer with intercalated proteins

¹**uni·va·lent** \ˌyü-ni-'vā-lənt\ *n* : a chromosome that lacks a synaptic mate

²**univalent** *adj* **1** : MONOVALENT 1 **2** : being a chromosomal univalent **3** *of an antibody* : capable of agglutinating or precipitating but not both : having only one combining group

universal antidote *n* : an antidote for ingested poisons having activated charcoal as its principal ingredient

universal donor *n* **1** : a person who has Rh-negative blood of the blood group O and whose blood can be donated to any recipient; *broadly* : a person with blood group O blood **2** : the blood or blood group of a universal donor

universal recipient *n* **1** : a person who has Rh-positive blood of the blood group AB and who can receive blood from any donor; *broadly* : a person with blood group AB blood **2** : the blood or blood group of a universal recipient

un·la·beled *or* **un·la·belled** \ˌən-'lā-bəld\ *adj* : not labeled esp. with an isotopic label ⟨~ DNA⟩

un·la·bored \ˌən-'lā-bərd\ *adj* : produced without exertion, pain, or undue effort ⟨~ breathing⟩

un·li·censed \-'lī-sᵊnst\ *adj* : not licensed; *esp, of a drug* : not approved for use by the appropriate regulating authority (as the Food and Drug Administration in the U.S.)

un·linked \-'liŋkt\ *adj* : not belonging to the same genetic linkage group ⟨~ genes⟩

un·my·elin·at·ed \ˌən-'mī-ə-lə-ˌnā-təd\ *adj* : lacking a myelin sheath ⟨~ axons⟩

Un·na's boot \'ü-nəz-\ *or* **Un·na boot** \-nə-\ *n* : a compression dressing for varicose veins or ulcers consisting of a paste made of zinc oxide, gelatin, glycerin, and water

Unna, Paul Gerson (1850–1929), German dermatologist.

Unna's paste boot *n* : UNNA'S BOOT

un·ni·hex·i·um \ˌyün-²l-'hek-sē-əm\ *n* : SEABORGIUM — symbol *Unh*

un·ni·len·ti·um \ˌyün-²l-'pen-tē-əm\ *n* : DUBNIUM — symbol *Unp*

un·nil·qua·di·um \ˌyün-²l-'kwä-dē-əm\ *n* : RUTHERFORDIUM — symbol *Unq*

un·of·fi·cial \ˌən-ə-'fi-shəl\ *adj* : not official; *specif* : of, relating to, or being a drug not described in the *U.S. Pharmacopeia* and *National Formulary* — compare NONOFFICIAL, OFFICIAL

un·op·posed \-ə-'pōzd\ *adj* : being or relating to estrogen replacement therapy in which a progestin (as medroxyprogesterone acetate) is not coadministered to reduce the potential risks (as endometrial cancer) associated with estrogen used alone

un·os·si·fied \-'ä-sə-ˌfīd\ *adj* : not ossified

un·ox·y·gen·at·ed \-'äk-si-jə-ˌnā-təd, -äk-'si-jə-\ *adj* : not oxygenated ⟨~ blood⟩

Unp *symbol* unnilpentium

un·paired \-'pard\ *adj* **1** : not paired: as **a** : not matched or mated **b** : being an electron that does not share its orbital with another electron **2** : situated in the median plane of the body; *also* : not matched by a corresponding part on the opposite side

un·pig·ment·ed \-'pig-mən-təd\ *adj* : not pigmented : having no pigment

un·pro·tect·ed \-prə-'tek-təd\ *adj* : not protected; *esp* : performed without measures to prevent pregnancy or sexually transmitted disease ⟨~ sex⟩

Unq *symbol* unnilquadium

un·re·ac·tive \-rē-'ak-tiv\ *adj* : not reactive ⟨pupils ~ to light⟩

un·re·solved \-ri-'zälvd, -'zȯlvd\ *adj* : not resolved : not having undergone resolution ⟨~ pneumonia⟩

un·re·spon·sive \ˌən-ri-'spän-siv\ *adj* : not responsive (as to a treatment or stimulus) — **un·re·spon·sive·ness** *n*

un·san·i·tary \-'sa-nə-ˌter-ē\ *adj* : not sanitary : INSANITARY ⟨~ facilities⟩

un·sat·u·rate \-'sa-chə-rət\ *n* : an unsaturated chemical compound

un·sat·u·rat·ed \-'sa-chə-ˌrā-təd\ *adj* : not saturated: as **a** : capable of absorbing or dissolving more of something ⟨an ~ solution⟩ **b** : able to form products by chemical addition; *esp* : containing double or triple bonds between carbon atoms ⟨~ oils⟩ — **un·sat·u·ra·tion** \ˌsa-chə-'rā-shən\ *n*

un·seg·ment·ed \-'seg-ˌmen-təd\ *adj* : not divided into or made up of segments

un·sound \-'saȯnd\ *adj* : not sound: as **a** : not healthy or whole ⟨an ~ limb⟩ **b** : not mentally normal : not wholly sane ⟨of ~ mind⟩ **c** : not fit to be eaten ⟨of ~ food⟩ — **un·sound·ness** *n*

un·sta·ble \-'stā-bəl\ *adj* : not stable: as **a** : characterized by frequent or unpredictable changes ⟨a patient in ~ condition⟩ **b** : readily changing in chemical composition or biological activity **c** : characterized by the lack of emotional control or stability

unstable angina *n* : angina pectoris characterized by sudden changes (as an increase in the severity or length of anginal attacks or a decrease in the exertion required to precipitate an attack) esp. when symptoms were previously stable

un·stri·at·ed muscle \ˌən-'strī-ˌā-təd-\ *n* : SMOOTH MUSCLE

un·struc·tured \-'strək-chərd\ *adj* : lacking structure : not formally organized ⟨~ psychological tests⟩

un·trau·ma·tized \-'traù-mə-ˌtīzd, -'trò-\ *adj* : not subjected to trauma

un·treat·ed \-'trē-təd\ *adj* : not subjected to treatment ⟨an ~ disease⟩ — **un·treat·able** \-'trē-tə-bəl\ *adj*

un·vac·ci·nat·ed \-'vak-sə-ˌnā-təd\ *adj* : not vaccinated ⟨~ children⟩

un·well \-'wel\ *adj* 1 : being in poor health : SICK 2 : undergoing menstruation

up·grade \'əp-ˌgrād\ *vb* **-grad·ed; -grad·ing** 1 : to assign a less serious status to 2 : to reclassify (as a cancer or concussion) to a more serious grade when the grades are numbered from least to most serious

¹**up·per** \'ə-pər\ *n* : an upper tooth or denture

²**upper** *n* : a stimulant drug; *esp* : AMPHETAMINE

upper airway *n* : any or all of the air-conducting passges of the respiratory system that extend to the larynx from the two external openings of the nose and from the lips through the mouth

upper GI series *n* : fluoroscopic and radiographic examination (as for the detection of gastroesophgeal reflux, hiatal hernia, or ulcers) of the esophagus, stomach, and duodenum during and following oral ingestion of a solution of barium sulfate — called also *upper gastrointestinal series*

upper jaw *n* : JAW 1a

upper respiratory *adj* : of, relating to, or affecting the upper respiratory tract ⟨upper respiratory infection⟩

upper respiratory tract *n* : the part of the respiratory system including the nose, nasal passages, and nasopharynx — compare LOWER RESPIRATORY TRACT

up·reg·u·la·tion \'əp-ˌre-gyə-ˈlā-shən, -gə-\ *n* : the process of increasing the response to a stimulus; *specif* : increase in a cellular response to a molecular stimulus due to increase in the number of receptors on the cell surface — **up·reg·u·late** \-'re-gyə-ˌlāt\ *vb*

up·set \'əp-ˌset\ *n* 1 : a minor physical disorder ⟨a stomach ~⟩ 2 : an emotional disturbance — **up·set** \(ˌ)əp-'set\ *vb* — **up·set** \'əp-ˌset\ *adj*

up·stream \'əp-'strēm\ *adv or adj* : in a direction along a molecule of DNA or RNA opposite to that in which transcription and translation take place and toward the end having a hydroxyl group attached to the position labeled 5′ in the terminal nucleotide — compare DOWNSTREAM

up·take \'əp-ˌtāk\ *n* : an act or instance of absorbing and incorporating something esp. into a living organism, tissue, or cell ⟨oxygen ~⟩

ur- *or* **uro-** *comb form* 1 : urine ⟨uric⟩ 2 : urinary tract ⟨urology⟩ 3 : urinary and ⟨urogenital⟩ 4 : urea ⟨uracil⟩

ura·chal \'yùr-ə-kəl\ *adj* : of or relating to the urachus ⟨a ~ cyst⟩

ura·chus \-kəs\ *n* : a cord of fibrous tissue extending from the bladder to the navel and constituting the functionless remnant of a part of the duct of the allantois of the embryo

ura·cil \'yùr-ə-ˌsil, -səl\ *n* : a pyrimidine base $C_4H_4N_2O_2$ that is one of the four bases coding genetic information in the polynucleotide chain of RNA — compare ADENINE, CYTOSINE, GUANINE, THYMINE

ur·ae·mia *chiefly Brit var of* UREMIA

ura·ni·um \yù-'rā-nē-əm\ *n* : a silvery heavy radioactive metallic element that exists naturally as a mixture of three isotopes of mass number 234, 235, and 238 — symbol *U*; see ELEMENT table

uranium 235 *n* : a light isotope of uranium of mass number 235 that when bombarded with slow neutrons undergoes rapid fission into smaller atoms with the release of neutrons and atomic energy

urate \'yùr-ˌāt\ *n* : a salt of uric acid

ure- *or* **ureo-** *comb form* : urea ⟨urease⟩

urea \yù-'rē-ə\ *n* : a soluble weakly basic nitrogenous compound CH_4N_2O that is the chief solid component of mammalian urine and an end product of protein decomposition and that is administered intravenously as a diuretic drug

urea·plas·ma \yù-'rē-ə-ˌplaz-mə\ *n* 1 *cap* : a genus of mycoplasmas (family Mycoplasmataceae) that are able to hydrolyze urea with the formation of ammonia and that include one (*U. urealyticum*) found in the human genitourinary tract, oropharynx, and anal canal 2 : a mycoplasma of the genus *Ureaplasma*

ure·ase \'yùr-ē-ˌās, -ˌāz\ *n* : an enzyme that catalyzes the hydrolysis of urea into ammonia and carbon dioxide

Ure·cho·line \ˌyùr-ə-'kō-ˌlēn\ *trademark* — used for a preparation of the chloride of bethanechol

ure·mia \yù-'rē-mē-ə\ *n* 1 : accumulation in the blood of constituents normally eliminated in the urine that produces a severe toxic condition and usu. occurs in severe kidney disease 2 : the toxic bodily condition associated with uremia — **ure·mic** \-mik\ *adj*

ure·ter \'yùr-ə-tər, yù-'rē-tər\ *n* : either of the paired ducts that carry away urine from a kidney to the bladder or cloaca and that in humans are slender membranous epithelium-lined flat tubes about sixteen inches (41 centimeters) long which open above into the pelvis of a kidney and below into the back part of the same side of the bladder — **ure·ter·al** \yù-'rē-tə-rəl\ *also* **ure·ter·ic** \ˌyùr-ə-'ter-ik\ *adj*

ure·ter·ec·ta·sis \ˌyùr-ə-tər-'ek-tə-səs, yù-ˌrē-tər-\ *n, pl* **-ta·ses** \-ˌsēz\ : dilation of a ureter

ure·ter·ec·to·my \ˌyùr-ə-tər-'ek-tə-mē, yù-ˌrē-tər-\ n, pl **-mies** : surgical excision of all or part of a ureter

ure·ter·i·cus — see TORUS URETERICUS

ure·ter·i·tis \ˌyùr-ə-tər-'ī-təs, yù-ˌrē-tər-\ n : inflammation of a ureter

uretero- comb form **1** : ureter ⟨ureterography⟩ **2** : ureteral and ⟨ureteroileal⟩

ure·ter·o·cele \yù-'rē-tə-rə-ˌsēl\ n : cystic dilation of the lower part of a ureter into the bladder

ure·ter·o·en·ter·os·to·my \yù-ˌrē-tə-rō-ˌen-tə-'räs-tə-mē\ n, pl **-mies** : surgical formation of an artificial opening between a ureter and the intestine

ure·ter·o·gram \yù-'rē-tə-rə-ˌgram\ n : an X-ray photograph of the ureters after injection of a radiopaque substance — **ure·ter·og·ra·phy** \yù-ˌrē-tə-'rä-grə-fē, yùr-ə-tə-\ n

ure·tero·il·e·al \yù-ˌrē-tə-rō-'i-lē-əl\ adj : relating to or connecting a ureter and the ileum

ure·tero·li·thot·o·my \yù-ˌrē-tə-rō-li-'thä-tə-mē\ n, pl **-mies** : removal of a calculus by incision of a ureter

ure·ter·ol·y·sis \ˌyùr-ə-tər-'ä-lə-səs, yù-ˌrē-tər-\ n, pl **-y·ses** \-ˌsēz\ : a surgical procedure to free a ureter from abnormal adhesions or surrounding tissue (as in retroperitoneal fibrosis)

ure·tero·neo·cys·tos·to·my \yù-ˌrē-tər-ō-ˌnē-ō-sis-'täs-tə-mē\ n, pl **-mies** : surgical reimplantation of a ureter into the bladder

ure·tero·pel·vic \yù-ˌrē-tə-rō-'pel-vik\ adj : of, relating to, or involving a ureter and the adjoining renal pelvis ⟨∼ obstruction⟩

ure·tero·plas·ty \yù-'rē-tə-rə-ˌplas-tē\ n, pl **-ties** : plastic surgery performed on a ureter

ure·tero·py·elog·ra·phy \yù-ˌrē-tə-rō-ˌpī-ə-'lä-grə-fē\ n, pl **-phies** : X-ray photography of a renal pelvis and a ureter following the injection of a radiopaque medium

ure·tero·py·elo·ne·os·to·my \yù-ˌrē-tə-rō-ˌpī-ə-lō-nē-'äs-tə-mē\ n, pl **-mies** : surgical creation of a new channel joining a renal pelvis to a ureter

ure·tero·py·e·los·to·my \-ˌpī-ə-'läs-tə-mē\ n, pl **-mies** : URETEROPYELONEOSTOMY

ure·ter·or·rha·phy \yù-ˌrē-tə-'ror-ə-fē, ˌyùr-ə-tə-\ n, pl **-phies** : the surgical operation of suturing a ureter

ure·ter·o·scope \yù-'rē-tə-rō-ˌskōp\ n : an endoscope for visually examining and passing instruments into the interior of the ureter

ure·ter·os·co·py \yù-ˌrē-tə-'räs-kə-pē, ˌyùr-ə-tə-\ n, pl **-pies** : visual examination of the interior of a ureter

ure·tero·sig·moid·os·to·my \yù-ˌrē-tə-rō-ˌsig-ˌmòi-'däs-tə-mē\ n, pl **-mies** : surgical implantation of a ureter in the sigmoid colon

ure·ter·os·to·my \ˌyùr-ə-tər-'äs-tə-mē, yù-ˌrē-tər-\ n, pl **-mies** : surgical creation of an opening on the surface of the body for the ureters

ure·ter·ot·o·my \ˌyùr-ə-tər-'ä-tə-mē, yù-ˌrē-tər-\ n, pl **-mies** : the operation of cutting into a ureter

ure·tero·ure·ter·os·to·my \yù-ˌrē-tə-rō-yù-ˌrē-tər-'äs-tə-mē\ n, pl **-mies** : surgical establishment of an artificial communication between two ureters or between different parts of the same ureter

ure·tero·ves·i·cal \yù-ˌrē-tə-rō-'ve-si-kəl\ adj : of or relating to the ureters and the urinary bladder

ure·thane \'yùr-ə-ˌthān\ or **ure·than** \-ˌthan\ n : a crystalline compound $C_3H_7NO_2$ that is used esp. as a solvent and in anesthetizing laboratory animals — called also ethyl carbamate

urethr- or **urethro-** comb form : urethra ⟨urethritis⟩ ⟨urethroscope⟩

ure·thra \yù-'rē-thrə\ n, pl **-thras** or **-thrae** \-(ˌ)thrē\ : the canal that carries off the urine from the bladder and in the male serves also as a passageway for semen — **ure·thral** \-thrəl\ adj

urethrae — see SPHINCTER URETHRAE

urethral crest n : a narrow longitudinal fold or ridge along the posterior wall or floor of the female urethra or the prostatic portion of the male urethra

urethral gland n : any of the small mucous glands in the wall of the urethra — see GLAND OF LITTRÉ

urethral sphincter n : SPHINCTER URETHRAE

urethral syndrome n : a group of symptoms (as urinary frequency, dysuria, and suprapubic pain) that resemble those of a urinary tract infection but for which no significant bacteriuria exists

ure·threc·to·my \ˌyùr-i-'threk-tə-mē\ n, pl **-mies** : total or partial surgical excision of the urethra

ure·thri·tis \ˌyùr-i-'thrī-təs\ n : inflammation of the urethra

ure·thro·cele \yə-'rē-thrə-ˌsēl\ n : a pouched protrusion of urethral mucous membrane in the female

ure·thro·cu·ta·ne·ous \yù-ˌrē-thrō-kyù-'tā-nē-əs\ adj : of, relating to, or joining the urethra and the skin

ure·thro·cys·tog·ra·phy \yù-ˌrē-thrō-sis-'tä-grə-fē\ n, pl **-phies** : radiography of the urethra and bladder that utilizes a radiopaque substance

ure·throg·ra·phy \ˌyùr-i-'thrä-grə-fē\ n, pl **-phies** : radiography of the urethra after injection of a radiopaque substance

ure·thro·pexy \yù-'rē-thrə-ˌpek-sē\ n, pl **-pex·ies** : surgical fixation to nearby tissue of a displaced urethra that is causing incontinence by placing stress on the opening from the bladder

ure·thro·plas·ty \yù-'rē-thrə-ˌplas-tē\ n, pl **-ties** : plastic surgery of the urethra

ure·thro·rec·tal \yu̇-ˌrē-thrō-ˈrekt-ᵊl\ *adj* : of, relating to, or joining the urethra and the rectum ⟨a ~ fistula⟩

ure·thror·rha·phy \ˌyu̇r-ə-ˈthrȯr-ə-fē\ *n, pl* **-phies** : suture of the urethra for an injury or fistula

ure·thro·scope \yu̇-ˈrē-thrə-ˌskōp\ *n* : an endoscope for viewing the interior of the urethra — **ure·thro·scop·ic** \-ˌrē-thrə-ˈskä-pik\ *adj* — **ure·thros·co·py** \ˌyu̇r-ə-ˈthräs-kə-pē\ *n*

ure·thros·to·my \ˌyu̇r-ə-ˈthräs-tə-mē\ *n, pl* **-mies** : the creation of a surgical opening between the perineum and the urethra

ure·throt·o·my \ˌyu̇r-ə-ˈthrä-tə-mē\ *n, pl* **-mies** : surgical incision into the urethra esp. for the relief of stricture

ure·thro·vag·i·nal \yu̇-ˌrē-thrō-ˈva-jən-ᵊl\ *adj* : of, relating to, or joining the urethra and the vagina ⟨a ~ fistula⟩

urge incontinence *n* : involuntary leakage of urine from the bladder when a sudden strong need to urinate is felt — compare STRESS INCONTINENCE

ur·gen·cy \ˈər-jən-sē\ *n, pl* **-cies** : a sudden compelling desire to urinate or defecate

ur·gin·ea \ər-ˈji-nē-ə\ *n* **1** *cap* : a genus of bulbous herbs native to the Old World and esp. to the Mediterranean region — see SQUILL **2** *often cap* : the sliced young bulb of an Asian plant of the genus Urginea (*U. indica*) with the same properties and uses as those of squill (*U. maritima*)

URI *abbr* upper respiratory infection

-uria \ˈyu̇r-ē-ə, ˈu̇r-\ *n comb form* **1** : presence of (a specified substance) in urine ⟨albumin*uria*⟩ **2** : condition of having (such) urine ⟨poly*uria*⟩; *esp* : abnormal or diseased condition marked by the presence of (a specified substance) ⟨py*uria*⟩

uric \ˈyu̇r-ik\ *adj* : of, relating to, or found in urine

uric- *or* **urico-** *comb form* : uric acid ⟨*urico*suric⟩

uric acid *n* : a white odorless and tasteless nearly insoluble acid $C_5H_4N_4O_3$ that is present in small quantity in human urine and occurs pathologically in renal calculi and the tophi of gout

uric·ac·id·uria \ˌyu̇r-ik-ˌa-sə-ˈdu̇r-ē-ə, -ˈdyu̇r-\ *n* : the presence of excess uric acid in the urine

uri·cae·mia *chiefly Brit var of* URICEMIA

uri·ce·mia \ˌyu̇r-ə-ˈsē-mē-ə\ *n* : HYPERURICEMIA — **uri·ce·mic** \-mik\ *adj*

uri·co·su·ria \ˌyu̇r-i-kə-ˈsu̇r-ē-ə, -ˈshu̇r-\ *n* : the excretion of uric acid in the urine esp. in excessive amounts

uri·co·su·ric \ˌyu̇r-i-kə-ˈsu̇r-ik, -ˈshu̇r-\ *adj* : relating to or promoting uricosuria — **uricosuric** *n*

uri·dine \ˈyu̇r-ə-ˌdēn\ *n* : a ribonucleoside $C_9H_{12}N_2O_6$ containing uracil in the form of phosphate derivatives that plays an important role in carbohydrate metabolism

urin- *or* **urino-** *comb form* : UR- ⟨*uri*nary⟩

urinae — see DETRUSOR URINAE

uri·nal \ˈyu̇r-ən-ᵊl\ *n* **1** : a vessel into which a bedridden patient urinates **2** : a container worn by a person with urinary incontinence

uri·nal·y·sis \ˌyu̇r-ə-ˈna-lə-səs\ *n, pl* **-y·ses** \-ˌsēz\ : chemical analysis of urine

uri·nary \ˈyu̇r-ə-ˌner-ē\ *adj* **1** : relating to, occurring in, or constituting the organs concerned with the formation and discharge of urine ⟨~ infections⟩ **2** : of, relating to, or used for urine **3** : excreted as or in urine

urinary bladder *n* : a distensible membranous sac that serves for the temporary retention of the urine, is situated in the pelvis in front of the rectum, receives the urine from the two ureters and discharges it at intervals into the urethra through an orifice closed by a sphincter

urinary calculus *n* : a calculus occurring in any portion of the urinary tract and esp. in the pelvis of the kidney — called also *urinary stone, urolith*

urinary system *n* : the organs of the urinary tract comprising the kidneys, ureters, urinary bladder, and urethra

urinary tract *n* : the tract through which urine passes and which consists of the renal tubules and renal pelvis, the ureters, the bladder, and the urethra

uri·nate \ˈyu̇r-ə-ˌnāt\ *vb* **-nat·ed; -nat·ing** : to discharge urine

uri·na·tion \ˌyu̇r-ə-ˈnā-shən\ *n* : the act of urinating — called also *micturition*

urine \ˈyu̇r-ən\ *n* : waste material that is secreted by the kidney, is rich in end products (as urea, uric acid, and creatinine) of protein metabolism together with salts and pigments, and forms a clear amber and usu. slightly acid fluid

uri·nif·er·ous tubule \ˌyu̇r-ə-ˈni-fə-rəs-\ *n* : a tubule of the kidney that collects or conducts urine

uri·no·ma \ˌyu̇r-ə-ˈnō-mə\ *n, pl* **-mas** *also* **-ma·ta** \-mə-tə\ : a cyst that contains urine

uri·nom·e·ter \ˌyu̇r-ə-ˈnä-mə-tər\ *n* : a small hydrometer for determining the specific gravity of urine

uro- — see UR-

uro·bi·lin \ˌyu̇r-ə-ˈbī-lən\ *n* : any of several brown bile pigments formed from urobilinogens and found in normal feces, in normal urine in small amounts, and in pathological urines in larger amounts

uro·bi·lin·o·gen \ˌyu̇r-ə-bī-ˈli-nə-jən, -ˌjen\ *n* : any of several chromogens that are reduction products of bilirubin

uro·ca·nic acid \ˌyu̇r-ə-ˈkä-nik-, -ˈka-\ *n* : a crystalline acid $C_6H_6N_2O_2$ normally present in human skin that is held to act as a screening agent for ultraviolet radiation

uro·dy·nam·ics \ˌyùr-ə-dī-ˈna-miks\ *n* : the hydrodynamics of the urinary tract — **uro·dy·nam·ic** \-mik\ *adj* — **uro·dy·nam·i·cal·ly** \-mi-k(ə-)lē\ *adv*

uro·ep·i·the·li·al \ˌyùr-ō-ˌe-pə-ˈthē-lē-əl\ *adj* : of or affecting the epithelium of the urinary tract ⟨∼ cells⟩ — **uro·ep·i·the·li·um** \-əm\ *n*

uro·er·y·thrin \ˌyùr-ō-ˈer-ə-thrən\ *n* : a pink or reddish pigment found in many pathological urines and also frequently in normal urine in very small quantity

uro·gas·trone \ˌyùr-ə-ˈgas-ˌtrōn\ *n* : a polypeptide that has been isolated from urine and inhibits gastric secretion — compare ENTEROGASTRONE

uro·gen·i·tal \ˌyùr-ō-ˈje-nə-tᵊl\ *adj* : of, relating to, affecting, treating, or being the organs or functions of excretion and reproduction : GENITOURINARY

urogenital diaphragm *n* : a double layer of pelvic fascia with its included muscle that is situated between the ischial and pubic rami, supports the prostate in the male, is traversed by the vagina in the female, gives passage to the membranous part of the urethra, and encloses the sphincter urethrae

urogenital sinus *n* : the ventral part of the embryonic mammalian cloaca that eventually forms the neck of the bladder and some of the more distal portions of the genitourinary tract

urogenital system *n* : GENITOURINARY TRACT

urogenital tract *n* : GENITOURINARY TRACT

uro·gram \ˈyùr-ə-ˌgram\ *n* : a radiograph made by urography

urog·ra·phy \yù-ˈrä-grə-fē\ *n, pl* **-phies** : radiography of a part of the urinary tract (as a kidney or ureter) after injection of a radiopaque substance — **uro·graph·ic** \ˌyùr-ə-ˈgra-fik\ *adj*

uro·gy·ne·col·o·gist \ˌyùr-ō-ˌgī-nə-ˈkä-lə-jəst\ *n* : a specialist in urogynecology

uro·gy·ne·col·o·gy \-ˈkä-lə-jē\ *n, pl* **-gies** : a branch of medicine concerned with the urological problems (as urinary incontinence) of women — **uro·gy·ne·co·log·ic** \-kə-ˈlä-jik\ *or* **uro·gy·ne·co·log·i·cal** \-ji-kəl\ *adj*

uro·ki·nase \ˌyùr-ō-ˈkī-ˌnās, -ˌnāz\ *n* : an enzyme that is produced by the kidney and is found in urine, that activates plasminogen, and that is used therapeutically to dissolve blood clots (as in the heart)

uro·lag·nia \ˌyùr-ō-ˈlag-nē-ə\ *n* : sexual excitement associated with urine or with urination

uro·lith \ˈyùr-ə-ˌlith\ *n* : URINARY CALCULUS

uro·lith·i·a·sis \ˌyùr-ə-li-ˈthī-ə-səs\ *n, pl* **-ia·ses** \-ˌsēz\ : a condition that is

characterized by the formation or presence of calculi in the urinary tract

urol·o·gist \yù-ˈrä-lə-jist\ *n* : a physician who specializes in urology

urol·o·gy \-jē\ *n, pl* **-gies** : a branch of medicine dealing with the urinary or urogenital organs — **uro·log·i·cal** \ˌyùr-ə-ˈlä-ji-kəl\ *also* **uro·log·ic** \-ˈlä-jik\ *adj*

uro·patho·gen·ic \ˌyùr-ō-ˌpa-thə-ˈje-nik\ *adj* : of, relating to, or being a pathogen (as some strains of E. coli) of the urinary tract — **uro·patho·gen** \-ˈpa-thə-jən\ *n*

urop·a·thy \yù-ˈrä-pə-thē\ *n, pl* **-thies** : a disease of the urinary or urogenital organs — **uro·path·ic** \ˌyùr-ə-ˈpa-thik\ *adj*

uro·pep·sin \ˌyùr-ō-ˈpep-sən\ *n* : a proteolytic hormone found in urine esp. in cases of peptic ulcers and other disorders of the digestive tract

uro·por·phy·rin \ˌyùr-ō-ˈpór-fə-rən\ *n* : any of four isomeric porphyrins $C_{40}H_{38}N_4O_{16}$ closely related to the coproporphyrins

uro·ra·di·ol·o·gy \ˌyùr-ō-ˌrā-dē-ˈä-lə-jē\ *n, pl* **-gies** : radiology of the urinary tract — **uro·ra·dio·log·ic** \-ˌrā-dē-ə-ˈlä-jik\ *adj*

uros·co·py \yùr-ˈäs-kə-pē\ *n, pl* **-pies** : examination or analysis of the urine

uro·sep·sis \ˌyùr-ō-ˈsep-səs\ *n, pl* **-sep·ses** \-ˌsēz\ : a toxic condition caused by the extravasation of urine into bodily tissues

uros·to·my \yù-ˈräs-tə-mē\ *n, pl* **-mies** : an ostomy for the elimination of urine from the body

ur·so·de·oxy·cho·lic acid \ˌər-sō-dē-ˌäk-sē-ˈkō-lik-\ *n* : URSODIOL

ur·so·di·ol \ˌər-sō-ˈdī-ˌól, -ˌól\ *n* : a bile acid $C_{24}H_{40}O_4$ stereoisomeric with chenodeoxycholic acid that is used to dissolve uncalcified radiolucent gallstones — called also *ursodeoxycholic acid*

ur·ti·ca \ˈər-ti-kə\ *n* **1** *cap* : a genus of widely distributed plants (family Urticaceae, the nettle family) comprising the nettles with leaves having stinging hairs **2** : NETTLE 1

ur·ti·car·ia \ˌər-tə-ˈkar-ē-ə\ *n* : HIVES — **ur·ti·car·i·al** \-ē-əl\ *adj*

urticata — see ACNE URTICATA

uru·shi·ol \yù-ˈrü-shē-ˌól, -ˌól\ *n* : an oily toxic irritant mixture present in poison ivy and some related plants of the genus *Rhus*

USAN *abbr* United States Adopted Names — used to designate officially recognized nonproprietary names of drugs as established by a joint committee of medical and pharmaceutical professionals

Ush·er syndrome \ˈə-shər-\ *also* **Ush·er's syndrome** \-shərz-\ *n* : a genetic disease that is characterized by congenital deafness or progressive hearing loss during childhood and by retinitis pigmentosa and that is inher-

799

ited chiefly as an autosomal recessive trait

Usher, Charles Howard (1865–1942), British ophthalmologist.

us·nic acid \'əs-nik-\ n : a yellow crystalline antibiotic $C_{18}H_{16}O_7$ that is obtained from various lichens (as *Usnea barbata*)

USP abbr United States Pharmacopeia

USPSTF abbr U.S. Preventive Services Task Force

uta \'ü-tə\ n : mucocutaneous leishmaniasis occurring in the highlands of Peru and Argentina — compare ESPUNDIA

ut dict abbr [Latin *ut dictum*] as directed — used in writing prescriptions

uter- or **utero-** \for 2, ‚yü-tə-rō\ comb form **1** : uterus ⟨*utero*salpingography⟩ **2** : uterine and ⟨*utero*placental⟩

uteri pl of UTERUS

uteri — see CERVIX UTERI, CORPUS UTERI

uter·ine \'yü-tə-rən, -‚rīn\ adj : of, relating to, occurring in, or affecting the uterus ⟨~ tissue⟩ ⟨~ cancer⟩

uterine artery n : an artery that arises from the internal iliac artery and supplies the uterus and adjacent parts and during pregnancy the placenta

uterine gland n : any of the branched tubular glands in the mucous membrane of the uterus

uterine plexus n : a plexus of veins tributary to the internal iliac vein by which blood is returned from the uterus

uterine tube n : FALLOPIAN TUBE

uterine vein n : any of the veins that make up the uterine plexus

utero–ovar·ian \‚yü-tə-ō-(‚)rō-ō-'var-ē-ən\ adj : of or relating to the uterus and the ovary ⟨~ blood flow⟩

utero·pla·cen·tal \-plə-'sent-ᵊl\ adj : of or relating to the uterus and the placenta ⟨~ circulation⟩

utero·sa·cral ligament \‚yü-tə-rō-'sa-krəl-, -'sā-\ n : a fibrous fascial band on each side of the uterus that passes along the lateral wall of the pelvis from the uterine cervix to the sacrum and that serves to support the uterus and hold it in place — called also *sacrouterine ligament*

utero·sal·pin·gog·ra·phy \-‚sal-‚piŋ-'gä-grə-fē\ n, pl **-phies** : HYSTEROSALPINGOGRAPHY

utero·ton·ic \‚yü-tə-rō-'tä-nik\ adj : stimulating muscular tone in the uterus ⟨a ~ substance⟩

utero·tub·al \-'tü-bəl, -'tyü-\ adj : of or relating to the uterus and fallopian tubes ⟨the ~ junction⟩

utero·vag·i·nal \-'va-jən-ᵊl\ adj : of or relating to the uterus and the vagina

utero·ves·i·cal pouch \-'ve-si-kəl-\ n : a pouch formed by the peritoneum between the uterus and the bladder

uter·us \'yü-tə-rəs\ n, pl **uteri** \-‚rī\ also **uter·us·es** : an organ in female mammals for containing and usu. for

nourishing the young during development prior to birth that has thick walls consisting of an outer serous layer, a very thick middle layer of smooth muscle, and an inner mucous layer containing numerous glands — called also *womb*; see CERVIX 2a, CORPUS UTERI, FUNDUS c

UTI \‚yü-‚tē-'ī\ n : a urinary tract infection

utilization review n : the critical evaluation (as by a physician or nurse) of health-care services provided to patients that is made esp. for the purpose of controlling costs and monitoring quality of care

utri·cle \'yü-tri-kəl\ n : a small anatomical pouch: as **a** : the part of the membranous labyrinth of the ear into which the semicircular canals open and that contains the macula utriculi — called also *utriculus* **b** : PROSTATIC UTRICLE — **utric·u·lar** \yü-'tri-kyə-lər\ adj

utriculi — see MACULA UTRICULI

utric·u·lo·sac·cu·lar duct \yü-‚tri-kyə-lō-'sa-kyə-lər-\ n : a narrow tube connecting the utricle to the saccule in the membranous labyrinth of the ear

utric·u·lus \yü-'tri-kyə-ləs\ n, pl **-li** \-‚lī\ : UTRICLE a

UV abbr ultraviolet

UVA \‚yü-‚vē-'ā\ n : radiation that is in the region of the ultraviolet spectrum which is nearest to visible light and extends from 320 to 400 nm in wavelength and from which comes the radiation that causes tanning and contributes to aging of the skin

UVB \-'bē\ n : radiation that is in the region of the ultraviolet spectrum which extends from 280 to 320 nm in wavelength and that is primarily responsible for sunburn, aging of the skin, and the development of skin cancer

UVC \-'sē\ n : radiation that is in the region of the ultraviolet spectrum which extends from 200 to 280 nm in wavelength and that is more hazardous than UVB but is mostly absorbed by the earth's upper atmosphere

uvea \'yü-vē-ə\ n : the middle layer of the eye consisting of the iris and ciliary body together with the choroid coat — called also *vascular tunic* — **uve·al** \'yü-vē-əl\ adj

uve·itis \‚yü-vē-'ī-təs\ n, pl **uve·it·i·des** \-'i-tə-‚dēz\ : inflammation of the uvea

uveo·pa·rot·id fever \‚yü-vē-ō-pə-'rä-təd-\ n : chronic inflammation of the parotid gland and uvea that is typically associated with sarcoidosis and is marked esp. by low-grade fever, facial swelling, and paralysis of the facial nerves — called also *Heerfordt's syndrome*

UV index n : a number on a scale which extends indefinitely upward from a baseline of 0 and whose values express the intensity of solar ultraviolet radiation at noon on a given day for a particular location with 0 indicating negligible ultraviolet exposure and values over 10 indicating very high ultraviolet exposure

uvu·la \'yü-vyə-lə\ *n, pl* **-las** \-ləz\ *or* **-lae** \-ˌlē\ **1** : the pendent fleshy lobe in the middle of the posterior border of the soft palate **2** : a lobe of the inferior vermis of the cerebellum located in front of the pyramid — **uvu·lar** \-lər\ *adj*

uvu·lec·to·my \ˌyü-vyə-'lek-tə-mē\ *n, pl* **-mies** : surgical excision of the uvula

U wave \'yü-ˌ\ *n* : a positive wave following the T wave on an electrocardiogram

V

V *symbol* vanadium

vac·ci·nal \'vak-sən-ᵊl, vak-'sēn-\ *adj* : of or relating to vaccine or vaccination ⟨∼ control of a disease⟩

vac·ci·nate \'vak-sə-ˌnāt\ *vb* **-nat·ed**; **-nat·ing** : to administer a vaccine to usu. by injection — **vac·ci·na·tor** \-ˌnā-tər\ *n*

vac·ci·na·tion \ˌvak-sə-'nā-shən\ *n* **1** : the act of vaccinating **2** : the scar left by vaccinating

vac·cine \vak-'sēn, 'vak-ˌ\ *n* : a preparation of killed microorganisms, living attenuated organisms, or living fully virulent organisms that is administered to produce or artificially increase immunity to a particular disease; *also* : a mixture of several such vaccines

vac·ci·nee \ˌvak-sə-'nē\ *n* : a vaccinated individual

vac·cin·ia \vak-'si-nē-ə\ *n* **1 a** : COW-POX : a reaction to smallpox vaccine prepared from live vaccinia virus that may involve a rash, fever, headache, and body pain **2** : a poxvirus of the genus *Orthopoxvirus* (species *Vaccinia virus*) that differs from but is closely related to the viruses causing smallpox and cowpox and that includes a strain of uncertain natural origin used in making vaccines against smallpox — called also *vaccinia virus* — **vac·cin·i·al** \-nē-əl\ *adj*

vac·u·o·lat·ed \'va-kyü-ō-ˌlā-təd\ *or* **vac·u·o·late** \-ˌlāt\ *adj* : containing one or more vacuoles

vac·u·o·la·tion \ˌva-kyü-ō-'lā-shən\ *n* : the development or formation of vacuoles ⟨neuronal ∼⟩

vac·u·ole \'va-kyü-ˌōl\ *n* **1** : a small cavity or space in the tissues of an organism containing air or fluid **2** : a cavity or vesicle in the cytoplasm of a cell usu. containing fluid — **vac·u·o·lar** \ˌva-kyü-'ō-lər, -ˌlär\ *adj*

vac·u·ol·i·za·tion \ˌva-kyü-ˌō-lə-'zā-shən\ *n* : VACUOLATION

vac·u·um aspiration \'va-(ˌ)kyüm-, -kyəm-\ *n* : a method of abortion performed in the later half of the first trimester of pregnancy by aspiration of the contents of the uterus through a narrow tube — **vacuum aspirator** *n*

VAD \ˌvē-(ˌ)ā-'dē\ *n* : an artificial device that is implanted in the chest to assist a damaged or weakened heart in pumping blood — called also *ventricular assist device*

vag- *or* **vago-** *comb form* : vagus nerve

va·gal \'vā-gəl\ *adj* : of, relating to, mediated by, or being the vagus nerve — **va·gal·ly** *adv*

vagal escape *n* : resumption of the heartbeat that takes place after stimulation of the vagus nerve has caused it to stop and that occurs despite the continuing of such stimulation

vagal tone *n* : impulses from the vagus nerve producing inhibition of the heartbeat

vagi *pl of* VAGUS

vagin- *also* **vagini-** *comb form* : vagina ⟨vaginectomy⟩

va·gi·na \və-'jī-nə\ *n, pl* **-nae** \-(ˌ)nē\ *or* **-nas** : a canal in a female mammal that leads from the uterus to the external orifice opening into the vestibule between the labia minora

vaginae — see SPHINCTER VAGINAE

va·gi·nal \'va-jən-ᵊl, və-'jī-nᵊl\ *adj* **1** : of, relating to, or resembling a vagina : THECAL **2 a** : of, relating to, or affecting the genital vagina ⟨∼ discharge⟩ ⟨∼ infection⟩ **b** : occurring through the birth canal ⟨a ∼ delivery⟩ ⟨a ∼ birth⟩ — **va·gi·nal·ly** *adv*

vaginal artery *n* : any of the several arteries that supply the vagina and that usu. arise from the internal iliac artery or the uterine artery

vaginal hysterectomy *n* : a hysterectomy performed through the vagina

Vaginalis — see PROCESSUS VAGINALIS, TUNICA VAGINALIS

vaginal process *n* **1** : a projecting lamina of bone on the inferior surface of the petrous portion of the temporal bone that is continuous with the tympanic plate and surrounds the root of the styloid process **2** : either of a pair of projecting laminae on the inferior surface of the sphenoid that articulate with the alae of the vomer

vaginal smear *n* : a smear taken from the vaginal mucosa for cytological diagnosis

801

vaginal thrush *n* : candidiasis of the vagina or vulva

vag·i·nec·to·my \ˌva-jə-ˈnek-tə-mē\ *n*, *pl* **-mies** : COLPECTOMY

vag·i·nis·mus \ˌva-jə-ˈniz-məs\ *n* : a painful spasmodic contraction of the vagina

vag·i·ni·tis \ˌva-jə-ˈnī-təs\ *n*, *pl* **-nit·i·des** \-ˈni-tə-ˌdēz\ **1** : inflammation of the vagina (as from bacterial or fungal infection, allergic reaction, or hormone deficiency) that may be marked by irritation and vaginal discharge — see ATROPHIC VAGINITIS, BACTERIAL VAGINOSIS, TRICHOMONIASIS **2** : inflammation of a sheath (as a tendon sheath)

vag·i·no·plas·ty \ˈva-jə-nə-ˌplas-tē\ *n*, *pl* **-ties** : plastic surgery of the vagina

vag·i·no·sis \ˌva-jə-ˈnō-səs\ *n*, *pl* **-no·ses** \-ˌsēz\ : an abnormal or diseased condition of the vagina; *specif* : BACTERIAL VAGINOSIS

vago- — see VAG-

va·go·lyt·ic \ˌvā-gə-ˈli-tik\ *adj* : PARASYMPATHOLYTIC ⟨~ effects⟩

va·got·o·my \vā-ˈgä-tə-mē\ *n*, *pl* **-mies** : surgical division of the vagus nerve — **va·got·o·mize** \-ˌmīz\ *vb*

va·go·to·nia \ˌvā-gə-ˈtō-nē-ə\ *n* : excessive excitability of the vagus nerve resulting typically in vasomotor instability, constipation, and sweating — compare SYMPATHICOTONIA — **va·go·ton·ic** \-ˈtä-nik\ *adj*

va·go·va·gal \ˌvā-gō-ˈvā-gəl\ *adj* : relating to or arising from both afferent and efferent impulses of the vagus nerve ⟨a ~ reflex⟩

va·gus \ˈvā-gəs\ *n*, *pl* **va·gi** \ˈvā-ˌgī, -ˌjī\ : VAGUS NERVE

vagus nerve *n* : either of the tenth pair of cranial nerves that arise from the medulla and supply chiefly the viscera esp. with autonomic sensory and motor fibers — called also *pneumogastric nerve, tenth cranial nerve, vagus*

Val *abbr* valine

val·a·cy·clo·vir \ˌva-lə-ˈsī-klō-ˌvir\ *n* : a prodrug of acyclovir that is administered orally in the form of its hydrochloride $C_{13}H_{20}N_6O_4$·HCl to treat shingles, genital herpes, and cold sores — see VALTREX

val·de·cox·ib \ˌval-də-ˈkäk-sib\ *n* : a COX-2 inhibitor $C_{16}H_{14}N_2O_3S$ used esp. to treat osteoarthritis, rheumatoid arthritis, and primary dysmenorrhea but withdrawn from sale by the manufacturer because of its link to cardiovascular events (as heart attack) and severe skin rashes — see BEXTRA

va·lence \ˈvā-ləns\ *n* **1** : the degree of combining power of an atom as shown by the number of electrons in its outermost energy level that are lost, gained, or shared in the formation of chemical bonds **2** : relative capacity to unite, react, or interact (as with antigens or a biological substrate)

-va·lent \ˈvā-lənt\ *adj comb form* : having (so many) chromosomal strands or homologous chromosomes ⟨*bivalent*⟩

va·le·ri·an \və-ˈlir-ē-ən\ *n* : a preparation of the dried rhizome and roots of a perennial herb (*Valeriana officinalis* of the family Valerianaceae, the valerian family) that is used as an herbal remedy esp. to relieve insomnia and anxiety — called also *valerian root*

valgum — see GENU VALGUM

val·gus \ˈval-gəs\ *adj* **1** : turned outward; *esp* : of, relating to, or being a deformity in which an anatomical part is turned outward away from the midline of the body to an abnormal degree ⟨~ deformity of the big toe⟩ ⟨a ~ heel⟩ — see CUBITUS VALGUS, HALLUX VALGUS, TALIPES VALGUS; compare GENU VALGUM, GENU VARUM **2** : VARUS 1 — used esp. in orthopedics of the knee — **valgus** *n*

va·line \ˈvā-ˌlēn, ˈva-\ *n* : a crystalline essential amino acid $C_5H_{11}NO_2$ — abbr. *Val*

val·in·o·my·cin \ˌva-lə-nō-ˈmīs-ᵊn\ *n* : an antibiotic $C_{54}H_{90}N_6O_{18}$ produced by a bacterium of the genus *Streptomyces* (*S. fulvissimus*)

Val·ium \ˈva-lē-əm, ˈval-yəm\ *trademark* — used for a preparation of diazepam

val·late \ˈva-ˌlāt\ *adj* : having a raised edge surrounding a depression

vallate papilla *n* : CIRCUMVALLATE PAPILLA

val·lec·u·la \va-ˈle-kyə-lə\ *n*, *pl* **-lae** \-ˌlē\ : an anatomical groove, channel, or depression: as **a** : a groove between the base of the tongue and the epiglottis **b** : a fossa on the underside of the cerebellum separating the hemispheres and including the inferior vermis — **val·lec·u·lar** \-lər\ *adj*

valley fever *n* : COCCIDIOIDOMYCOSIS

val·pro·ate \val-ˈprō-ˌāt\ *n* : a salt or ester of valproic acid; *esp* : SODIUM VALPROATE

val·pro·ic acid \val-ˈprō-ik-\ *n* : a carboxylic acid $C_8H_{16}O_2$ used as an anticonvulsant often in the form of its sodium salt $C_8H_{15}NaO_2$ — see DEPAKENE, SODIUM VALPROATE

Val·sal·va maneuver \val-ˈsal-və-\ *also* **Val·sal·va's maneuver** \-vəz-\ *n* : a forceful attempt at expiration when the airway is closed at some point; *esp* : a conscious effort made while holding the nostrils closed and keeping the mouth shut (as for the purpose of adjusting middle ear pressure or aborting supraventricular tachycardia) — called also *Valsalva*

A. M. Valsalva — see SINUS OF VALSALVA

val·sar·tan \val-ˈsär-ˌtan\ *n* : an antihypertensive drug $C_{24}H_{29}N_5O_3$ that blocks the action of angiotensin II — see DIOVAN

Val·trex \'val-ˌtreks\ *trademark* — used for a preparation of the hydrochloride of valacyclovir

val·va \'val-və\ *n, pl* **val·vae** \-ˌvē\ : VALVE

valve \'valv\ *n* **1** : a bodily structure (as the mitral valve) that closes temporarily a passage or orifice or permits movement of fluid in one direction only **2** : any of various mechanical devices by which the flow of liquid (as blood) may be started, stopped, or regulated by a movable part that opens, shuts, or partially obstructs one or more ports or passageways; *also* : the movable part of such a device

valves of Kerk·ring *or* **valves of Kerck·ring** \-'ker-kriŋ\ *n pl* : PLICAE CIRCULARES

 Kerck·ring \'ker-kriŋ\, **Theodor** (1640–1693), Dutch anatomist.

val·vot·o·my \val-'vä-tə-mē\ *n, pl* **-mies** : VALVULOTOMY

valvul- *or* **valvulo-** *comb form* : small valve : fold ⟨*valvul*itis⟩ ⟨*valvulo*tome⟩

val·vu·la \'val-vyə-lə\ *n, pl* **-lae** \-ˌlē, -ˌlī\ : a small valve or fold

valvulae con·ni·ven·tes \-ˌkä-nə-'ven-ˌtēz\ *n pl* : PLICAE CIRCULARES

val·vu·lar \'val-vyə-lər\ *adj* **1** : resembling or functioning as a valve **2** : of, relating to, or affecting a valve esp. of the heart ⟨~ heart disease⟩

val·vu·li·tis \ˌval-vyə-'lī-təs\ *n* : inflammation of a valve esp. of the heart

val·vu·lo·plas·ty \'val-vyə-lō-ˌplas-tē\ *n, pl* **-ties** : plastic surgery performed on a heart valve

val·vu·lo·tome \'val-vyə-lō-ˌtōm\ *n* : a surgical blade designed for valvulotomy or commissurotomy

val·vu·lot·o·my \ˌval-vyə-'lä-tə-mē\ *n, pl* **-mies** : surgical incision of a valve; *specif* : the operation of enlarging a narrowed heart valve by cutting through the mitral commissures with a knife or by a finger thrust to relieve the symptoms of mitral stenosis

vampire bat *n* : any of several Central and So. American bats (*Desmodus rotundus*, *Diaemus youngi*, and *Diphylla ecaudata*) that feed on the blood of birds and mammals and esp. domestic animals and that are sometimes vectors of disease and esp. of rabies; *also* : any of several other bats that do not feed on blood but are sometimes reputed to do so

va·na·di·um \və-'nā-dē-əm\ *n* : a grayish malleable ductile metallic element — symbol *V*; see ELEMENT table

Van·co·cin \'van-kə-ˌsin\ *trademark* — used for a preparation of vancomycin

van·co·my·cin \ˌvan-kə-'mīs-ᵊn\ *n* : an antibiotic $C_{66}H_{75}Cl_2N_9O_{24}$ derived from an actinomycete (*Amycolatopsis orientalis* syn. *Streptomyces orientalis* syn. *Nocardia orientalis*) that is effective against gram-positive bacteria and is used chiefly in the form of its hydrochloride $C_{66}H_{75}Cl_2N_9O_{24}·HCl$

against staphylococci resistant to methicillin — see VANCOCIN

van den Bergh test \'van-dən-ˌbərg-\ *also* **van den Bergh's test** \-ˌbərgz-\ *n* : a test indicating presence of bilirubin in the blood (as in jaundice)

 Van den Bergh, Albert Abraham Hijmans (1869–1943), Dutch physician.

van·il·lyl·man·de·lic acid \ˌva-nə-ˌlil-man-'dē-lik-\ *n* : a principal catecholamine metabolite $C_9H_{10}O_5$ whose presence in excess in the urine is used as a test for pheochromocytoma — abbr. *VMA*

van·il·man·de·lic acid \ˌvan-ᵊl-man-'dē-lik-\ : VANILLYLMANDELIC ACID

va·por \'vā-pər\ *n* : a substance in the gaseous state as distinguished from the liquid or solid state — **va·por·ize** \'vā-pə-ˌrīz\ *vb* — **va·por·iz·able** \ˌvā-pə-'rī-zə-bəl\ *adj*

va·por·iz·er \'vā-pə-ˌrī-zər\ *n* : one that vaporizes: as **a** : ATOMIZER **b** : a device for converting water or a medicated liquid into a vapor for inhalation

va·pour *chiefly Brit var of* VAPOR

Va·quez's disease \vä-'ke-zəz-\ *n* : POLYCYTHEMIA VERA

 Vaquez, Louis Henri (1860–1936), French physician.

Var \'vär\ *n* : a vaccine that protects against chicken pox — see VARIVAX

var·den·a·fil \vär-'de-nə-ˌfil\ *n* : a drug used in the form of its hydrated hydrochloride $C_{23}H_{32}N_6O_4S·HCl·3H_2O$ to treat erectile dysfunction — see LEVITRA

variable region *n* : the part of the polypeptide chain of a light or heavy chain of an antibody that ends in a free amino group $–NH_2$, that varies greatly in its sequence of amino acid residues from one antibody to another, and that prob. determines the conformation of the combining site which confers the specificity of the antibody for a particular antigen — called also *variable domain*; compare CONSTANT REGION

variant Creutzfeldt–Jakob disease *n* : a fatal prion disease that is held to be a variant of Creutzfeldt-Jakob disease caused by the prion associated with bovine spongiform encephalopathy and contracted by consuming infected beef or beef products — abbr. *vCJD*; called also *new variant Creutzfeldt-Jakob disease*, *variant CJD*

varic- *or* **varico-** *comb form* : varix ⟨*varic*osis⟩ ⟨*varico*cele⟩

var·i·ce·al \ˌvar-ə-'sē-əl, və-'ri-sē-əl\ *adj* : of, relating to, or caused by varices ⟨~ hemorrhage⟩

var·i·cel·la \ˌvar-ə-'se-lə\ *n* : CHICKEN POX

varicella zoster *n* : a herpesvirus that causes chicken pox and shingles — called also *varicella-zoster virus*

var·i·cel·li·form \ˌvar-ə-'se-lə-ˌfȯrm\ *adj* : resembling chicken pox

Var·i·cel·lo·vi·rus \,var-ə-'se-lə-,vī-rəs\ *n* : a genus of herpesviruses that includes the causative agents of chicken pox, infectious bovine rhinotracheitis, pseudorabies, rhinpneumonitis, and shingles

varices *pl of* VARIX

var·i·co·cele \'var-i-kō-,sēl\ *n* : a varicose enlargement of the veins of the spermatic cord producing a soft compressible tumor mass in the scrotum

var·i·co·cel·ec·to·my \,var-i-kō-sē-'lek-tə-mē\ *n, pl* **-mies** : surgical treatment of varicocele by excision of the affected veins often with removal of part of the scrotum

var·i·cose \'var-ə-,kōs\ *also* **var·i·cosed** \-,kōst\ *adj* **1** : abnormally swollen or dilated ⟨~ lymph vessels⟩ **2** : affected with varicose veins ⟨~ legs⟩

varicose vein *n* : an abnormal swelling and tortuosity esp. of a superficial vein of the legs — usu. used in pl.

var·i·co·sis \,var-ə-'kō-səs\ *n, pl* **-co·ses** \-,sēz\ : the condition of being varicose or of having varicose vessels

var·i·cos·i·ty \,var-ə-'kä-sə-tē\ *n, pl* **-ties 1** : the quality or state of being abnormally or markedly swollen or dilated **2** : VARIX

Var·i·dase \'var-ə-,dās\ *n* : a preparation containing a mixture of streptodornase and streptokinase — formerly a U.S. registered trademark

va·ri·ety \və-'rī-ə-tē\ *n, pl* **-et·ies** : any of various groups of plants or animals ranking below a species : SUBSPECIES

va·ri·o·la \və-'rī-ə-lə\ *n* : SMALLPOX; *also* : the poxvirus of the genus *Orthopoxvirus* (species *Variola virus*) that causes smallpox

variola major *n* : a severe form of smallpox characterized historically by a death rate of about 30 percent

variola minor *n* : a mild form of smallpox of low mortality — called also *alastrim*

var·i·o·la·tion \,var-ē-ə-'lā-shən\ *n* : the deliberate inoculation of an uninfected person with the smallpox virus (as by contact with pustular matter) that was widely practiced before the era of vaccination as prophylaxis against the severe form of smallpox

variola vac·cin·ia \-vak-'si-nē-ə\ *n* : COWPOX

var·i·ol·i·form \,var-ē-'ō-lə-,fórm\ *adj* : resembling smallpox

varioliformis — see PITYRIASIS LICHENOIDES ET VARIOLIFORMIS ACUTA

va·ri·o·loid \'var-ē-ə-,lóid, və-'rī-ə-,lóid\ *n* : a modified mild form of smallpox occurring in persons who have been vaccinated or who have had smallpox

Var·i·vax \'var-ə-,vaks\ *trademark* — used for a vaccine against chicken pox containing live attenuated varicella zoster

var·ix \'var-iks\ *n, pl* **var·i·ces** \'var-ə-,sēz\ : an abnormally dilated and lengthened vein, artery, or lymph vessel; *esp* : VARICOSE VEIN

Varolii — see PONS VAROLII

varum — see GENU VARUM

var·us \'var-əs\ *adj* **1** : of, relating to, or being a deformity in which an anatomical part is turned inward toward the midline of the body to an abnormal degree ⟨a ~ heel⟩ — see CUBITUS VARUS, TALIPES VARUS; compare GENU VALGUM, GENU VARUM **2** : VALGUS 1 — used esp. in orthopedics of the knee — **varus** *n*

vas \'vas\ *n, pl* **va·sa** \'vā-zə\ : an anatomical vessel : DUCT

VAS *abbr* visual analog scale

vas- *or* **vaso-** *comb form* **1** : vessel: as **a** : blood vessel ⟨*vasomotor*⟩ **b** : vas deferens ⟨*vasectomy*⟩ **2** : vascular and ⟨*vaso*vagal⟩

vasa ab·er·ran·tia \-,a-bə-'ran-chə, -chē-ə\ *n pl* : slender arteries that are only occas. present and that connect the axillary or brachial artery with an artery (as the radial artery) of the forearm or with its branches

vas ab·er·rans of Hal·ler \-'a-bə-,ranz . . . -'hä-lər\ *n, pl* **vasa ab·er·ran·tia of Haller** \-,a-bə-'ran-chə-, -chē-ə-\ : a blind tube occas. present parallel to the first part of the vas deferens

Haller, Albrecht von (1708–1777), Swiss biologist.

vasa deferentia *pl of* VAS DEFERENS

vasa ef·fer·en·tia \-,e-fə-'ren-chə, -chē-ə\ *n pl* : the 12 to 20 ductules that lead from the rete testis to the vas deferens and except near their commencement are greatly convoluted and form the compact head of the epididymis

va·sal \'vā-zəl\ *adj* : of, relating to, or constituting an anatomical vessel

vasa rec·ta \-'rek-tə\ *n pl* **1** : numerous small vessels that arise from the terminal branches of arteries supplying the intestine, encircle the intestine, and divide into more branches between its layers **2** : hairpin-shaped vessels that arise from the arteriole leading away from a renal glomerulus, descend into the renal pyramids, reunite as they ascend, and play a role in the concentration of urine

vasa va·so·rum \-vā-'sór-əm\ *n pl* : small blood vessels that supply or drain the walls of the larger arteries and veins and connect with a branch of the same vessel or a neighboring vessel

vascul- *or* **vasculo-** *comb form* : vessel; *esp* : blood vessel ⟨*vasculo*toxic⟩

vas·cu·lar \'vas-kyə-lər\ *adj* **1** : of, relating to, constituting, or affecting a tube or a system of tubes for the conveyance of a body fluid (as blood or lymph) **2** : supplied with or containing ducts and esp. blood vessels — **vas·cu·lar·i·ty** \,vas-kyə-'lar-ə-tē\ *n*

vascular bed *n* : an intricate network of minute blood vessels that ramifies through the tissues of the body or of one of its parts

vascular dementia *n* : dementia (as multi-infarct dementia) of abrupt or gradual onset that is caused by cerebrovascular disease

vascular endothelial growth factor *n* : a protein that promotes the growth of new blood vessels — abbr. *VEGF*

vascularis — see STRIA VASCULARIS

vas·cu·lar·i·za·tion \,vas-kyə-lə-rə-'zā-shən\ *n* : the process of becoming vascular; *also* : abnormal or excessive formation of blood vessels (as in the retina or on the cornea) — **vas·cu·lar·ize** \'vas-kyə-lə-,rīz\ *vb*

vascular resistance *n* : resistance to blood flow through blood vessels and esp. arterioles — see PERIPHERAL VASCULAR RESISTANCE

vascular tunic *n* : UVEA

vas·cu·la·ture \'vas-kyə-lə-,chùr, -,tyùr, -,tùr\ *n* : the arrangement of blood vessels in an organ or part

vas·cu·li·tis \,vas-kyə-'lī-təs\ *n, pl* **-lit·i·des** \-'li-tə-,dēz\ : inflammation of a blood or lymph vessel — **vas·cu·lit·ic** \,vas-kyə-'li-tik\ *adj*

vas·cu·lo·gen·ic \,vas-kyə-lō-'je-nik\ *adj* : caused by disorder or dysfunction of the blood vessels ⟨∼ impotence⟩ ⟨∼ migraine⟩

vas·cu·lo·tox·ic \,vas-kyə-lō-'täk-sik\ *adj* : destructive to blood vessels or the vascular system ⟨∼ effects⟩

vas def·er·ens \-'de-fə-rənz, -,renz\ *n, pl* **vasa def·er·en·tia** \-,de-fə-'ren-chə, -chē-ə\ : a sperm-carrying duct that is a small but thick-walled tube about two feet (0.6 meter) long that begins at and is continuous with the tail of the epididymis, runs in the spermatic cord through the inguinal canal, and descends into the pelvis where it joins the duct of the seminal vesicle to form the ejaculatory duct — called also *ductus deferens, spermatic duct*

va·sec·to·my \va-'sek-tə-mē, vā-'zek-\ *n, pl* **-mies** : surgical division or resection of all or part of the vas deferens usu. to induce sterility — **va·sec·to·mize** \-,mīz\ *vb*

Vas·e·line \,va-sə-'lēn\ *trademark* — used for a preparation of petroleum jelly

vaso- — see VAS-

va·so·ac·tive \,vā-zō-'ak-tiv\ *adj* : affecting the blood vessels esp. in respect to the degree of their relaxation or contraction — **va·so·ac·tiv·i·ty** \-ak-'ti-və-tē\ *n*

vasoactive intestinal polypeptide *n* : a protein hormone that consists of a chain of 28 amino acid residues, has been implicated as a neurotransmitter, and has a wide range of physiological activities (as stimulation of secretion by the pancreas and small intestine, vasodilation, and inhibition of gastric juice production) — abbr. *VIP;* called also *vasoactive intestinal peptide*

va·so·con·stric·tion \,vā-zō-kən-'strik-shən\ *n* : narrowing of the lumen of blood vessels esp. as a result of vasomotor action — **va·so·con·stric·tive** \-'strik-tiv\ *adj*

va·so·con·stric·tor \,vā-zō-kən-'strik-tər\ *n* : an agent (as a sympathetic nerve fiber or a drug) that induces or initiates vasoconstriction — **vasoconstrictor** *adj*

va·so·de·pres·sor \,vā-zō-di-'pre-sər\ *adj* : causing or characterized by vasomotor depression resulting in lowering of the blood pressure

va·so·di·la·tion \,vā-zo-dī-'lā-shən\ *or* **va·so·di·la·ta·tion** \-,dī-lə-'tā-shən, -,dī-\ *n* : widening of the lumen of blood vessels

va·so·di·la·tor \,vā-zō-'dī-,lā-tər\ *n* : an agent (as a parasympathetic nerve fiber or a drug) that induces or initiates vasodilation — **vasodilator** *also* **va·so·di·la·to·ry** \-'dī-lə-,tōr-ē, -'dī-\ *adj*

va·so·for·ma·tive \,vā-zō-'fòr-mə-tiv\ *adj* : functioning in the development and formation of vessels and esp. blood vessels ⟨∼ cells⟩

va·sog·ra·phy \vā-'zä-grə-fē\ *n, pl* **-phies** : radiography of blood vessels

va·so·li·ga·tion \,vā-zō-lī-'gā-shən\ *n* : surgical ligation of a vessel and esp. of the vas deferens

va·so·mo·tion \,vā-zō-'mō-shən\ *n* : alteration in the caliber of blood vessels

va·so·mo·tor \,vā-zō-'mō-tər\ *adj* : of, relating to, affecting, or being nerves or the centers (as in the medulla and spinal cord) from which they arise that supply the muscle fibers of the walls of blood vessels, include sympathetic vasoconstrictors and parasympathetic vasodilators, and by their effect on vascular diameter regulate the amount of blood passing to a particular body part or organ

vasomotor rhinitis *n* : chronic rhinitis that is not attributable to allergy or infection and is thought to be a hypersensitive reaction to various potentially irritating stimuli (as strong odors or air pollution)

va·so·oc·clu·sive \-ə-'klü-siv\ *adj* : relating to, resulting from, or caused by occlusion of a blood vessel ⟨a ∼ crisis characteristic of sickle-cell anemia⟩

va·so·pres·sin \,vā-zō-'pres-³n\ *n* : a polypeptide hormone that is secreted together with oxytocin by the posterior lobe of the pituitary gland, is also obtained synthetically, and increases blood pressure and exerts an antidiuretic effect — called also *antidiuretic hormone;* see ARGININE VASOPRESSIN, LYSINE VASOPRESSIN, PITRESSIN

¹va·so·pres·sor \-'pre-sər\ *adj* : causing a rise in blood pressure by exerting a vasoconstrictor effect

²vasopressor *n* : a vasopressor agent

¹va·so·re·lax·ant \-ri-'lak-sənt\ *adj* : relating to or producing vasorelaxation

²**vasorelaxant** *n* : a vasorelaxant agent
va·so·re·lax·ation \-,rē-,lak-'sā-shən\ *n*
: reduction of vascular tension
vasorum — see VASA VASORUM
va·so·spasm \'vā-zō-,spa-zəm\ *n*
: sharp and often persistent contraction of a blood vessel reducing its caliber and blood flow — **va·so·spas·tic** \,vā-zō-'spas-tik\ *adj*
Va·so·tec \'vā-zō-,tek\ *trademark* — used for a preparation of enalaprilat or the maleate of enalapril
va·sot·o·my \vā-'zä-tə-mē\ *n, pl* **-mies**
: surgical incision of the vas deferens
va·so·va·gal \,vā-zō-'vā-gəl\ *adj* : of, relating to, or involving both vascular and vagal factors
vasovagal syncope *n* : a usu. transitory condition that is marked esp. by fainting associated with hypotension, peripheral vasodilation, and bradycardia resulting from increased stimulation of the vagus nerve — called also *neurocardiogenic syncope*
va·so·va·sos·to·my \,vā-zō-vā-'zäs-tə-mē\ *n, pl* **-mies** : surgical anastomosis of a divided vas deferens to reverse a previous vasectomy
vas·tus in·ter·me·di·us \'vas-təs-,in-tər-'mē-dē-əs\ *n* : the division of the quadriceps muscle that arises from and covers the front of the shaft of the femur
vastus in·ter·nus \-in-'tər-nəs\ *n* : VASTUS MEDIALIS
vastus lat·er·a·lis \-,la-tər-'ā-ləs, -'a-\ *n* : the division of the quadriceps muscle that covers the outer anterior aspect of the femur, arises chiefly from the femur, and inserts into the outer border of the patella by a flat tendon — called also *vastus externus*
vastus me·di·a·lis \-,mē-dē-'ā-ləs, -'a-\ *n* : the division of the quadriceps muscle that covers the inner anterior aspect of the femur, arises chiefly from the femur and the adjacent intermuscular septum, inserts into the inner border of the patella and into the tendon of the other divisions of the muscle, sends also a tendinous expansion to the capsule of the knee joint, and is closely and in the upper part often inseparably united with the vastus intermedius — called also *vastus internus*
vault \'volt\ *n* : an arched or dome-shaped anatomical structure: as **a** : SKULLCAP, CALVARIUM ⟨the cranial ∼⟩ **b** : FORNIX d
VBAC \'vē-,bak\ *n* [*v*aginal *b*irth *a*fter *c*esarean] : delivery through the birth canal in a pregnancy subsequent to one in which delivery was by cesarean section
VCG *abbr* vectorcardiogram
vCJD *abbr* variant Creutzfeldt-Jakob disease
VD *abbr* venereal disease
VDRL \,vē-(,)dē-(,)är-'el\ *n* : VDRL TEST
VDRL *abbr* venereal disease research laboratory

VDRL slide test *n* : VDRL TEST
VDRL test *n* : a flocculation test for syphilis employing cardiolipin in combination with lecithin and cholesterol
¹**vec·tor** \'vek-tər\ *n* **1** : a quantity that has magnitude and direction and that is usu. represented by part of a straight line with the given direction and with a length representing the magnitude **2** : an organism (as an insect) that transmits a pathogen from one organism to another ⟨fleas are ∼s of plague⟩ — compare CARRIER 1a **3** : an agent (as a plasmid or virus) that contains or carries modified genetic material (as recombinant DNA) and can be used to introduce exogenous genes into the genome of an organism — **vec·to·ri·al** \vek-'tōr-ē-əl\ *adj*
²**vector** *vb* **vec·tored; vec·tor·ing** : to transmit (a pathogen or disease) from one organism to another : act as a vector for ⟨a disease ∼*ed* by flies⟩
vec·tor·car·dio·gram \,vek-tər-'kär-dē-ə-,gram\ *n* : a graphic record made by vectorcardiography — abbr. *VCG*
vec·tor·car·di·og·ra·phy \-,kär-dē-'ä-grə-fē\ *n, pl* **-phies** : a method of recording the direction and magnitude of the electrical forces of the heart by means of a continuous series of vectors that form a curving line around a center — **vec·tor·car·dio·graph·ic** \-dē-ə-'gra-fik\ *adj*
VEE *abbr* Venezuelan equine encephalitis; Venezuelan equine encephalomyelitis
veg·an \'vē-gən\ *n* : a strict vegetarian who consumes no animal food or dairy products — **vegan** *adj* — **veg·an·ism** \'vē-gə-,ni-zəm\ *n*
veg·e·ta·ble \'vej-tə-bəl\ *n* : a person whose mental and physical functioning is severely impaired and esp. one who requires supportive measures (as mechanical ventilation) to survive
veg·e·tar·i·an·ism \,ve-jə-'ter-ē-ə-,ni-zəm\ *n* : the theory or practice of living on a diet made up of vegetables, fruits, grains, nuts, and sometimes eggs or dairy products — **veg·e·tari·an** \-'ter-ē-ən\ *n or adj*
veg·e·ta·tion \,ve-jə-'tā-shən\ *n* : an abnormal outgrowth upon a body part; *specif* : any of the warty excrescences on the valves of the heart that are composed of various tissue elements including fibrin and collagen and that are typical of endocarditis
veg·e·ta·tive \'ve-jə-,tā-tiv\ *adj* **1 a** (1) : growing or having the power of growing (2) : of, relating to, or engaged in nutritive and growth functions as contrasted with reproductive functions ⟨a ∼ nucleus⟩ **b** : of, relating to, or involving propagation by nonsexual processes or methods **2** : affecting, arising from, or relating to involuntary bodily functions **3** : characterized by, resulting from, or being

a state in which there is a total loss of cognitive functioning typically indicated by a lack of awareness of oneself or one's environment and in which only involuntary bodily functions (as breathing or blinking of the eyes) are sustained 〈a ∼ state〉 — **veg·e·ta·tive·ly** adv

VEGF abbr vascular endothelial growth factor

ve·hi·cle \'vē-i-kəl, -,hi-\ n 1 : an inert medium in which a medicinally active agent is administered 2 : an agent of transmission 〈a ∼ of infection〉

vein \'vān\ n : any of the tubular branching vessels that carry blood from the capillaries toward the heart and have thinner walls than the arteries and often valves at intervals to prevent reflux of the blood which flows in a steady stream and is in most cases dark-colored due to the presence of reduced hemoglobin — **veiny** \'vā-nē\ adj

vein·ous \'vā-nəs\ adj 1 : having veins that are esp. prominent 〈∼ hands〉 2 : VENOUS

vela pl of VELUM

veli — see LEVATOR VELI PALATINI, TENSOR VELI PALATINI

ve·lo·pha·ryn·geal \,vē-lō-,far-ən-'jē-əl, -fə-'rin-jəl, -jē-əl\ adj : of or relating to the soft palate and the pharynx

Vel·peau bandage \vel-'pō-\ or **Velpeau's bandage** \-'pōz-\ n : a bandage used to support and immobilize the arm when the clavicle is fractured
   Velpeau, Alfred–Armand–Louis–Marie (1795–1867), French surgeon.

ve·lum \'vē-ləm\ n, pl **ve·la** \-lə\ : a membrane or membranous part resembling a veil or curtain: as a : SOFT PALATE b : SEMILUNAR CUSP

ven- or **veni-** or **veno-** comb form : vein 〈venipuncture〉

ve·na ca·va \,vē-nə-'kā-və\ n, pl **ve·nae ca·vae** \,vē-nē-'kā-(,)vē\ : either of two large veins by which the blood is returned to the right atrium of the heart: a : INFERIOR VENA CAVA b : SUPERIOR VENA CAVA — **vena caval** \-vəl\ adj

vena co·mi·tans \-'kō-mə-,tanz\ n, pl **venae co·mi·tan·tes** \-,kō-mə-'tan-,tēz\ : a vein accompanying an artery

venae cor·dis min·i·mae \-'kór-dəs-'mi-nə-,mē\ n pl : minute veins in the wall of the heart that empty into the atria or ventricles

vena vor·ti·co·sa \-,vór-tə-'kō-sə\ n, pl **venae vor·ti·co·sae** \-(,)sē\ : any of the veins of the outer layer of the choroid of the eye — called also vorticose vein

ve·neer \və-'nir\ n : a plastic or porcelain coating bonded to the surface of a cosmetically imperfect tooth

ve·ne·re·al \və-'nir-ē-əl\ adj 1 : resulting from or contracted during sexual intercourse 〈∼ infections〉 2 : of, relating to, or affected with venereal disease 〈a high ∼ rate〉 3 : involving

the genital organs 〈∼ sarcoma〉 — **ve·ne·re·al·ly** adv

venereal disease n : a contagious disease (as gonorrhea or syphilis) that is typically acquired in sexual intercourse — abbr. VD; compare SEXUALLY TRANSMITTED DISEASE

venereal wart n : GENITAL WART

ve·ne·re·ol·o·gy \və-,nir-ē-'ä-lə-jē\ also **ven·er·ol·o·gy** \,ve-nə-'rä-lə-jē\ n, pl **-gies** : a branch of medical science concerned with venereal diseases — **ve·ne·re·o·log·i·cal** \və-,nir-ē-ə-'lä-ji-kəl\ adj — **ve·ne·re·ol·o·gist** \və-,nir-ē-'ä-lə-jist\ n

venereum — see LYMPHOGRANULOMA VENEREUM, LYMPHOPATHIA VENEREUM

veneris — see MONS VENERIS

vene·sec·tion \'ve-nə-,sek-shən, 'vē-\ n : PHLEBOTOMY

Venezuelan equine encephalitis n : EQUINE ENCEPHALITIS c

Venezuelan equine encephalomyelitis n : EQUINE ENCEPHALITIS c

veni- — see VEN-

ve·ni·punc·ture \'vē-nə-,pəŋk-chər, 've-\ n : surgical puncture of a vein esp. for the withdrawal of blood or for administration of intravenous fluids or drugs

venisection var of VENESECTION

ven·la·fax·ine \,ven-lə-'fak-,sēn\ n : an antidepressant drug that is used in the form of its hydrochloride $C_{17}H_{27}NO_2 \cdot HCl$ and acts by inhibiting the reuptake of serotonin and norepinephrine by neurons — see EFFEXOR

veno- — see VEN-

ve·no·ar·te·ri·al \,vē-nō-är-'tir-ē-əl\ adj : relating to or involving an artery and vein

ve·noc·ly·sis \vē-'nä-klə-səs\ n, pl **-ly·ses** \-,sēz\ : clysis into a vein

ve·no·con·stric·tion \,vē-nō-kən-'strik-shən\ n : constriction of a vein

ve·no·gram \'vē-nə-,gram\ n : a radiograph made by venography

ve·nog·ra·phy \vi-'nä-grə-fē, vā-\ n, pl **-phies** : radiography of a vein after injection of an opaque substance — **ve·no·graph·ic** \,vē-nə-'gra-fik\ adj

ven·om \'ve-nəm\ n : poisonous matter normally secreted by some animals (as snakes, scorpions, or bees) and transmitted to prey or an enemy chiefly by biting or stinging

ven·om·ous \'ve-nə-məs\ adj 1 : POISONOUS 2 : having a venom-producing gland and able to inflict a poisoned wound 〈∼ snakes〉

ve·no·oc·clu·sive \,vē-nō-ə-'klü-siv\ adj : marked by occlusion or compression of small veins 〈∼ disease〉

venosum — see LIGAMENTUM VENOSUM

venosus — see DUCTUS VENOSUS, SINUS VENOSUS, SINUS VENOSUS SCLERAE

ve·not·o·my \vi-'nä-tə-mē\ n, pl **-mies** : PHLEBOTOMY

ve·nous \'vē-nəs\ *adj* **1 a** : full of or characterized by veins **b** : made up of or carried on by veins ⟨the ~ circulation⟩ **2** : of, relating to, or performing the functions of a vein ⟨a ~ inflammation⟩ **3** *of blood* : having passed through the capillaries and given up oxygen for the tissues and become charged with carbon dioxide and ready to pass through the respiratory organs to release its carbon dioxide and renew its oxygen supply : dark red from reduced hemoglobin — compare ARTERIAL 2

venous hum *n* : a humming sound sometimes heard during auscultation of the veins of the neck esp. in anemia

venous return *n* : the flow of blood from the venous system into the right atrium of the heart

venous sinus *n* **1** : a large vein or passage (as the canal of Schlemm) for venous blood **2** : SINUS VENOSUS

vent \'vent\ *n* : the external opening of the rectum or cloaca : ANUS

vent gleet *n* : CLOACITIS

ven·ti·late \'vent-ᵊl-ˌāt\ *vb* **-lat·ed; -lat·ing 1** : to expose to air and esp. to a current of fresh air for purifying or refreshing **2 a** : OXYGENATE, AERATE ⟨~ blood in the lungs⟩ **b** : to subject the lungs of (an individual) to ventilation **3** : to give verbal expression to (as mental or emotional conflicts)

ven·ti·la·tion \ˌvent-ᵊl-'ā-shən\ *n* **1** : the act or process of ventilating **2** : the circulation and exchange of gases in the lungs or gills that is basic to respiration — **ven·ti·la·to·ry** \'vent-ᵊl-ə-ˌtōr-ē\ *adj*

ven·ti·la·tor \'vent-ᵊl-ˌā-tər\ *n* : RESPIRATOR 2

Ven·to·lin \'ven-tᵊl-ən\ *trademark* — used for a preparation of albuterol

ventr- *or* **ventri-** *or* **ventro-** *comb form* **1** : abdomen ⟨*ventr*al⟩ **2** : ventral and ⟨*ventro*medial⟩

ven·tral \'ven-trəl\ *adj* **1** : of or relating to the belly : ABDOMINAL **2 a** : being or located near, on, or toward the lower surface of an animal (as a quadruped) opposite the back or dorsal surface **b** : being or located near, on, or toward the front or anterior part of the human body — **ven·tral·ly** *adv*

ventral column *n* : VENTRAL HORN

ventral corticospinal tract *n* : a band of nerve fibers that descends in the ventrolateral part of the spinal cord and consists of fibers arising in the motor cortex of the brain on the same side of the body — called also *anterior corticospinal tract, direct pyramidal tract*

ventral funiculus *n* : ANTERIOR FUNICULUS

ventral gray column *n* : VENTRAL HORN

ventral horn *n* : a longitudinal subdivision of gray matter in the anterior part of each lateral half of the spinal cord that contains neurons giving rise to motor fibers of the ventral roots of the spinal nerves — called also *anterior column, anterior gray column, anterior horn, ventral column, ventral gray column;* compare DORSAL HORN, LATERAL COLUMN 1

ventralis — see SACROCOCCYGEUS VENTRALIS

ventral median fissure *n* : ANTERIOR MEDIAN FISSURE

ventral mesogastrium *n* : MESOGASTRIUM 1

ventral root *n* : the one of the two roots of a spinal nerve that passes anteriorly from the spinal cord separating the anterior and lateral funiculi and that consists of motor fibers — called also *anterior root;* compare DORSAL ROOT

ventral spinocerebellar tract *n* : SPINOCEREBELLAR TRACT b

ventral spinothalamic tract *n* : SPINOTHALAMIC TRACT a

ventri- — see VENTR-

ven·tri·cle \'ven-tri-kəl\ *n* : a cavity of a bodily part or organ: as **a** : a chamber of the heart which receives blood from a corresponding atrium and from which blood is forced into the arteries **b** : any of a system of communicating cavities in the brain that are continuous with the central canal of the spinal cord — see FOURTH VENTRICLE, LATERAL VENTRICLE, THIRD VENTRICLE **c** : a fossa or pouch on each side of the larynx between the false vocal cords above and the true vocal cords below

ven·tric·u·lar \ven-'tri-kyə-lər, vən-\ *adj* : of, relating to, or being a ventricle esp. of the heart or brain

ventricular assist device *n* : VAD

ventricular fibrillation *n* : very rapid uncoordinated fluttering contractions of the ventricles of the heart resulting in loss of synchronization between heartbeat and pulse beat — abbr. *VF, V-fib*

ventricular folds *n pl* : FALSE VOCAL CORDS

ventricular septal defect *n* : a congenital defect in the interventricular septum — abbr. *VSD*

ventricular tachycardia *n* : tachycardia that is associated with the generation of electrical impulses within the ventricles and is characterized by an electrocardiogram having a broad QRS complex — abbr. *VT, V-tach*

ven·tric·u·li·tis \ven-ˌtri-kyə-'lī-təs\ *n* : inflammation of the ventricles of the brain

ven·tric·u·lo·atri·al \ven-ˌtri-kyə-lō-'ā-trē-əl\ *adj* **1** : of, relating to, or being an artificial shunt between a ventricle of the brain and an atrium of the heart esp. to drain cerebrospinal fluid (as in hydrocephalus) **2** : of, relating to, or being conduction from the ventricle to the atrium of the heart

ven·tric·u·lo·atri·os·to·my \-ˌā-trē-'äs-tə-mē\ *n, pl* **-mies** : surgical establishment of a shunt to drain cerebrospinal fluid (as in hydrocephalus) from a ventricle of the brain to the right atrium

ven·tric·u·lo·cis·ter·nos·to·my \-ₜsis-tər-'näs-tə-mē\ *n, pl* **-mies** : the surgical establishment of a communication between a ventricle of the brain and the subarachnoid space and esp. the cisterna magna to drain cerebrospinal fluid esp. in hydrocephalus

ven·tric·u·lo·gram \ven-'tri-kyə-lə-ₜgram\ *n* : an X-ray photograph made by ventriculography

ven·tric·u·log·ra·phy \ven-ₜtri-kyə-'lä-grə-fē\ *n, pl* **-phies** **1** : the act or process of making an X-ray photograph of the ventricles of the brain after withdrawing fluid from the ventricles and replacing it with air or a radiopaque substance **2** : the act or process of making an X-ray photograph of a ventricle of the heart after injecting a radiopaque substance — **ven·tric·u·lo·graph·ic** \-kyə-lō-'gra-fik\ *adj*

ven·tric·u·lo·peri·to·ne·al \ven-ₜtri-kyə-lō-ₜper-ə-tə-'nē-əl\ *adj* : relating to or serving to communicate between a ventricle of the brain and the peritoneal cavity ⟨a ∼ shunt⟩

ven·tric·u·los·to·my \ven-ₜtri-kyə-'läs-tə-mē\ *n, pl* **-mies** : the surgical establishment of an opening in a ventricle of the brain to drain cerebrospinal fluid esp. in hydrocephalus

ven·tric·u·lot·o·my \ven-ₜtri-kyə-'lä-tə-mē\ *n, pl* **-mies** : surgical incision of a ventricle (as of the heart)

ventro- — see VENTR-

ven·tro·lat·er·al \ven-ₜtrō-'la-tə-rəl\ *adj* : ventral and lateral — **ven·tro·lat·er·al·ly** *adv*

ven·tro·me·di·al \-'mē-dē-əl\ *adj* : ventral and medial — **ven·tro·me·di·al·ly** *adv*

ventromedial nucleus *n* : a medially located nucleus of the hypothalamus situated between the lateral wall of the third ventricle and the fornix

ve·nule \'vēn-(ₜ)yül, 'ven-\ *n* : a small vein; *esp* : any of the minute veins connecting the capillaries with the larger systemic veins — **ven·u·lar** \'ven-yə-lər\ *adj*

vera — see ALOE VERA, DECIDUA VERA, POLYCYTHEMIA VERA

ve·rap·am·il \və-'ra-pə-ₜmil\ *n* : a calcium channel blocker used in the form of its hydrochloride $C_{27}H_{38}N_2O_4 \cdot HCl$ esp. to treat hypertension and angina pectoris — see CALAN

ver·a·trine \'ver-ə-ₜtrēn\ *n* : a mixture of poisonous alkaloids that is obtained from the seeds of a Mexican plant (*Schoenocaulon officinalis*) of the lily family (Liliaceae) and has been used as a counterirritant in neuralgia and arthritis

ve·ra·trum \və-'rā-trəm\ *n* **1 a** *cap* : a genus of herbs having short poisonous rootstocks **b** : any hellebore of the genus *Veratrum* **2** : HELLEBORE 2b

ver·big·er·a·tion \(ₜ)vər-ₜbi-jə-'rā-shən\ *n* : continual repetition of stereotyped phrases (as in some forms of mental disorder)

verge — see ANAL VERGE

ver·gence \'vər-jəns\ *n* : a movement of one eye in relation to the other

vermes *pl of* VERMIS

vermi- *comb form* : worm ⟨*vermi*cide⟩ ⟨*vermi*form⟩

ver·mi·cide \'vər-mə-ₜsīd\ *n* : an agent that destroys worms; *esp* : ANTHELMINTIC

ver·mi·form \'vər-mə-ₜform\ *adj* : resembling a worm in shape

vermiform appendix *n* : a narrow blind tube usu. about three or four inches (7.6 to 10.2 centimeters) long that extends from the cecum in the lower right-hand part of the abdomen and represents an atrophied terminal part of the cecum

ver·mi·fuge \'vər-mə-ₜfyüj\ *n* : an agent that serves to destroy or expel parasitic worms : ANTHELMINTIC — **ver·mif·u·gal** \vər-'mi-fyə-gəl, ₜvər-mə-'fyü-gəl\ *adj*

ver·mil·ion border \vər-'mil-yən-\ *n* : the exposed pink or reddish margin of a lip

ver·mil·ion·ec·to·my \vər-ₜmil-yə-'nek-tə-mē\ *n, pl* **-mies** : surgical excision of the vermilion border

ver·min \'vər-mən\ *n, pl* **vermin** : small common harmful or objectionable animals (as lice or fleas) that are difficult to control

ver·min·ous \'vər-mə-nəs\ *adj* **1** : consisting of, infested with, or being vermin **2** : caused by parasitic worms

ver·mis \'vər-mis\ *n, pl* **ver·mes** \-ₜmēz\ **1** : either of two parts of the median lobe of the cerebellum: **a** : one slightly prominent on the upper surface — called also *superior vermis* **b** : one on the lower surface sunk in the vallecula — called also *inferior vermis* **2** : the median lobe or part of the cerebellum

vernal conjunctivitis *n* : conjunctivitis occurring in warm seasons as a result of exposure to allergens

Ver·ner–Mor·ri·son syndrome \'vər-nər-'mȯr-ə-sən-, -'mär-\ *n* : a syndrome characterized esp. by severe watery diarrhea and hypokalemia that is often due to an excessive secretion of vasoactive intestinal peptide from a vipoma esp. of the pancreas — called also *pancreatic cholera*

> **Verner, John Victor** (*b* 1927), American physician.
> **Morrison, Ashton Byrom** (*b* 1922), American pathologist.

ver·ni·er acuity \'vər-nē-ər\ *n* : the aspect of visual acuity that involves the ability to detect the alignment or lack of alignment of the two parts of a broken line

ver·nix \'vər-niks\ *n* : VERNIX CASEOSA

vernix ca·se·o·sa \-ˌka-sē-'ō-sə\ *n* : a pasty covering chiefly of dead cells and sebaceous secretions that protects the skin of the fetus

ver·o·nal \'ver-ə-ˌnȯl, -nəl\ *n, often cap* : a preparation of the sodium salt of barbital

ver·ru·ca \və-'rü-kə\ *n, pl* **-cae** \-ˌkē\ : a wart or warty skin lesion

verruca acu·mi·na·ta \-ə-ˌkyü-mə-'nä-tə\ *n* : GENITAL WART

verruca pla·na \-'plä-nə\ *n* : FLAT WART

verruca plan·ta·ris \-ˌplan-'tar-əs\ *n* : PLANTAR WART

verruca vul·ga·ris \-ˌvəl-'gar-əs\ *n* : WART 1; *esp* : one occurring on the back of the fingers and hands

ver·ru·cose \və-'rü-ˌkōs\ *adj* **1** : covered with warty elevations **2** : having the form of a wart ⟨a ~ nevus⟩

ver·ru·cous \və-'rü-kəs\ *adj* **1** : VERRUCOSE **2** : characterized by the formation of warty lesions ⟨~ dermatitis⟩

verrucous endocarditis *n* : endocarditis marked by the formation or presence of warty nodules of fibrin on the lips of the heart valves

ver·ru·ga \və-'rü-gə\ *n* **1** : VERRUCA **2** : VERRUGA PERUANA

verruga per·u·a·na \-ˌper-ə-'wä-nə\ *also* **verruga pe·ru·vi·ana** \-pə-ˌrü-vē-'a-nə\ *n* : the second stage of bartonellosis characterized by warty nodules tending to ulcerate and bleed

versicolor — see PITYRIASIS VERSICOLOR, TINEA VERSICOLOR

ver·sion \'vər-zhən, -shən\ *n* **1** : a condition in which an organ and esp. the uterus is turned from its normal position **2** : manual turning of a fetus in the uterus to aid delivery

ver·te·bra \'vər-tə-brə\ *n, pl* **-brae** \-ˌbrā, -(ˌ)brē\ *or* **-bras** : any of the bony or cartilaginous segments composing the spinal column that have a short more or less cylindrical body whose ends articulate by pads of elastic or cartilaginous tissue with those of adjacent vertebrae and a bony arch that encloses the spinal cord

¹ver·te·bral \(ˌ)vər-'tē-brəl, 'vər-tə-\ *adj* **1** : of, relating to, or being vertebrae or the spinal column : SPINAL **2** : composed of or having vertebrae

²vertebral *n* : a vertebral part or element (as an artery)

vertebral arch *n* : NEURAL ARCH

vertebral artery *n* : a large branch of the subclavian artery that ascends through the foramina in the transverse processes of each of the cervical vertebrae except the last one or two, enters the cranium through the foramen magnum, and unites with the corresponding artery of the opposite side to form the basilar artery

vertebral body *n* : the main anterior bony part of a vertebra that consists of the centrum, the ossified postero-lateral joints linking the centrum and each half of the neural arch, and part of the neural arch

vertebral canal *n* : a canal that contains the spinal cord and is delimited by the neural arches on the dorsal side of the vertebrae — called also *spinal canal*

vertebral column *n* : SPINAL COLUMN

vertebral foramen *n* : the opening formed by a neural arch through which the spinal cord passes

vertebral ganglion *n* : any of a group of sympathetic ganglia which form two chains extending from the base of the skull to the coccyx along the sides of the spinal column — compare SYMPATHETIC CHAIN

vertebral notch *n* : either of two concave constrictions of which one occurs on the inferior surface and one on the superior surface of the pedicle on each side of a vertebra and which are arranged so that the superior notches of one vertebra and the corresponding inferior notches of a contiguous vertebra combine to form an intervertebral foramen on each side

vertebral plexus *n* : a plexus of veins associated with the spinal column

vertebral vein *n* : a tributary of the brachiocephalic vein that is formed by the union of branches originating in the occipital region and forming a plexus about the vertebral artery in its passage through the foramina of the cervical vertebrae

vertebra pro·mi·nens \-'prä-mi-ˌnenz\ *n* : the seventh cervical vertebra characterized by a prominent spinous process which can be felt at the base of the neck

ver·te·brate \'vər-tə-brət, -ˌbrāt\ *n* : any of a subphylum (Vertebrata) of animals that have a spinal column including the mammals, birds, reptiles, amphibians, and fishes — **vertebrate** *adj*

ver·te·bro·ba·si·lar \ˌvər-tə-brō-'bā-sə-lər\ *adj* : of, relating to, or being the vertebral and basilar arteries

ver·te·bro·chon·dral rib \ˌvər-tə-brō-'kän-drəl-\ *n* : any of the three false ribs that are located above the floating ribs and that are attached to each other by costal cartilages

ver·te·bro·plas·ty \ˌvər-tə-brō-ˌplas-tē\ *n, pl* **-ties** : a medical procedure for reducing pain caused by a vertebral compression fracture (as that associated with osteoporosis) that involves injection of an acrylic cement into the body of the fractured vertebra for stabilization — compare KYPHOPLASTY

ver·te·bro·ster·nal rib \-'stər-nəl-\ *n* : TRUE RIB

ver·tex \'vər-ˌteks\ *n, pl* **ver·ti·ces** \'vər-tə-ˌsēz\ *also* **ver·tex·es 1** : the top of the head **2** : the highest point of the skull

vertex presentation *n* : normal obstetric presentation in which the fetal occiput lies at the opening of the uterus

ver·ti·cal \ˈvər-ti-kəl\ *adj* : relating to or being transmission (as of a disease) by genetic inheritance or by a congenital or perinatal route — compare HORIZONTAL 2 — **ver·ti·cal·ly** *adv*

vertical dimension *n* : the distance between two arbitrarily chosen points on the face above and below the mouth when the teeth are in occlusion

vertical nystagmus *n* : nystagmus characterized by up-and-down movement of the eyes

ver·tig·i·nous \(ˌ)vər-ˈti-jə-nəs\ *adj* : of, relating to, characterized by, or affected with vertigo or dizziness

ver·ti·go \ˈvər-ti-ˌgō\ *n, pl* **-goes** *or* **-gos** 1 : a sensation of motion which is associated with various disorders (as of the inner ear) and in which the individual or the individual's surroundings seem to whirl dizzily — see SUBJECTIVE VERTIGO 2 : disordered vertiginous movement as a symptom of disease in lower animals; *also* : a disease (as gid) causing this

ver·vet \ˈvər-vət\ *n* : GREEN MONKEY

very–low–density lipoprotein *n* : VLDL

vesicae — see TRIGONUM VESICAE, UVULA VESICAE

ves·i·ca fel·lea \ˈve-si-kə-ˈfe-lē-ə\ *n* : GALLBLADDER

¹**ves·i·cal** \ˈve-si-kəl\ *adj* : of or relating to a bladder and esp. to the urinary bladder ⟨∼ burning⟩

²**vesical** *n* : VESICAL ARTERY

vesical artery *n* : any of several arteries that arise from the internal iliac artery or one of its branches and that supply the urinary bladder and adjacent parts: as **a** : any of several arteries that arise from the umbilical artery and supply the upper part of the bladder — called also *superior vesical, superior vesical artery* **b** : one that arises from the internal iliac artery or the internal pudendal artery and that supplies the bladder, prostate, and seminal vesicles — called also *inferior vesical, inferior vesical artery*

vesical plexus *n* : a plexus of nerves that comprises preganglionic fibers derived chiefly from the hypogastric plexus and postganglionic neurons whose fibers are distributed to the bladder and adjacent parts

vesical venous plexus *n* : a plexus of veins surrounding the neck of the bladder and the base of the prostate gland

ves·i·cant \ˈve-si-kənt\ *adj* : producing or tending to produce blisters ⟨a ∼ substance⟩ — **vesicant** *n*

vesica uri·nar·ia \-ˌyùr-i-ˈnar-ē-ə\ *n* : URINARY BLADDER

ves·i·cle \ˈve-si-kəl\ *n* **1 a** : a membranous and usu. fluid-filled pouch (as a cyst or cell) in a plant or animal **b**

: SYNAPTIC VESICLE **2** : a small abnormal elevation of the outer layer of skin enclosing a watery liquid : BLISTER **3** : a pocket of embryonic tissue that is the beginning of an organ — see BRAIN VESICLE, OPTIC VESICLE

vesico- *comb form* : of or relating to the urinary bladder and ⟨*vesico*uterine⟩

ves·i·co·en·ter·ic \ˌve-si-kō-ən-ˈter-ik\ *adj* : of, relating to, or connecting the urinary bladder and the intestinal tract ⟨a ∼ fistula⟩

ves·i·cos·to·my \ˌve-si-ˈkäs-tə-mē\ *n, pl* **-mies** : CYSTOSTOMY

ves·i·co·ure·ter·al reflux \ˌve-si-kō-yù-ˈrē-tə-rəl-\ *n* : reflux of urine from the bladder into a ureter

ves·i·co·ure·ter·ic reflux \-tə-rik-\ *n* : VESICOURETERAL REFLUX

ves·i·co·uter·ine \ˌve-si-kō-ˈyüt-ə-ˌrīn, -rən\ *adj* : of, relating to, or connecting the urinary bladder and the uterus

ves·i·co·vag·i·nal \ˌve-si-kō-ˈva-jən-ᵊl\ *adj* : of, relating to, or connecting the urinary bladder and vagina

vesicul- *or* **vesiculo-** *comb form* **1** : vesicle ⟨*vesicul*ectomy⟩ **2** : vesicular and ⟨*vesiculo*bullous⟩

ve·sic·u·lar \və-ˈsi-kyə-lər, ve-\ *adj* **1** : characterized by the presence or formation of vesicles ⟨a ∼ rash⟩ **2** : having the form of a vesicle

vesicular breathing *n* : normal breathing that is soft and low-pitched when heard in auscultation

vesicular dermatitis *n* : a severe dermatitis esp. of young chickens and turkeys — called also *sod disease*

vesicular exanthema *n* : an acute virus disease primarily of swine that is caused by a calicivirus (species *Vesicular exanthema of swine virus* of the genus *Vesivirus*) and closely resembles foot-and-mouth disease

vesicular ovarian follicle *n* : GRAAFIAN FOLLICLE

vesicular stomatitis *n* : an acute virus disease esp. of horses and cows that resembles foot-and-mouth disease, is marked by erosive blisters in and about the mouth, and is caused by any of three rhabdoviruses (species *Vesicular stomatitis Alagoas virus*, *Vesicular stomatitis Indiana virus*, and *Vesicular stomatitis New Jersey virus* of the genus *Vesiculovirus*) which sometimes infect humans producing symptoms resembling influenza

ve·sic·u·la·tion \və-ˌsi-kyə-ˈlā-shən\ *n* **1** : the presence or formation of vesicles **2** : the process of becoming vesicular ⟨∼ of a papule⟩

ve·sic·u·lec·to·my \və-ˌsi-kyə-ˈlek-tə-mē\ *n, pl* **-mies** : surgical excision of a seminal vesicle

ve·sic·u·li·tis \və-ˌsi-kyə-ˈlī-təs\ *n* : inflammation of a vesicle and esp. a seminal vesicle

ve·sic·u·lo·bul·lous \və-ˌsi-kyə-lō-ˈbù-ləs\ *adj* : of, relating to, or being both vesicles and bullae ⟨a ∼ rash⟩

ve·sic·u·lo·gram \və-'si-kyə-lə-ˌgram\ *n* : a radiograph produced by vesiculography

ve·sic·u·log·ra·phy \və-ˌsi-kyə-'lä-grə-fē\ *n, pl* **-phies** : radiography of the seminal vesicles following the injection of a radiopaque medium

ve·sic·u·lo·pus·tu·lar \və-ˌsi-kyə-lō-'pəs-chə-lər\ *adj* : of, relating to, or marked by both vesicles and pustules

ve·sic·u·lot·o·my \və-ˌsi-kyə-'lä-tə-mē\ *n, pl* **-mies** : surgical incision of a seminal vesicle

Ves·prin \'ves-prən\ *trademark* — used for a preparation of triflupromazine

ves·sel \'ves-səl\ *n* : a tube or canal (as an artery, vein, or lymphatic) in which a body fluid (as blood or lymph) is contained and conveyed or circulated

ves·tib·u·lar \ve-'sti-byə-lər\ *adj* **1** : of or relating to the vestibule of the inner ear, the vestibular system, the vestibular nerve, or the vestibular sense **2** : lying within or facing the vestibule of the mouth ⟨the ~ side of a tooth⟩ — **ves·tib·u·lar·ly** *adv*

vestibular apparatus *n* : VESTIBULAR SYSTEM

vestibular folds *n pl* : FALSE VOCAL CORDS

vestibular ganglion *n* : a sensory ganglion in the trunk of the vestibular nerve in the internal auditory canal that contains cell bodies supplying nerve fibers comprising the vestibular nerve

vestibular gland *n* : any of the glands (as Bartholin's glands) that open into the vestibule of the vagina

vestibular ligament *n* : the narrow band of fibrous tissue contained in each of the false vocal cords and stretching between the thyroid and arytenoid cartilages

vestibular membrane *n* : a thin cellular membrane separating the cochlear duct and scala vestibuli — called also *Reissner's membrane*

vestibular nerve *n* : a branch of the auditory nerve that consists of bipolar neurons with cell bodies collected in the vestibular ganglion, with peripheral processes passing to the semicircular canals, utricle, and saccule, and with central processes passing to the vestibular nuclei of the medulla oblongata

vestibular neuronitis *n* : a disorder of uncertain etiology that is characterized by transitory attacks of severe vertigo

vestibular nucleus *n* : any of four nuclei in the medulla oblongata on each side of the floor of the fourth ventricle of the brain in which fibers of the vestibular nerve terminate — see INFERIOR VESTIBULAR NUCLEUS, LATERAL VESTIBULAR NUCLEUS, MEDIAL VESTIBULAR NUCLEUS, SUPERIOR VESTIBULAR NUCLEUS

vestibular sense *n* : a complex sense concerned with the perception of bodily position and motion, mediated by end organs in the vestibular system, and stimulated by alterations in the pull of gravity and by head movements — called also *labyrinthine sense*

vestibular system *n* : a complex system of the inner ear that functions in mediating the vestibular sense and consists of the saccule, utricle, and semicircular canals — called also *vestibular apparatus*

ves·ti·bule \'ves-tə-ˌbyül\ *n* : any of various bodily cavities esp. when serving as or resembling an entrance to some other cavity or space: as **a** (1) : the central cavity of the bony labyrinth of the ear (2) : the parts of the membranous labyrinth comprising the utricle and the saccule and contained in the cavity of the bony labyrinth **b** : the space between the labia minora containing the orifice of the urethra **c** : the part of the left ventricle of the heart immediately below the aortic orifice **d** : the part of the mouth cavity outside the teeth and gums

vestibuli — see FENESTRA VESTIBULI, SCALA VESTIBULI

ves·tib·u·lo·co·chle·ar nerve \ve-ˌsti-byə-lō-'kō-klē-ər-, -ˌkä-\ *n* : AUDITORY NERVE

ves·tib·u·lo·plas·ty \ve-'sti-byə-lō-ˌplas-tē\ *n, pl* **-ties** : plastic surgery of the vestibular region of the mouth

ves·tib·u·lo·spi·nal tract \ve-ˌsti-byə-lō-'spī-nəl-\ *n* : a nerve tract on each side of the central nervous system containing nerve fibers that arise from cell bodies in the lateral vestibular nucleus on one side of the medulla oblongata and that descend on the same side in the lateral and anterior funiculi of the spinal cord to synapse with motor neurons in the ventral roots

ves·tige \'ves-tij\ *n* : a bodily part or organ that is small and degenerate or imperfectly developed in comparison to one more fully developed in an earlier stage of the individual, in a past generation, or in closely related forms — **ves·tig·ial** \ve-'sti-jəl, -jē-əl\ *adj*

vestigial fold of Mar·shall \-'mär-shəl\ *n* : a fold of endocardium that extends from the left pulmonary artery to the more superior of the two left pulmonary veins

J. Marshall — see OBLIQUE VEIN OF MARSHALL

vet \'vet\ *n* : VETERINARIAN

vet·er·i·nar·i·an \ˌve-tə-rə-'ner-ē-ən, ˌve-trə-\ *n* : a person qualified and authorized to practice veterinary medicine

¹vet·er·i·nary \'ve-tə-rə-ˌner-ē, 've-trə-\ *adj* : of, relating to, or being the science and art of prevention, cure, or alleviation of disease and injury in animals and esp. domestic animals

²**veterinary** *n, pl* **-nar·ies** : VETERINAR-
IAN
veterinary surgeon *n, Brit* : VETERI-
NARIAN
VF *abbr* ventricular fibrillation
V–fib *abbr* ventricular fibrillation
vi·a·ble \ˈvī-ə-bəl\ *adj* **1** : capable of
living ⟨∼ cancer cells⟩; *esp* : having
attained such form and development
of organs as to be normally capable of
living outside the uterus ⟨a ∼ fetus⟩
2 : capable of growing or developing
⟨∼ eggs⟩ — **vi·a·bil·i·ty** \ˌvī-ə-ˈbi-lə-
tē\ *n*
Vi·ag·ra \vī-ˈa-grə\ *trademark* — used
for a preparation of the citrate of
sildenafil
vi·al \ˈvī-əl, ˈvīl\ *n* : a small closed or
closable vessel esp. for liquids —
called also *phial*
Vi antigen \ˈvē-ˈī-\ *n* : a heat-labile somatic antigen associated with virulence in some bacteria (as of the
genus *Salmonella*) and esp. in the typhoid fever bacterium
Vi·bra·my·cin \ˌvī-brə-ˈmīs-ᵊn\ *trademark* — used for a preparation of
doxycycline
vibration white finger *n, chiefly Brit*
: Raynaud's disease esp. when caused
by severe vibration
vi·bra·tor \ˈvī-ˌbrā-tər\ *n* : a vibrating
electrical apparatus used in massage
or for sexual stimulation
vib·rio \ˈvi-brē-ō\ *n* **1** *cap* : a genus of
motile gram-negative bacteria (family
Vibrionaceae) that are straight or
curved rods and include pathogens (as
V. cholerae) causing esp. gastrointestinal disease (as cholera) **2** : any bacterium of the genus *Vibrio*; *broadly* : a
curved rod-shaped bacterium
vib·ri·on·ic abortion \ˌvi-brē-ˈä-nik-\ *n*
: abortion in sheep and cattle associated with vibriosis
vib·ri·o·sis \ˌvi-brē-ˈō-səs\ *n, pl* **-o·ses**
\-ˌsēz\ **1** : an infectious disease of
sheep and cattle caused by a bacterium of the genus *Campylobacter*
(*C. fetus* syn. *Vibrio fetus*) and marked
esp. by infertility and abortion **2** : infection with or disease caused by a
bacterium of the genus *Vibrio*; *esp* : a
gastrointestinal illness of humans that
is caused by consuming raw or undercooked fish or shellfish contaminated
with a vibrio (as *V. parahaemolyticus*)
vi·bris·sa \vī-ˈbri-sə, və-\ *n, pl* **vi·bris-
sae** \vī-ˈbri-(ˌ)sē; və-ˈbri-(ˌ)sē, -sī\
: any of the stiff hairs growing within
the nostrils that serve to impede the
inhalation of foreign substances
vi·car·i·ous \vī-ˈkar-ē-əs, və-\ *adj* : occurring in an unexpected or abnormal
part of the body instead of the usual
one ⟨∼ menstruation manifested by
bleeding from the nose⟩
vice \ˈvīs\ *n* : an abnormal behavior
pattern in a domestic animal detrimental to its health or usefulness
Vi·co·din \ˈvī-kō-dən\ *trademark* —
used for a preparation of acetamino-

phen and the bitartrate of hydrocodone
vid·ar·a·bine \vi-ˈdär-ə-ˌbēn\ *n* : an antiviral agent $C_{10}H_{13}N_5O_4 \cdot H_2O$ derived
from adenine and arabinoside and
used esp. to treat keratitis and encephalitis caused by the herpes simplex virus — called also *adenine
arabinoside, ara-A*
Vi·dex \ˈvī-ˌdeks\ *trademark* — used
for a preparation of ddI
Vid·i·an artery \ˈvi-dē-ən-\ *n* : a branch
of the maxillary artery passing
through the pterygoid canal of the
sphenoid bone
Gui·di \ˈgwē-dē\, **Guido** (*Latin
Vidus Vidius*) (1508–1569), Italian
anatomist and surgeon.
Vidian canal *n* : PTERYGOID CANAL
Vidian nerve *n* : a nerve formed by the
union of the greater petrosal and the
deep petrosal nerves that passes forward through the pterygoid canal in
the sphenoid bone and joins the
pterygopalatine ganglion
vi·gab·a·trin \vī-ˈga-bə-trən\ *n* : an anticonvulsant drug $C_6H_{11}NO_2$
vil·lo·nod·u·lar \ˌvi-lō-ˈnä-jə-lər\ *adj*
: characterized by villous and nodular
thickening (as of a synovial membrane) ⟨∼ synovitis⟩
vil·lus \ˈvi-ləs\ *n, pl* **vil·li** \-ˌlī\ : a small
slender vascular process: as **a** : one of
the minute fingerlike processes of the
mucous membrane of the small intestine that serve in the absorption of
nutriment **b** : one of the branching
processes of the surface of the
chorion of the developing embryo of
most mammals that help to form the
placenta — **vil·lous** \ˈvi-ləs\ *adj*
vin·blas·tine \(ˌ)vin-ˈblas-ˌtēn\ *n* : an
alkaloid that is obtained from the
rosy periwinkle and is used esp. in the
form of its sulfate $C_{46}H_{58}N_4O_9 \cdot H_2SO_4$
to treat neoplastic diseases (as
Hodgkin's disease and testicular
carcinoma) — called also *vinca-
leukoblastine*
vin·ca \ˈviŋ-kə\ *n* : PERIWINKLE
vin·ca·leu·ko·blas·tine \ˌviŋ-kə-ˌlü-kə-
ˈblas-ˌtēn\ *n* : VINBLASTINE
Vin·cent's angina \ˈvin-sənts-, (ˌ)vanⁿ-
ˈsäⁿz-\ *n* : acute necrotizing ulcerative
gingivitis in which the ulceration has
spread to surrounding tissues (as of
the pharynx and tonsils) — called
also *trench mouth*
Vincent, Jean Hyacinthe (1862–
1950), French bacteriologist.
Vincent's infection *n* : ACUTE NECRO-
TIZING ULCERATIVE GINGIVITIS
Vincent's organisms *n pl* : a bacterium of the genus *Fusobacterium* (*F.
nucleatum*) and a spirochete of the
genus *Treponema* (*T. vincentii*) that
are sometimes found in necrotic tissue (as that of acute necrotizing ulcerative gingivitis or tropical ulcer)
vin·cris·tine \(ˌ)vin-ˈkris-ˌtēn\ *n* : an al-
kaloid that is obtained from the rosy
periwinkle and is used esp. in the

form of its sulfate $C_{46}H_{56}N_4O_{10} \cdot H_2SO_4$ to treat some neoplastic diseases (as acute leukemia) — called also *leurocristine;* see ONCOVIN

Vine·berg procedure \'vīn-ˌbərg-\ *n* : surgical implantation of an internal thoracic artery into the myocardium

Vineberg, Arthur Martin (1903–1988), Canadian surgeon.

vi·nyl chloride \'vīn-ᵊl-\ *n* : a flammable gaseous carcinogenic compound C_2H_3Cl

vinyl ether *n* : a volatile flammable liquid unsaturated ether C_4H_6O formerly used as an inhalation anesthetic

vi·o·my·cin \ˌvī-ə-'mīs-ᵊn\ *n* : a polypeptide antibiotic that is produced by several soil actinomycetes of the genus *Streptomyces* and is administered intramuscularly in the form of its sulfate $C_{25}H_{43}N_{13}O_{10} \cdot xH_2SO_4$ to treat tuberculosis esp. in combination with other antituberculous drugs

vi·os·ter·ol \vī-'äs-tə-ˌról, -ˌról\ *n* : CALCIFEROL

Vi·oxx \'vī-ˌäks\ *trademark* — used for a preparation of rofecoxib

VIP *abbr* vasoactive intestinal peptide; vasoactive intestinal polypeptide

vi·per \'vī-pər\ *n* : a common Eurasian venomous snake of the genus *Vipera* (*V. berus*) whose bite is usu. not fatal to humans; *broadly* : any of a family (Viperidae) of venomous snakes that includes Old World snakes (subfamily Viperinae) and the pit vipers

Vi·pera \'vī-pə-rə\ *n* : a genus of Old World venomous snakes (family Viperidae)

vi·po·ma \vī-'pō-mə, vi-\ *n* : a tumor of endocrine tissue esp. in the pancreas that secretes vasoactive intestinal polypeptide

Vi·ra·cept \'vī-rə-ˌsept\ *trademark* — used for a preparation of the mesylate of nelfinavir

vi·rae·mia *chiefly Brit var of* VIREMIA

vi·ral \'vī-rəl\ *adj* : of, relating to, or caused by a virus — **vi·ral·ly** *adv*

Vir·chow–Ro·bin space \'fir-ˌkō-rō-'baⁿ-\ *n* : any of the spaces that surround blood vessels as they enter the brain and that communicate with the subarachnoid space

Virchow, Rudolf Ludwig Karl (1821–1902), German pathologist, anthropologist, and statesman.

Robin, Charles–Philippe (1821–1885), French anatomist and histologist.

Virchow's node *n* : SIGNAL NODE

vi·re·mia \vī-'rē-mē-ə\ *n* : the presence of virus in the blood of a host — **vi·re·mic** \-mik\ *adj*

vir·gin \'vər-jən\ *n* : a person who has not had sexual intercourse — **vir·gin·i·ty** \(ˌ)vər-'ji-nə-tē\ *n*

vi·ri·ci·dal \ˌvī-rə-'sīd-ᵊl\ *adj* : VIRUCIDAL

vi·ri·cide \'vī-rə-ˌsīd\ *n* : VIRUCIDE

vir·ile \'vir-əl, -ˌīl\ *adj* **1** : having the nature, properties, or qualities of an adult male; *specif* : capable of functioning as a male in copulation **2** : characteristic of or associated with men : MASCULINE — **vir·il·i·ty** \və-'ri-lə-tē\ *n*

vir·il·ism \'vir-ə-ˌli-zəm\ *n* **1** : precocious development of secondary sex characteristics in the male **2** : the appearance of secondary sex characteristics of the male in a female

vir·il·ize \'vir-ə-ˌlīz\ *vb* **-ized; -iz·ing** : to make virile; *esp* : to cause or produce virilism in — **vir·il·i·za·tion** \ˌvir-ə-lə-'zā-shən\ *n*

vi·ri·on \'vī-rē-ˌän, 'vir-ē-\ *n* : a complete virus particle that consists of an RNA or DNA core with a protein coat sometimes with external envelopes and that is the extracellular infective form of a virus

vi·rol·o·gy \vī-'rä-lə-jē\ *n, pl* **-gies** : a branch of science that deals with viruses — **vi·ro·log·i·cal** \ˌvī-rə-'lä-ji-kəl\ *or* **vi·ro·log·ic** \-jik\ *adj* — **vi·ro·log·i·cal·ly** *adv* — **vi·rol·o·gist** \vī-'rä-lə-jist\ *n*

vi·ro·pause \'vī-rə-ˌpóz\ *n* : ANDROPAUSE

virtual dead space *n* : PHYSIOLOGICAL DEAD SPACE

vi·ru·cid·al \ˌvī-rə-'sīd-ᵊl\ *adj* : having the capacity to or tending to destroy or inactivate viruses (~ activity)

vi·ru·cide \'vī-rə-ˌsīd\ *n* : an agent having the capacity to destroy or inactivate viruses — called also *viricide*

vir·u·lence \'vir-yə-ləns, 'vir-ə-\ *n* : the quality or state of being virulent: as **a** : relative severity and malignancy **b** : the relative capacity of a pathogen to overcome body defenses — compare INFECTIVITY

vir·u·len·cy \-lən-sē\ *n, pl* **-cies** : VIRULENCE

vir·u·lent \-lənt\ *adj* **1 a** : marked by a rapid, severe, and malignant course (a ~ infection) **b** : able to overcome bodily defense mechanisms (a ~ pathogen) **2** : extremely poisonous or venomous : NOXIOUS

vi·rus \'vī-rəs\ *n* **1** : the causative agent of an infectious disease **2** : any of a large group of submicroscopic infective agents that are regarded either as extremely simple microorganisms or as extremely complex molecules, that typically contain a protein coat surrounding an RNA or DNA core of genetic material but no semipermeable membrane, that are capable of growth and multiplication only in living cells, and that cause various important diseases — see FILTERABLE VIRUS **3** : a disease caused by a virus

virus pneumonia *n* : pneumonia caused or thought to be caused by a virus; *esp* : PRIMARY ATYPICAL PNEUMONIA

viscer- *or* **visceri-** *or* **viscero-** *comb form* : visceral : viscera (*viscero*tropic)

viscera *pl of* VISCUS

vis·cer·al \'vis-sə-rəl\ *adj* : of, relating to, or located on or among the viscera — compare PARIETAL 1 — **vis·cer·al·ly** *adv*

visceral arch *n* : BRANCHIAL ARCH

visceral leishmaniasis *n* : KALA-AZAR

visceral muscle *n* : smooth muscle esp. in visceral structures

visceral pericardium *n* : EPICARDIUM

visceral peritoneum *n* : the part of the peritoneum that lines the abdominal viscera — compare PARIETAL PERITONEUM

visceral reflex *n* : a reflex mediated by autonomic nerves and initiated in the viscera

vis·cero·meg·a·ly \,vi-sə-rō-'me-gə-lē\ *n, pl* **-lies** : ORGANOMEGALY

vis·cero·mo·tor \,vi-sə-rō-'mō-tər\ *adj* : causing or concerned in the functional activity of the viscera

vis·cer·op·to·sis \,vi-sə-räp-'tō-səs\ *n, pl* **-to·ses** \-,sēz\ : downward displacement of the abdominal viscera

vis·cer·o·trop·ic \,vi-sə-rə-'trä-pik\ *adj* : tending to affect or having an affinity for the viscera ⟨∼ leishmaniasis⟩ — **vis·cer·ot·ro·pism** \,vi-sə-'rä-trə-,pi-zəm\ *n*

vis·cid \'vi-səd\ *adj* 1 : having an adhesive quality 2 : having a glutinous consistency

vis·com·e·ter \vis-'kä-mə-tər\ *n* : an instrument used to measure viscosity — **vis·co·met·ric** \,vis-kə-'me-trik\ *adj*

vis·co·sim·e·ter \,vis-kə-'si-mə-tər\ *n* : VISCOMETER — **vis·cos·i·met·ric** \vis-,kä-sə-'me-trik\ *adj*

vis·cos·i·ty \vis-'kä-sə-tē\ *n, pl* **-ties** : the quality of being viscous; *esp* : the property of resistance to flow in a fluid

vis·cous \'vis-kəs\ *adj* 1 : having a glutinous consistency and the quality of sticking or adhering : VISCID 2 : having or characterized by viscosity

vis·cus \'vis-kəs\ *n, pl* **vis·cera** \'vi-sə-rə\ : an internal organ of the body; *esp* : one (as the heart, liver, or intestine) located in the large cavity of the trunk

vis·i·ble \'vi-zə-bəl\ *adj* 1 : capable of being seen : perceptible to vision 2 : situated in the visible spectrum

visible spectrum *n* : the part of the electromagnetic spectrum to which the human eye is sensitive extending from a wavelength of about 400 nm for violet light to about 700 nm for red light

vi·sion \'vi-zhən\ *n* 1 : the act or power of seeing 2 : the special sense by which the qualities of an object (as color, shape, and size) constituting its appearance are perceived through a process in which light rays entering the eye are transformed by the retina into electrical signals that are transmitted to the brain via the optic nerve

vis·it \'vi-zət\ *n* 1 : a professional call (as by a physician to treat a patient) 2 : a call upon a professional person (as a physician or dentist) for consultation or treatment — **visit** *vb*

visiting nurse *n* : a nurse employed (as by a hospital or social-service agency) to perform public health services and esp. to visit and provide care for sick persons in a community — called also *public health nurse*

vis·na \'vis-nə\ *n* : ovine progressive pneumonia esp. as manifested by neurological symptoms

Vis·ta·ril \'vis-tə-,ril\ *trademark* — used for a preparation of hydroxyzine

vi·su·al \'vi-zhə-wəl\ *adj* 1 : of, relating to, or used in vision ⟨∼ organs⟩ 2 : attained or maintained by sight ⟨∼ impressions⟩ — **vi·su·al·ly** *adv*

visual acuity *n* : the relative ability of the visual organ to resolve detail

visual agnosia *n* : a form of agnosia characterized by inability to recognize familiar objects observed by sight — see PROSOPAGNOSIA

visual analog scale *n* : a testing technique for measuring subjective or behavioral phenomena (as pain) in which a subject selects from a gradient of alternatives (as from "no pain" to "worst imaginable pain") arranged in linear fashion — abbr. *VAS*

visual cortex *n* : a sensory area of the occipital lobe of the cerebral cortex receiving afferent projection fibers concerned with the sense of sight — called also *visual area*

visual field *n* : the entire expanse of space visible at a given instant without moving the eyes — called also *field of vision*

vi·su·al·i·za·tion \,vi-zhə-wə-lə-'zā-shən\ *n* 1 : formation of mental visual images 2 : the process of making an internal organ visible by the introduction (as by swallowing, by an injection, or by an enema) of a radiopaque substance followed by radiography — **vi·su·al·ize** \'vi-zhə-wə-,līz\ *vb*

vi·su·al·iz·er \-,lī-zər\ *n* : one that visualizes; *esp* : a person whose mental imagery is prevailingly visual — compare AUDILE, TACTILE

visual projection area *n* : STRIATE CORTEX

visual purple *n* : RHODOPSIN

vi·suo·mo·tor \,vi-zhə-wō-'mō-tər\ *adj* : of or relating to vision and muscular movement ⟨∼ coordination⟩

vi·suo·spa·tial \-'spā-shəl\ *adj* : of or relating to thought processes that involve visual and spatial awareness

vi·tal \'vīt-ᵊl\ *adj* 1 a : existing as a manifestation of life b : concerned with or necessary to the maintenance of life ⟨∼ organs⟩ 2 : characteristic of life or living beings 3 : recording data relating to lives 4 : of, relating to, or constituting the staining of living tissues — **vi·tal·ly** *adv*

vital capacity *n* : the breathing capacity of the lungs expressed as the number of cubic inches or cubic centimeters of air that can be forcibly exhaled after a full inspiration

vital function *n* : a function of the body (as respiration) on which life is directly dependent

vi·tal·i·ty \vī-'ta-lə-tē\ *n, pl* **-ties** : capacity to live and develop; *also* : physical or mental vigor esp. when highly developed

Vi·tal·li·um \vī-'ta-lē-əm\ *trademark* — used for a cobalt-chromium alloy of platinum-white color used esp. for cast dentures and prostheses

vi·tals \'vīt-ªlz\ *n pl* : vital organs (as the heart, liver, lungs, and brain)

vital signs *n pl* : signs of life; *specif* : the pulse rate, respiratory rate, body temperature, and often blood pressure of a person

vital statistics *n pl* : statistics relating to births, deaths, marriages, health, and disease

vi·ta·min \'vī-tə-mən\ *n* : any of various organic substances that are essential in minute quantities to the nutrition of most animals and some plants, act esp. as coenzymes and precursors of coenzymes in the regulation of metabolic processes but do not provide energy or serve as building units, and are present in natural foodstuffs or sometimes produced within the body

vitamin A *n* : any of several fat-soluble vitamins or a mixture of two or more of them whose lack in the animal body causes keratinization of epithelial tissues (as in the eye with resulting night blindness and xerophthalmia): as **a** : a pale yellow crystalline alcohol $C_{20}H_{29}OH$ that is found in animal products (as egg yolk, milk, and butter) and esp. in marine fish-liver oils (as of cod, halibut, and shark) — called also *retinol, vitamin A₁* **b** : a yellow viscous liquid alcohol $C_{20}H_{27}OH$ that contains one more double bond in a molecule than vitamin A₁ and is less active biologically in mammals and that occurs esp. in the liver oil of freshwater fish — called also *vitamin A₂*

vitamin A aldehyde *n* : RETINAL

vitamin A₁ \-,ā-'wən\ *n* : VITAMIN A a

vitamin A palmitate *n* : RETINYL PALMITATE

vitamin A₂ \-,ā-'tü\ *n* : VITAMIN A b

vitamin B *n* **1** : VITAMIN B COMPLEX **2** : any of numerous members of the vitamin B complex; *esp* : THIAMINE

vitamin B_c \-,bē-'sē\ *n* : FOLIC ACID

vitamin B complex *n* : a group of water-soluble vitamins (as biotin, niacin, and thiamine) found esp. in yeast, seed germs, eggs, meat, and green vegetables that have varied metabolic functions and include coenzymes and growth factors — called also *B complex*

vitamin B₁ \-,bē-'wən\ *n* : THIAMINE

vitamin B₁₇ \-,bē-,se-vən-'tēn\ *n* : LAETRILE

vitamin B₆ \-,bē-'siks\ *n* : pyridoxine or a closely related compound found widely in combined form and considered essential to vertebrate nutrition

vitamin B_T \-,bē-'tē\ *n* : CARNITINE

vitamin B₃ \-,bē-'thrē\ *n* : NIACIN

vitamin B₁₂ \-,bē-'twelv\ *n* **1** : a complex cobalt-containing compound $C_{63}H_{88}CoN_{14}O_{14}P$ found in animal products (as meat and eggs) that is essential to normal blood formation, neural function, and growth, and is used esp. in treating pernicious and related anemias and in animal feed as a growth factor — called also *cyanocobalamin* **2** : any of several compounds similar to vitamin B₁₂ in action but having different chemistry

vitamin B₂ \-,bē-'tü\ *n* : RIBOFLAVIN

vitamin C *n* : a water-soluble vitamin $C_6H_8O_6$ found in plants and esp. in fruits and leafy vegetables or made synthetically and used in the prevention and treatment of scurvy and as an antioxidant for foods — called also *ascorbic acid*

vitamin D *n* : any or all of several fat-soluble vitamins chemically related to steroids, essential for normal bone and tooth structure, and found esp. in fish-liver oils, egg yolk, and milk or produced by activation (as by ultraviolet irradiation) of sterols: as **a** : CALCIFEROL **b** : CHOLECALCIFEROL — called also *sunshine vitamin*

vitamin D₃ \-,dē-'thrē\ *n* : CHOLECALCIFEROL

vitamin D₂ \-,dē-'tü\ *n* : CALCIFEROL

vitamin E *n* : any of several fat-soluble vitamins that are chemically tocopherols, are essential in nutrition, are found esp. in wheat germ, vegetable oils, egg yolk, and green leafy vegetables or are made synthetically, and are used chiefly in animal feeds and as antioxidants; *esp* : ALPHA-TOCOPHEROL

vitamin G *n* : RIBOFLAVIN

vitamin H *n* : BIOTIN

vitamin K *n* **1** : either of two naturally occurring fat-soluble vitamins that are essential for the clotting of blood because of their role in the production of prothrombin in the liver and that are used in preventing and treating hypoprothrombinemia and hemorrhage: **a** : an oily naphthoquinone $C_{31}H_{46}O_2$ that is obtained esp. from alfalfa or made synthetically and that has a fast, potent, and prolonged biological effect — called also *phylloquinone, phytonadione, vitamin K₁;* see MEPHYTON **b** : a crystalline naphthoquinone $C_{41}H_{56}O_2$ that is obtained esp. from putrefied fish meal and is synthesized by various bacteria (as in the intestines) and that is slightly less active biologically than vitamin K₁ — called also *menaquinone, vitamin K₂* **2** : any of several synthetic compounds that are closely related chemically to vitamins K_1 and K_2 but are simpler in structure; *esp* : MENADIONE

vitamin K₁ \-,kā-'wən\ *n* : VITAMIN K 1a

vitamin K₃ \-,kā-'thrē\ *n* : MENADIONE

vitamin K₂ \-,kā-'tü\ *n* : VITAMIN K 1b

vitamin M *n* : FOLIC ACID

vi·ta·min·ol·o·gy \,vī-tə-mə-'nä-lə-jē\ *n, pl* **-gies** : a branch of knowledge dealing with vitamins, their nature, action, and use

vitamin PP \-,pē-'pē\ *n* : NIACIN

vitell- *or* **vitello-** *comb form* : yolk : vitellus ⟨*vitell*ogenesis⟩

vi·tel·lin \vī-'tel-ən, və-\ *n* : a phosphoprotein in egg yolk — called also *ovovitellin*

vi·tel·line \-'te-lən, -,lēn, -,līn\ *adj* : of, relating to, or producing yolk

vitelline duct *n* : OMPHALOMESENTERIC DUCT

vitelline membrane *n* : a membrane enclosing the egg proper and corresponding to the plasma membrane of an ordinary cell

vi·tel·lo·gen·e·sis \vī-,te-lō-'je-nə-səs, və-\ *n, pl* **-e·ses** \-,sēz\ : yolk formation — **vi·tel·lo·gen·ic** \-'je-nik\ *adj*

vi·tel·lus \vī-'te-ləs, və-\ *n* : the egg cell proper including the yolk but excluding any albuminous or membranous envelopes; *also* : YOLK

vit·i·li·go \,vi-tə-'lī-gō, -'lē-\ *n* : a progressive skin disorder that is a form of leukoderma caused by the localized or generalized destruction of melanocytes and marked by sharply circumscribed white spots of skin

vit·rec·to·my \və-'trek-tə-mē\ *n, pl* **-mies** : surgical removal of all or part of the vitreous body

¹vit·re·ous \'vi-trē-əs\ *adj* : of, relating to, constituting, or affecting the vitreous body ⟨~ hemorrhages⟩

²vitreous *n* : VITREOUS BODY

vitreous body *n* : the clear colorless transparent jelly that fills the eyeball posterior to the lens and is enclosed by a delicate hyaloid membrane

vitreous chamber *n* : the space in the eyeball between the lens and the retina that is occupied by the vitreous body

vitreous detachment *n* : separation of the posterior part of the vitreous body from the retina due to contraction of the vitreous body that typically occurs as part of the process of aging, that is usu. accompanied by the presence of floaters, and that may result in a torn retina or in retinal detachment — called also *posterior vitreous detachment*

vitreous humor *n* : VITREOUS BODY

vitro — see IN VITRO

vit·ro·nec·tin \,vi-trō-'nek-tən\ *n* : a glycoprotein of blood plasma that promotes cell adhesion and migration and is similar to fibronectin

Vi·vac·til \vī-'vak-til\ *trademark* — used for a preparation of protriptyline

vi·vax malaria \'vī-,vaks-\ *n* : malaria caused by a plasmodium (*Plasmodium vivax*) that induces paroxysms at 48-hour intervals — compare FALCIPARUM MALARIA

vivi- *comb form* : alive : living ⟨*vivi*section⟩

vi·vip·a·rous \vī-'vi-pə-rəs, və-\ *adj* : producing living young instead of eggs from within the body in the manner of nearly all mammals, many reptiles, and a few fishes — compare OVIPAROUS, OVOVIVIPAROUS — **vi·vi·par·i·ty** \,vī-və-'par-ə-tē, ,vi-\ *n*

vivi·sec·tion \,vi-və-'sek-shən, 'vi-və-,\ *n* : the cutting of or operation on a living animal usu. for physiological or pathological investigation; *broadly* : animal experimentation esp. if considered to cause distress or result in injury or death to the subject — **vivi·sect** \-'sekt\ *vb* — **vivi·sec·tion·ist** \,vi-və-'sek-sh(ə-)nəst\ *n*

vivo — see IN VIVO

VLDL \,vē-(,)el-(,)dē-'el\ *n* : a plasma lipoprotein that is produced primarily by the liver with lesser amounts contributed by the intestine, that contains relatively large amounts of triglycerides compared to protein, and that leaves a residue of cholesterol in the tissues during the process of conversion to LDL — called also *very-low-density lipoprotein*; compare HDL, LDL

VMA *abbr* vanillylmandelic acid

VMD *abbr* doctor of veterinary medicine

VNA *abbr* Visiting Nurse Association

VNTR \,vē-,en-,tē-'är\ *n, often attrib* [*variable number tandem repeat*] : a tandem repeat from a single genetic locus in which the number of repeated DNA segments varies from individual to individual and is used for identification purposes (as in DNA fingerprinting)

vo·cal \'vō-kəl\ *adj* **1** : uttered by the voice : ORAL **2** : having or exercising the power of producing voice, speech, or sound **3** : of, relating to, or resembling the voice — **vo·cal·ly** *adv*

vocal cord *n* **1** *pl* : either of two pairs of folds of mucous membrane of which each member of each pair stretches from the thyroid cartilage in front to the arytenoid cartilage in back, contains a band of fibrous or elastic tissue, and has a free edge projecting into the cavity of the larynx toward the contralateral member of the same pair forming a cleft which can be opened or closed: **a** : FALSE VOCAL CORDS **b** : TRUE VOCAL CORDS **2** : VOCAL LIGAMENT

vocal folds *n pl* : TRUE VOCAL CORDS

vo·ca·lis \vō-'kā-ləs\ *n* : a small muscle that is the medial part of the thyroarytenoid, originates in the lamina of the thyroid cartilage, inserts in the vocal process of the arytenoid cartilage, and modulates the tension of the true vocal cords

vo·cal·i·za·tion \ˌvō-kə-lə-ˈzā-shən\ *n* : the act or process of producing sounds with the voice; *also* : a sound thus produced — **vo·cal·ize** *vb*

vocal ligament *n* : the band of yellow elastic tissue contained in each true vocal cord and stretching between the thyroid and arytenoid cartilages — called also *inferior thyroarytenoid ligament*

vocal process *n* : the anterior angle of the arytenoid cartilage on each side of the larynx to which the vocal ligament of the corresponding side is attached

voice \ˈvȯis\ *n* **1** : sound produced esp. by means of lungs or larynx; *esp* : sound so produced by human beings **2** : the faculty of utterance : SPEECH

voice box *n* : LARYNX

void \ˈvȯid\ *vb* : to discharge or emit ⟨~ urine⟩

vol *abbr* volume

vo·lar \ˈvō-lər, -ˌlär\ *adj* : relating to the palm of the hand or the sole of the foot; *specif* : located on the same side as the palm of the hand

vol·a·tile \ˈvä-lə-təl, -ˌtīl\ *adj* : readily vaporizable at a relatively low temperature — **vol·a·til·i·ty** \ˌvä-lə-ˈti-lə-tē\ *n*

volatile oil *n* : an oil that vaporizes readily; *esp* : ESSENTIAL OIL

volitantes — see MUSCAE VOLITANTES

vo·li·tion \vō-ˈli-shən, və-\ *n* **1** : an act of making a choice or decision; *also* : a choice or decision made **2** : the power of choosing or determining — **vo·li·tion·al** \-ˈli-shə-nəl\ *adj*

Volk·mann's canal \ˈfȯlk-mənz-\ *n* : any of the small channels in bone that transmit blood vessels from the periosteum into the bone and that lie perpendicular to and communicate with the haversian canals

Volkmann, Alfred Wilhelm (1800–1877), German physiologist.

Volkmann's contracture *or* **Volkmann contracture** *n* : ischemic contracture of an extremity and esp. of a hand

volt \ˈvōlt\ *n* : the practical mks unit of electrical potential difference and electromotive force equal to the difference of potential between two points in a conducting wire carrying a constant current of one ampere when the power dissipated between these two points is equal to one watt

Vol·ta \ˈvȯl-tä\, **Alessandro Giuseppe Antonio Anastasio** (1745–1827), Italian physicist.

volt·age \ˈvōl-tij\ *n* : electrical potential or potential difference expressed in volts

voltage clamp *n* : stabilization of a membrane potential by depolarization and maintenance at a given potential by means of an electric current

from a source outside the living system — **voltage clamp** *vb*

voltage–gat·ed \-ˌgā-təd\ *adj* : permitting or blocking passage through a cell membrane in response to an electrical stimulus (as a potential difference across a cell membrane)

Vol·ta·ren \ˈvōl-tə-rən\ *trademark* — used for a preparation of the sodium salt of diclofenac

vol·un·tary \ˈvä-lən-ˌter-ē\ *adj* **1** : proceeding from the will or from one's own choice or consent **2** : of, relating to, subject to, or regulated by the will ⟨~ behavior⟩ — **vol·un·tari·ly** *adv*

voluntary hospital *n* : a private nonprofit hospital that is operated under individual, partnership, or corporation control

voluntary muscle *n* : muscle (as most striated muscle) under voluntary control

vol·vu·lus \ˈväl-vyə-ləs\ *n* : a twisting of the intestine upon itself that causes obstruction — compare ILEUS

vo·mer \ˈvō-mər\ *n* : a bone of the skull that in humans forms the posterior and inferior part of the nasal septum comprising a vertical plate pointed in front and expanding at the upper back part into lateral wings

vom·ero·na·sal \ˌvä-mə-rō-ˈnā-zəl, ˌvō-\ *adj* : of or relating to the vomer and the nasal region and esp. to the vomeronasal organ or the vomeronasal cartilage

vomeronasal cartilage *n* : a narrow process of cartilage between the vomer and the cartilage of the nasal septum

vomeronasal organ *n* : either of a pair of small blind pouches or tubes in many vertebrates that are situated one on either side of the nasal septum or in the buccal cavity and that are reduced to rudimentary pits in adult humans but are developed in reptiles, amphibians, and some mammals as chemoreceptors — called also *Jacobson's organ*

vomica — see NUX VOMICA

¹vom·it \ˈvä-mət\ *n* **1** : VOMITING **2** : stomach contents disgorged through the mouth — called also *vomitus*

²vomit *vb* : to disgorge the contents of the stomach through the mouth

vomiting *n* : an act or instance of disgorging the contents of the stomach through the mouth — called also *emesis*

vomiting center *n* : a nerve center in the medulla oblongata that initiates the act of vomiting when stimulated

vom·i·tus \ˈvä-mə-təs\ *n* : VOMIT

von Gier·ke disease \vän-ˈgir-kə-\ *or* **von Gier·ke's disease** \-kəz-\ *n* : a glycogen storage disease that is caused by a deficiency of glucose-6-phosphate, has a clinical onset at birth or during infancy, is characterized esp. by enlargement of the liver and kidney, hypoglycemia, hyperlipidemia, and stunted growth, and is inherited as an autosomal recessive trait

Gierke, Edgar Otto Konrad von (1877–1945), German pathologist.

von Grae·fe's sign \ˌvän-ˈgrä-fəz-\ *n* : the failure of the upper eyelid to follow promptly and smoothly the downward movement of the eyeball that is seen in Graves' disease

von Grae·fe \ˈfòn-ˈgre-fə\, **Albrecht Friedrich Wilhelm Ernst** (1828–1870), German ophthalmologist.

von Hip·pel–Lin·dau disease \ˌvän-ˈhi-pəl-ˈlin-ˌdaù-\ *n* : a rare genetic disease that is characterized by hemangiomas of the retina and cerebellum and often by cysts or tumors of the liver, pancreas, and kidneys and that is typically inherited as an autosomal dominant trait — called also *Lindau's disease*

von Hippel, Eugen (1867–1939), German ophthalmologist.

Lindau, Arvid Vilhelm (1892–1958), Swedish pathologist.

von Reck·ling·hau·sen's disease \-ˈre-kliŋ-ˌhaù-zənz-\ *n* : NEUROFIBROMATOSIS

F. D. Recklinghausen — see RECKLINGHAUSEN'S DISEASE

von Wil·le·brand factor \vän-ˈvi-lə-ˌbränt-\ *n* : a protein secreted esp. by endothelial cells that circulates in blood plasma, mediates platelet adhesion to collagen in subendothelial tissue at injury sites, and is often found complexed to factor VIII in plasma where it serves to protect it from degradation — see VON WILLEBRAND'S DISEASE

Willebrand, Erick Adolf von (1870–1949), Finnish physician.

von Wil·le·brand's disease \-ˌbränts-\ *n* : a genetic disorder that is caused by deficient or defective von Willebrand factor, is characterized by mucosal and petechial bleeding due to abnormal blood vessels, and is inherited chiefly as an autosomal dominant trait

vorticosa — see VENA VORTICOSA

vor·ti·cose vein \ˈvòr-tə-ˌkōs-\ *n* : VENA VORTICOSA

VO₂ max \ˌvē-ō-ˈtü-ˈmaks\ *n* : the maximum amount of oxygen the body can use during a specified period of usu. intense exercise that depends on body weight and the strength of the lungs — called also *maximal oxygen consumption, maximal oxygen uptake, max VO₂*

voy·eur \vòi-ˈyər, vwä-\ *n* : one obtaining sexual gratification from observing unsuspecting individuals who are partly undressed, naked, or engaged in sexual acts; *broadly* : one who habitually seeks sexual stimulation by visual means — **voy·eur·ism** \-ˌi-zəm\ *n* — **voy·eur·is·tic** \ˌvwä-(ˌ)yər-ˈis-tik, ˌvòi-ər-\ *adj*

VRE \ˌvē-ˌär-ˈē\ *n* [vancomycin-resistant enterococcus] : any of various bacterial strains of the genus *Enterococcus* (as *E. faecium* and *E. faecalis*) that are resistant to the antibiotic vancomycin, occur as part of the normal flora esp. of the gastrointestinal tract, and may cause serious infections typically in immunocompromised individuals in a hospital setting

VS *abbr* vesicular stomatitis

VSD *abbr* ventricular septal defect

VT *abbr* ventricular tachycardia

V–tach *abbr* ventricular tachycardia

vulgaris — see ACNE VULGARIS, ICHTHYOSIS VULGARIS, LUPUS VULGARIS, PEMPHIGUS VULGARIS, VERRUCA VULGARIS

vul·ner·a·ble \ˈvəl-nə-rə-bəl\ *adj* : capable of being hurt : susceptible to injury or disease — **vul·ner·a·bil·i·ty** \ˌvəl-nə-rə-ˈbi-lə-tē\ *n*

vul·sel·lum \vəl-ˈse-ləm\ *n, pl* -sel·la \-ˈse-lə\ : a surgical forceps with serrated, clawed, or hooked blades

vulv- *or* **vulvo-** *comb form* 1 : vulva 〈*vulvitis*〉 2 : vulvar and 〈*vulvo*vaginal〉

vul·va \ˈvəl-və\ *n, pl* **vul·vae** \-ˌvē, -ˌvī\ : the external parts of the female genital organs comprising the mons pubis, labia majora, labia minora, clitoris, vestibule of the vagina, bulb of the vestibule, and Bartholin's glands — **vul·val** \ˈvəl-vəl\ *or* **vul·var** \-vər\ *adj*

vulvae — see KRAUROSIS VULVAE, PRURITUS VULVAE

vul·vec·to·my \ˌvəl-ˈvek-tə-mē\ *n, pl* -mies : surgical excision of the vulva

vul·vi·tis \ˌvəl-ˈvī-təs\ *n* : inflammation of the vulva

vul·vo·vag·i·nal \ˌvəl-vō-ˈva-jən-ᵊl\ *adj* : of or relating to the vulva and the vagina 〈~ hematoma〉

vul·vo·vag·i·ni·tis \ˌvəl-vō-ˌva-jə-ˈnī-təs\ *n, pl* -nit·i·des \-ˈni-tə-ˌdēz\ : coincident inflammation of the vulva and vagina

Vy·tor·in \vī-ˈtòr-ən\ *trademark* — used for a preparation of ezetimibe and simvastatin

W *symbol* [German *wolfram*] tungsten

Waar·den·burg syndrome \ˈvär-dᵊn-ˌbərg-\ *or* **Waar·den·burg's syn·drome** \-ˌbərgz-\ *n* : a highly variable genetic disorder inherited as an autosomal dominant trait and marked esp.

by hearing loss, white hair and esp. a white forelock, widely spaced eyes, and heterochromia of the irises

Waardenburg, Petrus Johannes (1886–1979), Dutch ophthalmologist.

Wa·da test \'wä-də-\ n : a test that is used to determine whether the right or left cerebral hemisphere is dominant for speech and that typically involves injection of amobarbital into the internal carotid artery first on one side and then on the other so that transient aphasia results when the injection is made into the artery on the dominant side

Wada, Juhn Atsushi (b 1924), Canadian (Japanese-born) neurologist.

wad·ding \'wä-diŋ\ n : a soft absorbent sheet of cotton, wool, or cellulose used esp. in hospitals for surgical dressings

WAIS abbr Wechsler Adult Intelligence Scale

waist \'wāst\ n : the typically narrowed part of the body between the thorax and hips

waist·line \'wāst-ˌlīn\ n : body circumference at the waist

wake·ful \'wāk-fəl\ adj : not sleeping or able to sleep : SLEEPLESS — **wake·ful·ness** n

Wal·den·ström's macroglobulinemia \'väl-dən-ˌstremz-\ n : lymphoplasmacytic lymphoma marked by an elevated serum concentration of a monoclonal antibody of the class IgM and characterized esp. by hyperviscosity of blood, lymphadenopathy, hepatosplenomegaly, anemia, and peripheral neuropathy

Waldenström, Jan Gosta (1906–1996), Swedish physician.

Wal·dey·er's ring \'väl-ˌdī-ərz-\ n : a ring of lymphatic tissue formed by the two palatine tonsils, the pharyngeal tonsil, the lingual tonsil, and intervening lymphoid tissue

Wal·dey·er-Hartz \'väl-ˌdī-ər-'härts\, **Heinrich Wilhelm Gottfried von (1836–1921),** German anatomist.

walk·er \'wo-kər\ n : a framework designed to support a baby learning to walk or an infirm or physically disabled person

¹**walk–in** \'wok-ˌin\ adj : providing medical services to ambulatory patients without an appointment ⟨a ~ clinic⟩; also : being an individual who uses such services

²**walk–in** n : a walk-in patient

walk·ing \'wo-kiŋ\ adj : able to walk : AMBULATORY ⟨the ~ wounded⟩

walking cast n : a cast that is worn on a patient's leg and has a stirrup with a heel or other supporting device embedded in the plaster to facilitate walking

walking pneumonia n : a usu. mild pneumonia caused by a bacterium of the genus Mycoplasma (M. pneumoniae) and characterized by malaise, cough, and often fever

wall \'wol\ n : a structural layer surrounding a cavity, hollow organ, or mass of material ⟨the abdominal ~⟩ — **walled** \'wold\ adj

Wal·le·ri·an degeneration \wä-'lir-ē-ən-\ n : degeneration of nerve fibers that occurs following injury or disease and that progresses from the place of injury along the axon away from the cell body while the part between the place of injury and the cell body remains intact

Waller, Augustus Volney (1816–1870), British physiologist.

wall–eye \'wo-ˌlī\ n **1 a** : an eye with a whitish or bluish white iris **b** : an eye with an opaque white cornea **2 a** : strabismus in which the eye turns outward away from the nose — called also exotropia; compare CROSS-EYE 1 **b** pl : eyes affected with divergent strabismus — **wall-eyed** \-'līd\ adj

¹**wan·der·ing** \'wän-də-riŋ\ adj : FLOATING ⟨a ~ spleen⟩

²**wandering** n : movement of a tooth out of its normal position esp. as a result of periodontal disease

wandering cell n : any of various amoeboid phagocytic tissue cells

wandering pacemaker n : a back-and-forth shift in the location of cardiac pacemaking esp. from the sinoatrial node to or near the atrioventricular node

Wan·gen·steen apparatus \'waŋ-ən-ˌstēn-, -gən-\ n : the apparatus used in Wangensteen suction — called also Wangensteen appliance

Wangensteen, Owen Harding (1898–1981), American surgeon.

Wangensteen suction n : a method of draining fluid or secretions from body cavities (as the stomach) by means of an apparatus that operates on negative pressure

war·ble \'wor-bəl\ n **1** : a swelling under the hide esp. of the back of cattle, horses, and wild mammals caused by the maggot of a botfly or warble fly **2** : the maggot of a warble fly — **warbled** \-bəld\ adj

warble fly n : any of various dipteran flies (family Oestridae) whose larvae live under the skin of cattle and other mammals and cause warbles

ward \'word\ n : a division in a hospital; esp : a large room in a hospital where a number of patients often requiring similar treatment are accommodated ⟨a diabetic ~⟩

war·fa·rin \'wor-fə-rən\ n : an anticoagulant coumarin derivative $C_{19}H_{16}O_4$ related to dicumarol that inhibits the production of prothrombin by vitamin K and is used as a rodent poison and in medicine; also : its sodium salt $C_{19}H_{15}NaO_4$ used esp. in the prevention or treatment of thromboembolic disease — see COUMADIN

warm–blood·ed \'worm-'blə-dəd\ adj

: having a relatively high and constant body temperature relatively independent of the surroundings — **warm-blood-ed-ness** n

warm up vb : to engage in preliminary exercise (as to stretch the muscles) — **warm-up** \'wȯr-ˌməp\ n

war neurosis n : COMBAT FATIGUE

wart \'wȯrt\ n 1 : a horny projection on the skin usu. of the extremities produced by proliferation of the skin papillae and caused by any of numerous genotypes of the human papillomaviruses — called also *verruca vulgaris;* see FLAT WART, GENITAL WART, PLANTAR WART 2 : a skin lesion having the form of a wart but not caused by a human papillomavirus — **warty** \'wär-tē\ adj

War-thin–Star-ry stain \'wȯr-thən-'stär-ē-\ n : a silver nitrate stain used to show the presence of bacilli

　　Warthin, Aldred Scott (1866–1931), and Starry, Allen Chronister (b 1890), American pathologists.

¹**wash** \'wȯsh, 'wȧsh\ vb 1 : to cleanse by or as if by the action of liquid (as water) 2 : to flush or moisten (a bodily part or injury) with a liquid 3 : to pass through a liquid to carry off impurities or soluble components

²**wash** n : a liquid medicinal preparation used esp. for cleansing or antisepsis — see EYEWASH, MOUTHWASH

wash-able \'wȯ-shə-bəl, 'wä-\ adj 1 : capable of being washed without damage 2 : soluble in water

washings n pl : material collected by the washing of a bodily cavity

wash-out \'wȯsh-ˌau̇t, 'wäsh-\ n : the action or process of progressively reducing the concentration of a substance (as a dye injected into the left ventricle of the heart)

wasp \'wäsp, 'wȯsp\ n : any of numerous social or solitary winged hymenopteran insects (esp. families Sphecidae and Vespidae) that usu. have a slender smooth body with the abdomen attached by a narrow stalk, biting mouthparts, and in the females and workers an often painful sting

Was-ser-mann \'wä-sər-mən, 'vä-\ n : WASSERMANN TEST

Wassermann reaction n : the complement-fixing reaction that occurs in a positive complement fixation test for syphilis using the serum of an infected individual

　　Wassermann, August Paul von (1866–1925), German bacteriologist.

Wassermann test n : a test for the detection of syphilitic infection using the Wassermann reaction — called also *Wassermann*

¹**waste** \'wāst\ n 1 : loss through breaking down of bodily tissue 2 pl : bodily waste materials : EXCREMENT

²**waste** vb **wast-ed; wast-ing** : to lose or cause to lose weight, strength, or vitality : EMACIATE — often used with *away*

³**waste** adj : excreted from or stored in inert form in a living body as a by-product of vital activity

¹**wast-ing** \'wās-tiŋ\ adj : undergoing or causing decay or loss of strength

²**wasting** n : unintended loss of weight and lean body tissue characteristic of many disease (as cancer, tuberculosis, and AIDS) : gradual loss of strength or substance : ATROPHY

wa-ter \'wȯ-tər, 'wä-\ n 1 : the liquid that descends from the clouds as rain, is a major constituent of all living matter and that when pure is an odorless, tasteless, very slightly compressible liquid oxide of hydrogen H_2O, and freezes at 0°C (32°F) and boils at 100°C (212°F) 2 : liquid containing or resembling water: as **a** (1) : a pharmaceutical or cosmetic preparation made with water (2) : a watery solution of a gaseous or readily volatile substance — see AMMONIA WATER **b** : a watery fluid (as tears or urine) formed or circulating in a living body **c** : AMNIOTIC FLUID — often used in pl.; *also* : BAG OF WATERS

water balance n : the ratio between the water assimilated into the body and that lost from the body; *also* : the condition of the body when this ratio approximates unity

water blister n : a blister with a clear watery content that is not purulent or sanguineous

wa-ter-borne \'wȯ-tər-ˌbȯrn, 'wä-\ adj : carried or transmitted by water and esp. by drinking water

water brash n : regurgitation of an excessive accumulation of saliva from the lower part of the esophagus often with some acid material from the stomach — compare HEARTBURN

water–hammer pulse n : CORRIGAN'S PULSE

water hemlock n : a tall poisonous Eurasian perennial herb (*Cicuta virosa*) of the carrot family (Umbelliferae); *also* : any of several poisonous No. American plants of the same genus — compare POISON HEMLOCK

Wa-ter-house–Frid-er-ich-sen syn-drome \'wȯ-tər-ˌhau̇s-'fri-də-rik-sən-\ n : acute and severe meningococcemia with hemorrhage into the adrenal glands

　　Waterhouse, Rupert (1873–1958), British physician.

　　Friderichsen, Carl (1886–1979), Danish physician.

wa-ter-logged \-ˌlägd\ adj : EDEMATOUS

water moc-ca-sin \-'mä-kə-sən\ n : a venomous pit viper (*Agkistrodon piscivorus*) chiefly of the southeastern U.S. closely related to the copperhead — called also *cottonmouth, cottonmouth moccasin*

water on the brain n : HYDROCEPHALUS

water on the knee n : an accumulation of synovial fluid in the knee joint (as from injury or disease) marked esp. by swelling

water pick \-ˌpik\ *n* : a device that cleans teeth by directing a stream of water over and between the teeth

water pill *n* : a diuretic pill

water–soluble *adj* : soluble in water

Wa·ters' view \'wȯ-tərz-\ *n* : a radiographic image obtained by passing a beam of X-rays through the chin at an angle and used esp. to obtain diagnostic information in a single X-ray image about the bony structures of the front of the head

    Waters, Charles Alexander (1888–1961), American radiologist.

wa·tery \'wȯ-tə-rē, 'wä-\ *adj* 1 : consisting of or filled with water 2 : containing, sodden with, or yielding water or a thin liquid ⟨~ stools⟩

Wat·son–Crick \'wät-sən-'krik\ *adj* : of or relating to the Watson-Crick model ⟨the *Watson-Crick* helix⟩

    Watson, James Dewey (*b* **1928),** American molecular biologist.

    Crick, Francis Harry Compton (1916–2004), British molecular biologist.

Watson–Crick model *n* : a model of DNA structure in which the molecule is a double-stranded helix, each strand is composed of alternating links of phosphate and deoxyribose, and the strands are linked by pairs of purine and pyrimidine bases projecting inward from the deoxyribose sugars and joined by hydrogen bonds with adenine paired with thymine and with cytosine paired with guanine — compare DOUBLE HELIX

watt \'wät\ *n* : the mks unit of power equal to the work done at the rate of one joule per second or to the power produced by a current of one ampere across a potential difference of one volt

    Watt, James (1736–1819), British engineer and inventor.

wave \'wāv\ *n* 1 a : a disturbance or variation that transfers energy progressively from point to point in a medium and that may take the form of an elastic deformation or of a variation of pressure, electrical or magnetic intensity, electrical potential, or temperature b : one complete cycle of such a disturbance 2 : an undulating or jagged line constituting a graphic representation of an action ⟨an electroencephalographic ~⟩

wave·form \'wāv-ˌfȯrm\ *n* : a usu. graphic representation of the shape of a wave that indicates its characteristics (as frequency and amplitude) — called also *waveshape*

wave·length \-ˌleŋkth\ *n* : the distance in the line of advance of a wave from any one point to the next point of corresponding phase — symbol λ

wave·shape \'wāv-ˌshāp\ *n* : WAVE-FORM

wax \'waks\ *n* 1 : a substance secreted

by bees that is a dull yellow solid plastic when warm — called also *beeswax* 2 : any of various substances resembling beeswax: as a : any of numerous substances of plant or animal origin that differ from fats in being less greasy, harder, and more brittle and in containing principally compounds of high molecular weight b : a pliable or liquid composition used in uniting surfaces, making patterns or impressions, or producing a polished surface ⟨dental ~*es*⟩ 3 : a waxy secretion; *esp* : EARWAX

wax·ing *n* : the process of removing body hair with a depilatory wax

waxy \'wak-sē\ *adj* **wax·i·er; -est** 1 : made of, abounding in, or covered with wax 2 : resembling wax ⟨~ secretions⟩ ⟨a ~ complexion⟩

waxy flexibility *n* : a condition in which a patient's limbs retain any position into which they are manipulated by another person and which occurs esp. in catatonic schizophrenia

WBC *abbr* white blood cell

weal \'wēl\ *n* : WELT

wean \'wēn\ *vb* 1 : to accustom (as a young child) to take food otherwise than by nursing 2 : to detach usu. gradually from a cause of dependence or form of treatment

web \'web\ *n* : a tissue or membrane of an animal or plant; *esp* : that uniting fingers or toes at their bases — **webbed** \'webd\ *adj*

Web·er–Chris·tian disease \'we-bər-'kris-chən-\ *also* **Web·er–Chris·tian's disease** \-chənz-\ *n* : PANNICULITIS 2

    Weber, Frederick Parkes (1863–1962), British physician.

    H. A. Christian — see HAND-SCHÜLLER-CHRISTIAN DISEASE

We·ber–Fech·ner law \'we-bər-'fek-nər-, 'vā-bər-'fek-nər-\ *n* : an approximately accurate generalization in psychology: the intensity of a sensation is proportional to the logarithm of the intensity of the stimulus causing it — called also *Fechner's law*

    Weber, Ernst Heinrich (1795–1878), German anatomist and physiologist.

    Fechner, Gustav Theodor (1801–1887), German physicist and psychologist.

We·ber's law \'we-bərz-, 'vā-bərz-\ *n* : an approximately accurate generalization in psychology: the smallest change in the intensity of a stimulus capable of being perceived is proportional to the intensity of the original stimulus

    E. H. Weber — see WEBER-FECHNER LAW

We·ber test \'we-bər-, 'vā-\ *or* **We·ber's test** \-bərz-\ *n* : a test to determine the nature of unilateral hearing loss in which a vibrating tuning fork is held against the forehead at the midline and conduction deafness is indicated if the sound is heard more loudly in the affected ear and nerve deafness is indicated if it is heard more loudly in the normal ear

We·ber–Liel \'vā-bər-ˌlēl\, **Friedrich Eugen** (1832–1891), German otologist.

Wechs·ler Adult Intelligence Scale \'weks-lər-\ n : an updated version of the Wechsler-Bellevue test having the same structure but standardized against a different population to more accurately reflect the general population — abbr. *WAIS*

Wechsler, David (1896–1981), American psychologist.

Wechs·ler–Belle·vue test \-'bel-ˌvyü-\ n : a test of general intelligence and coordination in adults that involves both verbal and nonverbal tests and is now superseded by the Wechsler Adult Intelligence Scale — called also *Wechsler-Bellevue scale*

Wechsler Intelligence Scale for Children n : an intelligence test for children of elementary- and secondary-school age that involves verbal ability tests (as vocabulary and comprehension tests) and nonverbal performance tests (as assembly of an object given its parts) — abbr. *WISC*

wedge biopsy n : a biopsy in which a wedge-shaped sample of tissue is obtained; *also* : the tissue sample itself

wedge pressure \'wej-\ n : intravascular pressure that is measured by means of a catheter wedged into the pulmonary artery so as to block the flow of blood and that is equivalent to the pressure in the left atrium — called also *pulmonary capillary wedge pressure, pulmonary wedge pressure*

wedge resection n : any of several surgical procedures for removal of a wedge-shaped mass of tissue

WEE abbr western equine encephalitis; western equine encephalomyelitis

weep \'wēp\ vb **wept** \'wept\; **weeping** 1 : to pour forth (tears) from the eyes 2 : to exude (a fluid) slowly

Weg·e·ner's granulomatosis \'ve-gə-nərz-\ n : an uncommon disease of unknown cause that is characterized esp. by vasculitis of small vessels, by granuloma formation in the respiratory tract, and by glomerulonephritis

Wegener, F. (1907–1990), German pathologist.

weigh \'wā\ vb 1 : to find the heaviness of 2 : to measure or apportion (a definite quantity) on or as if on a scale 3 : to have weight or a specified weight

weight \'wāt\ n 1 : the amount that a thing weighs 2 : a unit of weight or mass

weight·less·ness \'wāt-ləs-nəs\ n : the state or condition of having little or no weight due to lack of apparent gravitational pull — **weight·less** adj

Weil–Fe·lix reaction \'vīl-'fā-liks-\ n : an agglutination test for various rickettsial infections (as typhus and scrub typhus) using particular strains of bacteria of the genus *Proteus* that have antigens in common with the rickettsiae to be identified — called also *Weil-Felix test*

Weil, Edmund (1880–1922), and **Felix, Arthur** (1887–1956), Austrian bacteriologists.

Weil's disease \'vīlz-, 'wīlz-\ n : a severe form of leptospirosis that is characterized by jaundice, chills, fever, muscle pain, anemia, and hepatomegaly and that is caused by a spirochete of the genus *Leptospira* (*L. interrogans*, esp. serotype *icterohaemorrhagiae*)

Weil, Adolf (1848–1916), German physician.

well \'wel\ adj 1 : free or recovered from infirmity or disease : HEALTHY 2 : completely cured or healed

well–adjusted adj : WELL-BALANCED 2

well–balanced adj 1 : nicely or evenly balanced, arranged, or regulated 〈a ~ diet〉 2 : emotionally or psychologically untroubled

Well·bu·trin \ˌwel-'byü-trin\ trademark — used for a preparation of the hydrochloride of bupropion

well·ness n : the quality or state of being in good health esp. as an actively sought goal

welt \'welt\ n : a ridge or lump raised on the body (as by a blow or allergic reaction)

wen \'wen\ n : SEBACEOUS CYST; broadly : an abnormal growth or a cyst protruding from a surface esp. of the skin

Wencke·bach period \'wen-kə-ˌbäk-\ n : WENCKEBACH PHENOMENON

Wenckebach, Karel Frederik (1864–1940), Dutch internist.

Wenckebach phenomenon n : heart block in which a pulse from the atrium periodically does not reach the ventricle and which is characterized by progressive prolongation of the P-R interval until a pulse is skipped

Werd·nig–Hoff·mann disease \'vert-nik-'hȯf-ˌmän-\ n : muscular atrophy that is caused by degeneration of the ventral horn cells of the spinal cord, is inherited as an autosomal recessive trait, becomes symptomatic during early infancy, is characterized by hypotonia and flaccid paralysis, and is often fatal during childhood — called also *Werdnig-Hoffmann syndrome*; compare KUGELBERG-WELANDER SYNDROME

Werdnig, Guido (1844–1919), Austrian neurologist, and **Hoffmann, Johann** (1857–1919), German neurologist.

Werl·hof's disease \'verl-ˌhȯfs-\ n : THROMBOCYTOPENIC PURPURA

Werlhof, Paul Gottlieb (1699–1767), German physician.

Wer·ner syndrome \'ver-nər-\ or **Werner's syndrome** \-nərz-\ n : a rare genetic disorder with onset during adolescence or early adulthood that is characterized by cessation of growth at puberty and by premature and accelerated aging with associated abnormalities (as muscle wasting, cataracts, osteoporosis, and hypogonadism) and that is inherited as an autosomal recessive trait

Werner, Otto (1879–1936), German physician.

Wer·nicke's aphasia \'ver-nə-kəz-\ *n* : SENSORY APHASIA; *specif* : sensory aphasia in which the affected individual speaks words fluently but without meaningful content

Wernicke, Carl (1848–1905), German neurologist.

Wernicke's area *n* : an area located in the posterior part of the superior temporal gyrus that plays an important role in the comprehension of language

Wernicke's encephalopathy *n* : an inflammatory hemorrhagic encephalopathy that is caused by thiamine deficiency, affects esp. chronic alcoholics, and is characterized by nystagmus, diplopia, ataxia, and degenerative mental disorders (as Korsakoff's psychosis)

Wert·heim operation \'vert-ˌhīm-\ *or* **Wert·heim's operation** \-ˌhīmz-\ *n* : radical hysterectomy performed by way of an abdominal incision

Wertheim, Ernst (1864–1920), Austrian gynecologist.

Wes·ter·gren erythrocyte sedimentation rate \'ves-tər-grən-\ *n* : sedimentation rate of red blood cells determined by the Westergren method — called also *Westergren sedimentation rate*

Westergren, Alf Vilhelm (1891–1968), Swedish physician.

Westergren method *n* : a method for estimating the sedimentation rate of red blood cells in fluid blood

Western blot *n* : a blot consisting of a sheet of a cellulose derivative or nylon that contains spots of protein for identification by a suitable molecular probe and is used esp. for the detection of antibodies — compare NORTHERN BLOT, SOUTHERN BLOT — **Western blotting** *n*

western black–legged tick *n* : BLACK-LEGGED TICK b

western equine encephalitis *n* : EQUINE ENCEPHALITIS b

western equine encephalomyelitis *n* : EQUINE ENCEPHALITIS b

West Nile encephalitis *n* : severe West Nile fever marked by encephalitis

West Nile fever *n* : illness caused by the West Nile virus

West Nile virus *n* : a virus of the genus *Flavivirus* (species *West Nile virus*) that causes an illness marked by fever, headache, muscle ache, skin rash, and sometimes encephalitis or meningitis, that is spread esp. from birds to humans by mosquitoes chiefly of the genus *Culex*, and that is closely related to the viruses causing Japanese B encephalitis and Saint Louis encephalitis; *also* : WEST NILE FEVER

wet \'wet\ *adj* : marked by the presence or abundance of fluid (as secretions or effusions)

wet dream *n* : an erotic dream culminating in orgasm and in the male accompanied by seminal emission

wet mount *n* : a glass slide holding a specimen suspended in a drop of liquid (as water) for microscopic examination; *also* : a specimen mounted in this way — **wet–mount** *adj*

wet nurse *n* : a woman who cares for and suckles young not her own

wetting agent *n* : a substance that promotes the spreading of a liquid on a surface or the penetration of a liquid into a material esp. by becoming adsorbed in such a way that the liquid is no longer repelled

Whar·ton's duct \'hwȯrt-ᵊnz-, 'wȯrt-\ *n* : the duct of the submandibular gland that opens into the mouth on a papilla at the side of the frenulum of the tongue

Wharton, Thomas (1614–1673), British anatomist.

Wharton's jelly *n* : a soft connective tissue that occurs in the umbilical cord and consists of large stellate fibroblasts and a few wandering cells and macrophages embedded in a homogeneous jellylike intercellular substance

wheal \'hwēl, 'wēl\ *n* : a suddenly formed elevation of the skin surface: as **a** : WELT; *esp* : a flat burning or itching eminence on the skin **b** : the transient lump occurring at the site of injection of a solution before the solution is normally dispersed — **whealing** *n*

wheat germ *n* : the embryo of the wheat kernel separated in milling and used esp. as a source of vitamins and protein

wheel·chair \'hwēl-ˌchar, 'wēl-\ *n* : a chair mounted on wheels esp. for the use of disabled individuals

¹**wheeze** \'hwēz, 'wēz\ *vb* **wheezed; wheez·ing** : to breathe with difficulty usu. with a whistling sound

²**wheeze** *n* : a sibilant whistling sound caused by difficult or obstructed respiration

whey \'hwā, 'wā\ *n* : the serum or watery part of milk that is separated from the coagulable part or curd, is rich in lactose, minerals, and vitamins, and contains lactalbumin and traces of fat

whip·lash \'hwip-ˌlash, 'wip-\ *n* : injury resulting from a sudden sharp whipping movement of the neck and head (as of a person in a vehicle that is struck head-on or from the rear by another vehicle)

Whip·ple operation \'hwi-pəl-, 'wi-\ *or* **Whip·ple's operation** \-pəlz-\ *n* : WHIPPLE PROCEDURE

Whipple procedure *or* **Whipple's procedure** *n* : PANCREATICODUO-DENECTOMY; *esp* : one in which there is complete excision of the pancreas and partial excision of the duodenum

Whipple, Allen Oldfather (1881–1963), American surgeon.

Whipple's disease *also* **Whipple disease** *n* : a rare malabsorption syndrome that is caused by an actinomycetous fungus (*Tropheryma whippelli*) in the mucous membrane of the intestine, that affects primarily the small intestine but becomes more generalized affecting esp. the joints, brain, liver, and heart, and that is marked by the accumulation of lipid deposits in the intestinal lymphatic tissues, diarrhea, weight loss, joint pain, mental confusion, and generalized lymphadenopathy — called also *intestinal lipodystrophy*

Whipple, George Hoyt (1878–1976), American pathologist.

whip·worm \'hwip-,wərm, 'wip-\ *n* : a parasitic nematode worm of the genus *Trichuris* having a body that is thickened posteriorly and is very long and slender anteriorly; *esp* : one (*T. trichiura*) of the human intestine

whirl·pool bath \'hwərl-,pül-, 'wərl-\ *n* : a therapeutic bath in which all or part of the body is exposed to forceful whirling currents of hot water — called also *whirlpool*

white blood cell *n* : any of the blood cells that are colorless, lack hemoglobin, contain a nucleus, and include the lymphocytes, monocytes, neutrophils, eosinophils, and basophils — called also *leukocyte, white blood corpuscle, white cell, white corpuscle;* compare RED BLOOD CELL

white coat hypertension *n* : a temporary elevation in a patient's blood pressure that occurs when measured in a medical setting (as a physician's office) and that is usu. due to anxiety on the part of the patient — called also *white coat effect*

white count *n* : the count or the total number of white blood cells in the blood usu. stated as the number in one cubic millimeter — compare DIF-FERENTIAL BLOOD COUNT

white fat *n* : normal fat tissue that replaces brown fat in infants during the first year of life

white·head \'hwīt-,hed, 'wīt-\ *n* : MIL-IUM

white light *n* : light that is composed of a wide range of electromagnetic frequencies and that appears colorless to the eye

white lotion *n* : a preparation made of sulfurated potash and zinc sulfate that is applied topically in the treatment of various skin disorders

white matter *n* : neural tissue esp. of the brain and spinal cord that consists largely of myelinated nerve fibers bundled into tracts, has a whitish color, and typically underlies the gray matter

white muscle disease *n* : a degenerative muscle disease of young domestic animals caused by a dietary deficiency of selenium or vitamin E — see STIFF-LAMB DISEASE

white noise *n* : a heterogeneous mixture of sound waves extending over a wide frequency range that has been used to mask out unwanted noise interfering with sleep — called also *white sound*

white ointment *n* : an ointment consisting of 5 percent white wax and 95 percent white petrolatum — called also *simple ointment*

white petrolatum *n* : decolorized petroleum jelly — called also *white petroleum jelly*

white piedra *n* : a form of piedra that affects esp. the facial hairs and is caused by a fungus of the genus *Trichosporan* (*T. beigelii*)

white pulp *n* : a parenchymatous tissue of the spleen that consists of compact masses of lymphatic cells and that forms the Malpighian corpuscles — compare RED PULP

white ramus *n* : RAMUS COMMUNI-CANS a

white ramus communicans *n* : RA-MUS COMMUNICANS a

whites *n pl* : LEUKORRHEA

white shark *n* : GREAT WHITE SHARK

white snake·root \-'snāk-,rüt, -,rüt\ *n* : a poisonous No. American herb (*Eupatorium rugosum* of the family Compositae) that is a cause of trembles and milk sickness

white sound *n* : WHITE NOISE

white squill *n* : SQUILL 2

Whit·field's ointment \'hwit-,feldz-, 'wit-\ *also* **Whit·field ointment** \-,fēld-\ *n* : an ointment that contains benzoic acid and salicylic acid and is used for its keratolytic effect in treating fungus skin diseases (as ringworm)

Whitfield, Arthur (1868–1947), British dermatologist.

whit·low \'hwit-,(,)lō, 'wit-\ *n* : a deep usu. suppurative inflammation of the finger or toe esp. near the end or around the nail — called also *felon;* compare PARONYCHIA

WHO *abbr* World Health Organization

whole \'hōl\ *adj* : containing all its natural constituents, components, or elements

whole blood *n* : blood with all its components intact that has been withdrawn from a donor into an anticoagulant solution for use to restore blood volume esp. after traumatic blood loss

whole–body *adj* : of, relating to, or affecting the entire body ⟨∼ radiation⟩

whole food *n* : a natural food and esp. an unprocessed one

whoop \'hüp, 'hùp, 'hwùp\ *n* : the crowing intake of breath following a paroxysm in whooping cough — **whoop** *vb*

whooping cough *n* : an infectious disease esp. of children caused by a bacterium of the genus *Bordetella* (*B. pertussis*) and marked by a convulsive spasmodic cough sometimes followed by a crowing intake of breath — called also *pertussis*

whorl \'hwórl, 'wórl, 'hwarl, 'warl\ *n* : a fingerprint in which the central papillary ridges turn through at least one complete turn

Wi·dal reaction \vē-'däl-\ *also* **Widal's reaction** \-'dälz-\ *n* : a specific reaction consisting in agglutination of typhoid bacilli or other salmonellae when mixed with serum from a patient having typhoid fever or other salmonella infection and constituting a test for the disease

  Widal, Georges–Fernand–Isidore (1862–1929), French physician and bacteriologist.

Widal test *also* **Widal's test** *n* : a test for detecting typhoid fever and other salmonella infections using the Widal reaction — compare AGGLUTINATION TEST

wide–spectrum *adj* : BROAD-SPECTRUM

wild type *n* : a phenotype, genotype, or gene that predominates in a natural population of organisms or strain of organisms in contrast to that of natural or laboratory mutant forms; *also* : an organism or strain displaying the wild type — **wild–type** *adj*

Wil·liams symdrome \'wil-yəmz-\ *n* : a rare genetic disorder marked esp. by hypercalcemia of infants, heart defects, characteristic facial features (as an upturned nose and pointed chin), a sociable personality, and mild to moderate mental retardation but a high verbal aptitude

  Williams, J. C. P (*fl* 1961), New Zealand cardiologist.

Wilms' tumor \'vilmz-\ *also* **Wilms's tumor** \'vilm-zəz-\ *n* : a malignant tumor of the kidney that primarily affects children and is made up of embryonic elements — called also *nephroblastoma*

  Wilms, Max (1867–1918), German surgeon.

Wil·son's disease \'wil-sənz-\ *n* : a genetic disease that is characterized by the accumulation of copper in the body (as in the liver or brain) due to abnormal copper metabolism associated with ceruloplasmin deficiency, that is inherited as an autosomal recessive trait, and that is marked esp. by liver dysfunction and disease and neurologic or psychiatric symptoms (as tremors or dementia) — called

also *hepatolenticular degeneration;* see KAYSER-FLEISCHER RING

  Wilson, Samuel Alexander Kinnier (1877–1937), British neurologist.

wind–bro·ken \'wind-,brō-kən\ *adj, of a horse* : affected with pulmonary emphysema or with heaves

wind·burn \'wind-,bərn\ *n* : irritation of the skin caused by wind — **windburned** \-,bərnd\ *adj*

wind·chill \-,chil\ *n* : a still-air temperature that would have the same cooling effect on exposed human skin as a given combination of temperature and wind speed — called also *chill factor, windchill factor, windchill index*

wind·gall \-,gól\ *n* : a soft tumor or synovial swelling on a horse's leg in the region of the fetlock joint

win·dow \'win-(,)dō\ *n* **1** : FENESTRA 1 **2** : a small surgically created opening : FENESTRA 2a **3** : a usu. narrow interval of time or range of values for which a certain condition or an opportunity exists — see THERAPEUTIC WINDOW

wind·pipe \'wind-,pīp\ *n* : TRACHEA

wind puff \-,pəf\ *n* : WINDGALL

wing \'win\ *n* **1** : one of the movable feathered or membranous paired appendages by means of which a bird, bat, or insect is able to fly **2** : a winglike anatomical part or process : ALA; *esp* : any of the four winglike processes of the sphenoid bone — see GREATER WING, LESSER WING — **winged** \'wind, 'win-əd\ *adj*

win·ter·green \'win-tər-,grēn\ *n* **1** : any plant of the genus *Gaultheria*; *esp* : a low white-flowered evergreen plant (*G. procumbens*) with spicy red berries **2** : OIL OF WINTERGREEN

wintergreen oil *n* : OIL OF WINTERGREEN

winter itch *n* : an itching disorder caused by prolonged exposure to cold dry air

winter tick *n* : an ixodid tick of the genus *Dermacentor* (*D. albipictus*) that is actively parasitic during the winter months on animals (as deer and moose) in parts of Canada and the northern and western U.S.

wire \'wīr\ *n* : metal thread or a rod used in surgery to suture soft tissue or transfix fractured bone and in orthodontic dentistry to position teeth — **wire** *vb*

Wir·sung's duct \'vir-,sùnz-\ *n* : PANCREATIC DUCT a

  J. G. Wirsung — see DUCT OF WIRSUNG

WISC *abbr* Wechsler Intelligence Scale for Children

wisdom tooth *n* : the third molar that is the last tooth to erupt on each side of the upper and lower jaws

wish–fulfillment *n* : the gratification of a desire esp. symbolically (as in dreams or neurotic symptoms)

Wis·kott–Al·drich syndrome \'vis-

,kät-'ôl-drich-\ *n* : a usu. fatal immunodeficiency disease of male children that is inherited as an X-linked recessive trait and is characterized esp. by thrombocytopenia, leukopenia, recurrent infections, eczema, and abnormal bleeding

Wiskott, Alfred (1898–1978), German pediatrician.

Aldrich, Robert Anderson (1917–1998), American pediatrician.

witch ha·zel \'wich-,hā-zǝl\ *n* **1** : a small tree or shrub (*Hamamelis virginiana* of the family Hamamelidaceae) of eastern No. America **2** : an alcoholic solution of a distillate of the bark of the witch hazel used as a soothing and mildly astringent lotion

with·draw·al \with-'drô-ǝl, with-\ *n* **1 a** : a pathological retreat from objective reality (as in some schizophrenic states) **b** : social or emotional detachment **2 a** : the discontinuance of administration or use of a drug **b** : the syndrome of often painful physical and psychological symptoms that follows discontinuance of an addicting substance **3** : COITUS INTERRUPTUS — **with·draw** \-'drô\ *vb*

withdrawal symptom *n* : one of a group of symptoms (as nausea, sweating, or depression) produced by deprivation of an addicting substance

with·drawn \with-'drôn\ *adj* : socially detached and unresponsive : exhibiting withdrawal : INTROVERTED

with·ers \'wi-thǝrz\ *n pl* **1** : the ridge between the shoulder bones of a horse **2** : a part corresponding to the withers in a quadruped other than a horse

Wit·zel·sucht \'vit-sǝl-,zụkt\ *n* : excessive facetiousness and inappropriate or pointless humor esp. when considered as part of an abnormal condition

wohl·fahr·tia \,vōl-'fär-tē-ǝ\ *n* **1** *cap* : a genus of dipteran flies (family Sarcophagidae) that deposit their larvae in wounds or on the intact skin of humans and domestic animals causing severe cutaneous myiasis **2** : any fly of the genus *Wohlfahrtia*

Wol·fart \'vōl-,färt\, **Peter (1675–1726),** German physician.

Wolff·ian body \'wôl-fē-ǝn-\ *n* : MESONEPHROS

Wolff \'vôlf\, **Caspar Friedrich (1734–1794),** German anatomist and embryologist.

Wolffian duct *n* : the duct of the mesonephros that persists in the female chiefly as part of the epoophoron and in the male as the duct system leaving the testis and including the epididymis, vas deferens, seminal vesicle, and ejaculatory duct — called also *mesonephric duct*

Wolff–Par·kin·son–White syndrome \'wôlf-'pär-kǝn-sǝn-'hwīt-, -'wīt-\ *n* : an abnormal heart condition characterized by preexcitation of the ventricle and an electrocardiographic

tracing with a shortened P-R interval and a widened QRS complex — called also *WPW syndrome*

Wolff, Louis (1898–1972), and **White, Paul Dudley (1886–1973),** American cardiologists.

Parkinson, Sir John (1885–1976), British cardiologist.

wol·fram \'wùl-frǝm\ *n* : TUNGSTEN

Wol·fram syndrome *or* **Wolfram's syndrome** \'wùl-frǝm-\ *n* : a rare hereditary disorder that is characterized esp. by type 1 diabetes, diabetes insipidus, optic atrophy, sensorineural deafness, and bladder dysfunction and that is inherited as an autosomal recessive trait

Wolfram, D. J. (*fl* **1938),** American physician.

womb \'wüm\ *n* : UTERUS

wonder drug *n* : MIRACLE DRUG

wood alcohol *n* : METHANOL

wooden tongue *n* : actinobacillosis or actinomycosis of cattle esp. when chiefly affecting the tongue

Wood's lamp \'wùdz-\ *also* **Wood lamp** \'wùd-\ *n* : a lamp for producing ultraviolet radiation that is used to detect various skin conditions (as some fungus infections) by the fluorescence induced in the affected areas by ultraviolet radiation

Wood, Robert Williams (1868–1955), American physicist.

Wood's light *also* **Wood light** *n* : WOOD'S LAMP; *also* : ultraviolet radiation produced by a Wood's lamp

wood tick *n* : any of several ixodid ticks: as **a** : ROCKY MOUNTAIN WOOD TICK **b** : AMERICAN DOG TICK

wool fat \'wùl-\ *n* : wool grease esp. after refining : LANOLIN

wool grease *n* : a fatty slightly sticky wax coating the surface of the fibers of sheep's wool that is used as a source of lanolin

wool·sort·er's disease \'wùl-,sôr-tǝrz-\ *n* : pulmonary anthrax resulting esp. from inhalation of bacterial spores from contaminated wool or hair

word–association test *n* : a test of personality and mental function in which the subject is required to respond to each of a series of words with the first word that comes to mind or with a word of a specified class of words

word blindness *n* : ALEXIA

word salad *n* : a jumble of extremely incoherent speech as sometimes observed in schizophrenia

work–related musculoskeletal disorder *n* : REPETITIVE STRAIN INJURY

work·up \'wǝr-,kǝp\ *n* : an intensive diagnostic study ⟨a gastrointestinal ∼⟩

work up \'wǝr-'kǝp, 'wǝr-\ *vb* : to perform a diagnostic workup upon

¹**worm** \'wǝrm\ *n* **1** : any of various relatively small elongated usu. naked and soft-bodied parasitic animals (as a grub, pinworm, or tapeworm) **2**

: HELMINTHIASIS — usu. used in pl. ⟨a dog with ~s⟩ — **worm-like** *adj*

²**worm** *vb* : to treat (an animal) with a drug to destroy or expel parasitic worms

worm-er \'wər-mər\ *n* : a worming agent used in veterinary medicine

Wor-mi-an bone \'wȯr-mē-ən-\ *n* : a small irregular inconstant plate of bone interposed in a suture between large cranial bones

Worm \'wȯrm\, **Ole** (*Latin* **Olaus Wormius**) (1588–1654), Danish physician.

worm-seed \'wərm-ˌsēd\ *n* : any of various plants (as of the genera *Artemisia* or *Chenopodium*) whose seeds possess anthelmintic properties

worm-wood \'wərm-ˌwu̇d\ *n* : any of various aromatic shrubs and herbs (genus *Artemisia* and esp. *A. absinthium* of the family Compositae)

wound \'wünd\ *n* **1 a** : a physical injury to the body consisting of a laceration or breaking of the skin or mucous membrane often with damage to underlying tissues **b** : an opening made in the skin or a membrane of the body incidental to a surgical operation or procedure **2** : a mental or emotional hurt or blow — **wound** *vb*

WPW syndrome \ˌdə-bəl-yü-ˌpē-'də-bəl-yü-\ *n* : WOLFF-PARKINSON= WHITE SYNDROME

wrench \'rench\ *n* : a sharp twist or sudden jerk straining muscles or liga-ments; *also* : the resultant injury (as of a joint) — **wrench** *vb*

Wright's stain \'rīts-\ *n* : a stain used in staining blood and parasites living in blood

Wright, James Homer (1869–1928), American pathologist.

wrin-kle \'riŋ-kəl\ *n* : a small ridge or furrow in the skin esp. when due to age, worry, or fatigue — **wrinkle** *vb*

wrist \'rist\ *n* : the joint or the region of the joint between the human hand and the arm

wrist-bone \-ˌbōn\ *n* **1** : a carpal bone **2** : the styloid process of the human radius that forms a prominence on the outer side of the wrist above the thumb

wrist–drop \-ˌdräp\ *n* : paralysis of the extensor muscles of the hand causing the hand to hang down at the wrist

wrist joint *n* : the articulation at the wrist

writer's cramp *n* : a painful spasmodic cramp of muscles of the hand or fingers brought on by excessive writing — called also *graphospasm*

wry-neck \'rī-ˌnek\ *n* : TORTICOLLIS

wt *abbr* weight

Wuch-er-e-ria \ˌwu̇k-kə-'rir-ē-ə\ *n* : a genus of filarial worms (family Dipetalonematidae) including a parasite (*W. bancrofti*) that causes elephantiasis

Wu-cher-er \'vu̇-kər-ər\, **Otto Eduard Heinrich (1820–1873)**, German physician.

X

x \'eks\ *n, pl* **x's** *or* **xs** \'ek-səz\ : the basic or haploid number of chromosomes of a polyploid series : the number contained in a single genome — compare N 1

x *symbol* power of magnification

Xal-a-tan \'za-lə-ˌtan\ *trademark* — used for a preparation of latanoprost

Xan-ax \'za-ˌnaks\ *trademark* — used for a preparation of alprazolam

xanth- *or* **xantho-** *comb form* : yellow ⟨*xanthoma*⟩

xan-than gum \'zan-thən-\ *n* : a polysaccharide produced by fermentation of carbohydrates by a bacterium (*Xanthomonas campestris*) and used as a thickening and suspending agent in pharmaceuticals and prepared foods — called also *xanthan*

xan-the-las-ma \ˌzan-thə-'laz-mə\ *n* : xanthoma of the eyelid

xanthelasma pal-pe-bra-rum \-ˌpal-ˌpē-'brar-əm\ *n* : XANTHELASMA

xan-thene dye \'zan-ˌthēn\ *n* : any of various brilliant fluorescent yellow to pink to bluish red dyes

xan-thine \'zan-ˌthēn\ *n* : a feebly ba-sic compound $C_5H_4N_4O_2$ that occurs esp. in animal or plant tissue, is derived from guanine and hypoxanthine, and yields uric acid on oxidation; *also* : any of various derivatives of this

xan-tho-chro-mia \ˌzan-thə-'krō-mē-ə\ *n* : xanthochromic discoloration

xan-tho-chro-mic \-'krō-mik\ *adj* : having a yellowish discoloration

xan-tho-ma \zan-'thō-mə\ *n, pl* **-mas** *also* **-ma-ta** \-mə-tə\ : a fatty irregular yellow patch or nodule on the skin that is associated esp. with disturbances of cholesterol metabolism

xan-tho-ma-to-sis \(ˌ)zan-ˌthō-mə-'tō-səs\ *n, pl* **-to-ses** \-ˌsēz\ : a condition marked by the presence of multiple xanthomas

xan-tho-ma-tous \zan-'thō-mə-təs\ *adj* : of, relating to, marked by, or characteristic of a xanthoma or xanthomatosis ⟨~ lesions⟩

xan-tho-phyll \'zan-thə-ˌfil\ *n* : any of several neutral yellow to orange carotenoid pigments that are oxygen derivatives of carotenes; *esp* : LUTEIN

xan·thop·sia \zan-'thäp-sē-ə\ *n* : a visual disturbance in which objects appear yellow

xan·tho·tox·in \'zan-thə-,täk-sən\ *n* : METHOXSALEN

xanth·uren·ic acid \,zanth-yə-'re-nik-\ *n* : a yellow crystalline phenolic acid $C_{10}H_7NO_4$ that is a tryptophan metabolite excreted in the urine

X chromosome *n* : a sex chromosome that usu. occurs paired in each female cell and single in each male cell in species in which the male typically has two unlike sex chromosomes — compare Y CHROMOSOME

X–disease *n* : any of various usu. virus diseases of obscure etiology and relationships; *esp* : MURRAY VALLEY ENCEPHALITIS

Xe *symbol* xenon

xen- or **xeno-** *comb form* **1** : strange : foreign ⟨*xeno*biotic⟩ **2** : HETER- ⟨*xeno*graft⟩

Xen·i·cal \'ze-ni-,kal\ *trademark* — used for a preparation of orlistat

xe·no·bi·ot·ic \,ze-nō-bī-'ä-tik, ,zē-, -bē-\ *n* : a chemical compound (as a drug or pesticide) that is foreign to a living organism — **xenobiotic** *adj*

xe·no·di·ag·no·sis \,ze-nō-,dī-ig-'nō-səs, ,zē-\ *n, pl* **-no·ses** \-,sēz\ : the detection of a parasite (as of humans) by feeding supposedly infected material (as blood) to a suitable intermediate host (as an insect) and later examining the intermediate host for the parasite — **xe·no·di·ag·nos·tic** \-'näs-tik\ *adj*

xe·no·ge·ne·ic \,ze-nō-jə-'nē-ik, ,zē-\ *also* **xe·no·gen·ic** \-'je-nik\ *adj* : derived from, originating in, or being a member of another species — compare ALLOGENEIC, SYNGENEIC

xe·no·graft \'ze-nə-,graft, 'zē-\ *n* : a graft of tissue taken from a donor of one species and grafted into a recipient of another species — called also *heterograft, heterotransplant, xenotransplant;* compare HOMOGRAFT — **xenograft** *vb*

xe·non \'zē-,nän, 'ze-\ *n* : a heavy, colorless, and relatively inert gaseous element — symbol *Xe*; see ELEMENT table

xe·no·phobe \'ze-nə-,fōb, 'zē-\ *n* : one unduly fearful of what is foreign and esp. of people of foreign origin — **xe·no·pho·bic** \,ze-nə-'fō-bik, ,zē-\ *adj*

xe·no·pho·bia \,ze-nə-'fō-bē-ə, ,zē-\ *n* : fear and hatred of strangers or foreigners or of anything that is strange or foreign

Xen·op·syl·la \,ze-näp-'si-lə\ *n* : a genus of fleas (family Pulicidae) including several (as the oriental rat flea) that are vectors of plague

xe·no·trans·plant \,ze-nə-'trans-,plant, ,zē-\ *n* : XENOGRAFT — **xenotransplant** *vb*

xe·no·trans·plan·ta·tion \-'trans-,plan-'tā-shən\ *n* : transplantation of an organ, tissue, or cells between two different species

xe·no·tro·pic \,ze-nə-'trä-pik, ,zē-nə-'trō-pik\ *adj* : replicating or reproducing only in cells other than those of the host species (∼ viruses)

xer- or **xero-** *comb form* : dry : arid ⟨*xero*derma⟩

xe·ro·der·ma \,zir-ə-'dər-mə\ *n* : a disease of the skin characterized by dryness and roughness and a fine scaly desquamation

xeroderma pig·men·to·sum \-,pig-mən-'tō-səm, -,men-\ *n* : a genetic condition inherited chiefly as a recessive autosomal trait that is caused by a defect in mechanisms that repair DNA damaged by ultraviolet light and is characterized by the development of pigment abnormalities and multiple skin cancers in body areas exposed to the sun — abbr. *XP*

xe·rog·ra·phy \zə-'rä-grə-fē, zir-'ä-\ *n, pl* **-phies 1** : a process for copying graphic matter by the action of light on an electrically charged surface in which the latent image is developed with a resinous powder **2** : XERORADIOGRAPHY — **xe·ro·graph·ic** \,zir-ə-'gra-fik\ *adj* — **xe·ro·graph·i·cal·ly** *adv*

xe·ro·mam·mog·ra·phy \,zir-ō-ma-'mä-grə-fē\ *n, pl* **-phies** : xeroradiography of the breast — **xe·ro·mam·mo·gram** \-'ma-mə-,gram\ *n*

xe·roph·thal·mia \,zir-,äf-'thal-mē-ə, -,äp-'thal-\ *n* : a dry thickened lusterless condition of the eyeball resulting esp. from a severe deficiency of vitamin A — compare KERATOMALACIA — **xe·roph·thal·mic** \-mik\ *adj*

xe·ro·ra·di·og·ra·phy \,zir-ō-,rā-dē-'ä-grə-fē\ *n, pl* **-phies** : radiography used esp. in mammographic screening for breast cancer that produces an image using X-rays in a manner similar to the way an image is produced by light in xerography — **xe·ro·ra·dio·graph·ic** \-,rā-dē-ō-'gra-fik\ *adj*

xe·ro·sis \zi-'rō-səs\ *n, pl* **xe·ro·ses** \-,sēz\ : abnormal dryness of a body part or tissue (as the skin)

xe·ro·sto·mia \,zir-ə-'stō-mē-ə\ *n* : abnormal dryness of the mouth due to insufficient secretions — called also *dry mouth*

xiph- or **xiphi-** or **xipho-** *comb form* : sword-shaped ⟨*xiphi*sternum⟩

xi·phi·ster·num \,zi-fə-'stər-nəm, ,zi-\ *n, pl* **-na** \-nə\ : XIPHOID PROCESS

xi·phoid \'zi-,fóid, 'zi-\ *n* : XIPHOID PROCESS — **xiphoid** *adj*

xiphoid process *n* : the smallest and lowest division of the human sternum that is cartilaginous early in life but becomes more or less ossified during adulthood — called also *ensiform cartilage, ensiform process*

x–ir·ra·di·a·tion \'eks-\ *n, often cap X* : X-RADIATION 1 — **x–ir·ra·di·ate** *vb, often cap X*

X–linked *adj* : located on an X chromosome ⟨an ~ gene⟩; *also* : transmitted by an X-linked gene ⟨an ~ disease⟩

XP *abbr* xeroderma pigmentosum

x–ra·di·a·tion *n, often cap X* **1** : exposure to X-rays **2** : radiation composed of X-rays

x–ra·di·og·ra·phy *n, pl* **-phies** *often cap X* : radiography by means of X-rays

x–ray \'eks-,rā\ *vb, often cap X* : to examine, treat, or photograph with X-rays

X-ray *n* **1** : any of the electromagnetic radiations of the same nature as visible radiation but of an extremely short wavelength that has the properties of ionizing a gas upon passage through it, of penetrating various thicknesses of all solids, of producing secondary radiations by impinging on material bodies, of acting on photographic films and plates as light does, and of causing fluorescent screens to emit light — called also *roentgen ray* **2** : a photograph obtained by use of X-rays ⟨a chest *X-ray*⟩ — **X-ray** *adj*

X–ray therapy *n* : medical treatment (as of cancer) by controlled application of X-rays

XTC \'ek-stə-sē\ *n* : ECSTASY 2

xy·la·zine \'zī-lə-,zēn\ *n* : a veterinary sedative, analgesic, and muscle relaxant administered in the form of its hydrochloride $C_{12}H_{16}N_2S \cdot HCl$

xy·lene \'zī-,lēn\ *n* : any of three toxic flammable oily isomeric aromatic hydrocarbons C_8H_{10}

xy·li·tol \'zī-lə-,tól, -,tōl\ *n* : a crystalline alcohol $C_5H_{12}O_5$ that is a derivative of xylose and is used as a sweetener

Xy·lo·caine \'zī-lə-,kān\ *trademark* — used for a preparation of lidocaine

xy·lo·met·a·zo·line \,zī-lə-,me-tə-'zō-,lēn\ *n* : a sympathomimetic agent with vasoconstrictive activity that is used in the form of its hydrochloride $C_{16}H_{24}N_2 \cdot HCl$ esp. as a topical nasal decongestant

xy·lose \'zī-,lōs, -,lōz\ *n* : a crystalline aldose sugar $C_5H_{10}O_5$

xy·lu·lose \'zīl-yü-,lōs, 'zil-lü-, -,lōz\ *n* : a ketose sugar $C_5H_{10}O_5$ of the pentose class that plays a role in carbohydrate metabolism and is found in the urine in cases of pentosuria

Y *symbol* yttrium

YAC *abbr* yeast artificial chromosome

Yas·min \'yaz-min\ *trademark* — used for a preparation of drospirenone and ethinyl estradiol

yaw \'yò\ *n* : one of the lesions characteristic of yaws

yawn \'yòn, 'yän\ *n* : an opening of the mouth wide while taking a deep breath often as an involuntary reaction to fatigue or boredom — **yawn** *vb*

yaws \'yòz\ *n sing or pl* : an infectious contagious tropical disease that is caused by a spirochete of the genus *Treponema* (*T. pertenue*) and that is characterized by a primary ulcerating lesion on the skin followed by a secondary stage in which ulcers develop all over the body and by a third stage in which the bones are involved — called also *frambesia, pian*

Yb *symbol* ytterbium

Y chromosome \'wī-\ *n* : a sex chromosome that is characteristic of male cells in species in which the male typically has two unlike sex chromosomes — compare X CHROMOSOME

yeast \'yēst\ *n* **1** : a unicellular chiefly ascomycetous fungus (as of the family Saccharomycetaceae) that has usu. little or no mycelium, that typically reproduces asexually by budding, and that includes forms (as *Saccharomyces cerevisiae*) which cause alcoholic fermentation and are used esp. in the making of alcoholic beverages and leavened bread **2** : a yellowish surface froth or sediment that occurs esp. in sugary fermenting liquids (as fruit juices) and consists chiefly of yeast cells and carbon dioxide **3** : a commercial product containing yeast cells in a moist or dry medium — **yeast·like** \-,līk\ *adj*

yeast artificial chromosome *n* : a chromosome that is used esp. to clone DNA segments longer than those capable of being cloned in bacteria and that is introduced for cloning into a yeast of the genus *Saccharomyces* (*S. cerevisiae*) — abbr. **YAC**

yeast infection *n* : an infection of the vagina with an overgrowth of a yeast-like fungus of the genus *Candida* (*C. albicans*) normally present in the vaginal flora that is characterized by vaginal discharge and vulvovaginitis; *broadly* : an infection (as thrush) caused by a yeast or yeastlike fungus

yellow body *n* : CORPUS LUTEUM

yellow fat disease *n* : a disease esp. of swine, cats, and mink that is associated with a deficiency of vitamin E and is marked by inflammation of the fatty tissue, subcutaneous edema, and varied visceral lesions — called also *steatitis, yellow fat*

yellow fever *n* : an acute infectious disease of warm regions (as sub-Saharan Africa and tropical So. America) marked by sudden onset, prostration, fever, and headache and sometimes albuminuria, jaundice, and hemorrhage and caused by a flavivirus (species *Yellow fever virus*) transmitted esp. by the yellow-fever mosquito

yellow–fever mosquito *n* : a small dark-colored mosquito of the genus *Aedes* (*A. aegypti*) that is the usual vector of yellow fever — called also *tiger mosquito*

yellow jacket *n* **1** : any of various yellow-marked social wasps (esp. genus *Vespula* of the family Vespidae) that usu. nest in the ground and can sting repeatedly and painfully **2** *slang* : pentobarbital esp. in a yellow capsule — usu. used in pl.

yellow marrow *n* : BONE MARROW a

yellow petrolatum *n* : petroleum jelly that has not been wholly or mostly decolorized

yel·lows \'ye-(ˌ)lōz\ *n sing or pl* : any of several diseases of domestic animals (as sheep) that are characterized by jaundice

yellow wax *n* : a wax obtained as a yellow to brown solid by melting a honeycomb with boiling water, straining, and cooling — called also *beeswax*

yer·ba san·ta \'yer-bə-'sän-tə, 'yər-, -'sän-\ *n* : an evergreen shrub (*Eriodictyon californicum* of the family Hydrophyllaceae) of California with aromatic leaves; *also* : ERIODICTYON

yer·sin·ia \yər-'si-nē-ə\ *n* **1** *cap* : a genus of enterobacteria that includes several important pathogens (as the plague bacterium, *Y. pestis*) formerly included in the genus *Pasteurella* — see PLAGUE 2 **2** : any bacterium of the genus *Yersinia*

Yer·sin \yer-'seⁿ\, **Alexandre– Emile–John** (1863–1943), French bacteriologist.

yer·sin·i·o·sis \yər-ˌsi-nē-'ō-səs\ *n* : infection with or disease caused by a bacterium of the genus *Yersinia*; *esp* : an infectious disease that is caused by a yersinia (*Y. enterocolitica*) transmitted chiefly in contaminated water and food (as raw or undercooked pork products) and is marked esp. by fever, abdominal pain, and diarrhea

Y ligament *n* : ILIOFEMORAL LIGAMENT

yo·ga \'yō-gə\ *n* **1** *cap* : a Hindu theistic philosophy teaching the suppression of all activity of body, mind, and will in order that the self may realize its distinction from them and attain liberation **2** : a system of physical postures, breathing techniques, and

meditation derived from Yoga but often practiced independently to promote bodily or mental control and well-being — see HATHA YOGA — **yo·gic** \-gik\ *adj*

yo·gurt *also* **yo·ghurt** \'yō-gərt\ *n* : a fermented slightly acid often flavored semisolid food made of milk and milk solids to which cultures of bacteria of the genus *Lactobacillus* (*L. bulgarius*) and *Streptococcus* (*S. thermophilus*) have been added

yo·him·be \yō-'him-bā\ *n* : a tropical African tree (*Pausinystalia yohimbe* syn. *Corynanthe yohimbe*) of the madder family (Rubiaceae) whose bark yields yohimbine; *also* : a preparation of the bark that is used esp. as an aphrodisiac

yo·him·bine \yō-'him-ˌbēn, -bən\ *n* : an alkaloid obtained from the bark of yohimbe that is a weak blocker of alpha-adrenergic receptors and has been used in the form of its hydrochloride $C_{21}H_{26}N_2O_3 \cdot HCl$ as a mydriatic and aphrodisiac and to treat impotence

yolk \'yōk\ *n* : material stored in an ovum that supplies food to the developing embryo and consists chiefly of proteins, lecithin, and cholesterol

yolk sac *n* : a membranous sac of most vertebrates that encloses the yolk, is continuous in most forms (as in humans) through the omphalomesenteric duct with the intestinal cavity of the embryo, and is supplied with blood vessels that transport nutritive yolk products to the developing embryo

yolk stalk *n* : OMPHALOMESENTERIC DUCT

Young–Helm·holtz theory \'yəŋ-'helm-ˌhōlts-\ *n* : a theory in color vision: the eye has three separate elements each of which is stimulated by a different primary color

Young, Thomas (1773–1829), British physician, physicist, and archaeologist.

Helmholtz, Hermann Ludwig Ferdinand von (1821–1894), German physicist and physiologist.

yo–yo dieting *n* : the practice of repeatedly losing weight by dieting and subsequently regaining it

yt·ter·bi·um \i-'tər-bē-əm\ *n* : a bivalent or trivalent metallic element — symbol Yb; see ELEMENT table

yt·tri·um \'i-trē-əm\ *n* : a trivalent metallic element — symbol Y; see ELEMENT table

yup·pie flu \'yə-pē-\ *n* : CHRONIC FATIGUE SYNDROME

za·fir·lu·kast \zə-ˈfir-lü-ˌkast\ *n* : a leukotriene antagonist $C_{31}H_{33}N_3O_6S$ that is administered orally in the treatment of asthma

zal·cit·a·bine \zal-ˈsi-tə-ˌbēn, -ˌbīn\ *n* : DDC

zal·e·plon \ˈza-lə-ˌplän\ *n* : a sedative and hypnotic drug $C_{17}H_{15}N_3O$ used in the treatment of insomnia — see SONATA

za·nam·i·vir \zə-ˈna-mə-ˌvir\ *n* : a neuraminidase inhibitor $C_{12}H_{20}N_4O_7$ used in the form of an inhalant against influenza A and B to prevent the spread of influenza virus from cell to cell in the lungs — see RELENZA

Zan·tac \ˈzan-ˌtak\ *trademark* — used for a preparation of the hydrochloride of ranitidine

Z–DNA \ˈzē-\ *n* : the left-handed uncommon form of double helix DNA in which the chains twist up and to the left around the front of the axis of the helix — compare B-DNA

ZDV \ˌzē-dē-ˈvē\ *n* : AZT

Zei·gar·nik effect \zī-ˈgär-nik-\ *n* : the psychological tendency to remember an uncompleted task rather than a completed one

    Zeigarnik, Bluma (1900–1988), Russian psychologist.

Zen·ker's diverticulum \ˈzeŋ-kərz-, ˈtseŋ-\ *n* : an abnormal pouch in the upper part of the esophagus in which food may become trapped causing bad breath, irritation, difficulty in swallowing, and regurgitation — called also *pharyngoesophageal diverticulum*

    Zenker, Friedrich Albert von (1825–1898), German pathologist and anatomist.

Zeph·i·ran \ˈze-fə-ˌran\ *trademark* — used for a preparation of benzalkonium chloride

Zes·tril \ˈzes-tril\ *trademark* — used for a preparation of lisinopril

Zet·ia \ˈze-tē-ə\ *trademark* — used for a preparation of ezetimibe

zi·con·o·tide \zī-ˈkä-nə-ˌtīd\ *n* : an analgesic $C_{102}H_{172}N_{36}O_{32}S_7$ that is a synthetic analog of a peptide found in a marine snail (*Conus magus*) and that is administered intrathecally to relieve chronic intractable pain

zi·do·vu·dine \zī-ˈdō-vü-ˌdēn, -vyü-\ *n* : AZT

Ziehl–Neel·sen stain \ˈtsēl-ˈnāl-sən-\ *n* : a stain used esp. for detecting the tubercle bacillus

    Ziehl, Franz (1857–1926), German bacteriologist.

    Neelsen, Friedrich Carl Adolf (1854–1894), German pathologist.

ZIFT *abbr* zygote intrafallopian transfer

zi·leu·ton \zī-ˈlü-tᵊn\ *n* : an antiasthma drug $C_{11}H_{12}N_2O_2S$ that is administered orally and acts by inhibiting the lipoxygenase catalyzing the formation of leukotrienes

zi·mel·i·dine \zi-ˈme-lə-ˌdēn\ *n* : a compound $C_{16}H_{17}BrN_2$ that functions as an SSRI but was withdrawn from use as an antidepressant because of its link to Guillain-Barré syndrome

zinc \ˈziŋk\ *n* : a bluish white crystalline bivalent metallic element that is an essential micronutrient for both plants and animals — symbol *Zn;* see ELEMENT table

zinc carbonate *n* : a crystalline salt $ZnCO_3$ having astringent and antiseptic properties

zinc chloride *n* : a poisonous caustic salt $ZnCl_2$ that is used as a disinfectant and astringent

zinc finger *n* : any of a class of proteins that typically possess fingerlike loops of amino acids with each loop containing a zinc-binding site that regulates transcription by binding to specific regions of a gene's DNA; *also* : one of the fingerlike amino acid loops of such a protein

zinc ointment *n* : ZINC OXIDE OINTMENT

zinc oxide *n* : a white solid ZnO used in pharmaceutical and cosmetic preparations (as in ointments and sunblocks)

zinc oxide ointment *n* : an ointment containing about 20 percent of zinc oxide and used in treating skin disorders

zinc peroxide *n* : any of various white to yellowish white powders that have the peroxide ZnO_2 of zinc as their chief ingredient and are used chiefly as disinfectants, astringents, and deodorants

zinc picolinate *n* : a biologically active salt $C_{12}H_8N_2O_4Zn$ of zinc complexed with picolinic acid that is used as a dietary supplement

zinc pyr·i·thi·one \-ˌpir-i-ˈthī-ˌōn\ *n* : an antibacterial and antifungal compound $C_{10}H_8N_2O_2S_2Zn$ that is nearly insoluble in water, possesses cytostatic activity against epidermal cells, and is the active ingredient in various shampoos used to control dandruff and seborrheic dermatitis — called also *pyrithione zinc*

zinc stearate *n* : an insoluble salt usu. of commercial stearic acid and usu. containing some zinc oxide that has astringent and antiseptic properties and is used as a constituent of ointments and powders

zinc sulfate *n* : a crystalline salt $ZnSO_4$ used in medicine as an astringent, emetic, and weak antiseptic

zinc un·dec·y·len·ate \-ˌən-ˌde-si-ˈle-ˌnāt\ *n* : a fine white powder $C_{22}H_{38}O_4Zn$ used as a fungistatic agent

zinc white *n* : ZINC OXIDE

zir·co·ni·um \ˌzər-ˈkō-nē-əm\ *n* : a strong ductile metallic element — symbol *Zr*; see ELEMENT table

zit \ˈzit\ *n, slang* : PIMPLE 1

Zith·ro·max \ˈzī-thrō-ˌmaks\ *trademark* — used for a preparation of azithromycin

Z line *n* : any of the dark thin lines across a striated muscle fiber that mark the junction of actin filaments in adjacent sarcomeres

Zn *symbol* zinc

zo- or **zoo-** *comb form* : animal ⟨zoonosis⟩

Zo·cor \ˈzō-ˌkòr\ *trademark* — used for a preparation of simvastatin

Zo·fran \ˈzō-ˌfran\ *trademark* — used for a preparation of the hydrated hydrochloride of ondansetron

-zo·ic \ˈzō-ik\ *adj comb form* : having a (specified) animal mode of existence ⟨saprozoic⟩

Zol·ling·er–El·li·son syndrome \ˈzä-liŋ-ər-ˈe-li-sən-\ *n* : a syndrome consisting of fulminant intractable peptic ulcers, gastric hypersecretion and hyperacidity, and the occurrence of gastrinomas of the pancreatic cells of the islets of Langerhans

   Zollinger, Robert Milton (1903–1992), American surgeon.
   Ellison, Edwin Homer (1918–1970), American surgeon.

zol·mi·trip·tan \ˌzōl-mi-ˈtrip-ˌtan\ *n* : a triptan $C_{16}H_{21}N_3O_2$ administered as an oral tablet or as a nasal spray to treat migraine headaches

Zo·loft \ˈzō-ˌlòft\ *trademark* — used for a preparation of the hydrochloride of sertraline

zol·pi·dem \ˈzōl-pə-ˌdem\ *n* : a sedative and hypnotic drug administered orally in the form of its tartrate $(C_{19}H_{21}N_3O)_2 \cdot C_4H_6O_6$ in the short-term treatment of insomnia — see AMBIEN

Zo·max \ˈzō-ˌmaks\ *n* : a preparation of zomepirac — formerly a U.S. registered trademark

zo·me·pir·ac \ˌzō-mə-ˈpir-ˌak\ *n* : a compound $C_{15}H_{13}ClNNaO_3 \cdot 2H_2O$ formerly used as an anti-inflammatory and analgesic agent but now withdrawn from use because of its link to life-threatening anaphylactic reactions — see ZOMAX

zo·na \ˈzō-nə\ *n, pl* **zo·nae** \-ˌnē, -ˌnī\ *or* **zonas** 1 : an anatomical zone or layer; *esp* : ZONA PELLUCIDA 2 : SHINGLES

zona fas·cic·u·la·ta \-fa-ˌsi-kyə-ˈlä-tə\ *n* : the middle of the three layers of the adrenal cortex that consists of radially arranged columnar epithelial cells

zona glo·mer·u·lo·sa \-ˌglō-ˌmer-yə-ˈlō-sə\ *n* : the outermost of the three layers of the adrenal cortex that consists of round masses of granular epithelial cells that stain deeply — called also *glomerulosa*

zona pel·lu·ci·da \-pə-ˈlü-sə-də\ *n* : the transparent more or less elastic noncellular outer layer or envelope of a mammalian ovum that is composed of glycoproteins

zona re·tic·u·lar·is \-re-ˌti-kyə-ˈlar-əs\ *n* : the innermost of the three layers of the adrenal cortex that consists of irregularly arranged cylindrical masses of epithelial cells

zone \ˈzōn\ *n* 1 : an encircling anatomical structure 2 : a region or area set off as distinct

zo·nu·la \ˈzōn-yə-lə\ *n, pl* **-lae** \-ˌlē\ *or* **-las** : ZONULE OF ZINN

zonula cil·i·ar·is \-ˌsi-lē-ˈar-əs\ *n* : ZONULE OF ZINN

zo·nu·lar \ˈzōn-yə-lər\ *adj* : of or relating to the zonule of Zinn

zon·ule \ˈzōn-ˌyül\ *n* : ZONULE OF ZINN

zonule of Zinn \-ˈtsin\ *n* : the suspensory ligament of the crystalline lens of the eye — called also *zonula, zonula ciliaris*

   J. G. Zinn — see LIGAMENT OF ZINN

zoo- — see ZO-

zo·ol·o·gy \zō-ˈäl-ə-jē\ *n, pl* **-gies** 1 : a branch of biology that deals with the classification and the properties and vital phenomena of animals 2 : the properties and vital phenomena exhibited by an animal, animal type, or group — **zoo·log·i·cal** \ˌzō-ə-ˈläj-i-kəl\ *also* **zoo·log·ic** \-ik\ *adj* — **zo·ol·o·gist** \zō-ˈäl-ə-jist\ *n*

-zo·on \ˈzō-ˌän, -ən\ *n comb form* : animal ⟨spermatozoon⟩

zoo·no·sis \ˌzō-ə-ˈnō-səs, zō-ˈä-nə-səs\ *n, pl* **-no·ses** \-ˌsēz\ : a disease communicable from animals to humans under natural conditions — **zoo·not·ic** \ˌzō-ə-ˈnä-tik\ *adj*

zoo·par·a·site \ˌzō-ə-ˈpar-ə-ˌsīt\ *n* : a parasitic animal

zoo·phil·ia \ˌzō-ə-ˈfil-ē-ə\ *n* : an erotic fixation on animals that may result in sexual excitement through real or imagined contact

zoo·pho·bia \ˌzō-ə-ˈfō-bē-ə\ *n* : abnormal fear of animals

zos·ter \ˈzäs-tər\ *n* : SHINGLES

zos·ter·i·form \zäs-ˈter-ə-ˌfòrm\ *adj* : resembling shingles ⟨a ~ rash⟩

Zos·trix \ˈzäs-triks\ *trademark* — used for a preparation containing capsaicin

Zo·vi·rax \zō-ˈvī-ˌraks\ *trademark* — used for a preparation of acyclovir

zox·a·zol·amine \ˌzäk-sə-ˈzä-lə-ˌmēn\ *n* : a drug $C_7H_5ClN_2O$ used esp. formerly as a skeletal muscle relaxant and uricosuric agent

ZPG *abbr* zero population growth

Z-plas·ty \ˈzē-ˌplas-tē\ *n, pl* **-ties** : a surgical procedure for the repair of constricted scar tissue in which a Z-shaped incision is made in the skin and the two resulting flaps are interposed

Zr *symbol* zirconium

Zy·ban \'zī-₁ban\ *trademark* — used for a preparation of the hydrochloride of bupropion

zyg- *or* **zygo-** *comb form* **1** : pair ⟨*zyg*apophysis⟩ **2** : union : fusion ⟨*zygo*genesis⟩

zyg·apoph·y·sis \₁zī-gə-'pä-fə-səs\ *n*, *pl* **-y·ses** \-₁sēz\ : any of the articular processes of the neural arch of a vertebra of which there are usu. two anterior and two posterior

zy·go·gen·e·sis \₁zī-gō-'je-nə-səs\ *n*, *pl* **-e·ses** \-₁sēz\ : reproduction by means of specialized germ cells or gametes : sexual reproduction

zy·go·ma \zī-'gō-mə\ *n*, *pl* **-ma·ta** \-mə-tə\ *also* **-mas 1** : ZYGOMATIC ARCH **2** : ZYGOMATIC BONE

¹**zy·go·mat·ic** \₁zī-gə-'ma-tik\ *adj* : of, relating to, constituting, or situated in the region of the zygomatic bone and the zygomatic arch

²**zygomatic** *n* : ZYGOMATIC BONE

zygomatic arch *n* : the arch of bone that extends along the front or side of the skull beneath the orbit and that is formed by the union of the temporal process of the zygomatic bone in front with the zygomatic process of the temporal bone behind

zygomatic bone *n* : a bone of the side of the face below the eye that forms part of the zygomatic arch and part of the orbit and articulates with the temporal, sphenoid, and frontal bones and with the maxilla of the upper jaw — called also *cheekbone, jugal, malar bone, zygoma*

zygomatic nerve *n* : a branch of the maxillary nerve that divides into a facial branch supplying the skin of the prominent part of the cheek and a temporal branch supplying the skin of the anterior temporal region

zygomatico- *comb form* : zygomatic and ⟨*zygomatico*facial⟩

zy·go·mat·i·co·fa·cial \₁zī-gə-₁ma-ti-kō-'fā-shəl\ *adj* **1** : of, relating to, or being the branch of the zygomatic nerve that supplies the skin of the prominent part of the cheek **2** : of, relating to, or being a foramen in the zygomatic bone that gives passage to the zygomaticofacial branch of the zygomatic nerve

zy·go·mat·i·co·max·il·lary \-'mak-sə-₁ler-ē\ *adj* : of, relating to, or uniting the zygomatic bone and the maxilla of the upper jaw ⟨the ~ suture⟩

zy·go·mat·i·co·tem·po·ral \-'tem-pə-rəl\ *adj* **1** : of, relating to, or uniting the zygomatic arch and the temporal bone ⟨the ~ suture⟩ **2 a** : of, relating to, or being the branch of the zygomatic nerve that supplies the skin of the anterior temporal region **b** : of, relating to, or being a foramen in the zygomatic bone that gives passage to the zygomaticotemporal branch of the zygomatic nerve

zygomatic process *n* : any of several bony processes that articulate with the zygomatic bone: as **a** : a long slender process of the temporal bone helping to form the zygomatic arch **b** : a narrow process of the frontal bone articulating with the zygomatic bone **c** : a rough triangular eminence of the maxilla of the upper jaw articulating with the zygomatic bone

zy·go·mat·i·cus \₁zī-gə-'ma-ti-kəs\ *n* **1** : ZYGOMATICUS MAJOR **2** : ZYGOMATICUS MINOR

zygomaticus major *n* : a slender band of muscle on each side of the face that arises from the zygomatic bone, inserts into the orbicularis oris and skin at the corner of the mouth, and acts to pull the corner of the mouth upward and backward

zygomaticus minor *n* : a slender band of muscle on each side of the face that arises from the zygomatic bone, inserts into the upper lip between the zygomaticus major and the levator labii superioris, and acts to raise the upper lip upward and laterally

zy·gos·i·ty \zī-'gä-sə-tē\ *n*, *pl* **-ties** : the makeup or characteristics of a particular zygote

zy·gote \'zī-₁gōt\ *n* : a cell formed by the union of two gametes; *broadly* : the developing individual produced from such a cell — **zy·got·ic** \zī-'gä-tik\ *adj* — **zy·got·i·cal·ly** *adv*

zygote intrafallopian transfer *n* : a method of assisting reproduction in cases of infertility in which eggs are obtained from an ovary and fertilized with sperm in vitro and the resulting fertilized eggs are inserted into a fallopian tube — abbr. *ZIFT;* compare GAMETE INTRAFALLOPIAN TRANSFER

zy·go·tene \'zī-gə-₁tēn\ *n* : the stage of meiotic prophase which immediately follows the leptotene and during which synapsis of homologous chromosomes occurs — **zygotene** *adj*

-zy·gous \'zi-gəs\ *adj comb form* : having (such) a zygotic constitution ⟨heterozygous⟩

zym- *or* **zymo-** *comb form* : enzyme ⟨*zymo*gen⟩

-zyme \₁zīm\ *n comb form* : enzyme ⟨lyso*zyme*⟩

zy·mo·gen \'zī-mə-jən\ *n* : an inactive protein precursor of an enzyme secreted by living cells and converted (as by a kinase or an acid) into an active form — called also *proenzyme*

zy·mo·gram \'zī-mə-₁gram\ *n* : an electrophoretic strip (as of starch gel) or a representation of it exhibiting the pattern of separated enzymes and esp. isoenzymes after electrophoresis

zy·mo·san \'zī-mə-₁san\ *n* : an insoluble largely polysaccharide fraction of yeast cell walls

Zy·prexa \zī-'prek-sə\ *trademark* — used for a preparation of olanzapine

Zyr·tec \'zər-₁tek\ *trademark* — used for a preparation of the dihydrochloride of cetirizine

SIGNS AND SYMBOLS

BIOLOGY

○ an individual, specif., a female—used chiefly in inheritance charts

□ an individual, specif., a male—used chiefly in inheritance charts

♀ female

♂ or ♂ male

× crossed with; hybrid

+ wild type

CHEMISTRY AND PHYSICS

(for element symbols see ELEMENT table)

α alpha particle

β beta particle, beta ray

λ wavelength

+ signifies "plus," "and," "together with"—used between the symbols of substances brought together for, or produced by, a reaction;

signifies a unit charge of positive electricity when placed to the right of a symbol as a superscript: Ca^{2+} or Ca^{++} denotes the ion of calcium, which carries two positive charges;

signifies a dextrorotatory compound when preceding in parentheses a compound name [as in (+)-tartaric acid]

– signifies removal or loss of a part from a compound during a reaction (as in $-CO_2$);

signifies a unit charge of negative electricity when placed to the right of a symbol as a superscript: Cl^- denotes a chlorine ion carrying a negative charge;

signifies a levorotatory compound when preceding in parentheses a compound name [as in (–)-quinine]

- signifies a single bond—used between the symbols of elements or groups which unite to form a compound (as in H–Cl for HCl and H–O–H for H_2O)

\> signifies separate single bonds from an atom to two other atoms or groups (as in the group >C=NNHR characteristic of hydrazone)

· used to separate parts of a substance regarded as loosely joined (as in $CuSO_4·5H_2O$);

also used to denote the presence of a single unpaired electron (as in H·)

= indicates a double bond;

signifies two unit charges of negative electricity when placed to the right of a symbol as a superscript (as in $SO_4^=$, the negative ion of sulfuric acid)

≡ signifies a triple bond or a triple negative charge

: signifies a pair of electrons belonging to an atom that are not shared with another atom (as in $:NH_3$);

sometimes signifies a double bond (as in $CH_2:CH_2$)

( ) marks groups within a compound [as in $(CH_3)_2SO$, the formula for dimethyl sulfoxide which contains two methyl groups (CH_3)]

— or — joins attached atoms or groups in structural formulas for cyclic compounds, as that for glucose

$$\longmapsto O \longmapsto$$

$CH_2OHCH(CHOH)_3CHOH$

1-, 2-, etc. used in names to indicate the positions of substituting groups, attached to the first, second, etc., of the numbered atoms of the parent compound (as in 5-fluorouracil or glucose-6-phosphate)

x, m, n used as subscripts following an atom or group in a chemical formula to indicate that the number of times the atom or group occurs is indefinite [as in $(C_6H_{10}O_5)_x$ for glycogen] or approximate [as in $C_{12}H_mAl_{16}O_nS_8$ for sucralfate where m and n are approximately 54 and 75]

R group—used esp. of an organic group

′ used to distinguish between different substituents of the same kind (as R′, R″, R‴ to indicate different organic groups)

MEDICINE

℞   take—used on prescriptions; prescription; treatment

☠   poison

☣   biohazard, biohazardous materials

☢ *or* ☢   radiation, radioactivity, radioactive materials

APOTHECARIES' MEASURES

℥   ounce

f ℥   fluid ounce

f ʒ   fluid dram

min *or* ♍   minim

APOTHECARIES' WEIGHTS

℔   pound

℥   ounce: as

   ℥ i *or* ℥ j, one ounce;

   ℥ ss, half an ounce;

   ℥ iss *or* ℥ jss, one ounce and a half;

   ℥ ij, two ounces

ʒ   dram

Ә   scruple